PEDIATRIC
CARDIOVASCULAR MEDICINE

JAMES H. MOLLER, MD

Professor and Head of Pediatrics

Paul F. Dwan Professor in Pediatric Cardiology

University of Minnesota Medical School

Minneapolis, Minnesota

JULIEN I. E. HOFFMAN, MD, FRCP

Professor of Pediatrics (Emeritus)

Senior Member of the Cardiovascular Research Institute

University of California

San Francisco, California

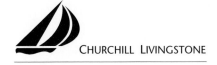

CHURCHILL LIVINGSTONE

A Harcourt Health Sciences Company
New York Edinburgh London Philadelphia

CHURCHILL LIVINGSTONE
A Harcourt Health Sciences Company

The Curtis Center
Independence Square West
Philadelphia, Pennsylvania 19106

Library of Congress Cataloging-in-Publication Data

Pediatric cardiovascular medicine / [edited by] James H. Moller, Julien I. E. Hoffman.—1st ed.

p.   cm.

ISBN 0–443–07677–4

1. Pediatric cardiology.   I. Moller, James H.   II. Hoffman, Julien I. E.
   [DNLM: 1. Heart Diseases—Child.   WS 290 P3719 2000]

RJ421.P43 2000

618.92'1—dc21   99–089085

Acquisitions Editor: Marc Strauss
Production Manager: Norman Stellander
Illustration Specialist: Robert Quinn

PEDIATRIC CARDIOVASCULAR MEDICINE   ISBN 0–443–07677–4

Printed in United States of America

Last digit is the print number: 9   8   7   6   5   4   3   2   1

Lindsey D. Allan, MD, FACE

Professor of Pediatrics, Columbia University, College of Physicians and Surgeons, New York, New York
Fetal Echocardiography

Kurt Amplatz, MD

Professor of Radiology, University of Minnesota School of Medicine, Minneapolis, Minnesota
Plain Film Diagnosis of Congenital Heart Disease

Page A. W. Anderson, MD

Professor of Pediatrics, Division of Pediatric Cardiology, Duke University School of Medicine and Medical Center, Durham, North Carolina
Developmental Cardiac Physiology and Myocardial Function

Robert H. Anderson, MD, FRCPath

Joseph Levy Professor of Paediatric Cardiac Morphology, Institute of Child Health, University College of London; Honorary Consultant Paediatric Cardiologist, Hospital for Sick Children, London, United Kingdom
Nomenclature and Classification: Sequential Segmental Analysis

Howard D. Apfel, MD

Assistant Professor of Pediatrics, Columbia University, College of Physicians and Surgeons; Assistant Attending Pediatrician, The New York Presbyterian Hospital, New York, New York
Patent Ductus Arteriosus and Other Aortopulmonary Anomalies

Michael Artman, MD

Professor of Pediatrics and of Physiology and Neuroscience, New York University School of Medicine; Director, Pediatric Cardiology, NYU Medical Center, New York, New York
Appendix: Drugs and Dosages

Marcelo Auslender, MD

Assistant Professor of Pediatrics, New York University School of Medicine; Director, Pediatric Critical Care Program, NYU Medical Center and Bellevue Hospital, New York, New York
Appendix: Drugs and Dosages

Elia M. Ayoub, MD

Distinguished Service Professor and Vice Chairman for Academic Affairs, Department of Pediatrics, University of Florida School of Medicine, Gainesville, Florida
Rheumatic Fever

Micael Berant, MD

Head, Non-Invasive Laboratory, Cardiology Institute, Schneider Children's Medical Center, Petach Tikva, Israel
Pulmonic Stenosis

Stephen M. Black, PhD

Associate Professor of Pediatrics, Molecular Pharmacology, and Biological Chemistry; Research Director, Neonatal Division, Northwestern Medical School, Chicago, Illinois
Control of Pulmonary Vasculature

Leonard C. Blieden, MB, BCh

Associate Professor of Cardiology (Pediatrics), Sackler School of Medicine, University of Tel Aviv, Tel Aviv; Director, Institute of Cardiology, Schneider Children's Medical Center, Petach Tikva, Israel
Pulmonic Stenosis

Elizabeth A. Braunlin, MD, PhD

Associate Professor of Pediatrics, University of Minnesota School of Medicine, Minneapolis, Minnesota
Complications in Chronic Cyanotic Heart Disease

J. Timothy Bricker, MD

Professor and Chief, Lillie Abercrombie Section of Cardiology, Baylor College of Medicine; Chief of Cardiology, Texas Children's Hospital; Chief, Department of Pediatric Cardiology, Texas Heart Institute, Houston, Texas
Pericardial Disease

Michael M. Brook, MD

Associate Professor of Clinical Pediatrics, University of California, San Francisco, School of Medicine; Attending Consulting Cardiologist, UCSF, San Francisco, California
Echocardiography

A. Louise Calder, MD, FRCP(C)
Pediatric Cardiologist, Green Lane Hospital, Auckland, New Zealand
Aortic Stenosis

Charles E. Canter, MD
Associate Professor of Pediatrics, Washington University School of Medicine; Medical Director, Pediatric Cardiac Transplant Program, St. Louis Children's Hospital, St. Louis, Missouri
Pediatric Cardiac Transplantation

Michael P. Carboni, MD
Senior Fellow, Pediatric Cardiology, Duke University Medical Center, Durham, North Carolina
Congestive Heart Failure

Adriano Carotti, MD
Associate in Pediatric Cardiac Surgery, Bambino Gesù Hospital, Rome, Italy
Malposition of the Heart

Michael W. Dae, MD
Professor of Radiology and Internal Medicine; Senior Member, Cardiovascular Research Institute, University of California, San Francisco, California
Nuclear Medicine in Pediatric Cardiology

Adnan S. Dajani, MD
Professor of Pediatrics, Wayne State University School of Medicine; Attending Staff Physician, Children's Hospital of Michigan, Detroit, Michigan
Infective Endocarditis

Thomas P. Doyle, MD
Assistant Professor of Pediatric Cardiology, Vanderbilt University School of Medicine; Director of Cardiac Catheterization Laboratory, Vanderbilt University Medical Center, Nashville, Tennessee
Tetralogy of Fallot and Pulmonary Atresia With Ventricular Septal Defect

David J. Driscoll, MD
Professor at Pediatrics and Head, Section of Pediatric Cardiology, Mayo Medical School; Consultant in Pediatric Cardiology, Mayo Clinic, Mayo Eugenio Litta Children's Hospital, Mayo Foundation, Rochester, Minnesota
Pediatric Exercise Testing

Adré J. du Plessis, MB,ChB, MPH
Assistant Professor of Neurology, Harvard Medical School; Assistant in Neurology, Children's Hospital, Boston, Massachusetts
Neurologic Problems in Childhood Heart Disease

Jesse E. Edwards, MD
Clinical Professor of Laboratory Medicine and Pathology, University of Minnesota Medical School, Minneapolis; Senior Consultant, Jesse E. Edwards Registry of Cardiovascular Disease, United Hospital, St. Paul, Minnesota
Cardiac Tumors

Benjamin W. Eidem, MD
Assistant Professor, Pediatrics, Loyola University School of Medicine; Director, Pediatric Echocardiography Laboratory, Loyola University Medical Center, Maywood, Illinois
Pediatric Exercise Testing

Fernando Eimbcke, MD
Auxiliary Professor of Pediatrics, School of Medicine, University of Chile; Pediatric Cardiologist, Cardiovascular Center, L. Calvo Mackenna Hospital, Santiago de Chile, Chile
Total Anomalous Pulmonary Venous Connection

Helen M. Emery
Professor of Pediatrics, University of California, San Francisco; Attending Rheumatologist, Moffitt-Long Hospitals, San Francisco, California
Cardiac Involvement in Vasculitis and Other Rheumatic Diseases

Gabriela Enríquez, MD
Chief of Echocardiography Department, Cardiovascular Center, L. Calvo Mackenna Hospital, Santiago de Chile, Chile
Total Anomalous Pulmonary Venous Connection

Michael L. Epstein, MD
Professor of Pediatrics, Wayne State University School of Medicine; Director of Cardiology, Children's Hospital of Michigan, Detroit, Michigan
Vascular Rings and Slings

Bonita Falkner, MD
Professor of Medicine and Pediatrics, Thomas Jefferson University, Philadelphia, Pennsylvania
Hypertension in Children and Adolescents

Robert H. Feldt, MD, MS
Emeritus Professor of Pediatrics, Mayo Medical School; Emeritus Consultant in Pediatric Cardiology, Mayo Clinic, Rochester, Minnesota
Ebstein Anomaly of the Tricuspid Valve

Jeffrey R. Fineman, MD
Associate Professor of Pediatrics, University of California, San Francisco, School of Medicine; Associate Investigator, Cardiovascular Research Institute, San Francisco, California
Control of Pulmonary Vasculature

Robert M. Freedom, MD, FRCPC

Professor of Pediatrics, Pathology, and Medical Imaging, The University of Toronto Faculty of Medicine; Director, Division of Cardiology, The Hospital for Sick Children, Toronto, Ontario, Canada

Angiography; Congenitally Corrected Transposition of the Great Arteries; Pulmonary Atresia and Intact Ventricular Septum

Thomas L. Gentles, MB,ChB, FRACP

Clinical Senior Lecturer, Department of Paediatrics, University of Auckland; Paediatric Cardiologist, Green Lane Hospital, Auckland, New Zealand

Aortic Stenosis

Welton M. Gersony, MD

Professor of Pediatrics, Columbia University, College of Physicians and Surgeons; Attending Pediatrician, The New York Presbyterian Hospital, New York, New York

Patent Ductus Arteriosus and Other Aortopulmonary Anomalies

Adriana C. Gittenberger-de Groot, PhD

Professor of Anatomy and Embryology, Department of Anatomy and Embryology, Leiden University Medical Center, Leiden, The Netherlands

Normal and Abnormal Cardiac Development

Oscar Gómez, MD

Adjunct Professor of Pediatrics, School of Medicine, University of Chile; Surgeon-in-Chief and Director of Cardiovascular Center, L. Calvo Mackenna Hospital, Santiago de Chile, Chile

Total Anomalous Pulmonary Venous Connection

Thomas P. Graham, MD

Ann and Monroe Carell Family Professor of Pediatric Cardiology, Vanderbilt University School of Medicine; Director of Pediatric Cardiology, Vanderbilt University Medical Center, Nashville, Tennessee

Tetralogy of Fallot and Pulmonary Atresia With Ventricular Septal Defect

Paolo Guccione, MD

Associate in Pediatric Cardiology, Bambino Gesù Hospital, Rome, Italy

Malposition of the Heart

Sheila Glennis Haworth, MD, FRCPath, FRCP, FACE

British Heart Foundation Professor of Developmental Cardiology, Institute of Child Health, University College and Hospital for Sick Children; Honorary Consultant Pediatric Cardiologist, Hospital for Sick Children, London, United Kingdom

Pulmonary Hypertension

Amy S. Hentges

Medical Student, University of Minnesota Medical School, Minneapolis, Minnesota

Connective Tissue Diseases

Michael A. Heymann, MD

Professor of Pediatrics (Emeritus), Senior Member, Cardiovascular Research Institute, University of California, San Francisco, California

Control of Pulmonary Vasculature

Julien I. E. Hoffman, MD, FRCP

Professor of Pediatrics (Emeritus), Senior Member of the Cardiovascular Research Institute, University of California, San Francisco, California

Physiology and Pathophysiology of Myocardial Blood Flow; Incidence, Prevalence, and Inheritance of Congenital Heart Disease; Coronary Arterial Abnormalities and Congenital Anomalies of the Aortic Root; Cardiac Involvement in Vasculitis and Other Rheumatic Diseases

Arno R. Hohn, MD

Professor of Pediatrics, University of Southern California; Head, Division of Cardiology, Children's Hospital of Los Angeles; Division of Pediatric Cardiology at LAC/USC, Los Angeles, California

Atrioventricular Septal Defect

Mark C. Johnson, MD

Assistant Professor, Department of Pediatrics, Washington University School of Medicine; St. Louis, Missouri

Genetic Control in Pediatric Cardiovascular Medicine

Carlo Kallfelz, MD, PhD, FESC

Professor of Pediatrics and Pediatric Cardiology (Emeritus), Children's Hospital, Paediatric Cardiology Section, Hannover Medical School, Hannover, Germany

Arteriovenous Fistulae and Allied Lesions

Hirohisa Kato, MD, DMSc

Professor and Chairman, Department of Pediatrics, Kurume University, Kurume, Japan

Kawasaki Disease

Ann Kavanaugh-McHugh, MD

Assistant Professor, Pediatrics, Division of Pediatric Cardiology, Vanderbilt University School of Medicine and Medical Center, Nashville, Tennessee

Tetralogy of Fallot and Pulmonary Atresia With Ventricular Septal Defect

Eduardo A. Kreutzer, MD

Professor of Pediatric Cardiology, University of Buenos Aires; Director, Pediatric Cardiology, Children's Hospital "Pedro de Elizalde," Buenos Aires, Argentina

Univentricular Heart

Guillermo O. Kreutzer, MD

Auxiliary Professor of Pediatrics, Division of Pediatric Cardiology; Head, Division of Cardiovascular Surgery, Children's Hospital, Buenos Aires, Argentina

Univentricular Heart

Jacqueline Kreutzer, MD
Instructor in Pediatrics, Harvard Medical School; Assistant in Cardiology, Children's Hospital, Boston, Massachusetts
Univentricular Heart

Thomas J. Kulik, MD
Associate Professor of Pediatrics and Communicable Diseases, University of Michigan Medical School; C. S. Mott Children's Hospital, and University of Michigan Hospitals, Ann Arbor, Michigan
Postoperative Problems

John Lane, MD
Instructor in Pediatrics, University of Southern California; Fellow, Critical Care Medicine, Children's Hospital of Los Angeles, Los Angeles, California
Atrioventricular Septal Defect

Larry A. Latson, MD
Professor of Pediatrics and Medicine, Ohio State University Medical School, Columbus; Chairman, Pediatric Cardiology, Cleveland Clinic Foundation, Cleveland, Ohio
Atrial Septal Defect

Ronald M. Lauer, MD
Professor of Pediatrics and Preventive Medicine, University of Iowa College of Medicine, Iowa City, Iowa
Hyperlipidemia in Children and Adolescents

Yves Lecompte, MD
Cardiac Surgeon, Hôpital Jacques Cartier, Massy, France
Transposition and Malposition of the Great Arteries With Ventricular Septal Defects

Jerome Liebman, MD
Professor of Pediatrics and Adjunct Professor, Biomedical Engineering, Case Western Reserve University Medical School; Pediatric Cardiologist, Rainbow Babies and Children's Hospital, University Hospitals of Cleveland, Cleveland, Ohio
Electrocardiography

Russell V. Lucas, Jr., MD
Emeritus Professor of Pediatrics, University of Minnesota Medical School, Minneapolis, Minnesota
Mitral Valve Prolapse

Susan G. MacLellan-Tobert, MD
Staff Pediatrician and Pediatric Cardiologist, Covenant Medical Center, Waterloo, Iowa
Ebstein Anomaly of the Tricuspid Valve

Bruno Marino, MD
Professor at Postgraduate School of Cardiology, Catholic University of Rome; Associate in Pediatric Cardiology, Bambino Gesù Hospital, Rome, Italy
Malposition of the Heart

Barry J. Maron, MD
Director, Cardiovascular Research, Minneapolis Heart Institute, Minneapolis, Minnesota
Sudden Cardiac Death in the Young Athlete and the Preparticipation Cardiovascular Evaluation

Doff B. McElhinney, MD
Resident in Pediatrics, Children's Hospital of Philadelphia, Philadelphia, Pennsylvania
Echocardiography

James J. McGovern, MD
Former Fellow, Pediatric Cardiology, Duke University Medical Center, Durham, North Carolina
Congestive Heart Failure

James H. Moller, MD
Professor and Head of Pediatrics, Paul F. Dwan Professor in Pediatric Cardiology, University of Minnesota Medical School, Minneapolis, Minnesota
Clinical History and Physical Examination

Kazuo Momma, MD, PhD, FACC
Professor and Chairman, Department of Pediatric Cardiology, The Heart Institute of Japan, Tokyo Women's Medical University, Tokyo, Japan
Approach to the Cyanotic Neonate

Ralph S. Mosca, MD
Associate Professor of Surgery, Pediatric Cardiovascular Surgery, Michigan Congenital Heart Center, University of Michigan Health Science System, Ann Arbor, Michigan
Postoperative Problems

Linda E. Muhonen, MD
Director of Preventive Cardiology, Pediatric Subspecialty Faculty, Children's Hospital of Orange County, Orange, California
Hyperlipidemia in Children and Adolescents

Charles E. Mullins, MD
Professor of Pediatrics, Baylor College of Medicine, Director Emeritus of Pediatric Cardiac Catheterization Labratory, Texas Children's Hospital, Houston, Texas
Cardiac Catheterization Hemodynamics and Intervention

John M. Neutze, MD, FRACP
Honorary Professor of Medicine, University of Auckland; Clinical Director and Pediatric Cardiologist (retired), Queen Lane Hospital, Auckland, New Zealand
Aortic Stenosis

Jane W. Newburger, MD, MPH
Associate Professor of Pediatrics, Harvard Medical School; Associate Cardiologist-in-Chief, Children's Hospital, Boston, Massachusetts
Neurologic Problems in Childhood Heart Disease

Michael R. Nihill, MB, BS

Professor of Pediatrics (Cardiology), Baylor College of Medicine, Houston, Texas
Cardiac Catheterization Hemodynamics and Intervention

Todd T. Nowlen, MD

Pediatric Cardiologist, Arizona Pediatric Cardiology Consultants, Phoenix, Arizona
Pericardial Disease

David G. Nykanen, MD

Assistant Professor of Paediatrics, University of Toronto; Assistant Director, Catheterization Laboratories, Hospital for Sick Children, Toronto, Ontario, Canada
Angiography

Mary Ella M. Pierpont, MD

Associate Professor of Pediatrics and Ophthalmology, University of Minnesota Medical School, Minneapolis, Minnesota
Connective Tissue Diseases

Robert E. Poelmann, PhD

Associate Professor of Anatomy and Embryology, Department of Anatomy and Embryology, Leiden University Medical Center, Leiden, The Netherlands
Normal and Abnormal Cardiac Development

P. Syamasundar Rao, MD

Professor of Pediatrics, St. Louis University School of Medicine; Director, Center for Transcatheter Treatment of Heart Defects in Children, Cardinal Glennon Children's Hospital, St. Louis, Missouri
Tricuspid Atresia

Larry A. Rhodes, MD

Assistant Professor of Pediatrics, University of Pennsylvania School of Medicine; Director of Electrophysiology, Children's Hospital of Philadelphia, Philadelphia, Pennsylvania
Syncope

Albert P. Rocchini, MD

Professor of Pediatrics, University of Michigan Medical College; Director, Pediatric Cardiology, C. S. Mott Children's Hospital, University of Michigan Health Systems, Ann Arbor, Michigan
Coarctation of the Aorta and Interrupted Aortic Arch

Amnon Rosenthal, MD

Professor of Pediatrics, C. S. Mott Children's Hospital, University of Michigan Health Care System, University of Michigan Medical School, Ann Arbor, Michigan
Hypoplastic Left Heart Syndrome

Abraham M. Rudolph, MD, FRCP, FRCPE

Professor of Pediatrics Emeritus, University of California, San Francisco, San Francisco, California
The Fetal Circulation and Its Adjustments After Birth

Robert H. Sadowski, MD

Assistant Professor of Clinical Pediatrics, Crozier-Chester Medical Center, Chester, Pennsylvania
Hypertension in Children and Adolescents

Daniel Sidi

Professor, University of Paris V René Descartes; Physician, Pediatric Cardiology, Hôpital Necker—Enfants Malades, Paris; Cardiac Surgeon, Hôpital Jacques Cartier, Massy, France
Complete Transposition of the Great Arteries; Transposition and Malposition of the Great Arteries With Ventricular Septal Defects

Norman H. Silverman, MD

Professor of Pediatrics and Radiology (Cardiology), University of California, San Francisco; Director, Pediatric Echocardiography Laboratory, San Francisco, California
Echocardiography

Linda Snetselaar, RD, PhD

Associate Professor in Preventive Medicine, University of Iowa School of Medicine, Iowa City, Iowa
Hyperlipidemia in Children and Adolescents

Jane Somerville, MD, FRCP, MB, BS(Lond), MRCS, LRCP

Emeritus Professor, Imperial College School of Medicine, London University; Emeritus Consultant Physician for Congenital Heart Disease, Royal Birmington and Harefield Trust; Consultant Cardiologist, GUCH Unit, Middlesex Hospital, Middlesex/UCL Medical School, London, United Kingdom
Cardiac Problems of Adults With Congenital Heart Disease

Julia Steinberger, MD

Assistant Professor of Pediatrics, Division of Pediatric Cardiology, University of Minnesota School of Medicine, Minneapolis, Minnesota
Cardiac Valvar Anomalies

Arnold W. Strauss, MD

Professor of Pediatrics and of Molecular Biology and Pharmacology, Washington University School of Medicine; Director, Pediatric Cardiology, St. Louis Children's Hospital, St. Louis, Missouri
Genetic Control in Pediatric Cardiovascular Medicine

Hiroyuki Suga, MD, PhD

Professor, Department of Physiology, Okayama University Medical School, Okayama, Japan
Cardiac Function

Norman S. Talner, MD

Clinical Professor of Pediatrics (Cardiology), Duke University Medical Center, Durham, North Carolina
Congestive Heart Failure

Kathryn A. Taubert, PhD

Associate Professor, University of Texas Southwestern Medical School; Senior Scientist, American Heart Association, Dallas, Texas

Infective Endocarditis

J. F. N. Taylor, MA, MD, FRCP, FRCPCH, FACC

Consultant Paediatric Cardiologist, Great Ormond Street Hospital for Children, London, United Kingdom

Persistent Truncus Arteriosus

Jack L. Titus, MD, PhD

Clinical Professor of Laboratory Medicine and Pathology, University of Minnesota Medical School, Minneapolis; Adjunct Professor of Pathology, Baylor College of Medicine, Houston, Texas; Director, Jesse E. Edwards Registry of Cardiovascular Disease, United Hospital, St. Paul, Minnesota

Cardiac Tumors

Jeffrey A. Towbin, MD

Professor of Pediatrics (Cardiology), Molecular and Human Genetics, and Cardiovascular Sciences; Texas Children's Hospital Foundation Chair in Pediatric Molecular Cardiology Research, Baylor College of Medicine; Director, Heart Failure and Transplantation Service, Texas Children's Hospital, Houston, Texas

Cardiomyopathies

Richard Van Praagh, MD

Professor of Pathology, Harvard Medical School; Director of the Cardiac Registry, Research Associate in Cardiology, and Research Associate in Cardiac Surgery, Children's Hospital, Boston, Massachusetts

Nomenclature and Classification: Morphologic and Segmental Approach to Diagnosis

Victoria Vetter, MD

Professor of Pediatrics, University of Pennsylvania School of Medicine; Chief, Division of Cardiology, Children's Hospital of Philadelphia, Philadelphia, Pennsylvania

Arrhythmias

James L. Wilkinson, MBChB, FRCP, FACC

Director of Cardiology, Royal Children's Hospital, Melbourne, Victoria, Australia

Ventricular Septal Defect

Nigel J. Wilson, MB,ChB, MRCP

Clinical Senior Lecturer, University of Auckland; Paediatric Cardiologist, Green Lane Hospital, Auckland, New Zealand

Aortic Stenosis

Pierre C. Wong, MD

Assistant Professor of Pediatrics and Director, Pediatric Echocardiographic Laboratory, Children's Hospital, Los Angeles, California

Atrioventricular Septal Defect

Benjamin Zeevi, MD

Lecturer, Sackler School of Medicine, University of Tel Aviv, Tel Aviv; Head, Cardiac Catheterization Laboratory, Schneider Children's Medical Center, Petach Tikva, Israel

Pulmonic Stenosis

Raúl Zilleruelo, MD

Assistant Professor of Pediatrics, School of Medicine, University of Chile; Chief of Cardiology, Cardiovascular Center, L. Calvo Mackenna Hospital, Santiago de Chile, Chile

Total Anomalous Pulmonary Venous Connection

PREFACE

With the growth and expansion of knowledge and methods of diagnosis and treatment of cardiac abnormalities that occur during childhood, the major textbooks on the subject have also expanded, often to multiple volumes. In our book, *Pediatric Cardiovascular Medicine*, we have attempted to be concise and focused in order to edit a single volume with contemporary knowledge of the discipline of pediatric cardiology. We have focused on the international aspect of pediatric cardiology, both in content and in the selection of a group of international experts in cardiology of the young. Authors from 12 countries have contributed chapters that are grouped into four sections: Scientific Background, Diagnostic Methods, Structural Heart Disease, and Miscellaneous Acquired Disease. In almost all of the 24 chapters on congenital heart disease, the organization and structure of the chapters are similar, making it easier for the reader. When appropriate, an indication of what happens to these patients in adult life is provided, and this information is supplemented by a chapter devoted to congenital heart disease in the adult. Two chapters on nomenclature and classification are included, one by Robert Anderson and the other by Richard Van Praagh, because most pediatric cardiologists and surgeons have a preference for one of these systems. An appendix on pharmacologic agents provides an overview of pharmacologic considerations in the treatment of particular conditions during childhood. Detailed information on a number of drugs is provided. The list of drugs is organized into categories based on principal use, such as, for example, diuretics or inotropes. As editors, we have sought to emphasize, whenever possible, pathophysiologic principles or understanding to help the reader comprehend and retain the information. Each chapter contains pertinent references, which we hope will enable the reader to explore further the fascinating area of pediatric cardiology.

We give grateful thanks to our secretaries, Ms. Mary Jo Antinozzi, Ms. Linda Boche, and Ms. Linda Chmielewski, for their interest in making this project a success. We appreciated working with Mr. Marc Strauss, Ms. Judith B. Gandy, and other staff at W. B. Saunders, whose advice and assistance were invaluable.

TABLE OF CONTENTS

SECTION IV
MISCELLANEOUS ACQUIRED DISEASE 707

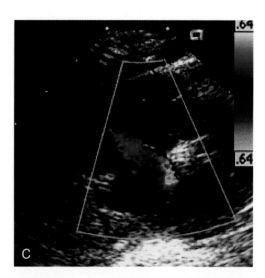

FIGURE 11-1

Continuous-wave, pulsed-wave, and color flow images of the same flow signal. *C,* Although color Doppler can measure broader areas, the Nyquist limit is low (0.6 m/sec). This leads to aliasing of the signal, shown by the blue central signal apparently going backward.

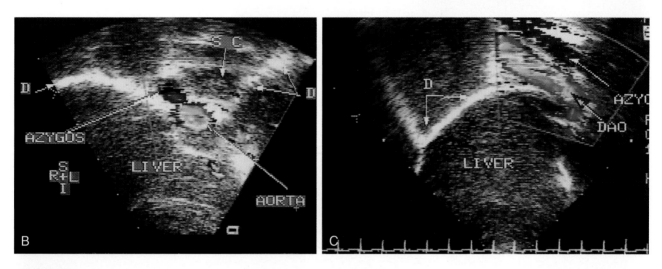

FIGURE 11-6

B, Subcostal coronal view shows the relation between the azygos vein and the aorta. D = diaphragm; SC = spinal canal. *C,* Image taken in a subcostal sagittal plane demonstrates the anteroposterior orientation. The descending aorta (DAO) is seen anterior to the azygos vein (AZYG). The central diaphragm (D) is seen separating the thorax from the liver below. (*B* from Silverman NH: Pediatric Echocardiography. Baltimore, Williams & Wilkins, 1993, p 310.)

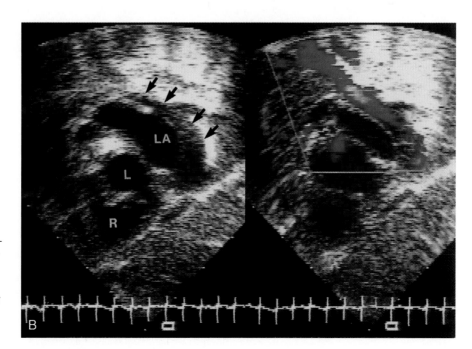

FIGURE 11-10

B, In this pair of images from the subcostal sagittal window, the left superior vena cava *(arrows)* seen coursing along the left atrium (LA) in the cross-sectional scan *(left)* is highlighted with Doppler color flow *(right),* which demonstrates flow moving toward the transducer. L = left ventricle; R = right ventricle.

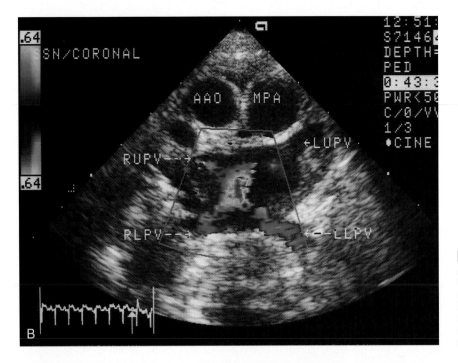

FIGURE 11–12

A suprasternal notch (SSN) coronal view shows the confluence of the right upper (RUPV), right lower (RLPV), left upper (LUPV), and left lower (LLPV) pulmonary veins entering the left atrium. The ascending aorta (AAO) and main pulmonary artery (MPA) are also seen in cross-section craniad to the left atrium.

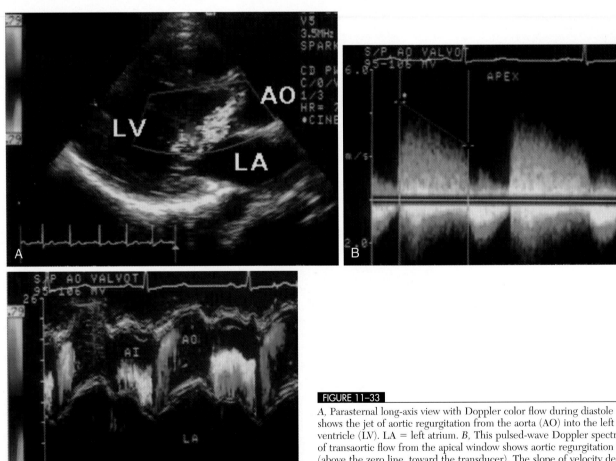

FIGURE 11–33

A, Parasternal long-axis view with Doppler color flow during diastole shows the jet of aortic regurgitation from the aorta (AO) into the left ventricle (LV). LA = left atrium. *B,* This pulsed-wave Doppler spectrum of transaortic flow from the apical window shows aortic regurgitation (above the zero line, toward the transducer). The slope of velocity decay is approximated with the descending white line between the two vertical lines during diastole. *C,* M-mode imaging with Doppler color flow shows regurgitant flow (AI) during diastole and aortic ejection (red) during systole. AI = aortic insufficiency; AO = aorta; LA = left atrium.

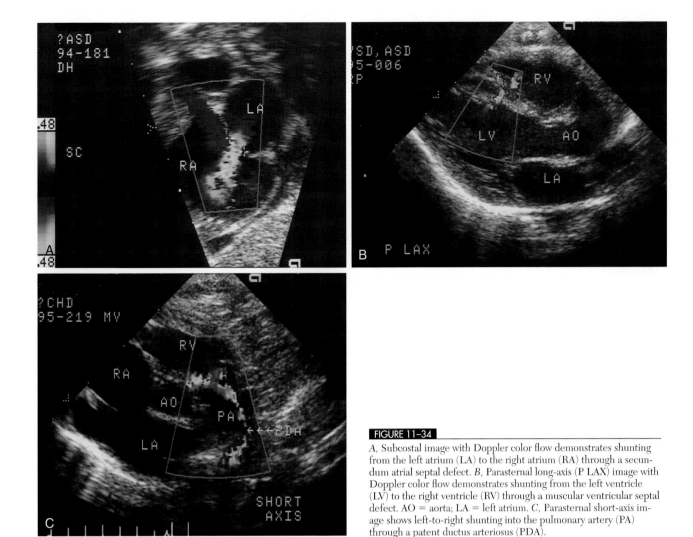

FIGURE 11-34

A, Subcostal image with Doppler color flow demonstrates shunting from the left atrium (LA) to the right atrium (RA) through a secundum atrial septal defect. *B*, Parasternal long-axis (P LAX) image with Doppler color flow demonstrates shunting from the left ventricle (LV) to the right ventricle (RV) through a muscular ventricular septal defect. AO = aorta; LA = left atrium. *C*, Parasternal short-axis image shows left-to-right shunting into the pulmonary artery (PA) through a patent ductus arteriosus (PDA).

FIGURE 11-36

Transgastric images in a patient with complete atrioventricular septal defect. The image on the left shows the left (LA, LV) and right (RA, RV) atria and ventricles, the common atrioventricular valve, and the large inlet ventricular septal defect. The Doppler color flow image on the right shows the inflow blood from the pulmonary veins (PV).

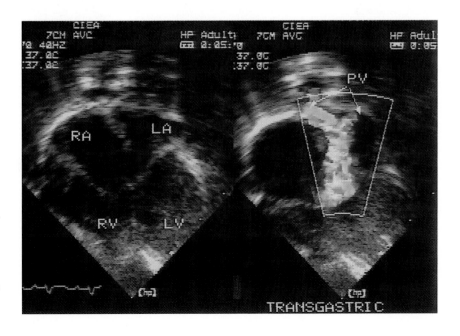

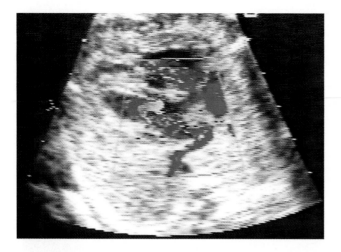

FIGURE 12–3

Blood flow from the left pulmonary vein is seen draining to the left atrium on color flow mapping.

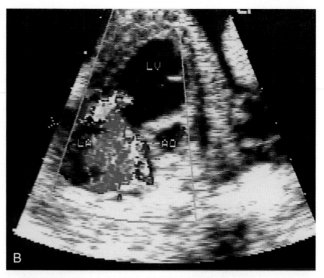

FIGURE 12–21

B, There is moderate mitral regurgitation on color flow mapping. There was forward flow in the ascending aorta with turbulence at the aortic valve. AO = aorta; LA = left atrium; LV = left ventricle.

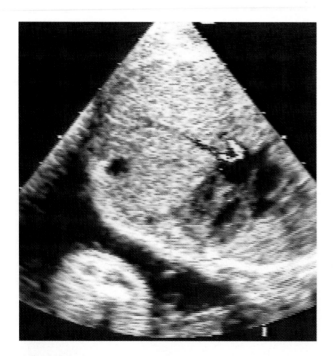

FIGURE 12–4

The hepatic veins are seen draining directly into the right-sided atrium on color flow mapping.

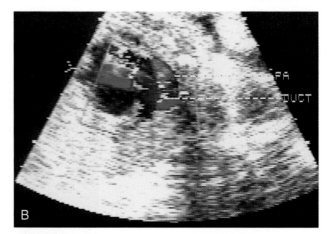

FIGURE 12–23

B, The color flow map revealed reverse flow (red flow) into the main pulmonary artery (PA) from the duct. The jet was then reflected off the atretic pulmonary valve to supply the branch pulmonary arteries (blue flow).

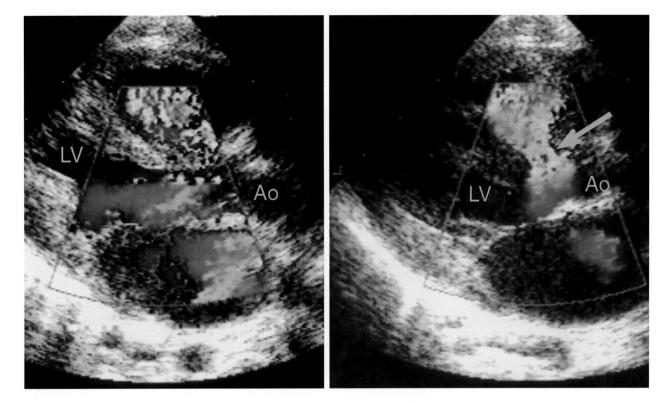

Echocardiogram, perimembranous ventricular septal defect. Medially rotated long-axis view shows a high-velocity jet through a moderate-sized perimembranous defect *(arrow)*. Ao = aorta; LV = left ventricle.

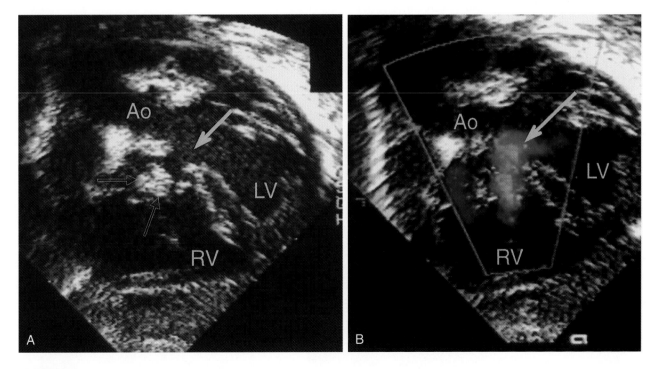

Echocardiogram, perimembranous defect. *A,* Subxiphoid view shows a ventricular septal defect *(solid arrow)* adjacent to the aortic valve, with tricuspid valve tissue on the right ventricular side *(open arrows)*. *B,* Similar view with color flow mapping shows a left-to-right shunt at low velocity through a large, nonrestrictive defect *(arrow)*. In this example, the aortic valve is seen to be above the ventricular septal defect, but the degree of malalignment is minor, with the aorta clearly originating from the left ventricle. Ao = aorta; LV = left ventricle; RV = right ventricle.

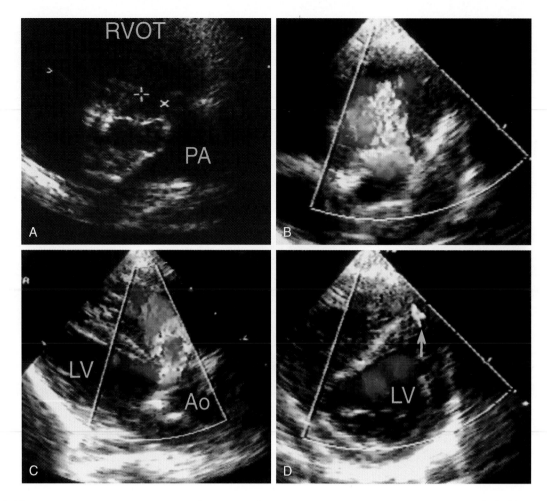

FIGURE 21–12

Echocardiogram, doubly committed subarterial and small additional muscular VSD. *A,* Short-axis scan at the level of the aortic valve shows a break with clear edges immediately below the right coronary leaflet and adjacent to the pulmonary valve leaflet. PA = pulmonary artery; RVOT = right ventricular outflow tract. *B,* View similar to *A* with color flow shows a high-velocity turbulent jet directed anteriorly into the right ventricular outflow tract. *C,* Long-axis scan with color shows a break in the septum with a high-velocity jet. The site of the defect is usually obvious in the conventional long-axis view, without the need to rotate the transducer medially (as is required to demonstrate a perimembranous defect). Ao = aorta; LV = left ventricle. *D,* Low short-axis scan in the same patient demonstrates a small apical muscular defect *(arrow)* apparent only from the turbulent jet on color flow mapping. LV = left ventricle.

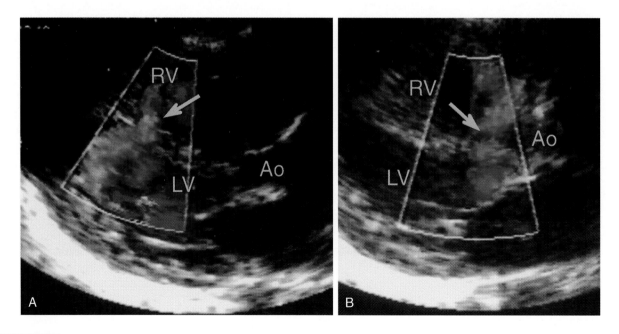

FIGURE 21–13

Echocardiogram, multiple defects. *A,* Long-axis view shows color flow through a midmuscular ventricular septal defect *(arrow)*. *B,* Medially rotated long-axis scan demonstrates large, nonrestrictive, perimembranous defect *(arrow)* in the same patient. Ao = aorta; LV = left ventricle; RV = right ventricle.

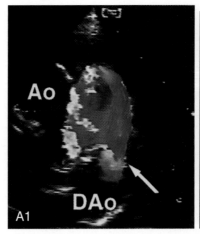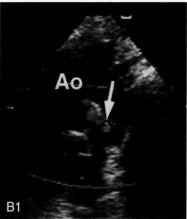

A, Two-dimensional echocardiographic parasternal short-axis view of a large, wide patent ductus arteriosus *(arrows).* Color flow Doppler imaging *(A1)* demonstrates left-to-right shunting at the large communication. *B,* Suprasternal arch view identifies a relatively narrow, tortuous ductus with left-to-right shunting on color flow imaging *(B1) (arrows).* Ao = aorta; DAo = descending aorta.

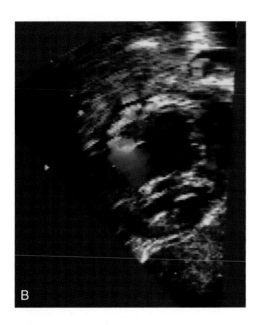

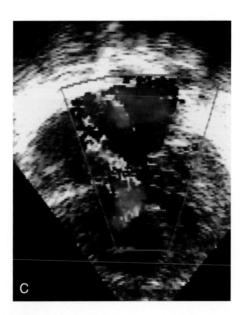

Subxiphoid short-axis view in a patient with a complete atrioventricular septal defect and right ventricular outflow tract obstruction (tetralogy of Fallot physiology). The infundibular septum is anteriorly malaligned, producing subpulmonary narrowing *(A),* and flow acceleration begins at this level *(B).*

Apical four-chamber view in a patient with a common atrioventricular septal defect. *C,* During systole, color flow Doppler mapping demonstrates a left ventricle–to–right atrium shunt.

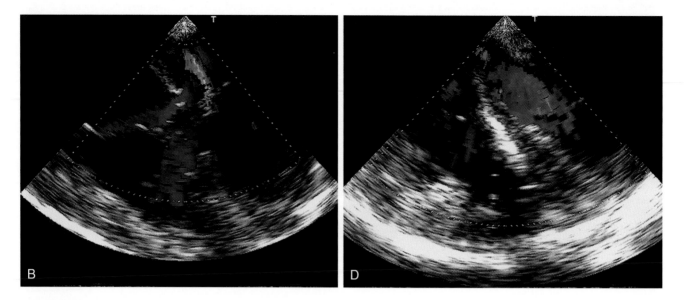

FIGURE 24–12

Transesophageal echocardiography performed in the operating room (*B*) shows a large complete atrioventricular septal defect with unobstructed left-to-right shunting at both atrial and ventricular levels. There is also a mild degree of mitral insufficiency. After surgery (*D*), the large patch can be well seen, and there is no left-to-right shunt.

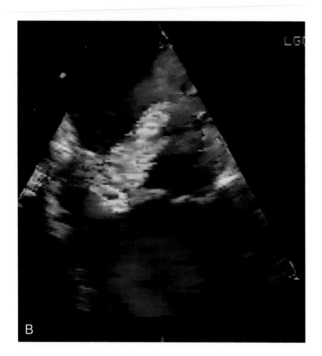

FIGURE 24–13

Intraoperative transesophageal echocardiography in an adult patient with a previously repaired atrioventricular septal defect who had subsequently developed significant mitral insufficiency. *B*, Color flow Doppler shows a prominent regurgitant jet.

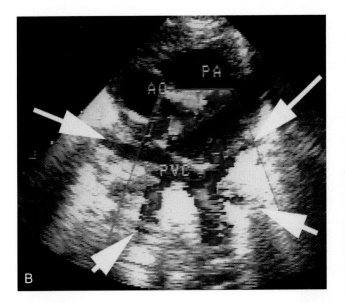

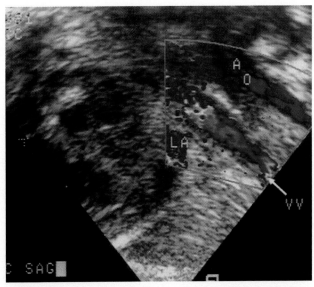

FIGURE 29–9

Infracardiac total anomalous pulmonary venous connection. *B,* Color Doppler image shows the four pulmonary veins *(arrows)* joining the common pulmonary vein that passes caudad (blue color). AO = aorta; LA = left atrium; PA = pulmonary artery; PVC = pulmonary venous confluence.

FIGURE 29–10

Infracardiac total anomalous pulmonary venous connection. Color Doppler image of a sagittal view shows the connection with the venous confluence (VV) parallel to the descending aorta (AO) and between it and the left atrium (LA). This large vessel cannot be the inferior vena cava, because the direction of flow is caudad.

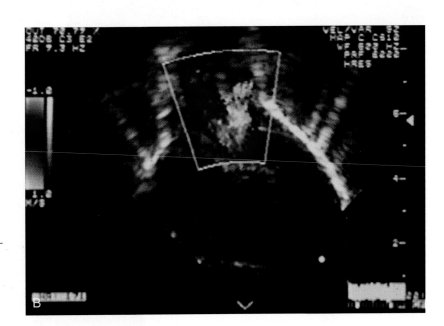

FIGURE 34–4

Truncus arteriosus, cross-sectional echocardiogram. *B,* Color Doppler image demonstrates turbulent flow into one pulmonary artery while there is laminar (blue) flow in the aorta. The plume of red color signifies flow toward the probe due to truncal valve incompetence.

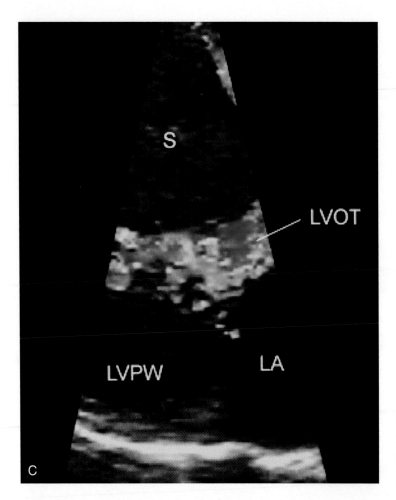

FIGURE 35–30

Echocardiographic systolic anterior motion of the mitral valve. *C*, Color Doppler image at midsystole demonstrates turbulence in the left ventricular outflow tract (LVOT). LA = left atrium; LVPW = left ventricular posterior wall; S = septum.

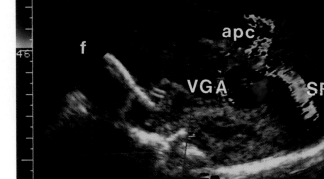

FIGURE 42–1

Vein of Galen aneurysmal malformation of the choroideal type. *A*, Cranial color flow Doppler image in a 6-week-old infant. Sagittal section demonstrates one feeding artery from above (arteria pericallosa [apc]), the ectatic vein of Galen (VGA), and the enlarged draining sinus rectus (SR). Note turbulent flow in all compartments. d = dorsal; f = frontal.

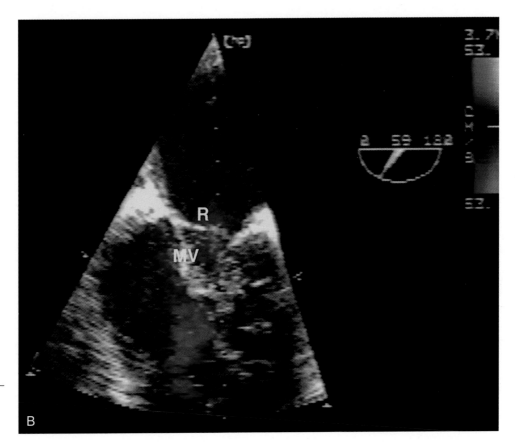

FIGURE 43–4

Supravalvar stenosing ring. *B*,
Color Doppler demonstrates that
turbulent flow begins at the ring.
MV = mitral valve; R = ring.

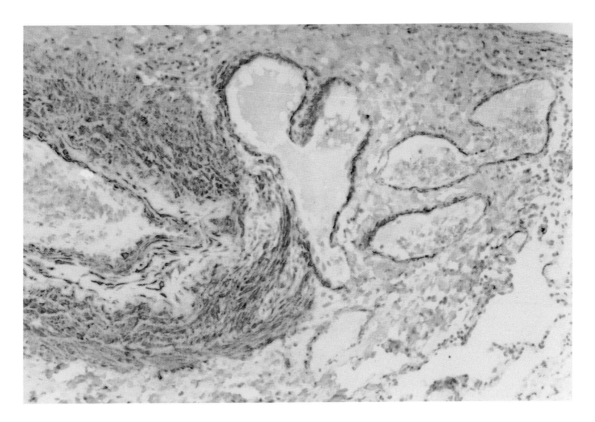

FIGURE 46–5

Photomicrograph of lung tissue from an explanted lung of a 15-year-old boy with a ventricular septal defect and Eisenmenger syndrome, showing inti-mal proliferation in the parent vessel and dilatation lesions. The smooth muscle cells in the media of the original vessel and in the walls of the dilatation lesions stain darkly with γ-actin, a contractile protein. Magnification ×250.

SECTION I
SCIENTIFIC BACKGROUND

CHAPTER 1
NORMAL AND ABNORMAL CARDIAC DEVELOPMENT

ADRIANA C. GITTENBERGER–DE GROOT   ROBERT E. POELMANN

In this chapter the main events of cardiac morphogenesis are discussed. We focus on both classic descriptions and new insights based on molecular biologic approaches that have modified our understanding of normal and abnormal cardiac development. More specific issues are discussed in Chapter 2 on genetic control of cardiovascular development.

ADVANCES AND LIMITATIONS IN STUDYING HUMAN DEVELOPMENT

Cardiac development begins with the formation of the cardiogenic plates and is completed essentially after formation of the coronary vascular system at about 8 weeks of development. A well-nourished organ that can cope with the extensive demands needed to ensure adequate circulation is formed. The earliest human intrauterine observations indicating normal or abnormal cardiac development can be made by ultrasonography and by echo Doppler techniques at 11 to 12 weeks' gestation.[1] These observations show mainly flow parameters and little morphologic detail until about 14 weeks' gestation. With improved knowledge and equipment, we will be able to identify cardiac morphology more clearly at younger ages.

Normal cardiovascular development of the human embryo in its crucial stages, between 2 and 8 weeks' gestation, has to be deduced from postmortem morphologic studies of abortion material, mainly spontaneous abortions. We do not know whether this material reflects normal morphogenesis. In addition, information on disturbed genes and chromosomes is provided by amniocentesis, chorionic biopsies, and subsequent FISH (fluorescent in situ hybridization analysis) with genetic markers. These studies are not performed, however, within the crucial first 8 weeks of development.

CORRELATION OF HUMAN DEVELOPMENT AND ANIMAL MODELS

Because of these limitations, our knowledge of detailed cardiac morphogenesis relies on an analysis of processes in animal species. Many animal species have been studied, the main embryonic models being avian (chick and quail) and rodent (mouse and rat). With the development of transgenic techniques, the mouse embryo has become very important. In this chapter we refer regularly to mouse embryo models when discussing certain abnormalities of cardiac development. An embryolethal phenotype after a gene knockout, as well as the absence of a phenotype in null mutants or overexpression models, might contribute little to the understanding of human cardiac malformations. The initial euphoria with regard to the possibilities of transgenic techniques is changing into a more realistic perspective.[2]

Biomechanical and hemodynamic factors have been undervalued in the research on cardiogenic programming. Their role in development of cardiac malformations has been acknowledged, however, and has led to a mechanistic classification.[3] A small number of publications link hemodynamics to cardiovascular developmental abnormalities,[4,5] including some reports on measurements made during normal and abnormal cardiac development.[6–9] However, the relationship among hemodynamic changes, gene expression, and cardiogenic patterning is far from clear.

FORMATION OF THE CARDIOGENIC PLATES AND THE CARDIAC TUBE

The developmental program of the heart starts with the formation within the splanchnic mesoderm of the bilateral cardiogenic plates, which give rise to the myocardium and probably to parts of the endocardium. The splanchnic mesoderm at the endoderm/mesoderm interface differentiates into the vascular endothelium[10] and supposedly into part of the endocardium.[11–13] The evidence for a cardiogenic plate origin of the endocardium supports a dual origin for this layer of the heart.[14,15]

The cardiogenic plates can be delineated early in embryonic life because several transcription factors and early developmental proteins are expressed in the bilateral asymmetric cardiogenic plates (Fig. 1–1). Only after the cardiogenic plates fuse does the cardiac tube develop.[12] At this stage it consists of an inner endocardial and an outer myocardial layer. The primitive cardiac endothelial network is remodeled into a single endocardial tube that connects the omphalomesenteric veins to the pharyngeal arch vasculature (Figs. 1–2 and 1–3A). The asymmetric cardiac jelly surrounding the endocardial tube formation suggests bilateral endocardial tubes, giving the wrong impression that in normal cardiac development there are two cardiac

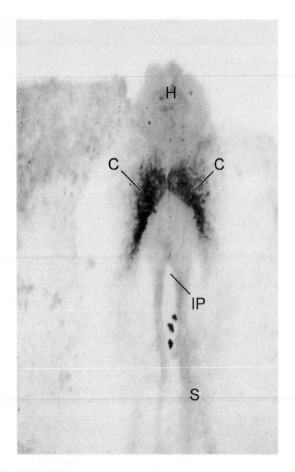

Whole mount of a quail embryo (stage HH 8) viewed from the ventral aspect, showing the bilateral cardiogenic plates (C) that have not yet fused across the midline. At this stage, the staining is done by a nonspecific neurofilament antibody. H = head region; IP = intestinal portal; S = somite.

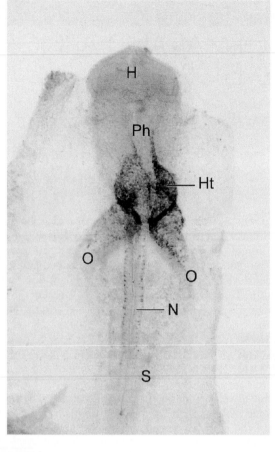

Whole mount of the fused heart tube (Ht) of a quail embryo (stage HH 10) viewed from the ventral aspect. The staining is by an anti-smooth muscle actin antibody, showing the myocardial lining of the tube. H = head region; Ph = pharyngeal region; O = omphalomesenteric vein; N = neural tube; S = somite.

tubes. From the onset, the endocardial tubes are, however, connected by endocardial cells that cross the midline.

Although this is the normal early course of development, real cardia bifida can occur spontaneously and can also be produced by experimental manipulation, such as retinoic acid overdose in the chicken embryo[16] or in a zebrafish mutational screen.[17] These studies show that each cardiogenic plate has the potential to give rise to an independent cardiac tube, implying that fusion of the cardiogenic plates is unnecessary for the onset of cardiac formation. Nevertheless, cardia bifida is lethal to the embryo as further cardiac development is hampered and no connection with the endothelium of the pharyngeal vascular system becomes established.

FORMATION OF A SEPARATE ARTERIAL AND VENOUS POLE

With the formation of the cardiac tube, the coelomic cavity becomes continuous across the midline, and the ventral mesocardium disappears. Thereafter, the cardiac tube is connected to the dorsal body wall or splanchnic mesoderm solely by the dorsal mesocardium that runs from the developing pharyngeal arches to the sinus venosus. This allows a connection between the intracardiac lining cells and the extracardiac endothelial cells. According to our studies in the quail embryo, which allow early detection of endothelial cells by the specific marker *QH1,* it is evident that this is an early, ill-understood connection between the heart and the extracardiac splanchnic mesoderm. This connection to the dorsal body wall is disrupted with the onset of cardiac looping. The dorsal mesocardium disappears in part, resulting in an arterial pole of the cardiac tube that is connected to the pharyngeal arch system and a venous pole that is connected to the dorsal body wall by what is still called the *dorsal mesocardium.* At this site the cardinal veins and the pulmonary veins gain entrance into the heart.

MOLECULAR BIOLOGIC DATA AND CONSEQUENCES FOR MALFORMATIONS

After mesoderm specification, for example by BMP4 (bone morphogenetic protein), the earliest known marker for the cardiogenic lineage in vertebrates is the homeobox *(HOX)*-containing gene *Nkx2.5* (homologue to *tinman* in *Drosophila*)[18,19] and the zinc finger–containing GATA 4/5/6 cluster of transcription factors.[20] An increasing number of genes coding for transcription factors that might regulate part of cardiac development are becoming known,[21]

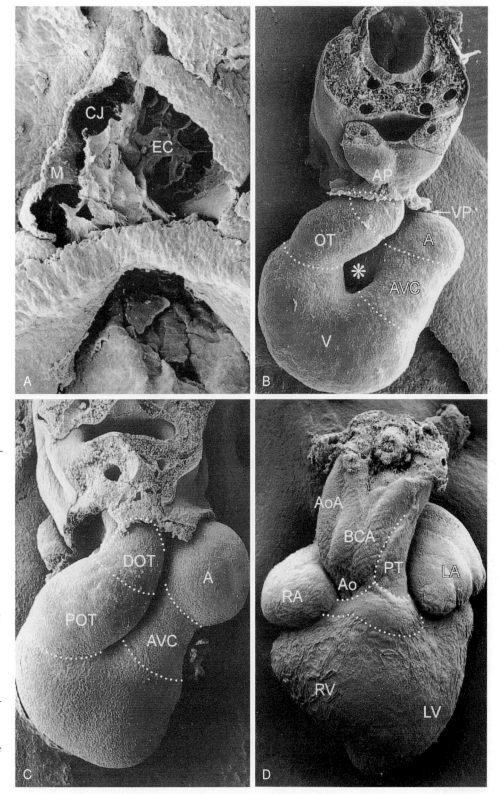

FIGURE 1–3

Scanning electron micrographs of the developing heart. *A,* The fused heart tube (see also Fig. 1–2) has been opened to show the endocardial cells (EC) inside the myocardium (M) and the cardiac jelly (CJ). *B,* The heart tube normally loops to the right showing a venous pole (VP) and an arterial pole (AP) and the inner curvature *(asterisk).* OT = outflow tract; A = atrium; V = ventricular loop; AVC = atrioventricular canal. *C,* As the inner curvature tightens, the outflow tract becomes positioned in front of the venous pole. DOT = distal outflow tract; POT = proximal outflow tract; AVC = atrioventricular canal; A = atrium. *D,* With completion of the looping process, the AP is wedged in between the atrioventricular orifices that connect the right atrium (RA) to the right ventricle (RV) and the left atrium (LA) to the left ventricle (LV). AoA = aortic arch (right sided in birds); BCA = brachiocephalic arteries; PT = pulmonary trunk; Ao = aortic root.

but a general organizational hierarchy, for example based on the clustered *HOX* genes,[19] is lacking.[2] Loss of function experiments with *tinman* in *Drosophila* resulted in embryos lacking a heart and thus in embryolethality.[18] The mammalian homologue *Nkx2.5* seems to code for a myosin light chain that is ventricular specific; at least, the heart fails to loop properly in homozygous null mutants.[22]

Data on development of the outflow tract of the heart and the role of the heart deformed *(hdf)* insertional mutation into the *versican* gene point toward a role of a potential anterior cardiac field.[23] This anterior area is responsible for adding an outflow tract segment to the early fused cardiac tube.[24] For more detailed data on molecular biology, see Chapter 2.

LOOPING OF THE CARDIAC TUBE

The single cardiac tube is never completely straight (see Fig. 1–2, 1–3A), as both cardiogenic plates have different dimensions.[15,25] In normal development, the cardiac tube loops to the right (D loop) (see Fig. 1–3B), whereas abnormalities such as L-loop and anterior-loop formation are related in the human embryo to ventricular inversion. Laterality problems are connected to abnormalities in the atrial situs.

The morphogenetic mechanism of looping can be divided into two processes, defined as *looping proper* and *wedging*. Looping proper is the mechanism of bending the originally (incompletely) straight cardiac tube into a U form that reaches out into in the third dimension by extension of the future right ventricular part (also referred to as *bulbus cordis*) to a more ventral position, while the venous and arterial poles remain fixed to the dorsal body wall. The venous pole becomes gradually hidden behind the cardiac loop. As the right atrial segment expands in concordance with expansion of the atrioventricular canal to the right, the arterial pole becomes positioned in front of the atrioventricular canal (see Fig. 1–3C). During outflow tract septation, the aorta and pulmonary trunk become separated, and by remodeling of the inner curvature of the cardiac tube (originally the site of disruption of the dorsal mesocardium), the aorta acquires a central position in the heart, and becomes positioned more distal and deeper into the base of the heart, as compared with the pulmonary orifice. This process is referred to as *wedging of the aorta* (see Fig. 1–3D).

MOLECULAR BIOLOGIC DATA AND CONSEQUENCES FOR MALFORMATIONS

The mechanisms underlying the primary looping direction are poorly understood, but a number of regulating genes are described, such as *sonic hedgehog, nodal,* and *activin receptor IIa.*[26] In mouse mutants *iv/iv* and *inv,* the laterality of the heart is affected. There is great clinical interest about the background of laterality problems and the heterotaxia syndromes in humans. The *iv* gene has been mapped to chromosome 12 in the mouse and is syntenic to chromosome 14q in the human. (see Chapter 2). In the human this specific abnormality is reflected in the heart by atrial isomerism and is referred to later in the section on atrial development and septation.

The proposed disturbed function of connexin43[27,28] in heterotaxia has not been substantiated in subsequent screenings of large patient-based populations. A detailed analysis of genes regulating cardiac looping as deduced from animal models and the relation to human heterotaxia syndromes is provided in Chapter 2.

SEGMENTAL SPECIFICATION AND TRANSITIONAL ZONES

It is tempting to postulate that in the early cardiac tube, or even in the prefused cardiogenic plates, an anteroposterior organization and specification are present, as demonstrated for other major parts of the embryo, such as the neural tube, the pharyngeal arches, and the somites. Until now, relatively few data have been found to substantiate this postulate. Some myosin-heavy chain genes show an anteroposterior orientation even in the cardiogenic plate,[29] and this gene expression pattern can be altered by various factors, such as retinoic acid. Other genes such as *hdf* are ascribed to specific parts of the cardiac tube.[23] This gene is initially expressed in the part that develops into the right ventricle and outflow tract. Several genes are expressed specifically in the future right ventricular part, later on spreading over the complete cardiac tube or disappearing altogether. This specific expression pattern does not reflect right-left asymmetry but rather an anteroposterior direction. Other genes like *GATA4*[20] are initially present in the complete myocardium, but during differentiation of the cardiac segments they become restricted or disappear. Unpublished data from several groups that study truncated promoter regions of cardiac-specific genes reveal temporal and spatial expression patterns more clearly. No direct effect of *HOX* patterning has been found in the normal development of the heart. Pardanaud and colleagues[10] have provided an excellent review of *Hox* genes and cardiac development, and they have shown that a number of paired, related genes such as *Prx1* and *Prx2,* as well as *Msx1* and *Msx2,* are expressed in the heart during certain stages of development.

SEGMENTATION OF THE CARDIAC TUBE

As indicated previously, the initial cardiac tube consists of myocardium with an inner lining of cardiac jelly and endocardium. Moorman and Lamers[30] described a number of genes (e.g., those responsible for coding acetylcholine esterase and SERCA [sarcoplasmic reticulum calcium^{2+} ATPase]) that are expressed in a gradient from the venous to the arterial pole. Later, several proteins and messenger RNAs are differentially expressed between the atrium and the ventricle. The expression of atrial and ventricular myosins as an exponent of fast longitudinal conduction areas alternates with areas that express atrial and ventricular myosins of slow conduction areas. The original cardiac tube with peristaltic contractions is succeeded by a more complex beating heart.

It is uncertain, however, when the cardiac segments and transitional zones can be unequivocally distinguished (Fig. 1–4A, B). From the inflow at the venous pole it is possible to distinguish the sinus venosus, the atrium, the atrioventricular canal lined by endocardial cushions, the trabeculated ventricular inflow segment, the primary fold, and the ventricular outflow segment that develops into a trabeculated part and a proximal and distal part lined by endocardial outflow tract cushions. Marker experiments with India ink and beads[24] show that the primary ventricular region of the cardiac tube becomes incorporated into the primary fold, forming the inner curvature and the ventricular septum. This supports the idea that the initial cardiac tube does not contain all the segments in miniature (like the homunculus in the sperm). On the contrary, various segments are added during differentiation and growth of the cardiac tube. Most experiments indicate an extension of the cardiac tube both cranially and caudally, the outflow tract being considered to be the last part formed. The endocardial

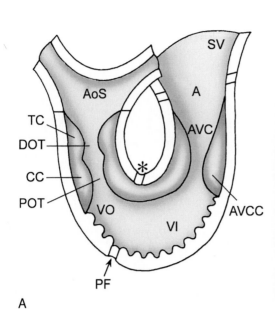

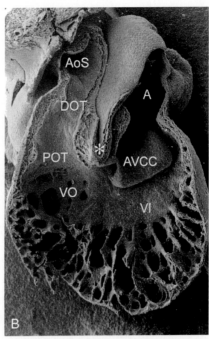

FIGURE 1–4

Diagram *(A)* and scanning electron micrograph *(B)* of a chick heart showing the segments and transitional zones in a developing heart before completion of septation. At the venous pole the heart starts with the sinus venosus (SV). Thereafter, it follows the atrial segment (A) that connects to the atrioventricular canal (AVC), a transitional zone that is lined by atrioventricular endocardial cushions (AVCC). The ventricular segment consists of an inflow (VI) and an outflow (VO) segment separated by the primary fold (PF). The outflow tract contains endocardial cushions, which in birds can be distinguished as conal cushions (CC) and truncal cushions (TC). The distal outflow tract (DOT) connects to the aortic sac (AoS). In the inner curvature *(asterisk)* the superior AVCC and one of the outflow tract conal endocardial cushions are continuous. This continuity disappears after proper septation. POT = proximal outflow tract.

cushion–lined transitional zones later form the atrioventricular and semilunar valves. The sinus venosus (in itself considered a transitional zone) and the primary fold, both lacking an endocardial cushion lining, are important for the formation of the future conduction system of the heart. All transitional zones are involved in septation of the heart into a four-chambered organ.

EXTRACARDIAC CONTRIBUTIONS

As mentioned previously, the early cardiac tube is connected by the mesocardium to the dorsal body wall, the connection sites persisting at the arterial and venous poles. Current research focuses primarily on the ectomesenchymal neural crest contribution to the heart. These initially pluripotent cells reach the heart and differentiate into various cell lineages comprising smooth muscle cells of the vessel wall and ganglionic cells of the autonomic nervous system, which are mainly parasympathetic ganglionic cells but also sympathetic nerve fibers. Last of all, neural crest cells take part substantially in outflow tract septation (Fig. 1–5A, B).

An understudied area is the venous connection to the body wall by the dorsal mesocardium. Through this portal, cells from an extracardiac origin migrate into the heart and merge with the inferior atrioventricular cushion and through the spina vestibula at the base of the primary atrial septum with the superior cushion (see Fig. 1–5B). This latter configuration plays an important part in atrial-to-

ventricular septation, closing the primary atrial septal foramen and septating the atrioventricular canal. The resultant septum is the atrioventricular septum. Last of all, the proepicardial organ[31–33] situated near the sinus venosus gives rise to the epicardium (see Fig. 1–12A) that grows over the myocardial cardiac tube. In the subepicardial tissue the endothelium of the coronary vasculature spreads out to form a vascular endothelium–lined network. Studies show that the smooth muscle cells of the media and the fibroblasts of the adventitia are also of epicardial origin.[34,35]

SINUS VENOSUS INCORPORATION AND ATRIAL SEPTATION

The sinus venosus in the developing heart is an intriguing structure that forms a transitional zone between the cardiac veins and the developing atrium proper. The musculature of the sinus venosus has its own gene expression pattern fitting with slow conduction.[30] On the basis of endothelial vascular patterns, scanning electron microscopic data, and immunohistochemical results, DeRuiter and colleagues[36] have shown that the sinus venosus is incorporated into both the dorsal wall of the right atrium and the dorsal wall of the left atrium (Fig. 1–6A, B). At the latter site, it encircles the entrance of the future pulmonary veins. The suggestion that the sinus venosus also contributes to the posterior wall of the left atrium has been substantiated from studies of the mouse embryo. Our own observations using

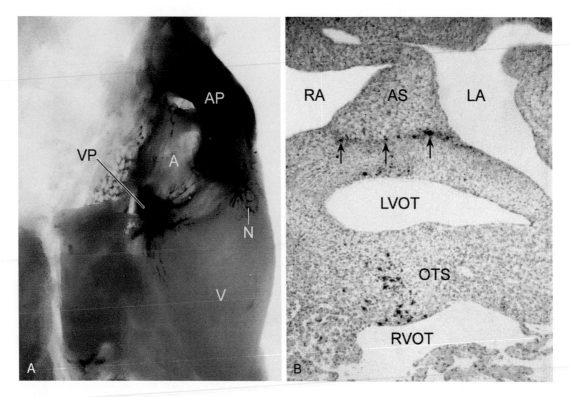

A, Whole mount staining of a chicken heart (stage HH 35) that shows the neural crest–derived cells after a retroviral transporter gene marker containing *lac-Z.* The neural crest cells are present at the arterial pole (AP) as smooth muscle cells in the vessel wall and over the heart as fine nerve fibers (N). The neural crest cells also reach the venous pole (VP) of the heart, where they enter the atrioventricular region through the dorsal mesocardium. *B,* A section through the inflow and outflow tract of a chicken heart in which the neural crest cells are seen in the outflow tract septum (OTS) as well as at the base of the atrial septum (AS) *(arrows),* where they have arrived through the dorsal mesocardium. The brown staining of the OTS neural crest cells by the TUNEL (TdT-mediated dUTP [deoxyuridine triphosphate] nick end labeling) technique detected apoptosis of these cells. A = atrium; V = ventricle; RA = right atrium; LA = left atrium; LVOT = left ventricular outflow tract; RVOT = right ventricular outflow tract.

an immunohistochemical technique show this to be true for the human embryo also.[36a] A publication on mouse development by Webb and associates[37] takes a somewhat different stance in which the pulmonary veins (pulmonary pit lined by pulmonary ridges) have their own origin, independent from the sinus venosus. The different explanations have a common feature, namely, that the veins are directly embedded in the mesenchyme of the dorsal body wall. In the fully developed human heart, this area is demarcated by the epicardial-pericardial fold, shaped like a halter.

The morphogenesis of the sinus venosus also provides new data on the septation of the atria. The primary atrial septum is a structure that consists of the atrial myocardium forming an arch that runs from posterior to anterior. In the posterior part, it attaches above the compressed sinus venosus. Also at this site, the extracardiac mesenchyme enters through the dorsal mesocardium to contribute to atrial-to-ventricular septation. The extracardiac mesenchyme provides cells to the inferior atrioventricular cushion and lines the lower rim of the primary atrial septum as the spina vestibula (see Figs. 1–5*B* and 1–6*B*). Closure of the primary atrial septal foramen is achieved by the fusion of the atrioventricular cushions with the spina vestibula.

The primary atrial septum itself becomes perforated and forms the foramen ovale (Fig. 1–7*A*). Further study of the development of the secondary atrial septum reveals that this septal component consists, in its basal and dorsal part, of sinus venosus (being the left venous valve) that has fused with the spina vestibula. The major anterior and superior parts of the secondary atrial septum are just a fold of the atrial myocardial wall.

MOLECULAR BIOLOGIC DATA AND CONSEQUENCES FOR MALFORMATIONS

Abnormal Pulmonary Venous Connection

Because the plexus from which the pulmonary veins originate has extensive connections to the cranial and caudal parts of the cardinal veins,[38] persistent connections can lead to a supracardiac or infracardiac pulmonary venous connection. The pulmonary veins do not grow out of the left atrial dorsal wall but are connected to the left atrial wall through incorporation of the sinus venosus into the left atrium. Supracardiac total abnormal pulmonary venous connection is often through a persistent left superior cardinal vein because in the early embryonic period the pulmonary veins are already connected to the sinus venosus. In a spatium pulmonale (i.e., no connection between the pulmonary veins and the atria), the incorporation of the sinus venosus has not taken place normally.

Atrial Septal Defects

The most common atrial septal defect (ASD) is the septum secundum ASD in which there is a discrepancy between the

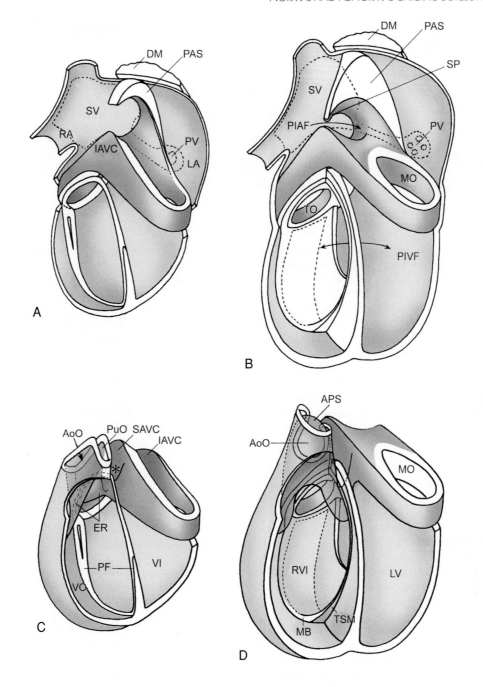

FIGURE 1–6

A. Schematic view of the developing heart after looping and before septation emphasizing the sinus venosus (SV) and the atrial segment. The atrioventricular cushions have not yet fused, and the atrial septation has just started. The sinus venosus *(dotted line)* is connected to both the right (RA) and the left (LA) atrium. In the LA, it encircles the pulmonary veins (PV). *B,* A depiction of stage in which septation is almost completed at both the ventricular and the atrial levels. There are still a primary interventricular foramen (PIVF) and a primary interatrial foramen (PIAF). The tissue of the dorsal mesocardium (DM) enters the heart at the venous pole at the site where the sinus venosus, atrium, and atrioventricular cushions (fused inferior [IAVC] and superior [SAVC]) meet in the posterior wall. Underneath the atrial septum, an endocardial cushion–like structure is present: the spina vestibula (SP), which is effective in closure of the PIAF. *C,* Figure comparable to *A,* focusing on the outflow tract. The borderline between the myocardium (lined on the inside by endocardial outflow tract ridges [ER]) and aortic sac is saddle shaped. In between the outflow tract and the atrioventricular canal there is the inner curvature *(asterisk).* The primary fold (PF) runs in this curvature and further separates the ventricular inlet (VI) and outlet (VO) segments. *D,* Ventricular inlet septation is partly affected by the outgrowth of the right ventricular inlet (RVI), resulting in a positioning of the tricuspid orifice above the right ventricle. The endocardial outflow tract ridges that contain the neural crest cells of the aortopulmonary septum (APS) form after fusion and myocardialization, the subpulmonary muscular infundibulum. This structure separates the right and left ventricular outflow tracts. This structure is remodeled into the subpulmonary muscular infundibulum. AoO = aortic orifice; PuO = pulmonary orifice; MO = mitral orifice; TO = tricuspid orifice; PAS = primary atrial septum; TSM = trabecula septomarginalis; MB = moderator band; LV = left ventricle.

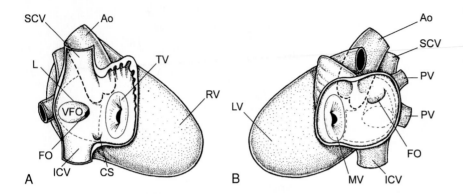

A, Schematic view of the atrial septum from the right side. In the original sinus venosus–derived compartment, the inferior (ICV) and superior (SCV) caval vein and the coronary sinus (CS) enter. The septum secundum, that in its upper part is a fold of the atrial wall, forms the limbus (L), which overlaps in part the valvula foraminis ovalis (VFO). Between both crescents the foramen ovale (FO) is present before birth. *B*, Left atrial view of the same structures as depicted in *A*. Ao = aorta; LV = left ventricle; MV = mitral valve; PV = pulmonary vein; RV = right ventricle; TV = tricuspid valve.

septum secundum (bordered on the right side by the limbus) and the free edge of the septum primum. In normal circumstances, they overlap as two crescents (see Fig. 1–7*A*, *B*) that become fused after birth. Defective development, including perforations, of the valve of the septum primum, the so-called valve of the foramen ovale, can lead to secundum defect. However, the septum secundum can also be deficient. The mechanisms leading to these abnormalities have not been adequately studied. Studies are needed to distinguish between retarded closure of the foramen ovale and a real secundum ASD. The development of a secundum ASD in an animal model on the basis of manipulation of transcription or growth factors has not been reported; it is difficult in the embryo to distinguish between a widely patent foramen ovale and a true ASD. Abnormalities in formation of the base of the atrial septum secundum can lead to a so-called sinus venosus ASD. In this defect, both the inferior and superior caval veins are closely related to the defect, and the right pulmonary veins are often abnormally positioned.

Atrioventricular Septal Defects

A completely different developmental sequence relates to the development of the atrioventricular septal defect. The origin of this anomaly has been considered to be an abnormal fusion of the atrioventricular cushions. When considering the extracardiac cellular contribution, abnormalities of this invading cell mass (like the neural crest in the outflow tract) may lead to deficient septation and the persistence of a primary ASD, as is typical for an atrioventricular septal defect.

There are some models, such as the trisomy 16 mouse, that show an atrioventricular septal defect[39] and a combination of both inflow and outflow anomalies. As chromosome 16 in the mouse is syntenic with chromosome 21 in the human, this mouse model is studied for correlation with trisomy 21 in humans. We refer to this model again when discussing the role of the neural crest in cardiac development. In humans, linkage analysis has shown that a form of familial secundum ASD maps to chromosome 5p.[40] Familial secundum ASD is considered to be a genetically heterogeneous disorder with low penetrance. Familial total anomalous pulmonary venous connection has been mapped to chromosome 4p13-q12.

DESIGNATION OF LEFT AND RIGHT ATRIA

Morphologists and clinicians are aware of the differences between the right and left atria. The easiest way of distinguishing them is to examine the auricles or the atrial appendages, which are blunt and short in the right atrium and crooked and finger-like in the left atrium. This specific morphology has been expanded by Anderson and associates[41] who described the posterior wall of the right atrium as trabeculated, whereas the left posterior wall was described as smooth (see Chapters 19 and 20). Atria are normally in situs solitus, implying that a morphologic right atrium is on the right and a morphologic left atrium is on the left. In abnormal hearts they can also be inverted, in mirror image, or even double right (right isomerism) or double left (left isomerism). Usually atrial situs correlates with the bronchial anatomy; the right bronchus leaves the trachea at a more acute angle and is longer than the left bronchus. Lung lobation, difficult to evaluate for the clinician, is less reliable. Another situs problem involves the spleen, polysplenia being common in left isomerism and asplenia in right isomerism (see also Chapters 2, 19, and 20).

MOLECULAR BIOLOGIC DATA AND CONSEQUENCES FOR MALFORMATIONS

Mouse mutations (*iv/iv* and *inv* mice) have shown that isomerism of the atria is similar to the human heterotaxia syndromes. Experiments using a truncated promoter of the *MLCIF/3F* gene[42] showed in expression studies that the right atrium, the atrioventricular canal, and the left ventricle in the early embryonic mouse heart form one entity that does not include the left atrium and the right ventricle. Crossing these mice with the *iv/iv* mouse showed that in right atrial isomerism both atria had the same pattern, indicating that the right and left atria temporarily present with their own genetic coding.

VENTRICULAR INFLOW TRACT SEPTATION AND THE FORMATION OF THE RIGHT VENTRICLE INLET

The mechanism of ventricular inflow tract septation is still under discussion.[14, 43–47] A muscular fold between the trabeculated ventricular inflow segment (the main part of the future left ventricle) and part of the ventricular outflow segment (trabeculated and part of the future right ventricle) is the main progenitor of the ventricular inflow tract septum. This fold, called the *primary fold,* is clearly recognized in human and mouse embryos (see Fig. 1–6*C*). In older literature,[14] the term *bulboventricular fold* has been used. The primary fold is considered to be a transitional zone, although it does not comply with the pattern of alternating slow and fast conduction segments,[48] because it always belonged to the fast conducting areas. This fold has received a great deal of attention, not only because it forms the major part of the ventricular inlet septum but also because it harbors the precursor of the atrioventricular conduction system in older embryos (see later).

The primary fold borders on the inner curvature of the heart where it coalesces with the right side of the atrioventricular canal (see Fig. 1–6C). The part of the primary fold close to the apex becomes part of the definitive septum, probably by condensation of the ventricular trabeculae and outgrowth of the trabeculated free wall of both left and right ventricles. Closure of the primary interventricular foramen between the right and left ventricles takes place by fusion of the inferior and superior atrioventricular cushions in combination with one of the outflow tract endocardial ridges that is connected to this superior cushion.

Confusion in terminology might easily arise about the use of the term *primary* (or *bulboventricular*) *foramen* encircled by the primary fold and the term *primary interventricular foramen*. The primary foramen is divided into right and left ventricular parts, and it remains widely patent as the connection between the right and left ventricular inlet and outlet segments.[49,50] The primary interventricular foramen is the embryonic connection between the left and the right ventricle that is closed during normal development, separating the primary foramen into the right and left ventricular parts (see Fig. 1–6B, D).

The role of the primary fold as progenitor of the main body of the ventricular septum deserves further attention. A proper septum is established only after a right ventricle, with its tricuspid valve and orifice, is formed. In the embryo, this is related to the formation of the right ventricular inlet compartment (see Fig. 1–6D). The right part of the atrioventricular canal with the adjoining part of the primary fold is transferred to the right. In our opinion, this is achieved by a splitting of the primary fold at the dorsal wall of the ventricular segment. Growth of the initially minute inflow part of the right ventricle allows for expansion of a right ventricular inlet with a new posterior wall of the right ventricle. In this way, the definitive right ventricle consists eventually of three parts, each with a different embryologic history: (1) the right ventricular inlet, bordered by the remnants of the primary fold (trabecula septomarginalis and moderator band) (see Fig. 1–6D); (2) the ventricular trabecular part (embryonic ventricular outlet segment); and (3) the part of the proximal and distal ventricular outlet segment underneath the pulmonary orifice, as described in the section on outflow tract separation.

When viewed from the right, the ventricular septum is composed of three parts. One part is the inlet septum that is formed during the expansion of the right ventricular inlet. This part is separated from the trabecular part of the septum by the crista supraventricularis and the moderator band. The muscular outflow tract septum or infundibulum derives its myocardium from the proximal and distal outflow tracts or conotruncal region lined by endocardial cushions. This part is discussed in the next section on outflow tract separation.

MOLECULAR BIOLOGIC DATA AND CONSEQUENCES FOR MALFORMATIONS

A number of abnormalities in human inflow tract septation may be elucidated by animal models.

Isolated or multiple muscular ventricular septal defects surrounded by myocardium can be the result of noncompaction of the myocardial trabeculae. There have been some mouse models that show this extensive spongy myocardium, but they become embryolethal before a malformation, supposedly comparable to that in humans, is reached.

Abnormal looping of the cardiac tube can prevent the tricuspid valve from being optimally placed above the right ventricle.[51,52] This can produce lesions ranging from a straddling tricuspid valve to a double inlet left ventricle. The cause for abnormal looping, also leading to the double outlet right ventricle, is variable, including retinoic acid induction in chicken embryos[51,53,54] as well as a growth factor null mutant (transforming growth factor β_2 [TGF-β_2]) mouse.[52] These embryos probably have a primary myocardial problem and not merely an abnormality of the formation of the septum itself.

Most perimembranous ventricular septal defects and outflow tract malalignment defects result from abnormal outflow tract septation and are discussed in the following paragraph.

The last interesting abnormality concerns the atrioventricular septal defect, described previously under the heading of atrial septation. We consider this anomaly to be the consequence of an abnormal fusion of the spina vestibula and the atrioventricular cushion mass. Whether the underlying problem is a failure of fusion of the cushion tissue, or a substantially diminished ventricular mass inclusive of the ventricular septum, or an abnormal cellular contribution through the dorsal mesocardium remains to be investigated. Several animal models, such as the trisomy 16 mouse,[39] comparable to the human trisomy 21, are useful. Both the trisomic human and mouse show outflow tract anomalies related to our observations in a reporter gene marked neural crest chick model.[55,56] We have traced neural crest cells to both the endocardial cushions in the outflow tract and the atrioventricular cushions in the inflow tract. The pathway to the latter area is considered to be through the dorsal mesocardium at the venous inflow.[56a]

VENTRICULAR OUTFLOW TRACT SEPARATION AND NEURAL CREST

Achieving outflow tract separation requires the participation of an extracardiac cell source such as the neural crest, just as septation of the venous pole (described in the section on atrial septation) requires a contribution of the extracardiac dorsal mesocardium.

We refer to the septation of this part as *separation*, because in the normal heart, the subpulmonary infundibular or muscular septum is mainly a free-standing sleeve of muscle. Outflow tract separation has been described for the human embryo by Bartelings and colleagues[49,57,58] and has proved to be essentially the same in animal species such as the chick and mouse.[14,56,59,60]

Separation starts in the distal outflow tract that is lined by endocardial cushion tissue arranged in two opposing spiraling ridges. One ridge runs in a dorsolateral direction to adjoin the myocardium of the primary fold at the future site of the ventriculoinfundibular fold in the full-grown heart. The other ridge runs in a ventroanterior direction to adjoin both the myocardium of the primary fold and the superior atrioventricular cushion in the inner curvature of the embryonic cardiac tube. This region is normally a site of remodeling, mainly shortening, a process referred to as *conus absorption*.[59]

The nomenclature of the endocardial outflow tract ridges is confusing. Some authors consider these ridges as being composed of proximal or conal ridges (leading after septation to the conal septum) and distal or truncal ridges (leading to a truncal septum). Pexieder[61] sorted out this nomenclature confusion. For this chapter the terms used are based on scanning electron micrograph studies showing ridges and boundaries in their full length (Fig. 1–8A). It is practical to distinguish between proximal and distal ridges, clearly visible as separate structures in the chicken embryo, but they are more continuous in humans and rodents (mouse and rat). The proximal ridges mainly form the muscular outflow tract septum, whereas the distal ridge area is subject to shortening and contributes to semilunar valve formation and the septation of the arterial orifice level.

Understanding the three-dimensional aspects of outflow tract separation starts with knowledge that the arterial orifice level, indicated by the mesenchymal (vessel wall)/ myocardial outflow tract boundary, is saddle shaped (see Figs. 1–8B and 1–6C, D). Even in the early embryo, this shape brings the future aortic orifice into a more lateral and lower position than the future pulmonary orifice. With normal cardiac looping, inclusive of wedging of the aorta, the aortic orifice is brought even deeper into the cardiac mass, resulting in the well-known difference in position and plane of both arterial orifices (see Fig. 1–8C, D). The highest (most distal) part of the saddle-shaped myocardium, always covered on the inside by endocardial cushion tissue, is positioned in the intersection between the sixth and fourth arch arteries (see Fig. 1–8A, B). It is exactly at this site that the condensation of extracardiac mesenchyme, derived from the neural crest, is located. In embryos before septation, two prongs of condensed mesenchyme enter the cushion tissue at these highest points. With the start of septation, this is followed by a central condensation just above the mesenchymal/myocardial outflow tract boundary. This is the aortopulmonary septum.[49,62]

In completing normal outflow tract separation, the myocardial outflow tract septum merges with the ventriculoinfundibular fold and the trabecula septomarginalis. The lower rim borders on the anterior tricuspid orifice and is called the *crista supraventricularis* in normal hearts. Eventually the right ventricular outflow tract is relatively long and surrounded by myocardium, whereas the left ventricular outflow tract is short and only partly surrounded

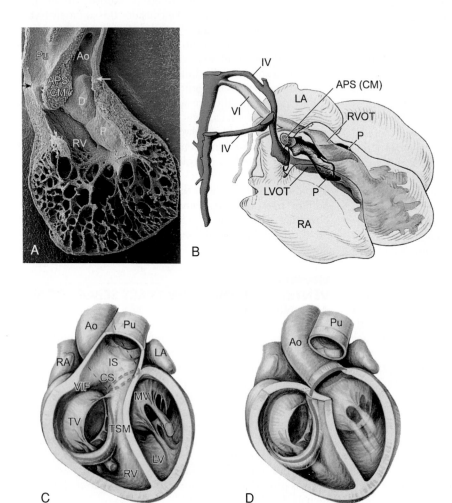

FIGURE 1–8

A, Scanning electron microscopic photograph of a preseptation chicken heart showing one set of the proximal (P) and distal (D) outflow tract ridges. The borderline between myocardium (lined on the inside by endocardial cushions) and arterial wall is indicated by *arrows*. The distal cushions remodel into semilunar valves. *B*, Septation of the outflow tract is achieved by fusion of the outflow tract ridges and an ingrowth of condensed mesenchyme (CM), also called the *aortopulmonary septum* (APS). The APS extends two prongs into the ridges. *C*, After septation of the outflow tract, a muscular subpulmonary infundibulum (IS) is formed, which separates the right ventricular outflow tract (RVOT) from the outside world and the aorta. In a normal heart the actual outflow tract septum separating the left ventricular outflow tract (LVOT) and RVOT is minimal. *D*, Depiction of the difference in length of the RVOT and the relative tilted position of the aortic and pulmonary orifice. Ao = aorta; Pu = pulmonary trunk; IV, VI = pharyngeal arch arteries; P = prong of CM; RA = right atrium; LA = left atrium; VIF = ventriculoinfundibular fold; TSM = trabecula septomarginalis; CS = crista supraventricularis; TV = tricuspid valve; MV = mitral valve; RV = right ventricle; LV = left ventricle.

by myocardium. In a normal heart, only a small stretch of musculature deserves to be called a septum between both outflow tracts (see Fig. 1–8C, D). This situation differs markedly from what is observed with disturbed outflow tract septation.

MOLECULAR BIOLOGIC DATA AND CONSEQUENCES FOR MALFORMATIONS

Our chicken-quail chimera studies and the reporter gene neural crest chick studies (Fig. 1–9) show this condensed mesenchyme to be mainly composed of neural crest cells.[14,56,63] These neural crest cells extend into the distal ridges and spread from here into the semilunar valves[56,64] as well as into the surrounding myocardium.[56] In the proximal ridges, the prongs continue to have a close approximation with the underlying myocardium of the primary fold. As in the distal ridge, the neural crest cells are observed within the myocardial/cushion boundary. Combining research from our group in which neural crest cells are marked by a reporter gene and concurrent application of a staining for apoptosis reveals that most of the neural crest cells at this level have gone into apoptosis. This is particularly prominent during the stage of myocardialization of what are, by now, the fused endocardial outflow tract ridges (see Fig. 1–5B). We postulate that the neural crest cell death program plays an active role in stimulating outflow tract myocardialization. This process is much less obvious at the distal valve level in which a lump of condensed mesenchyme persists and differentiates into a fibrous structure, the *conus tendon*.

Van Mierop and Kutsche[65] indicated the possible impact of the neural crest in outflow tract septation. With this in mind, the theory of hemodynamic modeling capacities and flow theories to explain intracardiac and arch malformations[66,67] have been given less prominence.

Kirby and associates[68] were the first to show experimentally the link between outflow tract malformations and the disturbed neural crest. They achieved this by ablating the neural crest in chicken embryos, ending up with a spectrum of outflow tract malformations ranging from a simple ventricular septal defect to double outlet right ventricle and, at the most extreme, a persistent truncus arteriosus (common arterial trunk). Studies with a variety of mutant and transgenic mice have refined this theory. It turns out that outflow tract septation is a very vulnerable process. Abnormalities can be evoked through all tissues in this area, including myocardium, endocardial cushion tissue, and neural crest. In this area of research, most transgenes that show a phenotype end up with some sort of outflow tract malformation.

Our own experience with a number of these models shows that neural crest ablation leads to a diminished number of neural crest cells in the outflow tract, but condensed mesenchyme can still be detected even in the most severe malformations, such as persistent truncus arteriosus. The condensed mesenchyme probably has a guiding function for coronary artery ingrowth.[69,70] With hemodynamic interference, as described in chicken venous clip experiments,[5] the muscular outflow tract septum is mesenchymal, lacking a normal myocardialized component. Neural crest cell tracing points toward an altered position of the condensed mesenchyme, containing neural crest as well as an

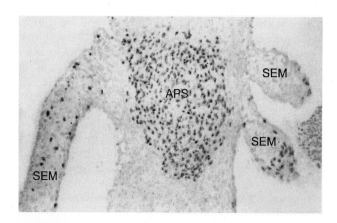

Section of the outflow tract of a chicken-quail cardiac neural crest chimera (stage HH 34). The quail cardiac neural crest cells (dark nuclei) fill almost completely the condensed mesenchyme of the aortopulmonary septum (APS). The semilunar valve leaflets (SEM) also show neural crest–derived cells.

altered apoptosis patterning. A mouse in which TGF-β_2 has been knocked out has a similar phenotype, with a spectrum ranging from simple ventricular septal defect to double outlet right ventricle.[52] Furthermore, myocardialization does not take place normally. Männer and colleagues[71] described several approaches that lead to outflow tract abnormalities, including overextension of the neck curvature of the embryo. Furthermore, teratogenic substances such as retinoic acid and knockout of the retinoic acid receptors can lead to a comparable spectrum.[72,73]

Yasui and coworkers[74] showed that carefully timed retinoic acid treatment of mouse embryos could lead to the above spectrum of lesions, including transposition of the great arteries. In the latter, the proximal outflow tract ridges had a straighter position. This fits nicely with the morphology of the heart in infants with transposition in which reversal of the great arteries is accompanied by a straighter outflow tract septum.[50]

Our current hypothesis is that the initial abnormality in most of the described models inclusive of the neural crest ablation[75] results from a hampered looping of the cardiac tube leading essentially to the aorta being too much to the right. During outflow tract separation, abnormalities of myocardium and endocardial outflow tract ridges as well as defective neural crest participation are added to formation of the outflow tract problems.

Study of this area in humans has received particular attention because a number of anomalies can now be brought together as the 22q11 deletion syndrome. Study of the DiGeorge critical region on human chromosome 22 by several groups[76,77] has provided a number of candidate genes. We are probably dealing with a contiguous gene syndrome, and a simple monogenic or neural crest disturbance is not to be expected at the present time; see also Chapter 2.

ATRIOVENTRICULAR AND SEMILUNAR VALVE FORMATION

All cardiac valves differentiate from the endocardial cushion tissue. The main difference is that the atrioventricular valves are connected to the ventricular wall by chordae tendineae and papillary muscles, whereas the semilunar valves do not have a tension apparatus.

Differentiation of the atrioventricular valves is not understood. The formation of a tricuspid and a mitral orifice, each encompassing part of the atrioventricular superior and inferior cushion mass, is shown in several studies[44, 78] and is referred to in this chapter in the section on inflow tract septation. The differentiation into fibrous leaflets has not received much attention. Wenink and Gittenberger-de Groot[43] postulated that for the human embryo the valves were mainly derived from undermined myocardium. More recent investigations by our group[79] have shown that the endocardial cushion tissue itself is remodeled into valve leaflets. This is also the opinion of Wessels and associates[80] who used immunohistochemical markers in the human embryo. Our studies show that the chordae tendineae are also derived from the endocardial cushion tissue and are not differentiated from the papillary muscles (Fig. 1–10A).

Semilunar valve development[81] occurs from the distal part of the endocardial outflow tract ridges on the borderline of mesenchyme and myocardium. Reconstructions of human stages[57, 58] showed that the orifice level is not located in one plane but has a saddle shape, whereby the future aortic orifice is tilted in a more dorsolateral and caudal position than the pulmonary side of the orifice. With septation of the outflow tract, the two main endocardial ridges are divided by the condensed mesenchyme of the aorto-pulmonary septum. The result is that four central cushion masses can be distinguished, two in each orifice. To achieve three valve leaflets in each orifice, two intercalated cushion swellings are present. These are positioned peripheral to the facing (see Fig. 1–10B) valve cushions. In the aorta, the intercalated valve swelling develops into the noncoronary cusp. The two facing semilunar valve sinuses receive the main stems of the right and left coronary arteries. For a proper attachment of the semilunar valve leaflets to the underlying myocardium and the vessel wall, a collagen ring is formed.[82] The mechanisms underlying the developmental processes of semilunar valve formation are still poorly understood.

MOLECULAR BIOLOGIC DATA AND CONSEQUENCES FOR MALFORMATIONS

Atrioventricular Valve Development

Extensive experimental work has been carried out on the differentiation of atrioventricular cushions, mainly by Markwald and coworkers.[83] They showed that substances excreted by the myocardium into the endocardial cushion tissue induce the endocardial/mesenchymal transformation necessary for the cellular composition of the future valves. One of the proteins involved in this process is ES130. The latter differentiation of the atrioventricular valve leaflets has received much less attention. Oosthoek and colleagues[79] showed in the developing valves of the

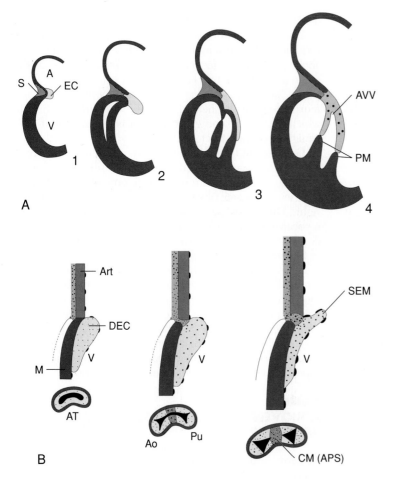

FIGURE 1–10

A, Schematic drawing of atrioventricular valve development. 1: Shows an initial continuation of atrial (A) and ventricular (V) myocardium. 2: Dissociation between A and V is seen with contact of subepicardial sulcus (S) tissue and the atrioventricular endocardial cushion (EC). 3: The myocardium inclusive of the EC is undermined, and a primitive atrioventricular valve (AVV) is formed. 4: The AVV is connected to the papillary muscles (PM) and the myocardial contribution has disappeared. *Dots* represent cells derived from epicardium. *B,* Schematic drawing of the formation of the semilunar valve (SEM) of the aortic (Ao) and pulmonary (Pu) orifice. The valve (V) is formed from the distal endocardial outflow tract ridge (DEC) that lines the myocardium (M). The Ao and Pu orifices are separated by the condensed mesenchyme (CM) of the aortopulmonary septum (APS) that is made up of neural crest cells that also migrate into the SEM (see Fig. 1–9). AT = arterial trunk; Art = artery.

chicken, mouse, and human embryos that the expression of differentiation markers in a number of layers differs on the atrial and the ventricular sides. This work[84] also provided new information on normal and abnormal papillary muscle formation, especially with regard to anomalous parachute mitral valve. In most parachute mitral valves, asymmetric formation occurs. Abnormal atrioventricular valve leaflets, such as in Ebstein malformation,[85] are still not easily explained from embryologic studies. The most likely explanation relates to incorrect undermining from the ventricular myocardium.

The valve leaflets in an atrioventricular septal defect are not abnormal in their tissue composition. This lesion is due to underdevelopment of the myocardium and a poorly septated inflow tract. A similar role can be assigned to the epicardium-derived cells (EPDCs) that migrate into the cushions from the subepicardial layer.[86]

Data from transgenic mice show that proteins comprising NF-ATc[87,88] and Sox-4[89] are specifically expressed in the endocardial cushion tissue. Null mutants show a spectrum from absence to underdevelopment of the mitral and tricuspid valves, as well as the semilunar valve leaflets. These models are embryolethal and have not been evaluated for disturbed valve formation. For the semilunar valve, a correlation has been found with human pathology in which aortic and pulmonary valves can be absent or very hypoplastic.[90] Absence of aortic leaflets is lethal for the human fetus, whereas absence of pulmonary valve leaflets is compatible with term delivery. We assume that absence of atrioventricular valve leaflets in the human embryo leads to early intrauterine death, as we have not seen this abnormality.

Semilunar Valve Abnormalities

A number of processes described for the atrioventricular cushions are also pertinent for the endocardial cushions in the outflow tract that develop into semilunar valve leaflets. Extracardiac cells also migrate into the valve anlagen, as proved for the neural crest cell population.[56,64] The mechanism underlying the formation of commissures and the sites of formation remain to be elucidated. Both genetic factors, as exemplified by a genetic hamster model of abnormal semilunar valve development,[91] and hemodynamic factors, as exemplified by rerouted venous flow in the chicken embryo,[5] can play a role.

DEVELOPMENT OF THE CONDUCTION SYSTEM

At 3 weeks of human development, the cardiac tube shows peristaltic contractions. The myocardial tube has alternating longitudinal areas of slow and fast conduction.[30] Thereafter, more specialized tracts differentiate, which guide the impulse from the base of the heart to the ventricular apex. The impulse is generated in a pacemaker, the sinoatrial node, situated in the right atrial wall at the base of the superior caval vein. It is still undecided whether to reach the atrioventricular node the impulse passes along specialized internodal atrial tracts,[92] or whether it takes preferential routes through an architectural array of myocardial fibers.

This atrioventricular node is situated in the triangle of Koch above the tricuspid orifice, next to the coronary sinus

orifice, and above the fibrous tissue separating atrial and ventricular myocardium. From this node the common bundle or bundle of His passes through the fibrous cardiac skeleton to reach the top of the ventricular septum, where it separates into right and left bundle branches. The right bundle branch consists of a compact bundle that runs through the trabecula septomarginalis to the moderator band of the right ventricle. The left bundle branch spreads out over the surface of the left ventricular septum. The central conduction system connects with a network of Purkinje's fibers.

The complete atrioventricular conduction system is considered to be derived from the embryonic myocardium. Wenink[93] postulated a role for so-called specialized rings situated at the transitional zones, between cardiac segments. In the human embryo, Wessels and coworkers[94] showed, with immunohistochemical techniques, that the primary fold between the developing ventricular inlet and outlet segment was the main source of the atrioventricular system. In this latter explanation, the development of the sinoatrial node and the atrial pathways remains unexplained. In a series of human embryos with the immunohistochemical marker HNK1,[36a,95] we have shown that the conduction system develops from the sinoatrial transition in combination with the primary fold. This developmental concept allows for an explanation of both the atrial and the atrioventricular conduction systems, inclusive of both nodes (Fig. 1–11A, B). It also provides a morphogenetic basis for a number of conduction system abnormalities.

A morphologic substrate for slow and fast conduction pathways is also provided by the presence of cell-cell interactions, as exemplified by the presence or absence of various connexins, such as connexin43.[96,97]

MOLECULAR BIOLOGIC DATA AND CONSEQUENCES FOR MALFORMATIONS

The description of the development of the conduction system in the human embryo is supported by a number of animal studies using various immunohistochemical markers.[14,98] HNK1, its counterpart in the rat and mouse Leu7, and other markers like PS NCAM[99] in the chicken embryo all show the described pathways. Until now, genetic models for conduction system abnormalities have been lacking, except for a zebrafish mutation with bradycardia.[100] The pathomorphology of the conduction system as seen in malpositioned nodes, anterior nodes, Kent's bundles, and Mahaim's fibers can be understood from the fact that the conduction system is more extensive in the embryo than in the fully differentiated system.[15] Our HNK1 investigations of the development of the atrial conduction system show that the sinus venosus encircles both the pulmonary veins and the coronary sinus and participates in the left and right venous valves (see Fig. 1–11A, B). These areas, which normally do not develop into specialized tracts, could be the site of abnormal atrial automaticity.

In the Wolff-Parkinson-White syndrome, early passage of conduction pulses occurs from the atria to the ventricles. This is not the result of persisting specialized myocardial pathways but of persisting working myocardial bundles that are not properly isolated during formation of the fibrous cardiac skeleton.

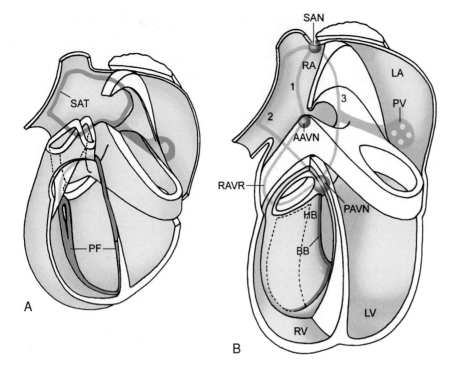

FIGURE 1–11

A, Schematic view of the looped heart tube (see also Fig. 1–6) in which the sinoatrial transition (SAT) and the primary fold (PF) are indicated as *grey lines.* From these areas of myocardium the conduction system develops. *B,* Schematic view of the midfetal (human) stage of conduction system development. With the use of immunohistochemical markers, three tracts can be distinguished in the atrium running from *1,* sinoatrial node (SAN) to an anterior nodal area (AAVN). Furthermore, there is a connection *(2)* over the lateral wall of the right atrium (RA) and one that runs along the basis of the atrial septum *(3).* These latter tracts connect the SAN and posterior AVN (PAVN). The PAVN is continuous with His' bundle (HB) and the right and left bundle branches (BB). In this early developmental stage, the coronary sinus (not shown) and the pulmonary veins (PV) are also encircled by tissue that stains identical to the central conduction system. RAVR = right atrioventricular ring bundle; LA = left atrium; LV = left ventricle; RV = right ventricle.

Data using the reporter gene neural crest model[56, 56a] show that neural crest cells enter the heart through the dorsal mesocardium and become positioned around the embryonic conduction system bundles (see Fig. 1–5A, B). The function of these cells remains obscure as they go into an apototic program, comparable to that in outflow tract septation.[56a] The data might explain the persisting rumors that neural crest cells form the conduction system proper.[101, 102] All our data point toward a myocardial origin of the conduction system.

DEVELOPMENT OF THE EPICARDIUM AND THE CORONARY VASCULATURE

The coronary vasculature is the last part of the developing heart that is essential for its survival as a beating pump. It provides nutrients to the cardiac wall, which cannot survive solely on diffusion. In a normal human embryo at about 6 weeks of development, the coronary arteries contact the two facing semilunar sinuses of the aorta (the right and left sinuses of Valsalva). These arteries spread over the heart. The left coronary artery splits into a left circumflex and anterior descending branch, whereas the right coronary artery usually perfuses the right ventricle and the posterior wall of the ventricles, including the septum and the atrioventricular node.

The coronary venous drainage is through the large veins accompanying the major coronary arteries. These end in the coronary sinus. A number of small anterior veins enter the anterior part of the right atrium. The development of this system has been followed in chicken-quail chimera studies and is explained later. In studying the human embryo, we have been unable to find an extensive, thebesian network connecting the ventricular lumen to the coronary veins. In the embryo, there is evidence, however, of an ex-tensive arteriovenous collateral network.[70, 103] The coronary veins have a myocardial media at their connection to the atria and only more distally is this replaced by a vascular wall composed of smooth muscle cells.

MOLECULAR BIOLOGIC DATA AND CONSEQUENCES FOR MALFORMATIONS

For understanding abnormal coronary vascular development, it is important to realize that the coronary arteries grow into the aortic wall and do not sprout from it (Fig. 1–12B). This has been shown in the quail embryo[104] and in the quail-chick chimera[30] using quail-specific endothelial markers. The question of why under normal circumstances only the two facing sinuses of the aorta harbor a coronary artery, leaving the nonfacing (noncoronary) cusp empty, is unanswered. The same holds for the pulmonary orifice not receiving a coronary artery. We hypothesize that a matrix or cell-adhesion mechanism designates this pattern. After neural crest ablation in the chick, it was shown in persistent truncus arteriosus that the coronary arteries enter only the aortic side of the orifice.[69] For the human, this could also be substantiated in a pathomorphologic study.[105]

The development of the coronary endothelial network takes place within the confinement of the subepicardial covering of the heart (see Fig. 1–12A). The epicardium grows out from the proepicardial organ[32, 33] and serves as a covering layer; the EPDCs also transform into the myocardiofibroblasts of the interstitium. These EPDCs also invade the atrioventricular cushions and play a role in the induction of the Purkinje fibers.[86] EPDCs also transform into smooth muscle cells and fibroblasts of the coronary vessel wall,[34, 35] implying that the coronary smooth muscle cells do not derive from the neural crest.[55]

Patterning of the main branches of the coronary arteries is largely guided by the underlying atrioventricular sulcus

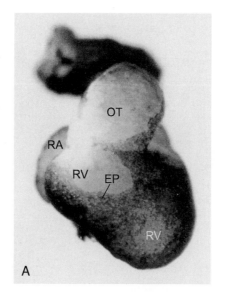

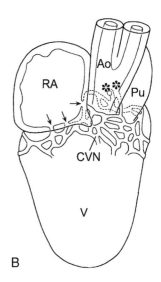

FIGURE 1–12

A, Cytokeratin whole mount staining of the epicardium (EP) of a quail heart (stage HH 24). The epicardium grows out from the epicardial organ at the sinus venosus and covers the outer part of the outflow tract (OT) and the right ventricle (RV). *B,* Schematic view of the coronary vascular network (CVN) at the peritruncal area underlying the epicardium. This network grows at a quail stage HH 32 into the aorta (two lumenized sprouts, *asterisks*) and into the anterior part *(arrows)* of the right atrium (RA). Ao = aorta; Pu = pulmonary trunk; V = ventricle.

and the position of the interventricular septum, even when these are abnormal in their position. The guidance for patterning from a developmental point of view is not understood. The variation in the main branching pattern at the orifice level seems to be related to the shortest distance to the area that has to be perfused. For the development of these main branches a peritruncal network of vessels is available that is remodeled into arteries and veins.[70]

An explanation for coronary arterial fistulae, which tend to be more common in the right ventricular wall, combined with diseased coronary arteries[106] is still unavailable. Data from the EPDC study[86] point toward transient connections between endocardium and epicardium through holes in the ventricular myocardium. If these connections persist, fistulae could develop. There are also some indications that during the fetal period large fistulae are a primary abnormality that can lead secondarily to atresia of the pulmonary orifice.[107]

DEVELOPMENT OF THE AORTIC ARCH SYSTEM AND PULMONARY ARTERIES

The aortic arch and its branches develop from an essentially bilateral symmetric arch system. This pharyngeal arch system is remodeled in the human embryo into a left aortic arch and prenatally a left ductus arteriosus. Figure 1–13 shows the basic embryonic to neonatal transformation of the arch system. The first and second arches are transformed into cranial arteries; the third arch provides the carotid arteries. The fourth arch is the first one that becomes asymmetric in that the left artery persists as the aortic arch, whereas the right artery forms a small segment of the right subclavian artery. The sixth arch arteries are very intriguing because they form a transient connection on both sides between the pulmonary trunk and the descending aorta. On the right side, the distal part of the sixth arch artery disappears. Studies on human embryos show that the pulmonary arteries might contact the aortic sac directly and are never inserted into the sixth arch artery. The right and left subclavian arteries have to move upward from the

seventh intersegmental level to the aortic arch, and in normal development, the left subclavian artery crosses over the ductus arteriosus entrance, thereby creating the isthmus (see Fig. 1–13).

MOLECULAR BIOLOGIC DATA AND CONSEQUENCES FOR MALFORMATIONS

The study of the pharyngeal arch system in the chicken neural crest ablation model[108] shows the significance of the neural crest for normal development of this region. Neural crest cells migrate from the cardiac neural crest, positioned between the otic placode and the third somite, to the third, fourth, and sixth pharyngeal arches and the outflow tract of the heart. The neural crest is obviously vulnerable in its complex differentiation and determination, as many experimental approaches show a combination of cardiac outflow tract and aortic arch anomalies. The neural crest indicator chick[55, 56, 63] shows that the smooth muscle cells of the great arteries, as well as the fibroblasts of the adventitia and the surrounding ganglionic cells, are of neural crest origin. Except for the nodose placode,[109] other parts of the neural crest can compensate for losses in the neural crest population, as has been demonstrated for the mesencephalic crest. Vessels not receiving neural crest cells are the subclavian arteries, the distal and intrapulmonary arteries, and the coronary arteries. The data from developmental studies in the avian embryo, in which neural crest cells can be traced,[55, 56, 63] cannot simply be transferred to the mouse or human embryo. In the latter, we do not have reliable neural crest cell markers that can be mapped to the various vessels and outflow tract. Whether the subsequent pharyngeal arch artery segments can be individually abnormal remains to be investigated. Each neural crest level spans several segments, allowing for compensation when the program of an individual segment is disturbed. Abnormalities of the aortic arch system, including those encompassed in the 22q11 deletion syndrome, show a phenotype that is paramount in certain parts of the arch system,[110] particularly as an interruption of part of the aortic arch (fourth arch derived) and

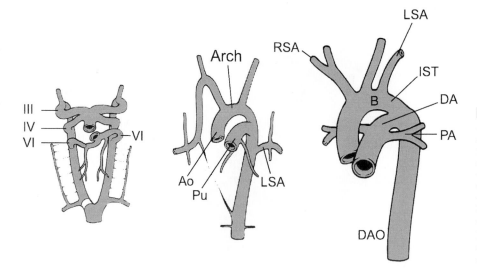

FIGURE 1–13

Schematic view of the remodeling thoracic arterial vasculature, from an almost symmetric system with a number of pharyngeal arch arteries (depicted are III, IV, and VI), to a left aortic arch. After the left subclavian artery (LSA) has migrated into its proper position the aortic arch has an isthmus (IST) and a segment B (vulnerable in the 22q11 deletion syndrome). Ao = aorta; Pu = pulmonary trunk; PA = pulmonary artery; DA = ductus arteriosus; DAO = dorsal aorta; RSA = right subclavian artery.

abnormalities of the ductus arteriosus/left pulmonary artery connection (sixth arch derived). The problem is more right sided than left sided. Explanations for the fact that the anomalies do not extend into the ascending aorta and left part of the arch system are still not provided.

The hypothesis that hemodynamics influence normal aortic arch development and may be responsible for malformations such as hypoplasia and coarctation[66, 111] cannot be refuted. The mechanism may, however, be more complicated, as shown in our venous clip experiments, in which the only insult was a rerouting of blood at the venous inflow, resulting in outflow tract malformations such as double outlet right ventricle and ventricular septal defect. In addition, extensive aortic arch malformations and abnormal semilunar valves occurred. Neural crest cell tracing showed a diminished number of neural crest cells in the outflow tract. The research focuses on shear stress influence and shear stress responsive genes, such as those that produce TGF-β and endothelin 1. Disturbed expression of these genes may initiate the cascade of abnormal formation.

CONCLUSION

This chapter offers information on the current status of knowledge of cardiac embryology. Great advances have been made with the use of experimental and transgenic animal models. We have also tried to indicate that much information directly relevant to the understanding of the human cardiac malformations is still missing. Theorizing on relevant mechanisms has moved from the morphologic level to the level of transcription factors and gene cascades. The area is intriguing and is widely open for future research with both unifying and highly diversifying morphogenetic concepts.

REFERENCES

1. van Splunder P, Stijnen T, Wladimiroff JW: Fetal atrioventricular flow velocity waveforms and their relation with arterial and venous flow velocity waveforms at 8–20 weeks of gestation. Circulation 94:1372, 1996.
2. Olson EN, Srivastava D: Molecular pathways controlling heart development. Science 272:671, 1996.
3. Clark EB: Pathogenetic mechanisms of congenital cardiovascular malformations revisited. Semin Perinatol 20:465, 1996.
4. Hogers B, DeRuiter MC, Baasten AMJ, et al: Intracardiac blood flow patterns related to the yolk sac circulation of the chick embryo. Circ Res 76:871, 1995.
5. Hogers B, DeRuiter MC, Gittenberger-de Groot AC, et al: Unilateral vitelline vein ligation alters intracardiac blood flow patterns and morphogenesis in the chick embryo. Circ Res 80:473, 1997.
6. Taber LA, Lin IE, Clark EB: Mechanics of cardiac looping. Dev Dyn 203:42, 1995.
7. Broekhuizen MLA, Mast F, Struijk PC, et al: Hemodynamic parameters of stage 20 to stage 35 chick embryo. Pediatr Res 34:44, 1993.
8. Broekhuizen MLA, Bouman HGA, Mast F, et al: Hemodynamic changes in HH stage 34 chick embryos after treatment with all-trans-retinoic acid. Pediatr Res 38:42, 1995.
9. Keller BB, Hu N, Serrino PJ, et al: Ventricular pressure-area loop characteristics in the stage 16 to 24 chick embryo. Circ Res 68:226, 1991.
10. Pardanaud L, Luton D, Prigent M, et al: Two distinct endothelial lineages in ontogeny, one of them related to hemopoiesis. Development 1221:1363, 1996.
11. DeRuiter MC, Poelmann RE, Mentink MMT, et al: Early formation of the vascular system in quail embryos. Anat Rec 235:261, 1993.
12. DeRuiter MC, Poelmann RE, VanderPlas-de Vries I, et al: The development of the myocardium and endocardium in mouse embryos. Fusion of two heart tubes? Anat Embryol (Berl) 185:461, 1992.
13. Wunsch AM, Little CD, Markwald RR: Cardiac endothelial heterogeneity defines valvular development as demonstrated by the diverse expression of JB3, an antigen of the endocardial cushion tissue. Dev Biol 165:585, 1994.
14. Gittenberger-de Groot AC, Bartelings MM, Poelmann RE: Overview: Cardiac morphogenesis. In Clark EB, Markwald RR, Takao A (eds): Developmental Mechanisms of Heart Disease. Mount Kisco, NY, Futura, 1995, pp 157–169.
15. Gittenberger-de Groot AC, Bartelings MM, DeRuiter MC, et al: Normal cardiac development. In Wladimiroff JW, Pilu G (eds): Ultrasound and the Fetal Heart. New York, Parthenon, 1996, pp 1–14.
16. Smith SM, Dickman ED, Thompson RP, et al: Retinoic acid directs cardiac laterality and the expression of early markers of precardiac asymmetry. Dev Biol 182:162, 1997.
17. Stainier DYR, Fouquet B, Chen J, et al: Mutations affecting the formation and function of the cardiovascular system in the zebrafish embryo. Development 123:285, 1996.
18. Bodmer R: Heart development in drosophila and its relationship to vertebrates. Trends Cardiovasc Med 5:21, 1995.
19. Kern MJ, Aragao EA, Potter SS: Homeobox genes and heart development. Trends Cardiovasc Med 5:47, 1995.

20. Laverriere AC, Macniell C, Mueller C, et al: GATA-4/5/6 a subfamily of three transcription factors transcribed in developing heart and gut. J Biol Chem 269:23177, 1994.

21. Doevendans PA, van Bilsen M: Transcription factors and the cardiac gene programme. Int J Biochem Cell Biol 28:387, 1996.

22. Lyons GE: Vertebrate heart development. Gene Dev 6:454, 1996.

23. Yamamura H, Zhang M, Markwald RR, et al: A heart segmental defect in the anterior-posterior axis of a transgenic mutant mouse. Dev Biol 186:58, 1997.

24. DeLaCruz MV, Castillo MM, Villavicencio GL, et al: Primitive interventricular septum, its primordium, and its contribution in the definitive interventricular septum: In vivo labelling study in the chick embryo heart. Anat Rec 247:512, 1997.

25. Gittenberger-de Groot AC, Poelmann RE, Bartelings MM: Embryology of congenital heart disease. *In* Freedom R (ed): Congenital Heart Disease. Philadelphia, Current Medicine, 1997, pp 1–10.

26. Levin M, Johnson AL, Stern CD, et al: A molecular pathway determining left-right asymmetry in chick embryogenesis. Cell 82:803, 1995.

27. Reaume AG, de Sousa PA, Kulkarni S, et al: Cardiac malformation in neonatal mice lacking connexin43. Science 267:1831, 1995.

28. Britz-Cunningham SH, Shah MM, Zuppan CW, et al: Mutations of the Connexin43 gap-junction gene in patients with heart malformations and defects of laterality. N Engl J Med 332:1323, 1995.

29. Yutzey C, Rhee JT, Bader D: Expression of the atrial-specific myosin heavy chain AMHC I and the establishment of anteroposterior polarity in the developing chicken heart. Development 120:871, 1994.

30. Moorman AFM, Lamers WH: Molecular anatomy of the developing heart. Trends Cardiovasc Med 4:257, 1994.

31. Poelmann RE, Gittenberger–de Groot AC, Mentink MMT, et al: Development of the cardiac coronary vascular endothelium, studied with antiendothelial antibodies, in chicken-quail chimeras. Circ Res 73:559, 1993.

32. Vrancken Peeters MP, Mentink MM, Poelmann RE, Gittenberger-de Groot AC: Cytokeratins as a marker for epicardial formation in the quail embryo. Anat Embryol (Berl) 191:503, 1995.

33. Viragh S, Gittenberger-de Groot AC, Poelmann RE, Kalman F: Early development of quail heart epicardium and associated vascular and glandular structures. Anat Embryol (Berl) 188:381, 1993.

34. Dettman RW, Denetclaw W, Ordahl CP, et al: Common epicardial origin of coronary vascular smooth muscle, perivascular fibroblasts, and intermyocardial fibroblasts in the avian heart. Dev Biol 193:169, 1998.

35. Vrancken Peeters MP, Gittenberger-de Groot AC, Mentink MMT, et al: Smooth muscle cells and fibroblasts of the coronary arteries derive from epithelial-mesenchymal transformation of the epicardium. Anat Embryol (Berl) 199:367, 1999.

36. DeRuiter MC, Poelmann RE, VanMunsteren JC, et al: Embryonic endothelial cells transdifferentiate into mesenchymal cells expressing smooth muscle actins in vivo and in vitro. Circ Res 80:444, 1997.

36a. Blom NA, DeRuiter MC, Poelmann RE, et al: Development of the cardiac conduction tissue in human embryos using HNK₁-antigen expression, relevance for understanding of abnormal atrial automaticity. Circulation 99:800, 1999.

37. Webb S, Brown N, Wessels A, et al: Development of the murine pulmonary vein and its relationship to the embryonic venous sinus. Anat Rec 250:325, 1998.

38. DeRuiter MC, Gittenberger-de Groot AC, Poelmann RE, et al: Development of the pharyngeal arch system related to the pulmonary and bronchial vessels in the avian embryo. Circulation 87:1306, 1993.

39. Webb S, Brown NA, Anderson RH: Cardiac morphology at late fetal stages in the mouse with trisomy 16: Consequences for different formation of the atrioventricular junction when compared to humans with trisomy 21. Cardiovasc Res 34:515, 1997.

40. Benson DW, Sharkey A, Fatkin D, et al: Reduced penetrance, variable expressivity and genetic heterogeneity of familial atrial septal defects. Circulation 97:2043, 1998.

41. Anderson RH, Webb S, Brown NA: Establishing the anatomic hallmarks of congenitally malformed hearts. Trends Cardiovasc Med 6:10, 1996.

42. Franco D, Kelly R, Lamers WH, et al: Regionalized transcriptional domains of myosin light chain 3f transgenes in the embryonic mouse heart: Morphogenetic implications. Dev Biol 188:17, 1997.

43. Wenink ACG, Gittenberger-de Groot AC: The role of atrioventricular endocardial cushions in the septation of the heart. Int J Cardiol 8:25, 1985.

44. Wenink ACG, Gittenberger-de Groot AC: Embryology of the mitral valve. Int J Cardiol 11:75, 1986.

45. Vuillemin M, Pexieder T: Normal stages of cardiac organogenesis in the mouse: I. Development of the external shape of the heart. Am J Anat 184:101, 1989.

46. Vuillemin M, Pexieder T: Normal stages of cardiac organogenesis in the mouse: II. Development of the internal relief of the heart. Am J Anat 184:114, 1989.

47. Lamers WH, Wessels A, Verbeek FJ, et al: New findings concerning ventricular septation in the human heart. Implications for maldevelopment. Circulation 86:1194, 1992.

48. Boheler KR, Moorman AF: Molecular aspects of myocardial differentiation. Eur Heart J 16(supp N):3, 1995.

49. Bartelings MM, Gittenberger-de Groot AC: The outflow tract of the heart—embryologic and morphologic correlations. Int J Cardiol 22:289, 1989.

50. Bartelings MM, Gittenberger-de Groot AC: Morphogenetic considerations on congenital malformations of the outflow tract. Part 2: Complete transposition of the great arteries and double outlet right ventricle. Int J Cardiol 33:5, 1991.

51. Bouman HGA, Broekhuizen MLA, Baasten AMJ, et al: Spectrum of looping disturbances in stage 34 chicken heart after retinoic acid treatment. Anat Rec 243:101, 1995.

52. Sanford LP, Ormsby I, Gittenberger-de Groot AC, et al: TGFbeta2 knockout mice have multiple developmental defects that are nonoverlapping with other TGFbeta knockout phenotypes. Development 124:2659, 1997.

53. Broekhuizen MLA, Wladimiroff JW, Tibboel D, et al: Induction of cardiac anomalies with all-trans retinoic acid in the chick embryo. Cardiol Young 2:311, 1992.

54. Gittenberger-de Groot AC, Poelmann RE: Principles of abnormal cardiac development. *In* Burggren W, Keller B (eds): Development of Cardiovascular Systems: Molecules to Organisms. Cambridge, Cambridge University Press, 1997, p 259.

55. Bergwerff M, Verberne ME, DeRuiter MC, et al: Neural crest cell contribution to the developing circulatory system. Implications for vascular morphology? Circ Res 82:221, 1998.

56. Poelmann RE, Mikawa T, Gittenberger-de Groot AC: Neural crest cells in outflow tract septation of the embryonic chicken heart: Differentiation and apoptosis. Dev Dyn 212:373, 1998.

56a. Poelmann RE, Gittenberger-de Groot AC: A subpopulation of apoptosis-prone cardiac neural crest cells targets to the venous pole. Multiple functions in heart development. Dev Biol 207:271, 1999.

57. Bartelings MM, Wenink ACG, Gittenberger-de Groot AC, et al: Contribution to the aortopulmonary septum to the muscular outlet septum in the human heart. Acta Morphol Need Scand 24:181, 1986.

58. Bartelings MM, Gittenberger-de Groot AC: The arterial orifice level in the early human embryo. Anat Embryol (Berl) 177:537, 1988.

59. Pexieder T: Development of the outflow tract of the embryonic heart. Birth Defects 14:29, 1978.

60. Thompson RP, Sumida H, Abercrombie M, et al: Morphogenesis of human cardiac outflow. Anat Rec 213:578, 1985.

61. Pexieder T: Conotruncus and its septation at the advent of the molecular biology era. *In* Clark EB, Markwald RR, Takao A (eds): Development Mechanisms of Heart Disease, Futura, 1995, pp 227–249.

62. Bharati S, McAllister HA, Lev M: Straddling and displaced atrioventricular orifices and valves. Am J Cardiol 43:364, 1979.

63. Noden DM, Poelmann RE, Gittenberger-de Groot AC: Cell origins and tissue boundaries during outflow tract development. Trends Cardiovasc Med 5:69, 1995.

64. Sumida H, Akimoto N, Nakamura H: Distribution of the neural crest cells in the heart of birds: A three dimensional analysis. Anat Embryol (Berl) 180:29, 1989.

65. Van Mierop LHS, Kutsche LM: Cardiovascular anomalies in DiGeorge syndrome and importance of neural crest as a possible pathogenetic factor. Am J Cardiol 58:133, 1986.

66. Moulaert AJ, Bruins CC, Oppenheimer-Dekker A: Anomalies of the aortic arch and ventricular septal defects. Circulation 53:1011, 1976.

67. Moene RJ, Gittenberger-de Groot AC, Oppenheimer-Dekker A, et al: Anatomic characteristics of ventricular septal defect associated with coarctation of the aorta. Am J Cardiol 59:952, 1987.

68. Kirby ML, Gale TF, Stewart DE: Neural crest cells contribute to normal aorticopulmonary septation. Science 220:1059, 1983.

69. Gittenberger-de Groot AC, Bartelings MM, Oddens JR, et al: Coronary artery development and neural crest. *In* Clark EB, Markwald RR, Takao A (eds): Development Mechanisms of Heart Disease, Mount Kisco, New York, Futura, 1995, p 291.

70. Vrancken Peeters MP, Gittenberger-de Groot AC, Mentink MMT, et al: Differences in development of coronary arteries and veins. Cardiovasc Res 36:101, 1997.

71. Männer J, Seidl W, Steding G: Formation of the cervical flexure: An experimental study on chick embryos. Acta Anat 152:1, 1995.

72. Mendelsohn C, Larkin S, Mark M, et al: RARP isoforms: Distinct transcriptional control by retinoic acid and specific spatial patterns of promoter activity during mouse embryonic development. Mech Dev 45:227, 1994.

73. Sucov HM, Dyson E, Gumeringer CL, et al: RXR alpha mutant mice establish a genetic basis for vitamin A signaling in heart morphogenesis. Genes Dev 8:1007, 1994.

74. Yasui H, Nakazawa M, Morishima M, et al: Morphological observations on the pathogenetic process of transposition of the great arteries induced by retinoic acid in mice. Circulation 91:2478, 1995.

75. Leatherbury L, Connuck DM, Kirby ML: Neural crest ablation versus sham surgical effects in a chick embryo model of defective cardiovascular development. Pediatr Res 33:628, 1993.

76. Scambler PJ: Deletions of human chromosome 22 and associated birth defects. Curr Opin Genet Dev 3:432, 1993.

77. Goldmuntz E, Driscoll D, Budarf ML, et al: Microdeletions of chromosomal region 22q11 in patients with congenital conotruncal cardiac defects. J Med Genet 30:807, 1993.

78. Wenink ACG, Gittenberger-de Groot AC, Brom AG: Developmental considerations of mitral valve anomalies. Int J Cardiol 11:85, 1986.

79. Oosthoek PW, Wenink ACG, Vrolijk BCM, et al: Development of the atrioventricular valve tension apparatus in the human heart. Anat Embryol (Berl) 198:317, 1998.

80. Wessels A, Markman MW, Vermeulen JL, et al: The development of the atrioventricular junction in the human heart. Circ Res 78:110, 1996.

81. Hurle JM, Colvee E, Blanco AM: Development of mouse semilunar valves. Anat Embryol (Berl) 160:83, 1980.

82. Hokken RB, Bartelings MM, Bogers AJJC, et al: Morphology of the pulmonary and aortic roots with regard to the pulmonary autograft procedure. J Thorac Cardiovasc Surg 113:453, 1997.

83. Markwald R, Eisenberg C, Eisenberg L, et al: Epithelial-mesenchymal transformations in early avian heart development. Acta Anat 156:173, 1996.

84. Oosthoek PW, Wenink ACG, Macedo AJ, et al: The parachute-like asymmetric mitral valve and its two papillary muscles. J Thorac Cardiovasc Surg 114:9, 1997.

85. Celermajer DS, Bull C, Till J, et al: Ebstein's anomaly: Presentation and outcome from fetus to adult. J Am Coll Cardiol 23:170, 1994.

86. Gittenberger-de Groot AC, Vrancken Peeters MP, Mentink MMT, et al: Epicardium-derived cells contribute a novel population to the myocardial wall and the atrioventricular cushions. Circ Res 82:1043, 1998.

87. De la Pompa JL, Timmerman LA, Takimoto H, et al: Role of the NF-ATc transcription factor in morphogenesis of cardiac valves and septum. Nature 392:182, 1998.

88. Ranger AM, Grusby MJ, Hodge MR, et al: The transcription factor NF-ATc is essential for cardiac valve formation. Nature 392:186, 1998.

89. Schilham MW, Oosterwegel MA, Moerer P, et al: Defects in cardiac outflow tract formation and pro-B-lymphocyte expansion in mice lacking Sox-4. Nature 380:711, 1996.

90. Hartwig NG, Vermeij-Keers C, De Vries HE, et al: Aplasia of semilunar valve leaflets: Two case reports and developmental aspects. Pediatr Cardiol 12:114, 1991.

91. Sans-Coma V, Cardo M, Thiene G, et al: Bicuspid aortic and pulmonary valves in the Syrian hamster. Int J Cardiol 34:249, 1992.

92. James TN: Cardiac conduction system: Fetal and postnatal development. Am J Cardiol 25:213, 1970.

93. Wenink ACG: Development of the human cardiac conducting system. J Anat 121:617, 1976.

94. Wessels A, Vermeulen JL, Verbeek FJ, et al: Spatial distribution of "tissue-specific" antigens in the developing human heart and skeletal muscle. III. An immunohistochemical analysis of the distribution of the neural tissue antigen GIN2 in the embryonic heart: Implications for the development of the atrioventricular conduction system. Anat Rec 232:97, 1992.

95. Luider TM, Bravenboer N, Meijers C, et al: The distribution and characterization of HNK-I antigens in the developing avian heart. Anat Embryol (Berl) 188:307, 1993.

96. Oosthoek PW, VanKempen MJA, Wessels A, et al: Distribution of the cardiac gap junction protein, connexin 43, in the neonatal and adult human heart. Muscle Motil Intercept 2:85, 1996.

97. Gourdie RG, Green CR, Severs NJ, et al: Immunolabelling patterns of gap junction connexins in the developing and mature rat heart. Anat Embryol (Berl) 185:363, 1992.

98. Ikeda T, Iwasaki K, Shjimokawa I, et al: Leu-7 immunoreactivity in human and rat embryonic hearts, with special reference to the development of the conduction tissue. Anat Embryol (Berl) 182:553, 1990.

99. Watanabe M, Timm M, Fallah-Najmabadi H: Cardiac expression of polysialylated NCAM in the chicken embryo: Correlation with the ventricular conduction system. Dev Dyn 194:128, 1992.

100. Baker K, Warren KS, Yellen G, et al: Defective "pacemaker" current (I_h) in a zebrafish mutant with a slow heart rate. Proc Natl Acad Sci U S A 94:1, 1997.

101. Gorza L, Schiaffino S, Vitadello M: Heart conduction system: A neural crest derivative? Brain Res 457:360, 1988.

102. Vitadello M, Matteoli M, Gorza L: Neurofilament proteins are coexpressed with desmin in heart conduction system myocytes. J Cell Sci 97:11, 1990.

103. Vrancken Peeters MP, Gittenberger-de Groot AC, Mentink MMT, et al: The development of the coronary vessels and their differentiation into arteries and veins in the embryonic quail heart. Dev Dyn 208:338, 1997.

104. Bogers AJJC, Gittenberger-de Groot AC, Poelmann RE, et al: Development of the origin of the coronary arteries, a matter of ingrowth or outgrowth. Anat Embryol (Berl) 180:437, 1989.

105. Bogers AJJC, Bartelings MM, Bökenkamp R, et al: Common arterial trunk, uncommon coronary arterial anatomy. J Thorac Cardiovasc Surg 106:1133, 1993.

106. Gittenberger-de Groot AC, Sauer U, Bindl L, et al: Competition of coronary arteries and ventriculo-coronary arterial communications in pulmonary atresia with intact ventricular septum. Int J Cardiol 18:243, 1988.

107. Chaoui R, Tennstedt C, Gijldner B, et al: Prenatal diagnosis of ventriculo-coronary communications in a second-trimester fetus using transvaginal and transabdominal color doppler sonography. Ultrasound Obstet Gynecol 9:194, 1997.

108. Kirby ML: Cardiac morphogenesis–recent research advances. Pediatr Res 21:219, 1987.

109. Kirby ML: Nodose placode provides extomesenchyme to the developing chick heart in the absence of cardiac neural crest. Cell Tissue Res 252:17, 1988.

110. Momma K, Kondo C, Matsuoka R: Tetralogy of Fallot with pulmonary atresia associated with chromosome 22q11 deletion. J Am Coll Cardiol 27:198, 1996.

111. Moene RJ, Oppenheimer-Dekker A, Moulaert AJ: The concurrence of dimensional aortic arch anomalies and abnormal left ventricular muscle bundles. Pediatr Cardiol 2:107, 1982.

CHAPTER 2
GENETIC CONTROL IN PEDIATRIC CARDIOVASCULAR MEDICINE

MARK C. JOHNSON   ARNOLD W. STRAUSS

The closing decade of the 20th century has witnessed an explosion of discoveries concerning genetic causes of congenital heart disease. These advances are based on a combination of clinical genetic studies of familial disease and a variety of molecular genetic techniques applied to humans and animal models. Single-gene causes have been proved or implicated in a wide variety of familial cardiac anomalies, and these studies are leading to more informative genetic counseling. Moreover, extension of these studies has identified a number of genetic mechanisms that may explain the apparent sporadic occurrence of cardiac malformations. These mechanisms include variable expression of mutations with lack of recognition of milder phenotypes (see CATCH-22); incomplete penetrance from nonmendelian mechanisms, such as triple repeats (see myotonic dystrophy); the unique genetics of mitochondrial mutations (see defects in oxidative phosphorylation); and de novo mutations (see hypertrophic cardiomyopathy). Ultimately, the identification of genes responsible for congenital heart defects will permit prenatal diagnosis and gene therapy to prevent them.

This chapter describes the investigative techniques of genetic studies and reviews current knowledge regarding the genetic causes of cardiac and vascular disease in children. The chapter concludes with a summary of general principles of genetic control of heart disease that have emerged. Genetic determinants of lipid disorders and systemic hypertension[1, 2] are important causes of cardiovascular disease not reviewed in this chapter.

INVESTIGATIVE TOOLS

A variety of genetic methods and molecular tools have been used to investigate the cause of congenital heart disease. Loci and candidate genes in humans with anomalies are identified by chromosome abnormalities visible by cytogenetic methods or through linkage analysis. At times, candidate genes are suspected on the basis of animal models with cardiac anomalies from naturally occurring mutations or targeted gene disruptions. In addition, animal models with targeted mutations are used to test the functional significance of candidate genes. A number of mouse mutants with cardiac abnormalities have already been studied[3] and are reviewed in this chapter.

Linkage analysis uses polymorphisms, normal DNA sequence variations found throughout the genome, to localize disease-causing genes in families with multiple affected members. If a polymorphic marker and the disease gene are close together, recombination is unlikely to occur, and the two sites will be linked together at a frequency greater than predicted by chance. With current mapping techniques, families with only 10 affected members may be informative. Computer analysis of DNA sequence data from the disease locus can identify candidate genes on the basis of homology of sequence data with previously studied genes in humans and animals.

After a disease gene or locus has been identified, the phenotypic variability associated with a mutation can be demonstrated by screening relatives of probands with techniques such as fluorescent in situ hybridization (FISH), restriction fragment analysis, or allele-specific oligonucleotide hybridization. FISH analysis detects chromosome deletions, whereas the other two techniques depend on identifying a specific disease-producing mutation.

The study of normal cardiac development in animals (see Chapter 1) has also identified genes and proteins that may be involved in the pathophysiologic process of cardiac malformations. The investigation of mutations that cause cardiac anomalies in animals such as *Drosophila* and zebrafish has identified potential models of congenital defects in humans. Studies to date suggest that mutations in genes that control cell-to-cell communication and adhesion may be responsible for a number of cardiac malformations.

CONGENITAL CARDIAC ANOMALIES

Reports of families with multiple relatives with a cardiac anomaly span the spectrum of structural anomalies. These kindreds support the theory that genetic abnormalities are the major cause of congenital cardiac defects. Table 2–1 is a partial list of anatomic cardiac malformations with reports of familial occurrence. Other families with a variety of cardiac phenotypes may have mutations that result in a lack of genetic control in an early stage of development analogous to the *iv/iv* mouse mutation (see later). Loss of control mutations at critical steps in cardiac development may lead to random pathways with phenotypes that range from lethal to clinically inapparent. Subsequent sections review potential mechanisms for structural cardiac abnormalities at differing stages of embryologic development; however, significant overlap among these sections occurs.

A single-gene defect can cause multiple cardiac anomalies that seem unrelated in the context of traditional anatomically based descriptions.

EARLY DEVELOPMENT

The establishment of cardiac myogenic lineage involves transcription factors that are distinct from the basic helix-loop-helix factors (*MyoD, myogenin, Myf5,* and *MRF4*) critical in skeletal muscle. Although some of the factors involved in cardiac myogenesis and morphogenesis have been identified, their roles in the development of clinically important cardiac anomalies have not been elucidated. Work in animals suggests that mutation of a transcription factor may interfere with cardiac morphogenesis at multiple stages.

The *HOX* (homeobox) genes encode DNA-binding proteins that regulate transcription. These genes are highly conserved across species in terms of DNA sequence homology and organization of multiple *HOX* in clusters on the genome. In *Drosophila, HOX* genes are involved in anterior-posterior and dorsal-ventral patterning. Knockout studies demonstrate that *HOX* genes also have important roles in specifying vertebrate body pattern formation.[22] Targeted interruption of the homeobox gene *Nkx2.5* in mice causes a lethal mutation with absent cardiac looping and disordered myocardial differentiation.[23]

Two basic helix-loop-helix transcription factors, *dHAND* and *eHAND*, are expressed in the developing mouse and chick heart. Treatment of chick embryos with antisense oligonucleotides to both *dHAND* and *eHAND* results in arrested cardiac development at the cardiac looping stage.[24] Specific and complementary expression of *dHAND* and *eHAND* in portions of the mouse cardiac tube that ultimately form the right and left ventricles is found before gross morphologic chamber differentiation is evident.[25] Lethal homozygous *dHAND*-null mutant mice initiate looping but develop a single morphologic left ventricle and a dilated aortic sac without primitive aortic arches.

The MEF2 transcription factors that interact with the basic helix-loop-helix factors may operate cooperatively with *dHAND* in these early stages of cardiac development. *MEF2C* homozygous null mutant mice demonstrate cardiac anomalies that are similar to the *dHAND*-null mice with absence of the right ventricle.[26] In contrast to the *dHAND* mutants, the *MEF2C* embryos do not initiate rightward looping. Furthermore, in the *MEF2C* mutants, *dHAND* expression is down-regulated at the time looping usually occurs. Thus, the *HAND* or *MEF2C* genes have an interrelated role in the specification of the ventricles and the outflow portions of the heart. Ultimately, mutations of these genes may be found to cause cardiac defects that include hypoplastic right or left ventricles and conotruncal defects.

Other candidate genes implicated in early cardiac development include N-*myc*,[27] a proto-oncogene, and the *GATA* transcription factors.[28] The *GATA4* transcription factor may have an important role in early development on the basis of the observation that *GATA4*-null embryo mice have two lateral cardiac tubes rather than a single central tube.[29] A downstream role for *GATA4* is suggested by the reduction of cardiac *GATA4* expression in the *dHAND*-deficient mice described before.[25]

CARDIAC TUBE LOOPING

Analysis of human kindreds and work in animal models suggest that a number of genetic factors are involved in cardiac tube looping. The human visceral heterotaxy syndromes, which involve abnormalities in organ symmetry and complex cardiac defects, represent a loss of control over right-left asymmetry. The asplenia and polysplenia syndromes include a spectrum of cardiac anomalies, abnormalities of thoracoabdominal organ situs, and splenic abnormalities. Multiple examples of asplenia, polysplenia, and situs inversus have been described in the same human kindred.[16, 30] Inheritance mechanisms in these kindreds include autosomal recessive, autosomal dominant, and X-linked recessive with linkage to Xq24-q27.1.

The *iv/iv* mouse is a single-gene recessive model for situs abnormalities and cardiac anomalies that maps to mouse chromosome 12, syntenic to 14q in humans.[31] Homozygotic *iv/iv* mice have randomization of atrial and visceral situs with a significant incidence of cardiac anomalies similar to those present in human heterotaxy syndromes.[31, 32] These mice demonstrate a high correlation of atrial arrangement (as determined by morphology of the appendages) with lung laterality.[32] The genetic complexity of situs determination is suggested by another recessive mouse mutation, *inv*, located on a different chromosome than the *iv* mutation, that results in abdominal situs inversus in 100% of homozygotes.[33]

Animal studies have identified a cascade of multiple genes that regulate lateral asymmetric development. RNA injection studies in *Xenopus* embryos suggest that differential protein processing of maternal *Vg1*, a transforming growth factor β molecule, may initiate left-right asymmetry.[34] Other genes from the transforming growth factor β family that may modulate left-right asymmetry include the mouse genes *lefty*,[35] *nodal*,[36] *activin*,[37] and *Xnr1* in *Xeno-*

pus.[34] *Lefty* and *nodal* are expressed transiently and asymmetrically in mouse embryos before cardiac tube looping. Inverted expression of *lefty* and *nodal* is found in the *iv* and *inv* mice embryos described before but is distinct and downstream from the mouse mutations.[35,36] Interference with other signaling molecules in the chick including sonic hedgehog[37] and a snail-related zinc finger transcription factor[38] can also lead to randomized heart tube looping. Mutations in homologous human genes are likely to be the cause of heterotaxy syndrome and other cardiac anomalies associated with situs abnormalities.

FUSION AND SEPTATION

The cardiac tube is divided into atria and ventricles by cellular differentiation, fusion of endocardial cushions, and growth of tissue that composes atrial and ventricular septa (Chapter 1). Many structural cardiac abnormalities are the result of disruption of these complex mechanisms. Defects that primarily involve the conal portion of the ventricular septum are discussed separately (see later).

Holt-Oram Syndrome

Holt-Oram syndrome, also known as heart-hand syndrome, is an autosomal dominant inherited disorder that causes anomalies of the upper limbs. Affected individuals frequently have a secundum atrial septal defect, muscular ventricular septal defect, and atrioventricular nodal disease. The severity of the phenotype is variable, with limb abnormalities that range from clinodactyly or limited supination to severe reduction defects.[39]

In 21 of 22 kindreds studied, Holt-Oram syndrome (heart-hand syndrome type I) has been linked to a locus on chromosome 12.[40] Linkage to this locus has been excluded in two additional kindreds with variant phenotypes. One family has skeletal anomalies with cardiac conduction disease but without septal defects (heart-hand syndrome type III). Another family is characterized by secundum atrial septal defect, first-degree atrioventricular block, but no skeletal abnormalities.[40]

Mutations in a candidate gene (*TBX5*) on chromosome 12 have been identified in five families and three sporadic patients with Holt-Oram syndrome.[41,42] The *TBX5* encodes a putative transcription factor that is expressed in the inflow portion of the human embryonic heart and forelimbs.[41]

Trisomy 21 and Atrioventricular Septal Defects

Atrioventricular septal (canal) defects are associated with divergent genetic syndromes, including heterotaxy syndromes described before, documenting that mutations in multiple loci can interfere with fusion of the endocardial cushions. Atrioventricular septal defects occur frequently in individuals with trisomy 21 but are uncommon in the general population. This suggests that genes on chromosome 21 have important roles in fusion of the endocardial cushions. The molecular mechanism by which aneuploidy leads to the phenotype of Down syndrome is unknown; however, phenotypic mapping of patients with partial trisomy for chromosome 21 has identified a critical locus that may contain genes responsible for cardiac malformations

in trisomy 21.[43] In this locus, two of the genes that code for collagen VI proteins are expressed in the fetal heart and are candidate genes for cardiac malformations in Down syndrome.[44]

The trisomy 16 mouse is a model for human trisomy 21 with many phenotypic features similar to Down syndrome, including atrioventricular septal defects. This mouse model suggests that failure of endocardial cushion fusion may result from a delay in cardiac mesenchyme cell formation. The endocardial cushions of trisomy 16 mice demonstrate altered temporal expression of fibronectin and cytotactin, two extracellular matrix proteins that are usually expressed at the time of cardiac mesenchyme formation.[45]

Other Candidate Loci and Genes for Canal Defects

Loci distinct from chromosome 21 can also interfere with normal fusion of the endocardial cushions. Aneuploidy of chromosomes 9 and 18 is associated with atrioventricular septal defects. In addition, nine patients with deletions on the short arm of chromosome 8 and atrioventricular septal defects have been described.[46,47] Conotruncal cardiac defects and mental retardation are also described in these patients with 8p deletion, suggesting that multiple contiguous genes in this region may affect cardiac and brain development. In the future, patients with 8p deletion and milder phenotypes (such as a cleft mitral valve) may be identified with FISH probes for this region.

Analysis of first-degree relatives of patients with an atrioventricular septal defect suggests that up to 50% of these cardiac anomalies are due to a single-gene defect.[6] Linkage analysis demonstrates genetic heterogeneity by excluding the 21q (Down syndrome) and 8p regions in kindreds with dominant inheritance of atrioventricular septal defects.[6,48] Linkage of atrioventricular septal defects to chromosome 1 in one family with incomplete penetrance and variable expression suggests the involvement of additional genes.[49]

Retinoid nuclear receptors are ligand-dependent transcription factors that play a significant role in vertebrate development.[50] These receptors may act by altering expression of the *HOX* genes described earlier.[50] Mice with homozygous knockout of the *RXRα* gene have a wide spectrum of cardiac malformations, including atrioventricular septal defect, muscular ventricular septal defect, and conotruncal defects. Heterozygous knockout mice exhibit fewer and less severe cardiac anomalies[51]; however, these anomalies would be clinically significant in humans. The similar spectrum of cardiac anomalies in humans with 8p deletions and these *RXRα* knockout mice raises the possibility of analogous genetic mechanisms. Because retinoid receptors regulate a variety of downstream genes, study of these mouse models may help identify candidate genes for a number of human cardiovascular malformations.

Other gene products that may be involved in fusion of the endocardial cushions and remodeling of the mitral and tricuspid valve include molecules from the transforming growth factor β family and some of the homeobox gene products (reviewed in reference 52).

Relatively little is known about genes that may be involved in later stages of atrioventricular valve development, which may be important in defects such as Ebstein's anomaly and mitral valve prolapse. The microfibril proteins fibrillin and fibulin are expressed during late stages of valve morphogenesis.[52] Marfan's syndrome, which can include mitral and tricuspid valve prolapse with regurgitation, is caused by mutations of fibrillin (see later).

CONOTRUNCAL AND AORTIC ARCH DEVELOPMENT

CATCH-22 Syndrome and the Neural Crest

Studies have begun to shed light on the genetic causes of cardiac anomalies that involve the conotruncal region of the heart and the aortic arch. The association of cardiac malformations with monosomy at the q11 site on chromosome 22 represents a clinically significant cause of heart disease in children. The acronym CATCH-22 (Cardiac defects, Abnormal facies, Thymic hypoplasia, Cleft palate, and Hypocalcemia with deletions in chromosome 22) has been used to encompass a variety of phenotypes previously classified as DiGeorge's syndrome, velocardiofacial syndrome (VCFS, Shprintzen's syndrome), and conotruncal anomaly face syndrome.

The CATCH-22 syndrome model illustrates how molecular and clinical genetic investigations of an uncommon and diverse set of syndromic associations have uncovered a common human mutation with significant clinical impact. The association of cytogenetically detected chromosome 22 deletions in patients with DiGeorge's syndrome was the first clue that opened up molecular analysis of the critical 22q11 region and clinical investigations that demonstrate a highly variable phenotype. Studies with FISH probes to ascertain small deletions not visible with standard cytogenetic analysis subsequently revealed CATCH-22 (22q11) deletions in 75 to 90% of patients with the classic DiGeorge, VCFS, or conotruncal anomaly face syndromes.[53,54]

Large prospective studies to establish the prevalence of CATCH-22 deletions in patients with specific cardiac anomalies have not been reported; however, a summary from several small prospective and retrospective reports in Table 2–2[47,55–59] demonstrates that deletions are frequent in some of the conotruncal and aortic arch anomalies. The CATCH-22 deletion may be one of the most common human deletion syndromes with an estimated prevalence of 1 per 4000 to 1 per 9700.[60] FISH screening should be considered in patients with cardiac defects with a high risk of deletion because careful physical examination may not reveal dysmorphic features in infancy.[47,58] Other major cardiac malformations reported with CATCH-22 deletions include ventricular septal defect (especially defects with hypoplasia of the infundibular septum or right aortic arch), coarctation of the aorta, and hypoplastic left heart. Minor anomalies of the aortic arch and branches observed more frequently in patients with CATCH-22 syndrome include right aortic arch, high or cervical aortic arch, aberrant subclavian arteries, and medial displacement of the internal carotid arteries.[47,61–63] CATCH-22 deletions in patients with tetralogy of Fallot/pulmonary atresia increase the risk of nonconfluent pulmonary arteries, absent ductus arteriosus, and major aortopulmonary collaterals.[61] A number of patients with typical features of CATCH-22 syndrome do not have deletions by FISH analysis.[59] Five patients have been identified with deletions on chromosome 10p, suggesting the presence of a second CATCH syndrome contiguous gene locus.[64] Ultimately, we may find that nondeletional mutations of critical genes within these loci may cause a similar phenotype.

Physicians caring for patients with CATCH-22 syndrome should be aware of the noncardiac anomalies, listed in Table 2–3, associated with this syndrome. Some patients may have severe hypocalcemia with seizures; others may have latent hypoparathyroidism with deficient secretory reserve.[65] A higher incidence of sudden, unexplained death in patients with this deletion has also been reported.[47] These findings suggest that in patients with CATCH-22 syndrome, calcium levels should be measured and hypocalcemia should be aggressively treated, especially at times of physiologic stress (e.g., surgery).

Significant immunodeficiency may affect the course of infants with CATCH-22 syndrome, leading to the recommendation for immunologic evaluation including lymphocyte subpopulation analysis.[66] Irradiated blood products should be used in these patients because of the risk of fatal graft-versus-host disease.[67]

The multiple clinical manifestations associated with CATCH-22 deletions together with evidence that the critical deletion region is at least 300 kilobases[68] suggest that this may be a contiguous gene syndrome in which deletion of specific genes is responsible for specific phenotypic features; however, an association between deletion size and phenotypic variability has not been demonstrated. Furthermore, family members with an apparently identical deletion demonstrate highly variable phenotypes.[69] Genes outside the deletion region or nongenetic factors may lead to variable expression of the CATCH-22 phenotype. Candidate genes in this region that are currently being investigated[68,70,71] include *TUPLE1* (or *HIRA*), a gene that is homologous to histone gene transcription repressors in the yeast.[68,70] Chick embryos with attenuated *TUPLE1* genes

TABLE 2–2			
PREVALENCE OF CATCH-22 DELETIONS IN CONOTRUNCAL AND AORTIC ARCH DEFECTS[47,55–57]			
	No. of Patients	Patients With Deletions	Prevalence (%)
Tetralogy of Fallot	347	28	8
Tetralogy of Fallot/pulmonary atresia	53	15	28
Absent pulmonary valve	11	7	64
Complete transposition	48	4	8
Interrupted aortic arch	25	10	40
Truncus arteriosus	29	3	10
Double-outlet right ventricle	33	0	0
Origin of branch pulmonary artery from aorta	3	2	67

NONCARDIAC FEATURES OF CATCH-22 SYNDROME

MINOR ANOMALIES
Prominent nose with squared nasal root, malar flatness
Nasal dimple
Narrow palpebral fissures
Retruded mandible
Ear anomalies
Slender hands and digits
Tortuous retinal vessels

ORAL
Cleft palate (overt or submucous)
Velopharyngeal insufficiency
Pharyngoesophageal dysmotility with feeding problems

IMMUNOLOGIC
Absent thymus
T lymphocyte deficiencies
Low immunoglobulin levels

ENDOCRINE
Hypoparathyroidism
Hypocalcemia
Short stature

NEUROLOGIC/PSYCHIATRIC
Speech disorder
Language delay and mental retardation
Sensorineural hearing loss
Attention deficit hyperactivity disorder
Bipolar disorder
Schizophrenia
Neural tube defects

---

have an increased incidence of incomplete cardiac looping, which may be a mechanism for the development of conotruncal anomalies.[72]

The notion that conotruncal malformations can result from a single-gene defect is supported by selective inbreeding of multiple generations of keeshond dogs.[73] Results from non-inbred keeshonds were thought to represent a multigenetic threshold model. However, analysis of more than 10 generations of inbred keeshonds established mendelian ratios consistent with a single-gene defect. Some of the affected animals had only mild subclinical anomalies of the crista supraventricularis detected at postmortem examinations. Familial disease in humans may be undetected because similar mild asymptomatic phenotypes are not recognized.

The clinical manifestations of CATCH-22 syndrome suggest that it arises from a defect of the embryologic third and fourth pharyngeal pouches. The neural crest plays an important role in the development of organs derived from these pharyngeal pouches. The role of the neural crest in congenital heart disease is confirmed by the occurrence of multiple cardiac anomalies, including truncus arteriosus, tetralogy of Fallot, double-outlet right ventricle, and interrupted aortic arch in chick embryos after portions of the neural crest are ablated.[74]

Animal Models of Conotruncal and Aortic Arch Anomalies

Animal experimentation points to several candidate genes that may play a role in human cardiac anomalies that are related to the neural crest. In these studies, animals with gene disruptions often have lethal fetal cardiac malforma-

tions. In humans, severe cardiac malformations may represent a common cause of fetal loss unrecognized because of limited pathologic examinations.[75]

Homozygous deletion of the *dHAND* gene (see early development) in mice results in a dilated aortic sac and complete absence of the primitive aortic arches as well as absence of the right ventricle.[25] Thus, mutations in the *HAND* genes may account for the frequent occurrence of ventricular arterial malalignment (double-outlet ventricles) and coarctation with a hypoplastic ventricle.

Disruption of the homeobox gene *Hox 1.5* in mouse stem cells leads to many of the anomalies noted in CATCH-22 syndrome, including facial malformations, absent thymus, and absent parathyroid glands.[76] *Hox 1.5*–deficient mice do not have conotruncal abnormalities; however, aortic arch abnormalities analogous to those in patients with CATCH-22 syndrome and semilunar valve abnormalities are found in these knockout mice.

The *Splotch* mouse mutant strain phenotype has abnormalities of neural crest derivatives, including limb musculature and the heart (truncus arteriosus). This mouse strain is characterized by multiple mutant alleles with mutations in the *Pax3* gene encoding a transcriptional regulator with homeobox DNA-binding motifs.[77] The dosage of these alleles and the size of the deletion within the allele affect the severity of the phenotype. For example, truncus arteriosus occurs in all mice homozygous for the Sp^{1H} allele, in none of the Sp^d homozygotes, and in only some of the double heterozygotes.[78] This model of genotype:phenotype correlations may partially explain the apparent sporadic occurrence of cardiac malformations in humans. Mutations of the homologous *Pax3* gene in humans cause Waardenburg's syndrome, a combination of deafness and pigmentary defects thought to be related to abnormalities of the neural crest.[79]

Mice with homozygotic disruption of the neurofibromatosis type 1 gene die in utero with cardiac anomalies, including ventricular septal defect and persistent truncus arteriosus, whereas heterozygotes do not have obvious cardiac anomalies.[80] The neurofibromin protein coded for by this gene is highly conserved, is expressed in the embryonic heart, and is a repressor of the Ras protein, an important regulator of cell proliferation.

Neurotrophin 3 is a growth factor that regulates neural crest cells and determines neuronal cell fate. Initial examinations of neurotrophin 3 knockout mice did not reveal cardiac anomalies; however, recent work describes tetralogy of Fallot, ventricular septal defect, truncus arteriosus, in utero closure of the ductus arteriosus, and myocardial thinning in neurotrophin 3–deficient mice.[81] Premature closure of the ductus arteriosus is thought to be a critical mechanism for absent pulmonary valve, a cardiac malformation in humans that is strongly associated with the CATCH-22 deletion.[82]

Mutations of the α subunit of the platelet-derived growth factor receptor[83] and endothelin-1[84] also produce some of the cardiac anomalies seen after ablation of the cardiac neural crest. Thus, animal studies demonstrate that mutations or knockout of multiple proteins that regulate gene transcription and cellular growth can lead to similar cardiac abnormalities. These studies may help identify mutations in downstream genes that cause isolated congenital anomalies.

Animal models have also identified candidate genes for isolated conotruncal and aortic arch malformations. Targeted mutation of connexin43, a gap junction protein, in the mouse causes lethal right ventricular outflow obstruction.[85] Gap junctions allow cell-to-cell communication through ions and other low-molecular-weight molecules.[86] Disruption of this communication pathway may lead to altered growth of adjacent cells in the developing heart. Thus, genes that code for the multiple proteins that make up gap junctions are possible candidates for congenital cardiac anomalies.

The zebrafish is a powerful model for the study of cardiac morphogenesis.[87] Zebrafish embryos are transparent, which allows direct observation of the developing vascular system including the multiple aortic arches that correspond to the primitive aortic arches of the human embryo. Multiple zebrafish mutations that affect cardiac morphogenesis, cardiac function, and cardiac rhythm have been identified.[88, 89] The classic hemodynamic theory for the etiology of coarctation of the aorta suggests that upstream anomalies that decrease anterograde aortic flow (ventricular septal defect, bicuspid aortic valve) cause inadequate growth of the aortic arch.[90] The recessive mutation *gridlock* in zebrafish is a potential model for a genetic cause of coarctation. These embryos develop a localized obstruction at the junction of the paired dorsal aorta with subsequent development of collateral vessels that bypass the obstruction.[91]

MUSCULAR VENTRICULAR SEPTUM

Some mutations of transcription factors that cause conotruncal anomalies (see earlier) also result in defects of the muscular septum. The retinoid receptor-α–deficient mice described before have muscular septal defects.[51] In addition to muscular ventricular septal defects and conotruncal anomalies, these homozygous mutant mice have hypoplasia of the compact zone of the ventricular myocardium and atrioventricular block.[51, 92] Models of isolated muscular ventricular septal defect have not been developed; however, genes regulated by retinoid receptors are potential candidates.

Another class of genes that may regulate cardiac morphogenesis are the *myc* proto-oncogenes. Myc proteins are basic helix-loop-helix proteins that regulate transcription by binding with DNA at specific sites. Overexpression of these factors is associated with a variety of tumors. Mouse embryos that are homozygous for the null mutation of the N-*myc* gene have severe cardiac malformations characterized by absence of endocardial cushions, atrial septum, and ventricular septum.[93] Compound heterozygotes for mutant N-*myc* alleles have hypoplasia of the compact zone of the ventricular myocardium[94] similar to that described in retinoid receptor knockout mice.

CARDIOMYOPATHIES

In the last decade, clinical studies have demonstrated a high prevalence of inherited cardiomyopathy (Chapter 49). At the same time, laboratory studies have characterized the genetic and molecular cause of disease in many of these familial cardiomyopathies. In a prospective study of patients with idiopathic dilated cardiomyopathy, evidence of familial disease was found in 24% of the 95 consecutive patients.[95] Ascertainment in this study included review of relatives' medical records and echocardiographic study of asymptomatic family members. Table 2–4 lists proven single-gene causes of cardiomyopathy. These diseases fall into two major pathophysiologic categories, (1) abnormalities of myocardial contractile and structural proteins and (2) disorders of cardiac energy metabolism. Other genetic causes of cardiomyopathy include myocardial infiltrative processes such as other glycogen storage diseases, mucopolysaccharidoses, and amyloidosis. Investigation of pa-

---

TABLE 2–4

HUMAN GENE DEFECTS CAUSING CARDIOMYOPATHY

Cardiac Manifestations	Genetic Defect or Syndromic Name
Hypertrophic cardiomyopathy	
Contractile protein mutations	β-Cardiac myosin heavy chain[98]
	α-Tropomyosin[103]
	Cardiac troponin T[103]
	Cardiac myosin–binding protein C[104]
	Regulatory myosin light chain proteins[105]
Metabolic enzyme defects	Very long chain acyl-CoA dehydrogenase deficiency[115, 116]
	Acid maltase deficiency (Pompe's disease)[97]
Dilated cardiomyopathy	
Fatty acid β-oxidation pathway defects	Long-chain 3-hydroxyacyl-CoA dehydrogenase deficiency (trifunctional protein deficiency)[97, 115]
	Very long chain acyl-CoA dehydrogenase deficiency[97, 115]
	Carnitine palmitoyltransferase II deficiency[77, 115]
Oxidative phosphorylation mitochondrial genome defects	Mitochondrial genome multiple or large deletions[96, 97, 115, 117]
	Mitochondrial leucyl-rRNA or lysine-tRNA[97, 115, 117]
Oxidative phosphorylation	Cytochrome *c* oxidase deficiency[97, 115]
Structural and other protein defects	Dystrophin (Duchenne's and Becker's muscular dystrophy)[98, 106–108]
	X-linked (Barth's syndrome and noncompaction of left ventricle)[109–113]
Arrhythmias with dilated cardiomyopathy	Mitochondrial DNA deletions (Kearns-Sayre syndrome)[96, 97, 115]
	Emery-Dreifuss muscular dystrophy[97]

Modified from Payne RM, Johnson MC, Grant JW, Strauss AW: Toward a molecular understanding of congenital heart disease. Circulation 91(2):494–504, 1995.

tients for these rare causes of cardiomyopathy is based on presenting clinical and laboratory features.[96, 97] Elucidation of the causes of cardiomyopathy has made the traditional distinction between dilated and hypertrophic disease less helpful because both clinical phenotypes can be caused by the same genetic mutation.

SARCOMERIC PROTEINS AND HYPERTROPHIC CARDIOMYOPATHY

Familial hypertrophic cardiomyopathy demonstrates an autosomal dominant pattern of inheritance with a high degree of penetrance and phenotypic variability. More than 50 different mutations, mostly missense, have been identified in the β-myosin heavy chain gene (located on chromosome 14q1) in families with hypertrophic cardiomyopathy.[98] Linkage studies confirm the relationship of the 14q1 region and disease in multiple kindreds. In addition, some sporadic examples of hypertrophic cardiomyopathy have similar missense mutations. Most of these mutations are located in the conserved globular head region of the protein and can interfere with actin-myosin interaction despite production of normal protein by the normal allele (a dominant negative mutation). Some of these mutations are associated with more severe disease, including a higher risk of sudden death.[98] Thus, identifying the mutation in a family may assist in counseling and medical management.

Animal models with mutations homologous to mutations in human kindreds facilitate an understanding of the pathophysiologic mechanisms of specific genotypes. Missense mutation of the α-myosin heavy chain in a heterozygous mouse model reproduces the cardiac anomaly and dysfunction seen in human disease.[99] Mouse models also demonstrate electrophysiologic abnormalities, including inducible ventricular ectopy.[100] Mutations of *Dictyostelium discoideum* myosin demonstrate decreased force generation between myosin and actin filaments that correlates with the phenotype severity of homologous human mutations.[101]

The clinical expression of mutations of contractile proteins may be modulated by genes coding for nonsarcomeric proteins. For example, in patients with either sporadic or familial hypertrophic cardiomyopathy, the D/D genotype of the angiotensin I–converting enzyme is associated with a greater degree of left ventricular hypertrophy.[102]

Family studies have identified five additional sarcomeric proteins with dominant negative mutations linked to hypertrophic disease: (1) α-tropomyosin encoded on chromosome 15q2 and (2) cardiac troponin T on chromosome 1q3 are components of the calcium-sensitive thin filament apparatus that regulates the interaction of actin and myosin[103]; (3) cardiac myosin–binding protein C on chromosome 11p13 is a thick filament protein that modulates myosin head interactions with thin filaments[104]; (4) essential and (5) regulatory myosin light chain proteins are thought to stabilize the α-helical neck of the myosin head.[105] Mutations in other sarcomeric proteins may be identified as further kindreds are investigated.

X-LINKED CARDIOMYOPATHY

The majority of patients with cardiomyopathy associated with Duchenne's and Becker's muscular dystrophy or X-linked cardiomyopathy without skeletal muscle disease have mutations of the dystrophin gene on Xp21, the largest gene identified in humans.[98, 106] Dystrophin is part of a multiprotein complex localized to the cytoplasmic face of the sarcolemma. This dystrophin complex appears to stabilize the contracting muscle fiber by linking the actin cytoskeleton to the extracellular matrix.[106, 107] Genes that code for other proteins in this complex are potential candidates for cardiomyopathies with non–X-linked inheritance patterns.

Disease severity in patients with Duchenne's and Becker's muscular dystrophy correlates with the type of mutation. Frameshift mutations that truncate the protein cause more severe disease, whereas in-frame mutations cause less disruption of the protein and milder disease.[108]

In families with X-linked cardiomyopathy but no skeletal muscle disease, deletions of the 5′ region of the dystrophin gene have been described.[109] These deletions may involve a cardiac specific promotor, the N-terminus of a cardiac isoform, or abnormal splicing of the mRNA. In one family, a point mutation in the 5′ splice site consensus sequence of the first intron was found in affected members.[110]

Barth's syndrome, also X-linked, is characterized by cardiac and skeletal myopathy but is distinguished from dystrophin-related diseases by onset in infancy with associated short stature, elevated concentrations of urinary organic acids, and neutropenia. Barth's syndrome is linked to mutations (premature stop codons or altered splice sites) of the *G4.5* gene that maps to Xq28.[111] A variant X-linked cardiomyopathy characterized by noncompaction of the left ventricular myocardium and ventricular dysrhythmias that lacks other features of Barth's syndrome has been linked to a missense mutation of the *G4.5* gene.[112, 113] The function of the *G4.5* gene products, called tafazzins, is unknown.

DISORDERS OF CARDIAC ENERGY METABOLISM

Because the heart uses energy at a high rate, disorders in energy metabolism can cause myocardial dysfunction. The process of oxidative phosphorylation that takes place in the mitochondria is the final step in the production of adenosine triphosphate for use by the myocardium. Reducing equivalents for oxidative phosphorylation are provided by glucose metabolism in the fetus. During the first day of life, the primary energy source shifts from glucose to β-oxidation of fatty acids, which also takes place in the mitochondria (Fig. 2–1). Mutations in genes encoding proteins of the β-oxidation spiral, proteins of the oxidative phosphorylation complexes, or proteins that transport fatty acids into the mitochondria can cause cardiomyopathy.

Fatty Acid Oxidation Disorders

Patients with abnormalities in proteins required for transport of fatty acids or fatty acid oxidation can present as neonates or infants with dilated or hypertrophic cardiomyopathy. Other clinical features include skeletal myopathy, fatty liver, sudden death (some with documented dysrhythmias), and hypoketotic hypoglycemia.[97, 114–116] Nondiagnostic laboratory findings that support the diagnosis of fatty acid oxidation disorders include reduced plasma car-

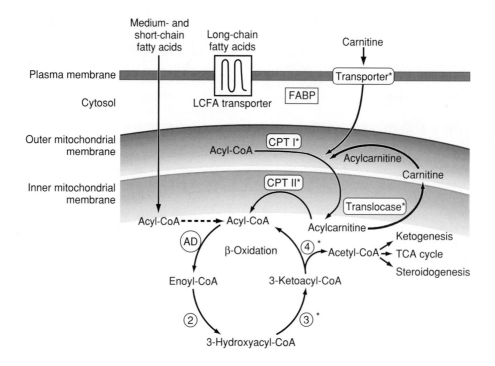

FIGURE 2–1

The import of fatty acids into mitochondria and the fatty acid β-oxidation spiral. Medium and short chain fatty acids are not thought to require active transport from plasma to the mitochondrial matrix, as indicated to the left of the figure. Long chain fatty acids (LCFAs) and carnitine are actively transported across the plasma membrane by integral membrane transporter proteins. Movement of LCFAs through the cytosol may require a fatty acid binding protein (FABP). Carnitine palmityl transferase (CPT) I and II shuttle long chain fatty acids across the inner mitochondrial membrane as carnitine-esters. The fatty acid oxidation spiral, shown in the bottom of the figure, includes an acyl-CoA dehydrogenase (AD) initial step followed by a 2,3-enoyl-CoA hydratase reaction (labeled 2), the 3-hydroxyacyl-CoA dehydrogenase step (labeled 3), and the thiolase cleavage reaction (labeled 4). For long chain fatty acids of 12 to 16 carbons in length, the acyl-CoA dehydrogenase step is catalyzed by very long chain acyl-CoA dehydrogenase and the last three steps are catalyzed by a complex, trifunctional protein, associated with the inner mitochondrial membrane. Cardiomyopathy is a prominent feature of very long chain AD deficiency and of trifunctional protein deficiency. "TCA" is the tricarboxylic acid cycle. The *asterisks* indicate steps in the fatty acid oxidation pathway for which human deficiency states have been described.

nitine (free and esterified acylcarnitine), hyperuricemia, hyperammonemia, and urinary excretion of specific metabolites such as dicarboxylic acids and acylglycines.[97,114] These inborn errors of metabolism are characterized by autosomal recessive inheritance. Missense and exon skipping mutations have been identified in kindreds with these disorders.[115,116]

Defects in Oxidative Phosphorylation

Most of the known disorders of oxidative phosphorylation are caused by mutations in mitochondrial DNA, resulting in a maternal inheritance and a highly variable phenotype due to varying amounts of abnormal mitochondrial DNA in different cells and tissues (heteroplasmy). The proportion of abnormal DNA can change as cells are replicated and may not reach the threshold level at which the abnormal phenotype is manifest in critical tissues. Thus, these disorders demonstrate another mechanism by which apparently sporadic cardiomyopathy can be due to a single-gene defect. Point mutations in mitochondrial transfer RNA genes and deletions of mitochondrial DNA have been described in families with these disorders.[115,117]

The most common cardiac phenotype in oxidative phosphorylation disorders is myocyte hypertrophy with decreased contractile function, but dilated cardiomyopathy is also described. The clinical presentation of these disorders

is variable (Table 2–5) but often includes skeletal myopathy.[97,115,117]

MYOTONIC DYSTROPHY

Cardiac manifestations of myotonic dystrophy include dilated cardiomyopathy, atrioventricular block, and ventricu-

TABLE 2–5

DEFECTS IN MITOCHONDRIAL OXIDATIVE PHOSPHORYLATION CAUSING CARDIOMYOPATHY

Defects presenting with cardiomyopathy and skeletal myopathy
  Lethal infantile cardiomyopathy
  Benign infantile mitochondrial myopathy and cardiomyopathy
  Maternally inherited myopathy and cardiomyopathy
  Inherited cardiomyopathy with multiple deletions of mitochondrial DNA
Defects involving multiple organ systems that may include cardiomyopathy
  Myoclonic epilepsy and ragged-red fiber disease
  Mitochondrial myopathy, encephalopathy, lactic acidosis, and stroke-like episodes
  Kearns-Sayre syndrome (with external ophthalmoplegia and heart block)

lar arrhythmias. Other features include myotonia, muscle wasting, cataracts, smooth muscle involvement, mental retardation, and male infertility. Inheritance is autosomal dominant with a marked variation in phenotype between and within families.

The molecular defect of myotonic dystrophy accounts for these inheritance patterns. Patients have an excessive number of unstable trinucleotide (CTG) repeats at the 3′ end of a protein kinase gene.[118] Disease severity, including the cardiac manifestations, is correlated with the number of trinucleotide repeats.[119] Expansion of the CTG repeats can occur as the gene is transmitted from parent to child, accounting for the increased disease severity and younger age at onset described in ensuing generations, a phenomenon termed genetic anticipation. The differing number of repeats in different tissues due to somatic instability may explain some of the phenotypic variability.[120]

The trinucleotide repeat mechanism of myotonic dystrophy is not seen in other species commonly used for genetic studies. This mechanism of mutation is described in other diseases (fragile X syndrome, spinobulbar muscular atrophy, Huntington's disease, spinocerebellar ataxia type 1, Friedreich's ataxia) and is a potential mechanism for other cardiac disorders with a highly variable phenotype.[121]

OTHER INHERITED CARDIOMYOPATHIES

Multiple additional loci have been linked to families with a variety of cardiac phenotypes (Table 2–6). Two of these phenotypes have dysrhythmias that usually precede the cardiomyopathy[122,123]; others have isolated dilated cardiomyopathy.[124–126] These studies suggest that most instances of idiopathic cardiomyopathy are due to a single-gene defect. Other genes and environmental factors may modulate the expression of these genes in apparently sporadic instances. Furthermore, rigorous family histories and study of asymptomatic family members may uncover familial disease.[95] The variable age at disease onset between and within kindreds suggests that genetic factors associated with aging, such as mitochondrial DNA mutation,

may have to reach a threshold before symptoms develop.[117] In some patients, myocarditis may be the trigger for cardiomyopathy in genetically susceptible hosts.[130]

A search for candidate genes at loci listed in Table 2–6 is ongoing. Tropomodulin, a protein that inhibits binding of myosin and actin, is a candidate gene in a large kindred with dilated cardiomyopathy linked to the 9q locus.[125] Connexin40, a gap junction protein, is encoded by one of the candidate genes in a kindred with dysrhythmias and dilated cardiomyopathy.[122] Mutations of this gene in affected family members have not yet been described.

Animal models of dilated cardiomyopathy will permit exploration of the pathophysiologic mechanism and genotype:phenotype correlations. Disruption of the *MLP* gene in mice results in a dilated left ventricle with reduced systolic function.[131] These hearts have disorganized cardiomyocyte cytoarchitecture similar to that described in human dilated cardiomyopathy.

VASCULOPATHIES

Vasculopathies can present in childhood with major vessel disease. The supravalvar aortic stenosis of Williams' syndrome is caused by monosomy for the elastin gene on chromosome 7. Marfan's syndrome is caused by mutations of the fibrillin gene on chromosome 15. Discovery of the causes of these syndromes has improved our understanding of normal vascular development and has led to the identification of genetic defects in sporadic, isolated vascular disease.

SUPRAVALVAR AORTIC STENOSIS AND WILLIAMS' SYNDROME

Discrete narrowing of the ascending aorta just distal to the sinuses of Valsalva can present in three clinical settings[132,133]: (1) almost half of them occur in families with autosomal dominant, isolated supravalvar aortic stenosis; (2) one third occur sporadically as a part of Williams' syndrome, which includes dysmorphic facial features, infan-

---

TABLE 2–6

LOCI LINKED TO AUTOSOMAL DOMINANT FAMILIAL CARDIOMYOPATHY

Locus	Cardiac Phenotype	Usual Age at Onset	Other Features
1p1–q1[122]	Dysrhythmias (atrial and heart block) Dilated cardiomyopathy	Adult	
3p22–p25[123]	Dysrhythmias (atrial and heart block) Dilated cardiomyopathy	Adolescence	Stroke
1q32[124]	Dilated cardiomyopathy	Childhood, adolescence	
9q13–q22[125]	Dilated cardiomyopathy	Adult	
10q21–q23[126]	Dilated cardiomyopathy Mitral valve prolapse	Adult	
12q22–qter[127]	Pulmonary stenosis Hypertrophic and restrictive cardiomyopathy	Childhood	Noonan's syndrome
14q23–q24[128]	Right ventricular dysplasia	Adult	
1q42–q43[129]	Ventricular tachycardia		

tile hypercalcemia, developmental delay, a behavioral disorder, and stenosis of other major vessels (pulmonary, carotid, coronary, and renal); (3) one quarter are sporadic and unassociated with anomalies of other organ systems. In all three settings, clinically important stenosis typically presents in early childhood, but severe stenosis occasionally occurs in neonates (see Chapter 35).

Elastin is a major protein of the extracellular matrix and is associated with vascular microfibrillar proteins (see next section on Marfan's syndrome). The first clues that mutations of the elastin gene caused supravalvar aortic stenosis came from linkage studies in families with autosomal dominant inheritance and a family with a unique chromosomal translocation that disrupted the elastin gene at 7q11.23.[134, 135] Subsequently, study of patients with Williams' syndrome showed that most were heterozygous for large deletions of chromosome 7 that include the elastin gene.[136] These results suggest that Williams' syndrome is a contiguous gene syndrome (see earlier section on CATCH-22 syndrome). The *LIM-kinase1* gene at the 7q11.23 locus is also deleted in Williams' syndrome patients. This gene is strongly expressed in the brain and is a candidate for the developmental and behavioral abnormalities seen in Williams' syndrome.[137]

Missense mutations, nonsense mutations, and intragenic deletions can also cause familial supravalvar aortic stenosis without other features of Williams' syndrome.[137] It is likely that similar de novo mutations will be identified as the cause of isolated, sporadic stenosis.

MARFAN'S SYNDROME

Microfibrils are composed primarily of fibrillin and are found in abundance in the elastic lamellae of the aortic wall. Marfan's syndrome, caused by mutations of the fibrillin-1 gene, is a pleiotropic disorder characterized by abnormalities of the skeleton, eye, skin, and cardiovascular system.[138] Death in the third to fifth decades occurs secondary to dilatation of the aortic root leading to aortic regurgitation and aortic dissection. A variant of this disorder can cause severe disease and death in early infancy.

Linkage analysis localized the gene responsible for Marfan's syndrome to chromosome 15q.[139] More than 50 different mutations, mostly missense, of the fibrillin-1 gene have subsequently been identified in patients with Marfan's syndrome.[140] Understanding of genotype:phenotype correlations is beginning to emerge. Mutations that allow higher expression of abnormal protein are associated with more severe disease, consistent with a dominant negative disease model.[141] Although mutations seem to be localized to a specific region in patients with severe disease in infancy, patients with late-onset disease also have mutations in this region.[141] Thus, other factors, genetic or environmental, probably modulate disease phenotype in Marfan's syndrome.

OTHER VASCULOPATHIES

Future studies may find that other types of vascular disease are caused by mutations in proteins that make up microfibrils. Alagille's syndrome is characterized by deep-set eyes, prominent forehead, corneal opacities, vertebral anomalies, intrahepatic bile duct hypoplasia, and peripheral pulmonary artery stenoses. Mutations of the human JAG1

gene, encoding a ligand in the Notch intercellular signalling pathway, have been linked to Alagilles syndrome in multiple families.[142]

The clinical manifestations of hereditary hemorrhagic telangiectasia (Osler-Rendu-Weber syndrome) include skin, mucosal, and visceral telangiectases with recurrent hemorrhage. This autosomal dominant disorder has been linked to loci at 9q3 and on chromosome 12.[143, 144] Mutations of endoglin, a transforming growth factor β–binding protein, are associated with disease in kindreds with the 9q3 locus.[143] Transforming growth factor β regulates several processes of endothelial cells including migration, adhesion, and proliferation. Heterozygous mutations identified in multiple affected patients are predicted to cause a truncated protein product as well as the normal protein, supporting a dominant negative disease model for Osler-Rendu-Weber syndrome.[145] Families with disease linked to the chromosome 12 locus have a lower incidence of pulmonary arteriovenous malformations than have families with chromosome 9 linkage.[144] Mutations of activin receptor–like kinase 1, a cell-surface receptor for the transforming growth factor β ligands, are reported in families with linkage to chromosome 12.[146]

INHERITED DYSRHYTHMIAS

Familial occurrence of dysrhythmias include long QT syndrome, re-entrant supraventricular tachycardias, heart block, and ventricular dysrhythmias with right ventricular dysplasia.

LONG QT SYNDROME

Long QT syndrome (Romano-Ward syndrome) is a disorder of repolarization with autosomal dominant inheritance. Elucidation of the genetics of this disease has helped characterize the electrophysiologic mechanism that underlies the clinical phenotype of prolonged QT interval, ventricular dysrhythmias, and sudden death.

Studies in multiple kindreds have linked long QT syndrome to more than 30 different mutations[147] in four different loci (Table 2–7). Voltage clamp studies suggest that mutations of the *HERG* (human *ether-a-go-go*–related) gene cause delay of the outward rectifier potassium current, thus prolonging action potential duration and the QT interval.[154] The deletions of *SCN5A* occur in a conserved region that is responsible for fast inactivation of this sodium channel.[149] Delayed sodium channel inactivation is predicted to prolong action potential duration.

Linkage to the *KVLQT1* potassium channel gene has also been shown in five families with the autosomal recessive disorder of long QT interval and congenital neural deafness (Jervell and Lange-Nielsen syndrome). Homozygous frameshift mutations in the *KVLQT1* gene were detected in four affected patients.[151, 152] In one kindred, family members with a heterozygous mutation have symptomatic long QT syndrome without deafness.[152] The *KVLQT1* gene is also expressed in the inner ear of mice and may play a role in endolymph homeostasis.

Knowledge of the genotype of long QT patients may alter therapeutic strategies. Short-term administration of potassium to patients with *LQT2* genotype corrects repo-

TABLE 2–7

GENETIC LOCI OF THE LONG QT SYNDROME

	Locus	Gene Product	Mutations
7q35–36	*(LQT2)*[148]	*Ether-a-go-go*–related (HERG) Cardiac potassium channel	Intragenic deletions Missense mutations
3p21	*(LQT3)*[149]	SCN5A Cardiac sodium channel	Intragenic deletions Missense mutations
11p15.5	*(LQT1)*[150–152*]	KVLQT1 Cardiac potassium channel	Intragenic deletions/insertions Missense mutations
4q25–27	*(LQT4)*[153]	??	??

*Kindreds with Jervell and Lange-Nielsen syndrome (autosomal recessive disease and deafness) have also been linked to this locus (see text).

larization abnormalities to a greater extent than do other therapies.[155] However, symptomatic response has not been tested with long-term trials. Patients with the *LQT3* genotype may benefit more from sodium channel blocking agents and cardiac pacing.[156]

The discovery that mutations of multiple genes with related functions can cause long QT syndrome is analogous to the story of inherited hypertrophic cardiomyopathy described before.

FAMILIAL HEART BLOCK

Autosomal dominant inheritance of heart block has been described in multiple kindreds. Two forms have been described. Familial heart block type I is defined as bundle branch block or complete heart block with broad QRS complexes, whereas the type II form is characterized by complete heart block with narrow QRS complexes. Inherited forms of heart block are associated with a high incidence of sudden death. Type I heart block has been linked to chromosome 19q in large South African and Lebanese kindreds.[157, 158]

ARRHYTHMOGENIC RIGHT VENTRICULAR DYSPLASIA

Arrhythmogenic right ventricular dysplasia is characterized pathologically by fibrous-fatty replacement of the right ventricular myocardium and clinically by ventricular tachycardia and sudden death. Occurrence in identical twins as well as autosomal dominant inheritance has been described with linkage to chromosome 14q in several families.[128] Linkage to a second locus on chromosome 1q has been demonstrated in a family with a milder phenotype characterized by effort-induced polymorphic ventricular tachycardia and no right ventricular enlargement.[129] α-Actinin genes, which code for sarcomeric proteins, map to the 14q and 1q loci. The candidacy of these genes in the pathogenesis of right ventricular dysplasia is supported by the role that other sarcomeric proteins play in familial hypertrophic cardiomyopathy (see earlier).

PRINCIPLES OF GENETIC CONTROL OF CONGENITAL HEART DISEASE

Several principles of genetic causes of cardiac malformations emerge from the studies reviewed in this chapter. These principles will guide clinical and basic investigators in coordinated studies that span the spectrum of congenital heart disease.

1. Single-gene defects, including de novo mutations, do cause cardiac malformations.

2. Heterogeneous mutations in one gene or mutations in multiple genes can cause a similar cardiac phenotype.

3. Multiple cardiac phenotypes, unrelated under traditional anatomic classification schemes, may be caused by mutations at a single locus.

4. The phenotypic expression of a mutation may be modulated by other genetic factors.

5. Deletion of contiguous genes may cause anomalies of multiple organs including the heart.

6. Determining the etiology of syndromic disorders that include cardiac anomalies can reveal their cause as an isolated lesion.

7. A careful search for subtle phenotypic variants in families of patients with apparently sporadic cardiac anomalies may reveal inherited disease.

8. Animal models may uncover genetic causes of lethal human cardiac malformations.

The pace of important molecular and clinical genetic discoveries is accelerating. We expect a detailed understanding of the cause of most congenital cardiac anomalies in the foreseeable future.

REFERENCES

1. Lifton RP: Molecular genetics of human blood pressure variation. Science 272:676, 1996.
2. Breslow JL: Genetics of lipoprotein disorders. Circulation 87(suppl):III-16, 1993.
3. Rossant J: Mouse mutants and cardiac development. Circ Res 78:349, 1996.
4. Rein AJJT, Sheffer R: Genetics of conotruncal malformations: Further evidence of autosomal recessive inheritance. Am J Med Genet 50:302, 1994.
5. Debrus S, Berger G, de Meeus A, et al: Familial non-syndromic conotruncal defects are not associated with a 22q11 microdeletion. Hum Genet 97:138, 1996.
6. Wilson L, Curtis A, Korenberg JR, et al: A large, dominant pedigree of atrioventricular septal defect (AVSD): Exclusion from the Down syndrome critical region on chromosome 21. Am J Hum Genet 53:1262, 1993.
7. Cousineau AJ, Lauer RM, Pierpont ME, et al: Linkage analysis of autosomal dominant atrioventricular canal defects: Exclusion of chromosome 21. Hum Genet 93:103, 1994.
8. David TJ: A family with congenital pulmonary valve stenosis. Humangenetik 21:287, 1974.

9. Henney AM, Tsipouras P, Schwartz RC, et al: Genetic evidence that mutations in the *COL1A1*, *COL1A2*, *COL3A1*, or *COL5A2* collagen genes are not responsible for mitral valve prolapse. Br Heart J 61:292, 1989.

10. Davidson HR: A large family with patent ductus arteriosus and unusual face. J Med Genet 30:503, 1992.

11. Glick BN, Roberts WC: Congenitally bicuspid aortic valve in multiple family members. Am J Cardiol 73:400, 1994.

12. Shokeir MHK: Hypoplastic left heart syndrome: An autosomal recessive disorder. Clin Genet 2:7, 1971.

13. Beekman RH, Robinow M: Coarctation of the aorta inherited as an autosomal dominant trait. Am J Cardiol 56:818, 1985.

14. Bleyl S, Nelson L, Odelberg SJ, et al: A gene for familial total anomalous pulmonary venous return maps to chromosome 4p13–q12. Am J Hum Genet 56:408, 1995.

15. Basson CT, Solomon SD, Weissman B, et al: Genetic heterogeneity of heart-hand syndromes. Circulation 91:1326, 1995.

16. Casey B, Devoto M, Jones KL, Ballabio A: Mapping a gene for familial situs abnormalities to human chromosome Xq24–q27.1. Nat Genet 5:403, 1993.

17. Driscoll DJ, Michels VV, Gersony WM, et al: Occurrence risk for congenital heart defects in relatives of patients with aortic stenosis, pulmonary stenosis or ventricular septal defect. Circulation 87(suppl):I-114, 1993.

18. Whittemore R, Wells JA, Castellsague X: A second-generation study of 427 probands with congenital heart defects and their 837 children. J Am Coll Cardiol 23:1459, 1994.

19. McIntosh N, Chitayat D, Bardanis M, Fouron JC: Ebstein anomaly: Report of a familial occurrence and prenatal diagnosis. Am J Med Genet 42:307, 1992.

20. Chitayat D, McIntosh, Fouron JC: Pulmonary atresia with intact ventricular septum and hypoplastic right heart in sibs. Am J Med Genet 42:304, 1992.

21. Gobel JW, Pierpont MEM, Moller JH, et al: Familial interruption of the aortic arch. Pediatr Cardiol 14:110, 1993.

22. Krumlauf R: *Hox* genes in vertebrate development. Cell 78:191, 1994.

23. Lyons I, Parsons LM, Hartley L, et al: Myogenic and morphogenetic defects in the heart tubes of murine embryos lacking the homeobox gene *Nkx2.5*. Genes Dev 9:1654, 1995.

24. Srivastava D, Cserjesi P, Olson EN: A subclass of bHLH proteins required for cardiac morphogenesis. Science 270:1995, 1995.

25. Srivastava D, Thomas T, Lin Q, et al: Regulation of cardiac mesodermal and neural crest development by the bHLH transcription factor, dHAND. Nat Genet 16:154, 1997.

26. Lin Q, Schwarz J, Bucana C, Olson E: Control of mouse cardiac morphogenesis and myogenesis by transcription factor MEF2C. Science 276:1404, 1997.

27. Moens CB, Stanton BR, Parada LF, Rossant J: Defects in heart and lung development in compound heterozygotes for two different targeted mutations at the N-*myc* locus. Development 119:485, 1993.

28. Arceci RJ, King AA, Simon MC, et al: Mouse GATA-4: A retinoic acid–inducible GATA-binding transcription factor expressed in endodermally derived tissues and heart. Mol Cell Biol 13:2235, 1993.

29. Molkentin JD, Lin Q, Duncan SA, Olson EN: Requirement of the transcription factor GATA4 for heart tube formation and ventral morphogenesis. Genes Dev 11:1061, 1997.

30. Niikawa N, Kohsaka S, Mizumoto M, et al: Familial clustering of situs inversus totalis, and asplenia and polysplenia syndromes. Am J Med Genet 16:43, 1983.

31. Brueckner M, D'Eustachio P, Horwich AL: Linkage mapping of a mouse gene, *iv*, that controls left-right asymmetry of the heart and viscera. Proc Natl Acad Sci USA 86:5035, 1989.

32. Seo JW, Brown NA, Ho SY, Anderson RH: Abnormal laterality and congenital cardiac anomalies: Relations of visceral and cardiac morphologies in the *iv/iv* mouse. Circulation 86:642, 1992.

33. Yokoyama T, Copeland NG, Jenkins NA, et al: Reversal of left-right asymmetry: A situs inversus mutation. Science 260:679, 1993.

34. Hyatt BA, Lohr JL, Yost HJ: Initiation of vertebrate left-right axis formation by maternal Vg1. Nature 384:62, 1996.

35. Meno C, Saijoh Y, Fujii H, et al: Left-right asymmetric expression of the TGFβ-family member lefty in mouse embryos. Nature 381:151, 1996.

36. Lowe LA, Supp DM, Sampath K, et al: Conserved left-right asymmetry of nodal expression and alteration in murine situs inversus. Nature 381:155, 1996.

37. Levin M, Johnson R, Stern C, et al: A molecular pathway determining left-right asymmetry in chick embryogenesis. Cell 82:803, 1995.

38. Isaac A, Sargent MG, Cooke J: Control of vertebrate left-right asymmetry by a snail-related zinc finger gene. Science 275:1301, 1997.

39. Newbury-Ecob RA, Leanage R, Raeburn JA, Young ID: Holt-Oram syndrome: A clinical genetic study. J Med Genet 33:300, 1996.

40. Basson CT, Solomon SD, Weissman B, et al: Genetic heterogeneity of heart-hand syndromes. Circulation 91:1326, 1995.

41. Li QY, Newbury-Ecob RA, Terrett JA, et al: Holt-Oram syndrome is caused by mutation in *TBX5*, a member of the Brachyury (T) gene family. Nat Genet 15:21, 1997.

42. Basson CT, Bachinsky DR, Lin RC, et al: Mutations in human cause limb and cardiac malformation in Holt-Oram syndrome. Nat Genet 15:30, 1997.

43. Korenberg JR, Chen XN, Schipper R, et al: Down syndrome phenotypes: The consequences of chromosomal imbalance. Proc Natl Acad Sci USA 91:4997, 1994.

44. Davies GE, Howard CM, Gorman LM, et al: Polymorphisms and linkage disequilibrium in the *COL6A1* and *COL6A2* gene cluster: Novel DNA polymorphisms in the region of a candidate gene for congenital heart defects in Down's syndrome. Hum Genet 90:521, 1993.

45. Hiltgen GG, Markwald RR, Litke LL: Morphogenetic alterations during endocardial cushion development in the trisomy 16 (Down syndrome) mouse. Pediatr Cardiol 17:21, 1996.

46. Digilio MC, Giannotti A, Marino B, Dallapiccola B: Atrioventricular canal and 8p– syndrome. Am J Med Genet 47:437, 1993.

47. Johnson MC, Hing A, Wood MK, Watson MS: Chromosome abnormalities in congenital heart disease. Am J Med Genet 70:292, 1997.

48. Amati F, Mari A, Mingarelli R, et al: Two pedigrees of autosomal dominant atrioventricular canal defect (AVCD): Exclusion from the critical region on 8p. Am J Med Genet 57:483, 1995.

49. Sheffield VC, Pierpont ME, Nishimura D, et al: Identification of a complex congenital heart defect susceptibility locus by using DNA pooling and shared segment analysis. Hum Mol Genet 6:117, 1997.

50. Kastner P, Mark M, Chambon P: Nonsteroid nuclear receptors: What are genetic studies telling us about their role in real life? Cell 83:859, 1995.

51. Gruber PJ, Kubalak SW, Pexieder T, et al: RXR-α deficiency confers genetic susceptibility for aortic sac conotruncal atrioventricular cushion and ventricular muscle defects in mice. J Clin Invest 98:1332, 1996.

52. Eisenberg LM, Markwald RR: Molecular regulation of atrioventricular valvuloseptal morphogenesis. Circ Res 77:1, 1995.

53. Driscoll DA, Salvin J, Sellinger B, et al: Prevalence of 22q11 microdeletions in DiGeorge and velocardiofacial syndromes: Implications for genetic counselling and prenatal diagnosis. J Med Genet 30:813, 1993.

54. Momma K, Kondo C, Matsuoka R, Takao A: Cardiac anomalies associated with a chromosome 22q11 deletion in patients with conotruncal anomaly face syndrome. Am J Cardiol 78:591, 1996.

55. Digilio MC, Marino B, Grazioli S, et al: Comparison of occurrence of genetic syndromes in ventricular septal defect with pulmonic stenosis (classic tetralogy of Fallot) versus ventricular septal defect with pulmonic atresia. Am J Cardiol 77:1375, 1996.

56. Takahashi K, Kido S, Hoshino K, et al: Frequency of a 22q11 deletion in patients with conotruncal cardiac malformations: A prospective study. Eur J Pediatr 154:878, 1995.

57. Melchionda S, Digiolo MC, Mingarelli R, et al: Transposition of the great arteries associated with deletion of chromosome 22q11. Am J Cardiol 75:95, 1995.

58. Trainer AH, Morrison N, Dunlop A, et al: Chromosome 22q11 microdeletions in tetralogy of Fallot. Arch Dis Child 74:62, 1996.

59. Webber SA, Hatchwell E, Barber JCK, et al: Importance of microdeletions of chromosomal region 22q11 as a cause of selected malformations of the ventricular outflow tracts and aortic arch: A three-year prospective study. J Pediatr 129:26, 1996.

60. du Montcel ST, Menidizabal H, Ayme S, et al: Prevalence of 22q11 microdeletion. J Med Genet 33:719, 1996.

61. Momma K, Kondo C, Matsuoka R: Tetralogy of Fallot with pulmonary atresia associated with chromosome 22q11 deletion. J Am Coll Cardiol 27:198, 1996.

62. Goldberg R, Motzkin B, Marion R, et al: Velo-cardio-facial syndrome: A review of 120 patients. Am J Med Genet 45:313, 1993.

63. Kumar A, McCombs JL, Sapire DW: Deletions in chromosome 22q11 region in cervical aortic arch. Am J Cardiol 79:388, 1997.

64. Daw SC, Taylor C, Kraman M, et al: A common region of 10p deleted in DiGeorge and velocardiofacial syndromes. Nat Genet 13:458, 1996.

65. Cuneo BF, Langman CB, Ilbawi MN, et al: Latent hypoparathyroidism in children with conotruncal cardiac defects. Circulation 93:1702, 1996.

66. Rhoden DK, Leatherbury L, Helman S, et al: Abnormalities in lymphocyte populations in infants with neural crest cardiovascular defects. Pediatr Cardiol 17:143, 1996.

67. Franklin RCG, Onuzo O, Miller PA, et al: Transfusion associated graft-versus-host disease in DiGeorge syndrome—index case report with survey of screening procedures and use of irradiated blood components. Cardiol Young 6:222, 1996.

68. Halford S, Wadey R, Roberts C, et al: Isolation of a putative transcriptional regulator from the region of 22q11 deleted in DiGeorge syndrome, Shprintzen syndrome and familial congenital heart disease. Hum Mol Genet 2:2099, 1993.

69. McLean SD, Saal HM, Spinner NB, et al: Velo-cardio-facial syndrome: Intrafamilial variability of the phenotype. Am J Dis Child 147:1212, 1993.

70. Lorain S, Demczuk S, Lamour V, et al: Structural organization of the WD repeat protein-encoding gene *HIRA* in the DiGeorge syndrome critical region of human chromosome 22. Genome Res 6:43, 1996.

71. Budarf ML, Collins J, Gong W, et al: Cloning a balanced translocation associated with DiGeorge syndrome and identification of a disrupted candidate gene. Nat Genet 10:269, 1995.

72. Hixon RL, Leatherbury L, Scambler P, et al: Morphologic and hemodynamic assessment of *tuple 1* gene attenuated chick embryos (Abstract). Pediatrics 98:534, 1996.

73. Patterson DF, Pexieder T, Schnarr WR, et al: A single major-gene defect underlying cardiac conotruncal malformations interferes with myocardial growth during embryonic development: Studies in the CTD line of keeshond dogs. Am J Hum Genet 52:388, 1993.

74. Kirby ML, Waldo KL: Role of neural crest in congenital heart disease. Circulation 82:332, 1990.

75. Hoffman JI: Incidence of congenital heart disease: II. Prenatal incidence. Pediatr Cardiol 16:155, 1995.

76. Chisaka O, Capecchi MR: Regionally restricted developmental defects resulting from targeted disruption of the mouse homeobox gene hox-1.5. Nature 350:473, 1991.

77. Epstein DJ, Vogan KJ, Trasler DG, Gros P: A mutation within intron 3 of the *Pax-3* gene produces aberrantly spliced mRNA transcripts in the Splotch mouse mutant. Proc Natl Acad Sci USA 90:532, 1993.

78. Franz T: The splotch *(Sp1H)* and splotch-delayed *(Spd)* alleles: Differential phenotypic effects on neural crest and limb musculature. Anat Embryol 187:371, 1993.

79. Tassabehji M, Read AP, Newton VE, et al: Waardenburg's syndrome patients have mutations in the human homologue of the *Pax-3* paired box gene. Nature 355:635, 1992.

80. Brannan CI, Perkins AS, Vogel KS, et al: Targeted disruption of the neurofibromatosis type-1 gene leads to developmental abnormalities in heart and various neural crest–derived tissues. Genes Dev 8:1019, 1994.

81. Donovan MJ, Hahn R, Tessarollo L, Hempstead BL: Identification of an essential nonneuronal function of neurotrophin 3 in mammalian cardiac development. Nat Genet 14:210, 1996.

82. Johnson MC, Strauss AW, Dowton SB, et al: Deletion within chromosome 22 is common in patients with absent pulmonary valve syndrome. Am J Cardiol 76:66, 1995.

83. Schatteman GC, Motley ST, Effmann EL, Bowen-Pope DF: Platelet-derived growth factor receptor α-subunit deleted patch mouse exhibits severe cardiovascular dysmorphogenesis. Teratology 51:351, 1995.

84. Kurihara Y, Kurihara H, Oda H, et al: Aortic arch malformations and ventricular septal defect in mice deficient in endothelin-1. J Clin Invest 96:293, 1995.

85. Reaume AG, de Sousa PA, Kulkarni S, et al: Cardiac malformation in neonatal mice lacking connexin43. Science 267:1831, 1995.

86. Kumar NM, Gilula NB: The gap junction communication channel. Cell 84:381, 1996.

87. Fishman MC, Stanier DY: Cardiovascular development. Prospects for a genetic approach. Circ Res 74:757, 1994.

88. Chen JN, Haffter P, Odenthal J, et al: Mutations affecting the cardiovascular system and other internal organs in zebrafish. Development 123:293, 1996.

89. Stainier DY, Fouquet B, Chen JN, et al: Mutations affecting the formation and function of the cardiovascular system in the zebrafish embryo. Development 123:285, 1996.

90. Hutchins GM: Coarctation of the aorta explained as a branch-point of ductus arteriosus. Am J Pathol 63:203, 1971.

91. Weinstein BM, Stemple DL, Driever W, Fishman MC: *Gridlock,* a localized heritable vascular patterning defect in the zebrafish. Nat Med 1:1143, 1995.

92. Dyson E, Sucov HM, Kubalak SW, et al: Atrial-like phenotype is associated with embryonic ventricular failure in retinoid X receptor α−/− mice. Proc Natl Acad Sci USA 92:7386, 1995.

93. Charron J, Malynn BA, Fisher P, et al: Embryonic lethality in mice homozygous for a targeted disruption of the N-*myc* gene. Genes Dev 6:2248, 1992.

94. Moens CB, Stanton BR, Parada LF, Rossant J: Defects in heart and lung development in compound heterozygotes for two different targeted mutations at the N-*myc* locus. Development 119:485, 1993.

95. Goerss JB, Michels VV, Burnett J, et al: Frequency of familial dilated cardiomyopathy. Eur Heart J 16(suppl O):2, 1995.

96. Johnson MC, Payne RM, Grant JW, Strauss AW: The genetic basis of paediatric heart disease. Ann Med 27:289, 1995.

97. Schwartz ML, Cox GF, Lin AE, et al: Clinical approach to genetic cardiomyopathy in children. Circulation 94:2021, 1996.

98. Marian AJ, Roberts R: Molecular basis of hypertrophic and dilated cardiomyopathy. Tex Heart Inst J 21:6, 1994.

99. Geisterfer-Lowrance AA, Christe M, Conner DA, et al: A mouse model of familial hypertrophic cardiomyopathy. Science 272:731, 1996.

100. Berul CI, Christe ME, Aronovitz MJ, et al: Electrophysiological abnormalities and arrhythmias in αMHC mutant familial hypertrophic cardiomyopathy mice. J Clin Invest 99:570, 1997.

101. Fujita H, Sugiura S, Mommomura S, et al: Characterization of mutant myosins of *Dictyostelium discoideum* equivalent to human familial hypertrophic cardiomyopathy mutants. J Clin Invest 99:1010, 1997.

102. Lechin M, Quinones MA, Omran A, et al: Angiotensin-I converting enzyme genotypes and left ventricular hypertrophy in patients with hypertrophic cardiomyopathy. Circulation 92:1808, 1995.

103. Thierfelder L, Watkins H, MacRae C, et al: α-Tropomyosin and cardiac troponin T mutations cause familial hypertrophic cardiomyopathy: A disease of the sarcomere. Cell 77:701, 1994.

104. Watkins H, Conner D, Thierfelder L, et al: Mutations in the cardiac myosin binding protein-C gene on chromosome 11 cause familial hypertrophic cardiomyopathy. Nat Genet 11:434, 1995.

105. Poetter K, Jiang H, Hassanzadeh S, et al: Mutations in either the essential or regulatory light chains of myosin are associated with a rare myopathy in human heart and skeletal muscle. Nat Genet 13:63, 1996.

106. Tinsley JM, Blake DJ, Zuelig RA, Davies KE: Increasing complexity of the dystrophin-associated protein complex. Proc Natl Acad Sci USA 91:8307, 1994.

107. Campbell KP: Molecular basis of three muscular dystrophies: Disruption of cytoskeleton-extracellular matrix linkage. Cell 80:675, 1995.

108. Chelly J, Gilgenkrantz H, Lambert M, et al: Effect of dystrophin gene deletions on mRNA levels and processing in Duchenne and Becker muscular dystrophies. Cell 63:1239, 1990.

109. Muntoni F, Cau M, Ganau A, et al: Deletion of the dystrophin muscle promoter region associated with X-linked cardiomyopathy. N Engl J Med 329:921, 1993.

110. Milasin J, Muntoni F, Severini GM, et al: A point mutation in the 5′ splice site of the dystrophin gene first intron responsible for X-linked cardiomyopathy. Hum Mol Genet 5:73, 1996.

111. Bione S, D'Adamo P, Maestrini E, et al: A novel X-linked gene, *G4.5,* is responsible for Barth syndrome. Nat Genet 12:385, 1996.

112. Bleyl SB, Mumford BR, Brown-Harrison M, et al: Xq28-linked noncompaction of the left ventricular myocardium: Prenatal diagnosis and pathologic analysis of affected individuals. Am J Med Genet 72:257, 1997.

113. Bleyl SB, Mumford BR, Thompson V, et al: Neonatal, lethal noncompaction of the left ventricular myocardium is allelic with Barth syndrome. Am J Hum Genet 61:868, 1997.

114. Hale DE, Bennett MJ: Fatty acid oxidation disorders: A new class of metabolic disorders. J Pediatr 121:1, 1992.

115. Kelly DP, Strauss AW: Inherited cardiomyopathies. N Engl J Med 330:913, 1994.

116. Strauss AW, Powell CK, Hale DE, et al: Molecular basis of human mitochondrial very-long-chain acyl-CoA dehydrogenase deficiency causing cardiomyopathy and sudden death in childhood. Proc Natl Acad Sci USA 92:10496, 1995.

117. Johns DR: Mitochondrial DNA and disease. N Engl J Med 333:638, 1995.

118. Brook JD, McCurrach ME, Harley HG, et al: Molecular basis of myotonic dystrophy: Expansion of a trinucleotide (CTG) repeat at the 3' end of a transcript encoding a protein kinase family member. Cell 68:799, 1992.

119. Melacini P, Villanova C, Menegazzo E, et al: Correlation between cardiac involvement and CTG trinucleotide repeat length in myotonic dystrophy. J Am Coll Cardiol 25:239, 1995.

120. Ashizawa T, Dubel JR, Harati Y: Somatic instability of CTG repeat in myotonic dystrophy. Neurology 43:2674, 1993.

121. Warren ST: The expanding world of trinucleotide repeats. Science 271:1374, 1996.

122. Kass S, MacRae C, Graber HL, et al: A gene defect that causes conduction system disease and dilated cardiomyopathy maps to chromosome 1p1–1q1. Nat Genet 7:546, 1994.

123. Olson TM, Keating MK: Mapping a cardiomyopathy locus to chromosome 3p22–p25. J Clin Invest 97:528, 1996.

124. Durand JB, Bachinski LL, Bieling LC, et al: Localization of a gene responsible for familial dilated cardiomyopathy to chromosome 1q32. Circulation 92:3387, 1995.

125. Krajinovic M, Pinamonti B, Sinagra G, et al: Linkage of familial dilated cardiomyopathy to chromosome 9. Am J Hum Genet 57:846, 1995.

126. Bowles KR, Gajarski R, Porter P, et al: Gene mapping of familial autosomal dominant dilated cardiomyopathy to chromosome 10q21–23. J Clin Invest 98:1355, 1996.

127. Jamieson CR, van der Burgt I, Brady AF, et al: Mapping a gene for Noonan syndrome to the long arm of chromosome 12. Nat Genet 8:357, 1994.

128. Rampazzo A, Vana A, Danieli GA, et al: The gene for arrhythmogenic right ventricular cardiomyopathy maps to chromosome 14q23–q24. Hum Mol Genet 3:959, 1994.

129. Rampazzo A, Nava A, Erne P, et al: A new locus for arrhythmogenic right ventricular cardiomyopathy (ARVD2) maps to chromosome 1q42–q43. Hum Mol Genet 4:2151, 1995.

130. Pinamonti B, Miani D, Sinagra G, et al: Familial right ventricular dysplasia with biventricular involvement and inflammatory infiltration. Heart 76:66, 1996.

131. Arber S, Hunter JJ, Ross J, et al: MLP-deficient mice exhibit a disruption of cardiac cytoarchitectural organization, dilated cardiomyopathy, and heart failure. Cell 88:393, 1997.

132. Beuren AJ: Supravalvular aortic stenosis: A complex syndrome with and without mental retardation. Birth Defects 8:45, 1972.

133. O'Connor WN, Davis JB, Geissler R, et al: Supravalvular aortic stenosis. Arch Pathol Lab Med 109:179, 1985.

134. Curran ME, Atkinson KL, Ewart AK, et al: The elastin gene is disrupted by a translocation associated with supravalvular aortic stenosis. Cell 73:159, 1993.

135. Ewart AK, Morris CA, Ensing GJ, et al: A human vascular disorder, supravalvular aortic stenosis, maps to chromosome 7. Proc Natl Acad Sci USA 90:3226, 1993.

136. Ewart AK, Morris CA, Atkinson D, et al: Hemizygosity at the elastin locus in a developmental disorder, Williams syndrome. Nat Genet 5:11, 1993.

137. Frangiskakis JM, Ewart AK, Morris CA, et al: LIM-kinase 1 hemizygosity implicated in impaired visuospatial constructive cognition. Cell 86:59, 1996.

138. Pyeritz RE: The Marfan syndrome in childhood: Features, natural history and differential diagnosis. Prog Pediatr Cardiol 5:151, 1996.

139. Kainulainen K, Puikkinen L, Savolainen A, et al: Location on chromosome 15 of the gene defect causing Marfan syndrome. N Engl J Med 323:935, 1990.

140. Nijbroek G, Sood S, McIntosh I, et al: Fifteen novel *FBNI* mutations causing Marfan syndrome detected by heteroduplex analysis of genomic amplicons. Am J Hum Genet 57:8, 1995.

141. Dietz HC: Molecular etiology, pathogenesis and diagnosis of the Marfan syndrome. Prog Pediatr Cardiol 5:159, 1996.

142. Li L, Krantz, ID, Deng Y, et al: Alagille syndrome is caused by mutations in human Jagged1, which encodes a ligand for Notch1. Nat Genet 16:243, 1997.

143. McAllister KA, Grogg KM, Johnson DW, et al: Endoglin, a TGF-β binding protein of endothelial cells, is the gene for hereditary haemorrhagic telangiectasia type 1. Nat Genet 8:345, 1994.

144. Johnson DW, Berg JN, Gallione CJ, et al: A second locus for hereditary hemorrhagic telangiectasia maps to chromosome 12. Genome Res 5:21, 1995.

145. McAllister KA, Baldwin MA, Thukkani AK, et al: Six novel mutations in the endoglin gene in hereditary hemorrhagic telangiectasia type 1 suggest a dominant-negative effect of receptor function. Hum Mol Genet 4:1983, 1995.

146. Johnson DW, Berg JN, Baldwin MA, et al: Mutations in the activin receptor–like kinase 1 gene in hereditary haemorrhagic telangiectasia type 2. Nat Genet 13:189, 1996.

147. Tanaka T, Nagai R, Tomoike H, et al: Four novel *KVLQT1* and four novel *HERG* mutations in familial long-QT syndrome. Circulation 95:565, 1997.

148. Curran ME, Splawski I, Timothy KW, et al: A molecular basis for cardiac arrhythmia: *HERG* mutations cause long QT syndrome. Cell 80:795, 1995.

149. Wang Q, Shen J, Splawski I, et al: *SCN5A* mutations associated with an inherited cardiac arrhythmia, long QT syndrome. Cell 80:805, 1995.

150. Wang Q, Curran ME, Splawski I, et al: Positional cloning of a novel potassium channel gene: *KVLQT1* mutations cause cardiac arrhythmias. Nat Genet 12:17, 1996.

151. Neyroud N, Tesson F, Denjoy I, et al: A novel mutation in the potassium channel gene *KVLQT1* causes the Jervell and Lange-Nielsen cardioauditory syndrome. Nat Genet 15:186, 1997.

152. Splawski I, Timothy KW, Vincent GM, et al: Molecular basis of the long-QT syndrome associated with deafness. N Engl J Med 336:1562, 1997.

153. Schott JJ, Charpentier F, Peltier S, et al: Mapping of a gene for long QT syndrome to chromosome 4q25–27. Am J Hum Genet 57:1114, 1995.

154. Sanguinetti MC, Jiang C, Curran ME, Keating MT: A mechanistic link between an inherited and acquired cardiac arrhythmia: *HERG* encodes the I_{kr} potassium channel. Cell 81:299, 1995.

155. Compton SJ, Lux RL, Ramsey MR, et al: Genetically defined therapy of inherited long-QT syndrome. Correction of abnormal repolarization by potassium. Circulation 94:1018, 1996.

156. Schwartz PJ, Priori SG, Locati EH, et al: Long QT syndrome patients with mutations of the *SCN5A* and *HERG* genes have differential responses to Na$^+$ channel blockade and to increases in heart rate. Circulation 92:3381, 1995.

157. Brink PA, Ferreira A, Moolman JC, et al: Gene for progressive familial heart block type I maps to chromosome 19q13. Circulation 91:1633, 1995.

158. de Meeus A, Stephan E, Debrus S, et al: An isolated cardiac conduction disease maps to chromosome 19q. Circ Res 77:735, 1995.

CHAPTER 3
DEVELOPMENTAL CARDIAC PHYSIOLOGY AND MYOCARDIAL FUNCTION

PAGE A. W. ANDERSON

The heart undergoes profound changes during development. After heart tube formation, however, the basic function of the heart is the same throughout life, sustaining an adequate cardiac output through developing pressure and ejecting blood. The dependencies of this basic function have been considered, somewhat artificially, as being separable: preload (e.g., ventricular end-diastolic volume), afterload (e.g., arterial pressure), and inotropy (e.g., an agent that increases the cytosolic calcium transient). Although these dependencies are found throughout development, the cellular and subcellular systems that support them undergo complex changes. The first of the following sections provides a general review of these systems and how they produce the active and passive properties of the myocardium. Subsequent sections deal with the developmental changes in these myocardial systems, ventricular function in utero and after birth, and the effects of birth on ventricular function.

MYOCARDIAL CONTRACTION

SARCOMERE

At all stages of development, the basic force-generating unit of the heart is the sarcomere.[1] The sarcomere contains a lattice of thin filaments, made up of coiled-coils of actin monomers, that surround in hexagonal arrays the thick filaments, made up of bundles of myosin dimers. The thin filaments are attached to the Z disks, and the thick filaments are centered between the flanking Z disks (Fig. 3–1). Interdigitation of the thick and thin filaments allows force-generating cross-bridges to form between myosin heads and their binding sites on actin. The chemical energy stored in adenosine triphosphate is transduced into mechanical work through movement of the myosin heads and sarcomere shortening against a load.[2–5]

MYOFILAMENT SENSITIVITY TO CALCIUM

The interaction of actin and myosin and cross-bridge formation are regulated through a thin filament–based complex of proteins made up of troponin and tropomyosin, in a calcium concentration–dependent manner.[2,3] The resulting sigmoidal relationship between cross-bridge formation and calcium is characterized by the relation between force

and pCa (negative log of calcium concentration), as shown in Figure 3–2.

The coiled-coil of actin filaments (the backbone of the thin filament) is wrapped by a coiled-coil of tropomyosin molecules, regularly decorated with troponin complexes that are made up of troponin I, troponin C, and troponin T.[3] Troponin I inhibits actin-myosin interaction. Troponin C binding of calcium disinhibits this interaction. Troponin T binds the troponin complex to tropomyosin and is essential for the calcium concentration dependence of force development and adenosine triphosphatase (ATPase) activity; in the absence of troponin T, calcium concentration changes over a broad range do not affect ATPase activity. On the other hand, with the complete troponin complex, increasing calcium concentration from diastolic levels (e.g., pCa 8.0 to 7.0) results in calcium binding to the troponin C low-affinity site, decreased strength of actin interaction with tropomyosin and troponin I, and increased strength of troponin I interaction with troponin T, resulting in a movement of tropomyosin that exposes myosin binding sites on actin and allows cross-bridge formation.[5] Maximal force and ATPase activity are achieved at saturating calcium concentrations. This calcium-dependent relation is present in embryonic, fetal, neonatal, and adult myocardium.

PRELOAD

In the intact heart, the dependency of force development on sarcomere length or preload (the load or stress the sarcomere is subjected to before activation) is characterized by the Frank-Starling relation (e.g., stroke volume increases with an increase in end-diastolic volume). This relation depends on the number of cross-bridge attachments that can be made at a given sarcomere length and the sarcomere length dependence of myofilament sensitivity to calcium (see Fig. 3–2).

The extent of overlap of the thin and thick filaments controls the total number of cross-bridge attachments.[6] In many striated muscles, the maximal number of cross-bridge interactions occurs at the sarcomere length of 2.0 to 2.2 μm, a consequence of a thick filament length of 1.5 μm, a thin filament length of 1 μm, and a 0.2-μm-long thick filament central bare region, which lacks myosin heads. At sarcomere lengths above 2.2 μm, the number of potential interactions between myosin heads and actin monomers decreases as the overlap of thick and thin fila-

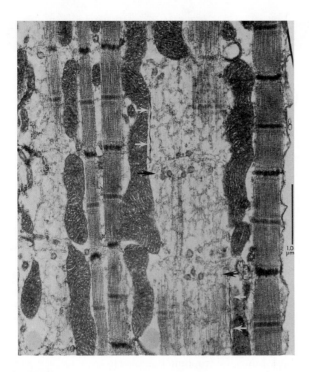

Electron micrograph of an isolated adult ventricular myocyte. This longitudinal section demonstrates the repetitive arrangement of the corbular *(black arrows)* and longitudinal *(white arrows, brackets)* sarcoplasmic reticulum (SR) typical of a mature ventricular myocyte. One myofibril passes slightly out of the section plane, revealing a ring of corbular SR at each Z disk from which extend the thin filaments (the I band of the sarcomere, 1 μm) and the lacy network of longitudinal SR that surrounds the A band of the sarcomere (which contains the electron-dense thick filaments). The corbular SR contains the ryanodine receptor (calcium release channel), and the longitudinal SR contains the SR ATPase. Transverse tubules, in cross-section with closely associated junctional SR, are seen at the level of the Z disks. (From Nassar R, Reedy MC, Anderson PAW: Developmental changes in the ultrastructure and sarcomere shortening of isolated rabbit ventricular myocyte. Circ Res 61[3]:465–483, 1987.)

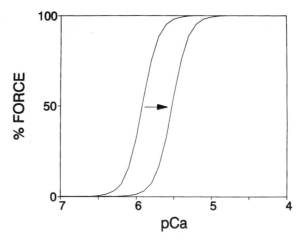

The effect of cytosolic calcium concentration on myocardial force development has a sigmoidal relation. This force-pCa (negative log of the calcium concentration) relation was obtained by chemically removing the cardiac membranes and exposing the skinned preparation to different buffered calcium concentrations. This relation, common to embryonic, fetal, neonatal, and adult myocardium, is affected by post-translational modifications, acidosis, and isoform expression of the sarcomere proteins. The rightward shift *(arrow)* of the relationship (a decrease in sensitivity of the myofilaments to calcium) exemplifies the effect of cAMP-dependent phosphorylation of cardiac troponin I (an effect of sympathomimetic stimulation).

ment decreases. At sarcomere lengths below 2.0 μm, double overlap of the thin filaments at the center of the sarcomere interferes with cross-bridge formation and decreases the force of contraction.[6]

The sarcomere length dependence of the sensitivity of the myofilaments to calcium may be the most important contributor to the Frank-Starling relation.[7] Specifically, the myofilaments are less sensitive to calcium at a shorter sarcomere length and require a relatively higher calcium concentration, compared with that at a longer sarcomere length, to achieve full activation (e.g., maximal force development and ATPase activity).

The Frank-Starling relation modulates the function of myocardium from the embryonic, fetal, neonatal, and adult heart.[8–10] At all ages, an increase in muscle length increases the force of myocardial contraction.

INOTROPY AND MYOFILAMENT FUNCTION

Inotropic interventions can produce their effects through changes in myofilament sensitivity to calcium. These effects can be described by shifts of the force-pCa relation.

For example, a decrease in sensitivity shifts the relation to the right (see Fig. 3–2), so that the pCa that generates half-maximal force (pCa$_{50}$ of 6 for many cardiac preparations) becomes smaller, that is, a higher calcium concentration is needed (recall that pCa 6 is 1 μM calcium, whereas pCa 5 is 10 μM calcium).

Myofilament sensitivity to calcium is modulated by adrenergic receptor stimulation. β-Adrenergic receptor agonist–induced increase in adenylate cyclase activity results in cyclic adenosine monophosphate (cAMP)–dependent protein kinase A phosphorylation of cardiac troponin I and the regulatory myosin light chain (MLC-2).[11] Phosphorylation of cardiac troponin I decreases myofilament sensitivity to calcium, and MLC-2 phosphorylation enhances sensitivity. In contrast, α-adrenergic receptor stimulation results in protein kinase C phosphorylation of other cardiac troponin I residues, decreased maximal ATPase activity, and no change in myofilament sensitivity.[12]

Pathophysiologic states (e.g., heart failure) have been described as increasing, decreasing, or having no effect on myofilament sensitivity to calcium. These apparently conflicting results may arise from heterogeneity in populations of patients, the disease processes, and methodologic differences and leave uncertain the effects of heart disease on myofilament sensitivity.[13–15]

Myofilament sensitivity to calcium is modulated by the expression of thin filament protein isoforms. For example, cardiac troponin T isoform expression affects troponin C binding of calcium (see later),[16] and troponin I isoform expression modulates the effects of respiratory acidosis.[17, 18] Although respiratory acidosis has a negative effect on myofilament sensitivity to calcium throughout development, the newborn is less affected.

INOTROPY AND CYTOSOLIC CALCIUM CONCENTRATION

The cytosolic calcium concentration transient that follows activation provides another important mechanism for modulating the force of contraction, enabling the heart to respond to changes in workload and disease processes and the effects of development. Many of the basic components of the system that control cell calcium are present throughout development. These components include the sarcolemma-based L (long)–type dihydropyridine (DHP)–sensitive calcium channel, Na^+-Ca^{2+} exchanger, Na^+,K^+-ATPase, and the sarcoplasmic reticulum (SR) Ca^{2+}-ATPase and Ca^{2+} release channel.[19–35]

With depolarization of the sarcolemma, the voltage-dependent calcium channels open. Two inward currents with different voltage dependencies, the L-type and T (transient)–type, have been identified in the heart.[19] The relative sizes of these currents differ among regions of the heart and with development.[19] The L-type current, however, is of central importance in supporting the cardiac contraction. In cardiac muscle, unlike in skeletal muscle, the movement of calcium through the DHP-sensitive channel is essential for calcium-induced calcium release (CICR) from the SR through its calcium release channels[20–22,35] (see Fig. 3–1); CICR amplifies the effect of the calcium current on cytosolic calcium concentration. In the absence of CICR, trans-sarcolemmal calcium flow results in a contraction whose peak force is only a fraction of that achieved in the presence of the amplification system. Triadin, a molecule closely associated with the L-type calcium channel and SR, has been found to have structural diversity, suggesting that it has a modulatory role in the interaction between the L-type channel and the SR.[23] The developmental acquisition of CICR functional importance is species dependent, apparently based on the level of maturation at birth.

CICR depends on SR removal of calcium from the cytosol by way of the SR Ca^{2+}-ATPase and SR calcium storage.[24–26] SR ATPase activity, like that of myofibrillar ATPase, is calcium concentration dependent. Consequently, the higher the calcium concentration transient is, the higher is the SR calcium ATPase activity, and the greater is the amount of calcium translocated into the SR. Another modulator of SR Ca^{2+}-ATPase is its closely associated inhibitor, phospholamban.[27,28] The cAMP-dependent phosphorylation of phospholamban removes its inhibitory effect and enhances ATPase activity. The important modulatory role of phospholamban has been characterized in transgenic animals (e.g., basal ventricular contractility is enhanced in the absence of phospholamban expression).[27,28]

The closely associated membranous complex that contains the L-type calcium channel and the SR calcium release channels (ryanodine receptor) has been named the junctional SR. In adult myocardium of large mammals such as the human, the junctional SR is primarily found in the sarcolemmal invaginations that make up the transverse tubule system (T-tubule, see Fig. 3–1). The T-tubule system is acquired with the maturational increase in myocyte size.[1] The sarcolemma-independent specialized region of the SR, the corbular SR, also contains the ryanodine receptor (see Fig. 3–1).[21,22] The junctional and corbular SR contain calsequestrin, a calcium-binding protein that appears to undergo a decrease in calcium affinity with calcium release channel opening.[29] In adult cardiac muscle, the junctional and corbular SR are anchored through the intermediate filaments to the Z disk, and so to the myofibrils. Extending from these specialized SR components is the longitudinal SR that contains the Ca^{2+}-ATPase. The lace-like tubular network of longitudinal SR surrounds the sarcomere, ensuring a coordinated increase and fall in calcium concentration, cross-bridge formation, and myocardial force.

The Na^+-Ca^{2+} exchanger[30–33,35] is integrated into the cell calcium control system as evidenced by its close anatomic relation to the DHP-sensitive calcium channel.[34] Multiple Na^+-Ca^{2+} exchanger isoforms with different exchange rates and stoichiometries are expressed.[31] The trans-sarcolemmal exchange of sodium for calcium during a contraction helps return cytosolic calcium concentration to diastolic levels. Importantly, the exchanger also provides a mechanism for increasing the calcium transient and the force of contraction. Specifically, when the myocyte depolarizes to a potential more positive than the Na^+-Ca^{2+} exchanger reversal potential, calcium enters the cell in exchange for sodium.[32–33] This "reverse" mode function of the Na^+-Ca^{2+} exchanger does not appear to induce CICR.[35] The contribution of reverse mode function to cardiac contraction appears to change with development and differ among species.

The dynamic ability of the heart to change its force of contraction from beat to beat through changes in cytosolic calcium concentration is demonstrated by altering the rate and pattern of stimulation (e.g., post-extrasystolic potentiation).[36,37] The extrasystole is less forceful than the contraction at the basic rate, and the post-extrasystolic contraction is more forceful (Fig. 3–3). When SR function is blunted by interfering with calcium uptake or release, post-extrasystolic potentiation is abolished, and the force of the extrasystole is increased, altering the restitution of contractility.[37] In the adult myocardium with normal SR function, extrasystolic force increases exponentially as the interval between the contraction at the basic rate and the extrasystole is increased (Fig. 3–4).[38] This relation is nearly eliminated by interfering with CICR.[37,39] The beat-to-beat changes in force may also be supported by changes in trans-sarcolemmal calcium movement (e.g., through the Na^+-Ca^{2+} exchanger).[32,33,35] The dependence of post-extrasystolic potentiation and restitution of contractility on the systems that control the calcium transient make these physiologic phenomena useful tools for examining how development affects these membrane systems and their function.

RECEPTOR-MEDIATED CHANGES IN INOTROPY

The components of the β- and α-adrenergic receptor systems and their role in modulating the cardiac contraction change with development, altering the functional effects of their agonists.[11,12,40–49] β-Adrenergic receptor stimulation modulates SR function by enhancing its SR Ca^{2+}-ATPase activity through cAMP-dependent phosphorylation of phospholamban and Ca^{2+}/calmodulin-dependent phos-

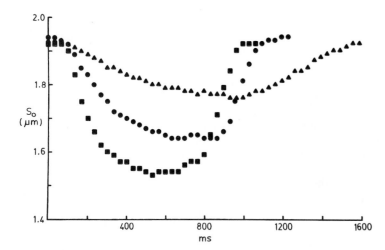

FIGURE 3–3

Post-extrasystolic potentiation: the effect of introducing an extrasystole on sarcomere shortening in an adult ventricular myocyte. The sarcomere waveforms of three consecutive contractions are superimposed: the contraction at the basic rate *(circles)*, the following extrasystole *(triangles)*, and the post-extrasystole *(squares)*. Amount and velocity of sarcomere shortening are smallest in the extrasystole and greatest in the post-extrasystolic contraction. (From Nassar R, Reedy MC, Anderson PAW: Developmental changes in the ultrastructure and sarcomere shortening of the isolated rabbit ventricular myocyte. Circ Res 61[3]:465–483, 1987.)

phorylation of the SR pump (see earlier).[27,50] These post-translational modifications markedly increase the amount of calcium taken up by, stored in, and available for release from the SR during subsequent contractions. This positive effect on contractility is opposite to the negative effect on myofilament sensitivity to calcium induced by β-adrenergic receptor stimulation–induced cardiac troponin I phosphorylation.[11] Other membrane components essential to CICR are also modulated by cAMP-dependent phosphorylation. For example, phosphorylation of the α_1 subunit of the L-type calcium channel increases the calcium current,[19] and the function of the ryanodine receptor and the Na^+-Ca^{2+} exchanger are modulated by phosphorylation.[22,51] The β-adrenergic receptor stimulation–induced phosphorylation of these membrane and myofilament proteins brings about the well-known effect of sympathetic stimulation on ventricular contraction, an enhancement in the rates of rise and fall of pressure, an increase in ventricular ejection, and a decrease in the duration of systole.

Other cardiac myocyte receptors include those for endothelin, angiotensin II, adenosine, adenosine triphosphate, opioids, thrombin, and histamine.[52–56] They affect the calcium transient and modify the response of the cardiac myofilaments to the transient and to adrenergic receptor stimulation. For example, endothelin increases the force of the cardiac contraction, whereas nitric oxide, adenosine, and the opioids decrease the calcium transient and contractility. Some of the ligands are expressed by cardiac myocytes and other myocardial cells and consequently have autocrine and paracrine actions that also affect cell division (hyperplasia) and hypertrophy.[57–60]

AFTERLOAD AND MYOCARDIAL SHORTENING

A fundamental property of the myocardium is its ability to shorten actively against a load imposed on the myocardium after activation and initiation of the contraction. At all stages of development, the heart ejects against an afterload that is made up primarily of the arterial pressure. This ability is essential for ventricular ejection and an adequate cardiac output. Afterload decreases myocardial shortening and stroke volume to an extent that is similar at all stages of development and in all cardiac preparations.[8,61,62] In the isolated cardiac myocyte, the higher the afterload, the smaller the amount and velocity of sarcomere shortening. Failure of the myocardium to shorten adequately results in death at any stage of development.[63]

The velocity of muscle shortening against a zero load, unloaded shortening velocity, has been used conceptually

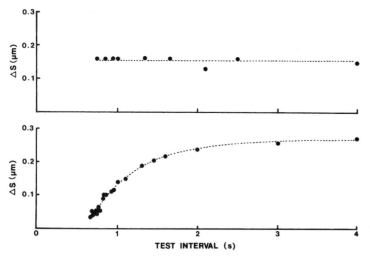

FIGURE 3–4

Restitution of sarcomere shortening in an immature ventricular myocyte *(upper)* is compared with that of an adult myocyte *(lower)*. Extrasystolic sarcomere shortening is plotted against the time interval between the stimulus that elicits the extrasystolic stimulus and that of the previous contraction at the basic paced rate (the test interval). In the adult cell *(lower)*, restitution is gradual *(dotted line* is monoexponential curve, time constant = 0.4 second); in the immature cell *(upper)*, the earliest extrasystole that can be elicited has the same amount of sarcomere shortening as the contraction at the regular rate (see response at test interval of 4 seconds). (From Nassar R, Reedy MC, Anderson PAW: Developmental changes in the ultrastructure and sarcomere shortening of the isolated rabbit ventricular myocyte. Circ Res 61[3]:465–483, 1987.)

to understand cross-bridge formation.[4] Unloaded sarcomere shortening cannot be measured in cardiac muscle (a load must be applied to the myocyte to achieve a rest sarcomere length greater than 1.9 μm). The velocity of cardiac muscle shortening does correlate with ATPase activity of myosin heavy chain isozymes,[64] suggesting that shortening velocity depends on the rate of cross-bridge breaking.

Although unloaded velocity of myocardial shortening can be conceptually useful, it is not relevant to the in vivo heart in which an afterload is always present. Consequently, the number of force-generating cross-bridge attachments is of central importance. In other words, when the myocardium contracts against an afterload, the greater the number of cross-bridges, the greater is the velocity of shortening.

TRANSDUCTION OF SARCOMERE FUNCTION TO CARDIAC CONTRACTION AND MYOCARDIAL COMPLIANCE

Myocardial contraction and ventricular ejection of blood require cross-bridge force to be transduced to ventricular wall stress and shortening.[65,66] The transduction system can be considered as having three components linked in series: starting from the sarcomere, they are the cytoskeleton, the sarcolemma-based integrin receptors that couple the cytoskeleton to the extracellular matrix, and the extracellular matrix.[67–70]

The cytoskeleton is a complex intracellular meshwork of filaments and tubules made up of titin, desmin, tubulin, and other structural proteins.[65–77] Titin, a large protein (>1 MDa), maintains a constant sarcomere length throughout the myofibril and thick filament centering within the sarcomere.[69,71,74,75] Titin is responsible for most of the passive tension-length relation of the cardiac myocyte[65] (and may also affect myofilament sensitivity to calcium). The titin molecule extends from its attachment in the Z disk to the end of the thick filament, independent of the thin filament, and extends from the end of the thick filament to the M-line. The portion of the titin molecule that lies between the Z disk and the thick filament extends when the cell is stretched.[69,75] The length of this extensible region varies among titin isoforms and correlates with stiffness differences among striated muscles. The centering of the thick filament and the transmission of tension follow from the thick filament's being attached at each end by titin molecules.

The function of the cytoskeleton also depends on desmin-containing intermediate filaments.[1,38,73,78] This meshwork connects one myofibril to another and the SR to the myofibrils at the Z disks. A scaffolding of microtubules connects the myofibrils and may modulate the force of contraction through altering the internal load against which the sarcomere shortens.[77,79] The cytoskeletal attachments maintain close anatomic relations among the myofibrils, sarcolemma, transverse tubules, mitochondria, and nuclei, ensuring that the force-generating myofibrils, the membrane systems that modulate the calcium transient, and the energy sources move in an integrated manner during the cardiac contraction.[38,76]

The sarcolemma-based integrin receptors, found at the level of the Z disk, are heterodimers of an α and a β sub-unit.[67,68,79–83] The integrin subunits are products of a large number of genes that also yield multiple isoforms through alternative splicing (Fig. 3–5). More than eight β subunits and 15 α subunits are expressed, and more than 20 different heterodimeric receptors have been identified (see Fig. 3–5).[80–82] The nonredundancy among α and β subunit isoforms is emphasized by embryonic death in the absence of integrin subunit isoforms. The integrins bind to both the cytoskeleton and extracellular matrix proteins (see Fig. 3–5). The receptors, in an α integrin isoform–specific manner, bind with different affinities to the various extracellular matrix proteins (e.g., laminin, collagen, and fibronectin).[84] The cytoplasmic domains of the β subunit are associated with the cytoskeletal proteins, which include talin, vinculin, and α-actinin. The Z disks of the myofibrils located immediately below the sarcolemma are attached by way of vinculin-containing costameres to the integrin receptors (see Fig. 3–5) and through the cytoskeleton to other myofibrils. The attachment of the integrins to the cytoskeleton and to the extracellular matrix

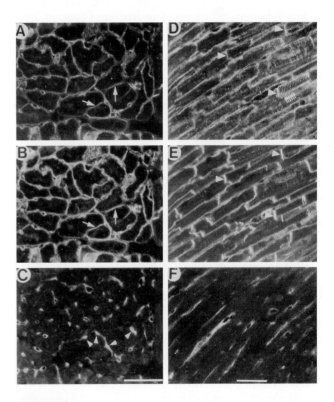

FIGURE 3–5

Comparison of localization and relative expression of two β integrin isoforms (β1D and β1A) and colocalization of vinculin, which connects the myofibril Z disk to the integrin receptor. The relative expression of the two isoforms changes with age. Serial transverse sections of mouse adult cardiac muscle (5-μm) stained with antibodies against β1D (*A*), vinculin (*B*), or β1A (*C*). *Arrows* mark the cardiomyocyte sarcolemma, *arrowheads* indicate nonmuscle cells, expressing β1A but lacking β1D integrin isoform. Longitudinal sections of mouse cardiac muscle (5-μm) were either double-stained with antibodies against β1D (*D*) and vinculin (*E*) or stained with antibody against β1A (*F*). *Small arrows* mark cardiomyocyte costameres, the site of vinculin localization. *Arrowheads* point to intercalated discs. Bar = 20 μm. (From Belkin AM, Zhidkova NI, Balzac F, et al: Beta 1D integrin displaces the beta 1A isoform in striated muscles: Localization at junctional structures and signaling potential in nonmuscle cells. Reproduced from The Journal of Cell Biology, 1996, volume 132, pages 211–226 by copyright permission of The Rockefeller University Press.)

provides the mechanism that transfers myofibril force generation to the extracellular matrix and to other cells and results in the smooth coordinated contraction of the ventricle (recall also the connexins that make up the gap junctions provide cell-to-cell coupling, which changes with development and connexin expression).[85] The integrins also transduce different kinds of signals in the opposite direction. These signals, which include various trophic and mitogenic peptides, are generated by the cardiac myocytes and fibroblasts and stored in the extracellular matrix.

The extracellular matrix components include the interstitial collagen types I and III, glycoproteins such as fibronectin and laminin, and the proteoglycans heparin sulfate and hyaluronic acid.[67,81,86] They make up the connective tissue network of the extracellular matrix that has been defined as containing four levels: epimysium, perimysium, endomysium, and the extracellular portion of the basement membrane of the cardiac myocyte. Figure 3–6 illustrates a model of the extracellular matrix found in the adult heart. The subepicardium and subendocardium make up the epimysium. The epimysial layer is connected to the endomysium by large cable-like bundles of collagen. The endomysial layer contains myocyte-myocyte connections, myocyte-capillary connections, and a weave network made of bundles of collagen that connect the adjacent myocytes and the myocytes to the capillaries and other components of the extracellular matrix. The fourth level of the extracellular matrix is composed of the specialized outer layer of the sarcolemma where collagen IV, laminin, fibronectin, and heparan sulfate are found.

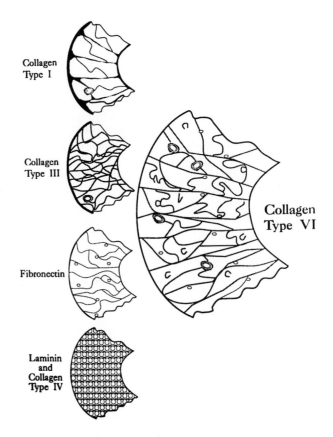

FIGURE 3–6

Diagram of the distribution of six cardiac extracellular matrix components in the adult left ventricular free wall, epicardium to the left and endocardium to the right. Collagen type I forms the major structural buttress of the myocardium and is present in large bundles or septa spanning the epicardium to the endocardium. Collagen type III is also found in these large bundles but is less prevalent than type I. Unlike type I, type III forms a major part of the finer septa and is prominent in the vascular adventitia. Collagen type VI and fibronectin extend from these finer septa to the connective tissue surrounding capillaries and to myocardial cells. In this pericellular location, they are likely to bind to basement membrane components (laminin and collagen type IV). This model suggests that the cardiac extracellular matrix proteins are organized in an architectural system in which load and stress are distributed in a hierarchical manner. The hierarchy in order of decreasing tensile strength and increasing pliability is as follows: type I → type III → type VI and fibronectin (and perhaps type V) → basement membranes. In this manner, changes induced by contraction and relaxation of myocardial cells can be distributed throughout the heart. (From Bashey RI, Martinez-Hernandez A, Jimenez SA: Isolation, characterization, and localization of cardiac collagen type VI. Associations with other extracellular matrix components. Circ Res 70[5]:1006–1017, 1992.)

MYOCARDIAL CONTRACTION AND DEVELOPMENT

FORCE OF CONTRACTION

Does myocardial ability to develop force and to shorten against a load increase with development, and if so, how? The answer to the first part of the question is yes,[8,87,88] as exemplified in Figure 3–7: the amount and velocity of sarcomere shortening in the immature myocardium are less than those of the adult myocyte.[38] The answer to the second part of the question has multiple components. For example, the developmental increase in myofibril amount and organization, myocyte number and size, and myocardial mass must contribute to this enhanced ability.

The developmental increase in the force of contraction, however, must be considered more broadly than as simply the ability to contract under one set of conditions. The heart must be able to modulate its ability to eject blood from moment to moment (e.g., with changes in state). The developmental dependence of this ability arises from changes in the systems that modulate cytosolic calcium concentration and myofilament sensitivity to calcium.

HYPERTROPHY AND HYPERPLASIA

Systemic arterial pressure and ventricular stroke volume increase with development. The ability of the myocardium to support this increased load follows, in part, from the developmental increase in ventricular mass.[89] In general, ventricular mass is matched to arterial pressure.

In utero, the developmental increases in right and left ventricular mass are closely matched, an apparent consequence of similar workloads.[90] In contrast, in the postnatal period, left ventricular weight (relative to body weight) increases markedly, whereas that of the right ventricle remains the same or decreases.[89] Neonatal increases in left ventricular stroke volume and systolic pressure increase left ventricular work, whereas the neonatal fall in pulmonary artery pressure and modest if any increase in right ventricular stroke volume result in decreased right ventricular work.

The responses of the heart to cardiac malformations and operative manipulations provide examples as to how age modulates the effects of workload on ventricular mass.

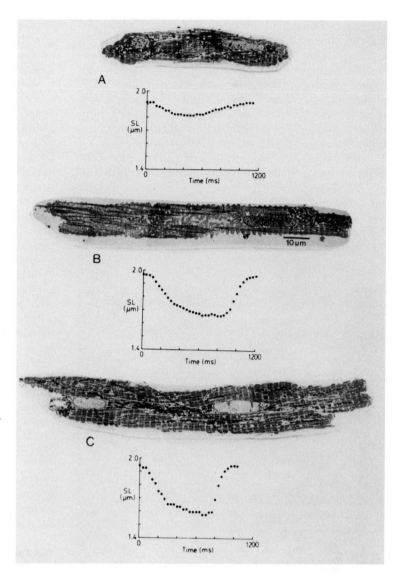

FIGURE 3–7

The contraction waveforms and longitudinal central sections of three isolated cardiac myocytes. Sarcomere contractions were measured and the cells then prepared for electron microscopy. Sarcomere length (SL) is plotted as a function of time (1 mM extracellular calcium). All cells in the figure are shown at identical magnification. *A,* An average-sized myocyte from a 3-week-old rabbit. *B,* A relatively small adult cell. *C,* An average-sized cell from an adult heart. (From Nassar R, Reedy MC, Anderson PAW: Developmental changes in the ultrastructure and sarcomere shortening of the isolated rabbit ventricular myocyte. Circ Res 61[3]:465–483, 1987.)

For example, in the infant with complete transposition being staged to an arterial switch, pulmonary artery banding produces a marked and rapid increase in left ventricular mass; but in the adolescent and young adult, this manipulation results in a much slower and smaller increase in left ventricular mass.[91]

One contributor to the fetal and neonatal increase in ventricular mass is myocyte division (i.e., hyperplasia).[89] During neonatal life, myocyte number of the left ventricle increases more rapidly than that of the right ventricle,[89] consistent with the more rapid neonatal increase in left ventricular mass and higher left ventricular workload. When neonatal cardiac myocyte hyperplasia ceases, aside from increases in nonmyocyte cell number and size, ventricular mass increases primarily through increasing myocyte size[89] (physiologic hypertrophy). The neonatal myocyte is approximately 40 μm in length and 5 μm in width, whereas the adult ventricular myocyte is usually more than 100 μm in length and 25 μm or more in width (see Fig. 3–7). The rate at which these increases occur are, in general, ventricle dependent, with left ventricular myocyte size increasing more rapidly. These changes in myocyte size are associated with changes in shape[38,92] and myofibril organization and distribution. Early during fetal life, the immature myocyte is spheroidal; but with maturation, the myocyte becomes longer, acquiring an ellipsoid shape with tapered ends, and in the months after birth achieves the complex three-dimensional shape of the adult myocyte (see Fig. 3–7).[38] The change from a spheroidal shape of the immature myocyte to the timber-like shape of the adult myocyte appears to result in a more effective shape for coupling sarcomere shortening to the development of ventricular wall tension and pressure.

How do neonatal life and increased workload induce greater hyperplasia, and what are the stimuli during the first weeks of neonatal life that suppress cardiac myocyte hyperplasia? The postnatal changes in a multitude of receptors, agonists, and effector systems make it likely that many candidates are involved in inducing hyperplasia, hypertrophy, and withdrawal of the cardiac myocyte from the cell cycle, and their contributions may differ from one stage of development to another.[60,93–97] Potential candidates have been identified. For example, acidic fibroblast growth factor (aFGF) stimulates myocyte proliferation and suppresses myocyte differentiation.[96] During postnatal life, myocardial levels of aFGF fall; transforming growth factor β increases, and myocyte hyperplasia ceases.[97] The fetal and neonatal cardiac myocytes express this mitogen and its receptor (Fig. 3–8) and excrete aFGF into the extracellular matrix, allowing this peptide to have an autocrine function. Interfering with its expression brings about cardiac myocyte differentiation and withdrawal from the cell cycle. The presence of the aFGF receptor in nonmyocyte and endothelial cells suggests that this peptide is important in neonatal angiogenesis (see Fig. 3–8).[96]

Neonatal cardiac myocyte hypertrophy is induced by norepinephrine, endothelin, basic fibroblast growth factor (bFGF), and other agents. For example, cardiac myocytes and fibroblasts express angiotensinogen, renin, angiotensin-converting enzyme, and the angiotensin II receptors (AT_1 and AT_2) and their subtypes.[57–60, 98] Through this system, angiotensin II acts in a paracrine and autocrine manner to play a role in neonatal left ventricular growth. In the adult heart, angiotensin-converting enzyme inhibition and AT_1 blockade prevent hypertrophy in response to pressure or volume overload. The complexity of the interactions that regulate this system is exemplified by subtype expression and the interactions, for example, among angiotensin II, bFGF, and insulin-like growth factor-1 (IGF-1).[53, 98–101]

The neonatal increase in circulating growth hormone levels provides another arm in the cascade that induces neonatal hypertrophy.[102] The growth hormone receptor gene is expressed in the heart. Stimulation of this receptor induces myocardial expression of IGF-1, and the extracellular increase in IGF-1 and the cardiac myocyte expression of the IGF-1 receptor stimulate myocyte hypertrophy and muscle-specific gene expression.

A well-characterized model of agonist-induced neonatal cardiac myocyte hypertrophy is based on α-adrenergic receptor stimulation.[103, 104] This process appears to be mediated through protein kinase C and is interrupted by α_1-adrenergic receptor blockade. In vivo overexpression of adrenergic receptor subtype α_{1b} induces hypertrophy, and in vitro hypertrophy is associated with repression of α_{1b} expression and induction of α_{1c} expression.[104] In contrast, the adult cardiac myocytes are little affected in vitro by norepinephrine.[114, 115] Explanations for this different response include greater neonatal α-adrenergic receptor expression and differences in G protein expression.[42, 105]

Developmental hypertrophy is normal and essential, but pathophysiologically induced hypertrophy is detrimental. How the regulation of the same ligand-based system (e.g., angiotensin II) brings about the normal hypertrophy of development and its positive effects and, in the mature heart, pathophysiologic hypertrophy and its negative effects remains to be determined.

MYOFIBRIL STRUCTURE AND ORGANIZATION

The myofibrils contain the basic contractile unit of the myofilament, the sarcomere. Consequently, changes in the myofibril must affect force development. Myofibril organization and amount are enhanced by development.[37, 38, 89, 92] During early fetal life, the myofibrils are distributed with no apparent orientation and are present at a low density compared with that of the adult myocyte. Later in fetal life and during neonatal life, when myocyte shape has changed from sphere-like to an ellipse of rotation, the myofibrils are oriented in the long axis of the cell. They are localized, however, in a shell only one or two myofibrils thick just inside the sarcolemma.[38] The immature myocardial contraction appears to be more dependent on trans-sarcolemmal calcium movement,[106] suggesting an intracellular calcium gradient.[38] In other words, calcium concentration is highest just beneath the sarcolemma and lowest at the center of the cell. On the basis of this model of the immature myocyte, subsarcolemmal localization of the myofibrils is essential if the sarcomeres are to be exposed to the highest cytosolic calcium concentration.

With further maturation, the cell organization changes into one in which layers of myofibrils alternate repetitively with layers of mitochondria from one side of the cell to an-

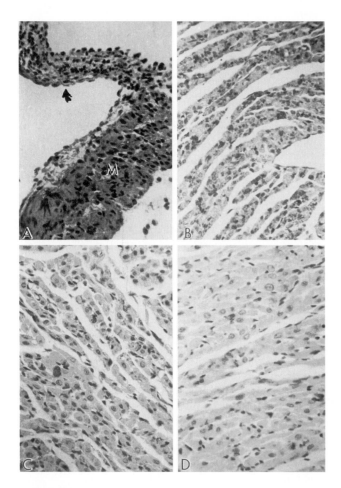

FIGURE 3–8

Photomicrographs showing immunohistochemical localization of acidic fibroblast growth factor receptor (*flg*) during heart development. Ventricular and neonatal tissues were isolated from embryonic (day 10 of gestation, *A*) and fetal (day 16 of gestation, *B*) Wistar-Kyoto rats and neonatal (*C*) and mature (*D*) spontaneously hypertensive rats. Fetal ventricular and atrial myocyte (day 20 of gestation) *flg* immunoreactivity is most intense during early development (*A, B*) and rapidly wanes in the neonatal (*C*) and mature (*D*) heart. In the neonate, the primary sites of immunoreactivity are in the small muscular arteries (*C*, 3-week-old rat) or the capillary bed (*D*, 5-week-old rat). (From Engelmann GL, Dionne CA, Jaye MC: Acidic fibroblast growth factor and heart development. Role in myocyte proliferation and capillary angiogenesis. Circ Res 72[1]:7–19, 1993.)

other (see Fig. 3–1). By this point in development, the SR, the extensive intracellular system for uptake and release of calcium, has been acquired (see Fig. 3–1), ensuring that intracellular calcium gradients do not occur and coordinated sarcomere shortening does. These changes in myofibril and membrane organization contribute to the developmental increase in the myocardial force of contraction. The timing and rate at which these changes occur with development vary among species, seemingly related to the degree of maturity at birth (e.g., the lamb running across the meadow versus the puppy hidden in the den).[8,89,92] The components of these changes, however, are common to all mammals, including the human.[90]

The myofibrils increase in length and in width throughout development. This ongoing construction and addition of more thick and thin filaments is evidenced by the fragmented myofilaments and many ribosomes seen in the immature myocyte. Sarcomeres in myofibrils undergoing this process probably contribute less effectively to force development than do those in the fully formed myofibrils of the adult heart.

The expression of the contractile proteins required for myofibrillogenesis is highly regulated. For example, a fixed stoichiometry of seven actin monomers to one tropomyosin, one troponin C, one troponin T, and one troponin I is found. The importance of this balance in transcription, translation, and myofibrillogenesis is evident in *Drosophila* indirect flight muscle mutants.[107] For example, a troponin T mutation that decreases the level of troponin T results in a concomitant decrease in expression of the other thin filament proteins and a decrease in myofibril size. Other thin filament protein mutants disrupt myofibrillogenesis.

DEVELOPMENTAL CHANGES IN CONTRACTILE PROTEIN EXPRESSION

The thin filament regulation of myocardial contraction, characterized by the force-pCa relation (see Fig. 3–2), suggests that developmental changes in the force of contraction may follow from contractile protein isoform expression, whereas a developmental increase in myocardial shortening velocity and myofibrillar ATPase activity suggests the differential effects of myosin isozyme expression. A search for isoforms of many of these proteins has been successful.[18,108–112]

Developmental and disease-associated changes in isoform expression have been found in many species, including the human. Some isoforms are products of alternative splicing of the primary transcript of a single gene, and others are products of multigene families. For example, cardiac troponin I and slow skeletal muscle troponin I, both expressed in the heart, are products of two genes,[18] whereas the multiple isoforms of cardiac troponin T arise from a single gene.[113] The expression of these and other isoforms often follows a temporally and chamber-specific complex pattern.[112,114] However, striking differences in these developmental patterns are found among species.[112,115]

The basis of the regulated cardiac expression of the contractile proteins remains to be defined. Present studies include the direct measurement of the effects of trophic agents on transcription and translation, and mutational analysis of potential promoter and enhancer regions. Such studies have been useful in coupling basic research to clinical observations. For example, the demonstration that thyroid hormone enhances α-myosin heavy chain expression, whereas only β-myosin heavy chain is expressed in the absence of thyroid hormone, stimulated the study of thyroid receptor gene binding and hormonal regulation of cardiac muscle transcription.[110] At the clinical level, these basic findings led to the recognition that neonatal cardiac surgery depresses thyroid-stimulating hormone and thyroxine levels, which may have negative effects on cardiac function.[116]

Mammalian myocardium expresses α- and β-myosin heavy chains,[110] which may be present in the thick filament as heterodimers or homodimers. The functional consequences are that myocardium containing primarily α-myosin heavy chain has the highest ATPase activity and shortening velocity, myocardium containing primarily β-myosin heavy chain has the lowest ATPase activity and shortening velocity, and myocardium containing the heterodimer has an intermediate activity and shortening velocity.[64] The study of myosin heavy chain expression was given impetus by the finding that changes in isozyme expression correlate with changes in myocardial function.[64,110,115] Before birth in the rodent, β-myosin heavy chain expression predominates, whereas in the adult ventricle, essentially only α-myosin heavy chain is expressed. The developmental increase in α-myosin heavy chain expression correlated with an increase in myocardial unloaded shortening velocity. Finally, in the rat, both hypertrophy and heart failure increase β-myosin heavy chain expression and decrease myocardial shortening velocity.[115,117]

These correlations led to the hypothesis that myosin heavy chain expression is central to developmental changes in myocardial function and the effects of disease. In the failing human heart, as in the rodent, myofibrillar ATPase activity is decreased.[118] In contrast to the rodent, however, in the human ventricle, β-myosin heavy chain is dominantly expressed from late fetal life through senescence, and its expression is little affected by heart failure.[112,115,119] Consequently, in the human, the decrease in myofibrillar ATPase activity with heart failure is unlikely to result from altered myosin heavy chain isozyme expression.

Isoform expression of two myosin light chains, which are bound to the myosin heavy chain head, appears to have a role in modulating myocardial function.[120,121] These proteins are the essential myosin light chain (MLC-1) and the regulatory myosin light chain (MLC-2). In smooth muscle, contraction is controlled by a calcium-regulated phosphorylation of MLC-2. Although this thick filament–based regulatory system remains to be demonstrated in cardiac muscle, the myosin light chains appear to modulate cardiac function. Their isoform expression follows a temporal and chamber-specific pattern. In the human, for example, the atrial MLC-1 isoform is expressed in the fetal ventricle but not in the adult ventricle.[120] However, in hypertrophied right ventricular muscle (e.g., in tetralogy of Fallot), the atrial MLC-1 isoform is re-expressed, and this expression correlates with enhanced contractility.[121] The regulatory myosin light chain, MLC-2, regulates function through its phosphorylation. This post-translational modification results in increased myofibrillar sensitivity to calcium. Another myosin-associated protein, protein C, has both structural and functional roles.[122] In addition to helping bind myosin into the thick filament, protein C modulates myofilament function through its cAMP-dependent phosphorylation. The functional effects of the isoforms of these myosin heavy chain–associated proteins continue to be explored.

Cardiac expression of α-actin isoforms is affected by development.[123, 124] In the bird and the rodent, the complex developmental pattern of expression of these actins, which make up the backbone of the thin filament, results in the sequential myocyte expression of vascular smooth muscle α-actin, skeletal muscle α-actin, and cardiac α-actin. In the adult rodent, ventricular pressure overload causes a transient re-expression of skeletal muscle actin. In contrast to these species, the human fetal heart predominantly expresses cardiac α-actin, and the hearts of the child and adult dominantly express skeletal α-actin.[124] Also, similar to human heart disease, which has little effect on myosin heavy chain isoform expression, hypertrophy or heart failure does not affect actin isoform expression in the human heart, that is, skeletal α-actin remains the dominantly expressed isoform.[124]

A functional consequence of the postnatal change in actin isoform expression in the human is suggested by a correlation in adult mouse heart between skeletal α-actin expression and ventricular contractility, described by dP/dt_{max}.[125] This positive correlation suggests that the human postnatal switch in actin isoform expression could increase contractility and support the function of the neonatal heart in its adaptation to the hemodynamic loads of a cardiac malformation and recovery from a cardiac operation.

Troponin C, whose binding to calcium disinhibits the effect of troponin I, is the only thin filament regulatory protein that does not undergo changes in isoform expression in the heart. From the earliest time in cardiac development, only cardiac troponin C is expressed, suggesting that its functional domain sequences are essential for cardiac-specific properties. One unresolved debate is whether cardiac troponin C confers onto cardiac muscle a greater sarcomere length dependence of myofilament sensitivity to calcium (which underlies the Frank-Starling relationship) than that of fast skeletal muscle, which expresses fast skeletal troponin C.[126] Functional differences among the troponin C isoforms are evidenced by transgenic expression of skeletal muscle troponin C in the heart, providing a protective effect against acidosis.[127] This functional effect suggests that inducing skeletal muscle troponin C expression in the heart will be clinically useful in disease states, such as ischemia.

Tropomyosin, the thin filament protein that binds the regulatory complex of troponin to actin, is expressed in the heart as products of two genes, whose developmental change in expression differs among species.[109, 128] (A third less well defined isoform, whose mutant is associated with nemaline rod disease, may also be expressed in the human heart.) The α and β isoforms are assembled into homodimers and heterodimers. In the human and in other large animals, some β-tropomyosin is expressed throughout development, but the adult and neonatal heart predominantly express α-tropomyosin. Functional correlations between these two isoforms suggest that α-tropomyosin allows more rapid relaxation, whereas β-tropomyosin expression is associated with slower contraction speeds. Transgenic overexpression of β-tropomyosin results in a slowing of diastolic relaxation,[128] increased sensitivity of the myofilaments to calcium,[129] and a decreased effect of cardiac troponin I cAMP-dependent phosphorylation on myofilament sensitivity to calcium. Although these isoform effects may prove valuable in understanding cardiac contraction, the dominant expression in the human heart of α-tropomyosin makes the tropomyosin isoforms less relevant than those of other contractile proteins (e.g., troponin I and troponin T) in understanding how disease and development affect human cardiac contractility.

Two isoforms of troponin I, the inhibitory component of the troponin complex, are expressed in the heart during development.[18] The switch in expression from slow skeletal muscle troponin I in the fetus to cardiac troponin I in the adult is common to the human and other species. A major sequence difference between these two isoforms (the N-terminal peptide of cardiac troponin I, in essence, a cardiac-specific extension of the troponin I molecule) has been found to have great functional importance in the response to β-adrenergic receptor stimulation.[130] Phosphorylation of this cardiac troponin I peptide's serines decreases myofilament sensitivity to calcium. In other words, after phosphorylation, a higher cytosolic calcium concentration is required to achieve the same level of activation (see Fig. 3–2).

The apparently counterintuitive effect of β-adrenergic stimulation on myofilament function is central to the integrated effects of sympathetic stimulation on the cardiac contraction. The decrease in myofibril sensitivity to calcium contributes to an enhanced rate of diastolic relaxation and a shortening of the contraction, a necessity given the β-agonist–induced increase in heart rate.[130] The predominant expression of slow skeletal muscle troponin I in the perinatal human heart[18] is likely to interfere with the integrated response to the normal marked perinatal increases in the level of circulating catecholamines that are further increased with stress. The potential consequences of this aspect of slow skeletal muscle troponin I expression on neonatal ventricular function remain to be identified.

Other cardiac troponin I residues are phosphorylated by α-adrenergic receptor stimulation and protein kinase C activation.[11, 12] In a protein kinase C isozyme–dependent manner, phosphorylation of these residues decreases maximal myofibrillar ATPase activity. This system does not appear to contribute to the decreased ATPase activity found in the failing human heart.[14]

Expression of slow skeletal muscle troponin I confers on the myocardium a relative resistance to respiratory acidosis.[17] Comparing myofilaments containing slow skeletal muscle troponin I with those containing cardiac troponin I mutants demonstrates that the cardiac troponin I N-terminal extension is not the basis of this increased resistance to acidosis. In the human, the high expression of slow skeletal muscle troponin I in the fetal and neonatal heart will decrease the negative effects of respiratory acidosis.

During the first few years of human postnatal life, the high level of slow skeletal muscle troponin I expression in the heart gradually wanes.[18] Later in life, human heart disease does not induce expression of slow skeletal muscle troponin I, just as it does not alter α-actin isoform expression.[14, 18, 124]

Cardiac troponin T, which binds the regulatory troponin complex to tropomyosin, is the only troponin T gene expressed in the heart. Combinatorial alternative splicing of the primary transcript yields multiple cardiac troponin T isoforms that are expressed in a developmentally and regionally regulated manner.[108, 113, 114, 131] The number of these isoforms varies among mammalian and avian species. In the human, four isoforms have been identified that differ through the variable presence of two N-terminal sequences. The largest isoform, $cTnT_1$, is most highly expressed in the fetal heart and contains both sequences; $cTnT_3$, expressed throughout development and dominantly in the adult heart, contains the shorter of the two sequences; and the smallest isoform, $cTnT_4$, is expressed during fetal life, is re-expressed with heart failure, and contains neither of the two alternatively spliced sequences.

The rich complex pattern of cardiac troponin T isoform expression suggests that these sequence differences have a functional significance. This possibility is supported by a range of observations.[16, 108, 132] For example, the sensitivity of the myofilaments to calcium is altered by its troponin T isoform content (Fig. 3–9A), and in the failing human heart, the increase in $cTnT_4$ expression is correlated with the fall in myofibrillar ATPase activity (Fig. 3–9B). Finally, human atrial expression of the cardiac troponin T isoforms is affected by the form of congenital cardiac anomaly and the presence of heart failure.[133] These correlations suggest that the N-terminal variability among these isoforms alters myofilament function and that modulating cardiac troponin T isoform expression would be useful as a therapeutic intervention in the human heart.

DEVELOPMENTAL CHANGES IN THE MEMBRANE SYSTEMS

The contraction of the immature myocardium is considered to be more dependent on extracellular calcium than that of the adult.[88, 106, 134] Potential contributions from changes in myofilament sensitivity to calcium aside, this dependence follows from changes in the multicomponent system that regulates cytosolic calcium concentration.

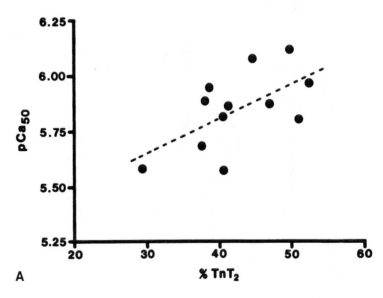

A

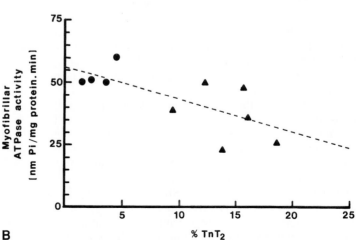

B

FIGURE 3–9

A, The pCa that induces half-maximal force for individual myocardial preparations (pCa$_{50}$) is shown as a function of their content of the cardiac troponin T isoform, TnT$_2$, a product of alternative combinatorial splicing in the primary transcript of two 5′ exons. Regression analysis (*dashed line,* r = 0.61, *P* = .037) demonstrates the correlation between TnT$_2$ content and myofilament sensitivity to calcium (the higher the pCa$_{50}$, the lower is the calcium concentration). (From Nassar N, Malouf NN, Kelly MB, et al: Force-pCa relation and troponin T isoforms of rabbit myocardium. Circ Res 69[6]:1470–1475, 1991.) *B,* Myofibrillar ATPase activities of normal (*circles*) and failing (*triangles*) human hearts are illustrated as a function of the percentage of troponin T composed of the smallest isoform (after the molecular identification of the human isoforms, this isoform was named cTnT$_4$). P$_i$ = inorganic phosphate. ATPase activity and cTnT$_4$(%) expression are inversely related (*dashed line,* r = 0.7, *P* < .02). (From Anderson PAW, Malouf NN, Oakeley AE, et al: Troponin T isoform expression in humans. A comparison among normal and failing adult heart, fetal heart, and adult and fetal skeletal muscle. Circ Res 69[5]:1226–1233, 1991.)

SARCOPLASMIC RETICULUM

The developmental acquisition of a decreased dependence on extracellular calcium suggests that in the adult myocyte, in comparison to the immature cardiac myocyte, a greater portion of the cytosolic calcium transient is provided by intracellular stores of calcium. The major intracellular site for uptake and storage of calcium is the SR. Its components (the junctional SR, corbular SR, and longitudinal SR), their specialized functions, and their relation with the L-type calcium channel are described earlier (see Fig. 3–1).[1]

All the maturational changes in the SR are consistent with these intracellular stores, providing in the adult a larger contribution to the cytosolic calcium transient.[24, 25, 38, 88, 135–137] For example, absolute and relative SR volumes increase with maturation, and the structural and functional differentiation of the SR components is acquired with maturation. In the immature myocardium, the dense material inside the corbular and junctional SR, a marker for calsequestrin, extends through a broad connection into the longitudinal SR, and the junctional and corbular SR calcium release channels extend onto the longitudinal SR.[38] The fixed SR relation with the myofibrils is also acquired with maturation. In the adult myocyte, the junctional and corbular SR are found at the level of the Z disk, but in the immature myocyte, these specialized components of the SR are scattered along the length of the sarcomere.[38] SR calcium release is also affected by maturation.[138] For example, ryanodine has little effect on the force of development of fetal (including that of the human) and newborn myocardium.

Although the different components of the SR are present in the immature myocyte, the lack of organization and restriction of structural characteristics to specific regions of the SR suggests that although the same basic calcium control processes are present at different stages of development, SR function is enhanced by development. There are increases in the expression of the single cardiac ATPase isoform SERCA2a (Fig. 3–10), SR ability to pump calcium, and SR Ca^{2+}-ATPase activity.[24, 25, 137, 139]

The physiologic consequences of these maturational SR changes appear to be reflected in the duration of the steady-state contraction and the responses to variations in the rate and pattern of pacing and β-adrenergic stimulation.[38, 135] For example, the amplitude and duration of the immature myocyte's contraction are smaller and longer, respectively, than those of the adult, and the rate of relaxation is slower. These effects are consistent with the immature myocyte's having a smaller, longer calcium transient, a potential consequence of the maturational differences in SR amount and effectiveness.

Consistent with the developmental changes in the SR, post-extrasystolic potentiation and restitution of contractility after a contraction change with development.[38, 87] These two physiologic phenomena depend on calcium-induced calcium release from the SR. For example, ryanodine, which disables the SR calcium release channel, and thapsigargin, which inhibits the SR Ca^{2+}-ATPase, blunt post-extrasystolic potentiation and restitution.[37, 39]

Restitution of contractility is acquired with maturation. In the isolated neonatal cardiac myocyte, the amount of

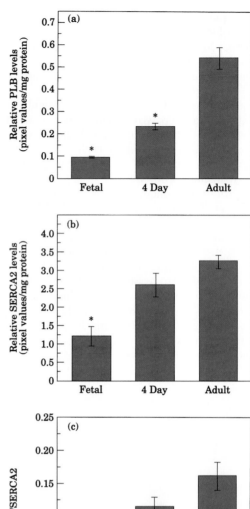

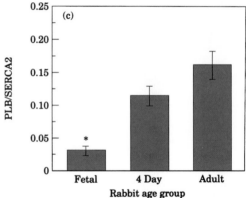

FIGURE 3–10

Western blot analysis of phospholamban (PLB, *a*) and cardiac sarcoplasmic ATPase (SERCA2, *b*) expression in hearts from fetal, 4-day-old, and adult rabbits. The relative ratio of phospholamban/SERCA2 (*c*) was determined for each age group. Expression of phospholamban and SERCA2 increases with age. However, in the fetal heart, SERCA2 is expressed at relatively higher levels than phospholamban is. *Bars* represent the mean ± SEM; asterisks show the significant differences from adult values. (From Szymanska G, Grupp IL, Slack JP, et al: Alterations in sarcoplasmic reticulum calcium uptake, relaxation parameters and their responses to beta-adrenergic agonists in the developing heart. J Mol Cell Cardiol 27:1819, 1995.)

sarcomere shortening in the premature extrasystole is essentially equal to that of the contraction at the basic rate, whereas in the myocyte from the adult heart, the amount of shortening increases exponentially from a small value in the most prematurely introduced extrasystole to achieve that of the contraction at the basic rate.[38]

Post-extrasystolic potentiation increases with maturation, also consistent with enhanced ability of the mature

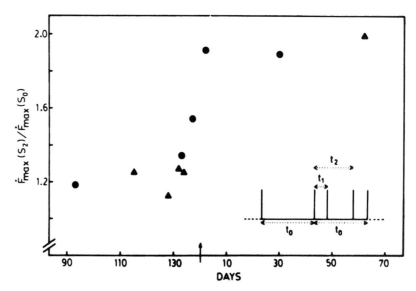

FIGURE 3–11

Post-extrasystolic potentiation increases with development. The ratio of the peak first derivative of force ($\dot{F}_{max}$) of the post-extrasystolic contraction and $\dot{F}_{max}$ of the previous contraction at the regular paced rate of isolated preparations from lamb hearts (*triangles,* trabeculae carneae; *circles,* moderator bands), as a function of age. The timing of the extrasystole was the same in each experiment (275 msec). *Inset,* The pacing pattern used to obtain these data: the basic pacing interval, t_0, 3000 msec; the times between the stimulus for the previous systole at the basic rate and the extrasystole, t_1, 275 msec; and the post-extrasystole, t_2, 2500 msec. (From Anderson PAW, Glick KL, Manning A, Crenshaw C Jr: Developmental changes in cardiac contractility in fetal and postnatal sheep: in vitro and in vivo. Am J Physiol 247:H371, 1984.)

SR to modulate cytosolic calcium concentration[87] (Fig. 3–11). Taken together, these findings are consistent with a maturational increase in the importance of SR calcium stores in supporting and modulating the cytosolic calcium transient and myocardial contractility.

The developmental difference in the effect of β-adrenergic stimulation is consistent with expression of SR ATPase being greater than that of phospholamban in perinatal myocardium (see Fig. 3–10).[135, 137] As reviewed before, β-adrenergic–induced phospholamban phosphorylation enhances SR Ca^{2+}-ATPase. As would be expected from the differences in expression of the ATPase and its inhibitor, β-adrenergic stimulation does not enhance the rate of diastolic relaxation in the fetal heart as greatly as it does in the adult (also recall that β-stimulation will not affect slow skeletal muscle troponin I, which is dominantly expressed in the perinatal heart). The developmental acquisition of cardiac sympathetic innervation[42, 45] is also teleologically consistent with a maturational increase in the importance of β-adrenergic stimulation on myofilament and SR function.

In general, the maturational changes in the SR enhance its effectiveness in removing calcium from the cytosol, storing calcium, and releasing it during subsequent contractions and so supporting the activation-induced calcium transient.

SARCOLEMMA

At all ages, extracellular calcium is required for the myocardial contraction. For example, in its absence, the adult myocyte will not contract. However, the developmental acquisition of an apparent decreased dependence of the force of contraction on extracellular calcium concentration has led to studies of how the sarcolemmal systems that control cell calcium change with maturation. These changes are complex and sometimes difficult to relate to the changes in this dependence.

The transverse (T)-tubule system, a complex membranous system made up of sarcolemmal invaginations that extend deep into the myocyte, is acquired with maturation (see Fig. 3–1).[1] In mammals that are mature at birth (e.g.,

the lamb and the guinea pig), a well-organized T-tubule system is present by the end of gestation, whereas in other species, the system is acquired during neonatal life.[1, 38, 92] Evidence of this system has been found in the fetal human heart.[90] The maturational acquisition of the T-tubule system appears to maintain a constant cell surface/volume ratio as cell size increases with development.[1] Thus, the acquisition of this system prevents intracellular ionic gradients, the consequence expected if a decrease in the surface/volume ratio occurred with maturation. Some mammalian species, however, do not acquire the T-tubule system with maturation (e.g., those species with small adult myocytes), yet these species demonstrate post-extrasystolic potentiation and restitution of contractility. Thus, the acquisition of the T-tubule system does not appear to play a role in modulating the calcium transient and the sensitivity of the myocyte to extracellular calcium.

CALCIUM CHANNELS. Changes in the dependency on extracellular calcium concentration might follow from changes in the trans-sarcolemmal calcium current. Two trans-sarcolemmal calcium currents are present in developing myocardium.[19] The L-type current is supported by the well-characterized DHP-sensitive calcium channel whose structure is known; the T-type current is supported by a DHP-insensitive channel whose structure remains to be solved. The relative contributions of these currents to calcium movement change with development. For example, in the chick heart, the T-type current density (density is used to correct for maturational increases in cell-surface area) is greatest during early embryonic life and exceeds the L-type current.[140] The developmental changes in the DHP-sensitive current differ in direction among species.[141] For example, L-type current density decreases during late avian embryonic development but increases during rat and mouse fetal development. During postnatal life, L-type current falls in the rat and, in contrast, increases in the rabbit.[47] What occurs in the human during development remains to be established.

These directionally opposite developmental time courses of L-type calcium channel current density among species appear even more complicated when the effects of organic calcium channel blockers are assessed.[19,142] For example, in both mature and immature myocardium, verapamil has a negative effect on the positive inotropic response to an increase in heart rate, whereas nitrendipine has a negative effect on this response to an increase in rate in the adult heart and a positive effect on the response in the immature heart.

These different effects may follow from developmentally regulated expression of isoforms of the subunits that make up the multimeric L-type calcium channel. Isoforms of two of the subunits, the α_1 and β subunits, are products of alternative splicing of the primary transcripts.[19,143] The functional consequences that follow from differences in isoform expression may underlie the various effects of calcium channel antagonists on different tissues and the various age-dependent effects of the organic calcium channel blockers.

Calcium channel function is affected by developmental changes in the expression of the trimeric guanosine triphosphate–binding (G) proteins.[42] These proteins transduce agonist stimulation of G-coupled receptors to post-translational calcium channel modifications, modifying the L-type calcium channel function. G protein isoform expression provides another richly complex system that alters calcium channel current density in response to α- and β-adrenergic and muscarinic receptor stimulation.[47] The developmental changes in the components of these effector systems are exemplified by β-stimulation, in the presence of muscarinic blockade, markedly increasing calcium current density in the immature cardiac myocyte but little affecting that of the adult myocyte. Another example is the developmental acquisition of an inhibitory G protein that results in α-agonist stimulation's slowing heart rate in the adult heart, in contrast to the same stimulation's increasing heart rate in the immature heart.[42,144] A similar developmental change from a positive to a negative response is seen in the inotropic response to α-adrenergic receptor stimulation of the mouse heart.[46] Against this background of physiologic changes must be considered the presence of three subtypes of each of the α-adrenergic receptor families (α_{1b}, α_{1c}, and α_{1d}; α_{2a}, α_{2b}, and α_{2c}) in addition to three β-adrenergic receptors. Although all α_1-adrenergic receptor subtypes activate phospholipase C, α_2-adrenergic receptors inhibit adenylate cyclase, and β-adrenergic receptor subtypes activate adenylate cyclase. Stimulation of the β_3-adrenergic receptor, which is not down-regulated by chronic stimulation in comparison to the two other β receptors, has a negative inotropic effect. These findings demonstrate that agonist stimulation at one stage of development may yield different effects at another time in development.

Na$^+$,K$^+$-ATPase. Na$^+$,K$^+$-ATPase, another sarcolemmal protein, helps maintain the relatively high intracellular potassium concentration and the resting potential of the myocyte through its 3:2 exchange rate.[145–148] The ATPase is made up of an α and a β subunit that are encoded by multiple genes, whose products produce multiple $\alpha\beta$ heterodimers.[145,146] Isoforms of the α subunit, the catalytic subunit, confer onto the pump differential affinities and oxidant sensitivities.[145,149] Small changes in α subunit primary structure have a large effect on the sensitivity of the pump to cardiac glycosides. For example, the α_2 and α_3 isoforms have a much lower affinity for sodium than does the α_1 subunit, whereas the α_2 and α_3 isoforms are much more sensitive to cardiac glycosides. The developmental expression of three α isoforms has been studied extensively in the rat heart with only α_1 and α_2 being expressed in the adult rat,[145,146] whereas all three isoforms are detected in the adult human. Relating the expression of these isoforms to human heart function is complicated by the levels of transcript and protein not being directly coupled to heterodimer assembly.

The Na$^+$,K$^+$-ATPase is the target of cardiac glycosides and so plays an important role in the pharmacologic treatment of heart failure.[148] The enhancement in cardiac contractility that follows from pump inhibition may be a consequence of increased cytosolic sodium concentration leading, through Na$^+$-Ca^{2+} exchange, to an increase in cell calcium content and greater myofilament force development.[147,148] Digoxin may also contribute to enhancement of cardiac contractility through sodium-independent mechanisms, such as activation of the SR calcium release channel, and may modulate heart failure signs and symptoms through reducing the neuroendocrine response to heart failure.[149]

The role of α subunit isoform expression in the sensitivity of human myocardium to cardiac glycosides at different stages of development remains to be established. The effects of development on subunit expression aside, at all ages human myocardium responds to digoxin with an increase in contractility. At all ages, digoxin toxicity through Na$^+$,K$^+$-ATPase inhibition increases serum potassium concentration while increasing cytosolic sodium concentration. Consequently, regardless of age, infusing calcium into a toxic patient has a deleterious and potentially fatal effect.

Na$^+$-Ca^{2+} EXCHANGER. The Na$^+$-Ca^{2+} exchanger controls calcium through trans-sarcolemmal exchange of Ca^{2+} for Na$^+$.[30–32] Its function is modulated by protein kinase C phosphorylation.[51] During diastole, the exchanger removes calcium from the cell. During systole, when membrane depolarization exceeds the reversal potential of the exchanger, sodium is extruded and calcium enters the cell, increasing the cytosolic calcium transient. The Na$^+$-Ca^{2+} exchanger, through reverse mode function during systole, provides a mechanism, in addition to the L-type calcium channel and the SR, for supporting myocardial contraction.

A greater trans-sarcolemmal contribution to the cytosolic calcium through reverse mode exchanger function in the neonate could explain a greater dependence of the immature heart on extracellular calcium. Indeed, in those species in which L-type calcium channel current density is lower in the neonate than in the adult (e.g., the rabbit), exchanger transcript, product, and current density are at their highest levels during perinatal life and fall subsequently to their nadir in the adult.[150] In contrast, in those species whose young flee the nest at birth (e.g., the guinea pig), these Na$^+$-Ca^{2+} exchanger measures do not differ between the neonate and the adult.[150] In the neonatal human, an important role is suggested by the marked sensitivity of cardiac contractility to a fall in extracellular calcium concentration after open heart surgery (recall the marked negative effect of L-type calcium channel blockade on ventricular function in the distressed lamb and the sick human neonate).

MATURATION AND PASSIVE MECHANICAL PROPERTIES

At all ages, the myocardium manifests a passive tension-length relation (Fig. 3–12). In contrast to the developmental increase in the strength of the myocardial contraction, the myocardium becomes less stiff (i.e., more compliant) with maturation.[8] The maturational increase in compliance, defined by the curvilinear passive tension-length or passive pressure-volume relation (see Fig. 3–12),[151] may follow from the developmental acquisition of the extracellular matrix, changes in expression of these matrix proteins and their isoforms, and changes in the amount and isoforms of the cytoskeletal proteins and their organization. The acquisition of greater myocardial compliance has significant consequences in terms of ventricular filling and interaction, which are also affected by neonatal and disease-associated changes in ventricular size and shape.[62,151,152]

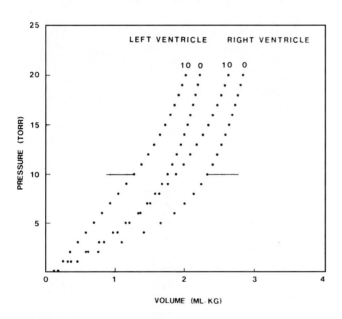

FIGURE 3–12

The effect of contralateral ventricular pressure on the ipsilateral ventricular passive pressure-volume relations of the fetal heart in vitro. Pressure-volume curves were determined with the pericardium in place and the opposite ventricular pressure at 0 or 10 mm Hg. The *horizontal lines* are two standard errors of the mean. Increasing pressure in the right ventricle from 0 to 10 mm Hg shifts the left ventricular pressure-volume relation to the left. This effect is greater in the fetal and neonatal heart than in the adult heart.[151] Changes in left ventricular end-diastolic pressure also affect right ventricular filling. The in vivo consequence of this ventricular interaction is, for example, that the higher the right ventricular diastolic pressure, the less the left ventricle will fill. These relations also demonstrate that the fetal right ventricular volume is larger than the left ventricular volume at comparable filling pressures, consistent with the greater contribution of the right ventricle to fetal cardiac output. (From Pinson CW, Morton MJ, Thornburg KL: An anatomic basis for fetal right ventricular dominance and arterial pressure sensitivity. J Dev Physiol 9:253, 1987.)

The proteins that make up the cytoskeleton and extracellular matrix and the organization of these systems change with maturation. Evidence of this extends from the maturational acquisition of the extracellular matrix to changes in the width of the Z disk,[38,153] the site of titin binding. The presence of multiple titin isoforms in skeletal and cardiac muscle suggests that the maturational increase in myocardial compliance could be a consequence of developmentally regulated expression of titin isoforms.[71,75]

The desmin-containing intermediate filaments also undergo a marked reorganization during perinatal development.[38,78] In the immature myocyte, a matrix of these filaments connects the myofibrils, found in a subsarcolemmal shell, to each other and the sarcolemma. A mass of mitochondria and nuclei, however, located in the center of the cell, prevents this matrix from extending from one side of the cell to the other. This organization appears to decrease the compliance and ability of the immature myocyte to contract. In contrast, in the adult myocyte, the intermediate filament system, which is connected to the integrin receptor, divides the cell into a much more efficient organization made up of repeating layers of myofibrils, membrane systems, and mitochondria (see Fig. 3–1).

The integrin receptor subunits also undergo developmental changes in expression that have functional importance given the differences among the β isoform cytoplasmic domains and α isoform binding specificity to extracellular matrix ligands.[154–156]

The organization of the extracellular matrix is acquired with maturation.[60,86,157] In some species, the first few weeks of neonatal life appear to be most important in matrix acquisition and progression to its adult structure (see Fig. 3–6).[86,157] Isoform expression of the proteins that make up the extracellular matrix (e.g., fibronectin, laminin, and collagen) is also affected by maturation.[157,158] During early cardiac development, for example, laminin is not expressed; later in embryonic and fetal development, laminin is localized to patches of the sarcolemma; and in the adult, laminin is identified along the entire length of the basement membrane (see Fig. 3–6).

Collagen is acquired with maturation.[86,93] With the postnatal increase in fibroblasts, collagen content increases rapidly. With further development in the human, the collagen/total cardiac protein ratio decreases toward that of the adult.[159] During human fetal and neonatal development, a relative change in collagen isoform expression occurs. The ratio of type I to type III collagen decreases, with type I collagen being stiffer and less flexible than type III.[159] These changes are likely to contribute to the developmental increase in myocardial compliance.[8]

VENTRICULAR FUNCTION AND DEVELOPMENT

Across development, the same variables modulate ventricular pressure development, stroke volume, and cardiac output.[9,10,61,62,87,160] They include end-diastolic volume (preload), heart rate, arterial pressure (afterload), and inotropic perturbations. At all stages of development, increasing muscle length, rate of stimulation, and other alterations in the inotropic state have a positive effect on the force of contraction, whereas increasing afterload has a negative effect on the velocity and amount of myocardial shortening. Thus, in vivo modulation of ventricular function through these dependencies is expected to be present throughout development.

A positive inotropic intervention, however, may have no effect in vitro or a negative one in vivo. For example, pacing the in vivo heart at a faster rate decreases stroke volume, whereas the force of contraction of the isolated myocardium increases with an increase in rate (the response of the fetal heart is also seen in the adult heart in vivo).[9, 160] These opposite effects follow from the difficulty in controlling in vivo the interaction of venous return, end-diastolic volume, inotropic state, heart rate, and afterload. In isolated myocardium, in contrast, experimental factors such as muscle length and afterload are straightforwardly controlled, thus preventing them from obscuring the functional effects of other perturbations. Attempts to control these factors in vivo are difficult, often requiring extensive instrumentation and the use of acutely instrumented animals, which may further complicate the findings through their negative effects on fetal well-being.

Differences in the in utero and postnatal circulations and the relative right and left ventricular outputs may further complicate the effects of failing to control one variable while altering another.[161] For example, increases in afterload have a much greater effect on fetal right ventricular function, apparently a consequence of the fetal right ventricle having relatively larger end-diastolic and stroke volumes (Figs. 3–13 and 3–14; see also Fig. 3–12). Apparent conflicts among experimental results can also be explained by methodologic differences and limitations. The following sections focus on results of studies that avoided the acute effects of surgery and instrumentation on ventricular function while monitoring measures of stroke volume, preload, and afterload.

HEART RATE

Heart rate has the same effect on ventricular output in the immature and adult heart.[160] The findings of studies that suggest a developmental acquisition of the modulation of cardiac output by heart rate result from experimental differences, such as whether the changes in heart rate are spontaneous, the result of pacing, or due to pharmacologic interventions.[160]

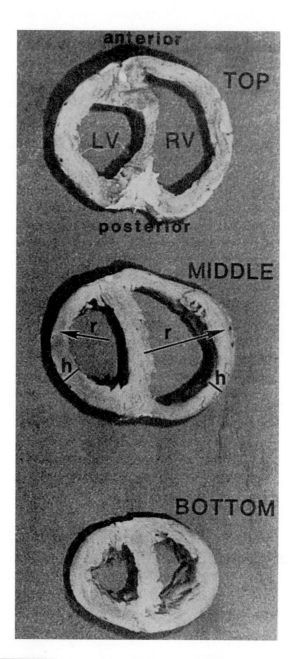

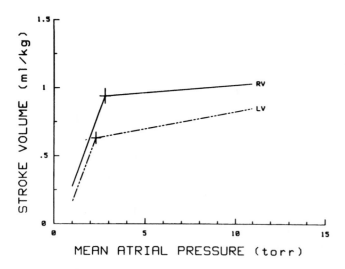

FIGURE 3–13

The average simultaneous ventricular function curves for a group of fetal lambs were determined for the right and left ventricles. These data demonstrate that the Frank-Starling relation is present in the fetal heart. The right ventricular (RV) function curve has a steep ascending limb similar to that of the left ventricular (LV) function curve. The plateaus differ significantly. (From Reller MD, Morton MJ, Reid DL, Thornburg KL: Fetal lamb ventricles respond differently to filling and arterial pressures and to in utero ventilation. Pediatr Res 22:621, 1987.)

FIGURE 3–14

Cross-sectional slices of fixed fetal lamb ventricles one fourth *(top)*, one half *(middle)*, and three fourths *(bottom)* of the distance from the atrioventricular valves to the ventricular apex are shown. Note the relatively larger right ventricular cavity and radius of curvature. LV = left ventricle; RV = right ventricle; r = radius; h = wall thickness. (From Pinson CW, Morton MJ, Thornburg KL: An anatomic basis for fetal right ventricular dominance and arterial pressure sensitivity. J Dev Physiol 9:253, 1987.)

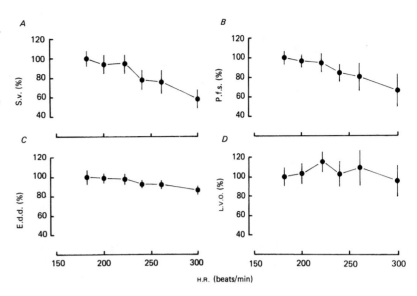

FIGURE 3–15

Effects of right atrial pacing on left ventricular end-diastolic volume and ejection in chronically instrumented in utero fetal lambs. Values are expressed as a percentage of the value obtained at the slowest rate, which is considered 100%. The paced rates range from 182 to 300 beats per minute. *A,* The percentage change in stroke volume (S.v.). *B,* The percentage change in percent fractional shortening [P.f.s. (systolic change in left ventricular diameter ÷ end-diastolic diameter) × 100%]. *C,* The percentage change in end-diastolic dimension (anterior ventricular free wall endocardium to posterior free wall endocardium, E.d.d.). *D,* The percentage change in left ventricular output (L.V.O.). The vertical bars represent two standard deviations of the mean. Left ventricular output is not affected by heart rate, whereas stroke volume, end-diastolic dimension, and percent fractional shortening fall significantly with an increase in rate. (From Anderson PAW, Glick KL, Killam AP, Mainwaring RD: The effect of heart rate on in utero left ventricular output in the fetal sheep. J Physiol [Lond] 372:557, 1986.)

THE EFFECTS OF ATRIAL PACING. An atrial pacing–induced increase in heart rate decreases several measures of ventricular function.[160] For example, stroke volume falls with an increase in heart rate, a consequence of decreasing end-diastolic filling time and end-diastolic volume (Figs. 3–15 and 3–16). Over a broad range of rates, the net effect on ventricular output is either no change or a fall in output. Consequently, ventricular output appears to be either independent of or negatively affected by a rate increase, in contrast to the inotropic effect of rate seen in isolated myocardium. This apparent independence of output on heart rate is common to the intact fetus and the adult.[160]

This in vivo confounding effect of an atrial pacing–associated decrease in ventricular diastolic filling time and end-diastolic volume can be circumvented; when longer paced intervals are introduced infrequently into the paced rate, ventricular systoles from the same end-diastolic volume can be compared against the background of different rates. By use of this approach to control end-diastolic volume, the positive inotropic effect of heart rate on stroke volume and output is clearly demonstrated[160] (Fig. 3–17).

These results, which reflect the modulation of stroke volume through the Frank-Starling relation and inotropy, also demonstrate how greatly fetal ventricular output can be increased.

The positive inotropic effect of an increase in fetal heart rate is reflected in the increase in maximal rate of rise of left ventricular pressure, dP/dt_{max}, over a broad range of rates despite a rate-induced fall in end-diastolic volume. This positive effect of rate on ventricular pressure development is found in the fetal, neonatal, and adult heart.[9, 162]

THE SITE OF ATRIAL PACING. The site of atrial pacing can alter the effect of an increase in heart rate.[160] For example, in the fetus when the left atrium is paced, left ventricular output falls with an increase in rate, whereas right ventricular output is unaffected over a broad range of rates (see Figs. 3–15 and 3–16).[160] The converse effect is seen with right atrial pacing. These site-dependent effects may follow from alterations in ventricular diastolic filling time, shunting through the foramen ovale, and the timing of atrial systole relative to ventricular systole.

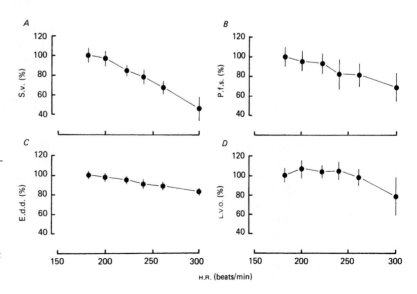

FIGURE 3–16

Effects of left atrial pacing on left ventricular end-diastolic volume and ejection in the same fetal lambs whose right atrial pacing data are presented in Figure 3–15. The paced rates range from 182 to 300 beats per minute. Left ventricular end-diastolic volume, stroke volume, and output fall significantly with an increase in heart rate. (From Anderson PAW, Glick KL, Killam AP, Mainwaring RD: The effect of heart rate on in utero left ventricular output in the fetal sheep. J Physiol [Lond] 372:557, 1986.)

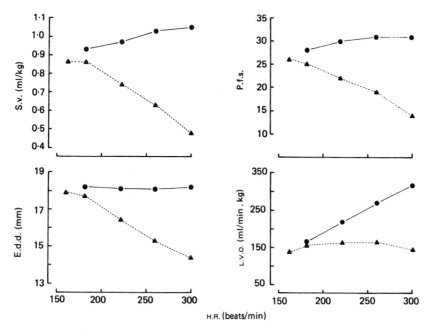

FIGURE 3–17

Left ventricular end-diastolic volume and ejection during right atrial pacing for systoles during pacing rates from 150 to 300 beats per minute *(triangles)* and the systoles that follow an interpolated longer pacing interval of 400 msec *(circles)*. Left ventricular end-diastolic dimensions (E.d.d.) after the longer paced intervals were within 0.1 mm, whereas the dimensions during continuous pacing at a constant rate became progressively smaller with each increase in rate. For the systoles with comparable end-diastolic dimensions *(circles)*, stroke volume (S.v., corrected for body weight), percent fractional shortening (P.f.s.), and left ventricular output (L.V.O., corrected for body weight) are larger, the faster the paced rate. The data were obtained from an in utero fetal lamb 10 days after surgery. (From Anderson PAW, Glick KL, Killam AP, Mainwaring RD: The effect of heart rate on in utero left ventricular output in the fetal sheep. J Physiol [Lond] 372:557, 1986.)

THE EFFECTS OF A SPONTANEOUS HEART RATE CHANGE. In both the fetus and the adult, a spontaneous increase in heart rate is usually associated with an increase in ventricular output.[160] The effects of a spontaneous heart rate change differ from those of a pacing-induced change because the underlying stimuli that induce the spontaneous rate change also affect inotropy, venous return, and afterload. For example, an increase in venous return that maintains end-diastolic volume despite a rate-induced shortening of diastolic filling can result in an increased stroke volume. Even if venous return is unchanged or falls and end-diastolic volume decreases, the stimulus that induces an increase in heart rate often increases contractility and, so, stroke volume. Exceptions to the positive effects of a spontaneous increase in heart rate on fetal right and left ventricular output can be explained by an increase in arterial pressure. The negative effect of afterload on ventricular ejection produces a fall in stroke volume and cardiac output (see later).[62]

PRELOAD

In the in vivo fetal and adult heart, ventricular output depends on end-diastolic volume (see Figs. 3–13 and 3–17).[9,10,62] However, differences of opinion exist about the relative importance of the Frank-Starling relation at different stages of development.[10,62,87,160,163] Differences in the effects of end-diastolic volume on ventricular ejection depend on the experimental intervention. For example, fetal volume infusions that achieve nonphysiologically high atrial pressures suggest little functional reserve in the fetal heart, whereas decreasing atrial pressure over a physiologic range (through blood withdrawal) decreases ventricular output.[10,62] These differences may follow from several factors, such as maturational differences in ventricular size, compliance, and interaction.[8,152,164] Volume infusions in the fetus also produce a relatively greater increase in afterload than in the adult. The consequent

negative effect of this increase in afterload on ventricular function may lead to the conclusion that the importance of the Frank-Starling relation in modulating cardiac output is acquired with maturation.

Another potentially confounding factor in the assessment of the Frank-Starling relation is the physiologic measure selected to estimate changes in end-diastolic volume. Studies whose results support maturational acquisition of a Frank-Starling reserve have often used indirect measures of ventricular volume (e.g., mean left atrial pressure). Recalling the passive pressure-volume relation of the intact ventricle (see Fig. 3–12), an increase in filling pressure from a high mean atrial pressure results in a small increase in ventricular volume. This relation has been demonstrated in the intact adult animal; when left ventricular end-diastolic pressure is high, only small increments in end-diastolic volume and stroke volume follow from a further increase in filling pressure. Consequently, given the greater stiffness of the immature myocardium, trivial increases in fetal end-diastolic volume are likely to follow increases in atrial pressure from what is already an elevated level.[8] In that the mean fetal atrial pressure is relatively low compared with that of the adult, a small increment in fetal stroke volume in response to what in the adult is a modest increase in atrial pressure from a low level might suggest to some the absence of a Frank-Starling relation in the fetus.

To better assess the effect of fetal ventricular end-diastolic volume on stroke volume, direct measures of ventricular end-diastolic volume (e.g., ultrasonic dimension transducers) are needed.[160] With use of such a measure, systolic minor axis shortening in the fetus increases with an increase in left ventricular end-diastolic dimension, and right and left ventricular stroke volume (Fig. 3–18) increases with an increase in end-diastolic volume.[160,165] These results are supported by the effects of an atrial pacing–induced change in heart rate on stroke volume that follow from the interaction of diastolic filling time and end-diastolic volume (see Figs. 3–15 to 3–17).

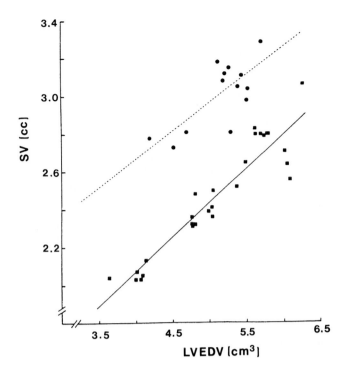

Relationship between fetal left ventricular stroke volume (SV) and end-diastolic volume (LVEDV) in a chronically instrumented fetal lamb. By altering heart rate through atrial pacing, a range of left ventricular end-diastolic volumes is obtained during a control state *(squares)* and during an infusion of isoproterenol *(circles)*. These data demonstrate that stroke volume depends on end-diastolic volume and inotropic state, exemplified by stroke volume being larger in the presence of isoproterenol for a given end-diastolic volume. Left ventricular end-diastolic volume is computed by measuring sonomicrometrically three left ventricular dimensions (two minor axes and one major axis). The computation was validated with in vitro calibration of the same heart.

AFTERLOAD

The function of the fetal and of the adult heart is negatively affected by an increase in afterload.[10, 62, 164] For example, in response to an increase in afterload, all measures of ventricular ejection are decreased, consistent with the in vitro finding that an increase in afterload decreases the velocity and amount of myocardial shortening at all stages of development.[8]

A quantitative maturational difference in the effects of afterload does exist. The fetal ventricle cannot eject against arterial pressures well tolerated by the adult heart, as would be expected from the weaker contraction of the immature myocardium (corrected for muscle cross-sectional area) and the thinner ventricular wall of the immature heart.[62]

Afterload, also, has a quantitatively different effect on right and left ventricular function. In the fetus and the adult, increases in arterial pressure have a much greater negative effect on stroke volume of the right ventricle than that of the left. In the fetus, this difference is a consequence of the relatively larger right ventricular stroke volume, end-diastolic volume, and free wall curvature in the presence of similar right and left ventricular free wall thicknesses (see Figs. 3–12 to 3–14).[160, 161, 164] Because of the Laplace relation, systolic wall stress of the right ventricle is greater than that of the left ventricle in the face of similar arterial pressures, which causes the right ventricular ejection to be more negatively affected by an increase in arterial pressure.

INOTROPY

For conceptual simplicity, inotropy is considered separately from preload, heart rate, and afterload. An intervention that does not alter preload or afterload yet increases the force of contraction or stroke volume is said to have a positive inotropic effect. This positive effect could arise from an increase in the sensitivity of the myofilaments to calcium or the cytosolic calcium transient. Given that myofilament sensitivity to calcium is increased by increasing sarcomere length, an increase in preload (i.e., an increase in sarcomere length) is an inotropic intervention comparable to increasing the cytosolic calcium transient.

Evidence for inotropic stimulation's enhancing fetal ventricular function depends on the experimental protocol and the measures used to characterize the effects of the intervention. For example, norepinephrine markedly enhances the force of contraction of isolated fetal myocardium, yet a norepinephrine infusion does not increase in utero fetal cardiac output.[8] The difference in the in vivo and in vitro responses is likely to arise from the dynamic properties of the intact cardiovascular system. For example, in the in vivo fetal study, the effects of afterload and heart rate, both of which are likely to be affected by norepinephrine, were not controlled.

In contrast, when a β-agonist, isoproterenol, which does not increase arterial pressure, is infused into the fetal lamb, stroke volume and cardiac output increase (see Fig. 3–18).[166] Just as in the adult animal, a β-agonist–induced increase in cardiac output is further enhanced by volume loading; in other words, in the fetus, an increase in preload amplifies an isoproterenol-induced increase in output.[61] This positive effect on output occurs when heart rate is controlled and is further amplified by an increase in heart rate.

Thus, the in vivo fetal heart responds to positive inotropic agents with an increase in left ventricular output. Considering the changes in the systems that support the force of contraction and ventricular pressure development and ejection, inotropic stimuli are likely to differ in their relative effects with development. The physiologic phenomenon of post-extrasystolic potentiation, for example, demonstrates such a maturational quantitative difference.

The value of using post-extrasystolic potentiation in measuring changes in inotropic state has been tested by examining the effects of preload and inotropy on potentiation in vitro and in vivo in the fetus, newborn, and adult. The amount of post-extrasystolic potentiation (dP/dt_{max} of the post-extrasystole divided by dP/dt_{max} of the preceding systole, controlling for heart rate and extrasystolic interval) is unaffected by a change in muscle length or ventricular volume (the end-diastolic volumes of the systole at the drive rate and the post-extrasystole being equal).[9] In contrast, a change in inotropy (e.g., an isoproterenol infusion) has a disproportionately greater effect on dP/dt_{max} of the systole at the basic heart rate, decreasing post-extrasystolic potentiation, as it does in vitro.[9] Other positive inotropic agents have been shown to increase postextrasystolic potentiation in vitro. The demonstration that post-extrasystolic potentiation is unaffected by ventricular volume while being affected by inotropic state led to its being used to evaluate the effects of maturation on contractility.

The use of post-extrasystolic potentiation to search for developmental changes in intrinsic myocardial and ventricular function was further stimulated by the limitations of other measures of ventricular function. For example, when left ventricular dP/dt_{max} is measured in the hearts of the fetus, child, and adult, no developmental change in inotropy is found[9,87,162] (dP/dt_{max} ranges between 1500 and 3000 mm Hg/sec in each group). In contrast to this developmental stability of dP/dt_{max}, left ventricular systolic pressure and stroke volume increase with development, whereas with the transition from fetal to postnatal life, right ventricular systolic pressure falls.

Post-extrasystolic potentiation is present in the fetal and adult heart in vivo and in vitro.[9,87,162] During in utero development, potentiation increases in vivo and in vitro[87] (see Fig. 3–11). This increase is likely to follow, at least in part, from the maturational acquisition of the SR. These findings support the conclusion that a developmental increase occurs in the range over which cytosolic calcium concentration is modulated.

VENTRICULAR COMPLIANCE AND VENTRICULAR INTERACTION

Ventricular compliance and interaction are affected by the maturational decrease in myocardial compliance and the increase in ventricular volume.[8] Figure 3–12 exemplifies the effects of ventricular end-diastolic volume on filling of the contralateral ventricle. These data obtained from the fetal lamb demonstrate that increasing right or left ventricular end-diastolic pressure decreases the filling of the contralateral ventricle.

Ventricular compliance increases with development. For example, the right ventricle of the adult is significantly more compliant than that of the fetus and the newborn, whereas at all ages, the right ventricle is more compliant than the left. In considering ventricular interaction, the influence of filling one ventricle on the distensibility of the other is most profound in the fetus, less in the newborn, and least in the adult. The maturational differences in compliance in ventricular interaction are likely to have profound effects in diseases of the neonate in which right ventricular systolic and diastolic loading are increased.

THE EFFECT OF BIRTH

Birth has large complex effects on the cardiovascular system. For example, left ventricular output is markedly enhanced with birth, whereas output of the right ventricle is little affected.[9,87,161] The neonatal increase in left ventricular output results from the combined effects of increases in heart rate, venous return, end-diastolic volume, and inotropy and its interaction with the right ventricle.[9,87]

Left ventricular end-diastolic volume and left atrial pressure increase with birth in response to the changes in the pulmonary and systemic circulation. Before ventilation with oxygen, the high pulmonary vascular resistance markedly limits pulmonary blood flow, and the majority of right ventricular output flows from the pulmonary artery through the ductus arteriosus into the aorta. With birth, pulmonary vascular resistance falls, and the direction of ductal flow is reversed. In utero ventilation with oxygen has effects that are analogous in some respects to birth.[161] After the initiation of in utero oxygen ventilation, pulmonary vascular resistance falls, pulmonary blood flow increases, and blood flow through the ductus arteriosus reverses with net flow going from the aorta to the pulmonary artery. These effects mimic the decrease in pulmonary vascular resistance and the increase in pulmonary venous return, left atrial pressure, and left ventricular filling that accompany birth. Altogether these changes result in a neonatal increase in left ventricular end-diastolic volume.

Neonatal ventricular filling may also be enhanced by the removal of in utero extracardiac restraints.[167] This possibility is supported by the effect of increasing left atrial pressure on ventricular stroke volume and output in the open chest neonatal lamb compared with the intact fetal lamb in utero.[62,168] In the neonate, increasing filling pressure enhances ventricular output to a much greater level, perhaps a consequence of the removal of the restraints imposed by the nonaerated lungs and the in utero environment. This possibility is supported by the finding that increasing blood volume during in utero liquid ventilation has little effect on left ventricular stroke volume in comparison to the positive effect on stroke volume of increasing blood volume during in utero oxygen ventilation.[161]

The neonatal increase in left ventricular end-diastolic volume and end-diastolic pressure and the accompanying increase in left ventricular stroke volume suggests that the reserves of the Frank-Starling relation may, in large part, be consumed by the effects of birth.[9,87] If so, the depletion must be transient. During the first neonatal day, left ventricular end-diastolic pressure falls and end-diastolic volume increases in the lamb, and left ventricular stroke volume and output of the preterm infant increase markedly in response to the volume loading of a patent ductus arteriosus.[87,169,170]

A postnatal acquisition of the Frank-Starling relation (or reacquisition in the context of birth-associated depletion in its reserves) has been suggested by volume infusion's having a greater effect on cardiac output in the older lamb, as defined by percentage change in output, than in the newborn lamb.[170] Of note, this approach amplifies the effect of volume loading in the older lamb because of the normal fall in left ventricular output per body weight during postnatal life. When the effects of volume loading are measured as a change in volume, rather than as a percentage, the 1-week-old increases its cardiac output by a greater amount than does the older lamb. Regardless of the measures used, the important conclusion is that the immature animal responds to an increase in circulating blood volume with an increase in left ventricular output.

The neonatal increase in left ventricular end-diastolic volume has an important effect on how a neonatal increase in heart rate affects left ventricular stroke volume. In the fetus, an increase in heart rate often results in a fall in end-diastolic and stroke volume because ventricular diastolic filling time is shortened, and left atrial pressure is not increased (see Figs. 3–15 and 3–16). In contrast, when this heart rate–induced fall in end-diastolic volume is prevented in utero, fetal stroke volume and ventricular output increase (see Fig. 3–17). The neonatal increase in pulmonary venous return and left atrial pressure enhance left ventricular filling and prevent or blunt the effect of a rate-induced decrease in diastolic filling time. Consequently, the neonatal increase in heart rate will enhance left ventricular output.

Inotropy also increases with birth. Left ventricular dP/dt_{max} increases with birth even when heart rate and left ventricular end-diastolic volume are controlled.[9, 87] The neonatal increase in contractility is also reflected in a neonatal fall in in vivo post-extrasystolic potentiation.[9, 87] These spontaneous changes in dP/dt_{max} and potentiation are evocative of an in utero infusion of isoproterenol.[9] Consistent with this analogy, circulating catecholamine levels increase with birth. All of these changes are consistent with the increase in inotropy after birth being a consequence of enhanced sympathetic stimulation. Thus, a neonatal increase in inotropy occurs, contributing to the neonatal increase in left ventricular output.

The importance of the in vivo environment on neonatal ventricular function is evident when the in vivo and in vitro responses to birth are examined by use of post-extrasystolic potentiation.[9, 87] In isolated myocardium, post-extrasystolic potentiation increases throughout the perinatal period. In contrast, in vivo post-extrasystolic potentiation increases in utero, until the hours immediately before parturition when post-extrasystolic potentiation begins, a fall that continues through the first days of neonatal life. The in vivo fall demonstrates the effect of endogenous inotropic stimulation (e.g., β-agonist stimulation), found in the intact neonate, that is absent in neonatal myocardium in vitro.

Enhanced inotropy through sympathetic stimulation appears to be more important in supporting the neonatal circulation than that of the adult. For example, the preterm infant's increase in left ventricular stroke volume in response to a patent ductus arteriosus is blunted by β-adrenergic receptor blockade, and the cardiac output of the stressed newborn is exquisitely sensitive to β-blockade.[163] When hypoxemia has been used to increase circulating catecholamine levels, isoproterenol and dobutamine further increase cardiac output.[171] These observations are consistent with a neonatal inotropic reserve that enables the neonate to respond to further neonatal stresses.

The contributions of other agonists and systems to the neonatal increase in cardiac contractility are suggested by the surge in endocrine activity that occurs with birth and the direct and indirect effects of other receptors on contractility. Enhanced neonatal thyroid function has been considered a potential contributor to the increase in cardiac output. Thyroidectomy at birth, however, does not prevent the neonatal increase in cardiac output.[172]

VENTRICULAR INTERACTION

Ventricular interaction must also contribute to the neonatal increase in cardiac output. Left ventricular filling and ejection are enhanced, for example, by a decrease in right ventricular afterload and end-diastolic volume (see Fig. 3–12). Consequently, the neonatal fall in right ventricular afterload, a result of the decrease in pulmonary vascular resistance, and the associated decrease in right ventricular end-diastolic volume will enhance left ventricular function (see Fig. 3–12). This enhancement may be blunted by many neonatal diseases. For example, those disease processes that increase right ventricular end-diastolic volume and pulmonary artery pressure will interfere with left ventricular filling and, consequently, decrease left ventricular stroke volume and output. Thus, neonatal diseases that seem to affect only the right ventricle are likely to have a negative effect on left ventricular function.

In summary, with birth, left ventricular output increases in response to increases in venous return and heart rate, increases of inotropic stimuli, removal of extracardiac restraints, and improvement of ventricular interaction. During neonatal life, cardiac output (indexed for body weight) gradually falls, dP/dt_{max} returns to its fetal levels, and post-extrasystolic potentiation and the inotropic response to β-adrenergic receptor stimulation increase.[87, 170] These changes suggest that the heart is acquiring greater functional reserves. These reserves will allow the heart to more effectively respond to stresses (e.g., the hemodynamic loading of cardiac defects) imposed during infancy.

REFERENCES

1. Sommer JR, Johnson EA: Ultrastructure of cardiac muscle. *In* Berne RM (ed): Handbook of Physiology, Vol 1. Bethesda, MD, American Physiological Society, 1979, p 113.
2. Weber A, Murray JM: Molecular control mechanisms in muscle contraction. Physiol Rev 53:612, 1973.
3. Zot AS, Potter JD: Structural aspects of troponin-tropomyosin regulation of skeletal muscle contraction. Annu Rev Biophys Biophys Chem 16:535, 1987.
4. Huxley HE: Molecular basis of contraction in cross-striated muscles. *In* Bourne GH (ed): The Structure and Function of Muscle, Vol 1, 2nd ed. New York, Academic Press, 1972, p 301.
5. Rayment I, Holden HM, Whittaker M, et al: Structure of the actin-myosin complex and its implications for muscle contraction. Science 261:58, 1993.
6. Robinson TF, Winegrad S: The measurement and dynamic implications of thin filament lengths in heart muscle. J Physiol (Lond) 286:607, 1979.
7. Wang Y-P, Fuchs F: Osmotic compression of skinned cardiac and skeletal muscle bundles: Effects on force generation, Ca^{2+} sensitivity and Ca^{2+} binding. J Mol Cell Cardiol 27:1235, 1995.
8. Friedman WF: The intrinsic physiologic properties of the developing heart. Prog Cardiovasc Dis 15:87, 1972.
9. Anderson PAW, Manring A, Glick K, et al: Biophysics of the developing heart. III. A comparison of the left ventricular dynamics of the fetal and neonatal lamb heart. Am J Obstet Gynecol 143:195, 1982.
10. Gilbert RD: Control of fetal cardiac output during changes in blood volume. Am J Physiol 238:H80, 1980.
11. Noland TA Jr, Guo X, Raynor RL, et al: Cardiac troponin I mutants: Phosphorylation by protein kinases C and A and regulation of Ca^{2+}-stimulated MgATPase of reconstituted actomyosin S-1. J Biol Chem 270:25445, 1995.
12. Venema RC, Kuo JF: Protein kinase C–mediated phosphorylation of troponin I and protein-C in isolated myocardial cells is associated with inhibition of myofibrillar actomyosin MgATPase. J Biol Chem 268:2705, 1993.
13. Wolff MR, Buck SH, Stoker SW, et al: Myofibrillar calcium sensitivity of isometric tension is increased in human dilated cardiomyopathies. J Clin Invest 98:167, 1996.
14. Bodor GS, Oakeley AE, Allen PD, et al: Troponin I phosphorylation in normal and failing adult human heart. Circulation 96:1495, 1997.

15. Schwinger RHG, Bohm M, Koch A, et al: The failing human heart is unable to use Frank-Starling mechanism. Circ Res 74:959, 1994.

16. McAuliffe JJ, Gao LZ, Solaro RJ, et al: Changes in myofibrillar activation and troponin C Ca^{2+} binding associated with troponin T isoform switching in developing rabbit heart. Circ Res 66:1204, 1990.

17. Solaro RJ, Lee JA, Kentish JC, et al: Effects of acidosis on ventricular muscle from adult and neonatal rats. Circ Res 63:779, 1988.

18. Hunkeler NM, Kullman J, Murphy AM: Troponin I isoform expression in human heart. Circ Res 69:1409, 1991.

19. Hille B: Calcium Channels. *In* Ionic Channels of Excitable Membranes, 2nd ed. Sunderland, MA, Sinauer Associates, 1991, p 83.

20. Fabiato A: Appraisal of the physiological relevance of two hypotheses for the mechanisms of calcium release from the mammalian cardiac sarcoplasmic reticulum: Calcium-induced release versus charge-coupled release. Mol Cell Biochem 89:135, 1989.

21. Ogawa Y: Role of ryanodine receptors. Crit Rev Biochem Mol Biol 29:229, 1994.

22. Valdivia HH, Kaplan JH, Ellis-Davies GC, et al: Rapid adaptation of cardiac ryanodine receptors: Modulation by Mg^{2+} and phosphorylation. Science 267:1997, 1995.

23. Peng M, Fan H, Kirley TL, et al: Structural diversity of triadin in skeletal muscle and evidence of its existence in heart. FEBS Lett 348:17, 1994.

24. Mahony L: Maturation of calcium transport in cardiac sarcoplasmic reticulum. Pediatr Res 24:639, 1988.

25. Fisher DJ, Tate CA, Phillips S: Development regulation of the sarcoplasmic reticulum calcium pump in the rabbit heart. Pediatr Res 31:474, 1992.

26. Chiesi M, Wrzosek A, Grueninger S: The role of the sarcoplasmic reticulum in various types of cardiomyocytes. Mol Cell Biochem 130:159, 1994.

27. Kadambi VJ, Ponniah S, Harrer JM, et al: Cardiac-specific overexpression of phospholamban alters calcium kinetics and resultant cardiomyocyte mechanics in transgenic mice. J Clin Invest 97:533, 1996.

28. Wolska BM, Stojanovic MO, Luo W, et al: Effect of ablation of phospholamban on dynamics of cardiac myocyte contraction and intracellular Ca^{2+}. Am J Physiol 271:C391, 1996.

29. Jorgensen AO, Shen AC, Campbell KP: Ultrastructural localization of calsequestrin in adult rat atrial and ventricular muscle cells. J Cell Biol 101:257, 1985.

30. Komuro I, Wenninger KE, Philipson KD, et al: Molecular cloning and characterization of the human cardiac Na$^+$/Ca^{2+} exchanger cDNA. Proc Natl Acad Sci U S A 80:4769, 1992.

31. Decollogne S, Bertrand IB, Ascensio M, et al: Na$^+$,K$^+$-ATPase and Na$^+$/Ca^{2+} exchange isoforms: Physiological and physiopathological relevance. J Cardiovasc Pharmacol 22(suppl 2):S96, 1993.

32. Levesque PC, Leblanc M, Hume JR, et al: Role of reverse-mode Na$^+$-Ca^{2+} exchange in excitation-contraction coupling in the heart. Ann N Y Acad Sci 639:386, 1991.

33. Leblanc PC, Hume JR: Sodium current-induced release of calcium from cardiac sarcoplasmic reticulum. Science 248:850, 1990.

34. Sacchetto R, Margreth A, Pelosi M, et al: Colocalization of the dihydropyridine receptor, the plasma-membrane calcium ATPase isoform 1 and the sodium/calcium exchanger to the junctional-membrane domain of transverse tubules of rabbit skeletal muscle. Eur J Biochem 237:483, 1996.

35. Sham JSK, Cleemann L, Morad M: Gating of the cardiac Ca^{2+} release channel: The role of Na$^+$ current and Na$^+$-Ca^{2+} exchange. Science 255:850, 1992.

36. Johnson EA: Force-interval relationship of cardiac muscle. *In* Berne RM (ed): Handbook of Physiology, Vol 1. Bethesda, MD, American Physiological Society, 1979, p 475.

37. Weir WG, Yue DT: Intracellular calcium transients underlying the short-term force-interval relationship in ferret ventricular myocardium. J Physiol (Lond) 376:507, 1986.

38. Nassar R, Reedy MC, Anderson PAW: Developmental changes in the ultrastructure and sarcomere shortening of the isolated rabbit ventricular myocyte. Circ Res 61:465, 1987.

39. Lewartowski B, Wolska BM: The effect of thapsigargin on sarcoplasmic reticulum Ca^{2+} content and contractions in single myocytes of guinea-pig heart. J Mol Cell Cardiol 25:23, 1993.

40. Lefkowitz RJ: Enhanced myocardial function in transgenic mice overexpressing the β$_2$-adrenergic receptor. Science 264:582, 1994.

41. Gauthier C, Tavernier G, Charpentier F, et al: Functional β$_3$ adrenoceptor in the human heart. J Clin Invest 98:556, 1996.

42. Robinson RB: Autonomic receptor-effector coupling during postnatal development (Review). Cardiovasc Res 31:E68, 1996.

43. Liu QY, Karpinski E, Pang PK: The L-type calcium channel current is increased by alpha-1 adrenoceptor activation in neonatal rat ventricular cells. J Pharmacol Exp Ther 271:935, 1994.

44. Picq M, Dubois M, Grynberg A, et al: Developmental differences in distribution of cyclic nucleotide phosphodiesterase isoforms in cardiomyocyte and the ventricular tissue from newborn and adult rats. J Cardiovasc Pharmacol 26:742, 1995.

45. Kojima M, Ishima T, Taniguchi N, et al: Developmental changes in β-adrenoceptors, muscarinic cholinoceptors and Ca^{2+} channels in rat ventricular muscles. Br J Pharmacol 99:334, 1990.

46. Tanaka H, Manita S, Matsuda T, et al: Sustained negative inotropism mediated by α-adrenoceptors in adult mouse myocardia: Developmental conversion from positive response in the neonate. Br J Pharmacol 114:673, 1995.

47. Osaka T, Joyner RW, Kumar R, et al: Postnatal decrease in muscarinic cholinergic influence on Ca^{2+} currents of rabbit ventricular cells. Am J Physiol 264:H1916, 1993.

48. Akita T, Joyner RW, Lu C, et al: Developmental changes in modulation of calcium currents of rabbit ventricular cells by phosphodiesterase inhibitors. Circulation 90:469, 1994.

49. Anderson PAW: Biophysics of the developing heart. *In* Elkayam U, Gleicher N (eds): Cardiac Problems in Pregnancy. New York, Alan R Liss, 1990, p 485.

50. Hawkins C, Xu A, Narayanan N: Sarcoplasmic reticulum calcium pump in cardiac and slow twitch skeletal muscle but not fast twitch skeletal muscle undergoes phosphorylation by endogenous and exogenous Ca^{2+}/calmodulin-dependent protein kinase. Characterization of optimal conditions for calcium pump phosphorylation. J Biol Chem 269:31198, 1994.

51. Iwamoto T, Pan Y, Wakabayashi S: Phosphorylation-dependent regulation of cardiac Na$^+$/Ca^{2+} exchanger via protein kinase C. J Biol Chem 271:13609, 1996.

52. Jones LG, Rozich JD, Tsutsui H, et al: Endothelin stimulates multiple responses in isolated adult ventricular cardiac myocytes. Am J Physiol 263:1447, 1992.

53. Smith RD, Timmermans PB: Human angiotensin receptor subtypes. Curr Opin Nephrol Hypertens 3:112, 1994.

54. Zheng JS, Boluyt MO, Long X, et al: Extracellular ATP inhibits adrenergic agonist–induced hypertrophy of neonatal cardiac myocytes. Circ Res 78:525, 1996.

55. Jiang TR, Kuznetsov V, Pak E, et al: Thrombin receptor actions in neonatal rat ventricular myocytes. Circ Res 78:553, 1996.

56. Xiao RP, Pepe S, Spurgeon HA, et al: Opioid peptide receptor stimulation reverses beta-adrenergic effects in rat heart cells. Am J Physiol 41:H797, 1997.

57. Beinlich CJ, Baker KM, White GJ, et al: Control of growth in the neonatal pig heart. Am J Physiol 261:3, 1991.

58. Dostal DE, Booz GW, Baker KM: Angiotensin II signalling pathways in cardiac fibroblasts: Conventional versus novel mechanisms in mediating cardiac growth and function (Review). Mol Cell Biochem 157:15, 1996.

59. Ruzicka M, Leenen FH: Relevance of blockade of cardiac and circulatory angiotensin-converting enzyme for the prevention of volume overload–induced cardiac hypertrophy. Circulation 91:16, 1995.

60. Booz GW, Baker KM: Molecular signalling mechanisms controlling growth and function of cardiac fibroblasts (Review). Cardiovasc Res 30:537, 1995.

61. Gilbert RD: Effects of afterload and baroreceptors on cardiac function in fetal sheep. J Dev Physiol 4:299, 1982.

62. Thornburg KL, Morton MJ: Filling and arterial pressures as determinants of left ventricular stroke volume in fetal lambs. Am J Physiol 251:H961, 1986.

63. Stainier DY, Fouquet B, Chen JN, et al: Mutations affecting the formation and function of the cardiovascular system in the zebrafish embryo. Development 123:285, 1996.

64. Pagani ED, Julian FJ: Rabbit papillary muscle myosin isozymes and the velocity of muscle shortening. Circ Res 54:586, 1984.

65. Granzier HL, Irving TC: Passive tension in cardiac muscle: Contribution of collagen, titin, microtubules, and intermediate filaments. Biophys J 68:1027, 1995.

66. Ohayon J, Chadwick RS: Effects of collagen microstructure on the mechanics of the left ventricle. Biophys J 54:1077, 1988.

67. Robinson TF, Factor SM, Capasso JM, et al: Morphology, composition, and function of struts between cardiac myocytes of rat and hamster. Cell Tissue Res 249:247, 1987.

68. Terracio L, Gullberg D, Rubin K, et al: Expression of collagen adhesion proteins and their association with the cytoskeleton in cardiac myocytes. Anat Rec 223:62, 1989.

69. Trombitas K, Jin JP, Granzier H, et al: The mechanically active domain of titin in cardiac muscle. Circ Res 77:856, 1995.

70. Craig SW, Pardo JV: Gamma actin, spectrin, and intermediate filament proteins colocalize with vinculin at costameres, myofibril-to-sarcolemma attachment sites. Cell Motil 3:449, 1983.

71. Kolmerer B, Olivieri N, Witt CC, et al: Genomic organization of M line titin and its tissue-specific expression in two distinct isoforms. J Mol Biol 256:556, 1996.

72. Pardo JV, Silicianno JD, Craig SW, et al: Vinculin is a component of an extensive network of myofibril-sarcolemma attachment regions in cardiac muscle fibers. J Cell Biol 97:1081, 1983.

73. Traub P: Intermediate Filaments. A Review. Berlin, Springer-Verlag, 1985, p 150.

74. Houmeida A, Holt J, Tskhovrebova L, et al: Studies of the interaction between titin and myosin. J Cell Biol 131:1471, 1995.

75. Gautel M, Lehtonen E, Pietruschka F: Assembly of the cardiac I-band region of titin/connectin: Expression of the cardiac-specific regions and their structural relation to the elastic segments. Muscle Res Cell Motil 17:449, 1996.

76. Danowski BA, Imanaka-Yoshida K, Sanger JM, et al: Costameres are sites of force transmission to the substratum in adult rat cardiomyocytes. J Cell Biol 118:1411, 1992.

77. DeTombe PP, Ter Keurs HEDJ: An internal viscous element limits unloaded velocity of sarcomere shortening in rat myocardium. J Physiol (Lond) 454:619, 1992.

78. van der Loop FT, Schaart G, Langmann H, et al: Rearrangement of intercellular junctions and cytoskeletal proteins during rabbit myocardium development. Eur J Cell Biol 68:62, 1995.

79. Tagawa H, Koide M, Sato H, et al: Cytoskeletal role in the contractile dysfunction of cardiocytes from hypertrophied and failing right ventricular myocardium. Proc Assoc Am Physicians 108:218, 1996.

80. Hynes RO: Integrins, a family of cell surface receptors. Cell 48:549, 1987.

81. Albelda SM, Buck CA: Integrins and other cell adhesion molecules. FASEB J 4:2868, 1990.

82. Carver W, Price RL, Raso DS, et al: Distribution of beta-1 integrin in the developing rat heart. J Histochem Cytochem 42:167, 1994.

83. Terracio L, Rubin K, Balog E, et al: Expression of collagen binding integrins during cardiac development and hypertrophy. Circ Res 68:734, 1991.

84. Borg TK, Rubin K, Lundgren E, et al: Recognition of extracellular matrix components by neonatal and adult cardiac myocytes. Dev Biol 104:86, 1984.

85. Kanter HL, Laing JG, Beyer EC, et al: Multiple connexins colocalize in canine ventricular myocyte gap junctions. Circ Res 73:344, 1993.

86. Borg TK, Terracio L, Lundgren E, et al: Connective tissue of the myocardium. *In* Ferrans VJ, Rosenquist GC, Weinstein C (eds): Cardiac Morphogenesis. New York, Elsevier, 1985, p 69.

87. Anderson PAW, Glick K, Manring A, et al: Developmental changes in cardiac contractility in fetal and postnatal sheep: In vitro and in vivo. Am J Physiol 247:H371, 1984.

88. Nakanishi T, Jarmakani JM: Developmental changes in myocardial mechanical function and subcellular organelles. Am J Physiol 246:H615, 1984.

89. Anversa P, Olivetti G, Load AV, et al: Morphometric study of early postnatal development in the left and right ventricular myocardium of the rat. I. Hypertrophy, hyperplasia, and binucleation of myocytes. Circ Res 46:495, 1980.

90. Kim HD, Kim DJ, Lee IJ, et al: Human fetal heart development after mid-term: Morphometry and ultrastructural study. J Mol Cell Cardiol 24:949, 1992.

91. Cochrane AD, Karl TR, Mee RB, et al: Staged conversion to arterial switch for late failure of the systemic right ventricle. Ann Thorac Surg 56:854, 1993.

92. Legato MJ: Cellular mechanisms of normal growth in the mammalian heart. II. A quantitative and qualitative comparison between the right and left ventricular myocytes in the dog from birth to five months of age. Circ Res 44:263, 1979.

93. Hudlicka O, Brown MD: Postnatal growth of the heart and its blood vessels. J Vasc Res 33:266, 1996.

94. Pennica D, King KL, Shaw KJ, et al: Expression cloning of cardiotrophin I, a cytokine that induces cardiac myocyte hypertrophy. Proc Natl Acad Sci U S A 92:1142, 1995.

95. Pasumarthi KBS, Kardami E, Cattini PA, et al: High and low molecular weight fibroblast growth factor-2 increase proliferation of neonatal rat cardiac myocytes but have differential effects on binucleation and nuclear morphology. Evidence for both paracrine and intracrine actions of fibroblast growth factor-2. Circ Res 78:126, 1996.

96. Engelmann GL, Dionne CA, Jaye MC: Acidic fibroblast growth factor and heart development. Role in myocyte proliferation and capillary angiogenesis. Circ Res 72:7, 1993.

97. Engelmann GL, Grutkoski PS: Coordinate TGFβ receptor gene expression during rat heart development. Cell Mol Biol Res 40:93, 1994.

98. Suzuki J, Matsubara H, Urakami M, et al: Rat angiotensin II (type 1A) receptor mRNA regulation and subtype expression in myocardial growth and hypertrophy. Circ Res 73:439, 1993.

99. Fischer TA, Ungureanu-Longrois D, Singh K, et al: Regulation of bFGF expression and ANG II secretion in cardiac myocytes and microvascular endothelial cells. Am J Physiol 272:H958, 1997.

100. Ikeda U, Maeda Y, Kawahara Y, et al: Angiotensin II augments cytokine-stimulated nitric oxide synthesis in rat cardiac myocytes. Circulation 92:2683, 1995.

101. Delafontaine P, Brink M, Du J: Angiotensin II modulation of insulin-like growth factor I expression in the cardiovascular system. Trends Cardiovasc Med 6:187, 1996.

102. Sacca L, Cittadini A, Fazio S: Growth hormone and the heart (Review). Endocr Rev 15:555, 1994.

103. Simpson P: Stimulation of hypertrophy of cultured neonatal rat heart cells through an α₁-adrenergic receptor and induction of beating through an α₁- and β₁-adrenergic receptor interaction: Evidence for independent regulation of growth and beating. Circ Res 56:884, 1985.

104. Rokosh DG, Stewart AF, Chang KC, et al: Alpha 1–adrenergic receptor subtype mRNAs are differentially regulated by alpha 1–adrenergic and other hypertrophic stimuli in cardiac myocytes in culture and in vivo. Repression of alpha 1B and alpha 1D but induction of alpha 1C. J Biol Chem 271:5839, 1996.

105. Felder RA, Calcagno PL, Eisner GM, et al: Ontogeny of myocardial adrenoceptors. II. Alpha adrenoceptors. Pediatr Res 16:340, 1982.

106. Boucek RJ, Citak M, Graham TP, et al: Effects of postnatal maturation on postrest potentiation in isolated rabbit atria. Pediatr Res 22:524, 1987.

107. Fyrberg E, Fyrberg CC, Beall C, et al: *Drosophila melanogaster* troponin-T mutations engender three distinct syndromes of myofibrillar abnormalities. J Mol Biol 216:657, 1990.

108. Anderson PAW, Malouf NN, Oakeley AE, et al: Troponin T isoform expression in humans: A comparison among normal and failing adult heart, fetal heart, and adult and fetal skeletal muscle. Circ Res 69:1226, 1991.

109. Wieczorek DF, Smith CW, Nadal-Ginard B: The rat α-tropomyosin gene generates a minimum of six different mRNAs coding for striated, smooth, and nonmuscle isoforms by alternative splicing. Mol Cell Biol 8:679, 1988.

110. Mahdavi V, Matsuoka R, Nadal-Ginard B, et al: Molecular characterization and expression of the cardiac α- and β-myosin heavy chain genes. *In* Ferrans VJ, Rosenquist GC, Weinstein C (eds): Cardiac Morphogenesis. New York, Elsevier, 1985, p 2.

111. Bishopric NH, Simpson PC, Ordahl CP: Induction of the skeletal α-actin gene in α₁-adrenoceptor–mediated hypertrophy of rat cardiac myocytes. J Clin Invest 80:1194, 1987.

112. Cummins P, Lambert SJ: Myosin transitions in the bovine and human heart. A developmental and anatomical study of heavy and light chain subunits in the atrium and ventricle. Circ Res 58:846, 1986.

113. Greig A, Hirschberg Y, Anderson PAW, et al: Molecular basis of cardiac troponin T isoform heterogeneity in rabbit heart. Circ Res 74:41, 1994.

114. Anderson PAW, Oakeley AE: Immunological identification of five troponin T isoforms reveals an elaborate maturational troponin T profile in rabbit myocardium. Circ Res 65:1087, 1989.

115. Schwartz K, Apstein C, Mercadier JJ, et al: Left ventricular isomyosins in normal and hypertrophied rat and human hearts. Eur Heart J 5:77, 1984.

116. Mainwaring RD, Lamberti JJ, Billman GF, et al: Suppression of the pituitary thyroid axis after cardiopulmonary bypass in the neonate [see comments]. Ann Thorac Surg 58:1078, 1994.

117. Swynghdauw B: Developmental and functional adaptation of contractile proteins in cardiac and skeletal muscle. Physiol Rev 66:710, 1986.

118. Pagani ED, Alousi AA, Grant AM, et al: Changes in myofibrillar content and Mg-ATPase activity in ventricular tissues from patients with heart failure caused by coronary artery disease, cardiomyopathy, or mitral valve insufficiency. Circ Res 63:380, 1988.

119. Bouvagnet P, Mairhofer H, Leger JO, et al: Distribution pattern of α and β myosin in normal and diseased human ventricular myocardium. Basic Res Cardiol 84:91, 1989.

120. Price KM, Littler WA, Cummins P: Human atrial and ventricular myosin light-chain subunits in the adult and during development. Biochem J 191:571, 1980.

121. Morano M, Zacharzowski U, Maier M, et al: Regulation of human heart contractility by essential myosin light chain isoforms. J Clin Invest 98:467, 1996.

122. Yamamoto K, Moos C: The protein-Cs of rabbit, red, white and cardiac muscles. J Biol Chem 258:8395, 1983.

123. Ruzicka DL, Schwartz RJ: Sequential activation of α-actin genes during avian cardiogenesis: Vascular smooth muscle α-actin gene transcripts mark the onset of cardiomyocyte differentiation. J Cell Biol 107:2575, 1988.

124. Boheler KR, Carrier L, de la Bastie D, et al: Skeletal actin mRNA increases in the human heart during ontogenic development and is the major isoform of control and failing adult hearts. J Clin Invest 88:323, 1991.

125. Hewett TE, Grupp IL, Grupp G, et al: Alpha-skeletal actin is associated with increased contractility in the mouse heart. Circ Res 74:740, 1994.

126. McDonald KS, Field LJ, Parmacek MS, et al: Length dependence of Ca^{2+} sensitivity of tension in mouse cardiac myocytes expressing skeletal troponin C. J Physiol (Lond) 483:131, 1995.

127. Palmer S, Kentish JC: The role of troponin C in modulating the Ca^{2+} sensitivity of mammalian skinned cardiac and skeletal muscle fibres. J Physiol (Lond) 480:45, 1994.

128. Muthuchamy M, Grupp IL, Grupp G, et al: Molecular and physiological effects of overexpressing striated muscle β-tropomyosin in the adult murine heart. J Biol Chem 270:30593, 1995.

129. Palmiter KA, Kitada Y, Muthuchamy M, et al: Exchange of beta- for alpha-tropomyosin in hearts of transgenic mice induces changes in thin filament response to Ca^{2+}, strong cross-bridge binding, and protein phosphorylation. J Biol Chem 271:11611, 1996.

130. Wattanapermpool J, Guo X, Solaro RJ: The unique amino-terminal peptide of cardiac troponin I regulates myofibrillar activity only when it is phosphorylated. J Mol Cell Cardiol 27:1383, 1995.

131. Malouf NN, McMahon D, Oakeley AE, et al: A cardiac troponin T epitope conserved across phyla. J Biol Chem 67:9269, 1992.

132. Nassar R, Malouf NN, Kelly MB, et al: Force-pCa relation and troponin T isoforms of rabbit myocardium. Circ Res 69:1470, 1991.

133. Saba Z, Nassar R, Ungerleider RM, et al: Cardiac troponin T isoform expression correlates with pathophysiological descriptors in patients who underwent corrective surgery for congenital heart disease. Circulation 94:472, 1996.

134. Chin TK, Friedman WF, Klitzner TS, et al: Developmental changes in cardiac myocyte calcium regulation. Circ Res 67:574, 1990.

135. Szymanska G, Grupp IL, Slack JP, et al: Alterations in sarcoplasmic reticulum calcium uptake, relaxation parameters and their responses to beta-adrenergic agonists in the developing rabbit heart. J Mol Cell Cardiol 27:1819, 1995.

136. Agata N, Tanaka H, Shigenobu K: Inotropic effects of ryanodine and nicardipine on fetal, neonatal and adult guinea-pig myocardium. Eur J Pharmacol 260:47, 1994.

137. Moorman AF, Vermeulen JL, Koban MU, et al: Patterns of expression of sarcoplasmic reticulum Ca^{2+}-ATPase and phospholamban mRNAs during rat heart development. Circ Res 76:616, 1995.

138. Penefsky ZJ: Studies on mechanism of inhibition of cardiac muscle contractile tension by ryanodine. Mechanical response. Pflugers Arch 347:173, 1974.

139. Anger M, Samuel JL, Marotte F, et al: In situ mRNA distribution of sarco(endo)plasmic reticulum Ca^{2+}-ATPase isoforms during ontogeny in the rat. J Mol Cell Cardiol 26:539, 1994.

140. Kawano S, DeHaan RL: Analysis of the T-type calcium channel in embryonic chick ventricular myocytes. J Membr Biol 116:9, 1990.

141. Davies MP, An RH, Doevendans P, et al: Developmental changes in ionic channel activity in the embryonic murine heart. Circ Res 78:15, 1996.

142. Artman M, Graham TP, Boucek RJ: Effects of postnatal maturation on myocardial contractile responses to calcium antagonists and changes in contraction frequency. J Cardiovasc Pharmacol 7:850, 1985.

143. Collin T, Wang JJ, Nargeot J, et al: Molecular cloning of three isoforms of the L-type voltage-dependent calcium channel β subunit from normal human heart. Circ Res 72:1337, 1993.

144. Drugge ED, Rosen MR, Robinson RB: Neuronal regulation of the development of the α-adrenergic chronotropic response in the rat heart. Circ Res 57:415, 1985.

145. Herrera VL, Emanuel JR, Ruiz-Opazo M: Three differentially expressed Na,K-ATPase α subunit isoforms: Structural and functional implications. J Cell Biol 105:1855, 1987.

146. Orlowski J, Lingrel JB: Tissue-specific and developmental regulation of rat Na,K-ATPase catalytic α isoform and β subunit mRNAs. J Biol Chem 263:10436, 1988.

147. Hanson GL, Schilling WP, Michael LH: Sodium-potassium pump and sodium-calcium exchange in adult and neonatal canine cardiac sarcolemma. Am J Physiol 264:H320, 1993.

148. McDonough AA, Wang J, Farley RA: Significance of sodium pump isoforms in digitalis therapy. J Mol Cell Cardiol 27:1001, 1995.

149. Xie Z, Jack-Hays M, Wang Y, et al: Different oxidant sensitivities of the alpha 1 and alpha 2 isoforms of Na$^+$/K$^+$-ATPase expressed in baculovirus-infected insect cells. Biochem Biophys Res Commun 207:155, 1995.

150. Artman M, Ichikawa H, Avkiran M, et al: Na$^+$-Ca^{2+} exchange current density in cardiac myocytes from rabbit and guinea pigs during postnatal development. Am J Physiol 268:H1714, 1995.

151. Romero T, Covell J, Friedman WF: A comparison of pressure-volume relations of the fetal, newborn and adult heart. Am J Physiol 222:1285, 1972.

152. Minczak BM, Wolfson MR, Santamore WP, et al: Developmental changes in diastolic ventricular interaction. Pediatr Res 23:466, 1988.

153. Schachat FH, Canine AC, Briggs MM, et al: The presence of two skeletal muscle α-actinins correlates with troponin-tropomyosin expression and Z-line width. J Cell Biol 101:1001, 1985.

154. Humphries MJ: The molecular basis and specificity of integrin-ligand interactions. J Cell Sci 97:585, 1990.

155. Thorsteinsdottir S, Roelen BA, Freund E, et al: Expression patterns of laminin receptor splice variants alpha 6A beta 1 and alpha 6B beta 1 suggest different roles in mouse development. Dev Dyn 204:240, 1995.

156. Yang JT, Rayburn H, Hynes RO: Cell adhesion events mediated by alpha 4 integrins are essential in placental and cardiac development. Development 121:549, 1995.

157. Samuel JL, Farhadian F, Sabri A, et al: Expression of fibronectin during rat fetal and postnatal development: An in situ hybridisation and immunohistochemical study. Cardiovasc Res 28:1653, 1994.

158. Farhadian F, Contard F, Corbier A, et al: Fibronectin expression during physiological and pathological cardiac growth. J Mol Cell Cardiol 27:981, 1995.

159. Marijanowski M, van der Loos CM, Mohrschladt MF, et al: The neonatal heart has a relatively high content of total collagen and type I collagen, a condition that may explain the less compliant state. J Am Coll Cardiol 23:1204, 1994.

160. Anderson PAW, Glick KL, Killam AP, et al: The effect of heart rate on in utero left ventricular output in the fetal sheep. J Physiol (Lond) 372:557, 1986.

161. Reller MD, Morton MJ, Reid DL, et al: Fetal lamb ventricles respond differently to filling and arterial pressures and to in utero ventilation. Pediatr Res 22:621, 1987.

162. Anderson PAW, Manring A, Serwer GA, et al: The force-interval relationship of the human left ventricle. Circulation 60:334, 1979.

163. Clyman RI, Teitel D, Padbury C, et al: The role of β-adrenergic receptor stimulation and contractile state in the preterm lamb's response to altered ductus arteriosus patency. Pediatr Res 23:316, 1988.

164. Pinson CW, Morton MJ, Thornburg KL, et al: An anatomic basis for fetal right ventricular dominance and arterial pressure sensitivity. J Dev Physiol 9:253, 1987.
165. Anderson PAW, Killam AP, Mainwaring RD, et al: In utero right ventricular output in the fetal lamb: The effect of heart rate. J Physiol (Lond) 387:297, 1987.
166. Anderson PAW, Fair EC, Killam AP, et al: The in utero left ventricle of the fetal sheep: The effects of isoprenaline. J Physiol (Lond) 430:441, 1990.
167. Grant DA, Kondo CS, Maloney JE, et al: Changes in pericardial pressure during the perinatal period. Circulation 86:1615, 1992.
168. Downing SE, Talner NS, Gardner TH: Ventricular function in the newborn lamb. Am J Physiol 208:931, 1965.
169. Shimada E, Kasai T, Konishi M, et al: Effects of patent ductus arteriosus on left ventricular output and organ blood flows in preterm infants with respiratory distress syndrome treated with surfactant. J Pediatr 125:270, 1994.
170. Klopfenstein HS, Rudolph AM: Postnatal changes in the circulation and responses to volume loading in sheep. Circ Res 42:839, 1978.
171. O'Laughlin MP, Fisher DJ, Dreyer WJ, et al: Augmentation of cardiac output with intravenous catecholamines in unanesthetized hypoxemic newborn lambs. Pediatr Res 22:667, 1987.
172. Breall JA, Rudolph AM, Heymann MA, et al: Role of thyroid hormone in postnatal circulatory and metabolic adjustments. J Clin Invest 73:1418, 1984.

CHAPTER 4

THE FETAL CIRCULATION AND ITS ADJUSTMENTS AFTER BIRTH

ABRAHAM M. RUDOLPH

The adult circulation is characterized by series blood flow. Blood is oxygenated in the lungs, returns through the pulmonary veins to the left atrium and ventricle, and is ejected into the arterial system to be distributed to the tissues. Some oxygen is extracted for metabolism, and carbon dioxide is taken up. The blood then returns through the venous system to the right atrium and ventricle, which ejects it into the pulmonary arteries.

In the fetus, oxygen uptake and carbon dioxide elimination occur in the placenta. Oxygenated blood flows to the fetus through the umbilical veins, which connect with the hepatic portal venous system and distribute blood to the liver. The ductus venosus, a connection between the umbilical vein and the inferior vena cava, allows some umbilical venous blood to bypass the hepatic vasculature and enter the central circulation directly. This well-oxygenated blood mixes with poorly oxygenated blood from the gastrointestinal tract in the portal veins or with venous blood from the lower body in the inferior vena cava. Unlike the adult, in whom there is a complete separation of oxygenated blood returning to the left side of the heart from the lungs and poorly oxygenated blood returning to the right side of the heart, there is some admixture in the fetus, and the blood distributed to the tissues is a mixture of well-oxygenated and poorly oxygenated blood.

In the fetus, the lungs do not serve the function of gas exchange as in the adult. Blood flow to the lung is limited by passage of blood through the ductus arteriosus, which connects the pulmonary trunk to the descending aorta. A third connection present in the fetus is the foramen ovale, which allows blood to enter the left atrium from the inferior vena cava and right atrium without having to be ejected by the right ventricle through the pulmonary circulation. The importance of these three fetal communications is discussed later.

COURSE OF THE FETAL CIRCULATION

The course of the circulation in the fetus has been studied by several methods. In 1906, Pohlman[1] injected starch granules in fetal veins and determined their distribution by exposing tissues to iodine. Barclay and colleagues[2] observed patterns of flow in fetal lambs exteriorized from the uterus by injecting radiographic contrast media into fetal veins in different sites. Dawes and associates[3] measured oxygen saturation in various vessels in fetal lambs and esti-

mated flow patterns from changes in the saturation. Mahon and coworkers[4] used indicator dilution techniques to examine flow patterns but also measured left and right ventricular output in fetal lambs. Those early studies were conducted in sheep or goats, with the ewe anesthetized and the fetus exteriorized. It was not known how these factors influenced the magnitude or patterns of blood flow.

Detailed analyses of the patterns of flow were accomplished in fetal lambs in utero, several days after recovery from surgery to insert catheters into limb vessels.[5] Radionuclide-labeled microspheres with different isotopic labels were injected into fetal vessels, and the specific isotopes as well as their quantity could be measured in various tissues. From these data, it was possible to calculate not only the patterns but also the magnitude of blood flows. As ultrasound techniques have improved, it has been possible to study flow patterns in the heart and vessels as well as the magnitude of flows, by Doppler techniques, in the human fetus.

Maternal arterial blood entering the uterine circulation has a PO_2 of about 100 mm Hg and an oxygen saturation close to 100%. Oxygen diffuses across the placental membrane into fetal arterial blood; in the sheep, blood entering the placenta from the umbilical artery has a PO_2 of about 20 to 23 mm Hg and an oxygen saturation of about 45 to 50%. Umbilical venous blood has a PO_2 of about 32 to 36 mm Hg and an oxygen saturation of about 80 to 90%. This high oxygen saturation at a relatively low PO_2 is due to the greater affinity of fetal hemoglobin for oxygen compared with that of adult hemoglobin; the P_{50} for fetal hemoglobin is about 25 to 28 mm Hg, compared with 35 to 38 mm Hg in the adult. Umbilical venous blood returns to the fetus through the umbilical vein, which enters the fetal abdomen and courses to the porta hepatis. It provides several branches to supply the left lobe of the liver, after which the ductus venosus arises and passes dorsally and cephalad to connect with the left side of the inferior vena cava just below the diaphragm. The umbilical vein then arches to the right side of the porta hepatis to connect with the portal vein.[6] The portal veins to the right lobe of the liver arise beyond this junction (Fig. 4–1).

Umbilical blood flow averages about 200 ml/min per kilogram of fetal weight in the sheep; this represents about 40% of the combined ventricular output (see later). About 50% of the umbilical venous blood is distributed to the left and right lobes of the liver, and the other half bypasses the liver through the ductus venosus.[6] Portal venous blood is

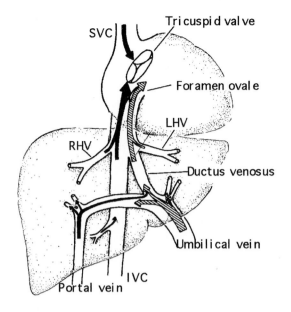

Diagram showing the patterns of blood flow in veins in the porta hepatis and the inferior and superior venae cavae entering the heart. IVC = inferior vena cava; LVH = left hepatic vein; RVH = right hepatic vein; SVC = superior vena cava.

almost completely distributed to the right lobe of the liver; only 5 to 10% passes through the ductus venosus, and none enters the left lobe of the liver. Thus, the left lobe of the liver receives almost exclusively well-oxygenated umbilical venous blood, whereas the right lobe receives umbilical venous blood as well as portal venous blood, which has a PO_2 of 12 to 14 mm Hg and an oxygen saturation of 20 to 25%. Because of these flow patterns, left hepatic venous blood has an oxygen saturation of 70 to 75%, whereas right hepatic venous blood oxygen saturation is 55 to 65%.

The inferior vena cava just below the diaphragm receives blood from four sources, all with different oxygen saturations, namely, umbilical vein, left and right hepatic veins, and distal inferior vena cava. The last has a PO_2 of 12 to 15 mm Hg with an oxygen saturation of 20 to 28%. The blood flowing from these four veins does not mix completely but shows differential streaming. The ductus venosus and left hepatic vein enter the inferior vena cava through a single orifice, which in the sheep is partly covered by a thin valve-like membrane. The blood from these two veins is well oxygenated, and it streams in the posterior and left portion of the inferior vena cava in the direction of the foramen ovale to enter the left atrium. This streaming related to the eustachian valve has been verified in humans.[7] The poorly oxygenated blood from the right hepatic vein joins blood returning from the distal inferior vena cava, and these stream along the anterior and right portions of the inferior vena cava toward the tricuspid valve to enter the right ventricle. Although these are the preferential patterns of flow, some of the blood derived from the ductus venosus does enter the tricuspid valve, and some blood from the distal inferior vena cava crosses the foramen ovale into the left atrium.

Blood returning to the heart through the superior vena cava has a PO_2 of 12 to 15 mm Hg and an oxygen saturation

of 20 to 30%. It is deflected by the tubercle of Lower in the right atrium in the direction of the tricuspid valve, and about 95% enters the right ventricle, whereas only 5% or less of superior vena caval blood passes across the foramen ovale into the left atrium.[5]

The preferential streaming of the venous blood returning to the heart results in blood of higher oxygen saturation in the left atrium than in the right ventricle and pulmonary artery. The blood entering the left atrium through the foramen ovale is joined by pulmonary venous blood. In the fetus, because there is no gas exchange in the lung, the oxygen saturation of pulmonary venous blood (about 50%) is slightly lower than that in the pulmonary artery. However, because pulmonary blood flow is low in the fetus and is considerably less than the volume of blood traversing the foramen ovale,[5] the oxygen saturation of mixed blood in the left atrium and left ventricle is only moderately lower than that of ductus venosus blood (left ventricular oxygen saturation of 65 to 70% versus ductus venosus blood oxygen saturation of 80 to 90%).

DISTRIBUTION OF CARDIAC OUTPUT

In the adult with a series circulation, the cardiac output is defined as the volume of blood ejected by each ventricle. These volumes are essentially similar, although small differences in left and right ventricular output may occur during short periods. The term *cardiac output* represents the volume of blood flow per unit time, through the series circulation.

In the fetus, as mentioned before, the blood from umbilical and systemic veins mixes to some extent and enters both the left and right sides of the heart. Blood ejected by each ventricle consists of a mixture of poorly oxygenated and well-oxygenated blood. The concept of cardiac output used for the adult circulation cannot be applied to the fetus. It has become customary to use the term *combined ventricular output* for the total volume of blood ejected by the fetal heart.[5] Combined ventricular output has been measured most definitively in fetal lambs by use of radionuclide-labeled microspheres[5] or electromagnetic flow transducers placed around the ascending aorta and pulmonary trunk.[5] Measurements in human fetuses have been more limited, but left and right ventricular output measurements have been reported with use of ultrasound techniques and application of the Doppler principle.[9, 10]

Figure 4–2B shows the proportions of the combined ventricular output returning to the heart through various veins and the proportions of blood ejected by each ventricle into the central arteries in the fetal lamb. Unlike in the adult, the volumes ejected by each ventricle are different. In the fetal lamb, the right ventricle ejects almost twice as much as the left ventricle: 65% of combined ventricular output compared with 35%. Combined ventricular output is fairly constant in relation to fetal body weight in the last trimester of gestation in the sheep: about 500 ml/kg fetal body weight per minute. Thus, right ventricular output is about 325 ml/kg/min and left ventricular output is about 175 ml/kg/min.

Because pulmonary vascular resistance is high in the fetus, only about 12% of blood ejected into the pulmonary

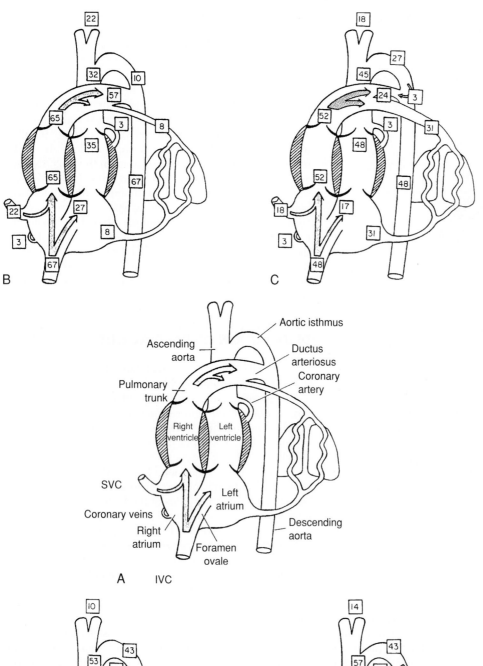

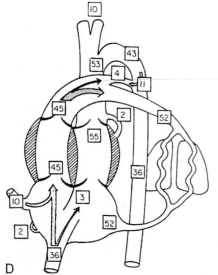

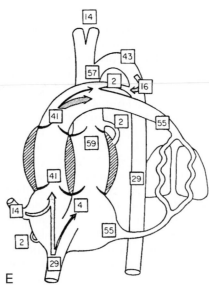

FIGURE 4–2

Distribution of the circulation in the fetal lamb. Percentages of combined ventricular output are shown in boxes. *A*, Anatomy of the fetal circulation. IVC = inferior vena cava; SVC = superior vena cava. *B*, Undisturbed state. *C*, After ventilation with 3% oxygen, so as not to alter fetal blood gases. *D*, After ventilation with oxygen. *E*, After ventilation with oxygen and umbilical cord occlusion.

trunk is distributed to the lungs; this represents about 8% of combined ventricular output or about 40 ml/kg of fetal body weight per minute. The remaining 88% of blood ejected by the right ventricle passes through the ductus arteriosus to the descending aorta. Thus, about 57% of combined ventricular output or about 285 ml/kg/min traverses the ductus arteriosus.

Of the blood ejected by the left ventricle into the ascending aorta, about 70% is distributed to the coronary circulation, the brain, the tissues of the head and neck, and the forelimbs, whereas only about 30% crosses the aortic isthmus to the descending aorta to join the blood traversing the ductus arteriosus from the pulmonary trunk. Of the 35% of combined ventricular output ejected by the left ventricle, about 22% is distributed to the forelimbs, heart, head, and brain, and only about 10% of combined ventricular output traverses the aortic isthmus to the descending aorta. This represents only about 50 ml/kg body weight per minute. This low flow explains why the aortic isthmus is the narrowest part of the aorta in the term infant and why lesions that alter ascending aortic flow in utero affect the diameter of the aortic isthmus and transverse aortic arch.

The left ventricle is filled by blood returning to the left atrium from the pulmonary veins (about 8% of the combined ventricular output) and through the foramen ovale (about 27% of combined ventricular output).

The descending aortic flow is about 67% of combined ventricular output, or 335 ml/kg/min. The umbilical-placental circulation receives about 40% of combined ventricular output, or about 200 ml/kg/min. The lower trunk, hind limbs, and abdominal organs receive about 27% of combined ventricular output, 135 ml/kg/min.

Measurements of left and right ventricular output have been made in human fetuses by use of the Doppler technique. A wide range of outputs has been reported. Right ventricular output was only 1.2 to 1.4 times the left ventricular output, compared with a ratio of 2:1 in the sheep.[9] This difference is probably related to the marked difference in brain size in the lamb and the human. The brain's blood supply is derived from branches of the ascending aorta. Therefore, left ventricular output is relatively higher in the human fetus. The greater volume of blood ejected from the left ventricle could be derived either from a higher pulmonary blood flow or by a larger flow across the foramen ovale. Measurements in human fetuses have recorded pulmonary blood flow of 85 to 100 ml/min per kilogram of estimated fetal weight.[11] This is about twice the pulmonary blood flow in fetal lambs, and it could account for the majority of the higher left ventricular output in human compared with lamb fetuses.

CIRCULATORY CHANGES AFTER BIRTH

Conversion of fetal to adult patterns of blood flow involves elimination of the umbilical-placental circulation, establishment of an adequate pulmonary circulation, and separation of the left and right sides of the heart by closure of fetal channels. The major events occurring at the time of birth include separation of the placental circulation and establishment of rhythmic ventilation. The umbilical cord is severed in animals by tearing or by biting by the mother,

and in humans usually by ligation. Ventilation comprises two components: physical expansion of the lungs with gas and elimination of fluid in the alveoli, and increase in alveolar oxygen concentration associated with breathing air.

CHANGES IN PATTERNS OF BLOOD FLOW

The changes at the time of birth normally occur almost simultaneously. It has been difficult to establish the role of individual events in inducing postnatal circulatory adjustments. To examine their contribution to these adjustments, we studied fetal lambs chronically instrumented in utero with a tracheal tube to ventilate the fetus, a balloon occluder around the umbilical cord to occlude the umbilical circulation, and various intravascular catheters to measure blood flows with radionuclide-labeled microspheres.[12] First, the lungs were ventilated with a gas with 3% oxygen, 5% carbon dioxide, and 92% nitrogen. This did not change fetal blood gases (PO_2 of about 21 mm Hg and PCO_2 of about 40 mm Hg). This rhythmic ventilation resulted in a marked reduction in pulmonary vascular resistance and increase in pulmonary blood flow (Fig. 4–2C). Subsequent ventilation with air or oxygen markedly increased systemic arterial PO_2, and pulmonary blood flow increased further (Fig. 4–2D). The magnitude of the change in pulmonary blood flow induced by physical expansion of the lung alone and by increase in oxygen concentration varied considerably in different fetuses.

During ventilation with 3% oxygen, the proportion of blood ejected by the right ventricle that entered the pulmonary circulation increased, whereas the volume traversing the ductus arteriosus from the pulmonary trunk to the descending aorta fell considerably. Although pulmonary vascular resistance fell, there was no significant fall in pulmonary arterial pressure, probably because the ductus arteriosus remained widely patent. Blood flow through the foramen ovale into the left atrium also decreased. The outputs of the left and right ventricles also became almost similar.

Ventilation with 100% oxygen produced a further fall in pulmonary vascular resistance, and with the greater rise in pulmonary blood flow, flow from the pulmonary trunk through the ductus arteriosus was negligible and there was a small left-to-right shunt from the aorta to the pulmonary artery. There was no flow through the foramen ovale into the left atrium. The left ventricular output increased and was slightly higher than that of the right ventricle. This was accounted for by the fact that there was a small left-to-right shunt through the ductus arteriosus. In association with these changes, left atrial mean pressure increased to levels 2 to 3 mm Hg higher than right atrial pressure. Pulmonary arterial pressure fell slightly in the first few minutes after ventilation with oxygen and subsequently fell slowly further. This was probably related to gradual constriction of the ductus arteriosus, leading to separation of the two sides of the heart.

Occlusion of the umbilical cord after ventilation with oxygen produced little further change. Systemic arterial pressure increased a small amount, and the left-to-right shunt through the ductus arteriosus increased slightly, but no further changes in pulmonary blood flow occurred (Fig. 4–2E).

On the basis of these studies, the reorientation of the circulation after birth can be accounted for largely by the onset of rhythmic ventilation with air. Even without elimination of the placental circulation, ventilation increases pulmonary flow and results in foramen ovale closure, and even though the ductus arteriosus does not close completely immediately after birth, flow from the pulmonary trunk to the aorta is almost completely eliminated.

Removal of the placental circulation abolishes umbilical venous return. Hepatic blood flow is reduced within the first few hours after birth but increases after portal blood flow is increased in association with feeding.[13] The elimination of umbilical venous blood flow reduces inferior vena caval return by 200 ml/kg/min. This facilitates closure of the foramen ovale and causes a small fall in right atrial pressure.

CHANGES IN PULMONARY CIRCULATION

During fetal life, pulmonary blood flow is low owing to the high pulmonary vascular resistance. This high resistance is related to both morphologic and functional features of pulmonary vessels. Pulmonary arterioles have a thick medial layer composed predominantly of smooth muscle cells. These vessels are extremely reactive; they constrict markedly with hypoxia and dilate with an increase in PO_2. Endothelial factors, such as endothelium-derived relaxing factor and nitric oxide, have an important role in regulating pulmonary vascular resistance (see Chapter 7).

The reduction in pulmonary vascular resistance after birth is associated with rhythmic ventilation and oxygenation. The mechanisms by which these events affect the pulmonary vessels have not been fully delineated. Studies in fetal lambs indicate that gaseous expansion of the lungs results in liberation of prostacyclin (prostaglandin I_2), a pulmonary vasodilator. A rise in PO_2 is thought to increase endothelial release of nitric oxide, which is also a potent vasodilator. Other vasoactive agents, such as endothelin, bradykinin, and angiotensin, possibly also have a role in affecting pulmonary vascular responses after birth.

Physiologic responses of the fetal pulmonary circulation and the mechanisms involved in the postnatal fall in pulmonary vascular resistance are discussed in detail in Chapter 7.

After the immediate fall in pulmonary vascular resistance that follows birth, morphologic changes in the pulmonary vessels result in a permanent fall in pulmonary vascular resistance. The most striking change is a decrease in the thickness of the smooth muscle layer in the arterioles. This results in a gradual further fall in pulmonary vascular resistance and pulmonary arterial pressure within 2 to 3 weeks after birth. The perinatal changes in morphology of the pulmonary vessels are presented in detail in Chapter 7.

CLOSURE OF THE DUCTUS ARTERIOSUS

The ductus arteriosus, normally widely patent in the fetus, constricts after birth. The current concept is that two factors are largely responsible for maintaining ductus patency in utero—the low oxygen tension of pulmonary arterial blood to which it is exposed, and the effect of circulating prostaglandin (prostaglandin E_2), which relaxes ductus arteriosus smooth muscle. Closure of the ductus after birth occurs at variable times in different species. In the lamb, it is usually closed within an hour of birth, but in the human, complete closure may be delayed for 10 to 15 hours. Constriction of the ductus arteriosus occurs with increase in arterial PO_2 associated with ventilation. After birth, there is a fall in plasma prostaglandin E concentrations. These two factors are thought to be the important mechanisms responsible for ductus constriction. Subsequently, permanent closure of the ductus is achieved by fibrosis. The initial process is thought to be dissolution of normal smooth muscle cells by hypoxia of the muscle associated with constriction. The ductus arteriosus is discussed in Chapter 23.

MYOCARDIAL PERFORMANCE

The myocardium undergoes numerous structural, biochemical, and functional changes during fetal development and postnatally. These are discussed in Chapter 3.

REFERENCES

1. Pohlman AG: The fetal circulation through the heart. Bull Johns Hopkins Hosp 18:409, 1907.
2. Barclay AE, Franklin KJ, Prichard MML: The Foetal Circulation and Cardiovascular System and the Changes that They Undergo at Birth. Oxford, UK, Blackwell Scientific Publications, 1944, p 275.
3. Dawes GS, Mott JC, Widdicombe JG: The foetal circulation in the lamb. J Physiol 126:563, 1952.
4. Mahon WA, Goodwin JW, Paul WM: Measurement of individual ventricular outputs in the fetal lamb by an indicator dilution technique. Circ Res 19:191, 1966.
5. Rudolph AM, Heymann MA: The circulation of the fetus in utero. Methods for studying distribution of blood flow, cardiac output and organ blood flow. Circ Res 21:163, 1967.
6. Edelstone DI, Rudolph AM, Heymann MA: Liver and ductus venosus blood flows in fetal lambs in utero. Circ Res 42:426, 1978.
7. Kiserud T, Eik-Nes SH, Blaas HG, Hellevik LR: Foramen ovale: An ultrasonographic study of its relation to the inferior vena cava, ductus venosus and hepatic veins. Ultrasound Obstet Gynecol 2:389, 1992.
8. Rudolph AM, Heymann MA: Cardiac output in the fetal lamb: The effects of spontaneous and induced changes of heart rate on right and left ventricular output. Am J Obstet Gynecol 124:183, 1976.
9. Kenny JF, Plappert T, Doubilet P, et al: Changes in intracardiac blood flow velocities and right and left ventricular stroke volumes with gestational age in the normal human fetus: A prospective Doppler echocardiographic study. Circulation 74:1208, 1996.
10. Sutton MS, Groves A, MacNeill A, et al: Assessment of changes in blood flow through the lungs and foramen ovale in the normal human fetus with gestational age: A prospective Doppler echocardiographic study. Br Heart J 71:232, 1994.
11. Rasanen J, Wood DC, Debbs RH, et al: Reactivity of the human fetal pulmonary circulation to maternal hyperoxygenation increases during the second half of pregnancy. Circulation 97:257, 1998.
12. Teitel D, Iwamoto HS, Rudolph AM: Effects of birth-related events on central blood flow patterns. Pediatr Res 22:557, 1987.
13. Townsend SF, Rudolph CD, Rudolph AM: Changes in ovine hepatic circulation and oxygen consumption at birth. Pediatr Res 25:300, 1989.

CHAPTER 5
CARDIAC FUNCTION

HIROYUKI SUGA

The heart is a pump, and the major determinants of its function are regarded (somewhat artificially) as the following: preload, represented by end-diastolic fiber length; afterload, represented by wall stress, the main component of which is arterial pressure; and contractility, a function of calcium (Ca^{2+}) entry into the myofiber and the sensitivity of the myofibrillar apparatus to Ca^{2+}. Because the heart pumps blood around the body, cardiac function interacts with the peripheral circulation, especially the compliance and resistance of the arterial and venous systems, and the total blood volume. For example, the low cardiac output (CO) in hypovolemia is due to reduced venous return (VR), not impaired cardiac function.

Cardiac function, however, is more than the ways intracardiac pressures and volumes determine CO. It includes the supply of oxygen (O_2) and substrate to cardiac muscle (see Chapter 6), the evaluation of myocardial oxygen consumption (MVO_2), and the use of O_2 to produce the energy that drives the contractile machinery.

BRIEF HISTORY OF VIEWS OF CARDIAC FUNCTION

COMPRESSION CHAMBER: FRANK'S VIEW

The heart was first viewed as a compression chamber by Frank in 1895 (Fig. 5–1A).[1–3] By experimenting with a frog heart with only one ventricle, Frank measured ventricular pressure development as a function of ventricular volume during isovolumic, isotonic, and auxobaric contractions. He obtained systolic pressure-volume (P-V) relation curves for the different modes of contraction and found them to be markedly different. The isovolumic end-systolic P-V relation (ESPVR) was convex upward and the highest, the isotonic ESPVR was less convex upward and the lowest, and the afterloaded isotonic and auxobaric ESPVRs were between the isovolumic and isotonic ESPVRs.

Although ventricular P-V loops could be obtained in humans by cineangiography in the 1940s, ESPVR curves were not investigated for a long time. In 1961, Monroe and French[4] used intraventricular volume plethysmography in the excised blood-perfused canine heart to show convincingly that Frank's ESPVRs did not apply to canine hearts. The isovolumic and variously auxobaric ESPVRs were relatively linear and practically superimposable in the left ventricle (LV). This observation led Suga in the late 1960s[5] to the discovery of the concept of maximum end-systolic

P-V ratio or elastance (Emax) as an index of ventricular contractility.[1, 6–8]

HYDRAULIC PUMP: STARLING'S AND SARNOFF'S VIEWS

Starling and coworkers used the canine heart-lung preparation developed by a Johns Hopkins physiologist, Newell Martin,[9] who discovered the importance of coronary circulation for the contraction of the mammalian heart as early as 1881, 14 years before the famous Langendorff preparation. Starling and associates discovered that cardiac output was first an increasing function of cardiac filling pressure but then began to decrease at higher pressures (see Fig. 5–1B).[10] Starling himself called this characteristic *the Law of the Heart*.[10, 11] His greatest insight was that he considered this law to be a manifestation of increasing "active surfaces" with increasing myocardial fiber length.[11] Although the mechanism responsible for this regulation was not revealed in his time, the Starling law had foreseen an underlying mechanism similar to the sliding filament theory.[12] Although the Starling law has often been correlated with cross-bridge mechanics,[13, 14] the underlying mechanism of the Starling effect is probably more complicated.[15]

Guyton[16] observed that the CO curve plateaued rather than descended when he raised venous pressure faster than Starling did. Guyton interpreted the descending limb as a composite curve of a working point falling from a higher to a lower CO curve with gradually increasing filling pressure. Therefore, the descending limb of the CO curve does not necessarily correspond to the descending limb of the force–sarcomere length relation.[14]

The CO curve describes only CO as an increasing function of cardiac filling pressure. This curve alone, however, does not specify the filling pressure or CO under in situ circulatory conditions. Guyton proposed that cardiac filling pressure and hence CO are determined by the intersection (circulatory equilibrium point) of the CO and VR curves[16] (see section on arterial and venous coupling and matching). The VR curve is the net expression of the peripheral circulatory parameters, consisting of the arterial and venous compliances and resistances, and the total blood volume.[16, 17] Therefore, CO cannot be determined by cardiac function per se but rather as the net result of cardiac function, peripheral circulation, and blood volume. In other words, CO cannot be increased simply by enhancing cardiac function. Nevertheless, the CO curve is helpful when combined with the VR curve.

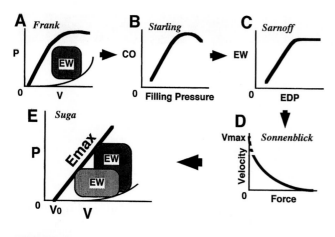

FIGURE 5–1

Schematic diagrams comparing different historical views of cardiac contraction. *A,* Frank's pressure-volume (P-V) diagram with a P-V loop and the maximally contracted P-V relation curve *(heavy line). B,* Starling's cardiac output curve *(heavy line). C,* Sarnoff's ventricular function curve *(heavy line). D,* Sonnenblick's hyperbolic force-velocity curve *(heavy line)* and Vmax as the velocity intercept of the extrapolated curve. *E,* Suga's P-V diagram with two P-V loops and the end-systolic P-V relation line *(heavy line).* P = ventricular pressure; V = ventricular volume; EW *(shaded area* within the P-V loop) = external work; CO = cardiac output; Filling Pressure = mean central venous pressure, mean right or left atrial pressure, or ventricular end-diastolic pressure; EDP = ventricular end-diastolic pressure; Vmax = maximum unloaded shortening velocity; Force = myocardial fiber force; Emax = maximum end-systolic pressure-volume ratio or elastance.

Starling, in fact, did not set out to measure CO; he wanted to quantify the total energy of cardiac contraction.[10,11] External work (EW) of the heart did not correlate with cardiac O_2 consumption,[18] and in those days, there was no concept of internal work (IW) or potential energy (PE). Starling thus gave up searching for the total energy of contraction and substituted CO at a given mean arterial pressure for the total energy of contraction.[10,11]

In the 1950s, Sarnoff considered that EW (stroke work) would be closer to the total energy of contraction than would CO. He proposed a family of ventricular function curves relating EW to end-diastolic pressure (see Fig. 5–1C).[19] However, because EW varies with end-diastolic fiber length rather than end-diastolic pressure and because EW varies as an inversely parabolic function of afterload, the ventricular function curve is not useful.

The preload-recruitable EW–end-diastolic volume relation is a practical modification of the ventricular function curve.[20] This measurement allows natural changes in arterial pressure and total peripheral resistance as the result of changes in CO. This relation seems generally linear and reflects the net response of the entire cardiovascular system. It sensitively reflects cardiac contractility, but its specificity to contractility remains to be tested under a variety of cardiovascular conditions.[21]

MUSCLE ASSEMBLAGE: SONNENBLICK'S VIEW

In the 1960s, Sonnenblick and associates viewed the heart as an assemblage of myocardial cells and evaluated contractility by the hyperbolic force-velocity curve (see Fig.

5–1D),[22] the cardiac version of the inverse force-velocity relation of skeletal muscle. They found that the maximum shortening velocity of unloaded contraction (Vmax) increased with positive inotropism. Because Vmax is considered to manifest the speed of adenosine triphosphate (ATP) hydrolysis, it was quickly accepted as a biochemically and physiologically sound index of myocardial contractility.[22]

Cardiologists attempted to measure myocardial Vmax-like shortening velocity in human in situ beating hearts, as well as in the excised beating hearts of animals.[22] Total mechanical unloading of the heart, however, was and is quite difficult. Therefore, mean circumferential shortening velocity (Vcf) was introduced as a substitute for Vmax.[22] Unfortunately, Vcf proved to be afterload dependent, and afterload is not directly measurable, although it can be calculated from ventricular P-V data by the Laplace law.[22] Moreover, the two- and three-element muscle models indicated that the shortening velocity of the contractile element must be measured from the muscle fiber shortening isotonically; otherwise, shortening velocity is contaminated by the shortening or stretching velocity of the series' elastic elements.[22] Besides, unlike Vmax of skeletal muscle, myocardial Vmax cannot be determined directly because cardiac muscle physiologically contracts in a twitch mode, unlike skeletal muscle, which can contract tetanically. Therefore, myocardial Vmax had to be obtained by extrapolating the limited force-velocity segment toward the shortening velocity axis. This extrapolated Vmax, however, was found to be preload dependent, and the force-velocity curve was not always hyperbolic.[23] For these reasons, Vmax eventually turned out to be an unreliable and, in practice, an inconvenient index of myocardial contractility in in situ hearts. Its use has become less popular since the 1970s.

Myocardial contractile function can also be characterized by the force-length (F-L) relation curve as the P-V relation for the cardiac chamber.[14,22] Here, length refers to either the myocardial fiber or the sarcomere. In both, the F-L relation curve shifts left and upward with positive inotropism and right and downward with negative inotropism.[14,22] The curve is convex upward at high Ca^{2+} concentrations, convex downward at low Ca^{2+} concentrations, and fairly linear at an intermediate concentration of Ca^{2+}.[14] Sarcomere length deviates from myocardial length by the extent of the lengthening and shortening of series elasticity by force, in which the series elasticity includes not only fibrous tissue but also damaged ends of the preparation.[13,14,22]

Currently, it is possible to measure directly the sliding speed and unitary force across myosin and actin molecules, as well as the rate of hydrolysis of ATP in an in vitro assay system.[24,25] There is an unloaded sliding excursion of 10 to 100 nm and a single cross-bridge force of 1 to 2 pN for each molecule of ATP hydrolyzed.[24,25] These results suggest that the number of cross-bridge on and off cycles for each molecule of ATP hydrolyzed varies usually between 1 and 10.[24,25] This suggestion contradicts the conventional view that hydrolysis of one molecule of ATP allows only one cross-bridge cycle, as tacitly assumed in the 1957 Huxley model of sliding filaments.[12]

OTHER VIEWS

Besides the previously discussed views of cardiac function and indices of contractility, many other indices of myocardial and ventricular contractility have different derivations. They include ejection fraction, shortening fraction, and dP/dt_{max}.[26] The preload and afterload dependence of these indices limits their utility.

In the late 1960s, Suga found that none of these views and contractility indices could satisfactorily answer the apparently naive question: How does the heart adjust blood ejection against varied afterloads within each beat? He then viewed the heart as a time-varying elastic chamber.[5,7,8] Although this view of cardiac function could be classified with Frank's view,[2] a substantial difference exists between the two views.[1,2,5-8] The remainder of this chapter has been developed from Suga's view of the P-V diagram (see Fig. 5–1E).[1]

ADVANTAGES OF THE PRESSURE-VOLUME DIAGRAM

P-V relations and P-V loops drawn in the P-V diagram have several advantages over other diagrams such as the Starling cardiac output curve,[10,11] the Sarnoff ventricular function curve,[19] and the Sonnenblick force-velocity curve (Fig. 5–2).[22] This difference comes from the different dimensions of the x and y coordinates and hence the different dimensions of the areas in their respective diagrams. These same advantages also hold for F-L and tension-area (T-A) diagrams,[27] as discussed later.

The first advantage of the P-V diagram is that the area within the P-V loop drawn in each contraction quantifies the EW produced by the contraction of any chamber (see Fig. 5–2A). Usually the P-V loop rotates counterclockwise, and EW is produced by the cardiac chamber. When the P-V loop is merely a vertical line in an isovolumic contraction, EW is zero. When the P-V loop becomes clockwise in

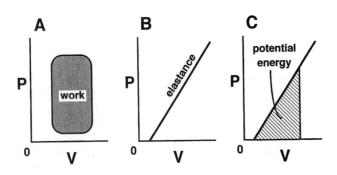

Advantages of the pressure-volume (P-V) diagram in cardiac function studies. *A*, P-V loop area of a contraction quantifies external or mechanical work of the cardiac chamber, whether atrial or ventricular and right or left. *B*, P-V line or curve drawn in the P-V diagram quantifies the elastance of the cardiac chamber. Linearity is not a prerequisite. *C*, Area (*hatched area*) under the elastance line or curve quantifies elastic or mechanical potential energy stored in the chamber. The advantage of *B* has led to the concept of Emax. Combining the advantages of *A* and *C* has led to the concept of the PVA.

abnormal contractions, the work is imposed from outside the cardiac chamber, and this work is called *negative* or *absorbed work*.

Another advantage is that a P-V relation line or curve drawn by changing a ventricular (or any chamber) volume in a certain contractile state represents an elastic property of the cardiac chamber (Fig. 5–2B). The steeper the P-V slope is, the greater the elastance of the chamber. (*Elastance* is defined as change of pressure divided by change of volume; it is the reciprocal of compliance.) As mentioned previously, this advantage led to the discovery of Emax as an index of ventricular contractility by Suga in the late 1960s.[5] A time-varying elastance concept emerged for the contracting ventricle, which has first a counterclockwise (in systole) and then a clockwise (in diastole) rotating P-V line or curve with respect to time within each cardiac cycle.[5,28,29]

The next advantage is that the area under a given P-V relation line or curve represents elastic PE (see Fig. 5–2C). This is easily understandable by considering a Hookean spring and its PE when extended. This energy concept holds whether the relation is linear or not. Steepening of the curve means that the PE has been increased, whether it comes from inside or outside. Flattening of the curve means that PE has been lost. This advantage led to the discovery of the systolic P-V area (PVA) as a measure of total mechanical energy by Suga in the 1970s.[6-8,30] PVA is developed during each ventricular contraction as the time-varying elastance increases. A variable part of this PE is convertible into EW.

CONTRACTILITY INDEX: EMAX

Figure 5–3 illustrates the basis that qualifies Emax as a ventricular contractility index. Physiologically and theoretically, the ESPVR as a whole, whether linear or curved, is important for understanding ventricular function.[1,5-8,28,29] If the ESPVR were as sensitively dependent on loading conditions, including afterload and contraction mode, in mammalian hearts as in the frog ventricle,[2,3] the simplicity of the ESPVR and hence its utility would be tremendously reduced. Fortunately, however, the ESPVR proved to be fairly linear and largely independent of loading conditions, as first discovered in the canine LV and gradually confirmed in the canine right ventricle and both atria.[1]

In addition to the ESPVR, the ventricular P-V relation at any intermediate time of contraction between the ends of diastole and systole proved to be fairly linear. It rotates counterclockwise during systole and clockwise during diastole, closely around a fulcrum point (V_0) on the volume axis.[1,5-8,28,29] More precisely, the true fulcrum volume point (V_d), which is positive (5 to 6 ml in a 50 to 80 g LV) is 10 to 20 mm Hg below the volume axis in the negative pressure range, and the volume-axis intercept shifts with contraction from the end-diastolic unstressed volume (V_u = 10 to 20 ml) to the end-systolic unstressed volume (V_0 = 6 to 8 ml).[31] During diastole, the volume-axis intercept shifts backward. This shift causes ventricular suction during the early ventricular filling phase, despite no posi-

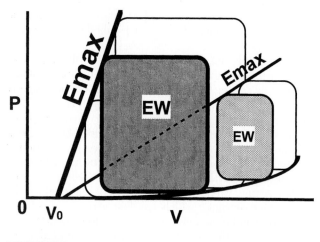

Ventricular pressure-volume (P-V) diagram with two end-systolic P-V relation lines with a high (larger letters) and low (smaller letters) Emax. The stronger ventricle with the larger Emax is considered to represent a greater recruitability of attached cross-bridges per unit increment in ventricular volume. The weaker ventricle with the smaller Emax is considered to represent a smaller recruitability of attached cross-bridges per unit increment in ventricular volume. Increasing ventricular volume extends sarcomeres leading to an increasing number of attached cross-bridges in the respective heart or contractile state. The same end-diastolic P-V relation is reasonably common to the same heart under acute inotropic interventions but may, however, vary with chronic inotropic interventions. EW = external work.

tive transmural filling pressure.[31] This family of rotating P-V relations supported the view that the ventricular chamber can be simulated as a time-varying elastic chamber. The entire time course of the time-varying elastance of the ventricle was denoted by $E(t)$.[1,5–8,28,29] $E(t)$ curves of isovolumic and physiologic contractions proved to be almost superimposable.[1,5–8,28,29] Emax is denoted as the peak of the $E(t)$ curve.

In the P-V diagram, the Emax corresponds to the slope of the linearized ESPVR of a cardiac chamber, whether a right ventricle, LV, or atrium. In adult canine hearts, the LV P-V loops under a stable inotropic background are located at various regions of the P-V diagram and have different heights, widths, and shapes, depending on preload (end-diastolic volume) and afterload (mainly arterial pressure). The left upper shoulders of these P-V loops, however, are on or close to a diagonal line, as shown in Figure 5–3. The relation appears linear or slightly curvilinear in adult canine heart chambers within physiologic loading and contractile conditions.[1,28,29] This relation is the ESPVR. Emax is the slope of the linearized ESPVR. For this reason, Emax is alternatively called end-systolic elastance (Ees), although there is a subtle difference of definition between the two terms.[1]

The ESPVRs we obtained in canine blood-perfused LVs, right ventricles, and both atria have usually been linear or slightly curvilinear in controlled, enhanced, or depressed contractile states.[1,28,29] When the relation is only slightly curvilinear, it can be approximated by a straight line, and hence its slope can be represented by Emax. It becomes, however, obviously convex upward with markedly enhanced contractility and convex downward with markedly depressed contractility in adult canine

LV.[1,32] In puppy LV, the ESPVR was convex upward in any of the controlled, enhanced, or depressed contractile states.[1,33] In rat LV, the ESPVR was convex upward in control contractility, but the convexity tended to decrease as contractility decreased.[34] The ESPVR was linear in a human LV with constrictive pericarditis when its P-V relation was measured directly in the excised, blood-perfused preparation.[35] When the ESPVR is far from linear, Emax cannot simply represent the entire ESPVR. If this happens, the position of the entire ESPVR, the slope and height parameters of its mathematical formula,[33] or the ESPVR height at a specified volume[34] can be used to judge contractility and its changes. For example, Teitel and associates[36] used V_{14} because 14 kPa was the starting mean arterial pressure of the lambs that they studied.

The linear ESPVR gives the remarkable advantage of allowing comparison of the global contractility of a cardiac chamber by a single index, Emax. When the ESPVR is curved, such an obvious advantage disappears, but the ESPVR as a whole still characterizes the upper boundary that P-V loops can reach. Moreover, the nonlinear ESPVR does not affect the physiologic significance of the energetic PVA concept, which derives from the $E(t)$ model,[33] as described later.

The ESPVR is not completely independent of the loading conditions.[1] The P-V loop tends to exceed the ESPVR when the ejection fraction is relatively low, a phenomenon known as *shortening activation* or *ejecting activation*. The P-V loop does not reach the ESPVR when the ejection fraction is relatively large, a phenomenon known as *shortening deactivation* or *ejecting deactivation*. The P-V loop tangentially touches the ESPVR at intermediate ejection fractions. As a whole, the isovolumic ESPVR appears largely linear in intermediate contractile states, and the ejecting ESPVR appears slightly sigmoidal around the linear ESPVR.[1] The shape of the ejecting ESPVR is slightly dependent on how afterload and preload are changed and fixed.[1] Nevertheless, these changes are usually smaller than the extent of the contractility-dependent shift of the ESPVR with positive and negative inotropic interventions.[1,28,29] The ejecting activation and deactivation seem to be caused by modulation of the Ca^{2+} responsiveness of the contractile machinery as a function of myocardial length and shortening velocity, but the mechanisms remain to be elucidated.

Acutely enhanced contractility is characterized by a steeper ESPVR and thus an increased Emax (see Fig. 5–3).[1,28,29] This means that end-systolic pressures at any volumes are increased. Such changes have been reported not only in canine hearts but also in the hearts of various other animal species, including humans.[1] The causes of enhanced contractility are varied, for example, β-receptor agonists (catecholamines), phosphodiesterase inhibitors, extracellular increased Ca^{2+}, Ca^{2+} channel agonists, Ca^{2+} sensitizers (new cardiotonic agents), paired pulse stimulation, postextrasystolic potentiation, Bowditch's (or staircase) phenomenon, and hypothermia.[26,37] Enhanced contractility is more directly caused by increased sarcoplasmic Ca^{2+} release, increased Ca^{2+} sensitivity (or responsiveness) of contractile proteins, or both.[26]

Chronic interventions, such as hypertensive hypertrophy, also increase Emax as long as concentric hypertrophy is maintained. Cardiac growth, however, tends to decrease Emax, despite increased normal myocardial mass. This is because the slope of the ESPVR decreases as the volume of the chamber increases with growth, so that Emax (as the ratio of pressure over the increased volume) decreases even without any decrease in myocardial contractility. In other words, Emax per se does not indicate myocardial contractility, although it characterizes ventricular contractility as a whole.[38] This aspect must be remembered when Emax values of different hearts with different sizes are compared.

Acutely depressed contractility is characterized by a less steep ESPVR and hence a decreased Emax. This means that end-systolic pressures at any given volume are decreased (see Fig. 5–3). Such changes have been reported not only in canine hearts but also in the hearts of various other animal species, including humans. The causes of depressed contractility include β-adrenergic blockade, Ca^{2+} antagonists, pentobarbital and other anesthetics, low coronary perfusion, increased asynchrony by ventricular pacing or intraventricular block, acidosis, postischemic or postacidotic stunning, hyperthermia, ryanodine, and thapsigargin.[26,37,39] In these failing hearts, the basic mechanisms are depression of Ca^{2+} handling or sensitivity and ATP production. Intracellular mechanisms underlying the depressed contractility are mostly opposite to those for enhanced contractility.

Chronic ventricular dilatation is accompanied by a considerably flattened ESPVR and thus a decreased Emax. These reductions are theoretically more than the decrease in myocardial contractility because increased myocardial volume itself reduces Emax, which is then further lowered by the decreased contractility.[38]

How can we compare Emax values of different hearts, or even the same hearts, before and after a change of cardiac mass? In normal growth, normalization of Emax for 100 g LV is reasonable. Because the unit of Emax is mm Hg/ml, its normalization for 100 g LV must be mm Hg/(ml/100 g) or mm Hg · ml^{-1} · 100 g, but not (mm Hg/ml)/100 g or mm Hg · ml^{-1} · 100 g^{-1}. This simple per unit weight normalization, however, does not guarantee Emax normalization when ventricular weight has been changed by hypertrophy, dilatation, or their regression. A theoretical solution would be to normalize Emax by V_0 to obtain Emax · V_0.[38] However, because the determination of V_0 is not always reliable, normalization remains a practical problem.

Regional ischemia depresses ventricular contractility as a whole. It does not, however, simply decrease the slope of ESPVR and Emax. Rather, it shifts the ESPVR to the right.[1,40] Therefore, the slope or Emax per se may erroneously characterize contractility in these regionally ischemic hearts. This strange response can be better understood by assuming that there are two components of the ventricle, one normal and the other depressed. Intraventricular pressures are the same in both compartments, and the ventricular volume is the sum of the volumes of the two compartments. By increasing ventricular volume, ventricular pressure is developed, but the distribution of the volume between the two compartments is not equal because the compliant compartment is more distended. As a whole, the depressed ESPVR becomes a downward con-

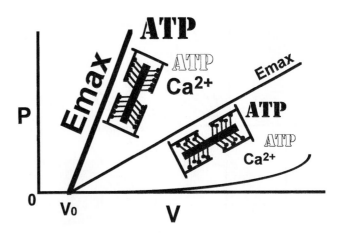

FIGURE 5–4

Ventricular pressure-volume (P-V) diagram with two end-systolic P-V relation lines with a high (larger letters) and a low (smaller letters) Emax. The stronger ventricle with the larger Emax can recruit more attached cross-bridges per unit increment in ventricular volume owing to a greater amount of released Ca^{2+} in the excitation-contraction (E-C) coupling. The weaker ventricle with the smaller Emax can recruit fewer attached cross-bridges per unit increment in ventricular volume owing to a smaller amount of released Ca^{2+} in the E-C coupling. Increasing ventricular volume extends sarcomeres, leading to increasing Ca^{2+} sensitivity of the contractile proteins and increasing number of attached cross-bridges in the respective heart or contractile state. More cross-bridge cycling and Ca^{2+} handling require more energy (ATP and oxygen consumption), as expressed by the letter size of ATP. The same end-diastolic P-V relation is reasonably common to the same heart under acute inotropic interventions but may vary with chronic inotropic interventions.

vex curve and is shifted to the right of the control ESPVR.[40]

What does Emax represent? Emax indicates the magnitude of the Starling effect or the incremental pressure per unit increment in volume in a cardiac chamber.[41] When the chamber volume is increased, myocardial fibers and thus sarcomeres are stretched. Contractile force increases as the sarcomere is stretched, as a consequence of an increased number of cross-bridges.[26] Therefore, Emax quantifies the degree of recruitment of cross-bridges per unit increment in ventricular volume (Fig. 5–4).[41] Thus, Emax has a physiologically sound basis in the contractile mechanism of muscle. A linear ESPVR and thus a constant Emax, however, do not mean that cross-bridge recruitment is a linear function of sarcomere length, because both the force-pressure relation (Laplace's law) and the sarcomere length-volume relation are nonlinear.

TOTAL MECHANICAL ENERGY: PRESSURE-VOLUME AREA

Up to this point, cardiac function has been characterized mechanically. Mechanical work production, however, requires energy from ATP and thus from metabolic substrates and O_2.[6] The two major ATP-consuming processes are cross-bridge cycling and ion (primarily Ca^{2+}) handling (see Fig. 5–4).

The time-varying elastance model of the LV theoretically deduced a new measure of total mechanical energy (PVA) as a new key concept of cardiac mechanoenergetics

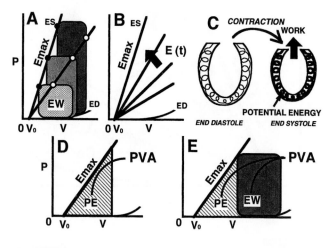

FIGURE 5–5

Deduction of the pressure-volume area (PVA) concept from the time-varying elastance model of the ventricle, which has also produced the Emax concept. *A,* Pressure-volume (P-V) diagram with three P-V loops. *Solid circles* on the left upper shoulders of the three P-V loops indicate end-systolic P-V points. The *diagonal line* whose slope is Emax connects the end-systolic P-V points and intercepts the volume axis at V_0. *Open circles* on the three loops are working P-V points at a specified time of systole. A diagonal line passes through these isochronal points and intercepts the volume axis at V_0. Emax = end-systolic P-V ratio or maximum elastance; ES = end systole; ED = end diastole; V_0 = volume-axis intercept of the Emax line; EW = external work. *B,* Time-varying P-V relation changes its slope as a function of time, *E(t).* Emax is the end-systolic maximum value of *E(t). C,* Time-varying elastance model of the ventricle. The elastance of the ventricular wall increases from an end-diastolic compliant level to the end-systolic stiff level. The increment in elastance (expressed as thickened spring) during contraction requires an increment in elastic potential energy and produces external work (EW) when ejection occurs against afterload. *D,* Triangular *(hatched)* area under the Emax line (or curve) on the origin side of an isovolumic P-V *line (vertical)* represents elastic potential energy (PE). The isovolumic PE represents the systolic PVA equivalent to the total mechanical energy generated by this isovolumic contraction. *E,* Total mechanical energy of an ejecting contraction consists of external work (EW; *shaded area*) within the P-V loop and elastic potential energy (PE; *hatched area*) under the Emax line on the origin side of the P-V loop. The sum of EW and PE represents the PVA of this ejecting contraction.

(Fig. 5–5).[6–8,30] The concept of PVA is related to the first and third advantages of the P-V diagram (see Fig. 5–1).

As discussed previously, Frank, Starling, and Sarnoff all tried and failed to equate EW to MVO_2.[2,10,11,19] The concept of IW became explicit only after Hill introduced the two- or three-element model of skeletal muscle (contractile element plus series and parallel elastic elements) into cardiac physiology.[22] IW is the mechanical work done on the series elastic element by contraction of the contractile element. To quantify IW, series elasticity was determined by quick release, usually of isolated muscle strips. The simple sum of EW and IW, however, did not correlate closely with MVO_2; instead, EW + nIW (where n = 2 or 3) showed a better correlation with MVO_2.[22] This greater energy requirement for IW than EW has been used as the explanation for greater O_2 use by pressure than volume work despite the same EW.[18] Nevertheless, the mechanism for this difference remained unexplained until the concept of PVA was introduced.[6,42]

PVA stands for a specific P-V area that is circumscribed by the ESPVR, the end-diastolic pressure-volume relation,

and the systolic P-V trajectory.[6,30] It consists of EW and a new area (PE) that was postulated to represent mechanical energy (see Fig. 5–5).[1,6,30] PE had not been given previous attention because the concept of PE required a specific model of the time-varying elastance of the cardiac chambers.[6,30] Although an original version of the time-varying elastance model of muscle had been proposed for skeletal muscle in the early 1900s, the model did not predict an important energetic feature called the *Fenn effect*, that is, an extra energy utilization for external mechanical work for a given tension development.[43] This failure totally eliminated the time-varying elastance concept in skeletal muscle physiology. The cardiac Fenn effect, however, proved to be substantially different from the skeletal one,[44] and the predicted energies from the cardiac time-varying elastance model matched the cardiac version of the Fenn effect.[45]

The PVA seems to be closest to the total energy of contraction that Starling sought.[10,11,41] Assuming that the time-varying elastic nature of the beating heart comes from cross-bridge cycling, PVA can be considered to represent the total mechanical energy produced by cross-bridge cycling (Fig. 5–6). For this reason, PVA was thought to be more likely than other methods to correlate with MVO_2.[6,30] In fact, PVA proved to be the most reliable predictor or determinant of MVO_2 in a huge series of experiments,[6,37,39] and this relation has been supported thermodynamically.[46,47]

PVA is a specific area in the P-V diagram, and hence its unit is mm Hg · ml.[6,30,37] Do not confuse this unit with the Emax unit of mm Hg/ml; the former is a unit of energy, whereas the latter is a unit of elastance. The unit mm Hg · ml may not appear to be a unit of energy, but it is the same as EW. Physically, 1 mm Hg · ml equals 1.33×10^{-4}J, where J (joule) is the standard unit of energy. Biochemically, 1 ml O_2 is equivalent to 19 to 21 J (average 20 J) in the myocardium.

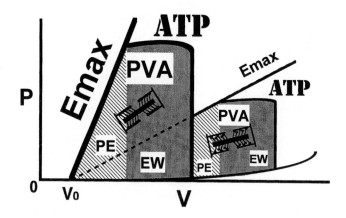

FIGURE 5–6

A stronger heart with a greater Emax can produce greater external work (EW) and systolic pressure-volume area (PVA) from a smaller end-diastolic volume against a higher afterload. A weaker heart with a smaller Emax produces smaller EW and PVA from a higher end-diastolic volume against a lower afterload. More ATP is consumed for the greater PVA. The same end-diastolic P-V relation is reasonably common to the same heart under acute inotropic interventions but may vary with chronic inotropic interventions. Sarcomeres and cross-bridges imply that PVA is their mechanical energy output. PE = potential energy.

The energetic equivalence of the PVA qualifies it to be a candidate to predict MVO_2. By contrast, none of the conventional predictors of MVO_2, such as tension, tension-time integral, peak pressure, pressure-time integral, double product, triple product, dP/dt_{max} $(dP/dt_{max})/IIT$ (integrated isometric tension), have a unit of energy.[1,26] The reason why these non–energy-related parameters were so eagerly used to predict MVO_2 was because EW had failed to be a useful predictor.

In studies of Emax and PVA, accurate pressure and volume measurements of the cardiac chamber are mandatory. The best preparation for these measurements seems to be the excised, cross-circulated heart.[1,29] This preparation can be made without myocardial ischemia. It is advantageous because the heart is independent of autonomic nervous regulation, and the LV does not have to support the peripheral circulation. When a balloon is fitted in the LV and filled with water, LV volume can be measured accurately and precisely controlled with a volume servopump.[1] This preparation can also be used in guinea pigs and rats.[48] The advent of the conductance catheter[36,49] has allowed accurate volume measurements to be made in intact hearts in a variety of species, including humans.

MYOCARDIAL OXYGEN CONSUMPTION–PRESSURE-VOLUME AREA–ELASTANCE RELATION

Figure 5–7 shows the MVO_2-PVA-Emax relationship established experimentally.[6] In this framework, MVO_2 is always per beat and not per minute. Canine blood-perfused LV experiments always showed high correlation and linear regression of MVO_2 per beat on PVA in a stable contractile state (see Fig. 5–7B).[6-8,37,39] The regression remained reasonably unique if preload and afterload varied widely, that is, no matter how the fractional PE or EW is varied in the PVA.[6] The MVO_2-PVA relations are virtually superimposable between isovolumic and ejecting contractions.[6] MVO_2 for the same PVA remains unchanged, even when pressure-time integral and force-time integral change widely with altered preload and afterload.[6,50] To test that PVA = EW + PE is the unique determinant of MVO_2, the correlation between MVO_2 and PVA = EW + kPE revealed that the correlation was maximal when k was virtually unity.[51] These features of PVA qualify it to be superior to any other conventional methods of predicting MVO_2.

When afterload pressure during relaxation was gradually unloaded, the LV continued ejection and produced EW even after end systole. Surprisingly, the amount of extra EW was nearly 100% of PE.[52] More surprisingly, MVO_2 for the same PVA remained constant, regardless of the amount of extra EW produced from what would otherwise have been the PE area.[52] Furthermore, when the EW area is eroded by advancing ventricular filling, PE increases without changing PVA and MVO_2.[53] These facts further support the value of PVA as a predictor or determinant of MVO_2.[6]

If one examines the MVO_2-PVA relation rigorously, an exception occurs with a relatively high afterload and preload and a relatively small ejection fraction.[54] Such an ejection exhibits ejecting activation, that is, a greater Emax

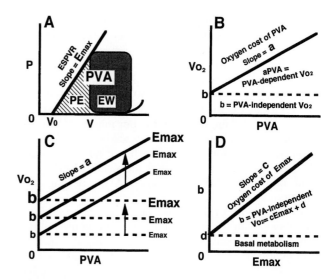

FIGURE 5–7

Diagrams of the standard oxygen (O_2) consumption (VO_2)-PVA-Emax relationship. *A,* Definitions of Emax and PVA (=PE + EW). Emax = slope of end-systolic P-V relation (ESPVR) line, end-systolic P/V ratio, or maximum elastance. V_0 = volume-axis intercept of the Emax line. PVA = systolic P-V area representing total mechanical energy. PE *(hatched area)* = elastic potential energy. EW *(shaded area)* = external work. *B,* VO_2-PVA relation. VO_2 = VO_2 per beat in steady-state (nonarrhythmic) beats. VO_2 consists of two fractions: PVA-dependent VO_2 (aPVA) *(upper, wedge)* and PVA-independent VO_2 (b) *(lower, band).* Slope a of the VO_2-PVA relation represents O_2 cost of PVA. *C,* Increases in Emax (ventricular contractility) elevate the VO_2-PVA relation in a parallel manner. Namely, b increases with Emax (as expressed by increasing letter sizes) but a does not change. *D,* PVA-independent VO_2 (=b = cEmax + d)-Emax relation. c = O_2 cost of Emax. d = basal metabolism. O_2 cost of Emax is constant for ordinary acute inotropic interventions, such as β-receptor stimulation, increased Ca^{2+}, phosphodiesterase inhibition, and high coronary perfusion (positive inotropism), or β-receptor blockade, Ca^{2+} channel blockade, low coronary perfusion, and anesthesia (negative inotropism). See text.

than expected from the isovolumic ESPVR.[1] When this occurs, MVO_2 is slightly but systematically smaller than expected from the PVA and Emax. The underlying mechanism may be related to modulation of Ca^{2+} handling by myocardial shortening due to a slight decrease in Ca^{2+} sensitivity during sarcomere shortening, followed by Ca^{2+} rebinding to troponin C.[54]

The empirical equation, as shown in Figure 5–7B,[1,6,37,39] for the reasonably unique and linear MVO_2-PVA relation is

$$MVO_2 = aPVA + b$$

where $aPVA$ is the PVA-dependent MVO_2, a is the O_2 cost of PVA (see later), and b is the PVA-independent MVO_2, which is assumed to be constant at any PVA that changes with preload.

MVO_2 is usually expressed in milliliters of O_2 per minute, because it is not directly measurable in each beat. It is better, however, to express MVO_2 in milliliters of O_2 per beat so that it can be correlated with PVA in mm Hg · ml/beat. Changes in heart rate from 80 to 220 beats/min do not affect the MVO_2-PVA relation per beat in the canine LV.[1,6,55] As the heart rate, however, decreases below 80 beats/min, the MVO_2-PVA relation tends to elevate.[56] This phenomenon can be explained by the fact that MVO_2 measured per beat includes basal metabolic MVO_2, which is fairly constant and independent of heart rate. As heart rate decreases, therefore, the proportion of basal metabolic MVO_2 gradually increases hyperbolically. This effect is relatively small at heart rates above 80 beats/min,[55] but it begins to elevate the MVO_2-PVA relation at heart rates below 80 beats/min. When, however, the per minute MVO_2-PVA relations at two different heart rates are compared, the relation is higher for the higher heart rate. Therefore, whether heart rate is a major determinant of MVO_2 depends on whether MVO_2 per beat or MVO_2 per minute is considered.

The MVO_2-PVA relation ascends in an enhanced Emax and descends in a depressed Emax when contractility is changed with conventional inotropic agents such as β-adrenergic receptor agonists and blockers, Ca^{2+} agonists and blockers, phosphodiesterase inhibitors, and pentobarbital (Fig. 5–8A, B; see Fig. 5–7C).[1,6,37] However, some exceptional inotropic interventions do not shift the MVO_2-PVA relation, which is expected from the changes in Emax (see Fig. 5–8C). These exceptions are discussed below.

These shifts of the MVO_2-PVA relation are ordinarily parallel with changes in b without a change in a, as shown in Figure 5–7C.[1,6,37] This indicates that inotropism primarily affects PVA-independent MVO_2 rather than the O_2 cost of PVA. Therefore, an empirical equation to describe a family of these MVO_2-PVA relation lines is

$$MVO_2 = aPVA + b = aPVA + cEmax + d$$

where $cEmax$ is Emax-dependent MVO_2, c is the O_2 cost of Emax, and d is basal metabolism.[6,37]

When the changes in PVA-independent MVO_2 are plotted against corresponding Emax values, a linear PVA-independent MVO_2-Emax relation is obtained, as in Figure 5–7D.[6,37] An empirical equation to describe this relation is

$$\text{PVA-independent } MVO_2 = b = cEmax + d$$

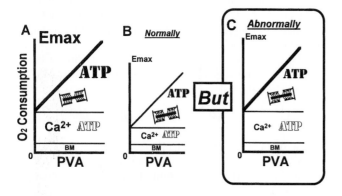

FIGURE 5–8

Normal and abnormal negative inotropic interventions and resultant O_2 consumption-PVA relations. A, Control contractile state. B, Normally depressed contractile state by ordinary negative inotropic agents. C, Abnormally depressed contractile state by postischemic stunning, postacidotic stunning, and acidosis, where the O_2 consumption-PVA relation does not descend, unlike the ordinary negative inotropism (B). Letter sizes of Emax, Ca^{2+}, and ATP show their quantitative differences. BM = basal metabolism; PVA = pressure-volume area.

where the slope c of this relation is fairly constant for conventional inotropic agents.[6,37] Conventional inotropic agents move a working b-Emax point upward along the standard b-Emax line, whereas conventional negative inotropic agents move the working point downward along the same line.

Exceptional instances (see Fig. 5–7C) in which PVA-independent MVO_2 does not decrease in proportion to depressed Emax include postischemic stunning,[57] postacidotic stunning,[58] and acidosis.[59]

OXYGEN COST OF PRESSURE-VOLUME AREA

The slope a of the MVO_2-PVA relation obtained under various preloading and afterloading conditions is fairly constant at any Emax level (see Figs. 5–7C and 5–8). This slope represents the O_2 cost of PVA because it indicates how much more O_2 a unit increment in PVA requires. It is on average 1.7×10^{-5} ml O_2/(mm Hg · ml), ranging from 1.4 to 2.0×10^{-5} ml O_2/(mm Hg · ml). This value is automatically normalized for LV mass. The value becomes 2.5 (dimensionless) after both 1 ml O_2 (at standard temperature 0°C and pressure 1 atm, dry) and 1 mm Hg · ml are converted to 20 J and 1.33×10^{-4} J respectively, to have the same units of energy.[6,37]

This value of 2.5 represents a contractile efficiency of 0.40 (=1/2.5) or 40%.[6,37,60–62] This efficiency is considered to consist of the chemochemical efficiency to produce ATP by consuming metabolic substrates and O_2, and the chemomechanical efficiency to produce mechanical energy by hydrolyzing ATP. The former efficiency reflects the oxidative phosphorylation efficiency (P:O ratio) of 3. The major metabolic substrates of the heart under aerobic conditions are lactate, glucose, and free fatty acids. Enthalpy values of consuming 1 ml O_2 for these substrates are 20 ± 1 J. Because the enthalpy of ATP is 48 kJ/mol in the myocardium, 6 mol of ATP have an enthalpy of 288 kJ. Dividing this enthalpy by the enthalpy of 44 kJ for 1 mol O_2 (=22.4 × 20) yields 0.64 or 64%.[60]

Dividing the contractile efficiency ($1/a$) of 0.40 or 40% by this O_2-to-ATP efficiency of 0.64 or 64% yields an ATP-to-PVA efficiency of 0.63 or 63%.[6,60] This resultant efficiency is reasonably attributable to the cross-bridge cycling in a twitch contraction. General constancy of the slope a of the MVO_2-PVA relation at any Emax level, therefore, seems to indicate general constancy of the efficiency of cross-bridge cycling.[6,37,60] One exception is a steeper slope of the MVO_2-PVA relation of the hyperthyroid rabbit LV in the standard excised cross-circulated heart preparation.[61] This increased slope suggests a decreased contractile efficiency, possibly due to the dominant V_1 type of isomyosin.[61] Another exception is a 10 to 20% decreased slope of the MVO_2-PVA relation of canine failing LV induced by acute and chronic interventions.[57–59] How these types of heart failure decrease the MVO_2-PVA slope remains to be determined. If the efficiency of cross-bridge cycling is actually increased in failing hearts, the underlying mechanisms would be most interesting because they might give insight into how to increase contractile efficiency.

CROSS-BRIDGE CYCLING

The contractile efficiency of 40% and the calculated cross-bridge cycling efficiency of 64% mentioned previously allow indirect estimation of the number of cross-bridge cycles in each contraction. The efficiency of 64% is only slightly smaller than the thermodynamic efficiency of cross-bridges.[47,60] This suggests that each cross-bridge effectively converts chemical energy of ATP into mechanical energy as assessed in terms of PVA, nearly all of which could be converted into EW.[52] The concentration of cross-bridges is about 150 μmol/kg wet weight of myocardium. If all these cross-bridges cycle once by hydrolyzing one ATP per cycle,[12] the amount of hydrolyzed ATP would be 150 μmol/kg wet weight. This, multiplied by the enthalpy of ATP of 48 kJ/mol and the efficiency of 64% yields mechanical energy of 7.2 J/kg or 0.72 J/100 g/beat, which corresponds to a PVA of 5400 mm Hg · ml. This PVA seems to be the maximum available value, as extrapolated from the routine maximal values obtained experimentally. This correspondence suggests that each cross-bridge cycles roughly about once or twice on average in each cardiac cycle.[60]

OXYGEN COST OF EMAX

The slope of the PVA-independent MVO_2-Emax represents the O_2 cost of Emax (Fig. 5–9).[6,37] The consistent linearity of this relation means constancy of this O_2 cost. It is largely constant for ordinary positive and negative inotropes in normal canine hearts.[6,37] Although Ca^{2+} sensitizers were expected to decrease the O_2 cost of Emax, they did not do so in normal hearts.[1,37]

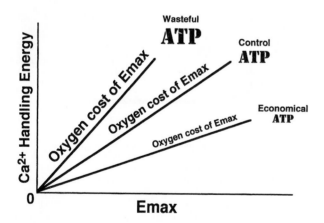

FIGURE 5–9

Ca^{2+} handling energy (or PVA-independent MVO_2 minus basal metabolism)-Emax relations and their slopes, O_2 cost of Emax in control, wasteful, and economic hearts. Control hearts have intermediate O_2 cost of Emax as represented by the intermediate letter size of adenosine triphosphate (ATP). Wasteful hearts such as postischemic stunned hearts, acidotic hearts, postacidotic stunned hearts, and hyperthermic hearts have a greater O_2 cost of Emax as represented by the large letter size of ATP. Economic hearts such as hypothermic hearts have a smaller O_2 cost of Emax as represented by the small letter size of ATP. A wasteful heart requires more O_2 consumption for a given Emax as well as for a given increment in Emax.

The O_2 cost of Emax, however, was increased 50 to 100% in failing hearts produced by hypercapnic acidosis as well as by stunning induced by either 15-minute ischemia followed by 1-hour reperfusion or acute correction of hypercapnic acidosis.[57–59] The increased O_2 cost of Emax means that the extra MVO_2 for each unit increment in Emax is increased. This increased O_2 cost of Emax is observed when Emax is enhanced with Ca^{2+} or epinephrine in these failing hearts. However, interestingly, Ca^{2+} sensitizers partially or largely correct this abnormally increased O_2 cost of Emax.[62] This beneficial effect is the one that has been expected from their pharmacologic action.[63]

When the LV is paced at different sites, Emax decreases as compared with normal atrioventricular conduction at a fixed heart rate, but PVA-independent MVO_2 remains unchanged.[64] Temperature changes of the heart affect the O_2 cost of Emax considerably; hypothermia to 30°C doubles Emax but does not elevate the MVO_2-PVA relation.[65] This indicates that the PVA-independent MVO_2 does not change despite the increase in Emax, namely, the O_2 cost of Emax is virtually zero.[65]

The greater O_2 cost of Emax as indicated by the steeper slope of the b-Emax relation means an ATP-wasteful heart. The smaller O_2 cost of Emax as indicated by the flatter slope of the b-Emax relation means an ATP-economical heart. The three diagonal lines in Figure 5–9 illustrate the mechanoenergetic differences of these hearts. The ordinate shows Ca^{2+} handling energy (or MVO_2) after basal metabolism is subtracted from the PVA-independent MVO_2.

CA^{2+} HANDLING ENERGY

Myocardial Ca^{2+} handling may remind most readers of Ca^{2+} transient or sarcoplasmic free Ca^{2+} concentration, which is of the order of 0.1 to 1 μmol/L.[63,66] The total amount of Ca^{2+}, however, released into the sarcoplasm and removed by consuming energy in each excitation-contraction coupling is of the order of 10 to 100 μmol/kg myocardial wet weight.[66] ATP consumption for this much Ca^{2+} handling is therefore of the order of 5 to 50 μmol/kg if all the calcium is assumed to be handled by the sarcoplasmic reticulum–Ca^{2+} pump, which removes Ca^{2+} with $2Ca^{2+}$:1ATP stoichiometry.[66] This ATP consumption would correspond at most to a third or half of the ATP consumption for cross-bridge cycling in normal beats.

Part of the total Ca^{2+} pump handling, however, is known to be processed by the trans-sarcolemmal route via the Na^+-Ca^{2+} exchange, Ca^{2+} pump, and Ca^{2+} channel (Fig. 5–10).[66] This external route has an overall stoichiometry of $1Ca^{2+}$:1ATP, half that of the sarcoplasmic reticulum Ca^{2+} pump.[66] Although no direct method is available yet to measure the total Ca^{2+} amount handled with each excitation-contraction coupling in the beating whole heart,[64] internal Ca^{2+} recirculation fraction as determined from the decay of postextrasystolic potentiation[67] enables us to quantitate the total handling and its internal and external fractions when the recirculation factor is combined with Ca^{2+} handling energy.[68] This new integrative approach may allow better understanding of the pathophysiologic Ca^{2+} handling in failing hearts with an abnormal O_2 cost of Emax.[68]

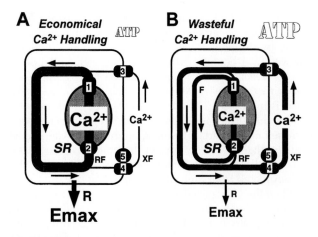

FIGURE 5–10

Economic Ca^{2+} handling *(A)* vs. wasteful Ca^{2+} handling *(B)*. In *A*, the major Ca^{2+} handling route is intracellular. Namely, most Ca^{2+} is released from the sarcoplasmic reticulum (SR) via its Ca^{2+} release channel *(1)* and sequestered by the SR via the Ca^{2+} pump ATPase *(2)*. Minor Ca^{2+} handling route is trans-sarcolemmal. Namely, some Ca^{2+} is extruded via the Na^+-Ca^{2+} exchange *(4)* and enters via the sarcolemmal Ca^{2+} channel *(3)*. The exchanged Na^+ is extruded by the Na^+/K^+ pump *(5)* in a steady-state beat for Na^+ homeostasis. The former fraction is internal recirculation fraction (RF) and the latter is extrusion fraction (XF). The internal route has a $2Ca^{2+}$: 1ATP stoichiometry, whereas the external route has a $1Ca^{2+}$: 1ATP stoichiometry, half of the former. The latter is therefore twice as wasteful or ATP consuming. When RF decreases and XF increases reciprocally, Ca^{2+} handling becomes more wasteful, as in *B*. In addition, if the SR becomes leaky to Ca^{2+}, Ca^{2+} is abnormally released from the SR and sequestered again by the SR Ca^{2+} pump. This Ca^{2+} cycling (F) is futile and energy wasting without contributing to contractility (Emax). When the reactivity (R) of Emax to total Ca^{2+} handling decreases, Ca^{2+} handling becomes also wasteful for Emax. Letter sizes of Emax, Ca^{2+}, ATP, and R show their quantitative differences.

ARTERIAL AND VENOUS COUPLING AND MATCHING

CIRCULATORY EQUILIBRIUM

Circulatory equilibrium, a key cardiovascular concept developed by Guyton, determines steady-state CO and VR as the circulatory equilibrium intersection of the CO and VR curves (Fig. 5–11).[16] Here the entire heart and the pulmonary circulation are lumped into a single heart-lung pump; the same concept is applicable to the right and left sides of the hearts separately.[1] The CO curve is an increasing function of cardiac filling pressure and the VR curve is a decreasing function of the same filling pressure on the common x axis. The CO curve characterizes the heart pump capability, whereas the VR curve characterizes the circulatory system other than the heart.[16] The circulatory equilibrium concept is mandatory for understanding cardiac function in situ and how CO is determined in situ.

EFFECTIVE ARTERIAL ELASTANCE

Ventricular contraction starts with a preload and ejects against an afterload, both of which are given by the circulatory equilibrium in steady state, although they can be assessed arbitrarily in transient beats. This ventriculoarterial

coupling is well described by the combination of Emax (or Ees) and effective arterial elastance (Ea).[1,69] Ea is the absolute value for the slope of the diagonal line connecting the end-diastolic volume point on the volume axis and the end-systolic P-V point of the ejecting P-V loop. Theoretically,

$$Ea = \text{end-systolic pressure/stroke volume}$$
$$= \text{end-systolic pressure/(CO/heart rate)}$$
$$= \text{total peripheral resistance} \times \text{heart rate}$$

with the same unit of mm Hg/ml as Emax. Different P-V loops with different preloads, afterloads, and stroke volumes could have the same Ea (see Fig. 5–11). What then determines a specific P-V loop when Ea is given is the circulatory equilibrium mentioned previously, as shown by the two arrows in Figure 5–11.

The ventriculoarterial coupling also determines the mechanical efficiency of EW from PVA and MVO_2.[1,70] EW/PVA is maximal at Ea/Emax = 1; EW/MVO_2 is maximal at an Ea/Emax variably smaller than 1. These Ea/Emax levels are considered to be optimal for the mechanoenergetic coupling of the heart with the afterload.[71] Ea/Emax ratio ranges around 0.5 to 1 in normal LVs but becomes greater than 1 in failing LVs.[71] Correction of

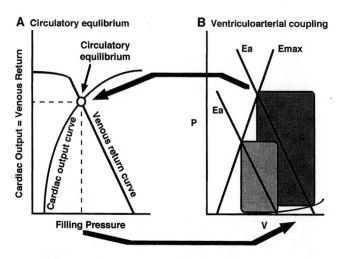

FIGURE 5–11

Circulatory equilibrium and ventriculoarterial coupling. *A* shows Guyton's circulatory equilibrium diagram. The increasing curve is a CO curve and the decreasing curve is a VR curve, both plotted against filling pressure. Their intersection indicates the circulatory equilibrium point that determines equilibrated cardiac output and filling pressure in steady state. *B* shows a ventricular P-V diagram with an Emax line, two Ea (effective arterial elastance) lines, and two P-V loops. In the ventricle with a given Emax, a variety of P-V loops with different combinations of ejection pressures (height) and stroke volume (width) and hence external work *(shaded area)* are possible. However, when Ea (=total peripheral resistance × heart rate) is given to the afterload, P-V loops are limited to those that match with Ea lines; namely, the absolute value for the slope of the line connecting end-systolic P-V point and end-diastolic volume on the volume (V) axis must be equal to Ea. The end-diastolic volume is given as a result of the equilibrated filling volume, as indicated by the *bottom arrow*. Then, stroke volume is given and hence the location and size of the P-V loop are specified. Stroke volume times heart rate specifies the equilibrated cardiac output, as indicated by the *top arrow*. Therefore, the ventriculoarterial coupling is a key determinant of the cardiac output curve.

the increased Ea/Emax to the normal level restores the optimal coupling.[72] The beauty of the Ea/Emax ratio is that it is dimensionless because Ea has the same unit as Emax.

MECHANOENERGETIC EQUIVALENCE IN CARDIAC WALL REGION AND MUSCLE

The greatest advantages of the P-V diagram and the mechanoenergetic concepts derived from it are their theoretically sound applicability to cardiac wall regions and muscles.[27,73,74] Cardiac wall regions and muscle are considered to be two-dimensional and one-dimensional muscle models, respectively, in contrast to a three-dimensional muscle model of the ventricle. As shown in Figure 5–12, the P-V diagram is equivalent to the T-A diagram of a wall region[27,74] and the F-L diagram of a muscle.[73] Here, T means surface-tension–like tension with units of circumferential force/circumferential length, whereas force simply has units of grams. The mentioned equivalence means that the areas within these P-V, T-A, and F-L diagrams all quantify mechanical work with energy units. This property derives from the ordinates of these three diagrams indicating stress and the abscissas, strain. An area in a stress-strain diagram quantifies work. Therefore, the mechanoenergetic properties developed on the basis of the P-V diagram are theoretically applicable to the T-A and F-L diagrams. In fact, by using a ventricular wall region and a papillary or trabecular muscle, the applicability of both Emax and PVA has been confirmed.[27,73,74] The end-systolic T-A and F-L relations become steeper with positive inotropism and become flatter with negative inotropism, although their end-systolic relations, which are called ESTAR and ESFLR, are usually curvilinear, and hence their slopes cannot simply be quantified by a single index such as Emax.

Furthermore, MVO$_2$ has been shown to correlate closely and linearly with not only PVA but also TAA (tension-area area) and FLA (force-length area).[27,73,74] Moreover, simply weight-proportional extrapolation of the MVO$_2$-TAA relation obtained in an LV wall region to the whole LV matches with the directly determined MVO$_2$-PVA in the LV.[27,74] The tension-ln(1/wall thickness) or T-ln(1/H) diagram has been shown to be equivalent to the T-A diagram.[75] Both T-A and T-ln(1/H) diagrams are useful to distinguish mechanoenergetics between normal and ischemic regions of the ventricular wall in a physiologically sound manner. The F-L diagram applied to a wall region may mislead us because L changes are not always isotropic. To incorporate the orthogonal L changes, the force-area diagram is used in place of the F-L or T-A diagram. However, the force-area diagram is inappropriate because the end-systolic force-area relation does not indicate a stress-strain relation, nor does the force-area represent mechanical work.[27,75]

SUMMARY

This chapter has emphasized a contemporary view for coherent understanding of cardiac function at the organ level. This view, however, is in the middle of the full spectrum of cardiac function studies ranging from genetic, molecular, and subcellular levels to whole body systems and environmental levels. The P-V diagram of the heart is therefore an excellent window to see how these microscopic and macroscopic or elementary and systemic levels interact and interfere with each other. The reader more interested in the details of the individual descriptions in this chapter is advised to read the author's review articles.[1,6–8,37,39,60,74]

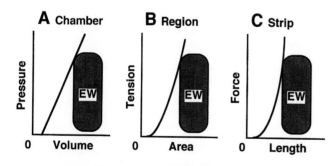

A Chamber **B** Region **C** Strip

Pressure / 0 Volume — Tension / 0 Area — Force / 0 Length — EW

FIGURE 5–12

Three theoretically equivalent diagrams in myocardial mechanoenergetics. *A*, Pressure-volume (P-V) diagram of a cardiac chamber. Units of the coordinates are usually mm Hg for pressure and ml for volume, and hence the unit of the area within the loop is mm Hg · ml. *B*, Tension-area diagram of a cardiac wall region. Units of the coordinates are usually g/cm for tension and cm^2 for wall area, and hence the unit of the area within the loop is g · cm. *C*, Force-length diagram of a cardiac muscle strip. Units of the coordinates are usually g for force and cm for length, and hence the unit of the area within the loop is g · cm. According to the convention of unit conversion, 1 g = 9.81×10^{-3} N (newton), and 1 mm Hg = 1.33×10^2 Pa (pascal = newton/m^2) = 1.36 g/cm^2. Hence 1 g = 9.81×10^{-5} J (joule), 1 mm Hg · ml = 1.33×10^{-4} J, or 1 J = 1.02×10^4 g · cm = 7.36×10^3 mm Hg · ml. EW = external work.

REFERENCES

1. Sagawa K, Maughan L, Suga H, Sunagawa K: Cardiac Contraction and the Pressure-Volume Relationship. New York, Oxford University Press, 1988.
2. Sagawa K, Lie RK, Schaefer J: Translation of Otto Frank's paper "Die Grundform des Arteriellen Pulses" Zeitschrift fur Biologie 37:483–526 (1899). J Mol Cell Cardiol 22:253, 1990.
3. Schmidt RF, Thews G (eds): Human Physiology. Berlin, Springer-Verlag, 1989.
4. Monroe RG, French GN: Left ventricular pressure-volume relationships and myocardial oxygen consumption in the isolated heart. Circ Res 9:362, 1961.
5. Suga H: Time course of left ventricular pressure-volume relationship under various enddiastolic volume. Jpn Heart J 10:509, 1969.
6. Suga H: Ventricular energetics. Physiol Rev 70:247, 1990.
7. Suga H: Paul Dudley White International Lecture: Cardiac performance as viewed through the pressure-volume window. Jpn Heart J 35:263, 1994.
8. Suga H: How we view systolic function of the heart: Emax and PVA. 1994 CSDS (Cardiac Systems Dynamics Society) Konrad Witzig lecture. *In* Ingels NB, Daughters GT, Baan J (eds): Systolic and Diastolic Function of the Heart. Burke, IOS Press, 1995.
9. Martin HN: A new method of studying the mammalian heart. Stud Biol Lab Johns Hopkins Univ 2:119, 1881.
10. Patterson SW, Piper H, Starling EH: The regulation of the heart beat. J Physiol (Lond) 48:465, 1914.
11. Starling EH: The Linacre Lecture on the Law of the Heart. London, Longmans, Green, 1918.
12. Huxley AF: Muscle structure and theories of contraction. Prog Biophys Chem 7:255, 1957.

13. CIBA Foundation Symposium 24 (new series): The Physiological Basis of Starling's Law of the Heart. Amsterdam, Elsevier, Excerpta Medica, North-Holland Associated Scientific Publishers, 1974.

14. ter Keurs HEDJ, Noble MIM: Starling's Law of the Heart Revisited. Dordrecht, the Netherlands, Kluwer Academic, 1988.

15. Prendergast BD, Sagach VF, Shah AM: Basal release of nitric oxide augments the Frank-Starling response in the isolated heart. Circulation 96:1320, 1997.

16. Guyton AC: Circulatory Physiology: Cardiac Output and Its Regulation. Philadelphia, WB Saunders, 1963.

17. Suga H: Incorporation of venous resistance in Togawa's four quadrant diagram for Guyton's circulatory equilibrium. Jpn Heart J 29:89, 1988.

18. Evans CL, Matsuoka Y: The effect of various mechanical conditions on the gaseous metabolism and efficiency of the mammalian heart. J Physiol (Lond) 49:378, 1915.

19. Sarnoff SJ, Mitchell JH: The control of the function of the heart. In Hamilton WF, Dow P (eds): Handbook of Physiology, Section 2: Circulation, Vol 1. Washington, DC, American Physiological Society, 1962, p 489.

20. Glower DD, Spratt JA, Snow ND, et al: Linearity of the Frank-Starling relationship in the intact heart: The concept of preload recruitable external work. Heart Vessels 10:57, 1995.

21. Takoakah H, Suga H, Goto Y, et al: Cardiodynamic conditions for the linearity of preload recruitable external work. Heart vessels *10*:57, 1995.

22. Braunwald E, Ross J, Sonnenblick EH: Mechanisms of Contraction of the Normal and Failing Heart, 2nd ed. Boston, Little, Brown, 1976.

23. Pollack GH: Maximum velocity as an index of contractility in cardiac muscle: A critical evaluation. Circ Res 26:111, 1970.

24. Ishijima A, Kojima H, Higuchi H, et al: Multiple- and single-molecule analysis of the actomyosin motor by nanometer-piconewton manipulation with a microneedle: Unitary steps and forces. Biophys J 70:383, 1996.

25. Sugi H, Pollack GH (eds): Mechanism of Myofilament Sliding in Muscle Contraction. Advances in Experimental Medicine and Biology Series, Vol 332. New York, Plenum, 1993.

26. Katz AM: Physiology of the Heart, 2nd ed. New York, Raven Press, 1992.

27. Goto Y, Igarashi Y, Yasumura Y, et al: Integrated regional work equals total left ventricular work in regionally ischemic canine heart. Am J Physiol 254:H894, 1988.

28. Suga H, Sagawa K, Shoukas AA: Load independence of the instantaneous pressure-volume ratio of the canine left ventricle and effects of epinephrine and heart rate on the ratio. Circ Res 32:314, 1973.

29. Suga H, Sagawa K: Instantaneous pressure-volume relationships and their ratio in the excised, supported canine left ventricle. Circ Res 35:117, 1974.

30. Suga H: Total mechanical energy of a ventricle model and cardiac oxygen consumption. Am J Physiol 236:H498, 1979.

31. Suga H, Yasumura Y, Nozawa T, et al: Pressure-volume relation around zero transmural pressure in excised cross-circulated dog left ventricle. Circ Res 63:361, 1988.

32. Burkhoff D, Sugiura S, Yue DT, Sagawa K: Contractility-dependent curvilinearity of end-systolic pressure-volume relations. Am J Physiol 252:H1218, 1987.

33. Suga H, Yamada O, Igarashi Y, et al: Left ventricular O_2 consumption and pressure-volume area in puppies. Am J Physiol 253:H770, 1987.

34. Tachibana H, Takaki M, Lee S, et al: New mechanoenergetic evaluation of left ventricular contractility in in situ rat hearts. Am J Physiol 272:H2671, 1997.

35. Burkhoff D, Flaherty JT, Yue DT, et al: In vitro studies of isolated supported human hearts. Heart Vessels 4:185, 1988.

36. Teitel DF, Klautz R, Steendijk P, et al: The end-systolic pressure-volume relationship in the newborn lamb: Effects of loading and inotropic interventions. Pediatr Res 29:473, 1991.

37. Suga H, Goto Y: Cardiac oxygen costs of contractility (Emax) and mechanical energy (PVA): New key concepts in cardiac energetics. In Sasayama S, Suga H (eds): Recent Progress in Failing Heart Syndrome. Tokyo, Springer-Verlag, 1991, p 61.

38. Suga H, Hisano R, Goto Y, Yamada O: Normalization of end-systolic pressure-volume relation and Emax of different sized hearts. Jpn Circ J 48:136, 1984.

39. Takaki M, Mataubara H, Araki J, et al: Mechanoenergetics of acute failing hearts characterized by oxygen costs of mechanical energy and contractility. In Sasayama S (ed): New Horizons for Failing Heart Syndrome. Tokyo, Springer-Verlag, 1996, p 133.

40. Sunagawa K, Maughan WL, Sagawa K: Effect of regional ischemia on the left ventricular end-systolic pressure-volume relationship of isolated canine hearts. Circ Res 52:170, 1983.

41. Suga H, Goto Y, Futaki S, et al: Systolic pressure-volume area (PVA) as the energy of contraction in Starling's law of the heart. Heart Vessels 6:65, 1991.

42. Suga H, Hisano R, Hirata S, et al: Mechanism of higher oxygen consumption rate: Pressure-loaded vs. volume-loaded heart. Am J Physiol 242:H942, 1982.

43. Fenn O: A quantitative comparison between the energy liberated and the work performed by the isolated sartorius muscle of the frog. J Physiol (Lond) 58:175, 1923.

44. Rall JA: Sense and nonsense about the Fenn effect. Am J Physiol 242:H1, 1982.

45. Nozawa T, Yasumura Y, Futaki S, et al: The linear relation between oxygen consumption and pressure-volume area can be reconciled with the Fenn effect in dog left ventricle. Circ Res 65:1380, 1989.

46. Mast F, Elzinga G: Heat released during relaxation equals force-length area in isometric contractions of rabbit papillary muscle. Circ Res 67:893, 1990.

47. Gibbs CL, Barclay CJ: Cardiac efficiency. Cardiovasc Res 30:627, 1995.

48. Takaki M, Tachibana H, Hata Y, et al: Mechanoenergetics of rat left ventricles in in situ and excised blood-perfused hearts and in unloaded rat left ventricular slices. Heart Vessels 12(suppl):100, 1997.

49. Burkhoff D, Van der velde ET, Kass D, et al: Accuracy of volume measurement by conductance catheter in isolated, ejecting canine hearts. Circulation 72:440, 1985.

50. Suga H, Goto Y, Nozawa T, et al: Force-time integral decreases with ejection despite constant oxygen consumption and pressure-volume area in dog left ventricle. Circ Res 60:797, 1987.

51. Suga H, Hayashi T, Shirahata M, et al: Regression of cardiac oxygen consumption on ventricular pressure-volume area in dog. Am J Physiol 240:H320, 1981.

52. Hata K, Goto Y, Suga H: External work during relaxation period does not affect myocardial oxygen consumption. Am J Physiol 261:H1778, 1991.

53. Suga H, Goto Y, Yamada O, Igarashi Y: Independence of myocardial oxygen consumption from pressure-volume trajectory during diastole in canine left ventricle. Circ Res 55:734, 1984.

54. Burkhoff D, de Tombe PP, Hunter WC, Kass DA: Contractile strength and mechanical efficiency of left ventricle are enhanced by physiological afterload. Am J Physiol 260:H569, 1991.

55. Suga H, Hisano R, Hirata S, et al: Heart rate-independent energetics and systolic pressure-volume area in dog heart. Am J Physiol 244:H206, 1983.

56. Harasawa Y, de Tombe PP, Sheriff DD, Hunter WC: Basal metabolism adds a significant offset to unloaded oxygen consumption per minute. Circ Res 71:414, 1992.

57. Ohgoshi Y, Goto Y, Futaki S, et al: Increased oxygen cost of contractility in stunned myocardium of dog. Circ Res 69:975, 1991.

58. Hata K, Takasago T, Saeki A, et al: Stunned myocardium after rapid correction of acidosis. Increased oxygen cost of contractility and the role of the Na^+-H^+ exchange system. Circ Res 74:794, 1994.

59. Hata K, Goto Y, Kawaguchi O, et al: Hypercapnic acidosis increases oxygen cost of contractility in the dog left ventricle. Am J Physiol 266:H730, 1994.

60. Suga H, Goto Y, Kawaguchi O, et al: Ventricular perspective on efficiency. Basic Res Cardiol 88(suppl 2):43, 1993.

61. Goto Y, Slinker BK, LeWinter MM: Decreased contractile efficiency and increased nonmechanical energy cost in hyperthyroid rabbit heart. Relation between O_2 consumption and systolic pressure-volume area or force-time integral. Circ Res 66:999, 1990.

62. Goto Y, Hata K: Mechanoenergetic effect of pimobendane in failing dog heart. Heart Vessels 12(suppl):103, 1997.

63. Lee JA, Allen DG: Modulation of Cardiac Calcium Sensitivity. A New Approach to Increasing the Strength of the Heart. Oxford, Oxford Medical, 1993.

64. Burkhoff D, Oikawa RY, Sagawa K: Influence of pacing site on canine left ventricular contraction. Am J Physiol 251:H428, 1986.

65. Suga H, Goto Y, Igarashi Y, et al: Cardiac cooling increases Emax without affecting relation between O_2 consumption and systolic pressure-volume area in dog left ventricle. Circ Res 63:61, 1988.

66. Bers D: Excitation-Contraction Coupling and Cardiac Contractile Force. Dordrecht, the Netherlands, Kluwer Academic, 1991.
67. Noble MIM, Seed WA (eds): The Interval-Force Relationship of the Heart. Bowditch Revisited. Cambridge, Cambridge University Press, 1992.
68. Shimizu J, Araki J, Mizuno J, et al: A new integrative method to quantify total Ca^{2+} handling and futile Ca^{2+} cycling in failing hearts. Am J Physiol 275:H2325, 1998.
69. Sunagawa K, Maughan WL, Burkhoff D, Sagawa K: Left ventricular interaction with arterial load studied in isolated canine ventricle. Am J Physiol 245:H773, 1983.
70. Burkhoff D, Sagawa K: Ventricular efficiency predicted by an analytical model. Am J Physiol 250:R1021, 1986.
71. Sugimachi M, Todaka K, Sunagawa K, Nakamura M: Optimal afterload for the heart vs optimal heart for the afterload. Front Med Biol Eng 2:217, 1990.
72. Asanoi H, Sasayama S, Kameyama T: Ventriculoarterial coupling in normal and failing heart in humans. Circ Res 65:483, 1989.
73. Hisano R, Cooper G: Correlation of force-length area with oxygen consumption in ferret papillary muscle. Circ Res 61:318, 1987.
74. Goto Y, Suga H: Left ventricular regional mechanics and energetics assessed in the wall tension—regional area diagram. *In* Sasayama S, Suga H (eds): Recent Progress in Failing Heart Syndrome. Tokyo, Springer-Verlag, 1991, p 117.
75. Nakano K, Sugawara M, Kato T, et al: Regional work of the human left ventricle calculated by wall stress and the natural logarithm of reciprocal of wall thickness. J Am Coll Cardiol 12:1442, 1988.

CHAPTER 6

PHYSIOLOGY AND PATHOPHYSIOLOGY OF MYOCARDIAL BLOOD FLOW

JULIEN I. E. HOFFMAN

DEFINITIONS AND UNITS OF MEASUREMENT

Coronary blood flow (flow passing through the coronary arteries) and myocardial flow (flow entering the myocardium) are usually similar, except for a small amount of myocardial flow that comes from pericardial and mediastinal vessels. In coronary-cameral or coronary-pulmonary arterial fistulas, not all the flow entering the coronary arteries goes into the myocardium.

Myocardial oxygen consumption or uptake is the amount of oxygen used by the myocardium. It may be measured in units of milliliters or micromoles of oxygen per beat or per minute for the whole heart and for the left ventricle or per unit mass of tissue (per gram or 100 g). Myocardial oxygen demand is the amount of oxygen that the heart needs. Normally, myocardial oxygen consumption and demand are equal as long as myocardial oxygen supply is unrestricted, but if supply falls below demand, there will be myocardial ischemia.

Ischemia is defined in many ways.[1] In general, ischemia represents an imbalance between oxygen supply and demand that leads to impaired myocardial oxidative metabolism and function. The impairment may be transient (stunning, hibernation) or permanent. If ischemia lasts more than several hours, cells die and are replaced by scar tissue.

BASIC PHYSIOLOGY

MYOCARDIAL OXYGEN DEMAND

The heart has one of the highest oxygen consumptions per unit mass of any organ in the body (Fig. 6–1). With exercise or other stresses, myocardial oxygen consumption and demand increase four- or five-fold above the resting level.

Most of the energy and oxygen consumption during muscle contraction is used to generate force (internal or contractile element work), and only 10% is used for shortening (external work). Another 15% is used for basal metabolism (protein synthesis, transport of sodium and potassium), and about 10% is used in activation, related to Na^+,K^+-ATPase and Ca^{2+}-ATPase. If contractility is in-

creased, myocardial oxygen consumption also increases.[3] In the whole heart, the major consumption of oxygen is incurred in generating pressure, with lesser amounts being used in ejection (shortening), basal metabolism, and activation. Sarnoff and colleagues[4] found that left ventricular myocardial oxygen consumption correlated with the area under the left ventricular pressure curve in systole (termed the tension-time index). However, ventricular systolic pressure is not synonymous with afterload. It is preferable to calculate circumferential wall stress, which, at the midwall, is a function of ventricular pressure, diameter, and wall thickness and is a better predictor of myocardial oxygen consumption than is pressure alone.[5]

Wall stress is based on the Laplace relationship:

$$\text{wall stress} = \frac{Pr}{2h}$$

where P is pressure, r is radius of curvature, and h is wall thickness. However, the left ventricle is not a regular sphere, particularly in systole, so that the Laplace formula is oversimplified. A simple, fairly accurate formula was developed by Grossman and coworkers[6]:

$$\text{wall stress} = \frac{1.35PD}{4h(1 + h/D)}$$

where P is pressure, D is left ventricular minor axis dimension, and h is wall thickness at the level of the minor axis.

Because changes in pressure and wall stress differ, indices that use pressure as a predictor of myocardial oxygen consumption are inaccurate, even though the two measures tend to change in the same direction. Therefore, tension-time index, double product (peak systolic pressure × heart rate), and triple product (double product × duration of ejection) are only rough predictors of myocardial oxygen consumption and cannot be relied on to indicate small differences in oxygen demand (see Chapter 5).

More recently, Suga and colleagues have done a series of studies in isolated hearts that show that left ventricular oxygen consumption can be predicted accurately by the area inside the pressure-volume loop (which represents external work) plus the area that represents end-systolic pressure energy (see Chapter 5).[7–9]

As heart rate rises, oxygen consumption per minute increases because of more contractions per minute and in-

Supported in part by Program Project Grant HL-25847 from the National Institutes of Health.

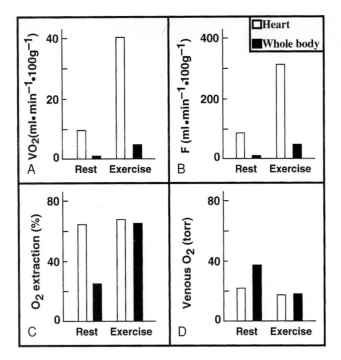

Comparison of left ventricle (*open columns*) and total body (*solid columns*) at rest and near maximal sustained exercise. Human data based on studies by Kitamura and coworkers.[2] *A,* Oxygen consumption. *B,* Blood flow. *C,* Oxygen extraction. *D,* Venous oxygen tension.

creased contractility. Increased contractility increases oxygen consumption per beat, but proportionally not as much in the intact heart as in the muscle strip because at the same time it decreases ventricular volume and thus wall stress.[10]

Virtually all studies predicting myocardial oxygen consumption have been done in healthy animals, and little has been done in hearts that are diseased, let alone in humans.

The right ventricle does not have a single draining vein. Some investigators have found oxygen extraction to be the same in the two ventricles, whereas others found lower extraction in the right ventricle.[3, 11]

Little is known about the regional distribution of myocardial oxygen consumption across the left ventricular wall. Weiss and colleagues[12] observed slightly greater oxygen extraction and oxygen consumption in the left ventricular subendocardial muscle than in the midwall or the subepicardial muscle. They also observed considerable variability of venous oxygen saturation within each layer.

MYOCARDIAL BLOOD FLOW

The high left ventricular myocardial oxygen consumption is associated with a high oxygen extraction even at rest, and although a little more oxygen can be extracted to meet increased oxygen demands, this amount is limited by the hemoglobin-oxygen dissociation curve if tissue hypoxia is to be avoided. Therefore, the high myocardial oxygen consumption must be met by a high myocardial blood flow in the resting subject, and when myocardial oxygen demands increase with exercise, they are normally supplied by an increase in myocardial blood flow (Fig. 6–1*B*). In the left

ventricle, flows in resting subjects are about 80 to 100 ml/min/100 g.[11] In dogs and pigs, conscious or anesthetized, right ventricular flows per unit mass have been 50 to 67% of those of the left ventricle.[11] The ventricular septum, although usually contracting as part of the left ventricle, has flow characteristics of both ventricles. The left side of the septum behaves like the left ventricular free wall, particularly its subendocardial region, whereas the right part of the septum has flows similar to those in the right ventricular free wall.

Flows in ventricular walls are inhomogeneous. If the left ventricular free wall is cut into concentric layers, flows tend to be less in the outermost third or quarter (subepicardial muscle) than in the innermost third or quarter (subendocardial muscle), particularly in conscious animals.[11] Therefore, the left ventricle's inner/outer (or subendocardial/subepicardial) ratio of flows per gram may normally be 1.2 to 1.4. In addition to this regional layer inhomogeneity, there is considerable small-scale inhomogeneity within each layer.[13, 14] In the right ventricle, the inner/outer flow ratio per gram is usually close to 1.[11]

What determines the regional distribution of myocardial blood flow? For a given coronary artery pressure, flow depends on the resistance that it meets; the lower the resistance, the higher the flow. In any region of the ventricle, there are three resistances to consider.[14, 15] The first is the minimal resistance (Rmin) of the vascular bed when it is maximally dilated and the heart is not contracting (long diastole, cardioplegia). The second is the added resistance (Rbeating) imposed when the heart beats and compresses the vessels. Finally, when the vessels have tone, this superimposes another resistance, Rtone.

Rmin is lower in left ventricular subendocardium than in subepicardium, so that in the arrested heart with maximally dilated vessels, subendocardial flow is much greater than subepicardial flow[11, 16]; the inner/outer flow ratio may be 2 or more. Within any layer, however, there is great variability of flow,[13, 14] presumably because of differences in the resistances of the vascular pathways to small regions of the ventricular wall. The flow patterns are not completely random. Regions with high or low flows are surrounded by other regions with high or low flows, respectively; the diameters of regions with similar flows are about 5 to 9 mm in the dog left ventricle.

With increasing heart rate, subendocardial flow per minute per gram decreases roughly linearly.[17] Because of the high intramyocardial pressures in the subendocardium in systole, there is probably no systolic perfusion of the subendocardial muscle. As heart rate increases, the duration of diastole per minute decreases, and therefore so does subendocardial blood flow. However, when the heart beats, subepicardial flow exceeds the flow in the arrested heart[18] for complex reasons. There are no high systolic intramyocardial pressures in the subepicardium, so that no obstruction to forward flow occurs in this region in systole or diastole. Studies performed with tiny flow transducers placed on small coronary arteries just before they enter the myocardium[18] have shown little if any forward flow, particularly if contractility is increased. Therefore, although about 20 to 25% of the coronary flow enters the origins of the coronary arteries in systole, most of this merely distends the extramural arteries and is stored there. On the other hand, microscopy of the superficial subepicardial vessels in the beating heart has shown continuous forward flow throughout the cardiac cycle.[19] The conclusions from these studies are that almost no flow enters the myocardium from the extramural vessels in systole and that systolic subepicardial forward flow comes from blood squeezed retrograde from the subepicardial vessels.[18]

When tone is added to the vessels, the flows are lower than when the vessels are maximally dilated. There is still great heterogeneity of flows, even within a layer, but no correlation exists between flows in the beating heart with and without vascular tone. The inner/outer flow ratio per gram remains about 1 to 1.4, but in small regions, flows are determined primarily by local metabolic demands rather than by intramyocardial pressures or static minimal vascular resistances.

AUTOREGULATION

When the heart is beating and the vessels have tone, each region regulates flow to match its metabolic needs. This can be studied by cannulating the left coronary artery so that its perfusing pressure can be raised or lowered without altering left ventricular pressure or heart rate, and thus with little alteration in myocardial oxygen consumption. When pressure is raised, flow immediately rises but then during 20 to 30 seconds returns to near its control value because the vessels constrict. When pressure is lowered, flow immediately decreases but then gradually returns to nearly normal because the vessels dilate. At high pressures (above about 120 mm Hg mean perfusing pressure in acute studies), the flows increase persistently, presumably because vasoconstriction has been overcome by the high pressure. Below a pressure of about 60 to 70 mm Hg in anesthetized dogs and about 40 mm Hg in conscious dogs,[20] flow begins to decrease, because some vessels cannot dilate further and so can no longer compensate for a reduced perfusion pressure. These vessels are then pressure dependent, and in them any fall in pressure decreases flow, or any increase in myocardial oxygen demand at a constant pressure cannot be met by an increased flow. In either event, ischemia will occur in the territory supplied by those vessels.

METABOLIC REGULATION

Myocardial oxygen demands are increased by tachycardia, increased pressure, and, to a lesser extent, volume work and an increase in contractility. Normal hearts can tolerate high heart rates, for example, 200 to 250 beats per minute, for short periods.[21, 22] The tachycardia decreases the total diastolic time per minute and the proportion of diastole per cycle.[23] It also decreases stroke volume, ventricular volume, and wall stress but increases contractility. Therefore, tachycardia increases myocardial oxygen consumption.[10] Increased wall stress due to higher pressure or volume work also increases myocardial oxygen demand, as does an increase in contractility. Even when myocardial oxygen demands are increased, however, autoregulation still occurs at the higher flow.

CORONARY FLOW RESERVE

At any given pressure, the flow when the vessels have tone is determined by the myocardial oxygen needs at that moment. When the vessels are maximally dilated, flow depends only on vascular resistance and myocardial contraction, independent of metabolism. If flow is measured at different perfusing pressures when the vessels have tone and then when they are maximally dilated, a typical coronary conductance diagram results (Fig. 6–2). (Conductance is the reciprocal of resistance. The higher the conductance, the greater the flow at any perfusion pressure.) The normal conductogram (Fig. 6–2A) shows a relatively horizontal line of autoregulated flow between perfusing pressures of 40 and 120 mm Hg; autoregulation fails outside those limits. When the vessels are maximally dilated, there is a steep pressure-flow line. The vertical difference between the two lines indicates the extra flow that can be attained at any given pressure by dilating the vessels and is termed the coronary flow reserve. Like the other flows, it is measured in milliliters per minute. It is also possible to derive a dimensionless coronary flow reserve ratio by dividing maximal flow by autoregulated flow; this is particularly useful if flows or velocities cannot be related to a particular tissue mass. Note that either form of flow reserve gets smaller as the perfusing pressure decreases.

What happens to flow reserve when, in the uncannulated preparation, aortic pressure rises? The increased pressure work increases the autoregulated flow, but the increased coronary perfusing pressure increases maximal flow. McGinn and colleagues[24] observed in humans that increases in mean arterial pressure of about 20 mm Hg increased autoregulated and maximal flows proportionally, so that the coronary flow reserve ratio was unaltered. What happens at higher pressure elevations is unknown.

Coronary flow reserve can be reduced by two types of changes. One is if maximal flow remains unchanged but autoregulated flow increases (Fig. 6–2B); the other is if autoregulated flow remains the same but maximal flows are reduced (Fig. 6–2C). The causes of increased or decreased autoregulated flows are shown in Tables 6–1 and 6–2.

Some factors like tachycardia may increase autoregulated flow and decrease maximal flow, and some diseases like cyanotic heart disease may elevate autoregulated flow (from hypoxemia) and decrease maximal flow (from polycythemia). Such combinations may decrease coronary flow reserve profoundly (Fig. 6–2D).

Note that when coronary flow reserve is reduced, because of either an increase in autoregulated flow or a decrease in maximal flow, the pressure at which autoregulation fails and pressure dependency starts shifts to the right, that is, toward higher pressures. This is a consequence of the slope of the line of maximal pressure-flow relations. As a result, autoregulation can fail at normal perfusing pressures (Fig. 6–2D).

REGIONAL CORONARY FLOW RESERVE

Loss of coronary reserve implies that the vessels are maximally dilated, and if perfusion time or pressure is inadequate, there will be ischemia. As described later, this fail-

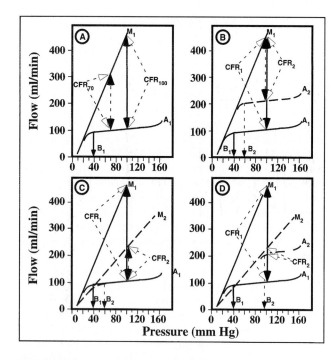

FIGURE 6–2

Coronary conductance diagrams: plots of left ventricular flow (milliliters per minute) against mean coronary perfusing pressure. Left ventricle has a mass of about 100 g. *A,* Normal. A1 is the control autoregulation line; when autoregulation fails, the curve turns downward at low pressures and turns upward at high pressures. M1 is the control maximal pressure-flow line. The two *vertical arrows* with solid heads show the coronary flow reserve at two different perfusing pressures, 70 mm Hg and 100 mm Hg; the *open arrows* and *dashed lines* demarcate the extent of the two flow reserves (CFR100 and CFR70). The *small arrow* B1 shows the approximate pressure at which autoregulation fails at low pressures in the conscious dog. *B,* Altered autoregulation. Superimposed on the normal coronary conductogram are *dashed lines* that indicate autoregulation at increased myocardial oxygen consumption (A2). Note that the lower pressure at which autoregulation fails is higher when myocardial oxygen consumption is increased (B2) than when it is normal (B1). Furthermore, the coronary flow reserve is reduced when myocardial oxygen consumption is increased (CFR2). Symbols as in *A.* The causes of increased autoregulated flow are given in Table 6–1. *C,* Decreased maximal pressure-flow line. The lower slope of the line of reduced maximal pressure-flow relations (M2) has reduced coronary flow reserve at 100 mm Hg perfusing pressure (CFR2) so that it is now less than the normal reserve (CFR1). Note, too, that the lower pressure at which autoregulation fails (B2) is higher than normal (B1) when the maximal pressure-flow line has a lower slope. Symbols as in *A.* The causes of decreased maximal flow are given in Table 6–2. *D,* Combined increased myocardial oxygen consumption and decreased maximal pressure-flow line. Note that coronary flow reserve is now small (CFR2) even at a perfusing pressure of 100 mm Hg. In this setting, autoregulation fails at about 95 mm Hg perfusing pressure (B2). This dire combination is what can be expected in a cyanotic patient with ventricular hypertrophy, arterial hypoxemia, and polycythemia. Symbols as in *A.*

ure of autoregulation occurs first in the subendocardial muscle, no matter what the cause may be. The loss of reserve is heterogeneous, even within a layer.[30]

PRESSURE-FLOW RELATIONS

When coronary perfusing pressure is progressively reduced, flow ceases at a pressure of about 45 mm Hg during autoregulation and at about 10 to 18 mm Hg when the vessels are maximally dilated. The mechanism is complex and

---

TABLE 6–1

CAUSES OF INCREASED AUTOREGULATED FLOWS[25–29]

Exercise
Fever
Tachycardia
Increased myocardial contractility
Thyrotoxicosis
Ventricular hypertrophy
Anemia
Hypoxemia
Left shift of oxyhemoglobin dissociation curve due to
    Fetal hemoglobin
    Alkalosis
    Carboxyhemoglobin
    Certain abnormal hemoglobins

not fully resolved.[31] Some investigators believe that there is vascular closure within the myocardium that causes this backpressure, whereas others believe that the zero flow pressure is a mixture of a vascular waterfall in the epicardial coronary veins and a time factor related to intramyocardial blood volume. (In a waterfall, raising the level of the water in the river below the fall does not change flow over the lip of the fall. Similarly, in a vascular waterfall, there is a discontinuity between pressure in the "waterfall" segment and more distal venous pressure, and increasing venous pressure will not alter flow in the vascular bed until it exceeds the waterfall pressure.[31])

What is clear is that under some circumstances, the zero flow pressure can rise and reduce the coronary driving pressure (the difference between inflow perfusion pressure and outflow or backpressure). This can certainly occur with pericardial tamponade and with high right or left ventricular diastolic pressures. A rise in backpressure, for whatever reason and mechanism, has the same effect in reducing coronary flow reserve as does a decrease in perfusing pressure.

TABLE 6–2

CAUSES OF DECREASED MAXIMAL FLOWS[25–29]

Increased blood viscosity
    Polycythemia
    Macroglobulinemia
Abnormal cardiac function
    High left ventricular diastolic pressure (congestive heart failure)
    Low aortic diastolic pressure (aortic incompetence)
    Pericardial tamponade
    Marked increase in myocardial contractility
    Tachycardia
    Ventricular hypertrophy
Small coronary vessel disease
    Systemic lupus erythematosus
    Aortic stenosis
    Systemic hypertension
    Hypertrophic cardiomyopathy
    Diabetes mellitus
    Idiopathic
Large coronary vessel disease
    Atherosclerosis
    Embolism
    Spasm

REGULATION OF MYOCARDIAL VASCULAR TONE

The heart cannot sustain anaerobic metabolism without becoming injured, so that myocardial oxygen supply must be tightly regulated. When myocardial oxygen demand increases, flow increases within 10 to 20 seconds to supply the extra oxygen; when myocardial oxygen demand decreases, flow decreases rapidly until oxygen supply and demand are once again in balance. The mechanisms involved in this adjustment are poorly understood. The first proposed mechanism concerned adenosine. When muscle contraction breaks down adenosine triphosphate (ATP), some of the adenosine monophosphate produced is degraded by 5′-nucleotidase to adenosine, a powerful coronary vasodilator. The more the muscle works, the more the amount of adenosine produced and the more the coronary vasodilatation. The increased myocardial oxygen supply therefore increases to match the demand. When muscle work decreases, so does the amount of adenosine produced, and the vessels constrict to decrease flow and oxygen supply appropriately. Although this mechanism has all the ingredients needed for a control system, there are some major arguments against its being the only or even the most important system. Virtual elimination of the interstitial adenosine by infusing low-molecular-weight adenosine deaminase does not alter autoregulation. Even with definite ischemia, as in reactive hyperemia, infusing adenosine deaminase reduces but does not abolish the hyperemic response.[3] More recently, many other potential regulators have been studied. These include potent vasodilators such as nitric oxide, substance P, prostacyclin, vasoactive intestinal peptide, ATP-dependent potassium channels, bradykinin, atrial natriuretic peptides, and calcitonin gene–related product as well as vasoconstrictors such as neuropeptide Y and endothelin, and also the adrenergic nerves with their transmitters. At least in the dog, nitric oxide, ATP-dependent potassium channels, and adenosine appear to be the major vasodilators.

GENERAL ASPECTS

When perfusing pressure decreases below the lower limit of autoregulation, the fall in flow occurs first in the subendocardium.[25, 28] Furthermore, the changes in flow are not uniform within each layer; some pieces of muscle retain reasonable flows, whereas others decrease their flow markedly.[30] Nevertheless, most low-flow regions are in the subendocardium, some are in the midwall, and few are in the subepicardium. A similar pattern of selective subendocardial ischemia was shown in experiments in noncannulated dogs in which severe supravalvar aortic stenosis, an arteriovenous fistula, or rapid ventricular pacing reduced the inner/outer ratio per gram to low values, even though the absolute subendocardial flow might not have been reduced. In these studies, some of the maneuvers increased myocardial oxygen demand throughout the heart, but the pathophysiologic changes prevented the appropriate increase in subendocardial blood flow. Common to all these experiments is the notion that once the vessels become maximally dilated, and this always occurs first in the subendocardium, subendocardial flow becomes pressure dependent. Therefore, an inadequate perfusion pressure or a reduced diastolic perfusion time for myocardial needs will cause subendocardial flow to either decrease or fail to increase appropriately and lead to a lowered inner/outer flow ratio per gram as well as functional and biochemical manifestations of subendocardial ischemia.

SPECIFIC LESIONS AND ABNORMAL STATES

Tachycardia

Heart rates above 250 beats per minute for an extended period may decrease inner/outer flow ratio owing to a shorter diastolic perfusion time, lowered aortic diastolic perfusing pressure, and perhaps a rise in left ventricular diastolic pressure. Although the absolute flows rise in all layers, coronary flow reserve becomes reduced in the inner half and, at high rates, may be absent. The subendocardial vessels become pressure dependent, and ischemia may result. The absolute subendocardial flow might be above normal but is not high enough to supply the needed oxygen to the muscle. The inner/outer flow ratio per gram is in these instances a better guide to subendocardial ischemia than is the actual subendocardial flow. If the ventricle is hypertrophied, tachycardia causes subendocardial ischemia much more readily, in fact, above heart rates of 200 beats per minute.[21, 22] Modest tachycardia at a rate of 200 beats per minute will cause subendocardial ischemia in dogs with coronary stenosis. Presumably, the tighter the stenosis, the less the heart rate increase required to cause subendocardial ischemia.

Ventricular Hypertrophy

In hypertrophy in adult animals, there is an increase in muscle mass but no corresponding increase in arteries and larger arterioles.[26, 28] In general, increased wall thickening tends to keep wall tension normal, so that myocardial oxygen consumption per unit mass remains at control values. However, because of a greater muscle mass, myocardial oxygen consumption per ventricle is increased in proportion to the increase in muscle mass. Flow increases to supply this increased amount of oxygen and does so by dilating the normal-sized myocardial vascular bed. On the other hand, maximal flow per ventricle is not increased (or may even be decreased if there is associated small-vessel medial hypertrophy or intimal disease). Therefore, coronary flow reserve is reduced.[32–34] Similar results have been found in humans.[32, 34] When hypertrophy is due to hypertension, the increased perfusion pressure may result in a normal coronary flow reserve, with both resting and maximal flows being increased in proportion.

Young animals, however, can increase the cross-sectional area of the myocardial vascular bed to keep pace with the increase in ventricular muscle mass, at least in the right ventricle.[26, 28]

Aortic Stenosis

In this lesion, subendocardial ischemia and fibrosis are prominent, both in children and in adults.[25, 28] The pressure load causes ventricular hypertrophy, which tends to normalize the wall stress. Therefore, flow per unit mass is relatively normal, but total flow is increased in proportion to the increased muscle mass. Because conducting intramyocardial coronary vessels do not increase in number or size, or do not increase enough to compensate for the increased muscle mass, coronary flow reserve is reduced and may even be absent in the subendocardium. Because the subendocardial vessels are the first to be affected, the effort angina that these patients get is accompanied by ST depression in the left precordial leads, and often there will be substantial subendocardial fibrosis and necrosis. If there are added obstructive changes in intramural arteries, the tendency to subendocardial ischemia is made worse. With significant aortic stenosis, subendocardial ischemia will be brought on earlier by added stresses like anemia, tachycardia, extramural coronary arterial disease, or anything that causes the ventricle to dilate and increase the wall stress. Injudicious use of catecholamines in the treatment of noncardiac disease in these patients may also be detrimental.

Aortic Insufficiency

With severe incompetence, left ventricular systolic pressure is elevated and there is ventricular hypertrophy, but with the associated increase in ventricular volume, the wall stress is elevated. Furthermore, the mean diastolic aortic perfusing pressure is reduced. These patients therefore have a much reduced coronary flow reserve, so that angina pectoris and subendocardial ischemic damage may occur. One notable difference from aortic stenosis is that with incompetence, tachycardia can improve cardiac function and subendocardial blood flow for at least two reasons. A faster heart rate reduces the time available for regurgitation and so reduces the degree of regurgitation and ventricular volume. Second, the shorter diastole raises mean diastolic perfusing pressure. This may be why clinically pacing about 15 to 20 beats per minute above the resting heart rate has produced major clinical improvement in patients with aortic incompetence and intractable cardiac failure.[35]

Anemia

Anemia increases cardiac output and thus myocardial oxygen consumption and at the same time decreases oxygen-carrying capacity of the blood. This is compensated for by an increased coronary blood flow, but at the expense of reducing coronary flow reserve.

Polycythemia

Polycythemia reduces resting blood flow because of its increased oxygen-carrying capacity and viscosity. Because maximal flows are decreased by the increased blood viscosity, coronary flow reserve is reduced. As for anemia, resting blood flow can be supplied (to a normal heart) at any hematocrit, perfusing pressure, and arterial oxygen saturation, but the demands of exercise cannot be met.

Hypoxemia

Hypoxemia increases coronary blood flow and reduces coronary flow reserve.

Coronary Arterial Stenoses

With a localized atheromatous lesion of a major branch of the left coronary artery, there will be a pressure drop at rest across the obstruction because of the increased resistance it offers to flow. This pressure drop is greater in diastole, when flow is highest, than in systole. Autoregulation causes the small intramural vessels to dilate and lower their resistance, so that myocardial oxygen demands can be met. Coronary flow reserve is, however, decreased in this distal bed. If the stenosis becomes more severe, whether acutely by spasm or hemorrhage into the plaque or chronically by growth in volume of the plaque, distal pressures may fall below the level at which autoregulation can compensate; coronary flow reserve will be absent. Consequently, there will be a decrease in flow below the amount needed to supply myocardial oxygen needs, particularly in the subendocardium, and the patient will have rest pain. Because rest pain indicates severely impaired coronary flow to a region that does not have an increased oxygen demand, it is a precursor of necrosis if it is allowed to persist.

If a mild obstruction gradually increases, resting flow remains at its previous value but coronary flow reserve becomes progressively reduced. Exercise that raises myocardial oxygen needs may then exhaust flow reserve and lead to subendocardial ischemia. These features are the basis for various types of exercise tests, with or without radionuclide scans to delineate ischemic regions.

REFERENCES

1. Hearse DJ: Myocardial ischaemia: Can we agree on a definition for the 21st century? (Editorial) Cardiovasc Res 28:1737, 1994.
2. Kitamura K, Jorgensen CR, Gobel FL, et al: Hemodynamic correlates of myocardial oxygen consumption during upright exercise. J Appl Physiol 32:516, 1972.
3. Hoffman JIE: Coronary physiology. In Garfein OB (ed): Current Concepts in Cardiac Physiology. New York, Academic Press, 1990, p 289.
4. Sarnoff SJ, Braunwald E, Welch GH Jr, et al: Hemodynamic determinants of oxygen consumption of the heart with special reference to the tension time index. Am J Physiol 192:148, 1958.
5. McDonald RH, Taylor RR, Cingolani HE: Measurement of myocardial developed tension and its relation to oxygen consumption. Am J Physiol 211:667, 1966.
6. Grossman W, Jones D, McLaurin LP: Wall stress and patterns of hypertrophy in human left ventricle. J Clin Invest 56:56, 1975.
7. Suga H, Hisano R, Hirata S, et al: Mechanism of higher oxygen consumption rate: Pressure-loaded vs. volume loaded heart. Am J Physiol 242:H942, 1982.
8. Hata K, Takasago T, Saeki A, et al: Stunned myocardium after rapid correction of acidosis. Increased oxygen cost of contractility and the role of the Na^+-H^+ exchange system. Circ Res 74:794, 1994.
9. Hata K, Goto Y, Kawaguchi O, et al: Hypercapnic acidosis increases oxygen cost of contractility in the dog left ventricle. Am J Physiol 266:H730, 1994.
10. Graham TP Jr, Covell JW, Sonnenblick EH, et al: Control of myocardial oxygen consumption: Relative influence of contractile state and tension development. J Clin Invest 47:375, 1968.
11. Feigl EO: Coronary physiology. Physiol Rev 63:1, 1983.
12. Weiss HR, Neubauer JA, Lipp JA, Sinha AK: Quantitative determination of regional oxygen consumption in the dog heart. Circ Res 42:394, 1978.
13. Hoffman JIE: Heterogeneity of myocardial blood flow. Basic Res Cardiol 90:113, 1995.
14. Austin RE Jr, Smedira NG, Squiers TM, Hoffman JIE: Influence of cardiac contraction and coronary vasomotor tone on regional myocardial blood flow. Am J Physiol 266:H2542, 1994.
15. Klocke FJ: Coronary blood flow in man. Prog Cardiovasc Dis 19:117, 1976.
16. Chilian WM: Microvascular pressures and resistances in the left ventricular subepicardium and subendocardium. Circ Res 69:561, 1991.

17. Domenech RJ, Goich J: Effect of heart rate on regional coronary blood flow. Cardiovasc Res 10:224, 1976.

18. Flynn AE, Coggins DL, Goto M, et al: Does systolic subepicardial perfusion come from retrograde subendocardial flow? Am J Physiol 262:H1759, 1992.

19. Ashikawa K, Kanatsuka H, Suzuki T, Takishima T: Phasic blood flow velocity pattern in epimyocardial microvessels in the beating canine left ventricle. Circ Res 59:704, 1986.

20. Canty JM Jr: Coronary pressure-function and steady-state pressure-flow relations during autoregulation in the unanesthetized dog. Circ Res 63:821, 1988.

21. Bache RJ, Vrobel TR, Arentzen CE, Ring WS: Effect of maximal coronary vasodilation on transmural myocardial perfusion during tachycardia in dogs with left ventricular hypertrophy. Circ Res 49:742, 1981.

22. Bache RJ, Vrobel TR, Ring WS, et al: Regional myocardial blood flow during exercise in dogs with chronic left ventricular hypertrophy. Circ Res 48:76, 1981.

23. Boudoulas H, Rittgers SE, Lewis RP, et al: Changes in diastolic time with various pharmacologic agents. Implications for myocardial perfusion. Circulation 60:164, 1979.

24. McGinn AL, White CW, Wilson RF: Interstudy variability of coronary flow reserve. Influence of heart rate, arterial pressure, and ventricular preload. Circulation 81:1319, 1990.

25. Hoffman JIE, Buckberg GD: Transmural variations in myocardial perfusion. *In* Yu P, Goodwin JW (eds): Progress in Cardiology, vol 5. Philadelphia, Lea & Febiger, 1976, p 37.

26. Marcus ML: The Coronary Circulation in Health and Disease. New York, McGraw-Hill Book Company, 1983.

27. Hoffman JIE: Regulation of myocardial blood flow and oxygen delivery during hypoxia. *In* Arieff AI (ed): Hypoxia, Metabolic Acidosis, and the Circulation. Clinical Physiology Series. Oxford, Oxford University Press, 1992, p 21.

28. Hoffman JIE: Transmural myocardial perfusion. Prog Cardiovasc Dis 39:429, 1987.

29. Hoffman JIE: Pediatric cardiovascular intensive care: Myocardial perfusion. Prog Pediatr Cardiol 4:117, 1995.

30. Coggins DL, Flynn AE, Austin RE Jr, et al: Nonuniform loss of regional flow reserve during myocardial ischemia in dogs. Circ Res 67:253, 1990.

31. Hoffman JIE, Spaan JAE: Pressure-flow relations in coronary circulation. Physiol Rev 70:331, 1990.

32. Strauer B-E: Hypertensive Heart Disease. New York, Springer-Verlag, 1980.

33. Wicker P: Coronary circulation and coronary reserve in the hypertensive heart. *In* Safar ME, Fouad-Tarazi FM (eds): The Heart in Hypertension. Norwell, MA, Kluwer Academic Publishers, 1989, p 253.

34. Strauer B-E: Myocardial oxygen consumption in chronic heart disease: Role of wall stress, hypertrophy and coronary reserve. Am J Cardiol 44:730, 1979.

35. Judge TP, Kennedy JW, Bennett LJ, et al: Quantitative hemodynamic effects of heart rate in aortic regurgitation. Circulation 44:355, 1971.

CHAPTER 7
CONTROL OF PULMONARY VASCULATURE

JEFFREY R. FINEMAN   STEPHEN M. BLACK   MICHAEL A. HEYMANN

In the fetus, gas exchange occurs in the placenta, not in the lung. Pulmonary vascular resistance is high, pulmonary blood flow is low (about 35 ml/min/kg fetal body weight in near-term fetal lambs), and right ventricular output is thereby directed toward the placenta for gas exchange. At the time of birth and the onset of pulmonary ventilation, pulmonary vascular resistance falls, and pulmonary blood flow rapidly increases approximately eight-fold, reaching a level of about 300 to 400 ml/min/kg body weight shortly after birth.[1] Failure of the pulmonary circulation to undergo this transition at birth results in persistent pulmonary hypertension of the newborn (PPHN), a condition that can result in significant morbidity and mortality. In addition, the status of the pulmonary vasculature is often the principal determinant of the clinical course and feasibility of surgical treatment for many cardiac anomalies. Many factors regulate pulmonary blood flow in these critical periods, including mechanical influences and the release of a variety of vasoactive substances. Evidence suggests that mediators produced and released by the pulmonary vascular endothelium, either locally or into the circulation (paracrine or endocrine function), are central to many of these phenomena.

This chapter discusses the current knowledge dealing with the regulation of blood flow in the normal fetal, transitional, and postnatal pulmonary circulations. Particular emphasis is placed on newer information relating to the role of the pulmonary vascular endothelium in the regulation of the pulmonary circulation. A great deal of our knowledge of fetal blood flow and distribution is based on animal studies. Data on human fetuses and newborns are sparse because of the invasive techniques that would be necessary to obtain them. Therefore, the applicability of these animal studies to humans should be questioned. Overlapping data obtained in animal and human studies on the pulmonary circulation have had excellent correlation, however.

MORPHOLOGIC DEVELOPMENT OF THE PULMONARY VASCULATURE

The morphologic development of the pulmonary circulation affects the physiologic changes that occur in the perinatal period. In the fetus and immediate neonate, small pulmonary arteries of all sizes have a thicker muscular coat compared with the external diameter of the vessels than do similar arteries in the adult. This greater muscularity is generally held responsible, at least in part, for the vasore-

activity and for the high pulmonary vascular resistance found in the fetus, particularly near term. In fetal lamb lungs fixed at perfusion pressures similar to those found normally in utero, the medial smooth muscle coat is most prominent in the smallest arteries (fifth- and sixth-generation arteries; external diameter, 20 to 50 μm). During the latter half of gestation, the medial smooth muscle thickness remains constant in relationship to the external diameter of the artery.[2] Similar observations using slightly different techniques have been made in human lungs.[3,4] After birth, particularly within the first several weeks, the medial smooth muscle involutes, and the thickness of the media of the small pulmonary arteries decreases rapidly and progressively.[5]

Toward the periphery of the lung, the completely encircling smooth muscle of the media gives way to a region of incomplete muscularization.[4] In these partially muscularized arteries, the smooth muscle is arranged in a spiral or a helix. More peripherally, the muscle disappears from arteries that are still larger than capillaries (nonmuscularized small pulmonary arteries). In these nonmuscular small pulmonary arteries, an incomplete pericyte layer is found within the endothelial basement membrane. In the nonmuscular portions of the partially muscular small pulmonary arteries, intermediate cells (i.e., cells intermediate in position and structure between pericytes and mature smooth muscle cells) are found.[6] These cells are precursor smooth muscle cells; under certain conditions, such as hypoxia, they may rapidly differentiate into mature smooth muscle cells.[6]

Small pulmonary arteries (20 to 50 μm in external diameter) are conveniently identified by their relationship to airways (Fig. 7–1). Preacinar pulmonary arteries lie proximal to or with terminal bronchioli. Intra-acinar pulmonary arteries course with respiratory bronchioli, with alveolar ducts, or within alveolar walls. In the fetus, during the last quarter of gestation, only about half of the pulmonary arteries associated with respiratory bronchioli (precapillary) are muscularized or partially muscularized, and the alveoli are free of muscular arteries.[3] In the adult, complete circumferential muscularization extends peripherally along the intra-acinar arteries so that the majority of small pulmonary arteries in relationship to alveoli are completely muscularized. Between birth and teenage years, the arteries undergo progressive peripheral muscularization, and the adult pattern is reached at about the time of puberty.

During growth in fetal lambs, the number of small arteries increases greatly, not only in absolute terms but also per unit volume of lung.[2] In the human, the main preaci-

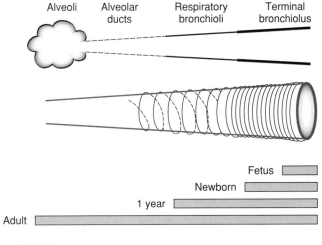

Alveoli Alveolar ducts Respiratory bronchioli Terminal bronchiolus

Fetus

Newborn

1 year

Adult

FIGURE 7–1

Diagrammatic representation of smooth muscle distribution in normal human pulmonary vessels. (Adapted from Reid LM: Structure and function in pulmonary hypertension. New perceptions. Chest 89:279, 1986.)

nar pulmonary artery branches that accompany the larger airways are developed by 16 weeks of gestation.[3] However, the development of the intra-acinar circulation relates more closely to the alveolar development that occurs late in gestation and perhaps even predominantly after birth.[5] As the alveoli multiply, so do the arteries, a process that is generally complete by 10 years of age. In the early period of postnatal life (first 2 years in humans), pulmonary artery growth is more rapid than alveolar growth.[5]

PHYSIOLOGY OF THE PULMONARY VASCULATURE

DETERMINANTS OF PULMONARY VASCULAR RESISTANCE

Pulmonary vascular resistance changes throughout gestation and after birth. The resistance of the pulmonary circulation at any time is related to several factors and can be estimated by applying the resistance equation and the Poiseuille-Hagen relationship.[7] The resistance equation (the hydraulic equivalent of Ohm's law) states that the resistance to flow between two points along a tube equals the decrease in pressure between the two points divided by the flow. For the pulmonary vascular bed, where Rp is pulmonary vascular resistance and $\dot{Q}p$ is pulmonary blood flow per minute, the decrease in mean pressure is from the pulmonary artery (Ppa) to the pulmonary vein (Ppv):

$$Rp = (Ppa - Ppv)/\dot{Q}p$$

Therefore, pulmonary vascular resistance increases when pulmonary arterial pressure increases, or when pulmonary venous pressure increases, because this causes an increase in pulmonary arterial pressure to maintain the driving pressure across the lungs. Similarly, pulmonary vascular resistance also increases when pulmonary blood flow decreases.

Other factors that affect pulmonary vascular resistance can be defined by applying a modification of the Poiseuille-

Hagen relationship, which describes the resistance (R) to the flow of a Newtonian fluid through a straight glass tube of constant cross-sectional area:

$$Rp = 8l\eta/\pi r^4$$

where l is the length of the tube, r is the internal radius of the tubes, and η is the viscosity of the fluid. If there are k tubes in parallel, the expression becomes $Rp = 8l\eta/k\pi r^4$. According to this relationship, increasing the viscosity of blood perfusing the lungs or decreasing the radius or cross-sectional area (πr^4) of the pulmonary vascular bed increases pulmonary vascular resistance. Early in gestation, pulmonary vascular resistance is much higher than that of the neonate or the adult because fewer pulmonary arteries are in the fetal lung, resulting in a decreased cross-sectional area. Secondary to the growth of new pulmonary arteries and the increase in cross-sectional area of the pulmonary vascular bed, pulmonary vascular resistance decreases during fetal life. However, pulmonary vascular resistance near term is still much higher than that after birth.

Because these equations describe steady, laminar flow of a Newtonian fluid in rigid glass tubes, differences between physical and biologic systems should be considered. First, blood is not a Newtonian fluid. However, this is probably of little importance at normal hematocrits.[8] The viscosity of blood is related to red cell number, fibrinogen concentration, and red cell deformability. An increased hematocrit (secondary to fetal hypoxemia, twin-to-twin or maternal-to-fetal blood transfusion, or delayed clamping of the umbilical cord) increases viscosity. Pulmonary vascular resistance increases logarithmically when the hematocrit increases. Second, pulmonary vessels are not rigid tubes. Their walls are deformable, and their size and shape are influenced by transmural pressure. For example, as either pulmonary blood flow or left atrial pressure increases, vessel diameter may change, and the recruitment of different pulmonary vessels may occur. Therefore, the fall in calculated pulmonary vascular resistance with increases in pulmonary blood flow is nonlinear.[9–11] However, the clinical importance of this alinearity is unclear, considering that the pressure-flow relationship remains linear with normal or increased flow.[9] Third, blood flow through the pulmonary circulation is pulsatile, not laminar, and the small pulmonary arteries are branched, curved, and tapered, not smooth. In addition, the small pulmonary arteries are in parallel, and the radii of these arteries may differ in different lung zones.

Despite these differences from physical models, the general effects of changes in physical factors, such as viscosity and radius, do apply. In fact, a change in luminal radius is the major factor responsible for maintaining a high pulmonary vascular resistance in the fetus.[1] Consideration of these factors, particularly viscosity and cross-sectional area of the vascular bed, is important in evaluating the pathophysiologic mechanism of PPHN.

NORMAL FETAL CIRCULATION

In the fetus, normal gas exchange occurs in the placenta, and pulmonary blood flow is low, supplying only nutritional requirements for lung growth and performing some metabolic functions. Pulmonary blood flow in near-term lambs is about 100 ml/100 g wet lung weight, representing between 8 and 10% of the total output of the heart.[12] In human fetuses near term, pulmonary blood flow is about 25% of total cardiac output.[13] Pulmonary blood flow is low despite the dominance of the right ventricle, which in the fetus ejects about two thirds of total cardiac output. Most of the right ventricular output is diverted away from the lungs and through the widely patent ductus arteriosus to the descending thoracic aorta, from which a large proportion reaches the placenta through the umbilical circulation for oxygenation. In young fetal lambs (about halfway through gestation), pulmonary blood flow is approximately 3 to 4% of the total combined left and right ventricular outputs of the heart (fetal cardiac output). This value increases to about 6% at about 80% of the way through gestation, corresponding temporally with the onset of the release of surface-active material into lung fluid. Then another progressive slow rise in pulmonary blood flow occurs, reaching about 8 to 10% near term.[12] Fetal pulmonary arterial pressure increases with advancing gestation. At term, mean pulmonary arterial pressure is about 50 mm Hg, generally exceeding mean descending aortic pressure by 1 to 2 mm Hg.[14] Pulmonary vascular resistance early in gestation is extremely high relative to that in the infant and adult, probably owing to the low number of small arteries. During the last half of gestation, new arteries develop, and cross-sectional area increases. Pulmonary vascular resistance falls progressively; however, baseline pulmonary vascular resistance is still much higher than after birth.[1,14]

REGULATION OF FETAL PULMONARY VASCULAR RESISTANCE

Pulmonary vascular resistance in the fetal lung is initially high and falls slightly throughout the final third of gestation. Many factors, including mechanical effects, state of oxygenation, and production of vasoactive substances, regulate the tone of the fetal pulmonary circulation. In unventilated fetal lungs, fluid filling the alveolar space compresses the small pulmonary arteries and thus increases pulmonary vascular resistance. In addition, the high pulmonary vascular resistance is associated with the normally low oxygen tension in pulmonary and systemic arterial blood. In fetal lambs, the pulmonary arterial PO_2 is 17 to 20 mm Hg (±2.6 kPa) and the femoral arterial PO_2 is 20 to 24 mm Hg. Reducing PO_2 to similar values in newborn lambs after birth produces a marked increase in pulmonary vascular resistance.[14] Similarly, fetal pulmonary vascular resistance is increased by decreasing fetal PO_2 either by maternal hypoxia or by compression of the umbilical cord.[15,16] Conversely, fetal pulmonary vascular resistance is decreased by increasing PO_2.[17] The exact mechanism and site of hypoxic pulmonary vasoconstriction in the fetal pulmonary circulation remain unclear. In isolated fetal pulmonary arteries, oxygen modulates the production of both prostacyclin (prostaglandin I_2, PGI_2) and endothelium-derived nitric oxide (EDNO), two potent vasoactive substances that may in part underlie the responses of the developing pulmonary circulation to changes in oxygenation.[18,19] In the intact fetal lamb, oxygen-induced pulmonary vasodilatation is mediated, in part, by the release

of EDNO.[17] Oxygen-related changes in pulmonary vascular resistance are also affected by pH; acidemia increases pulmonary vascular resistance and accentuates hypoxic vasoconstrictor responses.

In addition to the hypoxic environment, metabolites of arachidonic acid may be actively involved in the control of fetal pulmonary vascular resistance. Leukotrienes C_4 and D_4 are potent pulmonary vasoconstrictors synthesized from arachidonic acid by a 5'-lipoxygenase enzyme in pulmonary arterial tissue. Although their role as mediators of hypoxic pulmonary vasoconstriction in adults has been challenged, a role for them has been proposed in newborn lambs, and the possibility remains that they may be tonically active in utero.[20–22] In fetal lambs, end-organ antagonism (receptor blockade) or inhibition of leukotriene synthesis increases pulmonary blood flow about eight-fold, that is, to those levels that accompany normal ventilation after birth.[23,24] These observations have suggested a physiologic role for leukotrienes in maintaining pulmonary vasoconstriction and, thereby, a low pulmonary blood flow in the fetus. Leukotrienes have also been isolated from tracheal fluid of near-term fetal lambs and from lung lavage fluid of newborns with the syndrome of PPHN, further suggesting that leukotrienes may contribute to maintaining the high pulmonary vascular resistance in the fetus.[25,26] However, nonselectivity of leukotriene antagonists in the animal studies has brought into question these conclusions, and the physiologic role of leukotrienes remains unclear.[1,14] In some systems, leukotriene effects may be mediated by inducing the production of thromboxane A_2. However, this does not seem to apply to the fetal lamb because inhibiting thromboxane A_2 synthesis does not affect pulmonary vascular resistance or the response to leukotriene end-organ antagonism.[27]

In addition to producing vasoconstrictors, the fetal pulmonary circulation actively and continuously produces vasodilating substances that modulate the degree of vasoconstriction under normal conditions and may play a more active role during periods of fetal stress. These substances are mainly endothelium derived and include EDNO and PGI_2. EDNO is synthesized by the oxidation of the guanidino nitrogen moiety of L-arginine.[28] After certain stimuli, such as shear stress and the receptor binding of specific vasodilators (endothelium-dependent vasodilators), nitric oxide (NO) is synthesized and released from the endothelial cell by the activation of NO synthase (NOS). Once released from endothelial cells, NO diffuses into vascular smooth muscle cells and activates soluble guanylate cyclase, the enzyme that catalyzes the production of guanosine 3',5'-cyclic monophosphate (cGMP) from guanosine 5'-triphosphate. Activation of guanylate cyclase increases the concentrations of cGMP, thus initiating a cascade that results in smooth muscle relaxation (Fig. 7–2).[29] Endothelial production of NO and cGMP has been demonstrated in the fetal, neonatal, and adult pulmonary vasculature.[30] In the fetus, EDNO production is stimulated both by receptor-mediated mechanisms and by activation of adenosine triphosphate–dependent K^+ channels.[31] The latter pathway is thought to be stimulated by stretch or by increased shear forces on the pulmonary vascular endothelium. In fetal lambs, inhibiting EDNO synthesis produces marked increases in resting fetal pulmonary vascular resis-

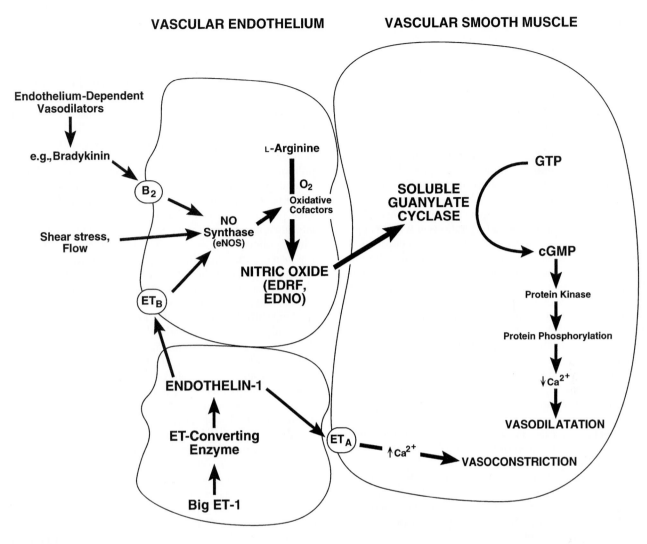

VASCULAR ENDOTHELIUM

VASCULAR SMOOTH MUSCLE

Endothelium-Dependent Vasodilators

e.g.,Bradykinin

B_2

Shear stress, Flow

ET_B

L-Arginine

O_2
Oxidative Cofactors

NO Synthase (eNOS)

NITRIC OXIDE (EDRF, EDNO)

ENDOTHELIN-1

ET-Converting Enzyme

Big ET-1

ET_A

SOLUBLE GUANYLATE CYCLASE

GTP

cGMP

Protein Kinase

Protein Phosphorylation

$\downarrow Ca^{2+}$

VASODILATATION

$\uparrow Ca^{2+}$ VASOCONSTRICTION

FIGURE 7–2

Schematic representation of the interactions, in vascular endothelial and smooth muscle cells, between the NO-cGMP cascade and ET-1 and its receptors in modulating pulmonary vascular tone. NO = nitric oxide; O_2 = oxygen; EDRF = endothelium-derived relaxing factor; EDNO = endothelium-derived nitric oxide; GTP = guanosine triphosphate; cGMP = cyclic guanosine monophosphate; ET_B = endothelin B receptor; ET_A = endothelin A receptor; B_2 = bradykinin receptor.

tance and inhibits the ventilation-induced decrease in pulmonary vascular resistance.[32,33] In addition, studies of intrapulmonary arteries and isolated lung preparations of the sheep reveal maturational increases in NO-mediated relaxation during the late fetal and early postnatal period.[34–38] For example, in intrapulmonary arteries, basal NO production rises two-fold from late gestation to 1 week of life and another 1.6-fold from 1 to 4 weeks of life.[36] Similarly, in rat lung parenchyma, both endothelial NOS (eNOS) and soluble guanylate cyclase gene expression rise during late gestation but fall postnatally.[37,38] This maturational increase in NO and cGMP production parallels the dramatic decrease in pulmonary vascular resistance that occurs at birth. These data suggest that NO activity mediates, in part, resting fetal pulmonary vascular tone, regulates the fall in pulmonary vascular resistance during the transitional pulmonary circulation, and maintains the normal low postnatal pulmonary vascular resistance. Data also suggest that NO (with the associated increase in cGMP) is

released in response to acute pulmonary vasoconstricting stimuli, such as acute alveolar hypoxia or thromboxane, to modulate the pulmonary hypertensive response in the postnatal pulmonary circulation.[39]

PGI_2 is synthesized primarily in vascular endothelial cells and produces vasodilatation by activating adenylate cyclase through receptor G protein–coupled mechanisms. Activation of adenylate cyclase increases adenosine 3′,5′-cyclic monophosphate (cAMP) concentrations, thus initiating a cascade that results in smooth muscle relaxation. Throughout gestation, there is a maturational increase in PGI_2 production that parallels the decrease in pulmonary vascular resistance in the fetal third trimester.[18] However, in vivo, prostaglandin inhibition does not markedly change resting pulmonary vascular resistance, questioning the importance of basal PGI_2 activity in mediating resting fetal pulmonary vascular tone.[40]

Endothelin-1 (ET-1), a 21–amino acid polypeptide also produced by vascular endothelial cells, has potent vasoactive properties.[41] The hemodynamic effects of ET-1 are mediated by at least two distinctive receptor populations, ET_A and ET_B. ET_A receptors are located on vascular smooth muscle cells and are likely to be responsible for the vasoconstricting effects of ET-1, whereas most ET_B receptors are located on endothelial cells and are likely to be responsible for the vasodilating effects of ET-1 (see Fig. 7–2).[42, 43] The predominant effect of exogenous ET-1 in the fetal and newborn pulmonary circulation is vasodilatation, mediated by ET_B receptor activation and NO release. However, the predominant effect in the juvenile and adult pulmonary circulation is vasoconstriction, mediated by ET_A receptor activation.[44, 45] This developmental alteration in the hemodynamic response to exogenous ET-1 is associated with developmental alterations in ET-1 receptor densities.[46] In fetal lambs, selective ET_A receptor blockade produces small decreases in resting fetal pulmonary resistance. This suggests a potential, minor role for basal ET-1–induced vasoconstriction in maintaining the high fetal pulmonary vascular resistance.[47] Although plasma concentrations of ET-1 are increased at birth, in vivo data suggest that basal ET-1 activity does not play an important role in mediating the transitional or resting postnatal pulmonary circulation.[48, 49]

Other vasoactive substances may also play a role in maintaining the high pulmonary vascular resistance in the fetus. Thromboxane A_2, synthesized from arachidonic acid by the cyclooxygenase enzymes, is a vasoconstrictor, as is platelet-activating factor. Both produce potent pulmonary vasoconstriction in newborn and adult animals. Several growth factors, particularly platelet-derived growth factor, which are involved in vascular smooth muscle growth and proliferation, also have vasoconstrictor effects. Whether any of these, or other compounds yet to be defined, contribute to maintaining the high pulmonary vascular resistance in the fetus is unknown.

Animal studies suggest that the autonomic nervous system plays little or no role in mediating normal resting control of the fetal pulmonary vascular resistance but, when stimulated, could alter pulmonary vascular resistance.[50, 51] The increased pulmonary vasomotor tone found in the fetus accentuates the responses to various stimuli. Whether these mechanisms are invoked during fetal stress or are involved in perinatal changes is not clear.

CHANGES IN THE PULMONARY CIRCULATION AT BIRTH

After birth, with initiation of ventilation by the lungs and the subsequent increase in pulmonary and systemic arterial blood oxygen tensions, pulmonary vascular resistance decreases and pulmonary blood flow increases by 8- to 10-fold to match systemic blood flow (300 to 400 ml/min/kg body weight). This large increase in pulmonary blood flow increases pulmonary venous return to the left atrium, increasing left atrial pressure. The valve of the foramen ovale then closes, preventing any significant atrial right-to-left shunting of blood. In addition, the ductus arteriosus constricts and closes functionally within several hours after birth, effectively separating the pulmonary and systemic circulations. Mean pulmonary arterial pressure decreases

and is approximately 50% of mean systemic arterial pressure by 24 hours of age. Adult values are reached 2 to 6 weeks after birth.[52–54]

The decrease in pulmonary vascular resistance with ventilation and oxygenation at birth is regulated by a complex and incompletely understood interplay between metabolic and mechanical factors, triggered by the ventilatory and circulatory changes that occur at birth (Fig. 7–3). Physical expansion of the fetal lamb lung without changing oxygen tension increases fetal pulmonary blood flow and decreases pulmonary vascular resistance, but not to newborn values.[55] A small proportion of this decrease relates to replacement of fluid in the alveoli with gas, which allows unkinking of the small pulmonary arteries, and to the changes in alveolar surface tension, which exert a negative dilating pressure on the small pulmonary arteries, maintaining their patency.[56] Physical expansion of the lung also releases vasoactive substances such as PGI_2, which increases pulmonary blood flow and decreases pulmonary vascular resistance in the fetal goat and lamb.[57] There is also net production of PGI_2 by the lung with the initiation of ventilation at birth.[57] In addition, inhibitors of prostaglandin synthesis (such as indomethacin and meclofenamic acid) not only block PGI_2 production but also attenuate the increase in pulmonary blood flow and decrease in pulmonary vascular resistance that occur with physical expansion of the fetal lung, although not the changes that occur with oxygenation.[58] Therefore, PGI_2 or perhaps, but less likely, another metabolite of arachidonic acid plays an important role in the increase in pulmonary blood flow and decrease in pulmonary vascular resistance that occur in association with the mechanical component (stretch) of ventilation at birth.

Other prostaglandins may also play a role in these circulatory changes. PGE_2, produced in the fetal vasculature and the placenta, not only maintains patency of the ductus arteriosus but also decreases pulmonary vascular resistance in fetal lambs and goats. However, both PGI_2 and PGE_2 also produce systemic vasodilatation in intact term fetal animals, whereas systemic vascular resistance normally increases soon after ventilation begins.[14] Therefore, they probably are not the only prostaglandins involved with pulmonary vasodilatation. Among the other prostaglandins, PGD_2 has attracted particular interest. PGD_2 given to newborn animals produces greater pulmonary than systemic vasodilatation.[59, 60] This differential effect is lost by about 12 to 15 days of age, when PGD_2 produces pulmonary vasoconstriction. A similar pattern of response follows the administration of histamine, which is a modest pulmonary vasodilator in the immediate perinatal period but subsequently becomes a pulmonary vasoconstrictor.[61] Both PGD_2 and histamine are released from mast cells. In fetal rhesus monkeys, mast cell numbers increase in the lungs during the last portion of gestation, and after birth, they decrease markedly.[62] Therefore, the stimulus of lung expansion may cause mast cells to degranulate and release PGD_2 and histamine, which contribute to the initial postnatal pulmonary vasodilatation.

Bradykinin, another vasoactive agent, is a potent vasodilator in the fetus.[63] After the lungs of fetal lambs are ventilated with oxygen or the fetuses are exposed to hyperbaric oxygen, the concentration of kininogen, the brady-

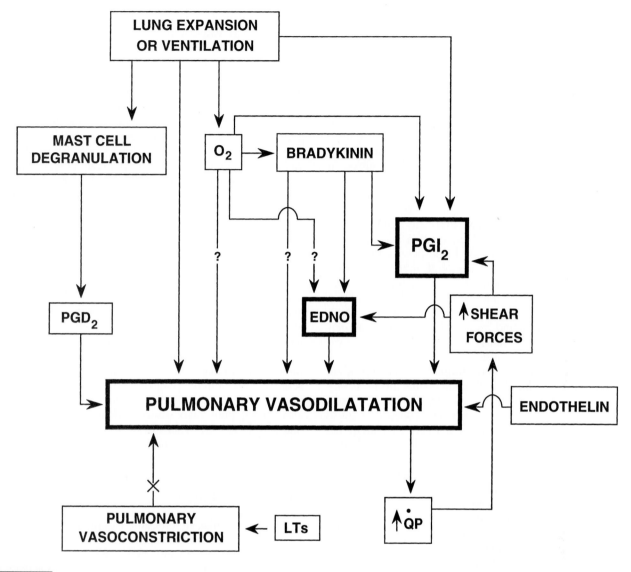

FIGURE 7–3

Factors likely to be responsible for the changes of pulmonary vascular resistance and pulmonary blood flow with ventilation with oxygen at birth. PGD_2 = prostaglandin D_2; EDNO = endothelium-derived nitric oxide; PGI_2 = prostacyclin; $\dot{Q}P$ = pulmonary blood flow per minute; LTs = leukotrienes; O_2 = oxygen.

kinin precursor, decreases and the concentration of bradykinin in blood increases.[63] Bradykinin stimulates PGI_2 production in intact fetal lungs and in pulmonary vascular endothelial cells in culture, which would enhance vasodilatation.[64] Bradykinin receptor blockade, however, does not change the increase in pulmonary blood flow and the decrease in pulmonary vascular resistance that occur with ventilation of the fetal lamb with oxygen.[65] Therefore, the role of bradykinin in the transitional circulation is questionable. Although ET-1 is a potent fetal pulmonary vasodilator and circulating levels of ET-1 are increased in the newborn period, in vivo data suggest that ET-1 activity does not play an important role in mediating the transitional pulmonary circulation.[44, 48, 49, 66]

Ventilation of the fetus without oxygenation produces partial pulmonary vasodilatation, whereas ventilation with air or oxygen produces complete pulmonary vasodilatation.

The exact mechanisms of oxygen-induced pulmonary vasodilatation during the transitional circulation remain unclear. The increase in alveolar or arterial oxygen tension may decrease pulmonary vascular resistance either directly by dilating the small pulmonary arteries or indirectly by stimulating the production of vasodilator substances such as PGI_2 or bradykinin. EDNO has been implicated as an important mediator of the decrease in pulmonary vascular resistance at birth in association with increased oxygenation. For example, inhibition of NOS attenuates the increase in pulmonary blood flow due to oxygenation of fetal lambs induced by either in utero ventilation with oxygen or maternal hyperbaric oxygen exposure.[17, 67] In utero ventilation without changing fetal blood gases increases eNOS gene expression in lung parenchyma of fetal lambs; this is further increased by ventilation with 100% oxygen.[68] Shaul and coworkers[36] have shown in cultured fetal and newborn pulmonary endothelial cells that there is a maturational rise in NO production from late gestation to 4 weeks of age.[36] In addition, this NO production appears to be modulated by oxygen.[19] Moreover, both acute inhibition and chronic inhibition of NOS before delivery significantly attenuate the normal increase in pulmonary blood flow at birth.[32,69] These data suggest an important role for EDNO activity during the transitional circulation. However, the immediate decrease in pulmonary vascular resistance minutes after birth is not attenuated by NO inhibition. Therefore, there are at least two components to the decrease in pulmonary vascular resistance with the initiation of ventilation and oxygenation. First, there is partial pulmonary vasodilatation caused by physical expansion of the lung and the production of prostaglandins (PGI_2 and PGD_2). This is probably independent of fetal oxygenation and results in a modest increase in pulmonary blood flow and decrease in pulmonary vascular resistance. Next, there is a further maximal pulmonary vasodilatation associated with fetal oxygenation, which is not necessarily dependent on prostaglandin production. This results in an increase in pulmonary blood flow and decrease in pulmonary vascular resistance to newborn values. This latter pulmonary vasodilatation is probably caused by the synthesis of EDNO, although the exact stimulus or stimuli for EDNO production are not yet defined. Both components are necessary for the successful transition to extrauterine life. An additional mechanism by which vasodilatation occurs relates to the stimulation by increased shear forces of endothelial cells to produce both EDNO and PGI_2. It is possible that after the initial fall in pulmonary vascular resistance, due to another mechanism, this particular mechanism acts to maintain pulmonary vasodilatation.

Additional vasoactive substances, such as adrenomedullin and calcitonin gene–related peptide, have been shown to be potent pulmonary vasodilators and should be considered possible physiologic mediators.[70,71] Control of the perinatal pulmonary circulation, therefore, probably reflects a balance between factors producing pulmonary vasoconstriction (low oxygen tension, leukotrienes, and other vasoconstricting substances) and those producing pulmonary vasodilatation (high oxygen tension, PGI_2, EDNO, and other vasodilating substances). The dramatic increase in pulmonary blood flow with the initiation of ventilation and oxygenation at birth reflects a shift from active pulmonary vasoconstriction in the fetus to active pulmonary vasodilatation in the neonate.

REGULATION OF POSTNATAL PULMONARY VASCULAR RESISTANCE

As stated before, mean pulmonary arterial pressure decreases to approximately 50% of mean systemic arterial pressure by 24 hours of age, and adult values are reached 2 to 6 weeks after birth.[51–53] Therefore, after the immediate postnatal state, the pulmonary circulation is maintained in a dilated, low-resistance state. In fact, most pulmonary vasodilators cannot further dilate the resting newborn pulmonary circulation.[9] Evidence suggests that basal release of NO, with the subsequent increase in smooth muscle cell concentrations of cGMP, mediates in part the low resting pulmonary vascular resistance of the neonate. For example, intravenous infusion of N^ω-nitro-L-arginine, an inhibitor of

EDNO synthesis, produces significant increases in the resting pulmonary vascular resistance of newborn lambs and pigs.[72] In addition, M&B 22948 (a cGMP-specific phosphodiesterase inhibitor, which prevents the breakdown of endogenous cGMP) is one of the few agents that can further dilate the resting pulmonary circulation of the newborn lamb.[73] The infusion of N^ω-nitro-L-arginine completely blocks M&B 22948–induced pulmonary vasodilatation, suggesting that the majority of endogenous cGMP is generated from the basal release of NO. Other vasoactive substances including histamine, 5-hydroxytryptamine, bradykinin, and metabolites of arachidonic acid by the cyclooxygenase and lipoxygenase pathways have been implicated in mediating postnatal pulmonary vascular tone. However, their roles, if any, are not well elucidated. Prostaglandin inhibition after the infusion of meclofenamic acid does not alter resting pulmonary vascular tone of the resting newborn lamb, minimizing the role of prostaglandins.[74]

Two of the most important factors affecting pulmonary vascular resistance in the postnatal period are oxygen concentration and pH. Decreasing oxygen tension or pH elicits pulmonary vasoconstriction of the resting pulmonary circulation.[75] The pulmonary vasoconstriction in response to acute alveolar hypoxia is probably greater in the younger animal than in the adult.[76] The mechanism of acute hypoxic pulmonary vasoconstriction remains unclear and is the subject of extensive review.[77] Acidosis potentiates hypoxic pulmonary vasoconstriction, and alkalosis reduces it.[75] The exact mechanism of pH-mediated pulmonary vasoactive responses also remains incompletely understood but appears to be independent of $PaCO_2$.[78]

METABOLIC FUNCTION

Pulmonary vascular endothelium can produce (e.g., PGI_2, EDNO, bradykinin, angiotensin II, ET-1) and remove (e.g., catecholamines, bradykinin, PGE_2, ET-1) many different vasoactive substances from the circulation. This activity is present in the fetus and changes at the time of transition to air breathing.[79,80] Concomitant with the increasing metabolic activity of the fetal lung (particularly increasing antioxidant enzyme and surfactant phospholipid synthesis) in the latter weeks of gestation, resting pulmonary blood flow in the fetal lamb increases (from about 4% of combined ventricular output to about 8%). After birth, in association with the dramatic increase in pulmonary blood flow, pulmonary vascular metabolic capacity also increases markedly, to a large extent because of a significant increase in pulmonary vascular endothelium functional surface area. Angiotensin I conversion to angiotensin II by the endothelial enzyme angiotensin-converting enzyme increases, and the same enzyme is responsible for the metabolic breakdown of the vasoactive peptide bradykinin. Metabolic removal of PGE_2 also increases, and this is an important component of the transition because PGE_2 is responsible for ductus arteriosus patency.

FAILURE OF PULMONARY VASCULAR RESISTANCE TO DECREASE AT BIRTH

Failure of pulmonary vascular resistance to decrease at birth is discussed in detail in Chapter 46.

ALTERED PULMONARY VASCULAR REGULATION SECONDARY TO INCREASED PULMONARY BLOOD FLOW

This is discussed in detail in Chapter 46.

ALTERED PULMONARY VASCULAR REGULATION AT ALTITUDE

Since Rotta and colleagues[81] first published data on right-sided heart catheterization of the natives of Morococha, Peru, it has been well established that the pulmonary circulation of high-altitude natives is altered as a result of the low oxygen tension. The most striking adaptation to altitude is the development of hypoxia-induced pulmonary hypertension. In spite of a great deal of research, the mechanisms of hypoxia-induced pulmonary vasoconstriction and pulmonary hypertension remain unclear.

Newcomers to altitude develop acute increases in pulmonary arterial pressure and pulmonary vascular resistance. This represents acute pulmonary vasoconstriction secondary to alveolar hypoxia and is quickly reversed by restoring normal alveolar oxygen tension. Both acclimatized lowlanders and high-altitude natives have chronic pulmonary hypertension and right ventricular hypertrophy that are not completely reversed by oxygen breathing. This is associated with not only active vasoconstriction but also substantial structural remodeling of the pulmonary circulation. The characteristic structural change of high-altitude natives is increased muscle in the small pulmonary arteries. Irreversible changes, such as occlusive intimal fibrosis, rarely occur. This is consistent with physiologic findings that the mean pulmonary arterial pressure of high-altitude natives is decreased by approximately 20% when oxygen is breathed and is halved after 2 years of residence at sea level.[82] Lowlanders exposed to altitude for 2 to 3 weeks develop pulmonary hypertension that is also not completely reversed by breathing 100% oxygen, suggesting that smooth muscle changes can occur within this time.[83] This is supported by animal studies. In fact, infants born at a high altitude show a persistent fetal muscularization of the pulmonary circulation that changes to the adult pattern only after a few weeks.[84]

REFERENCES

1. Heymann MA, Soifer SJ: Control of the fetal and neonatal pulmonary circulation. *In* Weir EK, Reeves JT (eds): Pulmonary Vascular Physiology and Pathophysiology. New York, Marcel Dekker, 1989, pp 33–50.
2. Levin DL, Rudolph AM, Heymann MA, Phibbs RH: Morphological development of the pulmonary vascular bed in fetal lambs. Circulation 53:144, 1976.
3. Hislop A, Reid LM: Intra-pulmonary arterial development during fetal life—branching pattern and structure. J Anat 113:35, 1972.
4. Reid LM: Structure and function in pulmonary hypertension. New perceptions. Chest 89:279, 1986.
5. Hislop A, Reid LM: Pulmonary arterial development during childhood: Branching pattern and structure. Thorax 28:129, 1973.
6. Meyrick B, Reid L: The effect of continued hypoxia on rat pulmonary arterial circulation: An ultrastructural study. Lab Invest 38:188, 1978.
7. Roos A: Poiseuille's law and its limitations in vascular systems. Med Thorac 19:224, 1962.
8. Agarwal JB, Paltoo R, Palmer WH: Relative viscosity of blood at varying hematocrits in pulmonary circulation. J Appl Physiol 29:866, 1970.
9. Rudolph AM, Auld PA: Physical factors affecting normal and serotonin-constricted pulmonary vessels. Am J Physiol 198:864, 1960.
10. Culver BH, Butler J: Mechanical influence on the pulmonary microcirculation. Annu Rev Physiol 42:187, 1980.
11. Permutt S, Caldini P, Maseri A, et al: Recruitment vs. distensibility in the pulmonary vascular bed. *In* Fishman AP, Hecht HH (eds): The Pulmonary Circulation and Interstitial Space. Chicago, University of Chicago Press, 1969, p 375–390.
12. Rudolph AM, Heymann MA: Circulatory changes during growth in the fetal lamb. Circ Res 26:289, 1970.
13. Rasanen J, Wood DC, Weiner S, et al: Role of the pulmonary circulation in the distribution of human fetal cardiac output during the second half of pregnancy. Circulation 94:1068, 1996.
14. Rudolph AM: Fetal and neonatal pulmonary circulation. Annu Rev Physiol 41:383, 1979.
15. Parker HR, Purves MJ: Some effects of maternal hyperoxia and hypoxia on the blood gas tension and vascular pressures in the fetal sheep. Q J Exp Physiol 12:205, 1967.
16. Soifer SJ, Kaslow D, Roman C, Heymann MA: Umbilical cord compression produces pulmonary hypertension in newborn lambs: A model to study the pathophysiology of persistent pulmonary hypertension of the newborn. J Dev Physiol 9:239, 1987.
17. Tiktinsky MH, Morin FC: Increasing oxygen tension dilates fetal pulmonary circulation via endothelium-derived relaxing factor. Am J Physiol 265:H376, 1993.
18. Shaul PW, Farrar MA, Magness RR: Oxygen modulation of pulmonary arterial prostacyclin synthesis is developmentally regulated. Am J Physiol 265:H621, 1993.
19. Shaul PW, Farrar MA, Zellers TM: Oxygen modulates endothelium-derived relaxing factor production in fetal pulmonary arteries. Am J Physiol 262:H355, 1992.
20. Ahmed T, Oliver W Jr: Does slow-reacting substance of anaphylaxis mediate hypoxic pulmonary vasoconstriction? Am Rev Respir Dis 127:566, 1983.
21. Schuster DP, Dennis DR: Leukotriene inhibitors do not block hypoxic pulmonary vasoconstriction in dogs. J Appl Physiol 65:1808, 1987.
22. Schreiber MD, Heymann MA, Soifer SJ: Leukotriene inhibition prevents and reverses hypoxic vasoconstriction in newborn lambs. Pediatr Res 19:437, 1985.
23. LeBidois J, Soifer SJ, Clyman RI, Heymann MA: Piriprost: A putative leukotriene synthesis inhibitor increases pulmonary blood flow in fetal lambs. Pediatr Res 22:350, 1987.
24. Soifer SJ, Loitz RD, Roman C, Heymann MA: Leukotriene end organ antagonists increase pulmonary blood in fetal lambs. Am J Physiol 249:H570, 1985.
25. Velvis H, Krusell J, Roman C, et al: Leukotrienes C_4, D_4, and E_4 in fetal lamb tracheal fluid. J Dev Physiol 14:37, 1990.
26. Stenmark KR, James SL, Voelkel NF, et al: Leukotriene C_4 and D_4 in neonates with hypoxemia and pulmonary hypertension. N Engl J Med 309:77, 1983.
27. Clozel M, Clyman RI, Soifer SJ, Heymann MA: Thromboxane is not responsible for the high pulmonary vascular resistance in fetal lambs. Pediatr Res 19:1254, 1985.
28. Palmer RMJ, Ashton DS, Moncada S: Vascular endothelial cells synthesize nitric oxide from L-arginine. Nature 333:664, 1988.
29. Fiscus RR: Molecular mechanisms of endothelium-mediated vasodilatation. Semin Thromb Hemost 14:12, 1988.
30. Shaul PW: Nitric oxide in the developing lung. Adv Pediatr 42:367, 1995.
31. Chang J, Moore P, Fineman JR, et al: K^+ channel pulmonary vasodilatation in fetal lambs: Role of endothelium-derived nitric oxide. J Appl Physiol 73:188, 1992.
32. Abman SH, Chatfield BA, Hall SL, McMurtry IF: Role of endothelium-derived relaxing factor during transition of pulmonary circulation at birth. Am J Physiol 259:H1921, 1990.
33. Moore P, Velvis H, Fineman JR, et al: EDRF inhibition attenuates the increase in pulmonary blood flow due to oxygen ventilation in fetal lambs. J Appl Physiol 73:2151, 1992.
34. Perreault T, De Marte J: Maturational changes in endothelium-derived relaxations in newborn piglet pulmonary circulation. Am J Physiol 264:H302, 1993.

35. Steinhorn RH, Morin FC III, Gugino SF, et al: Developmental differences in endothelium-dependent responses in isolated ovine pulmonary arteries and veins. Am J Physiol 264:H2162, 1993.

36. Shaul PW, Farrar MA, Magness RR: Pulmonary endothelial nitric oxide production is developmentally regulated in the fetus and newborn. Am J Physiol 265:H1056, 1993.

37. North AJ, Star RA, Brannon TS, et al: Nitric oxide synthase type I and type III gene expression are developmentally regulated in rat lung. Am J Physiol 266:L635, 1994.

38. Bloch KD, Filippov G, Sanchez LS, et al: Pulmonary soluble guanylate cyclase, a nitric oxide receptor, is increased during the perinatal period. Am J Physiol 272:L400, 1997.

39. Fineman JR, Chang R, Soifer SJ: EDRF inhibition augments pulmonary hypertension in intact newborn lambs. Am J Physiol 262:H1365, 1992.

40. Morin FC, Egan EA, Norfleet WT: Indomethacin does not diminish the pulmonary vascular response of the fetus to increased oxygen tension. Pediatr Res 24:696, 1988.

41. Yanagisawa M, Kurihara H, Kimura S, et al: A novel potent vasoconstrictor peptide produced by vascular endothelial cells. Nature 332:411, 1988.

42. Arai H, Hori S, Aramori I, et al: Cloning and expression of a cDNA encoding an endothelin receptor. Nature 348:730, 1990.

43. Sakurai T, Yanagisawa M, Takuwa Y, et al: Cloning of a cDNA encoding a non–isopeptide-selective subtype of the endothelin receptor. Nature 348:732, 1990.

44. Chatfield BA, McMurtry IF, Hall SL, Abman SH: Hemodynamic effects of endothelin-1 on ovine fetal pulmonary circulation. Am J Physiol 261:R182, 1991.

45. Wong J, Vanderford PA, Fineman JR, Soifer SJ: Developmental effects of endothelin-1 on the pulmonary circulation in sheep. Pediatr Res 36:394, 1994.

46. Hislop AA, Zhao YD, Springall DR, et al: Postnatal changes in endothelin-1 binding in porcine pulmonary vessels and airways. Am J Respir Cell Mol Biol 12:557, 1995.

47. Ivy DD, Kinsella JP, Abman SH: Physiologic characterization of endothelin A and B receptor activity in the ovine fetal pulmonary circulation. J Clin Invest 93:2141, 1994.

48. Nakamura T, Kasai K, Konuma S, et al: Immunoreactive endothelin concentrations in maternal and fetal blood. Life Sci 46:1045, 1990.

49. Winters J, Wong J, Van Dyke D, et al: Endothelin receptor blockade does not alter the increase in pulmonary blood flow due to oxygen ventilation in fetal lambs. Pediatr Res 40:152, 1996.

50. Colebatch HJH, Dawes GS, Goodwin JW, Nadeau RA: The nervous control of the circulation of the foetal and newly expanded lungs of the lamb. J Physiol 178:544, 1965.

51. Rudolph AM, Heymann MA, Lewis AB: Physiology and pharmacology of the pulmonary circulation in the fetus and newborn. In Hodson WA (ed): Lung Biology in Health and Disease. Vol 6: Development of the Lung. New York, Marcel Dekker, 1977, pp 497–523.

52. Iwamoto HS, Teitel D, Rudolph AM: Effects of birth-related events on blood flow distribution. Pediatr Res 22:634, 1987.

53. Rudolph AM: Distribution and regulation of blood flow in the fetal and neonatal lamb. Circ Res 57:811, 1985.

54. Reeves JT, Grover RF: High altitude pulmonary hypertension and pulmonary edema. Prog Cardiol 4:99, 1975.

55. Dawes GS, Mott JC, Widdicombe JG, et al: Changes in the lungs of the newborn lamb. J Physiol 121:141, 1953.

56. Enhorning G, Adams FH, Norman A: Effect of lung expansion on fetal lamb circulation. Acta Paediatr Scand 55:441, 1966.

57. Leffler CW, Hessler JR, Green RS: The onset of breathing at birth stimulates pulmonary vascular prostacyclin synthesis. Pediatr Res 18:938, 1984.

58. Velvis H, Moore P, Heymann MA: Prostaglandin inhibition prevents the fall in pulmonary vascular resistance as a result of rhythmic distension of the lungs in fetal lambs. Pediatr Res 30:62, 1991.

59. Cassin S, Tod M, Phillips J, et al: Effects of prostaglandin D2 in perinatal circulation. Am J Physiol 240:H755, 1981.

60. Soifer SJ, Morin FC III, Kaslow DC, Heymann MA: The developmental effects of prostaglandin D2 on the pulmonary and systemic circulations in the newborn lamb. J Dev Physiol 5:237, 1983.

61. Goetzman BW, Milstein JM: Pulmonary vascular histamine receptors in newborn and young lambs. J Appl Physiol 49:380, 1980.

62. Schwartz LS, Osborn BI, Frick OL: An ontogenic study of histamine and mast cells in the fetal rhesus monkey. J Allergy Clin Immunol 56:381, 1974.

63. Heymann MA, Rudolph AM, Nies AS, Melmon KL: Bradykinin production associated with oxygenation of the fetal lamb. Circ Res 25:521, 1969.

64. McIntyre TM, Zimmerman GA, Satoh K, Prescott SM: Cultured endothelial cells synthesize both platelet activating factor and prostacyclin in response to histamine, bradykinin, and adenosine triphosphate. J Clin Invest 76:271, 1985.

65. Banerjee A, Heymann MA: Bradykinin receptor blockade does not affect oxygen mediated pulmonary vasodilatation in fetal lambs. Pediatr Res 36:474, 1994.

66. Yoshibayashi M, Nishioka K, Nakao K, et al: Plasma endothelin levels in healthy children: High values in early infancy. J Cardiovasc Pharmacol 17:S404, 1992.

67. Cornfield DN, Chatfield BA, McQueston JA, et al: Effects of birth-related stimuli on L-arginine–dependent pulmonary vasodilatation in ovine fetus. Am J Physiol 262:H1474, 1992.

68. Black SM, Johengen MJ, Ma ZD, et al: Ventilation and oxygenation induce endothelial nitric oxide synthase gene expression in the lungs of fetal lambs. J Clin Invest 100:1448, 1997.

69. Fineman JR, Wong J, Morin FC, et al: Chronic nitric oxide inhibition in utero produces persistent pulmonary hypertension in newborn lambs. J Clin Invest 93:2675, 1994.

70. de Vroomen M, Takahashi Y, Gournay V, et al: Adrenomedullin increases pulmonary blood flow in fetal sheep. Pediatr Res 41:493, 1997.

71. Takahashi Y, de Vroomen M, Roman C, Heymann MA: Calcitonin gene–related peptide increases pulmonary blood flow in fetal sheep. Pediatr Res 41:269A, 1997.

72. Fineman JR, Heymann MA, Soifer SJ: N^{ω}-Nitro-L-arginine attenuates endothelium-dependent pulmonary vasodilatation in lambs. Am J Physiol 260:H1299, 1991.

73. Braner DAV, Fineman JR, Chang R, Soifer SJ: M&B 22948, a cGMP phosphodiesterase inhibitor, produces and augments pulmonary vasodilatation in the newborn lamb. Am J Physiol 264:H252, 1993.

74. Fineman JR, Wong J, Soifer SJ: Hyperoxia and alkalosis produce pulmonary vasodilatation independent of endothelium-derived nitric oxide synthesis in newborn lambs. Pediatr Res 33:341, 1993.

75. Rudolph AM, Yuan S: Response of the pulmonary vasculature to hypoxia and H^+ ion concentration changes. J Clin Invest 45:399, 1966.

76. Custer JR, Hales CA: Influence of alveolar oxygen on pulmonary vasoconstriction in newborn lambs versus sheep. Am Rev Respir Dis 132:326, 1985.

77. Cutaia M, Rounds S: Hypoxic pulmonary vasoconstriction. Physiologic significance, mechanism, and clinical relevance. Chest 97:706, 1993.

78. Schreiber MD, Heymann MA, Soifer SJ: Increased arterial pH, not decreased PaCO2, attenuates hypoxia-induced pulmonary vasoconstriction in newborn lambs. Pediatr Res 20:113, 1986.

79. Said SI: Metabolic functions of the pulmonary circulation. Circ Res 50:325, 1982.

80. Pitt BR: Metabolic functions of the lung and systemic vasoregulation. Fed Proc 43:2574, 1984.

81. Rotta A, Canepa A, Hurtado A, et al: Pulmonary circulation at sea level and at high altitude. J Appl Physiol 9:328, 1956.

82. Penaloza D, Sime F, Banchero N, Gamboa R: Pulmonary hypertension in healthy man born and living at high altitudes. Med Thorac 19:449, 1962.

83. Groves BM, Reeves JT, Sutton JR, et al: Operation Everest II: Elevated high-altitude pulmonary resistance unresponsive to oxygen. J Appl Physiol 63:521, 1987.

84. Ward MP, Milledge JS, West JB (eds): Cardiovascular system. In High Altitude Medicine and Physiology. Philadelphia, University of Pennsylvania Press, 1989, pp 148–160.

SECTION II
DIAGNOSTIC METHODS

CHAPTER 8
CLINICAL HISTORY AND PHYSICAL EXAMINATION

JAMES H. MOLLER

The history and physical examination form the keystone in the diagnostic process. After the completion of these two initial steps, the physician, in most instances, should have a major diagnosis or a narrow differential diagnosis and a focused approach to further diagnostic studies. As an example, in requesting an echocardiogram after the history and physical examination, the physician requesting the study should indicate a tentative diagnosis and the particular anatomic and hemodynamic information being sought.

HISTORY

The history provides four categories of information: (1) diagnostic, (2) severity assessment, (3) etiologic, and (4) effect on the child and family. In addition, while obtaining the history from the parents and the child (when it is age appropriate), the physician can allow the parents to express their concerns and questions and can assess the level of understanding about the child's condition. The medical interview is also an excellent time to provide information and allay anxiety.

DIAGNOSTIC INFORMATION

The medical history, although generally not specific for a particular diagnosis, can often lead to specific categories of conditions. Some of the important information is related to the onset of signs and symptoms.

The age at onset of congestive heart failure can provide information about diagnosis. Heart failure present at birth or in a fetus is rare and caused by paroxysmal tachycardia, myocardial abnormality, or a severely regurgitant valve (see Chapter 54). Failure occurring within the first 10 days of age is usually secondary to closure of the ductus arteriosus that unmasks a serious left-sided obstructive condition, such as aortic stenosis, aortic atresia, coarctation of the aorta, or interruption of the aortic arch.

Signs and symptoms related to cardiac failure presenting between 6 weeks and 3 months of age occur when a shunt is present at the level of the ventricles or great arteries. Examples are large ventricular septal defect, patent ductus arteriosus, and truncus arteriosus. In each of these, the volume of blood shunted is inversely related to the pulmonary vascular resistance. As the normal decline of pulmonary resistance occurs postnatally, the volume of pulmonary blood flow increases. The left ventricle is incapable of handling this excessive volume load, and failure ensues. Heart failure

occurring at an older age is most likely related to an acquired cardiac problem (see Chapter 54).

The age at which a murmur is first heard is also important. A systolic murmur heard on the first examination in the neonatal period usually reflects either semilunar valve stenosis or atrioventricular valve insufficiency or a small ventricular septal defect. Classically, the murmur of a large ventricular septal defect or patent ductus arteriosus is initially heard on the first examination after discharge from the nursery. Murmurs heard for the first time on preschool or school examinations are usually functional, but mild valvar stenosis, atrial septal defect, mitral valve prolapse, and hypertrophic cardiomyopathy may initially be recognized at this time.

The symptoms of cyanosis, blueness, or duskiness must be carefully assessed by history and physical examination to distinguish central (serious) from peripheral cyanosis (see Chapter 17). The age at onset of the cyanosis is also helpful diagnostically (see Chapter 17). Complete transposition is the most common cause of cyanosis appearing during the first day of life; more severe forms of tetralogy of Fallot, pulmonary atresia, and tricuspid atresia are others. The Ebstein malformation can also result in severe cyanosis at this age but becomes milder as pulmonary vascular resistance falls, allowing improved pulmonary blood flow (see Chapter 32).

Symptoms of stridor and dysphagia can point to a vascular ring or sling (see Chapter 41). Symptoms of stridor, noisy breathing, and hoarse voice appear in infancy and may improve with extension of the neck. Dysphagia can develop with the introduction of solid foods.

Chest Pain
Anginal chest pain occurs rarely in children with a cardiac abnormality and is associated usually with severe valvar aortic stenosis or supravalvar aortic stenosis (in the latter, coronary arterial abnormalities may coexist), cardiomyopathy, or pulmonary hypertension. The characteristics of angina in children are similar to those described in adults. The pain is typically substernal, pressing or constricting and of some duration, and may follow exertion. In adolescence, chest pain is not an infrequent complaint and is usually of musculoskeletal origin. Chest pain accounts for about 0.25% of clinic visits for children.[1,2] Because chest pain in adults is often associated with cardiac disease, its occurrence in a child causes parental anxiety. Careful history about the features of the pain can usually identify its cause. Most chest pain in children and adolescents originates in the chest wall and occurs from costochondritis,

trauma, myositis, and precordial catch syndrome. Such pain is abrupt in onset and may last for 15 minutes, but it usually lasts only a few seconds and is sharp and focal.

Other considerations for chest pain in children include the typical pain complexes of dissecting aortic aneurysm of Marfan's syndrome, pericarditis, pulmonary embolism, spontaneous pneumothorax, pleurisy, and ulcer disease.

Pneumonia and pleuritis cause chest pain by irritation of the pleura. The pain is sharp, accentuated by respiration or cough, and may be referred to the shoulder. Pneumonia, bronchitis, and other conditions associated with excessive coughing can irritate the chest wall. Gastritis and esophagitis may cause chest pain, but the history of relation to meals is helpful in identifying these conditions.

The symptom of syncope is discussed in Chapter 56 and of cyanosis in Chapter 17.

INFORMATION ABOUT SEVERITY OF CARDIAC CONDITION

Details about growth patterns, the presence of cyanosis, or congestive heart failure may provide information about the severity of the cardiac condition.

Growth

Growth is slowed in many infants and children with a cardiac malformation. Weight is more affected than is length, and head circumference is seldom affected by the severity of the cardiac anomaly.[3] An abnormally small head circumference can point to a potential cause of the cardiac malformation (e.g., a syndrome, or intrauterine growth retardation secondary to maternal viral infection).

Perhaps 20% of neonates with a cardiac malformation have a birth weight below 2500 g.[4] The frequency of low birth weight varies with the type of anomaly, being higher in ventricular septal defect and atrioventricular septal defect but rare in those with complete transposition. In fact, in complete transposition, the weight frequently exceeds 4.0 kg.

The explanation for delayed growth in utero is uncertain but could include hemodynamic effects of the anomaly on the developing fetus, the generalized effect of an etiologic agent (i.e., rubella), or the presence of a syndrome that in itself is associated with slow growth. Postnatal slow growth may be related to a combination of poor feeding and increased metabolic demands related to increased respiratory effort.

Congestive Heart Failure

The physiologic mechanisms associated with congestive heart failure are discussed in Chapter 54. The cardinal symptoms are slow feeding, rapid respiration, excessive perspiration, growth failure, and frequent respiratory infections. An infant with congestive heart failure is a "poor feeder." Although eager to eat, the infant soon tires from the fatigue of sucking. Heart failure indicates a severe cardiac malformation.

Cyanosis

Central cyanosis indicates a right-to-left shunt. The intensity of cyanosis reflects the magnitude of shunting and, when combined with knowledge of the anatomy of the malformation, allows estimation of the severity of factors influencing pulmonary blood flow or intracardiac mixing. See Chapter 17.

ETIOLOGIC FACTORS

Although the etiology of the condition cannot be discovered in most instances of congenital heart disease and many of acquired heart disease, the history and physical examination may provide clues not only of etiology but also about the underlying diagnosis and, at times, prognosis.

A careful history seeking information about siblings or other relatives with cardiac problems, neonatal deaths, "blue babies," and cardiac operations during childhood may provide clues. The recurrence rate of congenital heart disease is about 3% between siblings or between parent and child, and the concurrence rate for the type of defect is about 50% (see Chapter 18). Certain conditions, such as complete transposition, seem to have a low rate of recurrence. Others, such as coarctation of the aorta and aortic stenosis, have perhaps a 10% rate if careful screening is done to identify bicuspid aortic valves in relatives.

Many acquired conditions afflicting the heart follow mendelian patterns of inheritance. These are discussed in Chapter 2 (genetics), Chapter 49 (myocardial disease), Chapter 58 (connective tissue disorders), Chapter 35 (aortic stenosis relative to Williams' syndrome), and Chapter 36 (pulmonary stenosis relative to LEOPARD syndrome).

Perhaps as many as 50% of children with Down syndrome have a cardiac malformation. In patients with Down syndrome, atrioventricular septal defect and ventricular septal defect are the most common conditions. Less common but occurring in equal proportions are tetralogy of Fallot, patent ductus arteriosus, and atrial septal defect. Pulmonary vascular obstructive disease tends to develop early in life. Aortic stenosis and coarctation are rare. This syndrome results from additional copies of chromosome 21. The frequency of Down syndrome increases with maternal age, being 1 per 1925 women at age 20 years and 1 per 100 women at age 40 years, and trisomy is found in age-related Down syndrome. Chromosome analysis should be performed to identify familial translocation involving chromosome 21 or mosaicism. Half of the translocations arise de novo, and the other half are inherited from a carrier parent.

MATERNAL HISTORY

A history of acute illness during the pregnancy, especially within the first trimester, or a chronic condition may provide important etiologic information.

A viral infection during the first trimester may be an etiologic factor. Only rubella, which can cause the classic triad of cataracts, neurosensory deafness, and congenital heart disease (patent ductus arteriosus and peripheral pulmonary artery stenosis),[5] has been identified.

Maternal diabetes mellitus has been associated with a higher (about 3 times) occurrence rate of cardiac malformation.[6] Diabetes mellitus during pregnancy, even of gestational origin, has been associated with asymmetric septal hypertrophy that resolves in the months after delivery. About 30% of such infants of diabetic mothers have cardiomegaly, and cardiac failure occurs in 5 to 10%.

Maternal systemic lupus erythematosus and other collagen vascular disease cause complete heart block from the transplacental transfer of antibodies that attack this developing conduction system. (See Chapter 55.)

Excessive maternal alcohol ingestion is associated with fetal alcohol syndrome, in which ventricular septal defect is common.[7] The level of alcohol intake during the first trimester of pregnancy correlates with teratogenic risk.

Maternal medications may have a teratogenic effect as well. Phenytoin, trimethadione, and paramethadione have been associated with a higher rate of cardiac malformation, including congenital heart disease, although it remains controversial about the causative relationship of congenital heart disease in offspring. Lithium use in mothers has been associated with Ebstein malformation of the tricuspid valve. Thalidomide was found 30 years ago to cause truncus arteriosus and limb abnormalities in infants born of mothers who took this agent as a sedative. Major fetal abnormalities are related to isotretinoin,[8] including cardiovascular anomalies, and this drug must not be used in pregnant women.

PHYSICAL EXAMINATION

The approach to physical examination of a patient in the pediatric age range is determined by the patient's age and the setting of the examination. Most physicians who care for infants and children have developed particular techniques and sequences of the examination, so that all the necessary information is gathered and key data are not overlooked. Examination of neonates and infants receiving ventilatory assistance may be difficult because of interference with easy access to the patient. Often in these situations, it may be difficult to listen to the back, but this should be done if possible because cardiac murmurs may be heard louder or only over the back.

One- to 3-year-old children fear strangers. Having the child sit in the parent's lap is helpful. Begin the examination by inspection of the child and palpation of the peripheral pulses, before progressing to palpation of the thorax. Auscultation should be performed last. Examine from the patient's right side if you are right-handed, from the left side if you are left-handed.

In all patients, length and height must be measured and plotted on a growth chart. For those younger than 3 years, the occipital-frontal circumference should be measured and plotted. In infants and children, cyanosis or cardiac failure affects growth. Weight may be severely affected, but height is affected to a lesser degree. Head circumference is usually unaffected. When head circumference, height, and weight are each low or the severity of the cardiac condition is mild, the retarded growth should be attributed to another factor, such as familial factors or the presence of a chromosome anomaly.

GENERAL APPEARANCE

Take a moment to assess the general appearance of the infant or child. Is there distress or appearance of acute or chronic illness? Is the infant or child responsive? Most infants respond to others and are happy. Infants with cyanosis or congestive cardiac failure are frequently irritable.

SKIN COLOR

Particularly in neonates and infants, the color of the skin can provide a clue about the cardiovascular status. Is it pale, red, blue, or mottled?

Cyanosis may be difficult to note particularly in neonates, especially if the degree of hypoxemia is mild. The amount of ambient light, the examiner's experience, pigmentation, and other factors influence ability to detect cyanosis. Nurses or parents often use the term "dusky" to describe mild cyanosis. With the widespread availability of oxygen saturation monitors, milder degrees of hypoxemia can be detected and some quantification of hypoxemia obtained.

Cyanosis can be detected when approximately 5 g/dl of reduced hemoglobin is present in capillary beds. In a patient with a normal hemoglobin concentration, cyanosis can be detected when oxygen saturation is less than 88%.[9] With polycythemia, it should be possible to detect cyanosis at a higher oxygen saturation. Conversely, anemia makes it difficult to detect even more marked desaturation.

Cyanosis has been divided into two broad categories, peripheral and central. In peripheral cyanosis, also called acrocyanosis, the central oxygen saturation is normal, but because of sluggish peripheral circulation, cyanosis appears peripherally. The classic examples are the hands and feet of neonates or infants that appear blue when exposed to ambient temperature and the circumoral cyanosis that occurs in children who live in a cold climate. This form of cyanosis disappears with passive or active motion of the extremity or exposure to warmth. The trunk, abdomen, lips, and mucous membranes are not cyanotic. On occasion, generalized cyanosis occurs in a cardiac condition that is fundamentally acyanotic but has caused severe reduction in cardiac output. Diffuse cyanosis occurs then because of inadequate and slow tissue perfusion.

In central cyanosis, generalized cyanosis is present, including mucous membranes. In distinction to peripheral cyanosis, aortic oxygen saturation is reduced. Pulmonary, cardiac, and hematologic problems are associated with central cyanosis. Any condition that interferes with the transport of oxygen from the environment to the pulmonary capillary can reduce the oxygen saturation of blood exiting the pulmonary capillary bed. In neonates, the conditions range from choanal atresia to respiratory distress syndrome. Severe pneumonia and pulmonary edema are other examples of conditions interfering with oxygen transport.

Methemoglobinemia can cause cyanosis. Whether it is inherited or acquired, as from infant formula made with contaminated well water (with nitrates), the ferrous ion of hemoglobin is replaced with the ferric ion. The resultant hemoglobin cannot combine with oxygen, so cyanosis results. This condition can be suspected by finding a normal arterial PO_2 but reduced oxygen saturation value.

Finally, certain classes of cardiac malformation result in cyanosis. In common, they have a right-to-left shunt, so some of the blood reaching the aorta has not passed through the pulmonary capillary bed. There are two major groups of cyanotic cardiac conditions. In one, there is obstruction to pulmonary blood flow and an intracardiac shunt (e.g., tetralogy of Fallot and tricuspid atresia). In the other group are conditions in which mixing of systemic and pulmonary venous returns occurs within the heart (e.g., complete transposition, truncus arteriosus, and total anomalous pulmonary venous connections). A rare cause of cyanosis is pulmonary arteriovenous fistula.

In older infants and children, it is usually easy to determine from history and physical examination the organ system causing the cyanosis. In neonates, it may be difficult to do so. In this age group, the hemoglobin is elevated, which may give a ruddy appearance. The ductus arteriosus and foramen ovale may be patent and allow an intermittent right-to-left shunt if the neonate cries or there is pulmonary disease. Finally, a serious cardiac condition may be present without a murmur to point to the heart as being an issue.

In neonates, cyanosis requires a careful and directed assessment (this is discussed fully in Chapter 17). Measurement of oxygen saturation should be made in the right arm and a lower extremity in neonates to detect differential cyanosis,[10] indicating different levels of oxygen saturation in the upper and lower portions of the body. If the ductus is patent and blood flows from the pulmonary trunk to the descending aorta, a lower oxygen saturation is found in the lower than in the upper extremity. This pattern is a result of either increased pulmonary vascular resistance, due to causes ranging from pulmonary parenchymal disease to pulmonary venous obstruction (as from obstructed total anomalous pulmonary venous connection), or severe obstruction in the distal aortic arch (as from interruption of the aortic arch or coarctation of aorta). The pattern of differential cyanosis is reversed in a neonate with complete transposition and a patent ductus arteriosus, with flow of oxygenated blood from the pulmonary trunk to the descending aorta. Cyanosis in a single extremity is usually from interference to venous return, as may be associated with a vascular catheter.

Neonates may appear ruddy if hemoglobin or hematocrit is elevated, as from maternal-fetal transfusion or stripping of the umbilical cord.[11] In this situation, the arterial oxygen saturation is usually normal. Because hypervolemia is present, tachypnea and tachycardia are present and the chest radiograph shows cardiomegaly and increased pulmonary vascular markings. Distinction from a cardiac malformation may be difficult without the use of echocardiography.

Pallor or mottling of the skin indicates reduced cardiac output or cardiogenic shock. Sepsis, aortic atresia, and critical aortic stenosis or coarctation of the aorta are typical causes in neonates.

RESPIRATION

The respiratory pattern and effort should be assessed. In neonates and infants with pulmonary venous congestion from increased left ventricular filling pressure, edema develops in alveoli and bronchial and interstitial tissues. This leads to increased work of breathing manifested initially by tachypnea; but as the condition progresses, it becomes associated with flaring of the alae nasi and suprasternal and intercostal retractions. Wheezing and rales may become associated.

Hyperpnea is found in neonates and infants with reduced pulmonary blood flow and hypoxemia.

FEATURES OF SYNDROMES

A variety of syndromes associated with cardiac malformation are displayed in Table 8–1.

THORAX

The thorax is inspected for symmetry and precordial abnormalities. The posterior thorax is inspected throughout the respiratory cycle for symmetric movement and size. In patients with a hypoplastic lung, as in scimitar syndrome, the involved hemithorax (right) is smaller. Scoliosis can also cause asymmetry of the thorax. The presence of scoliosis should be sought, particularly in adolescence, and it can be brought out by asking the patient to stand and touch the toes. Although scoliosis may be more common in children with a cardiac malformation, all adolescents should be screened for it. Other causes of thoracic asymmetry and scoliosis include a Blalock-Taussig shunt, Marfan's syndrome, and muscular dystrophy.

The precordium is inspected for a bulge, a finding that signifies cardiac enlargement or right ventricular hypertrophy. In some patients, particularly with Marfan's syndrome, there may be pectus carinatum or pectus excavatum. The latter is also common in prematurely born neonates. Even if severe, it does not cause cardiac problems. The apex impulse, however, is displaced to the left; on chest radiography, the transverse diameter of the cardiac silhouette is increased, but it is narrow on a lateral film.

The precordium is palpated for the apex impulse, heaves, or thrills. The apex impulse is the most lateral spot on the thorax where the cardiac activity can be felt. This should be within the midclavicular line. It is located in the fourth interspace through age 4 years and in the fifth interspace thereafter. Displacement lateral to the site indicates cardiac enlargement or mediastinal shift. Dextrocardia can be identified by palpating the apex on the right side. On palpating the precordium with the palm of the hand, an outward movement along the left sternal border reflects right ventricular hypertrophy, and at the apex, left ventricular hypertrophy.

Thrills should also be sought with the palm of the hand rather than fingertips, because the palm is more sensitive to vibration. Thrills indicate a loud murmur, and their location helps identify the location of maximal intensity. The suprasternal notch should be palpated in addition to the precordium. Murmurs originating from the base of the heart, particularly the murmur from aortic stenosis, result in a thrill in this area. Pulmonary stenosis, coarctation of the aorta, and patent ductus arteriosus sometimes are associated with a thrill at this site, but ventricular septal defect is not. Aortic notch pulsations are prominent in patients with "aortic runoff," as in significant aortic or truncal regurgitation or a large systemic arteriovenous fistula or patent ductus arteriosus.

TABLE 8–1

MAJOR SYNDROMES ASSOCIATED WITH CARDIAC ANOMALIES

Disorder	Major Feature	Cardiovascular Abnormality	Etiology
CRANIOFACIAL SYNDROME			
Goldenhar's syndrome (oculoauriculovertebral dysplasia, hemifacial microsomia)	Facial asymmetry and hypoplasia, microtia, eartag, cleft lip/palate, hypoplastic vertebrae	(35%) VSD, T of F	?
DiGeorge's syndrome (velocardiofacial syndrome, Shprintzen's syndrome, familial conotruncal disease, CATCH-22 [see also Chapter 2])	Hypertelorism, short philtrum, down-slanting eyes, cleft palate, hypoplastic/absent thymus and parathyroid	IAA, type B; T of F ± pulmonary atresia, right aortic arch	Chromosome 22q11 deletion
Alagille's syndrome (arteriohepatic dysplasia)	Long thin face, intrahepatic bile duct paucity, butterfly vertebrae	Peripheral pulmonary arterial stenosis	Chromosome 20p11.2
Laurence-Moon-Biedl syndrome	Obesity, retinitis pigmentosa, syndactyly, polydactyly, hypoplastic genitalia, mental retardation, diabetes mellitus	Common atrium	Autosomal recessive
SYNDROMES WITH LIMB DEFECTS			
Holt-Oram syndrome (see also Chapter 2)	Upper limb deficiency—absent or triphalangeal thumb	ASD	Autosomal dominant
Aase's syndrome	Triphalangeal thumb, radial hypoplasia, hypoplastic anemia	CHD	?Autosomal recessive
Thrombocytopenia–absent radius (TAR) syndrome	Thrombocytopenia, absent radii	VSD	Autosomal recessive
ASSOCIATIONS			
VATER	Vertebral defects, anal atresia, tracheoesophageal fistula, radial dysplasia, renal dysplasia	VSD	
CHARGE	Coloboma, congenital heart defect, choanal atresia, growth and mental retardation, genitourinary anomalies, ear anomalies	CHD	
CARDIOFACIAL SYNDROMES			
Noonan's syndrome	Abnormal facies, hypertelorism, low-set ears, small stature, lymphedema, mental retardation	Pulmonary stenosis (often dysplasia), peripheral pulmonary artery stenosis, ASD, hypertrophic cardiomyopathy	Autosomal dominant
Williams' syndrome (see also Chapter 2)	Small stature, mental retardation, characteristic facies (epicanthal folds, anteverted nares, periorbital fullness), infantile hypocalcemia, stellate iris	Supravalvar aortic stenosis, peripheral pulmonary artery stenosis	Sporadic 7q23
Rubenstein-Taybi syndrome	Short stature, mental retardation, broad thumbs and toes, beaked nose, hypoplastic mandible	VSD	Microdeletion of 16p13.3
de Lange's syndrome	Prenatal growth retardation, microcephaly, limb reduction anomalies, hirsutism, synophrys, anteverted nares, down-turned lips	CHD	Some partial deletion of chromosome 3
MAJOR CHROMOSOME ABNORMALITIES			
Down syndrome (trisomy 21) (see also Chapter 2)	Characteristic facies, hypotonia, mental retardation, Brushfield's spots, simian crease, intestinal obstruction	40–50% AVSD, VSD; PDA, ASD, T of F, often PVOD; aortic stenosis, coarctation—rare	Trisomy 21, balanced translocation
Turner's syndrome	Short stature, webbed neck, lymphedema, gonadal dysgenesis	(20%) Coarctation of aorta–bicuspid aortic valve	Monosomy 45,X (50%); other abnormalities of sex chromosomes (50%)
Edward's syndrome (trisomy 18)	Low birth weight, microcephaly, micrognathia, rocker-bottom feet, closed fist with overlapping fingers	80% VSD with pulmonary hypertension	Trisomy 18
Patau's syndrome (trisomy 13)	Low birth weight, central facial anomalies, polydactyly, chronic hemangiomas, low-set ears, visceral and genital anomalies	80% VSD with pulmonary hypertension, dextrocardia	Trisomy 13
OTHER SYNDROMES DISCUSSED ELSEWHERE			
Tuberous sclerosis	See Chapter 59 (cardiac tumors)		
Marfan's syndrome	See Chapter 58 (connective tissue disease) and Chapter 2 (genetic disease)		
Ehlers-Danlos syndrome	See Chapter 58 (connective tissue disease)		

ASD = atrial septal defect; AVSD = atrioventricular septal defect; CHD = congenital heart disease; IAA = interruption of aortic arch; PDA = patent ductus arteriosus; PVOD = pulmonary vascular obstructive disease; T of F = tetralogy of Fallot; VSD = ventricular septal defect.

CARDIAC AUSCULTATION

With the attention directed to learning and applying a variety of diagnostic techniques, such as echocardiography, to evaluate the heart of children, the skills of auscultation are frequently considered to be less important. The skills of auscultation must be learned by supervised listening to a variety of heart sounds and murmurs and maintained by frequent practice.

Studies[12, 13] showed that physical examination is a highly sensitive and specific method of screening asymptomatic subjects for valvar heart disease. Newburger and associates[14] evaluated the ability of pediatric cardiologists to accurately detect the presence of a cardiac condition or a functional murmur by history and physical examination. They further determined the frequency that the initial categorization rate of abnormal or normal status was altered by subsequent investigative studies. They found that among 142 children considered to have a normal heart, 134 were still considered normal after testing; 5 had a possible anomaly; and only 3 had a cardiac anomaly, and these were considered minor anomalies. Among the 104 initially diagnosed with a cardiac anomaly, after investigation all 104 did have an abnormality. The study concluded that an experienced pediatric cardiologist can accurately distinguish normal from abnormal. Through training, experience, confidence in one's abilities, and a conviction that auscultation is a valuable diagnostic technique, physicians can correctly identify cardiac murmurs and avoid unnecessary costs and parental anxieties.

To gather the maximal amount of information from cardiac auscultation, particularly in neonates and infants, concerted effort, patience, and experience are required. Repeated examination may be necessary, particularly in neonates or critically ill infants and children, because of changes in cardiac rate or physiologic state. It is preferable to listen to neonates and infants when they are asleep, because the cardiac rate is slower and respirations are quieter. In neonates and infants, it is often preferable to listen through the clothing initially, before disturbing the infant by removal of the clothing, causing the infant to cry or have a faster cardiac rate. In children between the ages of 1 and 3 years, it is preferable to examine them while they sit on the parent's lap, because of the natural fear of strangers in this age group. A patient of this age should be approached slowly and in a nonthreatening way. Distraction with a toy or a light may be useful to have a chance to listen. In older children and adolescents, anxiety may cause tachycardia, which makes auscultation difficult.

Physicians should use their own stethoscopes rather than one available at the bedside or in the clinic. It should have short, thick tubing and snugly fitting earpieces. The metal tubing adjacent to the earpieces can be bent to create a firm fit. The stethoscope should have both a bell and a diaphragm. I use a 1-inch-wide diaphragm and ¾-inch bell. It is not necessary to use smaller sizes even when examining prematures; a smaller diaphragm may mask some high-pitched sounds. High-pitched murmurs, clicks, and cardiac sounds are heard better with a diaphragm. Low-frequency sounds and murmurs are heard better with the bell. Do not press the bell tightly against the skin, for this stretches the underlying skin, creating a diaphragm and diminishing low-frequency sounds.

The anterior and posterior thorax should be auscultated for murmurs. The back can be examined for both respiratory sounds and murmurs (e.g., coarctation) when the child sits, when an infant is held against the parent's chest, or when a neonate is prone. Frequently, I sit to the right side of the recumbent patient to perform auscultation. My head is positioned slightly above the level of the patient's head. Often I close my eyes to improve my concentration and open my mouth slightly because this improves hearing. Each of the four standard auscultatory areas (cardiac apex [mitral area], lower left sternal border [tricuspid area], upper left sternal border [pulmonary area], and upper right sternal border [aortic area]) should be systematically auscultated with both diaphragm and bell. The right anterior chest and both axillae should be auscultated as well, particularly in neonates and infants in whom peripheral pulmonary artery stenosis is common. If abnormalities are noted at a particular site, further exploration should extend outward from that site. In neonates with severe cardiac failure, auscultation over the head, liver, or other sites may identify an arteriovenous malformation. Attention must be directed to both the characteristic of the heart sounds and the features of murmurs.

Cardiac Sounds

The classic works of Wiggers[15] describe the relationship between electrical events, intracardiac pressure, and flow changes during the cardiac cycle. An understanding of these relationships is invaluable in understanding cardiac sounds and in interpreting murmurs on the basis of their location within the cardiac cycle (Fig. 8–1). The origin of heart sounds is uncertain, having been ascribed to valvar events, acceleration or deceleration of columns of blood, myocardial contractions, or a combination of these. Because both normal and abnormal heart sounds occur at approximately the same time as closure or opening of cardiac valves, it has been convenient to ascribe a causal relationship between the two, particularly in discussing cardiac auscultation as in this chapter. In 1958, Leatham[16] wrote an excellent article about cardiac auscultation, which is an extremely helpful review for understanding heart sounds and murmurs, even though it is more than a few decades old.

Heart sounds mark the transition of phases of the cardiac cycle (Fig. 8–1). In infants and children, four distinct heart sounds may normally be heard. These include a first heart sound, the aortic component of the second heart sound, the pulmonic component of the second heart sound, and a third heart sound (about 50% of children). These are described first, followed by abnormal heart sounds including systolic ejection click, mid to late systolic click, opening snap, and fourth heart sound. The normal characteristics and the alterations from normal are discussed.

FIRST HEART SOUND (S₁)

The first heart sound occurs at the time of closure of the mitral and tricuspid valves. Although consisting of several components, the first heart sound is single in most infants

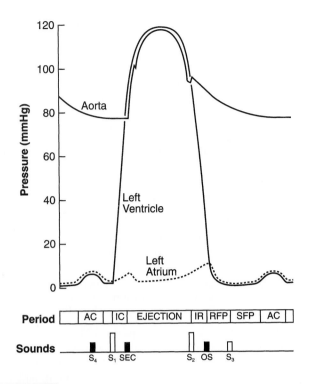

Modification of Wiggers' diagram.[15] Relationship between left-sided cardiac pressures, heart sounds, and phases of the cardiac cycle. AC = atrial contraction; IC = isovolumetric contraction; IR = isovolumetric relaxation; OS = opening snap; RFP = rapid filling phase; S_1 = first heart sound; S_2 = second heart sound; S_3 = third heart sound; S_4 = fourth heart sound; SEC = systolic ejection click; SFP = slow filling phase.

and children. It may be split, with the initial component reflecting the earlier closure of the mitral valve. Rarely is the first heart sound split in infancy. When it is, an Ebstein malformation of the tricuspid valve must be considered strongly.

The first heart sound is heard best at the cardiac apex and is louder than the second heart sound at this location. When the first heart sound is heard better along the lower left sternal border, an abnormality on the right side of the heart must be suspected.

The first heart sound may be either accentuated or diminished. The first heart sound may be accentuated in four conditions:

1. Increased blood flow across an atrioventricular valve. In patients with either increased pulmonary blood flow or regurgitation of an atrioventricular valve, the first heart sound may be accentuated. The first heart sound is accentuated at the cardiac apex in patients with increased anterograde flow across the mitral valve, as in ventricular septal defect, patent ductus arteriosus, or mitral insufficiency. The first heart sound is accentuated along the lower left sternal border (tricuspid area) in patients with increased anterograde flow across the tricuspid valve, as in atrial-level left-to-right shunt or tricuspid regurgitation.

2. Atrioventricular valvar stenosis. Both tricuspid and mitral stenosis are rare in children in many parts of the world. In areas with a high prevalence of rheumatic heart disease, mitral stenosis may be found in late childhood and

adolescence. In such patients, a high-pressure differential exists across the mitral valve at the end of the diastole. Thus, a higher than normal ventricular systolic pressure must develop before valve closure occurs. It is believed that because of the higher closure pressure, the first heart sound is accentuated. I have heard this accentuation in older children with congenital mitral stenosis but have not appreciated it in infants or young children with this condition.

3. Short PR interval. If the PR interval is short, as in Wolff-Parkinson-White syndrome, the interval between atrial contraction and onset of ventricular systole is also shortened. Presumably, this occurs at a time when the atrioventricular valves are maximally open, so the length of excursion of leaflets to closure is great. Thus, the first heart sound is loud.

4. Conditions with increased cardiac output. Increased cardiac output from conditions such as anemia and arteriovenous fistula is associated with increased anterograde flow across the atrioventricular valves, shortened diastole, and often increased contractility. These factors continue to increase loudness of the first heart sound.

The loudness of the first heart sound may be diminished from two general conditions:

1. Prolonged atrioventricular conduction. When the interval between atrial contraction and onset of ventricular systole is prolonged, the atrioventricular valve leaflets have been considered to have returned from their maximally opened position. Thus, the length of valvar excursion to closure is presumably decreased, and the first heart sound is soft.

2. Depressed myocardial function. In patients with depressed myocardial contractility, as in myocarditis, the first heart sound may be diminished.

SECOND HEART SOUND (S_2)

The normal second heart sound is composed of two sounds; the first, A_2, represents the earlier closure of the aortic valve, and the second, P_2, represents the later closure of the pulmonary valve. These sounds occur at the time of the incisura of aortic and pulmonary arterial pressure tracings and are generally coincidental with the transition between the end of ejection and the onset of isovolumetric relaxation. The components of the second heart sound are heard best in the second and third left intercostal spaces because the pulmonary valve, the most anteriorly located valve, lies immediately below this area.

The term *splitting of the second heart sound* is applied to the phenomenon of hearing two components of the second heart sound. Our studies have indicated that an interval of at least 20 or 25 milliseconds must be present between the two components before they can be heard as separate sounds by an experienced pediatric cardiologist. The degree of splitting normally varies with respiration, increasing with inspiration and decreasing with expiration, reflecting the variable volume of blood returning to the right ventricle with the phases of respiration. This phenomenon is termed *variable splitting*. In patients with tachycardia, particularly neonates and infants, it may be difficult to appreciate splitting or variability. In these patients, repeated auscultation when the heart rate is slower may allow clearer characterization of the second heart sound. Considerable diagnostic information can be obtained by careful attention to details of the second heart sound. Three aspects of the second heart sound must be assessed: loudness of individual components, degree of splitting, and variations in patterns of splitting.

Loudness of the components of the second heart sound depends on the level of pressure in the great arteries, position of the aortic and pulmonary valves within the thorax, and thickness of the anterior chest wall. In infants and children, P_2 is louder than A_2 because the pulmonary valve lies immediately below the chest wall, whereas the aortic valve is located centrally within the thorax. This difference occurs even though pulmonary arterial pressure is considerably lower than aortic pressure. In patients with transposition of the great arteries, the second heart sound is loud and single because the aortic valve, located beneath the chest wall, is closed with a high pressure.

The loudness of a component of the second heart sound depends on the pressure level at the time of the incisura, reflecting neither peak systolic nor diastolic arterial pressure. Because many forms of cardiac malformation are associated with pulmonary hypertension, care must be directed toward increased loudness of P_2, which reflects an elevation of pulmonary artery pressure.

The aortic valve is centrally placed, approximately behind the sternum at the level of the fourth space, and the ascending aorta comes closest to the chest wall to the right of the upper sternum. Therefore, A_2 is normally heard loudest at the upper right sternal border or equally loud at the upper right and left sternal borders. If A_2 is loudest at the left sternal border, it indicates an abnormal aortic position. Thus, in tetralogy of Fallot, with a dextroposed and dilated ascending aorta, A_2 is loudest to the left of the sternum in the fourth intercostal space. In both complete and corrected transposition, A_2 is loudest to the left of the sternum in the second intercostal space, and the same may be true in a truncus arteriosus. Other forms of malposition, including dextrocardia, also give an A_2 that is loudest at the upper left sternal border.

During the first two days of life, the second heart sound appears single because of the elevated pulmonary vascular resistance normally present at this stage of life. Subsequently, the second heart sound appears split. The presence of a single second heart sound beyond the immediate neonatal period indicates a serious cardiac anomaly. There may be only one semilunar valve, as in truncus arteriosus, or two valves in which one is either atretic or severely stenotic. The second heart sound is single (aortic component) in patients with pulmonary atresia, severe pulmonary stenosis, or tetralogy of Fallot. It may be single (pulmonary component) in aortic atresia or severe aortic stenosis. Unfortunately, these conditions cause severe symptoms in neonatal life, when S_2 normally appears single, so auscultation cannot allow identification of these conditions.

If the second heart sound is split but does not vary with respiration, the phenomenon is called *fixed splitting*. This usually coexists with wide splitting and indicates the presence of an atrial communication, as typically occurs in patients with an atrial septal defect.

In evaluating the second heart sound, attention should be directed to the degree of splitting. With experience, it is possible to identify wide splitting, indicating that this interval between the components of the second heart sound exceeds 60 milliseconds. If the second heart sound is easily heard to be split in a tachycardic neonate or infant, it should be considered widely split.

The second heart sound is widely split in patients with prolonged right ventricular ejection. Three types of abnormalities cause this:

1. Increased volume of right ventricular ejection. If the volume of blood ejected by the right ventricle across the pulmonary valve is increased, P_2 is delayed. This may result from pulmonary regurgitation or atrial-level shunt, such as atrial septal defect or anomalous pulmonary venous connection.

2. Obstruction to right ventricular outflow. In severe pulmonary stenosis or tetralogy of Fallot, right ventricular ejection is prolonged and P_2 delayed.

3. Complete right bundle branch block. In this condition, right ventricular depolarization is prolonged abnormally and so is right ventricular systole. Thus, P_2 is delayed.

Conditions that delay closure of the aortic valve can be identified because of paradoxical splitting of the second heart sound. Because A_2 is delayed and may occur after P_2, the degree of splitting narrows on inspiration and widens on expiration, a pattern opposite of normal. In my experience, paradoxical splitting is rare during childhood and adolescence. Three types of conditions associated with paradoxical splitting are (1) increase of left ventricular ejection volume, as in severe aortic regurgitation or patent ductus arteriosus; (2) obstruction to left ventricular outflow, as in severe aortic stenosis; and (3) complete left bundle branch block.

THIRD HEART SOUND (S_3)

A third heart sound is commonly heard in infancy. This low-frequency, broad sound occurs at the peak of ventricular inflow velocity and the transition between rapid and slow filling phases of diastole. This sound has been considered to arise in the ventricle from sudden deceleration of flow during rapid filling.[17,18] The third heart sound disappears in adulthood because the increased left ventricular wall thickness with age causes a decrease in the velocity of ventricular filling.[19]

Third heart sounds may originate from either the left or right ventricle, being heard better at the cardiac apex (mitral area) or lower left sternal border (tricuspid area), respectively. This sound is prominent in patients with conditions associated with increased volume of ventricular filling. These are conditions with increased pulmonary blood flow, valvar regurgitation, and anemia. In a patient with tachycardia from any cause, a third heart sound may become prominent and be interpreted as a gallop, a sound suggesting cardiac failure and myocardial dysfunction. In this situation, proceed carefully and reserve the term *gallop* for situations in which other findings support a diagnosis of cardiac failure.

SYSTOLIC EJECTION CLICK

A systolic ejection click may occur shortly after the first heart sound at the transition between isovolumetric contraction and the onset of ejection. It occurs at or shortly after the opening of a semilunar valve. During the first 24 hours of life, a click may be heard; but after that age, an ejection click is always abnormal. It indicates dilatation of either the ascending aorta or pulmonary trunk. Dilatation may occur from either aortic or pulmonary valvar stenosis (poststenotic dilatation) or from conditions associated with an enlarged major arterial trunk, such as truncus arteriosus, Marfan's syndrome, and pulmonary hypertension.

The mechanism for production of a click is unknown. It occurs at the time of maximal opening of a stenotic valve, suggesting that it may be valvar in origin. On the other hand, it may result from sudden tensing of the wall of a dilated great vessel in which elastic fibers are known to have degenerated so that the wall is supported mainly by indistensible collagen.

The characteristics of a systolic ejection click originating from a dilated pulmonary trunk allow distinction from those of a dilated ascending aorta. Pulmonary clicks are heard better with the diaphragm of the stethoscope. Pulmonary ejection clicks are heard best in the pulmonary area with the patient upright. They vary in loudness with respiration, being louder in expiration. Aortic ejection clicks are heard best at the cardiac apex and left lower back when the patient is reclining. They do not vary with the phase of respiration. They are lower pitched than pulmonary clicks and may be difficult to distinguish from the second component of a split first heard sound.

MID TO LATE SYSTOLIC CLICK

Mid to late systolic clicks occur with mitral valve prolapse. These sharp, high-pitched sounds are heard best at the cardiac apex. They vary considerably in loudness and location with maneuvers that alter left ventricular volume. They are louder when the patient is standing or sitting and become softer and later when the patient reclines or squats, because left ventricular volume is smaller in the former positions. They may also be heard (along the left sternal border) when a ventricular septal defect is being closed by a pseudoaneurysm.

OPENING SNAP

An opening snap is a rare auscultatory finding in children and adolescents of most parts of the world. It occurs in mitral valve stenosis, which is most commonly caused internationally by rheumatic heart disease. This sound is heard better with a diaphragm at the cardiac apex or lower left sternal border. This sound occurs shortly after the end of isovolumetric relaxation, at the time of maximum opening excursion of the anterior leaflet of the mitral valve. The mechanism for the sound production is unknown.

FOURTH HEART SOUND (S₄)

A fourth heart sound is low pitched, occurs during atrial contraction, and precedes peak atrial inflow velocity. It is associated with conditions that limit ventricular distensibility. It is a frequent finding in patients with coronary artery disease, cardiomyopathy, severe semilunar valve stenosis (either aortic or pulmonic), and hypertension (systemic or pulmonary). A fourth heart sound may be found in patients with increased cardiac output, such as anemia or arteriovenous fistula. It can also be heard in patients with second- or third-degree heart block. Fourth heart sounds originating

from the left ventricle are heard at the apex, those from the right ventricle along the lower left sternal border. These are common in adults and are infrequent in children.

Cardiac Murmurs

Cardiac murmurs result from turbulence of blood flow through the heart or major arteries. Reynolds' number has been used to understand the factors that cause turbulence in a system of laminar flow. Although blood flow is not necessarily laminar and homogeneous, the equation helps understand factors leading to turbulence. Reynolds[20] indicated that turbulence arises in a newtonian fluid of viscosity (μ) and density (ρ), flowing with a velocity V through a tube with diameter D according to the relationship Re = $DV\rho/\mu$, where Re is Reynolds' number. Reynolds' number is dimensionless, but when it exceeds a critical value, about 2000 for a viscous fluid, turbulence occurs. Thus, with a high velocity or low viscosity, for example, turbulence could occur.

Six characteristics of a murmur should be described, for each provides a specific type of information. These characteristics are

- Loudness, which may reflect severity of the anomaly
- Location within the cardiac cycle, which relates the murmur to hemodynamic events
- Location on the thorax, which relates the murmur to anatomic sites
- Radiation, which indicates direction of turbulent flow
- Pitch, which reflects the magnitude of the pressure difference
- Other characteristics meaningful to the examiner

Combining these characteristics, the examiner can characterize the underlying condition causing the murmur.

LOUDNESS

The loudness of murmurs is described in a system of grades. These are

- Grade 1/6: Soft and heard after an extended period of listening
- Grade 2/6: Soft but immediately heard
- Grade 3/6: Moderately loud, unassociated with a thrill
- Grade 4/6: Loud, usually associated with a thrill
- Grade 5/6: Loud, heard with stethoscope barely off thoracic wall
- Grade 6/6: Loud, heard with stethoscope off thoracic wall

This system is most useful to an individual examiner who has developed an internal sense of grading so that over time, murmurs of similar loudness receive the same grade. Even with experience, this is not always possible to achieve. I find it particularly difficult to apply grades 3/6 and 4/6 to systolic murmurs and grades 1/6 and 2/6 to diastolic murmurs.

The loudness of a murmur reflects the severity of a lesion and the amount of blood passing through the abnormal area.

1. In aortic or pulmonic regurgitation, the more severe the lesion, the greater the regurgitant volume and the louder the regurgitant murmur. If the regurgitant orifice is

small, there is a pressure gradient from the artery to the ventricle throughout the whole of diastole, and the murmur is long. If the regurgitant orifice is large, pressures tend to equalize in the artery and the ventricle so that the murmur tends to end early during diastole.

2. When the whole cardiac output passes through an abnormal region, as in aortic, pulmonic, or mitral valve stenosis, the more severe the stenosis, the greater the pressure drop across the valve, the greater the turbulent flow, and thus the louder the murmur. However, if the obstruction becomes so great that cardiac output is greatly reduced, the murmur becomes softer. Furthermore, the tighter the aortic or pulmonic stenosis, the higher the velocity of flow across it and thus the higher the frequency (or pitch) of the resulting murmur.

3. If a ventricular septal defect is small, with a large pressure drop from left to right ventricle, the shunt jet is turbulent and the murmur is loud. If the defect is large and there is a huge left-to-right shunt through it, the murmur is still loud, even though the pressures are similar on the two sides. An increased pulmonary vascular resistance (neonatal period, or after pulmonary vascular disease develops) allows only a small flow across the defect, and a small flow through a large defect produces little turbulence and only a soft murmur. Similarly, when the ventricular septal defect is small, perhaps less than 2 mm in diameter, so little blood crosses it that the murmur becomes high pitched and soft.

LOCATION IN THE CARDIAC CYCLE

Murmurs should be described according to when they occur in the cardiac cycle. Timing of murmurs has been broadly described as systolic, diastolic, or continuous. Each of these three categories can be further divided into more specific intervals of the cardiac cycle. In neonates, infants, and others with tachycardia, it may be difficult to categorize it beyond systolic, diastolic, or continuous, but other features may be helpful, such as location on the thorax or pitch.

SYSTOLIC MURMURS. There are three types of systolic murmurs: pan(holo)systolic, ejection systolic, and late systolic.

Pansystolic Murmur. Although the prefix *pan-* suggests all of systole, these murmurs do not necessarily extend to the second heart sound, but they do begin with the first heart sound. Therefore, pansystolic murmurs include the period of isovolumetric contraction, and this often makes it difficult to hear the first heart sound. During isovolumetric contraction, blood should not be moving within the heart. Only three conditions allow blood to move within the cardiac chambers at that time: ventricular septal defect, because the ventricles are in full communication throughout systole; mitral insufficiency; and tricuspid insufficiency. In the last two, the higher ventricular systolic pressure compared with lower atrial pressure causes blood to move from a ventricle to an atrium during isovolumetric contraction. Pansystolic murmurs are also called regurgitant murmurs, indicating regurgitation across an atrioventricular valve.

The murmur of mitral insufficiency is heard best at the cardiac apex, is high pitched, and has been described as "blowing." Tricuspid insufficiency is heard along the lower left sternal border, as is the much more frequently occurring ventricular septal defect.

Ejection Systolic Murmur. Ejection murmurs are limited to the ejection phase of systole and therefore begin after the isovolumetric contraction phase. This point is a key distinction between the two major types of systolic murmurs. In an ejection murmur, a short period exists between the first heart sound and the onset of the murmur.

Ejection murmurs result from turbulence either into or within the aorta or pulmonary trunk. These can be caused by outflow tract obstruction, by narrowing in large central arterial vessels, or from increased volume of blood across normal outflow tract structures. Respective examples are pulmonary or aortic stenosis (valvar, subvalvar, supravalvar), coarctation of the aorta or peripheral pulmonary artery stenosis, and atrial septal defect. Because there are only two avenues by which blood exits the heart, the maximal location of the murmur allows identification of whether obstruction lies in the right (pulmonary area) or left (aortic area) side of the heart.

Late Systolic Murmur. Late systolic murmurs occur with mitral valve prolapse. As the left ventricular volume becomes progressively smaller during systolic ejection, there comes a volume small enough so that typically the posterior leaflet prolapses into the left atrium, permitting regurgitation that increases as the ventricle continues to contract to the end of systole. Thus, the murmur is crescendo to the second heart sound. As discussed previously in this chapter, the murmur is introduced by a mid to late systolic click (see also Chapter 44).

DIASTOLIC MURMURS. There are three types of diastolic murmurs, early, mid, and late. The first follows S_2, the second represents a widening of the S_3, and the last reaches a peak where an S_4 would be heard.

Early Diastolic Murmur. Early diastolic murmurs immediately follow the second heart sound, occupy the period of isovolumetric relaxation, and may extend beyond that period. They result from insufficiency of either the aortic or pulmonary valve so that regurgitation takes place from the higher pressure great artery to the lower pressure ventricle. They have been called regurgitant murmurs. Note that all regurgitant murmurs, whether in systole or diastole, occupy isovolumetric periods.

Mid-Diastolic Murmur. Mid-diastolic murmurs occupy a period of time about the transition from rapid to slow filling phases of the cardiac cycle. They occur from increased volume of blood flow across anatomically normal atrioventricular valves. Usually, the anterograde flow must be about twice normal before a mid-diastolic murmur is heard. Mitral mid-diastolic murmurs are heard in conditions such as mitral insufficiency and shunts at the ventricular or great vessel level (ventricular septal defect, patent ductus arteriosus, truncus arteriosus). Tricuspid mid-diastolic murmurs occur in tricuspid regurgitation (as in the Ebstein malformation) and atrial-level shunt (atrial septal defect, total anomalous pulmonary venous connection). Mid-diastolic murmurs occur with mitral and tricuspid stenosis with presystolic accentuation. Because there is little diastolic pressure difference across the atrioventricular valves in these conditions, the murmurs are low pitched.

Late Diastolic Murmur. Murmurs occurring late in diastole have also been called protodiastolic or presystolic. They result from atrioventricular valve stenosis, which is usually the mitral valve. They are usually crescendo to the first heart sound as the gradient between the atrium and its respective ventricle increases and is accentuated by atrial contraction.

CONTINUOUS MURMURS. Continuous murmurs are those that begin in systole and continue into diastole, with the murmur having the same characteristics in both phases of the cardiac cycle. It is not a separate systolic and diastolic murmur. Continuous murmurs do not necessarily continue throughout the cardiac cycle but pass unaltered across the second heart sound. Continuous murmurs can be subdivided into two categories, depending on whether the murmur is louder in systole or in diastole.

Louder in Systole. A continuous murmur, louder in systole, indicates a communication between the arterial and venous systems. The classic example is patent ductus arteriosus, but others are bronchial collaterals in cyanotic patients and arteriovenous malformation. In a neonate, a continuous murmur over the upper chest often indicates pulmonary atresia, with patent ductus arteriosus being the major or sole source of pulmonary blood flow. In a neonate, continuous murmurs are also heard from arteriovenous malformations or fistulae and are heard best over their anatomic location. In a patent ductus arteriosus, the murmur is often crescendo in late systole because of the time taken for the pulse wave to reach the ductus.

Louder in Diastole. Continuous murmurs louder in diastole point to an abnormality of blood flow into major veins, because the volume of blood returning to the right atrium increases during diastole. The most frequent cause is a benign venous hum, but it can occur if there is increased blood flow in the superior caval system, as in total anomalous pulmonary venous connection to a supracardiac vein or cerebral arteriovenous fistula.

LOCATION ON THE THORAX
The location where a murmur is heard best provides an indication of the anatomic site of origin of the murmur, because sound is louder closer to its site of origin. Murmurs should be described by their anatomic location, such as upper right sternal border, upper left sternal border, lower left sternal border, or cardiac apex, rather than by the respective terms commonly used: aortic area, pulmonary area, tricuspid area, mitral area. Because of the array of cardiac malformations, the pulmonary artery and valve may not be located in the "pulmonary area," as in transposition of the great arteries, and a murmur in the "mitral area" may arise from an inverted tricuspid valve in congenitally corrected transposition of the great arteries.

In addition to the four traditional auscultatory sites, both axillae should be auscultated (peripheral pulmonary artery stenosis), as should the back, particularly the left paraspinal area (coarctation of the aorta). In patients with normally related great arteries, murmurs heard best along the upper left sternal border and beneath the left clavicle originate from the right ventricular outflow tract, and those along the midsternum to the area beneath the right clavicle originate from the left ventricular outflow tract.

Murmurs along the lower left sternal border commonly result from a ventricular septal defect, with less frequent conditions of obstructive cardiomyopathy or tricuspid insufficiency being heard in this area.

RADIATION
Not only the site where the murmur is heard maximally should be described, but also other locations where the murmur is heard. These secondary sites indicate radiation of the murmur and reflect the direction of turbulent blood flow. Murmurs from the right ventricular outflow tract radiate to the left upper back, because the left pulmonary artery is a direct extension of the pulmonary trunk that is directed posteriorly and to the left. In tetralogy of Fallot wherein the right ventricular outflow tract is oriented typically toward the right, this murmur is heard better over the right side of the back. Murmurs from the left ventricular outflow tract area are directed into the carotid arteries, particularly the right. In patients with a moderate or large ventricular septal defect or significant tricuspid regurgitation, radiation is toward the right sternal border and right anterior chest, reflecting the direction of turbulence. The murmur of mitral regurgitation classically extends to the left axilla and left lower back.

PITCH
The frequency or pitch of a murmur reflects the pressure that is creating the turbulence and murmur. High-pitched murmurs result when there is a large pressure difference, as in mitral regurgitation or aortic regurgitation. In contrast, the murmurs of tricuspid and pulmonary regurgitation are lower pitched because of lower right-sided cardiac pressures in normal individuals. Certainly the murmur of pulmonary regurgitation, for instance, can be higher pitched if pulmonary hypertension is present. Diastolic murmurs related to turbulent anterograde flow across an atrioventricular valve are low pitched.

High-pitched murmurs are heard better with the diaphragm of the stethoscope, low-pitched murmurs with the bell.

OTHER FEATURES
A variety of other terms are used commonly on rounds or in clinics to describe murmurs. These terms, such as harsh, blowing, musical, and to and fro, are less precise and perhaps are of greatest use to the individual examiner who has his or her own auditory concept of harsh, blowing, or musical.

Functional Murmurs

Sometime during childhood, most children have a murmur. These are often transient, appearing when the child has a fever or only on one examination, and occur in a structurally normal heart. Although these have been called functional or innocent murmurs, I prefer to call them normal murmurs when describing them to parents, to indicate that the heart is normal and that these murmurs are normal in children.

The clinical diagnosis of a functional (normal) murmur is a two-step process. The first is to distinguish whether the patient's murmur reflects a major cardiac condition or could represent a normal murmur. This step depends on whether the murmur is associated with five features common to all children with a functional murmur:

1. There are no cardiovascular symptoms.
2. The murmur is less than grade 3/6.
3. The heart sounds are normal. Particular attention must be directed at the second heart sound.
4. The heart size is normal. This can be assessed by palpation of the cardiac apex.
5. The murmur is usually short.

Because some patients with less severe cardiac malformations may meet these criteria, the normal murmur should be categorized into a specific type. Six distinct normal murmurs have been identified, and each must be distinguished from murmurs resulting from cardiac abnormalities that may have some similar features.

PULMONARY FLOW MURMUR

This soft, short systolic ejection murmur believed to result from turbulence in the right ventricular outflow tract and pulmonary trunk is heard along the upper left sternal border (pulmonary area). It is common with fever and anemia. The major condition it must be distinguished from is atrial septal defect. In atrial septal defect, the features of the second heart sound showing wide, fixed splitting are diagnostic. Also in atrial septal defect, in contrast to a functional pulmonary flow murmur, the tricuspid valve closure is loud, and a mid-diastolic murmur is common in the tricuspid area. Mild valvar pulmonary stenosis may have a similar murmur, but it is longer and preceded by an ejection click.

VIBRATORY, "TWANGY STRING," OR STILL'S MURMUR

This is a short, early midsystolic murmur heard best between the lower left sternal border and the cardiac apex. Like pulmonary flow murmur, it seldom persists beyond midsystole. It is uniform in frequency, thus its name vibratory. The murmur is believed to be related to turbulent flow out of the left ventricular outflow tract. In some children, an anomalous band has been found in the left or right ventricle.[21] In one study,[22] 76% of patients with this murmur had a band in the left ventricular outflow tract, compared with 14% of those without a murmur. Others,[23] in studies of these patients, suggest that the murmur is from the combination of a small aortic diameter and high aortic velocity. A report[24] and accompanying commentary[25] provide insight into this type of murmur as possibly originating from increased intraventricular velocities. The murmur may be heard in young infants and preschool-aged children.

The major differentiation is from ventricular septal defect. Because most ventricular septal defects are membranous, they are heard best along the left sternal border in the third and fourth interspace. The murmur of a muscular ventricular septal defect may be heard in the same area, but it is harsher.

VENOUS HUM

This is a continuous murmur, louder in diastole and heard best along the upper right sternal border. It results from turbulent flow in the jugular venous system. Thus, there may be a thrill posterior to the sternocleidomastoid muscle. The murmur is heard better when the patient is sitting and disappears on reclining. The murmur varies as the patient turns the head back and forth or when gentle pressure is applied over the base of the neck.

A similar murmur can be heard in an occasional patient with total anomalous pulmonary venous connection to the left superior vena cava. It may also be heard with a cerebral arteriovenous malformation.

CAROTID BRUIT

In virtually all children, an early systolic murmur may be heard over the bifurcation of the carotid arteries. It should not be confused with radiation of a murmur of aortic stenosis to the carotid arteries. Palpation of the suprasternal notch is helpful because with aortic stenosis, a thrill is palpated in this area.

CARDIOPULMONARY MURMUR

This noise is believed to result from compression of the lingula of the lung between the heart and anterior chest wall. I have heard a similar noise along the right sternal border. This noise is louder during midinspiration and midexpiration, becoming soft or absent on full inspiration or full expiration. It is heard better when the patient is sitting.

PERIPHERAL PULMONARY ARTERY STENOSIS

In some neonates, particularly those born prematurely, a midsystolic ejection murmur may be heard over both lung fields, including on the back, in the axillae, and beneath both clavicles, but not over the precordium. Present in the neonatal period, it usually disappears by 3 months of age and is always gone by 1 year of age. It results from turbulence produced by discrepancy of size between the large pulmonary trunk and small branch pulmonary arteries.

Mammary Souffle

In lactating women, a low-frequency background hum due to a large increase in blood flow to the breast through superficial blood vessels may be heard immediately above the breast. Gentle pressure over the area may diminish the loudness. Its importance is in distinguishing it from a patent ductus arteriosus or an arteriovenous fistula.

Variant Auscultatory Findings

In two groups of pediatric patients, neonates and athletes, the auscultatory findings vary.

NEONATES

The first heart sound is loud at birth and decreases in intensity during the first 48 hours of life. It may be split, with the second component being loud in the tricuspid area. A systolic ejection click along the left sternal border has been reported to occur in many neonates.[26] The second heart sound is single at birth presumably because of elevated pulmonary vascular resistance.[26, 27] By 2 days of age, it is split in all normal neonates.

Several studies of normal neonates have described the frequency and types of murmurs in neonates.[26–35] On careful auscultation, one third to three fourths of neonates have been described to have a murmur.

1. A continuous murmur in the pulmonary area heard best with the bell. In one series, this occurred in 37% of normal neonates,[29] was transient, and usually disappeared by 12 hours of age. Its frequency is higher in premature infants and those with asphyxia, in whom it may not disappear for several months, indicating delayed closure of the ductus arteriosus.

2. Crescendo systolic murmur in the pulmonary area. This grade 1 to 2/6 murmur is also believed to be related to flow through the ductus, because in some neonates this murmur represents a transition from a continuous to the crescendo murmur.

3. Pulmonary systolic ejection murmur. This grade 1 to 2/6 murmur may develop during the first day of life and last up to 6 days.

A high frequency of functional murmurs has been found in infants and, in one study, in 80% of prematurely born infants,[31] most frequently at 3 months of age. Many of these have characteristics of a vibratory murmur. Other authors have described a low incidence of functional murmurs in neonates and infants.[33–35]

In neonates, a significant murmur present at birth or during the first hours of life usually indicates either aortic stenosis or pulmonary stenosis (with either intact ventricular septum or a ventricular communication). Mitral and tricuspid insufficiency, both rare conditions in a neonate, result also in a systolic murmur. A small ventricular septal defect may be heard within days of birth. Large shunts at either the ventricular or great vessel level are not evident in the neonatal period because of the commonly elevated pulmonary arterial pressure and resistance that limits blood flow through the communication.

ATHLETES

In trained athletes, the resting cardiac rate is often low. Therefore, the stroke volume and end-diastolic volume are increased as a result of these physiologic adaptations, and certain changes occur on physical examination. Obviously, the pulse rate is lower than normal, and the peripheral pulses are strong. The pulse pressure is increased, reflecting an increase in systolic pressure from increased stroke volume and lowered diastolic pressure from prolonged diastole. The apex impulse may be slightly beyond the midclavicular line. An ejection systolic murmur is heard along the upper left sternal borders, and a third heart sound may be prominent.

ABDOMEN

Hepatic location and size are key components to be determined in the examination of an infant or child with a cardiac abnormality. Hepatic location helps identify visceral situs, which is important in understanding the nature of a cardiac malposition. Assessment of hepatic size aids in the recognition of congestive cardiac failure, for in this physiologic state, hepatomegaly is present and may change rapidly. The hepatic margin should be sought by palpation and its distance from the rib margin measured in the midclavicular line. The hepatic span is 6 cm in neonates[36]; it

may be palpated as far as 3 cm below the right costal margin,[37] and it is no longer palpable by 4 years. If the hepatic margin is palpable, the upper margin of the liver should be percussed because in patients with hyperexpanded lungs, the liver may be displaced into the abdomen. The upper extent of the liver is located in the fifth intercostal space in the midclavicular line.

The spleen tip may be palpable in infants and is rarely enlarged in pediatric patients with cardiac failure. It may be enlarged in those with infective endocarditis.

PERIPHERAL EDEMA

Peripheral edema is present in many normal neonates during the first 2 days of life. It may persist longer in premature infants.

Abnormal degrees of edema are found at birth from fetal hydrops and nonpitting lymphedema, often associated with Turner's syndrome. Cardiac causes are uncommon (supraventricular tachycardia being the most common); urinary tract obstruction and hepatic cirrhosis are other causes. The edema, being dependent, may be identified by observing puffy eyelids or edema over the back of a neonate.

Edema from cardiac causes is also uncommon after the neonatal period and is usually related to renal disease or exudative enteropathy. An unusual but important cause to recognize is constrictive pericarditis.

SKIN

Hypoxemia, even mild, may be associated with digital clubbing after 6 months of age. Early in the process, there is a loss in the angle between the base of the nail and the mantle. At this stage, there is redness or shininess of the terminal phalanx. Subsequently, there is widening and thickening of the distal phalanx of toes and fingers, and the nails become convex like the back of a spoon. In some infants and small children with a large left-to-right shunt, the fingertips and at times the palms become red. Nail beds should be inspected for splinter hemorrhages in patients with suspected infective endocarditis. In cyanotic patients, the scalp veins are often dilated. The skin should be inspected for hemangiomas, particularly of the strawberry type, in patients with a clinical picture that could represent multinodular hemangiomatosis.[38]

REFERENCES

1. Selbst SM, Ruddy RM, Clark BJ, et al: Pediatric chest pain: A prospective study. Pediatrics 82:319, 1988.
2. Tunaoglu FS, Olgunturk R, Akcaloay S, et al: Chest pain in children referred to a cardiology clinic. Pediatr Cardiol 16:69, 1995.
3. Linde LM, Dunn OJ, Shireson R, et al: Growth in children with congenital heart disease. J Pediatr 70:413, 1967.
4. Anderson RC, Moller JH: Ten year and longer follow-up of 1,000 consecutive children with cardiac malformations. The University of Minnesota Experience. *In* Engle MA, Perloff JK (eds): Congenital Heart Disease After Surgery. Chicago, Yorke Medical Books, 1983, p 49.
5. Hardy JB: Rubella as a teratogen. Birth Defects 7:64, 1971.
6. Rowland TW, Hubbell JP Jr, Nadas AS: Congenital heart disease in infants of diabetic mothers. J Pediatr 83:815, 1973.

7. Loser H: Human alcohol embryopathy and changes in the cardiovascular system (Abstract). Teratology 24:29A, 1981.

8. Stern RS, Rosa F, Baum C: Isotretinoin and pregnancy. J Am Acad Dermatol 10:851, 1984.

9. Goldman HI, Maralit A, Sun S, et al: Neonatal cyanosis and arterial oxygen saturation. J Pediatr 82:319, 1973.

10. Chesler E, Moller JH, Edwards JE: Anatomic basis for delivery of right ventricular blood into localized segments of the systemic arterial system. Relation to differential cyanosis. Am J Cardiol 21:72, 1968.

11. Gatti RA, Muster AJ, Cole RB, et al: Neonatal polycythemia with transient cyanosis and cardiorespiratory abnormalities. J Pediatr 69:1063, 1966.

12. Etchells E, Bell C, Rob BK: Does the patient have an abnormal systolic murmur? JAMA 277:572, 1997.

13. Rolden CA, Shively BK, Crawford MH: Value of the cardiovascular physical examination for detecting valvar heart disease in asymptomatic subjects. Am J Cardiol 77:1327, 1996.

14. Newburger JW, Rosenthal A, Williams RG, et al: Noninvasive tests in the initial evaluation of heart murmurs in children. N Engl J Med 308:61, 1983.

15. Wiggers CJ: Studies on the consecutive phases of the cardiac cycle: II. The laws governing the relative duration of ventricular systole and diastole. Am J Physiol 56:439, 1921.

16. Leatham A: Auscultation of the heart. Pediatr Clin North Am 5:839, 1958.

17. Vancheri F, Gibson D: Relation of third and fourth heart sounds to blood velocity during left ventricular filling. Br Heart J 61:144, 1989.

18. Ewing G, Magundar J, Goldblatt E, et al: A non-invasive study of the third heart sound in children by phono and echo-cardiography. Acta Cardiol 39:241, 1984.

19. Van de Werf F, Geboers J, Kesteloot H, et al: The mechanism of disappearance of the physiologic third heart sound of age. Circulation 73:877, 1986.

20. Reynolds O: An experimental investigation of the circumstances which determine whether the motion of water shall be direct or sinuous and the law of resistance in parallel channels. Philos Trans R Soc Lond 174:935, 1883.

21. Miao CY, Zuberbuhler JS, Zuberbuhler JR: Genesis of vibratory functional murmurs. Am J Cardiol 60:1198, 1987.

22. Darazs B, Hesdorffer GS, Butterworth AM, Ziady F: The possible etiology of the vibratory systolic murmur. Clin Cardiol 10:341, 1987.

23. Schwartz ML, Goldberg SJ, Wilson N, et al: Relation of Still's murmur, small aortic diameter and high aortic velocity. Am J Cardiol 57:1344, 1986.

24. Spooner PH, Perry MP, Brandenburg RO, Pennock GD: Increased intraventricular velocities. An unrecognized cause of systolic murmur in adults. J Am Coll Cardiol 32:1589, 1998.

25. Murgo JP: Systolic ejection murmurs in the era of modern cardiology. What do we really know? J Am Coll Cardiol 32:1596, 1998.

26. Craige E, Harned HS Jr: Phonocardiographic and electrocardiographic studies in normal newborn infants. Am Heart J 65:180, 1963.

27. Braudo M, Rowe RD: Auscultation of the heart—early neonatal period. Am J Dis Child 101:575, 1961.

28. Papadopoulos GS, Folger GM Jr: Transient solitary diastolic murmurs in the newborn. Clin Pediatr 22:548, 1983.

29. Burnard ED: A murmur from the ductus arteriosus in the newborn baby. Br Med J 1:806, 1958.

30. Clarkson PM, Orgill AA: Continuous murmurs in infants of low birth weight. J Pediatr 84:208, 1974.

31. Walsh SZ: The incidence of murmurs in healthy premature infants during the first 18 months of life. J Pediatr 62:480, 1963.

32. Hallidie-Smith KA: Some auscultatory and phonocardiographic findings observed in early infancy. Br Med J 1:756, 1960.

33. Lyon RA, Rauh LW, Stirling JW: Heart murmurs in newborn infants. J Pediatr 16:310, 1940.

34. Taylor WC: The incidence and significance of systolic cardiac murmurs in infants. Arch Dis Child 28:52, 1953.

35. Richards MR, Merritt KK, Samuels MH, et al: Frequency and significance of cardiac murmurs in the first years of life. Pediatrics 15:169, 1955.

36. Reiff MI, Osborn LM: Clinical estimation of liver size in newborn infants. Pediatrics 71:46, 1983.

37. Deligeorgis D, Yannakos D, Panayofou P, et al: The normal borders of the liver in infancy and childhood. Clinical and x-ray study. Arch Dis Child 45:702, 1970.

38. McLean RH, Moller JH, Warwick WJ, et al: Multinodular hemangiomatosis of the liver in infancy. Pediatrics 49:563, 1972.

CHAPTER 9
ELECTROCARDIOGRAPHY

JEROME LIEBMAN

The heart muscle is an electric generator. Because it lies in a conducting medium, currents flow within the torso, creating an electric field. A potential difference (in millivolts) is the measurement of the difference between two points in an electric field. The potential field is everywhere in the body, and what we see on the surface is the tip of the iceberg.[1,2] The electrical activity of the cardiac muscle cells (cardiac current sources) is projected onto the surface of the torso by the intervening conducting medium. The potentials recorded on the surface of the torso reflect *both* the cardiac generators and the surrounding volume conductor.

The cardiac current sources are distributed throughout the myocardium and can be specified by dipole elements in the heart. It is a crude approximation to represent the ventricles (as an example) electrically by a single dipole, the vector sum of all these dipole elements. It remains useful to interpret an electrocardiogram (ECG), including a vectorcardiogram, using this simplified representation as a single heart vector, but it is obviously distorted by proximity effects and ignores the effects of the complex and inhomogeneous conducting medium.

The intracellular potentials are directly related to the flow of ions across the cell membrane.[3,4] In the intracellular space are K^+ (140 mmol/L) and nondiffusible anion (120 mmol/L), along with Cl^- (30 mmol/L), Na^+ (10 mmol/L), and a trace of Ca^{2+}. In the extracellular space are Na^+ and Cl^- (140 and 100 mmol/L, respectively), with K^+ (4 mmol/L), Ca^{2+} (2 mmol/L), and nondiffusible anion (8 mmol/L). The resting transmembrane potential depends on K^+, which diffuses out of the cell, leaving the inner membrane negatively charged relative to the positive charge in the outer membrane. The resting transmembrane potential is therefore negative (about -92 mV) and constitutes an inward electrical force on potassium, thereby equilibrating the outward diffusional force. The action potential begins with a fast upstroke (phase 0, Fig. 9–1) when sodium permeability greatly increases and generates the depolarizing sodium current (I_{Na}). As a result, the membrane potential quickly moves toward the sodium equilibrium Nernst potential (V_{Na}). Because the extracellular sodium concentration is much greater than the intracellular concentration, sodium diffusion is inward. Equilibrium is established when the intracellular potential is positive relative to the extracellular (by about 60 mV), constituting an outward electric field that balances the inward diffusional force.

Sodium conductivity is then rapidly inactivated (phase 1), terminating depolarization. A prolonged plateau (phase 2) results from the balance of an inward calcium current (I_{Ca}) and two outward potassium currents (I_K, I_{K1}). Potassium conductance increases, and the reduction of sodium influx coupled with an increasing potassium efflux causes the transmembrane potential to become more negative until the cell recovers its initial potential (phase 4). Restoration of baseline concentrations requires a reverse ion movement against the passive gradients and requires expenditure of energy through the sodium-potassium pump, operated by the hydrolysis of adenosine triphosphate (ATP). Three sodium ions are pumped out for each potassium ion pumped in.

Neither the resting cell (phase 4) nor the fully depolarized cell (phase 2) contributes significantly to the extracellular potential. The major voltages from the normal cell occur only during phase 0 (the QRS) and phase 3 (the T wave).

Each specialized cell of the heart has a different transmembrane potential. The working atrial muscle cell has a shorter transmembrane potential than does the ventricular muscle cell, and its plateau is less flat. The working atrial and ventricular cells provide most of the electric field that makes up the ECG.

Cells in the sinus node do not maintain a resting potential but show slow spontaneous depolarization (rising phase 4) that, when a threshold is reached, leads to an action potential that rises more slowly than the action potential of working ventricular muscle cells. The result is a rhythmic behavior that makes the sinus node an ideal pacemaker.

Electrical activity initiated in atrial and ventricular working cells by the conduction tissue spreads contiguously in all directions. Because low-resistance junctions are found mainly at the ends of cells,[5,6] propagation along the cardiac fibers is more rapid than in a transverse direction. Conduction transversely depends on zigzag pathways that use the end-to-end low-resistance junctions. The greater number of junctions encountered by action currents in the transverse direction relative to the longitudinal direction is a factor explaining the slower transverse velocity.

The cardiac muscle fibers spiral around each cavity, and there is a continuous change in the fiber angle from circumferential (0 degrees) at midwall to approximately 75 degrees endocardially.[7] Stimulating the endocardium by the Purkinje system initiates activation over a broad region, with activation spreading from endocardium to epicardium in a cross-fiber direction. The excitation front is oriented, therefore, in the slow direction. This epicardial-endocardial obliqueness of fiber direction must be considered when interpreting the electricity generated by the heart.[8,9]

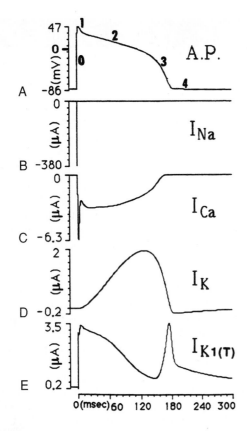

A cardiac ventricular action potential (*A*) and major membrane ionic currents that determine its shape (*B* through *E*). Bold numbers in *A* indicate phases during the action potential (A.P.). The fast kinetics and large amplitude of the sodium current I_{Na} (*B*) result in the upstroke of the action potential (phase 0). The inward calcium current I_{Ca} (*C*) supports the action potential plateau (phase 2) against the repolarizing potassium currents I_K (*D*) and $I_{K1(T)}$ (*E*). The large increase of I_K and the late peak of $I_{K1(T)}$ is the total time-independent potassium current that includes a plateau current, $I_{K1(T)}$4. *A* depicts the action potential as a function of time. The A.P. in space has a similar shape and is related to the temporal A.P. through the velocity of propagation.

EMBRYOLOGY, ANATOMY, AND PHYSIOLOGY OF THE CONDUCTION SYSTEM

THE ATRIA

In humans, the pacemaker portion of the sinus venosus becomes incorporated into the right atrium and into the regions of the ostia of the two venae cavae, the coronary sinus, the sinus intercavarum, the eustachian ridge, and most of the atrial septum. The right atrium is divided into the trabeculated portion, which contains none of the conduction system, and the smooth portion, which contains all of the conduction system.

SINUS NODE

The sinus node is at the lateral margin of the superior vena cava–right atrial junction and is composed primarily of P cells and transitional cells.[10,11] P cells occur densely in groups, especially in the central area, near the nutrient artery and nerves. The P cells are presumed to make up

the cardiac pacemaker.[12] They predominate in early life but decrease with aging. The transitional cells connect with P cells, other transitional cells, and working myocardial cells in the area of presumed internodal tracts. They become more common with increasing age from the neonatal period.

Before a definite sinus node can be identified in the human embryo, parasympathetic nerve fibers can be found in the region. At birth, parasympathetic innervation of the heart is almost complete, whereas sympathetic innervation is not fully functional for several months.[13] Therefore, in the neonatal period the autonomic control of the heart is predominantly cholinergic, so that activities that provoke vagal discharge, such as sucking or coughing, may cause profound slowing of the cardiac rate. There is, however, dispute about this concept.[14] It may be that both sympathetic and parasympathetic nerve fibers are immature, but the former are more so. Even without obvious vagal discharge, the sinus node in the neonatal period is unstable and the sinus pacemaker demonstrates wide swings of rate and rhythm.

INTERNODAL AND INTERATRIAL PATHWAYS

Three internodal and interatrial pathways exist.[10,15,16] They have no sheath and, unlike bundle branches, do not contain only Purkinje cells. Two of the three tracts pass through the atrial septum, and all pass through the smooth portion of the atrium. They merge in an intense decussation at the crest of the atrioventricular (AV) node. The posterior tract then mainly bypasses the bulk of the AV node to enter it inferiorly, near the bundle of His, although some of its fibers end blindly in the tricuspid ring. A few fibers from the anterior and middle pathways bypass the cells of the AV node to join the node more anteriorly.

Conduction velocity from the sinus node to the AV node is faster than is lateral spread to the atria, but whether there are specialized tracts is disputed.

ATRIOVENTRICULAR JUNCTION

The AV node in an infant is just above the septal leaflet of the tricuspid valve and anterior.[17] The node and the connecting bundle of His are proportionately larger and more chaotic in appearance in a neonate than in an adult.[17] Because the node contains more cells in the periphery, the anatomy is ideal for occurrence of re-entrant rhythm. Shortly after birth, the AV node and bundle of His undergo a resorptive process and become unusually compact.[18]

The AV node arises from the posterior invagination of the AV ring of specialized tissue, and the bundle of His arises separately astride the bulboventricular septum.[19] The two structures unite early in gestation. Fibrous discontinuity as a cause of AV block is easily understood, but there are other causes.[18,20]

BUNDLE OF HIS AND BUNDLE BRANCHES

The common bundle of His passes through the central fibrous body to reach the crest of the ventricular septum. It continues anteroinferiorly in the margin of the membranous septum. In 75 to 80% of human hearts, the bundle runs high along the left side of the septum, providing a wide origin for the left bundle branch. In the remaining 20 to 25%, the bundle of His courses high along the right side of the septum, so that the connection to the left bundle branch is by a narrow stem 1 mm in diameter.

The right bundle does not have a sheath and is functionally separate from the surrounding working myocardial tissue. The proximal third may have a short intramyocardial course before reaching the right septal subendocardium. The middle third is intramyocardial, passing along the inferior region of the septal band. The distal third is again subendocardial and courses through the moderator band to reach the anterior papillary muscle. From here, there is a thin septal branch to the right side of the ventricular septum one half to two thirds down the septum, as the moderator band continues, dividing into several branches to the right endocardium.

The left bundle fans out over the left septal surface. There is great variability in the normal anatomy of the left bundle[21]; there may be three main radiations of the left bundle instead of the usual two (anterior and posterior). Frequently a middle bundle travels to the midseptal region. The posterior branch usually provides a midseptal branch, or there is a complex interweaving of fasciculi from both anterior and posterior branches to the midseptum. The anterior branch extends to the base and medial portion of the anterior papillary muscle, and the posterior branch extends to the base of the posterior papillary muscle. The posterior free wall near the septum is also provided by branches of the posterior branch.

The left bundle branches are rich in Purkinje cells and have sheaths of connective tissue separating them from ventricular muscle. Only after reaching the papillary muscle[5] do extensive fine branches extend to the left side of the septum. The left posterior branch is responsible for most of the left-to-right septal activation, and the anterior branch is responsible for activation up the septum. There are fewer right septal branches than left septal branches.

ACTIVATION OF THE HEART

After the sinus node discharges, it takes about 80 milliseconds to activate right and left atria in the adult; less time is required in the infant. Propagation slows at the AV junction, which conducts at 0.1 m/sec, resulting in a delay of up to 200 milliseconds. Spread through the His-Purkinje system is then extremely rapid (1 to 3 m/sec), so that many points in the heart are activated nearly simultaneously.

If electrical activity is initiated within the myocardium, as in an ectopic beat, spread of activity to neighboring cells occurs because currents from one cell can flow into the neighboring cell through low-resistance gap junctions. Because the cells are staggered, lateral spread takes place as well as end-to-end spread along the fiber axis. However, the velocity is faster along the fiber direction than across the fiber axis by a factor of about 3:1.[22] Similar cell-to-cell conduction occurs when the right ventricle is stimulated by the left ventricle through the septum, as in right bundle branch block. Normal stimulation of the right ventricle via the bundle branches and the Purkinje system results in much faster conduction, as well as the normal endocardial-to-epicardial spread of activation.

Ventricular excitation begins in the septum at a broad, relatively well-delineated area about one half to two thirds the distance down the septum. Initial activation begins in five major areas: the left posterior septum, the left posterior free wall adjacent to the left posterior septum, the anterior superior portion of that septal area, the right septum, and the right ventricular endocardium (Fig. 9–2). All occur quite close in time, although in most humans activation begins a bit earlier on the left free wall.[23] The left posterior branch of the left bundle stimulates the left posterior portion of the septum as well as the adjacent posterior wall.[24] The right septum is stimulated by the septal branch of the right bundle, after the right bundle arrives in the moderator band at the base of the anterior papillary muscle. At the right septum, activation begins a little more inferior than at the left septum. Also, activation of the right ventricular endocardium may be even earlier than that of the right septum,[24] after which the entire endocardium then activates quite rapidly, including the apices. Almost as soon as septal activation begins, activation spreads slowly up the septum. The stimulus is from the left anterior branch of the left bundle. Although posterior spread in the left ventricle begins early in the cycle, most of the left ventricle is depolarized after apical depolarization is completed. The lateral walls of both ventricles are depolarized at about the same time, but activation of the right ventricular wall is completed before that of the left; presumably in neonates or in patients with right ventricular hypertrophy, this does not occur. The final areas to be depolarized are the posterior left ventricle followed by the posterobasal left ventricle, the anterior superior septum, and the right ventricular infundibulum. In normal children, one or more of these four areas can be the last to be depolarized.[25] The posterobasal left ventricle has less Purkinje tissue than does the remainder of the free wall of the left ventricle, providing one reason why it completes depolarization so late. The right side of the septum also has

Vector of Initial Activation

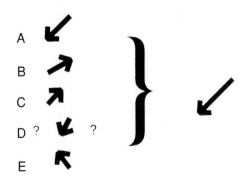

FIGURE 9–2

Diagrammatic representation of the five major areas that make up initial ventricular activation, considering only left-right and anterior-posterior directions. A, Left to right, posterior to anterior in the septum one half to two thirds down. B, Right to left, anterior to posterior in the posterior left ventricular free wall. C, Right to left, anterior to posterior in the right septum one half to two thirds down. D, Posterior to anterior, left to right and in the right ventricular anterior free wall. E, Left to right, anterior to posterior, up the septum.

less Purkinje tissue than does the left side, helping to explain why late depolarization of the superior septum is from left to right and posterior to anterior. Although much of the research on activation has been done in dogs, the classic detailed activation analysis of Durrer and colleagues was of the resuscitated human adult heart.[24] His group also studied the epicardial breakthrough in the resuscitated human fetal heart.[26] The earliest epicardial excitation wave was in the region of attachment of the right ventricular anterior papillary muscle, after which spread was radial and simultaneous in two waves in each ventricle. The result is a double envelopment of the epicardial surface to the upper septum.

RECOVERY

Activation and recovery of each cardiac cell are manifest in the same action potential but must be considered differently.[27, 28] During depolarization, the sources are reasonably confined to narrow regions defined by the rising phase of activation and are associated with isochrones. (An isochrone is an activation surface at the specific instant of time. Resting tissue is ahead of the isochrone, and active tissue is behind the isochrone.) In contrast, during recovery, the action potential duration is so great that the entire heart becomes a volume source for a time. The normal ST-T segment is not considered to be a propagated wave. Because activation begins at the endocardium, so does recovery. The action potential duration is longer at the endocardium than at the epicardium, so that recovery is completed earlier at the epicardium. Consequently, the gradient is in the opposite direction of that during activation, so that the QRS complex and the T wave have a similar direction. The sources during activation depend on the activation pattern, and the sources during recovery depend on both the activation pattern *and* the action potential duration. Therefore, in evaluating the time integral of QRS complex plus T wave, the activation contribution of the QRS complex cancels out that of the T wave. What is left depends only on the local recovery properties of the cardiac tissue and is called the *ventricular gradient*.[29] No statistical relationship was found between the spatial orientations of the QRS complex and T wave in normal children,[30, 31] but in abnormal children there was a definite statistical relationship between the QRS complex and the T wave.

In a normal subject, repolarization takes longer on the endocardial surfaces than on the epicardial surfaces, longer at the apex than at the base of the epicardium, and longer on the left side of the septum than on the right side.[32] Even in a normal subject, however, there may be differences from one part to another part, even in the same area of the heart. In an abnormal subject, data indicate even more complexity.

ELECTROCARDIOGRAM

FROM CELL TO BODY SURFACE

In describing the ECG, we have found the concept of the submergence of a battery in a conducting medium useful.[33] Current flows from the positive to the negative terminal. The quantity of current depends on the voltage and the resistivity of the medium. If the positive (source) and negative (sink) terminals are close together, the resulting current flow field is characteristic of a dipole field (Fig. 9–3), defined as a field resulting from two point sources of equal magnitude and opposite sign whose physical separation is small. This dipole field is different from a "dipole," which refers to the source-sink combination itself. The resultant dipole field depends on the source-sink orientation as well as the source and sink magnitudes, so that a vector is necessary to describe the dipole. By convention, the vector direction points from the negative to the positive pole. The maximal resulting voltage occurs along the dipole axis (see Fig. 9–3). There is angular dependence, the voltage being less than maximal depending on how far the dipole axis is located off the electrode so that at points perpendicular to the dipole axis the voltage is zero. There is also distance dependence; the farther away the electrode is located, the lower the voltage.

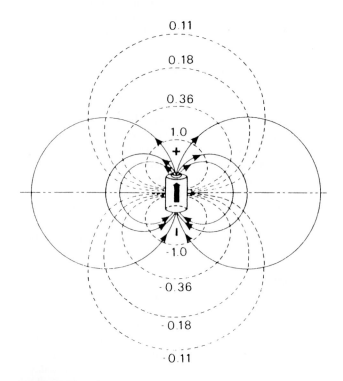

0.11

0.18

0.36

1.0

+

I

I

-1.0

-0.36

-0.18

-0.11

FIGURE 9–3

Dry cell battery submerged in conducting fluid. Current flows from the positive terminal and returns to the negative terminal along paths shown. Vector *(heavy central arrow)* shows orientation of battery and, correspondingly, of field. Under these conditions, because the battery provides a source-sink combination, it is characterized as a dipole. The vector representing this (dipole) property of the battery has orientation (from negative to positive within the battery) and magnitude (strength of the dipole related to the battery electromotive force). Several interrupted lines of equipotential and their relative values are shown. This physical example is analogous to the electrocardiograph in which the active muscle in the heart constitutes the dipole generator. Current flows away from the positive region (leaves the heart) into the torso volume conductor and returns to the negative region of the heart. Because the region of activity shifts from moment to moment, the dipole characterizing it is continually changing orientation and magnitude, and the current flow field and associated surface potential change concomitantly. (From Liebman J, Plonsey R: Basic principles for understanding electrocardiography. Pediatrician 2:251, 1973, with permission from S. Karger, Basel, Switzerland.)

In a depolarizing heart, dipole sources lie within the rising phase of the action potential (a 0.5-mm-thick *activation front*). The activation front can be considered as being infinitely thin and the dipole source can be considered as being on the surface.

Clinical ECG potentials arise from the primary sources in the contractile myocardial cells. The potentials on the thoracic wall, however, actually reflect both the volume conductor and the contribution of secondary sources. To study these problems, a model was developed by Rudy and coworkers.[34] This model consists of two eccentric sets of concentric spheres. The heart is represented as a sphere consisting of a central blood volume bounded by a spherical heart-muscle shell and pericardium. This heart is placed eccentrically within a spherical torso that includes a lung region bounded by spherical muscle and fat layers. The source of the field is a double-layer spherical cap lying concentrically within the myocardium, representing an activation wave. The direction of the double layer is radial, simulating the endocardial-to-epicardial spread of activation in the ventricles.

Geometric effects are separate from those related to inhomogeneities in conductivity. The cardiac position, the heart being in the left hemithorax, is crucial. Burger and Van Milaan,[35] in their scalene triangle model, showed major errors in Einthoven's equilateral triangle concept. Lead I is a poor lead, its R-L (x axis) characteristics being considerably and variably distorted by superior-inferior and anterior-posterior effects. Another critical aspect is that the closer the myocardium is located to the thoracic wall, the higher the voltage is. This effect, the proximity effect, is extremely important. In the preschool child in whom the heart is close to the thoracic wall, initial R wave voltages, particularly in the right chest leads (V_4R, V_1, V_2), are often quite high. The size of the heart creates another possible distortion. Individuals with cardiac disease with a dilated heart also project greater ECG potential than they would if the proximity effect were not present. For many reasons, including a greater effect of the blood cavity and perhaps an increase in the area of the double-layer source, dilatation of the heart augments the magnitude of the surface potentials.[34, 36] This problem is compounded in infants because the heart is large in relation to the size of the thorax. In addition, there are variations in voltage among various ethnic groups for which explanations are not available.[37]

The effects of the inhomogeneities do not change the general characteristics of the potential distribution but *do* increase the magnitude of the surface potential. A very important property of the volume conductor is the *smoothing effect*. In the model, when two activation waves are separated by 40 degrees or 80 degrees, the two waves appear as two peaks on the epicardium but as one peak on the simulated body surface. Only when the two waves are separated by more than 100 degrees are two discrete maxima present on the thoracic surface. The torso surface thus provides only a low-resolution picture of regional cardiac events. However, epicardial potentials do indeed reflect details of the underlying activation patterns and do not appear to be affected by the position of the heart within the thorax.[38, 39]

In the thorax, blood has the highest conductivity,[40] three times that of the myocardium. Therefore, intracavitary blood has a great effect (the Brody effect). Blood increases the magnitude of the potentials as a result of radial excitation from endocardium to epicardium, as in normal activation, and decreases the magnitude of the potentials as a result of excitation tangential to the blood cavity. An increase in blood conductivity occurs with a decrease in hematocrit, which therefore increases the magnitude of the ECG potentials. Conversely, an increase in hematocrit decreases conductivity, thus decreasing the magnitude of the potentials.[41] Although the clinical effects are important, they are not as great as the original studies indicated, because these studies involved only one inhomogeneity (blood) and an otherwise homogeneous medium. In our studies with the eccentric spheres model, with blood added to an otherwise homogeneous model, enhancement of the radially oriented surface potential was 72.0%, whereas when other inhomogeneities were included (lung, pericardium, skeletal muscle, fat) the enhancement was only 46.4%. Blood also "smooths out" the surface potential distribution. Obviously, in the neonatal period and in early infancy, when changes in hematocrit may be dramatic, or in cyanotic congenital cardiac anomalies and anemia, the effect of hematocrit is particularly important.

The pericardium provides the simplest clinical observation of the effect of an inhomogeneity. When a finite-thickness pericardium is used, the potential increases to a maximum of about twice the normal conductivity, but with continually increasing conductivities, the voltages actually decrease. The predicted behavior was observed experimentally by Manoach and colleagues,[42] who found decreases in potential magnitude when the pericardial sac of cats was filled with saline (high conductivity) or with olive oil (low conductivity). Our model demonstrates that with a pericardial effusion with the conductivity of plasma, magnitudes decrease by almost 50% relative to normal.

The most extensive inhomogeneity in the body is in the lungs, which have very low conductivity. The lungs envelop the heart, except for the posterior mediastinum, which also has a low conductivity, and the anterior region where the heart is close to the thoracic wall. The model demonstrates nonuniform behavior, reflecting the asymmetry of the lung compartment. The lung increases magnitudes anteriorly by 16% while decreasing potentials posteriorly only slightly. The reduced potentials for low lung conductivity are consistent with the low voltages found in patients with obstructive pulmonary disease.[43] Most important, increased residual volume and increased functional residual capacity are associated with an abnormally posterior vector in patients with cystic fibrosis. Such patients have emphysematous pulmonary tissue anteriorly and laterally, so that magnitudes are apparently enhanced posteriorly and diminished anteriorly and laterally. In fact, the abnormally posterior vector can be used to predict the lung volume roughly and is also used to explain the difficulty in interpreting right ventricular hypertrophy electrocardiographically. The diagrammatic representation of a transverse vector loop shown in Figure 9–4 is quite helpful in understanding such concepts.

High lung conductivity occurs in patients with pulmonary venous congestion or infiltration.[44] In patients with cardiomegaly and pulmonary venous congestion as a result of left ventricular failure, decreased ECG potentials are found.[44] Because both an enlarged heart and congested lungs can affect the ECG potentials, we obtained

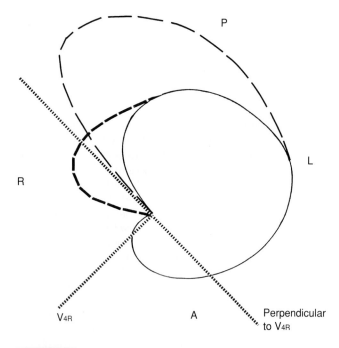

FIGURE 9–4

A diagrammatic representation of a transverse plane vector loop with two different terminal vectors. The V_4R lead axis is depicted as well as the perpendicular to the projection of the V_4R lead. Both terminal vectors extend about equally to the right, with the posterior *(lighter dashed lines)* slightly farther to the right. Note that the terminal vector with the *heavier dashed lines* crosses the perpendicular to the V_1 lead axis. Therefore, V_4R (and V_1) would project on the chest leads in V_4R and V_1 as rS complexes. P = posterior; L = left; R = right; A = anterior. (From Liebman J: Electrocardiography. *In* Moss AJ, Adams FH, Emmanouilides GC [eds]: Heart Disease in Infants, Children, and Adolescents. Baltimore, Williams & Wilkins, 1977, pp 183–221.)

scalar orthogonal ECG recordings and vectorcardiograms from human subjects undergoing pulmonary lavage of a whole lung, the air in the lung being replaced by high-conductivity physiologic saline. The result was a decrease in the ECG magnitude with the maximal decrease posteriorly, consistent with the fact that the largest part of the lung volume lies posterior to the heart. With high lung conductivity, most of the current flow is confined to the lung region. When the lung conductivity is decreased, more of the current flow is through the low-resistance surface muscle layer. Both changes result in a low voltage.[45]

The high-conductivity surface muscle layer has many effects, the primary being that of attenuating potential differences on the torso. The muscle layer is an important contributor to the smoothing effect of the volume conductor, the ECG magnitudes decreasing with increasing muscle conductivity. Type II glycogenosis (Pompe's disease) provides excellent clinical confirmation of the theory. Large quantities of glycogen, a very poor conductor, accumulate in the skeletal muscle, resulting in decreased conductivity. The clinical effect is that of remarkably high QRS voltages. The heart is also dilated and thus contributes to the QRS voltage, but, compared with the ECGs of other infants with the same size heart, the difference in QRS voltages is striking.

The subcutaneous fat layer, considered to be an important attenuator of ECG voltages, does not influence the surface potentials significantly as a result of its low conduc-

tivity. The proximity effect is the most likely explanation for reduced voltages in an obese patient because the electrodes are farther from the source.

Correlation exists between cardiac size and the magnitude of body surface potential[42, 46, 47]; an increase in magnitude results from the increase in volume of the blood compartment and an increase in the size of the source as a result of dilatation.

The thickness of the ventricular wall (hypertrophy) remains an enigma. No theory explains why hypertrophy increases ECG magnitudes. Studies show only minimal changes in magnitude despite large changes in thickness of the wall. In fact, when the thickness of the wall is doubled at the expense of the blood cavity size, the potentials decrease.

LEAD THEORY

The ECG potentials measured at the body surface reflect all cardiac sources, but for a particular lead (or, properly, lead pair) some sources have a greater effect. The word *lead* is best used to imply a lead pair because the ECG galvanometer requires connections to both the positive pole and the negative pole. Therefore, all leads are either bipolar or compound when more than two electrodes are involved. The unipolar leads of the standard ECG are compound leads, with a number of leads connected together and attached to the negative pole of the apparatus and an "exploring" electrode attached to the positive pole. Frequently, a passive network connects several electrodes designed to give a weighted sum in a particular direction. For example, the orthogonal (mutually perpendicular) lead systems are designed to measure the x, y, and z (right-left, superior-inferior, and anterior-posterior, respectively) components of the net cardiac vector.

Note that a lead vector of a given lead is a fixed vector and that the lead voltage is proportional to the projection of the cardiac vector on the lead vector. Orientation of the lead vector depends on the geometry of the leads, the presumed location of the cardiac vector, the body shape, and the torso inhomogeneities. Dipole elements close to a lead, where the lead vector field is expected to be greatest, will generally have stronger weighting than those located in distal regions. An important concept to visualize is that the orientation of the lead vector *within the heart* is not parallel to a line joining the leads or at a 60-degree angle to the horizontal. It is also nonuniform in the heart region and at an angle that varies between perhaps 20 degrees and 80 degrees to the horizontal.

The limb leads I, II, and III are simple lead pairs. *All other leads in standard electrocardiography are compound leads.* The Wilson central terminal is formed by connecting each electrode (right arm, left arm, left leg) to a 5000-ohm resistor and tying the distal resistor terminals together to form a single lead connected to the negative pole of the electrocardiograph. For leads VR, VL, and VF, Wilson connected the electrodes of the right arm, left arm, and left leg, in turn, to the positive pole. The resulting voltages were very small and not usable, but Goldberger[48] disconnected the connection of the central terminal to the right arm resistor when the right arm electrode was connected to the positive pole. The result was a large voltage, similar to that of leads I, II, and III, so that the lead was called aVR for augmented VR. The same augmentation was done for VL and VF so that leads aVL and aVF were also created. In the chest leads, the exploring electrode on the chest is connected to the positive pole. The lead vector of the precordial leads is roughly from the center of the torso to the specific electrode site on the precordium.

When a resistor network is connected to electrodes placed on the torso, it becomes, in a sense, an extension of the passive volume conductor. This property has been used in various compound lead systems designed to measure the x, y, and z components of the dipole source. Because these components are mutually perpendicular to each other, such lead systems are called orthogonal lead systems.[49,50] The most commonly used orthogonal system is that of Frank.

INSTRUMENTATION

Small, direct writing instruments are convenient and portable, but any recorder that uses a heated stylus system with waxed carbon paper has a low-frequency response.[51] To improve the quality of ECGs, a pen that provides a fine jet of quick-drying ink is used. Many of the electrode problems have been overcome to minimize skin resistance. Furthermore, active electrodes with built-in buffer amplifiers on each electrode, needing no electrode paste, are available; these electrodes are impedance transformers having a very high input impedance.[52] The newest disposable electrodes use built-in electrode paste, which is excellent for keeping skin resistance low.

The high-frequency components coming from the heart may be very important,[53] although most ECG information appears to be at less than 100 to 125 Hz.[51] To record frequency components of 100 to 125 Hz, an ECG system with a frequency response of at least twice that (250 cycles/sec) is needed.[54] Very few machines in commercial use provide this much frequency response.

There must also be a low-frequency cutoff in the range of 0.5 cycle/sec to allow accurate recording of low-frequency components on the ECG, the ST-T segment, and the U waves. All commercial machines provide the appropriate low-frequency response.

The term *electrocardiogram* refers to any technique by which the electrical activity from the heart is recorded, whether it is from an impaled cell, the epicardium, or the surface of the body (torso). In this chapter, I use the term to imply that it is from the torso, but I include *any* method on the torso, including the standard ECG, orthogonal ECG with or without vector display, or body surface potential mapping (BSPM). A *scalar recording* refers to one in which the recording device, while moving along the paper at a specific speed, records the magnitude of the potential, either up (positive) or down (negative) depending on the calibration. This is the type of ECG commonly employed. A vector display is a recording in which two or more scalars are measured simultaneously to obtain a vector, the sum total of all activity from the atrium or ventricle at an instant of time. When successive vectors are measured throughout the cardiac cycle, a continuous connection of the terminus of each vector results in the *vector loop*. When using scalar recording, there is no need to have it represent just one lead. In our own BSPMs we record the scalars from 180 electrodes simultaneously and then add their values to make one scalar, called the *magnitude function*.

The traditional ECG is actually two different lead systems, the frontal plane ECG (the limb leads) and the horizontal plane ECG (the chest leads). A different x axis or right-left lead is used in each lead system, lead I for the frontal plane and leads V_5 and V_6 for the horizontal plane. There is nothing magical about the term *vectorcardiography,* because it can and has used the limb leads of the standard ECG. Currently, in the Western hemisphere, only the orthogonal Frank system is used to any degree. The Frank system has seven electrodes and 13 different resistors to develop the x, y, and z axes. These axes (right-left, superior-inferior, and anterior-posterior, respectively) *can be* and *are* recorded as either scalars or vector loops. These scalars from one P, QRS, and T complex are recorded along with the horizontal, frontal, and often sagittal loops. In addition, the orthogonal scalar could be recorded as a long strip as in a standard ECG, to allow rhythm analysis. It is my practice to use orthogonal electrocardiography with vector display, because our group has shown it to be more accurate in diagnosing and quantifying abnormality than is the 12-lead ECG. However, because of physician demand, the regular ECG obtained in all patients is standard. Because, by chance, the chest leads of the standard ECG provide a reasonable approximation of the Frank orthogonal ECG's horizontal plane vector display, the chest lead scalars are readily translated into a vector loop. I find the technique of drawing the loops from the standard ECG very educational, and they also provide improved diagnostic ability. The chest scalars must be simultaneously inscribed, either as three leads at a time or as all six leads at a time, to draw these vector loops satisfactorily.

LEAD PLACEMENT

For the standard ECG, the limb lead electrodes are placed on the right arm, left arm, and left leg, with a ground electrode on the right leg. The extremities are relatively equipotential so that the measurements change very little when the electrodes are placed near the trunk. The left arm electrode is attached to the positive terminal for lead I with the right arm connected to the negative terminal. For leads II and III, the left foot is connected to the positive terminal, and the right and left arms are connected to the negative terminal, respectively. Lead I is considered to be an x axis lead with the deflection positive (upright) to the left, and the negative (downward) to the right. Unfortunately, there is so much distortion in the superior-inferior and anterior-posterior directions that it is not a very useful lead. Leads II and III are close to y axis leads, with lead II useful mainly because its lead vector best reflects atrial activation from the sinus node to the AV node. The result is a large P wave, facilitating rhythm analysis and the diagnosis of right atrial hypertrophy. Lead aVF is a particularly good lead, providing a very good y axis.[55] In lead aVF, a positive (upright) deflection is inferior, whereas a negative (inverted) deflection is superior.

The chest lead system's specific lead placements are as follows:

- V_1: Fourth intercostal space, right parasternal line.
- V_2: Fourth intercostal space, left parasternal line.

- V$_3$: Between fourth and fifth intercostal spaces, midway between V$_2$ and V$_4$.
- V$_4$: Fifth intercostal space, left midclavicular line.
- V$_5$: Same transverse level as V$_4$ (not along intercostal space), left anterior axillary line.
- V$_6$: Same transverse level as V$_4$ and V$_5$, left midaxillary line. In addition, as a routine, lead V$_3$R or V$_4$R is strongly recommended. V$_4$R is the lead most commonly used.
- V$_4$R: Fifth intercostal space, right midclavicular line.
- V$_3$R: Between fourth and fifth right intercostal spaces, midway between V$_1$ and V$_4$R. With some commercial equipment another lead is commonly used, especially V$_7$.
- V$_7$: Same transverse level as V$_4$, V$_5$, and V$_6$, left posterior axillary line.

When dextrocardia is present, equivalent right chest leads should be placed, but the limb leads should not be altered. Great accuracy should be used in placing the chest leads because minor electrode misplacement may cause considerable change.

Although vector loops for the Frank system and the standard ECG are qualitatively similar, in abnormal situations the Frank system and chest lead standard ECGs may be *very* different. There are many reasons for this in the standard ECG, including proximity potentials, which may represent as much as 30% of the magnitude of the complexes, particularly in the right chest leads.[56] Nonetheless, the principles of interpretation are the same regardless of the lead system. Therefore, I construct vector loops for frontal and horizontal planes of the standard ECG and make interpretations as I do for the Frank system with vector display.

The term *axis* refers to the mean vector in the frontal plane. Particularly because lead I is such a poor lead, construction of that mean vector is useless. Another related expression, an indeterminate axis, is also useless, because an indeterminate axis is merely a vector loop in which there are two main vectors that are quite far apart but determinable. Therefore, the term axis should be restricted to only the above-mentioned x, y, and z axes. The expression axis deviation is obviously also not to be used, nor should right axis deviation or the very incongruous left axis deviation. The last term, perhaps the worst term in electrocardiography, has been used whenever the mean vector in the frontal plane is abnormally superior.[57] Many electrocardiographers state that −80 degrees, for example, is a greater "left axis" than −40 degrees, even though −80 degrees is more to the right than −40 degrees. Obviously, such a vector is more to the right than is normal, making the term left axis incongruous. Our preferred term is *an abnormally superior vector* for, indeed, the large terminal vector is abnormally superior.

CONSTRUCTION OF THE VECTOR LOOP

As part of our methodology for QRS complex vector loop construction, I estimate mean vectors for the T wave but not the QRS. In drawing the QRS loop, however, I estimate the mean vector at each instant of time. A mean vector for the entire QRS has no meaning. For orientation only, I estimate a *main* vector for the entire QRS. In our method of construction, I use perpendiculars to the lead vectors, not the lead vectors themselves, because it makes an understanding of the projection much easier (Fig. 9–5). By using the perpendicular for a lead—for example, lead I—any aspect of the P, QRS, or T vector that is positive in the lead is to the left of the line, and any aspect that is negative is to the right of the line. Any aspect of the QRS vector that is positive in lead aVF is inferior, and any aspect that is negative in aVF is superior. The same holds for each lead.

Once the electrocardiographer learns how to draw the loops, they can be constructed rapidly.[58] Figure 9–6A represents an enlarged idealized six-channel standard ECG of the limb leads (frontal plane). The initial vector is negative in aVF (q wave) and positive in lead I. Therefore, the initial QRS vector is in the left upper quadrant (left superior) (see Fig. 9–6B). To delineate further the reasonably accurate position of the initial QRS vector, leads II and aVR are examined. Both begin negative, confining the initial QRS vector to between 300 and 330 degrees (see Fig. 9–6C). To analyze the entire QRS loop, each succeeding instant of time is similarly analyzed. Note the smooth QRS loop (see Fig. 9–6H), where the main and mean vectors are, by accident, the same. The method for estimating this vector is similar to that just described at each instant of time. The net value of leads I and aVF is positive, putting the mean vector in the left lower quadrant (left inferior). Lead aVL is isoelectric (equal negative and positive deflections) so that the mean vector is +60 degrees.

The method of constructing the chest lead (horizontal plane) vectors is similar, and the result is more valuable clinically. Leads V$_2$ and V$_5$ are approximately 90 degrees apart and are analyzed first, as were leads I and aVF for the frontal plane. In Figure 9–7A, the initial QRS vector is negative (to the right) in V$_5$, and positive (anterior) in V$_2$. Therefore, the initial QRS vector is in the right lower quadrant (right anterior) (see Fig. 9–7B). Because lead V$_4$ is initially positive, the initial QRS vector is between 90 and 130 degrees (see Fig. 9–7C). In following each instant of time, the loop rotates counterclockwise (see Fig. 9–7H). V$_5$ is mainly positive, and V$_2$ is predominantly negative, placing the mean QRS vector in the left upper quadrant (left posterior). Lead V$_4$ is isoelectric so that the mean vector is at 310 degrees (see Fig. 9–7G). The approximate main vector is the same. Figure 9–8A, B shows the timing of simultaneous events for the frontal and horizontal planes.

The mean T vector is derived similarly, for the same hypothetical ECG (Fig. 9–9). The mean T vector is positive in lead I and positive in lead aVF, placing the mean vector in the left lower quadrant. Lead III is then examined and is positive, putting the mean T vector between 30 and 90 degrees. Lead aVL is also positive, so that the estimated mean T vector is 45 degrees. The same technique is used for the horizontal plane. Lead V$_5$ is positive, and lead V$_2$ is negative, putting the T vector in the left upper quadrant. Lead V$_4$ is positive, so that the mean T vector is between 310 degrees and 0 degrees. The magnitudes of the T vector in leads V$_4$ and V$_2$ are about the same, so that the estimated mean T vector is 335 degrees in the horizontal plane.

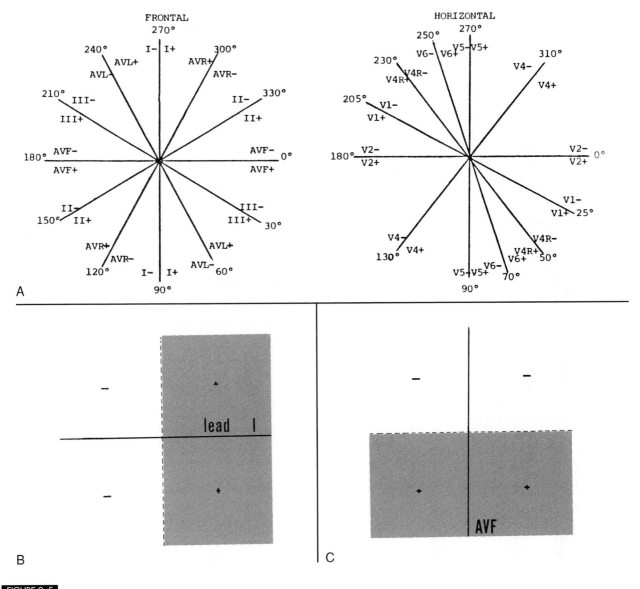

FIGURE 9–5

A, Lines drawn represent perpendiculars to leads as labeled. *B,* The *solid line* (lead I) and *dashed line* (its perpendicular) separate positive and negative sides. *C,* The *solid line* (lead aVF) and *dashed line* (its perpendicular) separate positive and negative sides. (*A–C* from Ravielle A, Liebman J: The methodological approach to the interpretation of the electrocardiogram. *In* Liebman J, Plonsey R, Gillette PC [eds]: Pediatric Electrocardiography. Baltimore, Williams & Wilkins, 1982, pp 60–75.)

After 6 weeks of age, the normal child shows a counterclockwise QRS vector in the horizontal plane. A tall brief R wave in lead V_2 is normal. A tall brief R wave in V_2 is also common in a normal 6-year-old child.

In the Frank system vectorcardiogram (Fig. 9–10), the horizontal plane contains the x and z scalars; the sagittal plane (not shown), the y and z scalars; and the frontal plane, the x and y scalars. The vector loops are traditionally interrupted at regular time intervals (usually at 20 or 25 milliseconds, but at 40 milliseconds in this tracing), allowing estimation of speed of conduction of the "vector" during the QRS complex. In this vectorcardiogram, conduction is slow early and late in the QRS complex but more rapid during the midportion. It is common in preschool children to have considerable proximity effect. That is why the anterior vector in the horizontal plane is much greater

than the posterior vector. In the standard ECG, the anterior and posterior vectors (see lead V_2) are equal. In teenage years and adulthood, the posterior vector is usually much greater than the anterior vector. Yet, on autopsy, the left-right ventricular wall thickness ratio is about 2:1 at 3 months of age and up to 3:1 in adulthood.

The vector loop as well as the scalar x and z leads can be analyzed in relation to the sequence of ventricular depolarization. The right ventricle is both anterior and to the right of the left ventricle, and initial activation, derived from five different activation areas, is directed to the right and anterior. The earliest activation of the free ventricular wall is in the right ventricle, which is anterior, and when the free wall of the left ventricle begins activating, it is also anterior. Soon, because the left ventricle has a thicker wall than does the right ventricle, the vector is directed to the left

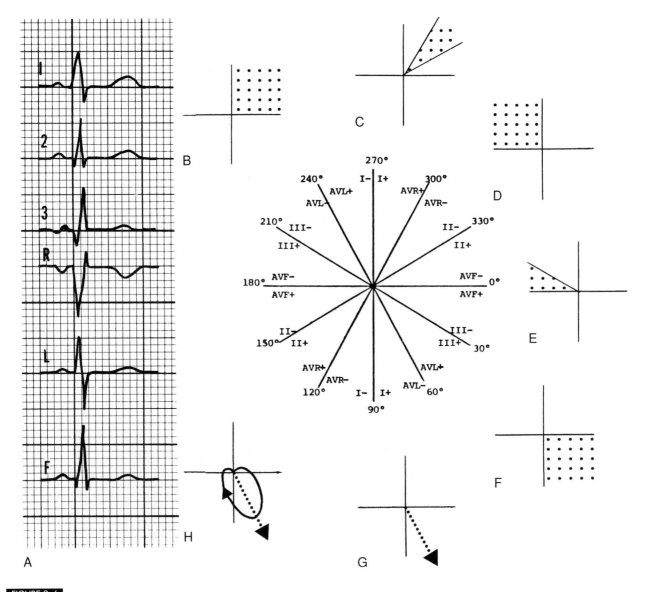

FIGURE 9–6

Interpretation of the ECG (see text). *A,* Single QRS complex from a frontal plane simultaneous six-channel ECG. *B,* Quadrant of the initial forces. *C,* Angle of the initial forces. *D,* Quadrant of the terminal forces. *E,* Angle of terminal forces. *F,* Quadrant of the mean vector. *G,* Angle of the mean vector. *H,* Frontal plane QRS vector loop. (*A–H* from Ravielle A, Liebman J: The methodological approach to the interpretation of the electrocardiogram. *In* Liebman J, Plonsey R, Gillette PC [eds]: Pediatric Electrocardiography. Baltimore, Williams & Wilkins, 1982, pp 60–75.)

and *still* anterior. When both lateral portions of the ventricles are depolarized, the vector is directed well to the left. Subsequently, the vector is posterior and to the left because the posterior portions of both ventricles are being depolarized. Finally, the terminal QRS vector is slightly to the right, because the last portions of the ventricles to be depolarized in children—the superior septum, the postero-basal left ventricle, and the right ventricular outflow tract—are all to the right of the vector of initial activation. Had the right ventricle been thicker, the main cardiac vector would have been less to the left and less posterior. Because of the considerable proximity effect associated with the anterior right ventricle,[34] had the right ventricle been as thick as the left ventricle, the main vector would have been directed to the right and anterior. If the left ventricle had been thicker than normal, the vector would have been of increased magnitude to the left and posterior.

Three standard ECGs (Figs. 9–11 to 9–13) are shown to demonstrate our method of analysis. In each, only part of the standard ECG is shown, including an enlargement of leads V_4R, V_2, and V_5. Leads V_2 and V_5 are approximations of the z and x axes, respectively, and lead V_4R almost bisects the other two axes. Therefore, an approximate construction of the horizontal plane vector is possible and is depicted.

In Figure 9–11, the activation sequence is normal for a teenager, although the maximal magnitudes on the x and z axes are much greater than normal. During the entire time that the free walls of the right and left ventricles are being depolarized, the vector is directed more to the left and posterior than normal. Therefore, left ventricular hypertrophy (LVH) is diagnosed.

In Figure 9–12, the activation sequence is not normal. The vector originates directly to the left and anterior.

Many conditions can cause this,[59] including left bundle branch block, ventricular inversion, fibrosis of the left side of the septum, left posterior free wall hypertrophy as in severe aortic stenosis,[60] and severe right ventricular hypertrophy (RVH) as in severe pulmonic stenosis,[61] as well as low-resistance total anomalous pulmonary venous connection and hypoplastic left ventricle syndrome. In the last two conditions, the initial QRS is often posterior as well because the septum is well to the left and posterior. As activation continues, at the time the posterior free walls of each ventricle are depolarized, the thick-walled right ventricle, the proximity effect, and the decreased potential from the left ventricle cause the vector to be well to the right and anterior. Finally, the terminal rightward vector is of considerable duration. An actual vectorcardiogram would probably rule out terminal slowing and thus right bundle branch block, so RVH is diagnosed. After the first three timed points, lead V_4R is always positive, and this does not fit with leads V_2 and V_5. Therefore, lead V_4R is demonstrating a considerable proximity effect so that this lead cannot be used in constructing the vector.

In Figure 9–13, the activation sequence is also abnormal. The initial vector is directed almost to the left, probably for similar reasons as in Figure 9–12. After the third point, the vectors are anterior instead of posterior, so that the loop has to become clockwise in orientation. The free wall of the right ventricle must be very thick to cause the larger leftward vector to be anterior and to cause the terminal vector to be far to the right, so RVH is the diagnosis.

NORMAL ELECTROCARDIOGRAM

The first deflection on the scalar tracing of the standard ECG is the P wave, which reflects the depolarization of the atrial muscle cells; electrical activity of the sinus node is

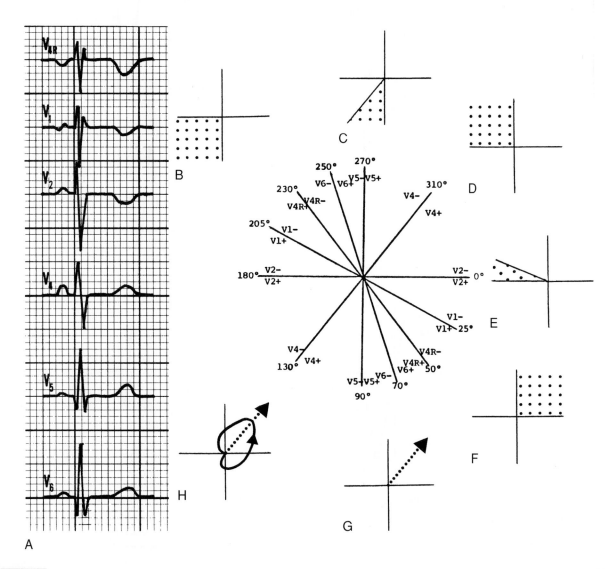

FIGURE 9–7

Interpretation of the ECG (see text). *A* to *H* show events similar to those described in Figure 9–6, but with horizontal leads. (From Ravielle A, Liebman J: The methodological approach to the interpretation of the electrocardiogram. (*A–H* from Ravielle A, Liebman J: The methodological approach to the interpretation of the electrocardiogram. *In* Liebman J, Plonsey R, Gillette PC [eds]: Pediatric Electrocardiography. Baltimore, Williams & Wilkins, 1982, pp 60–75.)

not of enough magnitude to be detected. Recovery of the atria is the T_a wave, always opposite in direction from the P wave. Much of the T_a wave is buried in the QRS complex, so that the wave may not be readily recognized. During the sinus tachycardia of exercise, the T_a wave frequently becomes more prominent so that the erroneous interpreta-

tions of ST segment depression may be made. Because of the T_a wave, measurements of P waves should be made from the preceding baseline. Electrical activity from the AV node (just as from the sinus node) is not of enough magnitude to be detected, nor can the bundle of His be seen using standard methods.

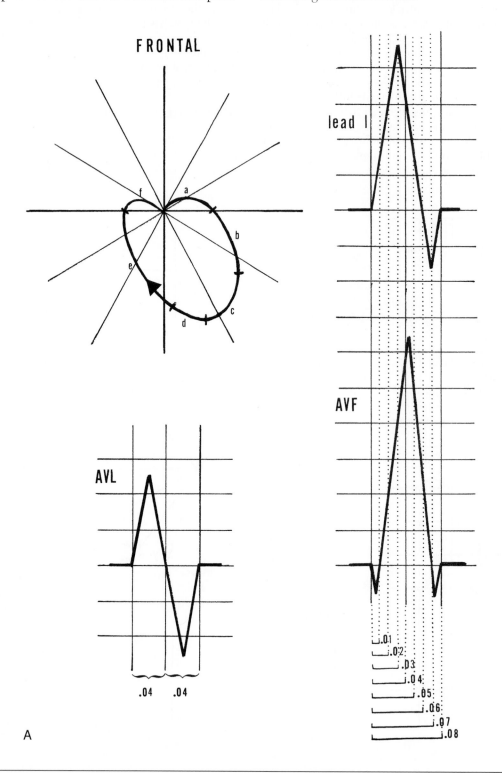

FIGURE 9–8

A, Interpretation of the ECG in the frontal plane. Enlargement of leads I, aVF, and aVL showing timing of simultaneous events: *(a)* 0 to 0.01 second, *(b)* 0.01 to 0.03 second, *(c)* 0.02 to 0.04 second, *(d)* 0.045 to 0.055 second, *(e)* 0.055 to 0.07 second, and *(f)* 0.07 to 0.08 second.

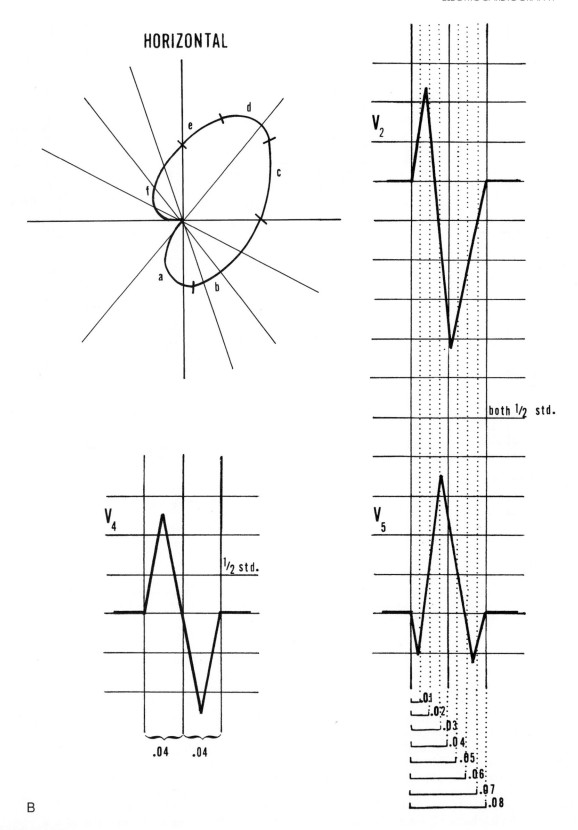

B, Interpretation of the ECG in the horizontal plane (see text). *(a)* 0 to 0.015 second, *(b)* 0.015 to 0.025 second, *(c)* 0.025 to 0.035 second, *(d)* 0.035 to 0.05 second, *(e)* 0.05 to 0.065 second, and *(f)* 0.065 to 0.08 second. (*A, B* from Ravielle A, Liebman J: The methodological approach to the interpretation of the electrocardiogram. *In* Liebman J, Plonsey R, Gillette PC [eds]: Pediatric Electrocardiography. Baltimore, Williams & Wilkins, 1982, pp 60–75.)

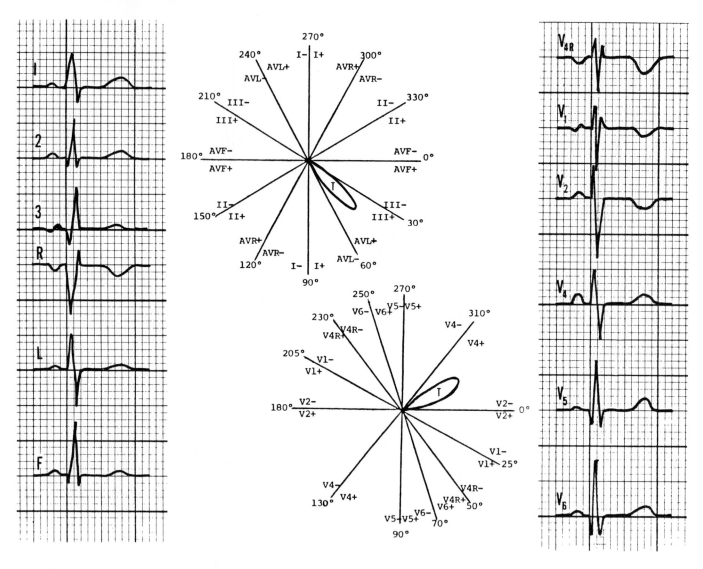

FIGURE 9–9

Interpretation of the ECG (see text). The frontal and horizontal leads and the T vector loops are as they would be drawn from the ECG. (From Ravielle A, Liebman J: The methodological approach to the interpretation of the electrocardiogram. *In* Liebman J, Plonsey R, Gillette PC [eds]: Pediatric Electrocardiography. Baltimore, Williams & Wilkins, 1982, pp 60–75.)

The next complex is the QRS, reflecting the electric field of the ventricles. Repolarization of the ventricles is represented by the ST segment and the T wave, properly called the ST-T segment. Repolarization actually occurs as soon as one ventricular cell depolarizes, so that repolarization begins at the beginning of the QRS complex. At times, there is so much repolarization near the end of the QRS complex that there is considerable distortion of the complex, as well as the early ST segment. Commonly, this is called *early repolarization,* an obvious misnomer. It is often difficult to determine the end of the T wave, which may appear to melt into the next wave, the U wave. The U wave is usually best seen in the midchest leads. Its etiology is unknown, although it is related to repolarization.

Specific Definitions and Intervals

- *PR interval:* Onset of the P wave to onset of the QRS complex

- *PR segment:* End of the P wave to onset of the QRS complex
- *QRS complex:* Beginning of the QRS complex (even if there is no Q wave) to the end of QRS
- *QT interval:* Beginning of the QRS complex to end of the T wave
- *QU interval:* Beginning of the QRS complex to end of the U wave
- *Q:* First downward deflection before an R wave
- *QS:* If only deflection is downward
- *R:* First upward deflection
- *S:* First downward deflection after an R wave (use q, r, and s rather than Q, R, and S when deflections are <0.5 mV)
- *r′ or R′:* Second upward deflection
- *s′ or S′:* Second downward deflection
- *J point:* Junction between the QRS complex and the ST segment

CONSIDERATIONS IN OBTAINING AN ELECTROCARDIOGRAM

Without kindness to the patient and attention to detail, proper recording of ECGs is impossible. *Electrode placement for the standard ECG and any other lead system must be exact,* and the skin must be prepared so that its resistance is low, unless the ECG machine is equipped with very high impedance buffer amplifiers. Electrode paste must be used, *not alcohol or saline,* although disposable electrodes with built-in electrode paste are in common use. The machine should ideally have a high-frequency response (at least 250 Hz) (although few such commercial machines are available) and a rapid enough sampling rate. The machine must be kept clean and maintained to make sure that the specifications are maintained.

The leads must be recorded simultaneously, preferably six at a time. If only three are recorded simultaneously, then the recommended groups are: I, II, III; aVR, aVL, aVF; V_4R, V_2, V_5; and V_1, V_4, V_6. There should also be a simultaneous set for P wave analysis, preferably leads II, V_1, V_2, and V_5 recorded at least double speed and at least double standard. With this type of recording, both components of the P wave can be analyzed, as in Figure 9–14.

Interpretation of the ECG data requires analysis of various measurements, both linear and angular.[30,62] Percentiles must be used in "defining normality," preferably the 2.5th and 97.5th percentiles.

Although large amounts of electrocardiographic data have been obtained for all age groups, large gaps remain. Furthermore, separate tables must be available for QRS tracings taken with a low-frequency recorder (most machines in use) and those taken with high-frequency optical or jet-pen writing recorders. Beginning with puberty, there should be separate tables for African Americans and Caucasians, as well as males and females, because African Americans appear to have higher voltages. In infants and prepubertal children, there are no known ethnic or sex differences (see the Appendix to this chapter).

ATRIAL ELECTROCARDIOGRAM (P WAVE)

ATRIAL DEPOLARIZATION. The atria, being thin-walled and virtually two-dimensional structures, activate at the endocardial and epicardial surfaces nearly simultaneously. Because very little of the right atrium is to the right

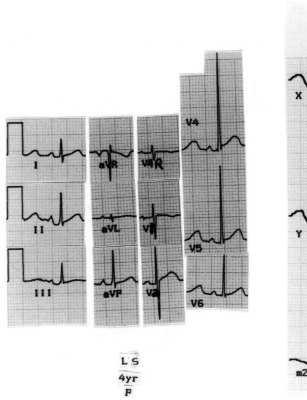
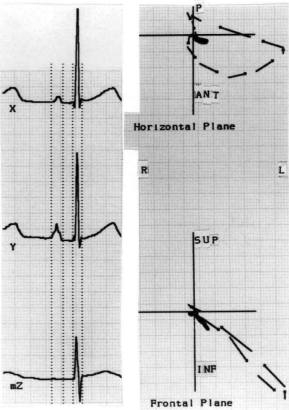

FIGURE 9–10

Standard ECG, orthogonal ECG, and horizontal and frontal vector loop of a 4-year-old normal girl. Note that in lead V_2 the brief anterior voltage is of equal magnitude to the posterior voltage (lead Z), and in the horizontal plane the loop is normally counterclockwise but is greater anterior than posterior. P = posterior; ANT = anterior; SUP = superior; INF = inferior. (From Ravielle A, Liebman J: The methodological approach to the interpretation of the electrocardiogram. *In* Liebman J, Plonsey R, Gillette PC [eds]: Pediatric Electrocardiography. Baltimore, Williams & Wilkins, 1982, pp 60–75.)

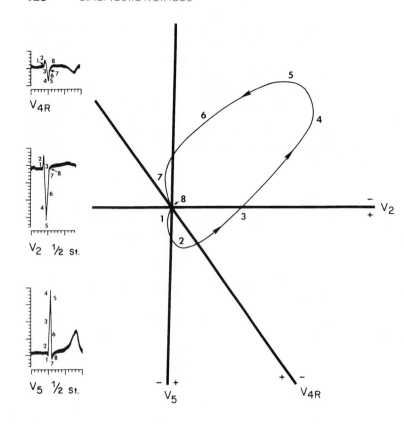

FIGURE 9–11

Enlargement of lead V_4R, V_2, and V_5 from a 16-year-old boy with left ventricular hypertrophy. At eight consecutive instants of time, a vector is projected on leads (perpendiculars to leads are depicted). The terminus of each vector forms a "loop." The direction of loop is normal, but vectors during activation of free walls of right and left ventricle are abnormally to left and posterior. Leads V_2 and V_5 are recorded at half standardization (½ St). (From Ravielle A, Liebman J: The methodological approach to the interpretation of the electrocardiogram. *In* Liebman J, Plonsey R, Gillette PC [eds]: Pediatric Electrocardiography. Baltimore, Williams & Wilkins, 1982, pp 60–75.)

of or posterior to the sinus node, the direction of activation is leftward, inferior, and anterior. The last part of the right atrium to be depolarized normally is the most anteroinferior, although occasionally the posteroinferior right atrium is activated quite late. Under any circumstances, depolarization then continues posteriorly. The left atrium begins depolarizing well before completion of the right atrium, by way of Bachmann's bundle[10] off the anterior internodal tract. Left atrial activation usually begins superiorly, near the right pulmonary veins. The spread occurs laterally, pos-

FIGURE 9–12

Enlargement of leads V_4R, V_2, and V_5 from a 5.5-year-old girl with mild right ventricular hypertrophy. At eight consecutive instants of time, a vector is projected on leads (perpendiculars to leads are depicted). The terminus of each vector forms a loop. The loop is very abnormal. The initial vector is to left. Vectors during the midportion are less posterior than average. Rightward vector has an abnormal duration. The considerable proximity effect in lead V_4R must be deleted in constructing the vector. Leads V_2 and V_5 are recorded at half standardization (½ St). (From Ravielle A, Liebman J: The methodological approach to the interpretation of the electrocardiogram. *In* Liebman J, Plonsey R, Gillette PC [eds]: Pediatric Electrocardiography. Baltimore, Williams & Wilkins, 1982, pp 60–75.)

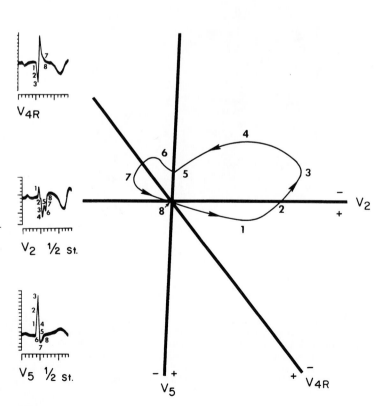

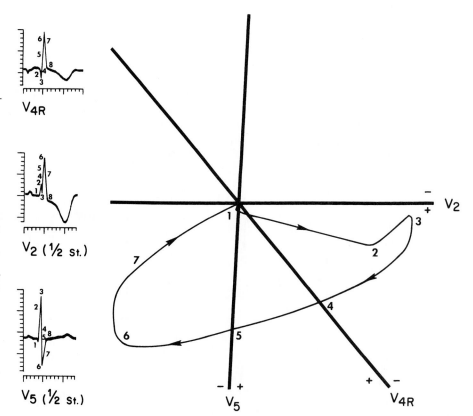

Right ventricular hypertrophy in an 8-year-old girl. Leads V_4R, V_2, and V_5 are enlarged. At eight consecutive instants of time, a vector is projected on leads (perpendiculars to leads are depicted). The terminus of each vector forms a loop. The loop is very abnormal. The initial vector is almost to the left, although points 2 and 3 are normal. However, all points after that are anterior, with late points also to the right. This can be caused in a child only by considerable right ventricular hypertrophy. When vectors are anterior at the time of depolarization of free wall, decreased left ventricular potential from infarction or from hypoplasia of the left ventricle is possible. In an 8-year-old child, right ventricular hypertrophy is diagnosed. Leads V_2 and V_5 are recorded at half standardization (½ St). (From Rudy Y: The effects of the thoracic volume conductor (inhomogeneities) on the electrocardiogram. *In* Liebman J, Plonsey R, Rudy Y [eds]: Pediatric and Fundamental Electrocardiography. The Hague, Netherlands, Martinus Nijhoff, 1987, p 49.)

teromedially, and finally posteroinferiorly near the left inferior pulmonary vein. Sometimes the left atrial appendage is the last portion to be depolarized.

The first portion of the P wave is formed from the right atrium. Usually, right atrial depolarization is completed before that of the left atrium. Puech[63] divided the P wave into thirds, the middle third representing activation of both atria and the first and last portions representing the right atrium and left atrium, respectively. Durrer's data[24] from reperfused human hearts indicated that left atrial activation began at 45 to 50% of P wave duration. In the ECG, even at high frequency, high gain, and high speed,

the three separate areas cannot be recognized; two distinct areas separated by a notch is the norm (see Fig. 9-14).

CRITERIA FOR DIAGNOSIS. In the ECG, atrial hypertrophy cannot be distinguished from atrial enlargement, so that the term *hypertrophy* indicates either condition or both conditions. The term *enlargement* is often used instead of hypertrophy.

Diagnostic criteria for right atrial hypertrophy (RAH) involve the use of the first part of the P wave and are reliable. Because an increased duration of right atrial activation is lost in the second portion of the P wave, only the magnitude

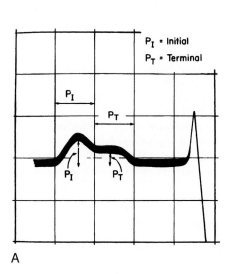

A

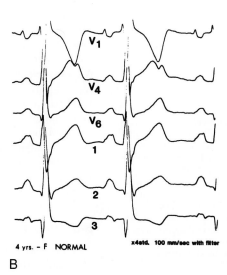

B

P wave analysis. *A*, Diagram of the P wave of lead V_1 with a normal notch. The first portion is called P_1 (P initial), and second part is called P_t (P terminal). Usually, the second portion of P is negative in lead V_1, although in lead II, both portions are positive. (From Morris JJ Jr, Estes EH Jr, Whalen RE, et al: P-wave analysis in valvular heart disease. Circulation 29:242–252, 1964, by permission of The American Heart Association, Inc.) *B*, Simultaneously recorded standard ECG of a normal 4-year-old girl for P wave analysis. Note two major portions of P wave, initially anterior and inferior, terminally posterior and inferior. (From Liebman J: The normal electrocardiogram. *In* Liebman J, Plonsey R, Gillette PC [eds]: Pediatric Electrocardiography. Baltimore, Williams & Wilkins, 1982, pp 134–139.)

of the P wave is used. The most important is a large-magnitude leftward inferiorly directed vector, as seen in lead II in the first part of the P wave (Fig. 9–15). The next criterion, just as reliable but not as frequently used, is a large-magnitude anteriorly directed vector in the first part of the P wave, observed especially in lead V_1 but also in lead V_2. *A large-magnitude inverted P wave in V_1 also commonly occurs in RAH and is often erroneously called left atrial hypertrophy (LAH).* To make the diagnosis of LAH when the P wave is inverted in lead V_1, the P wave must be inverted in

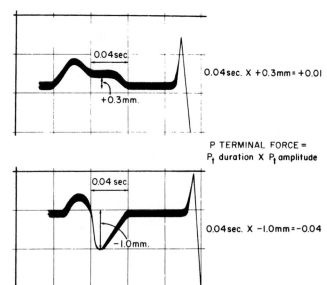

P TERMINAL FORCE =
P_t duration X P_t amplitude

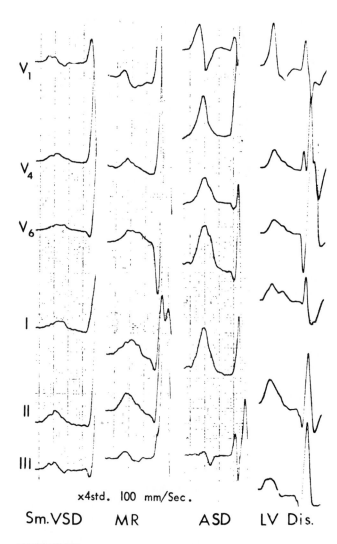

FIGURE 9–15

Four representative ECGs for P wave analysis. The simultaneous tracings of leads V_1, V_4, V_6, I, II, and III are recorded at four times standard and 100 mm/sec. In the first tracing from a patient with a small ventricular septal defect (Sm.VSD), the P waves are normal. In the tracing from a second patient with mitral regurgitation (MR), the second portion of the P wave is very prolonged, indicative of left atrial hypertrophy. In the third tracing from a patient with atrial septal defect (ASD), the first portion of the P wave has very high voltage anterior and inferior, indicative of right atrial hypertrophy. In the fourth tracing from a patient with left ventricular cardiomyopathy (LV Dis.), the first portion has a large voltage anterior and inferior, indicative of right atrial hypertrophy, and the second portion is very prolonged, indicative of left atrial hypertrophy. Thus, there is combined atrial hypertrophy. (From Liebman J: Atrial hypertrophy. *In* Liebman J, Plonsey R, Gillette PC [eds]: Pediatric Electrocardiography. Baltimore, Williams & Wilkins, 1982, pp 140–143.)

FIGURE 9–16

Diagram of calculation of P terminal force (P_t) in two different P waves from lead V_1. The P wave is divided into initial and terminal portions. Amplitude and duration are measured separately. The terminal duration × terminal amplitude = P terminal force. P_t force may be positive (as in the upper tracing) or negative (as in the lower tracing). The same measures are made for the initial portion of the P wave. Values are expressed in arbitrary units (millimeters per second). (From Morris JJ Jr, Estes EH Jr, Whalen RE, et al: P-wave analysis in valvular heart disease. Circulation 29:242–252, 1964, by permission of The American Heart Association, Inc.)

lead V_2 as well. If the large P wave is inverted in V_1 and upright in V_2, then it is anterior, and RAH is the diagnosis.

Diagnostic criteria for LAH involve the second portion of the P wave and are less reliable than those for RAH. Both magnitude and duration are important, especially the latter. The only magnitude of importance is an increased magnitude posteriorly, as seen in leads V_1 and V_2. The measured duration of the second portion of the P wave is a reliable criterion, is readily recognized with high-quality tracings, and is best seen in the left chest leads using simultaneous leads. The Macruz index[64] (the ratio of the duration of the P wave to the duration of the PQ segment) uses a measure of the unrelated AV node conduction. When the ratio is greater than 1.6 : 1, LAH is the diagnosis. The P terminal force measure of Morris[65] (P_t duration times P_t amplitude as measured in the second portion of the P wave in lead V_1) is also a good criterion (Fig. 9–16). A special measure, the time between peaks of the first and second portions of the P wave, is also useful and suggests LAH when the interval is greater than 0.02 second in infants and greater than 0.04 second in adolescents.[66]

Combined atrial hypertrophy (CAH) best uses the increased magnitude of the first portion plus one of the measures using increased duration of the second portion of the P wave. Simultaneous leads are essential for optimal interpretation.

The following criteria are the most helpful.

RAH: Standard Electrocardiography

1. Increased magnitude of first portion of P wave—lead II (mainly inferior)

2. Increased magnitude of first portion of P wave—lead V_1 (mainly anterior)

3. Increased negative magnitude of P wave— lead V_1 if P wave in lead V_2 is anterior

LAH: Standard Electrocardiography

1. Increased P terminal force (more than −0.03 mm)
2. Increased duration of second portion of P wave
3. Increased time between first and second peak of P wave

CAH: Standard Electrocardiography

1. Increased magnitude anteriorly (first part) and/or inferiorly plus increased duration of P wave (would be due to increased duration of second part of P wave)

2. Increased magnitude anteriorly (first part) and/or inferiorly plus increased magnitude posteriorly (second part)

3. Increased magnitude anteriorly and/or inferiorly plus increased P terminal force

4. Increased magnitude anteriorly and/or inferiorly plus increased time between first and second peaks of P wave

VENTRICULAR ELECTROCARDIOGRAM (THE QRS COMPLEX)

VENTRICULAR DEPOLARIZATION.   The ventricles are three-dimensional compared with the atria's essentially two-dimensional nature. Ventricular depolarization throughout the QRS complex is complicated and occurs in multiple areas simultaneously. Initial QRS activation occurs at five distinct areas (see Fig. 9–2). The net result, in a normal 10-year-old child, for example (remembering that because of proximity anterior vectors are greatly accentuated), is that the normal initial QRS vector is to the right, anterior, and superior. Understanding the five major areas of initial ventricular activation allows us to understand, among other things, how the initial QRS can change with specific pathology.

At the next instant of time there is considerable activation in the right ventricle, bringing the vector more anterior. Then the anterior walls of each ventricle are activated simultaneously, bringing the vector to the left and anterior, because the left ventricle has much more muscle mass than does the right. By this time also, because the left ventricle is inferior, the vector is also inferior, and remains there throughout the cardiac cycle. Activation is now very rapid and quickly reaches the lateral wall of each ventricle. The vector is now well to the left, and, as the posterior portions of each ventricle are activated, the vector remains to the left and rapidly goes very posterior. The final areas that could be potentially depolarized include the anterior superior septum, the right ventricular outflow tract, the posterobasal left ventricle, and the left ventricular posterior wall. In children, the posterior left ventricular wall is the least common to be depolarized as a terminal event, but each of the other three areas could terminate alone or at nearly the same time.[25] Importantly, each of the last three is directed toward the right of the site where activation began. The terminal vector, in addition to being directed to the right and posterior, may also be superior. The interpreter of ECGs must know this sequence and must understand the projection of the cardiac vector onto the surface of the torso at each instant of time.

In the frontal plane, the almost constant inferior vector contributes to a clockwise vector more often than to a counterclockwise vector. This is particularly evident in the standard ECG, in which the very inaccurate lead I distorts each instantaneous vector to the right. At each instant of time, an estimate of the portion of the ventricle being activated can be made. Although pathologic conditions may change activation sequences, data about such changes are unknown. By knowing the normal depolarization sequence, differences from normal can be estimated. An understanding of the various inhomogeneities and their modification of the vector also improves diagnostic accuracy.

A number of commonly used criteria for interpreting the QRS should be avoided:

- *Ventricular activation time and the intrinsicoid deflection:* These terms have been used by some to evaluate the QRS complex. The only intrinsicoid deflection is found in the electrogram from an impaled cardiac cell. The time from the onset of the QRS complex to the peak positive deflection (the so-called ventricular activation time) has nothing to do with the onset of ventricular activation, which began many milliseconds earlier. At the instant of the peak positive deflection in lead V_5 or V_6, or both, for example, the sum total of electrical activity from the entire heart is directed leftward.

- *Cardiac position:* A *vertical* heart has been defined electrocardiographically as one in which the mean frontal plane vector is near 90 degrees, and a *horizontal* heart is one near 0 degrees. When one has a vertical heart, it may mean only that there is even more distortion of lead I than usual. It also has nothing to do with tall, thin people or short, fat people.

- *Axis:* The only axes are the x, y, and z axes. As commonly used, the term axis indicates a mean vector and should be discarded. As an aside, mean QRS vectors per se have very little use as well.

- *Right axis deviation (mean frontal plane QRS vector to the right):* The word axis, of course, is a misnomer and should not be used, but the term *axis deviation* is ingrained in common usage. More important, because of the distortions of lead I, normal subjects commonly have a mean frontal plane vector directed to the right. In standard electrocardiography, the term is of no use. In orthogonal electrocardiography, a mean frontal plane vector to the right is a reliable indicator of RVH, but it is merely a manifestation of an abnormal terminal x component directed to the right (terminal x right), known to be an excellent criterion for RVH.

- *Left axis deviation (mean frontal plane QRS vector abnormally superior):* As described earlier, a mean vector to the left, as universally used, is likely to be more to the right than is normal. The proper term is *an abnormally superior vector.*

- *Anatomic rotation:* Clockwise rotation and counterclockwise rotation, the former in RVH, the latter in LVH, are used to imply actual anatomic rotation of the heart in hypertrophy. It is a different usage from that of the rotation of the vector loop. There is no evidence that such anatomic rotation occurs.

Criteria of use in interpretation of hypertrophy are described subsequently, although for detail the reader is referred to Liebman and Rudy.[56]

ELECTROCARDIOGRAM OF THE NEONATE

Until 31 weeks' gestation the left ventricle is significantly thicker than the right ventricle, the average ratio being 1.15:1.[67] After that, a gradual change occurs, reaching an average of 1.3:1 in favor of the right ventricle after 36 weeks. After birth,[68] the ratio of ventricular weights changes, so that by 1 month of age, the left ventricle is significantly larger than the right. By 3 to 6 months, the left ventricle has about twice the muscle mass of the right ventricle, approaching a teenage ratio of 2.5:1 or 3:1.

The ECG's right ventricular dominance of a full-term infant is well known,[69] but there is considerable variability. The change in the QRS complex during the first month of life is striking,[70] but the changes are not as great as would be expected from the changes of ventricle weight ratios. Furthermore, although at 1 month the weight ratio is similar to that of a teenager, the ECG is much different. The premature infant is also different after 1 month, because there is less of the full-term neonatal right ventricular dominance.[71] Major factors in the appearance of the newborn's QRS complex include the large size of the neonatal heart in relation to the thorax. The result is a considerable proximity effect[46] as well as maximal effects on nondipolar elements.

The change in hemodynamics at birth is not reflected in the QRS complex during the first days of life, but the striking variability of the T wave after birth probably is. Three distinct phases of T wave location occur (Fig. 9–17).[72,73]

1. Birth (0 to 5 minutes). The T wave vector is directed well to the left and anterior (as well as superior *or* inferior).[72]

2. Transient phase (1 to 6 hours after birth). The T wave is directed to the right, anterior and inferior.

3. Restitution phase (usually by 3 days, but always by 7 days). The T wave is again directed to the left, remains inferior, and reaches well posterior more slowly, usually by 48 to 72 hours. Occasionally, 7 days may pass before it becomes posterior. The T wave then remains posterior until the late teenage years or early adulthood, with very gradual anterior shift.

The reason for the marked rightward T vector in the first hours of life is likely related to the sudden increase in left ventricular work as the umbilical cord is clamped and the low-resistance placenta is out of the circuit. The restitution phase, with the T wave returning to the left and becoming well posterior, is presumably the result of the adjustment of the left ventricular myocardium to the workload (see Fig. 9–17).

The change in the QRS complex in normal neonates is quite rapid after 72 hours of age, although week-by-week analyses are unavailable for the standard ECG. During the first 72 hours, the horizontal plane is usually inscribed in a wide-open clockwise manner, although narrow loops with two main vectors may occasionally occur. In the Frank system, 60% are clockwise vectors, 25% are narrow crossed vectors, and 15% are narrow counterclockwise vectors. In the last two groups, usually the first vector is to the left anterior and the second is to the right posterior. The orientation is mainly anterior-posterior. By 1 month of age, the horizontal plane loop, in the orthogonal or standard ECG,

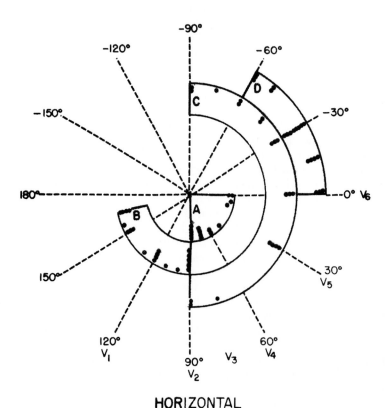

HORIZONTAL

FIGURE 9–17

Representation of mean direction of T waves of 20 normal full-term neonates in the horizontal plane of the standard ECG. Region A, at birth. Region B, at the end of a 6-hour transient phase. Region C, restitution at age 3 days. Region D, completion of restitution at age 7 days. (From Hait G, Gasul BM: The evolution and significance of T-wave changes in the normal newborn during the first seven days of life. Am J Cardiol 12:494, 1963.)

is either counterclockwise or narrow with two main vectors. A clockwise loop is rare, and when present it is very narrow. In most infants by 6 weeks of age, and in all by 2 months, the loop is counterclockwise, although there might be a small right posterior terminal projection. Nonetheless, most of the loop is anterior. The horizontal plane vector loop is mainly posteriorly directed by 1 to 2 years. From age 2 years until school age, a gradual change occurs, but a prominent, brief anterior projection is usual, as a result of the heart's anterior location. Throughout childhood, this anterior projection gradually decreases both in its magnitude and in the relative amount of the early QRS complex that is directed anteriorly.

The rotation of the frontal plane is not useful in neonates or infants, because even late in childhood the frontal plane loop is usually clockwise. Even the Frank system's frontal plane is rotated clockwise 85% of the time. Because of the poor lead I of the standard ECG, neither the frontal plane rotations nor the mean vector measurements are very useful. The main vector of the neonate of 135 degrees changes to 75 degrees by 1 to 3 months of age. After infancy, marked LVH may occasionally cause the frontal plane vector to be well to the left and to rotate counterclockwise.

Analysis of initial QRS activation, useful diagnostically, also reveals changes in hemodynamics. Approximately 10% of full-term neonates and 5% of premature neonates have the initial QRS vector directed to the left, presumably because of the right ventricular dominance. With aging, the normally small q wave in the left chest leads increases in magnitude, because the initial QRS vector is directed more to the right. The initial QRS vector can also be directed superiorly early in infancy and gradually decreases throughout childhood. The mechanism for the change is unknown.

Finally, spatial QRS (and T) vector voltages change throughout life. The mechanisms are unknown.

RIGHT VENTRICULAR HYPERTROPHY

A variety of congenital cardiac anomalies are associated with RVH. There is a spectrum of findings for RVH, but the concept of diastolic overloading as an ECG diagnosis as compared with systolic overloading is not useful. Any diagnostic criteria for these two patterns most likely indicate only differences in severity; for example, severe volume overloading may cause an ECG similar to that seen with moderate pressure overloading. A possible exception is the expected terminal right conduction delay, such as in right ventricular volume overload of atrial septal defect, although mild to moderate pulmonic stenosis may also have terminal right conduction delay. In RVH, there are frequently two main vectors. Commonly, the first is directed to the left and anterior, and the second is to the right and posterior. After 6 to 7 weeks of age, the presence of two main vectors provides a criterion for RVH. If the first vector is abnormally far to the left, then additional LVH is diagnosed.

Criteria for Right Ventricular Hypertrophy

A variety of criteria exist for RVH. Two criteria, an increased magnitude of the terminal vector to the right and

specific changes in the horizontal plane vector loop, are the most sensitive.

1. *Increased magnitude of terminal vector to the right.*
2. *Horizontal plane vector loop:* (a) initial QRS vector to the left anterior; (b) mean QRS vector to the right; (c) main QRS vector abnormally anterior, which by itself is an unreliable sign of RVH. The proximity effect, particularly in preschool children or in patients with chest deformities such as pectus excavatum, may cause overreading of RVH.
3. *Mean QRS vector in the frontal plane to the right.* This has been called right axis deviation. It is common in normal people to have a very large S wave in lead I as a result of superior-inferior distortion, as per Burger's scalene triangle.[35] In the standard ECG, this is quite unreliable.
4. *Increased magnitude of terminal rightward vector (increased terminal x, deep S wave in lead V_5).* This is a most reliable measurement criterion for RVH, made even more reliable if there is a deep S wave in V_6 as well.
5. *Terminal r or R wave in leads V_4R and V_1.* This has been the most used yet most misunderstood criterion for RVH and gives an example as to why "pattern reading" or the identification of a particular criterion in one lead may be fraught with error. A terminal r or R wave in V_4R and V_1 indicates only that the terminal projection crosses the perpendicular to the V_4R and V_1 lead vectors (see Fig. 9–4). A terminal vector to the right, when large, crosses the V_1 lead vector even though the vector is also far posterior. However, when the terminal right vector is not very posterior, only a small magnitude to the right is enough to cross the V_1 lead vector, helping to explain the "normal variant" rsr′. The rsr′ or rsR′ pattern has been called incomplete right bundle branch block (IRBBB) by most electrocardiographers. Usually, that diagnosis is in error. (To make sure that there is no confusion with the terminology of the past [even when IRBBB is truly present, as in many postoperative patients], we have discarded the term in favor of *partial right bundle branch block*.)
6. *Increased magnitude of anterior vector (increased z anterior, tall R wave in leads V_1 and V_2).* This is only a fairly good criterion. It is easy to overread RVH when there is a tall spiking R wave of brief duration as part of an RS complex. Most of the time, particularly in the preschool child, the cause is a proximity effect because the heart is so close to the thoracic wall at this age. To suggest the diagnosis of RVH, the duration of the initial R wave should be at least 30 milliseconds. An increased ratio of R to S in lead V_1 is commonly used to diagnose RVH, but the same cautions are needed. It is unreliable.
7. *Increased magnitude of inferior vector (increased y, tall R wave in lead aVF).* This may be part of severe RVH, although if it is present when all other criteria are normal, it usually indicates LVH.
8. *Increased magnitude of posterior vector (increased z posterior, deep S wave in leads V_1 and V_2).* This may be part of severe RVH as the terminal rightward posterior portion of a clockwise horizontal plane loop.
9. *Abnormal ratio of specific magnitudes.* Abnormal ratios of specific magnitudes—for example, an increased ratio of the magnitude of z anterior–z posterior and/or an increased ratio of the magnitude of x terminal right–x

left—are particularly useful in the presence of abnormally low voltage from various causes, including pulmonary disease, with the x terminal right–x left being more reliable.

10. *Increased magnitude of the terminal R wave in lead aVR.* This is reliable, but the diagnosis is usually obvious from other criteria.

11. *Increased magnitude of the maximal spatial vector to the right (MSVR).* MSVR = $\sqrt{x^2 + y^2 + z^2}$ at the time the terminal x of the orthogonal ECG is directed to the right. This is in general an excellent criterion.

12. *Abnormally prolonged QRS complex duration.* This criterion is only fair for diagnosing RVH. For example, even in atrial septal defect, in which there is a terminal right conduction delay, the total QRS complex duration is infrequently greater than normal.

13. *T wave abnormality.* In severe hypertrophy, with the QRS vector well anterior, the T vector may be abnormally posterior (inverted T waves in right precordial leads) and even to the right. The criterion cannot be used to diagnose RVH, but if RVH is clearly present, it indicates greater severity.

14. *ST segment abnormality.* As with the T waves, the abnormality occurs only with severe hypertrophy, the ST vector being posterior (depressed in right precordial leads) and very infrequently to the right as well.

15. *Anterior T vector.* If the T vector is anterior left after 72 hours of age (yields upright T waves in right precordial leads), RVH is present. There is no relationship to severity, and the mechanism is not known.

LEFT VENTRICULAR HYPERTROPHY

There are many criteria,[31,56,74] but the most sensitive is an increased magnitude of QRS vectors posterior with a normally directed horizontal plane vector loop and specific abnormalities in the vector loop (e.g., a counterclockwise horizontal plane vector loop in the newborn).

Criteria for Left Ventricular Hypertrophy

1. *Direction of inscription.* A wide-open counterclockwise vector in a neonate is indicative of LVH no matter what the voltage (Fig. 9–18), and LVH can be suspected on the basis of a vector loop different from normal without regard for voltage for 4 to 6 weeks. After that age, the loop in LVH may be exactly the same as normal, with the initial QRS vector directed to the right and anterior, followed by the vector being less anterior than normal, increased to the left, then well posterior, ending slightly to the right and posterior. The spatial voltage in LVH is greater than normal. Particularly in severe hypertrophy, the vector may extend to the posterior before terminating farther to the left. As a result, the terminal part of the loop is clockwise (Fig. 9–19). The genesis of this pattern is presumed to be an intraventricular condition abnormality, associated with fibrosis. When the initial QRS vector is directed to the left, it is impossible to distinguish from partial left bundle branch block.

   The direction of inscription in the frontal plane is usually clockwise in infants and children with LVH, although in older children with severe LVH the vector is occasionally counterclockwise.

2. *Initial QRS vector to the left and anterior.* This is a manifestation of several LVH (loss of q waves in left precordial leads).

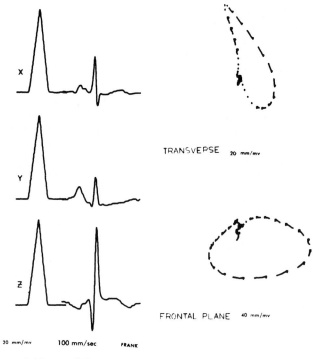

Z P=1.85mv 1day−m   PA

A Frank system vectorcardiogram (scalars at 20 mm/mV) of a 1-day-old infant with hypoplastic right ventricle and pulmonary atresia (PA). Note the wide-open counterclockwise horizontal plane vector loop. Although occasional full-term newborns have counterclockwise plane loops, such loops are usually quite narrow. Note also the inferior vector (whereas had the hypoplastic right ventricle been associated with tricuspid atresia instead of pulmonary atresia, there would usually be an abnormally superior vector because there is usually a ventricular septal defect [VSD] in the endocardial cushion defect position). Note also the large inferior magnitude of the first portion of the P wave in the y lead, indicative of right atrial enlargement. (From Liebman J: Ventricular hypertrophy. *In* Liebman J, Plonsey R, Gillette PC [eds]: Pediatric Electrocardiography. Baltimore, Williams & Wilkins, 1982, pp 144–171.)

3. *Increased magnitude of posterior vector (increased z posterior, deep S wave in leads V_1 and V_2).* An abnormally posterior vector with a normal activation sequence is probably the single best criterion for LVH (Fig. 9–20), although pulmonary parenchymal disease with a high residual volume may diminish the magnitude anterior and left because of the decreased conductivity of air and cause an abnormally posterior vector without LVH. In severe RVH, a clockwise horizontal plane vector loop may terminate abnormally posteriorly, probably because of late posterior right ventricular potentials after the left ventricle has completed activation. To diagnose LVH on that basis would be an error (Fig. 9–21).

4. *Increased magnitude of terminal rightward vector with an abnormally posterior vector.* It is not possible to distinguish between LVH with additional RVH and pure LVH, including the posterobasal segment. This ECG finding can indicate pure LVH.

5. *Abnormal ratios of specific magnitudes.* A decreased magnitude of the ratio of z anterior to z posterior is useful, although other ratios are less reliable. It is particularly useful in the presence of low voltage from various causes.

6. *Increased magnitude of the R wave in lead aVL.* This is a reliable criterion, but the diagnosis is usually obvious from other criteria. An important caution is that with an abnormally superior vector, the magnitude of the R wave in lead aVL is increased because the vector is along aVL's lead vector. If this occurs, therefore, the criterion cannot be used.

7. *Increased magnitude of the maximal spatial vector to the left (MSVL).* $MSVL = \sqrt{x^2 + y^2 + z^2}$ with the main vector to the left. This is an excellent criterion, but the measurement of z posterior by itself is simpler and probably just as good.

8. *Angle of the mean or main vector abnormally posterior.* This is only a fair sign of LVH because there is so much normal variability.

9. *Horizontal plane vector loop rapidly progressing from anterior to posterior.* If the vector is posterior before 2 milliseconds, the diagnosis may be anterior myocardial infarction, but the vector for patients with severe LVH (Fig. 9–22) may extend posterior before 2 milliseconds (Fig. 9–23). Anterior myocardial infarction in children is extremely rare. Therefore, the criterion, even if *before* 2 milliseconds, is very useful.

10. *Increased magnitude of leftward vector (increased x to the left, tall R wave in leads V_5 and V_6).* This is an excel-

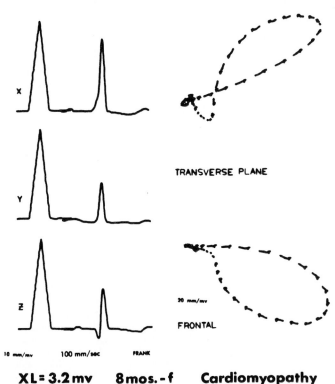

XL = 3.2 mv   8 mos. - f   Cardiomyopathy

FIGURE 9–19

Frank vectorcardiogram (scalars at 10 mm/mV) of an 8-month-old infant with congestive heart failure and idiopathic cardiomyopathy. Typical left bundle branch block (LBBB), although in the x lead (XL) a slow initial upstroke suggested Wolff-Parkinson-White syndrome. The vectorcardiogram shows only a small amount of initial QRS slow conduction. The T vector is 180 degrees from the QRS vector. The QRS duration suggests partial left bundle branch block. (From Liebman J: Interpretation of conduction abnormalities. *In* Liebman J, Plonsey R, Gillette PC [eds]: Pediatric Electrocardiography. Baltimore, Williams & Wilkins, 1982, pp 172–191.)

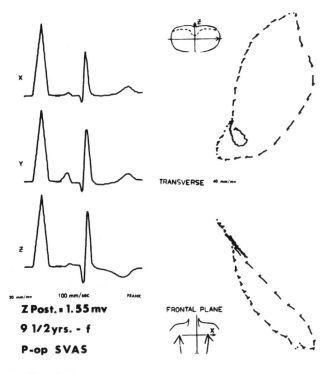

Z Post. = 1.55 mv

9 1/2 yrs. - f

P-op SVAS

FIGURE 9–20

A Frank vectorcardiogram (scalars at 20 mm/mV) of a 9.5-year-old girl who had been operated on for subvalvular aortic stenosis (SVAS) 5 years previously. The gradient across the subvalvular diaphragm had been 80 mm Hg. The QRS had indicated considerable left ventricular hypertrophy (LVH), and the T vector was abnormally anterior (but not to the right). The QRS activation sequences are now apparently normal with initial QRS to the right, anterior and superior, and the magnitudes of the leftward, posterior and inferior vectors normal. The only suggestion of LVH is that the angle of the maximal QRS vector is abnormally posterior (only a fair sign of LVH). However, the T vector remains anterior despite excellent surgery. (From Liebman J: Ventricular hypertrophy. *In* Liebman J, Plonsey R, Gillette PC [eds]: Pediatric Electrocardiography. Baltimore, Williams & Wilkins, 1982, pp 144–171.)

lent sign of LVH (see Fig. 9–22). In addition, if lead V_6 is greater than lead V_5, even though neither is above the 97.5 percentile, LVH should be considered. The projection is that of a large leftward vector that stays to the left a long time.

11. *Increased magnitude of inferior vector (increased y inferior, tall R wave in lead aVF).* With a normal horizontal vector loop and good left-sided chest potential, a large inferior vector (even if not abnormally high) suggests LVH. The left ventricle is the more inferior ventricle, but this criterion is only moderately reliable because of considerable variability in the magnitude of lead aVF and because significant RVH can also cause a large inferior vector.

12. *Abnormally prolonged QRS complex duration.* On average, the QRS complex is prolonged, but the usefulness of the criterion is only fair because the variation is so great.

13. *T wave abnormality.* There are two major types of T wave abnormality. The first, common in patent ductus arteriosus and other volume overloading lesions, is a large-magnitude T vector in the normal direction (increased left and/or inferior). By itself the criterion is not useful, because tall T waves can be present in many situations, including hyperkalemia, and are not an indication of severity. Although often present in volume overloading, tall T waves can also be present in patients with pressure

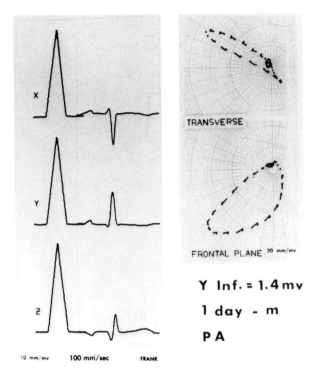

FIGURE 9–21

A Frank system vectorcardiogram of a 1-day-old male infant with maximal tetralogy (tetralogy with pulmonary atresia). Note the initial QRS to the left, the clockwise transverse plane loop, and the large terminal rightward posterior vector. This is severe right ventricular hypertrophy (RVH). In the standard ECG, there are deep S waves in the left chest leads. Leads V_1 and V_2 did not show a terminal R wave—only V_4R did. This is classic severe RVH; in a standard ECG, pattern reading analysis often misses the diagnosis. (From Liebman J: Ventricular hypertrophy. *In* Liebman J, Plonsey R, Gillette PC [eds]: Pediatric Electrocardiography. Baltimore, Williams & Wilkins, 1982, pp 144–171.)

overloading. The second type of T wave abnormality is that of a wide deviation of the T wave from the QRS complex, an indication of severity of the LVH. In the most severe instances, the T vector is so anteriorly directed that the T waves are upright in the right chest leads. If, in addition, the T vector is to the right, the T in the left chest leads is also negative. Although this type of T abnormality has been associated with severe pressure overload, it may be also present in pure severe volume overload. Severity of the hypertrophy, perhaps with fibrosis, seems to be the cause, rather than the type of hemodynamics (e.g., pressure versus volume overloading). A low-voltage T wave vector may have similar significance to that of a wide QRS-T angle.

14. *ST segment abnormality.* When the T wave abnormality is markedly abnormal, there is usually also marked ST segment abnormality. This severe ST segment abnormality may be manifested by depression in the x leads V_5 and V_6 and sometimes by elevation in leads V_4R and V_1. Depression inferiorly, as in lead aVF, may also be present. As in the T wave abnormality, ST segment abnormality has usually been associated with severe pressure overload, but severe volume overload, as in a large shunt patent ductus arteriosus, may also be responsible.

COMBINED VENTRICULAR HYPERTROPHY

There are several criteria for diagnosing combined ventricular hypertrophy (CVH).

1. *Direction of inscription of horizontal plane vector loops.* There are many variations of CVH in which the direction of inscription is particularly useful. (a) The presence of two main vectors in the horizontal plane often provides excellent evidence (Fig. 9–24). Usually the first vector is directed abnormally to the left and anterior or posterior and the second vector abnormally to the right

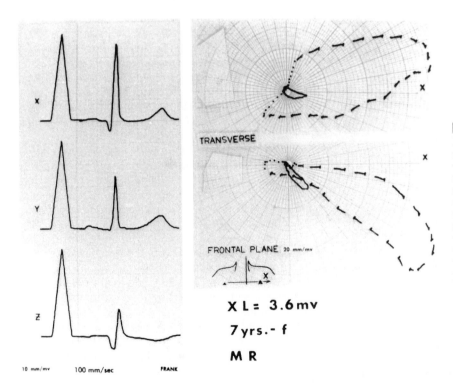

FIGURE 9–22

Frank vectorcardiogram (VCG) (scalars at 10 mm/mV) of 7-year-old girl with moderately severe mitral regurgitation (MR) and normal pulmonary artery pressures. The activation sequence in the horizontal plane is normal, and it is counterclockwise in the frontal plane. The magnitude of the x axis to the left (XL) is well above normal, so that the diagnosis of left ventricular hypertrophy (LVH) is definite. The vector magnitude posterior is only a little below normal, so that additional right ventricular hypertrophy (RVH) cannot be diagnosed. The magnitude of the initial QRS to the right is top normal, so that the diagnosis of possible left septal hypertrophy is also made. (From Liebman J, Rudy Y: Electrocardiography. *In* Moller JH, Neal WA [eds]: Fetal Neonatal and Infant Cardiac Disease. Norwalk, CT, Appleton & Lange, 1990, p 179. Reproduced with permission of The McGraw-Hill Companies.)

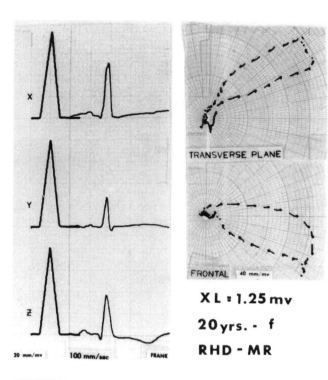

XL = 1.25mv

20 yrs. - f

RHD - MR

FIGURE 9–23

A Frank system vectorcardiogram (VCG) (scalars at 20 mm/mV) of a 20-year-old woman with severe mitral regurgitation (MR) as a result of rheumatic heart disease (RHD). Although the QRS rotates clockwise, the initial QRS is to the right and anterior, so that left bundle branch block cannot be diagnosed. Possibilities include lateral wall fibrosis and infarction. Cardiac catheterization did not demonstrate anomalous left coronary artery, and the left lateral wall of the left ventricle contracted normally. XL = x axis to the left. (From Liebman J, Rudy Y: Electrocardiography. *In* Moller JH, Neal WA [eds]: Fetal Neonatal and Infant Cardiac Disease. Norwalk, CT, Appleton & Lange, 1990, p 179. Reproduced with permission of The McGraw-Hill Companies.)

and anterior or posterior. After 1 month of life, RVH is definite, and LVH is additionally diagnosed if the leftward vector is of increased magnitude at any age. A very large anterior vector, followed by a very large posterior vector, may also be part of CVH. (b) The activation sequence may be exactly as normal, with a wholly counterclockwise loop and large-magnitude leftward and/or posterior projection. In the neonatal period, such a loop indicates LVH even without abnormal magnitudes. If the anterior projection is also quite large and prolonged, then additional RVH is diagnosed. In the same situation, if the terminal right magnitude is increased, RVH should also be suggested, but if the vector is abnormally posterior, then the large rightward vector may indicate posterobasal LVH rather than additional RVH. (c) If the horizontal plane is wholly clockwise, pure RVH is the usual diagnosis, but if it is also abnormally to the left, additional LVH should be considered. The diagnosis of additional LVH, however, can be an error, because a greatly dilated right ventricle can cause a considerable proximity effect on the lead projections on the left chest. A definite error is to diagnose additional LVH if, with a wholly clockwise horizontal plane loop, there is a large terminal rightward posterior projection. This terminal posterior projection is probably derived from the right ventricle after the left ventricle has completed activation and is a manifestation of severe RVH.

2. *Increased magnitude posterior and/or to the left, with a large terminal vector to the right.* These findings provide excellent criteria for CVH, but the terminal right posterior vector is a possible manifestation of posterobasal LVH instead of additional RVH. In a standard ECG the CVH may be missed. The abnormally posterior vector may cause the projection of the large terminal rightward vector not to cross the perpendicular projections to leads V_4R and V_1. In the standard ECG, there would be a deep S wave in leads V_1, V_2, V_5, and V_6 and the lack of a terminal r or R vector in leads V_4R and V_1.

FIGURE 9–24

A Frank vectorcardiogram (VCG) (scalars at 10 mm/mV) of a 4-month-old boy with a large ventricular septal defect (VSD) (two thirds systemic level pulmonary hypertension and large left to right shunt). There are two main vectors in the horizontal (transverse) and frontal planes with large leftward and rightward vectors, along with a clockwise QRS rotation. In the standard ECG, the voltages were extremely large to the left and to the right, but also the R and S waves in lead V_4 were of very large magnitude, totaling more than 60 mm. XL = x axis to the left. (From Liebman J, Rudy Y: Electrocardiography. *In* Moller JH, Neal WA [eds]: Fetal Neonatal and Infant Cardiac Disease. Norwalk, CT, Appleton & Lange, 1990, p 179. Reproduced with permission of The McGraw-Hill Companies.)

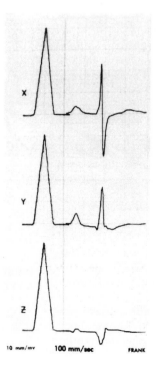

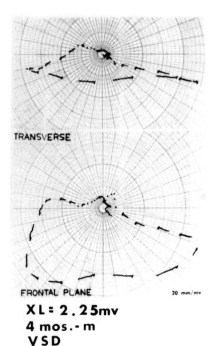

XL = 2.25mv

4 mos. - m

VSD

3. *Increased magnitude plus definite evidence for LVH.* The anterior portion provides only a soft sign for associated RVH. To make the diagnosis, the initial anterior forces should be broad and of at least 0.03 second's duration after infancy. A large initial rightward anterior could also be due to left septal hypertrophy, whereas a tall spiking initial anterior in the right chest leads is commonly due to a proximity effect, particularly in preschool children.

4. *Increased magnitude inferior vector (increased y inferior, tall r wave in aVF) in the presence of RVH as diagnosed in the horizontal plane.* With good left ventricular potentials and not very severe RVH, additional LVH can be considered with increased magnitude of the inferior vector. If there is severe RVH, however, the increased inferior magnitude should be presumed to be part of RVH.

5. *Increased magnitude anterior and posterior.* If there is a wholly counterclockwise horizontal loop, with the time elapsed anterior at least 0.03 second and an increased magnitude posterior, CVH is reliably diagnosed. This type of ECG is common in early infancy.

6. *Katz-Wachtel phenomenon.* This is an ECG "pattern" that is not generally useful, although it is commonly discussed in relation to ventricular septal defect. It was originally described as "tall R and S waves" in the midchest leads, together with tall R and S waves in two of the three "bipolar standard limb leads."[75] The biphasic nature of the QRS complex was believed to be due to the opening in the septum, but, of course, this is not true. The manifestation of CVH is that of a wide-open counterclockwise horizontal plane vector with the first vector far anterior and the second vector far posterior. Namin and Miller[76] have reported that R + S in the midprecordial leads over 60 mm indicates CVH. We have seen more than 100 mm (10 mV) total R + S in lead V_4 of the standard ECG in the presence of CVH.

7. *Mean QRS vector to the right in the frontal plane of the standard ECG in the presence of definite LVH (as recorded in the horizontal plane).* This is an artifact caused by the poor x axis in standard lead I and is not an indicator of CVH.

8. *Clockwise rotation of the frontal plane in the presence of definite LVH (as recognized in the horizontal plane).* Although these criteria have been used as an indicator of CVH, They are unreliable in the pediatric age group because of the clockwise frontal plane normally present in most children, including virtually all infants.

9. *Main QRS vector to the left (not superior) in the presence of RVH.* By itself this is a poor sign.

10. *Abnormally superior vector in the presence of RVH.* This is not a sign of CVH, because the abnormally superior vector (formerly called left axis deviation)[57] indicates a conduction defect involving the left anterior branch of the left bundle. The abnormally superior vector may also cause the projection in lead aVL to be of increased magnitude, so that this finding cannot be used either.

11. *Definite hypertrophy of one ventricle, with suggested evidence for hypertrophy of the other.* This nonspecific statement is usually good policy, and the interpretation should be stated as such.

12. *ST segment and T wave abnormalities.* In our present state of knowledge, ST segment and T wave abnormalities with combined hypertrophy, as diagnosed by other parameters, indicate severity, but they cannot be used to diagnose hypertrophy itself. Usually the severity is that of the LVH.

ST AND T ABNORMALITIES AS A RESULT OF PRIMARY CAUSES

The cardiac cell is the one type of cell in the body available for indirect analysis of primary changes that may affect the entire body. The tool for such analysis is the surface ECG. The ECG is useful for identifying electrolyte abnormalities. Low or high concentrations of certain chemicals, such as potassium and calcium, affect the ECG in special ways, but the effects are confounded by changes in sodium, magnesium, or bicarbonate levels or by acidosis or alkalosis. An excellent example of the ECG's usefulness is provided by two patients with a serum potassium level of 7 mEq/L who may have very different ECGs. One may have the classic tall peaked T waves, whereas the other ECG may be nearly normal. The patient whose ECG is nearly normal is at much less acute risk of the detrimental effects of hyperkalemia than is the patient whose ECG demonstrates tall peaked T waves. Therefore, the physician concerned with a patient whose serum potassium level is high is not obtaining all the information available when serum potassium levels are measured and ECGs are *not* being recorded. The reader is referred to three excellent reviews on this subject and related issues.[77–79]

The meanings of the ST segment and T wave, including the U wave, are being re-examined, including the concept of dispersion of repolarization.[80] Heterogeneities of repolarization occur in the ventricular myocardium's three-dimensional structure. The ventricular myocardium's M cells, in the midregion of the myocardial wall of the ventricle, have longer action potential duration than that of the endocardium or epicardium.[81] The M cell action potential is prolonged disproportionately in response to the slowing of heart rate as well as to certain agents that prolong action potential duration. The beginning of the T wave is caused by a more rapid decline of phase 2 of the action potential of the epicardium, which normally completes its repolarization at the time of the peak of the T wave. Repolarization of the endocardium is completed during the descending limb of the T wave, and the M region completes its repolarization at the end of the T wave.[82]

The U wave, particularly when prominent and in abnormal situations, may be related to abnormal M cell repolarization, but this is unclear; nor is the etiology of the normal U wave understood. The entire area of the prolonged QT (or Qu) and situations of presumed abnormal dispersion of repolarization are in the process of extensive investigation.[28, 77, 78] Our understanding and clinical use of the ST segment and T waves will ultimately be completely revamped.[83]

REFERENCES

1. Plonsey R: The biophysical basis for electrocardiography. *In* Liebman J, Plonsey R, Gillette PC (eds): Pediatric Electrocardiography. Baltimore, Williams & Wilkins, 1982, pp 1–14.

1a. Plonsey R: Activation of the heart. *In* Liebman J, Plonsey R, Gillette PC (eds): Pediatric Electrocardiography. Baltimore, Williams & Wilkins, 1982, pp 23–28.

1b. Plonsey R: Electrocardiographic lead theory and lead systems. *In* Liebman J, Plonsey R, Gillette PC (eds): Pediatric Electrocardiography. Baltimore, Williams & Wilkins, 1982, pp 29–39.

2. Rudy Y: The electrocardiogram and its relationship to excitation of the heart. *In* Sperelakis N (ed): Physiology and Pathophysiology of the Heart, 3rd ed. Boston, Kluwer Academic, 1995, p 201.

3. Woodbury FW: Cellular electrophysiology of the heart. *In* Hamilton WF, Dow P (eds): Handbook of Physiology, Section 2: Circulation, Vol 1. Washington, DC, American Physiological Society, 1962, p 237.

4. Luo C, Rudy Y: A model of the ventricular cardiac action potential: Depolarization, repolarization and their interaction. Circ Res 68:1501, 1991.

5. Lowenstein WR: Junctional intercellular communication: The cell-to-cell membrane channel. Physiol Rev 61:829, 1981.

6. Page E, Shibata Y: Permeable junctions between cardiac cells. Annu Rev Physiol 43:431, 1981.

7. Streeter DD: Gross morphology and fiber geometry of the heart. *In* Berne RM (ed): Handbook of Physiology, Section 2: The Cardiovascular System, Vol 1: The Heart. Baltimore, Williams & Wilkins, 1979, p. 61.

8. Taccardi B, Macchi E, Lux RL, et al: Effect of myocardial fiber direction on epicardial potentials. Circulation 90:3076, 1994.

9. Colli-Franzone P, Guerri L, Taccardi B: Spread of excitation in a myocardial volume. Simulation studies in a model of ventricular muscle activated by point stimulation. J Cardiovasc Electrophysiol 4:144, 1993.

10. James TN: The connecting pathways between the sinus node and A-V node and between the right and the left atrium in the human heart. Am Heart J 66:498, 1963.

11. James TN, Sherf L, Fine G, et al: Comparative ultrastructure of the sinus node in man and dog. Circulation 34:139, 1966.

12. Boineau JP, Schuessler RB, Mooney CR, et al: Multicentric origin of the atrial depolarization wave. The pacemaker complex. Relation to dynamics of atrial conduction, P-wave changes and heart rate control. Circulation 58:1036, 1978.

13. Mace SE, Levy MN: Neural control of heart rate: A comparison between puppies and adult animals. Pediatr Res 17:491, 1983.

14. Pickoff AS, Stolfi A: Postnatal maturation of autonomic modulation of heart rate. Assessment of parasympathetic and sympathetic efferent function in the developing canine heart. J Electrocardiol 29(suppl):215, 1966.

15. James TN: Sir Thomas Lewis redivivus: From pebbles in a quiet pond to autonomic storms. Br Heart J 52:1, 1984.

16. Liebman J: Anatomy of the cardiac conduction system. *In* Liebman J, Plonsey R, Gillette PC (eds): Pediatric Electrocardiography. Baltimore, Williams & Wilkins, 1982, p 15.

17. James TN, Sherf L: Ultrastructure of the human atrioventricular node. Circulation 37:1049, 1968.

18. Anderson RH, Wenich AC, Losekoot TG, et al: Congenitally complete heart block. Developmental aspects. Circulation 56:90, 1977.

19. Janse MK, Anderson RH, van Capelle FJ, et al: A combined electrophysiological and anatomical study of the human fetal heart. Am Heart J 91:556, 1976.

20. Lev M: The pathology of complete atrioventricular block. Prog Cardiovasc Dis 6:317, 1964.

21. Kulbertus HE: Advances in the understanding of conduction disturbances. Eur J Cardiol 8:271, 1978.

22. Spach MS, Miller WT III, Miller-Jones E, et al: Extracellular potentials related to intracellular action potentials during impulse conduction in anisotropic canine cardiac muscle. Circ Res 45:188, 1979.

23. Scher AM, Spach MS: Cardiac depolarization and repolarization and the electrocardiogram. *In* Hamilton WF, Dow P (eds): Handbook of Physiology, Section 2: Circulation, Vol 1: The Heart. Washington, DC, American Physiological Society, 1962, p 357.

24. Durrer D, Van Dam RT, Freud GE, et al: Total excitation of the isolated human heart. Circulation 41:899, 1970.

25. Liebman J, Thomas CW, Rudy Y, et al: Electrocardiographic body surface potential maps of the QRS in normal children. J Electrocardiol 14:249, 1981.

26. Durrer D, Buller J, Graaff P, et al: Epicardial excitation pattern as observed in the isolated revived and perfused fetal human heart. Circ Res 9:29, 1961.

27. Plonsey R: Recovery of cardiac activity. The T wave and ventricular gradient. *In* Liebman J, Plonsey R, Rudy Y (eds): Pediatric and Fundamental Electrocardiography. The Hague, Martinis Nijhoff, 1987, p 9.

28. Harumi K, Burgess MJ, Abildskov JA: A theoretic model of the T wave. Circulation 34:657, 1966.

29. Plonsey R: A contemporary view of the ventricular gradient of Wilson. J Electrocardiol 12:337, 1979.

30. Liebman J, Downs TD, Priede A: The Frank and McFee vectorcardiogram in normal children. A detailed quantitative analysis of 105 children between the ages of two and nineteen years. *In* Hoffman IZ (ed): Vectorcardiography 2. Amsterdam, North-Holland Publishing, 1971, p 483.

31. Lee MH, Liebman J, Mackay W: Orthogonal electrocardiography. Correlative study of 100 children with pure cardiac defects. *In* Hoffman I, Hamby RI (eds): Vectorcardiography 3. Amsterdam, North-Holland Publishing, 1976, p 181.

32. Burgess MJ, Green LS: Ventricular repolarization properties and their relation to the body surface electrocardiogram. *In* Liebman J, Plonsey R, Rudy Y (eds): Pediatric and Fundamental Electrocardiography. The Hague, Martinus Nijhoff, 1986, p 39.

33. Liebman J, Plonsey R: Basic principles of understanding electrocardiography. Paediatrician 2:251, 1973.

34. Rudy Y: The effects of the thoracic volume conductor (inhomogeneities) on the electrocardiogram. *In* Liebman J, Plonsey R, Rudy Y (eds): Pediatric and Fundamental Electrocardiography. The Hague, Martinus Nijhoff, 1987, p 49.

35. Burger HC, Van Milaan JB: Heart-vector and leads. Br Heart J 9:154, 1947.

36. Castini D, Vitolo E, Ornaghi M, Gentile F: Demonstration of the relationship between heart dimensions and QRS voltage amplitude. J Electrocardiol 29:167, 1996.

37. Rautaharju PM, Zhou SH, Calhoun HP: Ethnic differences in ECG amplitudes in North American white, black and Hispanic men and women. J Electrocardiol 27(suppl):20, 1994.

38. Gulrajani RM, Mailloux GE: A simulation study of the effects of torso inhomogeneities on electrocardiography potentials, using realistic heart and torso models. Circ Res 52:45, 1985.

39. Spach MS, Barr RC, Lanning CF: Experimental basis for QRS and T wave potentials in the WPW syndrome. The relation of epicardial to body surface potential distributions in the intact chimpanzee. Circ Res 42:103, 1978.

40. Rush S, Nelson CV: The effects of electrical inhomogeneity and anistropy of thoracic tissues on the field of the heart. *In* Nelson CV, Geselowitz DB (eds): The Theoretical Basis of Electrocardiography. Oxford, Clarendon, 1976, p 323.

41. Nelson CV, Rand PW, Angelakos ET, et al: Effect on intracardiac blood on the spatial vectorcardiogram. 1. Results in the dog. Circ Res 31:95, 1972.

42. Manoach M, Gitter S, Grossman E, et al: The relation between the conductivity of the blood and the body tissue and the amplitude of the QRS during heart filling and pericardial compression in the cat. Am Heart J 84:72, 1972.

43. Liebman J, Krause DA, Doershuk CF, et al: Orthogonal vectorcardiogram in cystic fibrosis: Diagnostic significance and correlation with pulmonary function tests: A four year follow-up. Chest 63:218, 1973.

44. Ishikawa K, Berson AS, Pipberger HV: Electrocardiographic changes due to cardiac enlargement. Am Heart J 81:635, 1971.

45. Rudy Y, Wood R, Plonsey R, et al: The effect of high lung conductivity on electrocardiographic potentials. Results from human subjects undergoing bronchopulmonary lavage. Circulation 65:440, 1982.

46. Rudy Y, Plonsey R: Comments on the effect of variations of the size of the heart on the magnitude of ECG potential. J Electrocardiol 13:79, 1980.

47. Manoach M, Gitter S, Grossman E, et al: Influence of hemorrhage on the QRS complex of the electrocardiogram. Am Heart J 82:55, 1971.

48. Goldberger E: A simple indifferent electrocardiographic electrode of zero potential and a technique of obtaining augmented, unipolar extremity leads. Am Heart J 23:483, 1942.

49. Frank E: An accurate, clinically practical system for spatial vectorcardiography. Circulation 13:736, 1956.

50. Brody DA, Arzbaecher RC: A comparative analysis of several corrected vectorcardiographic leads. Circulation 29:533, 1964.

51. Dower GE, Moore AD, Ziegler WG, et al: On QRS amplitude and other errors produced by direct-writing electrocardiographs. Am Heart J 65:307, 1963.

52. Ko WH, Hynacek J: Dry electrode and electrode amplifiers. *In* Miller HA, Harrison DC (eds): Biomedical Electrode Technology: Theory and Practice. New York, Academic, 1974, p 169.

53. Holcroft JW, Liebman J: Notching of the QRS complex in high frequency electrocardiograms of normal children and in children with rheumatic fever. J Electrocardiol 3:133, 1970.

54. Thomas CW: Electrocardiographic measurement response. *In* Liebman J, Plonsey R, Gillette PC (eds): Pediatric Electrocardiography. Baltimore, Williams & Wilkins, 1982, p 40.

55. Pipberger RV, Bialek SM, Perloff JK, et al: Correlation of clinical information in the standard 12-lead ECG and the corrected orthogonal 3-lead ECG. Am Heart J 61:34, 1961.

56. Liebman J, Rudy Y: Electrocardiography. *In* Moller JH, Neal WA (eds): Fetal Neonatal and Infant Cardiac Disease. Norwalk, CT, Appleton & Lange, 1990, pp 179–245.

57. Liebman J, Nadas AS: An abnormally superior vector (formerly called marked left axis deviation). Am J Cardiol 27:577, 1971.

58. Ravielle A, Liebman J: The methodological approach to the interpretation of the electrocardiogram. *In* Liebman J, Plonsey R, Gillette PC (eds): Pediatric Electrocardiography. Baltimore, Williams & Wilkins, 1982, pp 60–75.

59. Liebman J, Plonsey R, Ankeney JL: The initial QRS vector in ventricular hypertrophy. (Proceedings of the IXth International Congress on Electrocardiography, June 7–11, 1982, Tokyo, Japan.) Jpn Heart J 23(suppl):480, 1982.

60. Liebman J, Thomas CW, Rudy Y, Saltzberg R: The initial QRS in severe aortic stenosis–A body surface potential mapping study. *In* Macfarlane PW, de Padua F (eds): Electrocardiology '92. Singapore, World Scientific, 1993, p 33.

61. Liebman J, Saltzberg R, Thomas CW: The initial QRS in severe pulmonic stenosis as compared to severe aortic stenosis. A preliminary body surface potential mapping study. *In* Macfarlane PW, Rautaharju P (eds): Electrocardiology '93. Singapore, World Scientific, 1994, p 187.

62. Downs TD, Liebman J, Agusti R, et al: The statistical methods for vectorcardiographic directions. IEEE Trans Biomed Eng 16:87, 1969.

63. Puech P: The P wave: Correlation of surface and intra-atrial electrocardiograms. Cardiovasc Clin 6:43, 1974.

64. Macruz R, Perloff JK, Case RB: A method for the recognition of atrial enlargement. Circulation 17:882, 1958.

65. Morris JJ Jr, Estes EH Jr, Whalen RE, et al: P-wave analysis in valvular heart disease. Circulation 29:242, 1964.

66. Ishikawa K, Kini PM, Pipberger HV: P wave analysis in 2464 orthogonal electrocardiograms from normal subjects and patients with atrial overload. Circulation 48:565, 1973.

67. Emery JL, MacDonald MS: The weight of the ventricles in the latter weeks of intrauterine life. Br Heart J 22:563, 1960.

68. Emery JL, Mithal A: Weights of cardiac ventricles at and after birth. Br Heart J 23:313, 1961.

69. Guller B, Lau FY, Dunn RA, et al: Computer analysis of changes in Frank vectorcardiograms of 666 normal infants in the first 72 hours of life. J Electrocardiol 10:19, 1977.

70. Alimurung MM, Joseph LG, Nadas AS, et al: The unipolar precordial and extremity electrocardiogram in normal infants and children. Circulation 4:420, 1951.

71. Sreenivasan VV, Fisher BJ, Liebman J, et al: Longitudinal study of the standard electrocardiogram in the healthy premature infant during the first year of life. Am J Cardiol 31:57, 1973.

72. Hait G, Gasul BM: The evolution and significance of T-wave changes in the normal newborn during the first seven days of life. Am J Cardiol 12:494, 1963.

73. Liebman J: The normal electrocardiogram in newborns and infants (a critical review). *In* Cassels D, Ziegler RF (eds): Electrocardiography in Infants and Children. New York, Grune & Stratton, 1996, p 79.

74. Liebman J: Electrocardiography in congenital heart disease. *In* Macfarlane PW, Lawrie TDV (eds): Comprehensive Electrocardiology. New York, Pergamon, 1989, p 729.

75. Katz LN, Wachtel H: The diphasic QRS type of electrocardiogram in congenital heart disease. Am Heart J 13:207, 1937.

76. Namin EP, Miller RA: Pediatric electrocardiography and vectorcardiography. *In* Gasul BM, Arcilla RA, Lev M (eds): Heart Disease in Children—Diagnosis and Treatment. Philadelphia, JB Lippincott, 1966, pp 69–120.

77. Surawicz B: Relationship between electrocardiogram and electrolytes. Am Heart J 73:814, 1967.

78. Surawicz B: Primary and secondary T wave changes. Heart Bull 15:31, 1996.

79. Fisch C, Knoebel S, Feigenbaum H, Greenspan K: Potassium and the monophasic action potential, electrocardiogram, conduction and arrhythmias. Prog Cardiovasc Dis 8:387, 1966.

80. Han J, Moe GR: Non uniform recovery of excitability in ventricular muscle. Circ Res 14:44, 1964.

81. Antzelevitch C, Nesterenko VV, Shimuzu W, DiDiego JM: Electrophysiologic characteristics of the M cell. *In* Proceedings of the Symposium on Monophasic Action Potentials, Munich, 1997.

82. Antzelevitch C, Shimuzu W, Yan GX, Sicouri S: Cellular basis for QT dispersion. *In* Proceedings of the 22nd International Society for Computerization in Electrocardiology, April 26–May 1, 1997, Palm Coast, Florida. J Electrocardiol 30(suppl):168, 1998.

83. Surawicz B: Will QT dispersion play a role in clinical decision making? J Cardiovasc Electrophysiol 7:777, 1996.

APPENDIX

TABLE 9–1

QRS AND T MEAN VECTORS (DEGREES)

Age	QRS Mean Vector (Frontal Plane)					T Mean Vector (Frontal Plane)				
	Min.	5%	Prev. Dir.	95%	Max.	Min.	5%	Prev. Dir.	95%	Max.
0–24 hr	60	60	135	180	180	+340	0	70	140	180
1–7 days	60	80	125	160	180	+320	+320	25	80	100
8–30 days	0	60	110	160	180	+340	0	35	60	120
1–3 mo	20	40	80	120	120	0		35	60	80
3–6 mo	40	20	65	80	100	0		35	60	60
6–12 mo	20	0	65	100	120	+320	0			
1–3 yr	0	20	55	100	100	+340	0	30	80	80
3–5 yr	0	40	60	80	80	+340	0	30	60	60
5–8 yr	+340	40	65	100	100	+320	0	30	60	60
8–12 yr	0	20	65	80	120	+320	0	30	60	60
12–16 yr	+340	20	65	80	100	+320	0	35	60	60

Prev. Dir. = prevalent direction.

From Liebman J: Table of normal standards. *In* Liebman J, Plonsey R, Gillette PC (eds): Pediatric Electrocardiography. Baltimore, Williams & Wilkins, 1982, pp 82–133.

TABLE 9–2

AMPLITUDE LEAD V$_4$R (LOW-FREQUENCY DATA) (MM) (MV × 10)

Age	R Wave					S Wave				
	Min.	5%	Mean	95%	Max.	Min.	5%	Mean	95%	Max.
30 hr	3.5	4.0	8.6	14.2	15.0	0.0	0.2	3.8	13.0	12.0
1 mo	3.0	3.3	6.3	8.5	12.0	0.0	0.8	1.8	4.6	9.0
2–3 mo	0.5	1.1	5.1	10.1	15.0	0.0	0.0	3.4	9.3	15.0
4–5 mo	2.0	2.4	5.2	7.5	9.0	1.0	0.3	3.5	6.7	9.0
6–8 mo	2.0	1.3	4.4	7.1	7.0	0.0	0.2	3.9	11.7	10.0
9 mo–2 yr	1.0	0.2	4.0	6.6	8.0	0.0	0.8	4.9	8.1	10.5
2–5 yr	1.0	1.6	3.4	7.4	8.0	1.0	1.2	4.8	9.5	12.0
6–13 yr	0.2	0.6	2.5	5.7	7.0	0.5	0.9	5.8	12.5	20.0

From Liebman J: Table of normal standards. *In* Liebman J, Plonsey R, Gillette PC (eds): Pediatric Electrocardiography. Baltimore, Williams & Wilkins, 1982, pp 82–133.

TABLE 9–3

AMPLITUDE LEAD V$_1$ (LOW-FREQUENCY DATA) (MM) (MV × 10)

Age	R Wave					S Wave				
	Min.	5%	Mean	95%	Max.	Min.	5%	Mean	95%	Max.
30 hr	5.0	4.3	11.9	21.0	30.0	0.0	1.1	9.7	19.1	26.0
1 mo	4.0	3.3	11.1	18.7	20.0	0.0	0.0	6.1	15.0	15.0
2–3 mo	2.0	4.5	11.2	18.0	20.0	0.5	0.5	7.5	17.1	22.0
4–5 mo	3.0	4.5	11.2	17.4	21.0	1.0	1.0	8.6	16.8	17.0
6–8 mo	3.0	3.2	11.4	21.2	21.0	1.5	1.5	10.7	25.7	30.0
9 mo–2 yr	0.5	2.5	9.7	15.6	26.0	0.2	2.0	8.5	17.2	25.0
2–5 yr	0.5	2.1	7.5	13.9	20.0	1.0	2.1	10.9	21.6	25.0
6–13 yr	0.5	1.1	5.3	10.7	20.0	1.0	3.8	12.6	22.3	36.0

From Liebman J: Table of normal standards. *In* Liebman J, Plonsey R, Gillette PC (eds): Pediatric Electrocardiography. Baltimore, Williams & Wilkins, 1982, pp 82–133.

TABLE 9–4

AMPLITUDE LEAD V$_5$ (LOW-FREQUENCY DATA) (MM) (MV × 10)

Age	R Wave					S Wave				
	Min.	5%	Mean	95%	Max.	Min.	5%	Mean	95%	Max.
30 hr	2.0	3.1	9.4	16.6	20.0	0.5	2.4	9.5	18.5	22.0
1 mo	3.8	3.8	15.0	24.2	30.0	0.0	2.8	8.3	16.3	30.0
2–3 mo	6.0	9.5	20.7	26.2	32.0	1.0	1.2	7.9	14.4	28.0
4–5 mo	10.0	10.0	20.8	28.8	34.0	2.0	2.6	8.9	16.0	16.0
6–8 mo	12.0	12.0	20.1	29.0	38.0	1.5	1.5	7.9	19.6	25.0
9 mo–2 yr	4.0	7.3	17.4	28.4	34.0	0.0	0.6	5.4	10.5	18.0
2–5 yr	7.0	9.4	21.5	33.3	40.0	0.0	0.6	4.3	8.9	13.8
6–13 yr	5.0	12.4	22.0	33.0	46.0	0.0	0.0	4.0	9.2	17.0

From Liebman J: Table of normal standards. *In* Liebman J, Plonsey R, Gillette PC (eds): Pediatric Electrocardiography. Baltimore, Williams & Wilkins, 1982, pp 82–133.

TABLE 9–5

AMPLITUDE LEAD V₆ (LOW-FREQUENCY DATA) (MM) (MV × 10)

Age	R Wave					S Wave				
	Min.	5%	Mean	95%	Max.	Min.	5%	Mean	95%	Max.
30 hr	1.5	1.5	5.4	11.3	15.0	0.2	1.0	5.6	13.8	20.0
1 mo	1.0	1.0	10.8	16.2	22.0	0.0	0.0	4.8	9.5	18.0
2–3 mo	5.0	5.4	12.8	20.8	25.0	0.0	0.1	4.2	9.1	15.0
4–5 mo	4.0	4.4	13.9	22.4	26.0	0.0	0.0	3.5	8.0	12.0
6–8 mo	6.0	6.0	13.0	22.0	28.0	0.2	0.2	2.5	4.4	8.0
9 mo–2 yr	2.5	5.7	12.1	20.0	30.0	0.0	0.3	2.3	5.2	10.0
2–5 yr	4.0	6.4	14.4	22.1	28.0	0.0	0.0	1.5	3.7	7.0
6–13 yr	4.5	7.7	15.7	23.3	33.0	0.0	0.0	1.4	4.1	8.0

From Liebman J: Table of normal standards. *In* Liebman J, Plonsey R, Gillette PC (eds): Pediatric Electrocardiography. Baltimore, Williams & Wilkins, 1982, pp 82–133.

TABLE 9–6

AMPLITUDE T WAVES WHEN POSITIVE (HIGH-FREQUENCY DATA) (MM) (MV × 10)

Age	V₄				V₅				V₆			
	Mean	95%	Max.	SD	Mean	95%	Max.	SD	Mean	95%	Max.	SD
0–24 hr	4.3	7.2	8.5	0.95	3.3	6.3	7.5	1.62	2.4	3.9	4.5	0.63
1–7 days	4.4	7.7	8.5	1.39	4.9	7.3	7.5	1.44	2.9	4.2	4.5	0.67
8–30 days	5.3	8.1	8.5	1.49	5.3	7.5	10.5	1.50	3.5	5.3	7.5	1.01
1–3 mo	5.5	8.2	8.5	1.50	5.0	7.3	7.5	1.43	3.5	4.7	5.5	0.79
3–6 mo	5.5	8.2	8.5	1.50	6.0	9.5	10.5	1.64	3.7	6.9	7.5	1.42
6–12 mo	5.5	8.2	8.5	1.50	5.7	7.5	10.5	1.31	3.8	5.7	6.5	0.86
1–3 yr	6.3	10.7	11.5	2.23	6.0	10.1	13.5	1.85	4.2	6.7	7.5	1.09
3–5 yr	7.0	10.1	11.5	1.39	6.3	9.9	10.5	1.82	4.6	6.4	8.5	1.23
5–8 yr	7.7	11.5	14.5	2.51	7.5	12.5	13.5	2.44	4.9	7.9	8.5	1.49
8–12 yr	7.6	11.5	14.5	2.41	8.1	12.4	13.5	2.26	5.3	8.0	8.5	1.60
12–16 yr	9.1	13.9	14.5	2.82	7.8	12.4	13.5	2.43	4.9	7.5	8.5	1.46

SD = standard deviation.
From Liebman J: Table of normal standards. *In* Liebman J, Plonsey R, Gillette PC (eds): Pediatric Electrocardiography. Baltimore, Williams & Wilkins, 1982, pp 82–133.

TABLE 9–7

PREVALENT DIRECTION—QRS: PREMATURES

Age of Infants	Frontal Plane				First Horizontal Vector				Second Horizontal Vector			
	No. of Infants	Prevalent Direction	Percentile		No. of Infants	Prevalent Direction	Percentile		No. of Infants	Prevalent Direction	Percentile	
			5TH	95TH			5TH	95TH			5TH	95TH
24 hr	60	127	75	194	58	74	338	240	16	239		
72 hr	68	121	75	195	59	84	295	220	15	233		
1 wk	61	117	75	165	54	69	332	216	21	231	191	332
1 mo	42	80	17	171	35	58	340	115	13	232		
2 mo	30	63	345	105	30	46	340	60	8	231		
3 mo	24	59	352	105	23	51	346	108	2	223		
6 mo	15	58			16	30			1	240		
1 yr	18	46			18	12			2	253		

From Sreenivasan VV, Fisher BJ, Liebman J, Downs TD: Longitudinal study of the standard electrocardiogram in the healthy premature during the first year of life. Am J Cardiol 31:57–63, 1973.

TABLE 9–8

QRS MAGNITUDES (MM) (MV × 10): PREMATURES

Age of Infants	No. of Infants	R Wave	Percentile 5th	Percentile 95th	No. of Infants	S Wave	Percentile 5th	Percentile 95th
			LEAD V$_5$ (X AXIS)					
24 hr	64	6.5	2.0	12.6	61	6.8	0.06	17.6
72 hr	65	7.4	2.6	14.9	64	6.5	1.0	16.0
1 wk	61	8.7	3.8	16.8	56	6.8	0.00	15.0
1 mo	38	13.0	6.2	21.6	38	6.2	1.2	14.0
2 mo	30	18.3	12.1	31.5	29	7.0	0.96	15.0
3 mo	24	21.0	14.6	31.5	24	6.7	1.3	21.4
6 mo	16	20.3			16	6.8		
1 yr	18	17.5			17	3.0		
			LEAD aVF (Y AXIS)					
24 hr	63	6.7	0.85	16.6	28	0.96	0.00	4.5
72 hr	68	7.1	0.86	13.9	33	1.2	0.00	5.5
1 wk	61	7.6	1.3	14.1	30	0.98	0.00	3.3
1 mo	42	9.0	1.8	18.8	20	0.86	0.00	4.0
2 mo	30	10.0	1.2	21.7	13	0.90	0.00	5.3
3 mo	24	11.1	1.9	23.0	14	0.77	0.00	3.8
6 mo	16	12.0			9	0.53		
1 yr	18	9.1			9	0.56		
			LEAD V$_2$ (Z AXIS)					
24 hr	65	11.4	3.5	21.3	65	15.0	2.5	26.5
72 hr	66	11.9	5.0	20.8	66	13.5	2.6	26.0
1 wk	60	12.3	4.0	20.5	60	14.0	3.0	25.0
1 mo	41	15.0	8.3	21.0	41	14.0	5.1	26.3
2 mo	30	19.0	8.6	32.0	30	17.1	8.0	34.5
3 mo	23	20.1	13.3	30.0	23	16.1	6.0	37.6
6 mo	16	20.6			16	18.5		
1 yr	18	16.3			18	16.0		

From Sreenivasan VV, Fisher BJ, Liebman J, Downs TD: Longitudinal study of the standard electrocardiogram in the healthy premature during the first year of life. Am J Cardiol 31:57–63, 1973.

TABLE 9–9

P AMPLITUDE—LEAD II (MM) (MV × 10): PREMATURES

Age	No.	Mean Amplitude	Percentile 5th	Percentile 95th
24 hr	65	1.1	0.5	2.0
72 hr	69	1.3	0.5	2.0
1 wk	62	1.3	0.5	2.6
1 mo	40	0.8	0.3	1.5
2 mo	30	0.9	0.4	1.5
3 mo	24	1.0	0.5	1.9
6 mo	16	1.1		
1 yr	18	1.2		

From Sreenivasan VV, Fisher BJ, Liebman J, Downs TD: Longitudinal study of the standard electrocardiogram in the healthy premature during the first year of life. Am J Cardiol 31:57–63, 1973.

TABLE 9–10

HEART RATE AND DURATIONS: ADOLESCENTS

	Sex	Mean	SD	5%	50%	95%
A	M	69	11	52	70	90
	F	73	12	57	70	92
	B	71	12	55	70	90
B	M	0.09	0.02	0.06	0.08	0.11
	F	0.09	0.02	0.06	0.09	0.12
	B	0.09	0.02	0.06	0.09	0.11
C	M	0.15	0.03	0.10	0.15	0.20
	F	0.15	0.02	0.12	0.15	0.19
	B	0.15	0.02	0.11	0.15	0.20
D	M	0.08	0.01	0.06	0.08	0.10
	F	0.08	0.01	0.05	0.08	0.09
	B	0.08	0.01	0.06	0.08	0.10
E	M	0.38	0.04	0.32	0.38	0.42
	F	0.37	0.03	0.32	0.38	0.42
	B	0.37	0.04	0.32	0.38	0.43
F	M	0.21	0.06	0.16	0.20	0.35
	F	0.19	0.04	0.15	0.18	0.28
	B	0.20	0.05	0.15	0.20	0.31

A = heart rate; B = P wave duration; C = PR interval; D = QRS duration; E = QT interval; F = T wave duration; SD = standard deviation.

From Strong WB, Downs TD, Liebman J, Liebowitz R: The normal adolescent electrocardiogram. American Heart J 83:115–128, 1972.

CHAPTER 10
PLAIN FILM DIAGNOSIS OF CONGENITAL HEART DISEASE

KURT AMPLATZ

Plain film analysis used to be one of the most important diagnostic tools in the assessment of congenital heart disease. Previously, infants and children with a cardiac malformation underwent fluoroscopy, and films of the thorax in four projections were obtained. These four views of the heart were a key tool in the diagnostic process. With the development of ultrasonography, the importance of plain film findings has decreased, and currently only posteroanterior (PA) and lateral chest films are obtained. Chest radiography, however, remains a very simple, inexpensive method to obtain important information about cardiac size, pulmonary vasculature, concomitant pulmonary disease, bone abnormalities, situs, bronchomalacia, and other features. In many patients, the cardiac configuration is characteristic enough to allow a specific diagnosis.

Serial radiographs are also important to the physician because changes in heart size and pulmonary vasculature have important prognostic implications, particularly after an operation for the cardiac anomaly.

The radiation burden of chest x-rays to a child is minimal, as compared with cineangiography. A dose of 10 mR for PA and lateral chest radiography in a child compares very favorably with a dose of 10,000 mR/min for cineradiography, as carried out in a catheterization laboratory.

TECHNICAL FACTORS

To evaluate the pulmonary vasculature, the chest radiograph must be properly exposed, neither overpenetrated nor underpenetrated. On an overpenetrated radiograph, the thoracic spine is clearly visible through the cardiac silhouette, whereas on underpenetrated x-ray films, the spine is not visible. In general, overpenetrated radiographs are interpreted as decreased pulmonary vasculature because the vessels are "burned out." However, an underpenetrated radiograph emphasizes the pulmonary vasculature, which may lead to the erroneous diagnosis of "increased flow." Proper interpretation takes experience and is difficult for the novice because of these technical variations.

To analyze a chest radiograph intelligently physicians must be familiar with some principles of radiation and technical factors. The radiographic technique of a chest x-ray can dramatically change the appearance of the pulmonary vasculature. In general, low-kilovoltage films have more contrast, and, consequently, the lung fields appear blacker, giving an appearance of decreased pulmonary vasculature. Typically, radiographs of infants and children are taken with lower kilovoltage.

Another important factor affecting the appearance of the pulmonary vasculature is the exposure time. Exposure time is comparatively long with portable x-ray equipment, because such equipment has less power. With the rapid cardiac and respiratory rates of neonates, motion blurs vascular structures, which again may be interpreted as decreased pulmonary vasculature. Furthermore, the pulmonary arteries are quite small, particularly in premature infants, and their size approaches the resolution capability of the radiographic system.

The degree of inspiration is another technical factor affecting evaluation of pulmonary vasculature and cardiac size. During deep inspiration, the lung fields appear much darker because of the high content of air within the alveoli. Consequently, the tendency is to interpret such films as decreased pulmonary vasculature. In contrast, during expiration, a large amount of the air is expelled, and the lungs are denser. This appearance may be interpreted as increased vasculature, or even as pulmonary edema. The respiratory effort, therefore, is extremely important and is determined radiographically by counting the number of ribs posteriorly and relating them to the position of the diaphragm. A position of the diaphragm at the level of the ninth ribs posteriorly is considered to be an adequate respiratory effort. The degree of inspiration also has a profound influence on cardiac size. The heart is attached to the diaphragm by the cardiophrenic ligament and consequently follows diaphragmatic motion. In deep inspiration the heart assumes a midline vertical position, giving the appearance of a small heart. This phenomenon has also been named *drop heart*. In contrast, during expiration the heart assumes a more transverse position, simulating cardiomegaly. Three features must be assessed when interpreting a chest radiograph: pulmonary vasculature, cardiac size, and cardiac contour.

PULMONARY VASCULATURE

The pulmonary vasculature can be increased by distention of pulmonary arteries, pulmonary veins, or both. In radiographic terminology, one speaks, therefore, of *increased arterial* and *increased venous* pulmonary vasculature. The differentiation is sometimes difficult or impossible, but there are helpful secondary signs. If increased vascular markings are present, they are likely to be arterial because increased venous vasculature is comparatively rare in childhood. Furthermore, the appearance of increased pulmonary venous vasculature in infancy and childhood produces a very characteristic pattern that differs from increased arterial vasculature. Naturally, with increased pulmonary flow there is also distention of pulmonary veins. The cross-sectional area of the pulmonary veins, however, is much larger than that of the pulmonary arteries, because there are four pulmonary veins and only two pulmonary arteries.

What is observed radiographically is not increased pulmonary flow but the size of the pulmonary arteries. With increased flow, the pulmonary artery size enlarges, giving the radiographic appearance of increased pulmonary vasculature. Obviously, with enlargement of peripheral pulmonary arteries, an enlargement of the main pulmonary artery is also present, as evidenced by a prominent *pulmonary arterial segment,* if the great vessels are normally related (Fig. 10–1). When interpreting chest radiographs it is a good idea to use the term enlarged pulmonary arterial segment rather than enlarged pulmonary artery. One can never be certain that a particular bulge along the cardiac contour indeed represents a specific enlarged anatomic structure.

If the peripheral pulmonary vasculature is increased and the main pulmonary arterial segment is not prominent, it may be either overshadowed by thymic tissue, common in infancy, or in an abnormal intramediastinal position, as with transposition complexes (Fig. 10–2).

Increased pulmonary arterial vasculature may be difficult to diagnose in patients with a left-to-right shunt and normal pulmonary arterial pressure, as in patients with an atrial septal defect. Many patients with an atrial septal de-

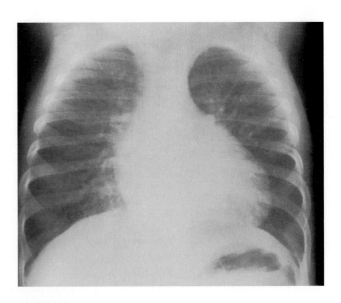

Posteroanterior radiograph showing transposition of the great arteries. The heart is enlarged, and the pulmonary vasculature is increased. The main pulmonary artery, which is also enlarged, does not form a prominent pulmonary arterial segment because it is in an abnormal intramediastinal position. The mediastinum is narrow because of the small thymus.

fect have radiographically normal pulmonary vasculature but usually have right-sided cardiac enlargement.

The radiographic diagnosis of increased arterial vasculature becomes much more obvious if pulmonary hypertension is also present, as occurs with a shunt located beyond the level of the atrioventricular (AV) valves. In these conditions, enlargement of the pulmonary arteries occurs by both increased flow and pressure (Fig. 10–3).

Increased pulmonary arterial pressure causes tortuosity of the pulmonary arteries, as evidenced by an increased number of arteries seen on end. With increased pulmonary arterial vasculature secondary to increased pulmonary blood flow, cardiac size is increased because of the volume overload of cardiac chambers. This is distinct from increased pulmonary venous vasculature, which is usually associated with a normal or minimally enlarged heart, because increased pulmonary resistance limits blood flow.

Increased pulmonary venous vasculature results in a characteristic radiographic appearance, particularly in infancy. A typical example of pulmonary venous obstruction is total anomalous pulmonary venous connection below the diaphragm. This condition results in a characteristic granular pattern throughout both lung fields. This granularity is due to edema of the interlobar septa, and sometimes a small pleural effusion may be present. In general, pleural effusions caused by pulmonary venous obstruction are exceedingly rare in infants and children, in distinction to adults, who develop large pleural effusions with increased pulmonary venous pressure (Fig. 10–4).

The radiographic appearance of pulmonary venous hypertension in neonates is indistinguishable from hyaline membrane disease. A small pleural effusion suggests venous obstruction, and pulmonary consolidation with an air bronchogram strongly favors the diagnosis of hyaline membrane disease.

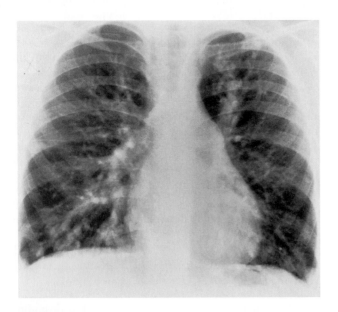

Typical left-to-right shunt with increased arterial vasculature. The arterial pattern is distinct. Numerous vessels are seen on end suggesting tortuosity, which, in turn, indicates increased pulmonary artery pressure. With increased pulmonary artery vasculature there must be enlargement of the main pulmonary artery, as seen here.

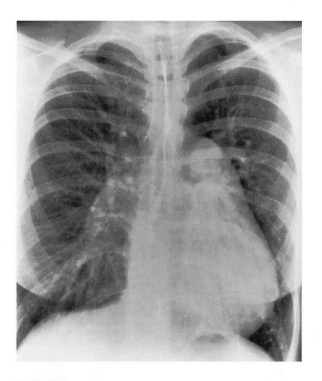

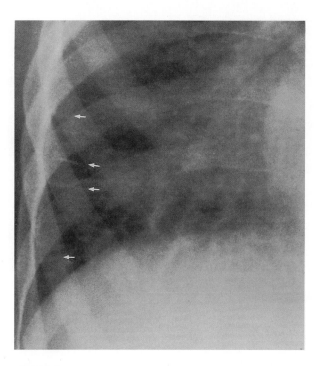

FIGURE 10–3

Posteroanterior radiograph of an intracardiac left-to-right shunt and pulmonary vascular disease. The main pulmonary artery is huge. Pulmonary arteries in the hila are prominent. The peripheral vasculature is normal to decreased, a characteristic of pulmonary vascular disease. This radiographic appearance has been described as "pruning" or "leafless tree." Numerous arteries are seen in cross-section because of tortuosity.

FIGURE 10–5

Close-up view of the right base. This shows typical horizontal lines (*arrows*) described as Kerley's B lines. This is good radiographic evidence for long-standing venous pulmonary hypertension with wedge pressures above 20 mm Hg.

In children who have chronic pulmonary venous hypertension, redistribution of blood flow occurs (see Fig. 10–4). In a healthy individual relatively little blood flows through the upper lobes because of the gravitation effect on pulmonary pressure. In pulmonary venous obstruction, preferential flow occurs through the upper lobes (redistribution of blood flow). The likely explanation for redistribution is increased resistance to flow through the lower lobes because of interstitial edema, alveolar hypoxia, or reflex vasoconstriction of arterioles.

Concurrently, or somewhat later, another characteristic and diagnostic finding appears, Kerley's B lines. These horizontal lines, best seen at the lung base and at the periphery of the lung, are caused by interstitial edema and later by fibrosis and hemosiderosis of the intralobular septa (Fig. 10–5). Kerley's B lines occur when the pulmonary wedge pressure exceeds 20 mm Hg. They are rarely seen in infants and young children.

Later in life, signs of pulmonary venous hypertension show a different radiographic pattern with transudation of fluid into alveoli. The pulmonary vasculature has an indistinct fluffy appearance; pulmonary edema may occur and opacify the lung fields (Fig. 10–6).

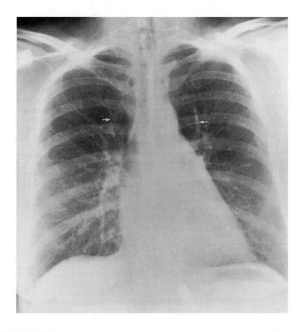

FIGURE 10–4

Posteroanterior radiograph of pulmonary venous hypertension showing the redistribution of blood flow (cephalization). The upper lobe pulmonary veins are distinctly seen (*arrows*). The heart is not enlarged, as is typical for left-sided obstruction proximal to the mitral valve.

DECREASED PULMONARY VASCULATURE

Decreased pulmonary vasculature is difficult to diagnose radiographically. Commonly, radiographs taken in an intensive care unit show decreased pulmonary vasculature, although the pulmonary flow may be normal because of

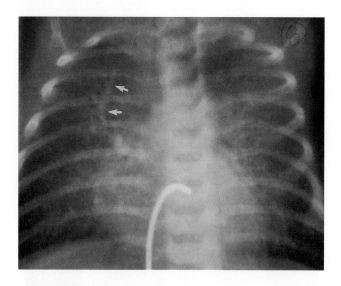

FIGURE 10–6

Posteroanterior radiograph of acute pulmonary venous obstruction. Diffuse haziness over both lung fields and indistinctness of the pulmonary vasculature indicate frank pulmonary edema. Marked prominence of the right upper lobe pulmonary vein *(arrows)* further confirms venous pulmonary obstruction.

technical factors discussed earlier. However, in a cyanotic patient the vasculature must be defined as either increased or decreased to establish a diagnosis.

BRONCHIAL VASCULATURE

In patients with pulmonary atresia and ventricular septal defect, as well as more complex conditions with pulmonary atresia, the lungs may be supplied with bronchial arteries that can be recognized on a plain chest radiograph. Normally, the pulmonary arteries form a characteristic shadow in the hila, but this density is absent in patients with pulmonary atresia. The pulmonary vasculature may not be decreased but has a bizarre appearance because numerous pulmonary vessels are seen on end. In contrast to pulmonary arteries, which have a characteristic regular fanlike pattern emanating from the hila, bronchial arteries lack regularity and are much more tortuous. Consequently, they are seen more frequently on end. Because bronchial arteries frequently pass behind the esophagus, posterior indentations of the posterior wall of the barium-filled esophagus may be found.

CARDIAC SIZE

The most important value of a chest radiograph is probably the evaluation of cardiac size. Proper interpretation requires an understanding of the technical factors and anatomy of the heart.

There are many causes of apparent cardiomegaly. First, a common technical problem is an anteroposterior (AP) rather than a PA projection. Because of the divergence of the x-ray beam emanating from the x-ray tube, structures that are further away from the radiographic film are magnified more than structures located closer to the film. Because the heart is located anteriorly in the thoracic cavity, it is magnified more on an AP projection than a PA projection. Because the chest of an infant is small, the projection is not as important in the evaluation of cardiac size; it is more convenient to take chest radiographs in an AP projection in most infants.

Second, the divergence of the x-ray beam is more pronounced when the x-ray tube is closer to the film. By increasing the film distance to 6 ft (2 m in Europe), the divergence of the x-ray beam can be minimized and a true nonmagnified image of the chest can be obtained. Portable x-ray machines use a 40-inch film distance. Therefore, a heart may appear enlarged with a portable machine at 40 inches but appears normal if a chest radiograph is obtained at 6 ft.

A third factor influencing cardiac size is the patient's position. When the patient is supine, the diaphragm tends to be higher than when the patient is in the upright position. Therefore, the cardiac silhouette appears larger on a supine chest radiograph than on an upright radiographic study.

Another important factor is the degree of inspiration. The heart is attached to the diaphragm by the cardiophrenic ligament and moves with the left hemidiaphragm. On deep inspiration the heart rotates into a left anterior oblique position, resulting in a small cardiac silhouette (Fig. 10–7A). On expiration it rotates into a right anterior oblique position, resulting in an apparent enlargement of the cardiac silhouette (see Fig. 10–7B). Typically, an individual with a low diaphragm, for example, a patient with asthma, has a *vertical heart*, which is pulled down by the low diaphragm; the cardiac silhouette appears radiographically small. However, a person with an elevated diaphragm, particularly an adult patient with obesity, shows an enlarged cardiac silhouette, although the heart may be normal in size. This variation in the radiographic appearance of the cardiac silhouette is a strong argument against the use of *cardiothoracic ratio*, in which the transverse diameter of the heart is related to the transverse diameter of the chest to assess cardiac size.

A final concept of the evaluation of cardiac size is the position of the heart within the thoracic cavity. The long axis of the heart passes obliquely to the sagittal plane of the thorax. Therefore, on a chest radiograph the long axis is foreshortened. Normally the cardiac axis is inclined about 45 degrees to the sagittal plane. If this angle is greater, the heart is rotated clockwise (as seen from below the diaphragm). If the angle is less, it is rotated counterclockwise. The long axis of the heart in relation to the sagittal plane, therefore, largely determines cardiac size on a chest radiograph. Clockwise-rotated hearts appear enlarged on a PA view (e.g., obese patients with high diaphragm or pectus excavatum deformity), and hearts with counterclockwise rotation (e.g., patients with pulmonary emphysema) appear small. On a right-angle view (lateral view) the clockwise-rotated heart, however, appears small, whereas the counterclockwise-rotated heart appears large. Consequently, cardiac size cannot be evaluated on a PA chest film alone, so the commonly used cardiothoracic ratio is inaccurate for evaluating cardiac size.

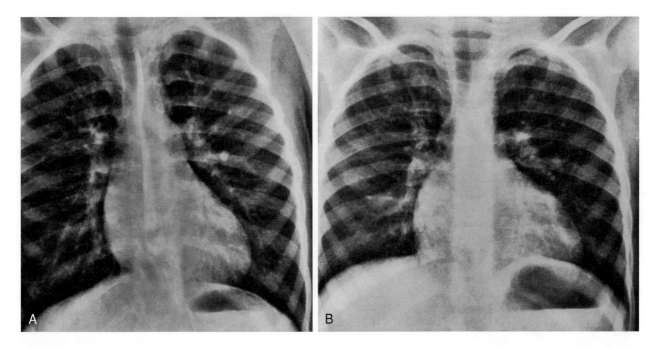

FIGURE 10–7

Posteroanterior radiograph of a small ventricular septal defect. *A,* No significant cardiomegaly (deep inspiration). *B,* During expiration the heart assumes a transverse position.

CHARACTERISTIC PLAIN FILM FINDINGS IN VARIOUS CONGENITAL CARDIAC MALFORMATIONS

Although examples of chest radiographs are shown in other chapters of this book, a synopsis is presented in the following section of this chapter. Emphasis is placed on the characteristic radiographic appearance rather than on radiographic evaluation of chamber size. The latter can be much better accomplished by ultrasonography. Furthermore, the well-known signs of chamber enlargement apply largely to acquired cardiac disease, in which an originally normal heart is altered by an acquired condition. In congenital heart disease, the heart has developed abnormally; consequently, radiographic assessment of chamber enlargement is often difficult or impossible. There are, however, fairly characteristic radiographic appearances of many cardiac malformations. For a more detailed description the reader is referred to *Radiology of Congenital Heart Disease* by Amplatz and Moller, Mosby–Year Book.

LEFT-TO-RIGHT SHUNTS

Significant left-to-right shunts have one common important radiographic finding, increased pulmonary arterial blood flow. This is evident on a chest radiograph by enlargement of the pulmonary arteries and the pulmonary trunk (see Fig. 10–1). In general only a shunt larger than 50% results in a radiographic appearance of increased pulmonary arterial vasculature. With a smaller shunt, the vasculature is normal. In some patients with an atrial septal defect and a large left-to-right shunt, the pulmonary vasculature also appears normal. No explanation for this phenomenon is available. All large left-to-right shunts result in cardiomegaly, with right-sided enlargement in atrial communications, and left atrial and left ventricular enlargement with shunts at the ventricular or great vessel level. The size of the left atrium and the volume of pulmonary blood flow correlate with the clinical finding of a diastolic flow murmur across the mitral valve.

In an extracardiac shunt, as in a large patent ductus arteriosus, blood flow is also increased through the ascending aorta, making the aorta more prominent, but this is not a reliable finding.

The differential diagnosis of various left-to-right shunts cannot be made with certainty by plain film analysis. However, some clues help to distinguish an atrial level communication from shunts occurring at ventricular or great vessel level. In an atrial communication only right-sided enlargement occurs (except for a left ventricular–right atrial shunt, which results in left-sided enlargement). In addition, the pulmonary vasculature is less distinct because the pulmonary arterial pressure is normal. The right atrial border may be prominent, and the ascending aorta and right superior vena cava are not seen because of clockwise rotation of the heart. Enlargement of the right ventricle is halted by the sternum, which may be bowed anteriorly in children with a large atrial septal communication. Because the right ventricle cannot further enlarge against the bony sternum, clockwise rotation of the heart ensues. This rotation pulls the ascending aorta medially. Therefore, it is inconspicuous or not seen at all on a PA film.

In one of the left-to-right shunts, namely the scimitar syndrome, the chest radiograph is diagnostic. With the complete syndrome asymmetry of the thorax is present. The right hemithorax is smaller than the left hemithorax because of hypoplasia of the right lung, which also causes elevation of the right hemidiaphragm. The density of the

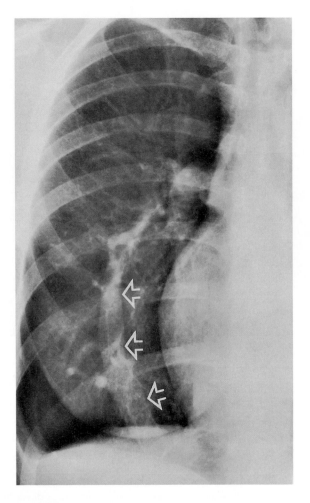

FIGURE 10–8

Posteroanterior radiograph of the right lung. Classic curved scimitar vein *(arrows)* empties into the inferior vena cava.

COARCTATION OF THE AORTA

The diagnosis of this lesion can be made in most patients from a PA and lateral chest radiograph with barium swallow. Cardiac size is normal or minimally enlarged. The aortic knob is absent because of commonly associated tubular hypoplasia of the isthmus and a dilated left subclavian artery (Fig. 10–9). The poststenotic segment of the thoracic aorta may be seen on a plain radiograph but is better visualized if a barium swallow is performed (Fig. 10–10). The esophagus is displaced, producing the characteristic "reversed figure 3" sign. In older children and adults intercostal collateral arteries enlarge, causing rib erosions, which are well demonstrated on a chest radiograph (see Fig. 10–9). Rib-notching indicates severe coarctation with well-developed collaterals. It is rarely seen below the age of 6 years.

In neonates and infants, severe left-sided obstructive lesions are not well tolerated and result in left ventricular decompensation. The radiograph in this age group shows a markedly enlarged heart. The cardiomegaly with pulmonary venous congestion is consistent with a left-sided obstructive lesion, of which coarctation of the aorta is most common in this age group.

PULMONARY VALVAR STENOSIS

This malformation can also be suspected from plain chest radiographs showing a normal-sized heart with enlargement of the main pulmonary trunk and usually left pulmonary artery. The latter two result from poststenotic dilatation. Because the left pulmonary artery is a continuation of the pulmonary trunk, the jet produced by the stenotic pulmonary valve extends into the left pulmonary

right pulmonary artery in the right hilum appears small because of hypoplasia of the right lung. The hallmark of scimitar syndrome is the visualization of a scimitar-like vein extending toward the right diaphragm (Fig. 10–8).

Radiographic findings in endocardial cushion defect are identical to those of other large left-to-right shunts, such as atrial shunts, but cardiomegaly may be greater because left AV valve insufficiency may coexist.

In patients with a shunt at the ventricular or great vessel level, the increased pulmonary arterial vasculature is more distinct and prominent, because pulmonary arterial pressure is elevated. The pulmonary arterial segment is prominent, and left atrial enlargement and left ventricular enlargement are present.

AORTIC VALVAR STENOSIS

Aortic stenosis can be suspected from a chest film showing a prominent ascending aorta, which results from poststenotic dilatation. As long as the left ventricle is compensated, the heart is normal or minimally enlarged. Left ventricular hypertrophy may result in a left ventricular configuration from counterclockwise rotation of the heart.

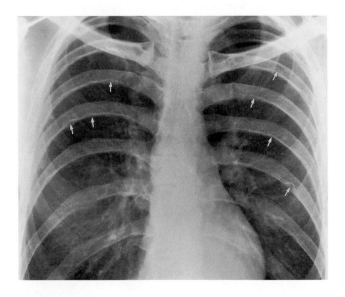

FIGURE 10–9

Posteroanterior radiograph demonstrating coarctation of the aorta. Note rib-notching *(arrows)*. In an older patient the heart is typically not enlarged. The aortic segment is most commonly not prominent as a result of tubular hypoplasia of the aortic isthmus.

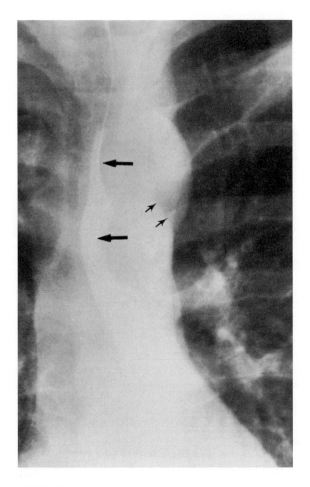

FIGURE 10–10

Barium swallow showing coarctation of the aorta. Two bulges are clearly demonstrated *(arrows)*. The upper one is the aortic arch, which is unusually large, and the lower one *(small arrows)* is the poststenotic dilatation. There is also displacement of the esophagus by the poststenotic dilatation forming the reversed 3 sign.

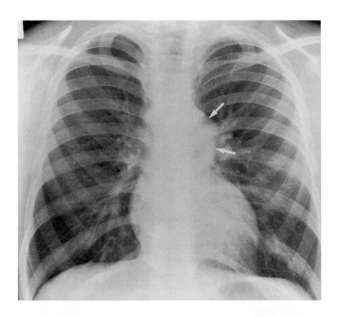

FIGURE 10–11

Posteroanterior radiograph of valvar pulmonary stenosis. The heart is not enlarged. Pulmonary vasculature is normal. There is marked prominence of the pulmonary arterial segment *(arrows)*.

artery causing it to dilate (Fig. 10–11). Exceptions are rare.

A chest radiograph does not allow full assessment of the size of the pulmonary artery because only the portion with an interface with the left lung is visible. Prominence of the pulmonary artery segment may be seen in healthy individuals, particularly in adolescents, but the left pulmonary artery is not enlarged.

CYANOSIS AND DECREASED PULMONARY ARTERIAL VASCULATURE

Several important conditions are associated with cyanosis and decreased pulmonary vasculature, the most common being tetralogy of Fallot. Tetralogy of Fallot can result in a characteristic radiographic appearance. The pulmonary vasculature is frankly decreased, and the heart assumes a boot-shaped, coeur en sabot configuration (Fig. 10–12). The apex of the heart is elevated, and the pulmonary arterial segment is concave because the pulmonary trunk is hypoplastic.

Another helpful finding is the location of the aortic arch, which is right-sided in approximately 25% of patients with tetralogy of Fallot. The location of the arch can be readily determined on a chest radiograph by observing the position of the trachea. The trachea invariably deviates away from the aortic arch. In a normal (left-sided) arch the trachea moves toward the right. With a right-sided aortic arch the trachea moves toward the left. This deviation can be emphasized by taking an expiration view of the thorax, which causes elevation of the heart with pronounced buckling of the trachea away from the aortic arch.

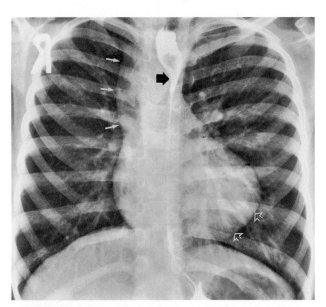

FIGURE 10–12

Posteroanterior radiograph showing the tetralogy of Fallot. The apex of the heart is elevated resulting in a boot-shaped configuration *(open arrows)*. The heart is not enlarged, and the pulmonary vasculature is at the lower limits of normal, suggesting a mild form of tetralogy of Fallot. There is displacement of the superior vena cava *(arrows)* by a right-sided aortic arch, which also displaces the esophagus toward the left *(black arrow)*.

A chest radiograph without deviation of the trachea is suggestive either of interruption of the aortic arch in which there is no arch, or of a double aortic arch in which the trachea is encircled and cannot shift.

TETRALOGY WITH PULMONARY ATRESIA

In tetralogy with pulmonary atresia the pulmonary vasculature tends to be more prominent than in classic tetralogy of Fallot or may appear normal if a large ductus arteriosus or large bronchial arteries are present. Bronchial arteries can be diagnosed by observing an increased number of vessels seen on end. These are evident as round circular densities. If a barium swallow is performed, the esophagus may be indented posteriorly by bronchial arteries, which almost invariably cross behind the esophagus.

In a variant of tetralogy of Fallot with absence of the pulmonary valve, a characteristic radiographic appearance is found. There is massive dilatation of the right pulmonary artery, which appears as a tumor-like density in the right lung (Fig. 10–13). Less commonly, the intramediastinal portion of either the right pulmonary artery or the left pulmonary artery is enlarged, resulting in a less classic radiographic appearance.

TRICUSPID ATRESIA

Tricuspid atresia is usually associated with a restrictive ventricular septal defect or pulmonary stenosis, either of which results in decreased pulmonary flow. Normal cardiac size or minimal cardiomegaly is present. The heart has a fairly characteristic configuration (Fig. 10–14). Because both the systemic venous return and the pulmonary venous return pass through the left ventricle, it enlarges, be-

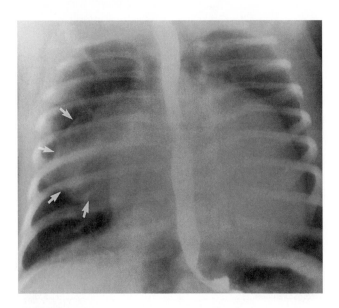

FIGURE 10–13

Posteroanterior radiograph of tetralogy of Fallot and absence of the pulmonary valve. Typically the right pulmonary artery shows massive dilatation (*arrows*). The heart is markedly enlarged because of the increased stroke volume of the right ventricle. Dilatation of the left pulmonary artery may occur but is much less common.

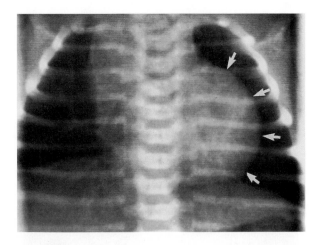

FIGURE 10–14

Posteroanterior radiograph of tricuspid atresia. Pulmonary vasculature is decreased because most patients have a restrictive ventricular septal defect and pulmonary stenosis. The heart is not significantly enlarged. Contrary to tetralogy of Fallot, the left ventricular contour has a typical rounded configuration (*arrows*).

comes rounded, and yields a typical radiographic appearance. The pulmonary arterial segment tends to be concave because pulmonary blood flow is reduced, and the main pulmonary artery is small.

PULMONARY ATRESIA WITH INTACT VENTRICULAR SEPTUM

In this condition, which is usually discovered shortly after birth, the heart tends to be greatly enlarged and the pulmonary vasculature markedly decreased unless a large ductus arteriosus is present (Fig. 10–15). Another condition resulting in severe cardiomegaly and markedly decreased pulmonary vasculature is Ebstein malformation.

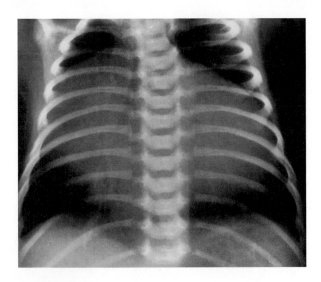

FIGURE 10–15

Posteroanterior radiograph of pulmonary atresia, intact septum, and marked tricuspid insufficiency. There is massive cardiomegaly. Lung fields show decreased vasculature. The radiographic appearance is indistinguishable from severe Ebstein abnormality.

EBSTEIN MALFORMATION

The radiographic findings in Ebstein malformation vary from a normal cardiac configuration to massive cardiomegaly with decreased vasculature. This spectrum reflects the variation in the degree of tricuspid regurgitation. Typically, the heart is huge in the advanced stage, and the pulmonary vasculature is severely decreased. The radiographic appearance is identical to that of pulmonary atresia with intact septum (see Fig. 10–15).

CYANOSIS AND INCREASED PULMONARY ARTERIAL VASCULATURE

TRANSPOSITION OF THE GREAT ARTERIES

The plain film findings of the transposition of the great arteries may be characteristic. Because this serious malformation causes hypoxic stress in neonates, typically thymic tissue is not seen.

Because the pulmonary artery is located medially in an intramediastinal position, the pulmonary arterial segment is absent. The heart is enlarged, and the pulmonary vasculature is increased. The classic cardiac configuration in transposition has been described as "egg on the side" or "apple on the string" (see Fig. 10–2). Immediately after birth, while the pulmonary vascular resistance is still elevated, the pulmonary vasculature may appear normal but increases with time as pulmonary vascular resistance decreases.

DOUBLE OUTLET RIGHT VENTRICLE

In contrast to complete transposition of the great arteries, double outlet right ventricle is radiographically indistinguishable from a left-to-right shunt, such as ventricular septal defect. The heart is enlarged, the pulmonary arterial segment is prominent, and the vasculature is increased.

CONGENITAL CORRECTED TRANSPOSITION

Most patients have a ventricular septal defect and pulmonary stenosis with a right-to-left shunt, as in tetralogy of Fallot. Depending on the degree of pulmonary stenosis, the pulmonary vasculature may be normal to decreased. The plain film findings are quite characteristic with a rounded upper left cardiac border that is formed by the inverted right ventricle and an absence of a pulmonary arterial density caused by the ascending aorta along the left heart border (Fig. 10–16).

TRUNCUS ARTERIOSUS

Radiographically, the appearance of truncus arteriosus is difficult to distinguish from double outlet right ventricle and sometimes from transposition of the great arteries. All patients with truncus arteriosus show cardiomegaly with in-

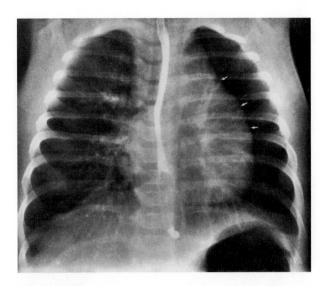

FIGURE 10–16

Posteroanterior radiograph demonstrates corrected transposition of the great arteries. The heart is not enlarged. The pulmonary vasculature is normal. The ascending aorta forms a large arch along the left heart border *(arrows)*. The pulmonary arterial segment is not evident.

creased pulmonary blood flow, unless there is concomitant stenosis of the pulmonary arteries. If the pulmonary artery arises from the left side of the truncus, the pulmonary arterial segment may be prominent. If the pulmonary arteries arise posteriorly from the truncus arteriosus, the pulmonary segment may be absent, and the radiographic appearance resembles complete transposition. A helpful plain film diagnostic finding is the position of the aortic arch because about 50% of patients with truncus arteriosus have a right-sided aortic arch. A history of cyanosis, cardiomegaly, increased flow, and deviation of the trachea to the left, as from a right-sided aortic arch, therefore, clinches the diagnosis of truncus arteriosus (Fig. 10–17).

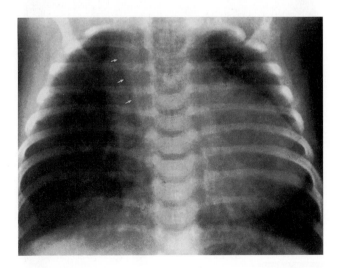

FIGURE 10–17

Posteroanterior radiograph of truncus arteriosus. The heart is massively enlarged. The pulmonary vasculature is increased, and there is a right-sided aortic arch *(arrows)*. A patient with cyanosis, increased pulmonary vasculature, and right-sided aortic arch very likely has truncus arteriosus.

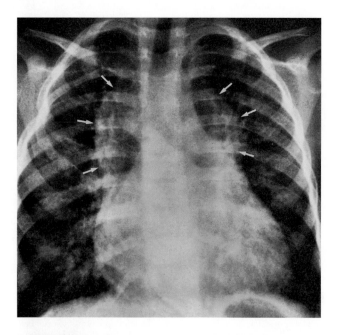

FIGURE 10–18

Posteroanterior radiograph of total anomalous pulmonary venous connection to the left superior vena cava. The heart is massively enlarged. The enlarged left superior vena cava (*arrows*) and right superior vena cava (*arrows*) form the characteristic figure 8 or snowman's heart configuration.

TOTAL ANOMALOUS PULMONARY VENOUS CONNECTION

In total anomalous pulmonary venous connection, the plain film findings are identical to those of left-to-right shunts at the atrial level. If connection of the pulmonary veins is to the left superior vena cava, a characteristic radiographic appearance ensues (Fig. 10–18), although not

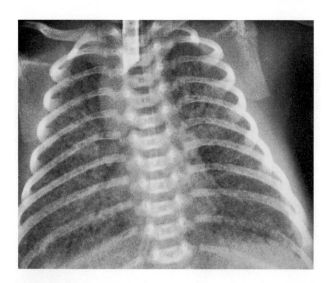

FIGURE 10–19

Posteroanterior radiograph of total anomalous pulmonary venous connection below the diaphragm. Typically, the heart is not enlarged. The lung fields have a diffuse granular appearance identical to hyaline membrane disease. Rarely, a small pleural effusion may be present.

usually until after 1 year of age. The enlarged left superior vena cava and right superior vena cava result in a "figure 8" or "snowman" configuration of the cardiac silhouette.

Total anomalous pulmonary venous connection below the diaphragm has a completely different radiographic appearance. It represents a venous obstructive lesion. Therefore, cardiac size is normal, and both lung fields show a characteristic granular appearance indistinguishable from hyaline membrane disease (Fig. 10–19).

PULMONARY ARTERIOVENOUS FISTULA

Arteriovenous fistulae of the pulmonary arteries have a characteristic radiographic appearance. They present as a single or multiple, lobulated mass lesions with an enlarged pulmonary arterial branch and vein leading to and from the malformation. The vascular nature of the malformation may not always be apparent on plain films but is readily identified by laminography and computed tomography.

CYANOSIS AND INCREASED VENOUS PULMONARY VASCULATURE

ATRESIA OF THE COMMON PULMONARY VEIN

The radiographic appearance is indistinguishable from other causes of pulmonary venous obstructions, such as the more common total anomalous pulmonary venous connection below the diaphragm. Cardiac size is normal, and the lung fields have a fine granular appearance identical to hyaline membrane disease. A small pleural effusion may be present.

In atresia of the right or left pulmonary veins, the involved side shows a smaller hemithorax with shift of the mediastinum toward the involved side and an accentuated venous pattern.

HYPOPLASTIC LEFT VENTRICLE SYNDROME

In this condition, the radiographic appearance varies considerably, depending on the hemodynamics. If the obligatory left-to-right shunt at the atrial level is not restrictive, marked cardiomegaly and increased pulmonary vasculature are present. The vascularization is mixed arterial and venous. With a small patent foramen ovale the cardiac silhouette is smaller or normal, but pulmonary venous obstruction is prominent.

MITRAL STENOSIS AND COR TRIATRIATUM

Both of these conditions obstruct pulmonary venous return and accentuate the pulmonary venous vasculature. On a barium swallow, the esophagus is displaced in patients with mitral stenosis but not with cor triatriatum. Cardiac size is normal or only slightly enlarged. Later in life, the venous obstructive pattern is characterized by redistribution of blood flow through the upper lobes and the appearance of Kerley's B lines at the lung bases (Fig. 10–20).

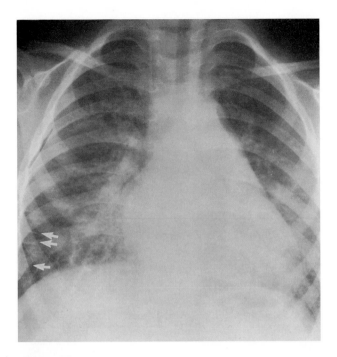

Posteroanterior radiograph of mitral stenosis. The heart is only slightly enlarged. The pulmonary vasculature is indistinct and somewhat accentuated as with pulmonary venous hypertension. Kerley's B lines are demonstrated at the right base *(arrows)*.

AORTIC ARCH ANOMALIES

In patients with clinical symptoms of stridor, a vascular cause must be excluded. A chest radiograph and barium swallow are simple and inexpensive techniques to exclude such abnormalities. A thoracic chest radiograph, in which the trachea is shifted toward the left, indicates a right-sided aortic arch. A right-sided aortic arch can also be diagnosed by a density along the right side of the spine representing the descending aorta. This type of right-sided aortic arch usually occurs with congenital heart disease, such as tetralogy of Fallot and truncus arteriosus, and is unassociated with tracheal compression (see Figs. 10–12 and 10–17). In a vascular ring or right-sided aortic arch with aberrent left subclavian artery, an arterial structure passes behind the upper esophagus.

Demonstration of a right-sided aortic arch without tracheal shift is consistent with some type of vascular ring that prevents shift of the trachea. A barium swallow shows a characteristic large indentation of the barium-filled esophagus from behind, because the retroesophageal portion of a double aortic arch is usually larger than the anterior arch (Fig. 10–21). The main virtue of a barium swallow examination is the exclusion of an aortic arch abnormality by the absence of a retroesophageal vascular structure.

VASCULAR SLING

The term *vascular sling* is applied to the origin of the left pulmonary artery from the right pulmonary artery. The left

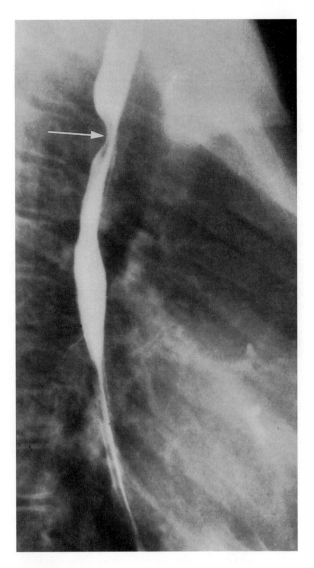

Lateral thoracic radiograph. Barium swallow shows an indentation of the esophagus from behind *(arrow)*. This can be due to an aberrant subclavian artery, a diverticulum of Kommerell, or a retroesophageal segment of a double aortic arch. In tetralogy of Fallot, bronchial arteries may indent the esophagus from behind, but these indentations are much smaller than those seen here.

pulmonary artery then passes between the trachea and esophagus to the left lung. Vascular sling can be diagnosed by a barium swallow, which demonstrates a vascular structure passing between the trachea and the esophagus (Fig. 10–22). No other vascular structure passes between the trachea and the esophagus, except rarely a bronchial artery may do so. A normal esophagogram does not completely rule out a vascular sling.

CARDIAC MALPOSITION

Chest radiography is an important method to determine cardiac malposition. Careful analysis of the chest radiograph allows determination of the situs. This is performed by correlating the position of the stomach, apex of the

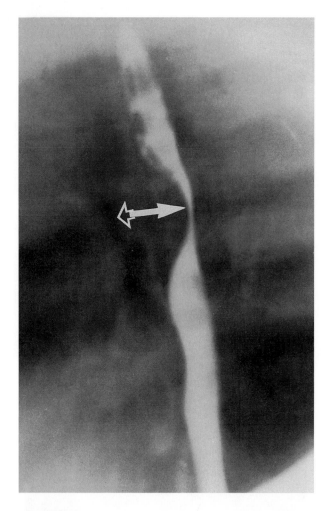

FIGURE 10–22

Lateral radiograph during barium swallow showing displacement of the esophagus anteriorly *(solid arrow)*. There is also displacement of the trachea *(open arrow)*. This appearance is diagnostic for a pulmonary sling passing between esophagus and trachea. No other vascular structure passes between the esophagus and trachea except, very rarely, a bronchial artery.

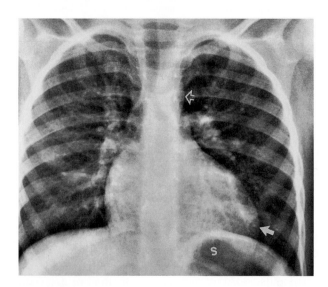

FIGURE 10–23

Posteroanterior radiograph of situs solitus. Aortic arch *(open arrow)*, apex of the heart *(solid arrow)*, and stomach (S) are concordant.

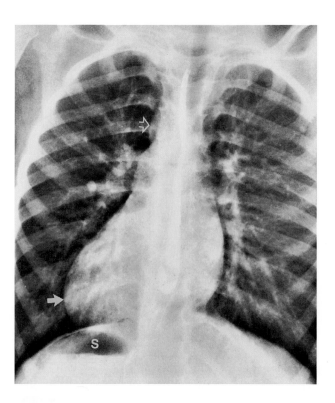

FIGURE 10–24

Posteroanterior radiograph of situs inversus totalis. Aorta *(open arrow)*, cardiac apex *(solid arrow)*, and stomach (S) are concordant but on the right side of the chest.

heart, and aortic arch. In normal visceral situs, the aortic arch, apex of the heart, and stomach are concordant (Fig. 10–23). In situs inversus the aortic arch, apex, and stomach are concordant but on the right side (Fig. 10–24). If the stomach and aortic arch are discordant, an ambiguous or indeterminate situs exists (Fig. 10–25). This is commonly

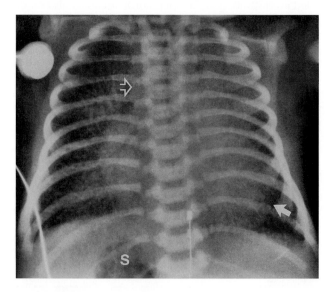

FIGURE 10–25

Posteroanterior radiograph in a patient with venous obstruction and ambiguous situs. Aortic arch *(open arrow)* and stomach (S) are concordant, but the cardiac apex *(solid arrow)* is on the left side.

present with a splenic abnormality such as asplenia and polysplenia. Cyanosis, decreased pulmonary blood flow, and a midline position of the liver strongly suggest the asplenia syndrome. Rarely, bilateral middle lobe fissures can be seen. In the differential diagnosis of asplenia and polysplenia, the patient's age is important. Asplenia is associated with severe cardiac anomalies and pulmonary stenosis or atresia. Consequently, these infants come to exami-

nation early in life. On the other hand, polysplenic syndrome has typically less severe cardiac anomalies and increased pulmonary flow. These patients often have an interrupted inferior vena cava with azygos continuation. Demonstration of what appears to be a double aortic arch is due to the density of the enlarged azygos vein and is an important diagnostic tool.

CHAPTER 11
ECHOCARDIOGRAPHY

DOFF B. McELHINNEY   MICHAEL M. BROOK   NORMAN H. SILVERMAN

The development of modern echocardiographic systems has drastically altered pediatric cardiology practice. No longer do children require catheterization to establish diagnosis before treatment. In fact, many children with congenital heart disease undergo a corrective operation solely on the basis of echocardiographic diagnosis. It has become the standard diagnostic tool and a required skill for all pediatric cardiologists. This chapter provides an overview of echocardiography, including physical principles, strategies of anatomic and physiologic examination, limitations of the technique, and a brief description of some newer technologies. It is not intended as a primer of the echocardiographic findings of the major congenital lesions; these findings are included in the relevant chapters.

PHYSICS

Despite the ability of the equipment to produce high-quality images, the operator still has significant input into the final result. This section focuses on those factors to which the operator has input essential for optimal imaging, which include selecting the proper transducer, using the proper mode of ultrasonography, and optimizing equipment settings for the appropriate application. Interested readers may wish to review more comprehensive literature.[1–3]

BASICS OF PULSED ULTRASONOGRAPHY

Ultrasound waves are generated by piezoelectric crystals. When an electrical signal is applied to the crystal, it vibrates, transmitting ultrasound waves at its natural frequency, generally between 2.5 and 10 MHz. Conversely, when the crystal is made to vibrate by coming in contact with ultrasound waves, it emits an electrical impulse. Thus, the crystal functions both as a transmitter and as a receiver of ultrasound energy. The intensity of the electrical signal generated by the transducer correlates with the density of acoustic waves received. Because the instrument knows the timing of the pulse, the speed of sound in the body, the timing of the signal's return, and the intensity of the returning signal, it can interpret the distance from the transducer and produce the appropriate image.

The primary mode of imaging in modern echocardiographic systems is two-dimensional scanning, in which images are produced as a sector. A sector is produced by aiming the ultrasound beam (usually electronically) in a particular direction, sending the pulse, and receiving the echoes returning from the body. The beam is then redirected, and the process is repeated. This produces individual scan lines, which are then displayed on the screen to represent the image. Most instruments acquire and display a sector of 128 scan lines, although this can be varied.

DETERMINANTS OF IMAGE QUALITY

The quality of the echocardiographic image is affected by many factors, some inherent to the ultrasound beam, some operator dependent. Penetration power, resolution, and artifacts are most affected by transducer selection and user-definable settings.

Penetration Power

Ultrasound waves, like all electromagnetic waves, are attenuated as they pass through the body. Some of the beam is reflected (or echoed) back to produce the image of each structure it comes in contact with, some is reflected off at an angle and cannot be detected by the transducer, and some is absorbed by the tissue. The degree of attenuation is inversely related to the frequency of the transducer. Higher frequency ultrasound transducers (7 to 10 MHz) begin to lose significant penetration beyond 6 to 8 cm, whereas lower frequency transducers (2.5 to 5 MHz) can easily penetrate to 20 cm. The attenuation can be minimized by manipulating the electronics of the system, but in general, the greater the depth, the lower the frequency of the optimal transducer.

Resolution

Image resolution is generally divided into three components: detail resolution, the ability to distinguish small structures; contrast resolution, the ability to distinguish differences in tissue density; and uniformity of the image throughout the sector display.[4] The last two are discussed only briefly, because no commercially available system allows the user to manipulate these parameters.

Detail resolution is the minimal distance by which two structures must be separated to be seen as two separate acoustic echoes. Resolution differs in each direction: axial resolution refers to the minimal distance along the direction of the beam, and lateral resolution is that perpendicular to the direction of the beam. Axial resolution is determined by the physical length of the pulse. If two objects are closer to each other than the length of the pulse, their echoes merge and produce one long echo. The physical length of the pulse depends on its wavelength and duration. The speed (*c*) of electromagnetic waves in the body is constant (roughly 1560 m/sec) and carries the formula

$$c = f \times l \qquad (1)$$

where *f* equals frequency of the wave in hertz (cycles per second) and *l* is the wavelength in meters. Therefore, wavelength is inversely proportional to the transducer frequency. The wavelength is the absolute limit to resolution, because structures must be separated by at least 1 wavelength. The wavelengths for standard ultrasound transducers are as follows:

Frequency (MHz)	Wavelength (mm)
2.0	0.80
3.5	0.45
5.0	0.30
7.5	0.20
10	0.16

The ultrasound pulse must also have length. Most systems produce a pulse that is 3 to 5 wavelengths long. Therefore, for a 5-MHz transducer with a pulse duration of 3 wavelengths, the physical length of the pulse is 3 × 0.3 = 0.9 mm. Two objects closer to each other than 1 mm are seen as one object. In practice, most systems can produce a pulse with a physical length of 1.5 mm at any frequency, somewhat smaller for higher frequency transducers. However, an axial resolution of 1 mm serves as a rough guide for most ultrasound systems.

Lateral resolution depends on the beam width. Two objects closer to each other than the beam width are seen as a single broad echo. Like all waves, the ultrasound beam diverges as it passes through the tissue. Therefore, lateral resolution also depends on the depth of the tissue. Modern transducers are able to focus the beam electronically to narrow it at the optimal distance, or focal zone. The width of the beam in millimeters at the focal zone is expressed as

$$\text{Width} = \frac{\lambda x}{d} \qquad (2)$$

where λ is the wavelength of the wave, *x* the distance to the structure, and *d* the diameter of the transducer. Therefore, minimal beam diameter and lateral resolution are directly related to transducer frequency and depth of the structure and inversely related to transducer size. An ideal transducer would then be of higher frequency and larger. However, because of the physics of beam formation, the beam has a wider diameter nearer to the focal zone (near field), and practical considerations limit the ability of large transducers to focus in the near field. In addition, in smaller patients, a large transducer may produce rib artifacts when the image is viewed from the parasternal planes. Therefore, in general, smaller, higher frequency transducers provide the best near-field resolution in smaller children, and larger, lower frequency transducers provide the best far-field resolution. For a standard size 5-MHz transducer, the minimal beam diameter at the focal zone is approximately 1.5 mm. In addition, better lateral resolution can be achieved by using a scan plane that brings the structure closer to the transducer.

Contrast resolution, the ability to distinguish differences in tissue density, applies particularly to the ability to distinguish faint structures next to brighter ones. The determinants of contrast resolution are similar to those for detail resolution, and axial resolution is better than lateral resolution. The development of computer-controlled image generation, or computed sonography, allows the manufacturer, but not the operator, to control these signals.

In early mechanically focused systems, the near-field and far-field images were indistinct as a result of problems with lateral resolution. With newer phased-array systems, the image quality is much more uniform with dynamic focusing. Because the system knows the depth from which echoes are returning (because of the constant speed of sound), it can continually adjust the focal zone to achieve maximal resolution for images at that particular depth. This allows the effective beam diameter to be fairly uniform throughout the scanning depth.

Artifacts

Artifacts can significantly degrade the image quality. The most commonly encountered artifacts are dropout of parallel structures, side-lobing, and shadowing. Images generated by waves echoed back to the transducer depend on an interface perpendicular to the ultrasound beam. Most structures are irregular so that even when they are nearly parallel to the beam, enough of the surface is perpendicular to generate an image. Smooth structures parallel to the ultrasound beam generate little echo back to the transducer and therefore generate weak signals, which can easily be lost. The best example of this is the atrial septum, which is parallel to the beam from the apical view and often drops out. From the subcostal view, however, the septum is perpendicular and easily seen.

Side-lobing and shadowing are both caused by dense structures that produce bright echoes. These structures, such as the pericardium, reflect a much greater proportion of the beam than do other structures. Side-lobing refers to the lateral spread of these bright echoes. They are a consequence of the divergence of the beam in the far field. Although we refer to beam diameter (see lateral resolution, earlier), the beam does not have distinct edges. Rather, the beam becomes less intense farther away from the centerline. High-intensity echoes are therefore wider than less intense ones and can appear to extend more laterally than they actually do. This is most often seen when a bright structure, such as the pericardium, appears to extend into the lumen of a nearby vessel.

Shadows are caused when extremely bright echoes allow little of the ultrasound beam to pass through them. Because images depend on echo transmission and reflection, this obscures structures behind a bright object, such as a prosthetic valve, which almost completely obscures all structures behind it because of an intense shadow effect.

DOPPLER ULTRASONOGRAPHY

Doppler ultrasonography is vital to modern echocardiography. Without it, the degree of obstruction, the size of shunts, and small defects would be beyond the scope of echocardiography. The Doppler principle states that the frequency of transmitted sound is altered if the source is moving, as in the classic example of the moving train. This principle applies if either the source or the receiver of the sound is moving. The frequency is altered according to the Doppler equation

$$f_d = \frac{2f_o V \cos \theta}{c} \qquad (3)$$

where f_d is the observed Doppler shift in hertz, f_o is the frequency of the source sound in hertz, V is the velocity of the object (source or receiver) in meters per second, θ is the intercept angle between the source and receiver in degrees, and c is the velocity of sound in the body (1560 m/sec).

In echocardiography, the Doppler shift is used to measure the velocity of blood as it moves through the heart. The frequency shift observed is usually about several kilohertz and produces an audible signal. The signal is also processed and displayed graphically as the component velocities (Fig. 11–1A, B). By convention, blood moving toward the transducer is shown as a signal above the baseline, that moving away as a signal below the baseline. If flow is laminar, nearly all of the blood is moving in parallel fashion at similar velocity. This produces a musical tone and a narrow band on the graphic display (Fig. 11–1B). However, if flow is turbulent, the audible signal is harsher, and the graphic display is "filled in."[5] The velocity can be calculated by solving Equation 3 for velocity:

$$V = \frac{cf_d}{2f_o \ \cos \theta} \qquad (4)$$

Therefore, the velocity is proportional to the frequency shift but inversely proportional to the originating frequency and the cosine of the angle of incidence. The angle of incidence provides the principal source of error in velocity measurements. Rarely is the blood flow parallel to the transducer beam, particularly in disturbed flow. In practice, if the angle of incidence is less than 20 degrees, the error is minimal. If the angle is greater, it should be minimized, preferably by use of a different view, but it can also be corrected in the instrument.

Three types of Doppler applications are commonly employed: continuous-wave, pulsed-wave, and color Doppler.

Continuous-Wave Doppler

Continuous-wave Doppler is the simplest of the modes. Two crystals are used, one as the transmitter, and the other as the receiver. Signals are sent continuously and thus received continuously. Because the signal is continuous, the instrument cannot calculate the depth of the returning signal. Therefore, signals are received from the entire path of the beam, which may contain multiple flows. However, Doppler shifts of any magnitude can be received. Sampling theory dictates that to display a signal of a given frequency, it must be sampled at least at twice that frequency. Because the sampling is continuous, any frequency can be sampled (Fig. 11–1A). Therefore, continuous-wave Doppler is accurate at any velocity but inaccurate with respect to location.

Pulsed-Wave Doppler

Pulsed-wave Doppler complements continuous-wave Doppler. A single crystal alternately transmits pulses and receives echoes. Echoes can be sampled within a time window established by the desired depth of sampling. Sampling must finish before the next pulse transmission. Therefore, the location can be accurately sampled in pulsed-wave Doppler. However, because the sampling frequency is limited by the pulse repetition frequency, only a limited range of frequencies and therefore a limited range of velocities can be sampled. This limit is the Nyquist limit. Velocities above the Nyquist limit cannot be resolved accurately and are therefore electronically cut off and "wrapped around," or aliased (Fig. 11–1B). From Equa-

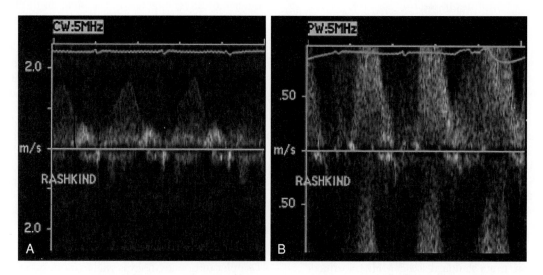

FIGURE 11–1

Continuous-wave, pulsed-wave, and color flow images of the same flow signal. *A,* With continuous-wave Doppler, continuous sampling allows measurement of higher velocities, but because multiple samples are being taken, the result is a "filled in" signal. *B,* With pulsed-wave Doppler, the limited sampling frequency prevents measurement of higher velocities, which leads to aliasing (wrapping around) of the signal. *C,* See Color Figure 11–1C.

tion 4, the velocity is inversely proportional to the transmitted frequency. Therefore, lower frequency transducers can resolve higher velocities for a given Doppler shift and thus are more useful in pulsed Doppler than are higher frequency transducers. A standard 5-MHz transducer has a Nyquist limit of 1 to 3 m/sec, depending on the depth of sampling.

Color Doppler

Color Doppler (Fig. 11–1C [see Color Plates]) is an implementation of pulsed Doppler in which a mean velocity for an area is calculated and a color is applied to the two-dimensional image to represent the velocity. Color Doppler has added tremendously to echocardiographic examination by allowing detection of small defects that are not possible to see by two-dimensional imaging alone.

Because color Doppler is a form of pulsed Doppler, it is subject to all the advantages and limitations of pulsed Doppler. However, it has some additional advantages and limitations. A much broader area can be sampled by color Doppler than by conventional pulsed Doppler. This allows much quicker determination of velocities across a larger area. However, the instrument must perform the same transmission/reception sequence for each Doppler sampling volume and also perform a transmission/reception sequence for the accompanying two-dimensional image. Therefore, the pulse repetition frequency is much lower, as is the Nyquist limit, or maximal detectable velocity. The same 5-MHz transducer that can sample 1 to 3 m/sec by pulsed Doppler can achieve only 0.5 to 1 m/sec by color Doppler. The Nyquist limit of color Doppler is affected by both the width and depth of the color sampling volume and also by the depth of the two-dimensional image. Decreasing the size of the sampling volume, a feature available on most commercial systems, can increase the Nyquist limit significantly.

EFFECTIVE USE OF ULTRASONOGRAPHY

In cross-sectional imaging, a higher frequency transducer generally produces better resolution, but a lower frequency transducer provides better penetration. In Doppler sampling, a lower frequency transducer allows more accurate determination of velocity in spectral displays and also provides more penetration for better color Doppler signals. Use of appropriate scan planes, particularly those that bring structures closer to the transducer, will significantly increase resolution, both by allowing use of higher frequency transducers and by improving lateral resolution and penetration.

ECHOCARDIOGRAPHIC EXAMINATION

The purpose of an echocardiographic examination is thorough morphologic and physiologic assessment of the heart and great vessels. Because of the asymmetric position of the heart in the chest, and the sonographic interference by the lungs and thoracic skeleton, several standard acoustic windows are typically employed during a study: the parasternal, apical, subcostal, and suprasternal. The transesophageal route is an alternative. Each of these views allows variable definition of cardiovascular structures, and together they provide consistent frames of reference for measurement and discussion (Fig. 11–2). These reference views, however, should be appreciated as the framework for a total scan of the heart and vessels, from top to bottom, side to side, and front to back. Modifying these windows may allow further definition of select structures in some patients, especially young infants in whom skeletal components are less osseous.

Because the major cardiac axes differ from those of the body, it is essential to understand the spatial relationship of the heart and great vessels relative to other thoracic structures to perform an echocardiographic study or appreciate an image (Fig. 11–3; see also Fig. 11–2).[6] The long axis of the heart runs from the apex to the base. In the body, this axis runs approximately from the left hypochondrium anteroinferiorly through to the tip of the right scapula posterosuperiorly. Several of the standard echocardiographic views, such as the parasternal and apical, are oriented with

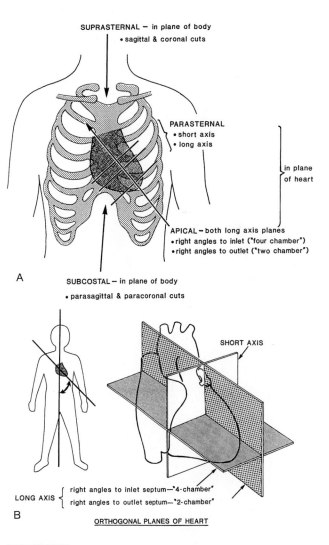

FIGURE 11–2

A, The standard echocardiographic windows on the body surface are oriented to the major axes of either the body or the heart. B, The standard reference planes for cardiac long-axis or short-axis imaging. (A, B from Silverman NH, Hunter S, Anderson RH, et al: Anatomical basis of cross sectional echocardiography. Br Heart J 50:421, 1983.)

respect to the cardiac axes, and orthogonal planes from these windows are described in terms of the cardiac long- and short-axis (parasternal) or two- and four-chamber (apical) views. Other windows, such as the subcostal and suprasternal, are more closely aligned with the major axes of the body and are thus described in terms of coronal, sagittal, and transverse (horizontal) planes (see Figs. 11–2 and 11–3).

An echocardiographic examination may be performed in a sequential view–oriented approach, with multiple views employed to obtain information that is then integrated to define the anatomy of the heart according to the segmental method, originally developed and presented by Van Praagh.[7] The morphologic information is complemented by physiologic information. In dedicated pediatric echocardiography textbooks, the sonographic evaluation of the heart and great vessels is often presented in terms of the standard views, an approach that lends itself to the technical performance and evaluation of an echocardiogram.[8,9] However, from the perspective of presenting the strengths and weaknesses of echocardiography in congenital heart disease, there is also merit in organizing a description in terms of the anatomic cardiac segments. In the following, morphologic evaluation is summarized according to a segmental approach, followed by physiologic evaluation and a presentation of special techniques, such as transesophageal, intravascular, and three-dimensional ultrasonography.

MORPHOLOGIC EVALUATION

Cross-sectional two-dimensional echocardiography allows excellent delineation of morphology and can be complemented with data obtained from Doppler color flow mapping, tissue tagging, and M-mode imaging. Morphologic evaluation in specific anomalies is presented in later chapters discussing the lesions, although select examples are given here to illustrate the capabilities of ultrasonography.

Systemic Veins

The relationships between the major abdominal systemic veins (inferior vena cava, hepatic veins, and azygos-hemiazygos system) and the abdominal aorta are of central importance in determining visceroatrial situs (Fig. 11–4). In situs solitus, the inferior vena cava is right-sided and to the right of the aorta, and the azygos and hemiazygos veins are more posterior in the right and left paravertebral spaces, respectively. These relationships are reversed in situs inversus. In patients with visceroatrial heterotaxia (atrial isomerism), these relationships are generally disturbed. The positions of the abdominal systemic veins can be evaluated from the subcostal window with both transverse and sagittal views. A coronal image can also be used to identify the intrahepatic segment of the inferior vena cava and the entrance of the hepatic veins (Fig. 11–5). The inferior vena cava must be imaged from below the liver to its junction with the right atrium to verify that it is truly the inferior vena cava and not a hepatic vein. When there is interruption of the inferior vena cava with azygos continuation, the intrahepatic segment of the inferior vena cava is absent, whereas the more posteriorly located azygos vein is of substantially increased caliber. Pulsed Doppler ultrasonography and color flow mapping can be used to characterize flow patterns, helping to confirm the identity of the vessel in question (Fig. 11–6 [see also Color Plates]). The course of the inferior vena cava can be imaged superiorly with progressive coronal angulation of the transducer.

The proximal superior vena cava and both cavoatrial junctions can be appreciated from subcostal coronal and sagittal views (Fig. 11–7). The tributaries of the superior vena cava are most readily imaged from the suprasternal notch and high parasternal windows, where the position of the left innominate vein relative to the aortic arch can be appreciated (Fig. 11–8). In small children, this vessel can be viewed with subcostal imaging, particularly the coronal view. High parasternal long-axis and subcostal sagittal views can be used to show the azygos vein running posteriorly and then over the right pulmonary artery to join the superior vena cava (Fig. 11–9). When a left superior vena cava is present, suprasternal notch, high parasternal, and subcostal views clearly identify its course and drainage (Fig. 11–10A), as can color flow Doppler (Fig. 11–10B [see Color Plates]). If drainage is to the coronary sinus, the coronary sinus is usually enlarged and can be identified as a large annular structure above the mitral valve (Fig.

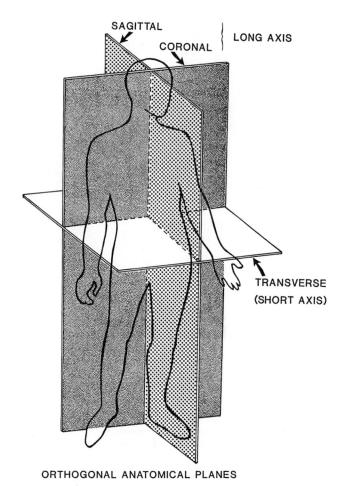

ORTHOGONAL ANATOMICAL PLANES

FIGURE 11–3

The three orthogonal planes of the body are the sagittal, coronal, and transverse planes. (From Silverman NH, Hunter S, Anderson RH, et al: Anatomical basis of cross sectional echocardiography. Br Heart J 50:421, 1983.)

Vascular arrangement in variations of body situs

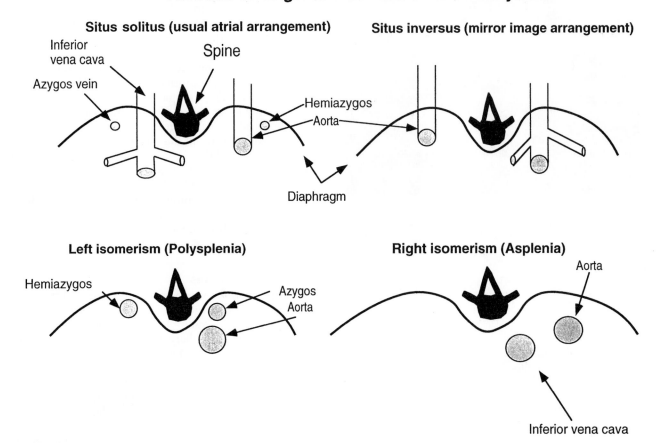

Situs solitus (usual atrial arrangement)

Inferior vena cava

Azygos vein

Spine

Hemiazygos
Aorta

Diaphragm

Situs inversus (mirror image arrangement)

Left isomerism (Polysplenia)

Hemiazygos

Azygos
Aorta

Right isomerism (Asplenia)

Aorta

Inferior vena cava

FIGURE 11–4

Diagrammatic representation of the probable positions of the aorta, inferior vena cava, and azygos veins in the four possible forms of atrial situs. In left isomerism, the inferior vena cava is interrupted, and drainage of lower extremity venous blood continues through either the azygos or hemiazygos. Left isomerism and right isomerism are both depicted here with the aorta and azygos–inferior vena cava on the left, although the vessels may be on the right as well. (Modified from Silverman NH: Pediatric Echocardiography. Baltimore, Williams & Wilkins, 1993, p 308.)

11–11). In this situation, a bridging vein is typically absent and cannot be imaged. The coronary sinus may be seen in transverse section from the parasternal long axis and in longitudinal section with posterior angulation from the apical four-chamber view. The coronary sinus can be distinguished from the descending aorta in the parasternal long axis by identifying the pericardium, which defines the coronary sinus as an intrapericardial structure (see Fig. 11–11). In addition, from the apical four-chamber view, the coronary sinus passes anterior to the left pulmonary veins, whereas the descending aorta is posterior to the left pulmonary veins.

Pulmonary Veins

The pulmonary veins can be defined from a number of windows, including parasternal, suprasternal, apical four-chamber, and subcostal views. A complete evaluation of the pulmonary veins requires that all four veins and their venoatrial connections be identified. With careful manipulation of the transducer in the suprasternal notch coronal view or high parasternal horizontal view, all four pulmonary veins can sometimes be visualized at their confluence with the left atrium in a single plane ("crab view," Fig.

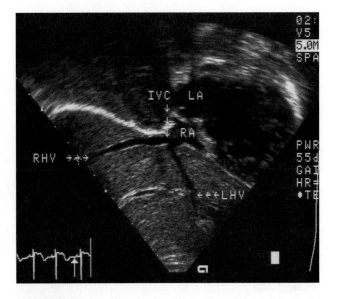

FIGURE 11–5

Subcostal coronal image demonstrates the confluence of the left (LHV) and right hepatic veins (RHV) with the inferior vena cava (IVC) just below the caval junction with the right atrium (RA). LA = left atrium.

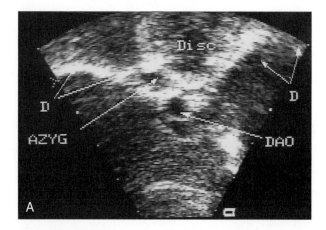

FIGURE 11–6

A, Subcostal transverse scan in an interrupted inferior vena cava with azygos (AZYG) continuation of flow in a patient with left isomerism. *B,* See Color Figure 11–6B. *C,* See Color Figure 11–6C. D = diaphragm; DAO = descending aorta. (*A, B* from Silverman NH: Pediatric Echocardiography. Baltimore, Williams & Wilkins, 1993, p 310.)

11–12 [see also Color Plates]), although slight rotation and angulation are more often necessary to display all of the pulmonary venoatrial junctions. In imaging the pulmonary veins from the apical four-chamber view, the descending aorta passes posterior to the left atrium between the left and right pulmonary veins and should not be confused with the left pulmonary veins (Fig. 11–13). As with examination of the systemic veins, pulsed Doppler interrogation and color flow mapping can be used to demonstrate flow and thus offer guidance regarding the anatomy of the pulmonary veins when their identity is otherwise not obvious.

Atria

As described before, the relationships of the major abdominal vessels and the connections of the systemic and pulmonary veins to the atria provide important information about atrial situs. The distinctive morphology of left and right atrial appendages can also be determined by images obtained from the parasternal and subcostal windows. The right atrial appendage is typically broad based and triangular (Fig. 11–14A), whereas the left atrial appendage is thin and "finger-like" with a narrow base (Fig. 11–14B).[10] Other typical features of the morphologic right atrium include the orifice of the coronary sinus, the limbus forming the superior border of the fossa ovalis on the right atrial aspect of the septum (Fig. 11–14C), and the eustachian valve. The interatrial septum is investigated from multiple windows, including the parasternal short-axis, apical four-chamber, and subcostal views, allowing all aspects of the septum to be identified (see Fig. 11–9).

Atrioventricular Valves

The atrioventricular valvar apparatus consists of the annulus (or basal attachment of the leaflets to the atrioventricular junction), the valve leaflets proper, the chordae tendineae, and the papillary muscles. The morphologic left (mitral) and right (tricuspid) atrioventricular valvar complexes are unique in each of these components and can be fully characterized by echocardiography.

The mitral valve and its tensor apparatus can be well defined with use of parasternal long- and short-axis views, together with the apical four-chamber and subcostal coronal and sagittal views. The mitral valve annulus and tensor apparatus can be identified clearly and measured from the parasternal long-axis and apical four-chamber views (Fig. 11–15). The valve leaflets are assessed by these as well as

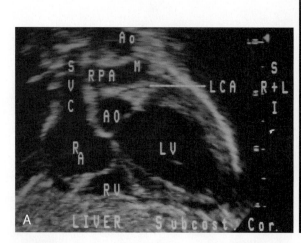

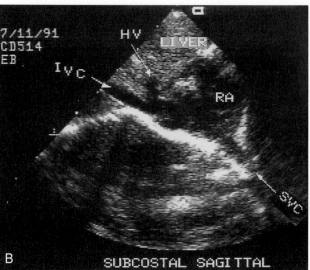

FIGURE 11–7

A, This frame is taken with slightly more anterior angulation to identify the position and course of the left main and left anterior descending coronary arteries (LCA) as they run from the aorta (AO) inferior to the right pulmonary artery (RPA) on the anterior surface of the right ventricle (RV). The superior vena cava (SVC) enters the right atrium (RA). LV = left ventricle, M = main pulmonary artery. *B,* In this subcostal sagittal view with cranial scanning, the relationship of the inferior vena cava (IVC), superior vena cava (SVC), right atrium (RA), and hepatic vein (HV) can be clearly traced. (*A, B* from Silverman NH: Pediatric Echocardiography. Baltimore, Williams & Wilkins, 1993, p 24.)

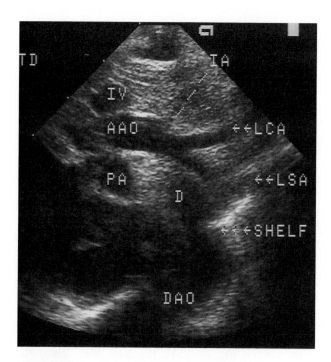

FIGURE 11–8

In this oblique scan from the suprasternal notch, the left innominate vein (IV) is identified running anterior to the ascending aorta (AAO). The innominate artery (IA), left common carotid artery (LCA), and left subclavian artery (LSA) can also be seen arising from the arch, which then continues into the descending aorta (DAO). A coarctation (shelf) is present at the level of the ductus arteriosus (D). PA = pulmonary artery.

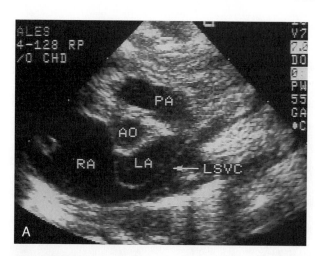

FIGURE 11–10

A, This image from the high parasternal window shows a left superior vena cava (LSVC) draining through the coronary sinus to the right atrium (RA). The left atrium (LA), aorta (AO), and pulmonary artery (PA) are also shown. B, See Color Figure 11–10B.

the parasternal short-axis and subcostal views. From the parasternal short-axis views, the image plane is directed through the mitral valve orifice, allowing assessment of orifice geometry as well as anomalous structures such as clefts and accessory orifices or tissue (Fig. 11–16).

The tricuspid valve and subvalvar apparatus are also investigated with a combination of views. From the parasternal short-axis and subcostal sagittal views, the valve can be investigated in the plane of the valve ring. The normal offset appearance of the mitral and tricuspid valves, wherein the atrioventricular septum separates the right atrium from the

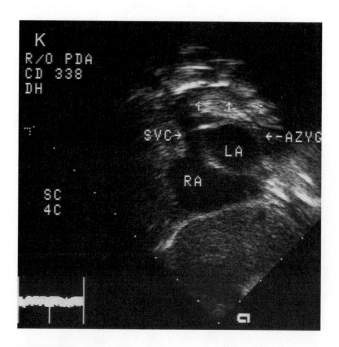

FIGURE 11–9

This subcostal sagittal scan demonstrates the azygos vein (arrows) draining above the right pulmonary artery and into the superior vena cava (SVC). The right atrial appendage can be seen as a separate bulge from the right atrium (RA), and the atrial septum is seen separating the right atrium from the left atrium (LA). (From Silverman NH: Pediatric Echocardiography. Baltimore, Williams & Wilkins, 1993, p 29.)

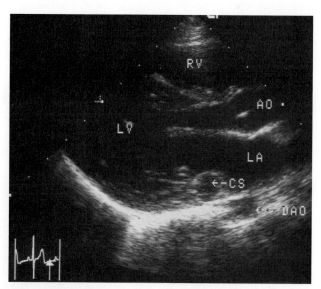

FIGURE 11–11

A parasternal long-axis view demonstrates a coronary sinus enlargement (CS) anterior to the descending aorta (DAO) in a patient with a superior vena cava–coronary sinus connection. AO = aorta; LA = left atrium; LV = left ventricle; RV = right ventricle. (From Silverman NH: Pediatric Echocardiography. Baltimore, Williams & Wilkins, 1993, p 516.)

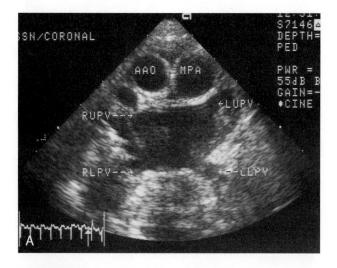

FIGURE 11-12

A suprasternal notch (SSN) coronal view shows the confluence of the right upper (RUPV), right lower (RLPV), left upper (LUPV), and left lower (LLPV) pulmonary veins entering the left atrium. The ascending aorta (AAO) and main pulmonary artery (MPA) are also seen in cross-section craniad to the left atrium. See also Color Figure 11–12B.

left ventricular outflow tract, can be appreciated from the apical four-chamber view (see Fig. 11–15B). The hinge points, thickness, and chordal attachments of the septal and anterosuperior leaflets are clearly distinguished from this view as well. Medial angulation of the transducer from the parasternal long-axis window cuts through the tricuspid valve in the plane of the anterosuperior and posteroinferior (or mural) leaflets and provides an opportunity to evaluate all components of the posteroinferior leaflet. All three leaflets can also be examined from the subcostal window. Anomalous attachments of tricuspid chordae, such as with straddling, may be seen from various windows, including the subcostal coronal and apical four-chamber views.

Ventricles

Ventricular morphology, size, and position can be well delineated by two-dimensional echocardiography using images from the parasternal, apical, and subcostal windows. The goal of examination is determination of ventricular morphology, chamber dimensions, and atrioventricular and ventriculoarterial connections. Almost all specific features of the left and right ventricles can be identified with echocardiography and synthesized to distinguish the morphologic left and right ventricles. The echocardiographic hallmarks of the morphologic right ventricle are septal attachment of the right atrioventricular (tricuspid) valve, the triangular shape of the ventricle, the trabecular septal surface, and the septomarginal trabeculation (Fig. 11–17). The characteristic features of the left ventricle are the lack of mitral valve chordal attachments to the septum (see Fig. 11–15A), smooth septal surface, conical shape of the ventricle, and aortic-mitral fibrous continuity, although the last is not always definable by echocardiography. The inlet, body, and outlet components of the left ventricle can be seen in a single plane from the parasternal long-axis, apical, and subcostal windows (Fig. 11–18; see also Fig. 11–15A). The inlet, body, and outlet components of the right ventricle can be depicted in a single subcostal plane with the transducer rotated into a position intermediate between sagittal and coronal cuts (Fig. 11–19).

Assessment of ventricular chamber size is based on geometric models that allow estimation of volume from one or more cross-sectional measurements (Fig. 11–20). Various models have been employed, primarily for calculation of left ventricular volume, which is more readily amenable to such models by virtue of its roughly symmetric dimensions. In our experience, the most reliable approach in children is to use the biplane Simpson's rule (method of disks), which can be applied irrespective of the shape of the chamber to be measured.[8] This method requires imaging in two orthogonal planes sharing a common long axis and reconstructs the chamber volume from the summed

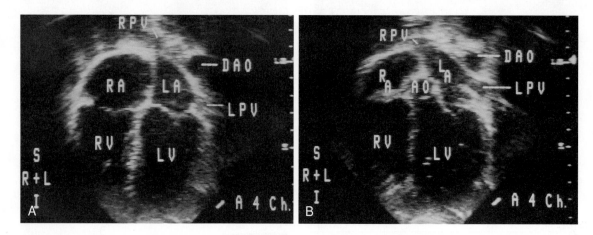

FIGURE 11-13

A, Apical posterior four-chamber view. B, Apical anterior five-chamber view. In both images, the right and left lower pulmonary veins (RPV, LPV) can be seen entering the left atrium (LA) and straddling the descending aorta (DAO). AO = aorta; LV = left ventricle; RA = right atrium; RV = right ventricle. (A, B from Silverman NH: Pediatric Echocardiography. Baltimore, Williams & Wilkins, 1993, p 17.)

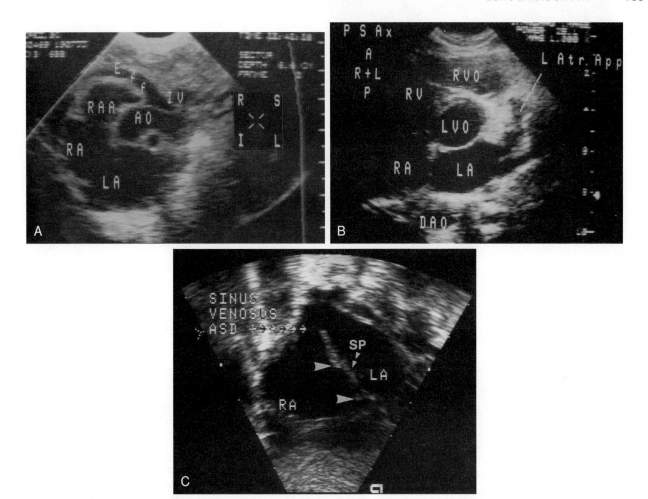

A, High parasternal long-axis view demonstrates the characteristic appearance of a right atrial appendage (RAA), which is broad and blunt with a wide connection to the body of the right atrium (RA). The ascending aorta can also be seen arising from the heart. The innominate vein (IV) is seen crossing anterior to the aorta (AO), and a small pericardial effusion (Eff) is present. LA = left atrium. Orientation: I, inferior; L, left; R, right; S, superior. *B,* Parasternal short-axis (P S Ax) view at the level of the left ventricular outflow tract (LVO) demonstrates the characteristic morphology of the left atrial appendage (L Atr. App.). The "finger-like" left atrial appendage joins the body of the atrium with a narrow connection. Other structures identified in this plane are the right ventricular outflow tract (RVO), right ventricular body (RV), right atrium (RA), left atrium (LA), and descending aorta (DAO). Orientation: A, anterior; L, left; P, posterior; R, right. *C,* This subcostal image in a patient with sinus venosus atrial septal defect (ASD) shows the limbus (above the upper broad arrow) on the right atrial (RA) surface of the interatrial septum (septum primum [SP], between the two broad arrows), forming the superior margin of the fossa ovalis. LA = left atrium. (*A, B* from Higgins CB: Congenital Heart Disease: Echocardiography and Magnetic Resonance Imaging. New York, Raven Press, 1990, p 81.)

volumes of multiple elliptical slices of equal thickness that are defined by the two orthogonal short-axis dimensions (see Fig. 11–20). For calculation of left ventricular volume, we use apical four- and two-chamber views as the orthogonal planes, although other views can be used as well. Estimation of right ventricular volume is more complex, both because the right ventricle has an irregular shape that fits no simple geometric model and because it lies close to the chest, which makes imaging of the entire ventricular outline difficult in older children.[11, 12] In children, however, orthogonal views of the right ventricle can be obtained easily from the subcostal window, and Simpson's rule can be applied for volume calculation from these images by using the common long axis from the diaphragmatic surface to the pulmonary artery and the area outlines of the right ventricle from orthogonal subcostal cuts, which may be best obtained from slightly oblique views rather than true sagittal and coronal images.[12]

Semilunar Valves

The semilunar valves are structures that consist functionally not only of the leaflets but of the annuli, the sinuses of Valsalva, and the sinotubular junctions as well. They can be imaged with two-dimensional echocardiography from a variety of windows, including the parasternal, apical, and subcostal views. The aortic root may be viewed in its long axis from the parasternal long-axis, apical two- and four-chamber, and subcostal coronal and sagittal views. The hinge points of the aortic valve leaflets as well as their thickness are appreciated with use of these cuts, as are the dimensions of the sinuses and sinotubular junction (see Figs. 11–15*A* and 11–18). The morphology of the aortic

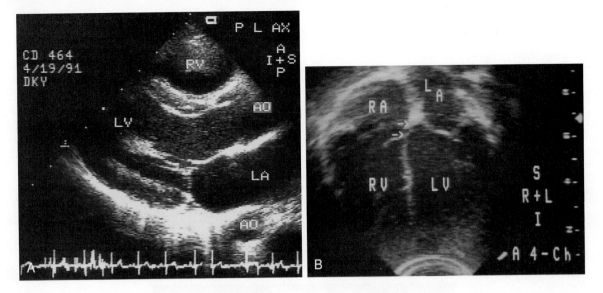

FIGURE 11–15

A, This parasternal long-axis (P L Ax.) view demonstrates the mitral valve between the left atrium (LA) and left ventricle (LV) during early systole. The ascending aorta and descending aorta (AO) are seen anterior (A) and posterior (P) to the left atrium. Orientation: I, inferior; S, superior. *B*, In this image from the apical four-chamber view, the atrioventricular septum (*arrows*) is seen between the left ventricular (LV) outflow tract and right atrium (RA). The mitral annulus is clearly demonstrated. The aortic leaflet of the mitral valve (or anterior leaflet) has been separated from the left ventricular outflow tract, and it and the septal leaflets of the tricuspid valve appear to arise from different levels. LA = left atrium; RV = right ventricle. (*A, B* from Silverman NH: Pediatric Echocardiography. Baltimore, Williams & Wilkins, 1993, p 7.)

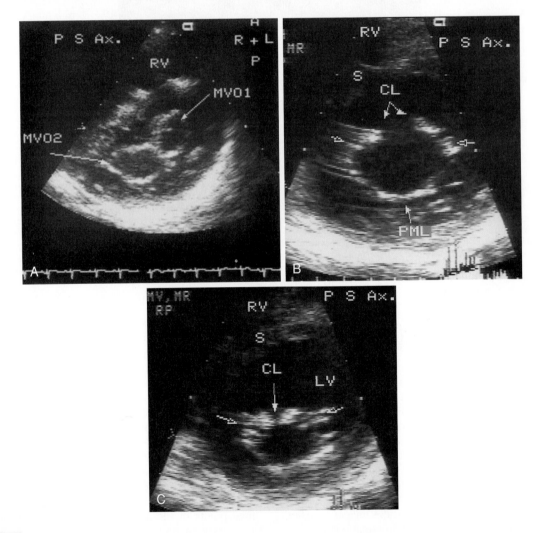

FIGURE 11–16

A, Parasternal short-axis (P S Ax.) view shows a double-orifice mitral valve, with two similar size openings (MVO1 and MVO2). The right ventricle (RV) is anterior (A) to the mitral valve. Orientation: L, left; P, posterior; R, right. (Reprinted from American Journal of Cardiology, Volume 76, Banerjee A, Kohl T, Silverman NH: Echocardiographic evaluation of congenital mitral valve anomalies in children, Pages 1284–1291, Copyright 1995, with permission from Excerpta Medica Inc.) *B, C*, This series of parasternal short-axis images shows a cleft (CL) in the anterior leaflet of the mitral valve. The valve is shown open during diastole in *B* and closing during early systole in *C*. The posterior mitral leaflet (PML) is also indicated, as are the left (LV) and right ventricles. S = septum.

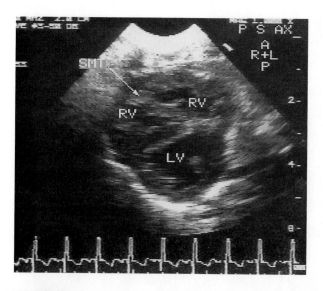

FIGURE 11–17

With cranial angulation and orientation of the transducer to concentrate on right ventricular structure, the septomarginal trabeculation (SMT) (*arrow*) can be seen lying within the right ventricular cavity adherent to the ventricular septum and dividing the right ventricle (RV) into inlet and outlet components. LV = left ventricle. (From Silverman NH: Pediatric Echocardiography. Baltimore, Williams & Wilkins, 1993, p 11.)

valve leaflets can be distinguished clearly from the parasternal short axis, in both systole and diastole, when the imaging plane passes through the sinuses of Valsalva (Fig. 11–21). The leaflets may be of unequal size. A bicuspid aortic valve, which typically results from fusion of the left coronary leaflet with either the right or noncoronary leaflet, may appear to be a normal tricuspid valve from this view, because the raphe of the fused commissure is visible.

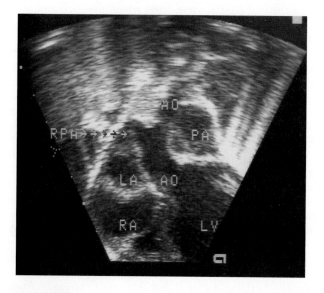

FIGURE 11–18

In this subcostal coronal view in a patient with anomalous origin of the right pulmonary artery (RPA) from the ascending aorta (AO), the aortic root dimensions are seen clearly. The left ventricle (LV), main pulmonary artery (PA), and right (RA) and left (LA) atria can also be identified.

However, the motion of this leaflet differs from the normal trileaflet configuration, and an asymmetric valvar orifice is typically present during systole and can be distinguished by two-dimensional and Doppler color flow imaging.

The pulmonary valve is imaged primarily from the parasternal and subcostal windows. As with the aortic valve, leaflet thickness, hinge points, and dimensions of the sinuses and sinotubular junction are evaluated in the long axis of the pulmonary artery. In the parasternal short axis, the pulmonary valve is seen at the level of the aortic valve, to which it is oriented almost perpendicularly (Fig. 11–22A). From the parasternal long axis, the pulmonary valve is brought into view with extreme leftward angulation (Fig. 11–22B). The pulmonary valve is viewed from the subcostal coronal window with anterior angulation and kept in view as the transducer is rotated into the sagittal plane.

Coronary Arteries

The coronary arteries can be evaluated from several echocardiographic windows, including the parasternal, apical four-chamber, and subcostal. Depending on the cardiac anatomy, techniques must be modified to define the coronary arteries. The acoustic plane remains stable while the heart shifts in position through the cardiac cycle, causing the coronary arteries to move in and out of the image plane. Because the coronary arteries lie on the surface of the heart and run in different planes, segments that are displayed during the various parts of the cycle will differ.

The coronary origins and proximal arteries are most reliably identified from the parasternal short axis and with anterior angulation from the apical four-chamber view (Fig. 11–23A, B). The bifurcation of the left main coronary artery into the left anterior descending and circumflex arteries can also be appreciated from these views (Fig. 11–23A, C). The right coronary and circumflex arteries run in the atrioventricular grooves and can be seen in longitudinal section when the scan plane is directed parallel to the atrioventricular grooves, either from the parasternal short-axis (Fig. 11–24A) or subcostal sagittal views or with posterior angulation from the apical four-chamber view (Fig. 11–24B). In addition, the right coronary artery can be demonstrated in the atrioventricular groove from the parasternal long-axis view with medial angulation. The anterior and posterior descending coronary branches are brought out in their long axis when the scan is directed parallel to the interventricular grooves, in which they run. The left anterior descending artery is imaged with extreme anterior angulation from the subcostal coronal and apical four-chamber views (see Fig. 11–23A) or with medial angulation from the parasternal long-axis view. The posterior descending branch of the right coronary artery, which runs posteriorly and along the diaphragmatic surface of the heart, is visible with extreme caudal angulation from the apical four-chamber view and from the subcostal plane by directing the scan plane just superior to the left hemidiaphragm (Fig. 11–24C, D).

Great Arteries

In evaluating the great arteries, it is important to determine size, morphologic anomalies or variations, and the ventriculoarterial connections. The aorta, arch vessels, and

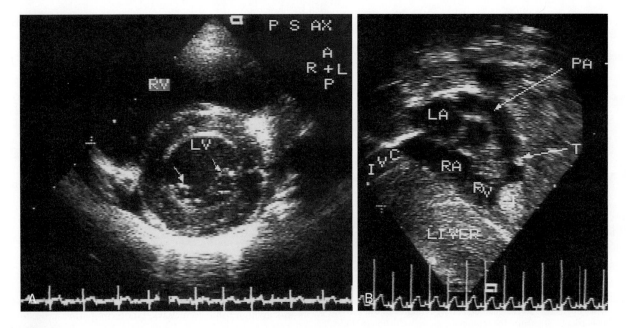

FIGURE 11–19

A, From the parasternal short-axis (P S AX) window, the most inferior cut is taken through the papillary muscle level (*arrows*) and demonstrates the circular left ventricle (LV) posteriorly with the right ventricle (RV) draped around it anteriorly. Orientation: A, anterior; R, right; L, left; P, posterior. Because the transducer is oriented slightly to the left, minor rotation of the short axis occurs, with the anterolateral and posteromedial papillary muscles being approximately in the 4 and 7 o'clock positions rather than the anatomic positions of 2 and 6 o'clock. (From Silverman NH: Pediatric Echocardiography. Baltimore, Williams & Wilkins, 1993, p 10.) *B,* In this subcostal oblique view in a patient with a right ventricular tumor (T), the right atrium (RA), entire right ventricle (RV), and outflow tract and pulmonary artery (PA) can be seen in a single plane. Also seen are the inferior vena cava (IVC) entering the right atrium (RA), the left atrium (LA), and the liver.

main and branch pulmonary arteries are effectively assessed from most echocardiographic windows. Characteristic features that help distinguish the aorta from the pulmonary trunk include the origins of the coronary arteries, the arch and its branches, and the bifurcation of the pulmonary trunk into two separate branch pulmonary arteries.

Two-dimensional imaging of the thoracic aorta is possible from parasternal, apical, subcostal, and suprasternal windows. The left ventricular origin of the ascending aorta and its proximal course can be demonstrated in the parasternal long-axis view, but a longer segment of ascending aorta can be seen from the subcostal and apical views in young children (Fig. 11–25A, B). The distal ascending aorta, arch, and proximal descending aorta are imaged from the high parasternal or suprasternal windows in the parasagittal plane. The full course of the arch can be developed with leftward angulation and clockwise rotation of the transducer or, if arch laterality is anomalous, by adjustment of the scan plane appropriately (Fig. 11–25C). Arch laterality is best demonstrated from the coronal view. The aorta is seen in cross-section, and with superior angulation, the innominate artery arises from the aorta and then proceeds either left or right (Fig. 11–25D). The arch is always on the side opposite the innominate artery and can also, with further superior angulation, be seen to course posterior, lateral to the trachea. Arch laterality can also be confirmed with progressive lateral angulation from the suprasternal sagittal view, which allows the transverse arch to be followed to either the left or the right of the trachea and esophagus. The innominate, carotid, and subclavian

arteries can also be identified from the suprasternal window, and their recognition is essential for confirmation of arch identity. Bifurcation of the innominate artery into the carotid and subclavian arteries may be demonstrated with coronal scanning from the suprasternal notch (Fig. 11–25C). The thoracic descending aorta is seen best from the subcostal sagittal view, from which the arch and isthmus can also be appreciated, especially in infants and small children.

The main pulmonary artery is imaged at its origin from the right ventricle in the parasternal short-axis, the parasternal long-axis with rightward angulation, and the subcostal sagittal and coronal views. The branching of the pulmonary trunk into left and right pulmonary arteries can be imaged in a single plane from the parasternal short-axis and sometimes from the subcostal coronal window (Fig. 11–26). From the subcostal coronal view, the branch pulmonary arteries can be followed peripherally beyond the level of the upper lobe artery origin in many patients. This view may be augmented by rotating the transducer into an oblique position that is more closely aligned with the posterior and lateral course of the central branch pulmonary arteries. Oblique views from the high parasternal and suprasternal views also enable delineation of the branch pulmonary arteries and are helpful for defining their relationship to the aortic arch and the upper extremity arteries.

Pericardium and Adnexa

The pericardium is present in most views of the heart. Pericardial effusion or thickening is best appreciated by evalua-

ALGORITHM	MODEL	FORMULA

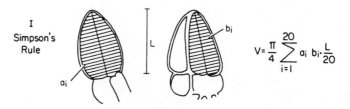

I
Simpson's
Rule

$$V = \frac{\pi}{4} \sum_{i=1}^{20} a_i \cdot b_i \cdot \frac{L}{20}$$

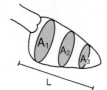

II
Simpson's
Rule

$$V = \left(\frac{A_1 + A_2}{2}\right)\frac{L}{3} + \left(\frac{A_2 + A_3}{2}\right)\frac{L}{3} + \frac{1}{3}A_3 \cdot \frac{L}{3}$$

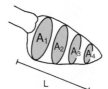

III
Simpson's
Rule

$$V = \frac{L}{4}\left(A_1 + \frac{A_2 + A_3}{2} + \frac{A_3 + A_4}{2} + \frac{1}{3}A_4\right)$$

IV
Biplane
Area
Length

$$V = \frac{8 A_1 \cdot A_2}{3 \pi L}$$
$$= \frac{0.85 \cdot A_1 A_2}{L}$$

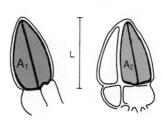

V
Hemisphere
Cylinder

$$V = A \cdot \frac{L}{2} + \frac{2}{3} A \cdot \frac{L}{2}$$
$$= \frac{5}{6} AL$$
$$= 0.83\ AL$$

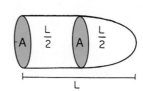

VI
Biplane
Area
Length

$$V = \frac{\pi}{6} D_1 D_2 \cdot L$$

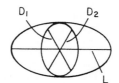

VII
Single Plane
Area Length

$$V = \frac{8(A)^2}{3 \pi L}$$
$$= 0.85 \frac{(A)^2}{L}$$

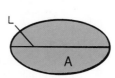

FIGURE 11–20

Schematic demonstration of various methods employing different geometric models to calculate chamber volumes from two-dimensional echocardiography. *I,* The biplane Simpson's rule based on orthogonal views in an apical two- and four-chamber view. The volume is calculated as the sum of volumes of ellipsoidal cylinders with the major and minor axes *a* and *b* and the height *L/n,* where *L* is the common long axis and *n* the number of segments chosen. In the example shown, *n* equals 20. *II, III,* The principle of Simpson's rule can be applied to a different method that calculates the chamber volume from three *(II)* or four *(III)* area measurements obtained in parasternal short axis; the height of the segments is taken from equivalents of the long axis measured from the apical window. The assumption, however, that all slices in the parasternal short axis are equidistant from each other and are perpendicular to the long axis is almost impossible to satisfy in practice. *IV,* With a biplane area-length method, the areas *A1* and *A2* are traced in apical two- and four-chamber views; the long axis *L* is taken from either plane. The formula used in this calculation is that for an ellipse, which may be reasonable for the left ventricle but not for the right ventricle. *V,* The hemisphere-cylinder (or bullet) model uses a cross-sectional area of the left ventricle in a parasternal short axis at the level of the tips of the papillary muscles and a length taken from an apical view. The formula considers the chamber volume as the sum of a hemisphere and a cylinder, which is also not valid for the right ventricle. *VI,* Biplane ellipsoidal method using the length *L* taken from an apical plane and the diameters *D1* (anteroposterior) and *D2* (lateral) taken from a parasternal short axis at the level of the tips of the papillary muscles. This model can also be used only for left ventricular volume calculation. *VII,* The single area-length method is similar to the biplane area-length method *(IV)* but assumes both orthogonal areas to be equal; either the apical two- or four-chamber view may be used with this method. (From Silverman NH, Snider AR: Two-Dimensional Echocardiography in Congenital Heart Disease. Norwalk, CT, Appleton-Century-Crofts, 1982, p 250.)

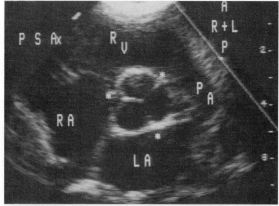

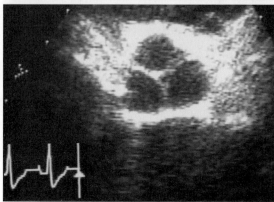

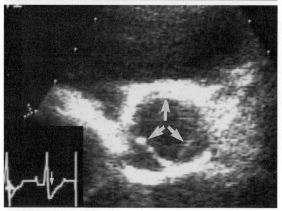

FIGURE 11–21

These frames demonstrate the aortic valve cusps within the aortic root from the parasternal short-axis (P S Ax) view. In the top frame, these are identified by asterisks adjacent to the junction of the commissures. In the middle frame taken with high-resolution magnification, the cusps are seen in diastole; in the lower frame in early systole, the cusps (*arrows*) are seen in their open position (see inset with ECG arrow for reference). LA = left atrium; PA = pulmonary artery; RA = right atrium; RV = right ventricle. (From Silverman NH: Pediatric Echocardiography. Baltimore, Williams & Wilkins, 1993, p 12.)

tion from multiple windows (Fig. 11–27). The parasternal short-axis view is the standard view for M-mode imaging of the pericardium. The diaphragm may be evaluated from the subcostal window with a combination of transverse, coronal, and sagittal views. Abdominal and mediastinal organs may be abnormal in certain forms of congenital heart disease, such as those occurring with DiGeorge's syndrome and atrial isomerism, respectively, and can be evaluated

during the echocardiographic examination. It is also important to be aware of the anatomic relationships between these structures and the heart and great vessels. The thymus is visible from the high parasternal window, or from the standard parasternal window in young children, in whom the thymus is typically large (see Fig. 11–26). The liver, stomach, and spleen can be evaluated from the subcostal window; it is important to visualize them in patients with forms of heart disease consistent with visceroatrial heterotaxia.

PHYSIOLOGIC EVALUATION

Ultrasonography can be used to define most aspects of cardiovascular function in children quite well. Spectral and color flow Doppler techniques have the most to offer in terms of characterizing blood flow patterns, and two-dimensional and M-mode techniques allow visualization of myocardial and valvar motion as well as the anatomic substrates of flow abnormalities. Contrast echocardiography is valuable for evaluating intracardiac or intrapulmonary shunts as well as anomalies of systemic venous return and certain forms of vascular obstruction that may otherwise be difficult to image. New technologies of Doppler tissue mapping and automated border detection are increasing the options for evaluation of ventricular function.

Ventricular Physiology

Ventricular performance is typically conceptualized in terms of systolic and diastolic function. Steady advances have been made in the noninvasive assessment of each of these components.

SYSTOLIC FUNCTION

The complex process of ventricular contraction and ejection is collectively referred to as systolic function. The shortening fraction and ejection fraction are the most-used methods of assessing function because of their simplicity.

The shortening fraction (SF) is the ratio of decrease in ventricular short-axis dimension relative to the diastolic dimension. The ventricular end-diastolic (EDD) and end-systolic (ESD) short-axis dimensions are measured in M-mode, and the ratio of shortening to end-diastolic dimension is obtained:

$$SF = 100 \frac{EDD - ESD}{EDD}$$

Ejection fraction (EF) is the change in ventricular volume from end diastole to end systole with use of M-mode or cross-sectional two-dimensional images. In M-mode measurements, a shape is assumed for the ventricle and a volume calculated on the basis of measurements obtained for the shortening fraction. End-diastolic volume (EDV) and end-systolic volume (ESV) are measured from one or two planes, either by manual tracing or by automated border detection, and the ejection fraction is obtained by dividing the volume difference (stroke volume) by end-diastolic volume and converting to percentage:

$$EF = 100 \frac{EDV - ESV}{EDV}$$

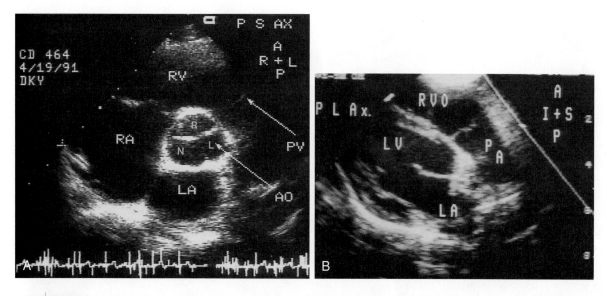

FIGURE 11-22

A, In this parasternal short-axis view at the level of the semilunar valve roots, the aortic root (AO) can be seen in the center of the plane. Within the aortic root, the characteristic V at the junction between the noncoronary (N) and right coronary leaflets and right (R) and left (L) coronary leaflets is shown by dense bright lines, and a faint echo is seen where the noncoronary and left coronary leaflets abut. LA = left atrium; PV = pulmonary valve; RA = right atrium; RV = right ventricle. *B,* Extreme leftward angulation from the parasternal long axis (P L Ax.) shows the pulmonary valve separating the right ventricular outflow tract (RVO) from the pulmonary artery (PA). The left atrium (LA), mitral valve, and left ventricle (LV) are also shown. Orientation: A, anterior; P, posterior; I, inferior; S, superior. (*A, B* from Silverman NH: Pediatric Echocardiography. Baltimore, Williams & Wilkins, 1993, p 11.)

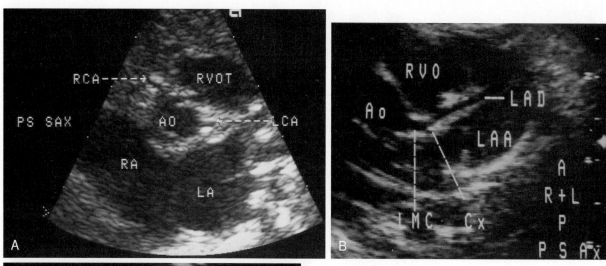

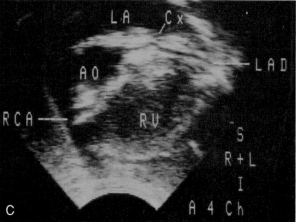

FIGURE 11-23

A, Parasternal short-axis (PS SAX) view at the level of the coronary ostia shows the right (RCA) and left (LCA) coronary arteries arising from the aortic root (AO). The right ventricular outflow tract (RVOT), right atrium (RA), and left atrium (LA) are also shown. *B,* This parasternal short-axis (P S Ax) view shows the left main coronary artery (LMC) dividing into the left anterior descending (LAD) branch, which then courses behind the pulmonary artery, and the circumflex (Cx). LAA = left atrial appendage; AO = aorta; RVO = right ventricular outflow tract. *C,* Anteriorly directed scan from the apical four-chamber view demonstrates the right (RCA) and left coronary arteries originating from the aortic root (AO). The left coronary can be seen dividing into left anterior descending (LAD) and circumflex (Cx) branches. LA = left atrium; RV = right ventricle. (*A–C* from Silverman NH: Pediatric Echocardiography. Baltimore, Williams & Wilkins, 1993, p 13.)

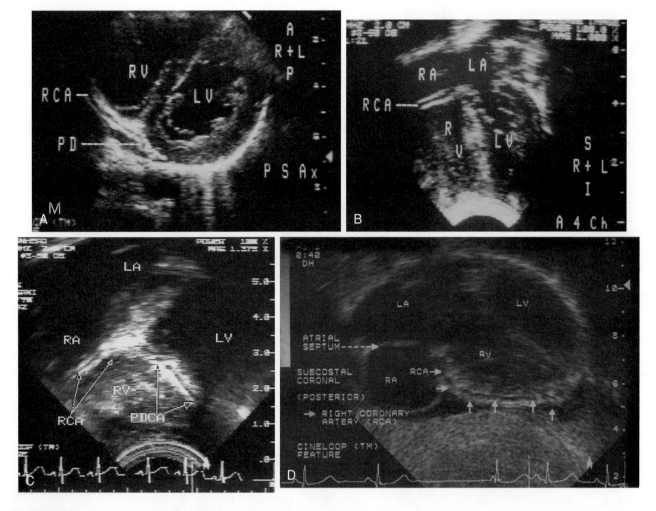

FIGURE 11-24

A, This view in the parasternal short axis (PSAx) concentrates on the right coronary artery (RCA) lying posterior to the right ventricle (RV) in the right coronary groove and its extension into the posterior descending coronary artery (PO). *B,* Apical four-chamber view with posterior angulation shows the right coronary artery (RCA) in the posterior atrioventricular groove. *C,* Extreme posterior angulation from the apical four-chamber view shows the right coronary artery (RCA) and posterior descending coronary artery (PDCA) as they course from a most posterior scanned plane near the crux of the heart. *D,* In this subcostal coronal cut, the right coronary artery (RCA) and its continuation as the posterior descending coronary artery *(arrows)* can be identified. LA = left atrium; LV = left ventricle; RA = right atrium; RV = right ventricle. (*A–D* from Silverman NH: Pediatric Echocardiography. Baltimore, Williams & Wilkins, 1993, p 18.)

Automated border detection with integrated ultrasonic backscatter may simplify and standardize this process[13, 14] for both left and right ventricular function. These indices are useful for simple estimation but are less reliable than other methods because they depend on heart rate, ventricular preload, and assumptions of ventricular geometry. M-mode measurements of ventricular size and function can be variable owing to a variability both in the position of the left ventricle from which the measurements are made and in the positioning of the measurement cursors. There is uncertainty of the exact position of the ventricular endocardial surface (as opposed to papillary muscles) and the timing of end systole and end diastole (relative to the R wave versus when the ventricle reaches its maximum or minimum). Therefore, M-mode measurements should be interpreted with respect to both this variability and the clinical situation, not viewed as absolutes on their own. Normal standards for children can be obtained from references 15 and 16.

Dividing the shortening fraction by the heart rate–adjusted ejection time (ET_C),

$$ET_C = \frac{\text{ejection time}}{\sqrt{\text{ECG R-R interval}}}$$

yields a rate-corrected mean velocity of circumferential fiber shortening (VCF_C). This is related to end-systolic wall stress (ESWS):

$$ESWS = \frac{1.35 D_{ES}\, P_{ES}}{4h\left(1 + \dfrac{h}{D_{ES}}\right)}$$

where D_{ES} is end-systolic dimension, P_{ES} is end-systolic pressure, and h is end-systolic posterior wall thickness. ESWS and VCF_C are inversely related in a linear fashion

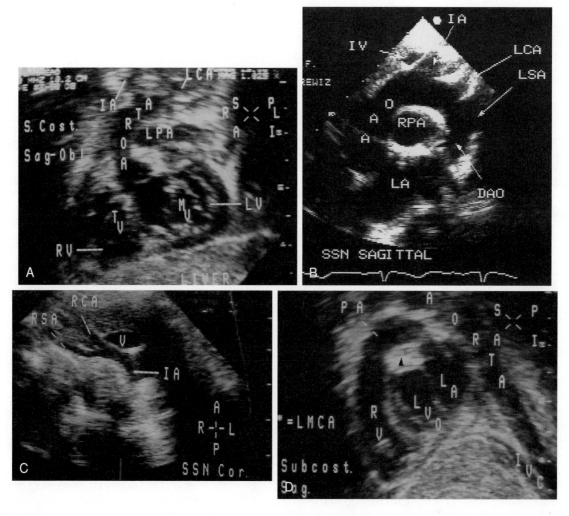

FIGURE 11–25

A, The relationship of the ascending aorta, left pulmonary artery (LPA), and left ventricle (LV) can be appreciated from this subcostal sagittal-oblique (Sag-Obl) view. The innominate artery (IA) and left carotid artery (LCA) can be identified superiorly. MV = mitral valve; RV = right ventricle; TV = tricuspid valve. *B,* Suprasternal notch sagittal view demonstrates the aortic arch, ascending aorta (AAO), innominate artery (IA), innominate vein (IV), left carotid and left subclavian arteries (LCA, LSA), and descending aorta (DAO). The left atrium (LA) can be seen lying inferior to the right pulmonary artery (RPA) and anterior to the descending aorta (DAO). *C,* In this view from the suprasternal notch coronal (SSN Cor.) plane, the innominate artery (IA) can be seen branching into the right subclavian (RSA) and right common carotid (RCA) arteries. The innominate vein is also shown (V). *D,* In this subcostal sagittal view, the body of the right ventricle (RV) can be seen to be continuous with the pulmonary artery (PA). The *asterisk* and *black arrow* indicate the position of the left main coronary artery (LMCA); the left ventricular outflow tract (LVO) lies immediately posterior to the ventricular septum, and the left ventricle is separated from the left atrium (LA) by the mitral valve. The entire descending thoracic and upper abdominal aorta can be seen posteriorly at this point. A small portion of the inferior vena cava (IVC) can be identified. (*A–D* from Silverman NH: Pediatric Echocardiography. Baltimore, Williams & Wilkins, 1993, p 28.)

in most physiologic ranges.[17,18] In addition, they depend less on preload and afterload than do other indices but require cumbersome data acquisition.

Doppler techniques for evaluating systolic ventricular function offer the advantage of being independent of ventricular geometry. Measurements from Doppler-derived aortic velocity curves that have been used to assess systolic function include peak velocity, acceleration time, ejection time, isovolumic contraction time, and velocity-time integral. Indices derived from these measures include peak rate of acceleration and mean acceleration (Fig. 11–28), which correlate with systolic performance.[19,20] The ratios of acceleration time to ejection time and of isovolumic contraction time to acceleration time may also be used as indices of ventricular function. Two other Doppler-based techniques for assessing ventricular function employ the continuity equation (flow = arterial cross-sectional area × mean velocity) to determine flow through the ascending aorta and by extension stroke volume and cardiac output. The area of the vessel is calculated from a measurement of the diameter, and mean systolic velocity is calculated by integrating the area under the velocity-time curve measured with spectral Doppler (velocity-time integral). The product of area and velocity-time integral is flow for one cardiac cycle, or stroke volume. This can be multiplied by the heart rate to yield cardiac output and divided by estimated body surface area to give the cardiac index, providing an estimate of cardiac performance.

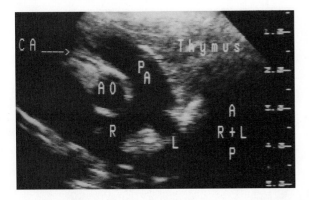

FIGURE 11–26

This parasternal short-axis view shows the main pulmonary artery (PA) branching into the left (L) and right (R) pulmonary arteries. The ascending aorta (AO) and right coronary artery (CA) are also seen. The highly echogenic mass anterior and lateral to the pulmonary artery is the thymus. (From Silverman NH: Pediatric Echocardiography. Baltimore, Williams & Wilkins, 1993.)

A number of novel techniques for more objectively evaluating ventricular function have been developed in recent years. Tissue Doppler imaging employs Doppler color flow technology to evaluate myocardial velocity with use of two-dimensional and M-mode echocardiography.[21, 22] Although this promising method has been shown to correlate with myocardial indices derived from pressure-volume loops,[23] it has not been well established in children. Another new technique, color kinesis imaging, is a visually enhanced mode of automated border detection in which sonographic backscatter analysis is used to color-code blood-myocardium interfaces that are then integrated over the cardiac cycle and analyzed to assess wall motion.[24] These, and other techniques in development, provide the prospect of an accurate, easily obtainable, reproducible echocardiographic assessment of systolic ventricular function.

DIASTOLIC FUNCTION

The process of ventricular relaxation and filling is collectively referred to as diastolic function. Diastole is much more complicated than systole and is less understood, so that all diastolic indices, both echocardiographic and invasive, are less developed than their systolic counterparts. However, there are several well-established methods of estimating diastolic function by echocardiography, and steady advances are being made. Ventricular diastole is composed of an isovolumic relaxation phase, during which intracellular calcium is resequestered in the sarcoplasmic reticulum by energy-dependent means, and a filling phase, during which venous return passes from the atria into the ventricles. Diastolic dysfunction can manifest as impaired isovolumic relaxation, impaired filling, or both. Isovolumic relaxation time is the interval from aortic valve closure to mitral valve opening, and it can be measured by Doppler techniques (Fig. 11–29).[25] Ventricular filling may be assessed with Doppler analysis of mitral and tricuspid valve diastolic inflow patterns, which are composed of three phases. Early (rapid) filling is represented by Doppler as the upslope of the E wave. After the peak early filling velocity is reached, there is a transition to slow filling, which is represented by the deceleration of the E wave and is measured as deceleration time. Atrial contraction produces late ventricular filling, represented by the A wave on the mitral-tricuspid inflow tracing. Pulmonary and hepatic venous flow Doppler velocity spectra can also provide insight into diastolic function, insofar as atrial inflow velocity is inversely related to pressure in the receiving chamber.

Echocardiographic assessment of diastolic function has been performed with use of all of these measures. Isovolumic relaxation time is typically increased when there is impaired ventricular relaxation and decreased when there is a

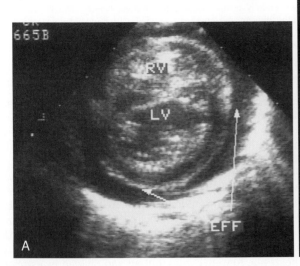

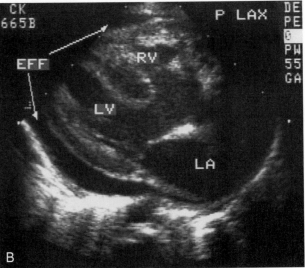

FIGURE 11–27

Pericardial effusion (EFF) can be appreciated from many views, including the parasternal short axis (A) and the parasternal long axis (B). LA = left atrium; LV = left ventricle; RV = right ventricle.

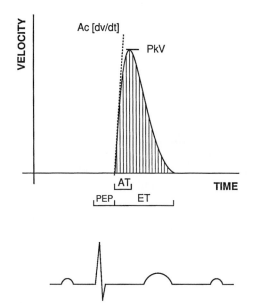

FIGURE 11-28

Graphic representation of an aortic velocity curve from which the peak velocity (PkV), the acceleration time (AT), the ejection time (ET), and the velocity-time integral *(shaded area)* can be measured. Indices of systolic left ventricular function that can be derived from these measurements include the peak rate of acceleration (Ac [*dv/dt*]), the mean acceleration (mAc = PkV/AT), and the ratio AT/ET. With the use of the electrocardiogram, the pre-ejection period (PEP) can also be measured, and the PEP/ET ratio can be calculated as another index of systolic left ventricular function. (From Silverman NH, Schmidt KG: The current role of Doppler echocardiography in the diagnosis of heart disease in children. Cardiol Clin 7:265, 1989.)

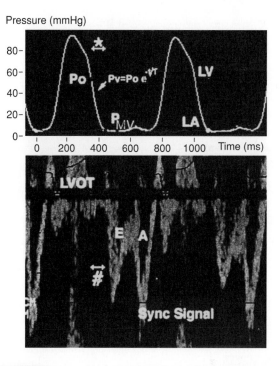

FIGURE 11-29

Combined display of left ventricular (LV) pressure and left atrial (LA) pressure *(top)* and their relationship to transmitral Doppler flow patterns. Instantaneous left ventricular pressure (Pv) follows an exponential pressure decay during early diastole (Pv = $Po e^{-t/\tau}$). Invasive isovolumic relaxation time (°) represents the period from peak $-dP/dt$ (Pv = Po) until mitral valve opening (Pv = P_{mv}). Doppler-derived isovolumic relaxation time (#) is the interval from the valve artifact at the end of the left ventricular outflow tract (LVOT) until the beginning of transmitral inflow (E). (From Scalia GM, Greenberg NL, McCarthy PM, et al: noninvasive assessment of the ventricular relaxation time constant (τ) in humans by Doppler echocardiography. Circulation 95[1]:151–155, 1997.)

restrictive pattern. The ratio of early filling to atrial filling (E/A), normally between 1.9 and 2.5 in children,[26] is decreased when there is impaired relaxation and increased when there is restrictive filling. Similarly, the deceleration time of the E wave is an indicator of ventricular compliance, being inversely related to the square of ventricular stiffness.[27] The area under the velocity-time curve of the Doppler inflow tracing correlates with diastolic changes in ventricular cavity dimension,[28] and hence volume.

Ventricular relaxation during the isovolumic relaxation interval is characterized by the maximal negative slope of ventricular pressure decay ($-dP/dt$) and by the relaxation time constant (τ), which is the inverse slope of the natural log of left ventricular pressure decay over time. The primary advantage of τ over isovolumic relaxation time and $-dP/dt$ as an indicator of diastolic function is its independence from heart rate and preload. Noninvasive estimates of these properties by use of Doppler technology correlate well with high-fidelity manometer-tipped catheter measurements.[25] More recently, color Doppler M-mode echocardiography of ventricular inflow has been proposed as a means of evaluating diastolic function, insofar as the slope of flow propagation in this mode is inversely related to $-dP/dt$ and τ.[29,30]

Tei and colleagues[31] have devised an index for assessing overall myocardial performance, including both systolic and diastolic components. Using pulsed-wave Doppler analysis of mitral valve inflow and left ventricular outflow, two intervals are measured: from cessation of mitral inflow

to onset of mitral inflow during the next cardiac cycle, and ejection time. The first represents the sum of isovolumic contraction time, ejection time, and isovolumic relaxation time. Ejection time is subtracted from this, and the difference is the sum of isovolumic contraction and relaxation times. The index of myocardial performance is the ratio of this duration (summed isovolumic contraction and relaxation times) to ejection time (Fig. 11–30). Although this index has not been assessed in children, it has been shown to correlate well with catheter-derived measurements of peak $-dP/dt$, $+dP/dt$, and τ and is likely to prove useful in a variety of populations of patients.

Valvar Physiology

Although cross-sectional methods are used to image the motion of the semilunar and atrioventricular valvar leaflets, Doppler technologies are the primary echocardiographic tools for evaluating valvar dysfunction, which can manifest as either stenosis or regurgitation.

VALVAR STENOSIS

Valvar obstruction is identified with continuous- or pulsed-wave Doppler analysis, which shows increased flow velocity during systole when the sample volume is placed distal to the stenotic orifice. Evaluation of the severity of flow ob-

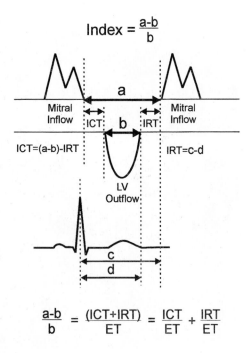

$$\text{Index} = \frac{a\text{-}b}{b}$$

$$\frac{a\text{-}b}{b} = \frac{(ICT+IRT)}{ET} = \frac{ICT}{ET} + \frac{IRT}{ET}$$

FIGURE 11–30

Schematic diagram of Doppler and electrocardiogram intervals used by Tei and colleagues[31] to determine a noninvasive index of myocardial performance. The index $(a - b)/b$ is calculated by measuring a (interval between cessation of and onset of mitral inflow) and b (ejection time [ET] of left ventricular [LV] outflow). The index is equivalent to the sum of isovolumic contraction time (ICT) and isovolumic relaxation time (IRT) divided by ejection time. Isovolumic relaxation time can be calculated as the difference between interval d (from the R wave of the electrocardiogram to cessation of left ventricular outflow) and interval c (from the R wave to onset of mitral inflow). Isovolumic contraction time can be calculated by subtracting isovolumic relaxation time from the quantity $a - b$. (Modified from Tei C, Nishimura RA, Seward JB, Tajik AJ: Noninvasive Doppler-derived myocardial performance index: Correlation with simultaneous measurements of cardiac catheterization measurements. J Am Soc Echocardiogr 10:169–178, 1997.)

struction has been standardized and greatly simplified by applying the simplified Bernoulli equation, which can be used to estimate the peak instantaneous pressure gradient from velocity measurements made with continuous- or pulsed-wave Doppler.

Based on the Bernoulli principle, the simplified Bernoulli equation holds that the pressure gradient between two points can be estimated as $P = 4(V_2^2 - V_1^2)$, where V_1 and V_2 are the proximal and distal flow velocities. For practical application in the echocardiography laboratory, proximal flow velocity is generally negligible (<1 m/sec) and this term is omitted, yielding the simplified equation $P = 4V_2^2$. This method is reasonably reproducible but requires an understanding of the principles of Bernoulli's law. Viscous forces are assumed to be minimal relative to inertial forces in the system being studied, which does not occur in long-segment stenoses or mild stenoses in a patient with increased blood viscosity (e.g., polycythemia in cyanotic patients). This technique, which yields an estimate of peak instantaneous gradient, requires consistent placement of the sample volume at the vena contracta (the point of maximal velocity at the midline of the jet immediately downstream from the stenotic orifice) because the velocity of the stenotic jet increases for some axial distance from the orifice. Continuous-wave Doppler can aid in minimizing variability due to sample volume placement, insofar as it detects the highest velocities as it passes axially along the jet length. The acoustic signal of the sample volume must also be aligned as closely as possible with the direction of the jet to optimize the sensitivity of the Doppler calculations. The sample volume is typically located with the aid of Doppler color flow mapping, which shows the direction of the jet as well as its dimensions. The simplified Bernoulli method tends to overestimate the pressure gradient of a stenosis relative to direct catheter measurements because of methodologic and physical factors[8, 32, 33]: catheterization measurements are of peak to peak pressure gradient (nonsimultaneous), whereas Doppler analysis estimates peak instantaneous gradient (Fig. 11–31); pressure is lower at the vena contracta than it is at the site of pressure recovery farther downstream, where catheter measurements are generally made owing to the difficulty of maintaining the catheter in the center of the jet; and sedation during the catheterization tends to decrease stroke volume in the basal state and hence flow velocity across the stenotic orifice. The mean systolic pressure gradient is less prone to systematic overestimation, but peak velocity measurements are less time-consuming and we use this approach in our practice.

Another useful method of calculating pressure drop is to measure acceleration time (the duration from valve opening to peak flow velocity), although other physiologic conditions (such as severe mitral regurgitation and ventricular dysfunction) can also cause the gradual rise in the velocity profile characteristic of more severe stenosis. Valvar orifice area, which may be used as an indirect indicator of function, can be estimated by a variety of techniques, including planimetry, M-mode echocardiography, the continuity equation, and measurement of pressure half-time. With an arterial level shunt, significant valvar obstruction may be indicated by diastolic flow reversal in the artery downstream from the affected valve. Color Doppler M-mode imaging may increase the temporal and spatial sensitivity for detecting flow disturbances and helping to break down complex outflow tract obstruction into its various components.

VALVAR REGURGITATION

With the advent of spectral Doppler and Doppler color flow imaging, it became possible to identify easily a regurgitant jet (reversed flow through the atrioventricular and semilunar valves during systole and diastole, respectively) even with trivial degrees of regurgitation. Unlike in stenotic lesions, however, quantification of valvar regurgitation is complicated by a number of factors. Initially, the degree of regurgitation was estimated by measuring the size of the regurgitant jet, and although this does allow gross characterization of the severity of regurgitation, it is difficult to make finer distinctions between grades with this method. Atrioventricular and semilunar valvar regurgitation pose different problems relating to quantification, primarily due to geometric features of the respective proximal and receiving chambers and to the flow dynamics in the proximal and receiving chambers.

In the ideal setting, a mitral or tricuspid regurgitant jet may be assumed to obey the laws of free jets. However,

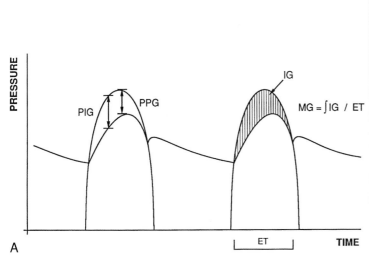
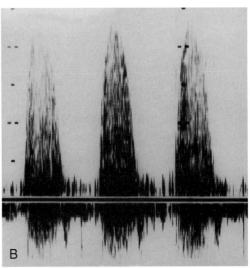

PRESSURE

TIME

A

B

A, Graphic representation of the relationship between the variables of pressure drop that can be measured at cardiac catheterization and by Doppler. The tracings represented schematically are those from ventricular and arterial pressures. Doppler measures peak instantaneous gradient (PIG), whereas it is conventional to measure the peak to peak gradient (PPG) at catheterization, even though peak ventricular and arterial pressures are not simultaneous. At catheterization and by Doppler, the mean gradient throughout systole (MG) is obtained by integrating the area of all instantaneous gradients (IG) and dividing by ejection time (ET). For measurement of the mean gradient, Doppler and manometric values are the same. *B*, Continuous-wave Doppler tracing recorded from a suprasternal notch position demonstrating an increased velocity in the ascending aorta in a patient with valvar aortic stenosis. The second and third complexes are most suitable for measurement because the envelopes are clean with well-marked appropriate peaks. Peak velocity is approximately 4.5 m/sec. By use of the modified Bernoulli equation, the instantaneous pressure drop is calculated to be 81 mm Hg. (*A*, *B* from Silverman NH: Pediatric Echocardiography. Baltimore, Williams & Wilkins, 1993, p 66.)

the shape and size of a regurgitant jet are influenced by numerous factors, only one of which is the severity of regurgitation.[34–37] Hemodynamic factors, such as the pressure in the receiving chamber, atrial counterflow, and cardiac function, influence the morphology of the jet. Geometric features of the proximal chamber, the valve itself, and the receiving chamber can have a significant impact on the flow pattern of the jet and on the Doppler color map.[34–36] In addition, instrument settings such as color gain, transducer frequency, velocity scale, and filtration can substantially alter the appearance of a regurgitant jet.[37]

To overcome these difficulties, a number of novel methods have been developed. The proximal isovelocity surface area method is based on the assumption that flow proximal to a regurgitant orifice accelerates along laminar radial streamlines and that this proximal zone is composed of concentric velocity isopleths (hemispheric shells of equal and accelerating velocities) that converge on the orifice.[38,39] When Doppler color flow mapping is used, flow accelerates into the orifice and is aliased at given distances from the orifice, depending on the Nyquist limit at which the system is set. The first flow alias forms a measurable hemisphere that reflects the boundary at which the velocity of the converging flow is equal to the Nyquist limit. Assuming that all flow entering the flow convergence region leaves the orifice as regurgitant flow, the continuity equation can be used to estimate regurgitant flow rate (Q) by multiplying the hemispheric area of the first alias shell ($2\pi r^2$, where r is radius) by the known velocity at this point (the Nyquist limit):

$$Q = 2\pi r^2 \times \text{Nyquist limit}$$

This can be performed with either two-dimensional or M-mode color Doppler imaging but is subject to systematic and physical limitations as mentioned before.

Another promising method of quantifying atrioventricular valvar regurgitation employs the laws of free jet physics. Free jets increase their mass by entraining surrounding particles and have a defined width based on an experimentally derived constant $k = 6.3$, such that the maximal width will be 6.3 times the orifice size. The larger the orifice, the broader the jet. Velocities along the central line of the jet are called the centerline velocities[40] that decay in proportion to orifice size, which can therefore be calculated from an equation relating the ratio of velocities at the orifice and at a distant point on the centerline, divided by the constant k:

$$V_m/V_o = 6.3 \times D/X$$

where V_o is the velocity at the orifice of the jet, D is the orifice diameter, and V_m is the centerline velocity at a given distance from the orifice X (Fig. 11–32). Rearranging the equation to solve for D ($D = V_m X/V_o 6.3$), orifice area can be calculated, assuming a circular orifice:

$$A = \frac{\pi}{4}(D^2)$$

The continuity equation (flow = $V \times A$) can then be employed to determine orifice flow rate (Q_o):

$$Q_o = V_o \frac{\pi}{4}\left(\frac{V_m X}{6.3 V_o}\right)^2$$

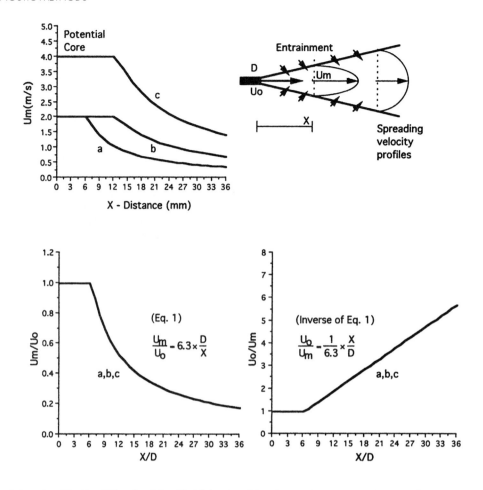

The principle of jet centerline decay is summarized by demonstration of the effects of orifice size and velocity on distal jet centerline velocity. Turbulent jets entrain fluid as they advance, causing the velocity profile to widen and the velocity to decay. At any given distance X, the maximal velocity (Vm) is on the centerline of the jet. In free jets of circular nozzle diameter (D), orifice velocity (Vo) remains constant for a short distance (defining the jet's potential core approximately = $6D$; that region of the jet where the centerline velocity is yet unaffected by the entrained mass) but hereafter decreases in a predictable fashion (Equation 1), where centerline velocity (Vm) decays with distance (X). Jet a originates from a 1-mm diameter orifice and jet b originates from a 2-mm orifice, but each has an orifice velocity of 2 m/sec. The potential core is twice as long in jet b, and after the potential core at any distance X, jet b has twice the velocity of jet a because the orifice is twice as large. Like jet b, jet c originates from a 2-mm diameter orifice, but jet c has twice the orifice velocity. The potential core is the same length for both jets, but at any distance X, jet c is twice as fast as jet b because it had twice the initial velocity. The effects of orifice size and velocity on distal jet centerline velocity are expressed compactly as Equation 1, because when jets a, b, and c are plotted as jet centerline velocity normalized to jet orifice velocity (Vm/Vo) versus distance from the orifice normalized to orifice diameter (X/D), all three jet centerline velocity curves collapse into one universal curve. The inverse of Equation 1 is a linear plot with slope = 1/6.3. (From Grimes RY, Hopmeyer J, Cape EG, et al: Quantification of mitral and tricuspid regurgitation using jet centerline velocities: An in vitro study of jets in an ambient counterflow. Echocardiography 13:357, 1996.)

Thus, flow rate can be calculated without a measure of orifice size.

Determining semilunar valvar regurgitation severity employs both color flow and spectral Doppler imaging as well. The regurgitant jet visualized during diastole with color flow Doppler is interrogated with continuous- or pulsed-wave Doppler at the center of the aortic or pulmonary valve (Fig. 11–33A, B [see Color Plates]). The velocity profile of the regurgitant jet reflects the diastolic aorta–left ventricle (or pulmonary artery–right ventricle) pressure gradient, and the velocity decay rate ($-dV/dt$) is a function of the gradient change over time. Accordingly, more severe regurgitation is reflected in a steeper velocity decay of the regurgitant jet, because the higher regurgitant volume leads to more rapid diminution of the ventriculoarterial pressure gradient (see Fig. 11–33B). Unfortunately, this method is not of great value in evaluating regurgitation in the pediatric population. A better indication of the severity of aortic regurgitation is the finding of retrograde diastolic flow in the descending aorta, which is evaluated from the subcostal sagittal view. Pulmonary regurgitation correlates best with the width of the regurgitant jet and right ventricular size. Methods for estimating atrioventricular valvar regurgitation according to the principles of free jet physics cannot be applied in the setting of semilunar valvar regurgitation, largely because the regurgitant volume originates as flow reversal after ejection in the restrictive confines of the great artery, which creates a nonideal proximal flow field. As with valvar stenosis, color Doppler M-mode imaging may be used to increase the sensitivity for detecting a regurgitant jet, whether it is atrioventricular or semilunar (Fig. 11–33C [see Color Plates]).

Vascular Physiology

Features of vascular physiology that can be evaluated with echocardiography include stenoses, compliance, abnormal connections or fistulae, flow volume, and other flow characteristics. Useful techniques include Doppler color flow, spectral Doppler, contrast echocardiography, cross-sectional imaging, and M-mode.

Vascular stenoses can be evaluated by the same techniques as described before for valvar obstruction. Doppler estimation of the peak instantaneous pressure gradient is the simplest and most common approach. The simplified Bernoulli equation is the standard method, although it may not be applicable when serial or long-segment stenoses are present. Because pressure is estimated by measuring flow velocity at a single point, with the assumption that velocity proximal to the stenosis is negligible, high-flow velocities distal to one stenosis and proximal to the next render this assumption invalid. Each successive stenosis must be measured separately, which is possible with continuous-wave Doppler, in which each separate point of acceleration appears as on the spectral display in a superimposed fashion. In addition, with long-segment stenoses, viscous forces may exert a substantial effect on the pressure drop, but these are ignored by the simplified Bernoulli equation. Arterial flow patterns distal to the obstruction, such as damping of the pulse wave and diastolic flow reversal, may also indicate significant stenosis.

Pulmonary arterial pressures and flows can be estimated with echocardiography, although not with sufficient precision to obviate catheterization when there is a concern about the state of the pulmonary vasculature. Pressure is estimated by subtracting the right ventricle–pulmonary artery gradient (predicted with Doppler imaging and the simplified Bernoulli equation) from the estimated right ventricular pressure. Right ventricular systolic pressure is calculated by determining the systolic right ventricle–right atrium pressure drop, which is estimated by applying the Bernoulli equation to the velocity of a tricuspid regurgitant jet (often pres-ent even in individuals without cardiac anomalies) and assuming a right atrial pressure of 5 to 10 mm Hg. Pulmonary arterial distensibility, which can be estimated by measuring the diastolic-systolic diameter change, may also contribute information regarding pulmonary arterial pressure. In patients with decreased pulmonary vascular compliance, late diastolic flow reversal may be evident with Doppler analysis.

Shunt Physiology

Doppler color flow mapping allows visualization of most shunts at the cardiac or great vessel level (Fig. 11–34 [see Color Plates]). The restrictiveness of a discrete anatomic shunt (such as a septal defect or patent ductus arteriosus) may be evaluated with spectral Doppler to estimate the pressure gradient according to the Bernoulli principle.

Shunts that may be more difficult to image with color flow, such as those from pulmonary or systemic arteriovenous malformations or small interatrial communications, can be analyzed by contrast echocardiography. Agitated saline is injected into a systemic vein (or artery), and the echogenic microbubbles pass through all vessels or cardiac defects larger than their diameter of 8 to 15 μm and appear downstream or in the receiving chamber (Fig. 11–35).[41]

Interchamber defects that are difficult to distinguish from valvar regurgitation with standard Doppler color flow may sometimes be clarified by increasing the color gain in the Doppler color flow mode to highlight the proximal flow convergence region approaching the low-velocity defect. The diagnosis of an arteriovenous shunt can be solidified by diastolic flow reversal in the descending aorta (distal to the shunt) in the absence of semilunar valvar regurgitation and by identifying high levels of output and associated chamber dilatation.

Shunt lesions that are most likely to be missed on echocardiographic examination are small defects that occur in conjunction with a larger, nonrestrictive defect, as in multiple muscular ventricular septal defects with a nonre-

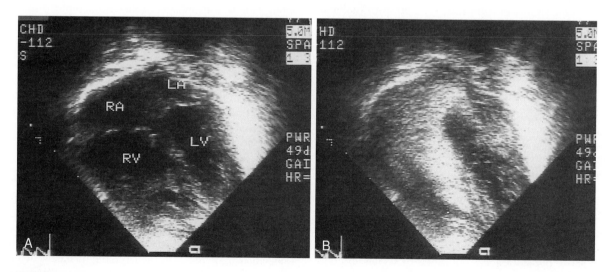

FIGURE 11-35

A, Apical four-chamber view showing right atrium (RA), left atrium (LA), right ventricle (RV), and left ventricle (LV). *B*, After injection of agitated saline into the right arm, microbubbles appear in the right atrium and enter the right ventricle. Microbubbles in the left atrium and obliteration of the atrial septum indicate a right-to-left interatrial communication. If there had been a left-to-right ventricular communication and mitral incompetence, the microbubbles would have appeared in the left ventricle before the left atrium.

strictive inlet or perimembranous defect. In these patients, there may be no pressure gradient between the chambers and no accelerative flow that can be seen with Doppler techniques.

SPECIAL TECHNIQUES

Stress Echocardiography

Echocardiography can be used to assess the effect of increased workload, or stress, on ventricular performance and hemodynamics (stress echocardiography). The increased workload is generated either by exercise[42] or by giving dobutamine.[43] Dobutamine is particularly useful in smaller patients who cannot exercise on demand. Stress echocardiography provides information about the coronary reserve, the ventricular function under increased output demands, and the response of ventricular outlet obstruction to increased output.

The procedure is similar to that performed in adults.[44,45] Images of the left ventricle are obtained from the parasternal short- and long-axis and from the apical two- and four-chamber views. These views allow visualization of the entire ventricular wall. Images are obtained at rest, at multiple levels of stress, and after recovery. The images are then compared for changes in regional wall motion (hypokinesis, akinesis, or dyskinesis). Wall motion abnormalities suggest impaired myocardial perfusion. Stress echocardiography compares favorably with nuclear medicine studies in adults.[44,45] In evaluating obstructive lesions, Doppler gradients are obtained at all stress levels and compared to assess the change in degree of obstruction. Response of the obstruction to stress is variable; some patients with minimal obstruction at rest can develop severe obstruction with stress. The increased cardiac motion, particularly combined with the motion of exercise, can make image acquisition difficult. Anterior wall segments are most affected by motion, because they are the most difficult to image even at baseline. In patients with obstructions, the examiner must measure both proximal and distal velocities; with increased output, the proximal velocity may increase to significantly greater than 1 m/sec. When this occurs, the longer version of the Bernoulli equation ($V_2^2 - V_1^2$) must be used to account for this increase.

Children who may benefit most from stress echocardiography include patients who have undergone coronary manipulation, such as after the arterial switch, the Ross procedure, or the Konno procedure[46]; those with coronary anomalies, as in Kawasaki syndrome; children with abnormal ventricular function, as in anthracycline cardiotoxicity[47]; and those with left-sided heart obstructions, such as aortic stenosis and coarctation.[48]

Transesophageal Echocardiography

The first report of transesophageal echocardiography in the pediatric population was published by Cyran and colleagues[49] in 1989, when they described their experience in patients with lower weight and age limits of 22 kg and 7 years, respectively. With the development of miniaturized transducers suitable for patients below 20 kg, the application of transesophageal scanning in children expanded rapidly.[50–55] These studies demonstrated the ability of transesophageal echocardiography to monitor intraoperative cardiac function and evaluate the adequacy of surgical repair, to demonstrate accurately most forms of normal and abnormal cardiac morphology, and to evaluate function with pulsed-wave Doppler and color flow Doppler features (Figs. 11–36 [see Color Plates] and 11–37).

The primary application of transesophageal echocardiography in children is intraoperative monitoring and evaluation of surgical repair.[54] Outside of the operating room and catheterization laboratory, transesophageal echocardiography may be valuable in larger children, adolescents, and the few smaller children who cannot be imaged completely with transthoracic transducers or when surgical dressings preclude noninvasive imaging. Compared with intraoperative epicardial echocardiography, the transesophageal approach has the advantages of not interrupting the surgical procedure and of providing multiple imaging windows for morphologic evaluation and Doppler analysis; it does not cause dysrhythmias, hypotension, or potential infectious complications associated with direct transducer contact with the epicardium. Aside from intraoperative studies, transesophageal echocardiography is not a substitute for precordial echocardiography. It is an invasive procedure reserved for patients in whom a thorough precordial examination has proved inadequate or for use during surgical and interventional cardiac catheterization procedures. Although the transesophageal approach has been a useful alternative for imaging the mitral valve in adult patients, it is less frequently necessary in infants and small children because complete precordial imaging of all important morphologic and flow phenomena is obtainable in the large majority of children.

The transducer employed for transesophageal echocardiography is mounted on a standard flexible endoscope. The pediatric transesophageal probe can be manipulated in three directions: advanced or withdrawn, anteflexed or retroflexed, and rotated either clockwise or counterclockwise relative to the sagittal plane (Fig. 11–38). Biplane and multiplane transesophageal echocardiography probes provide an additional control that allows lateral flexion. The approach to transesophageal imaging is not discussed in detail in this chapter. Scan planes differ from those of precordial imaging, but the same information can be acquired, especially in infants and children, whose hearts and thoracic dimensions are small relative to the depth resolution of the ultrasound technology used. For more detailed description of transesophageal echocardiography, the reader is referred to other sources.[9,54–57]

Intravascular Ultrasonography

Intravascular imaging employs advanced ultrasound technology to image the heart and vessels from within the lumen. A variety of transducer configurations are mounted on the tip of an endovascular catheter. The most commonly used designs provide 360-degree cross-sectional imaging at right angles to the catheter, by means of a rotating transducer or mirror or by an array of multiple crystals encircling the catheter with phased-array technology used to produce the image. Intravascular imaging is typically performed at frequencies of 20 to 30 MHz, which both allows much higher resolution than with other ultrasound techniques and limits the scanning depth substantially. As

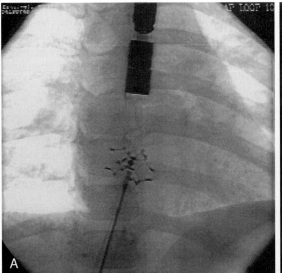

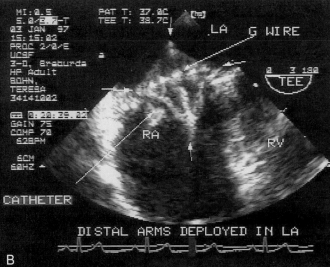

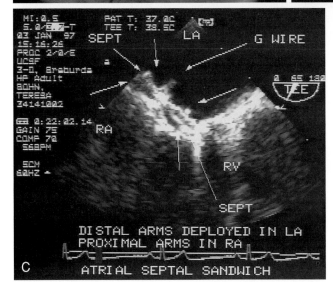

FIGURE 11–37

A, Fluoroscopy image taken during transcatheter device closure of an atrial septal defect shows the catheter in the right atrium attached to the device. *B,* A transverse transesophageal image taken during deployment of the device. The tip of the guide wire (G wire) can be seen at the center of the device, which has four arms indicated by the arrows. LA = left atrium; RA = right atrium; RV = right ventricle. *C,* Another transverse scan shows the device seated across the defect in the septum (sept), with the deployed arms indicated by the arrows.

such, currently available forms of this technology are most useful for demonstrating fine detail of vessels of relatively small caliber. With decreasing catheter/lumen diameter ratio, the potential for erroneous imaging is increased. Not only does this place the catheter at a greater distance from the arterial wall, where lateral resolution is decreased, but it also increases the likelihood of cross-sectional distortion due to non-coaxial orientation of the ultrasound catheter within the vessel (Fig. 11–39).

Intravascular ultrasound technologies offer unique advantages in terms of both morphologic and physiologic evaluation. Cross-sectional imaging can be used to distinguish the intimal, medial, and adventitial layers of an artery as well as calcifications, atheromatous plaques, thrombi, tumors, and foreign bodies. Precise measurements of luminal area are also possible. Blood flow velocity can be measured by Doppler velocimetry, by use of a flexible guide wire system with a piezoelectric Doppler crystal mounted in the tip. For simultaneous cross-sectional imaging and flow velocimetry, the ultrasound catheter may be either placed alongside or introduced over the Doppler guide wire.

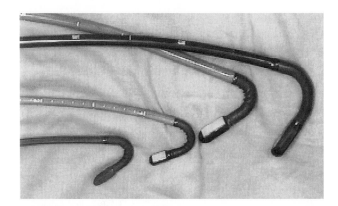

FIGURE 11–38

From top to bottom, this figure depicts adult omniplane, adult biplane, pediatric biplane, and pediatric single-plane transesophageal ultrasound transducers. The differences in transducer diameter, which range from 13 mm for the adult omniplane transducer to 8 mm for the pediatric single-plane transducer, can be appreciated, as can the increased flexion possible with pediatric transducers. The scale is indicated by the 5-cm markers on the probes.

Longitudinal View

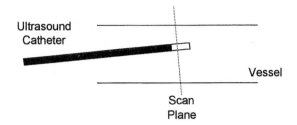

Ultrasound
Catheter

Vessel

Scan
Plane

Transverse View

FIGURE 11-39

Diagram represents the implications of an intravascular ultrasound catheter oriented in the vessel in a non-coaxial fashion (longitudinal view). The resulting transverse scan image appears as an ellipse rather than a circle.

The widest clinical and experimental application of intravascular ultrasonography has been in adult cardiology, wherein it is most often used to evaluate coronary arterial architecture before and after transcatheter dilatation, stenting, and atherectomy.[58] In children, intravascular ultrasonography has had limited clinical application. For the most part, it has been used to evaluate vascular and valvar lesions treated with transcatheter dilatation. In this setting, it may have several unique merits. The ability to visualize

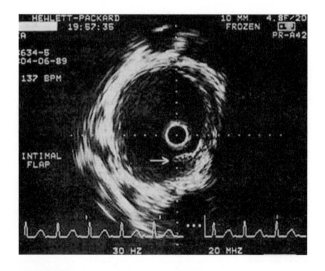

FIGURE 11-40

Intravascular ultrasound image after balloon dilatation of a native aortic coarctation showing an echogenic intimal flap (arrow). (From Sohn S, Rothman A, Shiota T, et al: Acute and follow-up intravascular ultrasound findings after balloon dilation of coarctation of the aorta. Circulation 90[1]:340–347, 1994.)

clearly intimal flaps after balloon dilatation of aortic coarctation or pulmonary arterial stenosis may help to define more clearly factors associated with successful dilatation and, ultimately, to guide the interventionalist in determining further management (Fig. 11–40).[59,60] Morphologic evaluation of the intermediate pulmonary arteries and the coronary arteries may also prove useful in certain circumstances, such as Williams' syndrome, postoperative pulmonary atresia with unifocalized aortopulmonary collaterals, and Kawasaki disease.[61,62]

Clinical use of intravascular Doppler velocimetry in pediatric cardiovascular disease has been limited to date. Nevertheless, this technology has the potential to augment currently available interventional techniques for physiologic evaluation. With current technology, intravascular ultrasound techniques are best suited for use in patients undergoing cardiac catheterization for other reasons.

Three-Dimensional Echocardiography

Cross-sectional two-dimensional echocardiography is used to create tomographic images of the heart that provide excellent morphologic detail. Because the heart is a complex three-dimensional structure, however, full appreciation of normal and pathologic anatomy requires multiple cross-sectional images to be obtained and integrated. This is usually adequate, but nevertheless, at times, three-dimensional images might improve our understanding of pathologic cardiac anatomy. Thus, it is natural that ultrasound technology would evolve to allow three-dimensional imaging. Advances in image acquisition and digital data processing technology have allowed reconstruction of three-dimensional images from cross-sectional scans. Reconstruction of real-time images is also possible, giving us dynamic three-dimensional echocardiography.

For the most part, three-dimensional echocardiography has been achieved with off-line reconstruction techniques that require acquisition of cross-sectional images from multiple cardiac cycles, with image acquisition gated to the electrocardiogram and respiratory cycle. A variety of scanning methods, including transthoracic, transesophageal, and intravascular, have been employed for this approach.[63,64] Equally spaced parallel scans can be captured with a transducer mounted on an automated sliding carriage. Images can also be obtained at equal angles across a fan-shaped sweep. A third technique is rotational imaging, in which the transducer rotates 180 degrees around the central axis of the scan plane, acquiring images every 2 seconds. These techniques, which use phased-array scanning, suffer from the need to acquire from multiple cardiac cycles and the time and manipulation required to reconstruct high-quality images. Investigators have started to experiment with parallel-array transducers to acquire equidistant parallel images from a single cardiac cycle, thus minimizing the time required for image acquisition and the error and artifact introduced from integrating data from multiple cardiac cycles.

To date, the clinical application of three-dimensional echocardiography in children has been limited. Although investigators have characterized the three-dimensional echocardiographic anatomy of various congenital heart defects,[64-68] circumstances in which three-dimensional imaging will prove practically superior have yet to be established. Even with relatively simple lesions, such as

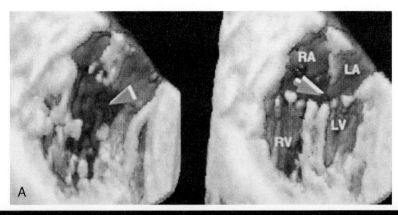

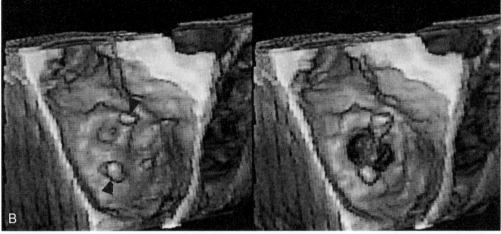

FIGURE 11–41

Select images obtained with three-dimensional echocardiography. *A,* Scans from the apical four-chamber view taken in a patient with complete atrioventricular septal defect. RA = right atrium; LA = left atrium; RV = right ventricle; LV = left ventricle. (Courtesy of Gerald R. Marx, MD.) *B,* These short-axis images show a mechanical mitral valve prosthesis in the closed *(left)* and open *(right)* positions. (Courtesy of Elyse Foster, MD.)

atrial and ventricular septal defects, defining the three-dimensional anatomy of the defect may allow more informed planning of interventional and surgical procedures (Fig. 11–41).[66–68] Another potentially useful capability of three-dimensional ultrasound technology that seems likely to extend the capabilities of echocardiography for physiologic evaluation is measurement of right ventricular volume and mass,[69, 70] which are difficult to calculate accurately with two-dimensional techniques and are of particular importance in congenital heart disease, in which the right side of the heart is frequently affected. The clinical applicability of three-dimensional imaging will likely be enhanced if scan time and accuracy are improved with the use of simultaneous parallel-array technology and if the time required for processing and image reconstruction can be reduced. For now, though, this technique is not an established component of clinical evaluation.

REFERENCES

1. Wells PNT: Biomedical Ultrasonics. London, Academic Press, 1977.
2. Hatle L, Angelsen B: Doppler Ultrasound in Cardiology: Physical Principles and Clinical Applications, 2nd ed. Philadelphia, Lea & Febiger, 1985.
3. Vermillion RP: Basic physical principles. *In* Snider AR, Serwer GA, Ritter SB (eds): Echocardiography in Pediatric Heart Disease. St. Louis, Mosby–Year Book, 1997, p 1.
4. Maslak SH: Computed sonography. *In* Sanders RC, Hill MC (ed): Ultrasound Annual 1985. New York, Raven Press, 1985.
5. Nishimura RA, Miller FA, Callahan MJ, et al: Doppler echocardiography: Theory, instrumentation, technique, and application. Mayo Clin Proc 60:321, 1985.
6. Silverman NH, Hunter S, Anderson RH, et al: Anatomical basis of cross sectional echocardiography. Br Heart J 50:421, 1983.
7. Van Praagh R: The segmental approach to diagnosis in congenital heart disease. Birth Defects 8:4, 1972.
8. Silverman NH: Pediatric Echocardiography. Baltimore, Williams & Wilkins, 1993.
9. Snider AR, Serwer GA, Ritter SB (eds): Echocardiography in Pediatric Heart Disease, 2nd ed. St. Louis, Mosby–Year Book, 1997.
10. Van Praagh S, Kreutzer J, Alday L, Van Praagh R: Systemic and pulmonary venous connections in visceral heterotaxy with emphasis on the diagnosis of the atrial situs: A study of 109 postmortem cases. *In* Clark EB, Takao A (eds): Developmental Cardiology, Morphogenesis and Function. Mt. Kisco, NY, Futura Publishing, 1990, p 671.
11. Silverman NH, Hudson S: Evaluation of right ventricular volume and ejection fraction in children by two-dimensional echocardiography. Pediatr Cardiol 4:197, 1983.
12. Shiraishi S, DiSessa TG, Jarmakani JM, et al: Two-dimensional echocardiographic assessment of right ventricular volume in children with congenital heart disease. Am J Cardiol 50:1368, 1982.
13. Helbing WA, Bosch HG, Maliepaard C, et al: On-line automated border detection for echocardiographic quantitation of right ventricular size and function in children. Pediatr Cardiol 18:261, 1997.

14. Perez JE, Waggoner AD, Barzilai B, et al: On-line assessment of ventricular function by automatic boundary detection and ultrasonic backscatter imaging. J Am Coll Cardiol 19:313, 1992.

15. Roge CL, Silverman NH, Hart PA, Ray RM: Cardiac structure growth pattern determined by echocardiography. Circulation 57:285, 1978.

16. Henry WL, Gardin JM, Ware JH: Echocardiographic measurements in normal subjects from infancy to old age. Circulation 162:1054, 1980.

17. Colan SD, Borow KM, Neumann A: Use of calibrated carotid pulse tracing for calculation of left ventricular pressure and wall stress throughout ejection. Am Heart J 109:1306, 1985.

18. Colan SD, Borow KM, Neumann A: Left ventricular end-systolic wall stress–velocity of fiber shortening relation: A load-independent index of myocardial contractility. J Am Coll Cardiol 4:715, 1984.

19. Isaaz K, Ethevenot G, Admant P, et al: A simplified normalized ejection phase index measured by Doppler echocardiography for the assessment of left ventricular function. Am J Cardiol 65:1246, 1990.

20. Sabbah HN, Khaja F, Brymer JF, et al: Noninvasive evaluation of left ventricular performance based on peak aortic blood acceleration measured with continuous-wave Doppler velocity meter. Circulation 74:323, 1986.

21. Rychik J, Tian ZY: Quantitative assessment of myocardial tissue velocities in normal children with Doppler tissue imaging. Am J Cardiol 77:1254, 1996.

22. Miyatake K, Yamagishi M, Tanaka N, et al: New method of evaluating left ventricular wall motion by color-coded tissue Doppler imaging: In vitro and in vivo studies. J Am Coll Cardiol 25:717, 1995.

23. Gorscan J, Strum DP, Mandarino WA, et al: Quantitative assessment of alterations in regional left ventricular contractility with color-coded Doppler echocardiography: Comparison with sonomicrometry and pressure-volume relations. Circulation 95:2423, 1997.

24. Mor-Avi V, Vignon P, Koch R, et al: Segmental analysis of color kinesis images: New method for quantification of the magnitude and timing of endocardial motion during left ventricular systole and diastole. Circulation 95:2082, 1997.

25. Scalia GM, Greenberg NL, McCarthy PM, et al: Noninvasive assessment of the ventricular relaxation time constant (τ) in humans by Doppler echocardiography. Circulation 95:151, 1997.

26. Snider AR: Prediction of intracardiac pressures and assessment of ventricular function with Doppler echocardiography. Echocardiography 4:305, 1987.

27. Thomas JD, Newell JB, Choong CY, Weyman AE: Physical and physiological determinants of transmitral velocity: Numerical analysis. Am J Physiol 260:H1718, 1991.

28. Snider AR, Gidding SS, Rocchini AP, et al: Doppler evaluation of left ventricular diastolic filling in children with systemic hypertension. Am J Cardiol 56:921, 1985.

29. Cohen GI, Pietrolungo JF, Thomas JD, Klein AL: A practical guide to assessment of ventricular diastolic function using Doppler echocardiography. J Am Coll Cardiol 27:1753, 1996.

30. Takatsuji H, Mikami T, Urasawa K, et al: A new approach for evaluation of left ventricular diastolic function: Spatial and temporal analysis of left ventricular filling flow propagation by color M-mode Doppler echocardiography. J Am Coll Cardiol 27:365, 1996.

31. Tei C, Nishimura RA, Seward JB, Tajik AJ: Noninvasive Doppler-derived myocardial performance index: Correlation with simultaneous measurements of cardiac catheterization measurements. J Am Soc Echocardiogr 10:169, 1997.

32. Levine RA, Jimoh A, Cape EG, et al: Pressure recovery distal to a stenosis: Potential cause of gradient "overestimation" by Doppler echocardiography. J Am Coll Cardiol 13:706, 1989.

33. Cape EG, Jones M, Yamada I, et al: Turbulent/viscous interactions control Doppler catheter pressure discrepancies in aortic stenosis: The role of the Reynolds number. Circulation 94:2975, 1996.

34. Pu M, Vandervoort PM, Greenberg NL, et al: Impact of wall constraint on velocity distribution in proximal flow convergence zone: Implications for color Doppler quantification of mitral regurgitation. J Am Coll Cardiol 27:706, 1996.

35. Simpson IA, Valdes-Cruz LM, Sahn DJ, et al: Doppler color flow mapping of simulated in vitro regurgitant jets: Evaluation of the effects of orifice size and hemodynamic variables. J Am Coll Cardiol 13:1195, 1989.

36. Maciel BC, Moises VA, Shandas R, et al: Effects of pressure and volume of the receiving chamber on the spatial distribution of regurgitant jets as imaged by color Doppler flow mapping: An in vitro study. Circulation 83:605, 1991.

37. Sahn DJ: Instrumentation and physical factors related to visualization of stenotic and regurgitant jets by Doppler color flow mapping. J Am Coll Cardiol 12:1354, 1988.

38. Aotsuka H, Tobita K, Hamada H, et al: Validation of the proximal isovelocity surface area method for assessing mitral regurgitation in children. Pediatr Cardiol 17:351, 1996.

39. Recusani F, Bargiggia GS, Yoganathan AP, et al: A new method for quantification of regurgitant flow rate using color Doppler flow imaging of the flow convergence region proximal to a discrete orifice: An in vitro study. Circulation 83:594, 1991.

40. Grimes RY, Hopmeyer J, Cape EG, et al: Quantification of mitral and tricuspid regurgitation using jet centerline velocities: An in vitro study of jets in an ambient counterflow. Echocardiography 13:357, 1996.

41. Van Hare GF, Silverman NH: Contrast two-dimensional echocardiography in congenital heart disease: Techniques, indications and clinical utility. J Am Coll Cardiol 13:673, 1989.

42. Pahl E, Sehgal R, Chrystof D, et al: Feasibility of exercise stress echocardiography for the follow-up of children with coronary involvement secondary to Kawasaki disease. Circulation 91:122, 1995.

43. Noto N, Ayusawa M, Karasawa K, et al: Dobutamine stress echocardiography for detection of coronary artery stenosis in children with Kawasaki disease. J Am Coll Cardiol 27:1251, 1996.

44. Huang PJ, Ho YL, Wu CC, et al: Simultaneous dobutamine stress echocardiography and thallium-201 perfusion imaging for the detection of coronary artery disease. Cardiology 88:556, 1997.

45. Takeuchi M, Miura Y, Toyokawa T, et al: The comparative diagnostic value of dobutamine stress echocardiography and thallium stress tomography for detecting restenosis after coronary angioplasty. J Am Soc Echocardiogr 8:696, 1995.

46. Kimball TR, Witt SA, Daniels SR: Dobutamine stress echocardiography in the assessment of suspected myocardial ischemia in children and young adults. Am J Cardiol 79:380, 1997.

47. De Wolf D, Suys B, Maurus R, et al: Dobutamine stress echocardiography in the evaluation of late anthracycline cardiotoxicity in childhood cancer survivors. Pediatr Res 39:504, 1996.

48. Cyran SE, Grzeszczak M, Kaufman K, et al: Aortic "recoarctation" at rest versus at exercise in children as evaluated by stress Doppler echocardiography after a "good" operative result. Am J Cardiol 71:963, 1993.

49. Cyran SE, Kimball TR, Meyer RA, et al: Efficacy of intraoperative transesophageal echocardiography in children with congenital heart disease. Am J Cardiol 63:594, 1989.

50. Ritter SB, Thys D: Pediatric transesophageal color flow imaging: Smaller probes for smaller hearts. Echocardiography 6:431, 1989.

51. Ritter SB: Transesophageal echocardiography in children: New peephole to the heart. J Am Coll Cardiol 16:447, 1989.

52. Stumper OF, Elzenga NJ, Hess J, Sutherland GR: Transesophageal echocardiography in children with congenital heart disease: An initial experience. J Am Coll Cardiol 16:433, 1989.

53. Kaulitz R, Stumper O, Geuskens R, et al: Comparative values of the precordial and transesophageal approaches in the echocardiographic evaluation of the atrial baffle function after an atrial correction procedure. J Am Coll Cardiol 16:686, 1990.

54. Muhiudeen IA, Roberson DA, Silverman NH, et al: Intraoperative echocardiography in infants and children with congenital cardiac shunt lesions: Transesophageal versus epicardial echocardiography. J Am Coll Cardiol 16:1687, 1990.

55. Roberson D, Muhiudeen I, Silverman NH: Transesophageal echocardiography in pediatrics: Technique and limitations. Echocardiography 7:699, 1990.

56. Muhiudeen IA, Silverman NH, Anderson RH: Transesophageal transgastric echocardiography in infants and children: The subcostal view equivalent. J Am Soc Echocardiogr 8:231, 1995.

57. Seward JB, Khandheria BK, Edwards WD, et al: Biplanar transesophageal echocardiography: Anatomic correlations, image orientation, and clinical applications. Mayo Clin Proc 65:1193, 1990.

58. Chou TM, Fitzgerald PJ, Yock PG, Sudhir K: Intravascular two-dimensional and Doppler ultrasound. In Parmley WW, Chatterjee K (eds): Cardiology. Philadelphia, Lippincott-Raven, 1996, Chapter 56.

59. Sohn S, Rothman A, Shiota T, et al: Acute and follow-up intravascular ultrasound findings after balloon dilation of coarctation of the aorta. Circulation 90:340, 1994.

60. Ino T, Okubo M, Akimoto K, et al: Mechanism of balloon angioplasty in children with arterial stenosis assessed by intravascular ultrasound and angiography. Am Heart J 129:132, 1995.

61. Rein AJJT, Preminger TJ, Perry SB, et al: Generalized arteriopathy in Williams syndrome: An intravascular ultrasound study. J Am Coll Cardiol 21:1727, 1993.

62. Sugimura T, Kato H, Inoue O, et al: Intravascular ultrasound of coronary arteries in children: Assessment of the wall morphology and the lumen after Kawasaki disease. Circulation 89:258, 1994.

63. von Birgelen C, Mintz GS, de Feyter PJ, et al: Reconstruction and quantification with three-dimensional intracoronary ultrasound: An update on techniques, challenges, and future directions. Eur Heart J 18:1056, 1997.

64. Pandian NG, Roelandt J, Nanda NC, et al: Dynamic three-dimensional echocardiography: Methods and clinical potential. Echocardiography 11:237, 1994.

65. Fyfe DA, Ludomirsky A, Sandhu S, et al: Left ventricular outflow tract obstruction defined by active three-dimensional echocardiography using rotational transthoracic acquisition. Echocardiography 11:607, 1994.

66. Rivera JM, Siu SC, Handschumacher MD, et al: Three-dimensional reconstruction of ventricular septal defects: Validation studies and in vivo feasibility. J Am Coll Cardiol 23:201, 1994.

67. Marx GR, Fulton DR, Pandian NG, et al: Delineation of site, relative size, and dynamic geometry of atrial septal defects by real-time three-dimensional echocardiography. J Am Coll Cardiol 25:482, 1995.

68. Magni G, Hijazi ZM, Pandian NG, et al: Two- and three-dimensional transesophageal echocardiography in patient selection and assessment of atrial septal defect closure by the new DAS-Angel Wings device: Initial clinical experience. Circulation 96:1722, 1997.

69. Jiang L, Siu SC, Handschumacher MD, et al: Three-dimensional echocardiography: In vivo validation for right ventricular volume and function. Circulation 89:2342, 1994.

70. Vogel M, Gutberlet M, Dittrich S, et al: Comparison of transthoracic three dimensional echocardiography with magnetic resonance imaging in the assessment of right ventricular volume and mass. Heart 78:127, 1997.

CHAPTER 12
FETAL ECHOCARDIOGRAPHY

LINDSEY D. ALLAN

Since the first reports of the prenatal identification of normal cardiac anatomy by ultrasonography in 1980, fetal echocardiography has become established as an essential part of pediatric cardiology. Accurate diagnosis of cardiac malformations can be made as early as 14 weeks' gestation,[1] although the usual timing for the examination is around 18 weeks, when all the cardiac connections can be seen in nearly every patient.

The incidence of congenital heart disease (CHD) in live births lies between 8 and 10 per 1000.[2] Some pregnancies are at increased risk of CHD in the fetus (Table 12–1). The risk of recurrence when a previous child has been affected is approximately doubled but depends on the lesion. There may be a higher rate of recurrence in the isomerism syndromes, for example, and in left-sided obstructive lesions.[3] Some authors suggest that there is a higher rate of recurrence of CHD if the mother, rather than the father, has or has had CHD.[4] Mothers with cyanotic CHD tend to be subfertile and, if they do conceive, have an increased risk of fetal loss. Maternal diabetes increases the risk of CHD by two-fold or three-fold. The risk is increased in insulin-dependent patients whether they are gestational or established nongestational diabetics. There is some debate as to whether poor diabetic control in early pregnancy increases this risk further.[5] Conotruncal malformations are said to be particularly frequent, but other malformations can occur.

FETAL PHYSIOLOGY

The fetal circulation differs from the postnatal circulation in both structural and functional characteristics. The fetal heart lies more horizontally in the thorax because of the large liver, which influences the orientation of cardiac sections in imaging of the heart. The right side of the heart is similar in size to the left side and ejects a slightly greater volume of blood throughout gestation.[6] The oxygenated blood from the placenta passes through the ductus venosus into the inferior vena cava (IVC). This stream of blood does not mix with the deoxygenated blood coming from the liver but is directed by the eustachian valve on the floor of the right atrium to the foramen ovale and left atrium.[7] Thus, the more oxygenated blood preferentially reaches the fetal brain. The ductus arteriosus connects the great arteries after their exit from the heart. Therefore, blood from the left and right ventricles mixes to pass down the descending aorta to the placenta and lower fetal body. This "open" system means that if there is change in the afterload or resistance faced by either ventricle, blood flow will be redirected to the other side of the heart. For example, obstruction to the left side of the heart lessens the shunt at the foramen or may even cause reversal of the interatrial flow.

The active tension generated by fetal myocardium is lower than that observed in adults. This may be due to a combination of a greater proportion of noncontractile protein, a difference in the activity of fetal myosin isoforms, less organization of myofibrils, and differences in myocyte function.[8] The fetal heart is less efficient in its relaxation phase and perhaps less compliant, both of which are suggested by pulmonary vein and atrioventricular valve flow patterns. Maturation in functional characteristics occurs as pregnancy advances. Systolic contraction, which can be measured by the shortening fraction of the left ventricle, is similar to that found in postnatal life. Ventricular filling is more dependent on atrial contraction (A wave) than it is in postnatal life, as evidenced from the higher A than E (passive filling) wave on the atrioventricular valve Doppler flow profile. This perhaps makes the fetus more susceptible to decompensation as a result of fetal arrhythmias. The human fetus has an intact Frank-Starling mechanism, although it may be functioning close to the end of the curve, limiting its reserve capacity. The preload of the right ventricle includes about 65% of the flow in the IVC and the flow from the superior vena cava (SVC) but will be influenced by the diastolic pressure of the left ventricle. The preload of the left ventricle depends on the foraminal flow (about 35% of IVC flow) and pulmonary vein flow and will also be influenced by right ventricular diastolic pressure. The pulmonary arteries receive about 20% of the combined ventricular output, which rises to 25% close to term,[9,10] unlike the pulmonary blood flow in the fetal lamb, which is less than 10% throughout gestation. Thus, pulmonary venous flow constitutes a significant proportion of left ventricular flow as evidenced by the small size of the left ventricle in total anomalous pulmonary venous connection.

Although each ventricle faces a different afterload (Table 12–2), the total resistance faced by each ventricle is similar in the fetus. Therefore, ventricular pressures are approximately equal, in contrast to postnatal life. Thus, a ventricular septal defect in utero shows a bidirectional shunt. Although the isthmus—the distal portion of the aortic arch—is the smallest part of the arch, there is no evidence of obstruction to blood flow at this level in the human fetus. In a normal fetus, there is forward flow in the aortic isthmus. If placental resistance rises (e.g., in placental insufficiency) or cerebral resistance falls (e.g., in a cere-

TABLE 12–1

TABLE 12–1

PREGNANCIES AT INCREASED RISK OF CONGENITAL HEART DISEASE

Maternal Factors	Risk (%)	Fetal Factors	Risk (%)
Family history of CHD			
Previous sibling	2	Fetal hydrops	25
2 previous siblings	10	Fetal arrhythmia	
Maternal	10	Heart block	50
Paternal	5	Tachycardia	2–3
Diabetes	2–3	Ectopic beats	2
Exposure to teratogens	2	Extracardiac	
		abnormality	30

CHD = congenital heart disease.

TABLE 12–2

CHARACTERISTICS OF FETAL CIRCULATION

PRELOAD OF RIGHT VENTRICLE	PRELOAD OF LEFT VENTRICLE
SVC flow	Foramen flow (35% IVC flow)
65% IVC flow	Pulmonary venous flow
Affected by LV diastolic function	Affected by RV diastolic function
AFTERLOAD OF RIGHT VENTRICLE	**AFTERLOAD OF LEFT VENTRICLE**
Pulmonary arterial bed	Cerebral resistance (dominant)
Ductus arteriosus	Upper body and aortic isthmus
Lower body	Lower body
Placenta (dominant influence)	Placenta

IVC = inferior vena cava; LV = left ventricle; RV = right ventricle; SVC = superior vena cava.

TABLE 12–3

POINTS TO NOTE IN FOUR-CHAMBER VIEW

Size	Heart occupies about ⅓ of thorax
Position	Most of the heart lies in left chest
	Interventricular septum is oriented at an angle of about 40 degrees to midline
Structures	Two atria of equal size
	Two ventricles of equal size and thickness
	Two atrioventricular valves
	Foramen ovale in atrial septum
	Intact cross at "crux" of heart
	Intact ventricular septum
Function	Atrioventricular valves open equally
	Ventricles contract equally

bral arteriovenous malformation), flow at this junction between the two sides of the heart reverses.

FETAL CARDIAC ANATOMY

The heart should be examined echocardiographically by sequential segmental analysis from the venous to the arterial poles. The easiest views are obtained in a transverse sweep of the fetus, from below the diaphragm to visualize the atrial situs, through all the cardiac structures, to the arch of the aorta in the inlet of the thorax. The most useful view is the four-chamber view, which images the pulmonary venous connection, both atria, the atrial septum, the atrioventricular junction and the atrioventricular valves, the ventricular septum, and both ventricles. The points to note in the four chamber-view are summarized in Table 12–3.

The connections of the fetal heart can be seen from as early as 14 weeks' gestation with currently available high-resolution (up to 9 MHz) vaginal transducers. These are in use for routine screening in some centers, although they are more commonly confined to high-risk pregnancies. In most patients at this early gestational age, reassurance can be offered on the normality of the cardiac connections, although a transvaginal scan should be followed by a later transabdominal scan, looking particularly for lesions that may develop later in pregnancy.[11] In general, fetal heart scanning is performed at 18 weeks' gestation. All the cardiac connections, including at least one pulmonary vein,

can be seen by this time. Rarely, in an obese patient, not all the connections are seen, and the patient needs to return a week or two later. The time taken for and the difficulty in scanning depend on the operator's experience. Most normal scans take a few minutes, but a complex difficult anomaly can take up to an hour to elucidate fully, although this is rare in my experience.

There are differing opinions on what constitutes a complete study. A study that shows color flow into the left atrium from at least one pulmonary vein, two equal-sized atria, the normal appearance of the foramen in the atrial septum, two patent atrioventricular valves, two equal-sized ventricles, two patent and normally connected great arteries, an apparently intact ventricular septum, and a normal junction of the aortic arch and the ductus arteriosus is satisfactory. Any view that shows these features is acceptable; not all possible cardiac "views" are essential. I rely on unaliased color flow mapping to ensure valve patency and do not routinely use M-mode, pulsed Doppler, or vessel or chamber measurement, although each is used in a targeted way to fully document a cardiac anomaly.

With the exception of the difficulty in excluding coarctation of the aorta in late pregnancy,[12] false-positive predictions are rare. To my knowledge, in my echocardiographic laboratory, we made a false-positive prediction in 2 of 12,000 scans since 1980; follow-up was almost complete. If the diagnosis is unclear, the scan should be repeated or the patient sent (or the videotape sent) to a more experienced observer. False-negative predictions occur but are usually related to minor anomalies, such as a small ventricular septal defect, mild aortic or pulmonary stenosis, or the milder forms of coarctation. Postnatal continued patency of the secundum atrial septum or ductus arteriosus is not diagnosable prenatally, of course. The quality of the images obtained in an individual study clearly influences the confidence one has in excluding minor lesions, but the cardiac connections should always be identifiable.

VENOUS-ATRIAL CONNECTION

Normal Anatomy

The IVC normally lies anterior and to the right of the aorta in the abdomen. It can be seen in a transverse section of the upper abdomen (see Fig. 11–4), and by moving the ultrasound beam cranially, it can be followed into the floor of the right atrium. The entry of the IVC and SVC into the right

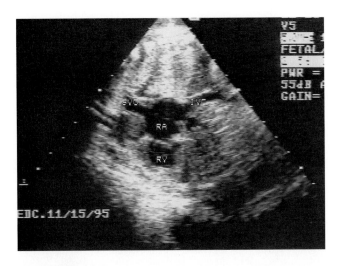

The fetus is imaged in a long-axis view to the right of the spine. The head lies to the left and the abdomen to the right in this image. The superior (SVC) and inferior caval (IVC) connections to the right atrium (RA) are seen. RV = right ventricle.

atrium can be seen in the long axis of the fetus (Fig. 12–1). The orientation of the heart in the thorax is different from that in postnatal life because of the size of the fetal liver, which extends into the left abdomen and pushes the apex cranially. Therefore, the four-chamber view is achieved in a transverse section of the thorax just above the diaphragm.

The lower left and right pulmonary veins are seen in a four-chamber view, entering the back of the left atrium on either side of the spine (Fig. 12–2). To confirm an apparently normal pulmonary venous connection to the left atrium, forward flow from the vein in the pulmonary parenchyma into the atrium should be documented on color flow mapping (Fig. 12–3 [see Color Plates]) and ideally pulsed wave Doppler in addition. As long as one pulmonary vein has been clearly identified as connected to the left atrium, this is usually sufficient for a normal fetal heart

scan. The normal pulmonary venous pulsed Doppler tracing shows forward flow throughout systole and early diastole with reversal of flow in late diastole (see Fig. 29–8). The flow pattern reflects left atrial events, the "suction" effect of atrial relaxation, followed by descent of the mitral valve orifice (late systole), passive opening of the mitral valve (early diastole), and atrial contraction causing flow reversal in late (ventricular) diastole.[13]

Abnormalities of the Venous-Atrial Connection

The normal relationship of the aorta and IVC in the abdomen is altered in left or right isomerism. In left isomerism, the IVC is usually interrupted above the level of the renal veins, and the venous return from the lower body continues instead in the azygous vein. No IVC will be found entering the right atrium. The hepatic veins enter the right atrium directly (Fig. 12–4 [see Color Plates]; also see Figs. 11–5 and 11–7B). The azygous vein lies behind the aorta and is usually seen as a prominent structure in the upper abdomen and lower thorax (see Figs. 11–6 and 11–9). The azygous vein connects to the right SVC or the left, if it is present, above the heart. In right isomerism, the IVC lies anterior but close to the aorta in the upper abdomen, usually on the same side of the fetus (see Fig. 11–4).

Abnormalities of pulmonary venous connection are not commonly recognized prenatally.[14] There is usually volume overload of the right side of the heart and dilatation of the right-sided heart structures. This diagnosis is part of the differential diagnosis when there is disproportion of the ventricular chambers. The left atrium is small, and the pulmonary veins are not seen connecting to the left atrium. The connection of the veins to the coronary sinus, or an ascending or descending vein, may be identifiable. Secondary features such as dilatation of the coronary sinus or SVC should be sought to confirm the diagnosis. A descending channel passing through the diaphragm with flow traveling caudally can sometimes be seen in anomalous connection to the IVC or portal venous system (see Fig. 29–10).

ATRIAL SEPTUM

Normal Anatomy

The atrial septum is best seen in a four-chamber view, dividing the atrial chambers in approximately equal parts (Fig. 12–5). The right atrium is anterior and the left posterior. The left atrium is related to the descending aorta posteriorly. The morphologic features of the atrial appendages are usually appreciable only when the atria are outlined by excessive pericardial fluid. The infolding of the atrial wall between the SVC and the right pulmonary veins can be seen forming the upper portion of the septum. The primum portion of the septum, which is attached to the ventricular septum at the atrioventricular junction, forms the lower part of the atrial septum. The foramen ovale occupies about one third of the atrial septum and is guarded by the flap valve that lies within the left atrium and is a marker for the left atrium. The flap valve has a biphasic motion during the cardiac cycle, partially closing at end systole and during atrial contraction (end diastole). Normally, the interatrial shunt is entirely right to left from the ductus venosus through a stream within the IVC.[7]

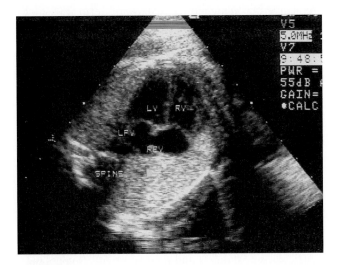

The heart is seen in a four-chamber view. The connections of the left and right pulmonary veins (LPV, RPV) to the left atrium are seen. LV = left ventricle; RV = right ventricle.

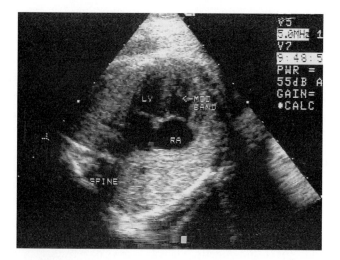

FIGURE 12–5

The heart is seen in the four-chamber view. The foramen ovale defect occupies about one third of the atrial septum. The differential insertion of the two atrioventricular valves can be seen with the tricuspid valve more apically positioned than the mitral. The moderator band also serves to distinguish the right from the left ventricle (LV). RA = right atrium.

Abnormalities of the Atrial Septum

It is impossible prenatally to detect the most common type of atrial septal defect, the secundum type, because the foramen ovale is normally widely patent. It is impossible to determine whether the foramen flap will be competent after birth. However, a large secundum defect or a primum defect is diagnosable (Fig. 12–6). An additional feature of a primum defect is the simultaneous insertion of the atrioventricular valves into the ventricular septum, with loss of the normal "offsetting." Detection of a sinus venosus atrial septal defect has not, to my knowledge, been described prenatally. In late pregnancy, it is common to see the flap of the foramen ovale "ballooning" into the left atrium (Fig. 12–7). This is a normal variant. It has been suggested that

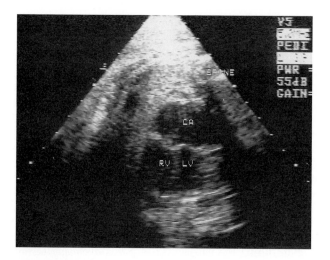

FIGURE 12–6

This fetus had left atrial isomerism and an interrupted inferior vena cava with azygous continuation. There was a large atrial septal defect and common atrium (CA). LV = left ventricle; RV = right ventricle.

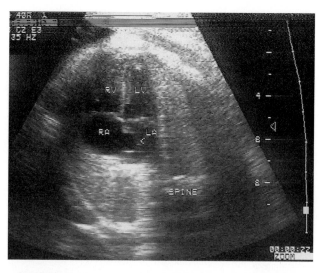

FIGURE 12–7

The flap valve of the atrial septum bulges into the left atrium (LA). LV = left ventricle; RA = right atrium; RV = right ventricle.

this causes atrial extrasystoles,[15] but both findings are common in late pregnancy.

ATRIOVENTRICULAR JUNCTION

Normal Anatomy

The atrioventricular junction is seen in a four-chamber view. The primum atrial septum can always be seen, with the septal leaflet of the tricuspid valve inserted lower in the septum than the mitral valve (differential insertion). The septal and free wall attachments of the tricuspid valve can often be differentiated from the purely free wall attachments of the mitral valve. The tricuspid valve and right ventricle lie anterior and to the right of the mitral valve and left ventricle. In the normal fetus, there is no atrioventricular valve regurgitation. The A wave, or atrial systolic wave, is higher than the E wave, or passive filling wave, in early pregnancy, becoming more equal toward term (Fig. 12–8). The ventricular septum is in line with the atrial septum and is at an angle of about 40 degrees to the midline of the thorax.[16] The right ventricular apex can be seen to be more heavily trabeculated than the left, and the moderator band is often prominent (see Fig. 12–5).

Abnormalities of the Atrioventricular Junction

Any variation from the normal features of the four-chamber view may indicate an abnormality of the atrioventricular junction.

TRICUSPID ATRESIA

This malformation can be readily detected on a four-chamber view (see Fig. 30–6). Muscular tissue forms the floor of the right atrium, and no patent valve exists between the right atrium and ventricle. There is nearly always a visible ventricular septal defect and right ventricular hypoplasia.

TRICUSPID STENOSIS

This rarely occurs as an isolated lesion. The tricuspid valve ring is small, and there is a degree of right ventricular hypoplasia.

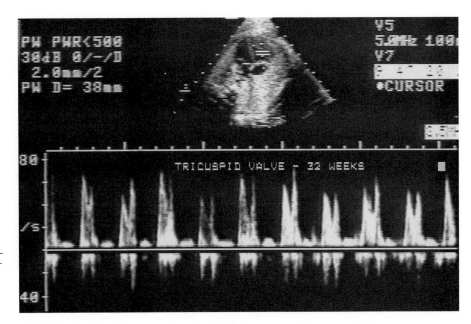

PW PWR<500
30dB 0/-/0
2.0mm/2
PW D= 38mm

TRICUSPID VALVE - 32 WEEKS

FIGURE 12–8

The typical biphasic pattern of atrioventricular valve flow is seen in the tricuspid valve. Toward the end of pregnancy, the E (early diastolic) wave and A (atrial) wave become equal.

EBSTEIN MALFORMATION

The septal leaflet of the tricuspid valve is displaced into the body of the right ventricle (Fig. 12–9). The severity of displacement is variable. There is commonly an atrial septal defect. Tricuspid regurgitation is common but variable in degree, and it can increase with advancing gestation. Right atrial dilatation is common and can be severe. If this results in severe cardiomegaly, there may be associated lung hypoplasia, which can be fatal in the immediate postnatal period.[17] Pulmonary stenosis and atresia are common associated features that tend to influence the prognosis adversely.

TRICUSPID DYSPLASIA

In this abnormality, the tricuspid valve is in a normal position, but the valve cusps are thickened and nodular. There is a variable degree of tricuspid regurgitation, which can be

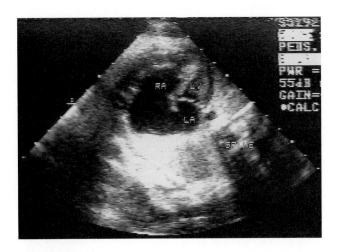

FIGURE 12–9

The right atrium (RA) is enlarged due to the downward displacement of the tricuspid valve into the right ventricle, indicating severe Ebstein malformation. There is only a small portion of right ventricle seen at the apex. LA = left atrium; LV = left ventricle.

massive. As with Ebstein's malformation, if cardiomegaly is severe, lung hypoplasia results and can be the cause of postnatal demise. There may also be associated pulmonary stenosis or atresia.

MITRAL ATRESIA

Mitral atresia can take the form of either muscular tissue at the site of the valve or a miniature imperforate mitral valve. A left-to-right shunt occurs at the atrial septum, and no forward flow occurs across the mitral valve. Mitral atresia is commonly associated with aortic atresia in the setting of the hypoplastic left heart syndrome, but it also occurs with a ventricular septal defect and a patent, normally connected aorta or with double-outlet right ventricle. The left ventricular cavity can be completely undetectable, small, and slit-like or small and globular, surrounded by echogenic hypertrophied walls (Fig. 12–10). The lesion is detectable on a four-chamber view.

MITRAL STENOSIS

This occurs rarely as an isolated lesion. The mitral valve ring is small, and there is a degree of left ventricular hypoplasia. If the atrial septum is restrictive, the left atrium is dilated.

COMMON ATRIOVENTRICULAR VALVE (ATRIOVENTRICULAR SEPTAL DEFECT)

This is one of the most common anomalies seen in the fetus, and it is readily detectable on a four-chamber view. There is a common atrioventricular valve bridging the atrial and ventricular septal defects. It can occur as an isolated cardiac malformation and is commonly associated with Down syndrome (Fig. 12–11). Alternatively, it can occur as part of a complex malformation associated with left or right atrial isomerism. In left isomerism, there is commonly an interrupted IVC with azygous continuation, complete heart block, and polysplenia. The orientation of the heart is frequently abnormal in left atrial isomerism, with the apex pointing either more centrally or more leftward. In this condition, the heart is dilated and thick walled. The

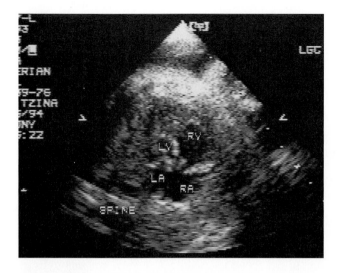

The right ventricle (RV) forms the apex of the heart. The left ventricle (LV) is a small globular cavity with echogenic walls. In the moving image, the mitral valve did not open, and there was no blood flow across the valve on color flow mapping. This, therefore, was mitral atresia. In this fetus, there was also aortic atresia, an element of the hypoplastic left heart syndrome. LA = left atrium; RA = right atrium.

natural history is for the atrial and ventricular rates to decrease and for hydrops to develop as pregnancy advances, leading to spontaneous intrauterine death. In contrast, in right atrial isomerism, there tends to be total anomalous pulmonary venous connection, double-outlet right ventricle with pulmonary stenosis or atresia, occurring in association with the atrioventricular septal defect and asplenia. These fetuses usually survive intrauterine life, but their high mortality postnatally is due to the complexity of the

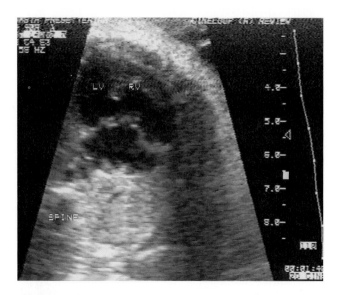

The normal "cross" appearance at the crux of the heart where the atrial and ventricular septa join the atrioventricular valves is lost in this fetus with a complete atrioventricular septal defect or canal defect. In this fetus, this was associated with trisomy 21. LV = left ventricle; RV = right ventricle.

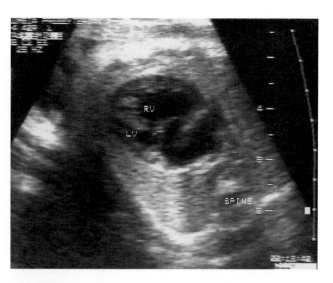

This is a complete atrioventricular septal defect with a dominant right ventricle (RV). In this fetus, there was right atrial isomerism, the aorta arose from the right ventricle, and there was pulmonary atresia. LV = left ventricle.

malformations. In fetal life, left isomerism is twice as common as right, the reverse of the ratio found postnatally, because of the high rate of fetal loss in left isomerism.

An atrioventricular septal defect with dominance of either the right or left ventricle is a common component of a complex cardiac malformation and may affect the surgical options (Fig. 12–12). This can be due to stenosis of one portion of the common valve, or the flow in the common valve can be directed more to one side of the heart than to the other.

Regurgitation of the common valve is frequent postnatally but less so prenatally. Its importance is difficult to predict in the fetus; it can remain constant, improve, or increase with advancing gestation.

DOUBLE-INLET CONNECTION

This condition can be detected in a four-chamber view because there is no ventricular septum dividing the heart into two equal parts. Both atrioventricular valves connect to a single ventricular chamber of either left or right morphology, the left being more common. In double-inlet left ventricle, the aorta usually arises from an outlet chamber on the upper border of the heart, which communicates with the main chamber through a ventricular septal defect of variable size. The pulmonary artery arises between the atrioventricular valves. In contrast, in double-inlet right ventricle, a rudimentary left ventricle is usually located posteriorly, and the two great arteries arise side-by-side from a double conus from the main chamber (Fig. 12–13).

DISCORDANT ATRIOVENTRICULAR CONNECTION

The morphologic right atrium connects to the morphologic left ventricle, and the left atrium connects to the right ventricle. There is reversal of the normal offsetting of the atrioventricular valves, with the lower atrioventricular valve insertion in the posterior left-sided ventricle. Ebstein malformation of the tricuspid valve (in the posterior ventri-

to-right shunting at the foramen ovale usually occurs in the fetus with coarctation.

VENTRICULAR SEPTUM

Normal Anatomy

The ultrasound beam should be swept from a four-chamber view cranially to image the origin of the aorta. The ventricular septum should appear intact from apex to crux and from the apex to the anterior wall of the aorta.

Abnormalities of the Ventricular Septum

In an apical four-chamber view, dropout can occur just below the atrioventricular valves, mimicking a ventricular septal defect (Fig. 12–14). To verify a ventricular septal defect, the defect must be seen in several projections, particularly in those perpendicular to the septum, and color flow must breach the septum in this orientation. There are usually "bright edges" to a true defect, whereas with dropout, the ventricular septum "fades" into the suspicious region. Defects may be seen in the inlet, trabecular, or outlet septum. Perimembranous defects are not commonly recognized prenatally.

Defects that are at least half the size of the aortic root are usually symptomatic in postnatal life. At 18 weeks, the mean aortic diameter is around 3 mm. A defect that is less than 1 to 2 mm in diameter is the lower limit of resolution of most ultrasound equipment and may not be detected. Thus, a moderate-sized defect could be missed in early pregnancy. Those undetected at later gestational ages, as the aorta reaches 6 to 10 mm in size, are likely to be less than 2 mm in diameter and therefore of no clinical significance. Lesions that cause an abnormal four-chamber view are listed in Table 12–4.

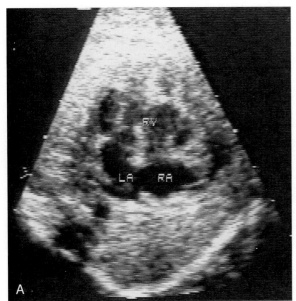
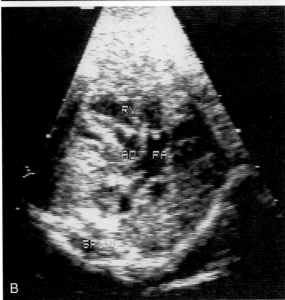

FIGURE 12–13

A, Both atrioventricular valves drain to a single ventricular chamber that was of right morphology. *B,* Both great arteries arise side-by-side from the single right ventricle (RV). In this fetus, the aorta (AO) lay to the left of the pulmonary artery (PA). LA = left atrium; RA = right atrium.

cle) is a common feature, and then the four-chamber view is noticeably abnormal. The orientation of the heart is also usually abnormal, with the ventricular septum lying at less of an angle to the midline than normal.

COARCTATION OF THE AORTA

This lesion can be inferred if there is a disproportion of the ventricular sizes with relative dilatation of the right ventricle in early pregnancy. During the last 10 weeks of pregnancy, the right ventricle appears larger than the left in a normal fetus. Further confirmation of coarctation should be sought by comparing the size of the aorta and pulmonary artery and examining the transverse arch.[12] Left-

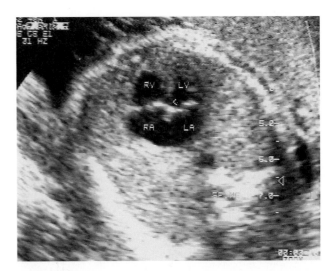

FIGURE 12–14

There appears to be a defect in the ventricular septum just below the atrioventricular valves. This artifact is due to the ultrasound beam's being parallel to the ventricular septum and the thin nature of the septum at this point. To confirm a real defect, it needs to also be seen when the beam is perpendicular to the septum as in Figure 12–24. LA = left atrium; LV = left ventricle; RA = right atrium; RV = right ventricle.

TABLE 12-4

ABNORMALITIES FOUND ON A FOUR-CHAMBER VIEW

Aortic atresia	Pulmonary atresia
Mitral atresia	Tricuspid atresia
Atrioventricular septal defect	Large septal defect
Ebstein malformation (severe)	Tricuspid dysplasia (severe)
Critical aortic stenosis	Critical pulmonary stenosis
Double-inlet ventricle	Coarctation of aorta (severe)

VENTRICULOARTERIAL JUNCTION

Normal Anatomy

The great artery connections to the ventricular chambers can be seen in a variety of projections. The easiest projections to obtain are the transverse views of the thorax. Moving cranially from a four-chamber view and maintaining a horizontal projection, the aorta can be seen arising from the posterior left ventricle (see Fig. 11–25). Moving cranial to this view, the pulmonary artery can be seen arising from the anterior right ventricle, crossing over the aortic origin to connect through the ductus arteriosus to the descending aorta (Fig. 12–15). Cranial to this view, the transverse aortic arch is seen curving from right to left to join the ductus just in front of the spine (see Fig. 11–25). By sweeping up and down the front of the thorax in this manner, the arterial connections can be identified. Alternatively, by turning the transducer into a long axis of the fetus, images more familiar to postnatal echocardiography can be seen, such as the short- and long-axis views of the left ventricle, the right ventricular outflow tract, and the aortic arch (Figs. 12–16 to 12–18). Whatever views are used to image the great arteries, certain details must be noted (Table 12–5).

For arterial Doppler studies, the transducer must be positioned so that the sample volume is placed parallel to the flow. If a satisfactory angle to the flow cannot be achieved for pulsed Doppler, nonturbulent unaliased flow across the two outflow tracts can be accepted as showing normal flow. The velocity of flow increases with gestational

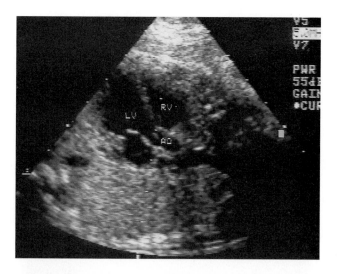

FIGURE 12-16

The transducer is tilted from the four-chamber view to image the origin of the aorta (AO) in the long axis of the left ventricle (LV). The aorta is wholly committed to the left ventricle with the anterior wall of the aorta continuous with the interventricular septum. RV = right ventricle.

age but is always a single peak in systole with no flow in diastole (Fig. 12–19). In the same fetus, the pulmonary velocity tends to be slightly lower than the aortic velocity. By use of the product of the valve area and mean velocity of flow, the ventricular output can be calculated on each side of the heart. The volume of right-sided heart output is always slightly greater than that of the left side, and both increase with advancing gestation.[10, 11]

Abnormalities of the Ventriculoarterial Junction

If the normal findings at the ventriculoarterial junction cannot be displayed, an abnormality should be suspected.

AORTIC ATRESIA

This may occur in the setting of mitral atresia in the hypoplastic left heart syndrome. The ascending aorta is small

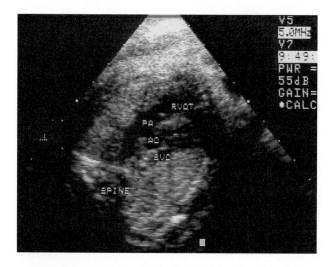

FIGURE 12-15

The origin of the pulmonary artery (PA) from the right ventricle (RVOT) is seen in a transverse section. The aorta (AO) and superior vena cava (SVC) lie to the right of the pulmonary artery.

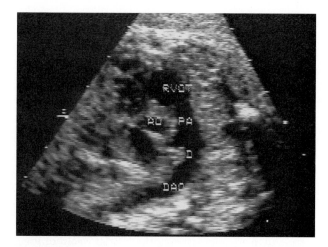

FIGURE 12-17

The fetus is imaged in a longitudinal plane to demonstrate the right ventricular outflow (RVOT) duct (D) and descending aorta (DAO). The aorta (AO) lies in the center of this scan plane. PA = pulmonary artery.

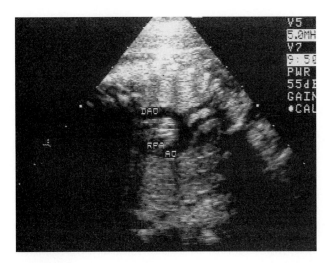

FIGURE 12–18

The aortic arch with the head and neck vessel origins is seen in a long-axis projection. The right pulmonary artery (RPA) lies between ascending (AO) and descending aorta (DAO).

or even thread-like, especially compared with the pulmonary artery, which appears "fat" in contrast (Fig. 12–20). There is no forward flow across the aortic valve, and there is reverse flow in the aortic arch. This can be seen on transverse or longitudinal views of the crest of the aortic arch and clinches the diagnosis of aortic atresia.

AORTIC STENOSIS

Critical aortic stenosis in utero produces a characteristic picture of left ventricular hypertrophy, dilatation, and dysfunction. There is commonly mitral regurgitation and left atrial dilatation (Fig. 12–21 [see also Color Plates]). The mitral regurgitation jet indicates higher than normal left ventricular systolic pressure. Left-to-right flow occurs through the foramen ovale. In some, the atrial septum is restrictive or intact. The left ventricular shortening frac-

TABLE 12–5

POINTS TO NOTE ON GREAT ARTERY VIEWS

Aorta arises from posterior left-sided ventricle
At its origin, aorta sweeps out of the heart toward the right
There is septal-aortic and mitral-aortic continuity
Aorta gives rise to arch, which gives off cranial branches
Pulmonary artery arises from anterior right-sided ventricle
Pulmonary artery crosses aortic origin
Pulmonary artery slightly larger than aorta in size
Pulmonary artery course is directly toward spine
Pulmonary artery branches laterally into ductus and branch pulmonary
    arteries
Ductus and aortic arch join just in front and to the left of spine

tion is reduced. The aorta is smaller than normal, and the aortic valve appears thickened and domes in systole. The velocity of flow across the valve is increased, but there is not the typical direct relationship between velocity and severity of stenosis that is found postnatally. This is partly because the blood has an "alternative route" through the foramen ovale to the right side of the heart in the presence of flow resistance in the left side and partly because once the left ventricle becomes dysfunctional, it can no longer produce a high gradient across the narrowed valve. In typical critical aortic stenosis, the maximal velocity of flow across the aorta is 2 m/sec, indicating a gradient of only 16 mm Hg, and there is reverse flow in the aortic arch. If the ventricle contracts well, a velocity of up to 4 or 5 m/sec can be found prenatally, and there is no reverse flow in the arch. The latter picture is much less common than the former, however, and despite the higher velocity represents less severe stenosis.

The natural history of fetal critical aortic stenosis is poor. If the aortic valve is critically obstructed early in pregnancy, it tends to become atretic with advancing gestation, and the left ventricle fails to grow normally, resulting in a typical hypoplastic left heart syndrome by term. Even if critical aortic stenosis becomes evident in late pregnancy, the chance of a successful two-ventricle repair is

FIGURE 12–19

The Doppler flow profile in the ascending aorta shows a single peak in systole at about 65 cm/sec with no diastolic flow. This is a normal velocity for this fetal age of 27 weeks.

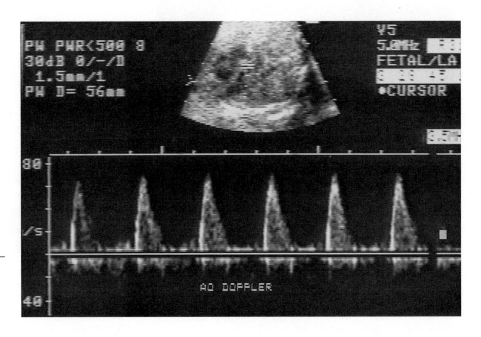

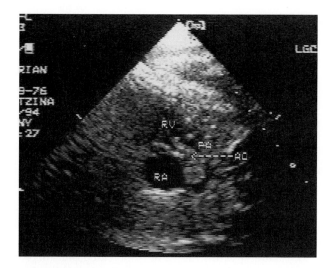

FIGURE 12–20

In the long-axis view of the fetus, the hypoplastic ascending aorta (AO) is seen. There was no forward flow within it on color flow mapping. The pulmonary artery (PA), which is a good size, is seen anterior to the aorta. RA = right atrium; RV = right ventricle.

poor. Indeed, these neonates are often impossible to stabilize in the first hours of life because of a combination of poor systemic output, restriction to pulmonary venous return, and diminished lung volume. The small lung volume is secondary to long-standing cardiomegaly from left atrial dilatation. For these reasons, prenatal balloon aortic valvoplasty has been attempted in affected fetuses in the hope of arresting the course of left ventricular damage. This can be performed by direct needle puncture of the left ventricular apex through the maternal abdomen and fetal chest wall. A balloon catheter is passed through the needle, positioned in the aortic valve orifice, and inflated. Of the fetuses in whom we attempted this technique, aortic valve dilatation was technically successful in two, and one has survived long term.[18]

PULMONARY ATRESIA

Pulmonary atresia can occur in the setting of tetralogy of Fallot, as a part of complex cardiac malformations, or as an isolated lesion with an intact ventricular septum. The last is described here. The tricuspid valve orifice is small and has little forward flow through it, and tricuspid regurgitation is often present. The velocity of regurgitation indicates the predicted right ventricular systolic pressure, which may be suprasystemic. The right ventricle is commonly hypertrophied and has a small cavity. It may contract poorly and show increased echogenicity of the walls (Fig. 12–22). If there is infundibular as well as valvar atresia, the cavity tends to be smaller, and sinusoids in the myocardium may be visible on color flow mapping. No forward flow occurs across the pulmonary valve, and flow in the duct is reversed (Fig. 12–23 [see also Color Plates]).

PULMONARY STENOSIS

Pulmonary stenosis can be of variable severity prenatally. The mild forms of pulmonary stenosis are not detectable. In moderate pulmonary stenosis, the only abnormal finding may be an increased Doppler velocity in the pulmonary artery. In some, right ventricular hypertrophy is evident. If pulmonary stenosis is severe, there is reverse flow through the duct. Severe pulmonary stenosis may progress to atresia as the pregnancy advances.[19] In addition, when there is a dilated, poorly contracting right ventricle, this can fail to grow normally with gestation, resulting in hypoplasia of the right ventricle by term. As with critical aortic stenosis, it may be beneficial to consider prenatal balloon pulmonary valvoplasty because once the pulmonary valve becomes atretic, the outlook is less favorable. Maintaining forward flow through the pulmonary valve prenatally may reduce the incidence of one-ventricle repair in this condition.

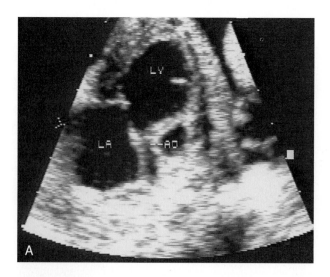

FIGURE 12–21

A, The heart is seen in the long-axis view of the left ventricle (LV). There was left atrial dilatation. The left ventricle is dilated and was poorly contracting in the moving image. The aorta (AO) was smaller than normal with increased echogenicity and poor excursion of the aortic valve. LA = left atrium. *B*, See Color Figure 12–21*B*.

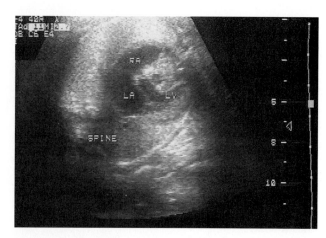

FIGURE 12–22

The heart is seen in the four-chamber view. There is a small cavity to the right ventricle with hypertrophy and increased echogenicity of the ventricular walls. This is typical of pulmonary atresia with intact septum. LA = left atrium; LV = left ventricle; RA = right atrium.

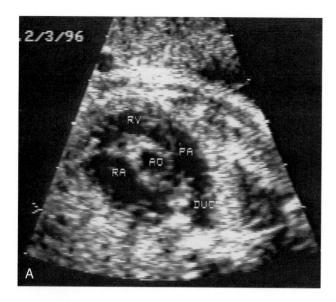

FIGURE 12–23

A, The right ventricular outflow tract (RV) and duct (DUCT) are seen anterior to the aorta (AO). On the moving image, the pulmonary valve did not appear to open although the infundibular region was widely patent. This is suggestive of membranous pulmonary atresia. PA = pulmonary artery; RA = right atrium. *B,* See Color Figure 12–23*B.*

TRANSPOSITION OF THE GREAT ARTERIES

When the great arteries are transposed, the four-chamber view is usually normal, but on great artery views, there is no "crossover" of the pulmonary artery over the aorta. The great arteries arise in parallel orientation, with the aorta from the right ventricle and the pulmonary artery from the left (Fig. 12–24). Because simple transposition has a different operative outlook in terms of both strategy and risk, for example, from transposition with a ventricular septal defect and pulmonary stenosis or transposition with a ventricular septal defect and coarctation, it is important to look carefully for additional features before counseling the parents. Simple transposition is rarely associated with extracardiac malformations or chromosome anomalies.

DOUBLE-OUTLET RIGHT VENTRICLE

In double-outlet right ventricle, the four-chamber view is also usually normal. The great arteries usually arise in parallel orientation from the right ventricle, but in some, the great arteries are normally related. Double-outlet right ventricle can coexist with a simple ventricular septal defect, an atrioventricular septal defect, mitral atresia, or hypoplasia of either ventricle. Pulmonary stenosis of variable severity is common and can progress during intrauterine life to atresia. Coarctation is less common but also occurs. The prognosis and operative management depend on the associated cardiac lesions. In addition, double-outlet right ventricle can be associated with extracardiac malformations and chromosome anomalies.

COMMON ARTERIAL TRUNK

The four-chamber view is normal, but only one great artery arises from the heart. The truncal valve is usually thickened and dysplastic and overrides the crest of the ventricular septum (Fig. 12–25). There is always a velocity of flow above the normal range for the aorta at about 1.5 m/sec,[20] but if it is higher than this, this implies a degree of truncal valve stenosis that has a high intrauterine or immediate postnatal mortality. There is commonly truncal regurgitation, but it varies in degree from trivial to severe. Severe truncal regurgitation becomes severe aortic regurgitation after repair.

In fetal life, the pulmonary artery can be seen arising from the common trunk. If the main pulmonary artery arises from the trunk or the branch pulmonary arteries arise close together, the repair seems to be easier than when the branch pulmonary artery origins are widely separated. Some surgeons use a pericardial tunnel to connect the right ventricle to the pulmonary arteries with the belief that this will not require as many revisions with growth of the child, but a conduit is usually used that will require two or more replacements. Common arterial trunk can be associated with a microdeletion of chromosome 22, which

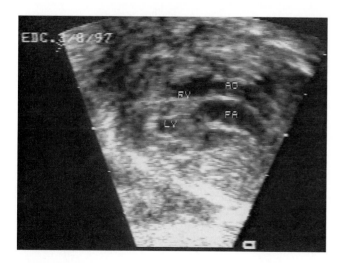

FIGURE 12–24

The two great arteries arise in parallel orientation with the aorta (AO) arising anteriorly from the right ventricle (RV) and the pulmonary artery (PA) from the left ventricle (LV).

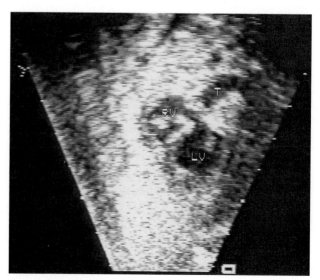

FIGURE 12–25

Only one great artery (T) arose from the heart astride the crest of the ventricular septum. The truncal valve was seen to be thickened and dysplastic. LV = left ventricle; RV = right ventricle.

can be detected on chromosome analysis of fluid from amniocentesis. These aspects need to be considered in evaluating a fetus before counseling of the parents.

TETRALOGY OF FALLOT WITH PULMONARY STENOSIS

The four-chamber view is normal, but aortic override is seen on examination of the left ventricular outflow tract. In addition, the pulmonary artery is smaller than the aorta, which is in contrast to a normal fetus. The aorta/pulmonary artery ratio is above the normal range.[20] The severity of pulmonary stenosis can progress during fetal life even to pulmonary atresia.[21] In addition, the growth of the branch pulmonary arteries fails to keep pace with the rest of fetal growth. Thus, branch pulmonary arteries that appeared of good size in early pregnancy can become hypoplastic by term. This is unpredictable, although in general, the smallest branch pulmonary arteries in early pregnancy tend to be the smallest at birth.

Complex forms of tetralogy such as those with the absent pulmonary valve syndrome are preferentially detected in fetal life. In addition, there is a high rate of association of tetralogy with extracardiac malformations such as omphalocele, tracheoesophageal atresia, and diaphragmatic hernia, often as part of VATER or CHARGE syndromes, and chromosome defects. The natural history of tetralogy of Fallot when it is detected initially in the fetus is much less favorable than the postnatal outlook.[22]

TETRALOGY OF FALLOT WITH PULMONARY ATRESIA

This more extreme form of tetralogy lacks a patent connection between the right ventricle and the pulmonary trunk. The pulmonary arteries are supplied by reverse flow in the ductus arteriosus or by collateral arteries, which can sometimes be detected in the fetus. In general, the smaller the ductus, the more likely there are to be collateral arteries. It is important to search for the pulmonary artery confluence in the mediastinum because patients with other nonconfluent or severely hypoplastic branch pulmonary arteries face much more difficult, often staged, operative procedures and have a poorer long-term outlook. This malformation can be associated with chromosome anomalies, particularly a microdeletion of chromosome 22.

AORTIC ARCH

Normal Anatomy

In a normal fetus, the aortic arch can be evaluated in both transverse and longitudinal views. The transverse view is more useful because the distal arch can be followed to its connection to the duct, and the two vessels can be directly compared in size—they should be equal in diameter. The longitudinal view shows the tight "hook" shape of the normal arch as it arises from the left ventricle and forms the arch. The right pulmonary artery and left atrium lie within the hook. Three brachiocephalic arteries can be seen arising from the crest of the arch.

Abnormalities of the Aortic Arch

The side of the aortic arch can be readily shown in fetal life, using the horizontal view of the arch. This is important to note in tetralogy of Fallot, because those with a right arch have an increased incidence of a microdeletion of chromosome 22. In addition, the side of the arch is impor-

tant in planning the placement of a Blalock-Taussig shunt in any malformation in which the pulmonary blood flow is reduced. Coarctation of the aorta is usually not detectable in the long-axis view of the arch, but hypoplasia of the transverse arch compared in size with the duct can suggest coarctation. The arch in fetuses with coarctation becomes progressively more hypoplastic with advancing gestation. In the fetus, coarctation of the aorta is frequently associated with chromosome anomalies. In counseling the parents of a fetus with coarctation, additional intracardiac defects, progression of the obstruction with gestation, and the possibility of chromosome anomalies must all be considered.

In interruption of the aortic arch, the ascending aorta is usually noticeably small, and the transverse arch is not in its usual position. The "V" sign or division of the aorta into two branches, in the most common interrupted arch type B, can be detected on fetal sections that would normally show the complete arch. Interrupted aortic arch type B is commonly associated with a microdeletion of chromosome 22.

ADDITIONAL MISCELLANEOUS ANOMALIES

A common finding in a four-chamber view is a bright echogenic spot (or "golf ball") within the ventricular cavity, most commonly on the left side (Fig. 12–26). This is due to calcium deposition within the papillary muscles, usually of the mitral valve, and has no cardiologic significance. It may be associated, however, with an increased risk of Down syndrome.[23, 24]

A cardiac tumor can present prenatally as a cardiac mass, ectopic beats, or tachycardia or with fetal hydrops. Rhabdomyomas are the most common.[25] Tumors are rarely seen before 20 weeks' gestation, even in an affected pregnancy. They tend to increase in size during fetal life under the influence of maternal hormones and shrink postnatally. They can obstruct inflow to, or outflow from, either ventricular chamber (Fig. 12–27). If multiple, they are likely to be associated with tuberous sclerosis. If the tumor mass is cystic

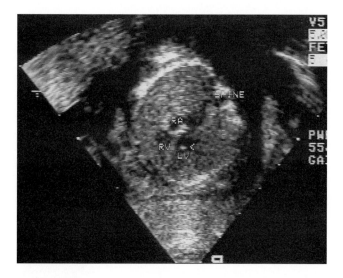

FIGURE 12–26

There is a bright echogenic "spot" (*arrow*) in the cavity of the left ventricle (LV). This has no cardiac significance but can be associated with chromosome defects. RA = right atrium; RV = right ventricle.

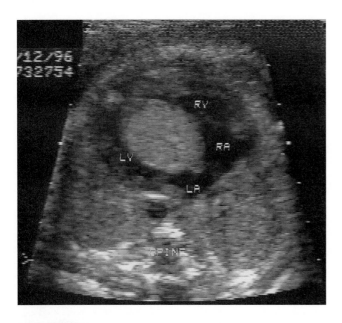

There is a large tumor in the interventricular septum. Despite its size, there was no acceleration to ventricular inflow or outflow on either side of the heart. LA = left atrium; LV = left ventricle; RA = right atrium; RV = right ventricle.

and pericardial, the diagnosis is usually teratoma. For all prenatal cardiac tumors, there is a high rate of spontaneous intrauterine death. The outlook in terms of neurologic development for associated tuberous sclerosis is poor.

Ectopia cordis is a rare anomaly in which the heart lies wholly outside the chest cavity. The heart appears to float freely in the amniotic cavity. Cardiac malformations are common, and successful repair is unlikely. A partial form of this anomaly is the pentalogy of Cantrell, which is more amenable to reparative operation.

Conjoint twins are a disorder of the twinning process. If they are joined at the thorax, they can share cardiac chambers. A complex malformation can result, and neither twin usually survives attempts to separate them.

MANAGEMENT AND COUNSELING

Management of the pregnancy concerns the option of termination or the timing, method, and place of delivery. The option of termination varies in different societies, but for fetal malformation, it is usually available before 24 weeks. It is a highly individual choice influenced by many social, religious, and personal factors too complex for discussion here. Medical factors to be considered include the gestational age at diagnosis, the presence of associated extracardiac malformations, and the cardiac diagnosis itself. In a continuing pregnancy, the fetus must have a thorough anatomic scan to exclude extracardiac malformations as far as this is possible. In most, karyotyping should be performed to exclude chromosome defects, although the risk is higher in some lesions, such as atrioventricular septal defect, than in others. In some cardiac malformations, such as interrupted aortic arch type B, tetralogy of Fallot, and common arterial trunk, a microdeletion of chromosome 22 must be specifically looked for in amniotic fluid.

TABLE 12–6
CARDIAC MALFORMATIONS THAT MAY BENEFIT FROM DELIVERY AT CARDIAC CENTER

Duct-dependent systemic circulation
    Aortic atresia
    Critical aortic stenosis
    Coarctation of aorta
    Interruption of aorta
Duct-dependent pulmonary circulation
    Pulmonary atresia (isolated or in complex CHD)
    Critical pulmonary stenosis
Potentially inadequate mixing situation
    Transposition of great arteries
    Total anomalous pulmonary venous connection

CHD = congenital heart disease.

The management of labor and delivery must be considered. It is not usually useful to deliver a fetus with congenital heart disease early unless the fetus shows signs of intrauterine deterioration. This might occur in critical aortic stenosis or in a fetus with hydrops, but it is unusual. A normal delivery should be expected in most, because the problem is usually structural rather than functional. Some perinatologists prefer to deliver a fetus with complete heart block by cesarean section, because the heart rate monitor cannot be used in this setting to indicate fetal distress. The place of delivery is important in some, although not all, fetal cardiac malformations. Those fetuses in whom the postnatal circulation is likely to be duct dependent should be delivered at or as near as possible to the site of intended cardiac operation (Table 12–6).

With practice and experience, the diagnosis of fetal congenital heart malformations is usually straightforward, although sometimes it is technically difficult. Much more challenging, however, is the counseling. This involves presenting a clear picture to the parents of what the anomaly is, what it means for the child's future, and what can be offered in terms of treatment. This should be done in an unbiased fashion, but the person offering counseling must have a clear idea of the natural history of fetal CHD, which is different from that seen in postnatal practice. The possible association with extracardiac malformations or chromosome defects must be considered. The potential for change or progression must be included in the counseling (Table 12–7). For example, progressive atrioventricular valve regurgitation, increasing valvar stenosis, and increasing hypoplasia of cardiac chambers or arterial vessels have been observed with advancing pregnancy. These changes alter the outlook for the fetus and the postnatal management. If the gestational age and the law allow, termination

TABLE 12–7		
LESIONS THAT CAN PROGRESS PRENATALLY		
Valvar stenosis	Mild to severe	
	Severe stenosis to atresia	
Growth failure	Ventricular chamber in aortic or pulmonary stenosis	
	Aorta or pulmonary artery in aortic or pulmonary stenosis	
	Aortic arch in coarctation	
Valvar incompetence	Ebstein's malformation or tricuspid dysplasia	
	Common valve	

TABLE 12–8

TYPES OF FETAL ARRHYTHMIA

	Cause	Risk of CHD (%)	Outcome
Irregular rhythm	PACs, PVCs	2	Good
Bradycardia	Coupled PACs	2	Good
	Isolated CHB	—	30% mortality
	CHB + CHD	100	90% mortality
Tachycardia	Re-entrant	2	Good if no cardiac failure
	Atrial flutter	2	Good if no cardiac failure

CHB = complete heart block; CHD = congenital heart disease; PACs = premature atrial contractions; PVCs = premature ventricular contractions.

of pregnancy must always be raised with the patient. It is the duty of the counselor to help the parents to reach a decision that is correct for them and their circumstances and to support their decision.

ARRHYTHMIAS

Three types of fetal rhythm disturbance are a source of referral—tachycardia, bradycardia, and an irregular rhythm (Table 12–8). Arrhythmias should be assessed by M-mode echocardiography positioned through the fetal heart to show the relationship between atrial and ventricular contractions (Fig. 12–28). Atrial contraction normally precedes ventricular contraction by 80 to 120 milliseconds at a normal fetal heart rate of 140 beats per minute. An irregular heart rhythm is the most common rhythm disturbance, and it is due to either atrial or ventricular premature contractions. These are found frequently, especially in the last 10 weeks of pregnancy, and are benign. They disappear spontaneously toward term. There is a slight increase in the risk of associated fetal cardiac malformation, so this should be excluded by a fetal echocardiogram. On occasion, coupled atrial premature contractions can be difficult to distinguish from complete heart block (Fig. 12–29). In

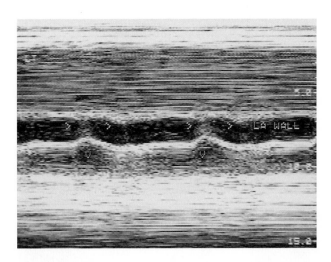

FIGURE 12–29

The atrial rate *(arrows)* in the left atrial (LA) wall is irregular, showing a sinus beat followed by an ectopic atrial beat, followed by a pause before the next sinus beat. The ventricle (V) is responding only to the sinus atrial contraction, and the ventricular rate is therefore about 80 beats per minute. This is an example of blocked atrial ectopic beats producing a bradycardia.

addition, the heart rate should be checked as the pregnancy continues for tachycardias that can occasionally be triggered by frequent premature beats.

Short episodes of fetal bradycardia are common in early pregnancy and of no significance. A sustained bradycardia, however, demands investigation. Sustained sinus bradycardia, with a one-to-one relationship between the atria and ventricles, can sometimes be seen in a preterminal fetus. There are usually other signs of impending death, such as fetal hydrops, lack of fetal movement, and fetal malformation. In complete heart block, the atrial contractions are usually at the normal rate of 140 beats per minute and unrelated to the slower ventricular rate (Fig. 12–30). In the fe-

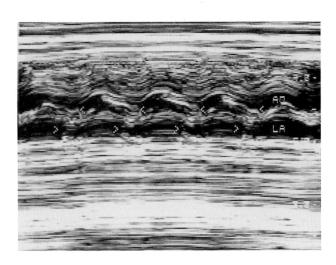

FIGURE 12–28

The M-mode cursor is positioned across the aortic root (AO) and left atrium (LA) posteriorly. Every opening of the aortic valve *(upper arrows)* is preceded by an atrial contraction *(lower arrows)* with a time interval of about 100 milliseconds. The heart rate is 140 beats per minute.

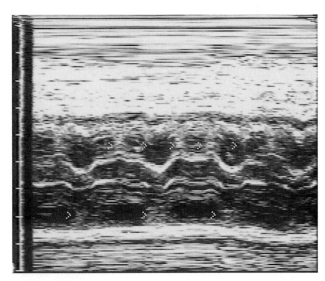

FIGURE 12–30

The M-mode tracing records atrial and ventricular contraction simultaneously. The atrial wall *(upper arrows)* contracts at about 140 beats per minute whereas the ventricular wall (LV) *(lower arrows)* contracts at 55 beats per minute, representing heart block.

tus, complete heart block occurs either as an isolated lesion or in association with a heart malformation.[26] When heart block is isolated, it usually occurs in association with maternal collagen disease, frequently subclinical, but with circulating anti-Ro antibody. These antibodies cross the placenta and damage the fetal conducting tissue. Complete heart block usually develops between 18 and 24 weeks of gestation, but it can develop later. When complete heart block is found, heart rate, cardiac size, arterial Doppler velocities, and left ventricular shortening fraction should be measured and followed sequentially. Most fetuses do well, and only about one third require pacing in early childhood. Some decompensate prenatally, however, and develop intrauterine cardiac failure that is associated with a poor outcome. These patients may benefit from the use of sympathomimetic agents, such as salbutamol or terbutaline, to increase the fetal heart rate.[27] When heart block is associated with cardiac anomalies, the outcome depends on the cardiac lesion. This is usually an atrioventricular septal defect with left atrial isomerism, for which there is a high mortality rate. Spontaneous intrauterine death usually occurs during the second or early third trimester of pregnancy.

Tachycardias are defined as a fetal heart rate above 200 beats per minute. Most fetuses have a supraventricular tachycardia at 240 beats per minute (Fig. 12–31), although atrial flutter or rarely ventricular tachycardias occur. The treatment and outcome depend on the type of tachycardia and the presence or absence of intrauterine cardiac failure. Elective premature delivery should be avoided until at least 36 weeks' gestation and should be a last resort after failure of medical therapy. In the nonhydropic fetus, treatment should be started with digoxin, 0.75 mg/day, given to the mother. If conversion to sinus rhythm has not occurred after 2 weeks with maternal serum levels at 2.0 μg/l, verapamil, 40 mg three times a day, increasing to a maximum of 240 mg/day, can be added. This will usually effect conversion in a fetus without heart failure.[28, 29] A hydropic fe-

tus, however, rarely converts with oral digoxin alone owing to poor placental transfer, although some workers suggest that intravenous digoxin administered to the mother is more effective.[30] Success has also been associated with the use of flecainide, 100 mg three times a day.[31] This drug is well transported across the placenta, even in a hydropic fetus, and has allowed clearance of hydrops and delivery at term in most fetuses treated. However, this drug has a recognized occurrence of sudden death. The risk is around 10% mortality. Alternative anti-arrhythmic therapy includes digoxin, adenosine, or amiodarone by direct fetal injection,[32] but cordocentesis probably carries the same risk of fetal loss as does oral maternal flecainide. There is also anecdotal evidence of the usefulness of quinidine, procainamide, or sotalol.

FUTURE DIRECTIONS

Within the next 10 years, skilled evaluation of the fetal heart at an early stage in every pregnancy will become the standard of practice. A greater number of parents will have information about complex cardiac malformation at a stage in pregnancy when interruption is a possible management option. This will increase the rate of termination of affected pregnancies, altering the spectrum of conditions presenting in infancy.[33] At the same time, operative results are likely to improve, such that more parents may be willing to continue with an affected pregnancy. It is difficult to predict how the debate over termination of pregnancy will proceed in the coming years, and it is likely to be different in different parts of the world. In general, as living standards improve, parents strive to ensure that their children are healthy, even if this involves the reluctant choice of interrupting an abnormal pregnancy. The movement is certainly toward more and better information so that they can be actively involved with management decisions. Early operative results are likely to be improved by optimizing perinatal management.[34] There is a small subsection of forms of CHD that may benefit from prenatal intervention, such as balloon valvoplasty or pacemaker insertion.[35] It seems unlikely that open uterus operations with the attendant maternal morbidity will establish a useful place in treatment. Endoscopic approaches to operative procedures are advancing rapidly and offer attractive possibilities for prenatal treatment, however.

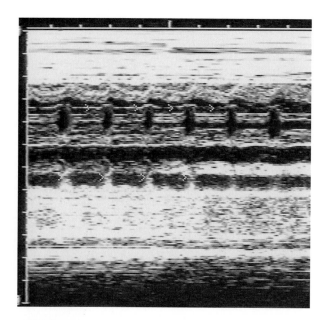

FIGURE 12–31

There is a one-to-one relationship between the atrial *(lower arrows)* and ventricular *(upper arrows)* wall motion. This is a supraventricular tachycardia at 240 beats per minute.

REFERENCES

1. Achiron R, Weissman A, Rotstein Z, et al: Transvaginal echocardiographic examination of the fetal heart between 13 and 15 weeks' gestation in a low-risk population. J Ultrasound Med 13:783, 1994.
2. Jackson M, Walsh KP, Peart I, Arnold R: Epidemiology of congenital heart disease in Merseyside—1979–1988. Cardiol Young 6:272, 1996.
3. Allan LD, Crawford DC, Chita SK, et al: The familial recurrence of congenital heart disease in a prospective series of mothers referred for fetal echocardiography. Am J Cardiol 58:334, 1986.
4. Nora JJ, Nora AH: Maternal transmission of congenital heart diseases: New recurrence risk figures and the questions of cytoplasmic inheritance and vulnerability to teratogens. Am J Cardiol 59:459, 1987.
5. Shield LE, Gan EA, Murphy HF, et al: The prognostic value of hemoglobin A$_{1c}$ in predicting fetal heart disease in diabetic pregnancies. Obstet Gynecol 81:954, 1993.

6. Kenny JF, Plappert E, Doubilet P, et al: Changes in intracardiac blood flow velocities and right and left ventricular stroke volumes with gestational age in normal fetuses: A prospective Doppler echocardiographic study. Circulation 74:1208, 1986.

7. Kiserud T, Eik-Nes SH, Blaas HG, Hellevik LR: Foramen ovale: An ultrasonographic study of its relation to the inferior vena cava, ductus venosus and hepatic veins. Ultrasound Obstet Gynecol 2:389, 1992.

8. Fouron JC: Fetal cardiac function and circulatory dynamics—the impact of Doppler echocardiography. Cardiol Young 6:120, 1996.

9. Rasanen J, Wood DC, Weiner S, et al: Role of the pulmonary circulation in the distribution of human fetal cardiac output during the second half of pregnancy. Circulation 94:1068, 1996.

10. Sutton MS, Groves A, MacNeill A, et al: Assessment of changes in blood flow through the lungs and foramen ovale in the normal human fetus with gestational age: A prospective Doppler echocardiographic study. Br Heart J 71:232, 1994.

11. Yagel S, Weissman A, Rotstein Z, et al: Congenital heart defects: Natural course and in utero development. Circulation 96:950, 1997.

12. Sharland GK, Chan K, Allan LD: Coarctation of the aorta: Difficulties in prenatal diagnosis. Br Heart J 71:70, 1994.

13. Better DJ, Kaufman S, Allan LD: The normal pattern of pulmonary venous flow on pulsed Doppler examination of the human fetus. J Am Soc Echocardiogr 9:281, 1996.

14. Allan LD, Sharland GK, Milburn A, et al: Prospective diagnosis of 1,006 consecutive cases of congenital heart disease in the fetus. J Am Coll Cardiol 23:1452, 1994.

15. Rice MJ, McDonald RW, Reller MD: Fetal atrial septal aneurysm: A cause of fetal atrial arrhythmias. J Am Coll Cardiol 12:1292, 1988.

16. Smith RS, Comstock CH, Kirk JS, Lee W: Ultrasonographic left cardiac axis deviation: A marker for fetal anomalies. Obstet Gynecol 85:187, 1995.

17. Sharland GK, Chita SK, Allan LD: Tricuspid valve dysplasia or displacement in intrauterine life. J Am Coll Cardiol 17:944, 1991.

18. Maxwell DJ, Allan LD, Tynan M: Balloon aortic valvoplasty in the fetus: A report of two cases. Br Heart J 65:256, 1991.

19. Rice MJ, McDonald RW, Reller MD: Progressive pulmonary stenosis in the fetus: Two case reports. Am J Perinatol 10:424, 1993.

20. Sharland GK, Allan LD: Normal fetal cardiac measurements derived by cross-sectional echocardiography. Ultrasound Obstet Gynecol 2:175, 1992.

21. Hornberger LK, Sanders SP, Sahn DJ, et al: In utero pulmonary artery and aortic growth and potential for progression of pulmonary outflow tract obstruction in tetralogy of Fallot. J Am Coll Cardiol 25:739, 1995.

22. Allan LD, Sharland GK: The prognosis in fetal tetralogy of Fallot. Pediatr Cardiol 13:1, 1992.

23. Sepulveda W, Cullen S, Nicolaidis P, et al: Echogenic foci in the fetal heart: A marker of chromosomal abnormality. Br J Obstet Gynaecol 102:490, 1995.

24. Simpson JM, Cook A, Sharland GK: The significance of echogenic foci within the fetal heart: A prospective study of 228 cases. Obstet Gynecol 8:225, 1996.

25. Groves AM, Fagg NLK, Cook AC, Allan LD: Cardiac tumours in intrauterine life. Arch Dis Child 67:1189, 1992.

26. Machado MVL, Tynan MJ, Curry PVL, Allan LD: Fetal complete heart block. Br Heart J 60:512, 1988.

27. Groves AM, Allan LD, Rosenthal E: Therapeutic trial of sympathomimetics in three cases of complete heart block in the fetus. Circulation 92:3394, 1995.

28. Maxwell DJ, Crawford DC, Curry PVM, et al: Obstetric importance, diagnosis and management of fetal tachycardias. Br Med J 297:107, 1988.

29. Van Engelen AD, Weijtens O, Brenner JI, et al: Management, outcome and follow-up of fetal tachycardia. J Am Coll Cardiol 24:1371, 1994.

30. Azancot-Benisty A, Jacqz-Algrain E, Guirgis NM, et al: Clinical and pharmacological study of fetal supraventricular tachyarrhythmias. J Pediatr 121:608, 1992.

31. Allan LD, Chita SK, Priestly K, et al: Flecanide in the treatment of fetal tachycardias. Br Heart J 65:46, 1991.

32. Gembruch U, Redel DA, Bald R, Hansmann M: Longitudinal study in 18 cases of fetal supraventricular tachycardia: Doppler echocardiographic findings and pathophysiologic implications. Am Heart J 125:1290, 1993.

33. Allan LD, Cook A, Sullivan I, Sharland GK: Changing birth prevalence of the hypoplastic left heart syndrome as a result of fetal echocardiography. Lancet 337:959, 1991.

34. Chang AC, Huhta JC, Yoon GY, et al: Diagnosis, transport and outcome in fetuses with left ventricular outflow obstruction. J Thorac Cardiovasc Surg 102:841, 1991.

35. Hanley FL: Fetal cardiac surgery. Adv Card Surg 5:47, 1994.

CHAPTER 13

CARDIAC CATHETERIZATION HEMODYNAMICS AND INTERVENTION

CHARLES E. MULLINS   MICHAEL R. NIHILL

Catheterization of the cardiovascular system developed as a method to understand the anatomy and physiology of the circulation. Modifications and improvements in operative, imaging, and catheterization techniques have changed the role of cardiac catheterization in the management of the infant and child with cardiovascular and pulmonary disease.[1] Cardiac catheterization is also a means of treating congenital cardiac abnormalities.

Noninvasive imaging by an experienced operator using high-resolution two-dimensional and Doppler echocardiography or magnetic resonance imaging can define most of the cardiovascular anatomy accurately in 95% of patients with congenital cardiovascular malformations.[2] Catheterization and angiography are necessary only for patients with unusual anatomy, unusual presentation of common anomalies, or inadequate echo windows. The resolution of echocardiography, however, does not yet approach that of angiocardiography. The need to obtain important detailed anatomic studies for an operation is decided by the treating cardiologists and surgeons.

INDICATIONS FOR DIAGNOSTIC CARDIAC CATHETERIZATION

At present, cardiac catheterization is the most reliable way to obtain data about the physiologic derangements caused by cardiovascular abnormalities. As the techniques for anatomic and physiologic correction of cardiac malformations continue to expand, there will be an increased need to evaluate the anatomic and hemodynamic results as thoroughly as possible on a long-term basis; cardiac catheterization and angiography continue to play an important part in the ongoing evaluation of these operative and medical treatments.

The various diagnostic procedures and data obtained during a cardiac catheterization are discussed later. The data that may be obtained by such procedures and their applicability to the treatment of the patient should be evaluated. Not all of the procedures are a required part of a cardiac catheterization in every patient; one must formulate a protocol and design the catheterization procedure to obtain the most useful information in the least traumatic manner.

PRECATHETERIZATION ASSESSMENT

Assessment of the patient's clinical problems before catheterization is essential to decide which catheterization procedure is to be used. Catheterization procedures should be goal oriented, planned to elucidate further the nature of the patient's problem and to set the background for future therapeutic maneuvers.

A thorough physical examination identifies the clinical condition of the patient; the state of hydration, cyanosis, and respiratory distress; and the adequacy of the peripheral circulation. Complementary laboratory investigations (such as a complete blood count, arterial blood gas analysis, and electrolyte measurements) determine whether the patient needs endotracheal intubation before the catheterization and whether other therapy (such as inotropic support, diuretics, or prostaglandins) should be started before catheterization.

An electrocardiogram is useful in evaluating arrhythmias, which may need to be controlled before the catheterization. The electrocardiogram can also reflect disturbances of electrolytes, pH, and blood glucose level.

Abnormalities of acid-base balance or electrolytes should be corrected as far as possible before the catheterization, because progressive acidemia and hypoglycemia often develop during catheterization of sick infants.[3] Hemoglobin and hematocrit should be measured before the catheterization, and blood volume or hemoglobin level should be corrected as necessary, using the arterial oxygen saturation (SaO_2) value as a guide to the optimal hemoglobin level. To predict the optimal hemoglobin value (g/dl) for cyanotic patients, we use the equation $38 - 0.25 \times SaO_2$.[4] The hematocrit level should be kept below 65% because the sharp rise in blood viscosity above this level reduces cardiac output and oxygen delivery. At least 20 ml/kg of blood should be typed, crossmatched, and available before the start of the catheterization in infants weighing less than 5 kg.

A current two-dimensional echocardiogram is reviewed before catheterization to evaluate the basic anatomy of the heart so that excessive use of contrast material is avoided. Anomalies of systemic venous return should be noted in planning the venous access route.[5] An echocardiogram is also useful in evaluating the contractility of the myocardium before catheterization. The patency of the ductus arteriosus can be determined and monitored in response to prostaglandin administration.[6]

A written outline or plan of the catheterization procedures should be made so that nothing is omitted during the course of the catheterization and the laboratory staff can prepare for the various procedures.

PREMEDICATION

Most neonates do not require sedatives or narcotics before cardiac catheterization. Infants are particularly susceptible to the depressant effects of narcotics on the central nervous system; morphine, in particular, may destabilize the hemodynamics of an infant with low cardiac output by producing vagotonic bradycardia and venous dilatation. Sedation of seriously ill patients should be administered under the direct supervision of the attending physician in the catheterization laboratory. Various combinations of analgesics, antihistamines, and sedatives have been used for premedication. Meperidine (Demerol, 1.5 to 2.0 mg/kg, up to 50 mg), promethazine (Phenergan, 1.0 mg/kg), and chlorpromazine (Thorazine, 1.0 mg/kg) are commonly used in combination as an intramuscular "lytic cocktail" and given 30 to 45 minutes before catheterization in older infants and children. Chlorpromazine is a potent vasodilator, especially when it is given intravenously, and it may cause unwanted changes in pulmonary or systemic vascular resistance. Premedication drugs that have significant effects on the cardiovascular system should be avoided in patients with obstruction of the ventricular outflow tract, tetralogy of Fallot, and pulmonary vascular disease.

Ketamine is commonly used during catheterization for supplemental sedation. It is a rapidly acting dissociative anesthetic and analgesic agent.[7] When it is given intravenously (0.5 to 1.0 mg/kg) in a period of 30 to 60 seconds, no significant change occurs in systemic or pulmonary hemodynamics. If ketamine cannot be given intravenously, 2 mg/kg intramuscularly sedates a child within 2 minutes. Moreover, ketamine does not lower systemic resistance and therefore is an excellent sedative for patients with tetralogy of Fallot, who are likely to have a hypercyanotic spell. Slow administration into the pulmonary circulation does not produce vasoconstriction. Ketamine does not depress pharyngeal or laryngeal reflexes. It promotes salivation in patients who have not been given drying agents, such as atropine or an antihistamine, and in whom suctioning of the hypopharynx may produce glottic spasm. Ketamine should be avoided as the sole sedative agent if endotracheal intubation is likely. Prophylactic antibiotics to prevent bacterial endocarditis are not recommended for cardiac catheterization.

MONITORING DURING CATHETERIZATION

The catheterization laboratory should be warmed to an ambient temperature of 80 to 85°F. Infants should be placed on some form of a warming device, and the body temperature should be constantly monitored.

If a patient is ventilated, the respirator must be easily accessible for adjustments and monitoring. The heart rate, electrocardiogram, blood pressure, temperature, respiratory rate, respirator settings, chest movement, and air entry and infusion sites are monitored during the catheterization. Soon after the arterial line is placed, arterial blood gas samples are drawn and analyzed to make sure that no significant deviation has occurred from the previous values. Two electrocardiographic leads are displayed, one for monitoring heart rate and one for diagnostic interpretation to observe the P waves and ST segments.

Excessive withdrawal of blood for blood gas measurements can be avoided by the use of a pulse oximeter placed over the toe, the palm of the hand, or the earlobe for constant monitoring during catheterization. Blood sampling should be carefully monitored, and excessive blood loss should be replaced with fresh packed red cells during the catheterization.

VASCULAR ACCESS

The percutaneous femoral route is the preferred approach for diagnostic catheterization in patients with congenital heart disease. Percutaneous insertion of a sheath into the femoral vein is now a standard procedure and allows multiple catheter exchanges with minimal trauma to the vein.[8] Relatively large sheaths can be used even in small infants; for example, a 7 French sheath can be used to insert a balloon septostomy catheter in infants as small as 1.5 kg. Smaller septostomy catheters that are now available can fit through a 5 or 6 French sheath. Exploration of the heart and cardiac vessels from the femoral vein is easier and allows much greater catheter control than access from the arm or neck.

The umbilical vein can usually be quickly cannulated and is often patent up to a week after birth.[9] This approach is useful for emergency atrial septostomy but does limit catheter maneuverability.

A brachial or axillary approach can be used if the femoral veins are not accessible. The axillary vein can be punctured percutaneously about 0.5 to 1.0 cm below the distal axillary crease. The vein usually lies medial to the axillary artery, but the position can vary. There is a greater risk of damaging the brachial plexus or axillary artery with a percutaneous approach because of the lack of supporting subcutaneous tissue. If an axillary approach is necessary, it may be more expedient and safer to perform a cutdown just distal to the distal axillary crease. The vein or artery can be cannulated with a needle and guide wire under direct vision to avoid incising these small vessels.

The anterior brachial vein can be entered percutaneously or by cutdown. However, in small neonates and premature infants, it is usually too small to accommodate even a 5 French catheter, and there is a greater risk of brachial vein spasm; it is more difficult to manipulate the catheter through the long course from the arm to the heart.

The right internal jugular vein can be entered percutaneously,[10] and a relatively large sheath can be placed into the superior vena cava; this can be useful for myocardial biopsies or pulmonary artery stenting. This approach requires a heavily sedated or anesthetized patient. Catheter manipulation from the jugular vein may be more difficult for operators accustomed to the femoral approach. A flow-guided balloon catheter is useful for this approach. Other routes of vascular access, such as carotid artery cutdown and left ventricular apical puncture, are used infrequently when other means of access are unavailable.

HEMOSTASIS AND ANTICOAGULANTS

Precatheterization clotting studies are performed on all neonates and on patients with a hematocrit above 60% who may have accelerated clotting and a consumptive co-agulopathy.[11] Phlebotomy with plasma replacement reduces this tendency.[12] Some neonates require vitamin K before catheterization. Other patients may have disorders of blood clotting or platelets because of infection or shock; fresh frozen plasma and fresh platelets should be given if clotting disorders are identified. One unit of fresh packed red cells, or at least 20 ml/kg, should also be available during catheterizations of infants who weigh less than 5 kg because of the relatively large blood loss in infants, compared with children, when exchanging catheters or sheaths.

Anticoagulants are not routinely used during venous catheterization. If a retrograde arterial catheterization is likely to take longer than 30 minutes, systemic heparinization at 50 U/kg should be instituted. The degree of anticoagulation is monitored by measuring an activated clotting time every 30 to 60 minutes.

POLYCYTHEMIA AND ANEMIA

Patients who are polycythemic have a marked elevation of blood viscosity when the hematocrit is above 65%, which has a significant effect on pulmonary and systemic vascular resistance.[13] If the precatheterization hemoglobin level is above 20 g/dl, a centrifuged hematocrit of venous blood is used to measure the true packed cell volume. To achieve a nearly normal arterial oxygen content, an oxygen-carrying capacity of 17 to 19 ml of oxygen per 100 ml of blood is desirable (assuming 95% saturation in a normal patient with 10 to 15 g of hemoglobin). If the hematocrit is 65% or greater, we recommend erythropheresis before angiography to reduce the centrifuged hematocrit to 60%. The amount of blood withdrawn is replaced with fresh plasma or 5% albumin solution, which has the same osmolality as plasma. Patients with secondary polycythemia have an elevated blood volume of the order of 90 to 100 ml/kg (average, 100) because of the increased red cell mass.[14]

Formula to Raise or Lower the Hemoglobin Level

It is prudent to do exchanges with 20 ml/kg, or if the child is in heart failure, with 10 ml/kg. Calculate the number of exchanges, N, by considering the initial hemoglobin, H_0; the target hemoglobin, H_t; the hemoglobin of the infused fluid, H_i, which might be zero for reducing hematocrit or above normal for packed cells; the volume infused per kilogram (U ml/kg); and the blood volume per kilogram (V = 90 ml/kg). Then we calculate N as

$$N = \ln[(H_i - H_t)(H_i - H_0)] \times (-V/U)$$

The symbol H could represent hemoglobin or hematocrit. A similar calculation can be used to increase the patient's

oxygen-carrying capacity if there is systemic hypoxemia and low oxygen-carrying capacity.

Reduction of the oxygen-carrying capacity and blood viscosity is performed cautiously in patients with obstruction to pulmonary blood flow, such as tetralogy of Fallot, or in those with high pulmonary resistance. In these patients with a relatively fixed obstruction to pulmonary blood flow, a reduction in blood viscosity results in a greater fall in systemic resistance than in pulmonary resistance, inducing more right-to-left shunting and systemic hypoxemia. However, with transposition physiology, systemic saturation improves with a reduction in hematocrit to 60%.[15]

HEMODYNAMIC CALCULATIONS

Physiologic Recordings

A minimum of four channels should be available to record two electrocardiograms and at least two simultaneous pressures. The pressure measuring and recording system should be evaluated before catheterization to optimize pressure signal recording and to minimize overdamping or underdamping.

Pressure waveforms are displayed and recorded at a gain to show the points of interest of the waveform in the middle of the screen. Each pressure recording is identified on the recording paper and in the procedure log, and a calibration signal is recorded for each pressure.

The recording device should produce an instantaneous record for immediate viewing; a permanent paper record of the pressure recordings should be generated and kept for review after the catheterization.

Blood Pressure Measurement

To obtain accurate and reproducible cardiovascular pressure measurements, one should have a well-balanced and optimally damped transducer, matched to the catheter size and length of the connection tubing if a fluid-filled measuring system is used. Catheters with both side and end holes are preferable. The most accurate measurements are made with a short and large catheter. Great care should be taken in using small, balloon-directed Swan-Ganz catheters,[16] which have only an end hole; the small lumen size and relatively long length of these multilumen catheters usually produce overdamped pressure tracings. Other factors that may influence the accuracy and reproducibility of the pressure recordings are severe airway obstruction with marked inspiratory and expiratory swings in intrathoracic pressure and high mean airway pressure produced by respirator settings necessary for adequate oxygenation.

Electronic catheter tip transducers should be used when extremely accurate blood pressure recordings are required, such as in deriving pressure-volume curves or the first derivative of the ventricular pressure to evaluate ventricular function.[17] Because these catheters are stiff, they are not often used in small infants. They can, however, be connected to the hub of a catheter with an adapter, thus avoiding the need to connect the catheter to the manometer by a long compliant tube and thereby improving the frequency response. Normal values for pressures, resistances, and oxygen saturations are given in references 18 and 19.

Calculation of Blood Flow and Shunts

Blood flow in the systemic and pulmonary circulation is difficult to measure directly. It can be measured by video densitometry, catheter-tipped velocity meters, or the more usual method of the indicator dilution principle.

THE INDICATOR DILUTION PRINCIPLE

Consider an organ with a constant flow of blood of F (ml/min) into its artery and out through its vein. The steady-state arterial and venous concentrations of an indicator are C_a and C_v, respectively. Concentration (C [mg/ml]) is a quantity (Q [mg]) divided by a volume (V [ml]), so that $Q = CV$. Then the quantity of indicator brought into the organ each minute (Q_a) is C_aV, where V is the volume entering the organ each minute. Because $V = F$ ml/min, then $Q_a = FC_a$; similarly $Q_v = FC_v$. Therefore, each minute, Q_a units of indicator enter the tissue and Q_v units leave it. Let the difference between these amounts be Q_x; the difference is positive if the indicator (e.g., oxygen in the tissues) is removed or negative if the indicator (e.g., oxygen in the lungs or indicator dye) is added. If we can measure this difference, we can measure flow as

$$Q_x = Q_a - Q_v = F(C_a - C_v)$$

so that $F = Q_x/(C_a - C_v)$. In cardiology, it is customary to use the symbol Q for flow and not to use a symbol for quantity.

Commonly used indicators are oxygen (the Fick principle), indocyanine green, and cold saline (thermodilution). When we use a foreign indicator such as indocyanine green and measure the output concentration, the input concentration C_a is zero. For oxygen and temperature, however, which are always present in the blood, we need to measure both the input and output concentrations. Oxygen consumption can be conveniently measured in children with a flow-through hood.[20]

Oxygen in the Blood

Oxygen-carrying capacity of blood =
13.6 ml O_2/g Hb/L blood (ml/L)

Dissolved oxygen =
0.03 ml O_2/L/mm Hg partial pressure of oxygen

Oxygen content of blood =
O_2 capacity (ml/L) $\times$ SaO_2 (%) + dissolved O_2 (ml/L)

This fits the definition of a concentration, because the volume of oxygen can be turned into a quantity in moles.

THE FICK PRINCIPLE

Blood flow =

$$\frac{O_2 \text{ added/min (oxygen consumption)}}{O_2 \text{ content (difference across body or lungs)}}$$

Pulmonary blood flow (Qp):

$$Qp \text{ (ml/min/m}^2) = \frac{O_2 \text{ consumption (}VO_2 \text{ ml/min/m}^2)}{PV \text{ content} - PA \text{ content (ml/L)}}$$

$$Qp \text{ (L/min/m}^2) = \frac{VO_2 \text{ (ml/min/m}^2)}{(PV \text{ sat} \times 13.6 \times Hb) - (PA \text{ sat} \times 13.6 \times Hb)}$$

Oxygen consumption, blood flow, and resistance should be expressed as indexed units in infants and children. To avoid mistakes, index VO_2 initially so that there is no need to index flow and resistance later on in the calculation.

Systemic blood flow (Qs):

$$Qs \text{ (L/min/m}^2) = \frac{VO_2 \text{ (ml/min/m}^2)}{(\text{aortic sat} \times 13.6 \times Hb) - (SVC \text{ sat} \times 13.6 \times Hb)}$$

Effective pulmonary blood flow (QeP), amount of blood that returns from the body to pick up oxygen:

$$QeP \text{ (L/min/m}^2) = \frac{VO_2 \text{ (ml/min/m}^2)}{(PV \text{ sat} \times 13.6 \times Hb) - (SVC \text{ sat} \times 13.6 \times Hb)}$$

The ratio of pulmonary blood flow to systemic blood flow (Qp/Qs):

$$Qp/Qs = \frac{\dfrac{VO_2 \text{ (ml/min/m}^2)}{(PV \text{ sat} \times 13.6 \times Hb) - (PA \text{ sat} \times 13.6 \times Hb)}}{\dfrac{VO_2 \text{ (ml/min/m}^2)}{(\text{aortic sat} \times 13.6 \times Hb) - (SVC \text{ sat} \times 13.6 \times Hb)}}$$

$$= \frac{\text{aortic saturation} - SVC \text{ saturation}}{PV \text{ saturation} - PA \text{ saturation}}$$

where PV is pulmonary vein; PA is pulmonary artery; SVC is superior vena cava; sat is saturation; and Hb is hemoglobin, measured in grams per liter.

For a quick calculation of pulmonary blood flow:

$$Qp = VO_2/[(\text{saturation } PV - \text{saturation } PA) \times 0.136 \times Hb]$$

$$\text{Left-to-right shunt} = Qp - QeP$$

$$\text{Right-to-left shunt} = Qs - QeP$$

CALCULATION OF SHUNTS AT MORE THAN ONE LEVEL

When there are left-to-right shunts at more than one level, such as with coexistent atrial septal defect (ASD), ventricular septal defect (VSD), and patent ductus arteriosus (PDA), it is important to calculate the amount of shunting at each level to determine which is the dominant lesion. An increase in saturation at the atrial level of 8 percentage points, at the ventricular level of 5 percentage points, and at the pulmonary artery level of 2 percentage points is considered significant and indicates a left-to-right shunt at that level.

Calculate the blood flow at each level as if the SaO_2 in that chamber is the final SaO_2 in the pulmonary artery, then subtract the flow from the proximal chamber.

ASD flow:

$$\text{"Qp"} = V_{O_2}/[(PV \text{ content} - RA \text{ content}) \times 0.136 \times Hb]$$
$$\text{Shunt through the ASD} = ASD \text{ flow} - Qs$$

VSD flow:

$$\text{"Qp"} = V_{O_2}/[(PV \text{ content} - RV \text{ content}) \times 0.136 \times Hb]$$
$$\text{Shunt through the VSD} = VSD \text{ flow} - ASD \text{ flow}$$

PDA flow:

$$\text{"Qp"} = V_{O_2}/[(PV \text{ content} - MPA \text{ content}) \times 0.136 \times Hb]$$
$$\text{Shunt through the PDA} = PDA \text{ flow} - VSD \text{ flow}$$

$$Qp = Qs + Qasd + Qvsd + Qpda$$

where PV is pulmonary vein; RA is right atrium; RV is right ventricle; and MPA is main pulmonary artery.

For example, a patient has an ASD, a VSD, and a PDA. Saturations at various sites are SVC = 70%, RA = 75%, RV = 80%, MPA = 85%, PV = 95%, aorta = 95%, Hb = 15 g/L, and V_{O_2} = 196 ml/min/m². The overall shunt calculation is Qs = 3.84 L/min/m²; Qp = 9.6 L/min/m²; Qp/Qs = 2.5 : 1.

ASD "flow" =
$$196/[(95 - 75) \times 0.136 \times 15] = 4.8 \text{ L/min/m}^2$$
ASD shunt (Qasd) = 4.8 − 3.84 (Qs) = 0.96 L/min/m²

VSD "flow" =
$$196/[(95 - 80) \times 0.136 \times 15] = 6.4 \text{ L/min/m}^2$$
VSD shunt (Qvsd) = 6.4 − 4.8 (Qasd) = 1.6 L/min/m²

PDA "flow" =
$$196/[(95 - 85) \times 0.136 \times 15] = 9.6 \text{ L/min/m}^2$$
PDA shunt (Qpda) = 9.6 − 6.4 = 3.2 L/min/m²

Qp =
Qs (3.84) + Qasd (0.96) + Qvsd (1.6) + Qpda (3.2) = 9.6 L/min/m²

Note that even though the increase in oxygen saturation percentage points is the same at each level, there is a much larger calculated shunt at the more distal sites because of the smaller arteriovenous difference. When the arteriovenous difference is small, greater errors in the calculation may occur because of the errors inherent in measuring oxygen saturation. For accurate shunt calculations, one should take duplicate samples or measure the oxygen content directly. These calculations also assume perfect mixing, which may not occur.

SHUNT CALCULATION AFTER ADMINISTRATION OF THE VASODILATOR OXYGEN

Many infants and children with increased pulmonary blood flow have a significant ventilation/perfusion defect that is made worse by sedation. The hypoxia and hypercapnia produced by hypoventilation raise pulmonary vascular resistance. To obtain a realistic calculation of pulmonary blood flow and pulmonary resistance, oxygen is adminis-tered to overcome the hypoventilation. Significant errors in these calculations can result if the increase in the oxygen dissolved in blood is not considered.

When the pulmonary artery saturation is high (large pulmonary blood flow), the arteriovenous difference is narrow, and small errors in measurement result in large errors of flow calculation.

Sample Shunt Calculations After Administration of the Vasodilator Oxygen

Patient = 10 kg; body surface area = 0.5 m²; Hb = 15 g/L; V_{O_2} = 196 ml/min/m²; oxygen capacity = 15 × 13.6 = 205 ml oxygen per liter of blood.

CONDITION 1: ROOM AIR ($FiO_2 = 0.21$)

Measure	MPA	PV	Aorta	SVC
SaO_2 (%)	85	95	95	75
Content (cap. × SaO_2)	173.4	193.8	193.8	153
PO_2 (mm Hg)	50	90	90	35
Dissolved O_2 (PO_2 × 0.03 ml)	1.5	2.7	2.7	1.05
Total O_2 content (cont. + dissolved)	174.9	196.5	196.5	154.05

Including dissolved O_2 (row 5):

$$Qp = \frac{196}{196.5 - 174.9} = 9.07 \text{ L/min/m}^2$$

$$Qs = \frac{196}{196.5 - 154.05} = 4.62 \text{ L/min/m}^2$$

$$Qp/Qs = 1.96 : 1$$

Disregarding dissolved O_2 (row 2):

$$Qp = \frac{196}{193.8 - 173.4} = 9.61 \text{ L/min/m}^2$$

$$Qs = \frac{196}{193.8 - 153} = 4.80 \text{ L/min/m}^2$$

$$Qp/Qs = 2 : 1$$

CONDITION 2: BREATHING 100% OXYGEN

Measure	MPA	PV	Aorta	SVC
SaO_2 (%)	95	100	100	80
Content (cap. × SaO_2)	193.8	204	204	163.2
PO_2 (mm Hg)	90	500	500	45
Dissolved O_2 (PO_2 × 0.03 ml)	2.7	15	15	1.35
Total O_2 content (cont. + dissolved)	196.5	219	219	164.6

Including dissolved O_2 (row 5):

$$Qp = \frac{196}{219 - 196.5} = 8.71 \text{ L/min/m}^2$$

$$Qs = \frac{196}{219 - 164.6} = 3.60 \text{ L/min/m}^2$$

$$Qp/Qs = 2.4:1$$

Disregarding dissolved O_2 (row 2):

$$Qp = \frac{196}{204 - 193.5} = 18.67 \text{ L/min/m}^2$$

$$Qs = \frac{196}{204 - 163.2} = 4.80 \text{ L/min/m}^2$$

$$Qp/Qs = 3.9:1$$

Resistance Calculations

Resistance (R) calculations are based on Ohm's law.

$$\text{Resistance} = \frac{\text{volts}}{\text{current (amps)}}$$

or

$$R = \frac{\text{pressure drop across lungs or body (mm Hg)}}{\text{blood flow through lungs or body (L/min/m}^2)}$$

$$R\ (U) = \text{mm Hg/L/min/m}^2 = \text{Wood units}$$

or

$$R\ (\text{dynes}) = \frac{\text{mm Hg}}{\text{L/min/m}^2} = \frac{\text{dynes/cm}^2}{\text{cm}^3 \cdot \text{sec}} =$$
$$\text{dyne} \cdot \text{sec/cm}^5 = \text{Wood units} \times 80$$

Total pulmonary resistance (TPR) does not consider wedge pressure:

$$TPR = \text{mean PaP}/Qp$$

Pulmonary arteriolar resistance (PAR):

$$PAR = \frac{\text{mean PaP} - \text{mean LAP or mean PaWedge}}{Qp}$$

Systemic vascular resistance (SVR):

$$SVR = \frac{\text{mean AoP} - \text{mean RAP}}{Qs}$$

where PaP is pulmonary arterial pressure; LAP is left atrial pressure; PaWedge is pulmonary artery wedge pressure; AoP is aorta pressure; and RAP is right atrial pressure.

To calculate Rp/Rs if Qp and Qs are unknown:

1. Assume Qs = 1.
2. Divide pulmonary perfusion pressure by Qp/Qs ratio.

For example:

$$\frac{\dfrac{\text{mean PaP} - \text{mean LAP}}{Qp/Qs} = \dfrac{40}{2}}{\dfrac{\text{mean AoP} - \text{mean RAP}}{1} = \dfrac{75}{1}} = \frac{20}{75} = 0.27:1$$

A major reason to calculate pulmonary vascular resistance is to assess the cross-sectional area of the pulmonary vascular bed to determine suitability for operative correction of a defect. In making this determination, the effects of hematocrit on viscosity must be considered. Figure 13–1 shows how viscosity changes with hematocrit, both relative to a hematocrit value of 45% and relative to plasma. Strictly speaking, the cross-sectional area of the vascular bed should be assessed by calculating *hindrance,* defined as

$$\frac{\text{resistance (mm Hg/L/min/m}^2)}{\text{absolute viscosity (poise)}}$$

Consider a pulmonary vascular resistance of 4 mm Hg/L/min/m² at hematocrit levels of 45%, 20%, and 75%, which have absolute viscosities of 0.04, 0.0205, and 0.0852 poise, respectively:

Hematocrit (%)	45	20	75
Resistance (mm Hg/L/min/m²)	4	4	4
Absolute viscosity (poise)	0.04	0.0205	0.0852
Hindrance (mm Hg/L/min/m²/ poise)	100	195	47

Then the respective hindrances are 100, 195, and 47 mm Hg/L/min/m²/poise, about a four-fold variation in a

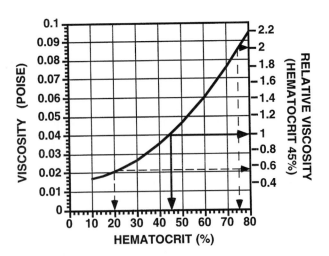

FIGURE 13–1

Viscosity changes with hematocrit, both relative to a hematocrit measurement of 45% and relative to plasma.

cross-sectional area. These differences could affect operative results; for example, a patient with this resistance having a Fontan-Kreuzer procedure would do well with a hindrance of 47 and perhaps poorly with one of 195.

Calculation of Valve Area

The pressure gradient across a cardiac valve is directly proportional to the flow across the valve and inversely proportional to the valve area. In patients with congestive heart failure or a low cardiac output secondary to an obstructive valve or vessel, the pressure gradient across the valve does not reflect the severity of the stenosis. This is particularly true in neonates in whom the myocardium tolerates poorly an acute increase in afterload. To evaluate the effectiveness of an intervention such as balloon valvoplasty, the cardiac output must be measured, and the valve area must be calculated. The valve area is indexed to the body surface area.

To calculate a valve area, one must know the cardiac output, the heart rate, and the pressure curves from each side of the stenotic valve. The Gorlin formula[21] is used to calculate the valve area.

$$\text{Aortic valve area (cm}^2) = \frac{\dfrac{\text{stroke volume (ml)}}{\text{systolic ejection period (sec)}}}{\text{correction factor} \times 44.3\sqrt{(\text{mean LV} - \text{aortic gradient}) \text{ mm Hg}}}$$

The number 44.3 is derived from the square root of the gravity acceleration factor × 2. The correction factor is 0.85 for the mitral valve and 1.0 for the tricuspid and semilunar valves. For atrioventricular valves, diastolic inflow replaces systolic ejection period. The accuracy of the Gorlin formula has been criticized because it assumes a steady flow rate, a constant valve area during systole, and the use of empirical constants. A modification of this formula has been proposed by Bache and colleagues[22]:

$$\text{Aortic valve area} = \frac{\text{stroke volume (ml)/systolic ejection period (sec)}}{36.4\sqrt{\text{maximal IPG}}}$$

where IPG = instantaneous pressure gradient between the left ventricle (LV) and aorta.

Measurement of Pump and Muscle Function

Methods used to evaluate cardiac pump and muscle function are discussed in Chapter 5.[23] These tests are usually used in a research study, and a full discussion of their merits and limitations is beyond the scope of this chapter. However, myocardial function, particularly of the right ventricle, is becoming an increasingly important factor in the assessment of patients with a functional single ventricle in deciding whether they should undergo a Fontan operation or cardiac transplantation. Methods currently used to assess right ventricular function are those used to assess left ventricular function, and they do not necessarily apply to a morphologically different right ventricle.

COMPLICATIONS OF CARDIAC CATHETERIZATION

The mortality and morbidity associated with cardiac catheterization are directly related to the underlying cardiopulmonary abnormality and the general condition of the patient, rather than to the age and size of the patient.[24] A moribund, acidotic, hypoxic neonate with poor perfusion, who has not responded to precatheterization medications and management, has a poor chance of survival with or without cardiac catheterization. Such neonates are likely to have complex or inoperable cardiopulmonary abnormalities and usually die in spite of, rather than because of, catheterization.

The incidence of complications and the number of deaths from cardiac catheterization have decreased sharply during the past 30 years. Cardiac catheterization techniques, vascular access, catheter design and materials, quality and type of imaging (including use of biplane cineangiography), and type of contrast materials used for imaging have undergone considerable refinements and have improved the quality and safety of cardiac catheterization and angiography. The indications for a cardiac catheterization have also changed with the introduction of other imaging modalities, such as two-dimensional echocardiography. This has reduced the need for catheterization in critically ill infants who have inoperable lesions or no cardiac anomaly.

Several reviews of catheterization complications from 1968 to 1978[25–27] revealed a significant decrease in diagnostic cardiac catheterization–related deaths in infants and children from 9.8 to 0.2%, and serious nonfatal complications have fallen 2 to 3%. The common types of complications are as follows:

Complications of Cardiac Catheterization

Ventricular tachycardia and fibrillation	Supraventricular tachycardia
Complete heart block	Cardiac perforation
Bleeding	Hypotension
Hypercyanotic spell	Seizures
Cerebral embolus and stroke	Arterial pulse loss
Sepsis	

THERAPEUTIC CARDIAC CATHETERIZATION

Treating cardiovascular lesions with a catheter or a catheter-delivered device has been the goal of cardiologists since the first cardiac catheterizations. The first attempt at a therapeutic catheter procedure for a congenital heart defect was the incision of the pulmonary valve with a wire at the tip of the catheter by Alvarez in 1953.[28] This procedure was so far before its time that it was not repeated, and its significance fell into oblivion. More than a decade later, the balloon atrial septostomy (BAS) procedure was introduced by William Rashkind in 1966.[29] This innovative and daring therapeutic catheter procedure saved many infants, and of equal importance, it demonstrated that intracardiac therapeutic procedures could be performed in a cardiac catheterization laboratory. This procedure provided the stimulus for the development of all subsequent therapeutic catheterization procedures.

In the years since Rashkind's dramatic and historic procedure, there has been an explosion in the development of catheter therapy of cardiac malformations and, in turn, a revolution in the management of patients with congenital heart disease. There are a number of procedures and devices undergoing, or just beginning to undergo, clinical studies, and they may be available for more general use in specialized centers by the time of this publication. The more promising of these are included in this chapter.

All therapeutic cardiac catheterization procedures require special skills and additional fellowship training. These procedures should be performed only in select centers by physicians with special training in those procedures. In addition to the operator requirements, because of the multitude of types of procedures and the ultimate size range of patients in a pediatric cardiac catheterization laboratory, these procedures require a separate, extensive inventory of specialized and expendable equipment. For these reasons, not every pediatric cardiologist, nor for that matter every pediatric cardiology center, should plan (or attempt) to perform every therapeutic catheterization procedure. An unsuccessful attempt by an untrained operator or even a skilled operator in an ill-equipped catheterization laboratory may, in fact, prevent or compromise the later successful completion of the same procedure by a skilled operator in a properly equipped laboratory.

BALLOON ATRIAL SEPTOSTOMY

BAS is one therapeutic catheterization procedure that should be available in all institutions caring for infants and children with a cardiac malformation. This procedure may be lifesaving and must often be performed immediately to be effective. As such, it should be available without having to transfer an infant to another institution. A BAS procedure is indicated in patients with an intact or nearly intact atrial septum and in whom further admixture of systemic and pulmonary venous blood would benefit the patient's oxygenation, cardiac output, or both. This indication includes all forms of arterial transposition physiology with or without other intracavitary or great artery communication. Unless the infant is actually en route to the operating room for an arterial switch procedure, BAS is indicated to prevent significant hypoxia and acidosis.

The most commonly used balloon for BAS is the Miller-Edwards balloon. This is a latex balloon on a single-lumen 5 French catheter, which requires a 7 French sheath for introduction. There is a new line of septostomy catheters with noncompliant balloons made of polyethylene. The balloons are on a 5 French double-lumen catheter and pass through a 6 French sheath. The double lumen allows the balloon catheter to pass over a wire and allows pressure measurements, blood sampling, or injection of contrast material through the catheter. Although the balloons are smaller, the noncompliant material makes them noncompressible so that theoretically the smaller balloon can be used to achieve the same result. In early trials, this does *not* seem to be true in *larger* patients, when a latex balloon inflated to 6 ml would normally be used.

When BAS is planned, start the catheterization procedure with an introducer sheath that accommodates the septostomy balloon. Frequently, the first sheath introduced produces venous spasm and prohibits the exchange to a larger sheath. Once inflated to the maximal tolerated diameter in the left atrium, the balloon catheter is rapidly and forcefully withdrawn across the septum with a snapping motion of only the fingers and wrist so that there is also rigid control of the distance on the withdrawal. The balloon pullthrough is usually repeated at least 3 times or until there is absolutely no further resistance to the balloon's passage across the atrial septum. When the procedure is performed properly and with a correct balloon size, an adequate ASD can be created in infants younger than 1 month. The BAS procedure for a neonate with transposition of the great arteries and intact ventricular septum is a lifesaving procedure and remains one of the few indications for an emergency cardiac catheterization in infancy.

BLADE ATRIAL SEPTOSTOMY

When balloon septostomy was extended to lesions in addition to transposition of the great arteries, particularly in infants and children older than 1 month, the results were less satisfactory and only temporary. In infants older than that age, the septum is usually too thick or tough, and the balloon stretches the existing hole temporarily, if at all. As a nonoperative solution to this problem, the Park blade septostomy catheter was developed.[30] The Park catheters have at the distal end of the catheter a small recessed blade that can be extended and retracted with a slide mechanism at the proximal end of the catheter. The blades come in three lengths—1.0 and 1.34 cm in a 6 French catheter and 2.0 cm in an 8 French catheter. The purpose of the blade is to first create a small incision in the septum, which can then be torn further with a standard BAS.

The blade catheter is positioned in the left atrium through a long sheath that has been passed into the left atrium either through a pre-existing opening or by a transseptal puncture.[31] The blade is opened carefully in the left atrium with the tip facing either the patient's right or left, but always anteriorly. The blade is withdrawn slowly but forcefully through the septum into the right atrium. The blade withdrawal is repeated one or more times, changing the angle of the blade with each withdrawal. When little or no resistance to the blade pullthrough is apparent, the blade procedure is followed by a BAS.

A trans-septal atrial puncture to introduce the blade catheter is necessary in patients with an intact atrial septum. The trans-septal technique is also useful in patients who have a pre-existing atrial communication, although it is inadequate to permit good mixing or venting. Small pre-existing atrial defects tend to elongate as a blade is withdrawn through them and, in turn, merely distort, rather than cut, with the blade withdrawal. A trans-septal puncture is performed in the adjacent intact septum a small distance (4 to 10 mm) in any direction away from the pre-existing defect where the needle can be engaged. The blade catheter is introduced through the trans-septal sheath in this new opening. The blade is withdrawn with the extended blade pointing in the direction of the diagnostic catheter in the pre-existing opening.

BALLOON DILATATION OF THE ATRIAL SEPTUM

One remaining problem with the catheter septostomy in an older patient concerns the toughness of the septum and its resistance to further "tearing" with a balloon septostomy catheter even after the "blading." In this situation, balloon *dilatation* catheters of the type for valve dilatations are used to extend the tear in the septum. The size of the balloon is chosen according to the size of the patient and the size of the defect to be created. The dilatation balloons have several advantages over the standard septostomy balloons besides overcoming the toughness of the septum. By using several dilatation balloons side by side, much larger openings can be created. The septum can be reached when the patient's trunk length is longer than the available standard-length septostomy balloon catheters, and the technique can be used from a superior vena caval approach when there is blockage of the femoral vessels or interruption of the inferior vena cava.

The combined blade and balloon septostomy using the various adaptations in the technique has proved safe, reliable, and effective in palliating these complex conditions. The combined blade and dilatation balloon septostomy procedure has extended the application of a catheter-produced septostomy to patients of all ages and sizes, including the rare adult patient requiring such palliation.[30] These patients usually have extremely complex cyanotic lesions for which there is no corrective operation available. In this category is the patient with long-standing pulmonary vascular disease regardless of the original etiology, but without intracardiac communications or right-sided heart failure and with symptoms due to low cardiac output. A carefully performed small atrial septostomy in these patients makes the patient cyanotic but, in turn, improves total venous return to the left atrium and increases systemic cardiac output.

DILATATION PROCEDURES

Andreas Gruntzig, in his report of the dilatation of coronary arteries in 1978,[32] introduced the concept of using a static dilatation balloon for intracardiac structures. For children with congenital cardiac anomalies, not much attention was given to this concept until Jean Kan, using a newly developed large dilatation balloon, reported the successful dilatation of a stenosed pulmonary valve in 1982.[33] This began a revolution in the management of valvar lesions. Techniques were developed and several reports appeared in short succession by Lababidi and colleagues[34] and Lock and associates[35] for the aortic and mitral valves as well as for the perfection of the technique for the pulmonary valve.

Early in the experience with the new dilatation techniques in congenital heart disease, the voluntary Valvuloplasty and Angioplasty of Congenital Anomalies (VACA) Registry of 27 centers performing these procedures was established. The main goal of the registry was to document the efficacy and safety of the dilatation procedures by tabulating the results and, of more importance, uncovering complications that might not become apparent in smaller individual series. The VACA Registry rapidly accumulated data on a large number of patients. This unique cooperative effort established that each of the procedures could be accomplished with relative safety and, certainly, that pulmonary valve dilatation was both efficacious and safe. Probably because of the relative ease of accomplishing the pulmonary valve dilatation and its status as the first valve to be attempted, the experience with pulmonary valve dilatation (and, in turn, valid data on the technique) was the most rapid to accumulate. By the end of 1986, more than 800 patients had been submitted to the VACA Registry.[36] Sufficient safety and efficacy of the procedure were demonstrated from these data to allow the Food and Drug Administration (FDA) to approve the particular balloon used in most of these patients for pulmonary valve dilatation in children.

The balloons for dilatation procedures are cylindrical, polyurethane or polyethylene, and noncompliant or static with the effective parallel walls tapering at both ends at the point of attachment to the catheter. The newer balloons come in a wide range of diameters, are on smaller shafts, have shorter tips, and taper yet fold into smaller and smoother profiles. The valvoplasty balloons, when inflated to their maximal recommended pressure of between 2.5 and 16 atm, reach a fixed and rigid diameter.[37]

Detailed descriptions of the techniques of dilating pulmonic, aortic, mitral, and tricuspid valves as well as coarctation of the aorta are given in their respective chapters.

SYSTEMIC VENOUS DILATATION

Stenoses of systemic veins or systemic venous channels are usually secondary to previous invasive procedures, the most notable being the stenoses within the venous baffles after a "venous" switch (Mustard's or Senning's) procedure for transposition of the great arteries. The increased risks of repeated operations are formidable, and the eventual results of repeated operations are unsatisfactory, so alternative therapy for these lesions is appealing.

Other obstructions of either central or more peripheral venous channels are usually asymptomatic and are found incidentally during attempts at repeated cardiac catheterization. When these obstructions are symptomatic with localized venous stasis proximal to the obstruction or when venous access is necessary to carry out further catheter interventions, dilatation of these venous obstructions may be indicated.

Dilatation of these channels can be performed with immediate success. The technique for systemic venous dilatation is straightforward. One or two guide wires are passed through the area of obstruction from the femoral veins, the internal jugular veins, or a combination of the two, depending on the site of obstruction and the access availability. One or two balloons are passed over the separate guide wires and positioned exactly within the obstruction. The balloon inflation is carried out carefully, observing the balloon positioning within the stenoses and the appearance and then disappearance of the waist in the balloons. Once the operator is satisfied with the dilatation, the balloon catheters are removed, and hemodynamic measurements and angiocardiograms are repeated.

Restenosis is common after dilatation of venous stenosis. The use of intravascular stents to support the dilated vessel enhances the long-term benefit of venous dilatation significantly. It is probably no longer justified to attempt dilatation of these structures without the concomitant implant of intravascular stents.

BRANCH PULMONARY ARTERY DILATATION

Branch pulmonary artery stenosis can occur as an acquired lesion after operation on the pulmonary arteries, as an isolated congenital defect in association with rubella and the Williams or Alagille syndromes, or as a combination of both congenital and acquired lesions. Operation for any of these branch pulmonary artery stenoses has been unsatisfactory, frequently resulting in a more severe stenosis than before the operation. Discrete and multiple areas of stenoses in both the congenital and acquired pulmonary artery lesions have been dilated acutely with some immediate benefit.[38] Unfortunately, all of these pulmonary artery lesions have unpredictable and generally unsatisfactory long-term results from dilatation alone. Congenital lesions seem to have the least satisfactory results and are definitely the more hazardous to dilate. The only lesions that do not seem to be acutely amenable to dilatation occur in those rare patients with true diffuse generalized hypoplasia of the entire pulmonary arterial bed, but until dilatation is attempted, it is impossible to distinguish these diffuse lesions from the multiple discrete lesions with secondary hypoplasia.

The technique for dilatation of branch pulmonary arteries involves positioning a super-stiff exchange-length guide wire far distal to the obstruction. A balloon diameter is chosen to be 3 to 4 times the diameter of the discrete narrowing but no more than 1.5 times the diameter of the vessel on either side of the narrowing. The balloon catheter is advanced over the prepositioned wire until at least the *parallel surfaces* of the balloon are well within the discrete area of obstruction. The balloon is inflated to its maximal recommended pressure or until the waist in the balloon disappears. If there is a persistent waist in the balloon at the site of discrete obstruction, the standard-pressure balloon is replaced with a high-pressure dilatation balloon of the same diameter, and the procedure is repeated. After dilatation, the pressures across the area of previous narrowing are recorded, and an angiocardiogram is performed to visualize the dilated area.

The success rate in the dilatation of branch pulmonary artery stenoses is between 30 and 70%, depending more on the criteria for successful dilatation than on the particular type or location of the branch stenoses.[39] Although most of these stenosed areas can be dilated acutely, they usually restenose, some as soon as the balloon is removed from the site and the others with time. The risk is greater for dilatation of branch pulmonary artery stenosis than with valve or other vessel dilatation. Because of the nature of the vessels and the need to overdilate the adjacent pulmonary arteries to acutely relieve the obstruction, vessel rupture and death from dilatation of pulmonary arteries is as high as 1 to 2%. With this combination of factors, dilatation alone of branch pulmonary arteries should probably be limited to patients for whom no alternative therapy exists. This would apply to patients who are too small for a safe and reasonable implant of an intravascular stent that can be dilated to adult pulmonary artery size and, at the same time, have systemic or near-systemic proximal pulmonary artery pressures or show signs of cardiac decompensation because of branch pulmonary artery stenosis.

PULMONARY VEIN DILATATION

Congenital pulmonary vein stenosis can be dilated, and immediately after dilatation, the veins appear to maintain adequate patency; however, in all instances (in as little as 1 month), these vessels restenose.[40] Except out of desperation, most centers have abandoned attempting this procedure. Discussion of technique is not warranted until further developments improve the outcome.

INTRAVASCULAR STENTS

A combination of factors dampened the enthusiasm for vessel dilatation procedures in centers truly interested in *correcting* the abnormalities. In the dilatation of both congenital and acquired vessel stenosis, there are many instances of successful acute dilatations with visual relief of the obstruction up to the diameter of the balloon or the adjacent normal vessel, but with recurrence of the stenosis either immediately with balloon deflation or within days or a few weeks after the dilatation. Acute dilatation proves that the vessels can be opened. The challenge is how long they can be maintained in the open state. A clinical trial for the use of the balloon expandable stent in pulmonary arteries and systemic veins in humans was begun under an FDA Investigational Device Exemption protocol in late 1989.[41] As of September 1995 and still under the only Investigational Device Exemption–approved protocol for this use in children and patients with a cardiac malformation, 418 stents were implanted in the branch pulmonary arteries and systemic veins in 211 patients. The results have been only short of spectacular. There have been minimal complications, particularly considering the severity of abnormalities of the cohort of patients in the study.

The delivery of the stents is similar for the branch pulmonary arteries and the systemic veins.[42] Unless the area of stenosis is extremely tight (less than 3 mm), the stenosis is *not* predilated before stent implant. A long 11 or 12 French sheath-dilator is advanced over a super-stiff exchange wire well past the stenotic lesion. The stent, mounted on a balloon of the desired diameter, is delivered over the wire and through the sheath to the desired location. The sheath is withdrawn from the balloon, and the balloon and stent are expanded to the predetermined diameter of the delivery balloon. If further dilatation of the stent is desired, the original balloon is replaced with a larger or higher pressure balloon, and the inflation is repeated.

Stents have been successfully implanted in tandem or simultaneously in bifurcation lesions with the same acute and midterm results. On late follow-up catheterization, stents have been further dilated to accommodate growth of the patient or of the particular stented vessel.[43] To not create future stenosis, which unequivocally would require further surgery, only stents demonstrated to be effective and strong enough to support the vessels in the intended areas and stents that are capable of being expanded to the adult size of the target vessel are used in the proximal pulmonary arteries and central venous channels. To date, this has required the use of the larger P308 ("iliac") stents in all proximal or central vascular channels. This has limited the use of the stents to patients who weigh more than 10 kg and preferably more than 15 kg. The P204 ("renal") stents have been used only in distal branch pulmonary arteries or very small systemic veins near or in an extremity. With modification of these particular stents or with development of different stents, these limitations should be overcome to extend the use to smaller patients. In spite of the favorable early and midterm results with these particular stents, a longer follow-up is necessary to determine the permanent effects of the intravascular stents in these locations.

OCCLUSION DEVICES AND TECHNIQUES

Nonoperative occlusion of vascular communications was first accomplished by the use of coil occlusion devices in lesions that were not unique to patients with cardiac malformations.[44] Specific devices for congenital lesions were first developed and used in the mid-1970s.[45, 46] Since then, newer and better devices specifically for PDA and ASD closure have been developed and extensively tested in clinical trials in the United States and the rest of the developed world. The various occlusion devices already developed or currently in clinical trials and the lesions for which they are applicable are discussed in the following section.

Coil Occlusion Devices

The original work in catheter occlusions was with the use of small embolization devices, particularly Gianturco coils, for the occlusion of feeder arteries to abnormal structures.[44, 47] These procedures were directed toward occluding vessels supplying tumor masses in which the goal was to infarct the distal organ or to occlude small vessels that had ruptured or were eroded and bled into other organs. These coils soon found extensive application in patients with congenital cardiac anomalies.

The Gianturco coils are segments of 0.025- to 0.038-inch spring wire that have filaments of nylon fabric embedded within the wire and are formed into coils of predetermined diameters between 2 and 15 mm. To use the occlusion coils, an end hole–only delivery catheter is positioned selectively in the vessel to be occluded. The straightened coil is pushed into and through the catheter with a standard spring guide wire. As the embolization coil is pushed from the delivery catheter, it assumes its predetermined coiled configuration. When properly sized for the vessel to be occluded, it should coil irregularly within the vessel and *not* form a "doughnut" shape. The combination of the irregular loops of the coiled wire and the attached fiber filaments initiates thrombosis in the area of the coil and in turn occludes the vessel. The Gianturco coils are effective in occluding systemic-to-pulmonary artery collaterals, which are particularly common in cardiac anomalies, such as pulmonary atresia with VSD, many postoperative caval–pulmonary artery single-ventricle repairs, and many atriovenous fistulae.

In addition to the Gianturco coil, there are smaller helical coils that can be delivered through tiny, flexible, and trackable catheters. The Tracker system has the advantage that the coils are delivered through much smaller and more tortuous feeder vessels to much more distal locations. The delivery system does have the disadvantages of being relatively complex to use, and except for a tiny marker at the tip of the catheter, the delivery catheter is nonopaque. These coils have a place for the occlusion of small abnormal vessels in distal circuitous locations. As an adjunct to this type of therapy, detachable miniballoons[48] and a long wire in a bag[49] were developed for the occlusion of abnormal vascular communications.

Bag Occlusion Device

For larger high-flow and tubular vessels, including a long tubular patent ductus, there is a device approved by the FDA and available in the United States. The Gianturco-Grifka Vascular Occlusion Device (GGVOD) consists of small nylon bags in diameters (sizes) of 3, 5, 7, and 9 mm; when implanted, the bags are *filled* according to diameters with specified long lengths of coreless spring guide wire.[49] The empty bag attached to the delivery catheter is delivered to the location within the vessel, which is to be occluded through a 7.5 French long delivery sheath. As the wire fills the bag, it forces the bag circumferentially against the vessel, which in turn fixes the bag in place in the vessel and occludes the vessel.

The GGVOD has the advantage of being adjustable and retrievable *before release*, if the initial location or size was inappropriate. Once fixed, because of its irregular configuration and the pressure against the wall of the vessel, the bag does not tend to migrate or move. The GGVOD has the disadvantages of being applicable only for long tubular vessels or communications, requiring a fairly large delivery system (especially for the arterial approach), and being relatively complex to position the release. Once released, it is difficult, if not impossible, to retrieve.

In the United States, only Gianturco coils, Target coils, and the GGVOD are available for vascular occlusions. The particular occlusion device used for a specific vascular communication depends on the type of communication, the origin of the feeder vessel, the size of the vessel, the area of discrete stenosis within the communication, and most important, the experience and choice of the operator.

Patent Ductus Arteriosus Occlusion Device

Werner Portsmann developed a device specifically for PDA occlusion in 1967.[50] William Rashkind performed transcatheter occlusion of the PDA with a different and more practical device in 1979.[46] Although the techniques were effective for PDA occlusion, the devices had disadvantages, neither gained wide acceptance, and both were abandoned. The first Rashkind occluder was modified into a "double umbrella" that could be delivered through either the venous or the arterial approach with an 8 French catheter.

Rashkind Occluding Device Used in Other Lesions

The Rashkind occluding device has been used successfully for the occlusion of rare or unusual communications, such as persistent ASD in postoperative patients with complex cardiac lesions, abnormal vena caval drainage into the left atrium, large systemic-to-pulmonary artery collateral vessels,[51] and even postmyocardial infarct VSD.[52] The Rashkind device has been used in combination with coils as a scaffold on which to stack the coils in unusually large and nonstenotic collaterals or other vascular communications. Although these uses for the ductus-occluding device probably will never become standard or routine, there will be increasing indications and demands for the use of this or similar devices in these complex lesions of usually critically ill patients and in anomalies that are difficult to repair by operation.

Non–Atrial Septal Defect Uses of Atrial Septal Defect Occlusion Devices

As with the PDA device, the original Clamshell ASD device was used for closure of other defects under a separate and special protocol. The other defects included the purposefully created fenestrations in the Fontan baffle, muscular VSDs, postacute myocardial infarction VSDs, residual unexpected postoperative communications, and miscellaneous intravascular communications in high-risk patients. Most of these uses proved effective although, with the nature of this population of patients, also much more difficult and hazardous. Even these more urgent uses had to be abandoned because of the eventual lack of availability of the devices.

Once proven safe and effective for human use in ASDs, certainly one or more of the new ASD devices now in development will have an application for some of these higher risk lesions or even larger PDAs.

FOREIGN BODY REMOVAL

The use of indwelling catheters for chemotherapy and hyperalimentation, in addition to the increasing number of therapeutic devices being implanted in the catheterization laboratory, all with the potential for embolization, necessitates that transcatheter removal of foreign bodies be included in the armamentarium of the interventional pediatric cardiologist. Techniques for removal of pieces of indwelling catheters have been available for several decades.[53] Most intravascular foreign bodies originate in the systemic venous circulation and lodge in the right side of the heart or pulmonary arterial bed. A high-resolution *biplane* imaging system is absolutely essential for foreign body removal. The operator must be able to localize the foreign body within millimeters and in three dimensions, particularly in the large areas of the lung fields. Without this capability, the likelihood of successful retrieval is small, and the radiation used in the attempt will be excessive.

A variety of catheter devices are available for intravascular foreign body removal. Most have been adapted from other specialties, particularly urology and radiology. The retrieval devices include snares and retrieval baskets in various diameters and configurations: Grabbers, bioptomes, tiny Jaws devices, and Amplatz deflector wires. Each device has a special application for different types of foreign bodies in different locations. All of the foreign body retrieval devices are used through a long Mullins-type sheath with a back bleed valve. The sheath should be large enough to accommodate the grasped foreign body. The sheath tip is positioned immediately adjacent to the foreign body, and the retrieval device is delivered to the foreign body through the sheath.

With the proper equipment and technique, virtually all intravascular foreign bodies should be retrievable in the cardiac catheterization laboratory without the need for operative intervention.

FUTURE OF THERAPEUTIC CATHETERIZATIONS

Newer devices for palliation and definitive treatment of specific anomalies are on the horizon. The success of the therapeutic catheterization procedures provides incentive for the continued introduction of still newer techniques and, we hope, support from manufacturers for the development of new devices. There seems to be no limit to lesions to which therapeutic catheterization procedures will be applicable.

At the same time, none of the corrective therapeutic catheterization procedures has stood the test of time. As more experience and follow-up become available, many of these procedures and those yet to be discovered will become established, whereas others will be restricted to limited circumstances or shown to be unacceptable. More significantly, with the giant strides in definitive noncatheterization diagnostic and imaging techniques, cardiac catheterization for cardiac malformations will be used predominantly for therapeutic procedures.

REFERENCES

1. Huhta JC, Glasow P, Murphy DJ, et al: Surgery without catheterization for congenital heart defects: Management of 100 patients. J Am Coll Cardiol 9:823, 1987.
2. Gutgesell HP, Huhta JC, Latson LA, et al: Accuracy of two-dimensional echocardiography in the diagnosis of congenital heart disease. Am J Cardiol 55:514, 1985.
3. Srouji MN, Rashkind WJ: The effects of cardiac catheterization on the acid-base status of infants with congenital heart disease. Pediatrics 75:943, 1969.
4. Gidding SS, Stockman JA: Erythropoietin in cyanotic heart disease. Am Heart J 116:128, 1988.
5. Huhta JC, Smallhorn JF, Macartney FJ, et al: Cross-sectional echocardiographic diagnosis of systemic venous return. Br Heart J 48:388, 1982.
6. Vick GW III, Huhta JC, Gutgesell HP: Assessment of the ductus arteriosus in preterm infants utilizing suprasternal two-dimensional/Doppler echocardiography. J Am Coll Cardiol 5:973, 1985.
7. Faithfull NS, Harder R: Ketamine for cardiac catheterization: An evaluation of its use in children. Anesthesia 26:318, 1971.
8. Takahashi M, Petry EL, Lurie PR, et al: Percutaneous heart catheterization in infants and children: Catheter placement and manipulation with guide wires. Circulation 42:1037, 1970.
9. Sapin SO, Linde LM, Emmanouilides GC: Umbilical vessel angiography in the newborn infant. Pediatrics 31:946, 1963.
10. Daily PO, Griepp RB, Shumway NE: Percutaneous internal jugular vein cannulation. Arch Surg 101:534, 1970.
11. Komp DM, Sparrow AW: Polycythemia in cyanotic congenital heart disease—a study of altered coagulation. J Pediatr 76:231, 1970.
12. Wedemeyer AL, Lewis JH: Improvement in hemostasis following phlebotomy in cyanotic patients with heart disease. J Pediatr 83:46, 1973.
13. Nihill MR, McNamara DG, Vick RL: The effects of increased blood viscosity on pulmonary vascular resistance. Am Heart J 92:65, 1976.
14. Rosenthal A, Button LN, Nathan DG: Blood volume changes in cyanotic congenital heart disease. Am J Cardiol 27:162, 1971.
15. Rosenthal A, Nathan DG, Marty A, et al: Acute hemodynamic effects of red cell volume reduction in polycythemia of cyanotic congenital heart disease. Circulation 42:297, 1970.

16. Swan HJC, Ganz W, Forrester J, et al: Catheterization of the heart in man with use of a flow-directed balloon-tipped catheter. N Engl J Med 283:447, 1970.
17. Mason DT, Braunwald E, Covell JW, et al: Assessment of cardiac contractility: The relation between the rate of pressure rise and ventricular pressure during isovolemic systole. Circulation 44:47, 1971.
18. Krovetz LJ, Goldbloom S: Normal standards for cardiovascular data. II. Pressure and vascular resistances. Johns Hopkins Med J 130:187, 1972.
19. Anderson RH, McCartney FJ, Shinebourne EA, et al: Cardiac catheterization and angiography. *In* Anderson RH (ed): Paediatric Cardiology. New York, Churchill Livingstone, 1987.
20. Lister G, Hoffman JIE, Rudolph AM: Oxygen uptake in infants and children: A simple method for measurement. Pediatrics 53:656, 1974.
21. Gorlin R, Gorlin SG: Hydraulic formula for calculation of the area of the stenotic mitral valve, other cardiac valves and central circulatory shunts. Am Heart J 41:1, 1951.
22. Bache RJ, Jorgenson CR, Yang Y: Simplified estimation of aortic valve area. Br Heart J 34:408, 1972.
23. Yang SS, Bentivoglio LG, Maranho V, et al (eds): From Cardiac Catheterization Data to Hemodynamic Parameters. Philadelphia, FA Davis, 1988.
24. Cohn HE, Freed MD, Hellenbrand WE, Fyler DC: Complications and mortality associated with cardiac catheterization in infants under one year. Pediatr Cardiol 6:123, 1985.
25. Braunwald E: Cooperative study on cardiac catheterization. Deaths related to cardiac catheterization. Circulation 37:III-17, 1968.
26. Stanger P, Heymann MA, Tarnoff H, et al: Complications of cardiac catheterization of neonates, infants and children: A three year study. Circulation 50:595, 1974.
27. Porter CJ, Gillette PC, Mullins CE, McNamara DG: Cardiac catheterization in the neonate. J Pediatr 93:97, 1978.
28. Rubio-Alvarez V, Limon RL, Soni J: Valvulotomias intracardiacas por medio de un cateter. Arch Inst Cardiol Mexico 23:183, 1953.
29. Rashkind WJ, Miller WW: Creation of an atrial septal defect without thoracotomy: A palliative approach to complete transposition of the great arteries. JAMA 196:991, 1966.
30. Park SC, Neches WH, Mullins CE, et al: Blade atrial septostomy: Collaborative study. Circulation 66:258, 1982.
31. Mullins CE: Transseptal left heart catheterization: Experience with a new technique in 520 pediatric and adult patients. Pediatr Cardiol 4:239, 1983.
32. Gruntzig AR: Transluminal dilation of coronary artery stenosis. Lancet 1:263, 1978.
33. Kan JS, White RIJ, Mitchell SE, Gardner TJ: Percutaneous balloon valvuloplasty: A new method for treating congenital pulmonary valve stenosis. N Engl J Med 307:540, 1982.
34. Lababidi Z, Wu JR, Walls TJ: Percutaneous balloon aortic valvuloplasty results in 23 patients. Am J Cardiol 53:194, 1984.
35. Lock JE, Khalilullah M, Shrivastava S, et al: Percutaneous catheter commissurotomy in rheumatic mitral stenosis. N Engl J Med 313:1515, 1985.
36. Stanger P, Cassidy SC, Girod DA, et al: Balloon pulmonary valvuloplasty: Results of the Valvuloplasty and Angioplasty of Congenital Anomalies registry. Am J Cardiol 65:775, 1990.
37. Abele JE: Balloon catheters and transluminal dilatation: Technical considerations. AJR Am J Roentgenol 135:901, 1980.
38. Hosking MC, Thomaidis C, Hamilton R, et al: Clinical impact of balloon angioplasty for branch pulmonary arterial stenosis. Am J Cardiol 69:1467, 1992.
39. Rothman A, Perry SB, Keane JF, Lock JE: Early results and follow-up of balloon angioplasty for branch pulmonary artery stenosis. J Am Coll Cardiol 15:1109, 1990.
40. Driscoll DJ, Hesslein PS, Mullins CE: Congenital stenosis of individual pulmonary veins: Clinical spectrum and unsuccessful treatment by transvenous balloon dilatation. Am J Cardiol 49:1767, 1982.
41. O'Laughlin MP, Perry SB, Lock JE, Mullins CE: Use of endovascular stents in congenital heart disease. Circulation 83:1923, 1991.
42. O'Laughlin MP, Slack MC, Grifka RG, et al: Implantation and intermediate-term follow-up of stents in congenital heart disease. Circulation 88:605, 1993.
43. Ing FF, Grifka RG, Nihill MR, Mullins CE: Repeat dilation of intravascular stents in congenital heart disease. Circulation 92:893, 1995.
44. Gianturco C, Anderson JH, Wallace S: Mechanical devices for arterial occlusion. AJR Am J Roentgenol 124:428, 1975.
45. King TD, Mills NL: Nonoperative closure of atrial septal defects. Surgery 75:383, 1974.
46. Rashkind WJ, Cuaso CC: Transcatheter closure of patent ductus arteriosus: Successful use in a 3.5 kilogram infant. Pediatr Cardiol 1:3, 1979.
47. Katzen BT: Interventional Diagnostic and Therapeutic Procedures. New York, Springer-Verlag, 1980.
48. Grinnell VS, Mehringer CM, Hieshima GB, et al: Transaortic occlusion of collateral arteries to the lung by detachable valved balloons in a patient with tetralogy of Fallot. Circulation 65:1276, 1982.
49. Grifka RG, Mullins CE, Gianturco C, et al: New Gianturco-Grifka vascular occlusion device. Initial studies in a canine model. Circulation 91:1840, 1995.
50. Porstmann W, Wierny L, Warnke H: Der Verschluss des Ductus arteriosus persistens ohne Thorakotomie (1 Mitteilung). Thoraxchir Vask Chir 15:199, 1967.
51. Lock JE, Cockerham J, Keane J, et al: Transcatheter umbrella closure of congenital heart defects. Circulation 75:593, 1987.
52. Lock JE, Block PC, McKay RG, et al: Catheter closure of post infarction/postoperative ventricular defects: Initial experience. Circulation 28:76, 1987.
53. Neches WH, Park SC, Zuberbuhler JR: Perspectives in Pediatric Cardiology. New York, Futura, 1991.

CHAPTER 14
ANGIOGRAPHY

DAVID G. NYKANEN   ROBERT M. FREEDOM

The standard mode of imaging for invasive cardiology is fluoroscopy aided by contrast medium–enhanced angiography. Although anatomic and functional information is provided by other imaging modes, such as echocardiography, computed tomography, magnetic resonance imaging, positron emission tomography, and nuclear medicine techniques, angiography has a complementary role.[1–7] In addition, interventional cardiology continues to flourish primarily in the catheterization laboratory. An understanding of the imaging chain and angiographic technique is essential for safe and effective practice.[8]

IMAGE PRODUCTION

EQUIPMENT AND PHYSICS

Since the late 1960s, considerable technological advances have occurred in the equipment that generates and processes x-rays. In addition, digital imaging modes are changing the means by which radiographic images are processed, stored, and accessed. Strict guidelines are mandated by governing bodies to limit radiation exposure to patients and to personnel in an effort to avoid genetic and stochastic side effects. Before one can consider creating angiographic images, one must have at least a basic understanding of how such images are made and stored. In addition, the cardiologist must be aware of the risks associated with cumulative radiation exposure to both the staff and the patient and the measures taken to reduce the risk as much as possible. This has particular relevance because many of the procedures currently undertaken in a catheter laboratory include both a diagnostic and an interventional component. Cineangiography, used primarily in cardiac imaging, bears particular relevance because the short cineangiographic exposure relative to total fluoroscopy time still results in as much as 25 to 35% of the total radiation dose because of the greater radiation energy required to generate the permanent image.

GENERATION OF X-RAYS

Current systems for generating x-rays consist of a rotating rhenium-tungsten anode target mounted to optimize dissipation of heat that is produced and decrease heat conduction to its bearings. In an effort to avoid the latter problem, at least one system uses an electromagnetic field to support the rotating anode rather than the more commonly used mechanical bearings. Another system uses fluid bearings.

The cathode consists of a tungsten filament housed in a focusing apparatus. Voltage and current from the generator heat the tungsten cathode; as a result, electrons are boiled off by thermo-ionic emission. The flow of electrons from the cathode to the anode describes the current in milliamperes (mA) and relates directly to the number of x-ray photons produced by the tube. The electrical potential across the x-ray tube is designated by kilovolts (kV) and relates to the penetrating power of each photon. Time of the exposure measured in milliseconds is often grouped with current and is designated by milliampere-seconds (mAS). Modern generators use microprocessors to control all aspects of the energy delivered to the x-ray tube (electric potential, current, duration) in an effort to achieve automatic exposure control using a photoelectric feedback system that responds to the density of light produced by the receptor of the x-ray photons after they pass through the patient.

Tungsten has a high melting temperature (3370°C), which is required by the high temperatures generated by a predominantly thermal interaction, with approximately 99.5% of the energy resulting in heat. The bombardment of the rotating anode by electrons that have boiled off the cathode results in the generation of x-ray photons by the anode tungsten atoms because of the rapid deceleration of electrons. The x-ray photons emitted are proportional to the electrical energy described by the voltage, current, and duration involved in the process. In general, increasing the kilovolts results in greater penetration of x-rays, whereas increasing the milliamperes increases both the image sharpness and the amount of scatter produced.

The electron beam generated by the cathode is fixed; however, the rotating anode is angled to allow for the creation of a larger apparent focal spot that is directed to the image intensifier. The apparent focal spot is thus larger than the effective focal spot, which is by definition "seen" at 90 degrees to the incident electron beam. Small focal spots allow for greater image sharpness but are limited in the amount of power they can handle, resulting in a high voltage–low current technique that blackens the cineangiogram with resultant loss of contrast. Most systems employ two focal spots, with the larger spot accommodating the increased power (kilowatts [kW]) required for larger patients or axially angulated views. Newer equipment, with the ability to pulse the fluoroscopy on and off rapidly to avoid flicker of the image perceptible to the human eye, while significantly decreasing the total radiation exposure to the patient and staff, may employ three focal spots. Pulsed fluoroscopy may either originate at the generator or be grid switched at the x-ray tube. Utilizing the larger focal spot sacrifices some image sharpness. *Blur* (unsharpness) tends to affect the margins of large images, whereas *contrast* affects the recognition of smaller details such as small guide wires or vessels. The x-ray is automatically collimated so that the beam is directed within the confines of the image intensifier on the opposite side of the patient. Further manual collimation confers the ability to cone the beam around the structure of interest, thus improving the image by decreasing the amount of stray radiation striking the intensifier. In general, the x-ray tube on modern systems is mounted such that the x-ray beam passes from under the patient to an intensifier above and from the right to left side of the patient in biplane systems.

RADIOGRAPHIC IMAGE

The generated x-rays are directed through the patient and are attenuated by tissues and contrast media. The emerging x-ray photons strike the intensifier screen to emit fluorescence (visible light), which is used to create an image whether analog or digitally processed. Image characteristics include blur, contrast, density, magnification, and noise. As discussed previously, the size of the focal spot contributes to image blur, observed by the loss of definition exhibited at the margins of an object. This is because the apparent focal spot has dimension rather than being a true point source and results in a halo effect. In addition, motion and the physical characteristics of the image receptor also contribute. In the laboratory, one can influence these minimally. Remember that these effects are increased by the magnification of the image produced by the distances between the source of the x-rays, the object (patient), and the image intensifier.

The air-space magnification can be reduced by decreasing the distance between the object (patient) and the image intensifier. The density of the image merely refers to the degree of light photon activity produced by the receptor receiving the x-ray after passing through the patient. The density of a good image is adjusted so that opacified smaller vessels are not obscured by too much energy, but the energy is not so weak as to merge soft tissues with the opacified image. In the voltage range of most equipment, density is doubled for every 10 kV increase in voltage. Current and time affect the radiographic density less; hence, if the amount of energy to be delivered is to remain the same, a decrease of 10 kV must be countered by a doubling of milliampere-seconds to preserve the same density. Current and duration of exposure, however, are limited by heat production at the anode that, if unchecked, could melt even the heat-resistant tungsten alloy. Heat is dissipated in part by rotation of the anode, with faster rotation favoring a cooler anode at the expense of bearing wear. An x-ray tube's *power rating*, which is the product of current and voltage expressed in milliwatts (mW), is defined by the point at which the tungsten alloy melts. Noise or quantum mottle is described by random fluctuations in density that may or may not be perceptible to the eye; however, current set too low results in a mottled image because of the influence of relatively greater noise. A higher current setting, although resulting in a sharper image, also increases the amount of radiation emitted. Point-to-point variations in density of the image define the contrast. The relationship of noise and contrast further defines the visibility of small objects.

One last physical concept, that of *tissue half thickness*,[9] is important to consider, particularly in a pediatric laboratory that must consider a variety of patient sizes in the setting of axially angled angiographic techniques. This concept describes a thickness, which is approximately 4 cm in humans, at which the attenuation of the x-ray beam is halved, thus decreasing the density of the image. In other words, for every 4 cm of tissue thickness introduced by either changing patient size or angulation of the patient relative to the x-ray beam, the kilovolts must be increased by 10 or the milliampere-seconds doubled to achieve the same density in the image produced. Increasing the kilovolts may require a larger focal spot, thus increasing the blur; however, increasing the current and duration of exposure also increases motion blur. Modern systems switch automatically between small and large focal spots to retain a constant density with changes in tissue half thickness introduced with changes in projection. A practical consideration involves long periods of fluoroscopy in axially angled projections for interventional procedures. These can significantly increase the radiation exposure to patients and staff.

Once the x-ray beam is generated, it consists of photons with different energies. Low-energy photons are attenuated by the tissues of the patient and do not participate in image production; they are filtered by a thin layer of aluminum before entering the patient. The collimated beam of x-rays is received by the image intensifier, which houses the primary image receptor and then converts x-ray photons to light. Before striking the receptor the x-rays pass through a lead grid that reduces the amount of scattered x-rays to improve the sharpness of the image.

The image intensifier increases the brightness of the produced image several thousand-fold. The x-rays strike an input phosphor (cesium iodide) that converts the x-ray to visible light. The light then strikes a photocathode and is converted to electrons that are projected and focused using electronic lenses via the anode to the smaller output phosphor (zinc cadmium sulfide) for reconversion to light. Most intensifiers have different input phosphor sizes available, with the larger sizes requiring less x-ray energy to produce equivalent images. In general, each incremental decrease in intensifier size approximately doubles the radiation exposure but increases magnification. The *inverse square law* dictates that each doubling of magnification requires a quadrupling of x-ray energy to achieve the same image density. Light output emitted from the output phosphor is then directed to the television camera or cinefilm if the system is so equipped. *Intensifier speed* refers to the amount of x-ray photons required to produce the image and is directly related to the size of phosphor crystals. Faster large crystals or thicker layers of phosphor require fewer x-ray photons for a given image density, but the trade-off for less x-rays is a relative increase in noise, resulting in decreased contrast. In addition, increased blur caused by diffusion of produced light is associated with these changes. The balance of these mutually exclusive effects is an important factor in performance.

The image intensifier is the key receptor in the system. It is capable in most systems of detecting a difference of 4 line pairs/mm in the smallest input sizes. Over time, the phosphor degrades, and the intensifiers require replacement as early as every 3 to 5 years depending on their use.

The light produced by the image intensifier in analog systems is electronically boosted and directed to a television camera using an optical lens to produce a uniform image. A mirror is present that is capable of directing a portion of the light to cinefilm for permanent recording of a cineangiogram pulsed at a rate of 15 to 60 frames/sec. As the phosphor emits a green light, cinefilm sensitive to this wavelength must be used.

In digital systems, the optical lens is replaced by megachips, thus dispensing with the need for cinefilm and mirror. Attention to the edge detail provided by video digital imaging systems is important when considering the quality of image produced. Most systems can offer 1024×1024 pixels at 30 frames/sec, which allow for approximately 3.9 line pairs/mm to be distinguished in the 13-cm image intensifier mode. Line pairs decrease to about 2 line pairs/mm as one approaches an intensifier mode of 23 to 25 cm. Although this is satisfactory for most situations, it is inferior to the capability of cinefilm, which ranges from 3.6 to 3.9 line pairs/mm in even the largest input phosphor sizes. The fact remains, however, that commercial production of television camera tubes is diminishing in the face of digital technology; hence, the demise of analog systems seems inevitable. Digital images also offer the advantage of subtraction technology and the ability to recall immediately data for online analysis that can be of advantage, particularly during interventional procedures. Archival and transfer of images have been standardized in the past to the medium of 35 mm film; however, the advent of digital systems has resulted in the standard medium to be defined in North America as DICOM-3 (Digital Imaging and COmmunication in Medicine) with the physical format of unfiltered CD-ROM. There are still many specific details to be resolved.[10, 11] In addition, digital systems offer the promise of remote accessibility, which has advantages with respect to immediate availability at point of care. Improvements in postacquisition digital processing should result in visually pleasing images with greater resolution at the work station.

RADIATION SAFETY

A working knowledge of the effects of radiation exposure and strategies for reduction are compulsory for an invasive cardiologist.[12] Direct primary exposure affects the patient for limited periods of time and cumulative secondary exposure describes the risk to personnel. Although cineangiography is associated with greater exposure per unit time than is fluoroscopy, the advent of interventional procedures has resulted in a greater proportion of time spent using fluoroscopy. Indeed, the catheterization laboratory represents one of the greatest sources of exposure to x-rays for patients and staff, relative to other x-ray diagnostic techniques.

Radiation exposure can be measured with ionization chambers, photographic film (badges), or thermoluminescent dosimeter salts. Units to describe radiation are difficult to conceptualize because of overlapping terminology, particularly as the unit of exposure (the roentgen) differs from the unit of protection that describes the absorbed dose.[12] The roentgen (R) is the ionization that the beam from an x-ray tube produces in air and is the amount of radiation that produces 2.58×10^{-4} coulombs/kg of air. Exposure (rad and gray) and equivalent (rem and Sievert) doses describe absorbed radiation and are essentially a semantic distinction as the factor to convert the former to the latter for x-rays is one. Essentially, the absorbed dose describes how much heating the x-rays produce in each unit of a specified material. The unit for absorbed dose is the familiar *rad*, which is 100 ergs of energy deposited in 1 g of tissue, with the SI unit being the gray (Gy), which is 1 joule/kg. The equivalent dose is the *rem*, which measures effective biologic radiation, and the analogous SI unit is the sievert (Sv). Equivalent doses are generally used in radiation protection as they describe the absorbed dose in biologic tissue. Fortunately, conversion between units is generally simplified in that under normal circumstances in the laboratory 1 R approximates 1 rad = 1cGy = 1 rem = 10 mSv.

The patient is exposed to radiation directly from the x-ray beam. Not surprisingly, soft tissues absorb less radiation than denser tissues such as bone. Only about 1% of the original x-ray beam reaches the image intensifier. In adults, the total equivalent absorbed dose ranges from 8.6 to 19.8 mSv for procedures ranging from diagnostic procedures to single stent implantation. This approximates 143 to 330 chest x-rays and is by far among the greatest for radiologic diagnostic procedures, surpassed only by myocardial scintigraphy.[12] In the pediatric population, the exposure has been estimated to be in the range of 50 x-rays for simple diagnostic procedures, and even simple interventional procedures can approach 1000 times the x-ray exposure.[13] Radiofrequency ablation procedures for arrhythmia management result in approximately 4 times the x-ray exposure.[14] In general, most nonpulsed systems require (for adults) about 30 mR/frame for cineangiography and 3 R/min for fluoroscopy. Roughly translated, the dose is at least 10 times greater per unit time for cineangiography. The advantages to the patient of a digital laboratory that obviates the need for cineangiography are obvious.[15] Pulsed fluoroscopy reduces the amount of radiation exposure to the patient by at least 35%.[16]

Staff exposed to ionizing radiation in a catheterization laboratory must wear a radiation dosimeter under lead garments at the waist, on the outside of garments at collar level, or both, depending on federal regulations.[17] Steps taken to lower exposure to the patient also decrease secondary scatter exposure to staff. The scatter is greatest at the entrance of the x-ray beam to the patient (i.e., at the level of the table) and rapidly decreases as one moves further from the patient because of the inverse square law. It is estimated that the assistant receives one third the dose of the primary operator.[13] In the era of intervention, operators in busy laboratories without pulsed fluoroscopy and still using cineangiography will approach maximum exposures when approaching 250 studies per year. Hence, attention to the details of radiation safety are relevant.

The effects of radiation are described as *stochastic* if they increase with cumulative doses but do not depend on individual dose. *Nonstochastic* effects occur when there is an all or none phenomenon. The average person receives approximately 2 to 3.5 mSv/yr from natural and unnatural (including medical) sources. North American individuals working in a catheterization laboratory are monitored for quarterly and yearly dose, whereas in some centers such as Sweden, the cumulative dose is monitored over the operator's working lifetime. Such cumulative monitoring allows for best estimates of the risk for stochastic effects. Somatic effects are related to the radiosensitivities of various tissues. The thyroid gland, gonads, bone marrow, lung, breast, and eye lens are more sensitive than are other tissues. Effects such as fibrosis, inflammation, atrophy, ulceration, decreased gametogenesis, and malignancy (especially of the thyroid and involving bone marrow) are described.[9, 12, 18] Genetic effects may present over two generations; however, the actual effect due to lifetime radiation exposure in the laboratory is difficult to distinguish from background mutation rates. The high gonadal doses required to increase the incidence of mutations result in other somatic effects of a more practical concern.[19] During the last decades, most regulatory agencies have decreased the permissible yearly doses of radiation, and the permissible dose will probably be further reduced in the future. When the cumulative and permanent effects of radiation exposure are considered, any measure to decrease exposure benefits both patients and staff. This has the added benefit of prolonging the life of the image intensifier, as radiation also degrades the phosphor responsible for converting the x-ray photon to visible light.

Measures to decrease radiation exposure start with the primary exposure to the patient. All equipment must be used in a specially designed suite that contains the radiation produced. The use of the minimum amount of x-ray energy to achieve an image is important for point source reduction. The equipment must be well maintained and calibrated regularly. Magnification should be used judiciously. If a digital system is utilized, postprocessing magnification is preferable to using a smaller intensifier. The use of pulsed fluoroscopy units should be encouraged. The x-ray should be collimated carefully with filters, and lead bars should be utilized to cone the beam around the area of interest. The image intensifier should be as close to the patient as possible. Importantly, every second of fluoroscopy should have a purpose, with intermittent fluoroscopy providing the additional benefit of prolonging the x-ray tube life. Digital review of previously saved fluoroscopy scenes can significantly reduce exposure. In addition, a carefully planned study that minimizes catheter exchanges and the use of catheters for multiple purposes also helps.[20] Similarly cineangiograms should be carefully planned with test injections of contrast agent under fluoroscopy replacing repeated angiograms to delineate anatomy. Short diagnostic angiograms are preferable, with the need for more than 6 to 8 seconds rarely indicated. Axial projections require more x-ray energy and are associated with more radiation scatter; hence, the operator must use these projections judiciously, especially during prolonged interventional procedures. Secondary exposure caused predominantly by scatter affects both the patient and the staff. However, the staff are exposed to cumulative long-term permanent doses of radiation. Shielding equivalent to 0.5 mm of lead decreases the exposure by a factor of 50; hence, its use over sensitive areas with aprons, shields

or collars, and glasses provides substantial protection. The protective equipment should be screened regularly for defects. Staff should be aware of the inverse square law (the radiation exposure decreases proportional to the inverse square of the distance from the x-ray beam) and should step away from the field during angiography, in addition to understanding the areas of greatest exposure to scatter.

The problem with radiation safety is that x-rays are not perceived at the time of exposure, so that attention to the details must be included as part of routine training in an effort to ensure that they are incorporated into the culture of the laboratory and its personnel.

CONTRAST MEDIA: PROPERTIES AND RELEVANCE

Most contrast agents for intravascular imaging are based on iodine and essentially function to increase the natural contrast that exists between tissues. Both positive effects and negative effects due to "wash in" of unopacified blood are of diagnostic importance (Figs. 14–1 and 14–2). Organic iodine derivatives with a benzoic acid ring were developed initially with only one iodide atom per ring. Subsequently, triiodide benzoic acid anions with sodium or methylglucamine cations were developed. Solubility, osmolality, and side effects of the agent are influenced by the side chains of the benzene ring. Radiodensity of the contrast media is related to the concentration of iodide atoms in the solution (usually 320 to 370 mg/ml). The standard high osmolality ionic agents (1797 to 2076 mOsm/kg water) have a viscosity of about 6 times that of blood and have

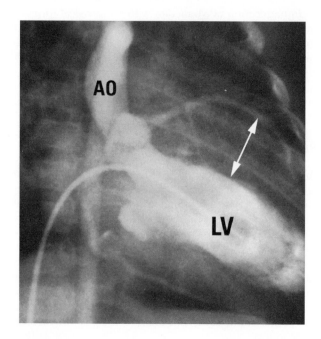

FIGURE 14-1

Hypertrophic cardiomyopathy. Right axial oblique projection of a left ventriculogram in a patient with muscular hypertrophy of the myocardium. Note the separation between the ventricular cavity and epicardial anterior descending coronary artery *(arrow)*. AO = aorta; LV = left ventricle.

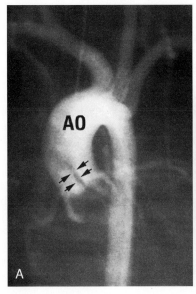
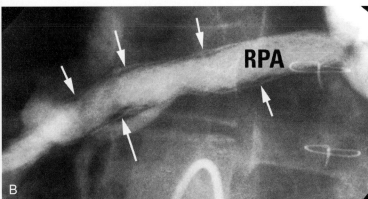

FIGURE 14-2

Utilization of negative contrast effects. *A*, Aortogram in a patient with significant aortic valve stenosis. In addition to the domed aortic valve and post-stenotic dilatation of the ascending aorta (AO), there is a narrow jet *(arrows)* of unopacified blood through the stenotic orifice. *B*, A negative intraluminal image *(arrows)* in the left pulmonary arteriogram immediately after balloon angioplasty suggests the presence of a thrombus. RPA = right pulmonary artery.

a higher incidence of mild to moderate side effects than have agents with lower osmolality or nonionic preparations (600 to 844 mOsm/kg water).[21–25] The osmolality of ionic contrast media was decreased by creating a benzene dimer that allowed six atoms of iodine to be present rather than three associated with the monomeric preparations. Notably, although described as low osmolality, these agents are still significantly more hypertonic than blood. A further development resulted in a nonionic benzene monomer that is water soluble and also of low osmolality but still more than that of blood. The last two classes of contrast media are considerably more costly than the more hyperosmolar compounds; however, increasingly, pediatric laboratories are using nonionic preparations, particularly in young neonates or patients with renal failure or significant ventricular dysfunction. In the latter, the cation load associated with the ionic preparations should be avoided.[26] Attention to fluid status and hydration in the latter patients is probably more important than choice of agent.[27] Debate exists in the literature as to the potential for increased thrombosis with the nonionic preparations and the effect of viscosity and temperature on injection rates; however, these issues are less of a practical concern given the disparate opinions.[28–33]

The viscosity and solubility of contrast media are of practical concern in angiography. The viscosity of a solution is conceptually the resistance of the fluid to deformation during flow. The greater the viscosity the more difficult it is to achieve a given flow. This can limit flow through a catheter as can the length and diameter of the catheter and the force of injection. Viscosity and solubility also contribute to the effects of streaming and layering. The mixture of contrast media in blood can layer similar to oil in water. When this occurs in a recumbent patient, some structures may not be visualized, similar to the failure to

opacify a coronary artery origin in a recumbent aortogram. This property can be useful to distinguish the anatomic relationship of many structures as well as in the form of wash in, wherein unopacified blood is visualized as a negative image on the cineangiogram.

Major side effects associated with contrast agents are low, with the incidence of death approaching 1/40,000 injections and the incidence of serious nonfatal reactions about 1/14,000.[34] Adverse and physiologic effects are related to both the hypertonicity of the agents and the intrinsic structure of the molecule. Pulmonary effects include an increase in pulmonary artery pressure and rarely edema. Vasospasm may result from local histamine release. Hyperosmolarity and chemotoxicity also result in peripheral vasodilatation and hypotension, which is augmented by decreased ventricular function. The agents also lengthen the QT interval. The hypertonicity of the agents draws water from red blood cells, which renders them less deformable and increases blood viscosity. Seizures may occur but tend to be related more to carotid artery studies in adults. Anaphylaxis does not appear to be an antibody/antigen-mediated phenomenon. Most cardiologists premedicate patients thought to be at high risk for anaphylaxis by using antihistamines, steroids, or both.

The total acceptable dose of contrast agent depends on both the clinical status of the patient and the duration of the study. Although absolute upper limits have not been clearly defined, one must exercise caution if more than 6 to 8 ml/kg of contrast medium are to be used for routine investigations. Digital subtraction technology can significantly decrease the contrast medium required for individual studies. The total amount given should be reduced in cyanotic polycythemic patients.

There have been several debates regarding the relative cost of contrast media with respect to the incidence of side effects. The incidence of major reactions to contrast media is low, even with high osmolality agents; hence, cost analysis usually favors contrast media rather than the considerably more expensive nonionic media.[35–37] Increasingly, however, issues of patient comfort with mild and moderate side effects are being considered, thus increasing the use of the more expensive agents. The decreased use of conventional high osmolality agents combined with the economic effect of a highly competitive multibillion dollar industry should result in a decreased discrepancy in price between the agents over time.

QUANTITATIVE ANGIOGRAPHY

MAGNIFICATION FACTOR CALCULATIONS

Many factors must be considered in the calculation of magnification for cineangiography.[38] The x-ray beam originates from a point source; hence, the size of the filmed object is increased when projected to the intensifier, and the image is further distorted by a pin cushion effect due to the nature of point source fluoroscopy wherein magnification factor increases in direct proportion to the radial distance from the isocenter. The image is then subjected to a decrease in magnification when filmed in 35 mm format and subsequently increased when projected. Digital systems similarly alter size when the image is projected to a monitor for viewing and analysis.

Essentially, a magnification factor is used to measure the size of a cardiac structure by comparing the measurement obtained with that of a known reference. The catheter diameter is frequently used. However, care must be taken to ensure that the reference catheter is reflected by the outer diameter and not by the contrast-filled inner diameter.[39–41] The catheter reference should be from a straight, not tapered or curved, portion to improve accuracy, and measurements should not be reported closer than to the nearest one half millimeter so as to avoid giving an impression of precision that does not exist due to limitations of the technique. In addition, care must be taken in measuring the size of large objects, such as valve orifices, using this technique in which small inaccuracies in measuring the catheter diameter result in large discrepancies between the measured and true sizes. Digital technology offers the possibility of immediate online measurement that can be of considerable benefit in interventional procedures. Many other techniques have been described to calculate a magnification factor for a larger object such as the ventricle, including the use of calibration-marked catheters, grids, vertebral bodies, and spheres.[42–44] The imprecise nature of the estimation of vertebral body size and the difficulties with foreshortening of the known linear distance between two marks on a catheter for biplane techniques render these alternatives less attractive for formal estimations. More precise and reproducible results are obtained by filming a reference grid, disk, or sphere placed in the same position relative to the x-ray tube and image intensifier as the cardiac chamber. With two-dimensional grids and disks, great care must be taken to film the reference at exactly 90 degrees to the x-ray beam and intensifier, preferably at the isocenter of the biplane system, to avoid foreshortening the reference. A sphere by definition offers the advantage of having its maximal diameter at 90 degrees to both image intensifiers, thus eliminating the need for time-consuming careful adjustment at the time of reference filming. This method allows the investigator to measure either linear diameter or planimetered area of the sphere for magnification factor correction. Although the so-called pin cushion effect of distortion introduced when filming objects out of the system isocenter may be better compensated by the area method, both methods result in comparable estimations.[38, 45, 46]

The range of chest sizes and ventricular orientations in pediatric patients with congenital heart disease has resulted in an increasing use of axial angiography.[47] Similarly, standard table heights and tube-intensifier distances used in the adult population are not practical for application to pediatrics. Thus, at the time of angiography, measurements of table height and intensifier to ventricle distances are often required to record the position accurately.

VENTRICULAR VOLUME CALCULATIONS

The estimation of ventricular volume provides a method of assessing cardiac structure and function and may have important application to the management of patients with cardiac malformations. Mathematical geometric models allow for an estimation of ventricular volume based on single and biplane cineangiography.[45, 48–51] An important consideration is the determination of a correction factor that compensates for the change in size of the imaged ventricle ultimately projected to a screen or digital monitor relative to the actual size of the ventricle. This calculation relies on the projection of a known dimension to the same medium.[38]

In the absence of clinically applicable imaging techniques with three-dimensional reconstruction capability, angiographic ventriculography remains the standard for estimating volumes in vivo. The technique, however, has significant limitations. The potential sources of error include overestimation of volume by the inclusion of trabeculae and papillary muscle in the tracing of the chamber, the morphology of the septum, the influence on septal position imposed by the hemodynamics of the opposing ventricle, the loading conditions of the ventricle including heart rate and patient size, and the projection chosen for angiography.[46, 52–56]

CATHETERS AND TECHNIQUES

The choice of catheter is influenced by the nature of the study and the information required. A carefully planned study results in efficient utilization of catheter resources and laboratory time. In general, important hemodynamic data should be obtained before angiography because contrast media, even the newer generation agents, have hemodynamic and electrophysiologic effects. The physical properties of angiographic catheters have been well reviewed.[57] Catheters are generally constructed by weaving or braiding plastic, incorporating a stainless steel braid and side holes. In a second method, extruded plastic is layered around a steel braid, and a nonbraided tip with punched-in holes is welded into position. In general, thick catheters allow for greater torque in achieving a position, and thin-walled catheters may allow for greater contrast delivery. Flow-directed catheters incorporate a balloon at the tip to facilitate positioning and to increase the safety of catheter manipulations by reducing the risk of perforation. In addition, the balloon can be quite useful in balloon occlusion angiography with injections exiting the catheter from distal or proximal holes.

Flow through a catheter is largely determined by Poiseuille's law, which relates maximum flow inversely to the length and internal diameter of the catheter. Added to this are features of the catheter such as smoothness of the internal bore (catheter coefficient of friction), tapered ends, and side holes that function to increase the maximum flow possible within limits. Maximum possible flow is affected by the viscosity of the contrast agent and the tensile strength of the catheter. Most catheters are designed to break outside the body at the hub in the event of too much pressure secondary to an excessive flow rate. In general, catheter choice is limited by the size of the patient; however, the shortest catheter with the largest internal diameter yields the most satisfying results. High-pressure injections contribute to ectopy in ventriculography and increase the risk of intramyocardial staining or vessel damage. Side holes decrease the velocity of the contrast jet exiting the catheter and stabilize the catheter from recoil during an injection. Before injection, the catheter tip must be confirmed to be in position and intraluminal, if perforation and dissection are to be avoided.

MANUAL AND POWER INJECTIONS

Angiograms may be undertaken by manual or power injection techniques. In general, catheters without side holes are unsuitable for a power injection due to the risk of perforation and problems with catheter recoil. Manual injections are utilized for small vessels such as coronary arteries or aortopulmonary collaterals, in addition to specialized techniques such as balloon occlusion pulmonary venous or arterial angiography. Small chambers, such as in a hypertensive right ventricle in pulmonary atresia and intact ventricular septum, may also require a manual injection. Power spring, lever pneumatic, or electrical injectors allow for a constant pressure or flow in delivering a greater amount of contrast material. The maximum force of injection is limited by the physical properties of the catheter. Automated injections are set to deliver a specific volume at a constant flow or pressure within specific limits. Some injectors allow for phase injections coordinated with the cardiac cycle; however, this is of limited use in infants and children. Many injectors are equipped to deliver contrast material with a gradual rise in pressure to avoid recoil; however, the physical properties of the injection system are such that a square-wave injection is not possible so that all are given with a "rise" regardless of setting. Flow and volume within the limits of pressure characteristics of a catheter define the quality of the angiocardiogram. In general, delivering the desired amount of contrast in the shortest time gives the best anatomic definition. One must carefully consider the purpose of the injection, particularly with ventriculography. Rapid high-contrast injections con-

tribute to ectopy in ventriculography so that injections undertaken for an assessment of volume, function, or wall motion should be delivered more slowly to avoid ectopic contractions. Conversely, ectopics in the setting of a high-contrast injection may provide valuable anatomic information, especially with respect to dynamic changes in structure associated with the cardiac cycle.

The volume of contrast medium delivered with each injection must be integrated carefully with expectations of the anatomy. In general, ventricular and large vessel injections should start with 1.0 ml/kg if no shunt is present. Anatomic definition is best if the contrast agent is delivered over a second, whereas an injection over 2 to 3 seconds is best for functional information. If a shunt is suspected, a larger volume is required. It is not necessary to exceed 2 to 3 ml/kg in any injection. Large vessels with high flows such as the aorta require 1.0 ml/kg given rapidly, over 0.5 to 1 second, but smaller vessels naturally require less contrast agent.

INJECTIONS OVER THE WIRE

Interventional catheterization often demands that catheter position be maintained during an injection. Postangioplasty assessment of a vessel often requires an immediate assessment of results of the intervention. The maintenance of wire position may also be important, especially with stent implantation in a large vessel. In this instance, injection over the wire by adapting a pigtail catheter and injecting through a "y" connector can be particularly useful.[58] Catheter stability is ensured, and wire position is maintained. The high pressure associated with flow through the side holes in this setting can damage vessels recently torn by balloon angioplasty.

ANGIOGRAPHIC PROJECTIONS

Initially all angiograms were obtained in the frontal and lateral projections. Flow over time provided important information with respect to connection of vessels and the segmental anatomy of the cardiac anomalies, but restriction in projection leads to suboptimal information, given the axial orientation of the heart in the thorax and the position of intracardiac structures. In the late 1960s, axial angiography was first recognized to be of benefit in patients with cardiac malformations[59] and was re-emphasized during the next two decades.[47, 60, 61]

Angiographic images are described by either using the recording device as a reference (view) or showing the direction of the x-ray beam from x-ray tube to the recording device (projection).[62] Hence, the familiar frontal view with the intensifier directly above the supine patient is the posteroanterior projection. Strictly speaking, the term *projection* is distinct from that of *view;* however, for practical purposes many use the terms interchangeably. The frontal position also carries the reference designation of 0 degrees. When the intensifier is moved to the left by 15 to 75 degrees, a left anterior oblique (LAO) view is defined, and similar angulation to the right results in a right anterior oblique (RAO) designation. A rotation of 90 degrees (usually to the left) designates the lateral view. Further rotation of the intensifier beyond 90 degrees is designated by some by substituting *posterior* for *anterior* (hence the designations LPO and RPO) to indicate that the projection defines an axial x-ray beam traveling from anterior to posterior. The x-ray beam can also be oriented to travel obliquely from head to toe, resulting in cranial or caudal tilt to the angiogram. By analogy, the projection can also be described as caudal-cranial or cranial-caudal angulations of the x-ray beam; however, this terminology tends to be cumbersome. Angulation in modern laboratories is achieved by mobile equipment. Most dedicated pediatric laboratories utilize biplane imaging to obtain information in two projections simultaneously in an effort to reduce contrast load. In some instances, only a single projection is possible owing to physical limitations in orientation of the equipment. Table 14–1 outlines some of the standard projections used in the study of cardiac malformations. These projections represent a guide. An experienced angiographer modifies these projections to obtain the maximum amount of information from each individual angiogram.

PROJECTIONS AND SEGMENTAL ANGIOGRAPHY

By far the most extensively utilized view is that of the cranially tilted LAO projection owing to the sigmoid nature of the interventricular septum.[63] The membranous septum is profiled best by a steep LAO with cranial tilt oriented such that approximately one third of the heart is projected over the vertebral bodies and cranially angulated so that the tip of the catheter in the apex of the ventricle is located at the bottom of the picture. The inlet of the ventricular septum is profiled using a less steep LAO view, thus projecting more of the cardiac silhouette to the left of the vertebral bodies.

In contrast, a steeper LAO projection profiles more of the outlet septum and moves the cardiac silhouette off the spine. Cranial angulation in this projection avoids overlapping with the lateral shoulder of the ventricle. The amount of cranial tilt can be estimated by considering the amount of the heart projected over the hemidiaphragms.

Systemic venoatrial connections can be identified by catheter course; however, where precise definition is required, angiography in frontal and lateral projections usually provides the necessary information. A careful approach is necessary to ensure that the entire systemic venous connection has been characterized when evaluating the patient before performing a cavopulmonary connection. Standard angiographic catheters can achieve this readily with an appropriate power injection from a distal location; however, manual injection utilizing a balloon occlusion technique with flow-directed catheters also provides the necessary information. Atrial appendage morphology, which provides the basis for defining the situs of the heart, can also be appreciated from this projection. The atrial septum is often best profiled using a shallow LAO view with cranial tilt. This view is often helpful in assessing the atrioventricular connection.

Pulmonary venous connections are variable, but selective injection into segmental portions of the lungs yields the best results during the levophase of the circulation. A shallow LAO view with cranial tilt often defines which side of the atrial septum the veins connect. Shallow RAO and LAO projections can provide important information after selective injection, especially when upper and lower veins are separated using some caudal tilt. The atrioventricular connection for concordant and discordant connections in addition to double inlet, common atrioventricular connections, and straddling atrioventricular valves can all be demonstrated with a shallow LAO projection.

Ventriculoarterial connections are best imaged in shallow RAO and LAO views with cranial tilt on the latter. When the ventricular septum is intact, the connections are evident; however, with a ventricular septal defect the connection may not be as obvious. One relies on an estimate of the relationship of the great vessel to the supporting ventricle by considering the imagined extension of the infundibular septum (RAO projection) and the perimembranous septum (LAO projection). Although inherently difficult to determine, a vessel is committed to the ventricle when greater than 50% of the vessel arises from the ventricle in two perpendicular projections.

The sigmoid nature of the ventricular septum must be considered. Injection into the high-pressure ventricle usually provides the best information about the septum. The most important projection is that of an axially angled LAO that elongates the long axis of the heart in most situations. This view also profiles the perimembranous ventricular septum. The base of the heart can be imaged with less LAO and cranial tilt, whereas the anterior high muscular septum is best profiled with an RAO view (Figs. 14–3 and 14–4).

Optimal aortography depends on the anatomic information required. The ventriculoarterial connection is often best studied using an LAO with cranial tilt and RAO at 90 degrees to the LAO. Removal of the cranial tilt may better

TABLE 14–1

COMMON CINEANGIOGRAPHIC PROJECTIONS

View	A Plane (Degrees)	B Plane (Degrees)
Posteroanterior and lateral	0	90 LAO
Long axial (LV and LPA)	30 RAO	60 LAO
		20 Cranial
Hepatoclavicular (four-chamber LV)	30 LAO	120 LAO
	40 Cranial	15 Cranial
Sitting up (cranial-caudal): RVOT, pulmonary arteries	0 to 7 LAO	90 LAO
	40 Cranial	
Right bidirectional cavopulmonary connection	30 to 40 RAO	90 LAO
	20 to 30 Caudal	
Atrial septal defect	30 LAO	Parked
	40 Cranial	
Down-the-barrel transposition of the great arteries	30 RAO	30 LAO
		45 Caudal
Selective biplane left coronary artery (No. 1)	30 RAO	60 LAO
Selective biplane left coronary artery (No. 2)	30 RAO	60 LAO
	30 Cranial	25 Cranial
Selective biplane left coronary artery (No. 3)	30 RAO	90 LAO
	30 Caudal	
Selective biplane right coronary artery (No. 1)	30 RAO	60 LAO
Selective biplane right coronary artery (No. 2)	30 LAO	Parked
	30 Cranial	

A plane = intensifier that records posteroanterior views; B plane = intensifier that records lateral or LAO views; LV = left ventricle; LPA = left pulmonary artery; RVOT = right ventricular outflow tract; LAO = left anterior oblique; RAO = right anterior oblique.

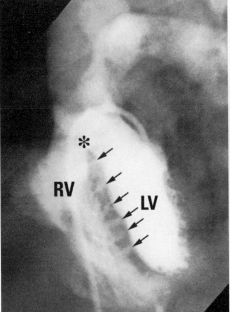

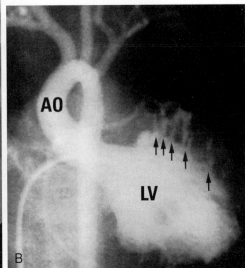

FIGURE 14–3

Imaging the ventricular septum. *A,* A cranially tilted left axial oblique view of a left ventriculogram results in projection of the heart over the spine and abdomen. The defect of the perimembranous septum is well profiled *(asterisk)* with multiple small defects present in the ventricular septum *(arrows). B,* A right axial oblique view in another patient demonstrates multiple defects of the anterosuperior interventricular septum *(arrows).* AO = aorta; LV = left ventricle; RV = right ventricle. (*A, B* from Freedom RM, Mawson JB, Yoo S-J, Benson LN [eds]: Congenital Heart Disease: Textbook of Angiocardiography, Vols I and II. Armonk, NY, Futura, 1997.)

identify the coronary ostia and sinuses of Valsalva. These projections also identify transverse arch anatomy. The aortic isthmus in a coarctation of the aorta can represent a challenge by virtue of the projection of the dilated descending thoracic aorta onto the coarctation area; hence, caudal or more rarely cranial angulation on the lateral and LAO views can be of considerable benefit to profile the coarctation for precise measurement in considering transcatheter intervention (Fig. 14–5).

Coronary arteries may be investigated utilizing aortography by an anterograde transvenous approach or retro-grade approach (Fig. 14–6). Improvements in catheter technology have resulted in the wide application of selective coronary injection, again by either approach (Fig. 14–7). Recently, the technique of balloon occlusion aortography in the "laid-back" or "down-the-barrel" views has received considerable attention in the neonate with discordant ventriculoarterial connections (Fig. 14–8). Coronary arteries may also be visualized by injection into the hypertensive ventricle with fistulous connections, as in pulmonary atresia with an intact ventricular septum. Details of coronary anatomy relevant to individual cardiac condi-

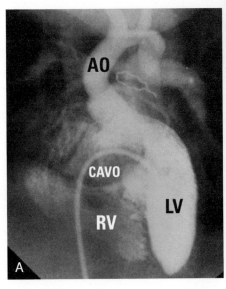

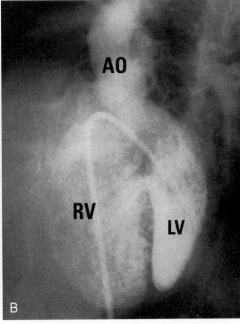

FIGURE 14–4

Hepatoclavicular view for the inlet septum. Steep cranial angulation of a left axial oblique projection demonstrates the relative size of the left (LV) and right (RV) ventricles in addition to obtaining a good profile of the inlet defect. *A,* The RV does not reach the apex, suggesting apical attenuation. *B,* Another patient with a smaller LV relative to the RV. The relative size of the ventricles must be considered in relation to the volume load. AO = aorta; CAVO = common atrioventricular valve orifice. (*A, B* from Freedom RM, Mawson JB, Yoo S-J, Benson LN [eds]: Congenital Heart Disease: Textbook of Angiocardiography, Vols I and II. Armonk, NY, Futura, 1997.)

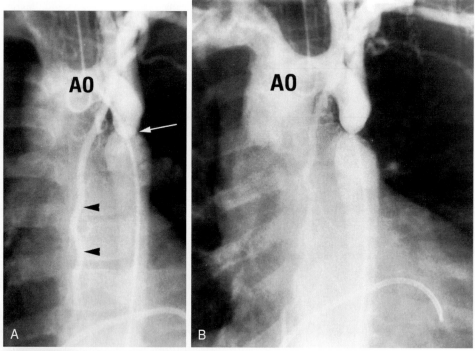

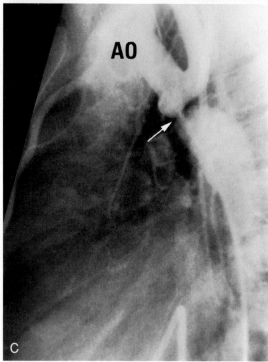

FIGURE 14–5

Aortography in coarctation of the aorta. A, A frontal projection superimposes the aortic isthmus on the dilated descending aorta (AO) *(white arrow)*. Note the enlarged left internal mammary artery *(arrowheads)*. B, Caudal angulation provides a better profile to assess the severity of the stenosis that is further defined in C, the lateral projection *(white arrow)*. (A–C from Freedom RM, Mawson JB, Yoo S-J, Benson LN [eds]: Congenital Heart Disease: Textbook of Angiocardiography, Vols I and II. Armonk, NY, Futura, 1997.)

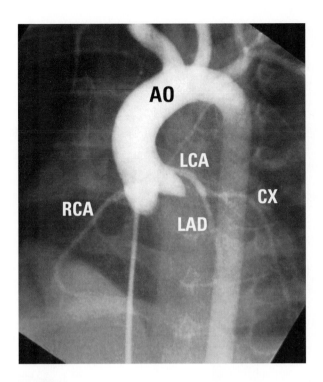

FIGURE 14-6
Aortography for coronary artery anatomy. Aortogram undertaken using a transfemoral approach to the right atrium and ventricle, through the ventricular septal defect, and into the ascending aorta (AO). Attention to detail of injection and catheter technique results in excellent opacification of the coronary arteries and no catheter-induced aortic insufficiency. CX = circumflex coronary artery; LCA = left main coronary artery; RCA = right coronary artery; LAD = left anterior descending coronary artery. (From Freedom RM, Mawson JB, Yoo S-J, Benson LN [eds]: Congenital Heart Disease: Textbook of Angiocardiography, Vols I and II. Armonk, NY, Futura, 1997.)

tions are discussed in the relevant chapters. Balloon occlusion descending aortography is also helpful in a neonate and young infant to identify aortopulmonary collateral arteries. Again, retrograde selective injections provide more detailed information.

Pulmonary arteriography is also tailored to the specific information required. The origins of the pulmonary arteries can often be imaged in the cranially angulated anteroposterior projection (Fig. 14–9). The main pulmonary artery and right ventricular outflow tract are often best seen with the lateral projection (Fig. 14–10), and caudal angulation can separate the origins of the right and left pulmonary arteries. The right pulmonary artery origin can be profiled in the RAO projection, whereas a cranially tilted LAO profiles the left (Figs. 14–11 and 14–12). Distal branches can best be seen in a lateral projection, and selective catheterization is preferable when detailed information is required (Fig. 14–13). In patients with pulmonary anatomy difficult to define by conventional angiography, pulmonary venous wedge injection may provide further anatomic definition (Fig. 14–14).

Specific projections and identification of complications in interventional procedures are discussed in the relevant chapters. Postoperative imaging must be prefaced by a knowledge of the surgical anatomy with an emphasis on obtaining the best axial projection to define a specific problem. As an example, the right-sided bidirectional cavopulmonary anastomosis is often created with the anastomosis superior and anterior so that the best information is often attained when one abandons the traditional anteroposterior view for one that is angled RAO with caudal tilt (Fig. 14–15).

Text continued on page 233

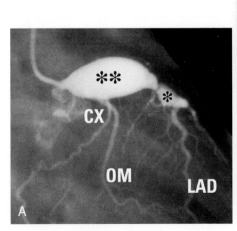
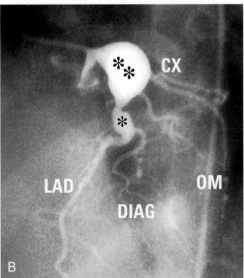

FIGURE 14-7
Selective coronary arteriograms in Kawasaki disease. Selective left coronary arteriogram in a patient with giant coronary aneurysms (*asterisks*) in the right oblique (A) and left axial oblique (B) projections with cranial tilt provides information on the extent of the aneurysm as well as defining possible stenosis. CX = circumflex coronary artery; DIAG = diagonal branch; LAD = left anterior descending coronary artery; OM = obtuse marginal coronary artery. (*A, B* from Freedom RM, Mawson JB, Yoo S-J, Benson LN [eds]: Congenital Heart Disease: Textbook of Angiocardiography, Vols I and II. Armonk, NY, Futura, 1997.)

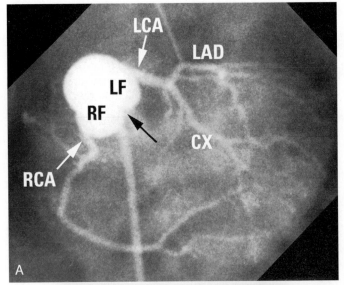

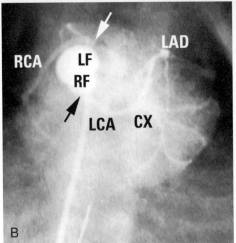

FIGURE 14–8

Balloon occlusion transvenous aortogram in a neonate with complete transposition. *A,* "Down-the-barrel" or "laid-back" aortogram demonstrates the usual origin and distribution of the coronary arteries in complete transposition. The shallow left axial oblique projection with extreme caudal tilt allows a view of the opacified aorta from the feet of the patient. Both facing sinuses and the interposed commissure are seen. *B,* Note the retropulmonary course of the LCA in another patient with inverted origins of the coronary artery origins. CX = circumflex coronary artery; LAD = left anterior descending coronary artery; LCA = left coronary artery; LF = left facing sinus; RCA = right coronary artery; RF = right facing sinus. (*A, B* from Freedom RM, Mawson JB, Yoo S-J, Benson LN [eds]: Congenital Heart Disease: Textbook of Angiocardiography, Vols I and II. Armonk, NY, Futura, 1997.)

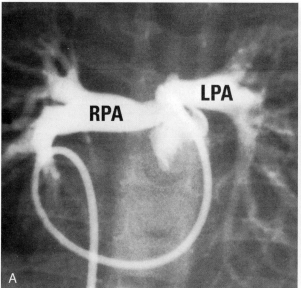
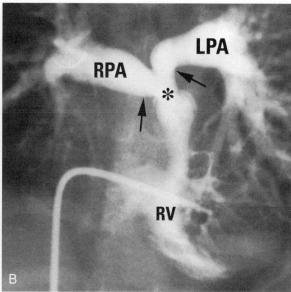

FIGURE 14–9

Cranial angulation improves pulmonary arteriography. *A,* Selective injection of the pulmonary arteries in a straight frontal projection does not delineate the nature of the main and proximal branch pulmonary arteries. *B,* Right ventriculogram in a cranially tilted frontal projection demonstrates anatomic detail, including proximal posteroanterior stenosis *(arrows)* and supravalvar pulmonary stenosis *(asterisk),* in the same patient. LPA = left pulmonary artery; RPA = right pulmonary artery; RV = right ventricle. (*A, B* from Freedom RM, Mawson JB, Yoo S-J, Benson LN [eds]: Congenital Heart Disease: Textbook of Angiocardiography, Vols I and II. Armonk, NY, Futura, 1997.)

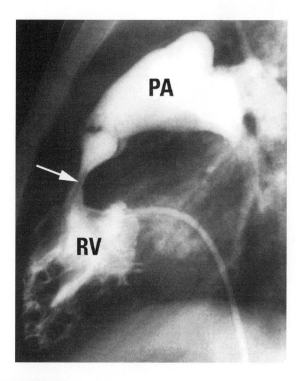

FIGURE 14–10

Right ventriculogram. The lateral projection provides an excellent view of the right ventricular outflow tract in this patient with dynamic muscular subpulmonary obstruction *(arrow)* in association with pulmonary valve stenosis. PA = pulmonary artery; RV = right ventricle. (From Freedom RM, Mawson JB, Yoo S-J, Benson LN [eds]: Congenital Heart Disease: Textbook of Angiocardiography, Vols I and II. Armonk, NY, Futura, 1997.)

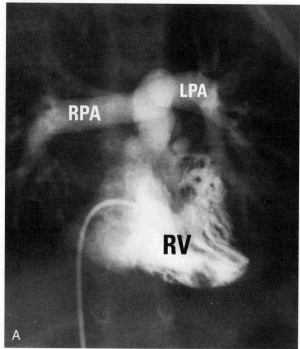

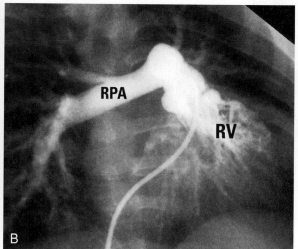

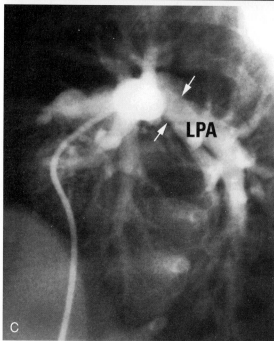

FIGURE 14–11

Pulmonary arteriography. The frontal right ventriculogram (*A*) superimposes the pulmonary artery origins, and the right axial oblique (*B*) and cranially tilted left axial oblique (*C*) views clearly demonstrate the anatomy with only mild stenosis of the left pulmonary artery (*white arrows*). LPA = left pulmonary artery; RPA = right pulmonary artery; RV = right ventricle. (*A–C* from Freedom RM, Mawson JB, Yoo S-J, Benson LN [eds]: Congenital Heart Disease: Textbook of Angiocardiography, Vols I and II. Armonk, NY, Futura, 1997.)

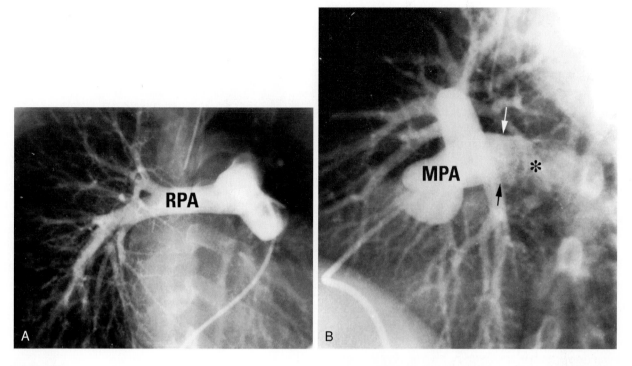

FIGURE 14–12

Pulmonary artery origins. The right axial oblique projection *(A)* defines the origin of the right pulmonary artery (RPA) complemented by a reciprocal left axial oblique projection *(B)* with cranial (long-axis) projection outlining the left pulmonary artery *(asterisk)* origin *(arrows)* illustrates the advantage of well-planned biplane imaging. MPA = main pulmonary artery. (*A, B* from Freedom RM, Mawson JB, Yoo S-J, Benson LN [eds]: Congenital Heart Disease: Textbook of Angiocardiography, Vols I and II. Armonk, NY, Futura, 1997.)

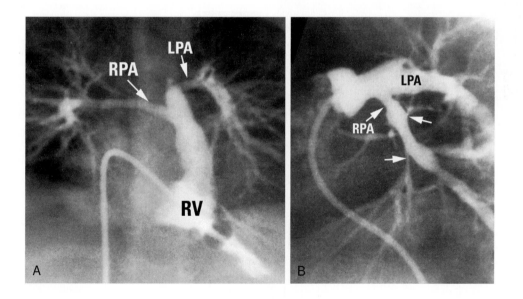

FIGURE 14–13

Imaging distal pulmonary artery stenosis. *A,* The frontal projection of a right ventricle (RV) angiogram demonstrates hypoplastic pulmonary arteries. *B,* The lateral projection more clearly defines stenosis of the origin of multiple arteries to the right lung *(arrows).* Caudal angulation of the lateral projection separates the origin of the pulmonary arteries, showing the left pulmonary artery (LPA) coursing superiorly and posteriorly and the right pulmonary artery (RPA) coursing inferiorly. (*A, B* from Freedom RM, Mawson JB, Yoo S-J, Benson LN [eds]: Congenital Heart Disease: Textbook of Angiocardiography, Vols I and II. Armonk, NY, Futura, 1997.)

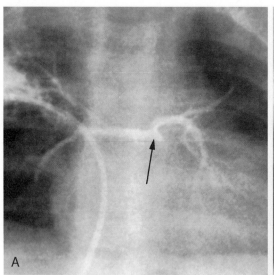

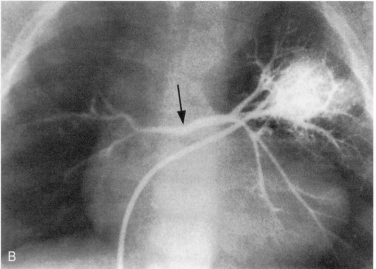

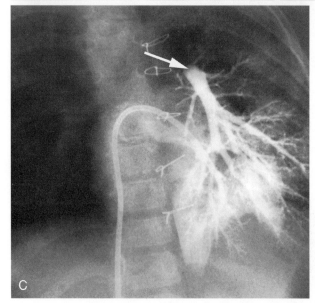

FIGURE 14–14

Pulmonary venous wedge angiography. Pulmonary vein wedge angiography from the right *(A)* and left *(B)* pulmonary vein demonstrates a hypoplastic and confluent pulmonary artery system filled by retrograde perfusion of the pulmonary capillary bed *(black arrows)*. *C,* Left lower pulmonary venous wedge angiogram outlines a well-developed pulmonary arterial system extending to the hilum of the left lung *(white arrow)*. (A–C from Freedom RM, Mawson JB, Yoo S-J, Benson LN [eds]: Congenital Heart Disease: Textbook of Angiocardiography, Vols I and II. Armonk, NY, Futura, 1997.)

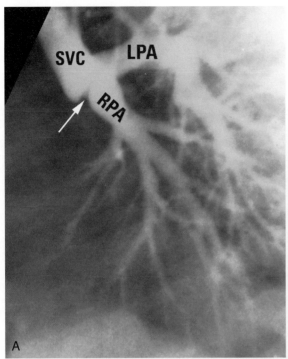

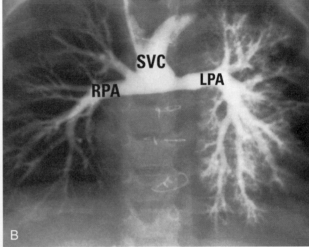

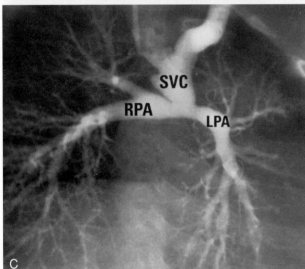

FIGURE 14–15

Angiography of a bidirectional cavopulmonary connection.
A, Lateral angiogram of a bidirectional cavopulmonary connection suggests an anterosuperior orientation to the connection *(arrow). B,* Frontal projection in the same patient superimposes the important aspect of the connection, thus obscuring the anatomy. *C,* The right axial oblique position and caudal tilt allows the details of the connection to be clearly profiled. LPA = left pulmonary artery, RPA = right pulmonary artery, SVC = superior vena cava. (*A–C* from Freedom RM, Mawson JB, Yoo S-J, Benson LN [eds]: Congenital Heart Disease: Textbook of Angiocardiography, Vols I and II. Armonk, NY, Futura, 1997.)

REFERENCES

1. Beekman RP, Filippini LH, Meijboom EJ: Evolving usage of pediatric cardiac catheterization. Curr Opin Cardiol 9:721, 1994.
2. Chung KJ, Simpson IA, Newman R, et al: Cine magnetic resonance imaging for evaluation of congenital heart disease: Role in pediatric cardiology compared with echocardiography and angiography. J Pediatr 113:1028, 1988.
3. Boothroyd AE, McDonald EA, Carty H: Lung perfusion scintigraphy in patients with congenital heart disease: Sensitivity and important pitfalls. Nucl Med Commun 17:33, 1996.
4. Hartnell GG, Meier RA: MR angiography of congenital heart disease in adults. Radiographics 15:781, 1995.
5. Ritchie JL, Bateman TM, Bonow RO, et al: Guidelines for clinical use of cardiac radionuclide imaging. A report of the American Heart Association/American College of Cardiology Task Force on Assessment of Diagnostic and Therapeutic Cardiovascular Procedures, Committee on Radionuclide Imaging, developed in collaboration with the American Society of Nuclear Cardiology. Circulation 91:1278, 1995.
6. Ritchie JL, Bateman TM, Bonow RO, et al: Guidelines for clinical use of cardiac radionuclide imaging. Report of the American College of Cardiology/American Heart Association Task Force on Assessment of Diagnostic and Therapeutic Cardiovascular Procedures (Committee on Radionuclide Imaging), developed in collaboration with the American Society of Nuclear Cardiology. J Am Coll Cardiol 25:521, 1995.
7. Sayad DE, Clarke GD, Peshock RM: Magnetic resonance imaging of the heart and its role in current cardiology. Curr Opin Cardiol 10:640, 1995.
8. Culham JAG, Freedom RM, Mawson JB, et al: Physical principles of image formation and projections in Angiocardiography. *In* Freedom RM, Mawson JB, Yoo S, Benson LN (eds): Congenital Heart Disease. Textbook of Angiocardiography, Vol 1. Armonk, NY, Futura, 1997.
9. Moore RJ: Imaging Principles of Cardiac Angiography. Bethesda, MD, Aspen, 1990.
10. Holmes DRJ: President's page. Cathet Cardiovasc Diagn 36:293, 1995.

11. Holmes DRJ: To compress or not, that is the question. Cathet Cardiovasc Diagn 36:382, 1995.

12. Aldridge HE, Chisholm RJ, Dragatakis L, Roy L: Radiation safety in the cardiac catheterization laboratory. Can J Cardiol 13:459, 1997.

13. Wu JR, Huang TY, Wu DK, et al: Radiation exposure of pediatric patients and physicians during cardiac catheterization and balloon pulmonary valvuloplasty. Am J Cardiol 68:221, 1991.

14. Kovoor P, Ricciardello M, Collins L, et al: Radiation exposure to patient and operator during radiofrequency ablation for supraventricular tachycardia. Aust N Z J Med 25:490, 1995.

15. Holmes DRJ, Wondrow MA, Gray JE: Isn't it time to abandon cine film? Cathet Cardiovasc Diagn 20:1, 1990.

16. Holmes DJ, Wondrow MA, Gray JE, et al: Effect of pulsed progressive fluoroscopy on reduction of radiation dose in the cardiac catheterization laboratory. J Am Coll Cardiol 15:159, 1990.

17. Balter S: Guidelines for personnel radiation monitoring in the cardiac catheterization laboratory. Laboratory Performance Standards Committee of the Society for Cardiac Angiography and Interventions. Cathet Cardiovasc Diagn 30:277, 1993.

18. Pratt TA, Shaw AJ: Factors affecting the radiation dose to the lens of the eye during cardiac catheterization procedure. Br J Radiol 66:346, 1993.

19. Miller SW, Castronovo FPJ: Radiation exposure and protection in the catheterization laboratories. Am J Cardiol 55:171, 1985.

20. Mannino SC, Scavina M, Palmer S: Modified multipurpose catheter enhances clinical utility for cardiac catheterizations. Cathet Cardiovasc Diagn 33:166, 1994.

21. Steinberg EP, Moore RD, Powe NR, et al: Safety and cost effectiveness of high-osmolality as compared with low-osmolality contrast material in patients undergoing cardiac angiography. N Engl J Med 326:425, 1992.

22. Matthai WJ, Hirshfeld JJ: Choice of contrast agents for cardiac angiography: Review and recommendations based on clinically important distinctions. Cathet Cardiovasc Diagn 22:278, 1991.

23. Vik MH, Rosland GA, Folling M, Danielsen R: Hemodynamic and electrocardiographic consequences of high- and low-osmolality contrast agents for left ventricular angiography. Cathet Cardiovasc Diagn 14:143, 1988.

24. Vik MH, Folling M, Barth P, et al: Influence of low osmolality contrast media on electrophysiology and hemodynamics in coronary angiography: Differences between an ionic (ioxaglate) and a nonionic (iohexol) agent. Cathet Cardiovasc Diagn 21:221, 1990.

25. Barrett BJ, Parfrey PS, Vavasour HM, et al: A comparison of nonionic, low-osmolality radiocontrast agents with ionic, high-osmolality agents during cardiac catheterization. N Engl J Med 326:431, 1992.

26. Hill JA, Winniford M, Cohen MB, et al: Multicenter trial of ionic versus nonionic contrast media for cardiac angiography. The Iohexol Cooperative Study. Am J Cardiol 72:770, 1993.

27. Solomon R, Werner C, Mann D, et al: Effects of saline, mannitol, and furosemide to prevent acute decreases in renal function induced by radiocontrast agents. N Engl J Med 331:1416, 1994.

28. Grabowski EF: A hematologist's view of contrast media, clotting in angiography syringes and thrombosis during coronary angiography. Am J Cardiol 66:23F, 1990.

29. Hill JA, Grabowski EF: Relationship of anticoagulation and radiographic contrast agents to thrombosis during coronary angiography and angioplasty: Are there real concerns? Cathet Cardiovasc Diagn 25:200, 1992.

30. Piessens JH, Stammen F, Vrolix MC, et al: Effects of an ionic versus a nonionic low osmolar contrast agent on the thrombotic complications of coronary angioplasty. Cathet Cardiovasc Diagn 28:99, 1993.

31. Parvez Z, Moncada R: Nonionic contrast medium: Effects on blood coagulation and complement activation in vitro. Angiology 37:358, 1986.

32. Rees CR, Merchun G, Becker GJ, et al: In vitro study of high-pressure catheters and various contrast agents. Radiology 166:53, 1988.

33. Roth R, Akin M, Deligonul U, Kern MJ: Influence of radiographic contrast media viscosity to flow through coronary angiographic catheters. Cathet Cardiovasc Diagn 22:290, 1991.

34. Lalli AF, Carswell HM: Nonionic agents extend safety of invasive agents. Diag Imaging 8:70, 1986.

35. Moore RD, Steinberg EP, Powe NR, et al: Frequency and determinants of adverse reactions induced by high-osmolality contrast media. Radiology 170:727, 1989.

36. Lasser EC, Berry CC, Talner LB, et al: Pretreatment with corticosteroids to alleviate reactions to intravenous contrast material. N Engl J Med 317:845, 1987.

37. Powe NR, Steinberg EP, Erickson JE, et al: Contrast medium-induced adverse reactions: Economic outcome. Radiology 169:163, 1988.

38. Sheeham FH, Mitten-Lewis S: Factors influencing accuracy in left ventricular volume determination. Am J Cardiol 61:441, 1989.

39. Reiber JHC, Kooijman CJ, Boer AD, Serruys PW: Assessment of dimensions and image quality of coronary contrast catheters from cineangiograms. Cathet Cardiovasc Diagn 11:521, 1985.

40. Leung W, Demopulos PA, Alderman EL, et al: Evaluation of catheters and metallic catheter markers as calibration standard for measurement of coronary dimension. Cathet Cardiovasc Diagn 21:148, 1990.

41. Jacobs JH, Bove AA, Smith HC, Chesebro JH: Use of a metal ring-marked catheter for geometric calibrations in quantitative angiography. Cathet Cardiovasc Diagn 15:121, 1988.

42. Pridie PB, Parnell B: The importance of magnification in left ventriculography. Br J Radiol 53:642, 1980.

43. Wagner HR, Teske DW, Sui TO: Cineangiographic measurements with the help of a vertebral grid system. Cathet Cardiovasc Diagn 2:353, 1976.

44. Kasser IS, Kennedy JW: Measurement of left ventricular volumes in man by single plane cineangiocardiography. Invest Radiol 4:83, 1969.

45. Dodge HT, Sandler H, Ballew DW, Lord JDJ: The use of biplane angiocardiography for the measurement of left ventricular volume in man. Am Heart J 60:672, 1960.

46. Lange PE, Onnasch D, Farr FL, Heintzen PH: Angiocardiographic left ventricular volume determination. Accuracy as determined from human casts, and clinical application. Eur J Cardiol 8:449, 1978.

47. Bargeron LM, Elliott LP, Soto B, et al: Axial cineangiography in congenital heart disease. Section 1: Concept, technical and anatomic considerations. Circulation 56:1075, 1977.

48. Green DG, Carlisle R, Grant C, Bunnel IL: Estimation of left ventricular volume by one plane cineangiography. Circulation 35:61, 1967.

49. Wynne J, Green LH, Mann T, et al: Estimation of left ventricular volumes in man from biplane cineangiograms filmed in oblique projections. Am J Cardiol 41:726, 1978.

50. Jones JW, Rackley CE, Bruce RA, et al: Left ventricular volumes in valvular heart disease. Circulation 29:887, 1964.

51. Chapman CB, Baker O, Reynolds J, Bonte FJ: Use of biplane cinefluorography for measurement of ventricular volume. Circulation 18:1105, 1958.

52. Ino T, Benson LN, Mikailian H, et al: Correlation of right ventricular volume using axial angulated ventriculography to known right ventricular cast volumes in infants and children with congenital heart disease. Am J Cardiol 61:161, 1988.

53. Ino T, Benson LN, Mikalian H, et al: Determination of left ventricular volumes by Simpson's rule in infants with congenital heart disease. Br Heart J 61:182, 1989.

54. Ino T, Benson LN, Mikailian H, et al: Correlation of left ventricular angiographic casts and biplane left ventricular volumetry in infants and children. Am J Cardiol 61:441, 1988.

55. Formanek A, Schey HM, Ekstrand KE, et al: Single versus biplane right and left ventricular volumetry: A cast and clinical study. Cathet Cardiovasc Diagn 10:137, 1984.

56. Glick G, Williams JFJ, Harrison DC, et al: Cardiac dimensions in intact unanaesthetized man: VI. Effects of changes in heart rate. J Appl Physiol 21:947, 1966.

57. Amplatz K, Moller JH: Radiology of Congenital Heart Disease. St. Louis, Mosby–Year Book, 1993.

58. Verma R, Keane JF: Use of cutoff pigtail catheters with intraluminal guidewires in interventional procedures in congenital heart disease. Cathet Cardiovasc Diagn 33:85, 1994.

59. Puyau FA, Burko H: The tilted left anterior oblique position in the study of congenital cardiac anomalies. Radiology 87:1069, 1966.

60. Soto B, Bargeron LM: Present status of axially angled angiocardiography. Cardiovasc Intervent Radiol 7:156, 1984.

61. Brant PWT: Commentary: Axially angled angiocardiography. Cardiovasc Intervent Radiol 7:166, 1984.

62. Grainger RG: Terminology for radiographic projections. Br Heart J 45:109, 1981.

63. Goor D, Lillehei CW, Edwards JE: The sigmoid septum. Variation in the contour of the left ventricular outlet. AJR Am J Roentgenol 107:366, 1969.

CHAPTER 15
NUCLEAR MEDICINE IN PEDIATRIC CARDIOLOGY

MICHAEL W. DAE

Cardiac catheterization and angiocardiography have long been definitive techniques for the anatomic and hemodynamic assessment of congenital heart disease. During the past decade, however, noninvasive imaging modalities such as two-dimensional echocardiography, magnetic resonance imaging, and radionuclide scintigraphy have led to a significant decrease in the need for invasive catheterization to evaluate congenital heart lesions.[1] Echocardiography and magnetic resonance imaging have emerged as the leading methods for the morphologic assessment of congenital heart disease; radionuclide imaging is used primarily for the assessment of cardiac physiology. Three major categories of radionuclide studies apply to the assessment of congenital lesions: (1) evaluation of shunts, (2) accurate determination of right and left ventricular function, and (3) assessment of myocardial perfusion.

ASSESSMENT OF LEFT-TO-RIGHT SHUNTS

Radionuclide methodology is currently most widely used in congenital heart disease for assessment of the presence and magnitude of left-to-right shunts. The method involves the rapid injection of a bolus of radionuclide (usually technetium Tc diethylenetriamine pentaacetic acid [Tc-DTPA]) into the circulation while transit through the heart and lungs is monitored with a gamma camera. For small infants (i.e., premature newborn infants), a butterfly needle can be used in a temporal scalp vein to deliver a compact bolus of activity to the central circulation. In older children and adults, either a butterfly needle or a small plastic catheter can be inserted into an external jugular vein. Antecubital veins can also be used. The delivery of a compact, nonfragmented bolus of activity is critical to allow accurate determination of the size of the shunt. With good technique, the success rate should be greater than 90%. It may be necessary to sedate infants and some children because crying simulates a Valsalva maneuver, which can impede entry into the thorax and lead to fragmentation of the bolus. As mentioned, Tc-DTPA is most commonly used for shunt studies. Doses are 200 μCi/kg of body weight, with a minimal dose of 2 mCi. The advantage of Tc-DTPA over other technetium-based agents is the fairly rapid renal excretion, which leads to prompt clearance of background activity. This becomes important if it is necessary to perform a second injection to improve the quality of the bolus. In general, no more than two sequential injections are done because of dosimetry limitations.

The study is done in the anterior projection with use of a converging collimator (which provides magnification) in infants and ideally a high-sensitivity parallel collimator (which maximizes count rate) in older children and adults. A dynamic acquisition with a sampling rate of two to four frames per second is adequate for evaluating shunts. If ejection fraction measurements are to be made by the first-pass method, a rate of at least 25 frames per second should be used. The sequential flow study is reviewed to provide useful information regarding chamber orientation and vascular connections. In the presence of normal anatomic relationships, right-sided heart structures appear, followed by the main pulmonary artery, the lungs, and subsequently the left ventricle (levophase) and descending aorta. Persistent pulmonary activity resulting in the absence of a distinct levophase is consistent with a moderate to large left-to-right shunt (Fig. 15–1). This appearance results from recirculation of activity from heart back to lungs and vice versa, across the shunt. This appearance has been called the smudge sign and generally indicates a left-to-right shunt with pulmonary-to-systemic flow (Qp/Qs) at least 1.6:1.

For quantification, time versus radioactivity curves are generated from regions of interest over the superior vena cava to assess the quality of the bolus and from the periphery of the right lung for shunt detection and magnitude (Fig. 15–2). A separate curve may be generated from a region over the left lung if differential shunting is expected (as may occur with a patent ductus arteriosus). The normal pulmonary artery curve has an ascending limb, reflecting the tracer's arrival in the pulmonary circulation, and a symmetric descending limb, reflecting the tracer's exiting the lungs and entering the left side of the heart. A late peak appears, reflecting systemic recirculation. In the presence of a left-to-right shunt, a shoulder will be present on the downslope, indicating recirculation of activity back to the lungs across the shunt. For shunt quantification, the shape of the pulmonary portion of the curve is approximated by an algebraic expression called a gamma variate function (Fig. 15–3).[2] In practice, the computer is given the coordinates of the upslope and initial downslope of the pulmonary curve, and a curve is generated that approximates the shape of the pulmonary curve. The area under this curve is proportional to pulmonary flow, Qp. This fitted curve is then subtracted from the initial time versus radioactivity curve, and another gamma variate fit is done on the remaining curve. The area under this second fitted curve is proportional to the shunt flow, Qsh. The difference between the two fitted curves is a measure of sys-

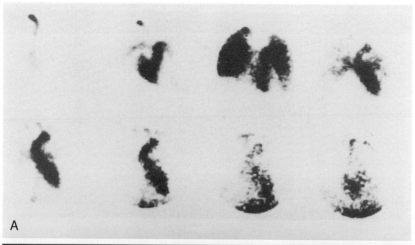

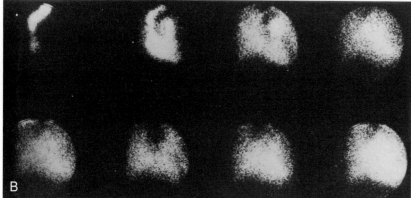

FIGURE 15–1

Radionuclide first-pass flow studies. Shown are radionuclide flow studies progressing left to right in a patient without left-to-right shunt *(A)* and in a patient with left-to-right shunt *(B)*. The absence of a levophase in *B* is consistent with a moderate to large shunt with a Qp/Qs above 1.5. (*A, B*, from Botvinick EH, Schiller NB: The complementary role of M-mode echocardiography and scintigraphy in the evaluation of adults with suspected left-to-right shunts. Additional observations on the role of two-dimensional echocardiography. Circulation 62[5]:1070–1079, 1980.)

temic flow, Qs. The resultant calculation of pulmonary to systemic flow, Qp/Qs, is performed as

$$Qp/Qs = Qp/(Qp - Qsh)$$

Ratios less than 1.2 : 1 are consistent with the absence of left-to-right shunts. The Qp/Qs calculation, by the gamma variate method, has shown excellent correlation with shunt size determined at cardiac catheterization over a clinically significant range of 1.2 : 1 to 3 : 1.[2] This relationship remains valid even in the presence of pulmonary hypertension, tricuspid regurgitation, and heart failure.[2,3] In these conditions, extensive dilution and slow flow lead to a slow downslope to the pulmonary curve. However, the upslope

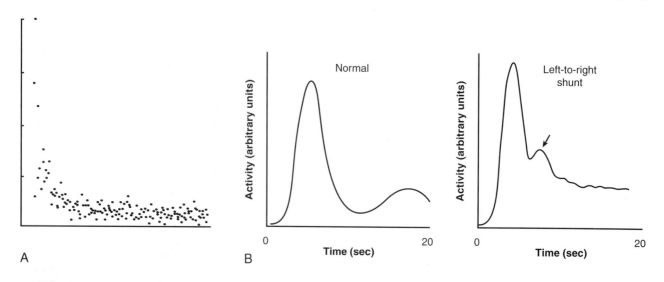

FIGURE 15–2

A, Time-activity curve from a region over the superior vena cava. The bolus of radiotracer is adequate because it produced a single peak. *B*, Pulmonary time-activity curves, normal *(left)* and left-to-right shunt *(right)*. (*B* from Treves S, Royal H, Babchyck B: Pediatric nuclear cardiology. *In* Engle MA [ed]: Pediatric Cardiovascular Disease. Philadelphia, FA Davis, 1981, pp 247–274.)

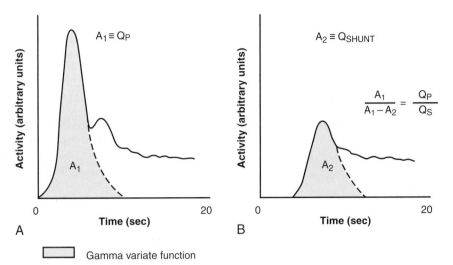

FIGURE 15–3

Calculation of pulmonary-to-systemic flow ratio (Qp/Qs) using pulmonary time-activity curves and the gamma variate model. *A*, Area under the first pass of tracer through the lungs as defined by a gamma variate extrapolation. Qp is pulmonary flow. *B*, Area under the portion of the curve corresponding to radiolabeled blood returning prematurely to the lung by the left-to-right shunt. Q shunt is shunt flow. A − B = Qs = systemic flow. (*A, B* from Treves ST: Pediatric Nuclear Medicine. New York, Springer-Verlag, 1985, p 252. Copyright Springer-Verlag GmbH.)

should be proportionately slowed and the curve fit method should generally apply. Nevertheless, caution should be exercised with long downslopes. Because the method depends on the full passage of the administered radionuclide through the lungs, left-to-right shunts will be overestimated in the presence of right-to-left shunts. Shunts with a ratio greater than 3:1 are difficult to fit by the gamma variate method owing to distortions in curve shape as a result of the large and torrential shunt flow. This is not a practical limitation, however, as any shunt with a Qp/Qs ratio greater than 3:1 is large. In general, a Qp/Qs ratio of 2:1 or greater is sufficient to warrant surgical correction.

With the anatomic detail provided by echocardiography, the hemodynamic correlates from Doppler examination, and the precise quantitation available from a radionuclide shunt study, it is sometimes possible to proceed directly to surgery without preoperative cardiac catheterization. This is particularly true with uncomplicated patent ductus and secundum atrial septal defect. In anomalous pulmonary venous return, the shunt size may be more accurately determined by radionuclide study than by oximetric methods at catheterization because of the inability to obtain a good mixed venous blood sample at catheterization.[4] The radionuclide method has also been used to measure changes in shunt magnitude in response to oxygen therapy for assessment of the reactivity of the pulmonary vascular bed in patients with large shunts and pulmonary hypertension.[5] This is an important consideration in determining operability in patients with moderate to large ventricular septal defects.

One of the leading indications for radionuclide shunt studies is the postoperative assessment of residual shunt size in patients with murmurs and echo Doppler evidence of persistent shunting after surgical correction of septal defects. Doppler quantification of shunt size is often not reliable after patch closure of defects because of the turbulence generated in the vicinity of the patch. In this situation, the radionuclide technique has been extremely helpful for assessing the need for repeated catheterization and possibly reoperation. It is possible to calculate the extent of left-to-right shunts by use of the equilibrium blood pool method. Stroke volume or amplitude images can be used to measure the difference in stroke volume between the ventricles, as is commonly performed for the evaluation of regurgitant lesions (Fig. 15–4).[6]

With a ventricular septal defect or a patent ductus arteriosus, the left ventricle handles the excess volume of the shunt flow. The left ventricular (LV) stroke volume is proportional to the pulmonary blood flow, and the right ventricular (RV) stroke volume is proportional to the systemic blood flow. The pulmonary-to-systemic flow ratio can be calculated as

$$Qp/Qs = LV \text{ stroke volume}/RV \text{ stroke volume}$$

where LV stroke volume equals LV end-diastolic volume minus end-systolic volume and RV stroke volume equals RV end-diastolic volume minus end-systolic volume.

For an atrial septal defect or anomalous pulmonary venous return, the right ventricle carries the excess shunt flow. The Qp/Qs can be calculated as

$$Qp/Qs = RV \text{ stroke volume}/LV \text{ stroke volume}$$

A good correlation ($r = .79$) has been noted between the shunt Qp/Qs ratio calculated from stroke volume ratios and oximetry.[7] This approach may be particularly useful when attempts at a good bolus injection are unsuccessful.

RIGHT-TO-LEFT SHUNT EVALUATION

Right-to-left shunts can be detected by inspection of the first-pass radionuclide angiogram, which reveals a premature appearance of radioactivity in the left-sided chambers or aorta. Time versus radioactivity curves generated from regions of interest over the carotid artery can be analyzed by curve fitting methods to quantify shunt size.[8] Intravenous injections of an inert radioactive gas, such as Xenon Xe 133 or krypton Kr 81m, can also be used for detecting right-to-left shunts.[9] Significant systemic activity of these agents, which should be totally extracted by the lungs and exhaled in the alveolar gas, indicates shunting.

The easiest and most commonly used method is the intravenous injection of ^{99m}Tc-labeled macroaggregated albumin particles, similar to those used for the assessment of pulmonary perfusion.[10] In the absence of right-to-left shunting, all of the particles are trapped in the lungs. When right-to-left shunting occurs at any level, particles enter the systemic circulation in proportion to the shunt flow, lodging in the capillary and precapillary beds of systemic organs (Fig. 15–5). A series of whole body images are taken to determine the percentage of right to left shunt as

$$\frac{\text{whole body counts} - \text{lung counts}}{\text{whole body counts}}$$

Pulmonary-to-systemic flow ratio can be calculated as

$$Qp/Qs = \text{lung counts/whole body counts}$$

A variation of this method is useful for assessing Qp/Qs in admixture lesions. Images in Figure 15–5 were obtained from a 16-year-old cyanotic patient who presented with a history of pulmonic atresia with intact ventricular septum and hypoplastic tricuspid valve. He received a Waterston aorta–right pulmonary artery shunt as a child. In addition, a left subclavian–central pulmonary shunt (Blalock-Taussig) was done, with flow primarily to the left lung. The procedure was done to assess the patency of the shunts. Although technically there is a left-to-right shunt of blood from the aorta to pulmonary artery, the major hemodynamic abnormality in this cyanotic lesion is complete admixture of systemic venous and pulmonary venous blood at the level of the left atrium. Both pulmonary blood and systemic blood arise from the aorta. Note the presence of brain and kidney uptake, consistent with right-to-left shunt. In this example, differential pulmonary perfusion is measured by determining relative counts in both lungs. Left lung activity represented 45% of total lung activity; right lung activity was 55% of total. These findings suggested that both the Waterston and Blalock-Taussig shunts were functioning. Additional important data were obtainable from this macroaggregated albumin particle study. The pulmonary-to-systemic flow ratio, Qp/Qs, was calculated as Qp equals lung counts, Qs equals whole body counts minus lung counts. This formula is applicable because the patient has an admixture lesion. There is complete mixing of the particles by the time the injected dose reaches the aorta. The particles are subsequently distributed in proportion to regional blood flow to the lungs and the body. The pulmonary-to-systemic flow ratio, Qp/Qs, is an important determinant of systemic arterial oxygen saturation in patients with admixture lesions.[11] In the example described here, the Qp/Qs was 1.6. This modest ratio suggested that pulmonary flow was not excessive, and increased systemic saturation would be likely to result with a slightly larger degree of pulmonary blood flow, that is, a larger Qp/Qs.

In spite of the general reluctance to administer particles to patients with known right-to-left shunts, the method has proved to be safe, accurate, and easy to perform.[10] The particle number should be kept below 50,000 in pediatric patients.

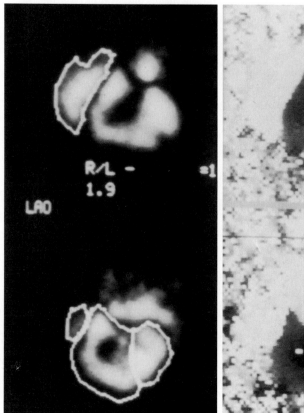
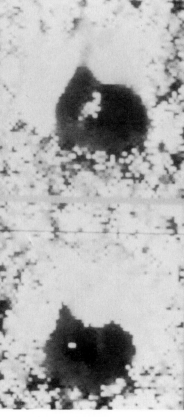

FIGURE 15–4

Amplitude and phase maps from the anterior projection (*upper*) and left anterior oblique projection (*lower*) from the same patient are illustrated. Note the increased amplitude (stroke volume) in the right ventricular region in the left anterior oblique projection. The amplitude ratio of the right ventricle to left ventricle, corrected for right atrial overlap with the right ventricle, is 1.9.

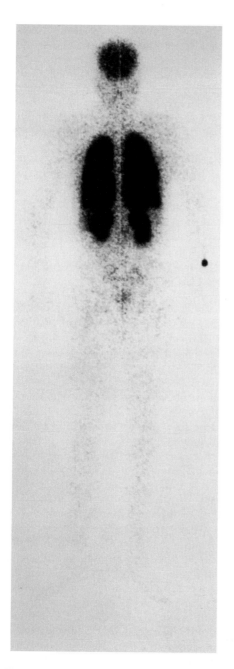

Shown is a posterior whole body image. Technetium-labeled macroaggregated albumin particles were injected intravenously and show localization to lungs, kidneys, and brain, indicating a right-to-left shunt.

ASSESSMENT OF VENTRICULAR FUNCTION

Radionuclide methods are well suited for assessing ventricular size and function in congenital heart lesions. Both first-pass and gated equilibrium methods for the determination of ejection fraction have been validated in the pediatric age group.[12, 13] Quantitative assessment of absolute ventricular volumes[14] and determination of regurgitant fraction have been reported in children as well.[15, 16] For infants, the imaging is optimized with the use of a converging collimator

to improve spatial resolution and increase the sensitivity. It is feasible to measure ejection fraction even in tiny premature infants with the use of the pinhole collimator.[17] Ventricular size and function evaluations are useful at rest and with dynamic stress in a variety of congenital lesions, both before and after surgical correction.[18, 19] Residual structural and functional abnormalities are common, and careful, long-term follow-up is important.

ASSESSMENT OF MYOCARDIAL PERFUSION

The primary abnormality leading to the onset of myocardial ischemia is inadequate myocardial blood flow to meet the metabolic demands of the heart. The heart has limited energy stores and requires constant delivery of oxygen and substrates and removal of metabolic wastes to function properly. Myocardial perfusion occurs by way of the coronary arteries. It is well appreciated that a fair degree of narrowing or stenosis is tolerated during the resting state without reductions in coronary flow (ischemia). As myocardial demands are increased (for instance, during exercise), however, the resulting augmentation in blood flow in a stenotic coronary artery is often not sufficient to maintain adequate function. The usual sequence of events in a patient with coronary disease during exercise is (1) a relative decrease in blood to a region of myocardium supplied by a stenotic vessel; (2) a sudden decrease in contractile function due to the rapid exhaustion of energy stores and the accumulation of metabolites; (3) electrocardiographic changes, primarily depression of the ST segments; and (4) the onset of chest pain.

If normal blood flow is quickly restored, the chest pain resolves, electrocardiographic changes return to baseline, and contractile function returns. If there is some delay in restoration of flow but it is eventually restored before the point of irreversible damage, contractile function may remain depressed for up to weeks (stunned myocardium). If blood flow is chronically reduced at rest, resulting in a chronic state of ischemia, contractile function may remain chronically depressed (hibernating myocardium). If blood flow is not restored, irreversible damage leads to myocardial necrosis and the eventual replacement of myocytes with scar. This regional territory then has permanent abnormalities in function, and if sufficient amounts of mass are involved, heart dilatation and failure ensue, and long-term prognosis is adversely affected.

It is because of these pathophysiologic changes that it is so important to be able to accurately evaluate one of the primary events, decreased myocardial perfusion. For this reason, myocardial perfusion imaging, or scintigraphy, has become an extremely useful clinical tool.

THALLIUM Tl 201

The most common agent for assessment of myocardial perfusion to date is thallium Tl 201. Thallium is a cyclotron-produced radionuclide with a half-life of 73 hours and predominant emission energy of 80 keV.

Thallium behaves physiologically like potassium and is transported into cells largely by the sodium-potassium

ATPase pump located on cellular membranes. The ability of the cells to transport thallium is probably related to the fact that the hydrated radius of thallium is similar in size to potassium and rubidium.[20] Myocardial cells extract thallium to a high degree. On the first exposure to the heart (first pass), more than 85% of the dose that reaches the myocardial cells is taken up. Hence, the extraction fraction is 85% or greater. As a result, the initial distribution of thallium provides a static map of myocardial perfusion at the time of injection. During an injection at rest, approximately 4% of the injected dose localizes in the heart, because the heart receives approximately 4% of the cardiac output. Thallium extraction by the myocardium depends on the delivery of the tracer (perfusion) and the presence of viable myocytes. Ischemic myocytes retain the ability to extract thallium (provided that some degree of perfusion is present). Only when ischemia is of sufficient severity and duration to lead to loss of membrane integrity (necrosis) will thallium not be extracted.[21]

Consider the situation in which one coronary vascular territory, the left anterior descending coronary artery, has a significant (>70%) stenosis. The two other major vessels (right coronary artery and left circumflex) are normal. In all likelihood, an injection of thallium in such a patient at rest would lead to a homogeneous distribution, as in normal subjects (Fig. 15–6). With increased coronary blood flow to maximal levels (generally up to 4 times baseline flow) by either maximal exercise or pharmacologically with a vasodilator such as dipyridamole, the delivery of thallium will be heterogeneous (see Fig. 15–6).

The resulting pattern of thallium uptake during vasodilatation would probably show diminished accumulation of thallium in the territory perfused by the stenotic left anterior descending coronary artery (septum and anterior wall) compared with the remaining myocardium perfused by the vessels without any stenosis. This relative heterogeneity of blood flow is the most important finding on a thallium image. The underperfused area, as in our example, represents normal but transiently underperfused or ischemic myocardium. An identical pattern would appear in a patient who has suffered a myocardial infarction involving the left anterior descending coronary artery. How can we distinguish between the two situations?

Thallium has another intrinsic physiologic property in the heart. It redistributes.[22] After the initial accumulation

in the heart, thallium slowly washes out into the blood until the washout rate from the heart and the excretion rate from the blood are in equilibrium. The tendency is for intracellular concentration gradients of thallium in the heart to equalize. As a result, regions with high blood flow and high concentrations of thallium wash out faster than do regions with lower blood flow or low concentrations of thallium. In fact, thallium may leave the normal areas of the heart and enter the areas of low concentration (ischemic territory) over time. The resultant delayed thallium image shows a more homogeneous distribution (see Fig. 15–6) if the initial region of reduced uptake represented ischemia in a region of viable myocytes. If the initial region of reduced uptake represented scar, a persistent defect appears on the delayed images.

TECHNETIUM Tc 99m–LABELED MYOCARDIAL PERFUSION TRACERS

Thallium 201 has gained widespread popularity as a useful myocardial perfusion agent. There are drawbacks, however. The relatively long half-life (72 hours) limits the amount of activity that can be injected because of dosimetry concerns. The low energy (80 keV) of the major photon emission poses potential problems because of soft tissue attenuation. Also, ^{201}Tl is cyclotron produced, which limits its availability. These features led to a continued search for myocardial perfusion tracers that could be labeled with technetium Tc 99m. Relative to ^{201}Tl, ^{99m}Tc has the advantage of higher energy (140 keV), leading to less attenuation; shorter half-life (6 hours), allowing the administration of larger doses; and ready availability because it is generator produced.

A number of myocardial perfusion tracers have been developed. Among these are sestamibi, teboroxime, furifosmin, tetrofosmin, and most recently NOET. Of these newer agents, sestamibi has been most extensively studied.

[99m]Tc-sestamibi, or Cardiolite, is a lipophilic, cationic complex of a class of compounds called isonitriles.[23] Sestamibi, like thallium, is delivered to the myocardium in proportion to blood flow. Its uptake is different from that of thallium, however. Sestamibi passively crosses the sarcolemmal membrane, and the driving force for uptake appears to be a large electrochemical gradient provided by the largely negative charge on mitochondria. Sestamibi has

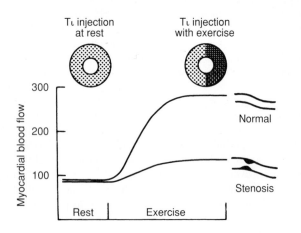

FIGURE 15–6

Diagrammatic illustration of the relationship between myocardial blood flow at rest and during exercise and regional myocardial ^{201}Tl uptake in zones perfused by normal and stenotic coronary arteries. When thallium is injected at rest, there is uniform distribution of the radionuclide throughout the myocardium (*upper left*). When thallium is injected during exercise, there is a relative diminution in thallium uptake in the zone perfused by the stenotic vessel (*middle panel*). Several hours after ^{201}Tl injection with exercise, there is "redistribution" and normalization of thallium uptake in normal and stenotic zones (*upper right*). (From Beller GA: Radionuclide evaluation before and after medical or surgical myocardial revascularization. *In* Gerson MC [ed]: Cardiac Nuclear Medicine. New York, McGraw-Hill, 1987, pp 349–369. Reproduced with permission of The McGraw-Hill Companies.)

been shown to bind tightly to mitochondria,[24] another major difference from thallium. Sestamibi shows little significant reversibility from the heart. This property led to earlier descriptions of sestamibi as a "chemical microsphere." A small amount of redistribution does exist; however, the amount is negligible within the first 60 minutes after injection. Separate injections of sestamibi are required for rest and stress assessment of myocardial perfusion.

The extraction fraction of sestamibi is lower than that of thallium (65% versus 85%).[25] The result is that sestamibi may underestimate myocardial blood flow at high flow rates (>2 ml/min/g) to a greater degree than does thallium.[25] In spite of this diffusion limitation, clinical results evaluating the sensitivity and specificity of thallium and sestamibi have been comparable.[26] Another property shared between sestamibi and thallium is the dependence on viable myocytes for extraction.[27] Sestamibi uptake has been shown to be markedly diminished in irreversibly injured myocytes.

APPLICATIONS OF PERFUSION SCINTIGRAPHY IN CONGENITAL HEART DISEASE

Myocardial perfusion scintigraphy has been applied extensively to adults and during recent years to children as well.[28] In the pediatric patient, perfusion imaging has been most widely used for the noninvasive identification of an anomalous left coronary artery[29, 30] (see Chapter 39). To evaluate patients for possible anomalous left coronary artery, ^{201}Tl is injected intravenously, at rest; images are acquired in multiple planar projections, or single-photon emission computed tomographic imaging is done. The usual anatomy in this rare disease is for the left main coronary artery to arise from the main pulmonary artery. This usually leads to regional ischemia and infarction of the left ventricle owing to low perfusion pressure from the pulmonary artery, which can create a coronary steal (Fig. 15–7). Thallium scintigraphy typically reveals a segmental perfusion abnormality at rest (Fig. 15–8). This pattern is useful for identifying an anomalous left coronary artery as opposed to myocarditis or cardiomyopathy as the cause of poor ventricular function in infants. The condition is often associated with Q waves on the electrocardiogram. Echocardiography is sometimes able to identify the aberrant origin of the left coronary artery, but catheterization is required for confirmation.

Another clinical condition for which perfusion scintigraphy may be useful is Kawasaki disease, or the mucocutaneous lymph node syndrome.[31] This syndrome is associated initially with persistent fevers, rash, adenopathy, and mucous membrane abnormalities. Before the introduction of intravenous immune globulin therapy, up to 20% of these patients developed aneurysms of the coronary arteries. Treatment with immune globulin within 10 days of the onset of the illness reduces the frequency of coronary aneurysms to about 4%. About 30 to 50% of such aneurysms spontaneously regress within the first 2 years of illness. The remaining aneurysms may later thrombose and cause myocardial ischemia and infarction. Bypass surgery has been advocated for some patients with objective evidence of ischemia. Perfusion abnormalities have also been induced with stress in adults with a variety of anomalous origins of the left coronary artery from the right. Evalua-

Myocardium at risk of
ischemia with the various
coronary thieves

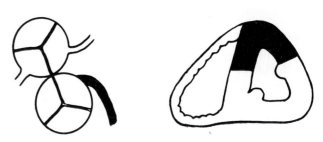

Left main from pulmonary trunk

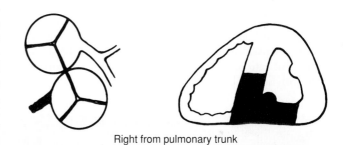

Left anterior descending from pulmonary trunk

Right from pulmonary trunk

FIGURE 15–7

Diagram showing the portion of left ventricular myocardium at risk for ischemia or necrosis when the left main, left anterior descending, or right coronary artery arises from the pulmonary trunk (PT). (From Roberts WC: Congenital coronary arterial anomalies unassociated with major anomalies of the heart or great vessels. *In* Roberts WC [ed]: Adult Congenital Heart Disease. Philadelphia, FA Davis, 1987, pp 583–629.)

tion of the resting pattern of ventricular perfusion and function can help differentiate a segmental pathologic process related to large-vessel coronary disease from other causes including cardiomyopathy, myocarditis, and small-vessel embolization. The pattern of thallium uptake can also suggest right and left ventricular hypertrophy and suggest the diagnosis of asymmetric septal hypertrophy.

Assessment of myocardial perfusion is becoming increasingly important in the evaluation and follow-up of patients with transposition of the great vessels who have undergone the arterial switch procedure[32–34] (see Chapter 25). The procedure consists of switching the great vessels to the proper ventricles and reimplantation of the coronary arteries to the newly formed aorta. The morphologic left ventricle then becomes the systemic pumping chamber for which it is better suited. Although technically demanding, the procedure is best performed during the neonatal period, before the regression of left ventricular mass as a result of the falling pulmonary vascular resistance that occurs after birth. Alternatively, the left ventricle can be conditioned to accept the high systemic vascular resistance by performing pulmonary banding as an initial procedure. Concerns have been raised since the inception of the arterial switch procedure about the possibility that distortion or growth failure of the newly implanted coronary arteries may result in myocardial ischemia and possibly infarction.

Some studies suggest that coronary artery manipulation and reimplantation do not cause late myocardial perfusion abnormalities, at least in those infants with successful initial results.[34] However, large perfusion abnormalities have been seen in the territories of occluded coronary arteries after the switch procedure.[28]

RADIONUCLIDE ASSESSMENT OF INFLAMMATION

A gallium scan from a neonate with cardiomegaly, pulmonary edema, sepsis, and disseminated intravascular coagulation is shown in Figure 15–9. Myocarditis was strongly suspected. As shown in Figure 15–9, the gallium scan was positive for myocardial localization, but the uptake showed a regional pattern with relatively greater uptake in the posterior lateral wall. This was more suggestive of myocardial infarction than of the diffuse pattern seen with myocarditis. A rest thallium perfusion study showed a dense perfusion abnormality in the posterior lateral wall, consistent with myocardial infarction. Catheterization subsequently showed normal coronary arteries and akinesis of

the posterolateral wall. The etiology of myocardial infarction was presumed to be thromboembolic.

Gallium citrate Ga 67 has been shown to accumulate in acute as well as in chronic inflammatory lesions of bacterial as well as of nonbacterial etiology.[35] Mechanisms leading to gallium uptake have been reviewed by Tsan.[35]

Gallium uptake has been described in a number of causes of inflammatory heart disease, including bacterial endocarditis, myocardial abscess, and pericarditis.[36] Animal studies have shown intense and uniform gallium accumulation in experimental myocarditis.[37] In addition, a high correlation between biopsy-proven myocarditis and gallium uptake has been found in patients.[38] In nearly all reported instances of gallium uptake in myocarditis, the pattern of uptake is diffuse. This diffuse pattern of uptake in myocarditis has been seen even in the presence of characteristic electrocardiographic changes that mimic myocardial infarction.[39] Antimyosin antibody cardiac imaging has also shown success in detecting biopsy-proven myocarditis.[40] Antimyosin localizes to regions of myocyte necrosis in myocarditis, as opposed to the localization of ^{67}Ga to the inflammatory component. Few studies have examined thallium uptake in myocarditis; however, focal perfusion defects have been reported.[41] These defects, however, tend to be in nonvascular distributions.

Experimental and clinical studies have confirmed that gallium accumulates in regions of acute myocardial infarction.[42, 43] In spite of the presence of normal coronary arteries, myocardial infarction is the most likely explanation for the scintigraphic findings and the etiology of the severe left ventricular dysfunction in the patient shown in Figure 15–9.

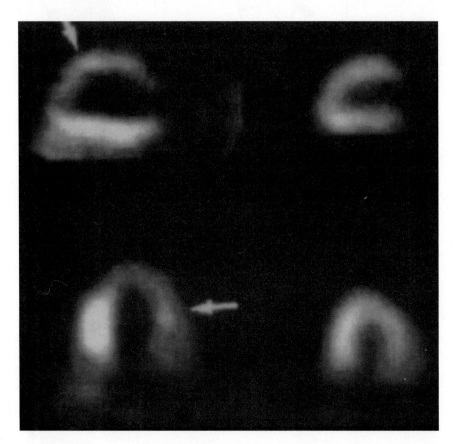

FIGURE 15–8

Shown are rest myocardial thallium uptake images by single-photon emission computed tomography from a 2-month-old infant presenting with a left coronary artery originating from the pulmonary artery. On the left are preoperative images showing markedly decreased perfusion to the anterior and lateral walls (*arrows*) and dilatation of the left ventricle. Postoperative images on the right show almost complete normalization of perfusion and a dramatic reduction in the chamber size. (From Fernandes J, Rutkowski M, Sanger JJ: Anomalous origin of the left coronary artery. Use of thallium perfusion scans in the evaluation of successful revascularization. Clin Nucl Med 17:177–179, 1992.)

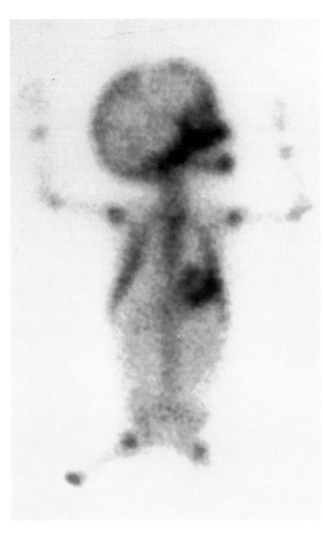

FIGURE 15–9

Anterior whole body gallium citrate Ga 67 scan.

Myocardial infarction in the neonatal period is rare and is associated with high mortality. It usually occurs in the absence of congenital heart disease. Congenital lesions associated with myocardial ischemia usually present with myocardial infarction in later infancy or in childhood.[44] In infants with structurally normal hearts and coronary arteries, the most common causes of myocardial infarction are perinatal asphyxia and thromboembolic occlusion. In the example of enteroviral infection with resulting disseminated intravascular coagulation (see Fig. 15–9), the associated myocardial infarction is most likely a result of thromboembolism. Interestingly, this patient survived the infarction, had gradually improved myocardial function, and presented with a normal ejection fraction 7 months after the acute event.

REFERENCES

1. Beekman R, Filippini L, Meijboom E: Evolving usage of pediatric cardiac catheterization. Curr Opin Cardiol 9:721, 1994.
2. Maltz OL, Treves S: Quantitative radionuclide angiocardiography. Determination of Qp/Qs in children. Circulation 476:1049, 1973.
3. Treves S, Kuruc A: Radionuclide evaluation of circulatory shunts. Cardiol Clin 1:427, 1983.
4. Baker E, Ellam S, Lorber A, et al: Superiority of radionuclide over oximetric measurement of left to right shunts. Br Heart J 53:535, 1985.
5. Fujii A, Rabinovitch M, Keane J, et al: Radionuclide angiographic assessment of pulmonary vascular reactivity in patients with left to right shunts and pulmonary hypertension. Am J Cardiol 49:356, 1982.
6. Dae M, Botvinick E, Schiller N, et al: Increased accuracy of valvar regurgitation using atrial corrected Fourier amplitude ratios. J Noninvasive Cardiol 1:155, 1987.
7. Rigo P, Chevigne M: Measurement of left to right shunts by gated radionuclide angiography: Concise communication. J Nucl Med 23:1070, 1982.
8. Peter C, Armstrong B, Jones R: Radionuclide quantitation of right-to-left shunts in children. Circulation 64:572, 1981.
9. Long R, Braunwald E, Morrow A: Intracardiac injection of radioactive krypton. Circulation 21:1126, 1963.
10. Sty J, Starshak R, Miller J: Particle body imaging in cardiopulmonary disorders. In Wagner HN (ed): Pediatric Nuclear Medicine. New York, Appleton-Century-Crofts, 1983, p 46.
11. Rudolph A: Congenital Diseases of the Heart. Chicago, Year Book Medical Publishers, 1974, p 124.
12. Baker E, Ellam S, Tynan M, Maisey M: First-pass measurement of left ventricular function in infants and children. Eur J Nucl Med 10:422, 1985.
13. Baker E, Ellam S, Maisey M, Tynan M: Radionuclide measurement of left ventricular ejection fraction in infants and children. Br Heart J 51:275, 1984.
14. Parrish M, Graham T, Born M, et al: Radionuclide ventriculography for assessment of absolute right and left ventricular volumes in children. Circulation 66:811, 1982.
15. Parrish M, Graham T, Born M, et al: Radionuclide stroke count ratios for assessment of right and left ventricular volume overload in children. Am J Cardiol 51:261, 1983.
16. Hurwitz RA, Treves S, Freed M, et al: Quantitation of aortic and mitral regurgitation in the pediatric population: Evaluation by radionuclide angiocardiography. Am J Cardiol 51:252, 1983.
17. Hannon D, Gelfand M, Bailey W, et al: Pinhole radionuclide ventriculography in small infants. Am Heart J 111:316, 1988.
18. Reduto L, Berger H, Johnstone D, et al: Radionuclide assessment of right and left ventricular exercise reserve after total correction of tetralogy of Fallot. Am J Cardiol 45:1013, 1980.
19. Hurwitz R, Papanicolaou N, Treves S, et al: Radionuclide angiography in evaluation of patients after surgical repair of transposition of the great arteries. Am J Cardiol 49:761, 1982.
20. Mullins LJ, Moor RD: The movement of thallium ions in muscle. J Gen Physiol 43:759, 1960.
21. Friedman BJ, Beihn R, Friedman JP: The effect of hypoxia on thallium kinetics in cultured chick myocardial cells. J Nucl Med 28:1453, 1987.
22. Pohost GM, Albert NM, Ingwall JS, Strauss HW: Thallium redistribution: Mechanisms and clinical utility. Semin Nucl Med 10:70, 1980.
23. Wackers FJ, Berman DS, Maddahi J, et al: Technetium-99m hexakis 2-methoxyisobutyl isonitrile: Human biodistribution, dosimetry, safety, and preliminary comparison to thallium-201 for myocardial perfusion imaging. J Nucl Med 30:301, 1989.
24. Carvalho PA, Chiu MC, Kronauge JF, et al: Subcellular distribution and analysis of technetium-99m-MIBI in isolated perfused rat hearts. J Nucl Med 33:11516, 1992.
25. DiRocco RJ, Rumsey WL, Kuczynski BL, et al: Measurement of myocardial blood flow using a co-injection technique for technetium-99m-teboroxime, technetium-96-sestamibi, and thallium-201. J Nucl Med 33:1152, 1992.
26. Kahn JK, McGhie I, Akers MJ, et al: Quantitative rotational tomography with ^{201}Tl and [99m]Tc 2-methoxyisobutyl-isonitrile: A direct comparison in normal individuals and patients with coronary artery disease. Circulation 79:1282, 1989.
27. Beanlands R, Dawood F, Wen W, et al: Are the kinetics of technetium-99m methoxyisobutyl isonitrile affected by cell metabolism and viability? Circulation 82:1802, 1990.
28. Bjorkhem G, Evander E, White T, Lundstrom N: Myocardial scintigraphy with 201-thallium in pediatric cardiology: A review of 52 cases. Pediatr Cardiol 11:1, 1990.
29. Findley J, Howman-Giles R, Gilday D, et al: Thallium-201 myocardial imaging in anomalous left coronary artery arising from the pul-

monary artery: Applications before and after medical and surgical treatment. Am J Cardiol 42:675, 1978.

30. Moodie D, Cook S, Gill C, et al: Thallium-201 myocardial imaging in young adults with anomalous left coronary artery arising from the pulmonary artery. J Nucl Med 2:1076, 1980.

31. Hijazi Z, Udelson J, Snapper H, et al: Physiologic significance of chronic coronary aneurysms in patients with Kawasaki disease. J Am Coll Cardiol 24:1633, 1994.

32. Hayes A, Baker E, Kakadeker A, et al: Influence of anatomical correction for transposition of the great arteries on myocardial perfusion: Radionuclide imaging with Tc^{99m} methoxy isobutyl isonitrile. J Am Coll Card 24:769, 1994.

33. Weindling S, Wernovsky G, Colan S, et al: Myocardial perfusion, function, and exercise tolerance after the arterial switch operation. J Am Coll Card 23:424, 1994.

34. Cohen D: Surgical management of congenital heart disease in the 1990's. Am J Dis Child 146:1447, 1992.

35. Tsan M: Mechanism of gallium-67 accumulation in inflammatory lesions. J Nucl Med 26:88, 1985.

36. Morguet A, Munz D, Emrich D: Scintigraphic detection of inflammatory heart disease. Eur J Nucl Med 21:666, 1994.

37. Reeves W, Jackson G, Flickinger F, et al: Radionuclide imaging of experimental myocarditis. Circulation 63:640, 1981.

38. O'Connell J, Henkin R, Robinson J, et al: Gallium-67 imaging in patients with dilated cardiomyopathy and biopsy-proven myocarditis. Circulation 70:58, 1984.

39. Folger G, Eltohami E, Hajar H: Acute myocardial-infarction-like findings with myocarditis in infancy. Angiology 45:737, 1994.

40. Dec G, Palacios I, Yasuda T, et al: Antimyosin antibody cardiac imaging: Its role in the diagnosis of myocarditis. J Am Coll Cardiol 16:97, 1990.

41. Tamaki N, Yonekura Y, Kadota K, et al: Thallium-201 myocardial perfusion imaging in myocarditis. Clin Nucl Med 10:562, 1985.

42. Kramer R, Goldstein R, Hirshfeld J, et al: Accumulation of gallium-67 in regions of acute myocardial infarction. Am J Cardiol 33:861, 1974.

43. Schor R, Massie B, Botvinick E, Shames D: Gallium-67 uptake in silent myocardial infarction. Radiology 129:117, 1978.

44. Bernstein D, Finkbeiner W, Soiffer S, Teitel D: Perinatal myocardial infarction: A case report and review of the literature. Pediatr Cardiol 6:313, 1986.

CHAPTER 16
PEDIATRIC EXERCISE TESTING

BENJAMIN W. EIDEM DAVID J. DRISCOLL

Exercise testing provides a quantitative and reproducible index of cardiorespiratory performance. In patients with congenital heart disease, exercise testing provides a means of assessing the physical limitations imposed by disease as well as of determining disease severity and response to therapeutic interventions.

Exercise testing is valuable for assessing the ability of an individual to perform work. Exercise involves the performance of work and the application of power. Work is defined as the application of force to move a specific mass a specified distance, such that work = force × distance. Power is defined as the amount of work performed per unit of time.

The amount of work performed during an exercise test has frequently been described as *exercise capacity* or *aerobic power*. Accurate reproducible quantitation of work performed has proved to be challenging. Maximal oxygen uptake ($\dot{V}O_2$max) during exercise has commonly been used as a measure of exercise performance. *Maximal aerobic power* can be defined as the highest achievable $\dot{V}O_2$ during exercise. Maximal oxygen uptake can be determined during exercise testing by determining the plateau of the $\dot{V}O_2$ curve that occurs during exercise despite continued work, with limited additional levels of work performed at the expense of anaerobic metabolism. The determinants of $\dot{V}O_2$ can be appreciated from the following relationship:

$$\dot{V}O_2 = (\text{cardiac output}) (\text{AV O}_2 \text{ difference})$$

or

$$\dot{V}O_2 = [(\text{HR}) (\text{SV})] [(\text{Hgb}) (1.36)]$$
$$(\text{arterial O}_2 \text{ saturation} - \text{mixed venous O}_2 \text{ saturation})]$$

or

$$\dot{V}O_2 = [(\text{HR}) (\text{LVEDV}) (\text{EF})] [\text{Hgb}] (1.36)]$$
$$(\text{arterial O}_2 \text{ saturation} - \text{mixed venous O}_2 \text{ saturation})]$$

where AV O_2 is arteriovenous oxygen content, HR is heart rate; SV is stroke volume, LVEDV is left ventricular end-diastolic volume, EF is ejection fraction, and Hgb is hemoglobin. From these equations, it is clear that changes in $\dot{V}O_2$ depend on changes in heart rate, LVEDV, ejection fraction, hemoglobin, and arterial and mixed venous blood oxygen saturation.

Assessment of exercise performance requires a subject to give a maximal effort during the study. Because of subjective discomfort at higher workloads, a maximal effort is seldom achieved during exercise studies for most children. Therefore, one must be careful when interpreting exercise performance because many children will not achieve true maximal aerobic power.

Subjects may stop exercise for a variety of reasons usually related to one of the major organ systems involved in exercise. As cardiovascular specialists, we hope that the subject terminates exercise because the cardiovascular system has been fully stressed and heart rate and stroke volume have reached a maximum. When this happens, further exercise is, by necessity, anaerobic, and generalized fatigue and discomfort compel the subject to discontinue exercise. In contrast, a subject with significant pulmonary disease, such as cystic fibrosis, may terminate exercise because of ventilatory insufficiency that occurs before cardiac function has become maximal. A patient with a skeletal myopathy or neuromuscular disorder may stop exercise because of muscle fatigue before reaching maximal cardiac or respiratory function. Some patients have psychological reasons for terminating exercise, and this may occur before any of the other organ systems involved in exercise reach a maximal state of performance. In many patients, more than one organ system may be abnormal, and one or all of the abnormal systems may contribute to reasons for termination of exercise. Examples of these include patients with intracardiac left-to-right shunts and pulmonary edema, patients with congenital heart disease and reactive airway disease, and patients with congenital heart disease and poor skeletal muscle strength secondary to chronic inactivity. The reason the subject terminated the test is important in interpreting the results of a clinical exercise test.

Maximal oxygen uptake can be influenced by several variables of the patient as well as by the specific exercise protocol used. Maximal oxygen uptake increases with body size. Boys have greater maximal oxygen uptake at all ages compared with girls of similar size. Because more muscle groups are used during treadmill exercise than during cycle exercise, generally $\dot{V}O_2$max is greater with use of a treadmill than with a cycle.

CARDIAC RESPONSE TO EXERCISE

HEART RATE

An increase in heart rate with exercise is a major determinant of increased cardiac output in normal individuals. Maximal heart rate with exercise is a function of age and underlying chronotropic response of the heart. Decreases in maximal heart rate have been shown to be a function of increasing age. In adults, maximal heart rate (HRmax) is predicted from the equation

$$HRmax = 210 - (0.65 \times age)$$

In children 5 to 20 years old, maximal heart rate is between 195 and 215 beats per minute.[1–3] Maximal heart rate determination in children younger than 5 years is limited by the difficulty in achieving a true maximal exercise test in this young age group.

Whether a patient achieves a maximal predicted heart rate during exercise has often been used as a determinant of a maximal cardiorespiratory effort. However, maximal heart rate response to exercise depends on many interrelated factors, any one of which may limit the heart rate response achieved. Maximal heart rate will vary depending on the type of exercise performed and the specific protocol used. Individuals performing treadmill exercise will achieve a higher maximal heart rate than will those performing cycle exercise. Maximal heart rate may not be a useful index of maximal cardiorespiratory effort in patients with congenital heart disease because many of these patients have significant chronotropic insufficiency, thus limiting achievement of their maximal predicted heart rate.

BLOOD PRESSURE

Blood pressure response to exercise is influenced by several factors. Systolic blood pressure increases during isotonic exercise, but diastolic blood pressure remains relatively unchanged.[4–6] In contrast, both systolic and diastolic blood pressure increase with isometric exercise.[7] Males have a higher peak systolic blood pressure than that of females of similar age and body size. Black children have a greater exercise blood pressure response than do white children. Larger children have higher systolic blood pressure response to exercise than do children of similar age but smaller body surface area.[5,6]

CARDIAC OUTPUT

Cardiac output increases linearly in response to increasing workload or oxygen uptake. Increase in cardiac output with exercise depends on increases in stroke volume and heart rate. Changes in stroke volume are dependent on ventricular end-diastolic volume and myocardial contractility. Stroke volume increases to its maximum early during exercise. Therefore, continued increases of cardiac output during sustained exercise result from increases in heart rate.

VENTILATORY RESPONSES TO EXERCISE

MINUTE VENTILATION

Minute ventilation increases with increasing exercise. $\dot{V}E$ increases by increases in respiratory frequency and tidal volume. The relative increments in respiratory frequency and tidal volume vary from subject to subject. In normal individuals, ventilation at peak exercise is approximately 65 to 80% of resting maximal voluntary ventilation. Achieve-

ment of less than 65% maximal voluntary ventilation suggests a submaximal cardiorespiratory effort.

Ventilation increases in a linear fashion relative to oxygen uptake during exercise. However, the slope of this line changes. Above the ventilatory anaerobic threshold, the slope is greater than it is below the anaerobic threshold. Indeed, the change in the slope of this line is one of the indications of having reached the ventilatory anaerobic threshold.

VENTILATORY EQUIVALENT FOR OXYGEN

The ventilatory equivalent for oxygen ($\dot{V}E/\dot{V}O_2$)' is the ratio of minute ventilation and oxygen uptake. Essentially it is the volume of air breathed each minute relative to the volume of oxygen used each minute. At rest, this value is 30 to 40. Shortly after exercise is begun, the value declines; as exercise continues, the value increases to reach about 35 at peak exercise. The initial decline of $\dot{V}E/\dot{V}O_2$ is due to improvement in gas exchange early in exercise that results from more uniform pulmonary perfusion. The level of $\dot{V}O_2$ at which $\dot{V}E/\dot{V}O_2$ begins to increase during exercise indicates the ventilatory anaerobic threshold.

SYSTEMIC ARTERIAL BLOOD OXYGEN SATURATION

In normal subjects, systemic arterial blood oxygen saturation is 95 to 99% at rest and during exercise. Although oxygen saturation may decrease below 90 to 94% in well-trained, highly fit individuals during intense exercise, such a reduction of oxygen saturation is usually abnormal.

FITNESS, DECONDITIONING, AND DISEASE

It is frequently impossible to distinguish between deconditioning and cardiac disease by use of exercise testing only. One can think of deconditioning as a disease of inactivity that negatively affects cardiac function. As one becomes more fit through a conditioning program, resting heart rate decreases and more work can be performed at a given level of heart rate, stroke volume, and oxygen uptake.

CONTRAINDICATIONS TO EXERCISE TESTING

Specific contraindications to exercise testing in pediatric patients with congenital heart disease are listed in Table 16–1.[8]

TABLE 16–1
CONTRAINDICATIONS TO EXERCISE TESTING IN PATIENTS WITH CONGENITAL HEART DISEASE
Uncontrolled congestive heart failure
Right ventricular hypertension in the absence of a ventricular septal defect
Severe aortic stenosis
Significant primary pulmonary hypertension
Uncontrolled hypertension
Acute rheumatic fever
Acute myocarditis or pericarditis
Bacterial endocarditis
Acute myocardial infarction
Acute febrile illness
Acute renal, hepatic, or thyroid disorder
Thrombophlebitis
Acute drug toxicity

EXERCISE RESPONSE IN PATIENTS WITH CONGENITAL HEART DISEASE: INDICATIONS AND CLINICAL APPLICATIONS

The role of exercise testing in specific lesions is found in the individual chapters, but some general remarks are in order.

Minor left-to-right shunts, or regurgitant or obstructive lesions, have little or no effect on maximal aerobic power. Therefore, if a patient with such a minor lesion has symptoms and has decreased maximal aerobic power in an exercise test, it would be well to look for other causes of symptoms like exercise-induced bronchospasm, anemia, hypothyroidism, or a decreased blood volume.

Large left-to-right shunts decrease maximal aerobic power[9] because a ventricle that at rest has a much increased stroke volume has a limited ability to increase that stroke volume further. In addition, if left atrial pressure rises with exercise, pulmonary congestion may impair the ventilatory response.

Significant obstructive lesions, normally asymptomatic, increase ventricular pressures on exercise.[9] For the more severe lesions, the ventricular muscle may not be able to maintain an adequate cardiac output, so that on exercise the systemic blood pressure may not increase appropriately, and decreased peripheral muscle blood flow may lead to premature fatigue. These effects will be intensified if the lungs become congested or the myocardium becomes ischemic.

In cyanotic lesions, the arterial hypoxemia tends to increase cardiac output and decrease mixed venous oxygen saturation, thereby limiting the usual increments in stroke volume and oxygen extraction that occur with exercise. Furthermore, these patients have an increased minute ventilation and ventilatory equivalent for oxygen at rest and on exercise. This is probably because the blood that bypasses the lungs cannot participate in gas exchange, and minute ventilation increases so as to decrease pulmonary venous carbon dioxide tension and maintain a normal systemic arterial carbon dioxide tension.[10] In this way, ventilatory as well as cardiac mechanisms may limit maximal aerobic power.

After recovery from surgical correction of the defect, the ability to exercise depends on whether there are residual lesions or myocardial damage. For many congenital heart lesions, however, normal exercise tolerance is expected. The exception to this occurs in those who have a single-ventricle repair, namely, the Fontan-Kreuzer operation or one of its variants.

FUNCTIONAL SINGLE VENTRICLE BEFORE AND AFTER THE FONTAN OPERATION

Exercise aerobic capacity is significantly decreased in patients with a functional single ventricle before and after the Fontan operation. Maximal aerobic power is significantly reduced before operation in patients with a functional single ventricle. There is an inverse relationship between aerobic power and age.[11] After a successful Fontan palliation, maximal aerobic power improves but remains significantly decreased compared with normal.[11,12] Decreased maximal

heart rate response to exercise and persistent deconditioning contribute to decreased maximal aerobic capacity after the Fontan operation.

Systemic arterial blood oxygen desaturation is a prominent factor contributing to decreased exercise capacity in preoperative patients with a functional single ventricle. Investigators have reported mean arterial blood oxygen saturations of 84 ± 6% at rest and 61 ± 14% at peak exercise in these preoperative patients.[11] After the Fontan palliation, systemic arterial blood oxygen saturation is significantly increased but remains slightly less than normal at rest and at peak exercise. Causes of persistent mild desaturation include small persistent intracardiac shunts, diversion of coronary sinus blood flow into the physiologic left atrium, and pulmonary ventilation-perfusion mismatch.

Systolic blood pressure in preoperative patients with a functional single ventricle is normal at rest and at peak exercise. Diastolic blood pressure at rest is slightly decreased compared with normal.[11] Postoperatively, systolic blood pressure is reduced compared with normal at peak exercise.

Cardiac output does not increase normally during exercise after the Fontan operation.[11–13] This results, in part, from reduced pulmonary blood flow, chronotropic insufficiency, and impaired ventricular contractility.[14]

Abnormal ventilation is present in patients who are cyanotic and have a functional single ventricle. Minute ventilation and respiratory frequency are increased at rest, and the ventilatory equivalent for oxygen is increased both at rest and at peak exercise. After a successful Fontan palliation, ventilation parameters tend to normalize at rest but remain significantly altered at peak exercise. Minute ventilation and the ventilatory equivalent for oxygen and carbon dioxide remain greater than normal.[15] Therefore, ventilation appears to have a significant impact on exercise limitation in patients before and after the Fontan operation.

Cardiac arrhythmias are common in patients both before and after the Fontan operation. Investigators have reported an incidence of arrhythmia of 14% and 21% of patients at rest before and after the Fontan operation, respectively. With exercise, 28% of preoperative patients and 38% of postoperative patients were noted to have arrhythmias.[11]

REFERENCES

1. Anderson K, Seliger B, Rutenfranz J, Berndt I: Physical performance capacity of children in Norway. II: Heart rate and oxygen pulse in submaximal and maximal exercises: Population parameters in a rural community. Eur J Appl Physiol 33:197, 1974.
2. Bar-Or O, Shephard R, Allen C: Cardiac output of 10- to 13-year-old boys and girls during submaximal exercise. J Appl Physiol 30:219, 1971.
3. Wilmore J, Sigerseth PO: Physical work capacity of young girls 7 to 13 years of age. J Appl Physiol 22:923, 1967.
4. Fixler D, Laird W, Browne R, et al: Response of hypertensive adolescents to dynamic and isometric exercise stress. Pediatrics 64:579, 1979.
5. Riopel D, Taylor A, Hohn A, et al: Blood pressure, heart rate, pressure rate product, and electrocardiographic changes in healthy children during treadmill exercise. Am J Cardiol 44:697, 1979.
6. Strong W, Miller M, Striplin M, et al: Blood pressure response to isometric and dynamic exercise in healthy black children. Am J Dis Child 132:587, 1978.
7. Asmussen E, Heebøll-Nielsen K: A dimensional analysis of physical performance and growth in boys. J Appl Physiol 7:593, 1955.

8. Driscoll DJ: Diagnostic use of exercise testing in pediatric cardiology: The noninvasive approach. *In* Bar-Or MD (ed): Advances in Pediatric Sport Sciences, Volume III: Biological Issues. Champaign, IL, Human Kinetics Books, 1989, p 223.

9. Driscoll DJ, Wolfe R, Gersony W, et al: Cardiorespiratory responses to exercise of patients with aortic stenosis, pulmonary stenosis, and ventricular septal defect. Circulation 87(suppl):I-102, 1993.

10. Strieder D, Mesko Z, Zaver A, Gold W: Exercise tolerance in chronic hypoxemia due to right-to-left shunt. J Appl Physiol 34:853, 1973.

11. Driscoll D, Danielson G, Puga F, et al: Exercise tolerance and cardiorespiratory response to exercise after the Fontan operation for tricuspid atresia or functional single ventricle. J Am Coll Cardiol 7:1087, 1986.

12. Zellers T, Driscoll D, Mottram C, et al: Exercise tolerance and cardiorespiratory response to exercise before and after the Fontan operation. Mayo Clin Proc 64:1489, 1989.

13. Ben Shachar G, Fuhrman B, Wang Y, et al: Rest and exercise hemodynamics after the Fontan procedure. Circulation 65:1043, 1982.

14. Gellwig MH, Lundstrom UR, Bull C, et al: Exercise responses in patients with congenital heart disease after Fontan repair: Patterns and determinants of performance. J Am Coll Cardiol 15:1424, 1990.

15. Grant G, Mansell A, Garofano R, et al: Cardiorespiratory response to exercise after the Fontan procedure for tricuspid atresia. Pediatr Res 24:1, 1988.

CHAPTER 17
APPROACH TO THE CYANOTIC NEONATE

KAZUO MOMMA

RECOGNITION OF CYANOSIS[1–3]

A neonate's skin is blue in color at birth but becomes pink with the onset of effective ventilation. Most neonates have pink bodies and lips but cyanotic hands and feet by 90 seconds after birth. A blue or dusky hue in a newborn infant is frequently brought to the attention of the physician by an experienced nurse. It may also be noticed first by a grandmother after the infant's discharge from the hospital.

Cyanosis is a serious sign in neonates and one to be treated with respect. Generalized cyanosis more than 90 seconds after birth occurs with low cardiac output, polycythemia, methemoglobinemia, cyanotic congenital heart disease, and pulmonary diseases. When a neonate remains cyanotic after a period in oxygen, the clinician must perform a rapid and systemic evaluation to determine whether a cardiac malformation is present so that potentially lifesaving measures can be instituted and the patient will be in an optimal hemodynamic and metabolic state to undergo an operation.

REDUCED HEMOGLOBIN CONCENTRATION AND CYANOSIS

Cyanosis is a blue color of the skin and mucous membranes caused by a reduced hemoglobin level of at least 4 to 6 g/dl in capillary beds. The oxygen content of capillary blood depends on hemoglobin level, oxygen saturation of arterial blood, and blood flow. Central cyanosis is detectable at higher arterial oxygen saturations when the hemoglobin concentration is elevated. On the other hand, with severe anemia, as for example of 10 g/dl, central cyanosis may not be evident until the arterial oxygen saturation falls to nearly 70%. The recognition of central cyanosis and its monitoring have been greatly simplified with the development of reliable pulse oximeters.

CENTRAL VERSUS PERIPHERAL CYANOSIS

Neonates suspected of being cyanotic are best examined when they are quiet or sleeping under a white light, preferably daylight. Central cyanosis is noticed in the tongue, mucous membranes, and nail beds. A comparison of the patient's nail beds with those of the examiner may clarify the presence or absence of cyanosis. In central cyanosis, the oxygen saturation of arterial blood is reduced, and this may be either physiologic or pathologic. Peripheral cyanosis is noticed best in the nail beds. It results from reduced peripheral blood flow. There is a normal arterial oxygen saturation. Peripheral cyanosis may be either physiologic or pathologic. Note that perioral cyanosis is common in infants owing to the virtual absence of tissue between the blood vessels and the skin; it is not a sign of central or peripheral cyanosis. Clinical confirmation that cyanosis of the extremities is peripheral in origin may be obtained by warming the baby's hand in a warm, moist towel; vasodilatation occurs, and the hand becomes pink.

Direct evidence is obtained by analyzing an arterial blood sample. Arterial blood may be obtained from various sites. A 3 or 5 French feeding tube or small catheter may be placed in the umbilical artery and left for sequential sampling. Central cyanosis should be considered to be present if arterial PO_2 is below 75 mm Hg at 24 hours of age or if arterial oxygen saturation is below 94%.

Differential cyanosis (i.e., a pink upper and blue lower part of the body or the reverse) always indicates a serious cardiac malformation, which includes interruption of the aortic arch, severe coarctation of the aorta, and transposition of the great arteries with a ductus arteriosus.

PHYSIOLOGIC CENTRAL CYANOSIS

Normal neonates appear cyanotic for a few minutes after birth. Most neonates, however, have a pink tongue and mucous membranes and an arterial PO_2 exceeding 50 mm Hg 10 minutes after their birth. Crying may cause a decrease in arterial oxygen saturation in a neonate with hypoventilation and a right-to-left shunt through a foramen ovale.

PATHOLOGIC MECHANISMS OF CENTRAL CYANOSIS

When a neonate at rest has central cyanosis that persists longer than 20 minutes after birth, further diagnostic studies are indicated. Cardiac and pulmonary conditions are two major categories of neonatal cyanosis:

- Major cardiac malformations include conditions associated with either pulmonary atresia or stenosis; complete transposition of the great arteries; admixture lesions, such as single ventricle, total anomalous pulmonary venous connection, or truncus arteriosus; left ventricular outflow obstruction and ductus-dependent systemic circulation; and persistent pulmonary hypertension or persistent fetal circulation.
- Pulmonary conditions include primary lung disease and mechanical interference with ventilation.

Other conditions causing neonatal cyanosis include central nervous system disease, methemoglobinemia, hypoglycemia, polycythemia, shock, and sepsis.

DIAGNOSTIC APPROACH TO CENTRAL CYANOSIS[1–3]

If a neonate has central cyanosis as determined by examination of the tongue or direct measurement of PaO_2, it is necessary to determine the cause. Often, definitive diagnosis may be made by clinical observation, chest radiography, blood gas values, and electrocardiography. Echocardiography is an extremely powerful tool in the diagnosis of neonatal cyanotic cardiac anomalies. The problem of differentiating between pulmonary and cardiac conditions arises frequently among neonates. Successful initial evaluation of the cyanotic neonate begins with careful observation of the breathing pattern. Certain clinical and laboratory findings favor either pulmonary or cardiac conditions (Table 17–1).

RESPIRATORY PATTERN

The respiratory rate of a sleeping neonate after 2 hours of life does not exceed 45 breaths per minute. A marked increase in respiratory rate in a cyanotic neonate suggests a pulmonary cause, left-sided heart failure, or pulmonary overcirculation. Cyanosis with increased depth of respiration suggests a cardiac malformation with decreased pulmonary blood flow. Intercostal retractions suggest airway obstruction or reduced lung compliance. Cyanosis with marked periodic breathing or apneic spells suggests central nervous system abnormalities with alveolar hypoventilation. Flaring of the alae nasi and grunting occur predominantly in idiopathic respiratory distress syndrome and pneumonia.

TABLE 17–1

DIAGNOSTIC FEATURES USEFUL TO DISTINGUISH CARDIAC FROM PULMONARY CAUSES OF CYANOSIS

	Suggest Heart Disease	Suggest Lung Disease
BIRTH HISTORY		
Prematurity, postmaturity, small for gestational age		+
Fetal distress, especially meconium staining, birth asphyxia, low Apgar score		+
MOVEMENT, RESPIRATION		
Flaccid, apathetic, little spontaneous movement; apneic spells	+	+
Deep sighing respiration, tachypnea with no other signs of respiratory distress	+	
Respiratory distress: tachypnea with intercostal retractions, grunting, flaring alae nasi	+	+
CARDIOVASCULAR EXAMINATION		
Cardiomegaly, hepatomegaly, murmurs	+	
CYANOSIS, BLOOD GAS VALUES, AND pH		
Marked generalized cyanosis, $PaO_2 < 25$ mm Hg, $PaCO_2$ normal or reduced	+	
Generalized cyanosis, $PaO_2 < 35$ mm Hg, $PaCO_2 > 45$ mm Hg		+
Differential cyanosis	+	+
pH < 7.2	+	+
RESPONSE TO OXYGEN OR VASODILATORS		
PaO_2 low on room air, <150 mm Hg with 100% oxygen	+	
PaO_2 low on room air, >250 mm Hg with 100% oxygen		+
Increased pH and PaO_2 with inhaled nitric oxide or infused tolazoline		+
MISCELLANEOUS LABORATORY FINDINGS		
Hypoglycemia	+	+
Hematocrit >65%	+	+
CHEST RADIOGRAPHY		
Clearly increased or decreased pulmonary vascular markings	+	
Snowstorm or reticular or granular pattern	+	+
Blotchy appearance consistent with aspiration		+
ELECTROCARDIOGRAPHY		
Moderate right ventricular hypertrophy	+	+
Gross abnormality	+	
ECHOCARDIOGRAPHY		
Normal cardiac structures		+
Abnormal chambers or great vessels	+	

SPONTANEOUS MOVEMENT

Lethargy and lack of adequate spontaneous movement suggest an intracranial lesion, shock, or sepsis. Neonates with advanced cyanosis, however, may become acidotic, hypotonic, and lethargic.

RESPONSE TO 100% OXYGEN BREATHING

The hyperoxia test is one method of distinguishing cyanotic congenital heart disease from pulmonary disease (Table 17–2). In many cyanotic neonates with pulmonary disease, cyanosis disappears with inhalation of 100% oxygen. It is commonly stated that if the neonate becomes pink in 100% oxygen, the hypoxemia is pulmonary in origin, whereas if blueness persists, it is cardiac in origin. This is an oversimplification. More accurately, a dramatic response to oxygen breathing suggests alveolar hypoventilation or severe ventilation/perfusion unevenness. Lack of visible response favors a large intracardiac or intrapulmonary shunt that may be caused by either a primary cardiac anomaly or primary lung disease.

If right radial artery blood samples are taken while 100% oxygen is administered for 5 to 10 minutes, a PO_2 value exceeding 250 mm Hg effectively excludes cyanotic forms of congenital heart disease. Failure of this value to rise above 150 mm Hg strongly suggests a cyanotic cardiac malformation, although it can also occur in severe pulmonary disease, particularly respiratory distress syndrome and pulmonary hypertension (persistent fetal circulation). As a single discriminator, radial blood gas sampling (when a patient's inspired oxygen concentration is high: $FIO_2 > 80\%$) is more useful than an electrocardiogram or chest film in deciding whether an infant has cyanotic rather than acyanotic heart disease or pulmonary disease. An elevated PCO_2 may be further evidence of primary pulmonary disease.

OTHER LABORATORY TESTS

A neonate with polycythemia may appear cyanotic, and anemia may inhibit the appearance of cyanosis. Measurement of hematocrit allows detection of the hyperviscosity syndrome. An elevated leukocyte count may point to sepsis. A Dextrostix test provides a screening test for hypoglycemia as a contributing factor to central cyanosis. Methemoglobinemia may be suspected by failure of blood to become red when it is placed on a slide and exposed to room air or when the PO_2 is normal but arterial oxygen saturation is below 94%. Confirmation is obtained by absorption spectrometry. Patients with methemoglobinemia are usually slate gray rather than blue. Electrolyte abnormalities may help identify dehydration, adrenocortical hyperplasia, and adrenal insufficiency. Adrenal insufficiency may mimic cyanotic congenital heart disease.

RADIOGRAPHIC FEATURES

A chest film of a cyanotic neonate is useful in assessing cardiac size and contour and the status of the pulmonary vasculature. Abnormal placement of the heart or abdominal organs may be evident. The radiographic approach to the differential diagnosis of congenital heart disease is discussed in Chapter 10. Various conditions affecting the lung are also evident: respiratory distress syndrome, bronchopulmonary dysplasia, congenital lymphangiectasia, diaphragmatic hernia, lung cyst, hypoplastic or absent lung, pneumonia, pneumothorax, and chylothorax. All of these give characteristic radiographic appearances and can be associated with cyanosis.

ECHOCARDIOGRAPHIC FEATURES[4–6]

Echocardiography provides major information for the diagnostic process. Two-dimensional recordings can be made without disturbing the neonate. Echocardiography can also identify almost all types of cyanotic heart disease and has supplemented and often replaced other diagnostic methods, including cardiac catheterization and angiography in sick neonates. Doppler interrogation is an essential part of echocardiography. Pulsed and continuous-wave Doppler blood flow velocimetry is applied to cardiac evaluation. Dynamic real-time color Doppler flow mapping equipment is available. Critically ill neonates with cardiac malformations can be managed without catheterization, provided that requisite skill in ultrasound imaging and the diagnostic experience are available. All of the standard views (discussed in Chapter 11) can be used, but the sub-

---

TABLE 17–2

RESPONSE TO 100% OXYGEN BREATHING IN CYANOTIC NEONATES

Category and Pathophysiologic Process	Response to 100% Oxygen Breathing
CHD with right-to-left shunt and decreased pulmonary blood flow	Little response because pulmonary capillary blood is almost completely saturated. Response is due to increased oxygen dissolved in plasma.
CHD with common mixing and increased pulmonary blood flow	Little response because pulmonary capillary blood is almost completely saturated.
CHD with severe heart failure; shunt or no shunt; alveolar hypoventilation	Response is usually good because alveolar hypoventilation is overcome.
Primary lung disease with alveolar hypoventilation, intrapulmonary right-to-left shunt, V/Q unevenness, or diffusion barrier	Response is unpredictable. Lack of response indicates intrapulmonary or intracardiac right-to-left shunting as a major factor.
Mechanical interference with lung function with alveolar hypoventilation	Response is usually good because alveolar hypoventilation is often the major mechanism of cyanosis.
Persistent pulmonary hypertension with right-to-left shunt through foramen ovale and ductus arteriosus	Response is variable depending on the severity of vasoconstriction and intracardiac right-to-left shunting.

CHD = congestive heart disease.
Adapted from Lees MH, Sunderland CO: Heart disease in the newborn. *In* Adams FH, Emmanouilides GC (eds): Moss' Heart Disease in Infants, Children, and Adolescents, 3rd ed. Baltimore, Williams & Wilkins, 1983, pp 658–669.

TABLE 17–3

ECHOCARDIOGRAPHIC FINDINGS IN IMPORTANT NONCARDIAC CAUSES OF CYANOSIS

PULMONARY HYPERTENSION

Persistent pulmonary hypertension (PPHN)	Patent foramen ovale, patent ductus arteriosus (PDA)	Right-to-left shunt through foramen ovale and ductus, tricuspid regurgitation with high velocity, suggesting high right ventricular pressure

NONCARDIAC CAUSES OF CYANOSIS

Neonatal asphyxia	Structurally normal heart, decreased ventricular motion	Tricuspid or mitral regurgitation ($+$ or $-$)
Infant of the diabetic mother	Disproportionate hypertrophy of ventricular septum	No shunt
Methemoglobinemia	Normal heart	No shunt
Polycythemia	Normal heart	No shunt
Pulmonary hypoplasia (secondary PPHN)	Normal heart, patent foramen ovale	Right-to-left shunt through foramen ovale ($\pm$PDA)
Sepsis and pulmonary hypertension (secondary PPHN)	Normal heart, patent foramen ovale	Right-to-left shunt through foramen ovale ($\pm$PDA)

costal four-chamber view is particularly helpful because each chamber and their relationships can be seen. Table 17–3 indicates findings in important noncardiac causes of cyanosis. Cardiac causes are described in detail in their respective chapters.

TREATMENT[3, 7–9]

Treatment of a cyanotic neonate should be tailored individually according to the underlying condition. Pulmonary and thoracic diseases should be treated as such. A clinician caring for a cyanotic neonate should not hesitate to start a prostaglandin E_1 infusion for a possible cardiac malformation in which the ductus is essential for either pulmonary or systemic circulation if a cardiac malformation is suspected on clinical grounds alone. Almost all cyanotic cardiac anomalies can be treated operatively with fairly good results. Therefore, a neonate with a cyanotic cardiac condition must be referred to a cardiac center in stable and satisfactory condition.

Profound hypoxemia leading to metabolic acidosis is a frequent complication of a cyanotic cardiac malformation. Metabolic acidosis must be treated by methods to improve oxygenation and with sodium bicarbonate. Metabolic acidosis clears relatively rapidly once an arterial oxygen saturation of 75 to 85% is attained by infusion of prostaglandin E_1.

OXYGEN

Oxygen is the first supportive measure readily available for a hypoxic neonate. Virtually all cyanotic neonates should be given oxygen to maintain an arterial Po_2 of about 50 mm Hg. Even in neonates with a cyanotic cardiac malformation with fully saturated pulmonary venous blood on breathing room air, administration of high concentrations of oxygen can increase the amount of dissolved oxygen in pulmonary venous blood, and this will result in a small but definite increase in arterial oxygen saturation. Later, after the infant's cardiovascular status has stabilized, attention should be directed to pulmonary problems that may result from prolonged inhalation of concentrations of oxygen greater than 40%.

In some cardiac conditions (Table 17–4), inhalation of 100% oxygen may induce congestive heart failure, pulmonary edema, and shock by dilating the pulmonary arterial vasculature; for instance, in hypoplastic left heart syndrome, inhalation of increased oxygen concentration dilates the pulmonary vasculature, and the increased Po_2 in ductus and aortic blood constricts the ductus arteriosus. As a result, pulmonary blood flow increases, systemic blood flow decreases, and shock ensues. In total anomalous pulmonary venous connection with pulmonary venous obstruction, inhalation of increased oxygen concentration increases pulmonary blood flow and causes pulmonary edema. Therefore, prostaglandin E_1 is the therapy of

TABLE 17–4

THERAPEUTIC INDICATIONS FOR 100% OXYGEN INHALATION AND INFUSION OF PROSTAGLANDIN E_1 IN CYANOTIC NEONATES WITH A CARDIAC MALFORMATION

Congenital Heart Disease	Oxygen	Prostaglandin E_1
Lesions with severe pulmonary stenosis or atresia	+	++
Total anomalous pulmonary venous connection	−	±
Single ventricle with increased pulmonary blood flow	−	−
Hypoplastic left heart syndrome with ductus arteriosus	−	++
Interrupted aortic arch with ventricular septal defect	−	++
Coarctation of aorta with ventricular septal defect	−	+
Complete transposition of great arteries	−	++

choice in a cyanotic neonate with ductus-dependent pulmonary or systemic circulation.

CONTROLLED RESPIRATION

Endotracheal intubation and mechanical ventilatory support are indicated in a cyanotic neonate with an admixture lesion, increased pulmonary blood flow, and severe respiratory distress. Single ventricle, tricuspid atresia, truncus arteriosus, and hypoplastic left heart syndrome—each without pulmonary stenosis—are included in this category. In these conditions, the most stable hemodynamic state is obtained with nearly equal pulmonary and systemic blood flows and an aortic oxygen saturation of 75 to 85%. These conditions are, however, usually associated with excessive pulmonary blood flow, high aortic oxygen saturation (exceeding 85%), and congestive heart failure. Hyperventilation lowers pulmonary vascular resistance. The lowering effect of hypocapnia on pulmonary vascular resistance is mediated by changing pH and not by PCO_2. In neonates with an admixture lesion, arterial blood gas should be checked and pulmonary blood flow controlled by adjusting the frequency and tidal volume of the mechanical ventilator.

PROSTAGLANDIN E₁

Prostaglandin E_1 can dilate a constricted ductus arteriosus. In a normal fetus, the ductus arteriosus is maintained patent by prostaglandin E_1 in ductal tissue and circulating plasma and the lower oxygen content of blood flowing through the ductus. After birth, tissue and plasma prostaglandin concentrations decline and oxygen content in ductal blood increases, and the ductus constricts (see Chapter 23).

Ductus-dependent pulmonary circulation is present in a variety of cardiac malformations associated with pulmonary atresia or severe stenosis, in which almost all pulmonary blood flow occurs through the ductus arteriosus (see Table 17–4). Postnatal constriction of the ductus in the hours or days after birth causes severe hypoxemia. Intravenous infusion of prostaglandin E_1 can open the ductus, increasing pulmonary blood flow and decreasing hypoxemia. Once a neonate is thought to be dependent on a ductus arteriosus as the source of pulmonary blood flow, an infusion of prostaglandin E_1 should be begun to maintain its patency. The neonate can then be transferred to a cardiac center with a continuous infusion of prostaglandin E_1.

Ductus-dependent systemic circulation is present in hypoplastic left heart syndrome, aortic interruption, severe coarctation of the aorta, and severe aortic stenosis. In hypoplastic left heart syndrome and severe aortic stenosis, all or almost all of the systemic blood flows through the ductus arteriosus. In interruption and severe coarctation, the blood flow to the lower part of the body is supplied through the ductus arteriosus. Postnatal constriction of the ductus arteriosus causes pulmonary hypertension, increased pulmonary blood flow, and decreased blood flow through the ductus into the aorta. Affected neonates deteriorate within a few days of birth and show mild hypoxemia, severe metabolic acidosis, anuria, and shock. Infusion of prostaglandin E_1 can dilate the ductus arteriosus, resulting in increased systemic perfusion, recovery from metabolic acidosis, and improved urine output.

Complete transposition is another cyanotic condition that benefits from prostaglandin E_1 administration. In complete transposition with an intact ventricular septum, a neonate survives with a bidirectional shunt through the foramen ovale. Dilatation of the ductus arteriosus by prostaglandin E_1 increases the blood flow from the aorta into the pulmonary artery. The shunt at the atrial level becomes left to right, and aortic oxygen saturation increases. In complete transposition with a ventricular septal defect, dilatation of the ductus arteriosus by prostaglandin E_1 and increased pulmonary blood flow augments the left-to-right shunt through the ventricular septal defect, and aortic oxygen saturation improves.

Prostaglandin E_1 is infused intravenously with an infusion pump. The initial dose is 0.05 to 0.1 µg/kg/min. The effect appears within 30 minutes. At the same time, adverse effects of this drug may appear. These effects are apnea, diarrhea, twitching, and temperature elevation. Prostaglandin E_1 must be infused through a secure intravenous line. If ductus patency does not become apparent within an hour of initiation of prostaglandin infusion in a neonate younger than 1 week, it should be assumed until proven otherwise that there is either a dosage error or a technical problem with delivery of the medication into the central blood stream. In a neonate with a right aortic arch, failure to improve may indicate absence of the ductus arteriosus.

Apnea resulting from prostaglandin E_1 may necessitate intubation of the neonate and use of controlled respiration. Once the ductus is dilated with prostaglandin E_1, a smaller dose can maintain ductal patency, and the dose may be reduced to 0.01 to 0.03 µg/kg/min.

PULSE OXIMETRY[10]

A pulse oximeter is an easy way to monitor arterial oxygen saturation noninvasively. It is widely used in neonatal intensive care units and has replaced transcutaneous PO_2 for routine monitoring. It is particularly useful in neonates with cyanotic forms of congenital heart disease. The devices are not significantly more expensive than transcutaneous PO_2 electrodes and are much easier to use. They do not require calibration, do not injure the skin, and give more or less instantaneous results. This last feature is of particular benefit during treatment with oxygen and prostaglandin E_1. The machines are relatively inaccurate, having an accuracy of 2% in the range from 70 to 100% saturation.

REFERENCES

1. Lees MH: Cyanosis of the newborn infant. Recognition and clinical evaluation. J Pediatr 77:484, 1970.
2. Jones RWA, Baumer JH, Joseph MC, Shinebourne EA: Arterial oxygen tension and response to oxygen breathing in differential diagnosis of congenital heart disease in infancy. Arch Dis Child 51:667, 1976.
3. Lees MH, Sunderland CO: Heart disease in the newborn. *In* Adams FH, Emmanouilides GC (eds): Moss' Heart Disease in Infants, Chil-

dren, and Adolescents, 3rd ed. Baltimore, Williams & Wilkins, 1983, pp 658–669.

4. Musewe NN, Dyke JD, Smallhorn JF: Echocardiography and the neonate with real or suspected heart disease. *In* Freedom RM, Benson LN, Smallhorn JF (eds): Neonatal Heart Disease. London, Springer-Verlag, 1992, pp 135–148.

5. Sanders SP: Echocardiography. *In* Long WA (ed): Fetal and Neonatal Cardiology. Philadelphia, WB Saunders, 1990, pp 301–329.

6. Bernstein D: Evaluation of the clinically ill neonate with cyanosis and respiratory distress. *In* Behrman RE, Kliegman RM, Arvin AM (eds): Nelson's Textbook of Pediatrics, 15th ed. Philadelphia, WB Saunders, 1996, pp 1310–1311.

7. Corbet AJ: Medical manipulation of the ductus arteriosus. *In* Garson A Jr, Bricker JT, Fisher DJ, Neish SR (eds): The Science and Practice of Pediatric Cardiology, 2nd ed. Philadelphia, Lea & Febiger, 1998, pp 2489–2514.

8. Momma K, Takao A, Sone K, Tasiro M: Prostaglandin E_1 treatment of ductus-dependent infants with congenital heart disease. Int Angiol 3(suppl):33, 1994.

9. Momma K: Ductus arteriosus and cardiovascular system in the neonate. *In* Curtis-Prior PB (ed): Prostaglandins. Biology and Chemistry of Prostaglandins and Related Eicosanoids. Edinburgh, Churchill Livingstone, 1988, pp 476–489.

10. Roberton NRC: Oxymetry. *In* Greenough A, Milner AD, Roberton NRC (eds): Neonatal Respiratory Disorders. London, Arnold, 1996, pp 159–160.

SECTION III
STRUCTURAL HEART DISEASE

CHAPTER 18

INCIDENCE, PREVALENCE, AND INHERITANCE OF CONGENITAL HEART DISEASE

JULIEN I. E. HOFFMAN

INCIDENCE

DEFINITIONS

Congenital heart disease refers to structural heart disease present at birth. Most studies adopt the definition of Mitchell and colleagues[1]: Congenital heart disease is "a gross structural abnormality of the heart or intrathoracic great vessels that is actually or potentially of functional significance." This definition excludes abnormalities of the great veins, such as persistent left superior vena cava, or aortic arch branches, such as a combined brachiocephalic–left carotid arterial trunk. Most studies of the incidence of congenital heart disease also exclude mitral valve prolapse, the bicuspid aortic valve (occurring in 2 to 3% of all live births[2]), and the patent ductus arteriosus of prematurity.

The incidence of congenital heart disease is the rate that refers to the number of children born with congenital heart disease related to the total number of births during a period, usually but not always one calendar year. It is usually expressed as a proportion of the number of children with congenital heart disease per 1000 or 1,000,000 births. It is important to define the denominator of such a rate, because there are big differences between rates based on all conceptions and those based merely on total or live births.[3]

Prevalence is the proportion that refers to all people with a given disease in the population at any time, and it includes all survivors with that disease, no matter when they were born.

FACTORS AFFECTING THE ACCURACY OF ASCERTAINMENT OF CONGENITAL HEART DISEASE

To determine the incidence of congenital heart disease, we need accurate diagnoses of *all* children who have the disease, and several factors may lead us to underestimate incidence. Important among these are prenatal deaths of children with congenital heart disease, inadequate access to medical care, and inadequate ascertainment and diagnostic methods.

Effect of Prenatal Death on Incidence Rates

The incidence of congenital heart disease is much higher in fetuses who die before birth than in liveborn infants.[3] Consequently, incidence rates based on liveborn infants underestimate the true incidence from the time of conception. Now that fetal echocardiograms are being done relatively early in most pregnancies, detecting these added lesions will alter our estimates of the incidence of congenital heart disease.

In two studies of a large number of early pregnancies,[4,5] 22 to 33% ended early before they were detected clinically, and another 10 to 12% ended later in clinically recognizable spontaneous abortions. A high proportion of these early fetal losses is associated with chromosome defects,[6] and 95% (range, 85 to 100%) of these chromosome defects are aneuploidies. Of these, about 25% are triploidies and tetraploidies (which are always lethal in utero), about 50% are autosomal trisomies, and about 18% are monosomy X; only 1% of these last two survive to term.[3] Berg and coworkers[7] calculated that cardiovascular malformations associated with four types of aneuploidy (trisomies 13, 18, and 21 and 45X) in the Baltimore-Washington Infant Study would have increased from 188 to 289 if fetal echocardiography had been done routinely at 18 weeks' gestation. Fetal echocardiography done even earlier, for example, at 14 weeks, would yield an even higher incidence of congenital heart disease, provided that high diagnostic accuracy could be achieved.

In general, stillborn infants and abortuses have an incidence of ventricular septal defects, many of them tiny, similar to that of liveborn infants. In contrast, in prenatal deaths, there is a higher incidence of coarctation of the aorta, double-inlet left ventricle, hypoplastic left heart syndromes (mainly aortic and mitral atresia), persistent truncus arteriosus, double-outlet right ventricle, and atrioventricular septal defect.[3] Pulmonary and aortic stenosis are disproportionately infrequent. The results obtained in 1006 fetuses with congenital heart disease detected in midpregnancy by fetal echocardiography[8] agree with the autopsy studies.

Adding the increased incidence of congenital heart disease in abortuses and stillborn children gives a total incidence for congenital heart disease that is about 5 times the incidence found in liveborn children alone. For example, of 100,000 pregnancies that last at least 4 weeks, there are likely to be about 21,800 spontaneous abortions, 1900 stillbirths, and 76,000 live births.[9] If the incidence of con-

Supported in part by Program Project Grant HL-25847 and NIH Training Grant HL-07544.

genital heart disease in each group, respectively, is 20% (assumed), 10%, and 1% (the latter incidences from Hoffman and Christianson[10]), the total incidence of congenital heart disease will be 4360 + 190 + 763 = 5313. By ignoring the incidence of congenital heart disease in prenatal deaths, the potential importance of genetic and chromosomal factors is grossly underestimated. Even the importance of environmental teratogens may be incorrectly assessed.[11]

Effect of Diagnostic Methods and Access to Medical Care

There has to be an efficient medical system to allow diagnoses of these lesions to be made by skilled, well-equipped pediatric cardiologists and to allow access to these cardiologists by the whole population. For these reasons, data collected long ago will be less accurate and complete than data collected more recently. Indeed, it is only with the advent of excellent echocardiography that accurate diagnostic evaluations can be made in populations of children with mild disease.

The completeness of ascertainment of the incidence of congenital heart disease in a population varies widely, depending on the methods used to detect and diagnose these patients. Children having lesions with prominent signs and symptoms like tetralogy of Fallot or large ventricular septal defects almost invariably come to medical attention and are diagnosed. On the other hand, those with minimal pulmonary stenosis, bicuspid aortic valves, or small atrial or ventricular septal defects are asymptomatic and often have inconspicuous physical signs. Such children may be missed by ordinary clinical examination and not included in any series. Most of them will not have any problems from their minimal heart disease, but failing to include them in any series underestimates the teratogenic factors that may be operating to cause them. On the other hand, some lesions that are lethal soon after birth may also not be included in a study, thereby leading to an underestimate of these severe lesions.

STUDIES ON INCIDENCE OF CONGENITAL HEART DISEASE

Determining the incidence of congenital heart disease by examining birth or death certificates is simple and inexpensive but inaccurate. Congenital heart disease is often not manifest by the time the birth certificate is filled in,[12–14] and indeed only one third or fewer of known congenital anomalies were listed on the birth certificates.[9, 15] Death certificates may also be inaccurate. Abu-Harb and coworkers[16] observed that 30% of infants who died with congenital heart disease had not been diagnosed before death. Because most congenital heart lesions do not cause early death, retrospective detection of cohorts of children born in a given region with congenital heart disease by examining death certificates is impossible.

Early studies of the incidence of congenital heart disease reported to Registries of Congenital Malformations active between 1940 and 1960 yielded what we now believe to be falsely low incidence rates of 3 to 5 per 1000 live births.[17] More recent studies have yielded an incidence of congenital heart disease in liveborn infants of 4.05 to 12.3

per 1000; the lower incidence figures probably represent considerable underascertainment of congenital heart disease. The highest incidences are reported from studies done in a localized region in which all children suspected of having congenital heart disease are referred to a single group of pediatric cardiologists and in which echocardiography is used extensively (Fig. 18–1A). The highest individual incidence of 12.3 per 1000 live births reported from Florence,[18] Italy, seems to be due principally to their high incidence of ventricular septal defects related to intensive study of newborn infants with echocardiography. Because these defects are the most common forms of congenital heart disease, inclusion of many who have tiny defects at birth will greatly influence the total incidence figure (Fig. 18–1B). In fact, Roguin and colleagues[19] detected 56 small muscular ventricular septal defects in 1053 (53.2 per 1000) consecutive neonates studied by Doppler echocardiography. If these are added to the other congenital heart lesions, the total incidence approaches 6% of live births, and this rises to about 8% if bicuspid aortic valves are included as well.

The effect of better diagnostic methods and the consequence of better ascertainment for the incidence of congenital heart disease are illustrated well by apparent changes in the incidence of ventricular septal defects. An increased incidence of ventricular septal defects during several years was first reported by Carlgren.[20, 21] He attributed the increased incidence during the second decade of the study to failure to include in the first decade small defects that closed early by themselves. Since then, there has been good evidence that the increase in incidence was due to better ascertainment of these small defects. In the counties around Albany, New York, Spooner and associates[22] showed that with the passing years, the median age at diagnosis decreased and the incidence of spontaneous closure increased. The increase in incidence applied to only the milder examples of ventricular septal defects, whereas the incidence of severe or complex ventricular septal defects remained steady. Perhaps most telling in their study there was a sudden increase in incidence after the introduction of echocardiography. Meberg and colleagues[23] noted that the increasing incidence of congenital heart disease in Vestfold County, Norway, was specifically due to the inclusion in later years of small muscular ventricular defects that were detected echocardiographically and that closed spontaneously by 1 year of age. Hiraishi and coinvestigators[24] studied term newborn infants with muscular ventricular septal defects, usually detected within 10 days of birth. The defects represented 2% of a consecutively studied population, 76% of them closed by 12 months after birth, and 42% of them had no murmurs. This was confirmed by Colloridi and associates,[25] who observed that 48.5% of all ventricular septal defects were in the muscular septum and that 69% of these closed before 1 year of age. Roguin and colleagues[19] detected 56 small muscular ventricular septal defects in 1053 (53.2 per 1000) consecutive neonates studied by Doppler echocardiography; about 90% of these closed spontaneously by 10 months of age. Failure to include these infants will therefore underestimate the incidence of ventricular septal defects and thus congenital heart disease as a whole. Similarly, studies in Dallas County, Texas,[26] and in the

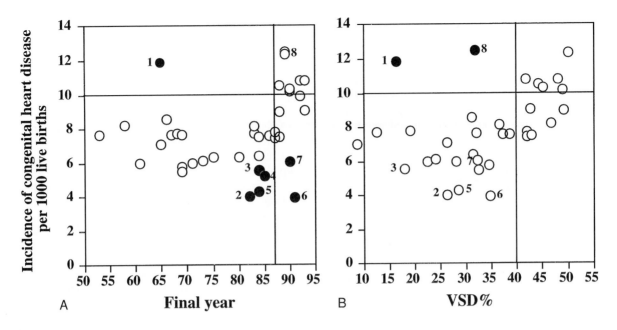

FIGURE 18–1

A, Incidence of congenital heart disease per 1000 births plotted against the final year of the study. An arbitrary horizontal line is drawn at a value of 10 per 1000 births; a vertical line indicates 1987 to show that the highest incidence rates, with one exception, occur in studies ending in or after 1987. Seven outliers are in solid circles. The rates for Alberta (3) and New South Wales (5) are low because they refer to only the first year of life, and the latter to only symptomatic lesions. The other low rates (2, Baltimore-Washington Infant Study; 4, Oviedo; 6, India; and 7, Guadaloupe) and the one high rate (1, Szolnok County) are unexplained, but note that the Baltimore-Washington Infant Study has the lowest proportion of ventricular septal defects of any series (see *B*) and that the proportion of ventricular septal defects was low in the studies in India and Guadaloupe, suggesting that many with small defects were not included in those studies. (Using the year of the midpoint of the study rather than the final year does not change the figure materially.) Those with the highest rates made extensive use of echocardiography in diagnosis. *B,* The percentage of ventricular septal defects (VSD) plotted against the incidence of all congenital heart disease per 1000 births. This figure shows that in general, the higher total incidence rates are associated with the highest proportions of ventricular septal defects, which thus play a major part in determining total incidence. The solid circles indicate two high outliers: 1 (Szolnok County) and 8 (Canadian Maritimes) have high total incidence rates despite a relatively low proportion of ventricular septal defects; 2 (Baltimore-Washington Infant Study), 3 (Alberta), 5 (New South Wales), 6 (India), and 7 (Guadaloupe) have low proportions of ventricular septal defects, possibly because follow-up was for only 1 year in Alberta and New South Wales and perhaps patients with small defects were not included in any of these studies. For detailed references, see Hoffman.[14]

Baltimore-Washington region[27] confirmed that the increased incidence of ventricular septal defects was restricted to the milder forms of the defect. For example, Fixler and coworkers[26] observed that between 1971 and 1984 in Dallas County, Texas, the incidence of all ventricular septal defects increased from 1.5 to almost 4 per 1000 live births. In contrast, the incidence of severe defects (defined as those having cardiac catheterization, surgery, or autopsy) remained steady at about 0.5 per 1000 live births throughout the period. Better ascertainment was probably also responsible for the increase in prevalence of ventricular septal defects per 1000 live births in Florence, Italy, from 4.7 in 1975–1980 to 8.6 in 1981–1984; all infants suspected of having heart disease received echocardiograms after 1980.[18]

This tendency for an increased incidence in the milder forms of congenital heart disease can be extended to other lesions as well. Fixler and colleagues[26] found that during the 14-year duration of the study, the incidence of mild forms of congenital heart disease tended to increase, whereas the incidence of severe forms of congenital heart disease remained constant. Bower and colleagues[12, 28] noted that with the use of echocardiography, the incidence of congenital heart disease in western Australia rose from 7.65 per 1000 in 1980–1989 to 10.4 per 1000 in 1990, largely owing to inclusion of more with minor ventricular

septal defects and pulmonary stenosis. Similar increases in these incidences with time were also ascribed to better ascertainment in the Canadian Maritimes[29] and in Arizona.[30]

The duration of follow-up also affects the incidence rate. Because a small percentage of patients are diagnosed late, the later years of a study tend to have a lower incidence rate for congenital heart disease compared with the earlier years. For example, in southern Australia, Haan and colleagues[13] observed incidence rates per 1000 births of 11.9 in 1986–1988, and these rates decreased year by year to reach 8.2 in 1993.

Those with mild pulmonary stenosis may also be underrepresented. It may be difficult to distinguish the murmur of a mild pulmonary stenosis from an innocent pulmonary flow murmur, and unless Doppler echocardiography or cardiac catheterization studies are done, the correct diagnosis may not be made.

There has been an increase in the incidence of patency of the ductus arteriosus with time.[31, 32] Anderson and coworkers,[31] in the Birth Defect Monitoring Study, observed a three-fold increase in this incidence between 1970 and 1975 nationwide and in metropolitan Atlanta. In Atlanta, the increase was associated with an increase in the numbers of patent ductus arteriosus in premature infants of low birth weight and an increase in those diagnosed in the first week of life. Depending on how many of these infants are included in a series on congenital heart disease, the total figures for incidence may vary considerably.

Given the limitations discussed, the incidence rate does not appear to vary consistently from country to country. However, in western Australia, the incidence rate of congenital heart disease was higher in aboriginal than in nonaboriginal children.[12] This finding is unlikely to have been due to increased access to medical care by aboriginal children.

INCIDENCES OF SPECIFIC LESIONS

The reported data are summarized in Figure 18–2. The incidences reported from numerous studies are more notable for their similarities than their differences.[14] They differ moderately in the incidences of the most common lesion, ventricular septal defect, because as mentioned before, the smallest defects were not included in several of the studies. In fact, because the incidence of ventricular septal defects was so high in the study from Florence,

Italy,[18] the effect was to decrease by about 35% the percentage of all the other lesions in the series. Conversely, studies reporting a small percentage of ventricular septal defects tend to have higher percentages for the remaining lesions. On the other hand, data on the absolute incidence of each lesion per 1,000,000 live births (Fig. 18–2) are not subject to how frequently small ventricular septal defects are found. Differences in the incidences of the rare lesions are probably explained by variation due to the small sample sizes in each series. The incidence of atrioventricular septal (endocardial cushion) defect varies about three-fold in different series, possibly related to differences in maternal age of those included in the study. Older mothers have an increased incidence of trisomy 21[33–35] in liveborn children and in spontaneous abortions[36,37]; about 50% of children with trisomy 21 have congenital heart disease,[38–40] and about 25 to 60% of the congenital heart disease that these children have is atrioventricular septal defect.[39,40] The inclusion of more of the older mothers in any series will therefore increase the incidence of atrioventricular septal defect in that series.

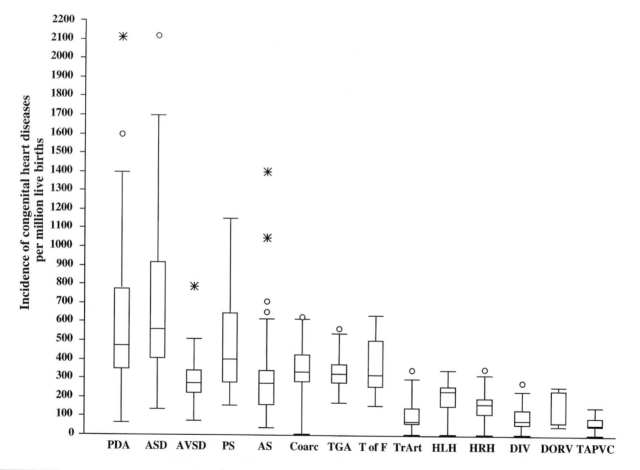

FIGURE 18–2

For major congenital heart lesions, the absolute incidences per million liveborn children are shown. Because there are about 4,000,000 live births per year in the United States, multiplying the absolute incidence figures by 4 gives the approximate number of children with each lesion who are born in the United States each year. In these box plots, the upper and lower ends of the rectangles are the upper and lower quartiles, respectively. The lines inside the rectangle are the median; the short horizontal lines terminating the vertical lines are the highest and lowest values for each set, except for circles (minor outliers) and asterisks (major outliers). PDA = patent ductus arteriosus; ASD = atrial septal defect; AVSD = atrioventricular septal defect; PS = pulmonic stenosis; AS = aortic stenosis; Coarc = coarctation of the aorta; TGA = complete transposition of the great arteries; T of F = tetralogy of Fallot; TrArt = truncus arteriosus; HLH = hypoplastic left heart; HRH = hypoplastic right heart; DIV = double-inlet left ventricle; DORV = double-outlet right ventricle; TAPVC = total anomalous pulmonary venous connection.

No intensive population studies have been done of various types of congenital heart disease in different indigenous racial groups in Australia, Asia, North America, Africa, and Greenland.[14] Ascertainment is incomplete, partly because access to medical care is limited and partly because cultural factors may prevent infants from receiving medical care or may not permit autopsies. Serious cardiac lesions like complete transposition of the great arteries and aortic atresia that cause early death, and mild or asymptomatic lesions like atrial septal defects, therefore may be underrepresented in reported series, which tend to have inflated incidences for lesions like tetralogy of Fallot that do not usually cause death in early infancy but are conspicuous enough to be diagnosed. Perhaps the most interesting differences from more intensively studied populations are the relatively low proportions of aortic coarctation and aortic stenosis, a deficit commented on by Anderson,[41] who studied Native Americans and who cited similar low proportions of these lesions reported from Japan, Korea, and Thailand. He regarded the low proportions of these two lesions as indicating some common genetic feature, but others[42, 43] speculated that the deficit might be due to inadequate medical care and ascertainment. This issue, however, cannot be considered closed. A markedly low incidence of coarctation of the aorta and aortic stenosis has been reported in Taiwanese,[44, 45] in a well-studied population in Hong Kong,[46] and in an Asian population studied in Birmingham, England.[47] Similarly, in the Baltimore-Washington Infant Study,[48] in Louisiana,[49] and in Dallas,[50] black children (and, in Dallas, Mexican Americans) had a relative deficiency of aortic stenosis and coarctation of the aorta as well as differences in some other lesions.

The incidence of ventricular septal defects in the outflow septum (e.g., doubly committed subarterial defects), either alone or associated with aneurysm of the sinus of Valsalva, appears much more frequently in patients from China and Japan than in the Western world.[45, 51]

PREVALENCE

At any time, the total number of people with congenital heart disease represents the total number born with congenital heart disease less those who have died or have cured themselves spontaneously. The affected people consist of those who need observation but no surgery, are awaiting surgery, or have had surgery. These, in turn, include some with little need for further medical care, others who need prolonged medical supervision, and still others who need further surgical procedures. The prevalence figures in any country are useful for planning medical services but fluctuate as the birth rate varies, indications for surgery change, or new forms of treatment with a lower mortality rate are introduced. Thus, whereas the numbers of surviving patients with complete transposition used to be low, the advent of successful surgical procedures has greatly increased their prevalence.

The prevalence of major congenital heart lesions in the United States was assessed by Roberts and Cretin.[52] Beginning with figures for the incidence of congenital heart disease estimated for 1975, they projected the numbers of live births and congenital heart disease to 1995 and then devised rough life tables for each of the seven selected lesions. Their estimates of surgical mortality were taken from reported data. They concluded that in 1995 in the United States, there will be nearly 300,000 children younger than 21 years with congenital heart disease, 38% of whom would have had one or more surgical procedures. As surgical mortality falls, the number of surviving children will rise, thereby increasing the numbers of consumers of cardiologic services. The prevalence figures obtained by Roberts and Cretin should be increased to reflect the better outlook for these children today, when about 90% of them survive to reach adult life.[53–56] On this basis, then, the prevalence of congenital heart disease in patients younger than 20 years in the United States will be about 643,000 rather than the 300,000 cited.

Because medical and surgical mortality were much higher 20 years ago, the prevalence of congenital heart disease in those older than 20 years is lower than the figures quoted. One estimate is that about 400,000 adults older than 21 years in the United States have congenital heart disease.[57] This includes those with or without previous treatment. There is about a 5% increase per year in this number. More than 90% of these people are capable of working but still require medical supervision.

INHERITANCE

This has been discussed in detail elsewhere.[58, 59] In general, the risk of recurrence of congenital heart disease in subsequent siblings varies from 1 to 6% if specific chromosomal or genetic syndromes are excluded; the risk is higher for more common than for rarer lesions. The risk of transmission to children from a parent with congenital heart disease varies from about 3 to 10% and is higher if the affected parent is the mother. If a sibling or a child has congenital heart disease, about 75% of the time the disease is concordant with the disease in the sibling or the parent. That is, the lesions are likely to be of the same type. This statement must be interpreted broadly. A bicuspid aortic valve and an aortic atresia are both in the family of left-sided heart obstructive lesions, and a pulmonic stenosis and a tetralogy of Fallot are both right ventricular outflow tract lesions. On the other hand, if the propositus has aortic or pulmonic stenosis, the next affected child is unlikely to have lesions as dissimilar as a truncus arteriosus or a complete transposition of the great arteries.

REFERENCES

1. Mitchell SC, Korones SB, Berendes HW: Congenital heart disease in 56,109 births. Incidence and natural history. Circulation 43:323, 1971.
2. Roberts WC: The congenitally bicuspid aortic valve. A study of 85 autopsy cases. Am J Cardiol 26:72, 1970.
3. Hoffman JIE: Incidence of congenital heart disease. II. Prenatal incidence. Pediatr Cardiol 16:155, 1995.
4. Miller JF, Williamson E, Glue J, et al: Fetal loss after implantation. A prospective study. Lancet 2:554, 1980.
5. Wilcox AJ, Weinberg CR, O'Connor JF, et al: Incidence of early loss of pregnancy. N Engl J Med 319:189, 1988.

6. Burgoyne PS, Holland K, Stephens R: Incidence of numerical chromosome anomalies in human pregnancy estimation from induced and spontaneous abortion data. Hum Reprod 6:555, 1991.

7. Berg KA, Clark EB, Astemborski JA, Boughman JA: Prenatal detection of cardiovascular malformations by echocardiography: An indication for cytogenetic evaluation. Am J Obstet Gynecol 159:477, 1988.

8. Allan LD, Sharland GK, Milburn A, et al: Prospective diagnosis of 1,006 consecutive cases of congenital heart disease in the fetus. J Am Coll Cardiol 23:1452, 1994.

9. Bierman JM, Siegel E, French FE, Simonian K: Analysis of the outcome of all pregnancies in a community: Kauai pregnancy study. Am J Obstet Gynecol 91:37, 1965.

10. Hoffman JIE, Christianson R: Congenital heart disease in a cohort of 19,502 births with long-term follow-up. Am J Cardiol 42:641, 1978.

11. Stein Z, Susser M, Warburton D, et al: Spontaneous abortion as a screening device. The effect of fetal survival on the incidence of birth defects. Am J Epidemiol 102:275, 1975.

12. Bower C, Ramsay JM: Congenital heart disease: A 10 year cohort. J Paediatr Child Health 30:414, 1994.

13. Haan E, Chan A, Byron-Scott R, Scott H: The South Australian Birth Defects Register, Annual Report 1993. Report from the Women's and Children's Hospital, Adelaide, S. Australia, 1995.

14. Hoffman JIE: Incidence of congenital heart disease. I. Postnatal incidence. Pediatr Cardiol 16:103, 1995.

15. Lilienfeld AM, Parkhurst E, Patton R, Schlesinger ER: Accuracy of supplemental medical information on birth certificates. Public Health Rep 66:191, 1951.

16. Abu-Harb M, Hey E, Wren C: Death in infancy from unrecognised congenital heart disease. Arch Dis Child 71:3, 1994.

17. Hoffman JIE: Natural history of congenital heart disease. Problems in its assessment with special reference to ventricular septal defects. Circulation 37:97, 1968.

18. Manetti A, Pollini I, Cecchi F, et al: Epidemiologia delle malformazioni cardiovascolari. III. Prevalenza e decorso in 46.895 nati vivi all Maternità di Careggi, Firenze, nel periodo 1975–1984. G Ital Cardiol 23:145, 1993.

19. Roguin N, Du Z-D, Barak M, et al: High prevalence of muscular ventricular septal defect in neonates. J Am Coll Cardiol 26:1545, 1995.

20. Carlgren LE: The incidence of congenital heart disease in children born in Gothenburg 1941–1950. Br Heart J 21:40, 1959.

21. Carlgren LE: The incidence of congenital heart disease in Gothenburg. Proc Assoc Eur Cardiol 5:2, 1969.

22. Spooner EW, Hook EB, Farina MA, Shaher RM: Evaluation of a temporal increase in ventricular septal defects: Estimated prevalence and severity in Northeastern New York, 1970–1983. Teratology. 37:21, 1988.

23. Meberg A, Otterstad JE, Frøland G, Sørland S: Barn med medfødt hjertefeil i Vestfold 1982–88. Tidsskr Nor Laegeforen 110:354, 1990.

24. Hiraishi S, Agata Y, Nowatari M, et al: Incidence and natural course of trabecular ventricular septal defects: Two-dimensional echocardiography and color Doppler flow imaging study. J Pediatr 120:409, 1992.

25. Colloridi V, Ventriglia F, Bastianon V, et al: Natural history of ventricular septal defects by serial color-flow Doppler echocardiographic studies. Cardiol Young 3(suppl I):140, 1993.

26. Fixler DE, Pastor P, Chamberlin M, et al: Trends in congenital heart disease in Dallas county births 1971–1984. Circulation 81:137, 1990.

27. Martin GR, Perry LW, Ferencz C: Increased prevalence of ventricular septal defect: Epidemic or improved diagnosis. Pediatrics 83:200, 1989.

28. Bower C, Rudy E, Ryan A, et al: Report of the Birth Defects Registry of Western Australia 1980–1991. Health Department of Western Australia, Statistical Series/32, 1992.

29. Roy DL, McIntyre L, Human DG, et al: Trends in the prevalence of congenital heart disease: Comprehensive observations over a 24-year period in a defined region of Canada. Can J Cardiol 10:821, 1994.

30. Mayberry JC, Scott WA, Goldberg SJ: Increased birth prevalence of cardiac defects in Yuma, Arizona. J Am Coll Cardiol 16:1696, 1990.

31. Anderson CE, Edmonds LD, Erickson JD: Patent ductus arteriosus and ventricular septal defect: Trends in reported frequency. Am J Epidemiol 107:281, 1978.

32. Edmonds LD, James LM: Temporal trends in the incidence of malformation in the United States, selected years, 1970–71, 1982–83. MMWR 34:1SS, 1985.

33. Hook EB: Estimates of maternal age-specific risks of a Down's syndrome birth in women aged 34–41. Lancet 2:33, 1976.

34. Hook EB: Rates of Down's syndrome in livebirths and at mid trimester amniocentesis. Lancet 1:1053, 1978.

35. Ferguson-Smith MA, Yates JRW: Maternal age specific rates for chromosome aberrations and factors influencing them: Report of a collaborative European study on 52 965 amniocenteses. Prenat Diagn 4 (special issue):5, 1984.

36. Hassold T, Chiu D: Maternal age-specific rates of numerical chromosome abnormalities with special reference to trisomy. Hum Genet 70:11, 1985.

37. Byrne J, Warburton D, Kline J, et al: Morphology of early fetal deaths and their chromosomal characteristics. Teratology 32:297, 1985.

38. Stoll C, Alembik Y, Dott B, Roth M-P: Epidemiology of Down syndrome in 118,265 consecutive births. Am J Med Genet Suppl 7:79, 1990.

39. Bhatia S, Verma IC, Shrivastava S: Congenital heart disease in Down syndrome: An echocardiographic study. Indian Pediatr 29:1113, 1992.

40. Wells GL, Barker SE, Finley SC, et al: Congenital heart disease in infants with Down's syndrome. South Med J 87:724, 1994.

41. Anderson RC: Congenital heart malformations in North American Indian children. Pediatrics 59:121, 1977.

42. Hernandez FA, Miller RH, Schiebler GL: Rarity of coarctation of the aorta in the American Negro. J Pediatr 74:623, 1969.

43. Van der Horst RL, Gotsman MS: Racial incidence of coarctation of the aorta. Br Heart J 34:289, 1972.

44. Lue HC, Chen CM, Hsu JY, Chen CL: The prevalence and types of congenital heart diseases in Chinese. J Formos Med Assoc 75:53, 1976.

45. Lien WP, Chen JR, Chen JH, et al: Frequency of various congenital heart diseases in Chinese adults: Analysis of 926 consecutive patients over 13 years of age. Am J Cardiol 57:840, 1986.

46. Sung RY, So LY, Ng HK, et al: Echocardiography as a tool for determining the incidence of congenital heart disease in newborn babies: A pilot study in Hong Kong. Int J Cardiol 30:43, 1991.

47. Sadiq M, Stümper O, Wright JGC, et al: Influence of ethnic origin on the pattern of congenital heart defects in the first year of life. Br Heart J 73:173, 1995.

48. Correa-Villasenor A, McCarter R, Downing J, Ferencz C: White-black differences in cardiovascular malformations in infancy and socioeconomic factors. Am J Epidemiol 134:393, 1991.

49. Storch TG, Mannick EE: Epidemiology of congenital heart disease in Louisiana: An association between race and sex and the prevalence of specific cardiac malformations. Teratology 46:271, 1992.

50. Fixler DE, Pastor P, Sigman E, Eifler CW: Ethnicity and socioeconomic status: Impact on the diagnosis of congenital heart disease. J Am Coll Cardiol 21:1722, 1993.

51. Chen JJ, Lien WP, Chang FZ: Ruptured congenital aneurysm of the right sinus of Valsalva into the right ventricle: With special reference to pathoanatomic and hemodynamic characteristics in symptomless cases. Jpn Circ J 44:87, 1980.

52. Roberts NK, Cretin S: The changing face of congenital heart disease. A method for predicting the influence of cardiac surgery upon the prevalence and spectrum of congenital heart disease. Med Care 18:930, 1980.

53. Morris CD, Menashe VD: 25-year mortality after surgical repair of congenital heart defect in childhood. A population-based cohort study. JAMA 266:3447, 1991.

54. Moller JH, Patton C, Varco RL, Lillehei CW: Late results (30 to 35 years) after operative closure of isolated ventricular septal defect from 1954 to 1960. Am J Cardiol 68:1491, 1991.

55. Moller JH, Anderson RC: Natural history of congenital heart disease. 1000 consecutive children with cardiac malformations with 26–37 year follow-up. Am J Cardiol 70:661, 1992.

56. Garson AJ, Begley CE: A model state funding program for adults with congenital heart disease. Cost-benefit analysis of job training and payback. J Am Coll Cardiol 19:355A, 1992.

57. Perloff J: Bethesda Conference 22: Congenital heart disease after childhood: An expanding patient population. J Am Coll Cardiol 18:311, 1991.

58. Burn J: The aetiology of congenital heart disease. In Anderson RH, Macartney FJ, Shinebourne EA, Tynan M (eds): Paediatric Cardiology. London, Churchill Livingstone, 1987, p 15.

59. Hoffman JIE: Congenital heart disease: Incidence and inheritance. Pediatr Clin North Am 37:25, 1990.

CHAPTER 19

NOMENCLATURE AND CLASSIFICATION: SEQUENTIAL SEGMENTAL ANALYSIS

ROBERT H. ANDERSON

Why do we need a system for nomenclature if congenitally malformed hearts themselves have not changed since their initial descriptions? The reason is that the number of individual lesions that can coexist within any malformed heart is considerable. Add to this the possibilities for combinations of lesions, and the problem of providing "pigeonholes" for each entity becomes immense. We all recognize the nature of straightforward lesions, such as septal deficiencies and valvar stenoses. Almost always, these entities are encountered in otherwise normally structured hearts. It is when the hearts containing the lesions are themselves built in grossly abnormal fashion that difficulties are produced. We can no longer be satisfied with a "wastebasket" category for so-called complex lesions because the recognition of apparent complexity does nothing to determine diagnosis or optimal treatment. If approached in simple and straightforward fashion, these abnormally structured hearts need not be difficult to understand and describe.

The simplicity comes when we recognize that, basically, all congenitally malformed hearts, like normal hearts, have three building blocks, namely, the atria, the ventricular mass, and the arterial trunks (Fig. 19–1). A system for description and categorization based on recognition of the limited potential for variation in each of these cardiac segments was developed independently in the 1960s by two groups, one based in the United States and led by Richard Van Praagh,[1,2] the other from Mexico City and headed by Maria Victoria de la Cruz.[3] Both of these systems concentrated on the different topologic arrangements of the individual components within each cardiac segment. For example, when Van Praagh introduced the concept of concordance and discordance between atria and ventricles,[4] he was concerned primarily with the harmony or disharmony to be found between atrial and ventricular "situs," placing no emphasis in segmental notation on the manner in which the cavities of the atrial and ventricular chambers were joined across the atrioventricular junctions. A similar approach, which concentrated on relationships of the great arterial trunks, was taken by de la Cruz and coworkers[5] in formulating their concept of arterioventricular concordance and discordance. Because it was often difficult, using the diagnostic techniques available at that time, to determine precisely how the cavities of adjacent structures were linked, these approaches were understandable. The advent of cross-sectional echocardiography changed all that. Since the mid-1970s, it has been possible with precision to determine how the myocardial structure of the atria is, or is not, joined to the

ventricular mass and to establish the precise morphology of the ventriculoarterial junctions. Because the system of nomenclature developed by myself and my colleagues, and to be discussed in this chapter, evolved concomitantly with the development of echocardiography, our approach has been to concentrate on the variations possible across the atrioventricular and ventriculoarterial junctions.[6,7] In making such analysis, it should not be thought that the segments themselves are ignored. Indeed, junctional connections cannot be established without knowledge of segmental topology.[8,9]

Our system, throughout its evolution, has followed the same basic and simple rules. From the outset, we have formulated our categories on the basis of recognizable anatomic facts, avoiding any speculative embryologic assumptions. Again, from the start, we have emphasized the features of morphology, connections, and relations of the segmental components as three different facets of the cardiac makeup. It still remains an undisputed fact that any system that separates these features, does not use one to determine another, and describes them with mutually exclusive terms must perforce be unambiguous. The clarity of the system, then, depends on its design. Some argue that brevity is an important feature and have constructed codifications to achieve this aim.[10] My opinion is that in the final analysis, clarity is more important than brevity.[11] We do not shy, therefore, from using several words in the place of one symbol or sequence of symbols. Wherever possible, we also strive to use words that are as meaningful in their systematic role as in their everyday use. It has been this desire to achieve optimal clarity that has led to several changes in our descriptions through the years, most notably in the use of the term *univentricular heart*. No apologies are made for these changes, because their formulation, in response to valid criticisms, has eradicated initially illogical points from our system to its advantage. It is our belief that the system now advocated is entirely logical.[9] We hope it is simple. Should further illogicalities become apparent, they would be extirpated as completely as was the univentricular heart from our lexicon as an appropriate descriptor for hearts that possess one big and one small ventricle.[8,11]

SEQUENTIAL SEGMENTAL ANALYSIS: BASIC CONCEPTS

The system[9] depends first on the establishment of the arrangement of the atrial chambers (situs). Next, attention

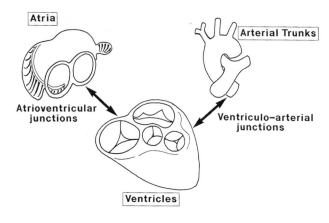

The three primary cardiac segments delineated anatomically by the discrete atrioventricular and ventriculoarterial junctions.

is concentrated on the anatomic nature of the junctions between the atrial myocardium and the ventricular myocardial mass. This feature, which is described as a type of connection, is separate from the additional feature of the morphology of the valve or valves that guard the junctions. There are two atrioventricular valves in the normally constructed heart, each guarding a separate atrioventricular junction, but the junction can be a common structure guarded by a common valve. To achieve proper analysis of the atrioventricular junctions, it is necessary also to identify the structure, topology, and relationships of the chambers within the ventricular mass. When the atrioventricular junctions have been dealt with in this fashion, the ventriculoarterial junctions are similarly analyzed in terms of the arrangement of the connections of ventricles with arterial trunks and the morphology of the arterial valves guarding them. Separate attention is directed to the morphology of the outflow tracts and to the relationships of the great arterial trunks. A catalogue is then made of all associated cardiac (and, when pertinent, noncardiac) malformations. Included in this final category are such features as the location of the heart and the arrangement of the other thoracic and abdominal organs. Each system is analyzed in its own right and is not designated according to changes observed in other systems.

Implicit in the system is the ability to distinguish the morphology of the individual atria and ventricles and to recognize the types of arterial trunks taking origin from the ventricles. This is not as straightforward as it may seem, because often in congenitally malformed hearts, these chambers or arterial trunks may lack some of the morphologic features that most obviously characterize them in the normal heart. For example, the most obvious feature of the morphologically left atrium in the normal heart is its connection to the pulmonary veins. But in hearts with totally anomalous pulmonary venous connection, these veins connect in extracardiac fashion, yet it is still possible to recognize the remnant of the left atrium. It is considerations of this type that prompted the concept now used for recognition of the cardiac chambers and great arteries. Dubbed by Van Praagh and colleagues[12] the *morphologic method* and based on the initial work of Lev,[13] the principle states that chambers should be recognized in terms of their in-

trinsic myocardial morphology, one part of the heart not being defined in terms of other structures that are themselves variable.

When this eminently sensible concept is applied to the atrial chambers, the connections of the great veins are immediately disqualified as markers of morphologic rightness or leftness because, as discussed before, the veins do not always connect to their usual atria. Lev[13] placed great stress on septal morphology as a distinguishing feature. Septal morphology, however, is of little help when the septum itself is absent. Similarly, the atrial vestibule is ruled out as a marker because it is usually lacking in hearts with atrioventricular valvar atresia. Fortunately, there is another component of the atrial chambers that, in our experience, has been almost universally present and, on the basis of the myocardial morphology of its junction with the remainder of the chambers, has enabled us always to distinguish between morphologically right and left atria. This is the appendage.[14] The morphologically right appendage has the shape of a blunt triangle and joins over a broad junction with the remainder of the atrium. The junction is marked externally by the terminal groove and internally by the terminal crest. The most significant feature, however, is that the pectinate muscles lining the appendage extend all around the parietal atrioventricular junction (Fig. 19–2). The morphologically left appendage, in contrast, is much narrower and tubular. It has a narrow junction with the remainder of the atrium that is marked by neither terminal groove nor muscular crest. The pectinate muscles are confined within the morphologically left appendage, with the posterior aspect of the morphologically left vestibule being smooth-walled as it merges with the pulmonary venous component (see Fig. 19–2).

The morphologic method also shows its value when it is applied to the ventricular mass, which extends from the atrioventricular to the ventriculoarterial junctions. Thus, the boundaries of the ventricular musculature are the fibrous tissue plane separating the atrial and ventricular muscle masses at the atrioventricular junction and the point at the ventricular outlets where the musculature changes to the typical fibroelastic structure of the walls of the great arterial trunks. Within the ventricular mass, as thus defined, there are almost always two ventricles. Description of ventricles, no matter how malformed they may be, is facilitated if they are analyzed as possessing three components. These are (1) the inlet, extending from the atrioventricular junction to the distal attachment of the atrioventricular valvar tension apparatus; (2) the apical trabecular component; and (3) the outlet component, supporting the leaflets of the arterial valve. Of these three components, it is the apical trabecular component that is most universally present in normal as well as in malformed and incomplete ventricles. Furthermore, it is the pattern of the apical trabeculations that differentiates morphologically right from left ventricles (compare Figs. 19–3 and 19–4). This is so even when the apical components exist as the basis of incomplete ventricles that lack either an inlet or an outlet component (or sometimes both of these components). When the morphology of individual ventricles is identified according to the apical myocardium, all hearts with two ventricles can readily be analyzed according to the way that the inlet and outlet components are shared between the apical trabecular components.

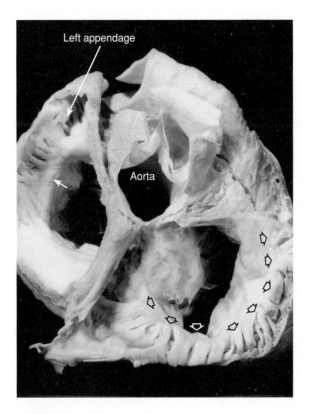

FIGURE 19–2

The short-axis view of the atrioventricular junctions from above shows the extent of the pectinate muscles, the feature that most reliably differentiates morphologically right from left atrial appendages *(long arrow)*. The muscles in the right atrium extend around the orifice of the tricuspid valve *(open arrows)*. Those in the left atrium are confined anterosuperiorly *(short arrow)*.

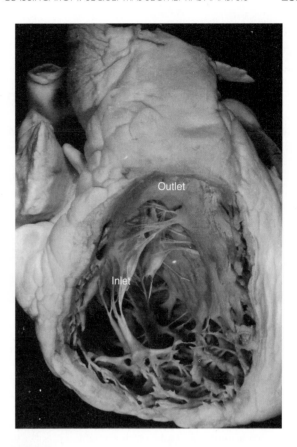

FIGURE 19–3

The characteristic features of the normal morphologically right ventricle. The typically coarse trabeculations occupy the entire apex beyond the tension apparatus of the tricuspid valve. The outlet (infundibulum) is smooth-walled.

To describe any ventricle fully, account must also be taken of its size. It is then necessary to describe the way that the two ventricles themselves are related within the ventricular mass. This feature is described in terms of ventricular topology, because two basic patterns are found that cannot be changed without physically taking apart the ventricular components and reassembling them. The two patterns are mirror images of each other and can be conceptualized in terms of the way that, figuratively speaking, the palmar surface of the hands can be placed on the septal surface of the morphologically right ventricle. In the morphologically right ventricle of the normal heart, irrespective of its position in space, only the palmar surface of the right hand can be placed on the septal surface such that the thumb occupies the inlet and the fingers fit into the outlet (Fig. 19–5). The palmar surface of the left hand then fits in comparable fashion within the morphologically left ventricle, but it is the right hand that is taken as the arbiter for the purposes of categorization. The usual pattern, therefore, can be described as right-hand ventricular topology.[15] The other pattern, the mirror image of the right-hand prototype, is then described as left-hand ventricular topology. In this left-hand pattern, seen typically in the mirror-image normal heart or in the variant of congenitally corrected transposition found with usual atrial arrangement, it is the palmar surface of the left hand that fits on the septal surface of the morphologically right ventricle with the thumb in the inlet and the fingers in the outlet. These two topologic patterns can always be distinguished, irrespective of the location occupied in space by the ventricular mass itself. A left-hand pattern of topology, therefore, is readily distinguished from a ventricular mass with right-hand topology in which the right ventricle has been rotated to occupy a left-sided position. Component makeup, trabecular pattern, topology, and size are independent features of the ventricles. On occasion, each may need a separate description if hearts are to be analyzed without confusion.

Only rarely will hearts be encountered with a solitary ventricle. Sometimes this may be because a right or left ventricle is so small that it cannot be recognized with usual clinical investigatory techniques. There is, nonetheless, a third pattern of apical ventricular morphology found in hearts possessing a truly single ventricle. This is when the apical component is of neither right nor left type but is coarsely trabeculated and crossed by multiple large muscle bundles. Such a solitary ventricle has an indeterminate morphology. Analysis of ventricles on the basis of their apical trabeculations precludes the need to use illogically the terms *single ventricle* or *univentricular heart* for description of those hearts that have one big and one small ventricle. All chambers that possess apical trabecular components can be described as ventricles, whether they are big or small and incomplete or complete. Any attempt to dis-

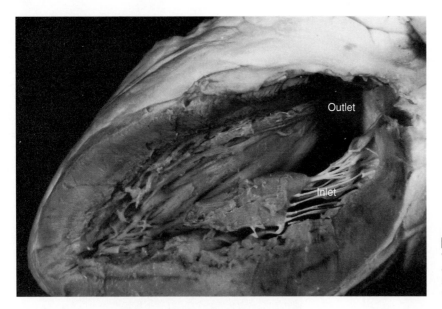

FIGURE 19–4

The normal morphologically left ventricle has overlapping inlet and outlet components, a smooth septal surface, and fine crisscrossing apical trabeculations.

qualify such chambers from ventricular status must lead to a system that is artificial. Only hearts with a truly solitary ventricle need be described as univentricular, albeit that the connections of the atrioventricular junctions can be univentricular in many more hearts.[9, 11]

In determining the morphology of the great arteries, there are no intrinsic features that enable an aorta to be distinguished from a pulmonary trunk or from a common or solitary arterial trunk. The branching pattern of the trunks themselves, nonetheless, is sufficiently characteristic to permit these distinctions (Fig. 19–6). Thus, the aorta gives rise to at least one coronary artery and the bulk of the systemic arteries. The pulmonary trunk gives rise directly to both, or one or other, of the pulmonary arteries. A common trunk directly supplies the coronary, systemic, and pulmonary arteries. A solitary arterial trunk exists in the absence of the proximal portion of the pulmonary trunk. In such circumstances, it is impossible to state with certainty whether the persisting trunk is common or aortic. Even in the rare instances that transgress one of these rules, examination of the pattern of branching usually permits distinction of the nature of the arterial trunks.

ATRIAL ARRANGEMENT

The cornerstone of any system of sequential analysis must be accurate establishment of atrial arrangement, because this is the starting point for subsequent analysis. Some argue that according to the venoatrial connections, all hearts have either usual or mirror-image arrangements.[16] This approach is a direct abrogation of the morphologic method, however, because it seeks to define one variable (atrial arrangement) on the basis of another (venoatrial connections). It also takes no account of myocardial morphology, which, as rightly emphasized by Van Praagh and associates,[17] is the cornerstone of proper analysis.

When arrangement of the atria is assessed according to the morphology of the junction of the appendages with the

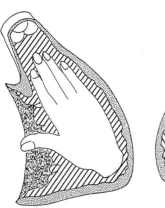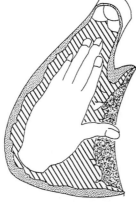

Right-Hand Topology   Left-Hand Topology

FIGURE 19–5

Ventricular topology is conceptualized in terms of the way in which the right and left hands can be placed on the septal surface of the morphologically right ventricle. All hearts with biventricular atrioventricular connections then have either right-hand or left-hand topology.

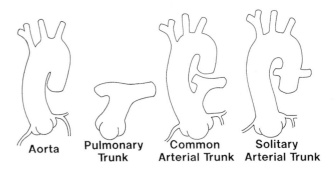

Aorta   Pulmonary   Common   Solitary
          Trunk   Arterial Trunk   Arterial Trunk

FIGURE 19–6

The four basic patterns of arterial trunks distinguished according to the nature of their branching. The solitary trunk exists in the complete absence of any intrapericardial pulmonary arteries.

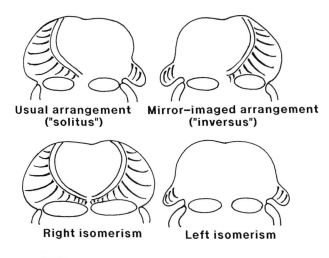

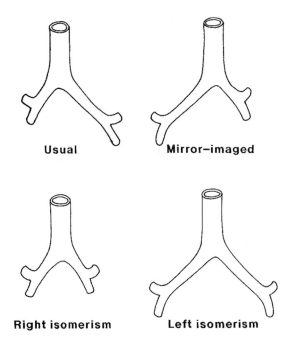

The four possible arrangements of the atrial chambers based on the morphology of the junction of the atrial appendages with the remainder of the atria.

The four patterns of bronchial morphology, which almost without exception are coincident with the arrangement of the atrial appendages.

rest of the atria,[14] in other words, on the basis of myocardial morphology, there are four possible patterns of arrangement because all hearts have two atrial appendages, each of which can only be of morphologically right or left type (Fig. 19–7). The most common is the usual arrangement (so-called situs solitus), in which the morphologically right appendage is right-sided and the morphologically left appendage is left-sided. The second arrangement, very rare, is the mirror image of the usual and is often called atrial situs inversus. In these two arrangements, the appendages are lateralized, with the morphologically right appendage being to one side and the morphologically left appendage to the other. The two other arrangements do not show such lateralization. Instead, there is isomerism of the atrial appendages. Thus, both appendages are mirror images of each other with morphologic characteristics, at their junctions with the rest of the atria on both sides, of either right or left type.

RECOGNITION OF ATRIAL ARRANGEMENT

The arrangement of the appendages is ideally recognized by direct examination of the extent of the pectinate muscles around the vestibules. This feature should now be recognizable with use of cross-sectional echocardiography, particularly from the transesophageal window. In most clinical situations, however, it is rarely necessary to rely only on direct identification. This is because, almost always, the morphology of the appendages is in harmony with the arrangements of the thoracic and abdominal organs. In patients with lateralized arrangements (usual and mirror image), it is exceedingly rare for there to be disharmony between the location of the organs. When the appendages are isomeric, in contrast, usually there is so-called heterotaxia of the abdominal organs. Even when there is abdominal heterotaxia, the lungs and bronchial tree are almost always symmetric, and it is rare for the bronchial arrangement to be disharmonious with the morphology of the appendages.[18] In suspicious circumstances, therefore, isomerism can almost always be inferred from the bronchial anatomy.[19, 20] The key is that the morphologically left bronchus is long and branches only after it has been crossed by the pulmonary artery, which supplies the lower lobe (making the bronchus hyparterial). In contrast, the morphologically right bronchus is short and is crossed by the lower lobe pulmonary artery only after it has branched (eparterial branching pattern). The four bronchial patterns (usual, mirror image, right isomerism, and left isomerism; Fig. 19–8) are then almost always in harmony with the arrangement of the atrial appendages.

Inferences similar to those provided from bronchial arrangement can also usually be obtained noninvasively by using cross-sectional ultrasonography to image the abdominal great vessels.[21] These vessels bear a distinct relation to each other and to the spine, which generally reflects body arrangement, although not as accurately as does bronchial anatomy. When the atria are lateralized then, almost without exception, the inferior caval vein and aorta lie to opposite sides of the spine, with the caval vein on the side of the morphologically right appendage. When there is right isomerism, the great vessels usually lie to the same side of the spine, with the caval vein anterior. In the setting of left isomerism, an azygos vein carrying the inferior caval venous blood on the same side, and posterior to, the abdominal aorta is a good indicator but does not differentiate usual or mirror-image arrangement with interrupted inferior caval vein.

Generally speaking, right isomerism is associated with absence of the spleen (asplenia), whereas left isomerism is associated with multiple spleens (polysplenia). Patients with isomerism of the atrial appendages are thus frequently grouped together, from the cardiac standpoint, under the banner of the "splenic syndromes." This approach is much less accurate than describing the syndromes directly in terms of isomerism of the atrial appendages, because the correlation between right isomerism and asplenia and between left isomerism and polysplenia is far from perfect.[22,23] In reality, it is necessary to describe both splenic status and the morphology of the appendages, but it is the latter feature that serves to concentrate attention on the heart.

THE ATRIOVENTRICULAR JUNCTIONS

In the normal heart, the atrial myocardium is contiguous with the ventricular mass around the orifices of the mitral and tricuspid valves. Electrical insulation is provided at these junctions by the fibrofatty atrioventricular grooves, other than at the site of the penetration of the bundle of His. In abnormal hearts, to analyze the morphology of the atrioventricular junctions accurately, it is first necessary to know the atrial arrangement. Equally, it is necessary to know the morphology of the ventricular mass to establish which atrium is connected to which ventricle. With this information, it is then possible to define the pattern of the muscular atrioventricular connections around the atrioventricular valvar orifices and to determine the morphology of the valves that guard the junctions. In hearts with complex malformations, it is also necessary on occasion to describe the precise topology of the ventricular mass and to specify the relationships of the ventricles themselves.

TYPES OF ATRIOVENTRICULAR CONNECTION

As already described, the term *atrioventricular connections* accounts for the patterns of the junctions of the myocardium of both atria with the ventricular myocardium around the entirety of the atrioventricular valvar orifices, the atrial and ventricular muscle masses being separated electrically by the fibrous rings other than at the site of the atrioventricular bundle. In every heart, because there are two atrial chambers, there is the possibility for two atrioventricular connections, which will be right-sided and left-sided (Fig. 19–9, *top left*). This is irrespective of whether the connections are guarded by two valves (Fig. 19–9, *top right*) or a common valve (Fig. 19–9, *bottom left*). One of the connections as thus defined may be blocked by an imperforate valvar membrane, but this does not alter the fact that in such a setting, there are still two atrioventricular connections present (Fig. 19–9, *center left*). In some hearts, in contrast, this possibility is not fulfilled because one of the connections is completely absent. Then, the atrial myocardium on that side has no connection with the underlying ventricular myocardium, being separated from the ventricular mass by the fibrofatty tissues of the atrioventricular groove. This arrangement is the most common pattern producing atrioventricular valvar atresia (Fig. 19–9, *bottom right*).

When atrioventricular connections are defined in this way, all hearts fit into one of three groups.[9] In the first group, by far the most common, each atrial chamber is connected actually or potentially, but separately, to an underlying ventricle (Figs. 19–10 and 19–11). The feature of the second group[24] is that only one of the ventricles (if indeed two are present) is connected to the atria (Fig.

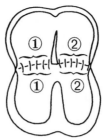
**Two AV Connections
- Valves not shown**

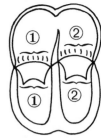
**Two AV Connections
- Two AV Valves**

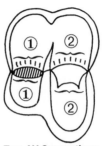
**Two AV Connections
- Imperforate Right-sided
AV Valve**

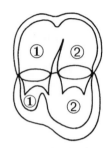
**Two AV Connections
- One Overriding and
Straddling Valve**

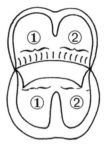
**Two AV Connections
- Common AV Valve**

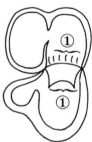
**One AV Connection
- Absent Right-sided
AV Connection**

FIGURE 19–9

The existence of two atrioventricular (AV) connections (*top left*, {1,1}, {2,2}) is not affected by the presence of either two valves (*top right*), one of which may be imperforate (*center left*) or straddling and overriding (*center right*), or a common (*bottom left*) atrioventricular valve. "Absent connection," however, means what it says (*bottom right*), namely, that only one atrium is connected to the ventricular mass. Although only an imperforate right-sided valve, a straddling and overriding right-sided valve, or an absent right-sided connection is illustrated, the same morphology can be found on the left side of the heart.

19–12). There is then an even rarer third group, which is seen when one atrioventricular connection is absent and the solitary atrioventricular junction is connected to two ventricles by a straddling valve. This arrangement is uniatrial but biventricular.[25]

There are three possible arrangements in hearts with each of the atria connected to its own ventricle, that is, three types of biventricular atrioventricular connections. These depend on the morphology of the chambers connected. The first pattern is seen when the atria are connected to morphologically appropriate ventricles, irrespective of the topology or relationship of the ventricles or of

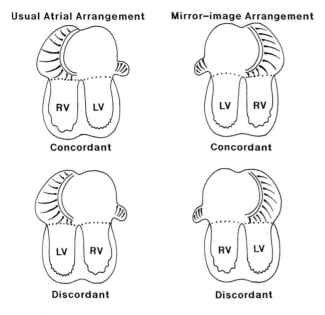

FIGURE 19–10

The concordant and discordant patterns of biventricular atrioventricular connections. RV = right ventricle; LV = left ventricle.

the morphology of the valves guarding the junctions. This arrangement is described as producing concordant atrioventricular connections. The second arrangement is the reverse of the first and is again independent of relationships or valvar morphology. It produces discordant atrioventricular connections. These first two arrangements (see Fig. 19–10) are found when the atrial appendages are lateralized. The other biventricular atrioventricular arrangement, in which each atrium is connected to a separate ventricle, is found in hearts with isomeric appendages,

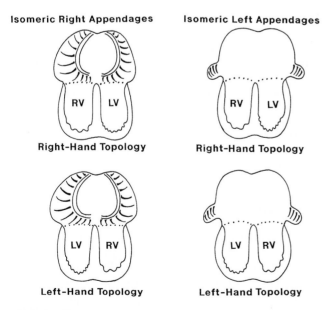

FIGURE 19–11

The atrioventricular connections are biventricular but ambiguous when hearts with isomeric appendages have each atrium connected to its own ventricle. The ventricular mass can show right-hand or left-hand topology. RV = right ventricle; LV = left ventricle.

whether they are of right or left morphology. Because of the isomeric nature of the appendages, this third arrangement cannot accurately be described in terms of concordant or discordant connections. It is a discrete biventricular pattern in its own right, which we consider to be ambiguous.[6, 7] It too is independent of ventricular relationships and atrioventricular valvar morphologies but in this instance requires specification of ventricular topology to make the description complete (see Fig. 19–11).

There are also three possible junctional arrangements that produce univentricular atrioventricular connections (see Fig. 19–12). The first is when the cavities of right-sided and left-sided atrial chambers are connected directly to the same ventricle. This is called double-inlet atrioventricular connection, irrespective of whether the right-sided and left-sided atrioventricular junctions are guarded by two atrioventricular valves or a common valve. The other two arrangements exist when one atrioventricular connection is absent, giving absent right-sided or absent left-sided atrioventricular connection. The group of univentricular atrioventricular connections is different from the group of biventricular connections in that it is not only independent of ventricular relationships and valvar morphology, but it is also independent of atrial and ventricular morphologies. Hearts with concordant or discordant atrioventricular connections can exist only when usually arranged or mirror-image atrial chambers are each connected to separate ventricles. A heart with ambiguous connection can be found only when each of two atrial chambers having isomeric appendages is connected to a separate ventricle. In contrast, double-inlet, absent right-sided, or absent left-sided atrioventricular connection can be found with usually arranged, mirror-image, or isomeric atrial appendages. Each type of univentricular atrioventricular connection can also be found with the atria connected to a dominant right ventricle, a dominant left ventricle, or a morphologically indeterminate ventricle. Ventricular morphology must always, therefore, be described separately in this group of hearts with univentricular atrioventricular connections.[24]

Although, in these hearts, only one ventricle is connected to the atria, a second ventricle is present in most of them. This second ventricle, of necessity rudimentary and incomplete, is of complementary trabecular pattern to the dominant ventricle. Most frequently, the dominant ventricle is a left ventricle, and the rudimentary and incomplete ventricle possesses right ventricular apical trabeculations. More rarely, the dominant ventricle is morphologically right, with the rudimentary and incomplete ventricle being morphologically left. Even more rarely, hearts will be found with a solitary ventricular chamber of indeterminate morphology. In clinical practice, apparently solitary left or right ventricles may be encountered when the complementary incomplete ventricle is too small to be demonstrated.

MODES OF ATRIOVENTRICULAR CONNECTION

Description of the type of atrioventricular connection accounts only for the way in which the atrial musculature is joined to the ventricular mass. The morphology of the valves guarding the overall atrioventricular junctional area

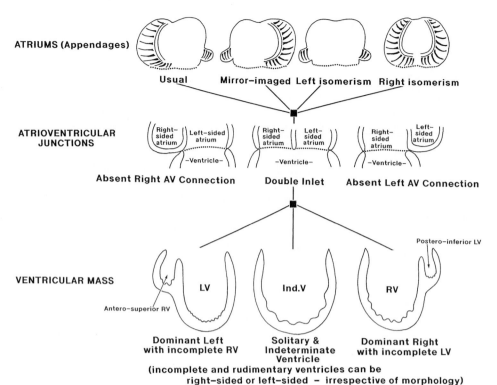

ATRIUMS (Appendages)

Usual   Mirror-imaged   Left isomerism   Right isomerism

ATRIOVENTRICULAR
JUNCTIONS

Right-sided atrium | Left-sided atrium
–Ventricle–

Right-sided atrium | Left-sided atrium
–Ventricle–

Right-sided atrium | Left-sided atrium
–Ventricle–

Absent Right AV Connection   **Double Inlet**   **Absent Left AV Connection**

Postero-inferior LV

VENTRICULAR MASS

LV   Ind.V   RV

Antero-superior RV

**Dominant Left
with incomplete RV**   **Solitary &
Indeterminate
Ventricle**   **Dominant Right
with incomplete LV**

**(incomplete and rudimentary ventricles can be
right-sided or left-sided – irrespective of morphology)**

FIGURE 19–12

The combinations of atrial arrangement and ventricular morphology that produce univentricular atrioventricular (AV) connections. LV = left ventricle; RV = right ventricle.

is independent of this feature, within the constraints imposed by the connection itself. Thus, when the cavities of both atria are connected directly to the ventricular mass, the right-sided and left-sided atrioventricular connections may be guarded by two patent valves, by one patent valve and one imperforate valve, by a common valve, or by straddling and overriding valves (see Fig. 19–9). These arrangements of the valves, therefore, can be found with the concordant, discordant, ambiguous, or double-inlet type of connection. Either the right-sided or left-sided valve may be imperforate, producing atresia, but in the setting of a potential as opposed to an absent atrioventricular connection. A common valve guards both right-sided and left-sided atrioventricular connections, irrespective of its morphology. A valve straddles when its tension apparatus is attached to both sides of a septum within the ventricular mass. It overrides when its annulus is connected to ventricles on both sides of a septal structure. A right-sided valve, a left-sided valve, or a common valve can straddle, can override, or can straddle and override. Rarely, both right-sided and left-sided valves may straddle or override in the same heart.

When one atrioventricular connection is absent, the possible modes of connection are greatly reduced. This is because there is, of necessity, a solitary right-sided or left-sided atrioventricular connection and, hence, a solitary atrioventricular valve. This single valve is usually committed in its entirety to one ventricle. More rarely, it may straddle, override, or straddle and override. These patterns produce the extremely rare group of uniatrial but biventricular connections.

A valve that overrides has an additional influence on description because the degree of commitment of the overriding atrioventricular junction to the ventricles on either side of the septum determines the precise nature of the atrioventricular connections. Hearts with two valves in which one valve is overriding are anatomically intermediate between those with, on the one hand, biventricular and, on the other hand, univentricular atrioventricular connections. There are two ways of describing such hearts. One is to consider the hearts as representing a special type of atrioventricular connection.[26] The alternative is to recognize the intermediate nature of such hearts in a series of anomalies and to split the series, depending on the precise connection of the overriding junction. For the purposes of categorization, only the two ends of the series are labeled, with hearts in the middle being assigned to one or the other endpoint. Our preference is for the second option.[7] When most of an overriding junction is connected to a ventricle that already receives the other atrioventricular connection, we designate the connection as being double inlet. If the overriding junction is connected mostly to a ventricle not itself connected to the other atrium, each atrium is categorized as though it is connected to its own ventricle (concordant, discordant, or ambiguous connection).

In describing atrioventricular valves, the adjectives mitral and tricuspid are strictly accurate only in hearts with biventricular atrioventricular connections having separate junctions, each guarded by its own valve. In this context, the tricuspid valve is always found in the morphologically right ventricle, the mitral valve in the morphologically left ventricle. In hearts with biventricular atrioventricular connections but with a common junction, in contrast, it is incorrect to consider the common valve as having mitral and tricuspid components, even when it is divided into right and left components. These right-sided and left-sided components, particularly on the left side, bear scant resemblance to the normal atrioventricular valves. In hearts with double inlet, the two valves are again better considered right-sided and left-sided valves rather than mitral or tricuspid. Similarly, when one connection is absent, although it is usually possible to deduce the presumed nature of the remaining solitary valve from concepts of morphogenesis, this is not always practical or helpful. The valve can always accurately be described as being right-sided or left-sided. Potentially contentious arguments are thus defused when the right-sided or left-sided valve straddles in the absence of the other atrioventricular connection (uniatrial but biventricular connections). The straddling valve seen in this setting may have features remarkably reminiscent of a common valve, but because it drains only one atrium, it is more accurately described as a left-sided or a right-sided valve.

VENTRICULAR TOPOLOGY AND RELATIONSHIPS

Even in the normal heart, the ventricular spatial relationships are complex. The inlet portions are more or less to the right and left, with the posterior part of the muscular ventricular septum lying in an approximately sagittal plane. The outlet portions are more or less anteroposteriorly related, with the septum between them in an approximately frontal plane. The trabecular portions extend between these two components, with the trabecular muscular septum spiraling between the inlet and outlet components. It is understandable that there is a desire to have a "shorthand" term to describe such complex spatial arrangements. We use the concept of ventricular topology for this purpose (see Fig. 19–5). In persons with usually arranged atria and discordant atrioventricular connections, for example, the left ventricular mass almost always shows left-hand topologic pattern, whereas right-hand ventricular topology is usually found with the combination of mirror-image atria and discordant atrioventricular connections. Although these combinations are almost always present, exceptions do occur.[27] In noting such unexpected ventricular relationships as a feature independent of the topology, it may be necessary to account for right-left, anterior-posterior, and superior-inferior coordinates. Should it be necessary, the position of the three ventricular components may be described separately and relative to each other.

Hearts with disharmonious combinations of atrial arrangement and ventricular topology produce one of the variants of so-called crisscross hearts. The crisscross pattern is usually a consequence of ventricular rotation in the setting of segmental harmony.[28] In such crisscross hearts with usual atrial arrangement and concordant atrioventricular connections, the ventricular rotation places the morphologically right ventricle in left-sided position. With extreme rotation, the inlet of the morphologically right ventricle may also be left-sided in association with concordant atrioventricular connections, but the rotation does not disguise the fact that there is still right-hand topology. Provided that relationships are described accurately, and separately, from both the connections and the ventricular topology, none of these unusual hearts will be difficult either to diagnose or to categorize.

In addition to these problematic crisscross hearts, it has already been discussed how analysis of ventricular topology is essential in accounting for the combination of isomeric appendages with ambiguous and biventricular atrioventricular connections. This is because, in this situation, the same terms would appropriately be used to describe the heart in which the left-sided atrium is connected to a morphologically right ventricle as well as the heart in which the left-sided atrium is connected to a morphologically left ventricle. The arrangements are differentiated simply by also describing the ventricular topology (see Fig. 19–11).

It is equally important to describe both the position and relationships of incomplete ventricles in hearts with univentricular atrioventricular connections. Here, the relationships are independent of both the connections and the ventricular morphology. Thus, whereas the rudimentary right ventricle is usually anterior and right-sided in classical tricuspid atresia, it can be anterior and left-sided without in any way altering the clinical presentation and hemodynamic findings. Similarly, in hearts with double-inlet ventricle, the position of the incomplete ventricle plays only a minor role in determining the clinical presentation. Although an argument can be made for interpreting such hearts with univentricular atrioventricular connections on the basis of presumed morphogenesis in the settings of right-hand or left-hand topologies, there are sufficient exceptions to make this approach unsuitable in the clinical setting. In accounting for the position of incomplete ventricles, therefore, it is best to account for their location relative to the dominant ventricle, taking note, when necessary, of right-left, anterior-posterior, and superior-inferior coordinates.

THE VENTRICULOARTERIAL JUNCTIONS

As with problems with other aspects of terminology, most previous polemics concerning the ventriculoarterial junctions devolved on the failure to distinguish between connections, relations, and infundibular morphology.[29,30] In this context, it is the prerogative of those who choose to define transposition in terms of an anterior aorta to speak rightly of "double outlet with transposition." For those choosing this approach, "posterior transposition" would be an impossibility.[29] This is not so when transposition is defined on the basis of ventriculoarterial connections. Such problems in the qualification of transposition are avoided when the term is not used as a descriptor for any single facet of the ventriculoarterial junctions, but instead connections, infundibular morphology, and relationships are described separately. Following a similar approach, it is possible also to defuse controversies concerning the role of the "bilateral conus" in the diagnosis of double-outlet right ventricle.

When connections, infundibular morphology, and arterial relationships are described independently, with mutually exclusive terms, there is no confusion. As with the atrioventricular junctions, it is necessary to account separately for the type and the mode of ventriculoarterial connections.

TYPES OF VENTRICULOARTERIAL CONNECTION

There are four types of connection. Concordant ventriculoarterial connections exist when the aorta arises from a morphologically left ventricle and the pulmonary trunk from a morphologically right ventricle, whether the ventricles are complete or incomplete. The arrangement whereby the aorta arises from a morphologically right ventricle or its rudiment, and the pulmonary trunk from a morphologically left ventricle or its rudiment, produces discordant ventriculoarterial connections. Double-outlet connection is found when both arteries are connected to the same ventricle, which may be of right ventricular, left ventricular, or indeterminate ventricular pattern. As with atrioventricular valves, overriding arterial valves (see later) are assigned to the ventricle supporting the greater parts of their circumference.

The fourth ventriculoarterial connection is single outlet from the heart. This may take one of four forms. A common trunk exists when both ventricles are connected by a common arterial valve to one trunk that gives rise directly to the coronary arteries, at least one pulmonary artery, and the majority of the systemic circulation. A solitary arterial trunk exists when it is not possible to identify any remnant of an atretic pulmonary trunk within the pericardial cavity. The other forms of single outlet are single pulmonary trunk with aortic atresia and single aortic trunk with pulmonary atresia. These two categories describe only those arrangements in which, by use of clinical techniques, it is not possible to establish the precise connection of the atretic arterial trunk to a ventricular cavity. If its connection can thus be established but is found to be imperforate, the appropriate connection is described, and the imperforate valve is then categorized as a mode of connection (see later). It is also necessary in hearts with single outlet to describe the ventricular connection of the arterial trunk. This may be exclusively from a right or a left ventricle, but more usually the trunk overrides the septum, being connected to both ventricles.

MODES OF VENTRICULOARTERIAL CONNECTION

There are fewer modes of connection at the ventriculoarterial than at the atrioventricular junctions. A common arterial valve is not considered a mode of connection because it can exist only with a specific type of single outlet, namely, a common arterial trunk. Straddling of an arterial valve is impossible because it has no tension apparatus. Thus, the possible modes of connection are two perforate valves (one or both of which may override) and one perforate and one imperforate valve. As with overriding atrioventricular valves, the degree of override of an arterial valve determines the ventriculoarterial connections present, the overriding valve (or valves) being assigned to the ventricle supporting the greater part of its circumference. For example, if more than half of an overriding pulmonary valve is connected to a right ventricle, the aorta being connected to a left ventricle, the ventriculoarterial connections are appropriately described as concordant. If more than half the overriding aortic valve is connected to the right ventricle in this situation, there are double-outlet ventriculoarterial connections. This approach again avoids the need for intermediate categories.

INFUNDIBULAR MORPHOLOGY

The infundibular regions are no more and no less than the outlet components of the ventricular mass. When recognized in this fashion, and their morphology described as

such, they, too, provide no problems in recognition and description. The morphology of the ventricular outlet portions is variable for any heart. Potentially, each ventricle can possess a complete muscular funnel as its outlet portion, and then each arterial valve can be said to have a complete infundibulum.

Considered as a whole, the outlet portions of the ventricular mass in the setting of bilateral infundibula have three discrete parts. Two of the parts form the anterior and posterior halves of the funnels of muscle supporting the arterial valves. The anterior parietal part is the free anterior ventricular wall. The posterior part is the inner heart curvature, a structure that separates the leaflets of the arterial from those of the atrioventricular valves; this component is the ventriculoinfundibular fold. The third part is the muscular septum that separates the two subarterial outlets, the outlet (or infundibular) septum. The dimensions of the outlet septum are independent of the remainder of the infundibular musculature. Indeed, it is possible, albeit rarely, for both arterial valves to be separated from both atrioventricular valves by the ventriculoinfundibular fold but for the arterial valves to be in fibrous continuity with one another because of the absence of the outlet septum. In most hearts, however, some part of the infundibular musculature is effaced so that fibrous continuity occurs between the leaflets of one of the arterial valves and the atrioventricular valves. Most frequently, it is the morphologically left ventricular part of the ventriculoinfundibular fold that is attenuated, so there is fibrous continuity between the leaflets of the mitral valve and the arterial valve supported by the left ventricle.

Whether the arterial valve is aortic or pulmonary depends on the ventriculoarterial connections present. In the usual arrangement, the morphologically right ventricular part of the ventriculoinfundibular fold persists so that there is tricuspid-arterial valvar discontinuity. Thus, depending on the integrity of the outlet septum, usually there is a completely muscular outflow tract, or infundibulum, in the morphologically right ventricle. When both arterial trunks are connected to the morphologically right ventricle, most frequently the ventriculoinfundibular fold persists in its entirety, and there is bilateral atrioventricular-arterial valvar discontinuity.

Many hearts in which both arterial valves are connected unequivocally to the right ventricle have atrioventricular-arterial valvar continuity. How is the ventriculoarterial connection of such hearts to be described if not as double-outlet right ventricle? This is another example of the controversy generated when one feature of cardiac morphology is determined from a second, unrelated, feature. The findings reinforce the need to follow the morphologic method. Returning to the basics of outlet morphology, when both outlet portions are connected to the morphologically left ventricle, the tendency is for there to be continuity between both arterial valves and both atrioventricular valves. Even then, the ventriculoinfundibular fold can persist in part or in its whole. It is the state of the ventriculoinfundibular fold, therefore, that determines the infundibular morphology. Ignoring the rare situation of complete absence of the outlet septum, and considering morphology from the standpoint of the arterial valves, there are then four possible arrangements. First, there may be a complete subpulmonary infundibulum with aortic-atrioventricular valvar continuity. Second, there may be a complete subaortic infundibulum with pulmonary-atrioventricular valvar continuity. Third, there may be bilateral infundibula without any arterial-atrioventricular valvar continuity. Fourth, there may be bilaterally deficient infundibula with bilateral arterial-atrioventricular continuity. In themselves, these terms are nonspecific. For specificity, it is necessary to know which arterial valve is connected to which ventricle. This emphasizes the fact that infundibular morphology is independent of the ventriculoarterial connections.

ARTERIAL RELATIONSHIPS

The final feature of the ventriculoarterial junctions requiring description is the relationships of the great arteries and their valves. Relationships are usually determined at the level of the arterial valves, and many systems for nomenclature have been constructed on this basis. Initially, the position of the arterial valves was held to reflect ventricular topology (the "loop rule").[1,2] In reality, arterial valvar position is a poor guide to ventricular topology.[31] Furthermore, describing arterial valvar position in terms of leftness and rightness takes no cognizance of anteroposterior relationships, a surprising omission because an anterior position of the aorta was, for many years, the cornerstone for definitions of transposition.[29] It is best, therefore, to describe arterial valvar relationships in terms of both right-left and anterior-posterior coordinates. Such description can be accomplished with as great a degree of precision as is required. A good system is the one that describes aortic position in degrees of the arc of a circle constructed around the pulmonary valve.[15] It is simpler to describe aortic valvar position relative to the pulmonary trunk in terms of eight positions of a compass, using the simple terms left, right, anterior, posterior, and side-by-side in their various combinations as the adjectives. As long as it is remembered that these terms describe only arterial valvar relations and convey no information about either connections or morphology, there can be no fear of producing confusion.

The positions of the arterial trunks are also important. In this respect, the pulmonary trunk spirals around the aorta as it ascends, or else the two trunks ascend in parallel fashion. It is rarely necessary to describe these relationships. Spiraling trunks are usually associated with concordant ventriculoarterial connections, parallel trunks with discordant or double-outlet connections, but again, there is no predictive value in these relationships. In almost all hearts, the aortic arch crosses superiorly to the bifurcation of the pulmonary arteries. The side of the aortic arch is determined by whether it passes to the right or left of the trachea. The position of the descending aorta is defined relative to the vertebral column.

ASSOCIATED MALFORMATIONS

Most patients seen with congenital heart disease have normal intersegmental connections together with normal morphology and relations. In such a setting, the associated malformation will be the major anomaly. The body of this book is concerned with describing the specific morphologic and clinical features of these anomalies. Consideration must also be given, nonetheless, to the position (within the chest) of the heart itself and of the cardiac apex (or, for that matter, identification of a heart positioned outside the thoracic cavity—ectopia cordis). An abnormal position of the heart within the chest is best considered as an associated malformation, and the cardiac malposition should not be promoted as a prime diagnosis. This is not to decry the importance of cardiac malposition (if only to interpret an electrocardiogram), but knowing that the heart is malpositioned gives no information concerning its internal architecture. Full sequential segmental analysis is needed to determine this analysis, not the other way around.

There are three basic positions for the heart: mostly in the left hemithorax, mostly in the right hemithorax, and centrally positioned in the mediastinum. There are also three basic positions for the cardiac apex: pointing to the left, to the right, or to the middle. Apical direction is independent of cardiac position. Both of these are independent of the arrangement of the atrial appendages and of the thoracic and abdominal organs. As with other aspects, if all the features are described separately, there can be no confusion.

ACKNOWLEDGMENTS

This chapter is abridged from the corresponding section on terminology that will appear in the second edition of *Paediatric Cardiology*, edited by R.H. Anderson, E.J. Baker, F.J. Macartney, M.L. Rigby, E.A. Shinebourne, and M. Tynan. This book is to be published by Churchill Livingstone, and I am indebted to them for permitting me to reuse the material. I am also indebted to Dr. Siew Yen Ho, who prepared most of the illustrative material. The work is supported by ongoing grants from the British Heart Foundation together with the Joseph Levy Foundation.

REFERENCES

1. Van Praagh R, Ongley PA, Swan HJC: Anatomic types of single or common ventricle in man: Morphologic and geometric aspects of sixty necropsied cases. Am J Cardiol 13:367, 1964.
2. Van Praagh R, Van Praagh S, Vlad P, Keith JD: Anatomic types of congenital dextrocardia. Diagnostic and embryologic implications. Am J Cardiol 13:510, 1964.
3. de la Cruz MV, Nadal-Ginard B: Rules for the diagnosis of visceral situs, truncoconal morphologies and ventricular inversions. Am Heart J 84:19, 1972.
4. Van Praagh R: The segmental approach to diagnosis in congenital heart disease. Birth Defects 8:4, 1972.
5. de la Cruz MV, Berrazueta JR, Arteaga M, et al: Rules for diagnosis of arterioventricular discordances and spatial identification of ventricles. Br Heart J 38:341, 1976.
6. Shinebourne EA, Macartney FJ, Anderson RH: Sequential chamber localization: The logical approach to diagnosis in congenital heart disease. Br Heart J 38:327, 1976.
7. Tynan M, Becker AE, Macartney FJ, et al: Nomenclature and classification of congenital heart disease. Br Heart J 41:544, 1979.
8. Anderson RH, Becker AE, Freedom RM, et al: Sequential segmental analysis of congenital heart disease. Pediatr Cardiol 5:281, 1984.
9. Anderson RH, Ho SY: Sequential segmental analysis—description and categorization for the millenium. Cardiol Young 7:98, 1997.

10. Van Praagh R: Tetralogy of Fallot {S,D,I}: A recently discovered malformation and its surgical management. Ann Thorac Surg 60:1163, 1995.

11. Anderson RH: How should we optimally describe complex congenitally malformed hearts? Ann Thorac Surg 62:710, 1996.

12. Van Praagh R, David I, Wright GB, Van Praagh S: Large RV plus small LV is not single LV. Circulation 61:1057, 1980.

13. Lev M: Pathologic diagnosis of positional variations in cardiac chambers in congenital heart disease. Lab Invest 3:71, 1954.

14. Uemura H, Ho SY, Devine WA, et al: Atrial appendages and venoatrial connections in hearts with patients with visceral heterotaxy. Ann Thorac Surg 60:561, 1995.

15. Bargeron LM Jr: Angiography relevant to complicating features. *In* Becker AE, Losekoot TG, Marcelletti C, Anderson RH (eds): Paediatric Cardiology, Vol 3. Edinburgh, Churchill Livingstone, 1981, pp 33–47.

16. Van Praagh R, Van Praagh S: Atrial isomerism in the heterotaxy syndromes with asplenia, or polysplenia, or normally formed spleen: An erroneous concept. Am J Cardiol 66:1504, 1990.

17. Van Praagh R, Wise JR Jr, Dahl BA, Van Praagh S: Single left ventricle with infundibular outlet chamber and tricuspid valve opening only into outlet chamber in 44-year-old man with thoracoabdominal ectopia cordis without diaphragmatic or pericardial defect: Importance of myocardial morphologic method of chamber identification in congenital heart disease. *In* Van Praagh R, Takao A (eds): Etiology and Morphogenesis of Congenital Heart Disease. Mount Kisco, New York, Futura Publishing, 1980, p 410.

18. Caruso G, Becker AE: How to determine atrial situs? Considerations initiated by 3 cases of absent spleen with a discordant anatomy between bronchi and atria. Br Heart J 41:559, 1979.

19. Partridge JB, Scott O, Deverall PB, Macartney FJ: Visualization and measurement of the main bronchi by tomography as an objective indicator of thoracic situs in congenital heart disease. Circulation 51:188, 1975.

20. Deanfield J, Leanage R, Stroobant J, et al: Use of high kilovoltage filtered beam radiographs for detection of bronchial situs in infants and young children. Br Heart J 44:577, 1980.

21. Huhta IC, Smallhorn JF, Macartney FJ: Two dimensional echocardiographic diagnosis of situs. Br Heart J 48:97, 1982.

22. Anderson C, Devine WA, Anderson RH, et al: Abnormalities of the spleen in relation to congenital malformations of the heart: A survey of necropsy findings in children. Br Heart J 63:122, 1990.

23. Uemura H, Ho SY, Devine WA, Anderson RH: Analysis of visceral heterotaxy according to splenic status, appendage morphology, or both. Am J Cardiol 76:846, 1995.

24. Anderson RH, Becker AE, Tynan M, et al: The univentricular atrioventricular connection: Getting to the root of a thorny problem. Am J Cardiol 54:822, 1984.

25. Anderson RH, Rigby ML: Editorial note. The morphologic heterogeneity of "tricuspid atresia." Int J Cardiol 16:67, 1987.

26. Liberthson RR, Paul MH, Muster AJ, et al: Straddling and displaced atrioventricular orifices and valves with primitive ventricles. Circulation 43:213, 1971.

27. Anderson RH, Smith A, Wilkinson JL: Disharmony between atrioventricular connections and segmental combinations; unusual variants of "crisscross" hearts. J Am Coll Cardiol 10:1274, 1987.

28. Anderson RH: Criss-cross hearts revisited. Pediatr Cardiol 3:305, 1982.

29. Van Mierop LHS: Transposition of the great arteries. Clarification or further confusion? (Editorial) Am J Cardiol 28:735, 1971.

30. Van Praagh R: Transposition of the great arteries. II. Transposition clarified. Am J Cardiol 28:739, 1971.

31. Carr I, Tynan MJ, Aberdeen E, et al: Predictive accuracy of the loop rule in 109 children with classical complete transposition of the great arteries (Abstract). Circulation 38:V-1, 1968.

CHAPTER 20

NOMENCLATURE AND CLASSIFICATION: MORPHOLOGIC AND SEGMENTAL APPROACH TO DIAGNOSIS

RICHARD VAN PRAAGH

MORPHOLOGIC ANATOMY

The myocardial morphologic method of diagnosing and designating cardiac chambers was introduced by Lev in 1954.[1] This method, fundamental to diagnosis, terminology, and classification, may be stated as follows.[1–3]

Cardiac chambers are identified and named in terms of their gross myocardial morphologic characteristics, not in terms of relative position (such as right-sided or left-sided), nor in terms of hemodynamics (such as venous or arterial), nor in terms of the valve or vessel of entry or exit, because all of these considerations are variables in congenital heart disease.

The diagnostic problem posed by congenital heart disease is that the morphologically or anatomically right atrium, left atrium, right ventricle, and left ventricle can—from the positional standpoint—be "anywhere."

For brevity, the morphologic anatomic features of the cardiac chambers are presented graphically: the morphologically right atrium (Fig. 20–1A, B),[4] the morphologically left atrium (Fig. 20–1C, D),[4] the morphologically right ventricle (Fig. 20–2A, B),[4] and the morphologically left ventricle (Fig. 20–2C, D).[4]

SEGMENTAL ANATOMY

The cardiac segments[5,6] are the anatomic and developmental "building blocks" of which all hearts, normal and abnormal, are made. The three main cardiac segments are (1) the atria, (2) the ventricles, and (3) the great arteries. The two connecting cardiac segments are (1) the atrioventricular canal or junction and (2) the infundibulum or conus arteriosus.

MAIN CARDIAC SEGMENTS

The Atria

There are two main types of visceroatrial situs (*situs* meaning the pattern of anatomic organization) (Fig. 20–3)[5,6]:

1. *situs solitus*, the usual and hence normal pattern of anatomic organization in which the right atrium is right-sided and the left atrium is left-sided; and
2. *situs inversus*, the inverted or mirror-image pattern in which the right atrium is left-sided and the left atrium is right-sided. In anatomy, *inversion* is defined as mirror imagery: right-left reversal, without anteroposterior or superoinferior change.

Situs "ambiguus" (Fig. 20–3)[5,6] indicates that the type of visceroatrial situs is anatomically uncertain or indeterminate, as can occur in the heterotaxy syndromes with asplenia or polysplenia and occasionally with a normally formed spleen. Situs ambiguus is not a third type of visceroatrial situs; instead, it merely indicates that the type of visceroatrial situs is undiagnosed. [Note that *ambiguus* is correct Latin spelling, appropriate with *situs,* which is also Latin. *Ambiguous* is correct English spelling.]

The type of visceral situs and the type of atrial situs are almost always the same (Fig. 20–3): both solitus, both inversus, or both ambiguous. The visceroatrial concordances can be helpful diagnostically in atrial localization.

Atrial-level isomerism or mirror imagery is an erroneous concept.[7–11] Neither bilateral right atria nor bilateral left atria have been documented. Bilateral right atrial appendages and bilateral left atrial appendages are also erroneous concepts.[7,9,11] Just as each human being has only one left ventricle and one right ventricle, so too each human being has only one right atrium and one left atrium and only one right atrial appendage and one left atrial appendage.

The realization that the old concept of atrial-level isomerism is erroneous facilitates the diagnosis of the atrial situs in the heterotaxy syndromes. My colleagues and I are now able to diagnose the atrial situs in virtually all of our postmortem polysplenia syndromes and in most of our autopsied asplenia syndromes.[11]

To summarize, the atrial situs is either solitus, or inversus, or undiagnosed (Fig. 20–3).

The Ventricles

There are two types of ventricular situs (Fig. 20–4)[2–6]:

1. *D-loop ventricles,* that is, solitus or noninverted ventricles in which the right ventricle is typically right-sided relative to the left ventricle, and the right ventricle is right-handed (Fig. 20–5A)[12]; and
2. *L-loop ventricles,* that is, inverted or mirror-image ventricles in which the right ventricle is typically left-sided relative to the left ventricle, and the right ventricle is left-handed (Fig. 20–5B).[12]

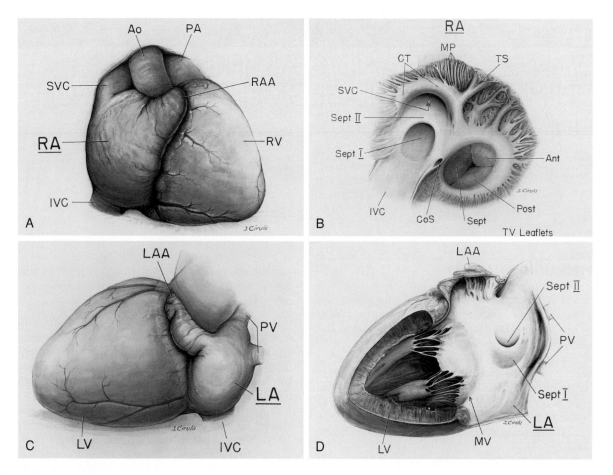

FIGURE 20–1

A, Exterior of morphologically right atrium (RA), which is broad and triangular. Ao = ascending aorta; IVC = inferior vena cava; PA = pulmonary artery; RAA = morphologically right atrial appendage; RV = morphologically right ventricle; SVC = superior vena cava. *B,* Interior of right atrium. Ant = anterior leaflet of the tricuspid valve (TV); CoS = ostium of coronary sinus; CT = crista terminalis (terminal crest); MP = musculi pectinati (pectinate muscles); Sept = septal leaflet of TV; Sept I = septum primum (the flap valve of the foramen ovale); Sept II = superior limbic band of septum secundum; TS = tinea sagittalis. *C,* Exterior of morphologically left atrium (LA), which has a long thin appendage. LAA = left atrial appendage; LV = morphologically left ventricle; PV = pulmonary veins. *D,* Interior of left atrium. MV = mitral valve. (*A–D* reprinted with the permission of Simon & Schuster from HEART DISEASE IN INFANCY AND CHILDHOOD 3/e by John D. Keith, Richard D. Rowe, Peter Vlad. Copyright © 1978 Macmillan Publishing Company.)

The Great Arteries

The great arteries may be either normally related or abnormally related.

There are two anatomic types of normally related great arteries (Fig. 20–6)[2–6]:

1. *solitus normally related,* the usual normal; and
2. *inverted normally related,* the inverted or mirror-image normal.

There are three anatomic types of abnormally related great arteries (Fig. 20–6)[2–6]:

1. *D-transposition or D-malposition of the great arteries,* in which the transposed or malposed aortic valve lies to the right (Latin *dextro* or D) relative to the transposed or malposed pulmonary valve;
2. *L-transposition or L-malposition of the great arteries,* in which the transposed or malposed aortic valve lies to the left (Latin *levo* or L) relative to the transposed or the malposed pulmonary valve; and
3. *A-transposition or A-malposition of the great arteries,* in which the transposed or malposed aortic valve lies

directly anterior (Latin *antero* or A) relative to the transposed or malposed pulmonary valve.

Transposition of the great arteries means[13, 14] that the great arteries are placed across the ventricular septum (Latin *trans,* across, and *ponere,* to place) and thus arise above the morphologically inappropriate ventricles (Fig. 20–7)[15]: aorta above the right ventricle, and pulmonary artery above the left ventricle.

Malposition of the great arteries[13, 14] is a broad, nonspecific term indicating that the great arteries are malposed but without specifying the anatomic type of ventriculoarterial malalignment that is present. There are four different anatomic types of malposition of the great arteries (Fig. 20–7):

1. *transposition of the great arteries,*[13, 14, 16] defined before;
2. *double-outlet right ventricle,*[17] in which both great arteries originate entirely or predominantly above the right ventricle;
3. *double-outlet left ventricle,*[18] in which both great arteries originate entirely or predominantly above the left ventricle; and

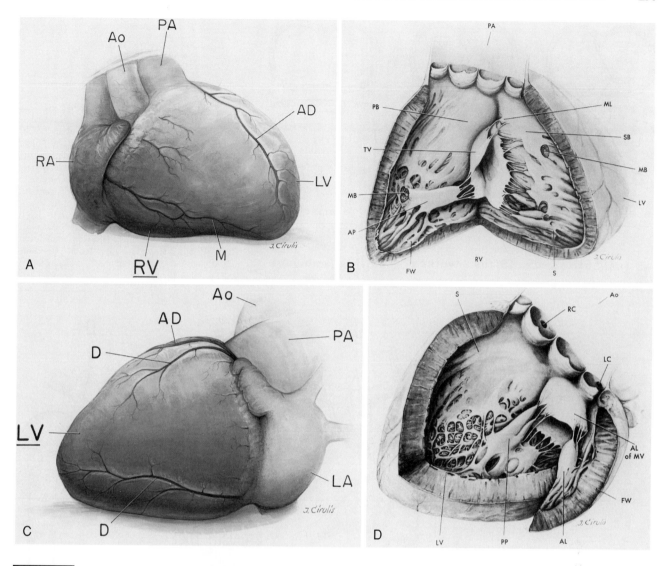

FIGURE 20–2

A, Exterior of right ventricle (RV). AD = anterior descending branch of left coronary artery; M = marginal branch of right coronary artery. *B*, Interior of right ventricle. AP = anterior papillary muscle; FW = free wall; MB = moderator band; ML = muscle of Lancisi or muscle of Luschka; PA = pulmonary artery; PB = parietal band; S = septum; SB = septal band. *C*, Exterior of left ventricle (LV). D = diagonal or obtuse marginal coronary artery. *D*, Interior of left ventricle. AL = anterolateral papillary muscle; AL of MV = anterior leaflet of mitral valve; LC = left coronary ostium; PP = posteromedial papillary muscle; RC = right coronary ostium. Other abbreviations as in Figure 20–1. (*A–D* reprinted with the permission of Simon & Schuster from HEART DISEASE IN INFANCY AND CHILDHOOD 3/e by John D. Keith, Richard D. Rowe, Peter Vlad. Copyright © 1978 Macmillan Publishing Company.)

4. *anatomically corrected malposition of the great arteries*,[19,20] in which the great arteries are malposed but arise nonetheless above the anatomically correct ventricles: aorta above the left ventricle, and pulmonary artery above the right ventricle.

CONNECTING CARDIAC SEGMENTS

The Atrioventricular Canal or Junction

The atrioventricular valves correspond to the ventricles of entry, not to the atria of exit. For example, if a patient has visceroatrial situs solitus and L-loop ventricles, as in classical physiologically corrected transposition (Fig. 20–7, *row 5, column 2*), the right-sided atrioventricular valve is a mitral valve—corresponding to the ventricle of entry (the right-sided left ventricle) and not corresponding to the atrium of exit (the right-sided right atrium). The left-sided atrioventricular valve is a tricuspid valve—corresponding to the ventricle of entry (the left-sided right ventricle) and not corresponding to the atrium of exit (the left-sided left atrium).

Thus, *the atrioventricular valves correspond to the type of ventricular loop that is present,* not to the type of atrial situs that coexists. This principle applies not only to *single-inlet each ventricle* (as earlier) but also to *double-inlet left ventricle and right ventricle.* For example, in double-inlet left ventricle with a ventricular D-loop, the right-sided atrioventricular valve is the tricuspid valve and the left-sided atrioventricular valve is the mitral valve. The tricuspid valve is "septophilic," often inserting into the ventricular septal remnant or into the infundibular outlet chamber. The mitral valve is "septophobic," seldom inserting into the ventricular septum or its remnant. The morphologic approach should be applied to the atrioventricular valves,

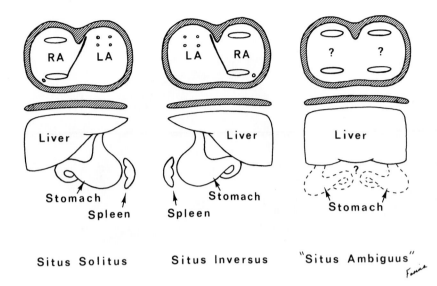

FIGURE 20–3

Types of visceroatrial situs: situs solitus (the usual and hence normal pattern of anatomic organization) and situs inversus (the mirror-image pattern). "Situs ambiguus" is the ambiguous pattern of anatomic organization in which the basic type of visceroatrial situs is undiagnosed (?), as can occur in the heterotaxy syndromes with asplenia or polysplenia and occasionally with a normally formed spleen. RA = right atrium; LA = left atrium. (From Van Praagh R, Weinberg PM, Matsuoka R, Van Praagh S: Malpositions of the heart. *In* Adams FH, Emmanouilides GC [eds]: Moss' Heart Disease in Infants, Children and Adolescents, 3rd ed. Baltimore, Williams & Wilkins, 1983, pp 422–458.)

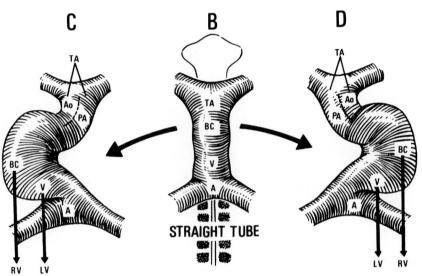

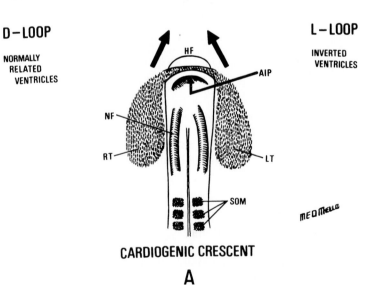

FIGURE 20–4

The two types of ventricular situs: ventricular D-loop with solitus or noninverted ventricles and ventricular L-loop with inverted or mirror-image ventricles. *A*, Cardiogenic crescent, ventral view. AIP = anterior intestinal portal; HF = head fold; LT = left side of the cardiogenic crescent of precardiac mesoderm; NF = neural fold; RT = right side of cardiogenic crescent; SOM = somites. *B*, Straight heart tube (preloop phase). A = atrium; BC = bulbus cordis; TA = truncus arteriosus; V = ventricle. *C*, D-Loop formation, in which the BC (future RV) lies to the right of the V (future LV). *D*, L-loop formation, in which the BC (future RV) lies to the left of the V (future LV). Ao = ascending aorta; PA = pulmonary artery; LV = left ventricle; RV = right ventricle. (*A–D* from Van Praagh R, Weinberg PM, Matsuoka R, Van Praagh S: Malpositions of the heart. *In* Adams FH, Emmanouilides GC [eds]: Moss' Heart Disease in Infants, Children and Adolescents, 3rd ed. Baltimore, Williams & Wilkins, 1983, pp 422–458.)

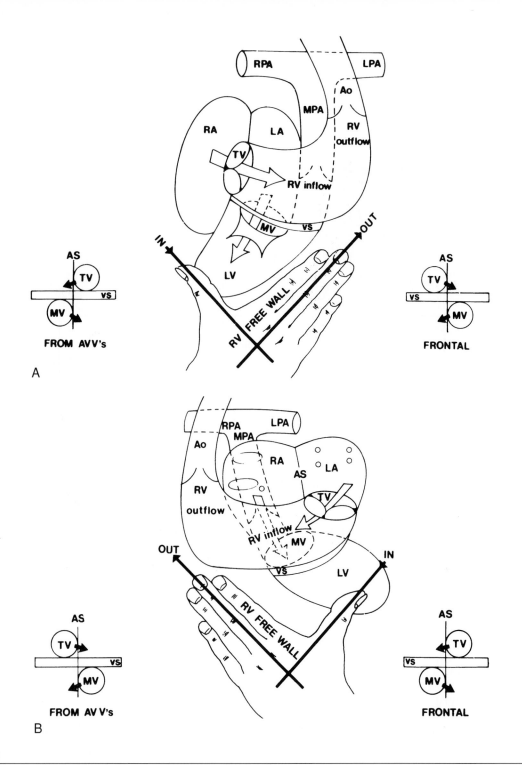

FIGURE 20–5

A, The right-handed right ventricle of D-loop ventricles. The thumb of one's right hand passes (literally or figuratively) through the tricuspid valve (TV). The fingers of the right hand are placed (literally or figuratively) in the RV outflow tract (RV outflow). The palm of only the right hand faces the RV septal surface. The dorsum of only the right hand faces the RV free wall. Hence, the D-loop RV may be described as right-handed. Note also that the atrioventricular (AV) alignments are concordant: RA to RV, and LA to LV. In this example of physiologically uncorrected transposition of the great arteries {S,D,L} with superoinferior ventricles and crisscross AV relations, the RV is both right-sided and left-sided, and so too is the LV. Thus, the conventional definition of ventricular noninversion/inversion in terms of the presence or absence of right/left reversal does not apply. However, the RV is right-handed, indicating that D-loop or solitus ventricles are present. Note that the atrial septum (AS) is approximately vertical, and the ventricular septum (VS) is approximately horizontal. As viewed from the front (FRONTAL), the TV is superior to and to the right of the MV. The right-sided location of the TV also indicates that D-loop ventricles are present. The posterior view from the atrioventricular valves (FROM AVV's) is the surgeon's view. *Arrows* indicate the crisscross directions of the AV inflow tracts. LPA = left pulmonary artery; MPA = main pulmonary artery; RPA = right pulmonary artery. *B*, The left-handed right ventricle of L-loop ventricles. The thumb of one's left hand goes through the TV. The fingers of the left hand pass out the RV outflow tract. The palm of only the left hand faces the RV septal surface. The dorsum of only the left hand faces the RV free wall. Hence, the L-loop RV may be described as left-handed. Note also that the AV alignments are discordant: RA to LV, and LA to RV. In this example of congenitally physiologically corrected transposition of the great arteries {S,L,D} with superoinferior ventricles and crisscross AV relations, the RV is both left-sided and right-sided, and the LV is both right-sided and left-sided. Hence, the conventional definition of ventricular noninversion/inversion does not apply. However, the RV is left-handed, indicating that L-loop or inverted ventricles are present. Note the left-sided location of the TV relative to the MV, also indicating L-loop ventricles. *Arrows* indicate the crisscross directions of the AV inflow tracts. Other abbreviations as in Figure 20–1. (*A, B* from Van Praagh R, David I, Gordon D, et al: Ventricular diagnosis and designation. *In* Godman M [ed]: Paediatric Cardiology. Edinburgh, Churchill Livingstone, 1981, pp 153–168.)

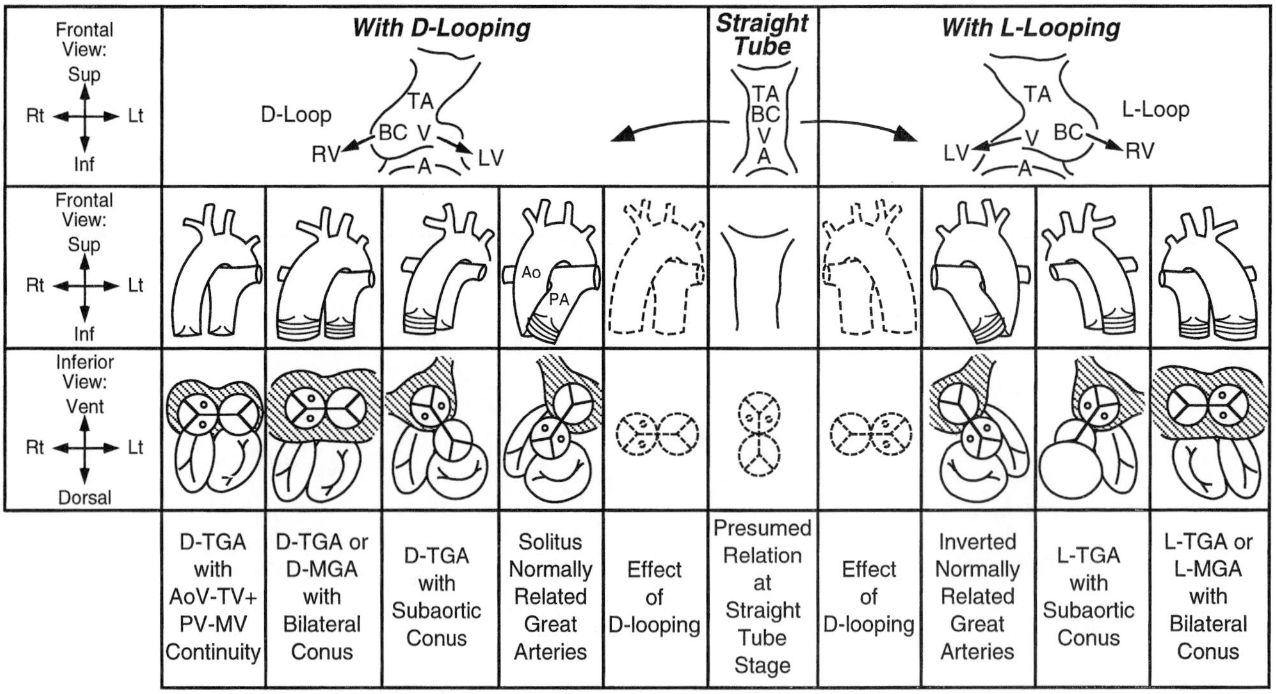

Frontal View: Sup Rt ← → Lt Inf	With D-Looping D-Loop	Straight Tube	With L-Looping L-Loop
Frontal View: Sup Rt ← → Lt Inf			
Inferior View: Vent Rt ← → Lt Dorsal			
	D-TGA with AoV-TV+ PV-MV Continuity	D-TGA or D-MGA with Bilateral Conus	D-TGA with Subaortic Conus	Solitus Normally Related Great Arteries	Effect of D-looping	Presumed Relation at Straight Tube Stage	Effect of D-looping	Inverted Normally Related Great Arteries	L-TGA with Subaortic Conus	L-TGA or L-MGA with Bilateral Conus

FIGURE 20–6

Variations in infundibular and great arterial anatomy with D-loop and L-loop ventricles. Subsemilunar conal musculature is indicated by *cross-hatching*. The tricuspid valve (TV) has three leaflets; the mitral valve (MV) has two leaflets. The aortic valve (AoV) is indicated by coronary ostia; the pulmonary valve (PV) has no coronary ostia. *Broken lines* indicate aorta (Ao) and pulmonary artery (PA) and AoV and PV at an early stage before aortopulmonary septation, diagrammed as septated for clarity. Note that solitus normally related great arteries and inverted normally related great arteries both have a subpulmonary conus and aortic-mitral fibrous continuity. D-Transposition of the great arteries (D-TGA) and L-transposition of the great arteries (L-TGA) both typically have a subaortic conus and pulmonary-mitral fibrous continuity. A bilateral conus beneath both the aortic valve (AoV) and the pulmonary valve (PV), preventing semilunar valve–AV valve fibrous continuity, occurs both with D-loop ventricles and D-TGA or D-malposition of the great arteries (D-MGA) (such as with double-outlet right ventricle) and with L-loop ventricles and L-TGA or L-malposition of the great arteries (L-MGA) (such as with double-outlet right ventricle, left-sided). Rarely, a bilaterally deficient conus can occur in D-TGA, resulting in aortic valve–tricuspid valve (AoV-TV) and pulmonary valve–mitral valve (PV-MV) fibrous continuity. The effect of D-loop formation is to carry the future aortic valve to the right of the future pulmonary valve *(shown in broken lines)*. The effect of L-loop formation is to carry the future aortic valve to the left of the future pulmonary valve *(broken lines)*. Many more conotruncal variations exist than are shown in this diagram. Inf = inferior; Sup = superior. A = atrium; BC = bulbus cordis; TA = truncus arteriosus; V = ventricle. (From Van Praagh R, Weinberg PM, Matsuoka R, Van Praagh S: Malpositions of the heart. *In* Adams FH, Emmanouilides GC [eds]: Moss' Heart Disease in Infants, Children and Adolescents, 3rd ed. Baltimore, Williams & Wilkins, 1983, pp 422–458.)

just as to the atria and the ventricles. "Right" atrioventricular valve and "left" atrioventricular valve are morphologically meaningless designations. The diagnostic questions are: Which is the right-sided atrioventricular valve? Is it the tricuspid valve or the mitral valve? Similarly, which is the left-sided atrioventricular valve (tricuspid valve or mitral valve)?

The Infundibulum or Conus Arteriosus

There are four anatomic types of conus (see Fig. 20–6)[2–6, 21–23]:

1. *subpulmonary,* with normally related great arteries (solitus and inversus) and with nearly normally related great arteries, such as tetralogy of Fallot;

2. *subaortic,* as with typical transposition of the great arteries (D- and L-);

3. *bilateral,* that is, subaortic and subpulmonary, as with double-outlet right ventricle; and

4. *absent or deficient,* as with double-outlet left ventricle.

The anatomic type of conus largely determines the presence or absence of *semilunar-atrioventricular fibrous continuity* (see Fig. 20–6)[21–23]:

1. A subpulmonary conus prevents pulmonary-atrioventricular fibrous continuity but permits aortic-atrioventricular fibrous continuity.

2. A subaortic conus prevents aortic-atrioventricular fibrous continuity but permits pulmonary-atrioventricular fibrous continuity.

3. A bilateral (subaortic and subpulmonary) conus typically prevents semilunar-atrioventricular valve fibrous continuity.

4. Absence or marked deficiency of the subsemilunar part of the conus typically permits aortic and pulmonary to atrioventricular valve fibrous continuity.

SEGMENTAL SETS OR COMBINATIONS

One of the charms (or frustrations) of congenital heart disease is that virtually any combination of atria, ventricles, and great arteries that one can imagine occurs. A simplified schema is shown in Figure 20–7.[15]

The columns are organized in terms of atrioventricular concordance or discordance. Columns 1 and 2 show atrioventricular concordance and discordance, respectively, in visceroatrial situs solitus. Columns 3 and 4 show atrioventricular concordance and discordance, respectively, in visceroatrial situs inversus.

For ease of expression, the main cardiac segments may be expressed as the members of a set: {atria, ventricles, great arteries}. Braces are mathematical symbols meaning "the set of." The members of the set are separated by commas, this being conventional set notation. Situs solitus of the viscera and atria may be symbolized as S, situs inversus as I. Situs ambiguus, A, is omitted for simplicity (see Fig. 20–7).

Hence, the segmental sets begin as {S,–,–} or as {I,–,–}, indicating visceroatrial situs solitus or situs inversus, respectively (see Fig. 20–7).

The type of ventricular loop is symbolized as D- or L-, for D-loop and L-loop, respectively (see Fig. 20–7): {–,D,–} and {–,L,–}.

Thus, {S,D,–} in column 1 (see Fig. 20–7) indicates a concordant (appropriate) atrioventricular alignment with right atrium opening into right ventricle and left atrium opening into left ventricle. However, {S,L,–} in column 2 (see Fig. 20–7) indicates a discordant (inappropriate) atrioventricular alignment with right atrium opening into left ventricle and left atrium opening into right ventricle.

Similarly, in visceroatrial situs inversus, {I,L,–} indicates a concordant atrioventricular alignment, and {I,D,–} denotes a discordant atrioventricular alignment (see Fig. 20–7).

Parenthetically, we prefer the concept of concordant or discordant atrioventricular alignments to that of concordant or discordant atrioventricular connections. Why? Because the atria and the ventricles do not connect muscle-to-muscle, except at the atrioventricular bundle of His, owing to the interposition of the fibrous atrioventricular junction. The functions of the atrioventricular junction include connecting, and separating, and electrically insulating the atrial and the ventricular segments from each other. If the atria and the ventricles do connect muscle-to-muscle, except at the His bundle, these abnormal atrioventricular connections may permit ventricular pre-excitation, resulting in the Wolff-Parkinson-White syndrome. Thus, the concept of atrioventricular *alignments* (not connections) is preferred.

The rows in Figure 20–7 are organized in terms of ventriculoarterial concordance and discordance. For ease of expression, solitus normally related great arteries are symbolized as S, as in {–,–,S}. Inverted normally related great arteries are symbolized as I, as in {–,–,I}. D-Transposition or D-malposition of the great arteries is symbolized as D, as in {–,–,D}. L-Transposition or L-malposition of the great arteries is symbolized as L, as in {–,–,L}. A-Transposition or A-malposition of the great arteries is symbolized as A, as in {–,–,A}, which was omitted from Figure 20–7 for simplicity.

We prefer the concept of ventriculoarterial alignments to that of ventriculoarterial connections because the ventricular sinuses and the great arteries do not connect tissue-to-tissue owing to the interposition of the conal connector. The concept of ventriculoarterial *alignments* is

anatomically accurate, whereas the concept of ventriculoarterial connections is not.

The approach to diagnosis that is diagrammed in Figure 20–7 is *morphologic* (right atrium, left atrium, right ventricle, left ventricle), *segmental* {atria, ventricles, great arteries}, and *sequential* (in blood flow sequence—from atria, to ventricles, to great arteries).

NOTATION

The situs of the three main cardiac segments may be written out in full or may be abbreviated by segmental symbols.[3, 24] Because the words and the symbols are synonyms, both approaches are equivalent, neither being inherently superior to the other.

For example, the solitus normal heart is {S,D,S} (Fig. 20–7, *row 1, column 1*). The inverted normal heart is {I,L,I} (Fig. 20–7, *row 1, column 3*). Classical physiologically uncorrected transposition of the great arteries is TGA {S,D,D} (Fig. 20–7, *row 5, column 1*). Typical congenitally physiologically corrected transposition of the great arteries is TGA {S,L,L} (Fig. 20–7, *row 5, column 2*). The most common form of double-outlet right ventricle is DORV {S,D,D} (Fig. 20–7, *row 7, column 1*).

Whether one prefers the clarity of words or the convenience of symbols is a matter of personal preference. Although we have long referred to this method of diagnosis as the segmental approach (Fig. 20–7),[5, 6] it is also a morphologic[1–6] and a sequential approach.[3–6] Diagnoses are made in venoarterial sequence—from atria, to ventricles, to great arteries. It has also been called the systematic approach to diagnosis.[25]

The advantages of this method of diagnosis and classification have long been appreciated worldwide, and this method has been built by many hands.[1–29]

TYPES OF HEART: SEGMENTAL SETS AND ALIGNMENTS

To become familiar with many of the different anatomic types of human heart, that is, with many of the different segmental combinations (sets) and segmental alignments that can occur, the reader is urged to study Figure 20–7 and its legend with care.

GUIDING PRINCIPLES

1. Terminology and classification should be *morphologic, segmental,* and *sequential* (Fig. 20–7).

2. Terminology and classification should *not be atrial situs–dependent*. For example, when used in an atrial situs–dependent fashion, ventricular inversion or atrioventricular discordance means one thing in visceroatrial situs solitus (L-loop ventricles), the opposite thing in visceroatrial situs inversus (D-loop ventricles), and nothing in visceroatrial situs ambiguus—because the atrial situs, which is the frame of reference in older methods, itself is unknown.

3. The anatomic status of the ventricles and the great arteries should be diagnosed *primarily and specifically* (e.g., D-loop ventricles/L-loop ventricles; D-TGA/L-TGA),

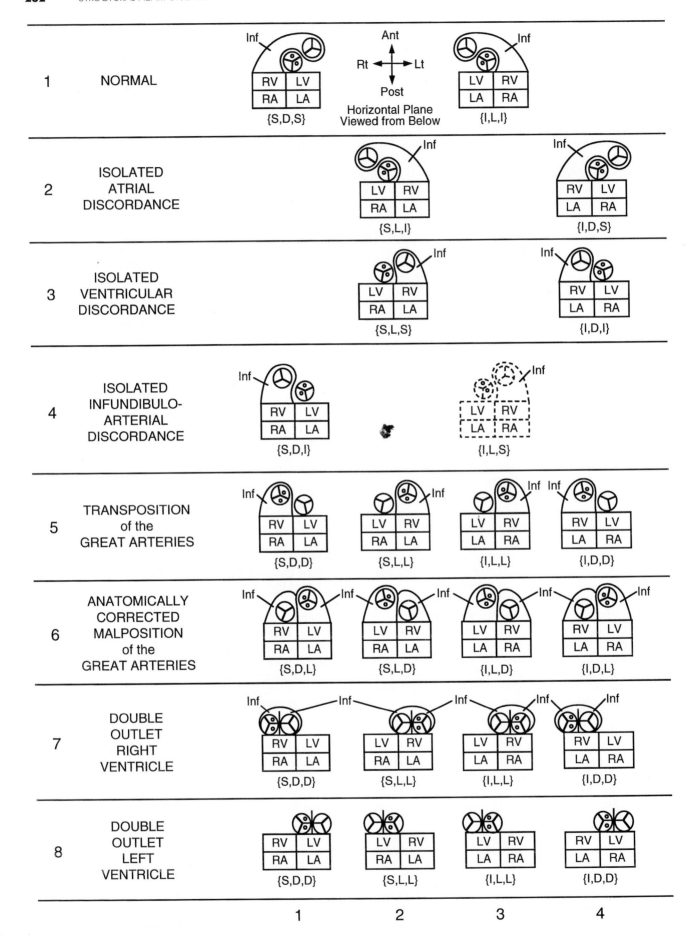

not secondarily and inferentially from the atrioventricular alignments and connections. Attempts to diagnose the anatomic status of the ventricles secondarily and inferentially by means of the atrioventricular alignments and connections often does not work (e.g., with straddling atrioventricular valves, double-inlet ventricle, and atrial situs ambiguus). The atrioventricular alignments and connections can even predict the ventricular situs wrongly: solitus atria and L-loop ventricles can have concordant atrioventricular alignments; and solitus atria and D-loop ventricles can have discordant atrioventricular alignments.[12, 30]

4. The meanings of the diagnostic terms used to describe the ventricles and the great arteries should be *constant* (unchanging) to facilitate diagnostic analysis in large series of complex hearts.[31] D-loop/L-loop ventricles and D-/L-TGA fulfill these criteria and were introduced[2, 3] to facilitate diagnostic data analysis. For example, D-loop ventricles always means the same thing (Figs. 20–5A and 20–7), no matter what the visceroatrial situs or any other variable may be.

5. Attempts to diagnose the anatomic status of the ventricles (such as the ventricular situs or a single ventricle) in terms of the atrioventricular valves are *violations of the myocardial morphologic method of ventricular diagnosis and designation* presented at the beginning of this chapter. The only uniformly successful method of diagnosing the anatomic status of the ventricles (e.g., the ventricular situs or a single ventricle) is to examine the myocardial morphology of the ventricular part of the heart (see Fig. 20–2). The myocardial morphologic method applies equally to the diagnosis and designation of the atria (see Fig. 20–1).

FIGURE 20–7

Types of human heart: segmental sets and alignments. Only some types of human heart are diagrammed here. They are shown from below, similar to a two-dimensional subxiphoid echocardiogram. ant = anterior; post = posterior; Rt = right; Lt = left.

Hearts shown in *column 1* have atrioventricular (AV) concordance with solitus atria and D-loop ventricles, that is, {S,D,–}. Hearts shown in *column 2* have AV discordance with solitus atria and L-loop ventricles, that is, {S,L,–}. Hearts diagrammed in *column 3* have AV concordance in visceroatrial situs inversus with L-loop ventricles, that is, {I,L,–}. Hearts shown in *column 4* have AV discordance with inversus (inverted) atria and D-loop ventricles, that is, {I,D,–}. Visceroatrial situs ambiguus is omitted for simplicity but is represented as {A,D,–} and as {A,L,–} with D-loop and L-loop ventricles, respectively.

The rows are organized in terms of the ventriculoarterial (VA) alignments. *Row 1* has normal VA alignments. The heart shown in row 1 and column 1, that is, *diagram 1,1*, depicts the solitus normal heart that has the segmental set of {S,D,S} with concordant AV and VA alignments. The inverted normal heart shown in *diagram 1,3* has a segmental set of {I,L,I} with concordant AV and VA alignments. *Row 2* also has concordant VA alignments. *Diagram 2,2* shows a heart with the segmental set of {S,L,I} with discordant AV alignments and concordant VA alignments. In classical terminology, this is ventricular inversion with inverted normally related great arteries in visceroatrial situs solitus. Because there is one segmental alignment discordance (at the AV level), the circulations are physiologically uncorrected. An atrial switch operation (Senning or Mustard) achieves physiologic and anatomic repair (the left ventricle supplies the aorta, and the right ventricle ejects into the pulmonary artery). *Diagram 2,4* has a segmental set of {I,D,S} with AV discordance and VA concordance. In classical terminology, this anomaly is ventricular noninversion with normally related great arteries in visceroatrial situs inversus. Because there is one segmental alignment discordance (at the AV level), the circulations are physiologically uncorrected. An atrial switch operation results in a physiologic and anatomic repair. *Row 3* also has VA concordance. *Diagram 3,2* shows a heart with a segmental set of {S,L,S} with AV discordance and VA concordance. In classical terminology, this is isolated ventricular inversion; only the ventricles are inverted, whereas the atria and the great arteries are not inverted. Because there is one segmental alignment discordance, the circulations are physiologically uncorrected. An atrial switch operation achieves physiologic and anatomic repair. *Diagram 3,4* has a segmental set of {I,D,I} with discordant AV alignments and concordant VA alignments. In classical terminology, this rare malformation might be called isolated ventricular noninversion; only the ventricles are noninverted, whereas the atrial and the great arterial segments both are inverted. *Row 4* also has VA concordance. *Diagram 4,1* has a segmental set of {S,D,I} with AV and VA concordance. In classical terminology, this rare anomaly is known as isolated infundibuloarterial inversion; only the infundibulum and the great arteries are inverted, whereas the atria and the ventricles are not inverted. Because AV and VA concordance are present, one might assume that no hemodynamic abnormality results. However, almost all known examples of {S,D,I} have had tetralogy of Fallot involving the inverted subpulmonary infundibulum and great arteries, resulting in tetralogy of Fallot {S,D,I}.[15, 55] *Diagram 4,3* in broken lines has not as yet been documented. *Row 5* depicts some of the known forms of transposition of the great arteries (TGA). All diagrams have VA discordance, that is, TGA. *Diagram 5,1* shows TGA {S,D,D} with AV concordance, this being the classical form of physiologically uncorrected (complete) TGA. *Diagram 5,2* depicts TGA {S,L,L} with AV discordance, this being the classical form of congenitally physiologically corrected TGA. *Diagram 5,3* is TGA {I,L,L} with AV concordance, this being typical physiologically uncorrected TGA in visceroatrial situs inversus. *Diagram 5,4* shows TGA {I,D,D} with AV discordance, this being typical congenitally physiologically corrected TGA in situs inversus. *Row 6* presents anatomically corrected malposition of the great arteries (ACM), in which the great arteries are malpositioned but nonetheless originate above the anatomically correct ventricles: aorta (indicated by the coronary ostia) above the left ventricle, and pulmonary artery (no coronary ostia) above the right ventricle. A bilateral infundibulum or conus (Inf) is often present (subaortic and subpulmonary). Note that the direction of ventricular looping and the twisting of the great arteries are always opposites. *Diagram 6,1* presents ACM {S,D,L} with AV concordance and VA concordance (by definition). Such patients often have a ventricular septal defect. *Diagram 6,2* shows ACM {S,L,D} with AV discordance. Because there is one segmental alignment discordance (at the AV level), the circulations are physiologically uncorrected. An atrial switch procedure (Senning or Mustard) results in physiologic and anatomic repair. *Diagram 6,3* presents ACM {I,L,D} with AV concordance. Because there are no segmental alignment discordances, the only hemodynamic abnormalities are related to associated malformations, such as ventricular septal defect and pulmonary outflow tract stenosis or atresia. *Diagram 6,4* shows ACM {I,D,L} with AV discordance. Because of one segmental alignment discordance (at the AV level), such patients need an atrial switch operation to achieve a physiologic and an anatomic repair. *Row 7* depicts some of the anatomic types of double-outlet right ventricle (DORV), which means that both great arteries arise entirely or predominantly above the morphologically right ventricle. *Diagram 7,1* depicts DORV {S,D,D} with AV concordance. *Diagram 7,2* shows DORV {S,L,L} with AV discordance. *Diagram 7,3* presents DORV {I,L,L} with AV concordance. *Diagram 7,4* shows DORV {I,D,D} with AV discordance. Associated malformations, such as subaortic or subpulmonary ventricular septal defect and the presence or absence of pulmonary outflow tract obstruction, are omitted from this schema for simplicity and clarity. *Row 8* shows some of the anatomic types of double-outlet left ventricle (DOLV), which means that both great arteries arise entirely or predominantly above the morphologically left ventricle. *Diagram 8,1* shows DOLV {S,D,D} with AV concordance. *Diagram 8,2* represents DOLV {S,L,L} with AV discordance. *Diagram 8,3* depicts DOLV {I,L,L} with AV concordance. *Diagram 8,4* shows DOLV {I,D,D} with AV discordance. (From Foran RB, Belcourt C, Nanton MA, et al: Isolated infundibuloarterial inversion {S,D,I}: A newly recognized form of congenital heart disease. Am Heart J 116:1337–1350, 1988.)

One variable (such as the anatomic status of the ventricular part of the heart) *must be defined primarily in terms of itself, not primarily in terms of any other variable* (such as the atrioventricular valves) no matter how important the other variable may be. Trying to define one variable primarily in terms of another variable is an error in logic.

6. *New terms* should be introduced if there is *no existing term* for the entity in question or if the existing term is *factually inaccurate.* New terms should be *morphologic.* Nonmorphologic anatomic terminology (e.g., "primitive" ventricle, "trabeculated pouch," "outlet chamber," "main chamber") should be avoided because these terms are morphologically meaningless. New terms should be introduced only if they are *essential.*

SPECIFIC EXAMPLES

Single Ventricle

There are two anatomic types of single ventricle[2, 32, 33]:

1. *absence of the right ventricular sinus* (body or inflow tract) (Fig. 20–8A), resulting in *single left ventricle with an* *infundibular outlet chamber* and double-inlet or common-inlet left ventricle; and

2. *absence of the left ventricular sinus* (body or inflow tract) (Fig. 20–8B), resulting in *single right ventricle* with double-inlet or common-inlet right ventricle.

With single left ventricle, the infundibular outlet chamber is not a "rudimentary right ventricle."[33] The conus is not an intrinsic, inseparable part of the right ventricle. The subsemilunar conus can be located *predominantly above the left ventricle,* as in anatomically corrected malposition of the great arteries[19, 20] and as in double-outlet left ventricle.[18] Rudimentary right ventricle is an erroneous nonmorphologic diagnosis: the infundibulum typically is not rudimentary, and the right ventricular sinus is absent, not rudimentary. The sine qua non of the right ventricle is the right ventricular sinus (the main segment), not either of the connecting segments (the atrioventricular canal component or the conal component).[34] For a right ventricle to be present, the sinus—the main pumping portion—must be present, and the same is true of the left ventricle. The infundibulum or conus forms the outflow tract of *both* ventricles.

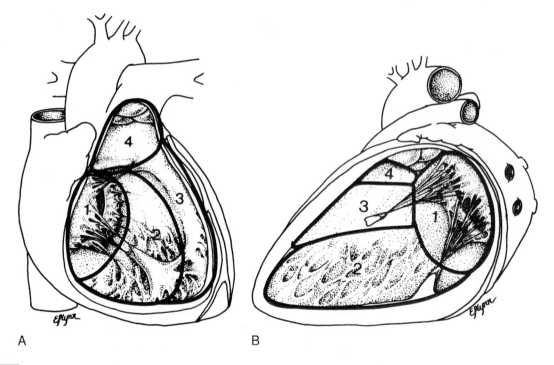

A   B

FIGURE 20–8

A, The four parts of the right ventricle. *Component 1* is the atrioventricular canal portion. *Component 2* is the right ventricular sinus, body, or inflow tract—the main pumping portion and the sine qua non of the right ventricle. *Component 3* is the septal band and moderator band portion—the proximal or apical part of the conus on which the right bundle branch runs. *Component 4* is the conal septum and parietal band portion—the distal or subsemilunar part of the conus. *The right ventricular inflow tract* consists of components 1 and 2. *The right ventricular outflow tract* consists of components 3 and 4. Ventricular septal defects (VSDs) occur within and between these four main components. *B,* The four parts of the left ventricle. *Component 1* is the atrioventricular canal portion. *Component 2* is the finely trabeculated left ventricular sinus, body, or inflow tract—the main pumping portion of the left ventricle that develops from evagination or outpouching. Component 3 is the smooth (nontrabeculated) superior portion of the left ventricular septum on which the left bundle branches run. Component 3 is confluent with the septal band on the right ventricular septal surface (Fig. 20–8A). *Component 4* is the distal or subsemilunar part of the conus, normally forming the conal septum beneath the right coronary leaflet of the aortic valve. *The left ventricular inflow tract* consists of components 1 and 2. *The left ventricular outflow tract* consists of components 3 and 4, and also of component 1, because the anterior leaflet of the mitral valve also is part of the left ventricular outflow tact. VSDs occur within and between these four main components, explaining the many possible locations of VSDs. For example, *VSDs of the atrioventricular canal type* (atrioventricular septal defects) involve component 1. *Muscular VSDs* involve component 2 and can occur between components 2 and 3, resulting in midmuscular VSDs. *Conoventricular VSDs* occur between components 4 and 3, with or without hypoplasia or malalignment of component 4. (*A, B* from Van Praagh R, Geva T, Kreutzer J: Ventricular septal defects: How shall we describe, name and classify them? Reprinted with permission from the American College of Cardiology [Journal of the American College of Cardiology, 1989, Volume 14, pages 1298–1299].)

Below the atria, there are *three* chambers, but only two of them are ventricles: (1) the left ventricular sinus, (2) the right ventricular sinus, and (3) the conus arteriosus. The conus is the connector between both ventricles and the great arteries. Finding only two chambers in the ventricular mass (instead of the normal three) should suggest that one chamber may be missing.

Univentricular atrioventricular connection is a recent restatement of the old unsatisfactory definition of single ventricle in terms of the atrioventricular valves. Exceptions to this old unsatisfactory definition are as follows:

1. With single left ventricle, the tricuspid valve can open predominantly or entirely into the infundibular outlet chamber, an anomaly known as *the Lambert heart*[35]: double-inlet left ventricle is not present (the atrioventricular connection is not univentricular).

2. *Double-inlet right ventricle* is usually *not* a single right ventricle because a small left ventricular sinus is typically present. Thus, although a univentricular atrioventricular connection is present (double-inlet right ventricle or common-inlet right ventricle), a single right ventricle is *not* present. This is the most frequent and the most glaring illustration of the fact that *the old definition of single ventricle, that is, univentricular atrioventricular connection, does not work and should be abandoned.* The solution is not to say that single ventricle does not exist. Instead, the solution is to define single left ventricle and single right ventricle with myocardial morphologic accuracy (as before).[36–40]

In conclusion, the confusion evident in the literature concerning single ventricle is readily resolved by an understanding of and adherence to the *gross myocardial morphologic method* of chamber identification and designation, specifically prohibiting the use of the atrioventricular valves for this purpose, which does not work because it represents an error in logic.

Common Atrioventricular Canal

Common atrioventricular canal is preferred to atrioventricular septal defect because common atrioventricular canal involves much more than just an atrioventricular septal defect; typically, in addition, there is a cleft in what normally is the anterior leaflet of the mitral valve and a deformity of the leaflets of what normally is the tricuspid valve. In other words, common atrioventricular canal involves a prominent *leaflet and valvar malformation* (common atrioventricular valve, cleft mitral valve, deformed tricuspid valve); it is not just a septal defect.

Also, there are partial forms of common atrioventricular canal that do not have a ventricular septal defect of the atrioventricular canal type; hence, *atrioventricular septal defect is not a satisfactory common denominator.*

Moreover, atrioventricular septal defect has been used for a defect in the atrioventricular portion of the membranous septum, resulting in left ventricular–to–right atrial shunt (the Gerbode defect).[41–43] Thus, the usage of atrioventricular septal defect is confused. Consequently, we prefer the term and concept of common atrioventricular canal.

Paramembranous or Juxtamembranous Ventricular Septal Defect

"Perimembranous" ventricular septal defect does not exist, accurately speaking. Paramembranous or juxtamembranous ventricular septal defect is what is meant.[44] *Peri* is a Greek word meaning around. No ventricular septal defect extends all around the membranous septum. If it did, the membranous septum would be floating freely in space, unattached to any adjacent structure. By analogy, the *parathyroid* gland means the gland "beside the thyroid." A "perithyroid" gland would extend all around the thyroid. Similarly, a *paravalvar* leak means a leak "beside the valve," but a *perivalvar* leak would be a leak all around the valve—a very different thing indeed. *Paramembranous*[44] ventricular septal defect means beside the membranous tissue, that is, confluent with the tricuspid valve (Greek *para*, beside). *Juxtamembranous*[45] ventricular septal defect also means beside the membranous tissue (Latin *juxta*, beside).

Parietal Band

The parietal band[46, 47] is the extension of the conal septum out onto the parietal (free) wall of the right ventricle (see Fig. 20–2B). This structure is known to be conal. Some wish to rename this structure the ventriculoinfundibular fold, a new term that raises several questions: Is the "ventriculoinfundibular" fold a ventricular structure, or is it an infundibular structure? Is it both? We think that the correct answer is an infundibular structure, at the ventriculoinfundibular junction.

We prefer a more specific approach. In the Taussig-Bing malformation,[48, 49] for example, the conus clearly displays three parts:

1. *the conal septum,* between the aortic and the pulmonary outflow tracts, beneath the aortopulmonary septum;

2. *the subaortic conal free wall,* the conal musculature remote from the conal septum, beneath the nonseptal (noncoronary) leaflet of the aortic valve; and

3. *the subpulmonary conal free wall,* the conal musculature remote from the conal septum, beneath the nonseptal leaflet of the pulmonary valve that is not confluent with the aortopulmonary septum.

With use of the aforementioned method, it is readily possible to specify exactly what part of the subsemilunar conus one is talking about. This is important. For example, the conal anomaly that results in transposition of the great arteries is growth and development of the subaortic conal *free wall.*[21] Although much attention has in the past been focused on the conotruncal septum in transposition of the great arteries, the essential defect appears to involve the growth and development of the subaortic conal free wall.

Septal and Moderator Bands

The septal and moderator bands are the standard designations[46, 47] of the proximal conal structures within the right ventricle (see Fig. 20–2B) that some of our colleagues wish to rename the trabecula septomarginalis or the septomarginal trabeculation. The trabecula septomarginalis is an old Latin designation for the moderator band: Latin *trabecula,* little beam, and *septomarginalis,* from the septum to the margin, meaning from the septum to the acute margin of the right ventricle. Septomarginal trabeculation is now used by some to mean the septal band and the moderator band. We prefer plain English terms whenever possible, rather than long Latin synonyms, particularly when they are more specific in meaning—such as *septal band* and *moderator band.*

Quadripartite Concept of the Ventricles

The quadripartite concept of the ventricles indicates that the right ventricle and the left ventricle each consists of four main parts (see Fig. 20–8),[44] not three. We prefer this four-part concept because it shows how the ventricular septum really "comes apart," explaining why ventricular septal defects occur where they do.

Transposition of the Great Arteries

Transposition of the great arteries[12–14, 16] is the standard term that some are endeavoring to replace with "ventriculoarterial discordance." Philologists point out that a common error in linguistics is to confuse a *term* with its *definition.* In the present example, *transposition* is the term and *ventriculoarterial discordance* is the definition.

Tricuspid Atresia

Tricuspid atresia[50, 51] is the standard term that some have tried to replace with "univentricular heart of the left ventricular type with absent right atrioventricular connection." Apart from its verbosity, this is a definition, not a term.

Plurals

The plural of *atrium* is *atria* (not "atriums"), and the plural of *septum* is *septa* (not "septums").

The 50% Rule

The 50% rule is a convenience, but it is not a basic concept. One cannot decide whether a chamber is or is not a ventricle according to whether an atrioventricular valve opens 51% into it (then it is a "ventricle") or 49% into it (then it is a "trabeculated pouch" or an "outlet chamber"). This use of the 50% rule *at the atrioventricular junction* is erroneous and a violation of the gross myocardial morphologic method[1–6] mentioned heretofore.

At the ventriculoarterial junction, the 50% rule can be useful, but it is not a basic concept. The 50% rule does *not* apply well to normally related great arteries. The aortic valve normally sits mainly above the ventricular septum, to the right of the left ventricular cavity. The pulmonary valve normally sits mostly above the infundibular septum, to the left of the right ventricular cavity. Because the so-called 50% rule does not apply well to the normal, this concept is not fundamental and hence should not be used to reclassify congenital heart disease:

In tetralogy of Fallot, considerable aortic overriding often occurs. Should the 50% rule be used to reclassify tetralogy of Fallot into those hearts with double-outlet right ventricle and those hearts without double-outlet right ventricle? We think the answer is no. As long as there is aortic-mitral fibrous continuity, we make the diagnosis of tetralogy of Fallot, and we describe the degree of aortic overriding. However, we do not make the diagnosis of tetralogy of Fallot with double-outlet right ventricle. This we regard as an error in diagnostic formulation. For pragmatic reasons, *diagnoses should be specific and mutually exclusive:* tetralogy of Fallot *or* double-outlet right ventricle (not tetralogy of Fallot *and* double-outlet right ventricle).

In transposition of the great arteries, typically there is pulmonary-mitral fibrous continuity. The pulmonary artery can override the ventricular septum to a considerable degree. As long as there is pulmonary-mitral fibrous continuity, we make the diagnosis of transposition of the great arteries (not transposition of the great arteries *and* double-outlet right ventricle).

These, then, are the two situations in which we ignore the 50% rule:

1. tetralogy of Fallot with considerable aortic overriding, but with aortic-mitral fibrous continuity; and
2. transposition of the great arteries with considerable pulmonary overriding, but with pulmonary-mitral fibrous continuity.

Accurate Diagnosis and Classification

- Accurate diagnosis and classification require the full segmental set.

We never should make a diagnosis such as L-TGA. Why not? Because you have to know *all of the segmental anatomy.* Although L-TGA typically is TGA {S,L,L}[16,52] (Fig. 20–7, *row 5, column 2*), it can be TGA {S,D,L}[16,53] (not shown in Fig. 20–7) or TGA {I,L,L}[16,31] (Fig. 20–7, *row 5, column 3*).

- Accurate diagnosis and classification require statement of the abnormal ventriculoarterial alignment.

We never make a diagnosis such as {S,D,D}. Why not? Because you have to know what type of ventriculoarterial alignment is present. The patient may have TGA {S,D,D} (Fig. 20–7, *row 5, column 1*), or DORV {S,D,D} (Fig. 20–7, *row 7, column 1*), or DOLV {S,D,D} (Fig. 20–7, *row 8, column 1*).

- Accurate diagnosis and classification may or may not require statement of the atrioventricular alignment.

For example, in typical TGA {S,D,D} (Fig. 20–7, *row 5, column 1*), we customarily omit the diagnosis of atrioventricular concordance because this is understood from the segmental anatomy: {S,D,D}. However, if the atrioventricular alignment is not as expected, for example, if there is straddling tricuspid valve, this must be stated specifically: TGA {S,D,D} with small right ventricle, ventricular septal defect of the atrioventricular canal type, and straddling tricuspid valve.

Terminology

In terminology, we should be conservative. Change is inevitable; indeed, change is one of the few constants that we know. But in language, change must be slow to avoid chaos. Although many of the neologisms of the recent past may seem nonessential, in the long eye of time they will probably be seen as *enrichments* of our scientific language. In our increasingly global society, there are about 2700 living languages, and although *terms* are important, even more important are *meanings.* The same things can be said satisfactorily in many different languages—English, French, German, Spanish, Italian, Greek, Russian, Japanese, Chinese, and others—by using different terms that have the same meanings. Consequently, we should focus on precise meaning and accurate understanding, changing our terminology as little as possible in the interests of clarity of communication and continuity of understanding.

CONCLUSION

The terminology and classification of congenital heart disease summarized here have been used at the Children's Hospital in Boston and at other medical centers worldwide for more than 30 years. This method[1–6,54–56]—which is morphologic, segmental, and sequential—has stood the test of time and has required few changes. This approach, developed by many colleagues, is brief, is convenient, and always works.

REFERENCES

1. Lev M: Pathologic diagnosis of positional variations in cardiac chambers in congenital heart disease. Lab Invest 3:71, 1954.
2. Van Praagh R, Ongley PA, Swan HJC: Anatomic types of single or common ventricle in man, morphologic and geometric aspects in sixty autopsied cases. Am J Cardiol 13:367, 1964.
3. Van Praagh R, Van Praagh S, Vlad P, Keith JD: Anatomic types of congenital dextrocardia, diagnostic and embryologic implications. Am J Cardiol 13:510, 1964.
4. Van Praagh R, Vlad P: Dextrocardia, mesocardia, and levocardia. The segmental approach to diagnosis in congenital heart disease. *In* Keith JD, Rowe RD, Vlad P (eds): Heart Disease in Infancy and Childhood, 3rd ed. New York, Macmillan, 1978, pp 638–695.
5. Van Praagh R: The segmental approach to diagnosis in congenital heart disease. Birth Defects 8:4, 1972.
6. Van Praagh R, Weinberg PM, Matsuoka R, Van Praagh S: Malpositions of the heart. *In* Adams FH, Emmanouilides GC (eds): Moss' Heart Disease in Infants, Children and Adolescents, 3rd ed. Baltimore, Williams & Wilkins, 1983, pp 422–458.
7. Van Praagh R, Van Praagh S: Atrial isomerism in the heterotaxy syndromes with asplenia, or polysplenia, or normally formed spleen: An erroneous concept. Am J Cardiol 60:1504, 1990.
8. Rubino M, Van Praagh S, Kadoba K, et al: Systemic and pulmonary venous connections in visceral heterotaxy with asplenia: Diagnostic and surgical considerations based on seventy-two autopsied cases. J Thorac Cardiovasc Surg 110:641, 1995.
9. Van Praagh S, Kakou-Guikahue M, Kim H-S, et al: Atrial situs in patients with visceral heterotaxy and congenital heart disease: Conclusions based on findings in 104 postmortem cases. Coeur 19:484, 1988.
10. Van Praagh S, Kreutzer J, Alday L, Van Praagh R: Systemic and pulmonary venous connections in visceral heterotaxy, with emphasis on the diagnosis of the atrial situs: A study of 109 postmortem cases. *In* Clark EB, Takao A (eds): Developmental Cardiology: Morphogenesis and Function. Mt. Kisco, NY, Futura Publishing, 1990, pp 671–728.
11. Van Praagh S, Santini F, Sanders SP: Cardiac malpositions with special emphasis on visceral heterotaxy (asplenia and polysplenia syndromes). *In* Fyler DC (ed): Nadas' Pediatric Cardiology. Philadelphia, Hanley & Belfus, 1991, pp 589–608.
12. Van Praagh R, David I, Gordon D, et al: Ventricular diagnosis and designation. *In* Godman M (ed): Paediatric Cardiology. Edinburgh, Churchill Livingstone, 1981, pp 153–168.
13. Van Praagh R, Pérez-Treviño C, López-Cuellar M, et al: Transposition of the great arteries with posterior aorta, anterior pulmonary artery, subpulmonary conus and fibrous continuity between aortic and atrioventricular valves. Am J Cardiol 28:621, 1971.
14. Van Praagh R: Transposition of the great arteries. II. Transposition clarified. Am J Cardiol 28:739, 1971.
15. Foran RB, Belcourt C, Nanton MA, et al: Isolated infundibuloarterial inversion {S,D,I}: A newly recognized form of congenital heart disease. Am Heart J 116:1337, 1988.
16. Van Praagh R: Transposition of the great arteries: History, pathologic anatomy, embryology, etiology, and surgical considerations. Cardiac Surgery: State of the Art Reviews 5:7, 1991.
17. Van Praagh S, Davidoff A, Chin A, et al: Double-outlet right ventricle: Anatomic types and developmental implications based on a study of 101 autopsied cases. Coeur 13:389, 1982.
18. Van Praagh R, Weinberg PM, Srebro J: Double outlet left ventricle. *In* Adams FH, Emmanouilides GC, Riemenschneider TA (eds): Moss' Heart Disease in Infants, Children and Adolescents, 4th ed. Baltimore, Williams & Wilkins 1989, pp 461–485.
19. Van Praagh R, Van Praagh S: Anatomically corrected transposition of the great arteries. Br Heart J 29:112, 1967.
20. Van Praagh R, Durnin RE, Jockin H, et al: Anatomically corrected malposition of the great arteries {S,D,L}. Circulation 51:20, 1975.
21. Van Praagh R, Layton WM, Van Praagh S: The morphogenesis of normal and abnormal relationships between the great arteries and the ventricles: Pathologic and experimental data. *In* Van Praagh R, Takao A (eds): Etiology and Morphogenesis of Congenital Heart Disease. Mt. Kisco, NY, Futura Publishing, 1980, pp 271–316.
22. Van Praagh R: Congenital heart disease: Embryology, anatomy, and approach to diagnosis. Cardiovascular Pathophysiology, Harvard Medical School 27:1, 1986.
23. Pasquini L, Sanders SP, Parness IA, et al: Conal anatomy in 119 patients with D-loop transposition of the great arteries with ventricular septal defect: An echocardiographic and pathologic study. J Am Coll Cardiol 21:1712, 1993.
24. Melhuish BPP, Van Praagh R: Juxtaposition of the atrial appendages, a sign of severe cyanotic congenital heart disease. Br Heart J 30:269, 1968.
25. Rao PS: Systematic approach to differential diagnosis. Am Heart J 102:389, 1981.
26. Otero Coto E, Quero Jimenez M: Aproximacion segmentaria al diagnostico y clasificacion de las cardiopatias congenitas. Fundamentos y utilidad. Rev Esp Cardiol 30:557, 1977.
27. Stanger P, Rudolph AM, Edwards JE: Cardiac malpositions, an overview based on study of sixty-five necropsy specimens. Circulation 56:159, 1977.
28. Calcaterra G, Anderson RH, Lau KC, Shinebourne EA: Dextrocardia—value of segmental analysis in its categorization. Br Heart J 42:497, 1979.
29. Ando M, Santomi G, Takao A: Atresia of tricuspid or mitral orifice: Anatomic spectrum and morphogenetic hypothesis. *In* Van Praagh R, Takao A (eds): Etiology and Morphogenesis of Congenital Heart Disease. Mt. Kisco, NY, Futura Publishing, 1980, pp 421–487.
30. Van Praagh R: When concordant or discordant atrioventricular alignments predict the ventricular situs wrongly. I. Solitus atria, concordant alignments, and L-loop ventricles. II. Solitus atria, discordant alignments, and D-loop ventricles. J Am Coll Cardiol 10:1278, 1987.
31. Van Praagh R, Weinberg PM, Calder AL, et al: The transposition complexes: How many are there? *In* Davila JC (ed): 2nd Henry Ford Hospital International Symposium on Cardiac Surgery. New York, Appleton-Century-Crofts, 1977, pp 207–213.
32. Van Praagh R, Plett JA, Van Praagh S: Single ventricle: Pathology, embryology, terminology, and classification. Herz 4:113, 1979.
33. Dobell ARC, Van Praagh R: The Holmes Heart: Historical associations and pathologic anatomy. Am Heart J 132:437, 1996.
34. Van Praagh R, David I, Van Praagh S: What is a ventricle? The single ventricle trap. Pediatr Cardiol 2:79, 1982.
35. Lambert EC: Single ventricle with a rudimentary outlet chamber, case report. Bull Johns Hopkins Hosp 88:231, 1951.
36. Van Praagh R, Wise JR, Dahl BA, Van Praagh S: Single left ventricle with infundibular outlet chamber and tricuspid valve opening only into outlet chamber in 44-year-old man with thoraco-abdominal ectopia cordis without diaphragmatic or pericardial defect: Importance of myocardial morphologic method of chamber identification in congenital heart disease. *In* Van Praagh R, Takao A (eds): Etiology and Morphogenesis of Congenital Heart Disease. Mt. Kisco, NY, Futura Publishing, 1980, pp 379–420.
37. Edwards JE: Congenital malformations of the heart and great vessels. A. Malformations of the atrial septal complex. *In* Gould SE (ed): Pathology of the Heart and Blood Vessels. Springfield, IL, Charles C Thomas, 1968, pp 262–279.
38. Rastelli GC, Kirklin JW, Titus JL: Anatomic observations on complete form of persistent common atrioventricular canal with special reference to atrioventricular valves. Mayo Clin Proc 41:296, 1968.
39. Bharati S, Lev M: The spectrum of common atrioventricular orifice (canal). Am Heart J 86:553, 1973.

40. Bharati S, Lev M, McAllister HA, Kirklin JW: The surgical anatomy of the atrioventricular valve in the intermediate type of common atrioventricular orifice. J Thorac Cardiovasc Surg 79:884, 1980.

41. Van Praagh R, Papagiannis J, Bar-El YI, Schwint OA: The heart in Down syndrome, pathologic anatomy. *In* Marino B, Pueschel SM (eds): Heart Disease in Persons with Down Syndrome. Baltimore, Paul H. Brookes Publishing, 1996, pp 69–110.

42. Ferencz C: Atrioventricular defect of the membranous septum, left ventricular–right atrial communication with malformed mitral valve simulating aortic stenosis. Bull Johns Hopkins Hosp 100:209, 1957.

43. Taguchi K, Matsura Y, Yoshizaki E, Tamura M: Surgery of atrioventricular septal defects with left ventricular–right atrial shunt, report of 23 cases. J Thorac Cardiovasc Surg 56:265, 1968.

44. Gerbode F, Hultgren H, Melrose D, Osborn J: Syndrome of left ventricular–right atrial shunt: Successful surgical repair of defect in 5 cases with observation of bradycardia on closure. Ann Surg 148:433, 1958.

45. Van Praagh R, Geva T, Kreutzer J: Ventricular septal defects: How shall we describe, name, and classify them? J Am Coll Cardiol 14:1298, 1989.

46. Soto B, Ceballos R, Kirklin JW: Ventricular septal defects: A surgical viewpoint. J Am Coll Cardiol 14:1291, 1989.

47. Lev M: Dissection and examination of the congenitally abnormal heart. *In* Lev M: Autopsy Diagnosis of Congenitally Malformed Hearts. Springfield, IL, Charles C Thomas, 1953, pp 3–12.

48. Bharati S, Lev M: Dissection of the heart. *In* Bharati S, Lev M: The Pathology of Congenital Heart Disease: A personal Experience With More Than 6,300 Congenitally Malformed Hearts. Armonk, NY, Futura Publishing, 1996, pp 15–20.

49. Taussig HB, Bing RJ: Complete transposition of aorta and levoposition of pulmonary artery. Am Heart J 37:551, 1949.

50. Van Praagh R: What is the Taussig-Bing malformation? Circulation 38:445, 1968.

51. Edwards JE, Burchell HB: Congenital tricuspid atresia: A classification. Med Clin North Am 33:1177, 1949.

52. Keith JD, Rowe RD, Vlad P (eds): Heart Disease in Infancy and Childhood. New York, Macmillan, 1967, pp 644–681.

53. Van Praagh R: What is congenitally corrected transposition? N Engl J Med 282:1097, 1970.

54. Houyel L, Van Praagh R, Lacour-Gayet F, et al: Transposition of the great arteries {S,D,L}: Pathologic anatomy, diagnosis, and surgical management of a newly recognized complex. J Thorac Cardiovasc Surg 110:613, 1995.

55. Pasquini L, Sanders SP, Parness I, et al: Echocardiographic and anatomic findings in atrioventricular discordance with ventriculoarterial concordance. Am J Cardiol 62:1256, 1988.

56. Santini F, Jonas RA, Sanders SP, Van Praagh R: Tetralogy of Fallot {S,D,I}: Successful repair without a conduit. Ann Thorac Surg 59:747, 1995.

CHAPTER 21
VENTRICULAR SEPTAL DEFECT

JAMES L. WILKINSON

HISTORICAL BACKGROUND

Anatomists and pathologists have documented defects in the ventricular septum for many centuries. Isolated defects excited little attention until recent times. Defects associated with more major malformations have been described or referred to in numerous publications during the last 200 years—especially in association with right ventricular outflow tract obstruction (pulmonary stenosis or atresia).[1,2] During the latter part of the 19th century, two widely different and highly significant publications drew attention to some of the clinical consequences of ventricular septal defect (VSD). First, the characteristic harsh and strikingly loud systolic murmur present in many affected patients was described, and the remarkable absence of symptoms experienced by such individuals was recognized.[3] Since this publication appeared, the term *maladie de Roger* has been widely used to imply a small asymptomatic VSD. Second, the development of cyanosis in adult life was attributed to a large VSD with associated aortic overriding, although this feature was believed to be the explanation of the cyanosis.[4] The defect described in this publication (large VSD with aortic override) came to be known as Eisenmenger's anomaly, and when cyanosis appeared in adolescence or adult life, the combination has been referred to as *Eisenmenger's complex*. According to Abbott, who coined the latter term, Dalrymple had described the same malformation in 1847.[5] The current use of the term *Eisenmenger's syndrome* to describe patients who have a wide range of malformations with pulmonary hypertension and who develop late cyanosis because of pulmonary vascular damage is a more recent (and probably inappropriate) use of the eponym. Recognition of pulmonary arteriolar disease as the cause of the cyanosis came long after the original description![6,7]

During the current century, two views of the significance of a VSD have emerged. These were the direct results of teachings based on Roger's observation[3] that most patients were asymptomatic and the recognition that large defects led to early symptoms or death or to late cyanosis due to Eisenmenger's complex. In many authoritative circles, there was a widely held view until the 1970s that most VSDs would, if unrepaired, inevitably lead to pulmonary hypertension and the Eisenmenger syndrome if they did not lead to uncontrollable heart failure and death in infancy or early childhood.[8] This belief was fostered by the heavy bias toward larger defects in the experience of most pediatric cardiologists and pathologists

and in the literature of patients who had been submitted to cardiac catheterization and hence had the diagnosis "proved." Epidemiologic data have recently shown that more than 70% of all VSDs are small and clinically asymptomatic and that a high proportion of defects close spontaneously during infancy or early childhood.[9,10] This perspective has been further clarified by the recent demonstration by echocardiography with color flow mapping in fetal life of many tiny VSDs, some of which close before birth.[11] There is also demonstration by echocardiography with color flow mapping of a substantial incidence of extremely small defects in the neonatal period or later in infancy. These are often clinically silent and would in the past have gone undetected (probably closing spontaneously in the early weeks or months of life in the majority).[12] Increasing awareness of such defects has led to the strong suspicion that the incidence of VSD may have been significantly underestimated in most epidemiologic series and that the proportion of all VSDs that are clinically important and require treatment may be relatively small.

INCIDENCE

Epidemiologic studies of the incidence of congenital cardiac anomalies suggest a frequency of 6 to 10 per 1000 total births,[10,13,14] with VSD accounting for at least 30% of all cardiovascular malformations (see Chapter 18). This implies an incidence for VSD of around 20 to 30 per 10,000 births. Data from routine fetal echocardiography and reports from experience with color Doppler echocardiography in "normal" neonates certainly suggest that the true incidence is likely to be very much higher. A study documented 56 neonates with muscular VSDs (almost all clinically silent) in a cohort of 1053 asymptomatic neonates.[12]

RACIAL VARIATIONS

Epidemiologic studies in different populations around the world have not demonstrated a significant variation in the incidence of congenital heart disease as a whole or of VSD. The frequency of different types of VSD does vary between racial groups, however; subpulmonary defects (doubly committed subarterial VSD, supracristal VSD) are substantially more common in Asian populations, and muscular and multiple VSDs are less frequent in the same groups.[15,16] In the experience of cardiac surgeons in

Japan, Hong Kong, and Indonesia, the frequency of sub-pulmonary (doubly committed) defects is at least 30% in patients requiring repair compared with an incidence of around 5% in white patients having an operation for VSD in North America, Europe, and Australasia. By contrast, muscular VSDs account for at least 30% of operated defects in the Western world but are uncommon in Asian populations, and multiple VSDs are reportedly extremely rare in the same groups although found in around 10% of patients needing an operation for VSD in the West.

ANATOMIC TYPES

The ventricular septum may be considered as having four components (Fig. 21–1). Three of these correspond to the three major parts of the ventricles, and the fourth is the area close to the central fibrous body, the membranous septum, at which the other components meet.

The component that separates the ventricular inlets (which contain the atrioventricular valves and their tension apparatus) is referred to as the inlet septum. Defects in this part of the septum are relatively uncommon (except in atrioventricular septal defects; see Chapter 24). These defects fall into two categories. Some are completely surrounded by muscle of the ventricular septum and hence are called *inlet muscular defects* (Fig. 21–2). Others lie immediately below the conjoined annuluses of the atrioventricular valves and abut the central fibrous body at the anterior end of the defect; these are termed *inlet perimembranous defects* (or, in other nomenclatures, atrioventricular canal type or subtricuspid) (Fig. 21–3).

The septum separating the outlet portions of the ventricles is called the outlet or infundibular septum. Defects in this area may abut the arterial valves, being referred to as *doubly committed subarterial defects* (or, in other nomenclatures, subpulmonary or supracristal) (Fig. 21–4; see Fig. 21–2), or they may be surrounded completely by muscle, *outlet muscular defects*.

The third component of the ventricular septum, which separates the body and the apices of the two ventricles, is called the trabecular septum. Defects in this area are re-

ferred to as *trabecular muscular* (see Fig. 21–2) or, when they extend to the central fibrous body, *perimembranous trabecular defects*. Muscular defects are variously referred to as central, anterior, or apical, depending on their location within the relatively extensive trabecular septum. When there are two or more (multiple) defects, they commonly involve the trabecular part of the septum (Fig. 21–5; see Figs. 21–3, 21–12, and 21–16).

The membranous septum is the smallest component of the ventricular septum, lying close to the central fibrous body and at the junction of the other three parts of the septum (see Fig. 21–1). It separates a small part of the left ventricle, immediately below the aortic valve, and is related to the commissure between the right coronary and

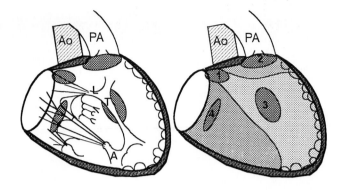

FIGURE 21–2

Illustration of major VSD sites as they relate to the right ventricular surface of the septum. *Left,* The tricuspid valve tension apparatus is shown, including the trabecula septomarginalis (T), the anterior papillary muscle (A), and the papillary muscle of the conus, muscle of Lancisi (L). Ao = aorta; PA = pulmonary artery. *Right,* The relationship of the different defects to the components of the septum is depicted (see Fig. 21–1): *1,* perimembranous defect (adjacent to medial commissure of tricuspid valve and close to aortic valve); *2,* doubly committed subarterial defect (adjacent to both pulmonary and aortic valves); *3,* trabecular muscular defect (often having several exit points around trabeculae on the right ventricular side); *4,* inlet muscular defect (often hidden under the septal leaflet of the tricuspid valve).

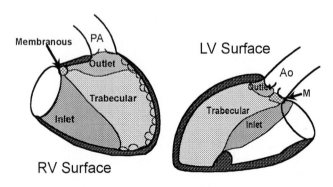

FIGURE 21–1

Diagram showing the four components of the ventricular septum as viewed from the right ventricular (RV) surface of the septum *(left)* and the left ventricular (LV) surface *(right)*. Because of septal curvature, the right ventricular surface is considerably more extensive than the left side. Ao = aorta; M = mitral valve; PA = pulmonary artery.

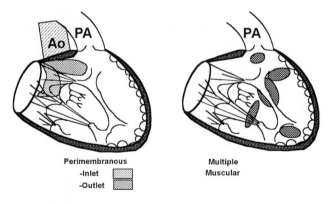

FIGURE 21–3

Left, Diagram showing relationships of inlet perimembranous defect, which lies largely beneath the septal leaflet of the tricuspid valve, and outlet perimembranous defect, which is adjacent to the aortic valve. *Right,* The various sites of some multiple muscular defects are shown (e.g., apical, anterior muscular, outlet muscular, central and inlet muscular). Ao = aorta; PA = pulmonary artery.

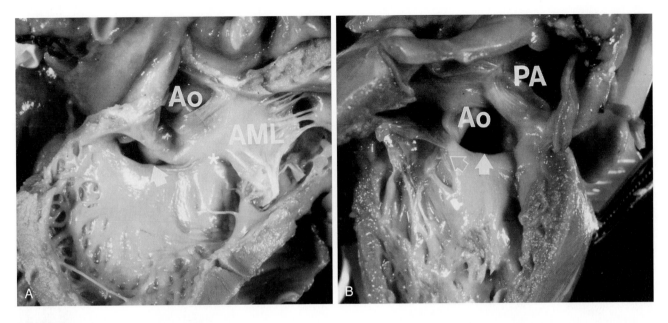

FIGURE 21-4

Anatomy, doubly committed subarterial VSD. *A,* Left ventricular view showing defect *(arrow),* which is separate from the membranous septum *(asterisk). B,* Right ventricular view of the same specimen showing the defect *(arrow)* adjacent to both aortic and pulmonary valves and involving the outlet part of the septum and Lancisi's muscle *(open arrow)* (see Figs. 21–1 and 21–2). AML = anterior leaflet of mitral valve; Ao = aorta; PA = pulmonary artery.

the noncoronary leaflets of the aortic valve, and the part of the right ventricle adjacent to the septal commissure of the tricuspid valve. Defects involving this area are termed *perimembranous* (Fig. 21–6). They are close to both the aortic and the tricuspid valves (see Figs. 21–2 and 21–3). When such defects extend anterosuperiorly, they tend to lie in an immediately "subaortic" position (being some-

times referred to as subaortic defects). Such defects usually excavate the outlet septum to a degree and are called *perimembranous outlet defects* (see Fig. 21–3). When the aorta overrides such a defect, the term *malalignment VSD* is sometimes applied (as is seen in tetralogy of Fallot). Perimembranous defects may, alternatively, excavate the inlet septum (see inlet perimembranous defects) and then

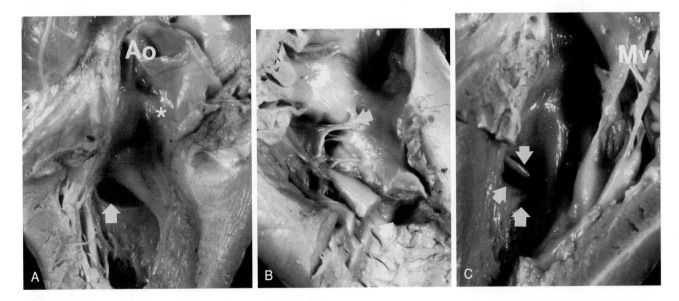

FIGURE 21-5

Anatomy, muscular VSD. *A,* Left ventricular view of large midmuscular defect *(arrow),* which is well separated from the membranous septum *(asterisk)* and aortic valve (Ao). *B,* Right ventricular view in the same specimen as in *A,* with septal trabeculae cut away to show the right ventricular end of the defect *(lower arrow).* Note position of medial commissure *(upper arrow). C,* Specimen similar to *A* but with multiple entry points in the left ventricle *(arrows).* The right ventricular exit points formed a spray around multiple trabeculae. These defects often present a formidable surgical problem because the right ventricular end of the defect is often difficult to define, being buried beneath multiple muscular trabeculae. Mv = mitral valve.

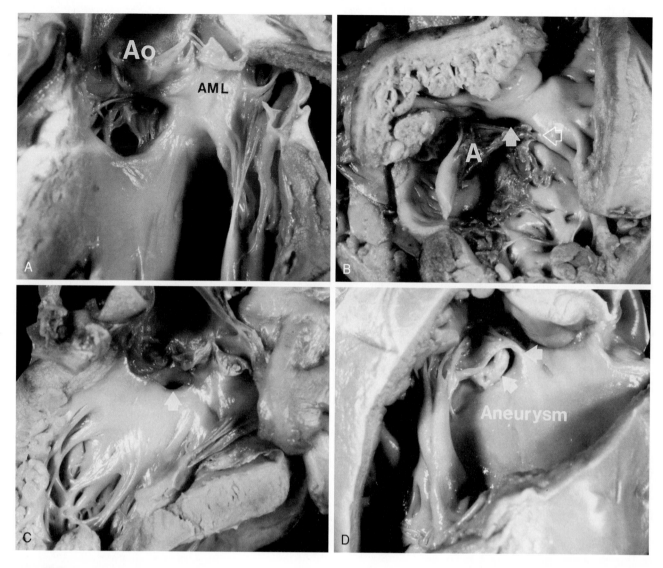

FIGURE 21–6

Anatomy, perimembranous VSD. *A,* Specimen showing large (confluent) perimembranous defect viewed from the left ventricle. The relationship to both the aortic valve (Ao) and the anterior leaflet of the mitral valve (AML) is well shown, with both being immediately adjacent to the defect. Tricuspid valve leaflets and chords are seen through the defect. *B,* Right ventricular view of the same specimen. The defect *(arrow)* is largely concealed by the tricuspid valve apparatus, but its relationship to the medial end of the anterior leaflet (A) and to the medial commissure *(open arrow)* is easily seen. *C,* Left ventricular view of small to moderate perimembranous VSD *(arrow).* This defect is not immediately adjacent to the aortic valve leaflets. *D,* Right ventricular view of the same specimen as in *C.* There is a small aneurysmal pouch of accessory tricuspid leaflet tissue partially covering the defect, adjacent to the medial commissure *(arrows).*

lie below the tricuspid septal leaflet (see Fig. 21–3), sometimes being associated with overriding or straddling of the tricuspid valve. Large perimembranous defects may excavate into all three of the muscular parts of the septum and are sometimes referred to as *confluent defects.*[17–20]

Part of the membranous septum separates the left ventricular outflow tract, adjacent to the commissure between the right and noncoronary leaflets of the aortic valve, from an area just above the annulus of the tricuspid valve and close to the septal commissure of the tricuspid valve, in the right atrium. This curious feature of the complex anatomy of this part of the heart results from the fact that the anterior part of the annulus of the septal tricuspid leaflet is actually attached across the middle of the membranous septum,[21, 22] thus separating it into an atrioventricular and an

interventricular component. Further posteriorly, behind the membranous septum, the annulus of the septal tricuspid leaflet is also attached at a lower level, at the inferior margin of the atrial septum, than is the mitral valve on the opposite side. This results in the characteristic offsetting of the two septal leaflets, which is readily seen on echocardiography in the four-chamber view. Such offsetting depends on an intact ventricular septum in this area, and a perimembranous VSD extending into the inlet septum (inlet perimembranous defect) is usually associated with loss of normal offsetting.

A defect involving the atrioventricular component of the membranous septum allows direct communication between the left ventricle and the right atrium, a so-called Gerbode VSD.[23] In practice, this is not the only situation in which a shunt from the left ventricle to the right atrium may occur. More commonly, a shunt through a perimembranous VSD that is directly related to the septal commissure of the tricuspid valve may jet, through the commissure, into the right atrium. Alternatively, there may be a defect in the septal leaflet at the area of the membranous septum, with lack of the normal annular attachment across the septum at this point, allowing the defect to communicate with both the right atrium and the right ventricle. All these types of defects fall within the spectrum of Gerbode defects.

ASSOCIATED ANOMALIES

Although VSDs are present in a wide range of more complex malformations (e.g., tetralogy of Fallot, tricuspid atresia, transposition), the only associated anomalies discussed here are those in which the combination of abnormalities present does not fall within any category dealt with elsewhere in this book. Associated atrial septal defect or persistent ductus arteriosus is relatively common although often clinically masked by and less significant than the VSD. On the other hand, associated aortic arch obstruction (e.g., coarctation or aortic arch interruption), which also occurs frequently, is usually of major clinical importance and may dominate the clinical picture—the VSD being of less significance, at least in the early neonatal period.

Associated left ventricular outflow tract obstruction, either valvar or subvalvar aortic stenosis, may compound the clinical problem and add to the complexity of management. By contrast, associated right ventricular outflow tract obstruction (valvar pulmonary stenosis or infundibular stenosis) may be well tolerated and often tends to diminish the effects of the VSD, especially if the septal defect is large. The development of increasing infundibular obstruction, which occurs in about 5% of patients with VSD, is probably related to progressive hypertrophy of anomalous muscle bundles in the right ventricle. This may progress during several months, leading to tight infundibular stenosis, resembling that associated with tetralogy of Fallot.

Other obstructive lesions of the left side of the heart, such as subaortic stenosis[24, 25] or mitral or supramitral stenosis, may also occur with VSD. The extent to which they aggravate the effects of the VSD depends on the severity of the associated obstruction.

Important but uncommon associated anomalies include those in which the mitral or the tricuspid valve overrides or straddles the VSD, because of malalignment between the atrial and the ventricular septa.

So-called aneurysms of the membranous septum are found in a high proportion of patients with a perimembranous defect, in which a fibrous sack around the right ventricular side of the VSD may partially occlude even a moderately large hole (see Fig. 21–4). These "aneurysms" are usually derived from tricuspid leaflet tissue, either of the septal leaflet or from accessory leaflet material, adherent to the rim of the VSD. The process of adhesion to the edge of the defect often progresses during months or years, leading to spontaneous diminution in size or closure in many patients.[26–30]

Aortic valve prolapse may be found in patients with a subarterial VSD; the aortic valve leaflet adjacent to the defect may be "sucked" into the septal defect with each ventricular contraction, as blood jets at high pressure through the hole into the right ventricle. This phenomenon is particularly characteristic of doubly committed defects, in which the prolapsing leaflet (the right coronary leaflet) may partially occlude the VSD, creating the impression clinically that the defect is small. Some perimembranous defects are associated with prolapse of the noncoronary or the right coronary leaflet. Prolapse tends, in months or years, to lead to progressively increasing aortic incompetence (see Fig. 21–18).[31–34]

CARDIAC CONDUCTION SYSTEM

An understanding of the location of the cardiac conduction system is essential for a cardiac surgeon, if damage to this pathway is to be avoided in operating on defects that involve related parts of the heart.[35–41] Details of the normal anatomy are given in Chapter 9 and Figure 21–7.

The position of the conducting system in relation to VSDs is easily understood when the site of the defect is viewed in relation to anatomic landmarks. Those defects that directly abut the area of the membranous septum and central fibrous body (perimembranous defects) always have the conducting tissue at the posteroinferior margin of the VSD and related to the crest of the trabecular part of the ventricular septum (see Fig. 21–7). With inlet perimembranous defects, the atrioventricular node and His bundle are posteriorly displaced, and the bundle pursues a longer than normal course on the crest of the ventricular septum (as occurs with atrioventricular septal defects). With other types

Conducting system and VSD sites

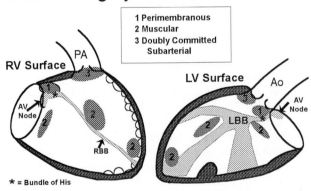

FIGURE 21–7

Diagram showing the relationship of the atrioventricular (AV) node, bundle of His *(asterisk)*, and main bundle branches to the common sites of VSDs: *1,* perimembranous—the bundle of His runs close to the posteroinferior margin of such defects; *2,* muscular defects—inlet defects lie posterior to the bundle of His and bundle branches; midmuscular and anterior or apical defects may lie between ramifications of the left bundle branch but are usually well separated from the bundle of His and the AV node; *3,* doubly committed subarterial defect—well separated from the bundle of His, unless the defect extends posteriorly to involve the membranous septum. Ao = aorta; PA = pulmonary artery; RV = right ventricle; LV = left ventricle; RBB = right bundle branch; LBB = left bundle branch.

of perimembranous defects, the position of the His bundle tends to be more nearly normal, with a short course for the bundle before bifurcation immediately below the aortic valve on the left side of the crest of the trabecular septum. Inlet muscular defects lie consistently below and behind the conducting pathways. Trabecular defects usually open into the right ventricle anterior to the right bundle branch and into the left ventricle at a variable point, often with the radiations of the left bundle branch running around the anterior and the posterior margins of the defect. Most such defects are distant from the bundle of His, although those that are close to the atrioventricular junction may have only a thin rim of muscle separating the defect from the bundle, which may therefore be vulnerable (see Fig. 21–7). Outlet defects (muscular or doubly committed) are usually separated from the area of the membranous septum, although some may have only a slender muscle bar between the defect and the membranous septum. Almost always, the conducting system is at a distance from the margins of the hole and relatively safe from operative damage.

Thus, the surgeon needs to know that with a perimembranous defect, the conducting system is likely to lie at the posteroinferior margin of the defect, where it is vulnerable. With muscular defects, the bundle of His is usually less likely to be damaged, lying in the anterosuperior rim of the defect with inlet defects and posterior to or inferior to most trabecular and outlet defects (see Fig. 21–7).[35, 36, 39–42]

EMBRYOLOGY

The development of the ventricular septum is complex; at least three separate but interlinked processes contribute. After looping of the cardiac tube, the area on the outer convexity of the ventricular loop, at the junction of the primitive ventricle and the bulbus cordis, starts to fold inward at the same time as the trabecular pouches of the primitive ventricle and the bulbus start to expand outward. As the ventricular cavities are enlarging, this infolding initiates the formation of a ridge on the inside of the loop that then extends progressively toward the inner curvature of the loop, forming the primary ventricular septum. Experimentally, labeled cells at the bulboventricular junction have been shown to migrate inward as the ventricular septum increases in size—moving from the distal part of the septum toward its crest.[43] With this process, the bulboventricular foramen becomes clearly delineated.

Simultaneously with this process, the atrioventricular canal expands to the right, allowing a direct connection between the right side of the early atrial cavity and the bulbus cordis. Within the atrioventricular canal, the endocardial cushions appear, and as the anterior and posterior cushions enlarge, they become aligned with the primary ventricular septum. Fusion of the anterior and posterior cushions with one another and with the posterior end of the ventricular septum partitions the ventricular inlets. This closes off the posterior end of the bulboventricular foramen, which now lies at the anterior margin of the fused cushions.

At the same time, the outlet septum is being formed by the cushions in the outlet part of the bulbus cordis, an area that itself is moving inward and to the left so that the arterial outlets (still undivided) can connect in part to the primitive ventricle. This is permitted by realignment of the bulboventricular foramen from a more or less sagittal plane to an oblique transverse plane. Separation of the outlets, by fusion of the outlet cushions with one another and with the anterior end of the primary septum, leaves the more posterior arterial outlet (the aorta) connected to the developing left ventricle (derived from the primitive ventricle). On the other hand, the anterior (pulmonary) artery is connected to the developing right ventricle (derived from the bulbus cordis). The remaining communication between the two ventricles lies between the three components of the septum. It is demarcated apically by the primary septum, anterosuperiorly by the outlet septum, and posteroinferiorly by the atrioventricular cushions. With further development, this area becomes progressively smaller and finally seals off with fibrous tissue, forming the membranous septum. The bulboventricular foramen itself persists as the left ventricular outlet to the aorta. Thus, the contributing parts of the developing septum correspond, more or less, to the components of the septum of the mature heart.

Septal defects may be the consequence of several factors. Failure of complete formation of the primary septum may contribute to trabecular defects, although it is likely that many muscular defects in the trabecular septum result from excessive undermining beneath and between trabeculae, during formation of the trabecular part of the septum, leaving defects between trabeculae. Failure of fusion of the atrioventricular cushions, with each other or with the primary septum, may leave an inlet defect (either as part of an atrioventricular septal defect or as an isolated defect). Malalignment or poor development of the outlet cushions contributes to outlet defects, as has been demonstrated experimentally.[44] Finally, failure of complete closure of the area that forms the membranous septum leaves a perimembranous defect. Many defects in this area are much larger than the membranous septum and are likely to result from incomplete development of one or other components of the muscular septum. This leaves a communication of such a substantial size that the normal mechanism for formation of the membranous septum is unable to effect complete closure.

PHYSIOLOGY

As the pulmonary circulation increases immediately after birth, with expansion of the lungs and pulmonary vasodilatation, pulmonary artery pressure drops from the slightly suprasystemic prenatal levels to subsystemic levels. With the closure of the ductus arteriosus in the early hours of postnatal life, an increasing discrepancy develops between pulmonary and systemic pressures and resistances. Subsequently, during several weeks, growth and maturation of the intra-acinar arterioles in the pulmonary circulation are associated with a continuing fall in vascular resistance. This process of growth and remodeling, with multiplication of intra-acinar arterioles in parallel with alveolar multiplication, continues for many months, so that the adult state of the lung vasculature is not reached for several years.[45] As these changes take place, the effects of a VSD on the circulation, and the clinical manifestations thereof, gradually evolve. Immediately after birth, there may be little shunting with a moderate or large defect. As pulmonary vascular resistance drops, however, a left-to-right shunt develops. With a small (restrictive) defect, the shunt is small, with little effect on either pulmonary blood flow or pressure. With each ventricular contraction, a small part of the left ventricular stroke volume is ejected into the right ventricle. The volume of the shunt is determined by the size of the defect and the systolic pressure difference between the ventricles. The amount of turbulence generated by the shunt is closely related to the pressure difference between the ventricles and the shunt volume—the larger the shunt and the higher the pressure gradient, the greater the resultant turbulence. The clinical manifestations of a VSD are closely linked to the size of the shunt (symptoms) and the amount of turbulence generated (which determines the loudness of the associated murmur). With a small defect, the shunt is small and symptoms are absent. The amount of turbulence, however, may be substantial (because of a large pressure difference between the ventricles), and the murmur may be loud and of relatively high frequency.

With a larger defect, the size of the left-to-right shunt increases progressively as pulmonary resistance falls during many weeks. In many patients, pulmonary artery pressure remains elevated because of the large shunt and a "nonrestrictive" VSD, which results in the systolic pressure in the two ventricles being at similar levels. The persistence of high pulmonary arterial pressure postnatally results in vasoconstriction in the pulmonary arterioles and retards the process of growth and maturation of the intra-acinar arterioles.[46,47] Both factors slow the extent to which pulmonary vascular resistance falls postnatally and hence reduce the size of the shunt, at least during the early weeks of life. Nonetheless, in most patients, the shunt volume increases to the point that within 2 to 3 weeks of birth, at least 50% (and often substantially more) of the left ventricular stroke volume is ejected through the VSD into the right ventricle and pulmonary circulation. A shunt of this size, especially when it is associated with significant elevation of pulmonary artery pressure (as often occurs), usually leads to the onset of symptoms, with dyspnea, tachypnea, and poor feeding being prominent. In the early weeks of life, before symptoms develop, the auscultatory signs may be unimpressive, with only a soft, nonspecific murmur or sometimes no murmur. In patients with a large, nonrestrictive VSD, there is no significant pressure gradient between the ventricles during systole. Therefore, the amount of turbulence generated by shunting may be small until the shunt becomes large enough to produce significant symptoms.

CLINICAL FEATURES

SYMPTOMS

Most infants with a VSD are asymptomatic at the time of presentation and come to notice when a murmur is detected on auscultation, either in the neonatal period or subsequently. At least 75% of affected patients have a defect that is small and have a small left-to-right shunt.[9] Such infants remain asymptomatic, feeding and thriving normally. If careful assessment of such patients confirms that the shunt is small and that the heart is not subjected to a significant hemodynamic disturbance, there is little likelihood of symptoms developing, and the family may be reassured accordingly. In those who have a larger defect, the shunt is often restricted during the first 2 weeks of life by the high pulmonary vascular resistance. While the left-to-right shunt remains small, the baby shows few symptoms. As pulmonary resistance falls, however, the increased pulmonary blood flow returning to the left atrium leads to the onset of pulmonary venous congestion with tachypnea, dyspnea, and feeding difficulties. Further rise in pulmonary blood flow, as resistance continues to drop, frequently produces more severe symptoms of high-output cardiac failure. The increased calorie demands resulting from the combination of high cardiac output and increased respiratory effort, coupled with reduced calorie intake due to difficulty feeding, lead to poor weight gain (failure to thrive). The onset of symptoms is usually between 2 and 6 weeks of age. The physiologic anemia of early infancy adds to the cardiac difficulties.

Associated abnormalities may alter the symptoms substantially. For instance, coexistent coarctation of the aorta usually leads to earlier symptoms, often in the first 2 weeks of life, with dyspnea, poor feeding, and rapid progression to severe manifestations of cardiac or respiratory failure. Conversely, the coexistence of infundibular pulmonary stenosis, even with a large unrestrictive VSD, limits the left-to-right shunt so that symptoms are absent and the baby may thrive normally. Later in infancy, if the infundibular obstruction progresses to the point that pulmonary blood flow is reduced, cyanosis becomes manifest owing to right-to-left shunting across the VSD (a combination that may represent a form of tetralogy of Fallot).[48]

Older children with a significant shunt have reduced exercise duration. With exercise, too, uniform premature ventricular contractions are frequent, and multiform premature contractions and couplets occasionally occur.

SIGNS

In the early neonatal period, a small defect, despite being restrictive, does not always produce a typical murmur; the murmur may be of medium frequency and occur in early to mid systole rather than being high-pitched and pansystolic in timing. In the early weeks of life, the murmur becomes characteristic of a small VSD, becoming harsher, higher pitched, and of longer duration during systole (usually pansystolic). There are usually few if any other abnormal findings. The peripheral pulses are normal, as is the cardiac impulse. A thrill is present when the murmur is of sufficient loudness. The murmur and thrill are most evident along the left sternal border, although the site of maximal intensity varies, being most often in the third and fourth interspaces but sometimes as high as the second space (which often indicates a high anterior muscular or outlet VSD). An apical muscular defect may produce a murmur that is best heard toward the apex and may be mistaken for the murmur of mitral regurgitation.

Some small defects are associated with a shorter decrescendo murmur, starting at the first sound and fading by mid or late systole. These high-pitched, early systolic murmurs are particularly characteristic of a small muscular defect. As with other types of VSD, the physical signs may be atypical during the early weeks of life, although in later childhood, this type of murmur (very high pitched, early systolic, localized) is typical. It is easily recognized by an experienced observer, and the diagnosis may be made with a high degree of confidence on clinical grounds alone.

With a larger VSD, the signs are often different. In the early neonatal period and for several weeks, there may be no murmur or only a soft, nonspecific ejection murmur. As the shunt increases with gradual fall in pulmonary vascular resistance, the murmur becomes louder, often becoming longer and more pansystolic. At the same time, with the increasing size of the left-to-right shunt, accompanied as it is (with a large VSD) by pulmonary hypertension, the heart becomes increasingly hyperdynamic. This is associated with a palpable systolic impulse at the left sternal edge due to the dilated and hypertensive right ventricle. During several weeks, the infant may develop precordial prominence. At the apex, a mid-diastolic murmur due to high flow across the mitral valve becomes audible.

During this time, most infants become increasingly dyspneic and tachypneic and may manifest marked intercostal and subcostal recession. Bilateral Harrison's sulci may appear because of distortion of the thoracic cage at the sites of the diaphragmatic attachments. Poor weight gain may be seen in some patients.

The loudness of the pulmonary component of the second heart sound (P_2) is often assumed to be a reliable indicator of pulmonary hypertension. Accentuation of the pulmonary closure sound, however, is greatly influenced by pulmonary artery diastolic pressure (rather than systolic pressure). Many infants with systolic pulmonary hypertension of severe degree, due to a large, nonrestrictive VSD, have little accentuation of P_2 in the early months of life because pulmonary vascular resistance is low. Subsequently, they develop an obviously loud second sound, by which time pulmonary vascular disease may be well established. Thus, to wait until P_2 is clearly loud may be to risk the development of significant pulmonary vascular damage.

NATURAL COURSE

SPONTANEOUS DIMINUTION IN SIZE AND CLOSURE

Many VSDs become smaller or close spontaneously. Muscular defects often close by a process of ingrowth of muscle at the margins. Some perimembranous defects diminish in size by accretion of fibrous tissue at the edges and progressive adhesion of tricuspid leaflet tissue, or accessory leaflet tissue, to the septum around the defect; this process often produces a pouch of fibrous/leaflet tissue, which has usually been referred to as an aneurysm of the membranous septum. The presence, on echocardiography or angiography, of such an aneurysm is usually a favorable prognostic sign that spontaneous diminution in size of the VSD is occurring or is likely to take place.[29,49-53] There are, however, exceptions to this course.

Some VSDs are unlikely to diminish in size. These include defects in which semilunar leaflets of the aortic or pulmonary valve form the basal margin of the VSD, as occurs with many malalignment defects and doubly committed subarterial defects. Defects of the latter type may appear to be partially closed (and may be clinically small or trivial) by the distorted aortic sinus (usually the right coronary sinus) or semilunar leaflet tissue, which is entrapped in and partially occludes the septal defect (see later section on aortic valve prolapse).

The frequency with which VSDs close spontaneously is unknown. At least 70% of defects present at birth will probably undergo closure, usually within the first year or two of life.[50,52,53] Because many tiny VSDs are undetected clinically (being found only with echocardiography, when it is performed for other reasons), the actual rate of closure may never be completely documented. Of defects that are clinically apparent, the rate of spontaneous closure has been estimated as being up to 75%.[50] Whereas most defects that undergo spontaneous closure are small, some larger and clinically significant defects diminish in size so that they are of little clinical significance or even close completely.

PULMONARY VASCULAR DISEASE

Large defects, associated with pulmonary hypertension, may lead to progressive pulmonary vascular obstructive disease if operation is delayed and pulmonary hypertension persists beyond infancy. The pulmonary vascular changes, which have been documented in infants and children with pulmonary hypertension, compose two distinct but overlapping processes. The first set of abnormalities represents acute responses to the elevation of pressure that is present with a large septal defect after birth, at a time when pulmonary artery pressure normally falls rapidly. In the presence of a high pulmonary blood flow, pulmonary arterial and venous muscularity increases, muscle extends into more peripheral arteries than normal, and there is a reduction in size and number of intra-acinar arteries. Occluded alveolar wall arteries are seen on electron microscopic examination, probably secondary to the hyperplasia and hypertrophy of differentiating smooth muscle cells in small, normally thin-walled precapillary segments. Quantitative morphometry has demonstrated poor growth and reduced branching of arterioles within the acinus in the early months. As a consequence, the total capacity of the arteriolar circulation is progressively reduced.[47,54,55] These changes are probably reversible if the pulmonary hypertension resolves before about 6 months because of spontaneous diminution in size of the VSD or operative repair thereof. Infants who are operated on at a later age may be left with a permanent reduction in the total capacity of their pulmonary arteriolar tree. This is probably the explanation for the well-documented phenomenon that pulmonary artery pressure, when measured years after operation, may increase to markedly abnormal levels as cardiac output rises with exercise.[56]

The second process through which changes develop in the pulmonary vasculature appears gradually during many months or years. Intimal thickening, coupled with pre-existing medial hypertrophy, is followed by progressive occlusion (by intimal lesions and intravascular thrombosis). Intimal proliferation tends to develop toward the end of the first year and fibrosis during the third year of life. Patients with severe pulmonary hypertension should thus be operated on before the age of 2 years and preferably before the age of 1 year. Intimal abnormalities gradually worsen with age and resistance increases. Progressive obstruction of the preacinar arterial lumen is associated with a reduction in intra-acinar arterial muscularity in the more distal arteries. Progression is relatively slow in the majority of children with this abnormality, and grade IV pulmonary vascular disease seldom occurs in young children with a VSD. In the minority of children who have severe obstructive intimal proliferation early, the arteries beyond the intimal obstruction have a relatively normal medial thickness, there is no generalized arterial dilatation or other stigmata of grade IV pulmonary vascular disease, and the pulmonary arteriolar resistance can exceed 6 units/m^2. In one study, these predilatation features were present in 62% of patients who either died at operation or had postoperative pulmonary hypertension. These observations suggest that a relatively low peripheral pulmonary arterial muscularity in patients with a VSD and severe pulmonary hypertension (mean pulmonary arterial pressure higher than 40 mm Hg after 6 months of age) represents a predilatation phase and that the severity of proximal luminal obstruction may prejudice the outcome of intracardiac repair.

New vessel formation around areas of vascular occlusion creates complex vascular lesions (plexiform lesions).[6,7] As pulmonary vascular obstructive disease progresses, there is a gradual increase in pulmonary vascular resistance. This may initially bring about clinical improvement as the left-to-right shunt decreases. Symptoms of a large shunt (poor weight gain, breathlessness) may disappear, and a false impression may be given that the heart problem is improving. Later, usually after several years, the shunt may become balanced, with little shunt in either direction, as pulmonary and systemic resistances become equal. Eventually, as pulmonary resistance continues to rise, shunt reversal develops and cyanosis begins to appear, producing the features of Eisenmenger's syndrome. Some cardiologists believe that children with Down syndrome are prone to early pulmonary vascular disease and tend to operate on these children earlier than they would on a child with normal chromosomes.

VENTRICULAR SEPTAL DEFECT IN ADULT LIFE

An unrepaired VSD, persisting in adult life, is relatively frequent. Surprisingly, its course and natural history remain inadequately documented. Many small defects persist into middle adult life and beyond without causing symptoms. Some undergo spontaneous closure, even in advanced adult life. Infective endocarditis (see later) occurs with greater frequency than in the childhood years.[57]

Gradual decompensation, with increasing effort intolerance and ventricular dilatation, is a familiar sequence of events in middle adult life but probably affects only those individuals who have had a moderate-sized shunt throughout life (e.g., Qp/Qs ratio of 1.5 to 2.0 or larger). Some degree of pulmonary hypertension may be present in these

patients, although this may be, at least in part, the consequence of left-sided heart failure.

Those individuals who survive to adult life with an unrepaired large defect and pulmonary hypertension almost always present the clinical features of Eisenmenger's syndrome. Shunt reversal, secondary to obliterative pulmonary vascular disease, occurs during adolescence or early adult life, unless progression of the pulmonary vascular changes was unusually rapid and led to earlier shunt reversal during childhood. Cyanosis is slowly progressive, with development of finger clubbing, compensatory polycythemia, and increasing exercise intolerance. Effort syncope may occur. Sudden death, especially during exercise, is relatively common, and death during pregnancy is a major risk among affected women, who should be strongly advised against becoming pregnant.[58] Most patients who develop the Eisenmenger syndrome die during their third, fourth, or fifth decade of life, although a few may live longer.[59-61] Lung or heart-lung transplantation offers good-quality short-term to medium-term palliation for some affected individuals.

COMPLICATING PROBLEMS

AORTIC VALVE PROLAPSE

Defects adjacent to the semilunar leaflets of the aortic valve may be associated with a phenomenon referred to as aortic valve prolapse. In this condition, the aortic sinus, which forms the roof of the defect, becomes distorted or dilated (sometimes developing an aneurysm of the sinus of Valsalva), and the leaflet starts to herniate into the VSD. In some patients, there is systolic displacement of the leaflet into the VSD, associated with a jet of blood passing at high pressure through the defect (Venturi effect). In other instances, the distorted aortic sinus fills in a large part of the defect, without systolic displacement of the leaflet itself. The type of VSD in which aortic prolapse occurs is usually the doubly committed subarterial ventricular septal defect.[31-34] However, a perimembranous defect may also be associated with a similar problem, if the VSD lies immediately adjacent to the aortic valve, with no intervening septal remnant. With a doubly committed defect, the right coronary sinus is involved; with a perimembranous defect, either the right or the noncoronary sinus is affected (or rarely both are).

Aortic valve prolapse is a consequence of the anatomic relationship between the aortic valve and the VSD. It usually develops during the first 5 to 10 years of life but can occasionally appear later. Aneurysms of an aortic sinus tend to appear during teenage years or later.[62] Increasing aortic regurgitation gradually develops after an interval and progresses, unless the defect is repaired. The clinical manifestations of the VSD are usually unaffected by prolapse (except for the fact that the prolapsing leaflet may partially obstruct the VSD and lessen the effects of the VSD). The diagnosis is made by echocardiography or by angiography (see Figs. 21–17 and 21–18).

Patients with a VSD, either repaired or otherwise, are at increased risk for development of gradually progressive aortic incompetence in adulthood, even in the absence of aortic valve prolapse.[63]

INFUNDIBULAR STENOSIS

Infundibular stenosis associated with a VSD is observed in 5 to 7% of patients. Obstruction results from gradual hypertrophy of anomalous right ventricular muscle bundles. Such abnormal muscle bundles are probably an associated abnormality and not due to hypertrophy of the right ventricle alone (with otherwise normal architecture). In contrast, pure right ventricular hypertrophy, as occurs with severe pulmonary stenosis, leads to secondary infundibular stenosis, but not with anomalous muscle bundles. The obstruction restricts the shunt and reduces symptoms when the VSD is large.

As infundibular stenosis progresses with time, the clinical picture and hemodynamic disturbance evolve. The infundibular stenosis is often unsuspected clinically, because the murmur of the obstruction tends to be overshadowed and masked by that from the VSD. The obstruction is frequently mild initially and the shunt across the VSD substantial, producing the signs and symptoms of a large VSD. Later, as the stenosis increases, the clinical picture changes with a reduction in symptoms and evidence of a smaller shunt.[48] The murmur may become harsher, suggesting that the VSD is becoming smaller. A clue to the diagnosis may be found on the electrocardiogram, which often shows disproportionate right ventricular hypertrophy. Doppler echocardiography demonstrates that the gradient across the right ventricular outflow tract is substantial (with velocities often of 4 m/sec or greater) and that the VSD is still large. If the obstruction becomes tight enough to reduce pulmonary blood flow, cyanosis appears, and the clinical picture and the hemodynamics become identical with tetralogy of Fallot.[48]

INFECTIVE ENDOCARDITIS

The risk of infective endocarditis with a small VSD is relatively high; it is probably lower with a larger defect. Also at risk are patients who have had VSD repair, especially if the defect is incompletely closed. The risk of endocarditis with VSD is of the order of 2.5 per 1000 patient-years.[64–67] This is equivalent to 2.5% for each 10 years of follow-up. The risk is lower during childhood and increases in adolescence and adult life. Patients with a small VSD, who have had a proven episode of endocarditis, are probably at increased risk of a recurrent infection.

LABORATORY STUDIES

ELECTROCARDIOGRAPHY

The electrocardiogram in patients with a VSD reflects the severity and nature of the hemodynamic disturbance. With a small defect, the tracing may be normal, and the absence of any abnormality is indirect evidence that the VSD is hemodynamically unimportant. Left axis deviation occurs in a small number of patients and may reflect abnormal distribution of the left bundle branch.[68] Without other electrocardiographic abnormalities, it is usually of no sinister significance, but if partial or complete right bundle branch block coexists, an atrioventricular septal defect needs to be excluded.

With a moderate or large shunt, the electrocardiogram manifests evidence of combined ventricular hypertrophy with increased left ventricular voltages along with prominent right ventricular forces or large combined voltages $(R + S)$ in the midchest leads (V_3, V_4) (Katz-Wachtel phenomenon).[69] Left atrial enlargement is also found in some patients.

Voltage evidence of left ventricular hypertrophy alone occurs, especially in later childhood, in patients with an unrepaired VSD with a significant shunt and nearly normal pulmonary arterial pressure.

Isolated right ventricular hypertrophy is a feature of infants with associated infundibular stenosis (similar to tetralogy of Fallot) or of patients with severe established pulmonary vascular disease (Eisenmenger's syndrome)

CHEST RADIOGRAPHY

Like the electrocardiogram, the chest radiograph reflects the hemodynamic disturbance. If cardiac size and the lung fields appear normal, there is a minor left-to-right shunt and a hemodynamically unimportant defect.

An increase in the transverse cardiac diameter usually indicates a significant shunt (Fig. 21–8). The left ventricular apex is displaced laterally and inferiorly (associated with left ventricular dilatation). Right ventricular dilatation may lead to the appearance of a smooth convexity on the left upper cardiac border, extending upward from the left ventricular silhouette and continuing onto an enlarged pulmonary conus. The left atrium may also be enlarged, producing flattening (upward displacement) of the left main bronchus and sometimes a double shadow over the right atrium. The lateral projection may also provide evidence of right ventricular enlargement and left atrial dilatation. Interpretation of pulmonary vascular markings must be made cautiously, because many factors discussed in Chap-

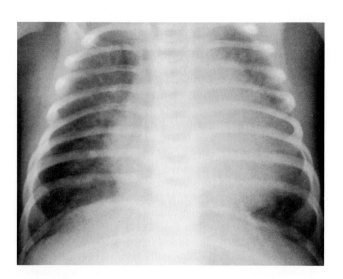

FIGURE 21–8

Chest film showing cardiac enlargement and pulmonary plethora from an infant with a large VSD with associated aortic coarctation.

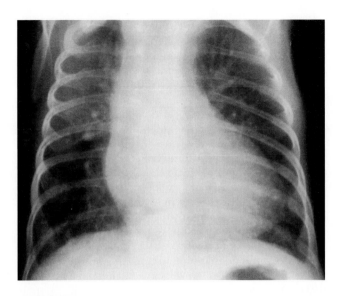

Chest film showing mild cardiac enlargement and slight increase in vascular markings. This infant actually had a large, nonrestrictive VSD, illustrating the fact that the x-ray appearance may be misleading and may suggest that the defect is much smaller than it actually is.

ter 10 will affect the appearance and can give a false impression of increased (or reduced) pulmonary vascularity. Increased pulmonary arterial markings are evident as vessels seen in cross-section in the hilar regions, which are distinctly larger than their accompanying bronchi. Prominent vessels are usually seen well out into the middle and upper zones of the lung, whereas such markings are seen only in the lower zones (particularly on the right side) in the normal chest radiograph.

Hyperinflation is frequently seen in an infant with a large shunt and probably reflects altered pulmonary compliance. Pulmonary congestion with interstitial edema may appear, and infective changes may be superimposed. The size of the cardiac silhouette and the extent of the pulmonary vascular changes are, in general, a good guide to the size of the shunt through the VSD. An occasional patient, however, seems to have a large shunt even without much cardiac enlargement (Fig. 21–9).

Development of pulmonary vascular obstructive disease in later childhood may be associated with a reduction in cardiac size toward normal. The central pulmonary vascular markings become prominent, but the peripheral pulmonary vasacularity (beyond the hilar areas) becomes reduced ("pruned").

ECHOCARDIOGRAPHY

Diagnosis of VSD depends mainly on a combination of cross-sectional images and color flow mapping.[70] M-mode and conventional Doppler imaging are used to obtain additional quantitative information—mainly reflecting hemodynamic effects of the VSD.[71–74]

The conventional scanning planes used to image the ventricular septum may each provide data about defects at different sites. Because the septum is a complex structure and is curved to different degrees at different levels (from apex to base), a combination of views is needed to study the entire septum. Individual patients vary markedly in the extent to which the various echocardiographic windows offer good imaging. It is easier to obtain satisfactory pictures from younger children than from older children or adults (especially from the subcostal window).

Imaging of a VSD should always be performed from more than one view; dropout may give an impression in one plane of a defect that cannot be confirmed when the same area is viewed in a different plane. A genuine defect usually has a clearly defined echogenic edge when the plane of section is at right angles to the margin of the defect. By contrast, areas of dropout tend to have "fuzzy" edges. With color flow mapping, it is almost always possible to confirm a suspicion of a VSD by demonstrating a color jet passing across the defect. Failure to obtain color evidence of a shunt usually implies that the defect, shown on imaging, is not real.

With many small VSDs, color flow mapping may provide the first clue (sometimes the only evidence) of a defect. The apparent presence of a VSD, indicated by a color jet, should be confirmed by conventional Doppler if imaging does not demonstrate any apparent defect at the site in question. This should demonstrate high-velocity flow at the site of the jet if a defect is genuinely present.

Parasternal long-axis and short-axis views are useful for imaging many VSDs. A perimembranous defect is often not well seen in the standard long-axis plane but usually can be identified in high short-axis planes. The jet may be identified, just below the aortic valve, by use of color flow mapping in a short-axis scan and in a medially rotated long-axis plane (Fig. 21–10 [see Color Plates]).

These defects are usually well seen from an apical four-chamber view by tilting the transducer forward toward the aortic root (Fig. 21–11 [see Color Plates]). A subcostal four-chamber view provides a slightly different view of this area. Aneurysmal tissue around such a VSD is best seen from the apical and subxiphoid views but may also be identified in short-axis planes.

A doubly committed subarterial defect may be seen in a conventional long-axis view (Fig. 21–12 [see Color Plates]) and in a high short-axis plane. In this view, the site of the defect, adjacent to the pulmonary valve (as well as the aortic valve), may be readily identified by the direction of the color jet with color flow mapping (see Fig. 21–12). The jet is oriented anteriorly and slightly toward the patient's left. The defect is immediately adjacent to both arterial valves, in distinction to the jet through a perimembranous defect, which is directed mainly to the patient's right and slightly anteriorly.

Such defects are well demonstrated by subxiphoid views with the transducer in a more or less sagittal view, with a little rotation to produce an oblique plane from left anterior to right posterior. This demonstrates the defect below the arterial valves and confirms that the pulmonary and aortic valves are immediately adjacent to one another and at the same level, without an infundibular (outlet) septum separating the ventricular outlets below the valves.

A malalignment defect, of the type in tetralogy of Fallot, is usually seen in long-axis planes, high short-axis planes, and apical or subxiphoid four-chamber views angled toward the aortic valve. The outlet septum, which is usually well formed, is characteristically deviated or rotated away from the trabecular septum, which allows the aortic valve to sit astride the VSD (overriding). Significant overriding of the aortic valve, with the rightward wall of the aorta deviated away from the line of the septum, suggests that there is malalignment. With an isolated perimembranous defect, by contrast, although part of the aortic sinus adjacent to the VSD may form the superior margin of the defect, the aortic wall is in line with the ventricular septum (see Fig. 21–11). In such defects, the extent to which the aortic lumen "overrides" the VSD is minor (being purely a consequence of the obliquity of the left ventricular outflow tract rather than malalignment).

Muscular VSDs may occur at almost any site within the muscular septum (Fig. 21–13 [see Color Plates]; see also Figs. 21–2, 21–3, and 21–12). A midmuscular defect may be imaged in conventional long-axis or short-axis planes. It is also well seen in apical and subxiphoid four-chamber views with angulation forward toward the aortic root. Inlet muscular defects are best seen in four-chamber planes, from the apex. Short-axis views and subxiphoid planes are also useful. An apical defect is often best seen in low short-axis views (see Fig. 21–12) and in subxiphoid views. A range of nonstandard oblique planes may be required to obtain satisfactory imaging, and in some patients, color flow mapping provides the only clear evidence of defects at this site, especially if they are small.

Defects in the anterior septum and in the outlet septum can be difficult to assess. Such defects are sometimes multiple and provide a great challenge to the echocardiographer and to the surgeon. A full range of conventional and intermediate views is required to examine this area comprehensively, and even then some defects of significant size may escape detection.[75–78]

Small muscular VSDs have been difficult to confirm echocardiographically in the past. With the advent of color flow mapping, however, these defects can generally be demonstrated convincingly, even when imaging shows no definite break in the septum. Nonetheless, there remain a small number of children with clear-cut signs of a small defect (e.g., a high-pitched, localized, early systolic murmur) in whom no defect can be demonstrated on echocardiography. This probably indicates that the defect is in an unusual site in the septum, which is difficult to access with either imaging or color flow mapping. This is a less frequent phenomenon in most major centers than the finding of a tiny muscular VSD, clearly shown on color flow mapping and confirmed with conventional Doppler, in a patient without clinical evidence of a septal defect being scanned for some other reason.[12]

With color flow mapping, small multiple defects are seen much more frequently now than previously. This may indicate that the frequency of such multiple VSDs (particularly small ones) is higher than has been documented in the past with use of other diagnostic modalities.[79]

Once the site and size of the VSD have been identified with cross-sectional imaging and color flow mapping, the severity of the hemodynamic disturbance may be evaluated with M-mode echocardiography and conventional Doppler, coupled with evidence from imaging of other structures.

Dilatation of the left ventricle and of the left atrium is evidence of a significant left-to-right shunt. Doppler interrogation of the VSD jet, using the color flow/imaging information to align the Doppler probe with the jet, allows an estimate of the systolic pressure difference between left ventricle and right ventricle.[80] By measuring arm blood pressure to assess systemic arterial systolic pressure, the level of the right ventricular and pulmonary artery systolic pressure can be estimated (provided that there is no coexisting aortic stenosis). Alternatively, right ventricular systolic pressure may be estimated by measuring the velocity of a tricuspid regurgitant jet (if one can be found) and adding the expected level of right atrial pressure to the calculated pressure gradient. By these means, it is usually possible to get a clear indication of the extent to which right ventricular systolic pressure is elevated in the individual patient. Measurement of pulmonary artery diastolic pressure is less useful, although the velocity of a pulmonary regurgitant jet may provide useful information.

Assessment of the size of shunts has been attempted by a wide range of methods.[81] The principle of all such calculations is to obtain quantitative data about valve area and mean flow across cardiac valves, with each cardiac cycle, and hence to derive figures for the ratio of pulmonary and systemic blood flows. Pulmonary flow may be estimated by studying flow across the pulmonary valve (subject to errors if the VSD jet is close to the pulmonary valve) or the mitral valve (subject to errors if there is an atrial shunt). Systemic flow may be estimated by measurements at the aortic valve or tricuspid valve. Unfortunately, these measurements are time-consuming and operator dependent, and the figures derived correlate only crudely with shunts calculated at cardiac catheterization, using the Fick method, or by radionuclide angiography.[82–84]

CARDIAC CATHETERIZATION AND ANGIOGRAPHY

Although echocardiography is now the main tool by which patients with a VSD are assessed, a number of questions may be difficult to answer precisely without cardiac catheterization. Shunt size and pulmonary artery pressure cannot be estimated accurately by noninvasive means. Pulmonary vascular resistance can only be inferred by indirect and imprecise means. Fortunately, most infants with a large defect and pulmonary hypertension do not need precise estimates of these variables, because the pulmonary vascular changes during the first 3 to 4 months are almost always reversible. On the other hand, after the first 6 months, patients presenting late with a large VSD merit cardiac catheterization to measure pulmonary pressure and resistance.

In some patients, it is difficult to be confident about the severity of the hemodynamic disturbance on clinical and echocardiographic grounds. In such children (e.g., the asymptomatic child with mild cardiomegaly and plethora or electrocardiographic changes), cardiac catheterization may be helpful in deciding whether it is safe to postpone an operation in the hope that the defect may become smaller or close. Additional abnormalities may also make catheterization and angiography desirable.

The question of which patients may be referred for operation without catheterization remains controversial.

Some centers continue to submit all symptomatic patients and those with a suspicion of pulmonary hypertension to catheter studies. Others, recognizing that the extent of the hemodynamic disturbance is often of secondary importance and that the child merits operation, do not perform catheterization provided there is only one VSD in a position that is accessible surgically. On the other hand, infants with a defect in an inaccessible site (e.g., apical muscular) or in whom there are multiple defects or additional problems may need catheterization and angiography. In an older child, depending on policy for surgical closure of a smaller defect, there may be a need to perform catheter studies to quantify the shunt. In many centers, it remains the policy not to recommend repair of a small defect (with a pulmonary-to-systemic flow ratio of less than 1.5:1). In borderline patients, precise measurement of the shunt is desirable.

Hemodynamic measurements at the catheter study include oxygen saturations from the superior vena cava (SVC), inferior vena cava (IVC), pulmonary vein (or left atrium, if it can be entered through a patent foramen or atrial septal defect), aorta, and pulmonary artery, including the main and branch pulmonary arteries. Additional saturation measurements may be obtained from other sites. In calculating a Qp/Qs ratio, a decision needs to be made whether to use the SVC saturation alone as representing "mixed venous" saturation or to use a formula to allow for the mixture of SVC and IVC and coronary sinus blood. I employ the formula

$$\text{mixed venous} = (3 \times \text{SVC} + 1 \times \text{IVC})/4$$

which provides a good approximation of mixed venous saturation.[85, 86]

Pressure measurements required include phasic and mean pressure in the right atrium, left atrium (and pulmonary artery wedge pressure), main pulmonary artery, and aorta and phasic pressures in the left ventricle and right ventricle.

Oxygen consumption should be measured in patients when calculation of pulmonary resistance is important. If equipment to measure oxygen is not available, assumed oxygen consumptions may be used.[86] However, measured oxygen consumption is frequently widely different from that which might be assumed, and large errors in calculation of pulmonary resistance result.[87]

In patients with elevated pulmonary vascular resistance, it is often desirable to test pulmonary vascular lability. This may be achieved by allowing the patient to breathe—or, if the patient is receiving general anesthesia, to be ventilated with—100% oxygen for at least 5 minutes, then repeating the hemodynamic measurements. Calculations of pulmonary/systemic blood flow and resistance, when the patient is receiving increased concentrations of oxygen, need to consider dissolved oxygen (see Chapter 13). A further fall in pulmonary vascular resistance may be achieved, in some patients, by adding nitric oxide (up to 80 ppm) to the inspired oxygen.[88, 89]

Decisions about suitability for repair in the presence of elevated pulmonary resistance depend on the level of resting resistance, the evidence of lability, and the patient's age. In my institution, levels exceeding 8 $U \cdot m^2$ (mm Hg/L/min/m^2) are regarded as strongly indicative of irreversible pulmonary vascular disease after the first year of life; hematocrit must be taken into account (see Chapter 13). Significant lability, with the level falling to less than 6 $U \cdot m^2$ in 100% oxygen, or with nitric oxide, and young age (e.g., <1 year), however, are features that in otherwise borderline patients might allow a decision to be made in favor of operation (or to seek further information on the extent of pulmonary vascular damage by performing a lung biopsy). Fortunately, few patients in developed countries now present with a VSD at a late stage, when the problem of pulmonary vascular disease is likely to be an issue.

Angiography

Angiographic delineation of VSDs has, until the last decade, been regarded as the "gold standard" in judging the relative merits of different diagnostic tools. Despite the dramatic improvements in imaging, made possible with advances in echocardiographic technology, and the availability of other emerging technologies (e.g., gated magnetic resonance imaging), angiography continues to be perceived by many cardiac surgeons as the most reliable modality, although most pediatric cardiologists with expertise in echocardiography would probably disagree!

Because of the complex shape of the ventricular septum and because septal defects occur at many sites, effective angiographic demonstration of VSDs requires a detailed understanding of the anatomy of the ventricular septum in the normal heart and with a range of cardiac malformations. The use of axial oblique views to profile the different parts of the ventricular septum accurately has made a major difference.[90-92] The radiographic projection used must be in line with the ventricular septum at the site of the VSD, so that contrast medium passing across the defect is seen in profile. It is usually possible to identify the site or sites of VSDs with echocardiography before cardiac catheterization, which makes the choice of projection much simpler.

Defects close to the membranous septum are best demonstrated by a left anterior oblique projection (40 to 45 degrees from lateral) with moderate craniocaudal tilt (20 degrees) (Fig. 21–14). This is not the conventional long-axial projection recommended for the demonstration of a perimembranous VSD. The conventional projection (30 degrees left anterior oblique with 15 degrees craniocaudal tilt) is more useful for showing trabecular muscular (Figs. 21–15 and 21–16), anterior muscular, or outlet muscular defects.

The so-called four-chamber view (16 degrees left anterior oblique with 30 degrees craniocaudal tilt) is used for profiling inlet defects and is particularly useful for demonstrating atrioventricular septal defects. A right anterior oblique projection is usually necessary to demonstrate doubly committed subarterial VSDs (Fig. 21–17). When biplane angiography is used, the second plane produces a right oblique projection when the first plane is recorded in a long-axial, four-chamber, or intermediate projection. Thus, if an appropriate projection is obtained to exclude defects in the midmuscular, anterior muscular, outlet muscular, or perimembranous areas, the second projection will

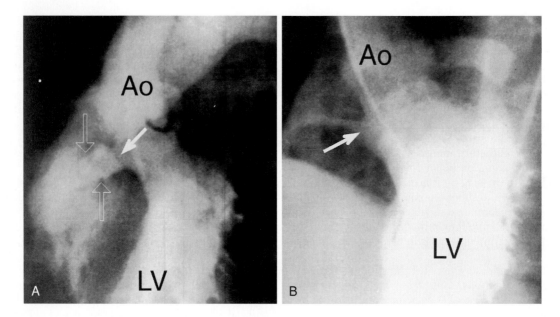

Angiogram, perimembranous defect. *A,* Left ventricular angiogram (left anterior oblique [LAO] projection of 45 degrees, craniocaudal [CC] tilt of 20 degrees) shows perimembranous defect *(arrow)* with some aneurysmal tissue on the right ventricular side *(open arrows)* and moderately large shunt. This defect is immediately related to the aortic valve. *B,* Left ventricular angiogram (LAO 45 degrees, CC 25 degrees) shows small perimembranous defect *(arrow),* which is separated from the aortic valve. Ao = aorta; LV = left ventricle.

usually demonstrate a doubly committed subarterial defect. The right oblique projection needed for defects of this type has been described by some authors as a "120-degree left anterior oblique." This seems an inappropriate description because left anterior oblique projections are those that lie between left lateral and anteroposterior (encompassing only 90 degrees). There is no uniformity in the way that cardiologists or radiologists describe oblique projections. Some use "30 degrees left anterior oblique" to describe a projection that is 30 degrees to the left of anteroposterior. Others, by contrast, use the same term to refer to a projection that is 30 degrees anterior of left lateral. In the descriptions used before, the oblique angulation is always counted from the lateral projection (e.g., 30 degrees left anterior oblique is 30 degrees from the lateral).

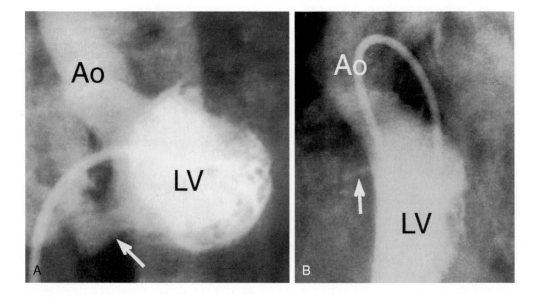

Angiogram, muscular VSD. *A,* Large midmuscular defect *(arrow)* is demonstrated on left ventricular angiogram (LAO 60 degrees, CC 20 degrees). *B,* Small midmuscular defect *(arrow)* is demonstrated on left ventricular angiogram (LAO 35 degrees, CC 15 degrees) (long-axial projection). Ao = aorta; LV = left ventricle.

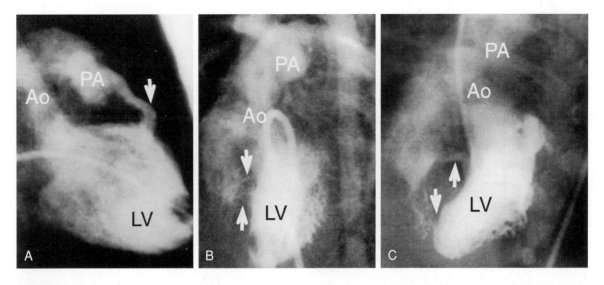

FIGURE 21–16

Angiogram, muscular and multiple VSDs. *A,* Left ventricular angiogram in right anterior oblique (RAO) view (RAO 45 degrees) shows moderate anterior muscular defect *(arrow)* with a tortuous course to the right ventricular outflow tract. *B,* Left ventricular angiogram (LAO 30 degrees, CC 15 degrees) shows multiple small trabecular defects (between the arrows). This angiogram was from the same patient as in *A. C,* Apical *(lower arrow)* and midmuscular *(upper arrow)* defects are demonstrated on left ventricular angiogram (LAO 45 degrees, CC 20 degrees). Ao = aorta; LV = left ventricle; PA = pulmonary artery.

As with good-quality echocardiography, the main requirement for angiography of VSDs relates to the need to identify multiple defects. Such defects can present a substantial challenge, both to the echocardiographer and to the cardiologist performing angiography. Multiple small muscular defects in the trabecular septum ("Swiss cheese" defects) are usually well demonstrated in a long-axial view (see Fig. 21–16). In some patients, however, there are several large defects at relatively distant sites within the septum. A moderate or large perimembranous VSD may be accompanied by muscular defects at the apex or in the anterior muscular septum. Multiple axial oblique projections may be required to adequately demonstrate all the defects. A limiting factor, which may be difficult to surmount, is the equalization of ventricular pressures, so that shunting across the several defects may not be sufficient to outline each of the defects satisfactorily.

The angiographic study should not neglect coexistent cardiovascular abnormalities that may require angiographic demonstration. Problems such as aortic coarctation or aortic regurgitation may necessitate an aortogram, which will also help to confirm aortic valve prolapse (Fig. 21–18) and exclude an associated patent ductus arteriosus. Right ventricular outflow obstruction (infundibular stenosis) or abnormalities of the pulmonary arteries, such as branch pulmonary artery stenosis, may necessitate a right ventricular angiogram or pulmonary arteriogram.

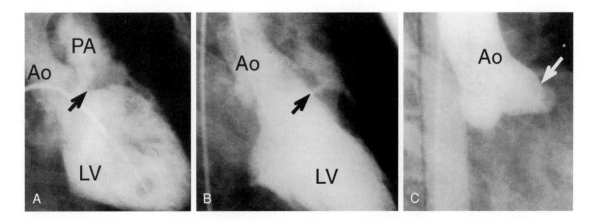

FIGURE 21–17

Angiogram, doubly committed subarterial defect. *A,* Left ventricular angiogram in RAO projection (RAO 60 degrees) shows jet of contrast agent passing into the right ventricular outflow tract and pulmonary artery through a moderately large defect *(arrow). B,* Left ventricular angiogram in RAO projection (RAO 60 degrees) shows a small defect *(arrow)* jetting into the right ventricular outflow tract. *C,* Aortogram from the same patient as in *B* (RAO projection) shows distorted and prolapsing right coronary sinus *(arrow),* which is largely occluding the VSD, but with no aortic incompetence. Ao = aorta; LV = left ventricle; PA = pulmonary artery.

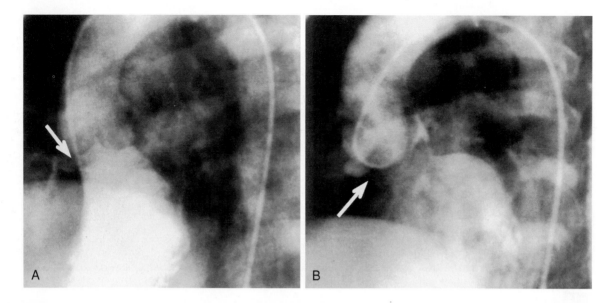

FIGURE 21–18

Angiogram, aortic valve prolapse. *A,* Left ventricular angiogram (LAO 30 degrees, CC 20 degrees) shows a small perimembranous VSD *(arrow)* adjacent to the aortic valve. *B,* Aortogram from the same patient demonstrates systolic prolapse of the right coronary leaflet *(arrow)* and moderate aortic regurgitation.

TREATMENT

MEDICAL

The medical management of children with a VSD is largely limited to treatment of congestive heart failure and prophylaxis of infective endocarditis.

In the early months of life, an infant with clinical manifestations of a large VSD associated with evidence of cardiac failure requires diuretic therapy with or without digoxin, the usefulness of which remains contentious.[93] Fluid restriction also often helps (e.g., ≤120 ml/kg/24 hr), although reduced volume of feeds may need to be compensated for by increased calorie content. Vasodilators may also be helpful (especially angiotensin-converting enzyme inhibitors, such as captopril).[94,95] Anticongestive therapy frequently relieves symptoms such as dyspnea and allows the infant to gain weight in the ensuing weeks. Most affected infants who require anticongestive therapy need to be evaluated with a view to surgery by the age of 3 to 6 months. Because such infants frequently have significant pulmonary hypertension, it is undesirable to postpone operative repair beyond the age of 6 months. Infants who fail to respond well to anticongestive therapy should be considered for early operation. In many institutions, the risks of repair of a VSD are not significantly different at 4 weeks than at 8 or 12 weeks. In such centers, little is to be gained by postponing operation, except in low-birth-weight infants.[96] On the other hand, there are many centers, especially in the developing nations, where corrective operation in infants may be unavailable or may present prohibitive risks. In such situations, the option of pulmonary artery banding deserves consideration (see later). The appropriate timing of this is similar to that for operative repair, and it is undesirable to postpone intervention beyond the age of 6 months if significant pulmonary hypertension is present.

INDICATIONS FOR OPERATION

Operation for moderate (or large) VSDs, in infancy, is frequently deferred for several months because there is a substantial chance (15 to 30%) that the defect will become smaller or close spontaneously. There are, however, several reasons for not waiting for this to occur.

1. Early and intractable congestive cardiac failure and failure to gain weight despite maximal medical therapy, including blood transfusion to raise hematocrit to about 50%: continuation of medical therapy is indicated if the infant can gain weight, even though complete remission of heart failure may not occur.

2. If such an infant goes home but then has several readmissions to the hospital, often with minor viral infections, and has shown no improvement during several weeks, early surgery is indicated.

3. A few infants show slow improvement but are so difficult to handle at home (often needing 2-hourly feeds) that the family becomes severely stressed and other children in the family are neglected.

4. On occasion, a child who might otherwise be managed medically lives far from medical care, or the family neglects frequent follow-up and the child's life is at risk.

5. An occasional child who is managing fairly well with medical treatment shows marked retardation of head growth. Such children are usually below the 5th percentile for weight and below the 10th percentile for height but will show catch-up growth when the defect is closed.[97] Head circumference, however, does not show catch-up

growth after 6 to 12 months but may return to normal if the defect is closed before 6 months of age.

After the age of 6 months, the risks of pulmonary vascular disease with a large VSD begin to rise, so that whereas conservative treatment is often worth pursuing in the early months, after 6 months there has to be a reason not to operate on a large defect. Any signs that pulmonary vascular resistance is increasing demand immediate investigation. These infants often show clinical improvement: lower heart rate, less tachypnea, better appetite and weight gain, lower requirements for anticongestive medications, quieter hearts, and less pulmonary plethora on chest x-ray examination. These changes could indicate decrease in size of the defect (usually indicated by the presence of an increasingly harsh, high-pitched systolic murmur) but might also be due to increasing pulmonary vascular resistance or, less often, the development of infundibular stenosis of the right ventricle. The differentiation between these outcomes cannot always be made reliably on clinical grounds; echocardiography and cardiac catheterization may be needed to reach the correct conclusion.

An occasional child with a large left-to-right shunt but normal pulmonary arterial pressure poses a problem. At one time, many cardiologists were conservative in the hope that the defect would get smaller or even close spontaneously. More recently, there is evidence that a chronically dilated and hypertrophied left ventricle does not function normally after the defect has been closed, in contrast to a similar ventricle in which the defect has been closed before 1 year of age. This argues for earlier closure of these defects. There remains controversy about the size of shunt that justifies surgical intervention in such patients. Most cardiologists and surgeons would not withhold surgical repair for patients who have a pulmonary-to-systemic flow ratio (Qp/Qs) greater than 2:1.

Chronic moderate left-to-right shunts may also justify closure, although not necessarily until later in childhood or adolescence. Many would recommend repair with a flow ratio (Qp/Qs) of 1.8:1. Some teams now use a figure of 1.5:1 as their threshold. Because of potential errors in calculating these ratios and because of errors in measurement of arteriovenous oxygen difference, clinical features must be considered as well. The age of the patient and the duration of follow-up during which the size of the shunt has remained static deserve to be taken into account. So also may such factors as cardiac enlargement on the chest film, electrocardiographic evidence of ventricular hypertrophy, or echocardiographic evidence of persisting left ventricular dilatation. Certainly patients who have reached adolescence with a significant shunt and no evidence of change in the size of the VSD during several years should have their defect repaired.

Additional indications for surgery include associated abnormalities such as aortic valve prolapse, with or without aortic incompetence, and infundibular pulmonary stenosis. In aortic valve prolapse, the site of the associated VSD and the severity of the distortion of the aortic valve affect the question of whether surgery should be recommended if the shunt through the VSD is small and there is no pulmonary hypertension. When the VSD is adjacent to the pulmonary valve (doubly committed subarterial VSD), there is a widespread consensus that the defect should be closed if there is clear evidence of aortic valve prolapse. The object of closing the VSD, in such patients, is to prevent the development of progressive aortic incompetence. If the VSD is perimembranous, the recommendation for operation depends more on the extent of the deformity of the aortic sinus/leaflet or associated aortic regurgitation. If the aortic valve is competent and the deformity is minor, many cardiologists and surgeons would not recommend intervention unless there were other indications for operation.

A documented episode of infective endocarditis may be regarded as an indication to close a VSD, even if there is no other reason to recommend surgery.[98] The endocarditis should usually be completely treated with appropriate antibiotic therapy before repair of the VSD is arranged, unless the endocarditis leads to serious immediate consequences (e.g., severe aortic incompetence), which themselves require urgent surgery.

OPERATIVE MANAGEMENT

PULMONARY ARTERY BANDING

Operation for infants and children with a VSD began when the important protective effect of pulmonary stenosis in patients with a large VSD was publicized.[99] Two years later, the use of pulmonary artery banding to create pulmonary stenosis in patients with a cardiac malformation associated with elevated pulmonary pressure and blood flow was reported.[100] For the next 20 years, this procedure became the standard initial management of most small infants with a severely symptomatic, large VSD. It remains the operation of choice in many parts of the world where the option of primary repair in early infancy is unavailable or presents an unacceptably high risk. The object of pulmonary artery banding is to reduce pulmonary pressure and blood flow toward normal levels. Some residual increase in pulmonary blood flow and pressure, in the early period after banding, allows growth and is usually well tolerated. As the infant grows, in the subsequent months, pulmonary flow and pressure tend to fall progressively, with the band offering a fixed resistance to right ventricular ejection, because the band becomes relatively tighter as the child gets bigger.

Major disadvantages of pulmonary banding include significant immediate mortality (about 15% in several series) and difficulty in adjusting the band to an appropriate degree to produce the required level of stenosis. Patients frequently have a band that is either ineffective (too loose) or so tight that they rapidly become cyanosed and need additional operation within a few days or weeks. Furthermore, unless the band is effectively fixed with sutures to the wall of the pulmonary trunk, the band can migrate to the pulmonary bifurcation, impinging on the origins of one or both branch pulmonary arteries; this can produce severe distortion or stenosis of the affected artery (particularly the right pulmonary artery), which greatly complicates later repair of the VSD.

In most institutions in the developed world, pulmonary banding is no longer the preferred initial option because direct repair of the VSD with use of cardiopulmonary bypass is now a low-risk procedure for most infants, for whom there is seldom any advantage in deferring definitive repair. There remain a small number of infants for whom banding may be considered, notably those with multiple VSDs (e.g., Swiss cheese defects) or a large VSD at the ventricular apex, which may be inaccessible or difficult to close effectively. Some low-birth-weight infants (e.g., below 1.5 kg) may be managed with a pulmonary artery band, if they are severely symptomatic and resistant to medical management. In some institutions, infants with associated aortic arch obstruction (coarctation or aortic arch interruption) have been managed with arch repair and pulmonary artery banding. Repair of the VSD and debanding are performed at a later procedure. At major centers, the arch repair is performed on bypass, through a sternotomy, and the VSD is closed at the same time. Currently, this approach carries a mortality of 5 to 10% or less in the best centers, significantly better than that achievable with use of a two-stage approach.

VENTRICULAR SEPTAL DEFECT REPAIR

Although the first successful repair of VSD was accomplished as early as 1954 with use of cross-circulation (three of five infants and three older children survived repair),[101] this operation did not become widespread until some 5 to 10 years later. By that time, heart-lung bypass had become adequately established to allow safe access for intracardiac repair in many centers in the Western world. Profound hypothermia with circulatory arrest, which was developed in the 1960s, encouraged primary repair in small infants, for whom conventional heart-lung bypass was technically difficult with available perfusion equipment. Subsequently, with improved bypass equipment, the feasibility of performing primary repair on full-flow or low-flow bypass with moderate hypothermia has meant that neonates, even of low birth weight, can be operated on with low risk. Nonetheless, some surgeons still employ deep hypothermia with circulatory arrest, especially in small infants.

In the early era, a VSD was usually approached through a right ventriculotomy. However, most surgeons attempt to avoid a ventriculotomy and gain access through an atriotomy, approaching the defect through the tricuspid valve or, in infants with a subpulmonary defect (doubly committed subarterial VSD), the pulmonary artery and pulmonary valve. The only defects that are likely to be inaccessible through either of these routes are those at, or close to, the ventricular apex or multiple defects in the muscular septum. Some such defects can be adequately visualized only through a right (or left) ventriculotomy, and the option of device closure, either in the cardiac catheter laboratory or intraoperatively, becomes attractive (see later).

High-risk or difficult repairs of a VSD are fortunately relatively uncommon; the risk of VSD closure, even in the early months of life, is now low in the major centers, with mortality of 1% or less. Thus, primary repair can be recommended as the treatment of choice for symptomatic infants who fail to respond rapidly to medical management,

and there is little reason to defer operation in those who are not gaining weight well.

Interventional Catheterization and Device Closure

The use of double-umbrella devices to close VSDs in the cardiac catheter laboratory was first performed in humans by Lock and associates[102] after experimental work in animals.[103] The devices used in the initial procedures were Rashkind PDA devices; in a subsequent group of patients, clamshell devices were employed.[104, 105] The defects that were closed by these methods were muscular or apical. Subsequently, other groups performed device closure of perimembranous defects.[106] The technique for closing VSDs in the catheter laboratory is complex. An end-hole balloon catheter (Swan-Ganz type) is passed to the left ventricle, either by the arterial route or, alternatively, from a venous approach and across the atrial septum, through an associated atrial septal defect or patent foramen ovale or by a trans-septal puncture. With the balloon inflated, an attempt is made to pass the catheter across the VSD. A guide wire passed through the catheter, into the right ventricle, right atrium, or pulmonary artery, is snared from a percutaneous right femoral vein or internal jugular vein catheter. A long introducer is then fed over the guide wire from the femoral or internal jugular vein through the right atrium, tricuspid valve, right ventricle, and VSD until the tip is in the left ventricle. The device is then introduced and deployed across the VSD.

Practical problems with this technique include the necessity to use a large sheath (8 or 11 French) that is relatively stiff and may tend to splint the ventricles. The guide wire itself can also produce hemodynamic instability and, particularly in small infants, may produce serious impairment of ventricular function.[107] Even with transesophageal echocardiographic monitoring, correct placement of the device may be extremely difficult. Perforation of the ventricular apex can occur. Damage to the atrioventricular valves may also result, and experience with device closure of perimembranous defects has shown aortic incompetence to be a significant complication.[106] Because of these various problems, relatively few centers have attempted this procedure. With improvements in the available devices and other changes in the technique of device placement, the use of transcatheter closure of VSDs will increase. For the foreseeable future at least, the defects that will be closed by this method will be limited to muscular and apical VSDs, which are inaccessible or difficult to close operatively.

Intraoperative Device Closure

The option of device closure of some muscular and multiple VSDs in the operating theater is also of importance. The practical difficulties with device closure in the catheter laboratory have already been mentioned. On the other hand, placement of a clamshell or Rashkind device under direct vision in the operating theater, with the patient on heart-lung bypass, offers an attractive alternative, especially when there are multiple muscular defects in the trabecular septum.[108, 109] Some patients with defects of this kind have an additional perimembranous VSD or have had pulmonary artery banding in infancy. Because the cardiac operation will be required to deal with these additional problems, the option of intraoperative device closure is particularly attractive, especially in view of the major problems with device closure in the catheter laboratory.

RESULTS OF OPERATION

Follow-up after VSD repair reveals 10 to 25% of patients with residual defects—usually with a shunt at one margin of the original VSD, where the patch has been inadequately attached to the edge of the defect or a stitch has pulled through in the perioperative period. In most patients, such defects are small and hemodynamically unimportant. Some such small defects close spontaneously in the early months after surgery. About 1 to 2% of children, however, may have a large enough residual shunt to merit reoperation, either early after their initial repair or later. This is more common among infants or children with multiple defects, which can be difficult to close completely. In some of these patients, the option of device closure of inaccessible or residual defects deserves consideration.

Most patients after VSD repair have minimal if any residual cardiac problems. Most grow normally, even if failure to thrive has been a major problem preoperatively, returning to the growth percentiles that would have been expected had they not had any cardiac abnormality (e.g., exhibiting catch-up growth).[97]

Some residual abnormalities may be demonstrable late after operation. These include persistent left ventricular dilatation and abnormal ventricular function, which are usually completely asymptomatic during childhood, although the longer term significance of these changes remains unknown. More significant is the development in some patients of gradually progressive aortic incompetence, which may be unrelated to the presence of aortic valve prolapse.[63]

Conduction abnormalities after operative repair are uncommon in the present era but still occur. Damage to the right bundle branch, leading to right bundle branch block, occurs in approximately 5 to 10% of patients having VSD repair. Transient complete block, in the immediate perioperative period, occurs in 1 to 5% of infants, who usually recover rapidly. Permanent complete atrioventricular block, resulting from surgical damage to the atrioventricular node or His bundle, now occurs in less than 1% of patients with isolated VSD, although occasional patients may develop block late postoperatively. Implantation of a permanent pacemaker is indicated for these relatively rare patients.

The question of whether postoperative patients require endocarditis prophylaxis after repair of an isolated VSD remains controversial. Some increase in risk of endocarditis is present, in many patients, because of the relatively high incidence of small residual VSDs (mentioned earlier). In addition, tricuspid valve abnormalities are frequent, either as a natural coexistent anomaly or as the consequence of operative attachment of the patch to the tricuspid valve. Furthermore, aortic valve abnormalities related to both aortic valve leaflet prolapse and later development of aortic incompetence put patients at risk. Although most postoperative endocarditis has occurred in patients with residual defects, the risk of endocarditis is not completely eliminated by VSD surgery. This is evidently different from the situation after closure of an isolated secundum atrial septal defect or ligation of a patent ductus arteriosus. For this reason, some pediatric cardiologists continue to recommend lifelong endocarditis prophylaxis, although current American Heart Association guidelines do not recommend coverage for patients in whom the defect has been completely closed and there is no demonstrable residual defect.[110]

REFERENCES

1. Farre JR: Malformations of the Human Heart. London, Hurst, Orme, Brown, 1814.
2. Fallot A: Contribution a l'anatomie pathologique de la maladie bleue (cyanose cardiaque). Marseille Med 25:77, 1888.
3. Roger H: Recherches cliniques sur la communication congenitale des deux coeurs, par inocclusion du septum interventriculaire. Bull Acad Med Paris 8:1074, 1879.
4. Eisenmenger V: Die angeborenen Defecte der Kammersscheidewand des Herzens. Z Klin Med 32(suppl):1, 1897.
5. Abbott ME: Congenital Heart Disease. New York, Thomas Nelson, 1932.
6. Heath D, Edwards JE: The pathology of hypertensive pulmonary vascular disease: A description of six grades of structural changes in the pulmonary arteries with special reference to congenital cardiac septal defects. Circulation 18:533, 1958.
7. Heath D, Helmholz HF Jr, Burchell HB, et al: Graded pulmonary vascular changes and hemodynamic findings in cases of atrial and ventricular septal defect and patent ductus arteriosus. Circulation 18:1155, 1958.
8. Campbell M: Natural history of ventricular septal defect. Br Heart J 33:246, 1971.
9. Dickinson DF, Arnold R, Wilkinson JL: Ventricular septal defect in children born in Liverpool 1960 to 1969. Br Heart J 46:47, 1981.
10. Hoffman JIE, Christianson R: Congenital heart disease in a cohort of 19,502 births with long term follow up. Am J Cardiol 42:641, 1978.
11. DeVore GR, Horenstein J, Siassi B, Platt LD: Fetal echocardiography. VII. Doppler color flow mapping: A new technique for the diagnosis of congenital heart disease. Am J Obstet Gynecol 156:1054, 1987.
12. Roguin N, Du ZD, Barak M, et al: High prevalence of muscular ventricular septal defect in neonates. J Am Coll Cardiol 26:1545, 1995.
13. Mitchell SC, Korones SB, Berendes HW: Congenital heart disease in 56,109 births. Circulation 43:323, 1971.
14. Dickinson DF, Arnold R, Wilkinson JL: Congenital heart disease among 160,480 liveborn children in Liverpool 1960–1969. Implications for surgical treatment. Br Heart J 46:55, 1981.
15. Tatsuno K, Ando M, Takao A, et al: Diagnostic importance of aortography in conal ventricular septal defect. Am Heart J 89:171, 1975.
16. Lue H, Takao A: Subpulmonic Ventricular Septal Defect. Proceedings of the Third Asian Congress of Pediatric Cardiology. New York, Springer-Verlag, 1986.
17. Anderson RH, Wilcox BR: The surgical anatomy of ventricular septal defects associated with overriding valvar orifices (Review). J Card Surg 8:130, 1993.
18. Anderson RH, Wilcox BR: The surgical anatomy of ventricular septal defect (Review). J Card Surg 7:17, 1992.
19. Soto B, Becker AE, Moulaert AH, et al: Classification of ventricular septal defects. Br Heart J 43:332, 1980.
20. Becker AE, Anderson RH: Classification of ventricular septal defects: A matter of precision. Heart Vessels 1:1, 1985.
21. Restivo A, Smith A, Wilkinson JL, Anderson RH: Normal variations in the relationship of the tricuspid valve to the membranous septum in the human heart. Anat Rec 226:258, 1990.
22. Restivo A, Smith A, Wilkinson JL, Anderson RH: The medial papillary muscle complex and its related septomarginal trabeculation. A normal anatomical study on human hearts. J Anat 163:231, 1989.

23. Gerbode F, Hultgren H, Melrose D, Osborn J: Syndrome of left ventricular–right atrial shunt: Successful surgical repair of defect in five cases, with observation of bradycardia on closure. Ann Surg 148:433, 1958.

24. Kitchiner D, Jackson M, Malaiya N, et al: Morphology of left ventricular outflow tract structures in patients with subaortic stenosis and a ventricular septal defect. Br Heart J 72:251, 1994.

25. Lauer RM, DuShane JW, Edwards JE: Obstruction of left ventricular outlet in association with ventricular septal defect. Circulation 22:110, 1960.

26. Wu MH, Wu JM, Chang CI, et al: Implication of aneurysmal transformation in isolated perimembranous ventricular septal defect. Am J Cardiol 72:596, 1993.

27. Beerman LB, Park SC, Fischer DA, et al: Ventricular septal defect associated with aneurysm of the membranous septum. J Am Coll Cardiol 5:118, 1985.

28. Ramaciotti C, Keren A, Silverman NH: Importance of (perimembranous) ventricular septal aneurysm in the natural history of isolated perimembranous ventricular septal defect. Am J Cardiol 57:268, 1986.

29. Varghese PJ, Izukawa T, Celermajer J, et al: Aneurysm of the membranous ventricular septum. A method of spontaneous closure of small ventricular septal defect. Am J Cardiol 24:531, 1969.

30. Chesler E, Korns ME, Edwards JE: Anomalies of the tricuspid valve, including pouches, resembling aneurysm of the membranous ventricular septum. Am J Cardiol 21:661, 1968.

31. Mori K, Matsuoka S, Tatara K, et al: Echocardiographic evaluation of the development of aortic valve prolapse in supracristal ventricular septal defect. Eur J Pediatr 154:176, 1995.

32. Craig BG, Smallhorn JF, Burrows P, et al: Cross-sectional echocardiography in the evaluation of aortic valve prolapse associated with ventricular septal defect. Am Heart J 112:800, 1986.

33. Menahem S, Johns JA, del Torso S, et al: Evaluation of aortic valve prolapse in ventricular septal defect. Br Heart J 56:242, 1986.

34. Ando M, Takao A: Pathological anatomy of ventricular septal defects associated with aortic valve prolapse and regurgitation. Heart Vessels 2:117, 1996.

35. Bharati S, Lev M, Kirklin JW: Cardiac Surgery and the Conduction System, 2nd ed. Mt. Kisco, NY, Futura Publishing, 1992.

36. Lev M, Fell EH, Arcilla R, Weinberg MH: Surgical injury to the conduction system in ventricular septal defect. Am J Cardiol 14:464, 1964.

37. Titus JL, Daugherty GW, Kirklin JW, Edwards JE: Lesions of the atrioventricular conduction system after repair of ventricular septal defect. Circulation 28:82, 1963.

38. Kulbertus HE, Coyne JJ, Hallidie-Smith KA: Conduction disturbances before and after surgical closure of ventricular septal defect. Am Heart J 77:123, 1969.

39. Lev M: The architecture of the conduction system in congenital heart disease. III. Ventricular septal defect. Arch Pathol 70:529, 1960.

40. Truex RC, Bishof IK: Conduction system in human hearts with interventricular septal defects. J Thorac Surg 35:421, 1958.

41. Milo S, Ho SY, Wilkinson JL, Anderson RH: Surgical anatomy and atrioventricular conduction tissues of heart with isolated ventricular septal defects. J Thorac Cardiovasc Surg 79:244, 1980.

42. Kurosawa H, Becker AE: Modification of the precise relationship of the atrioventricular conduction bundle to the margins of the ventricular septal defects by the trabecula septomarginalis. J Thorac Cardiovasc Surg 87:605, 1984.

43. Harh JH, Paul MH: Experimental cardiac morphogenesis. I. Development of the ventricular septum in the chick. J Embryol Exp Morphol 33:13, 1975.

44. Patterson DF, Pyke RL, Van Mierop LHS, et al: Hereditary defects of the conotruncal septum in Keeshond dogs: Pathological and genetic studies. Am J Cardiol 34:187, 1974.

45. Haworth SG, Hislop AA: Pulmonary vascular development: Normal values of peripheral vascular structure. Am J Cardiol 52:578, 1983.

46. Wagenvoort CA: The pulmonary arteries in infants with ventricular septal defects. Med Thorac 19:354, 1962.

47. Haworth SG, Sauer U, Buhlmeyer K, Reid L: Development of the pulmonary circulation in ventricular septal defect: A quantitative structural study. Am J Cardiol 40:781, 1977.

48. Gasul BM, Dillon RF, Vrla V, Hait G: Ventricular septal defects: Their natural transformation into those with infundibular stenosis or into the cyanotic or non-cyanotic type of tetralogy of Fallot. JAMA 164:847, 1957.

49. Ruangritnamchai C, Khowsathit P, Pongpanich B: Spontaneous closure of small ventricular septal defect first six months of life. J Med Assoc Thai 76(suppl)2:63, 1993.

50. Alpert BS, Mellitis ED, Rowe RD: Spontaneous closure of small ventricular septal defects: Probability rates in the first five years of life. Am J Dis Child 125:194, 1973.

51. Anderson RH, Lenox CC, Zuberbuhler JR: Mechanisms of closure of perimembranous ventricular septal defect. Am J Cardiol 52:341, 1983.

52. Alpert BS, Cook DH, Varghese PJ, Rowe RD: Spontaneous closure of small ventricular septal defects: Ten-year follow-up. Pediatrics 63:204, 1979.

53. Moe DG, Guntheroth WG: Spontaneous closure of uncomplicated ventricular septal defect. Am J Cardiol 60:674, 1987.

54. Bush A, Busst CM, Haworth SG, et al: Correlations of lung morphology, pulmonary vascular resistance, and outcome in children with congenital heart disease. Br Heart J 59:480, 1988.

55. Juaneda E, Gittenberger de Groot A, Oppenheimer-Dekker A, Haworth SG: Pulmonary arterial development in infants with large perimembranous ventricular septal defects associated with overriding of the aortic valve. Int J Cardiol 7:223, 1985.

56. Hallidie-Smith KA, Hollman A, Cleland WP, et al: Effects of surgical closure of ventricular septal defects upon pulmonary vascular disease. Br Heart J 31:246, 1969.

57. Corone P, Doyan F, Gaudeau S, et al: Natural history of ventricular septal defect: A study involving 790 cases. Circulation 55:908, 1977.

58. Presbitero P, Somerville J, Stone S, et al: Pregnancy in cyanotic congenital heart disease. Outcome of mother and fetus. Circulation 89:2673, 1994.

59. Wood P: The Eisenmenger syndrome. Br Med J 2:755, 1958.

60. Clarkson PM, Frye RL, DuShane JW, et al: Prognosis for patients with ventricular septal defect and severe pulmonary vascular obstructive disease. Circulation 38:129, 1968.

61. Warnes CA, Boger JE, Roberts W: Eisenmenger ventricular septal defect with prolonged survival. Am J Cardiol 54:460, 1984.

62. Momma K, Toyama K, Takao A, et al: Natural history of subarterial infundibular ventricular septal defect. Am Heart J 108:1312, 1984.

63. Otterstad JE, Ihlen H, Vatne K: Aortic regurgitation associated with ventricular septal defects in adults. Acta Med Scand 218:85, 1985.

64. Gersony WM, Hayes CJ, Driscoll DJ, et al: Bacterial endocarditis in patients with aortic stenosis, pulmonary stenosis, or ventricular septal defect. Circulation 87 (suppl):I-121, 1993.

65. Gersony WM, Hayes CJ: Bacterial endocarditis in patients with pulmonary stenosis, aortic stenosis, or ventricular septal defect. Circulation 56:84, 1977.

66. Shah P, Singh WSA, Rose V, Keith JD: Incidence of bacterial endocarditis in ventricular septal defects. Circulation 34:127, 1966.

67. Morris CD, Raller MD, Menashe VD: Thirty-year incidence of infective endocarditis after surgery for congenital heart disease. JAMA 279:599, 1998.

68. Gumbiner CH, Gillette PC, Garson A (eds): Pediatric Cardiac Dysrhythmias. New York, Grune & Stratton, 1981, pp 405–419.

69. Katz LN, Wachtel H: The diphasic QRS type of electrocardiogram in congenital heart disease. Am Heart J 13:202, 1937.

70. Ortiz E, Robinson PJ, Deanfield JE, et al: Localisation of ventricular septal defects by simultaneous display of superimposed colour Doppler and cross sectional echocardiographic images. Br Heart J 54:53, 1985.

71. Feigenbaum H: Echocardiography, 3rd ed. Philadelphia, Lea & Febiger, 1981.

72. Gutgesell HP, Paguet M: Atlas of Pediatric Echocardiography. Hagerstown, MD, Harper & Row, 1978.

73. Silverman NH, Snider AR, Rudolph AM: Evaluation of pulmonary hypertension by M-mode echocardiography in children with ventricular septal defect. Circulation 61:1125, 1980.

74. Goldberg SJ, Sahn DJ, Allen HD, et al: Evaluation of pulmonary and systemic blood flow by 2-dimensional Doppler echocardiography using fast Fourier transform spectral analysis. Am J Cardiol 50:1394, 1982.

75. Bierman FZ, Fellows K, Williams RG: Prospective identification of ventricular septal defects in infancy using subxiphoid two dimensional echocardiography. Circulation 62:80, 1980.

76. Sutherland CA, Godman MJ, Smallhorn JF, et al: Ventricular septal defects. Two-dimensional echocardiography and morphological correlation. Br Heart J 437:316, 1982.

77. Cheatham JP, Latson LA, Gutgesell HP: Ventricular septal defect in infancy: Detection with two-dimensional echocardiography. Am J Cardiol 47:85, 1981.

78. Capelli H, Andrade JL, Somerville J: Classification of the site of ventricular septal defect by 2-dimensional echocardiography. Am J Cardiol 51:1474, 1983.

79. Ludomirsky A, Huhta J, Vick G, et al: Color Doppler detection of multiple ventricular septal defects. Circulation 74:1317, 1986.

80. Murphy DJ, Ludomirsky A, Huhta JC: Continuous-wave doppler in children with ventricular septal defect: Noninvasive estimation of interventricular pressure gradient. Am J Cardiol 57:428, 1986.

81. Barron JV, Sahn DJ, Valdes-Cruz LM, et al: Clinical utility of two-dimensional Doppler echocardiographic techniques for estimating pulmonary to systemic blood flow ratios in children with left-to-right shunting atrial septal defect, ventricular septal defect or patent ductus arteriosus. J Am Coll Cardiol 3:169, 1984.

82. Askenazi J, Ahnberg DS, Korngold E, et al: Quantitative radionuclide angiocardiography: Detection and quantitation of left to right shunts. Am J Cardiol 37:382, 1976.

83. Anderson PAW, Jones RH, Sabiston DC: Quantitation of left-to-right cardiac shunts with radionuclide angiography. Circulation 49:512, 1974.

84. Flamm MD, Cohn KE, Hancock EW: Measurement of systemic cardiac output at rest and exercise in patients with atrial septal defect. Br Heart J 23:258, 1969.

85. Miller HC, Brown DJ, Miller GAH: Comparison of formulae used to estimate oxygen saturation of mixed venous blood from caval samples. Br Heart J 36:446, 1974.

86. LaFarge CG, Miettinen OS: The estimation of oxygen consumption. Cardiovasc Res 4:23, 1970.

87. Lundell BPW, Casas ML, Wallgren CG: Oxygen consumption in infants and children during heart catheterization. Pediatr Cardiol 17:207, 1996.

88. Winberg P, Lundell BP, Gustafsson LE: Effect of inhaled nitric oxide on raised pulmonary vascular resistance in children with congenital heart disease. Br Heart J 71:282, 1994.

89. Roberts JD Jr, Lang P, Bigatello LM, et al: Inhaled nitric oxide in congenital heart disease. Circulation 87:447, 1993.

90. Bargeron LM Jr, Elliott LP, Soto B, et al: Axial cineangiography in congenital heart disease: Section I. Concept, technical and anatomic considerations. Circulation 56:1075, 1977.

91. Elliott LP, Bargeron LM Jr, Beam PR, et al: Axial cineangiography in congenital heart disease. Section II. Specific lesions. Circulation 56:1084, 1977.

92. Green CE, Elliott LP, Bargeron LM Jr: Axial cineangiographic evaluation of the posterior ventricular septal defect. Am J Cardiol 48:331, 1981.

93. Berman W Jr, Yabek SM, Dillon T, et al: Effects of digoxin in infants with congested circulatory state due to a ventricular septal defect. N Engl J Med 308:363, 1983.

94. Shaw NJ, Wilson N, Dickinson DF: Captopril in heart failure secondary to a left to right shunt. Arch Dis Child 63:360, 1988.

95. Scammell AM, Arnold R, Wilkinson JL: Captopril in treatment of infant heart failure: A preliminary report. Int J Cardiol 16:295, 1987.

96. Castaneda AR, Mayer JE Jr, Jonas RA, et al: The neonate with critical congenital heart disease: Repair—a surgical challenge. J Thorac Cardiovasc Surg 98:869, 1989.

97. Weintraub RG, Menahem S: Early surgical closure of a large ventricular septal defect: Influence on long-term growth. J Am Coll Cardiol 18:552, 1991.

98. L'Ecuyer TJ, Embrey RP: Closure of hemodynamically insignificant ventricular septal defect after infective endocarditis. Am J Cardiol 72:1093, 1993.

99. Civin WH, Edwards JE: Pathology of the pulmonary vascular tree 1. A comparison of the intrapulmonary arteries in Eisenmenger's complex and in stenosis of ostium infundibuli associated with biventricular origin of the aorta. Circulation 2:545, 1950.

100. Muller WH Jr, Dammann JF Jr: The treatment of certain congenital malformations of the heart by the creation of pulmonic stenosis to reduce pulmonary hypertension and excessive pulmonary blood flow: A preliminary report. Surg Gynecol Obstet 95:213, 1952.

101. Lillehei CW, Cohen M, Warden HE, et al: The results of direct vision closure of ventricular septal defects in eight patients by means of controlled cross circulation. Surg Gynecol Obstet 101:447, 1955.

102. Lock JE, Block PC, McKay RG, et al: Transcatheter closure of ventricular septal defects. Circulation 78:361, 1988.

103. Rashkind W, Cuaso C: Transcatheter closure of atrial and ventricular septal defects in the experimental animal. Eur J Cardiol 5:297, 1977.

104. Perry SB, van der Velde ME, Bridges ND, et al: Transcatheter closure of atrial and ventricular septal defects (Review). Herz 18:135, 1993.

105. Goldstein SAN, Perry SB, Keane JF, et al: Transcatheter closure of congenital ventricular septal defects. Semin Perinatol 15:240A, 1990.

106. Rigby ML, Redington AN: Primary transcatheter umbrella closure of perimembranous ventricular septal defect [see comments]. Br Heart J 72:368, 1994.

107. Laussen PC, Hansen DD, Perry SB, et al: Transcatheter closure of ventricular septal defects: Hemodynamic instability and anesthetic management. Anesth Analg 80:1076, 1995.

108. Fishberger SB, Bridges ND, Keane JF, et al: Intraoperative device closure of ventricular septal defects. Circulation 88(suppl):II-205, 1993.

109. Chaturvedi RR, Shore DF, Yacoub M, Redington AN: Intraoperative apical ventricular septal defect closure using a modified Rashkind double umbrella. Heart 76:367, 1996.

110. Dajani AS, Taubert KA, Wilson W, et al: Prevention of bacterial endocarditis. Recommendations by the American Heart Association (Review). JAMA 277:1794, 1997.

CHAPTER 22
ATRIAL SEPTAL DEFECT

LARRY A. LATSON

The interatrial septum is more than a simple wall between the left and right atria. It is a structure that develops from two separate primitive septal ridges that must migrate, coalesce with the endocardial cushions and sinus venosus, and partially resorb to function normally in fetal and postnatal life. In normal fetal development, there must continuously be an interatrial communication to allow right-to-left shunting of oxygenated blood from the placenta to the left side of the heart. Postnatal persistence of a pathway for blood flow between the atria due to a deficiency of one or more components of the atrial septum, however, constitutes an atrial septal defect (ASD). The most common type of ASD is the secundum defect in the region of the fossa ovalis. Defects in the inferior portion of the atrial septum, primum ASDs, represent a form of endocardial cushion defect and are discussed in Chapter 24. Three percent to 10% of ASD are sinus venosus defects.[1–3] These are usually located posterosuperiorly near the orifice of the superior vena cava, but they are rarely located inferiorly near the entrance of the inferior vena cava. Persistent patency of the foramen ovale due to incomplete fusion of the valve of the foramen ovale to the septum secundum after birth represents only a potential interatrial communication under normal circumstances. At least a small patent foramen ovale can be identified in up to 30% of the adult population at autopsy.[4] When it is not associated with a detectable left-to-right shunt or deficiency of septal tissue, patent foramen ovale is considered a variation of normal rather than a pathologic defect.

Abnormal interatrial communications were described as early as 1875 by Rokitansky, but the clinical features were not elucidated in detail until 1941.[5] A specific genetic etiology for secundum ASD has not been identified, and most of them occur sporadically. ASD is the major cardiac abnormality in 5 to 10% of patients with congenital heart disease and is usually considered the fourth or fifth most common type of cardiac malformation.[6] Females are affected approximately twice as often as are males. Autosomal dominant inheritance of ASD has been documented in some families. Associated anomalies in some of these families have included abnormalities of the radius or radial portion of the hand (Holt-Oram syndrome) and abnormal prolongation of atrioventricular (AV) conduction.[7,8]

PATHOLOGIC ANATOMY

The normal interatrial septum is composed of derivatives of the embryologic septum primum, septum secundum, and right horn of the sinus venosus. The septum primum normally forms the inferior portion of the atrial septum and the flap-like valve of the foramen ovale. The septum secundum forms the anterior and posterior rims of the limbus fossa ovalis, which demarcates the foramen ovale, and much of the superior portion of the interatrial septum. The smooth-walled posterolateral portion of the right atrium is the remnant of the right horn of the sinus venosus. Abnormal incorporation of this structure into the right atrium results in a sinus venosus defect near the orifice of the superior or inferior vena cava.

A secundum ASD occurs in the region of the foramen ovale (Fig. 22–1). It can result from an abnormally short valve of the foramen ovale, an unusually large foramen ovale that is not completely covered by a normal valve, or fenestrations in the valve of the foramen ovale. Approximately two thirds of secundum ASDs requiring closure occur in the central portion of the foramen ovale. Twenty percent of secundum ASDs result from multiple fenestrations of the valve of the foramen ovale or a single large defect with multiple smaller fenestrations.[9] Most clinically evident secundum ASDs are at least 1 cm in diameter in children or adults.[10] A sinus venosus ASD is located in the smooth-walled region of the atrium posterior to the fossa ovalis (Fig. 22–1). It usually occurs superiorly near the orifice of the superior vena cava, but an inferior sinus venosus defect occasionally occurs near the orifice of the inferior vena cava. Unroofing or absence of the coronary sinus with persistence of the ostium into the right atrium is a rare defect known as a coronary sinus ASD.

Functional abnormalities of the mitral valve are commonly seen in patients with an ASD. When there is detectable mitral insufficiency, the mitral valve is usually normally formed but prolapses. It is controversial whether the mitral valve prolapse is simply secondary to deformation of the mitral apparatus by an enlarged right ventricle or an inherent abnormality of mitral valve tissue.[11,12] Rarely, the anterior leaflet of the mitral valve may be cleft and associated with mitral insufficiency. A small to moderate pressure gradient across the pulmonary valve is common with a large left-to-right shunt through an ASD. In most instances, the gradient is secondary to increased flow, but anatomic pulmonary valvar stenosis is found in 5% of patients. Eighty percent to 90% of patients with a superior sinus venosus defect also have partial anomalous pulmonary venous connection of the right pulmonary veins to the right atrium or superior vena cava.[13] Persistent left superior vena cava to the coronary sinus occurs in 10% of patients. It inserts directly to the left atrium in patients with a coronary sinus ASD.[13]

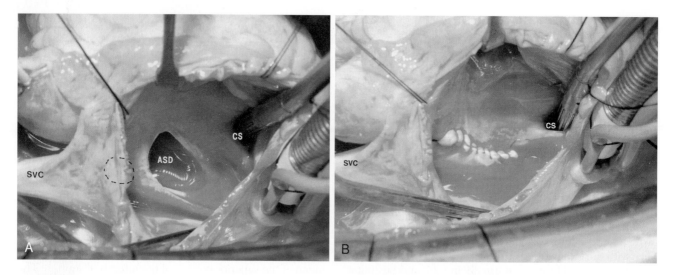

A, Surgical view of the interatrial septum in a patient with a secundum atrial septal defect (ASD). The right atrium has been opened to expose the right side of the atrial septum. The ASD is seen in the central portion of the atrial septum. The thickened tissue along the superior and anterior portions of the ASD is the limbus fossa ovalis. The *dotted circle* indicates the area where a sinus venosus ASD would be located. The ASD in this patient results from an abnormally short valve of the foramen ovale. SVC = superior vena cava; CS = coronary sinus. *B,* The secundum ASD has been surgically corrected by direct suture closure of the defect.

HEMODYNAMICS

In the fetus, oxygenated blood from the placenta returns to the inferior vena cava, and pulmonary blood flow is low compared with the normal postnatal pattern. High flow through the placenta, low left atrial pressure because of low pulmonary blood flow, and the orientation of the eustachian valve all contribute to the normal pattern of right-to-left shunting through the foramen ovale before birth. Early after birth, flows in the pulmonary and systemic circulations equalize with expansion of the lungs and removal of the placenta from the circulation. In the neonate, compliance of the left and right ventricles is similar, atrial pressures are relatively equal, and flow through an ASD may be bidirectional with little net left-to-right or right-to-left shunt.[14]

During infancy, the right ventricle gradually becomes more compliant than the left ventricle because of the markedly lower pressure and resistance in the pulmonary circulation compared with the systemic circuit. Because the increasingly compliant right ventricle more readily accepts excess volume, more blood is diverted from the left atrium to the right atrium through the ASD. Normal homeostatic mechanisms preserve systemic cardiac output to the brain, kidneys, and other vital organs under resting conditions. Pulmonary blood flow, consisting of systemic venous return plus the volume of blood that shunts from the left atrium to the right atrium, is thus increased. The pulmonary-to-systemic flow ratio usually exceeds 1.5:1 and often exceeds 2.5:1 in patients with a clinically evident ASD. Atrial level left-to-right flow enlarges the right atrium and right ventricle; this enlargement can be detected radiographically and clinically after infancy. Under normal circumstances, flow through an ASD is nearly all left-to-right, but there is a phasic variation. Maximal left-to-right flow occurs in late systole and early diastole. There is usually a small and transient right-to-left shunt near the end of the QRS.[15]

For a given size ASD, the volume and direction of shunting through the ASD largely depend on the relative compliance of the right and left ventricles. Thus, patients with right ventricular hypertrophy secondary to conditions such as pulmonary stenosis or pulmonary hypertension have a smaller left-to-right shunt. Severe right ventricular hypertrophy results in a net right-to-left shunt and cyanosis in the presence of an ASD or a patent foramen ovale. Conditions that reduce left ventricular compliance, such as aging and hypertrophy, may result in an increase in left-to-right shunting in late adulthood.

Congestive cardiac failure in an ASD might be thought to affect only the overloaded right ventricle, but the cardiac failure is atypical in that both ventricles have equally raised diastolic pressures, even though the left ventricle is not dilated. In the past, this has been attributed to left ventricular muscle failure. More recently, the raised left ventricular diastolic pressure has been ascribed, at least in part, to compression of the left ventricle by a hugely dilated right ventricle, much as ventricular diastolic pressures are raised by pericardial tamponade.

NATURAL HISTORY

Patients with an ASD are generally asymptomatic through infancy and childhood. Rarely, symptoms of pulmonary overcirculation, frequent respiratory infections, and congestive heart failure are seen in infants who have no other identified cardiac abnormality.[16,17] The heart failure in these infants is biventricular. Spontaneous closure of the ASD in such patients may occur during the first several years of life in as many as 40% of such infants if they respond to medical management.[18] Echocardiographic study has suggested that a secundum ASD less than 3 mm in diameter in the first 3 months of life nearly always closes, and one greater than 8 mm in diameter is unlikely to close.[19]

Patients diagnosed later in childhood often come to the attention of a cardiologist because of a relatively inconspicuous murmur. Although they do not have overt symptoms, they may appear asthenic in build.[10] Symptoms become progressively more common after the age of 20 years. Early symptoms are predominantly dyspnea on exertion, fatigue, palpitations, and sustained atrial arrhythmias. By the age of 40 years, 90% of untreated patients have one or more of these "minor" symptoms. More severe symptoms, such as congestive cardiac failure, angina, and cyanosis, develop in approximately 35% of the patients older than 40 years.[20] Beyond 50 years of age, congestive cardiac failure may be associated with massive mitral regurgitation. An ASD also allows possible paradoxical embolization of thrombus, air, or other material to the systemic circulation. Paradoxical embolism can result in stroke or ischemic damage to the extremities or major organs.[21] The risk of paradoxical embolization may be increased with pregnancy, especially in the peripartum period. Pregnancy is otherwise well tolerated. Infective endocarditis is rare in patients with an ASD in the absence of other cardiovascular abnormalities such as mitral insufficiency. Rarely, thrombosis of major pulmonary arteries may occur.

Each of the commonly occurring complications of ASD increases in frequency with age, but in slightly different patterns. Pulmonary hypertension occurs in less than 10% of children with an ASD, and an ASD in this age group is usually coincidental with primary pulmonary hypertension. Pulmonary artery pressure, however, does gradually increase with age in patients with an ASD. Approximately half of patients older than 30 years have a pulmonary artery mean pressure greater than 20 mm Hg but only mild elevation of pulmonary arterial resistance.[22, 23] Atrial arrhythmias become increasingly common with advancing age. More than 50% of patients older than 45 years have intermittent or chronic atrial fibrillation.[24, 25] The onset of atrial fibrillation or flutter is a common cause of relatively rapid deterioration in a previously minimally symptomatic adult. The degree of left-to-right shunting may also increase in adults because of decreasing left ventricular distensibility that can result from systemic hypertension or coronary artery disease.[26]

Survival of patients with a clinically detectable ASD into adulthood is expected, with more than 75% of patients surviving into their 30s. Campbell,[27] however, estimated that approximately 75% of patients do not survive past the age of 50 years, and only 10% survive past the age of 60 years. These estimates may be overly pessimistic and apply accurately only to patients with a large, easily detectable ASD, however, because Campbell's patients were identified before the widespread availability of current sensitive diagnostic tests. There are numerous reports of patients with an ASD surviving past the age of 80 years.[28]

HISTORY AND PHYSICAL EXAMINATION

The clinical history in most young patients with an ASD may be relatively unremarkable. It may be possible to elucidate a minor difference in exercise tolerance or growth compared with siblings, but it is unusual to have failure to thrive or clearly reduced exercise tolerance. On the other hand, exercise tolerance increases after closure of the defect. In adult patients, symptoms of overt congestive cardiac failure including peripheral edema become more common.[20] Palpitations are a frequent complaint, and the appearance of atrial fibrillation or flutter may precipitate the definitive evaluation and diagnosis. A small percentage of patients may be found to have an ASD or patent foramen ovale on cardiac evaluation after a stroke.

The physical findings of an ASD may be relatively subtle to the noncardiologist and were not described until the 1940s.[5] Examination of a patient suspected of having an ASD begins with inspection. Patients with a large left-to-right shunt may have mild left chest prominence. Careful evaluation of the jugular venous pulse typically shows equalization of the a and v waves instead of the normal large a wave.[28] The presence of deformities of the radial portions of the arm should significantly raise the index of suspicion for Holt-Oram syndrome, which may have an associated ASD.[7]

On palpation, there is a right ventricular lift (especially in expiration) along the sternal border if there is a large left-to-right shunt. This may be more prominent during inspiration in the subxiphoid area. The first heart sound is typically split, but not usually significantly more than normal. The second heart sound, however, is characteristically altered in nearly all patients with a large shunt. The second heart sound is widely split and the respiratory variation is greatly reduced, leading to the perception of fixed splitting. Multiple explanations for these findings have been put forth. The most detailed evaluations suggest that the wide splitting of the second heart sound is secondary to increased capacitance of the pulmonary bed leading to the elongation of the hangout time.[29, 30] The *hangout time* is the interval between the descending limbs of the pulmonary arterial and right ventricular pressure pulses. The fixed splitting may be explained by offsetting of the normal inspiratory increase in right ventricular volume by a reduction in the left-to-right shunt at this time. Thus, there is no significant net change in relative ejection volumes between the left and right ventricles.[31] The right ventricle ejects more than the left ventricle with each contraction, and the relative volumes do not change significantly with respiration.

The physical finding most readily apparent to noncardiologists is the relatively soft systolic murmur that occurs with ejection of increased blood flow through the pulmonary valve. The murmur is usually grade 3 or less unless there is a concomitant abnormality of the pulmonary valve. The murmur is typically maximal at the mid to upper left sternal border and radiates to the lung fields posteriorly. Patients with a large left-to-right shunt (Qp/Qs above 2 : 1) often have along the lower left sternal border a mid-diastolic flow rumble that is due to the increased diastolic flow through the tricuspid valve.[32] Pulmonary hypertension may result in accentuation of the pulmonary component of the second heart sound as well as normalization of the respiratory variation in the second heart sound. With severe pulmonary hypertension, murmurs of pulmonary insufficiency and tricuspid insufficiency may appear.[33]

ELECTROCARDIOGRAPHY

The electrocardiogram may be helpful in the diagnosis of ASD in children and young adults. In infancy, there is normally a pattern of right ventricular dominance, and infants with an ASD (other than primum ASDs) do not show diagnostic changes. The normal regression of relative right ventricular forces with age does not occur, however, and a typical pattern of persistent right-axis deviation and right ventricular enlargement becomes identifiable in early childhood. The QRS duration is usually at the upper limit of normal or mildly prolonged, with an rSr′ or rsR′ pattern seen in the right precordial leads (Fig. 22–2). In older children and adults, this pattern of complete or incomplete right bundle branch block is seen in 90% of patients referred for operation.[34] A notch in the R wave in the inferior limb leads may be especially prominent in patients with a large shunt.[34] This notch may disappear more quickly than the incomplete right bundle branch block pattern in lead V_1 after closure of the defect. In the rare patient with severe pulmonary hypertension associated with an ASD, the electrocardiographic pattern may be more typical of pure pressure overload with an rR or tall monophasic R wave preceded by a small Q wave in lead V_1.[28]

Conduction abnormalities and arrhythmias become increasingly apparent with age in patients with an ASD. The P waves frequently become tall and peaked as the right atrium enlarges. This may result in a slight prolongation of the PR interval. Detailed intracardiac electrophysiologic studies have indicated that abnormalities of the atrial-His interval increased to 40% in children 10 to 16 years of age, and abnormalities of corrected sinus node recovery time occurred in more than 90% of children in this age group.[35] These abnormalities are only rarely clinically significant, however. An advanced first-degree atrioventricular block progressing to a second-degree block or a complete atrioventricular block may be seen in a familial pattern associated with secundum ASDs.[7,8] Atrial arrhythmias clearly become more common with age. The most common is atrial fibrillation, but atrial flutter and supraventricular tachycardia can also develop. These arrhythmias are unusual in children and become gradually more common in teenagers. Past the age of 40 years, more than half of patients with an ASD have atrial fibrillation.[25]

CHEST RADIOGRAPHY AND MAGNETIC RESONANCE IMAGING

The chest radiograph may be helpful for the diagnosis of ASD in patients with a large left-to-right shunt. The typical appearance is of enlargement of the right atrium, right ventricle, and pulmonary trunk with a small-appearing ascending aorta (Fig. 22–3). The right atrial enlargement is most easily seen on the posteroanterior view. Right ventricular enlargement may be most easily seen in the lateral view with reduction in the normal retrosternal clear space. Overall pulmonary vascularity is increased along with enlargement of the main pulmonary artery segment. In patients with a sinus venosus ASD associated with anomalous

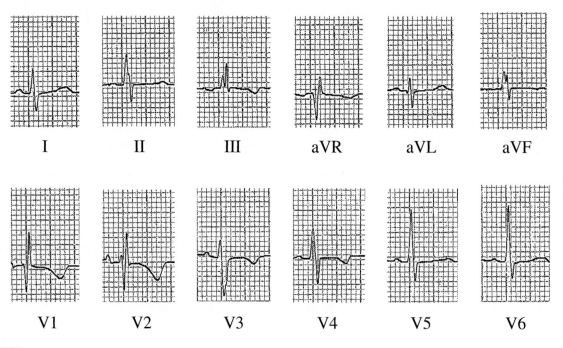

I II III aVR aVL aVF

V1 V2 V3 V4 V5 V6

FIGURE 22–2

Typical electrocardiogram of a teenager with a secundum ASD. Notice the rsR′ pattern in lead V_1. There is also a notch in the R wave in leads III and aVF.

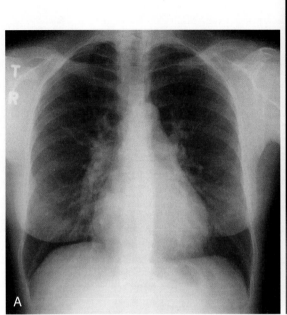
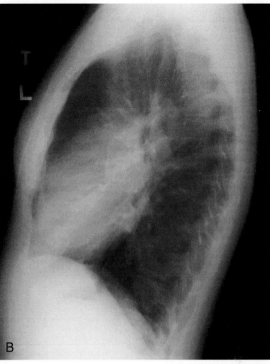

FIGURE 22–3

Chest film of a patient with secundum ASD. *A,* Posteroanterior projection. There is mild cardiomegaly with right atrial enlargement. The main pulmonary artery is enlarged, and pulmonary vascular markings are increased consistent with abnormally high pulmonary blood flow. The ascending aorta appears relatively small in comparison to the main pulmonary artery. *B,* Lateral chest film. There is right ventricular enlargement noted especially in the retrosternal area and no evidence of left atrial enlargement.

connection of the right pulmonary veins, the right hilar vessels may be especially prominent because the pulmonary veins are at the same level as the pulmonary artery.[10] With pulmonary hypertension, the peripheral pulmonary vascularity may gradually become decreased along with increasing size of the central pulmonary arteries. In adult patients with congestive cardiac failure, especially associated with atrial fibrillation or flutter, the pulmonary veins may be prominent and the left atrium may become enlarged.[28]

Magnetic resonance imaging (MRI) is another noninvasive modality that may be useful in patients with an ASD, especially older patients who may have suboptimal echocardiographic imaging windows. MRI can demonstrate the size and location of the ASD as well as anomalous connections of the pulmonary veins (Fig. 22–4). Flow quantitation can estimate the pulmonary-to-systemic flow ratio noninvasively.

ECHOCARDIOGRAPHY

Echocardiography has become the primary method of diagnosis and evaluation of ASDs. Transthoracic two-dimensional echocardiography can demonstrate the size and location of an ASD as well as the expected secondary changes of right atrial and right ventricular enlargement. Parasternal views typically demonstrate enlargement of the right ventricle with the appearance of flattening of the left ventricle in the long-axis view. Short-axis views are helpful in demonstrating that the intraventricular septum typically maintains a normal rounded contour in systole but is flattened or even concave in diastole because of the right ventricular volume overload (Fig. 22–5). The best views to visualize and measure an ASD are from the subxiphoid or subcostal location. In these views, the atrial septum is nearly perpendicular to the imaging axis, and measurements of the defect are most accurate. Secundum ASDs are seen in the central portion of the atrial septum and may extend anteriorly to the aortic root. Sinus venosus ASDs are typically more difficult to image than secundum ASDs. They are located in the superior atrial septum near the orifice of the superior vena cava. The finding of a sinus venosus ASD should prompt thorough evaluation of the right-sided pulmonary veins because partial anomalous drainage of one or more right-sided pulmonary veins is seen in 90% of affected patients (Fig. 22–6).[2] ASD may also be seen in the apical four-chamber view, but in this view, the atrial septum is nearly parallel to the imaging axis so that there may be areas of apparent dropout of the atrial septum even in the absence of an ASD. The apical view is excellent, however, to evaluate the relative size of the right and left atria and right and left ventricles.

Color Doppler echocardiography is helpful in confirming flow through an apparent atrial defect on two-dimensional echocardiography. In the normal situation, left-to-right flow is relatively laminar and can be easily seen. In patients with a small and restrictive ASD, the left-to-right flow may be identified as a higher velocity turbulent jet extending from the atrial septum into the right

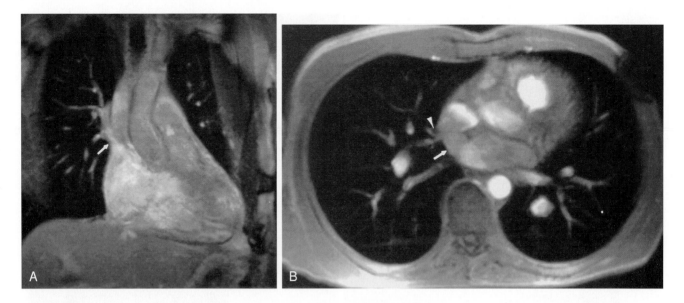

FIGURE 22–4

Cine-gradient-echo MRI in patient with sinus venosus ASD. *A,* Oblique coronal view. The *arrow* indicates anomalous connection of the right upper pulmonary vein to the right atrium at the base of the superior vena cava. The ASD is not well seen in this view. *B,* Transaxial projection. The *arrow* indicates the location of the sinus venosus ASD. The *arrowhead* indicates the anomalous connection of a pulmonary vein to the right atrium adjacent to the sinus venosus ASD. (Images provided by Dr. Scott Flamm, Cleveland Clinic Foundation.)

atrium. In patients with right ventricular hypertrophy from pulmonary stenosis or pulmonary hypertension, there may be little left-to-right flow, and right-to-left flow may predominate. Patients who will be sent for an operation without cardiac catheterization should have complete evaluation of all intracardiac structures as well as the pulmonary veins and systemic veins. In patients with suboptimal transthoracic echocardiographic windows, transesophageal echocardiography may be needed. Coronal and longitudinal views of the atrial septum can be used to identify and measure an ASD. Four-chamber views can demonstrate relative sizes of the right- and left-sided chambers.

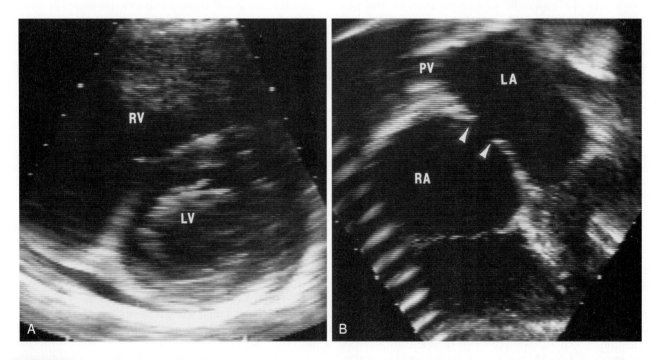

FIGURE 22–5

Two-dimensional echocardiogram of a patient with secundum ASD. *A,* Parasternal view. The right ventricle is enlarged. The left ventricle is flattened in diastole, and the interventricular septum is relatively straight rather than having the normal rounded contour. *B,* Subcostal two-dimensional echocardiographic view of ASD. The *arrowheads* indicate the edges of a relatively small secundum ASD. RV = right ventricle; LV = left ventricle; RA = right atrium; LA = left atrium; PV = right upper pulmonary vein.

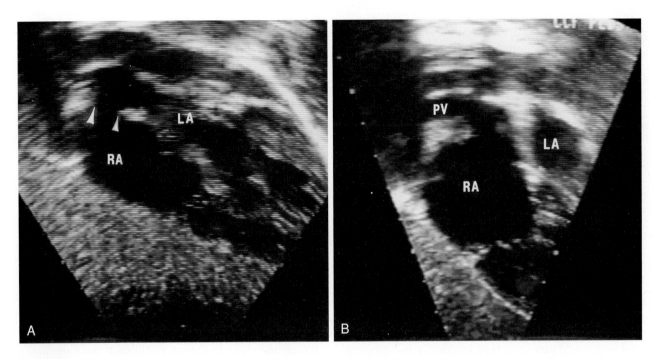

FIGURE 22–6

Subcostal two-dimensional echocardiogram of a patient with sinus venosus ASD. *A,* The *arrowheads* indicate the edges of the ASD in the superior portion of the atrial septum. *B,* View of posterior atrial septum. The right pulmonary vein is seen to enter the right atrium at the base of the superior vena cava. The sinus venosus defect itself is not well seen in this view. RA = right atrium; LA = left atrium; PV = right upper pulmonary vein.

CARDIAC CATHETERIZATION AND ANGIOGRAPHY

In most centers, cardiac catheterization is no longer indicated in most patients with typical clinical and echocardiographic features of ASD. Catheterization may sometimes be needed to evaluate associated abnormalities such as pulmonary valvar stenosis, pulmonary hypertension, or exact sites of connection of the pulmonary veins. In older adult patients, catheterization is indicated preoperatively to exclude concomitant coronary artery disease.

The size of an ASD can be evaluated by several methods in the cardiac catheterization laboratory. Oximetry is useful in estimating the relative pulmonary/systemic blood flows (Qp/Qs) by the Fick principle, but the inability to obtain a true mixed venous saturation introduces a significant source of error in the calculations. Saturations should be obtained in the high superior vena cava or innominate vein if there is suspicion of an anomalous right or left pulmonary vein to the normal right superior vena cava or to an anomalous left vertical vein. An increase in saturation is found in the area of left-to-right shunting of pulmonary venous blood. The estimated Qp/Qs frequently exceeds 2 : 1, but values as small as 1.5 : 1 may be associated with right atrial and right ventricular enlargement. Systemic arterial saturation is generally normal, as is systemic cardiac output measured by the Fick method. Thermodilution cardiac outputs by the usual technique do not accurately reflect systemic cardiac output. If the catheter tip is located in the pulmonary artery, the thermal bolus is diluted by the ASD flow.

Right and left atrial pressures are usually similar in patients with a moderate or large defect. The *v* wave in the right atrium may be more prominent than normal. The catheter can generally be passed through a secundum ASD in the midportion of the atrial septum to the left atrium. If there is a sinus venosus defect, the catheter passes into the left atrium near the base of the superior vena cava. A pulmonary arteriogram should be performed to delineate the sites of pulmonary venous connection if the pulmonary veins are not entered directly or the oxygen saturation values are inconsistent. If it is necessary to delineate the ASD angiographically, an injection of contrast agent in the right upper pulmonary vein is preferred because flow from the vein is directed along the atrial septum. The best view is usually obtained with the angiographic camera in a left anterior oblique and cranial orientation (Fig. 22–7).

MANAGEMENT

The management of a patient with an ASD is based on multiple factors including the age, symptoms, size of the defect, and magnitude of the shunt. Asymptomatic infants with a secundum ASD less than 8 mm in diameter should be observed expectantly. Endocarditis prophylaxis precautions are not necessary unless there are coexisting valvar abnormalities. More than three fourths of such secundum ASDs close spontaneously before 18 months of age. Spontaneous closure can occur in infancy even among patients who have signs of congestive cardiac failure.[19] If medical management is difficult, however, operative closure of the defect may be warranted even in children younger than 1 year.[16] I generally recommend elective closure of a moderate to large ASD in a patient who is asymptomatic, but who

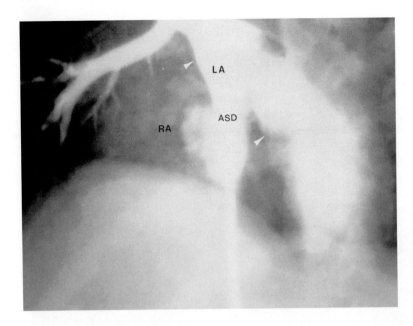

FIGURE 22–7

Left atrial angiogram in a patient with secundum atrial septal defect (ASD). The catheter tip is in the proximal right upper pulmonary vein. The *arrowheads* indicate the upper and lower limits of the atrial septum. Contrast material can be seen flowing through a secundum ASD in the midportion of the atrial septum. RA = right atrium; LA = left atrium.

has definite right atrial and right ventricular enlargement, at 3 to 5 years of age. Studies have shown no long-term benefit to earlier closure.[36]

Because most children and adolescents are asymptomatic and the physical findings may be relatively subtle, the diagnosis of ASD is frequently not made until past the age of 5 years. In older children and young adults, elective closure is recommended by nearly all authorities shortly after diagnosis if there is evidence of right atrial and right ventricular enlargement. Cardiac catheterization is rarely required in this age group because noninvasive evaluations are typically adequate to demonstrate the presence, location, and secondary effects of an ASD. Associated anomalies can also usually be adequately visualized noninvasively, and coronary arteriography is not needed routinely in this age group. Endocarditis prophylaxis precautions are not necessary in patients with an isolated ASD and no valvar dysfunction.

The management of an older adult patient with an ASD is more controversial. Such patients may have a higher operative risk (especially if they have significant pulmonary hypertension), and the incidence of atrial arrhythmias and even stroke may not be reduced in comparison to similar older adult ASD patients who are treated medically.[25, 37] The mortality risk for operation in the modern era should be less than 2%, however, and more than 80% of symptomatic adult patients have improved functional capacity after ASD closure.[24, 38, 39] Cardiac catheterization is recommended if there are risk factors for coronary artery disease or findings suggestive of pulmonary hypertension. Arrhythmia management is an important issue in patients with an ASD. Although an ASD is a potential pathway for paradoxical embolization, more than 90% of strokes in adult ASD patients occur in those who have atrial fibrillation.[40] Operative closure of an ASD in an older patient does not significantly reduce the incidence of late strokes because the incidence of atrial fibrillation is not reduced.[37, 38] Patients should therefore be monitored for the appearance of atrial fibrillation, and if the rhythm does not return to sinus rhythm, anticoagulation therapy should be

considered strongly. Symptomatic sinus node dysfunction and atrioventricular block may occur in ASD patients and may require pacemaker implantation.[36, 40]

Postoperative atrial arrhythmias are common in surgery patients following repair of ASD, with atrial fibrillation occurring in approximately 25% of patients older than 20 years compared with 5% of patients younger than 20 years.[40] The incidence of postoperative atrial arrhythmias has correlated with the increasing age of the patient, the left-to-right shunt size, and the degree of pulmonary hypertension.[41, 42] After ASD repair, 14% of patients develop new postoperative arrhythmias, especially sinus node dysfunction, which occurs more commonly after sinus venosus than after secundum ASD repair.[43, 44] The incidence of persistent late postoperative arrhythmias varies from 2 to 9% in children and 2 to 33% in adults.[40, 42] These late arrhythmias include junctional escape rhythms, sick sinus syndrome, AV block, and atrial flutter or fibrillation.[43] Similar arrhythmias occur after repair of total anomalous pulmonary venous connection.

Operative closure is accomplished by either direct suture closure or placement of a prosthetic patch over the defect with use of cardiopulmonary bypass. Direct suture is usually preferred if the defect is not too large because of concern about the possibility of thrombus formation on patch material, but no clear data exist regarding the superiority of one technique over the other. Operative mortality in younger patients should be less than 1%, but significant transient complications, such as pericardial or pleural effusion requiring treatment, pneumonia, or sepsis, may occur in 10 to 15% of patients in the immediate postoperative period.[45] The average time of hospitalization for ASD closure has been reduced to 4 days or less in some institutions.[46]

A midline sternotomy incision provides the best exposure of the atrial septum and the best opportunity to deal with potential unexpected findings, such as partial anomalous pulmonary venous connection. Other incisions, such as the submammary incision in women, are frequently used because of the potentially better cosmetic result. Operative closure of a sinus venosus ASD essentially always requires a prosthetic patch. The patch usually needs to be directed to the orifice of the superior vena cava because of the partial anomalous pulmonary venous connection to this area. In some patients, the superior vena cava may need to be enlarged with a patch or transected and relocated to the roof of the right atrium to ensure unobstructed drainage.

Patients with a small ASD unassociated with right ventricular and right atrial enlargement do not generally require an operation unless there is a high risk of paradoxical embolization. A patient with an ASD associated with severe pulmonary hypertension and severely elevated pulmonary vascular resistance must be evaluated carefully. In this situation, the ASD may be an associated defect in conjunction with primary pulmonary hypertension rather than the cause of Eisenmenger's reaction. Patients with severe primary pulmonary hypertension may survive longer and have better exercise tolerance if a small ASD is present, and creation of a small ASD has even been used as a form of palliation in this situation.[47]

PROGNOSIS

The prognosis for patients with an ASD is relatively good, especially if the diagnosis is made early and the defect is closed. Patients with an unrepaired ASD associated with a significant left-to-right shunt have an age-related increase in symptoms of dyspnea proceeding to congestive cardiac failure, development of atrial arrhythmias, and increased incidence of stroke. Closure of an isolated ASD is associated with a low mortality risk (<2%). Operative risk is substantially increased in the presence of increased pulmonary vascular resistance (>7 units/m^2) and is probably contraindicated if pulmonary vascular resistance is greater than 15 units/m^2.[48] Symptoms associated with a large left-to-right shunt are generally reversible even if operation is undertaken after the age of 60 years. Exercise tolerance frequently improves even in patients who did not complain of overt symptoms preoperatively.[24] Survival for the 25 years after operative closure in patients younger than 25 years at the time of closure is no different from survival in a normal population. Late cardiovascular events, including endocarditis, symptomatic arrhythmias, pacemaker implantation, and valvar surgery, however, have been seen in approximately 15% of such ASD patients.[40, 49] For the population of patients in whom ASD is not diagnosed until after the age of 25 years, overall long-term survival is decreased compared with that of the normal population regardless of whether the ASD is operatively closed.[40] This does not mean, however, that such patients should not undergo closure of their ASD. Late operative closure may or may not lengthen survival in comparison to patients with an unrepaired ASD but clearly results in improvement of symptoms.[24, 25, 37]

Because ASD closure in early childhood was not commonly practiced until the late 1960s, it is not certain whether early correction will eliminate complications such as atrial fibrillation, stroke, and mitral insufficiency that are not typically seen until later adult life in patients with an unrepaired ASD. The incidence of such complications increases dramatically after age 40 years. It will be at least

another 10 to 15 years before it can be definitively determined that operation in early childhood reduces the risk of these late problems to the rate of occurrence seen in the normal population. Preliminarily, approximately 10% of patients treated operatively before age 15 years develop atrial arrhythmias by age 45 years.[36, 49] This is probably less than the rate of atrial fibrillation in patients with an unrepaired ASD, but definitive data cannot be gleaned from presently available studies. The appearance of atrial fibrillation is serious because it may result in symptomatic deterioration and greatly increases the risk of stroke. It is not yet known whether modern methods of treatment of atrial fibrillation and systemic anticoagulation will improve the long-term outlook of affected patients. Young patients who undergo uneventful ASD closure have an excellent outlook for survival for the next 30 years but should be evaluated periodically.

FUTURE DIRECTIONS

A significant advance in the treatment of ASD may be the development of transcatheter techniques for percutaneous closure. Several devices have been developed and have demonstrated safety and moderate efficacy for ASD closure.[50, 51] The current devices are applicable only to secundum ASD with an adequate septal rim. All of the devices are associated with a higher rate of a small residual leak than is operative closure. Nearly complete closure of an ASD and resolution of the clinical and echocardiographic findings of ventricular enlargement may be achieved, however, in approximately 90% of patients. There may be no need to close residual defects that are only 2 to 3 mm in diameter, and benefits of transcatheter closure may outweigh the relatively inconsequential effects of a small left-to-right shunt. It remains to be seen whether the use of transcatheter devices will reduce the long-term incidence of late atrial arrhythmias.[52] The availability of transcatheter closure with less than 24-hour hospitalization, rapid recovery, and no residual thoracic scar is an exciting possibility in the next 10 years.

ATRIAL SEPTAL DEFECT OCCLUSION DEVICES. In 1974, King and Mills developed a catheter-delivered double umbrella device for occluding ASDs.[53] Although it was used successfully in several patients, it required a large delivery system, and its usage was complicated. The next clinically used device was developed by William Rashkind. This was a self-expanding umbrella device with hooks on the ends of the support arms. Although this device was used successfully in a small number of patients, the Rashkind ASD device had several major disadvantages and was never promoted to widespread use.

The success with the basic structure of the Rashkind ASD device and Rashkind PDA occluder (see Chapter 13) stimulated James Lock to develop a hookless double umbrella device large enough for ASD occlusion.[54] This device, the Clamshell device, was similar in design to the Rashkind PDA occluder with an additional spring joint in the center of each arm that optimized the device for closure of an opening in a septal surface instead of a tubular vessel. The Clamshell device was used in 545 patients in five centers. The safety and efficacy of the device and delivery system for closure of ASDs that are less than 20 mm in diameter proved to be excellent.[55] The implant rate was 98% and the effective closure rate 85%. In spite of the gratifying early success, fractures of the arms of the larger devices were detected as incidental findings on follow-up radiographs. Few clinical complications arose from these unexpected fractures; however, their presence led to withdrawal of the device from elective clinical trials in 1991.

Although the Clamshell device was abandoned by the original manufacturer, it did serve to stimulate a marked interest in nonsurgical correction of ASD. In 1998, no transcatheter ASD occlusion devices were approved for general use in the United States. However, at least five devices for ASD closure were in clinical trials to ascertain their safety and efficacy, in hopes of securing Food and Drug Administration (FDA) approval. The devices under evaluation are as follows:

CARDIOSEAL ASD DEVICE. The Clamshell materials and design were modified by a new manufacturer to develop the CardioSEAL device. The CardioSEAL device still consists of two opposing woven Dacron umbrellas attached at the centers. Each of the four legs of the umbrellas now has two joints along each leg. A new alloy that is more flexible and resistant to fracture is used in the manufacture of the CardioSEAL device. The delivery system and implant procedure, which were tested and proved to be safe and effective with the Clamshell device, are essentially unchanged. The CardioSEAL device began FDA trials in the United States in the fall of 1996, and the device is approved for use in many countries outside the United States.

SIDERIS BUTTON DEVICE. The Button ASD Occluder was developed during the trials of the Clamshell device, has undergone an FDA pilot study in the United States, and has been used extensively in most of the rest of the world. The left atrial portion of the device is a single square sheet of polyurethane foam supported by two wires in an "X" configuration. The left atrial umbrella is held in place with the aid of a counter occluder bar that the operator delivers separately and fastens to the center of the device by a unique button mechanism. This device is delivered through a slightly smaller delivery sheath than the CardioSEAL delivery system. The button device has been used extensively outside the United States with reported good results. It has undergone several modifications and improvements and is being used in the United States only in FDA clinical trials.

ANGEL WINGS ASD DEVICE. The Angel Wings device for ASD occlusion represents a different concept. It consists of two opposing square umbrellas or surfaces of stretchy Dacron. Each umbrella is supported circumferentially by a square frame of Nitinol wire. The two flat umbrella surfaces are sewn together at their centers with no rigid central connection. This central fabric attachment serves as a self-centering mechanism. The device is delivered through a long sheath with an elaborate delivery and release mechanism. This device is being evaluated in an FDA clinical trial in the United States and is available in several countries outside of the United States.

ASDOS (ATRIAL SEPTAL DEFECT OCCLUDER SYSTEM). The ASDOS device was developed in Germany and clinically tested successfully in Europe. It consists of two separate umbrella occluder portions that are made of a polyurethane membrane attached to a radiating Nitinol frame. This device has a relatively complex delivery system that requires the placement of a guide wire rail that extends from a femoral artery, through the heart, and out a femoral vein. Both umbrellas are delivered through a long sheath from the femoral vein. When the two umbrellas are in good position, they are screwed together to provide a clamping attachment to the atrial septum. The rail system is primarily for control of the umbrellas with the capability of adjustment of the device position on the septum. This device is completely retrievable until the device is screwed together and finally released. In 1998, limited FDA clinical trials were under way in the United States.

AMPLATZER ASD OCCLUSION DEVICE. This is the newest type of device undergoing significant trials in the United States in 1998 for ASD occlusion. The device is constructed of a weave of relatively fine Nitinol wire. It is filled with thrombogenic fabric. The device can be pulled into a delivery catheter and resumes its intended shape as it is extruded from the catheter. The intended shape is that of two relatively flat, round disks connected by a central portion of large diameter that provides self-centering and stenting to maintain the device in position. The device is particularly attractive because it can be easily withdrawn and repositioned before release. The design requires relatively accurate sizing of the ASD. The Amplatzer device is used in many countries outside of the United States and is under FDA trials in this country.

REFERENCES

1. Bedford DE: The anatomical types of atrial septal defect. Their incidence and clinical diagnosis. Am J Cardiol 6:568, 1960.
2. Davia JE, Cheitlin MD, Bedynek JL: Sinus venosus atrial septal defect: Analysis of 50 cases. Am Heart J 85:177, 1973.
3. Feldt RH, Weidman WH: Defects of the atrial septal and endocardial cushion. In Emmanouilides GC, Riemenschneider TA (eds): Moss's Heart Disease in Infants, Children and Adolescents, 4th ed. Baltimore, Williams & Wilkins, 1989, p 170.
4. Hagen PT, Scholz DG, Edwards WD: Incidence and size of patent foramen ovale during the first 10 decades of life: An autopsy of 965 normal hearts. Mayo Clin Proc 59:17, 1984.
5. Bedford D, Papp C, Parkinson J: Atrial septal defect. Br Heart J 3:37, 1941.
6. Fyler DC, Buckley LP, Hellenbrand WE, et al: Report of the New England regional infant cardiac program. Pediatrics 65(suppl):375, 1980.
7. Basson CT, Solomon SD, Weissman B, et al: Genetic heterogeneity of heart-hand syndromes. Circulation 91:1326, 1995.
8. Bjornstad PG: Secundum type atrial septal defect with prolonged PR interval and autosomal dominant mode of inheritance. Br Heart J 36:1149, 1974.
9. Chan KC, Godman MJ: Morphologic variations of fossa ovalis atrial septal defects (secundum): Feasibility for transcutaneous closure with the clam-shell device. Br Heart J 69:52, 1993.
10. Nadas AS, Fyler DC: Communications between systemic and pulmonary circuits with predominantly left-to-right shunts. In Nadas AS, Fyler DC: Pediatric Cardiology, 3rd ed. Philadelphia, WB Saunders, 1972, p 317.
11. Schreiber TL, Feigenbaum H, Weyman AE: Effect of atrial septal defect repair on left ventricular geometry and degree of mitral valve prolapse. Circulation 61:888, 1980.

12. Speechly-Dick ME, John R, Pugsley WB, et al: Secundum atrial septal defect repair: Long term surgical outcome and the problem of late mitral regurgitation. Postgrad Med J 69:912, 1993.
13. Raghib G, Ruttenberg HD, Anderson RC, et al: Termination of the left superior vena cava in left atrium, atrial septal defect, and absence of coronary sinus. A developmental complex. Circulation 31:906, 1965.
14. Mathew R, Thilenius OG, Arcilla RA: Comparative response of right and left ventricles to volume overload. Am J Cardiol 38:209, 1976.
15. Levin AR, Spach MS, Boineau JP, et al: Atrial pressure-flow dynamics in atrial septal defects (secundum type). Circulation 37:476, 1968.
16. Bull C, Deanfield J, deLeval M, et al: Correction of isolated secundum atrial septal defect in infancy. Arch Dis Child 56:784, 1981.
17. Dimich I, Steinfield L, Park SC: Symptomatic atrial septal defect in infants. Am Heart J 85:601, 1973.
18. Mahoney LT, Truesdell SC, Krzmarzick TR, et al: Atrial septal defects that present in infancy. Am J Dis Child 140:1115, 1986.
19. Radzik D, Davignon A, vanDoesburg N, et al: Predictive factors for spontaneous closure of atrial septal defects diagnosed in the first three months of life. J Am Coll Cardiol 22:851, 1993.
20. Hamilton WT, Haffajee CI, Dalen JE, et al: Atrial septal defect secundum: Clinical profile with physiologic correlates. In Roberts WC (ed): Adult Congenital Heart Disease. Philadelphia, FA Davis, 1987, p 395.
21. Loscalzo J: Paradoxical embolism: Clinical presentation, diagnostic strategies, and therapeutic options. Am Heart J 112:141, 1986.
22. Cherian G, Uthaman CB, Durairaj M, et al: Pulmonary hypertension in isolated secundum atrial septal defect: High frequency in young patients. Am Heart J 105:952, 1983.
23. Anderson M, Moller I, Lyngborg K, et al: The natural history of small atrial septal defect: Long-term follow-up with serial heart catheterizations. Am Heart J 92:302, 1976.
24. Craig RJ, Selzer A: Natural history and prognosis of atrial septal defect. Circulation 37:805, 1986.
25. Gatzoulis MA, Redington AN, Somerville J, et al: Should atrial septal defects in adults be closed? Ann Thorac Surg 61:657, 1996.
26. Shah D, Azhar M, Oakley CM, et al: Natural history of secundum atrial septal defect in adults after medical or surgical treatment: A historical prospective study. Br Heart J 71:224, 1994.
27. Campbell M: Natural history of atrial septal defect. Br Heart J 32:820, 1970.
28. Perloff JK: Atrial septal defect. In Dreibelbis D, Boehme JE (eds): The Clinical Recognition of Congenital Heart Disease, 3rd ed. Philadelphia, WB Saunders, 1987, p 272.
29. O'Toole JD, Reddy PS, Curtiss EI, et al: The mechanism of splitting of the second heart sound in atrial septal defect. Circulation 56:1047, 1977.
30. Shaver JA, O'Toole JD: The second heart sound: Newer concepts. Mod Concepts Cardiovasc Dis 46:7, 1977.
31. Berry WB, Austen WG: Respiratory variations in the magnitude of the left-to-right shunt in experimental interatrial communications. Am J Cardiol 14:201, 1964.
32. Nadas AS, Ellison RC: Phonocardiographic analysis of diastolic flow murmur in secundum atrial septal defect and ventricular septal defect. Br Heart J 29:684, 1967.
33. Perloff JK: Auscultatory and phonocardiographic manifestations of pulmonary hypertension. Prog Cardiovasc Dis 9:303, 1967.
34. Heller J, Hagege AA, Besse B: "Crochetage" (notch) on R wave in inferior limb leads: A new independent electrocardiographic sign of atrial septal defect. J Am Col Cardiol 27:877, 1996.
35. Kano Y, Abe T, Tanaka M: Electrophysiological abnormalities before and after surgery for atrial septal defect. J Electrocardiol 26:225, 1993.
36. Meijboom F, Hess J, Szatmari A, et al: Long-term follow-up (9 to 20 years) after surgical closure of atrial septal defect at a young age. Am J Cardiol 72:1431, 1993.
37. Konstantinides S, Geibel A, Olschewski M, et al: A comparison of surgical and medical therapy for atrial septal defect in adults. N Engl J Med 333:469, 1995.
38. Horvath KA, Burke RP, Collins JJ, et al: Surgical treatment of adult atrial septal defect: Early and long-term results. J Am Coll Cardiol 20:1156, 1992.
39. Willfort A, Gabriel H, Heger M, et al: Surgical versus conservative treatment for atrial septal defects in adults (Abstract). Circulation 94(suppl):309, 1996.
40. Murphy JG, Gersh BJ, McGoon MD, et al: Long-term outcome after surgical repair of isolated atrial septal defect: Follow-up at 27 to 32 years. N Engl J Med 323:1645, 1990.
41. Bink-Boelkens MTE, Meuzelaar KJ, Eygelaar A: Arrhythmias after repair of secundum atrial septal defect: The influence of surgical modification. Am Heart J 115:629, 1988.
42. Reid JM, Stevenson JC: Cardiac arrhythmias following successful surgical closure of atrial septal defect. Br Heart J 29:742, 1967.
43. Kyger ER, Frazier OH, Cooley DA, et al: Sinus venosus atrial septal defect: Early and late results following closure in 109 patients. Ann Thorac Surg 25:44, 1978.
44. Bink-Boelkens MTE, Velvis H, Van der Heide JJ, et al: Dysrhythmias after atrial surgery in children. Am Heart J 106:125, 1983.
45. Galal MO, Wobst A, Halees Z, et al: Peri-operative complications following surgical closure of atrial septal defect type II in 232 patients—a baseline study. Eur Heart J 15:1381, 1994.
46. Laussen PC, Reid RW, Stene RA, et al: Tracheal extubation of children in the operating room after atrial septal defect repair as part of a clinical practice guideline. Anesth Analg 82:988, 1996.
47. Austen WG, Morrow AG, Berry WB: Experimental studies of the surgical treatment of primary pulmonary hypertension. J Thorac Cardiovasc Surg 48:448, 1964.
48. Steele PM, Fuster V, Cohen M, et al: Isolated atrial septal defect with pulmonary vascular obstructive disease—long term follow-up and prediction of outcome after surgical correction. Circulation 76:1037, 1987.
49. Mandelik J, Moodie DS, Sterba R, et al: Long-term follow-up of children after repair of atrial septal defects. Clev Clin J Med 61:29, 1994.
50. Sideris EB, Rao PS: Transcatheter closure of atrial septal defects: Role of buttoned devices. J Invas Cardiol 8:289, 1996.
51. Latson LA: Percatheter ASD closure. Pediatr Cardiol 19:86, 1998.
52. Schenck MH, Sterba R, Foreman CK, et al: Improvement in non-invasive electrophysiologic findings in children after transcatheter atrial septal defect closure. Am J Cardiol 76:695, 1995.
53. King TD, Mills NL: Non-operative closure of atrial septal defects. Surgery 75:383, 1974.
54. Lock JE, Rome JJ, David R, et al: Transcatheter closure of atrial septal defects: Experimental studies. Circulation 79:1091, 1989.
55. Latson LA, Benson LN, Hellenbrand WE, et al: Early results of multicenter trial of the Bard Clamshell Septal Occluder. Circulation 84:2161a, 1991.

CHAPTER 23
PATENT DUCTUS ARTERIOSUS AND OTHER AORTOPULMONARY ANOMALIES

WELTON M. GERSONY   HOWARD D. APFEL

PATENT DUCTUS ARTERIOSUS

The ductus arteriosus connects the pulmonary trunk with the descending aorta and, like the proximal pulmonary artery, evolves from the sixth aortic arch. Persistent patency of the ductus after birth as an isolated defect in a term infant causes a classic left-to-right shunt, the volume of which depends on the size of the communication in the presence of normal pulmonary resistance. However, with associated anatomic and physiologic abnormalities, the patent ductus arteriosus results in far more complex interactions. The ductus arteriosus contributes to left ventricular volume loading when it occurs either as an isolated anomaly or with other sources of left-to-right shunt, such as atrial or ventricular septal defect. With pulmonary vascular disease, a balanced or right-to-left shunt occurs. When it is associated with lesions that include severe right ventricular outflow tract obstruction and cyanosis, the ductus may serve as the primary source of pulmonary blood flow. In severe left ventricular obstruction in the critically ill neonate, the patent ductus provides the major or only outlet of blood from the right side of the heart to the systemic circulation, allowing cardiac output to be sustained. In these circumstances, prostaglandin E has been extremely useful in the management of neonates who require persistent ductus patency for survival until more specific operative interventions can be carried out.

Persistence of patency of the ductus arteriosus in the first weeks of life results in important hemodynamic complications in a premature infant, especially in association with respiratory distress syndrome. Closure of the patent ductus arteriosus in a premature infant by giving indomethacin to block prostaglandin E production uniquely uses a pharmacologic intervention to replace operation during the first weeks of life. Ductus patency with right-to-left shunting occurs in conditions associated with increased pulmonary vascular resistance in a neonate, most often related to perinatal hypoxemia (known as persistent pulmonary hypertension of the newborn or persistence of the fetal circulation).

Closure of a patent ductus arteriosus was the first operative intervention for congenital heart disease 60 years ago, and ligation and division of a patent ductus arteriosus is still widely used throughout the world; some centers use video thoracoscopic techniques. Closure of a patent ductus arteriosus by interventional catheterization has recently become common.

Newer imaging methods have allowed recognition of an extremely small patent ductus arteriosus that in the past would not have been recognized clinically. Management of a tiny "echo ductus" has become controversial in terms of whether to close such a small communication. This represents another area of medicine in which new observations with use of sensitive noninvasive imaging instruments have revealed subclinical abnormalities, thus creating new management questions.

Patent ductus arteriosus is not always simply an isolated anatomic abnormality easily managed by surgical intervention. It occurs under varied circumstances, and its presence has stimulated a number of new techniques in surgery, interventional catheterization, and neonatal pharmacology. This has led to a number of management options for physicians caring for patients in whom the patent ductus arteriosus is an integral part of a complex disease process.

PATHOLOGIC ANATOMY

The ductus arteriosus evolves from the sixth aortic arch and by 4 months of gestation can be demonstrated to differ histologically from aortic and pulmonary artery tissues.[1] The ductus arteriosus contains elastic tissue only between the intima and the media, whereas the media of arteries is composed totally of elastic fibers. The ductus wall consists of a large amount of ground substance interspersed with smooth muscle cells in a spiral arrangement and containing few elastic fibers. The mucoid substance in the media layer of the ductus is not present in other arterial tissues. Under normal conditions, when the smooth muscle of the ductus wall contracts soon after birth, the mucoid substance and the wall coalesce, and intimal cushions protrude into the lumen of the ductus. When flow reaches a critically low level, there is impaired nutrition into this region, and cytolytic necrosis ensues. Intimal cushions proliferate and ultimately meet, sealing the ductus completely. Fibrous tissue eventually replaces the media and intima, resulting in a fibrotic structure referred to as the ligamentum arteriosum.[2]

In a normal full-term human infant, the ductus is completely closed in the first weeks of life. The mechanisms responsible for postnatal ductus closure have been well described, although some questions remain. Exposure to increased PO_2 as occurs with initial ventilation after birth constricts the ductus arteriosus, but increased oxygen tension[3–5] alone does not initiate the process that results in total obliteration of the lumen. Ductus patency is regulated by endogenously produced prostaglandin as well as by low oxygen tension. Prostaglandin E_2 appears to be the prostaglandin responsible for regulating ductus arteriosus patency, but whether this substance is produced in ductus tissue itself or by the pulmonary vasculature is not clear. The combination of low oxygen tension in the fetus (PO_2 18 to 28 mm Hg) and high plasma levels of prostaglandin E_2 serves to keep the ductus open during fetal life. In the final trimester, however, the ductus appears less responsive to the relaxing effect of prostaglandin, and its sensitivity to oxygen increases, resulting in the conditions encouraging constriction and functional closure within the first day or two of life. In a premature infant, a patent ductus arteriosus at birth usually continues to have the anatomic and physiologic potential for complete closure because the anatomic features of the structure are normal and will respond to changes in postnatal arterial oxygen tension and to increasing circulating prostaglandin E_2 levels. Therefore, later closure is expected on a physiologic basis. In contrast, full-term infants with persistent patent ductus arteriosus have a primary anatomic defect of the ductus wall, so that normal constriction does not occur. These infants have a genetically determined deficiency in the amount of ductus smooth muscle and an increase in elastic tissue similar to the adjacent aorta. Therefore, late spontaneous closure of a patent ductus arteriosus does not occur.[4,5]

HEMODYNAMICS

Isolated Patent Ductus Arteriosus

The hemodynamics of an established patent ductus arteriosus results in a left-to-right shunt from the aorta to the pulmonary artery. The magnitude of shunting depends on the size of the ductus orifice and the relationship between systemic and pulmonary vascular resistance. In an uncomplicated patent ductus arteriosus with normal pulmonary vascular resistance, the size of the left-to-right shunt eventually depends on the size of the ductus orifice. The ductus may be as large as the pulmonary artery or aorta in some patients, because this structure originally represented an aortic arch in fetal life. This could occur if there was no constriction of the ductus whatsoever. When the ductus constricts, usually beginning at the junction with the left pulmonary artery, a smaller shunt is present, ranging from moderate to inconsequential.

In a large ductus, shunts greater than 3 to 1 occur, and because there is little or no restriction of blood flow between the great arteries, pulmonary artery pressure is similar to systemic pressure, and the left ventricle is subject to a large volume load. This results in congestive heart failure. As with any intraventricular or great artery communication, elevated pulmonary vascular resistance in a neonate limits the shunt for days or weeks after birth, but when pulmonary vascular resistance regresses toward normal, left ventricular failure ensues. With smaller shunts, pulmonary hypertension is less prominent; and with a markedly restricted patent ductus arteriosus, pulmonary pressure may be normal, and the patient is asymptomatic.[6,7]

Patent Ductus Arteriosus With Other Left-to-Right Shunts

Ductus patency may be present in patients with an atrial septal defect, ventricular septal defect, or other less common left-to-right shunts. As with an uncomplicated patent ductus arteriosus, ductus flow from the aorta to the pulmonary artery relates to the size of the communication. However, with a large proximal left-to-right shunt that results in virtually maximal capacitance of the pulmonary circulation, a potential large ductus left-to-right shunt may be masked. Under these circumstances, before the era of echo Doppler technology, a large patent ductus could be easily missed without an aortic arch angiogram. With multiple significant shunting sites, pulmonary blood flow is unrestricted and pulmonary artery pressure is markedly elevated.[8,9] In some patients, however, small shunts at multiple levels may be found in relatively asymptomatic patients.

Patent Ductus Arteriosus With Severe Right Ventricular Outflow Tract Obstruction

Among neonates with particular cardiac malformations, such as pulmonary atresia with intact ventricular septum or extreme tetralogy with pulmonary atresia, a patent ductus arteriosus can be necessary for survival. Without significant pulmonary artery collateral flow in a neonate (rare with pulmonary atresia with intact ventricular septum, but more common with extreme tetralogy), systemic oxygenation totally depends on collaterals, and ductus closure results in rapid hypoxemia and death. Although low arterial oxygen tension might be suspected to stimulate persistent ductus patency, normal decrease in circulating prostaglandins almost always results in marked ductal constriction and closure, albeit delayed for some hours or days. Management of neonates with severe limitation of right ventricular outflow tract blood flow (e.g., pulmonary atresia, tricuspid atresia, severe tetralogy) focuses on pharmacologic treatment with prostaglandin to maintain ductal patency and preserve pulmonary blood flow until an appropriate operation can be performed.[10]

Patent Ductus Arteriosus and Severe Left Ventricular Outflow Tract Obstruction

Neonates with hypoplastic left heart syndrome, critical aortic stenosis, or severe coarctation of the aorta depend on right-to-left ductus blood flow to preserve cardiac output. Although this type of hemodynamic state, by definition, causes peripheral arterial desaturation, ductus flow can preserve adequate systemic blood flow until an operation can be carried out. In a symptomatic neonate with aortic stenosis, a right-to-left ductus shunt is strong evidence of inadequate cardiac output from the left ventricle. Such neonates are managed with prostaglandin therapy until an operation is carried out. If an infant with aortic stenosis has a left-to-right shunt through the ductus, the systemic blood flow is being provided by the left ventricle, suggesting a better prognosis for adequate left ventricular outflow after valvotomy.[11]

Patent Ductus Arteriosus With Transposition of the Great Arteries

Among neonates with transposition of the great arteries and intact ventricular septum, mixing at the atrial level is critical to allow survival until balloon septostomy or an arterial switch procedure can be done urgently. In a severely hypoxic infant, patency of the ductus arteriosus improves mixing. Therefore, prostaglandin E$_1$ is administered in an attempt to raise PaO$_2$ to the degree that fatal hypoxemia does not occur during transfer to a cardiology center, and preparations are made for balloon atrial septostomy or an arterial switch operation.[10–14] However, during the first day or two of life, when pulmonary arterial resistance is virtually identical to systemic resistance, additional bidirectional shunting at the ductus level is minimal, and PaO$_2$ does not increase as much as might be expected. As pulmonary resistance declines, more significant left-to-right shunting occurs across the ductus, and because an equal right-to-left shunt must occur at the foramen ovale level, oxygenation improves to a greater degree.

NATURAL HISTORY

Patent Ductus Arteriosus in a Term Infant

Because of the abnormal structure of the ductus arteriosus in term infants with persistent patency, spontaneous closure is extremely rare. A large patent ductus arteriosus leads to early congestive heart failure, which untreated can result in death. If the ductus is not eliminated, the development of pulmonary vascular disease in surviving patients with relatively unrestrictive communications is variable. Patients with a large patent ductus arteriosus, unrepaired during infancy or even childhood, may still have relatively normal pulmonary vascular resistance and improve with ligation at an older age. On the other hand, some individuals have progressive pulmonary vascular disease resulting in diminution of signs of left-sided heart failure, development of a right-to-left shunt, and eventual right-sided heart decompensation.[15] However, individuals with patent ductus and associated pulmonary vascular obstructive disease from early childhood are occasionally recognized in the pediatric age range or by history later in adolescence or young adulthood.

A small patent ductus arteriosus with diagnostic but minimal clinical signs is well tolerated. When pulmonary-to-systemic flow ratios are small, patients remain asymptomatic into adulthood but are at risk for bacterial endocarditis.[16] A few older individuals develop accelerated congestive heart failure with a relatively small ductus when late acquired myocardial disease occurs. Heart failure may be exaggerated by the requirement for increased cardiac output, however marginal, that occurs with a ductus.

A tiny subclinical ductus may be more common than is generally realized. A trivial patent ductus with no clinical manifestations cannot be recognized by physical examination. It is only discovered in patients who have echocardiograms for reasons unrelated to the clinical findings associated with a patent ductus. There is no evidence that there is a significant risk of endocarditis with the "silent" ductus, identifiable only by a tiny Doppler jet. It is possible that many such trivial ductus will eventually close on the basis of stasis.

Patent Ductus Arteriosus in the Premature Infant

In premature babies, persistence of ductus patency is common. Most undergo spontaneous closure as the premature infant matures and the effects of diminishing circulating prostaglandin on the natural closure mechanisms become manifest in the first months of life.[17] However, persistent patency may nevertheless occasionally occur. In recent years, an extremely small premature infant managed with ventilation, surfactant replacement therapy, and other therapies for respiratory distress syndrome is more likely to survive the first days of life, after which a large patent ductus arteriosus may play an increasingly important role in the infant's clinical course. Early right-to-left shunts are seen in premature infants with severe respiratory distress syndrome, based on elevated pulmonary vascular resistance at birth. This may evolve to a large left-to-right shunt and congestive heart failure as pulmonary resistance falls. Although a ductus under these circumstances may eventually close spontaneously, severe clinical manifestations require pharmacologic or operative closure during the first weeks of life to prevent overwhelming congestive heart failure, pulmonary failure, and death.[18]

CLINICAL EVALUATION

History

The medical history of a term infant with patent ductus arteriosus depends on the size of the left-to-right shunt. Infants with a large ductus display manifestations of left-sided heart failure similar to that seen for other ventricular or great artery communications. Varying degrees of tachypnea, decreased oral intake, and failure to thrive are the classic clinical manifestations. Less severe symptoms are noted with a moderate shunt, and a small patent ductus arteriosus has no effect on an infant's clinical course. A cardiac murmur is usually heard by the primary physician. Signs of congestive heart failure with a significant patent ductus arteriosus may be difficult to ascertain in the context of pulmonary disease in a premature infant, although a large left-to-right shunt may contribute to respiratory symptoms and may affect the patient's early clinical course.[19]

Older patients with a patent ductus arteriosus are almost always asymptomatic because larger communications are more likely to be identified in infancy. An older child with chronic congestive heart failure secondary to a large left-to-right shunt through a patent ductus arteriosus is rarely encountered in developed nations. A few patients with patent ductus arteriosus and pulmonary vascular disease have been identified who have no history of early symptoms or clinical findings. Such patients probably have a primary form of pulmonary artery hypertension, and it is unknown whether the ductus is an associated lesion or is somehow involved in the original etiology.[9] Older children with patent ductus arteriosus and pulmonary vascular obstructive disease can display lower body cyanosis in the late phase, but this is rarely diagnosed clinically.

Physical Examination

Neonates, both term and premature, with patent ductus arteriosus may present with a "clicky," "rolling dice" quality systolic murmur along the left mid and upper sternal border. The diastolic component is absent because there is less diastolic shunting when pulmonary hypertension is present. In babies not undergoing operative repair, this finding evolves into a more classic continuous bruit. The clinical examination of an older child with a significant patent ductus arteriosus includes an active precordium with a left ventricular impulse; a second sound partially obscured by the murmur; a continuous murmur at the left mid and upper sternal border with a classic machinery quality; and if the ductus is at least moderately large, widened pulse pressure and bounding peripheral pulses. A systolic thrill may accompany the murmur at the left mid and upper sternal border. A separate mid-diastolic rumble of increased flow across the mitral valve may be identified at the apex when a large left-to-right shunt is present. Patent ductus arteriosus in the context of associated congenital heart disease in which the pulmonary blood flow or systemic blood flow depends on patency of the ductus does not have the usual manifestations on physical examination and cannot be diagnosed by clinical examination.

Patients with a patent ductus arteriosus and pulmonary vascular obstruction have only a short systolic ejection murmur at the left mid and upper sternal border; the murmur becomes less prominent as pulmonary vascular resistance increases. The second sound becomes single and loud. With severe vascular disease and right-to-left ductus shunting, usually there are no striking murmurs audible. A soft diastolic murmur of pulmonary insufficiency may be noted (Graham Steell's murmur).

Electrocardiography

The electrocardiogram in a patient with a small patent ductus arteriosus is normal. With a large communication, left ventricular hypertrophy, occasionally with ST-T wave changes typical of left ventricular strain, is noted. When pulmonary artery hypertension is present, biventricular hypertrophy is apparent. In older patients with pulmonary vascular disease and a right-to-left shunt, right ventricular hypertrophy is prominent. Infants with patent ductus arteriosus and associated congenital lesions as well as infants with duct-dependent systemic or pulmonary blood flow display electrocardiograms more typical of the underlying cardiac malformation.

Chest Radiography

The chest film usually shows a prominent main pulmonary artery segment and cardiac enlargement related to the size of the left-to-right shunt. If the ductus is large, pulmonary vascular markings are increased and left atrial enlarge-

ment is noted. Patients with pulmonary vascular obstruction disease and patent ductus arteriosus show typical Eisenmenger-type radiographs with a small heart, prominent right ventricle, and tapering pulmonary blood vessel markings.

Echocardiography

The echocardiogram is useful in identifying a patent ductus arteriosus and also defines or excludes associated cardiac conditions. Documentation of a patent ductus is most easily accomplished by imaging in a high left parasternal short-axis view. A large wide ductus can be visualized throughout its course, but a smaller, more narrow ductus may require color flow Doppler mapping for identification. The long tortuous ductus requires multiple imaging planes for complete delineation. Careful angulation of the transducer from the suprasternal notch view of the aortic arch can demonstrate the entire course of the ductus from the distal main pulmonary artery–left pulmonary artery junction to the lesser curvature of the aorta, just distal to the left subclavian artery (Fig. 23–1 [see also Color Plates]). In instances of multiple systemic to pulmonary artery collateral connections, identification of the "true" ductus arteriosus may be difficult.

Doppler color flow mapping can be useful in determining the direction of flow within the ductus throughout the cardiac cycle. Continuous-wave Doppler examination can estimate pulmonary artery pressure by indicating the pressure difference between aorta and pulmonary artery. Ideally, the Doppler beam should be positioned parallel to ductus flow; this may be impossible in a large and tortuous ductus.

Echocardiography can also be helpful in estimating the hemodynamic significance of a patent ductus by showing left atrial or left ventricular enlargement. In increased vascular resistance, right-to-left shunting can be documented by color flow Doppler interrogation across the ductus. Bidirectional shunting is usually present until pulmonary vascular disease is severe. Other echocardiographic signs of pulmonary hypertension, such as right ventricular hypertrophy, systolic flattening of the interventricular septum, and right ventricular and pulmonary artery enlargement, can be demonstrated by the two-dimensional imaging.

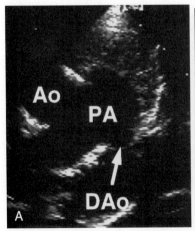
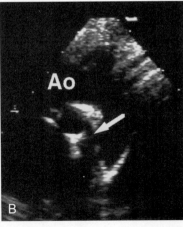

FIGURE 23–1

A, Two-dimensional echocardiographic parasternal short-axis view of a large, wide patent ductus arteriosus *(arrow).* Color flow Doppler imaging demonstrates left-to-right shunting at the large communication. (See also Color Figure 23–1*A*1.) *B,* Suprasternal arch view identifies a relatively narrow, tortuous ductus with left-to-right shunting on color flow imaging *(arrow).* (See also Color Figure 23–1*B*1.) Ao = aorta; DAo = descending aorta; PA = pulmonary artery.

Transesophageal echocardiography generally adds little to the assessment of this lesion in infants and small children. In adults, however, transesophageal echocardiography may complement information provided by transthoracic recordings and may identify a small patent ductus arteriosus missed by transthoracic imaging.[20] Transesophageal echocardiography during catheter closure of the patent ductus does not appear to enhance this procedure.[21] In contrast, transthoracic imaging before the interventional procedure is useful in estimating the size and morphology of the ductus, and it may play a role in evaluating the appropriateness of attempting coil closure (generally, more than 5 mm in diameter is too large) and predicting the difficulty of the procedure on the basis of the morphologic subtype.[22, 23]

Cardiac Catheterization

Cardiac catheterizations are today rarely performed in patients with isolated patent ductus arteriosus, given the specificity of the physical examination and echocardiogram. When a study is carried out, the patent ductus arteriosus is confirmed in a number of ways. First, the catheter may directly pass from the pulmonary artery through the ductus into the descending aorta. Catheters that enter the aorta through a ventricular septal defect or aortopulmonary window pass through the ascending aorta to the carotid arteries or around the aortic arch. Oxygen data indicate an increase in saturation from the right side of the heart to the distal pulmonary arteries, and when both peripheral left and right arterial saturations are similar, pulmonary blood flow can be measured and left-to-right shunts calculated on the basis of the Fick principle. The distal pulmonary artery oxygen saturations are most exact because streaming aberrations depending on where the ductus enters the pulmonary artery may result in misleading formulations.[7] In patients with pulmonary valve insufficiency, increases in oxygen saturations from the right atrium to the right ventricle may falsely suggest a coexistent ventricular septal defect. When more proximal atrial or ventricular communications with large left-to-right blood flow are present, the expected increase in oxygen saturation at the pulmonary artery level may be masked, and it becomes important to document the ductus patency by other imaging methods or direct observations in the operating room.

The presence and severity of pulmonary hypertension depend on the size of the ductus and pulmonary vascular resistance. A large ductus with massive pulmonary blood flow results in hyperkinetic pulmonary hypertension that resolves almost immediately after ductus ligation. If pulmonary vascular resistance is high, vascular obstructive pulmonary hypertension will be present even with a small left-to-right shunt, or in later stages of the disease, with a balanced or right-to-left shunt.

Selective angiography nicely illustrates the anatomy and size of a patent ductus arteriosus. Contrast material is injected into the ascending aorta immediately distal to the aortic side of a potential patent ductus arteriosus. The injection can be carried out either by a venous catheter that passes from the right side of the heart through the pulmonary artery to the aortic side of the ductus or by retrograde aortography. The ductus is best seen in a straight lateral projection, but various angulations may be helpful when a ductus appears to have an atypical course.

MANAGEMENT

The Premature Infant

General supportive measures in a premature infant with a clinically significant patent ductus arteriosus include maintaining an adequate hematocrit and restricting fluids to avoid volume overload. With the advent of a pharmacologic method for closure of the patent ductus in preterm infants in 1976, it appeared that the management of this lesion would be significantly simplified.[24] Yet, despite numerous clinical trials and different treatment strategies, the specific indications and timing for closure remain controversial.

Early studies in the late 1970s established the critical beneficial role of operative closure of a patent ductus with a significant left-to-right shunt in symptomatic neonates.[25–27] In the early 1980s, with the development of pharmacologic closure, most reports concentrated on comparison of treatment with indomethacin versus medical management with backup treatment with indomethacin if needed.[28, 29] One multicenter randomized double-blind collaborative trial compared three treatment strategies in 405 infants who had a "hemodynamically significant patent ductus arteriosus."[29] One strategy involved immediate administration of a three-dose course of intravenous indomethacin in addition to the usual medical therapy; the second strategy was the usual medical therapy initially with indomethacin as a backup; and the third approach was the usual medical management with operation as backup. There were no differences in mortality or morbidity between the three treatment regimens at 1-year follow-up. On the basis of this information, the recommended mode of therapy for premature infants with a hemodynamically significant patent ductus arteriosus was a trial of medical therapy at the time of diagnosis, with indomethacin used 24 to 48 hours later for infants with persistent severe symptoms.

Although it was carefully defined in the collaborative study, the term *clinically significant* may be subject to individual bias. To some physicians, any deterioration after fluid restriction or institution of diuretic therapy constitutes an indication for intervention to remove the ductus shunt. Others require the additional need for longer and more aggressive ventilatory support as sufficient indication of hemodynamic significance to warrant intervention.[30] This ambivalence led to comparisons of treatment of early symptomatic patients (i.e., when early clinical signs first appear at age 1 to 3 days) versus treatment only when signs of overt congestive heart failure appear (approximately 7 to 12 days).[31, 32] Merritt and coworkers,[31] in a relatively small randomized blinded trial (24 patients), provided support for the notion that even mildly symptomatic patients should be treated as early as the third day of life. However, other investigators examining similar treatment groups failed to demonstrate significant differences in mortality and morbidity rates.[32]

In the late 1980s and 1990s, a fourth treatment strategy has received considerable attention: the prophylactic use of indomethacin even before the onset of symptoms. This approach was considered in very low birth weight infants (i.e., the group at highest risk for symptomatic patent ductus arteriosus) as early as 1981.[33] Several studies have shown that the incidence of grade III or grade IV intraventricular and pulmonary hemorrhage can be significantly reduced in a prophylactically treated group.[34–36] No firm evidence has emerged, however, to support this treatment strategy as effective in preventing mortality or respiratory morbidity related to patent ductus arteriosus in premature infants. Furthermore, Couser and coauthors[37] evaluated multiple outcome variables, including incidence of intraventricular hemorrhage, survival, duration of stay in the intensive care unit, overall hospital stay, ventilation and oxygen requirements, and bronchopulmonary dysplasia, and found no significant difference between early indomethacin-treated and placebo-treated infants.

A meta-analysis of treatment strategies for the ductus in premature infants showed that early treatment of a symptomatic patent ductus arteriosus may significantly reduce the risk of pulmonary and necrotizing enterocolitis morbidity.[38] Furthermore, prophylactic therapy reduced the chances for development of a symptomatic patent ductus arteriosus. The author did not advocate routine prophylaxis, because most premature infants would not have become symptomatic even with treatment. Thus, on a risk/benefit basis, most premature babies can be observed for the development of symptoms. Prophylactic indomethacin treatment may be appropriate, however, when the risk for either grade III or grade IV intracranial hemorrhage or severe pulmonary hemorrhage is considered to be high.

A second course of indomethacin treatment is occasionally necessary to achieve adequate ductus closure. In a study of 77 premature infants, Weiss and colleagues[39] showed a 21% reopening of the ductus after clinical closure with indomethacin. The infants with residual luminal flow on echocardiography despite "complete clinical closure" were more likely to have subsequent clinical reopening than were those with no luminal flow. However, even those with apparent complete obliteration of ductus flow may have reopening.

It is essential to be certain of the absence of a ductus-dependent lesion before initiating indomethacin therapy to close this structure. Although reports have documented reopening of the ductus with prostaglandin after closure with indomethacin, irreversible clinical damage may occur under these circumstances before urgent salvage therapy.

Term Infants
LARGE DUCTUS ARTERIOSUS
Full-term infants who present with signs of congestive heart failure should undergo corrective closure of the patent ductus soon after diagnosis. Medical treatment with delay of definitive therapy is not recommended because the chances of late spontaneous closure are small, and the risk of corrective procedures is extremely low at any age. Indomethacin therapy is ineffective in a term infant.

Ligation is the procedure of choice at many institutions because of the high success rate for complete closure.[40] Furthermore, a hemodynamically significant ductus (greater than 5 mm in diameter) is often too large to be considered for transcatheter closure with use of the cur-

rently available stainless steel coils. Multiple coil techniques have only recently been introduced and are rarely used in the setting of a hemodynamically significant ductus.[41] Other ductus closure devices, such as the Rashkind double umbrella, have been used for large ducts but have several drawbacks, including the requirement of a large delivery catheter (greater than 7 French) and relatively high residual shunt rates.[42–44] Some institutions have successfully undertaken thoracoscopic ligation of the patent ductus.[45] This approach eliminates the postoperative scar and may reduce the postoperative convalescence period. Potential drawbacks include difficulty controlling intraoperative bleeding and the requirement for surgeons to learn a new technical skill. More experience with this technique will determine whether it can be done safely and effectively on a universal basis.

SMALL DUCTUS ARTERIOSUS
Closure of a patent ductus detectable by auscultation in an asymptomatic patient is recommended because of the risk of infectious endocarditis.[16] In contrast to a symptomatic ductus, however, intervention for a clinically apparent (i.e., audible) but hemodynamically insignificant ductus can be delayed at least until the end of the first year of life. There are two approaches for achieving ductus closure. Although many cardiologists recommend percutaneous catheter closure with use of stainless steel coil embolization or other devices designed specifically for ductus occlusion, others continue to prefer ligation. There are specific advantages and disadvantages to each approach (see sections on surgical repair and catheter closure). The particular approach at a given institution is guided by local practice patterns and parental preference.

SURGICAL CLOSURE OF THE DUCTUS. A ductus may be either divided or simply ligated at operation with excellent efficacy and only minimal associated risk. Typically, the ductus is approached through a left posterior thoracotomy. The patent ductus arteriosus is identified and dissected free without the use of cardiopulmonary bypass. The ductus is then ligated at both the pulmonary arterial and aortic ends and may be divided between the sutures. Well-documented examples of recanalization or incomplete initial ligation have influenced some surgeons to prefer transection to simple suture ligation.[46] On the other hand, although division offers the obvious advantage of definitive correction, the risk of hemorrhage particularly in large short ductus has reduced the popularity of this approach. With modern operative techniques, ligation alone suffices in most children with few residual shunts. Extremely rare complications associated with ligation include injury to the recurrent laryngeal nerve; disruption of the thoracic duct with chylothorax; and accidental ligation of the left pulmonary artery, descending aorta, or carotid artery.[47] Theoretical disadvantages to an operative approach, even in an uncomplicated ductus, include the need for general anesthesia, postoperative pain, thoracotomy scar, occasional need for chest tubes, and prolonged hospital stay.

CATHETER CLOSURE OF A DUCTUS. Closure of a patent ductus by nonoperative means was first reported by Porstmann in 1971.[48] Because this technique required a large arterial delivery system, its use was limited mainly to older children and adults. Another type of percutaneous catheter closure technique, applicable to children, was introduced by Rashkind in 1979. He constructed a small umbrella device using a catheter delivery system.[49] Subsequent modifications of the device and technique by Bash and Mullins[50] led to more widespread use of the procedure. By the early 1990s, several shortcomings of this and similar devices were being described, including a significant incidence of residual shunting and the need for a large delivery system.[51] The candidates for catheter closure were limited to patients with a large ductus, and some investigators advocated techniques designed to enlarge the ductus to fit in the device for vessel occlusion.[52] Other reported complications of early devices included "Waring blender"–induced hemolysis, injury to the tricuspid and pulmonary valves, and device embolization.[53, 54]

In an extensive collaborative study, the Rashkind PDA Occlusion Device was demonstrated to be both effective and safe.[49] In 1991, after accumulation of data on more than 700 patients during 10 years, the study was discontinued and the device was permanently withdrawn by the manufacturer from trials or use in the United States. The Rashkind occluder is an accepted device for patent ductus arteriosus closure with a *total* occlusion rate of approximately 83%. There were no deaths and no complications with permanent sequelae from the device or the procedure.

The Rashkind occluding device has two opposing umbrellas either 12 or 17 mm in diameter attached at the centers by a spring mechanism. Although the device can be delivered from either the arterial or venous approach, the venous approach is used for the delivery of most Rashkind PDA occluders. Once the size and shape of the ductus are determined, an appropriate diameter (8 or 11 French) long Mullins trans-septal sheath/dilator set is passed over an exchange wire into the descending aorta. The delivery catheter with the loaded occlusion device is introduced into the previously positioned sheath and advanced to the area of the tricuspid valve. The delivery wire is advanced carefully until the distal legs of the occluding device spring open in the aorta. The sheath, the delivery catheter, and the delivery wire are all then withdrawn as a single unit into the aortic isthmus of the ductus. With the delivery wire and catheter fixed at this position, the sheath alone is withdrawn several centimeters from the still-attached device, allowing the proximal legs of the device to open. The release mechanism of the delivery catheter is activated to release the device in the ductus.

The Rashkind ductus-occluding device is not and probably will not be approved for clinical use in the United States. In most other parts of the world, it is still used for correcting both a large and a very short patent ductus arteriosus. Gianturco coils, particularly with their significantly reduced expense, have replaced the Rashkind device for most small ductus even where the Rashkind device is available. Where the Rashkind device and the adjunct devices such as coils and Gianturco-Grifka vascular occlusion devices (see Chapter 13) are available and can be used selectively or in conjunction with each other, operative repair of a patent ductus arteriosus is being relegated to a historical procedure. Patients who have undergone transcatheter oc-

clusion of a patent ductus arteriosus are allowed to return to full, unlimited physical activity on the day after the occlusion. Because of the time required for complete endothelialization of the device, these patients should receive antibiotics for endocarditis prophylaxis for 6 months after complete occlusion with the device implant.

In response to the lack of universal availability of the Rashkind device, a new technique for ductus closure using coil embolization was introduced by Cambier and coworkers in 1991.[55] Stainless steel coils had been in use for occlusion of collateral vessels and arteriovenous malformations since 1975, and the technique was modified for ductus occlusion.[56] The procedure involves initial right-sided heart catheterization to assess the degree of shunting at the ductus level. This is followed by an aortogram to measure minimum ductus diameter and to assess ductus morphology (Fig. 23–2). A coil is chosen that has a diameter twice the diameter of the narrowest point in the ductus. A 4 or 5 French delivery catheter is passed from the femoral artery and through the patent ductus into the pulmonary artery. The coil is partially extruded from the catheter, and the delivery catheter with the coil is withdrawn until the exposed circle of coil is against the pulmonary end of the ductus. As the catheter is withdrawn further through the ductus and into the aorta, the remainder of the coil is *simultaneously* extruded into the aortic ampulla of the ductus. If complete occlusion has not occurred within a few minutes after implant, additional coils are implanted during the same procedure or at a later procedure.[57] In the United States, where other more specifically designed ductus devices are not available, the use of the coils for ductus occlusion has become the standard procedure for closure of a patent ductus arteriosus.[57, 58]

In the original report by Cambier and coworkers, closure by the coil technique was limited to ductus less than 2.5 mm in size. Several variations and modifications of the coil closure technique have subsequently led to use for larger ducts. Technique modifications have included a reduction in the size of the delivery system to 4 French[41]; the use of multiple coils to close ducts up to 5 mm size[41]; the use of coil-filled sac for an even larger ductus[59]; and the use of a snare technique to hold and manipulate the coil as it is delivered,[60] improving accuracy of placement and reducing the incidence of peripheral embolization. In a report describing early and intermediate results, Shim and coauthors[58] showed actuarial residual shunt rates in 75 patients of $6 \pm 5\%$ in 20 months. Of 14 patients with residual shunts, 5 had closure with a second coil. They reported no incidence of recanalization, endarteritis, acquired coarctation, or left pulmonary artery stenosis at early follow-up.

DUCT OCCLUDER DEVICE. The Redel Duct-Occlud device was developed specifically for patent ductus arteriosus.[61] The occlusion device is a semistiff spring wire specifically shaped into double cones of various sizes. This wire cone has no added thrombogenic materials (fibers) and depends on the tight coil of the wire itself to occlude the ductus. It is delivered with an elaborate attach/release system that allows retraction of the device if, once delivered, it is not in perfect position. This Duct-Occlud has had satisfactory clinical trials in Europe. As with the other catheter-delivered ductus occlusion devices, the initial occlusion

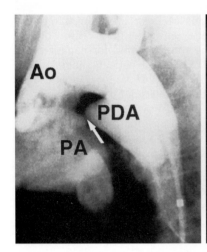
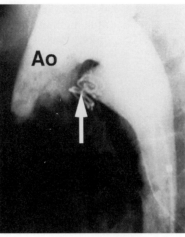

FIGURE 23-2

Left, Ascending aortogram (Ao) demonstrates filling of the pulmonary artery (PA) from the ductus arteriosus (PDA), which narrows toward the pulmonary arterial end *(arrow). Right,* A coil *(arrow)* has been placed inside the ductus toward its narrow end. Note that the pulmonary artery is no longer filled from the aortic angiogram.

rate is less than 100%; however, additional devices can be added to complete the occlusion. We hope that this device will be entering clinical investigational device exemption trials in the United States to add to the nonoperative armamentarium for correction of patent ductus arteriosus.

The advantages of ductus closure by the coil method include lack of a need for general anesthesia, shorter hospital stay and convalescent period, and elimination of a thoracotomy scar. Disadvantages and potential complications include an incidence of residual leaks, peripheral coil embolization, hemolysis (rare), left pulmonary artery turbulence or actual stenosis, and femoral vessel occlusion. The issue of coil placement complicating future magnetic resonance imaging has been raised. Strouse and coworkers[62] have concluded that the magnetic forces exerted on an implanted coil or other metallic device were small compared with the forces experienced secondary to heart motion and blood pressure in healthy individuals. Nevertheless, they cautioned that devices demonstrating substantial deflections not be imaged if in place for less than 5 to 6 weeks.

A SILENT DUCTUS

With the advent of color flow Doppler echocardiography, large numbers of tiny native ductus undetectable by conventional auscultation have been recognized. These were usually recognized when an echocardiogram was carried out to evaluate a nondescript heart murmur. In addition, with increasing use of transcatheter closure techniques for a significant ductus, a small residual silent leak is encountered.

There are no data regarding the risk of endocarditis in patients with a silent ductus compared with those with a clinically diagnosed patent ductus arteriosus or other cardiac anomalies. There has been one published report.[63] Furthermore, late closure of these tiny channels may well occur. Most pediatric cardiologists do not recommend intervention for the tiny nonclinical patent ductus. It is generally agreed that subacute bacterial endocarditis prophylaxis for appropriate procedures and follow-up examinations are prudent for a child with a silent ductus.

Management of Ductus-Dependent Lesions

When pulmonary or systemic blood flow depends on continued patency of the ductus arteriosus, continuous infusion of prostaglandin E_1 is essential. In a severely ill neonate presenting with critical left ventricular outflow obstruction, ductus patency improves systemic perfusion; pulmonary congestion is relieved, renal blood flow is established, and severe acidosis can be corrected. In extremely cyanotic infants with inadequate pulmonary blood flow, ductus dilatation allows stabilization of the patient before palliation by a systemic–pulmonary artery shunt placement. Prostaglandin therapy can be maintained for several months if needed, as in neonates and infants with hypoplastic left heart syndrome awaiting cardiac transplant.[64]

The initial dose of prostaglandin E_1 is 0.05 µg/kg/min, and it may be increased as needed to 0.15 µg/kg/min or more by continuous infusion. Potential acute complications include apnea and hypotension. Ductus responsiveness to prostaglandin E_1 has been reported as late as 11 months of age.[65] Effectiveness of initial treatment, however, diminishes with increasing postnatal age in full-term infants, and successful re-establishment of ductus flow using prostaglandin E_1 is rare in full-term infants after the first month of life.

AORTOPULMONARY WINDOW

Aortopulmonary window is a rare cardiac malformation consisting of a defect in the wall (spiral septum) between the ascending aorta and the main pulmonary artery. A distinct aortic valve and pulmonic valve are always present. This anomaly occurs in isolation in approximately half of patients; associated lesions include aortic coarctation, type A interruption of the aortic arch, tetralogy of Fallot, and aortic origin of the right pulmonary artery.[66]

Aortopulmonary windows vary in size and proximity to the semilunar valves; they are usually large. Early in infancy, the postnatal fall in pulmonary resistance often results in congestive heart failure. Correction of large windows is warranted relatively early in the first year of life.

PATHOLOGIC ANATOMY

Mori and coworkers[67] and later Kutsche and Van Mierop[68] identified three subtypes of windows, and the latter authors suggested that a different developmental mechanism was responsible for each type. The first subtype was circular and midway between the semilunar valves and pulmonary artery bifurcation. A second had a location similar to that of type 1, but the border was helical in shape. The third type displayed complete absence of the aortopulmonary posterior border. These authors also noted that aortopulmonary window is not associated with DiGeorge's syndrome or with certain cardiac anomalies that are often associated with truncus arteriosus. This suggests that the two entities are pathogenetically unrelated, despite similar location of the defect.

HEMODYNAMIC AND CLINICAL PRESENTATION

The hemodynamic effects depend on the size of the aortic-pulmonary communication. The clinical findings of a large aortopulmonary window resemble those of other large left-to-right shunts, with symptoms often appearing in the first weeks of life. Physical examination reveals tachypnea, subcostal retractions, and hepatomegaly. In a moderate or large defect, pulses may be bounding, similar to the findings in a large patent ductus arteriosus. Auscultatory findings depend on the size of the communication. The less common small defect can mimic the classic continuous machinery-type murmur of a patent ductus, but the bruit is often louder at the right sternal border. In a larger defect, a systolic ejection murmur is usually heard over the left upper sternal border. With significant pulmonary hypertension, a loud second heart sound may be noted, and when left-to-right flow is significant, a mid-diastolic rumble is present at the apex.

ELECTROCARDIOGRAPHY, CHEST RADIOGRAPHY, AND ECHOCARDIOGRAPHY

The electrocardiographic and chest radiographic findings are similar to those described for a hemodynamically significant patent ductus. Two-dimensional echocardiography with color flow Doppler mapping should identify all aortic-pulmonary windows, and it is particularly useful in differentiating this condition from a clinically suspected patent ductus arteriosus (Fig. 23–3). The diagnosis may be missed when it is not suspected in the presence of other significant heart disease. Therefore, care should be taken to exclude this possibility in patients with aortic arch interruption, coarctation, "pink tetralogy" and subpulmonary ventricular septal defect with aortic insufficiency, or concomitant patent ductus arteriosus.

The defect may be visualized in a parasternal short-axis view. The aorta–pulmonary artery communication is clearly demonstrated above the pulmonary valve. Suprasternal long-axis imaging may assist in identifying the exact location of the window relative to the aortic valve. Color Doppler easily marks the presence and direction of shunting.[69] Retrograde diastolic flow from the descending to ascending aorta is often present and should raise suspicion in patients in whom aortic-pulmonary window was not initially suspected, such as when tetralogy of Fallot or inter-

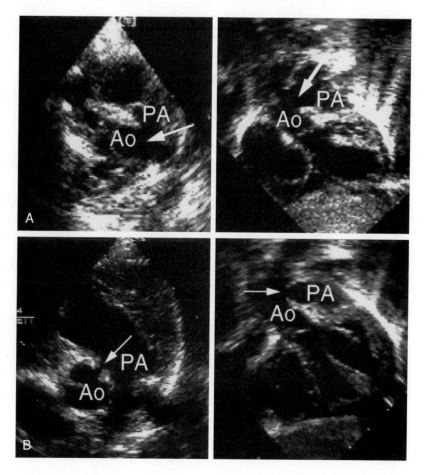

FIGURE 23–3

A, Two-dimensional echocardiographic parasternal short-axis view *(left)* and subxiphoid long-axis view *(right)* demonstrate a large aortopulmonary window *(arrows). B,* Same views demonstrate an unusual small defect *(arrows).* Ao = aorta; PA = pulmonary artery.

rupted aortic arch is present. Subcostal long-axis and parasternal views help differentiate aortic-pulmonary window from anomalous origin of the right pulmonary artery from the aorta.

MANAGEMENT

Repair of aortopulmonary window is indicated for symptoms of congestive heart failure refractory to medical therapy as well as to prevent irreversible pulmonary vascular changes from developing. Although it is unusual in this era of early echocardiographic diagnosis, an older patient with aortopulmonary window who has significant pulmonary hypertension may require catheterization to assess operability based on pulmonary-to-systemic resistance and shunt ratio.

Repair generally requires cardiopulmonary bypass; however, closure of a small window by hemoclip without the use of extracorporeal circulation has been reported.[70] Various operative techniques have been employed, depending on the specific location and morphology of the defect. In some patients, the defect can be closed by direct suturing, but a large window requires patch closure with use of cardiopulmonary bypass. In patients who have undergone repair appropriately, outcomes have been excellent with no specific long-term complications.[71]

Transcatheter occlusion of a small aortopulmonary window with use of a double-umbrella occluding device has been reported, but experience is limited.[72]

ANOMALOUS ORIGIN OF THE PULMONARY ARTERY FROM THE ASCENDING AORTA

Anomalous origin of one of the pulmonary arteries from the ascending aorta in the presence of a normal right ventricular outflow tract is rare. This anomaly is sometimes referred to as hemitruncus, a term that is inappropriate if there is a true pulmonary artery arising from the right ventricle supplying the contralateral lung. Anomalous right pulmonary artery is four times more common than the anomalous left.[73]

HEMODYNAMICS AND CLINICAL PRESENTATION

Infants with anomalous origin of the pulmonary artery from the ascending aorta without an associated anomaly usually present in severe congestive heart failure within the first month of life. The hemodynamics of this lesion are unique. The lung perfused by the anomalous pulmonary artery has systemic pulmonary pressure. Flow may be limited in the first days of life by the usual high pulmonary vascular resis-

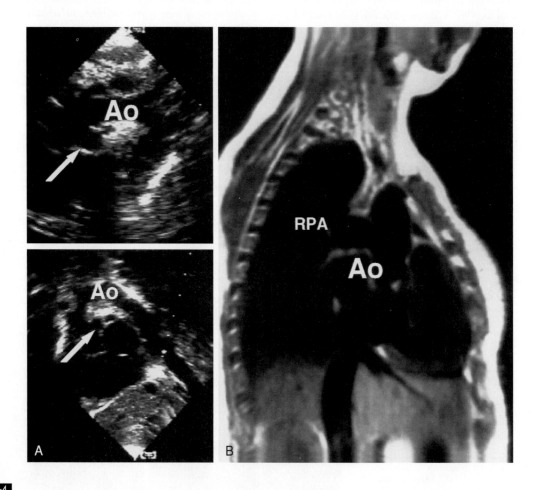

FIGURE 23-4

A, Rightward angulated suprasternal view *(above)* and subxiphoid short-axis view *(below)* demonstrate the right pulmonary artery (RPA) *(arrows)* originating from the proximal ascending aorta (Ao). *B,* Magnetic resonance imaging of the same patient in a right parasagittal cut.

tance found in the neonate. The pressures are initially elevated in the contralateral pulmonary artery on the same basis. During the first weeks of life as pulmonary vascular resistance falls, increased pulmonary blood flow and systemic pressure are noted in the ipsilateral lung. For reasons that are not immediately obvious, pulmonary artery pressures are also at systemic levels or greater in the lung supplied by the right ventricle. In the absence of an intracardiac or great vessel communication between the systemic and pulmonary circulations, the only explanation for this phenomenon is persistent severe pulmonary vascular constriction in the contralateral pulmonary vessels. Early severe biventricular failure results from a combination of high left ventricular preload due to the increased pulmonary blood flow in the affected lung and severe afterload on the right ventricle secondary to the pulmonary vascular constriction.[74]

Clinical presentation is usually that of an acutely ill neonate or young infant with symptoms and signs of congestive heart failure. A cardiac murmur is usually not prominent. Findings related to associated cardiac anomalies (aortopulmonary window, tetralogy of Fallot, interrupted aortic arch/coarctation) may dominate the clinical findings. The chest film most often reveals differential pulmonary blood flow, but this may not be obvious in the first day or two of life. Later, the lung perfused by the anomalous pulmonary artery from the aorta has increased pulmonary vascular markings compared with the contralateral lung. The diagnosis is made by echocardiography, but errors may be made if the right pulmonary artery is not carefully imaged to show that it emerges posteriorly from the aorta. Imaging in multiple planes usually allows a specific diagnosis of an aberrant right pulmonary artery to be made.[75] The origin of the left pulmonary artery laterally is less likely to result in a misdiagnosis (Fig. 23–4). Cardiac catheterization indicates pulmonary hypertension in both pulmonary arteries, sometimes greater in the pulmonary artery that arises normally. Aortic angiography defines the origin of the abnormal pulmonary artery from the ascending aorta and also determines the presence or absence of other anomalies.

MANAGEMENT

Management of an anomalous pulmonary artery from the ascending aorta is operation. The abnormal artery is divided from the aorta and reanastomosed to the main pulmonary artery. In some patients, a graft is required that may need replacement later. Operation should be carried out immediately after diagnosis. The contralateral sympathetic vasoconstrictive response usually resolves immediately after repair, and hemodynamic parameters return to normal; pulmonary artery pressure rapidly decreases to normal.[76] If repair is not carried out early, patients with anomalous origin of the pulmonary artery from the aorta develop irreversible pulmonary artery hypertension on the basis of chronic pulmonary vascular obstruction.

REFERENCES

1. Gittenberger-de-Groot AC: Histological observations. *In* Godman MJ, Marquis RM (eds): Pediatric Cardiology: Heart Disease in the Newborn. New York, Churchill Livingstone, 1979, p 4.

2. Jager BV, Wollenman OJ: An anatomical study of the closure of the ductus arteriosus. Am J Pathol 18:595, 1942.
3. Kennedy JA, Clark SL: Observations on the physiological reactions of the ductus arteriosus. Am J Physiol 136:140, 1942.
4. Kovalik V: The response of the isolated ductus arteriosus to oxygen and anoxia. J Physiol 169:185, 1963.
5. Starling MB, Elliott RB: The effects of prostaglandins, prostaglandin inhibitors and oxygen on closure of the ductus arteriosus, pulmonary arteries and umbilical vessels in vitro. Prostaglandins 8:187, 1974.
6. Rudolph AM, Scarpelli EM, Golinko RJ, Gootman N: Hemodynamic basis for clinical manifestations of patent ductus arteriosus. Am Heart J 68:447, 1964.
7. Rudolph AM, Mayer FE, Nadas AS, Gross RE: Patent ductus arteriosus: A clinical and hemodynamic study of patients in the first year of life. Pediatrics 22:892, 1958.
8. Espino-Vela J, Cardenas N, Cruz R: Patent ductus arteriosus. With special reference to patients with pulmonary hypertension. Circulation 38(suppl):45, 1968.
9. Gersony WM: Neonatal pulmonary hypertension: Pathophysiology, classification and etiology. Clin Perinatol 11:517, 1984.
10. Freed MD, Heymann MA, Lewis AB, et al: Prostaglandin E$_1$ in infants with ductus arteriosus dependent congenital heart disease. Circulation 64:899, 1981.
11. Fisher EA, Levitsky S: Prostaglandin E$_1$ infusion in newborns with hypoplastic left ventricle and aortic atresia. Pediatr Cardiol 2:95, 1982.
12. Henry CG, Goldring D, Hartmann A, et al: Treatment of d-transposition of the great arteries: Management of hypoxemia after balloon atrial septostomy. Am J Cardiol 47:299, 1981.
13. Benson LN, Olley PM, Patel RG, et al: Role of prostaglandin E$_1$ infusion in management of transposition of great arteries. Am J Cardiol 44:691, 1979.
14. Lang P, Freed MD, Bierman FZ, et al: Use of prostaglandin E$_1$ in infants with transposition of the great arteries and intact ventricular septum. Am J Cardiol 44:76, 1979.
15. Hoffman JE, Rudolph AM, Heymann MA: Pulmonary vascular disease with congenital heart lesions: Pathologic features and causes. Circulation 64:873, 1981.
16. Daher AH, Berkowitz FE: Infective endocarditis in neonates. Clin Pediatr 34:198, 1995.
17. Cotton RB, Stahlman MT, Kovar I, et al: Medical management of small preterm infants with symptomatic patent ductus arteriosus. J Pediatr 92:467, 1978.
18. Dudell GG, Gersony WM: Patent ductus arteriosus in neonates with severe respiratory disease. J Pediatr 104:915, 1984.
19. Jacob J, Gluck L, Disessa T, et al: The contribution of PDA in the neonate with severe RDS. J Pediatr 96:79, 1980.
20. Andrade A, Vargas-Barron J, Rijlaarsdan M, et al: Utility of transesophageal echocardiography in the examination of adult patients with patent ductus arteriosus. Am Heart J 130:543, 1995.
21. Stumper O, Witsenburg M, Sutherland GR, et al: Transesophageal echocardiographic monitoring of interventional cardiac catheterization in children. J Am Coll Cardiol 18:1506, 1991.
22. Hiraishi S, Horiguchi Y, Fujino N, et al: Two-dimensional and Doppler echocardiographic assessment of variably shaped ductus arteriosus by the parasternal approach. Pediatr Cardiol 12:6, 1991.
23. Krichenko A, Benson LN, Burrows P, et al: Angiographic classification of the isolated, persistently patent ductus arteriosus and implications for percutaneous catheter occlusion. Am J Cardiol 63:877, 1989.
24. Friedman WF, Hirschklan MJ, Printz MP, et al: Pharmacologic closure of patent ductus arteriosus in the premature infant. N Engl J Med 295:526, 1976.
25. Cotton RB, Stahlman MT, Berdio HW, et al: Randomized trial of early closure of symptomatic patent ductus arteriosus in small preterm infants. J Pediatr 93:647, 1978.
26. Merritt TA, White CL, Jacob J, et al: Patent ductus arteriosus treated with ligation or indomethacin: A follow-up study. J Pediatr 95:588, 1979.
27. Thibeault DW, Emmanouilides GC, Nelson RJ, et al: Patent ductus arteriosus complicating the respiratory distress syndrome in preterm infants. J Pediatr 86:120, 1975.
28. Yanagi RM, Wilson A, Newfeld EA, et al: Indomethacin treatment for symptomatic patent ductus arteriosus: A double-blind control study. Pediatrics 67:647, 1981.

29. Yeh TF, Luken JA, Tholji A, et al: Intravenous indomethacin therapy in premature infants with persistent ductus arteriosus: A double-blind controlled study. J Pediatr 98:137, 1981.

30. Gersony WM: Patent ductus arteriosus in the neonate. Pediatr Clin North Am 33:545, 1986.

31. Merritt TA, Harris JP, Roghmann K, et al: Early closure of the patent ductus arteriosus in very low birth weight infants: A controlled trial. J Pediatr 99:281, 1981.

32. Gersony WM, Peckham GJ, Ellison RC, et al: Effects of indomethacin in premature infants with patent ductus arteriosus: Results of a collaborative study. J Pediatr 102:895, 1983.

33. Mahony L, Violetta C, Brett C, et al: Prophylactic indomethacin therapy for patent ductus arteriosus in very low birth weight infants. N Engl J Med 306:506, 1982.

34. Bada HS, Green RS, Poureyrous M, et al: Indomethacin reduces the risk of severe intraventricular hemorrhage. J Pediatr 115:631, 1989.

35. Ment LR, Duncan CC, Ehrenkranz RA, et al: Randomized low-dose indomethacin trial for prevention of intraventricular hemorrhage in very low birth weight neonates. J Pediatr 112:948, 1988.

36. Garland J, Buck R, Weinberg M: Pulmonary hemorrhage risk in infants with a clinically diagnosed patent ductus arteriosus: A retrospective cohort study. Pediatrics 94:719, 1994.

37. Couser RJ, Ferrera TB, Wright GB, et al: Prophylactic indomethacin in the first 24 hours of life for the prevention of patent ductus arteriosus in preterm infants treated with prophylactic surfactant in the delivery room. J Pediatr 128:631, 1996.

38. Clyman RI: Recommendation for the postnatal use of indomethacin: An analysis of four separate treatment strategies. J Pediatr 128:601, 1996.

39. Weiss H, Cooper B, Brook M, et al: Factors determining reopening of the ductus arteriosus after successful clinical closure with indomethacin. J Pediatr 127:466, 1995.

40. Jones JC: Twenty-five years experience with the surgery of patent ductus arteriosus. J Thorac Cardiovasc Surg 50:149, 1965.

41. Hijazi ZM, Geggel RL: Results of anterograde transcatheter closure of patent ductus arteriosus using single or multiple Gianturco coils. Am J Cardiol 74:925, 1994.

42. Hosking MCK, Benson LN, Musewe MN, et al: Transcatheter occlusion of the persistently patent ductus arteriosus: Forty month follow-up and prevalence of residual shunting. Circulation 84:2313, 1991.

43. Nykaren DG, Hayes AM, Benson LN, Freedom RM: Transcatheter patent ductus arteriosus occlusion: Application in the small child. J Am Coll Cardiol 23:1666, 1994.

44. Dessy H, Hermus JP, van den Henvel F, et al: Echocardiographic and radionuclide pulmonary blood flow patterns after transcatheter closure of patent ductus arteriosus. Circulation 94:126, 1996.

45. Rothenberg SS, Chang JH, Toews WH, Washington RL: Thorascopic closure of patent ductus arteriosus: A less traumatic and more cost effective technique. J Pediatr Surg 30:1057, 1995.

46. Sorenson KE, Kirstensen BO, Hansen OK: Frequency of occurrence of residual ductal shunt after surgical ligation by color flow mapping. Am J Cardiol 67:653, 1991.

47. Kirklin JW, Barratt-Boyes BG: Patent ductus arteriosus. In Cardiac Surgery, 2nd ed. New York, Churchill Livingstone, 1993, p 854.

48. Portsmann W, Wierny L, Warnke H, et al: Catheter closure of patent ductus arteriosus: 62 cases treated without thoracotomy. Radiol Clin North Am 9:203, 1971.

49. Rashkind WJ, Mullins CE, Hellenbrand WE, Tait MA: Nonsurgical closure of patent ductus arteriosus: Clinical application of the Rashkind PDA Occluder System. Circulation 75:583, 1987.

50. Bash SE, Mullins CE: Insertion of patent ductus arteriosus occluder by transvenous approach: A new technique. Circulation 70(suppl):11–285, 1984.

51. Musewe NN, Benson LN, Smallhorn JF, Freedom RM: Two-dimensional echocardiographic and color flow Doppler evaluation of ductal occlusion with the Rashkind prosthesis. Circulation 80:1706, 1989.

52. Benson LN, Freedom RM: Balloon dilatation of the very small patent ductus arteriosus in preparation for transcatheter occlusion. Cathet Cardiovasc Diagn 80:1706, 1989.

53. Khan A, Yousef SA, Mullins CE, Sawyer W: Experience with 205 procedures of transcatheter closure of ductus arteriosus in 182 patients with special reference to residual shunts and long term follow up. J Thorac Cardiovasc Surg 104:1721, 1992.

54. Ottenkamp J, Hess J, Talsma MD, Buis-Liem TN: Protrusion of the device: A complication of the catheter closure of the patent ductus arteriosus. Br Heart J 68:301, 1992.

55. Cambier PA, Kirby WC, Wortham DC, Moore JW: Percutaneous closure of the small (<2.5 mm) patent ductus arteriosus using coil embolization. Am J Cardiol 69:815, 1992.

56. Gianturco C, Anderson JH, Wallace S: Mechanical devices for arterial occlusion. AJR Am J Roentgenol 124:428, 1975.

57. Lloyd TR, Fedderly R, Mendelsohn AM, et al: Transcatheter occlusion of patent ductus arteriosus with Gianturco coils. Circulation 88:1412, 1993.

58. Shim D, Fedderly RT, Beekman RH, et al: Follow-up of coil occlusion of patent ductus arteriosus. J Am Coll Cardiol 28:207, 1996.

59. Grifka RG, Ing FF, McMahon WS, et al: Transcatheter occlusion of patent ductus arteriosus and aorto-pulmonary collaterals using the Gianturco-Grifka occlusion device (Abstract). J Am Coll Cardiol 29:172A, 1997.

60. Sommer RJ, Gutierrez A, Wyman WL, Parness IA: Use of preformed nitinol snare to improve transcatheter coil delivery in occlusion of patent ductus arteriosus. Am J Cardiol 74:836, 1994.

61. Le TP, Redel DA, Neuss MB, et al: Deutsche multicenter Studie zum transkatheter Verschluss des PDA mittels der replazierbaren spirale Duct-Occlud, eine zwischen Bilamz. Z Kardiol 84:753, 1995.

62. Strouse PJ, Beekman RH: Magnetic deflection forces from atrial septal defect and patent ductus arteriosus—occluding devices, stents and coils used in pediatric aged patients. Am J Cardiol 78:490, 1996.

63. Blazer DT, Spray TL, McMullin O, et al: Endarteritis associated with a clinically silent patent ductus arteriosus. Am Heart J 125:1192, 1993.

64. Bailey LL, Concepcion W, Shattack H, et al: Method of heart transplantation for treatment of hypoplastic left heart syndrome. J Thorac Cardiovasc Surg 92:1, 1986.

65. Kashani IA, Schmunk GA, Merritt TA, et al: Prostaglandin E$_1$ responsive ductus at 11 months of age. Pediatr Cardiol 5:19, 1984.

66. Bertdini A, Dalmonte P, Bava GL, et al: Aortopulmonary septal defects, a review of the literature and report of ten cases. J Cardiovasc Surg 35:207, 1994.

67. Mori K, Ando M, Takao A, et al: Distal type of aortopulmonary window: Report of 4 cases. Br Heart J 40:681, 1978.

68. Kutsche LM, Van Mierop LH: Anatomy and pathogenesis of aortopulmonary septal defect. Am J Cardiol 59:443, 1987.

69. Balaji S, Burch M, Sullivan ID: Accuracy of cross-sectional echocardiography in diagnosis of aortopulmonary window. Am J Cardiol 67:650, 1991.

70. Kawata H, Kishimoto H, Ueno T, et al: Repair of aortopulmonary window in an infant with extremely low birth weight. Ann Thorac Surg 62:1843, 1996.

71. Van Son JA, Puga FJ, Danielson GK, et al: Aortopulmonary window: Factors associated with early and late success after surgical treatment. Mayo Clin Proc 68:128, 1993.

72. Stamato T, Benson LN, Smallhorn JF, Freedom RM: Transcatheter closure of an aortopulmonary window with a modified double umbrella occluder system. Cathet Cardiovasc Diagn 35:165, 1995.

73. Kutsche LM, Van Mierop LHS: Anomalous origin of a pulmonary artery from the ascending aorta: Associated anomalies and pathogenesis. Am J Cardiol 61:850, 1988.

74. Kean JF, Maltz D, Bernhard WF, et al: Anomalous origin of one pulmonary artery from the ascending aorta: Diagnostic, physiological and surgical considerations. Circulation 50:588, 1974.

75. King DH, Huhta JC, Gutgesell HP, et al: Two-dimensional echocardiographic diagnosis of anomalous origin of the right pulmonary artery from the aorta: Differentiation from aortopulmonary window. J Am Coll Cardiol 4:351, 1984.

76. Penkoske PA, Castaneda AR, Fyler DC, et al: Origin of pulmonary artery branch from ascending aorta: Primary surgical repair in infancy. J Thorac Cardiovasc Surg 85:537, 1983.

CHAPTER 24

ATRIOVENTRICULAR SEPTAL DEFECT

JOHN LANE   PIERRE C. WONG   ARNO R. HOHN

Atrioventricular septal defects (AVSDs) are a group of cardiac anomalies that commonly cause early cardiac distress and even death. These defects are characterized by abnormal development of the anlage of the atrioventricular (AV) valves and persistence of the atrial ostium primum and secondary ventricular septal opening. An AVSD is found in about 17% of fetuses examined by echocardiography.[1] Through fetal wastage, the frequency of AVSDs is apparently reduced to about 3 to 5% of congenital cardiac defects[2,3] after birth.

A strong genetic influence is known. AVSDs are often found in association with syndromes like Down, DiGeorge, and Ellis–van Creveld. In particular, about 40% of those with Down syndrome are afflicted with cardiac malformations, and 40% of these are AVSDs. Recent work has located the gene loci for the defect. Race and sex do not appear to play a role in the occurrence of the defect. Operative repair of AVSD offers optimistic long-term outlook to most of those with the disorder; those with the partial form of AVSD have an especially favorable prognosis. As with many cardiac anomalies, early diagnosis and treatment are imperative to avoid the complications known to occur with heart failure and to prevent pulmonary hypertensive vascular disease.

PATHOLOGIC ANATOMY

Practically, AVSDs fall into four broad groups: (1) *partial* and (2) *intermediate* or *transitional* defects in which there are two separate AV valves; (3) *complete* AVSD, defined by a common valve; and (4) *common atrium,* in which atrial septation is completely or nearly completely lacking and there is a common AV valve. These defects may be complicated by association with other serious anomalies like tetralogy of Fallot or visceral heterotaxia. All share a similar embryology with respect to endocardial cushion development and septation.

Within the spectrum of AVSDs, great anatomic variation exists. At one end of the spectrum are mild AV valve abnormalities, as typified by clefts in the anterior leaflet of the mitral valve or septal leaflet of the tricuspid valve. At the other end are the large primitive malformations known as complete AVSD, characterized by extensive defects of the atrial and ventricular septa and a large, undivided, common AV valve. Between these two ends of this spectrum, any combination of defects involving atrial septum, ventricular septum, and AV valves can occur, some associated with other cardiac abnormalities.

Typically, when AVSDs involve atrial or ventricular septa, there are large defects in the posterior portion of the involved septum. These parts of the septum correspond roughly to the embryologic derivations of the endocardial cushions, which explains why AVSDs are also labeled endocardial cushion defects. As noted in the embryology section of this chapter, however, this association is not universally accepted.[4-6]

To provide an anatomic schema that unifies partial and complete defects, some investigators have proposed that the difference between the two types resides in the position and attachment of the AV valves.[7] In both types, there is a large defect involving the posterior aspect of the atrial and ventricular septa (the endocardial cushion portion). In the complete form of AVSD, the large common AV valve has failed to divide and separate into two AV valves, leaving the large communication between the atrial and ventricular chambers. In the partial form, however, the AV valves are more completely formed, with AV valve tissue attaching to the crest of the interventricular septum.[8] Intervening AV valve tissue produces varying degrees of ventricular occlusion. When there is complete absence of a ventricular shunt, the residual atrial communication is termed an ostium primum atrial septal defect (ASD). When a small ventricular defect remains, the defect is called a transitional or intermediate AVSD. Complicating this classification is the fact that certain forms of AVSDs can exist with just a ventricular septal defect (VSD), called an AV canal–type VSD, and no atrial level defect. In addition, the most minor forms of AVSDs may have defects only of the AV valves and no abnormality of atrial or ventricular septum.

Regardless of whether AVSDs are partial or complete, certain anatomic hallmarks typify this class of lesions. First, because of the large deficiency in the ventricular septum, the attachments of the left AV valve are lower than in normal hearts. This produces a mismatch between the inflow and outflow portions of the left ventricle, with the mitral annulus–left ventricular apex length considerably less than the aortic annulus–left ventricular apex length (Fig. 24–1).[9] Second, the aortic valve is not wedged between the mitral and tricuspid valves as in a normal heart. Instead, it is shifted anteriorly relative to the two AV valves. The "sprung" left ventricular outflow tract is longer, more anterior, and usually narrower than normal, producing the "gooseneck" deformity seen on angiography. Third, the lack of AV valve differentiation also prevents the normal development of the longitudinal "offset" between mitral and tricuspid valves. Finally, the posterior portion of the

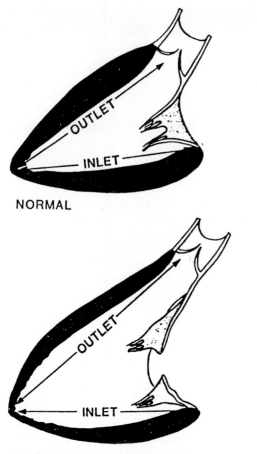

NORMAL

ATRIOVENTRICULAR SEPTAL DEFECT

FIGURE 24–1

Left ventricular aspect of the septum in hearts with normal *(upper panel)* and deficient *(lower panel)* atrioventricular septation. (From Anderson RH, Baker EJ, Ho SY, et al: The morphology and diagnosis of AVSDs. Cardiol Young 1:290, 1991.)

atrial and ventricular defects interferes with the development and placement of the normal pathways of AV conduction, specifically the AV node and bundle of His. Therefore, in AVSDs, the conduction system courses posterior to the ventricular defect, which probably accounts (at least in part) for the unusual QRS axis seen on the electrocardiogram.[9] This course also has important implications for operative repair.

PARTIAL AVSDS

Partial AVSDs can include any combination of atrial, ventricular, and AV valve abnormalities. The most commonly encountered constellation of defects is a large primum ASD and cleft mitral valve, with fibrous continuity remaining between the superior and inferior leaflets of the common AV valve. There is a defect in the posterior portion of the atrial septum, immediately adjacent to the AV valves. This defect varies in size but is usually large. In addition, there can be coexisting secundum ASD. Rarely, secundum and primum defects can coalesce so that there is virtual absence of the atrial septum, producing, in effect, a common atrium. The anterior leaflet of the mitral valve is in-

variably cleft and may or may not be competent. When left-sided AV valve regurgitation is present, it generally occurs through the cleft; regurgitant jets can often pass from the left ventricle to left atrium as well as from left ventricle to right atrium. The latter is possible because the ostium primum ASD extends directly to the AV valve septal insertions, thus allowing regurgitant flow from the cleft easy entry to the right atrium. Rarely, abnormalities of the right-sided AV valve can also occur, including a cleft in the septal leaflet or even a gap at the commissure of the medial and anterior leaflets.[10] As in the left AV valve, a right AV valve with these abnormalities may not be competent.

Although the ostium primum ASD with cleft valve represents the most common form of partial AVSD, other combinations of lesions do exist. Rarely, there is no atrial level defect, but a large posterior, AV canal–type VSD is present. This defect occupies the most posterior aspect of the ventricular septum and is often termed an inlet muscular VSD. Also, a cleft mitral valve can sometimes be the only manifestation of an AVSD. This type of cleft must be distinguished from isolated congenital mitral valve clefts seen in patients without an AVSD because there are important differences in the mitral valve's orientation and morphology and in the papillary muscle's position.[11, 12]

COMPLETE AVSD

In complete AVSD, there is a large deficiency in the posterior portion of the atrial and ventricular septa as well as a large, primitive, common AV valve. The superior and inferior leaflets of the AV valve are not in fibrous continuity. The large AV valve can be well balanced over both ventricles, or there can be varying degrees of malalignment of the ventricular septum favoring one ventricle over the other (so-called unbalanced AVSD). In more extreme examples, one ventricle can be so hypoplastic that it cannot serve as an isolated pumping chamber, and the patient must be committed to single-ventricle management. In these lesions, one side of the common AV valve is so poorly developed (or even "atretic") that the valve cannot be divided into two, further precluding biventricular repair.

The large common AV valve generally has five leaflets: two confined to the right ventricle; one exclusively in the left (the posterior or mural leaflet); and two crossing the ventricular septum, with attachments to both ventricles, known as superior and inferior bridging leaflets. Both superior and inferior bridging leaflets exhibit marked anatomic variability, and the variation in superior bridging leaflet morphology was used by Rastelli and coworkers[13] to devise a widely used classification of complete AVSD:

- Type A: The superior bridging leaflet is divided into two portions, both attached medially to the muscular septum. The membranous septum has formed, and the interventricular communication does not extend to the vicinity of the aortic cusps.
- Type B: The superior bridging leaflet is divided into two portions, unattached to the septum, but both portions are attached medially to an anomalous papillary muscle in the right ventricle adjacent to the septum.
- Type C: The superior bridging leaflet is undivided and unattached to the septum, floating freely above it. The

interventricular communication is complete under the common anterior leaflet and extends to the proximity of the aortic cusps.

In each type, the inferior leaflet is usually rudimentary and exhibits anatomic arrangements similar to those described for the superior leaflet. Of the three types, type A is the most common; type C is the second most common, and type B is rarely encountered. There is some controversy as to whether type A[14,15] or type C is most often seen with trisomy 21. Type C is also frequently associated with more complex malformations, such as conotruncal malformations and visceral heterotaxia. Because of superior bridging leaflet attachments to the crest of the ventricular septum, type A defects are far more likely to have left ventricular outflow tract obstruction.

ASSOCIATED ABNORMALITIES

Obstruction to left or right ventricular outflow can be seen in patients with an AVSD. *Left ventricular outflow obstruction* is more common. As mentioned before the left ventricular outflow tract is elongated and narrow, and subaortic obstruction can result from AV valve tissue attaching to the crest of the ventricular septum and partially occluding left ventricular outflow. This type of obstruction can be seen in both partial and complete forms of AVSDs. Outflow obstruction can also result from posterior malalignment of the infundibular septum, often occurring in association with a right dominant complete AVSD, with a hypoplastic left ventricle and sometimes atresia of the left side of the common AV valve.

When *right ventricular outflow obstruction* is associated with AVSDs, it generally occurs with anterior malalignment of the infundibular septum. This produces dynamic subpulmonary stenosis analogous to classic tetralogy of Fallot physiology. Indeed, such patients often behave like those with standard tetralogy. They may be acyanotic at birth, but with time, increasing infundibular hypertrophy leads to increased subpulmonary obstruction and more pronounced cyanosis. These patients can have hypercyanotic spells ("tet spells"). The combination of AVSD and right ventricular outflow obstruction may pose a surgical challenge.

Abnormalities of the left-sided AV valve tensor apparatus and papillary muscles can occur in some patients with AVSDs. In some, there may be only one papillary muscle. In most patients, there are two papillary muscles, but these are abnormally positioned. The usual anterolateral and posteromedial relation is changed, the muscles being closer together and aligned in an anterior-posterior relation. These two closely spaced muscles form a potential parachute mitral valve.[16–18] Sometimes the chordae tendineae can be divided similar to a double-orifice mitral valve.[19] While the anterior cleft is open, there is no obstruction to the left-sided inflow. Operative closure of the cleft, however, can produce anatomic and functional mitral stenosis.[20,21]

Complete AVSDs may be associated with almost any type of congenital malformation.[22] Such *anomalies* include persistent left superior vena cava to the coronary sinus, patent ductus arteriosus, pulmonary valve stenosis, and aortic coarctation. In addition, the coronary sinus can be short, with the orifice entering into the left atrium. AVSDs can also be seen as part of a complex constellation of cardiac anomalies; this is often in the setting of visceral heterotaxia (asplenia or polysplenia). Typically, asplenia (right atrial isomerism) patients have a large common AVSD, underdeveloped or absent left ventricle, large double-outlet right ventricle, and varying degrees of pulmonary outflow obstruction due to a subpulmonary conus.[23] Most of such patients cannot undergo biventricular repair. In contrast, patients with polysplenia (left atrial isomerism) tend to have a large complete AVSD in combination with normally related great arteries and left ventricular and aortic underdevelopment.[23] A much greater proportion of these patients can undergo successful biventricular repair.[24]

EMBRYOLOGY

Abnormalities of embryologic development of endocardial cushions are considered the cause of AVSDs. Debate remains about the role of endocardial cushions. The classic view that AVSDs were solely due to endocardial cushion defects had been questioned.[4–6,25] On the basis of studies of embryos with AVSDs, a theory was suggested that endocardial cushions serve only as "glue" for structures in the AV canal; thus, endocardial cushions provide no tissue for creating structures in the canal, and AVSDs are due to abnormalities in formations other than the endocardial cushions.[4–6] However, new techniques, such as monoclonal antibody staining, have shown that endocardial cushions actually do contribute tissue for the structures of the AV canal.[26]

By the time the embryo is 4.5 weeks old, the heart tube has completed the cardiac looping phase, but it is far from completing its development. The heart is composed of three layers: a one-cell thick layer of endothelium; an outer layer of myocardium two to three cells thick; and a layer of extracellular matrix, the cardiac jelly, separating the cell layers. Not only are the components of the heart primitive, but the pump action and flow of blood through the heart are rudimentary. In this sense, the heart is still just a contractile tube, and the blood flow is in series. Blood flows from the atrium to the left ventricle through the AV canal, then through the interventricular foramen to the right ventricle and out the conotruncus to the aortic arches. With further development, the AV canal shifts medially so that the atria empty directly into both ventricles (Fig. 24–2).[27]

Around this time, endothelial cells migrate into the cardiac jelly to form the myocardium. Endocardial cushions begin to form through this same process. The control of endocardial cushion formation is incompletely understood, but recent investigations have defined some of the factors involved. The endothelium has some influence over endocardial cushion formation because there is a subset of endothelial cells lining only the regions where cushions are formed (the outflow tract and the AV canal).[28,29] The myocardium exerts some influence because the endothelial cells that migrate into the jelly are transformed into mesenchymal cells by chemical signals produced by the overlying myocardium.[28,30,31] By whatever mechanism it

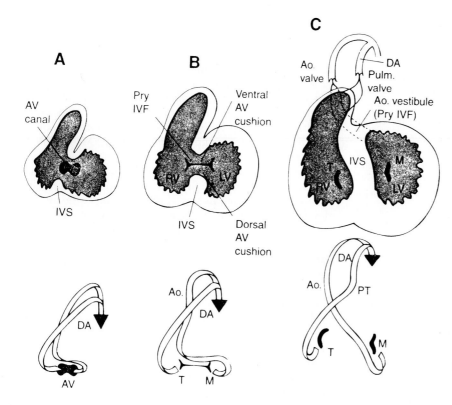

FIGURE 24–2

Sections through the heart at 4.5, 5, and 6 weeks. In *A*, the common atrioventricular (AV) canal has shifted to the midline. The fusion of endocardial cushions gives rise to the mitral and tricuspid orifices in *B* and *C*. The course of the circulation is shown in the lower row. Ao = aorta; ventral AV cushion = superior endocardial cushion; dorsal AV cushion = inferior endocardial cushion; DA = ductus arteriosus; IVS = interventricular septum; M = mitral orifice; Pry IVF = primary interventricular foramen; PT = pulmonary trunk; RV = right ventricle; T = tricuspid orifice. (From Moore KL, Persoud TVN: The Developing Human. Philadelphia, WB Saunders, 1998.)

is controlled, the major collections of cushion tissue that line the AV canal grow out from the superior and inferior aspects of the canal, fuse in the midline, and divide the canal into right and left AV orifices (Fig. 24–3).[32] There are also smaller cushions, the lateral cushions, that form and provide tissue for the AV valves.

The fused cushions initially function as valves for the AV orifices in the embryonic heart, but their role is not limited to this function.[33] Because of their location, the endocardial cushions are intimately involved in the septation of the heart and AV valve formation. The fused cushion arches superiorly and anteriorly to combine with the atrial septum

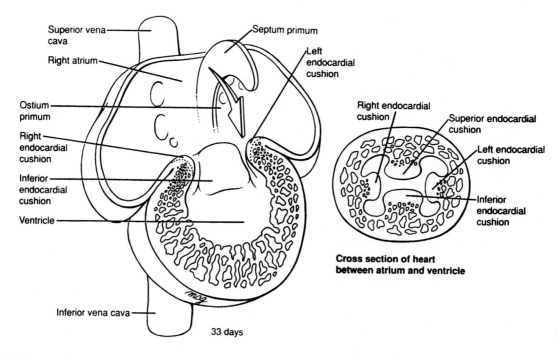

FIGURE 24–3

Embryo at 33 days showing the superior, inferior, right, and left endocardial cushions. The superior and inferior cushions have yet to fuse in the midline and divide the AV orifice in two. The right and left endocardial cushions contribute to AV valve formation. (From Larsen WJ: Human Embryology. New York, Churchill Livingstone, 1993, p 145.)

primum and close the ostium primum. The right side of the inferior margin of the arch merges with the muscular ventricular septum and conus septal tissue to complete the formation of the ventricular septum. Endocardial cushion tissue also contributes to the creation of the AV valve leaflets, especially the anterior mitral and septal tricuspid leaflets. The lateral endocardial cushions are involved in the formation of the other mitral and tricuspid leaflets.

Defective endocardial cushion formation results in AVSDs. The fact that there are different types of AVSDs is due to variation in the degree of defects in the endocardial cushions. Because of the prominent role they play in septation and AV valve formation, any defect in the endocardial cushions will produce abnormalities in these areas even though the other tissue components may be normal.[4] In a partial AVSD, endocardial cushions form and fuse in the midline of the canal, but further development stops. Because the fused cushion does not arch adequately, the atrial septum cannot combine with it to close the ostium primum, and a primum ASD results. There are separate AV orifices, but because of inadequate tissue for valve formation, there may be clefts in the AV valves, particularly the anterior mitral leaflet. The conus tissue and muscular ventricular septum are usually still able to combine with fibrous tissue and close the ventricular septum.[33] In the complete form of AVSD, the endocardial cushions may not form at all. There is a persistent ostium primum and a deficiency in the ventricular septum. If the AV valves attach to the crest of the septum, however, there may be no VSD.[4] Usually, however, there is a common AV orifice with abnormal AV valve leaflets. Typically, there is a five-leaflet AV valve with two leaflets bridging across the ventricular septum.

HEMODYNAMICS

The pathophysiologic mechanism of an uncomplicated AVSD is basically that of a shunt lesion. With the partial form of AVSD, the shunt circulatory dynamics are those of increased volume in the right ventricle and pulmonary bed. In many instances, AV valve regurgitation leads to left ventricular dilatation and augmented atrial level shunt. The volume load in the ventricles leads to elevation of pulmonary pressure, which may be made worse by the AV valve regurgitation. Pulmonary artery pressure rises, but pulmonary vascular resistance is usually normal, and congestive heart failure is uncommon.

In contrast, those with complete AVSD generally have hemodynamics resembling a large VSD and pulmonary hypertension, common AV valve regurgitation, and an atrial level shunt. Pulmonary arterial pressure is at systemic levels, and heart failure ensues from left ventricular volume overload. Those with Down syndrome seem particularly prone to development of severe pulmonary hypertension and pulmonary vascular disease in early life. Prompt operative treatment may avoid this devastating development.

On the other hand, if pulmonary outflow obstruction coexists, pulmonary blood flow may be reduced, and the clinical picture is that of tetralogy of Fallot. Other variants involve unbalanced septal placement. For example, in right ventricular dominant AVSD, the associated underdevelopment of the left ventricle and aortic arch leads to the pathophysiologic process of hypoplastic left heart syndrome. Asplenia or polysplenia and heterotaxia syndromes may add other complications, such as anomalous pulmonary venous return. Major hemodynamic features of the various types of AVSD are summarized in Table 24–1.

NATURAL HISTORY

Fetal survival is poor. More than two thirds of those with AVSD do not survive pregnancy.[1] Fetal echocardiograms showing the AVSD associated with a hypoplastic left ventricle, or reversed atrial or ductus shunting, have an especially poor outlook.[34]

The course of a patient with an AVSD depends on the extent of the AV canal, ventricular size, degree of AV valve insufficiency, obstruction to ventricular outflow, and associated syndromes. Because of early surgical intervention, the natural history of untreated AVSD is seldom seen. Of the various forms of AVSD, those with the *partial* form of AVSD fare the best without treatment.[1,3,35] Nevertheless, 50% die before 20 years of age, and only 25% survive beyond 40 years of age.[35] In that study of unrepaired primum ASDs, Somerville[35] noted that atrial arrhythmias, especially fibrillation, were the most common cause of later life disability and death. Acquired complete heart block was particularly deleterious. In contrast to those with complete AVSD, pulmonary hypertension was found to be an uncommon complication. A review debated the merits of

TABLE 24–1

HEMODYNAMIC FEATURES OF ATRIOVENTRICULAR SEPTAL DEFECT

Type	Qp	AV Valve Regurgitation	Ppa	Rp	Oxygen Saturation	CHF
Partial	Increased	Common	Normal to high	Usually normal	Normal	Uncommon
Complete						
Balanced	Increased	In most	Usually high	Usually high	Normal to decreased	Common
Right dominant	Decreased	May have	High	Normal to high	Decreased	Common
Left dominant	Decreased	May have	Low	Low	Decreased	Infrequent
Common atrium	Increased	Common	High	Normal to high	Normal to decreased	Common
Complicated						
Heterotaxia	Often increased	Common	Often high	May be high	Often decreased	Common
Right ventricular outflow obstruction	Decreased	May have	Low	Low	Decreased	Seldom

AV = atrioventricular; CHF = congestive heart failure.

operative repair of the partial defect past the age of 40 years[36]; one of the individuals cited lived to age 89 years in spite of the defect. Of course, if the partial defect is associated with a syndrome such as Down syndrome, the natural course is more like that of the syndrome.

On the other hand, those with uncomplicated *complete* forms of the defect commonly have symptoms of cardiac compromise and failure. They often succumb in the first or second year of life[3,37] if left untreated. Others with uncomplicated and untreated complete AVSD may develop pulmonary hypertensive vascular disease and survive into the third or fourth decade.

In infants with an AVSD, cellular intimal proliferation develops earlier and is more severe than in those with an isolated VSD, but it develops more slowly than in those with transposition and a VSD. Severe medial hypertrophy and intimal proliferation can be present by 6 or 7 months of age, and intracardiac repair should be carried out in early infancy. Pulmonary vascular structure can be particularly difficult to evaluate in complete AVSD because of the varying degree of incompetence of the left AV valve. When this is severe, the vein walls are abnormally thick and perivascular connective tissue deposition is excessive, particularly around the capillary bed and small veins.

When found today, the individuals with pulmonary vascular disease are mainly those with the Down syndrome from the era when early diagnosis and treatment were not universal, or they have arrived from developing countries where access to tertiary medical care was limited. These unfortunate individuals passed through a period when an operation could have been performed. Cardiac shunting is minimal as a result of balanced right- and left-sided heart pressures and outflow resistances. Then, in the teen years, the shunt reverses, and they become progressively cyanotic. Those so afflicted develop marked polycythemia and profound cyanosis and clubbing. Their hemoglobin levels are often above 20 mg/dl, and they may require phlebotomy to prevent strokes. Unless treated by lung or heart-lung transplantation, these individuals generally succumb in their third to fourth decades of hypoxic events or heart failure.

Complicated forms of complete AVSD pose special problems. When anatomic complications exist, like pulmonary stenosis or atresia, the course parallels that of tetralogy of Fallot. If the AVSD is unbalanced, the course is that of a single ventricle. Because of these outcomes, surgical intervention is universally recommended.[38] Operative outcomes vary with the form of the defect but average about 83% survival when all forms of AVSD are considered.[39]

HISTORY AND PHYSICAL EXAMINATION

The cardiac anomalies of AVSDs are often found as a component of a genetic syndrome. Accordingly, careful attention has to be paid to the cardiac examination in "syndrome" patients. A classic example is the Down syndrome; about 20% of infants affected with Down syndrome have an AVSD type of anomaly. Other syndromes, such as Ellis–van Creveld syndrome and Pallister-Hall syndrome, are also frequently associated with AVSDs. Patients with heterotaxia often have AVSDs as part of their complex cardiac anomaly.

Because there are a variety of anomalies that compose AVSDs, there are also a variety of symptoms and findings. The symptoms depend on the degree of anatomic anomalies and resultant hemodynamics. At one end of the anatomic spectrum, there is *partial or intermediate AVSD* with primum ASD. These patients are usually asymptomatic during infancy and do not develop congestive heart failure in childhood. Their symptoms may be minimal and vary with the amount of mitral insufficiency present in addition to the primum ASD shunt. At most, such patients may have respiratory symptoms or slow growth. Congestive heart failure may, however, appear in the neonatal period if the mitral insufficiency is severe.[40] Examination of patients with a partial AVSD usually reveals a pulmonary ejection systolic murmur, usually grade 3/6 or less. If a large shunt is present, there is a grade 1–2/6 mid-diastolic flow rumble at the mid to left sternal border and a right ventricular impulse in the same area. The first heart sound is accentuated in the tricuspid area. The second heart sound in the pulmonic area is widely split and fixed. P_2 is accentuated, depending on the level of pulmonary arterial pressure. The anterior leaflet of the mitral valve is frequently cleft, producing some mitral insufficiency and, at the apex, a high-pitched pansystolic murmur that radiates to the lower left sternal border and axilla. Should the insufficiency produce a volume load on the left ventricle, there may be an apical thrust and an apical mid-diastolic murmur as well. Often there is no ventricular shunting because the chordae tendineae of this valve are fused to the crest of the ventricular septum.

At the other end of the anatomic spectrum is the *complete AVSD*, in which there is one AV annulus and one AV valve. Shunting occurs at both the atrial and ventricular levels. There is often severe AV valve regurgitation. Patients with complete AVSDs are symptomatic in infancy because of left ventricular dilatation from increasing pulmonary blood flow and mitral regurgitation. Significantly, pulmonary hypertension is regularly present. Congestive cardiac failure, failure to thrive, and frequent upper respiratory tract infections appear soon after the pulmonary vascular resistance starts to fall. Because congestive cardiac failure is so predictable, if a patient is known to have a complete AVSD and has no congestive cardiac failure, the patient probably has pulmonary stenosis or pulmonary vascular disease.[41] On physical examination, the precordium is hyperactive, S_1 is usually single, S_2 is narrowly split, P_2 is loud, and there may be an S_3 gallop. There is at the apex a holosystolic murmur that radiates to the left axilla because of mitral insufficiency. There is frequently a mid-diastolic murmur heard at the lower left sternal border and apex from ventricular inflow through the AV valve. In contrast to patients with a partial AVSD, these patients usually have peripheral pulses that are less strong. Mild cyanosis is not uncommon, but if moderate cyanosis is found with a loud pulmonic murmur, associated right ventricular outflow obstruction must be suspected.

ELECTROCARDIOGRAPHY

Nearly all patients with an AVSD have similar electrocardiographic findings, regardless of the form of AVSD. Because of the location of the defects, the course of the conduction system is almost always abnormal. The AV node is

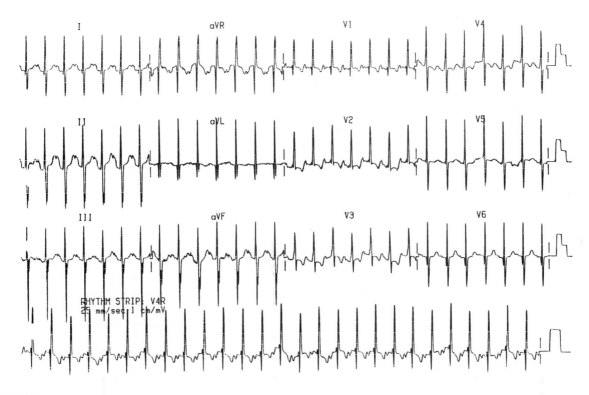

FIGURE 24–4

Reproduction of an electrocardiogram from a 6-month-old infant with a complete AVSD showing sinus rhythm with incomplete right bundle branch block, left axis deviation, and combined ventricular hypertrophy.

displaced inferiorly relative to its usual position near the coronary sinus.[42] The bundle branches are also abnormal: the right bundle branch is longer than usual, and the left bundle is posteroinferiorly displaced. As a result, the depolarization of the ventricles proceeds from a right inferior position to a left superior position, producing "left axis deviation" on a surface electrocardiogram. The deviation is often more prominent in a complete AVSD. Another common finding on electrocardiography is first-degree heart block, presumably caused by the increased time it takes to conduct through the enlarged atria (Fig. 24–4).[43] An rSr' in the right precordial leads is common and related to right ventricular enlargement, with the height of the r' wave increasing with increasing levels of right ventricular systolic pressure. If the left ventricle is significantly enlarged, a pattern of left ventricular hypertrophy is found as well.

ECHOCARDIOGRAPHY

Echocardiography has become the preferred modality for diagnosis of AVSDs, especially in neonates, infants, and small children. This is because of its superior definition of intracardiac anatomy, particularly AV valve and chordal morphology.[44–46] Visualization and characterization of anatomic anomalies are often so precise that operation can be performed solely on the basis of echocardiographic information.[47] This places greater reliance on the echocardiographer to ascertain all aspects of anatomy and physiology as accurately as possible. Accurate assessment, in turn, demands a detailed and thorough knowledge of the anatomy of AVSDs (see section on anatomy), including anatomic variations and associated abnormalities.

The following sections detail echocardiographic assessment of AVSDs by standard M-mode, transthoracic, transesophageal, and fetal two-dimensional echocardiography. Regardless of type of echocardiographic imaging, certain fundamental anatomic questions must be addressed in both partial and complete AVSDs. These questions, adapted from Snider and Serwer,[48] are listed in Table 24–2. The echocardiographer should always attempt to answer these questions systematically in any patient with suspected or known AVSD.

M-MODE ECHOCARDIOGRAPHY

The hallmark of both partial and complete AVSDs is apparent diastolic movement of the mitral valve through the plane of the ventricular septum.[49] Whether a defect is clas-

TABLE 24–2

KEY ANATOMIC QUESTIONS TO BE ANSWERED BY ECHOCARDIOGRAPHY

Extent of atrial communication

Extent of ventricular communication; nature of the tissue separating the atrioventricular valves from the trabecular septum

Anatomy of the atrioventricular valves and their chordal attachments

Degree of atrioventricular valve insufficiency

Distribution of the atrioventricular valves between the two ventricles

Degree of ventriculoatrial septal malalignment, and resultant sizes of the ventricular inflow tracts

Presence or absence of outflow tract obstruction

Associated lesions (e.g., systemic-pulmonary venous anomalies, patent ductus arteriosus, coarctation of aorta)

Adapted from Snider AR, Serwer, GA: Echocardiography in Pediatric Heart Disease. Chicago, Year Book Medical, 1990, p 154.

sified as partial or complete depends on the degree of ventricular septal dropout. Other characteristic M-mode findings include inferior displacement of the mitral valve, narrowing of the left ventricular outflow tract, an enlarged right ventricle, and multiple systolic and diastolic echoes of the mitral valve. Largely because of the diagnostic superiority of two-dimensional imaging as well as technical advances in two-dimensional echocardiographic images, M-mode imaging has almost entirely been replaced by two-dimensional echocardiography.

TWO-DIMENSIONAL ECHOCARDIOGRAPHY

Echocardiographic assessment of AVSDs begins with an examination of systemic and pulmonary venous connections. This is particularly important when visceral heterotaxia is suspected, because of the high incidence of systemic and pulmonary venous connection anomalies.[50–52] *Subxiphoid long- and short-axis planes* are useful in determining venous connections, although suprasternal notch examination is often necessary to image superior vena caval connection. During subxiphoid long-axis (four-chamber) imaging, as the transducer is angled more anteriorly, large ostium primum defects can be seen (Fig. 24–5). These defects are posterior, located just above the coronary sinus and adjacent to the AV valves. Doppler color flow imaging demonstrates left-to-right atrial level shunting. In addition, the remainder of the atrial septum must also be examined; ostium secundum atrial defects commonly accompany large ostium primum defects.

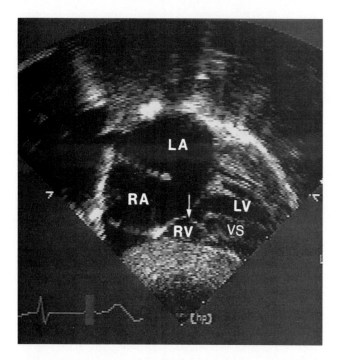

Echocardiogram of the subxiphoid long-axis (four-chamber) view of the atrial septal defect in a partial AVSD (also known as an ostium primum atrial septal defect). The AV valve has septated into mitral and tricuspid valves, and chordal tissue attaches to the crest of ventricular septum *(arrow)*, preventing ventricular level shunting. LA = left atrium; LV = left ventricle; RA = right atrium; RV = right ventricle; VS = ventricular septum.

In both the subxiphoid long- and short-axis views, the course, size, and mouth of the coronary sinus can also be seen. A dilated coronary sinus generally indicates a persistent left superior vena cava emptying directly into the coronary sinus, and with leftward angulation of the transducer in the subxiphoid short-axis plane, the left superior vena cava can sometimes be seen entering the coronary sinus. Because of its very posterior location, a dilated coronary sinus can sometimes be erroneously mistaken for a large primum ASD; care must taken to distinguish these two structures. Also, the precise origin of the mouth of the coronary sinus should be determined; there is occasionally a short coronary sinus, with the orifice draining into the left atrium.

As the transducer sweeps anteriorly (from subxiphoid long-axis view), more information becomes available about the AVSD, specifically whether there is a VSD component, the general morphology of the AV valves, and the size and morphology of the left ventricular outflow tract. Often, the characteristic gooseneck deformity can be seen with this view (Fig. 24–6). When a subxiphoid short-axis sweep (from right to left) is performed, the AV valves can be viewed en face, and the degree of septation and attachments of the superior bridging leaflet can be clearly seen (Fig. 24–7). The subxiphoid short-axis view is also helpful in evaluating the right ventricular outflow tract for obstruction (Fig. 24–8 [see also Color Plates]) and for visualizing the number and spacing of left ventricular papillary muscles.

The *apical four-chamber view* is one of the most important views to examine AVSDs; it is also the most easily understandable view for nonechocardiographers. From this view, the extent of the atrial and ventricular septal communications can be appreciated, as can the position of the AV valves in relation to the defects (Fig. 24–9). In partial AVSD, the lack of mitral-tricuspid valve offset becomes apparent. The relative size of both ventricles[53] and degree of malalignment of the AV valves (in relation to the ventricles) can be determined. Color flow Doppler interrogation clearly shows the location and degree of tricuspid and mitral regurgitation and also whether left ventricular–to–right atrial shunting is present (Fig. 24–9C [see Color Plates]). Tricuspid regurgitation can be quantified by pulsed and continuous-wave Doppler. With posterior angulation of the transducer, the course of the coronary sinus can be shown. With anterior angulation, the left ventricular outflow tract can be seen along with any subaortic obstruction. This view also affords an excellent angle for Doppler interrogation of the left ventricular outflow tract and aortic valve.

Parasternal long- and short-axis views offer excellent views of the AV valves, specifically leaflet morphology and chordal anatomy. On the parasternal long-axis view, the mitral valve appears to point more anteriorly than normal (Fig. 24–10). The submitral tensor apparatus can also be seen well. The left ventricular outflow tract can also be examined closely for possible chordal or discrete membranous subaortic obstruction.[54] When the transducer is angled rightward, the nature and extent of the ventricular level component can be determined. Chordae tendineae can also be visualized as they attach to the ventricular septum. Ventricular shunting (if any) can be shown by

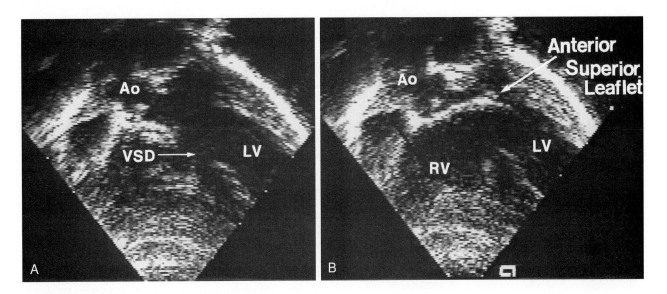

A, More superior angulation in the echocardiogram of the subxiphoid long-axis view demonstrates the large ventricular septal defect (VSD). *B,* The "gooseneck" deformity produced by inferior displacement of the AV valve, which leads to mismatch between the inflow and outflow lengths of the left ventricle. Ao = aorta; LV = left ventricle; RV = right ventricle.

Doppler color flow mapping. If tricuspid regurgitation is present, the rightward-angled parasternal long-axis view also provides a good angle of interrogation for quantitation of the jet. The parasternal short-axis view displays the AV valves en face similar to the subxiphoid short-axis (parasagittal) plane. The cleft of the anterior leaflet of the mitral valve can be demonstrated (Fig. 24–11), and Doppler color flow mapping demonstrates more precisely the site of any AV valve regurgitation. With a slow sweep into the ventricles, the tensor apparatus can be inspected for evidence of abnormalities (e.g., parachute or double-

orifice mitral valve). The number and spacing of the left ventricular papillary muscles can also be seen, and any additional muscular ventricular septal defects can be identified. With a superior sweep to the branch pulmonary arteries, a patent ductus arteriosus (if present) can be identified inserting into the main pulmonary artery. Right ventricular outflow obstruction can also be seen.

The *suprasternal notch views* are important for determining aortic arch sidedness and size of the transverse arch and for excluding coexistent coarctation of the aorta. Blood flow in the right superior vena cava can be exam-

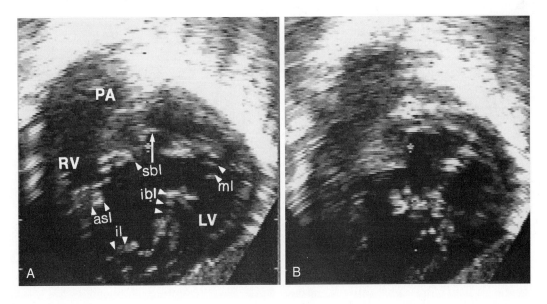

Echocardiogram of the subxiphoid short-axis view in a patient with complete AVSD in diastole *(A)* and systole *(B).* This view shows very well the orifice of the common AV valve, as well as the degree of valve septation and attachments of the superior bridging leaflet (see the Rastelli classification in the text). asl = [right] anterosuperior leaflet; ibl = inferior bridging leaflet; il = [right] inferior leaflet; LV = left ventricle; ml = mural leaflet; PA = pulmonary artery; RV = right ventricle; sbl = superior bridging leaflet.

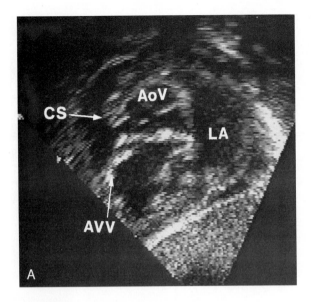

FIGURE 24–8

Echocardiogram of the subxiphoid short-axis view in a patient with a complete AVSD and right ventricular outflow tract obstruction (tetralogy of Fallot physiology). Note the lack of attachment of the anterior leaflet (AVV) to the conal septum (CS). The infundibular septum is anteriorly malaligned, producing subpulmonary narrowing (A), and flow acceleration begins at this level (B). (See Color Figure 24–8B.) AoV = aortic valve; AVV = common AV valve; CS = conal (infundibular) septum; LA = left atrium.

ined, and a persistent left superior vena cava (if present) can be seen. A patent ductus arteriosus can also be well seen from this view.

TRANSESOPHAGEAL ECHOCARDIOGRAPHY

Because of the proximity of the esophagus to the left atrium, transesophageal echocardiography (TEE) provides superb imaging and Doppler color flow mapping of intracardiac anatomy, particularly the atrial and ventricular septa and AV valves. This makes it especially well suited for the evaluation of AVSDs.[55] Virtually all available TEE views[56,57] are useful to visualize AVSDs (Fig. 24–12 [see also Color Plates]).

With the availability of the newer, smaller pediatric probes (with biplane imaging capability), TEE can be successfully performed in smaller children and infants as small as 2.0 kg. However, its semi-invasive nature and the excellent quality of transthoracic images generally obtainable in infants and children have restricted the use of TEE to specialized clinical settings. Its primary use is intraoperative—to monitor operative repair of the defects. In this setting, both a preoperative and postoperative study are performed. The preoperative assessment is used to confirm the intracardiac anatomy, including the nature and extent of the septal defects, the location and degree of AV valve regurgitation, and the presence or absence of right and left ventricular outflow obstruction. The postoperative assessment is important to evaluate for a residual atrial or ventricular shunt and to assess the status of the AV valve repair (Fig. 24–13 [see also Color Plates]). Of particular interest is the integrity of the mitral valve, especially the repaired cleft of the anterior leaflet. Postoperative ventricular function can also be easily assessed. In some patients, intraoperative TEE information alters or refines operative therapy and occasionally dictates an immediate reoperation to repair residual defects.[58]

TEE also has applications as an outpatient procedure and in the intensive care unit. In the outpatient setting, TEE serves as a useful diagnostic tool for large children and young adults with inadequate transthoracic echo windows.[59] It can be used preoperatively to confirm diagnostic findings or postoperatively to assess status of the repair. Outpatient TEE is particularly useful in evaluating pa-

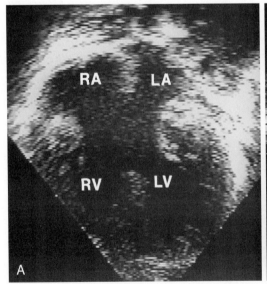
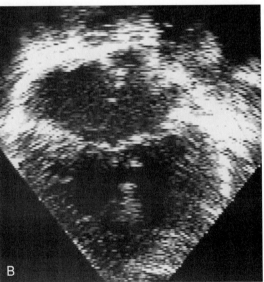

FIGURE 24–9

Echocardiogram of the apical four-chamber view during diastole (A) and systole (B) in a patient with common AVSD. Note the large atrial and ventricular septal defects and the lack of mitral-tricuspid offset. In this patient, the AV valve is well balanced over both ventricles. LA = left atrium; LV = left ventricle; RA = right atrium; RV = right ventricle. C, See Color Figure 24–9C.

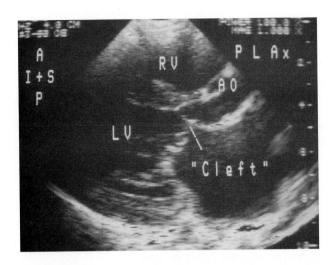

FIGURE 24–10

Echocardiogram of the parasternal long-axis view in a patient with an ostium primum atrial septal defect. The mitral valve leaflets point more anteriorly than normal, toward the ventricular septum. AO = aorta; LV = left ventricle; RV = right ventricle.

tients who have undergone mitral valve replacement with an artificial prosthesis (e.g., St. Jude), in whom transthoracic echocardiography notoriously produces unsatisfactory, often incomplete imaging. Similarly, TEE is useful in the intensive care setting when there are poor or inaccessible transthoracic echo windows; this particularly applies to patients with an open chest.[60,61]

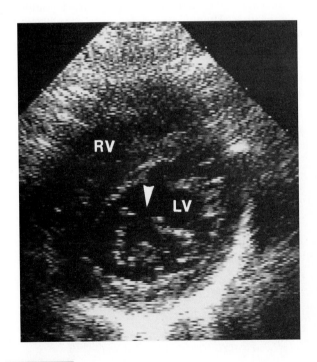

FIGURE 24–11

Echocardiogram of the parasternal short-axis view in a patient with an ostium primum atrial septal defect, showing the cleft in the anterior leaflet of the mitral valve (arrow). LV = left ventricle; RV = right ventricle.

FETAL ECHOCARDIOGRAPHY

AVSDs can be accurately diagnosed in utero by fetal echocardiography.[62,63] Distinctive morphologic characteristics are present as early as 12 to 16 weeks of gestation. A complete AVSD is readily apparent: the characteristic atrial and ventricular defects and common AV valve produce a large defect in the center of the heart, well seen in the four-chamber plane (which is used commonly by obstetricians to screen for congenital heart defects). A partial AV defect can also be identified by visualization of the ostium primum atrial defect and the recognition of two separate valve orifices (both at the same level). Doppler color flow mapping demonstrates left-to-right shunting and, when it is present, AV valve regurgitation.[64] Recognition of a complete AVSD in the fetus should prompt a thorough

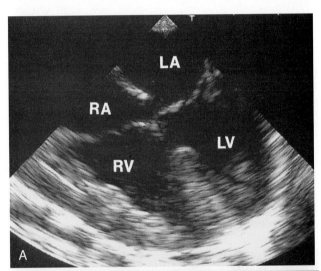

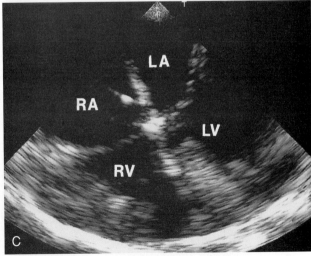

FIGURE 24–12

Transesophageal echocardiography performed in the operating room (A, B) shows a large complete AVSD with unobstructed left-to-right shunting at both atrial and ventricular levels. (See also Color Figure 24–12B.) There is also a mild degree of mitral insufficiency. After surgery (C, D), the large patch can be well seen, and there is no left-to-right shunt. (See also Color Figure 24–12D.) LA = left atrium; LV = left ventricle; RA = right atrium; RV = right ventricle.

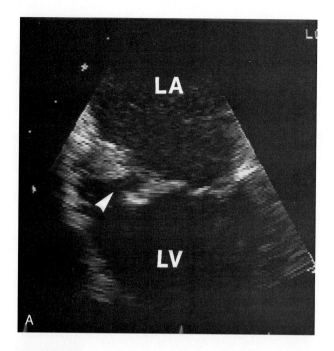

FIGURE 24–13

Intraoperative transesophageal echocardiography in an adult patient with a previously repaired AVSD who had subsequently developed significant mitral insufficiency. *A*, A residual cleft in the anterior leaflet of the mitral valve is clearly depicted *(arrow)*. LA = left atrium; LV = left ventricle. *B*, See Color Figure 24–13*B*.

search for other cardiac anomalies, especially visceroatrial heterotaxia. An amniocentesis is also indicated because of the frequent association of AVSD with Down syndrome and other chromosome abnormalities.[1]

RADIOGRAPHY

Although a chest film is not diagnostic, it furnishes information about the severity of the defect, especially about volume loading of the heart. The anatomic defect determines the radiographic findings. In a partial AVSD, with little or no mitral insufficiency, chest radiographic findings resemble those in patients with a secundum ASD: with significant atrial shunting, both right-sided chambers may be enlarged, and there is increased pulmonary vascularity (Fig. 24–14). If the patient has mitral insufficiency, there is even more cardiomegaly, and the left ventricle is enlarged because of the increased volume load. The left atrium remains small because it is decompressed by the ASD. In patients with a complete AVSD, there is often a marked increase in pulmonary vascularity, but the cardiomegaly present is out of proportion to the vascularity (Fig. 24–14).[65]

CARDIAC CATHETERIZATION

Cardiac catheterization is seldom required for most forms of AVSD. In most instances, the echocardiographic findings not only provide the anatomic features in the individual patient but also allow hemodynamic estimation of flows and resistances necessary to assess operability. At our hospital, less than 10% of patients with an AVSD undergo catheterization before operation. When the echocardiogram is not satisfactory to evaluate the hemodynamics or does not exclude associated anomalies, cardiac catheterization is performed. Catheterization provides data so that pulmonary vascular resistance can be calculated to detect pulmonary vascular disease. Others may need catheterization for verification of systemic or pulmonary venous connection. Left ventricular outflow obstruction, such as subaortic stenosis,[66] or right ventricular outflow obstruction, such as tetralogy of Fallot,[67] may require definition by catheterization. Altered visceral situs may complicate the interpretation of echocardiographic findings and is yet another reason for catheterization.

Catheterization for *partial AVSD* in childhood is not needed unless the defect is associated with abnormal visceral situs. In that rare instance, the catheterization

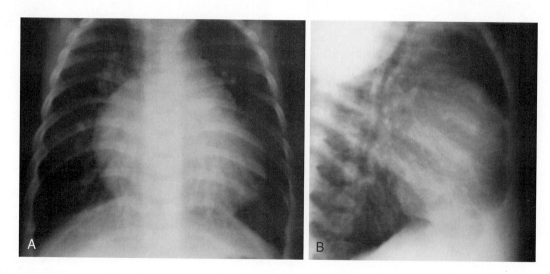

FIGURE 24–14

Chest film of a 5-month-old with complete AVSD demonstrates the posteroanterior (*A*) and lateral (*B*) views. Left atrial enlargement with cardiomegaly and increased lung vascularity are present.

demonstrates the atrial shunt and is likely to show some degree of mitral valve regurgitation. Pulmonary arterial pressures are normal or slightly elevated, and calculated pulmonary vascular resistance is normal. The reasons for cardiac catheterization in *intermediate or transitional AVSD* are similar to those for the partial form of AVSD. Once again, most patients do not require such investigation. If catheterization is performed, however, the findings are usually those of the partial defect with atrial shunting combined with AV valve regurgitation and some ventricular shunting. Pulmonary flows and pressures may be modestly increased, but pulmonary resistance is generally normal.

For *complete AVSD*, the findings are those of atrial or ventricular shunts that may be bidirectional. There is often a large increase in oxygen saturation in the right atrium, with a further increase in the right ventricle. The changes are due to left-to-right shunting at both atrial and ventricular levels. At the left ventricular level, there is a decrease in oxygen saturation, indicating a concomitant right-to-left shunt. The shunts are often large and frequently associated with pulmonary hypertension. Total pulmonary blood flow is markedly increased, resulting in elevated pulmonary artery pressure and usually an increased calculated pulmonary vascular resistance.

As previously noted, concern for elevated pulmonary vascular resistance is the reason for the cardiac catheterization in most such patients. Those with elevated pulmonary vascular resistance beyond 10 units/m^2, in the absence of significant AV valve insufficiency, are generally deemed inoperable. The keys, then, are both the pulmonary flow with its influence on the vascular bed and the function of the AV valves. Although AV valve regurgitation is best assessed on echocardiography, it can also be inferred from atrial pressure waves with a large regurgitant wave (*v* wave) as well as be seen on angiocardiography.

Common atrium is infrequent, but at catheterization, nearly complete atrial mixing of systemic and pulmonary venous returns is found. Oxygen saturations are generally the same in both ventricles and great arteries. Because of high pulmonary flows, the saturations are often about 90%. Pulmonary arterial pressure is commonly elevated, but pulmonary resistance is not.

Patients with a *complicated AVSD* may have tetralogy of Fallot type physiology; coarctation of the aorta, without or with septal malalignment (the latter may result in hypoplastic left or right ventricle); and abnormalities of venous return, or visceral situs. They frequently undergo cardiac catheterization to delineate these features and their effect on pulmonary anatomy and physiology. Often, oxygen saturations progressively increase at the right atrial and ventricular levels. These left-to-right shunt findings are coupled with decreased saturation in the left ventricle and aorta and indicate bidirectional shunting at the ventricular level. There is systemic pressure in the right ventricle with a pressure drop across the right ventricular outflow and pulmonary valve. The low left atrial mean pressure and low normal pulmonary artery pressure suggest minimal valve regurgitation. In fact, the clinical situation is that of tetralogy of Fallot with AVSD. With this information, an effective operative repair can be carried out.

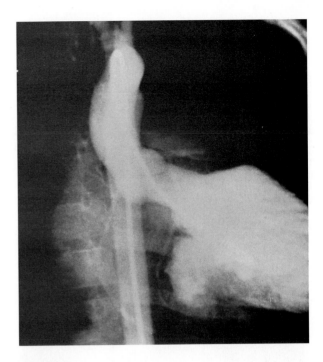

FIGURE 24–15

Cineangiocardiogram frame reproduction from a patient with AVSD. Contrast dye has been injected into the left ventricle. The elongated outflow tract gives rise to the gooseneck appearance typical of the defect. The distance between the aortic valve and the apex (off the picture) is clearly greater than that from the cleft mitral valve to the apex (i.e., outlet length greater than inlet length).

ANGIOCARDIOGRAPHY

The angiographic hallmark of an AVSD is the gooseneck appearance on left ventricular injection of contrast medium (Fig. 24–15). The AV valves are abnormal both in structure and in position. Even in a partial AVSD with two distinct valve orifices, the valves are abnormally low and at the same level (normally, the mitral valve is superior to the tricuspid). As a result, the inlet length of the left ventricle is less than the outlet length. Combined with an abnormally high aortic valve, the left ventricular outflow tract is longer and narrower, producing a gooseneck deformity. Varying degrees of AV valve insufficiency may be seen, as well as atrial and ventricular shunting. Angled oblique views (Fig. 24–16) may show the AVSD best. When there are associated abnormalities, especially of the great vessels, angiography clearly demonstrates the anatomy. The pulmonary vascular bed, in particular, is seen well with appropriate injections.

MANAGEMENT

The treatment of a patient with an AVSD depends on age at discovery, form of the defect, and symptoms. The goal of management is surgical correction, with closure of the defects, competency of the AV valves without stenosis, and an intact conduction system. After correction, the hope is for normal pulmonary vascular resistance. A number of those

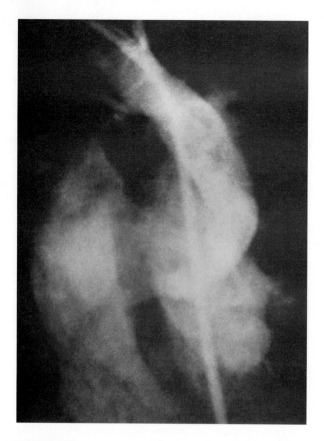

Angled oblique cineangiocardiogram frame reproduction showing the ventricular septum, two "balanced" ventricles, and the AVSD.

with partial forms of the defect may be asymptomatic. Others, more likely with transitional and complete forms of AVSD, require treatment for heart failure or intercurrent respiratory infections. They may also fail to thrive. Still others with complex forms are cyanotic. Well-known and often-used medical methods for symptomatic treatment of these findings are applicable to those with an AVSD.

Early operative repair of a symptomatic infant with an AVSD is preferred. In certain small, very sick infants, however, pulmonary artery banding may provide safe relief of pulmonary circulatory overload.[68] Operative repair of symptomatic AVSDs is often performed between 3 and 6 months of age. Earlier repair is feasible but may carry a higher risk. Delay often results in marked failure to thrive, recurrent pneumonias, and chronic lung disease. Delay also has the hazard of development of pulmonary vascular disease, especially in those with Down syndrome.

In those with an asymptomatic partial AVSD, repair at about age 1 to 2 years is commonly advocated. Current operative techniques avoid surgical complications of heart block, AV valve insufficiency, and stenosis that plagued the initial era of surgery for AVSD.[69] Currently used septal patch materials minimize hemolysis from residual jets from AV valve regurgitation striking the atrial septum (the "Waring blender" syndrome). If there is marked hemolysis, conservative management with supplemental iron and, if needed, transfusions may tide the patient over until the

hemolysis subsides. Rarely, reoperation is required to abolish the regurgitant jet or redirect it away from the atrial septum.

There is considerable variation in the exact technique for operative repair of an AVSD. The septal defects may be closed with either one or two patches if the ventricular component is large. Bridging leaflets may be split or left intact. The left AV valve may be left either tricuspid or bicuspid. The AV node and His bundle are avoided by suturing well below the rim of the ventricular defect from either the left or right side. Attachment of the patch to leaflet tissue may be accomplished by direct suture or pledgets or sandwich methods. Special operative considerations are needed for anatomic variants like absence of atrial septum, accessory AV valve orifices, single papillary muscle, septal malalignment (hypoplasia of left or right ventricle), double-outlet right ventricle or tetralogy of Fallot, transposition of the great arteries, and unroofed coronary sinus with left superior vena cava. Operative techniques for management of major categories of AVSD have been proposed by Kirklin and Barratt-Boyes[70] and are listed in Table 24-3.

Operative outcomes vary with the type of AVSD and the degree of preoperative AV valve incompetence. For the most part, results are good if the defect is uncomplicated. Those with Down syndrome are likely to do well because their thick redundant AV valves lend themselves to repair. The non-Down patient with AVSD may have thin and deficient valve tissue for adequate reconstruction, and these children may have progressive postoperative left AV valve regurgitation. If they are symptomatic, further valve repair or even replacement will be required, usually within several years of the first operation. In this instance, mechanical valves are the prostheses of choice with placement technique such as to avoid subvalvar aortic outflow obstruction. A hazard of AVSD valve replacement is interruption of conduction pathways with resultant complete heart block. Although heart block is much less common with present-day surgical techniques, a few patients will require pacemakers for surgically induced block. Those with

TABLE 24-3

AVAILABLE SURGICAL TECHNIQUES FOR SPECIFIC VARIANTS OF ATRIOVENTRICULAR SEPTAL DEFECT

Repair of complete atrioventricular (AV) canal defect with little or no bridging of the left superior and left inferior leaflets: Rastelli type A
Repair of complete AV canal defect with bridging of the left superior leaflet: Rastelli type B or C
Repair of partial AV canal defect with little or no left AV valve incompetence
Repair of AV canal defect with small interchordal interventricular communications
Repair of AV canal defect with common atrium
Repair of complete or partial AV canal defect with moderate or severe left AV valve incompetence
Right AV valve considerations
Right superior leaflet–left superior leaflet and right inferior–left inferior commissures
Repair with tetralogy of Fallot
Repair with double-outlet right ventricle
Repair with transposition of the great arteries
Repair of left ventricular outflow tract obstruction
Replacement of the left AV valve

AVSD requiring an operation on certain associated complicating defects, like extremely dominant right ventricle or other major defect, fare less well. On the other hand, there is a high degree of success for patients with tetralogy of Fallot. Early survival (for the first week after operation) is about 96% for all types of AVSD.

PROGNOSIS AFTER SURGERY

Information about long-term survival after operative repair is fragmentary. The survival rate for a partial AVSD (ostium primum defect) is about 80% at 30 years after operation.[34,70–75] The survival after operation for a complete AVSD is about 70% after 20 years.[36,37,70,71,76] Late mortality is mainly related to left AV valve insufficiency or stenosis as well as associated defects or syndromes. The percentage of patients who have event-free survival (that is, are functionally well and have not needed reoperation) may be only half of the percentage who survive. Reoperation may be needed to repair or replace mitral or tricuspid valves and occasionally to relieve subaortic stenosis. Arrhythmias, including complete AV block, are common and might be expected to become more frequent as the subjects age.

REFERENCES

1. Cook AC, Allan LD, Anderson RH, et al: AVSD in fetal life—a clinicopathological correlation. Cardiol Young 1:334, 1991.
2. Mitchell SC, Korones SB, Berendes HW: Congenital heart disease in 56,109 births. Incidence and natural history. Circulation 43:323, 1971.
3. Samanek M: Prevalence at birth, "natural" risk and survival with AVSD. Cardiol Young 1:285, 1991.
4. Wenink ACG, Zevallos JC: Developmental aspects of AVSDs. Int J Cardiol 18:65, 1988.
5. Allwork SP: Anatomical-embryological correlates in AVSD. Br Heart J 47:419, 1982.
6. Wenink ACG, Gittenberger-deGroot AC, Brom AG: Developmental considerations of mitral valve anomalies. Int J Cardiol 11:85, 1986.
7. Gutgesell HP, Huhta JC: Cardiac septation in AV canal defects. J Am Coll Cardiol 8:1421, 1986.
8. Piccoli GP, Gerlis LM, Wilkinson JL, et al: Morphology and classification of AV defects. Br Heart J 42:621, 1979.
9. Anderson RH, Baker EJ, Ho SY, et al: The morphology and diagnosis of AVSDs. Cardiol Young 1:290, 1991.
10. Bharati S, Lev M: Common AV orifice—intermediate type. In Bharati S, Lev M: The Pathology of Congenital Heart Disease. Armonk, NY, Futura Publishing, 1996, p 597.
11. Sigfusson G, Ettedgui JA, Silverman NH, et al: Is a cleft in the anterior leaflet of an otherwise normal mitral valve an AV canal malformation? J Am Coll Cardiol 26:508, 1995.
12. Kohl T, Silverman NH: Comparison of cleft and papillary muscle position in cleft mitral valve and AVSD. Am J Cardiol 77:164, 1996.
13. Rastelli GC, Kirklin JW, Titus JL: Anatomic observations on complete form of persistent common AV canal with special reference to AV valves. Mayo Clin Proc 41:296, 1966.
14. Tenckhoff L, Stamm SJ: An analysis of 35 cases of the complete form of persistent common AV canal. Circulation 48:416, 1973.
15. Silverman NH, Zuberbuhler JR, Anderson RH: AVSDs: Cross-sectional echocardiographic and morphologic comparisons. Int J Cardiol 13:309, 1986.
16. Chin AJ, Bierman FZ, Sanders SP, et al: Subxiphoid 2-dimensional echocardiographic identification of left ventricular papillary muscle anomalies in complete common AV canal. Am J Cardiol 51:695, 1983.
17. David I, Castenada AR, Van Praagh R: Potentially parachute mitral valve in common AV canal: Pathologic anatomy and clinical importance. J Thorac Cardiovasc Surg 84:178, 1982.
18. Tandon R, Moller JH, Edwards JE: Single papillary muscle of the left ventricle associated with persistent common AV canal: Variant of parachute mitral valve. Pediatr Cardiol 7:111, 1986.
19. Warnes C, Somerville J: Double mitral valve orifice in AV defects. Br Heart J 49:59, 1983.
20. Piccoli GP, Ho SY, Wilkinson JL, et al: Left-sided obstructive lesions in AVSDs. J Thorac Cardiovasc Surg 83:453, 1982.
21. Ilbawi MN, Idriss FS, DeLeon SY, et al: Unusual mitral valve abnormalities complicating surgical repair of endocardial cushion defects. J Thorac Cardiovasc Surg 85:697, 1983.
22. Fyler DC: Endocardial cushion defects. In Fyler DC (ed): Nadas' Pediatric Cardiology. Philadelphia, Hanley & Belfus, 1992, p 577.
23. Van Praagh S, Antoniadis S, Otero-Coto E, et al: Common AV canal with and without conotruncal malformations: An anatomic study of 251 postmortem cases. In Nora JJ, Takao A (eds): Congenital Heart Disease: Causes and Processes. Mt. Kisco, NY, Futura Publishing, 1984, p 599.
24. Hirooka K, Yagihara T, Kishimoto H, et al: Biventricular repair in cardiac isomerism: Report of seventeen cases. J Thorac Cardiovasc Surg 109:530, 1995.
25. Van Mierop LHS, Alley RD, Kausel HW, et al: The anatomy and embryology of endocardial cushion defects. J Thorac Cardiovasc Surg 43:71, 1962.
26. Lamers WH, Viragh S, Wessels A, et al: Formation of the tricuspid valve in the human heart. Circulation 91:111, 1995.
27. Moore KL, Persoud TVN: The Developing Human. Philadelphia, WB Saunders, 1993.
28. Eisenberg LM, Markwald RR: Molecular regulation of AV valvuloseptal morphogenesis. Circ Res 77:1, 1995.
29. Wunsch AM, Little CD, Markwald RR: Cardiac endothelial heterogeneity defines valvular development as demonstrated by the diverse expression of JB3, an antigen of endocardial cushion tissue. Dev Biol 165:585, 1995.
30. Runyan RB, Potts JD, Sharma RV, et al: Signal transduction of a tissue interaction during embryonic heart development. Cell Regul 1:301, 1990.
31. Wittee DP, Aronow BJ, Dry JK, et al: Temporally and spatially restricted expression of apolipoprotein J in the developing heart defines discrete stages of valve morphogenesis. Dev Dyn 201:290, 1994.
32. Larsen WJ: Human Embryology. New York, Churchill Livingstone, 1993.
33. Van Mierop LHS, Kutsche LK: Embryology of the heart. In Hurst JW, Schlant RC, Rackley CE (eds): The Heart, Arteries and Veins, 7th ed. New York, McGraw-Hill, 1990, p 3.
34. Berning RA, Silverman NH, Villegas M, et al: Reversed shunting across the ductus arteriosus or atrial septum in utero heralds severe congenital heart disease. J Am Coll Cardiol 27:481, 1996.
35. Somerville J: Ostium primum defect: Factors causing deterioration in the natural history. Br Heart J 27:413, 1965.
36. Bergin ML, Warnes CA, Tajik AJ, Danielson GK: Partial AV canal defect: Long-term follow-up after initial repair in patients ≥ 40 years old. J Am Coll Cardiol 25:1189, 1995.
37. Keith JD, Rowe RD, Vlad P: Heart Disease in Infancy and Childhood. New York, Macmillan, 1958, p 271.
38. Michielon G, Stellin G, Rizzoli G, Casarotto DC: Repair of complete common atrioventricular canal defects in patients younger than four months of age. Circulation 96(suppl II):316, 1997.
39. Najm HK, Coles JG, Endo M, et al: Complete AVSDs. Results of repair, risk factors, and freedom from reoperation. Circulation 96(suppl II):311, 1997.
40. Feldt RH, Edwards WD, Hagler DJ, Puga FJ: Endocardial cushion defects. In Moller JH, Neal WA (eds): Fetal, Neonatal, and Infant Cardiac Disease. Norwalk, CT, Appleton & Lange, 1990, p 411.
41. Vick GW, Titus JL: Defects of the atrial septum including the AV canal. In Garson A, Bricker JT, McNamara DG (eds): The Science and Practice of Pediatric Cardiology. Philadelphia, Lea & Febiger, 1990, p 1023.
42. Ih S, Fukuda K, Okada R, et al: Histopathological correlation between the QRS axis and disposition of the AV conduction system in common AV orifice and its related anomalies. Jpn Circ J 47:1368, 1983.
43. Feldt RH, Porter CJ, Edwards WD, et al: AVSDs. In Emmanouilides GC, Allen HD, Riemenschneider TA, et al (eds): Heart Disease in

Infants, Children, and Adolescents, 5th ed. Baltimore, Williams & Wilkins, 1995, p 704.

44. Hagler DJ, Tajik AJ, Seward JB, et al: Real-time wide-angle sector echocardiography: AV canal defects. Circulation 59:140, 1979.

45. Smallhorn JF, Tommasini G, Anderson RH, Macartney FJ: Assessment of atrioventricular septal defects by two dimensional echocardiography. Br Heart J 47:109, 1982.

46. Lange DJ, Sahn DJ, Allen HD, et al: Subxiphoid cross-sectional echocardiography in infants and children with congenital heart disease. Circulation 59:513, 1979.

47. Lipshultz SE, Sanders SP, Mayer JE, et al: Are routine preoperative cardiac catheterization and angiography necessary before repair of ostium primum atrial septal defect? J Am Coll Cardiol 11:373, 1988.

48. Snider AR, Serwer GA: Echocardiography in Pediatric Heart Disease. Chicago, Year Book Medical, 1990, p 154.

49. Williams RG, Rudd M: Echocardiographic features of endocardial cushion defects. Circulation 49:418, 1974.

50. Rose V, Izukawa T, Moes CAF: Syndrome of asplenia and polysplenia: A review of cardiac and non-cardiac malformations in 60 cases with special reference to diagnosis and prognosis. Br Heart J 37:840, 1975.

51. Ruttenberg HD: Corrected transposition of the great arteries and splenic syndromes. In Adams FH, Emmanouilides GC (eds): Moss' Heart Disease in Infants, Children and Adolescents, 3rd ed. Baltimore, Williams & Wilkins, 1983, p 333.

52. Van Praagh S, Kreutzer J, Alday L, et al: Systemic and pulmonary venous connections in visceral heterotaxy, with emphasis on the diagnosis of atrial situs: A study of 109 postmortem cases. In Clark E, Takao A (eds): Developmental Cardiology: Morphogenesis and Function. Mt. Kisco, NY, Futura Publishing, 1990, p 671.

53. Mehta S, Hirschfeld S, Riggs T, et al: Echocardiographic estimation of ventricular hypoplasia in complete AV canal. Circulation 59:888, 1979.

54. Heydarian M, Griffith BP, Zuberbuhler JR: Partial AV canal associated with discrete subaortic stenosis. Am Heart J 109:915, 1985.

55. Smallhorn JF, Perrin D, Musewe N, et al: The role of transesophageal echocardiography in the evaluation of patients with AVSD. Cardiol Young 1:324, 1991.

56. Seward JB, Khandheria BJ, Oh JK, et al: Transesophageal echocardiography: Technique, anatomic correlations, implementation, and clinical applications. Mayo Clin Proc 63:649, 1988.

57. Seward JB, Khanderia BK, Edwards WD, et al: Biplanar transesophageal echocardiography: Anatomic correlations, image orientation, and clinical applications. Mayo Clin Proc 65:1193, 1990.

58. Roberson DA, Muhiudeen KA, Silverman NH, et al: Intraoperative transesophageal echocardiography of AVSD. J Am Coll Cardiol 18:357, 1991.

59. Marcus BM, Steard DJ, Khan NR, et al: Outpatient transesophageal echocardiography with intravenous propofol anesthesia in children and adolescents. J Am Soc Echocardiogr 6:205, 1993.

60. Wolfe LT, Rossi A, Ritter SB: Transesophageal echocardiography in infants and children: Use and importance in the cardiac intensive care unit. J Am Soc Echocardiogr 6:286, 1993.

61. Marcus BM, Wong PC, Wells WJ, et al: Transesophageal echocardiography in the postoperative child with an open sternum. Ann Thorac Surg 58:236, 1994.

62. Machado MV, Crawford DC, Anderson RH, Allan LD: AVSDs in prenatal life. Br Heart J 59:352, 1988.

63. Gembruch U, Knopfle G, Chatteree M, et al: Prenatal diagnosis of AV canal malformations with up-to-date echocardiographic technology: Report of 14 cases. Am Heart J 121:1489, 1991.

64. Allan LD, Sharland GK, Cook AC: Color Atlas of Fetal Cardiology. London, Mosby-Wolfe, 1994, p 49.

65. Amplatz K, Moller JH: Endocardial cushion defect. In Amplatz K, Moller JH: Radiology of Congenital Heart Disease. St. Louis, Mosby–Year Book, 1993, p 365.

66. Van Arsdell GS, Williams WG, Boutin C, et al: Subaortic stenosis in the spectrum of AVSDs. J Thorac Cardiovasc Surg 110:1534, 1995.

67. Gatzoulis MA, Shore D, Yacoub M, Shinebourne EA: Complete AVSD with tetralogy of Fallot: Diagnosis and management. Br Heart J 71:579, 1994.

68. Williams WH, Guyton RA, Michalik RE, et al: Individualized surgical management of complete AV canal. J Thorac Cardiovasc Surg 86:838, 1983.

69. Studor M, Blackstone EH, Kirklin JW, et al: Determinants of early and late results of repair of AV septal (canal) defects. J Thorac Cardiovasc Surg 84:523, 1982.

70. Kirklin JW, Barratt-Boyes BG: AV canal defect. In Kirklin JW, Barratt-Boyes BG: Cardiac Surgery, 2nd ed. New York, Churchill Livingstone, 1993, p 693.

71. Kirklin JW, Blackstone EK, Bargeron LM Jr, et al: The repair of AVSDs in infancy. Int J Cardiol 13:333, 1986.

72. McMullan MH, McGoon DC, Wallace RB, et al: Surgical treatment of partial AV canal. Arch Surg 107:705, 1973.

73. Goldfaden DM, Jones M, Morrow AG: Long-term results of repair of incomplete persistent AV canal. J Thorac Cardiovasc Surg 82:69, 1981.

74. Lukács L, Szántó G, Kassai I, Lengyel M: Late results after repair of partial AVSD. Tex Heart Inst J 19:265, 1992.

75. Burke RP, Horvath K, Landzberg M, et al: Long-term follow-up after surgical repair of ostium primum atrial septal defect in adults. J Am Coll Cardiol 27:696, 1996.

76. Meehan JJ, Delius RE, Behrendt DM, et al: Long term outcome following repair of incomplete AVSDs. Circulation 94(suppl I):117, 1996.

CHAPTER 25
COMPLETE TRANSPOSITION OF THE GREAT ARTERIES

DANIEL SIDI

Complete transposition of the great arteries (TGA) is a common and life-threatening cardiac malformation characterized by isolated ventriculoarterial discordance. Neonatal survival depends on shunts between the two parallel circulations, mainly through the foramen ovale. Ductus arteriosus patency (natural or by prostaglandin E_1 [PGE_1] infusion) can also influence clinical tolerance but to a less extent and not always favorably.

About two thirds of the neonates have no other cardiac abnormalities apart from a patent foramen ovale and a small patent ductus arteriosus. The remainder may have a ventricular septal defect, a large atrial septal defect, a large patent ductus arteriosus, or significant subpulmonic stenosis. The first group and those with only a small ventricular septal defect are often termed simple TGA. The rest are included in the group of complex TGA, which also includes those with pulmonic or tricuspid atresia and various types of double-outlet ventricles (see Chapter 26). Other terms that are used include d-TGA, aortopulmonary transposition, and transposition of the great vessels.

KEY POINTS

- Every cyanotic neonate without respiratory distress should be considered as possibly having TGA until two-dimensional echocardiography has shown the relation between the great vessels and the ventricles to be normal.
- TGA is usually fatal soon after birth, and neonates can be saved by an early balloon atrioseptostomy (the Rashkind procedure).
- Prenatal diagnosis is possible. Deterioration soon after birth can be predicted from the size of the foramen ovale in utero, and delivery should be organized at a center where an early Rashkind procedure can be performed with two-dimensional echocardiographic guidance in the delivery room.
- Atrial repair leaving the ventriculoarterial discordance but adding atrioventricular discordance (the Mustard or Senning procedure) gives good immediate and midterm results but leads to frequent rhythm disturbances, and right ventricular failure may occur in the long term.
- Anatomic repair (arterial switch) gives excellent long-term results with a low perioperative mortality, but it can be performed only in a neonate while the left ventricle is still able to develop systemic pressures. Long-term

follow-up is necessary to be sure that the fate of the great arteries and coronary arteries will allow a normal life.

EMBRYOLOGY AND EPIDEMIOLOGY

This lesion represents about 5% of congenital heart disease or occurs in about 1 in 3000 liveborn infants (see Chapter 18). TGA, especially simple TGA, has a marked male preponderance.[1,2] Extracardiac malformations or chromosome anomalies are uncommon[1,2]; in particular, there is no association with microdeletion of chromosome 22. The etiology is unknown, and the low recurrence rate in siblings and the low transmission rate to offspring[1,3] suggest that genetic effects play little role. Overt diabetes has been associated with TGA.[1]

The embryology is discussed in Chapter 1.

PATHOLOGIC ANATOMY

In TGA, the aorta rises from the right ventricle above an infundibulum, so that there has not been resorption of the subaortic conus. The pulmonary artery rises from the left ventricle and is usually in continuity with the mitral valve, indicating complete resorption of the subpulmonic conus (Fig. 25–1) (see Chapters 1, 19, and 20). This means that TGA has a discordant ventriculoarterial connection. The pulmonary artery rather than the aorta is situated in the center of the heart in continuity with both atrioventricular valves (see Chapter 26). The aorta is usually positioned anteriorly and to the right of the pulmonary artery (d-TGA), but the aorta can be in front of or beside the pulmonary artery; rarely, it can be located to the left of or posterior to the pulmonary artery, even though it is connected to the right ventricle.

The atria are normal, and there is almost always a patent foramen ovale, seldom a true secundum atrial septal defect. The ventricles are also normal, but the wedging of the pulmonary artery into the center of the heart produces a small central fibrous body and atrioventricular and membranous interventricular septa that are smaller than normal.[4,5] The ventricular septum, if intact, is relatively straight rather than sigmoid, so that the right and left ventricular outflow tracts are parallel. After about 2 months of age, there is often a functional subpulmonic obstruction owing to bulging

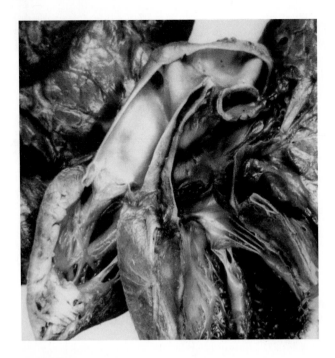

FIGURE 25-1

Pathology to show discordant ventriculoarterial connections.

of the ventricular septum into the left ventricular outflow tract where it is apposed to the septal leaflet of the mitral valve.[4-10] A ridge of endocardial thickening may be found where the mitral valve edge contacts the septum. The ob-

struction usually disappears after the arterial switch repair but persists after the atrial baffle repair.

There may be minor anomalies of the mitral and tricuspid valves, but these are clinically important in less than 5% of patients with simple TGA.[4,5,11]

The conduction system is normal except that the left bundle originates more distally than usual from the bundle of His and as a single cord rather than as a sheaf of fibers.[12]

The coronary arterial anatomy is of great importance. The posterior commissure of the aorta is usually aligned with the anterior commissure of the pulmonary artery, and the coronary arteries arise from the posterior sinuses (never from the anterior sinus). The origin and distribution of the coronary arteries are important for the surgeon intending to perform an arterial switch, because they have to be moved to the new aortic root. The right coronary artery is nearly always dominant. The left circumflex artery comes frequently (25%) from the right coronary artery (Fig. 25–2). The two coronary ostia usually rise laterally from the two posterior sinuses, but they can rise in between the vessels from a single ostium or from two ostia near the posterior commissure; the latter pattern is often associated with an intramural left coronary artery (usually the left anterior descending). Multiple classifications have been used to describe the coronary arterial origin and distribution,[11, 13–15] the first and still most commonly used being the Yacoub classification[13] shown in Figure 25–2. The sinus node artery usually originates from the proximal right coronary artery and courses upward and to the right, being partly embedded in the upper part of the limbus of the atrial septum.[11]

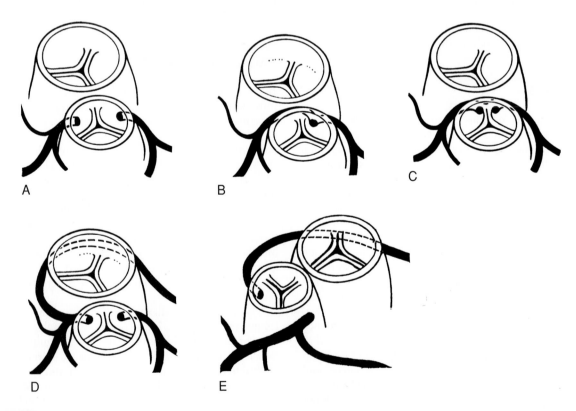

A   B   C

D   E

FIGURE 25-2

Yacoub classification of coronary arteries. (From Yacoub MH, Radley-Smith R: Anatomy of the coronary arteries in transposition of the great arteries and methods for their transfer in anatomical connection. Thorax 33:418, 1978.)

Although there is no structural abnormality of the cardiac chambers in complete TGA, the function and the mass of the right and left ventricles are normal only in the neonatal period just after fetal life when both ventricles had similar afterloads. After birth, the right ventricle facing a systemic afterload will grow more and quicker than the left ventricle because the left ventricle supports the low pressure of the pulmonary circulation. Thus, after a few weeks, the left ventricle becomes unable to sustain a systemic pressure unless it is prepared for it by an artificial increased afterload (pulmonary arterial banding) that leads to preoperative hypertrophy.

In some patients, without clear pathophysiologic reasons, pulmonary vascular disease occurs. This complication is rare before 3 months of age,[16–19] but it may occur in 25% of patients younger than 1 year and in 15 to 67% of patients older than 12 months.[11,16–19] As a rule, these pulmonary vascular changes are mild and do not cause profound pulmonary hypertension, but rarely (~1%) they may do so.[17] When pulmonary hypertension is significant, it does not react to oxygen or nitric oxide, and the small arteries histologically resemble classic pulmonary vascular disease, although sometimes numerous microthrombi are seen.

HEMODYNAMICS AND PATHOPHYSIOLOGY

THE FETUS

The fetus with TGA appears to have no disability. Because the pattern of streaming of the venous return is normal in these fetuses, the left ventricle receives much of its blood from the umbilical circulation (see Chapter 4), as in normal subjects, but then this blood, with an oxygen tension of about 24 mm Hg, is distributed to the lungs and through the ductus arteriosus to the lower body (Fig. 25–3). The heart and brain, on the other hand, receive blood with an oxygen tension of about 18 mm Hg. There might possibly be greater flows through the lungs (less hypoxemia to cause vasoconstriction) and the heart and brain (autoregulation because of more hypoxemia). Whether these changes cause differences in vascular development of the organs is unknown.

Normal development of the cardiac chambers is expected in a fetus with TGA, because atrial and ductus communications equalize preload and afterload of the ventricles. The respective volumes and outputs of the two ventricles should be identical in a normal fetus and a fetus with TGA. On the other hand, the sizes of the great arter-

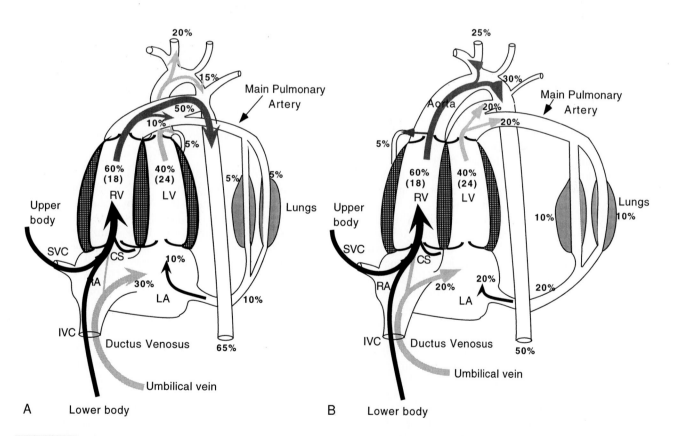

FIGURE 25–3

Fetal circulation in a normal subject *(A)* and one with TGA *(B)*. The percentages shown are proportions of the combined ventricular output coming from each ventricle and being distributed to various regions of the body. The figures in parentheses in the ventricles are the oxygen tensions (mm Hg). In *A*, the desaturated blood returning from the lungs and body is shown by *dark arrows.* The better oxygenated blood returning from the umbilical vein is shown by the *pale arrow,* and it is distributed to the head, coronary arteries, and aortic isthmus, which is the narrowest part of the aortic arch. The lungs and descending aorta receive blood of intermediate saturation. In *B*, note that in TGA, the aorta, main pulmonary artery, and aortic isthmus are wider than in the normal subject and that the foramen ovale and the ductus arteriosus are smaller. The distribution of well and poorly saturated blood differs from the normal. CS = coronary sinus; IVC = inferior vena cava; LA = left atrium; LV = left ventricle; RA = right atrium; RV = right ventricle; SVC = superior vena cava. (Courtesy of Dr. David F. Teitel.)

ies and of the foramen ovale that depend on the flow through them during fetal life are likely to be different (see Fig. 25–3). Fetuses with TGA are likely to have a larger ascending and transverse aorta and a larger aortic isthmus because of the higher right ventricular output, and the ductus arteriosus and the foramen ovale should be smaller because the higher pulmonary blood flow (due to a higher than normal PaO$_2$ in the pulmonary artery) decreases the amount of blood that passes through these structures during fetal life (see Fig. 25–3). These factors may explain the rarity of coarctation of the aorta in simple TGA, and they may also explain the devastating postnatal course due to inadequate shunting of blood between the two circulations in the absence of treatment with prostaglandins and balloon atrial septostomy.

There are increased number and size of pancreatic islet cells and an increased weight of the adrenal cortex; both of these findings resemble those found in infants of diabetic mothers.

THE NEONATE

Without communications between systemic and pulmonary circulations, an infant with TGA cannot survive more than a few minutes after the neonatal "placental-pulmonary switch." Because the two circulations are in parallel, blood oxygenated in the lungs would return exclusively to the lungs, whereas the desaturated systemic blood would go back through the aorta to the systemic tissues. Survival is possible only through one or more communications that allow some oxygenated blood to cross from the left side of the heart or the pulmonary artery to the right side of the heart or the aorta and the same amount of desaturated blood to cross back from the right side of the heart to the left side (Fig. 25–4). Of necessity, the same amount of blood must cross in each direction; otherwise, one circulation would empty into the other. It is only this shunted blood that allows some oxygen uptake in the lungs and some oxygen transport to the tissues.

Initially, there may be bidirectional shunts through the ductus arteriosus and across the atrial septum. At birth, the ductus arteriosus is open, and aortic and pulmonary arterial pressures are similar. During systole, left ventricular ejection imparts enough kinetic energy to the blood that some oxygenated blood passes through the ductus arteriosus into the descending aorta. In diastole, aortic blood may enter the pulmonary artery with its lower vascular resistance. Then, with the rise in systemic vascular resistance that follows removal of the placenta and a decrease in pulmonary vascular resistance, pulmonary-to-aortic shunting ceases. The flap (Vieussens valve) of the foramen ovale (that is intended to close the atrial septum when the pressures become higher in the left compared with the right atrium) usually crosses through a foramen ovale distended by the increased pulmonary blood flow and allows a left-to-right atrial shunt; in addition, the rise in right atrial pressure due to the increased systemic vascular resistance helps to keep the valve of the foramen ovale open. In early ventricular diastole, blood shunts from the right to the left atrium because of the lower resistance to filling of the left ventricle.[20] In ventricular systole, blood shunts from the left to the right atrium because the left atrium has higher pressures and is

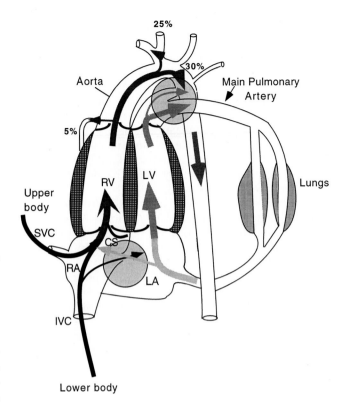

FIGURE 25–4

Diagram to show where shunts essential for survival *(gray circles)* after birth take place in simple TGA. It is possible for bidirectional shunting to occur through the ductus arteriosus, but the amounts are small. The least saturated blood is indicated by the *darkest arrows,* the best saturated blood by the *lightest arrows.* Intermediate saturations are suggested by intermediate shades of gray. CS = coronary sinus; IVC = inferior vena cava; LA = left atrium; LV = left ventricle; RA = right atrium; RV = right ventricle; SVC = superior vena cava.

less distensible. Respiration will also influence atrial shunting because inspiration increases the caval venous return to the right atrium. These atrial shunts explain why most neonates with TGA do well at birth with an adequate flow through the ductus arteriosus from aorta to pulmonary artery (shunt of desaturated blood destined for the lungs) associated with a quantitatively equivalent left-to-right atrial flow of oxygenated blood destined for the body.

The ductus arteriosus, smaller than normal in TGA, becomes progressively smaller soon after birth. When this happens, the infant's survival depends on bidirectional shunting at the atrial level. If, however, the foramen ovale is too small or the flap is too large and closes the foramen ovale instead of crossing it, the atrial communication is absent or restrictive. This situation is poorly tolerated because the shunt is inadequate (severe hypoxemia); any shunting that occurs is possible only with a high left atrial pressure (due to increased pulmonary flow) and a resulting high capillary pressure that can cause pulmonary edema.

After the neonatal period, with adequate atrial shunting through a natural or post-Rashkind atrial communication, the hemodynamic status usually improves. There is an increased pulmonary blood flow (Qp/Qs ~2) and adequate shunting (about half of systemic flow) so that aortic saturation is approximately 70%, the pulmonary arterial saturation is approximately 85%, and mixed venous caval blood saturation is approximately 40%. With a normal decrease of pulmonary vascular resistance, pulmonary arterial pressure is low, and the pathophysiologic process resembles a simple atrial septal defect but with obligatory cyanosis from blood going directly from the caval veins to the aorta. The major consequence of this fall in pulmonary arterial pressure is that the left ventricle in a neonate or infant will behave like a right ventricle in a normal circulation with an atrial septal defect. The left ventricle stops growing, progressively loses (perhaps forever) the ability to develop a normal systemic pressure, and will probably lose adequate coronary vascular bed growth.

Collateral circulation from the aorta to the pulmonary artery by bronchial arteries and from pulmonary veins to azygos vein can also play a role in the physiologic circulation in TGA. It can ensure some shunting in patients with closed foramen ovale, but the amount is insufficient to compensate for inadequate shunting at atrial and ductus levels. The collateral circulation complicates the evaluation of pulmonary blood flow and vascular resistance by the Fick method during catheterization because it alters the oxygen saturation proximally in the caval veins and distally in the pulmonary artery.

About half of the children with TGA have a greater than normal distribution of blood flow to the right lung, as shown by chest radiography, angiography, or radionuclide lung scans.[21] This effect is thought to be due to the abnormal rightward inclination of the main pulmonary artery that causes the blood flow to be directed toward the right pulmonary artery. This diversion probably does not have major physiologic effects, but it may explain associated hypoplasia of the left pulmonary arterial vessels and the occasional report of unilateral (always left-sided) pulmonary vein hypoplasia or stenosis.[22, 23]

NATURAL HISTORY

The natural history of untreated simple TGA is bleak; less than 5% survive more than 2 months.[2, 11, 24] Some with a large atrial septal defect may survive longer, but only 5 to 10% of them reach their first birthday. Death is usually from hypoxemia and acidosis, sometimes complicated by pulmonary edema.

PHYSICAL EXAMINATION

These infants are usually of normal birth weight, although reports of underweight and overweight exist, especially in the complex group.[1] The infants are initially well but may look dusky rather than overtly cyanotic. At this stage, pulses and breathing patterns are normal, as is activity. The heart is not enlarged and has the expected normal neonatal right ventricular lift. The first heart sound is normal. The second sound is usually single and heard with greatest intensity at the upper left sternal border because of the high position of the anterior aortic valve above the conus. A soft pulmonic closing sound is occasionally heard. No other sounds or clicks are present. There may be no murmurs or only the soft murmur of a ductus arteriosus or a short midsystolic murmur along the midsternal border.

As hours or days pass, the ductus closes and shunting at ductus and atrial levels becomes inadequate. The neonate becomes deeply cyanotic, and this is usually equal in fingers and toes. Respiration becomes deep but without retractions, and there is usually no tachypnea unless there is acidosis. With the onset of severe acidosis, activity becomes reduced.

In older children who have not undergone surgical correction, there may be a soft ejection murmur along the upper left sternal border to indicate mild subpulmonic stenosis.

ELECTROCARDIOGRAPHY

This shows merely the expected right ventricular dominance of the newborn term infant. After the first week, however, persistent upright T waves in the right precordial leads suggest abnormal right ventricular hypertrophy, as do decreased r waves in the left precordial leads. Should left forces be prominent (tall R waves in leads V_5 and V_6), some cause for a high left ventricular pressure, like pulmonary vascular disease or severe subpulmonic stenosis, should be sought.

CHEST RADIOGRAPHY

The pulmonary vascular markings are increased because pulmonary blood flow is usually increased. The heart is slightly enlarged, and the characteristic oval shape is due to absence of the pulmonary artery segment. As a rule, the thymus, although present, is notably small, so that the narrow mediastinal shadow gives an "egg on its side" or "apple on a string" appearance that is almost pathognomonic (see Fig. 10–2). The aortic arch is almost invariably left sided. On occasion, the chest film lacks these diagnostic features immediately after birth. It is important not to exclude the diagnosis of TGA because of a nonspecific x-ray picture.

ECHOCARDIOGRAPHY

IN THE FETUS

TGA is well tolerated by the fetus, and the diagnosis can be made on two-dimensional echocardiography if the screening is not limited to the four-chamber view (that is normal in TGA) but includes the great vessels (see Chapter 12). It is crucial to check on the size of the foramen ovale and on the anatomy of the atrial flap to predict early closure of the atrial septum at birth with the need for an early or immediate Rashkind procedure.

IN THE NEONATE

Two-dimensional echocardiography with Doppler interrogation is the major diagnostic method. It confirms the diagnosis by demonstrating a normal heart architecture but with two great vessels arising in parallel from the ventricles instead of crossing early after their origins (Fig. 25–5). The anterior vessel that arises from the right ventricle above an

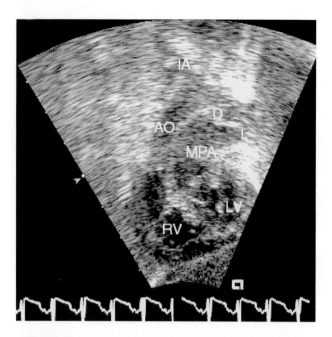

FIGURE 25–5

Echocardiogram, subcostal view, from a neonate with simple TGA. The left ventricle (LV) gives rise to the pulmonary artery (MPA), which divides into the left pulmonary artery (L) and ductus arteriosus (D). The right ventricle (RV) gives rise to the aorta (AO) from which the innominate artery (IA) originates. (Courtesy of Dr. Norman H. Silverman.)

infundibulum is the aorta because it is directed anteriorly and gives off the neck vessels, and the posterior vessel arising from the left ventricle in continuity with the mitral valve is a pulmonary artery because it is directed posteriorly and bifurcates or trifurcates into two branches and the ductus arteriosus. The two outflow tracts are parallel to each other. On a transverse view, the aorta is usually lo-

cated anterior and to the right of the pulmonary artery, and there is usually a good alignment between the commissures of the aorta and pulmonary artery with coronary arteries arising always from the posterior sinuses of the anterior vessel (Fig. 25–6).

It is especially important to look at the atrial septum (subxiphoid view) and the ductus view, which are the sites of shunting in TGA. Although the need for the Rashkind procedure is primarily indicated on a clinical basis, it should also be performed early when the foramen ovale is obstructed by the flap as shown by a high Doppler velocity (>1 m/sec). Conversely, if the atrial communication is large and the patient is not doing well, echocardiography helps to find a reason for the symptoms (e.g., high pulmonary vascular resistance, or associated cardiovascular anomalies like coarctation of the aorta or subpulmonic stenosis).

It is particularly helpful to look at the atrial shunting. If there is an exclusive left-to-right atrial shunt, there must always be another communication at the ventricular or the ductus level; if it is not at the ductus level, it must be elsewhere (ventricular septal defect or collateral circulation). If there is a bilateral shunting at the atrial level, it means that there is no other significant communication and that the ductus arteriosus is closed. If the ductus is widely patent with bilateral atrial shunting, it means that pulmonary vascular resistance is high.

Echocardiography helps to assess the hemodynamics by looking at the velocity of flow across the ductus arteriosus and the foramen ovale and at septal geometry. (Left ventricular deformation is related to the difference in pressure between the ventricles.)

Finally, the coronary artery ostial origins and course should be examined. It is important to note an unfavorable distribution, for example, if one coronary artery passes between the great vessels and especially if it is located in the wall of a great artery.

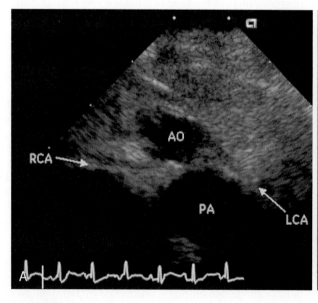
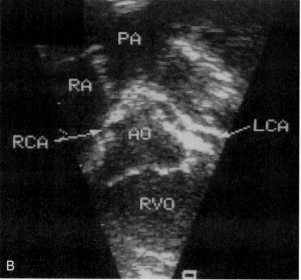

FIGURE 25–6

Echocardiograms showing the origin of the coronary arteries in TGA. *A,* The left coronary (LCA) and right coronary (RCA) arteries arise from the facing aortic (AO) sinuses. PA = pulmonary artery. *B,* Long intramural course of the LCA. RA = right atrium; RVO = right ventricular outflow tract. (*A, B* courtesy of Dr. Norman H. Silverman.)

CARDIAC CATHETERIZATION

Cardiac catheterization is useful only when a Rashkind procedure is indicated. Rarely is it used to look for associated abnormalities like a trabecular ventricular septal defect, collateral circulation, abnormal coronary arteries, or a small aortic isthmus if a coarctation is suspected.

The technique of cardiac catheterization is standard, except that special maneuvers are needed to enter the pulmonary artery from the left ventricle.[24, 25]

Calculations of flows by the Fick method are inexact because it is difficult to have mixed pulmonary arterial saturation samples if the ductus is open and when there is bronchial circulation (common). Pulmonary arterial samples are taken proximal to the entry of the bronchial collaterals that contain desaturated blood, so that a true mixed pulmonary arterial blood sample cannot be obtained. If bronchial collateral blood flow is only 10% of total pulmonary blood flow, there could be a 40% overestimate of pulmonary blood flow.[17] Another complication is that the arteriovenous difference of oxygen saturation across the pulmonary vascular bed is usually small, so that a tiny measurement error is translated into a large error in estimating pulmonary blood flow (see Chapter 13). Comparison of pulmonary blood flows measured by angiographic and Fick techniques suggests that pulmonary flows as calculated by the Fick method are about twice the true flows.[26] This means that pulmonary blood flow is usually overestimated, and pulmonary vascular resistance is underestimated. Nevertheless, in simple TGA, pulmonary blood flow is usually almost twice that in normal children, even in the absence of a large shunt.

DIFFERENTIAL DIAGNOSIS

In a cyanotic neonate without respiratory distress, TGA must be the diagnosis until two-dimensional echocardiographic–Doppler examination shows a normal position of the great arteries. The differential diagnosis therefore concerns the distinction between simple and complex TGA in which a ventricular septal defect, an abnormality of the great vessels (pulmonary artery stenosis, coarctation of the aorta), an anomaly of the atrioventricular or semilunar valves, or an abnormality of size or function of the ventricles is present.

Three major diagnostic difficulties exist:

1. Detection of a muscular ventricular septal defect especially at the apex, because this lesion may be difficult to see on echocardiography. Such a ventricular septal defect should be sought when there is left ventricular hypertension that is not explained by a widely patent ductus arteriosus or when there is an exclusive left-to-right atrial shunt with a closed ductus arteriosus (see earlier).

2. An associated coarctation of the aorta when the ductus is open, especially if the right ventricle is smaller than the left ventricle and the pulmonary artery is much larger than the aorta. It may be useful to stop PGE$_1$, so that the ductus arteriosus closes, and then evaluate the femoral pulses and the aortic isthmus. Catheterization may be needed to decide whether a coarctation repair should be done with the arterial switch.

3. An organic subpulmonic stenosis when an abnormal pulmonary arterial gradient cannot be explained by bulging of the ventricular septum. Particular attention should be paid to the mitral valve insertions on the septum.

CLINICAL COURSE

Without a good atrial communication, death occurs early with metabolic acidosis. With a good atrial communication (natural or after a Rashkind procedure), the infant with TGA survives with only mild or moderate cyanosis for years. These patients will be exposed to the complications of hypoxemia and polycythemia, mainly brain abscess or infarction (see Chapter 63) and progressive right ventricular failure. Some survive into adulthood, but most have problems by the age of 5 years (an age chosen in the 1960s and early 1970s for the Mustard operation). Progressive subpulmonic stenosis due to the bulge of the septum (pushed by the systemic right ventricle) under the pulmonary valve causes a systolic ejection murmur and left ventricular hypertrophy.[6–10]

MEDICAL MANAGEMENT

Medical therapy at birth is based on balloon atrial septostomy (the Rashkind procedure) and dilatation of the ductus arteriosus by PGE$_1$ infusion. These therapies have greatly improved the outcome of neonatal TGA.

When TGA is diagnosed prenatally, delivery should be performed at a center where a Rashkind procedure can be performed safely and quickly (Fig. 25–7; see Chapter 13 for details of the procedure). This can be done under two-dimensional echocardiographic guidance via the umbilical vein (through the ductus venosus) even in the delivery room.

If prenatal diagnosis was not made and severe hypoxemia occurs in the delivery room, PGE$_1$ should be infused and an emergency transfer organized to the nearest pediatric cardiology center that is able to do the Rashkind procedure.

PGE$_1$ infusion may be useful in the hypoxic neonate before the Rashkind procedure to allow some mixing and avoid (sometimes but not always) metabolic acidosis and death. It can also be useful after the Rashkind procedure to improve mixing (decrease hypoxemia) and increase pulmonary arterial and left ventricular pressure in preparation for an anatomic repair.

PGE$_1$ infusion has its drawbacks, however, because it can lead to apnea (with the need for artificial ventilation) and to pulmonary edema by the increase in pulmonary blood flow and pressure (especially if the foramen ovale is restrictive before or after a Rashkind procedure). It is also responsible for an increased water content in the tissues, including the vessel wall, that may complicate surgery (more bleeding at the anastomotic sites). This is why we (in Paris) do not routinely use PGE$_1$; we reserve its use for a neonate who does not tolerate hypoxemia and try to stop the infusion 2 days before surgery.

Rashkind Procedure

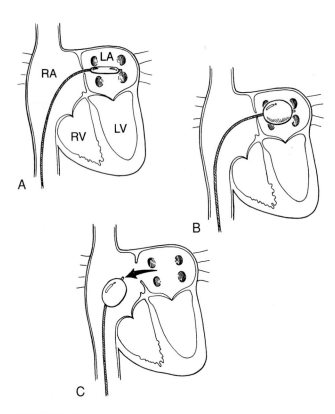

FIGURE 25–7

Diagram of Rashkind balloon atrial septostomy. *A*, The catheter with the balloon deflated is passed from the right atrium (RA) through the foramen ovale into the left atrium (LA). *B*, The balloon is inflated. *C*, The inflated balloon is jerked back into the right atrium, tearing the atrial septum. RV = right ventricle; LV = left ventricle.

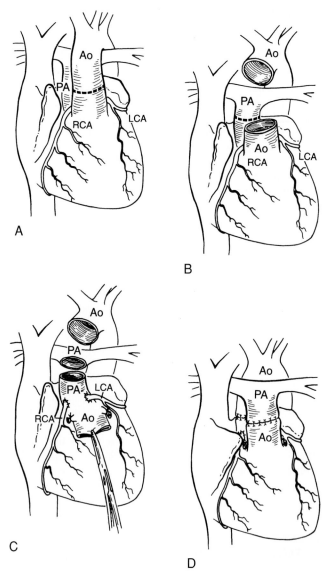

FIGURE 25–8

Diagram of arterial switch operation. *A*, The anterior aorta is shown giving off the coronary arteries. The *dashed line* shows where the ascending aorta is transected. *B*, The posterior pulmonary artery. The *dashed line* shows where the main pulmonary artery is transected. *C*, The coronary arteries have been removed from the aorta and implanted into the old pulmonary root, now the neoaortic root. The holes left in the aorta are patched. *D*, The distal pulmonary arteries are brought anteriorly after cutting the ligamentum arteriosum or the ductus arteriosus (Lecompte maneuver) and anastomosed to the old aortic root, now the neopulmonary arterial root. The pulmonary artery now receives blood from the right ventricle. The distal aorta has been anastomosed to the neoaortic root behind the pulmonary artery, and it receives blood from the left ventricle. Ao = aorta; LCA = left coronary artery; PA = pulmonary artery; RCA = right coronary artery.

Neonates with TGA are also at risk for hypoglycemia (they have pancreatic hyperplasia and increased insulin secretion) and necrotizing enterocolitis (the gut is perfused with a higher PO_2 in utero than after birth). Therefore, these patients benefit from parenteral alimentation with high glucose concentrations for the first day of life and for the 24 hours after a Rashkind procedure.

SURGICAL MANAGEMENT

Surgery is the only solution for these patients. Their natural history is catastrophic in the short term unless they have a large atrial septal defect, and even then they are exposed to serious neurologic and myocardial complications in the long term because of the chronic cyanosis.

There are two options for treating TGA. The first is the anatomic option consisting of correcting the ventriculoarterial discordance by an arterial switch of the great vessels above the sinuses of Valsalva (Fig. 25–8). Both arterial roots and sigmoid valves have similar sizes, shapes, and histologic features, at least at birth. The coronary arteries that arise from the aortic sinuses of Valsalva need to be moved to the new aortic root to perfuse the myocardium at high pressure with fully oxygenated blood. Second is the "physiologic" or atrial repair consisting of creation of an atri-oventricular discordance (by intra-atrial rerouting) to correct the physiologic consequences of the ventriculoarterial discordance (Fig. 25–9).

In most pediatric cardiologic centers, anatomic repair is the choice in neonates. It restores the left ventricle to its normal systemic function and avoids extensive atrial surgery that is responsible for subsequent rhythm disturbances.

The arterial switch is a challenging operation (see Fig. 25–8) because it is a long procedure in a neonate and has a

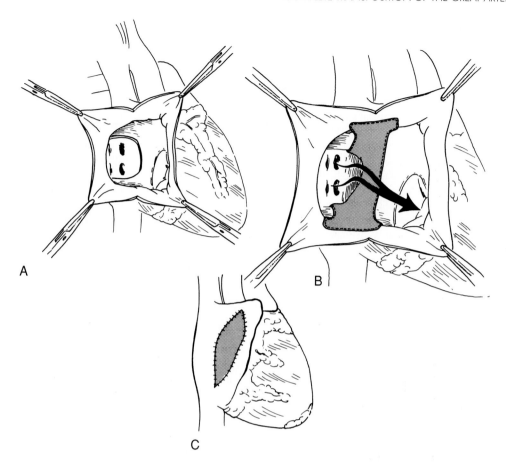

FIGURE 25–9

Diagram of atrial switch operation. *A*, The right atrium has been opened. The four pulmonary veins and the tricuspid valve can be seen. *B*, A patch made of pericardium (the Mustard procedure) or a displaced atrial septum (the Senning procedure) is shown in the shaded structure. It is placed to direct the drainage from the superior and inferior venae cavae through the mitral valve into the left ventricle, thence into the pulmonary artery (not shown, but posterior to the patch). At the same time, the patch directs the pulmonary venous return through the tricuspid valve into the right ventricle and thence into the aorta *(arrow)*. This diagram does not show the precise anatomy of the patch. *C*, The right atrium is closed with a patch to enlarge it and minimize the risk of obstruction to the pulmonary venous drainage.

long aortic cross-clamping time (usually performed without circulatory arrest). The surgeon must switch the great arteries without a conduit. This is done by applying the Lecompte maneuver[27] in which the distal aorta is brought beneath the bifurcation of the pulmonary trunk, which is moved anteriorly. The distal pulmonary trunk is anastomosed to the previous aortic root so that the lungs now receive blood from the right ventricle. The distal aorta is anastomosed to the previous pulmonary root so that the distal aorta receives blood from the left ventricle. These procedures are relatively easy. It is more difficult to transfer the coronary arteries from the old to the new aortic root without kinking or distortion. This transfer may be particularly difficult when the coronary artery has an intramural path.

The perioperative mortality, in excellent centers,[28,29] is below 5%; most deaths are due to ischemia from inadequate coronary artery transfer. Beyond the perioperative period, mortality and morbidity are extremely low.[11] Morbidity concerns the fate of three structures:

1. The new pulmonary artery. When the coronary arteries are removed from the aortic root, large buttons of aortic tissue are taken so as not to encroach on the coro-

nary ostia. Large pericardial patches are used to fill the holes made by the harvesting of the coronary arteries. Thus, the previous aortic root (new pulmonary root) is the great artery that has had the most damage during the arterial switch operation.[30]

Mild supravalvar pulmonary stenosis is the rule after an arterial switch (with systolic gradients around 30 mm Hg). Some patients (about 10% in our experience) need an operation before adult life to relieve this stenosis. Percutaneous balloon dilatation of the stenotic pulmonary trunk may relieve the obstruction, but this procedure is successful in only one third of patients. Stenting may improve the percutaneous results, but it is essential to check that the dilatation before the stenting does not compress the left coronary artery, which is usually close to the pulmonary trunk. If the artery is compressed, ST changes develop during dilatation. Before reoperation on the pulmonary trunk, we recommend a selective coronary angiogram to ascertain that no coronary arterial branches run in front of the pulmonary artery (commonly there is a right coronary artery in type E distribution).

Pulmonary regurgitation is common after the switch operation, but it is usually mild and well tolerated by the right ventricle.

2. The new aorta. Dilatation of the new aortic root and minor leak of the new aortic valves is the rule after a neonatal switch operation. In our experience, it has always been mild and well tolerated, and it has never justified medical or surgical treatment during a 15-year follow-up. In patients from the late 1970s or early 1980s who had pulmonary artery banding before the arterial switch, aortic regurgitation can be moderate or even severe. We have twice had to change the valves and the aortic root in such patients.

3. The coronary arteries. The major long-term concern after the arterial switch operation is left ventricular myocardial perfusion. Indeed, left ventricular coronary perfusion may be impaired by acquired lesions of the coronary arterial ostia resulting from surgical transfer, for example, stenosis or atresia by torsion or compression by the pulmonary artery or by fibrous tissue. This is the major cause of operative and early postoperative mortality and morbidity of the arterial switch procedure.

Late coronary ostial stenosis or atresia is rare after an arterial switch, but most of the centers have not looked carefully at the fate of the coronary arteries after the switch. The assumption has been made that if clinical, electrocardiographic, or echocardiographic signs of ischemia did not develop after the operation and before discharge from the hospital, the coronary arteries were normal and would remain normal and grow normally. Coronary arterial damage, however, has been responsible for late deaths.[31] In Paris, by performing selective coronary arterial angiograms in postoperative patients, we found coronary arterial anomalies in about 5% of patients who apparently had no evidence of postoperative ischemia.[32, 33] Most of them had minor signs of ischemia on electrocardiography and echocardiography, but some had no ischemia at all even on a myocardial perfusion thallium scan. Selective coronary arterial angiograms found coronary arterial stenosis or complete obstruction almost always in the left coronary artery (except one in the right coronary artery), usually with adequate collateral circulation from the right coronary arterial bed. A few (six in 1998) of these patients with reversible ischemia underwent reoperation, four with a successful coronary angioplasty and two with coronary artery bypass by internal mammary artery. The others do not have ischemia but are left with only one coronary artery; they may in the long term develop coronary arterial disease sooner and more often than will the normal population. Even without coronary artery stenosis, myocardial reserve may be impaired by inadequate position of the ostia for perfect diastolic filling, because of the high implantation of the coronary artery on the upper part of a dilated sinus of Valsalva, or by endothelial damage from the operation (cannulation and cold blood flushing). In theory, there could be a constitutional inadequacy of the left ventricular coronary circulation because the right coronary artery is nearly always dominant in TGA, and the left circumflex or left anterior descending artery is frequently small. We do not have information on myocardial reserve in these patients, but positron emission tomographic scanning with dipyridamole (Persantine) in a few patients suggests that myocardial reserve may be decreased.

Despite these concerns, however, with a mean follow-up of more than 8 years, almost all these children after an arterial switch live a normal life, including participation in competitive sports.

Our patients are followed up every year in the outpatient clinic with clinical history and examination, two-dimensional echocardiography–Doppler study, and an electrocardiogram; after 5 years of age, they have formal exercise testing. If ischemia is suspected, a coronary angiogram is indicated. In Paris, we check the coronary arteries systematically by a selective coronary angiogram by the age of 6 years. With a normal exercise test result and coronary angiogram, the children are allowed to participate in all sports, including competition.

BEYOND THE NEONATAL PERIOD

The arterial switch can be performed only in the neonatal period while the left ventricle is still competent to develop systemic pressures. Until recently, on the basis of echocardiographic characteristics of the thickness and shape of the left ventricle,[34] the upper age limit for the arterial switch was set at 3 to 4 weeks. The belief was that if the left ventricle was much thinner than the right ventricle, and if the ventricular septum bulged into the lower pressure left ventricle, the left ventricle would not be able to support systemic arterial pressures and flows. However, some centers have observed that the arterial switch can be performed safely up to 8 weeks of age, no matter what the shape of the left ventricle and the interventricular septum.[35, 36] Beyond that age, only patients with left ventricles that are still at high systolic pressure (because of an open ductus or subpulmonic stenosis) are good candidates.

For patients who do not meet these criteria, the arterial switch can be performed safely only if the left ventricle is prepared by an afterload challenge (usually pulmonary artery banding). If this causes severe hypoxemia, the patient may also need an aortopulmonary shunt. This two-stage surgery with a quick (about 10 days) left ventricular preparation before the arterial switch has been successful in some centers.[37] It is not an easy procedure, however, and in our experience it has some mortality and morbidity. Furthermore, the left ventricular myocardium may have inadequate fiber quality and decreased coronary reserve; there is little evidence for growth of coronary arteries after the newborn period (see Chapter 6). Therefore, many centers (like ours in Paris) perform an "atrial repair" rather than an arterial switch.

ATRIAL REPAIR: THE MUSTARD AND SENNING OPERATIONS

When the left ventricle has lost its systemic competence or when the surgical team has too high a mortality with the arterial switch, an atrial baffle repair can correct the physiologic abnormalities by rerouting the venous return. This is done by directing systemic venous drainage toward the mitral valve and pulmonary venous drainage toward the tricuspid valve by placing pericardial patches around the caval veins, as in the Mustard operation[38] introduced in 1963, or by moving the atrial septum in the Senning operation,[39] which was described in 1959 but subsequently modified and made easier to perform in 1977.[40]

These operations can be performed at any age and have a low mortality. Most of the patients (80 to 90%) are doing well with a follow-up of more than 20 years.[41] There are, however, three major problems or theoretical concerns with this procedure.

1. The atrial channels can become obstructed, leading to caval or pulmonary venous hypertension. These uncommon complications can usually be treated or improved by interventional catheterization with dilatation and stents. They rarely require reoperation. When the stenosis is limited to the superior vena caval channel, there is usually an efficient rerouting of the blood by the azygos or hemiazygos veins toward the inferior vena cava. When the pulmonary venous channel is obstructed, the clinical picture resembles cor triatriatum or mitral stenosis with pulmonary edema and postcapillary hypertension. In some patients, this pulmonary arterial hypertension "prepared" the left ventricle for a late switch procedure.

2. The incidence of atrial dysrhythmias is high, probably because of damage to the sinus node or its artery, or the internodal tracts, during the operation. The dysrhythmias can be severe and difficult to treat, with a risk of sudden death even after pacemaker implantation. Abnormal sinus node dysfunction was reported first in 1972.[42] Sinus node dysfunction progresses over time,[43–45] and 10 years after operation, only about 14% of these children remain in normal sinus rhythm.[45] The others have a tendency for bradycardia and junctional rhythm, sometimes with a restored sinus rhythm during exercise. These passive bradycardias are usually benign and rarely symptomatic, but about 10 to 20% need a pacemaker. Dysrhythmias can also be "active" in these patients with the appearance of ectopic atrial tachycardia, atrial flutter, or even atrial fibrillation.[46] A high proportion of these patients have inducible atrial flutter during electrophysiologic studies postoperatively,[47] and many of these later develop spontaneous atrial flutter. On electrocardiographic examination, the atrial flutter is atypical, with rates often from 180 to 260 beats per minute, frequently with 1:1 atrioventricular conduction. The flutter waves are of low amplitude and may be difficult to see. In fact, any patient after an atrial baffle repair with a resting heart rate above 100 beats per minute should be checked carefully to exclude atrial flutter with 2:1 or 3:1 atrioventricular block.

These active tachycardias or arrhythmias are dangerous for the patients and for right ventricular function. They can lead to serious myocardial or neurologic complications and even sudden death.[48] They are difficult to treat because they are associated with a weak or damaged sinus node, and antiarrhythmic drugs may be hazardous because of the risk of severe bradycardia. That is why the treatment of these atrial tachycardias often requires pacemaker implantation.

3. The long-term function of a right ventricle and a tricuspid valve working at systemic pressure is uncertain.[49] Some of these patients develop heart failure after 10, 20, or 30 years. The example of patients with double discordance (corrected transposition) shows that the long-term failure of a systemic right ventricle is not a certainty (some patients can live to 70 years without heart failure). Most of those with an atrial baffle, however, will probably develop heart failure, perhaps in part owing to inadequate myocardial protection during surgery (especially in the early days of this repair) and in part owing to associated anomalies of rhythm and atrioventricular conduction.

When the right ventricle begins to dilate, the attachments of the tricuspid valve to the septum are pulled laterally, thereby inducing tricuspid incompetence that increases the ventricular dilatation. A vicious circle is thus established. Furthermore, because the regurgitant blood enters the new pulmonary venous atrium, tricuspid incompetence causes pulmonary venous hypertension and eventually pulmonary edema.

When right ventricular failure develops after a Senning or Mustard procedure, chronic dysrhythmia may be the mechanism. If right ventricular failure is present without dysrhythmia, nonspecific medical therapy with diuretics, converting enzyme inhibitors, and digoxin (with care for sinus node dysfunction) can be tried but are seldom successful for long. The only possibility other than cardiac transplantation is conversion of the right ventricle into a subpulmonary ventricle by performing an arterial switch procedure and taking down the atrial baffle to reroute the venous returns to their original ventricles.[50] For this transformation, the left ventricle must be prepared for the arterial switch by an afterload challenge (pulmonary arterial banding).

This procedure of late preparation is different from the two-stage preparation done in the older infant with TGA and a low-pressure left ventricle. After a Mustard or Senning procedure, the heart has a circulation in series with no hypoxemia, and the banding will directly affect only the left ventricle, although it may indirectly affect the preload of the right ventricle. The severe hypoxemia attendant on preparing the left ventricle in the infant with TGA is not a problem. The preparation of an older left ventricle cannot be obtained in few days, however, and it needs a long and uncertain process (during several years in some patients) before getting adequate left ventricular mass. There is little information about the quality of the fibers and the coronary reserve. This situation is identical to the problem of treating a patient with double discordance or congenitally corrected transposition with a failing right ventricle and an abnormal regurgitant tricuspid valve. The issues concern fundamental unanswered questions about postnatal ventricular growth and coronary artery angiogenesis.

Experience has shown, however, that pulmonary arterial banding changes the septal geometry in some patients, pushing the septum back toward the right ventricle, and improves right ventricular and tricuspid valve function by decreasing tricuspid regurgitation. Often two or three banding adjustments may be needed to prepare the left ventricle during several years, while avoiding left ventricular failure. Thus, it is crucial to check the right ventricular function in the follow-up of these patients and not wait for severe dysfunction with heart failure before "retraining" a left ventricle.

REFERENCES

1. Malformations of the cardiac outflow tract. *In* Ferencz C, Loffredo CA, Correa-Villasenor A, Wilson PD (eds): Perspectives in Pediatric Cardiology, Vol 5: Genetic and Environmental Risk Factors of Major Cardiovascular Malformations. Armonk, NY, Futura, 1997, p 59.
2. Liebman J, Cullum L, Belloc NB: Natural history of transposition of the great arteries: Anatomy and birth and death characteristics. Circulation 40:237, 1969.

3. Burn J: The aetiology of congenital heart disease. *In* Anderson RA, Macartney FJ, Shinebourne EA, Tynan M (eds): Paediatric Cardiology. Edinburgh, Churchill Livingstone, 1987, p 15.

4. Smith A, Wilkinson JL, Anderson RH, et al: Architecture of the ventricular mass and atrioventricular valves in complete transposition with intact ventricular septum compared with the normal. I: The left ventricle, mitral valve, and interventricular septum. Pediatr Cardiol 6:253, 1986.

5. Smith A, Wilkinson JL, Anderson RH, et al: Architecture of the ventricular mass and atrioventricular valves in complete transposition with intact ventricular septum compared with the normal. II: The right ventricle and tricuspid valve. Pediatr Cardiol 6:299, 1986.

6. Aziz KU, Paul MH, Idriss FS, et al: Clinical manifestations of dynamic left ventricular outflow tract stenosis in infants with d-transposition of the great arteries with intact ventricular septum. Am J Cardiol 44:290, 1979.

7. Crupi G, Anderson RH, Ho SY, Lincoln C: Complete transposition of the great arteries with intact ventricular septum and left ventricular outflow tract obstruction. Surgical management and anatomical considerations. J Thorac Cardiovasc Surg 78:730, 1979.

8. Sansa M, Tonkin IL, Bargeron LM Jr, Elliott LP: Left ventricular outflow tract obstruction in transposition of the great arteries: An angiographic study of 74 cases. Am J Cardiol 44:88, 1979.

9. Chui I-S, Anderson RH, Macartney FJ, et al: Morphologic features of an intact ventricular septum susceptible to subpulmonary obstruction in complete transposition. Am J Cardiol 53:1633, 1984.

10. Yacoub MH, Arensman FW, Keck E, Radley-Smith R: Fate of dynamic left ventricular outflow tract obstruction after anatomic correction of transposition of the great arteries. Circulation 68(suppl II):56, 1983.

11. Kirklin JW, Barratt-Boyes BG: Complete transposition of the great arteries. *In* Kirklin JW, Barratt-Boyes BG (eds): Cardiac Surgery, 2nd ed. London, Churchill Livingstone, 1993, p 1383.

12. Bharati S, Lev M: The conduction system in simple, regular (D), complete transposition with ventricular septal defect. J Thorac Cardiovasc Surg 72:194, 1976.

13. Yacoub MH, Radley-Smith R: Anatomy of the coronary arteries in transposition of the great arteries and methods for their transfer in anatomical connection. Thorax 33:418, 1978.

14. Gittenberger de Groot AC, Sauer U, Oppenheimer-Dekker A, Quaegebeur J: Coronary arterial anatomy in transposition of the great arteries: A morphological study. Pediatr Cardiol 4(suppl 1):15, 1983.

15. Mayer JE Jr, Sanders S, Jonas R, et al: Coronary artery pattern and outcome of arterial switch operation for transposition of the great arteries. Circulation 82(suppl IV):139, 1990.

16. Wagenvoort CA, Nauta J, van der Schaar PJ, et al: The pulmonary vasculature in complete transposition of the great arteries, judged from lung biopsies. Circulation 38:746, 1968.

17. Lakier JL, Stanger P, Heymann MA, et al: Early onset of pulmonary vascular obstruction in patients with aortopulmonary transposition and intact ventricular septum. Circulation 51:875, 1975.

18. Clarkson PM, Neutze JM, Wardill JC, Barrett-Boyes BG: The pulmonary vascular bed in patients with complete transposition of the great arteries. Circulation 53:539, 1976.

19. Newfeld EA, Paul MH, Muster AJ, Idriss FS: Pulmonary vascular disease in transposition of the great vessels and intact ventricular septum. Circulation 59:525, 1979.

20. Carr I: Timing of bidirectional atrial shunts in transposition of the great arteries and atrial septal defect. Circulation 44(suppl II):70, 1971.

21. Muster AJ, Paul MH, van Grondelle A, Conway JJ: Asymmetric distribution of the pulmonary blood flow between the right and left lungs in d-transposition of the great arteries. Am J Cardiol 38:352, 1976.

22. Lock JE, Lucas RV Jr, Amplatz K, Bessinger FB Jr: Silent unilateral pulmonary venous obstruction: Occurrence after surgical correction of transposition of the great arteries. Chest 73:224, 1978.

23. Vogel M, Ash J, Rowe RD, et al: Congenital unilateral pulmonary vein stenosis complicating transposition of the great arteries. Am J Cardiol 54:166, 1984.

24. Paul MH, Wernovsky G: Transposition of the great arteries. *In* Emmanouilides GC, Allen HD, Riemenschneider TA, Gutgesell HP (eds): Heart Disease in Infants, Children, and Adolescents Including the Fetus and Young Adult. Baltimore, Williams & Wilkins, 1995, p 1154.

25. Anderson RA, Macartney FJ, Shinebourne EA, Tynan M: Complete transposition. *In* Anderson RA, Macartney FJ, Shinebourne EA, Tynan M (eds): Paediatric Cardiology. Edinburgh, Churchill Livingstone, 1987, p 829.

26. Keane JF, Ellison RC, Rudd M, Nadas AS: Pulmonary blood flow and left ventricular volumes in transposition of the great arteries and intact ventricular septum. Br Heart J 33:521, 1973.

27. Lecompte Y, Zannini L, Hazan E, et al: Anatomic correction of transposition of the great arteries: New technique without the use of a prosthetic conduit. J Thorac Cardiovasc Surg 82:629, 1981.

28. Castaneda AR, Norwood WI, Jonas RA, et al: Transposition of the great arteries and intact ventricular septum: Anatomical repair in the neonates. Ann Thorac Surg 38:438, 1984.

29. Sidi D, Planché C, Kachaner J, et al: Anatomic correction of simple transposition of the great arteries in 50 neonates. Circulation 75:429, 1987.

30. Paillole C, Sidi D, Kachaner J, et al: Fate of the pulmonary arteries after anatomic correction of simple transposition of the great arteries in newborn infants. Circulation 78:870, 1988.

31. Tsuda E, Imatika M, Yagilhara T, et al: Late death after arterial switch operation for transposition of the great arteries. Am Heart J 124:1551, 1992.

32. Bonhoeffer P, Bonnet D, Piechaud JF, et al: Coronary artery obstruction after the arterial switch operation for transposition of the great arteries in newborn. J Am Coll Cardiol 29:202, 1997.

33. Bonnet D, Bonheoffer P, Piechaud JF, et al: Long term fate of the coronary arteries after arterial switch operation in newborns with transposition of the great arteries. Heart 76:274, 1996.

34. Danford DA, Huhta JC, Gutgesell HP: Left ventricular wall stress and thickness in complete transposition of the great arteries. Implications for surgical intervention. J Thorac Cardiovasc Surg 89:610, 1985.

35. Davis AM, Wilkinson JL, Karl TR, Mee RB: Transposition of the great arteries with intact ventricular septum. Arterial switch repair in patients 21 days of age or older. J Thorac Cardiovasc Surg 106:111, 1993.

36. Foran JP, Sullivan ID, Elliott MJ, de Leval MR: Primary arterial switch operation for transposition of the great arteries with intact ventricular septum in infants older than 21 days. J Am Coll Cardiol 31:883, 1998.

37. Boutin C, Wernovsky G, Sanders SP, et al: Rapid two-stage arterial switch operation. Evaluation of left ventricular systolic mechanics late after an acute pressure overload stimulus in infancy. Circulation 90:1294, 1994.

38. Mustard WT: Successful two-stage correction of transposition of the great vessels. Surgery 55:469, 1964.

39. Senning A: Surgical correction of transposition of the great vessels. Surgery 50:773, 1959.

40. Quaegebeur JM, Rohmer J, Brom AG: Revival of the Senning operation in the treatment of transposition of the great arteries. Preliminary report on recent experience. Thorax 32:517, 1977.

41. Williams WG, Trusler GA, Kirklin JW, et al: Early and late results of a protocol for simple TGA leading to an atrial (Mustard) repair. J Thorac Cardiovasc Surg 95:717, 1988.

42. El-Said, Rosenburg HS, Mullins CE, et al: Dysrhythmias after Mustard's operation for transposition of the great arteries. Am J Cardiol 30:256, 1972.

43. Saalouke MG, Rios J, Perry LW, et al: Electrophysiologic studies after Mustard's operation. Am J Cardiol 41:1104, 1978.

44. Flinn CJ, Wolff GSS, Dick M: Cardiac rhythm after the Mustard operation for transposition of the great arteries. N Engl J Med 310:1635, 1984.

45. Hayes CJ, Gersony WM: Arrhythmias after the Mustard operation for transposition of the great arteries. J Am Coll Cardiol 7:133, 1986.

46. Vetter VL, Tanner CS, Horowitz LN: Electrophysiologic consequences of the Mustard repair of d-transposition of the great arteries. J Am Coll Cardiol 10:265, 1987.

47. Vetter VL, Tanner CS, Horowitz LN: Inducible atrial flutter after the Mustard repair of complete transposition of the great arteries. Am J Cardiol 61:428, 1988.

48. Garson A Jr, Bink-Boelkens M, Hesslein PS: Atrial flutter in the young: A collaborative study of 380 cases. J Am Coll Cardiol 6:871, 1985.

49. Martin RP, Qureshi SA, Ettedgui JA, et al: An evaluation of right and left ventricular function after anatomical correction and intra-atrial repair for complete transposition of the great arteries. Circulation 82:808, 1990.

50. Helvind MH, McCarthy JF, Imamura M: Ventriculo-arterial discordance: Switching the morphologically left ventricle into the systemic circulation after 3 months of age. Eur J Cardiothorac Surg 14:173, 1998.

CHAPTER 26

TRANSPOSITION AND MALPOSITION OF THE GREAT ARTERIES WITH VENTRICULAR SEPTAL DEFECTS

DANIEL SIDI   YVES LECOMPTE

INTRODUCTION: A NEW APPROACH BASED ON SURGERY

Conventionally, pediatric cardiology books have different chapters for transposition of the great arteries with ventricular septal defects and double-outlet ventricles (especially double-outlet right ventricle). This is because the usual approach in pediatric cardiology is to classify malformations into subgroups according to their anatomy and hemodynamics and then apply the surgical technique appropriate for each subgroup. This approach, however, does not work well for this group of malformations because of their extreme anatomic polymorphism and because of the difficulty in defining surgically helpful subgroups based on classical definitions. In addition, there are controversies about the definitions of some malformations, for example, double-outlet right ventricle, that are based by some authors on embryology (the double infundibulum, regardless of the malposition of the vessels or the location of the ventricular septal defects), by others on anatomy focusing on the malalignment between the vessels and the presumed septum, and by yet others on hemodynamic and surgical features depending on the position of the ventricular septal defect relative to the great arteries.

Our group therefore decided to put these malformations together under the global appellation of either "malposition of the great arteries" or "abnormal ventriculoarterial connection with ventricular septal defect" and base our approach in a nonconventional way on the different surgical options rather than on the different anatomic subgroups. We first describe the different surgical techniques and their anatomic and hemodynamic requirements, then look at the malformations to determine the best match between the repair and the malformation. We believe that this group of malformations deserves a "tailor-made" operation and not an operation "off the peg."

KEY POINTS

- This group of lesions includes a large variety of malformations with different embryologic origins and different pathologic definitions but a common surgical approach.

- The clinical presentation and surgical indications are based on the presence or absence of pulmonic stenosis and the position of the great arteries with respect to the ventricular septal defect and the annuli of the atrioventricular valves.
- Surgery is based on anatomic correction by constructing a tunnel between the left ventricle and the aorta (or the switched pulmonary artery) and reconstructing a right ventricle–pulmonary artery communication (or a communication to the switched aorta), if possible without prosthetic material. Despite the apparent complexity, with pertinent indications and when the ventricular septal defect is perimembranous (below the infundibula of the great arteries) without added malformations of ventricular sizes or atrioventricular valves, the surgical results and the prognosis are good.

EPIDEMIOLOGY

These lesions represent about 5% of congenital malformations and 20% of conotruncal malformations. Unlike tetralogy of Fallot, pulmonary atresia with ventricular septal defect, or truncus arteriosus, these malformations are rarely (except in heterotaxia syndromes) associated with extracardiac malformations or chromosome abnormalities and have a low recurrence rate.

EMBRYOLOGY, PATHOLOGY, AND DEFINITIONS

Cardiac malformations involving the ventriculoarterial connection are linked to the fate of the subarterial conus (infundibulum) during the later part of cardiac embryogenesis (see Chapter 1). Because conotruncal resorption participates not only in the spatial relationship between the aorta, the pulmonary artery, and the atrioventricular valves but also in the closure of the ventricular septum in the perimembranous and infundibular portion, the association of the three anomalies is frequent and logical. The association will result in an extreme polymorphism of malformations, however, because the three anomalies will not always combine in a logical embryologic pattern. The ventricular septal defect is usually in the perimembranous part of the septum just beneath the infundibulum of the great arteries (often persisting below both great arteries) and is often the consequence of malalignment between the infundibular septum and the rest of the ventricular septum (trabecular septum).[1-6] This malalignment will eventually produce subpulmonic stenosis when the infundibular septum is deviated toward the pulmonary artery (as in tetralogy of Fallot)[1,4,6] or subaortic stenosis when the infundibular septum is deviated toward the aorta (as in coarctation of the aorta or an interrupted aortic arch).[7] As a result of the obstruction, the fetal growth of the corresponding great artery is impaired, producing a small aorta or pulmonary trunk (but with normal intrapulmonary branches).

The other major intracardiac consequence of a persistent conus is that it maintains the arterial orifice at a distance from the atrioventricular annulus, and depending on the length of the infundibulum, the great vessels will rise near or far from the atrioventricular valve annulus (Fig. 26–1). In addition, if there is an asymmetric infundibulum, the distance from the artery to the mitral valve and the tricuspid valve will be different.

To understand the wide spectrum of these malformations and why there are difficulties and debates about defining and classifying some of them (namely, the wide spectrum of the malformation called double-outlet right ventricle), it is necessary to go back to the normal relationships between the great arteries and the ventricles and to realize that there is a big difference between concordance and alignment. The normal heart is characterized by an aorta that with the resorption of its infundibulum moves posteriorly into the center of the heart, in continuity with the annuli of the atrioventricular valves and the ventricular septum, whereas the pulmonary artery stays at a distance above its persisting infundibulum in discontinuity with the atrioventricular valves (Figs. 26–2 and 26–3). In addition, there is torsion between the upper part of the heart (the origin of the great arteries) and its apical part (determined by the axis of the trabecular septum). This torsion explains why, in a normal heart, the aorta rises from the left ventricle but above the right ventricle and the pulmonary artery rises

from the right ventricle but above the left ventricle (Fig. 26–4). Therefore, concordance does not go along with alignment even in the normal heart. When the septum is intact, however, concordance is evident, nobody pays attention to the "physiologic anatomic malalignment," and there is no controversy about the connections of a normal heart or the ventriculoarterial discordance of a complete transposition of the great arteries. When there is a large subarterial ventricular septal defect, the question of connection and alignment is much more difficult to answer because the origin of the great artery depends on the supposed situation of the upper part of the ventricular septum (Fig. 26–5).

This is precisely the problem with double-outlet right ventricle, a congenital anomaly in which both great arteries arise wholly or principally from the right ventricle. This definition is clear only in theory. In reality, this definition leads to controversies when there is a large ventricular septal defect beneath the infundibula of the great arteries.

Most pathologists (see Chapter 19) insist on the alignment of the great arteries in relation to the ventricle; if more than half of the artery is over one ventricle, it is considered to arise from this ventricle, regardless of atrioventricular discontinuity (or subarterial conus).[4,8,9] Because septal alignment is not physiologic, even in the normal heart, we believe that this definition is misleading, particularly when the two great arteries are above a ventricular septal defect. Indeed, the origin of the vessel depends entirely on the way the ventricular septal defect is closed at the upper edge of the septum, and this is not constant (see Fig. 26–5). If the upper part of the septum is the conus between the aorta and the pulmonary artery, each artery arises from a different ventricle and there is no double-outlet right ventricle (see Fig. 26–5B). If the upper part of the septum is at the lateral edge of the conus, the two arteries arise from the right ventricle if the septum is at the left edge of the conus (double-outlet right ventricle) (see Fig. 26–5C). On the other hand, if the septum is at the right edge of the conus, the heart will end up with a double-outlet left ventricle (see Fig. 26–5A).[10] In addition, what matters for the patient is not which part of the per-

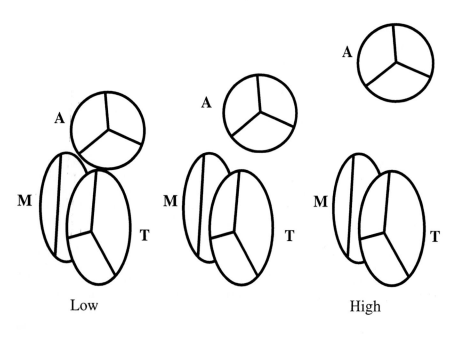

FIGURE 26–1

Diagram to show differing relationships of the annulus of a great artery (A, shown by the upper circle with the triradius in it) to the mitral valve annulus (M) and the tricuspid valve annulus (T). *Left,* Close relationship. *Center,* The great artery annulus is farther away, but its distances to both atrioventricular annuli are equal. *Right,* Not only is the great artery annulus far away, but its distances from the mitral and tricuspid valve annuli are unequal.

Low   High

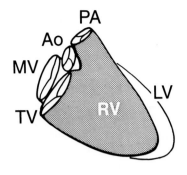

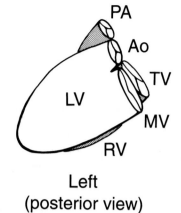

Right
(anterior view)

Left
(posterior view)

Diagram of normal heart to show aortic annulus in center of heart, closely associated with the annuli of the other three valves. *Left,* Right ventricular (RV) view. *Right,* Left ventricular (LV) view. Ao = aortic valve annulus; MV = mitral valve annulus; PA = pulmonic valve annulus; TV = tricuspid valve annulus.

sisting infundibulum is really the upper septum, but what difficulty the surgeon has in closing the ventricular septal defect in a correct position and allowing normal ventriculoarterial concordance or discordance without obstruction.

Other pathologists (see Chapter 20) require for the definition of double-outlet right ventricle a double infundibulum, regardless of the septal alignment.[6] This may have interesting embryologic or etiologic implications (in the chicken, various kinds of double-outlet right ventricle are created by stopping the embryologic process just before completion), but surgically speaking, it is not helpful or can even be misleading because the malformation is not completely identified by the conus abnormality alone. Some double-outlet right ventricles are nearly like a simple ventricular septal defect despite a long subaortic infundibulum. Others with subpulmonary stenosis resemble a tetralogy of Fallot or a transposition of the great arteries with ventricular septal defect with or without pulmonary stenosis. Some even resemble a more complex malformation like a single ventricle if atrioventricular valve abnormalities, significant differences in ventricular cavity sizes, or even multiple ventricular septal defects are present.

This dilemma cannot be solved by the recommendation of Lev and colleagues[9] to identify double-outlet right ventricle by the position of the ventricular septal defect relative to the great arteries: subaortic, subpulmonary, doubly committed, or noncommitted. The problem with this classification is that it is impossible to define clearly the extreme polymorphism of these malformations by this method alone because the polymorphism is determined by three independent variables (Fig. 26–6). More important, there is no strict correlation between the commitment of the ventricular septal defect to one or the other artery and the surgical options. Repair in many patients with double-outlet right ventricle and a subpulmonary ventricular septal defect can be achieved by intraventricular rerouting, as for a subaortic ventricular septal defect, without an arterial switch or displacement of the pulmonary artery. Conversely, some subaortic ventricular septal defects may require other types of repair than just an intraventricular patch or a tunnel between the left ventricle and the aorta.

Double-outlet left ventricle is less controversial because this rare malformation is characterized almost always by complete resorption of the two infundibula, which brings the two great arteries into continuity with the atrioventricular valves above a large perimembranous ventricular septal defect.[10] Pulmonic stenosis is usually present, there being a small annulus with a stenosed valve. The relation between the vessels and the atrioventricular valves and the

Diagram of normal heart to show continuity between the aortic valve annulus (Ao) and the annuli of the tricuspid valve (TV) and the mitral valve (MV). It also shows the discontinuity between the pulmonic valve annulus (PA) and the annuli of the tricuspid and mitral valves. Note that the pulmonary artery is anterior. *A,* Cross-sectional view. *B,* Longitudinal section. RV = right ventricle; LV = left ventricle; RA = right atrium; LA = left atrium.

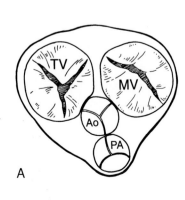

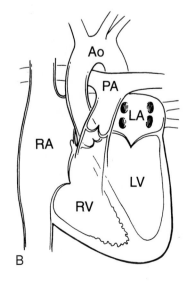

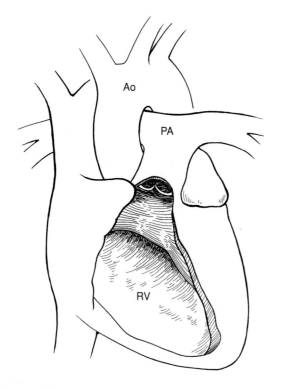

FIGURE 26–4

Diagram to show the normal spiral relationship of the aorta (Ao) and pulmonary artery (PA) to the right ventricle (RV).

presence or absence of pulmonic stenosis determine the best surgical strategy by the same rules as for any "malposition with a ventricular septal defect."

Malposition of the great arteries can be present also in complex malformations like atrioventricular canal or a large inlet ventricular septal defect, particularly in heterotaxia syndromes.

The problem with any anatomic definition of these malpositions with ventricular septal defect is that the malformation cannot be fully characterized by identifying the re-

lationship between the great arteries alone, or the relation of the arteries with the atrioventricular valves alone, or the location of the ventricular septal defect alone, because the three anomalies play independent roles. It is necessary to consider each of the three anatomic components, because they determine an infinite variety of anatomic malformations with different hemodynamics and surgical strategies. To summarize, in the conditions discussed in this chapter, if neither the clinician nor the surgeon is able to classify the individual patient into a single clear category, the patients may receive a standardized but nonoptimal operation based on an incomplete anatomic description. Furthermore, the medical community cannot evaluate the results because it is difficult to know from the literature which anatomic lesion was operated on with each particular technique.

We think that the only way to achieve appropriate surgical decisions is not to classify subgroups of patients anatomically but to consider each patient with malposition and ventricular septal defect as unique.[11] Then we need to determine whether the cardiac anatomy and hemodynamics fit with one of the possible anatomic repairs. If more than one surgical option exists for any given patient, one should choose the best and least risky procedure. It is therefore necessary for the pediatric cardiologist to know in detail the surgical requirements for the different operations. *Then the cardiologist checks by constructing mentally and on the echocardiography screen what the outflows of the two ventricles will be after repair.*

SURGICAL OPTIONS AND PREOPERATIVE SCREENING

ANATOMIC REPAIR

We call anatomic repair a surgical procedure that allows the left ventricle to be connected to the aorta and the right ventricle to be connected to the pulmonary artery as directly as possible, preferably without a prosthetic conduit.

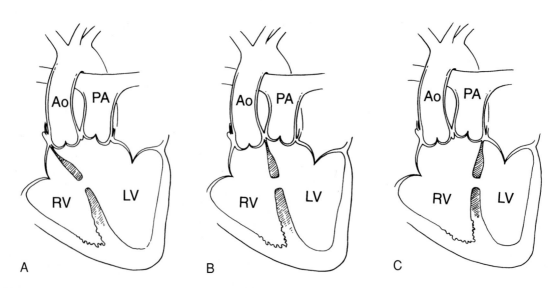

FIGURE 26–5

Diagram to show how the position of the infundibular septum determines whether there is a double-outlet left ventricle *(A)*, a normal connection *(B)*, or a double-outlet right ventricle *(C)*. Ao = aorta; PA = pulmonary artery; RV = right ventricle; LV = left ventricle.

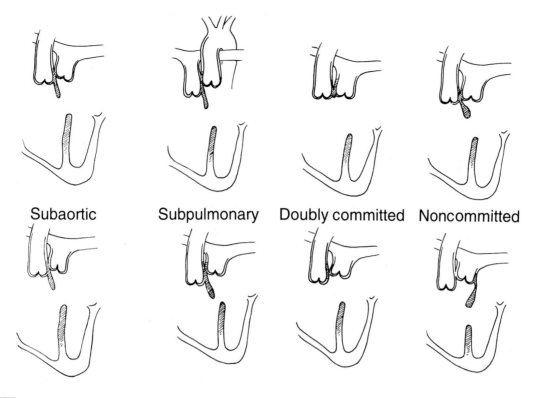

Subaortic   Subpulmonary   Doubly committed   Noncommitted

FIGURE 26–6

Diagram to show how the simple classification of Lev[9] *(top row)* becomes less useful once variations in the position of the infundibular septum occur *(bottom row)*.

Before the different surgical options are described, it is necessary to remember certain important facts:

1. The infundibular septum can be removed with no risk of atrioventricular block if the ventricular septal defect is perimembranous,[8, 12, 13] even when there are tricuspid insertions on the septum.

2. The great arteries can be switched if there is no organic subpulmonic stenosis and if the pulmonary valve is normal, regardless of the coronary artery distribution (see Chapter 25).

3. The pulmonary artery can be connected to the right ventricle without a prosthetic conduit (Lecompte maneuver, see Chapter 25) if the pulmonary artery branches are not fixed because of previous surgery (aortopulmonary shunts).[11, 14–17] This maneuver, however, goes along with sacrifice of the pulmonary valve and therefore can be applied only if the pulmonary vascular resistance is low, pulmonary arteries are of adequate size without stenoses, and postcapillary hypertension (due to left ventricular or mitral valve dysfunction) is absent.

On the basis of these considerations, there are three fundamental types of anatomic repair.

Intraventricular Repair

Intraventricular repair (IVR) consists of building an intraventricular patch to direct the left ventricular blood toward the aortic orifice (Fig. 26–7). The operation resembles simple closure of an isolated ventricular septal defect, but if the aorta is far removed from the mitral valve, the operation requires a long intracardiac tunnel that passes posterior to the right ventricular outflow tract. The fundamental consideration is that the right ventricular outflow tract should not be obstructed by the tunnel, and this depends mainly on the position of the pulmonary artery in relation to the tricuspid valve. If the distance between the tricuspid valve and the pulmonary artery is long enough (equal or greater than the distance to the aortic annulus), the left ventricular-to-aortic tunnel will not obstruct the right ventricular outflow tract regardless of the length of the tunnel (see Fig. 26–7A). If the distance from the pulmonary artery to the tricuspid valve is less than to the aortic annulus, either the pulmonary artery must be removed (see Fig. 26–7B; see later section on REV) or the tunnel must be constructed from the left ventricle to the pulmonary artery in association with a switch of the great arteries (see Fig. 26–7C; see later section on arterial switch).

To avoid left ventricular-to-aortic obstruction and to make this tunnel as short as possible (to avoid diminishing the size of the right ventricular cavity), the infundibular septum should be removed whenever it is in the way, that is, posterior to the aorta. If the ventricular septal defect is perimembranous, there is no theoretical risk of atrioventricular block. If the tricuspid valve is inserted onto the infundibular septum, the septum is not resected but mobilized posteriorly and reinserted on the patch. The only contraindication to this operation is insertion of the mitral valve on the infundibular septum.

Arterial Switch With Ventricular Septal Closure

This operation consists of building an intraventricular patch to direct the left ventricular blood toward the pulmonary artery, which will become an aorta after the arterial switch (see Fig. 26–7C). This is possible when the pul-

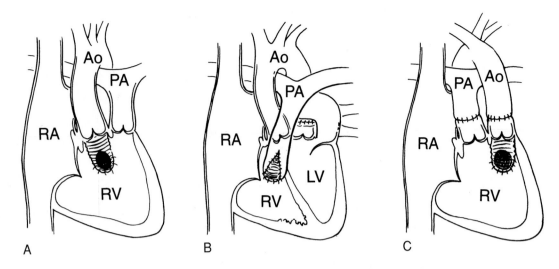

Diagram to show factors affecting the type of surgery for double-outlet right ventricle. *A,* A long tunnel connects the left ventricle to the aorta without obstructing the outflow to the pulmonary artery. *B,* If the tricuspid valve annulus is closer to the pulmonary artery than to the aortic annulus, the pulmonary artery can be removed and inserted into the anterior wall of the right ventricle in the REV operation. *C,* Alternatively, the great arteries can be switched, and a tunnel connects the left ventricle to the pulmonary artery. Ao = aorta; LV = left ventricle; PA = pulmonary artery; RA = right atrium; RV = right ventricle.

monic valve is normal and when there is no subpulmonic organic obstruction due to musculofibrous pulmonary valve tissue or mitral valve insertion in the subpulmonic region. As in IVR, the patch should not obstruct the future right ventricular outflow tract. In this respect, the same rules as for IVR are applied, and the infundibular septum should be resected if it is anterior to the pulmonary artery (future aorta).

Intraventricular Repair With Reposition of the Pulmonary Artery on the Right Ventricle (REV)

This operation, named REV (réparation étage ventriculaire) by its developer, Y. Lecompte, consists of a left ventricular-to-aortic tunnel associated with removal of the pulmonary artery from its position and its direct reimplantation onto the right ventricle (see Fig. 26–7B). It differs from the Rastelli procedure by the resection of the infundibular septum and the absence of a prosthetic conduit. The resection of the infundibular septum (Kawashima) is especially important because it is crucial to make the tunnel as short as possible to avoid any decrease in volume of the right ventricle. Otherwise, the right ventricle will also be damaged by the large ventriculotomy needed to insert the pulmonary artery, and it will eventually have to accommodate increased volume due to pulmonic regurgitation (because there is no pulmonic valve in REV) and perhaps later tricuspid regurgitation. Resection of the infundibular septum also improves left ventricular function by avoiding a large septal patch that will dilate the left ventricular outflow tract and act like a diverticulum or even an aneurysm.

NONANATOMIC REPAIR

We consider a repair nonanatomic when the operation results in the right ventricle's being located beneath the aorta or when each ventricle does not receive the correct venous return. We also need to differentiate between the

one-ventricle repair (total cavopulmonary circulation equivalent to the repair of a single ventricle) and the "1½-ventricle repair," in which only part of the caval venous return (usually from the inferior vena cava) enters the right ventricle while the other part (usually from the superior vena cava) goes directly to the lungs (partial cavopulmonary anastomosis).

PREOPERATIVE ANATOMIC EVALUATION

Each patient must be regarded as unique, and all anatomic and hemodynamic aspects important to the operation must be investigated. The pediatric cardiologist must, like an architect, construct the tunnel mentally and use echocardiography to assess whether there is potential outflow tract obstruction after the anatomic repair (left ventricle to future aorta and right ventricle to future pulmonary artery). It is useful to perform the two-dimensional echocardiogram with the surgeon present to clarify particular anatomic details. Three-dimensional echocardiography will be particularly helpful in the future in this group of malformations. The examination must evaluate the feasibility of an anatomic repair and, if it is possible, the feasibility of IVR. The echocardiographer must look carefully at the position of the ventricular septal defect and search for multiple ventricular septal defects, especially at the apex; the relative position of the great arteries and above all their relation to the atrioventricular valves; the function and the insertions of the atrioventricular valves; and the size of the ventricles.

Feasibility of an Anatomic Repair
Anatomic repair requires adequacy of both ventricles to assume their future workload. Therefore, both ventricles must be of adequate size and function; there is usually concern with the size of the left ventricle in malpositions with pulmonic stenosis (and reduced pulmonary venous return)

and with the size of the right ventricle in malposition with coarctation of the aorta. Abnormal ventricular size or function, however, also occurs with a restrictive ventricular septal defect[18,19] or an inlet ventricular septal defect with an overriding atrioventricular valve. We believe that the best index of ventricular size is the size of the atrioventricular valve annulus (in the absence of an overriding or straddling valve). An atrioventricular annulus size more than 2 SD below normal is considered a contraindication to anatomic repair. Assessment of ventricular function is based on ventricular contractility, knowing that the ventricle should be hyperkinetic if the afterload is low (increased pulmonary blood flow or atrioventricular valve incompetence) or have adaptive hypertrophy secondary to valvar or subvalvar aortic obstruction or secondary to a restrictive ventricular septal defect that functions like a subaortic stenosis if both great arteries originate from the right ventricle.[18,19]

Both atrioventricular valves should be inspected carefully, not only for size and function but also for the subvalvar apparatus (chordae and papillary muscles), particularly any abnormal insertion on the subarterial infundibula. Tricuspid valve chordal attachments on the infundibular septum or even straddling it are not a contraindication because the valve can be repaired adequately and be sufficient for a low-pressure subpulmonic ventricle. Conversely, abnormal attachments of the mitral valve are usually a contraindication unless the valve is competent and the surgeon can avoid touching it during surgery without creating obstruction.

Multiple trabecular ventricular septal defects (Swiss cheese) or an inlet ventricular septal defect may lead to serious complications.

A restrictive ventricular septal defect can be a problem not only if it affects normal growth and function of the left ventricle (see earlier) but also if the position of the ventricular septal defect is not in the perimembranous part of the septum. If it is not at this site, any enlargement of the defect is dangerous for the conduction system (although anterior extension of the ventricular septal defect is theoretically safe).

Finally, the afterload of both ventricles must be acceptable. We should pay particular attention to pulmonary arterial stenosis, especially after an aortopulmonary anastomosis, and to pulmonary hypertension. With pulmonic stenosis, the criteria are similar to those applied to tetralogy of Fallot. With pulmonary hypertension, assessment of pulmonary vascular resistance is necessary, just as for a simple ventricular septal defect. It is these afterload factors that may justify cardiac catheterization.

Feasibility of an Intraventricular Repair

For this repair, the crucial point is to determine whether it is possible to construct a left ventricular-to-aortic tunnel between the tricuspid and pulmonic orifices. This is possible if the tricuspid-to-pulmonic distance is equal to or longer than the diameter of the aortic annulus. This is best seen on a subxiphoid right anterior view (Fig. 26–8). If the pulmonary artery is above a well-developed infundibulum with a tricuspid-to-pulmonic distance greater than to the aortic annulus, an IVR is possible regardless of the size of the aortic infundibulum. On the left anterior subxiphoid view (Fig. 26–9), we can best see the infundibular septum that may need to be resected to construct a nonobstructed tunnel if the aorta is anterior (and the infundibular septum is posterior to the aorta) because it stands in the way from the posterior left ventricle to the anterior aorta. Conversely, when the aorta is posterior to the pulmonary artery, the infundibular septum is anterior to both the aorta and the left ventricular-to-aortic tunnel and may even constitute part of its wall.

If, however, the tricuspid-to-pulmonic distance is short (less than aortic annulus size), a simple IVR is not feasible. The choice is then between a tunnel from the left ventricle to the pulmonary artery in association with an arterial switch and a tunnel from the left ventricle to the aorta with occlusion of the pulmonic orifice and direct right ventricle–pulmonary artery continuity (REV) or a right ventricle–pulmonary artery conduit (Rastelli).

SURGICAL CLASSIFICATION

1. *Malposition that can be treated by IVR:* IVR is possible when the pulmonary artery annulus is far from the tricuspid valve annulus (see Fig. 26–7A), regardless of the position of the aorta, for that determines only the length of the tunnel. If there is pulmonic or subpulmonic stenosis, the operation is similar to that for a tetralogy of Fallot with the same concerns about the coronary artery distribution (see Chapter 28).

2. *Malposition that can be treated by a tunnel from the left ventricle to the pulmonary artery in association with an arterial switch:* This operation is possible when there is no pulmonic or subpulmonic stenosis and when the aortic annulus is far from the tricuspid valve annulus. This distance allows a nonobstructive right ventricular outflow

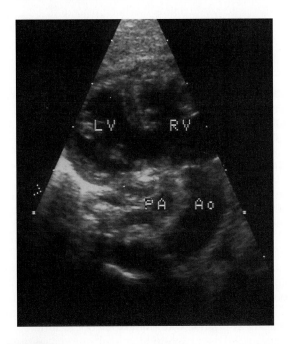

FIGURE 26–8

Two-dimensional echocardiogram in subxiphoid view (oblique left anterior). This echocardiogram shows where a tunnel from the left ventricle (LV) to the aorta (Ao) would have to be for an intraventricular repair. RV = right ventricle; PA = pulmonary artery.

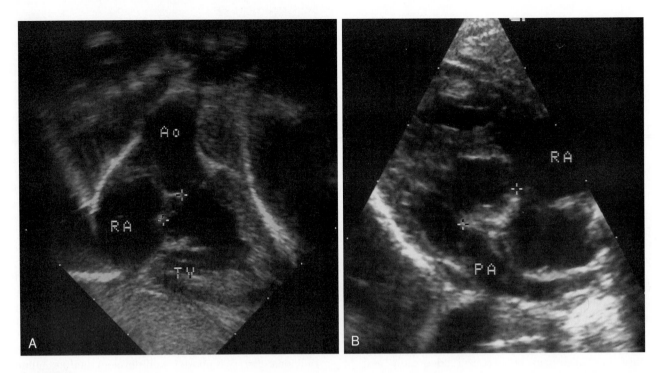

FIGURE 26–9

Two-dimensional echocardiograms in subxiphoid view (right anterior) of same patient as in Figure 26–8. Because the distances from the tricuspid annulus to the aortic and pulmonary artery annuli cannot be seen in the same plane, two different views are needed. *A,* The crosses show the distance between the tricuspid valve (TV) annulus and the annulus of the aorta (Ao). In this patient, the distance is 6.2 mm. *B,* The crosses show the distance between the tricuspid valve annulus and the annulus of the pulmonary artery (PA). In this patient, the distance is 10.1 mm. Because the size of the subpulmonic conus is too short for an IVR, the appropriate correction would be a REV operation (see text). RA = right atrium.

tract connection to the pulmonary artery (previous aorta) anterior to the left ventricular-to-aortic (previous pulmonary artery) tunnel (see Fig. 26–7C).

3. *Malposition that can be treated by a left ventricular-to-aortic tunnel in association with the displacement of the pulmonary artery (REV):* This operation can be done if there is a pulmonic stenosis (valvar or subvalvar) that contraindicates an arterial switch and when the pulmonary artery annulus is near the tricuspid annulus, which would lead to pulmonary artery obstruction by a left ventricular-to-aortic tunnel (see Fig. 26–7B). The pulmonary annulus and valves are sacrificed, and the junction between the right ventricle and the pulmonary artery is made either by a conduit (Rastelli operation) or better by the translocation of the pulmonary artery anteriorly onto the right ventricle (REV).

4. *Complex malpositions that cannot lead to a "simple" biventricular repair:* Biventricular repair usually cannot be performed when the ventricular septal defect (inlet or trabecular) is not committed to a great artery because placing a tunnel from the left ventricle to one of the great arteries is difficult when both arise from the right ventricle. It can also be difficult to repair these malformations when there are anomalies of the ventricles or the atrioventricular valves or when the conal septum cannot be removed because of mitral attachments.

These complex malpositions need careful discussion before a decision is made between a palliative operation (see Chapter 33) and corrective surgery with a high risk of atrioventricular block, atrioventricular valve replacement, or ventricular damage.

One interesting option in some patients is a 1½-ventricle repair (see earlier) when the right ventricle is too small initially or when it becomes too small after the left ventricular-to-aortic tunnel has been placed.

For clinical assessment, natural history, and pathophysiology, it is necessary to distinguish patients with and without pulmonary artery stenosis.

MALPOSITION WITH VENTRICULAR SEPTAL DEFECT WITHOUT RIGHT VENTRICULAR OUTFLOW TRACT OBSTRUCTION

PATHOPHYSIOLOGY

The absence of right ventricular outflow tract obstruction leads (as in simple ventricular septal defect) to pulmonary artery hypertension with increased pulmonary blood flow and a long-term risk of developing pulmonary vascular obstructive disease.

As in ventricular septal defect, because the pulmonary vascular resistance decreases slowly after birth, pulmonary blood flow is not excessive in the neonatal period and heart failure does not occur unless there is aortic obstruction, usually in association with coarctation of the aorta.[20]

Because of the malposition, some hypoxemia is present, depending on the relative position of the great arteries with respect to the ventricles and on the streaming patterns. Hypoxemia is never severe because of the increased pulmonary blood flow and adequate shunting through the ventricular septal defect (right ventricle to pulmonary artery in systole and left to right ventricle in diastole).

CLINICAL FINDINGS, DIAGNOSIS, AND MANAGEMENT

In the fetus, malposition of the great arteries with a ventricular septal defect is well tolerated. Diagnosis can be made on two-dimensional echocardiography if the screening includes exploration of the outlet septum and vessels and is not limited to the four-chamber view that can be normal.

In the neonate, there is usually mild cyanosis without respiratory distress and a systolic murmur (not constant) in an otherwise apparently healthy infant. If there is early heart failure, arterial pulses are usually diminished in the legs because of an associated coarctation of the aorta. After a few weeks, because of the increased pulmonary flow and left ventricular volume overload, congestive heart failure develops, manifested by dyspnea, liver enlargement, nutritional difficulties, and failure to gain weight. The clinical picture is that of a large ventricular septal defect with mild cyanosis.

Chest Radiography
The chest film shows cardiomegaly and increased lung vascularity. The thymus is present, and there is usually a left aortic arch.

Electrocardiography
The electrocardiogram shows right ventricular hypertrophy, sometimes with right axis deviation, depending on the location of the ventricular septal defect and the course of the conduction pathways.

Echocardiography
Two-dimensional echocardiography with Doppler study is the major examination.

Echocardiography confirms the diagnosis, demonstrating the ventricular septal defect and the abnormal position of the great arteries. These have to be assessed independently. There is no correlation between the relative positions of the great arteries and the position of the ventricular septal defect.[17]

It evaluates pulmonary vascular resistance (if the patient is older than 3 months) by evaluating left ventricular dimensions, looking at left ventricular dilatation as a sign of increased pulmonary blood flow and low pulmonary vascular resistance. It may be possible to estimate pulmonary artery diastolic pressure from the velocity of a pulmonary artery regurgitant jet.

It indicates the likely type of surgery. As explained before, it is crucial to analyze precisely the relationship of the aortic and pulmonary artery annuli to the atrioventricular valve annuli as well as the size and position of the ventricular septal defect. The two-dimensional echocardiographic subxiphoid view allows visualization of a tunnel between the left ventricle and one of the great arteries to see what it looks like (see Figs. 26–8 and 26–9). The examination also identifies any valvar attachment to the conal septum that would be removed at surgery.

Cardiac Catheterization
Catheterization is usually not needed to define anatomic details except if there is a doubt on two-dimensional echocardiography about pulmonary artery branches or an associated trabecular ventricular septal defect. Cardiac catheterization is useful for evaluating pulmonary vascular resistance in older children. In particular, it is the only way to assess the streaming patterns and to determine pulmonary artery oxygen saturation and therefore the arteriovenous difference in oxygen content that allows calculation of pulmonary vascular resistance.

EVOLUTION

Natural History
Pulmonary vascular disease can develop as soon as 3 months of age and be manifested by increased cyanosis and decreased congestive heart failure.

In some patients, the ventricular septal defect becomes smaller and creates an obstruction for the left ventricle if both vessels originate from the right ventricle, especially if there is no atrial septal defect. If there is a large atrial septal defect, there will be a rerouting of the blood and a progressive exclusion of the left ventricle from the circulation, as a result of which the left ventricle will not grow properly.

Treatment and Results
Medical treatment is nonspecific and based on the hemodynamics; the purpose is to improve the circulation and stabilize the infant so that an operation can be performed soon. As in all patients with a ventricular septal defect and heart failure, improvement can usually be obtained by diuretics, blood transfusion in anemic patients (to improve arterial oxygen content and decrease lung flow by increasing pulmonary vascular resistance through increased viscosity), vasodilators, and eventually digoxin. If a neonate has cardiac failure, usually in association with coarctation of the aorta, prostaglandin E_1 (PGE_1) infusion, artificial ventilation, and inotropic support with dobutamine are helpful. If there is inadequate mixing or a high left atrial pressure, with increased flow and a functional gradient across the mitral valve, a Rashkind atrioseptostomy is indicated to improve the clinical status (heart failure and cyanosis) before surgery.

Surgery is mandatory before 3 months of age to protect the lungs from developing pulmonary vascular disease.

Pulmonary artery banding may be indicated to protect the small pulmonary arteries, either if there is no straightforward anatomic repair or to wait until the infant is larger and healthier before undergoing an operation that may be difficult (e.g., if the tunnel will be long, if the tricuspid valve is attached to the infundibular septum, or if the right ventricle will be small after surgery). The banding is done by thoracotomy, improves congestive heart failure, but increases hypoxemia and may hinder an eventual arterial switch by dilating the pulmonary sinuses of Valsalva and altering the future aortic leaflets.

Corrective surgery with anatomic repair is usually possible (see the surgical classification earlier) either by a tunnel from the left ventricle to the aorta (IVR) if the pulmonary annulus is far enough from the tricuspid valve annulus or by a tunnel from the left ventricle to the pulmonary artery in association with an arterial switch if the aortic annulus is far from the tricuspid valve annulus.

With coarctation of the aorta, most surgical teams perform corrective surgery at once in the neonatal period rather than go through a coarctation repair and pulmonary artery banding as a first-stage procedure.

Hospital mortality for correction is around 10% with excellent results. The patient needs an annual evaluation with two-dimensional echo Doppler examination to assess the left and right ventricular outflow tracts and the growth of the two great arteries. If an arterial switch has been performed, a coronary artery angiogram should be considered. Obstruction of the left ventricular–aortic junction is rare when the surgery has involved adequate removal of the conal septum. Usually, the heart grows in harmony, close to normal anatomy.

The long-term follow-up and results of IVR are similar to those for isolated ventricular septal defect, because left ventricular-aortic obstructions are rare (none in the Lecompte series). When an arterial switch is added, complications of the switch procedure may be encountered (see Chapter 25) with common but rarely severe supravalvar pulmonic stenosis, common aortic dilatation with minimal (color Doppler) aortic regurgitation, and a few ischemic complications or potential complications due to the association of the coronary artery transfer with coronary ostial stenosis. When coarctation of the aorta is present, the follow-up should include the search for residual aortic obstruction and systemic hypertension at rest or during exercise. A scan or magnetic resonance imaging of the aorta may be useful to check the aortic isthmic anatomy after the aortoplasty.

When anatomic repair is not possible, the situation is similar to a single ventricle with pulmonary hypertension. It is imperative to protect the pulmonary arteries by banding with the intent of later creating a cavopulmonary circulation (see Chapter 33).

MALPOSITION WITH VENTRICULAR SEPTAL DEFECT AND PULMONIC STENOSIS

PATHOPHYSIOLOGY

The pathophysiologic features of this combination are similar to those in tetralogy of Fallot with more hypoxemia for the same degree of pulmonic stenosis because some of the oxygenated blood may return to the lungs as a result of streaming. There are usually no hypoxic spells because the subpulmonic stenosis is less muscular (especially if the vessels are transposed). The pulmonary artery branches are usually of normal size without stenosis (either at their origin or distally).

If there is a higher saturation in the pulmonary artery than in the aorta, hypoxemia can be treated by creating an atrial septal defect by a Rashkind procedure (see Chapters 13 and 25).

CLINICAL FINDINGS, DIAGNOSIS, AND MANAGEMENT

In the fetus, malposition of the great arteries with ventricular septal defect and pulmonic stenosis is well tolerated. The diagnosis can be made on two-dimensional echocar-diography if the outlet septum and vessels are examined and the screening is not limited to the four-chamber view that can be normal.

In the neonate, cyanosis is present and is associated with a rough systolic ejection murmur in an otherwise apparently healthy infant. With severe pulmonic stenosis or even pulmonary atresia, cyanosis can be severe in the neonate, who may need early intervention by PGE$_1$ to maintain patency of the ductus arteriosus, followed by an early operation (usually a palliative shunt, but eventually a balloon dilatation). Cyanosis increases rapidly because of the increased oxygen consumption and decrease in pulmonary flow.

Chest Radiography

The chest film shows normal cardiac size and variable lung vascularity. A thymus is present, and the aortic arch is usually left sided.

Electrocardiography

The electrocardiogram shows nonspecific right ventricular hypertrophy.

Echocardiography

Two-dimensional echocardiography with Doppler study is the major examination.

It confirms the diagnosis, demonstrating the ventricular septal defect, the abnormal position of the vessels, and the pulmonic stenosis.

It evaluates the degree and the type of the pulmonic stenosis, which is usually subvalvar and valvar and only rarely has anomalies of the pulmonary artery branches.

It helps establish the type of surgery. As explained before, it is crucial to analyze precisely the relationship of the aortic and pulmonary annuli with the atrioventricular valve annuli as well as the size and position of the ventricular septal defect. The two-dimensional echocardiographic subxiphoid view allows the physician to visualize the tunnel between the left ventricle and the aorta. The examination can also identify any valvar attachment to the conal septum that might need to be removed at surgery.

Cardiac Catheterization

Catheterization is usually unnecessary except to assess pulmonary artery branches after a previous shunt or if there is a doubt on two-dimensional echocardiography about the pulmonary artery branches, associated trabecular ventricular septal defect, or coronary artery disposition if there is to be a Fallot-type repair. Pressures in the pulmonary arteries (taken directly or through an occluded pulmonary vein) may also be useful in the decision about incorporating a valve in the right ventricle–pulmonary junction.

EVOLUTION

Natural History

Cyanosis increases, polycythemia occurs, and there will be increased collateral circulation from the aorta to the pulmonary arteries.

Treatment and Results

If a neonate has severe hypoxemia, usually in association with pulmonic atresia or severe stenosis, PGE$_1$ infusion maintains ductal flow. A Rashkind procedure is often useful to improve the mixing of the blood.

Balloon dilatation may be useful if there is a valvar component to the pulmonic stenosis to avoid or delay an aortopulmonary anastomosis or defer corrective surgery. Balloon dilatation is especially effective when oxygen saturation is lower in the pulmonary artery than in the aorta (as in tetralogy of Fallot). This situation is common when the aorta is near the left ventricle, but it may occur even when the great arteries are transposed because of the streaming patterns due to the location (especially the angulation) of the infundibulum with respect to the outflow tracts of the ventricles.

Surgery

Aortopulmonary anastomosis can be performed to delay corrective surgery until the infant is larger and healthier. The anastomosis is usually done by thoracotomy, and although it improves hypoxemia, it may hinder later corrective surgery by distorting and fixing a pulmonary artery branch that will be difficult to mobilize for the REV.

Corrective surgery is usually possible (see the surgical classification earlier) by a tunnel from the left ventricle to the aorta, either by an IVR associated with removal of a right ventricular tract obstruction, as in a tetralogy of Fallot repair, or by mobilizing the pulmonary artery in an REV or Rastelli repair when the distance from the pulmonary artery annulus to the tricuspid valve annulus is less than to the aortic annulus. When the pulmonary artery is near the tricuspid valve annulus, the pulmonary artery is closed above the valve, and the distal pulmonary artery is mobilized and translocated on the right ventricle in an REV operation or connected to the right ventricle by a prosthetic tube in a Rastelli operation.

Most surgical teams would try to wait for at least a year to perform an REV operation and for several years for a Rastelli repair. They would start by a Rashkind procedure and an aortopulmonary anastomosis or a balloon dilatation.

Mortality is around 10% with excellent results. Annual follow-up is needed as in tetralogy of Fallot for IVR or REV and as in truncus arteriosus for a Rastelli procedure.

REFERENCES

1. Neufeld HN, DuShane JW, Edwards JE: Origin of both great vessels from the right ventricle. II: With pulmonary stenosis. Circulation 23:603, 1961.

2. Neufeld HN, DuShane JW, Wood EH, et al: Origin of both great vessels from the right ventricle. I: Without pulmonary stenosis. Circulation 23:399, 1961.

3. Neufeld HN, Lucas RV Jr, Lester RG, et al: Origin of both great vessels from the right ventricle without pulmonary stenosis. Br Heart J 24:393, 1962.

4. Anderson RH, Wilkinson JL, Arnold R, et al: Morphogenesis of bulboventricular malformations. II. Observations on malformed hearts. Br Heart J 36:948, 1974.

5. Sridaramont S, Feldt RH, Ritter DG, et al: Double-outlet right ventricle: Hemodynamic and anatomic correlations. Am J Cardiol 38:85, 1976.

6. Van Praagh S, Davidoff A, Chin A, et al: Double-outlet right ventricle: Anatomic types and developmental implications based on a study of 101 cases. Coeur 12:389, 1982.

7. Lev M, Rimoldi HJA, Eckner FAO, et al: The Taussig-Bing heart: Qualitative and quantitative anatomy. Arch Pathol 81:24, 1966.

8. Wilcox BR, Ho SY, Anderson RH, et al: Surgical anatomy of double-outlet right ventricle with situs solitus and atrioventricular concordance. J Thorac Cardiovasc Surg 82:405, 1981.

9. Lev M, Bharati S, Meng L, et al: A concept of double-outlet right ventricle. J Thorac Cardiovasc Surg 64:271, 1972.

10. Hagler DJ, Edwards WD: Double-outlet left ventricle. In Emmanouilides GC, Allen HD, Riemenschneider TA, Gutgesell HP (eds): Heart Disease in Infants, Children and Adolescents: Including the Fetus and Young Adult, 5th ed. Baltimore, Williams & Wilkins, 1995, p 1270.

11. Lecompte Y, Batisse A, DiCarlo D: Double-outlet right ventricle: A surgical synthesis. Adv Card Surg 4:109, 1993.

12. Kawashima Y, Fujita T, Miyamoto T, Manabe H: Intraventricular rerouting of blood for the correction of Taussig-Bing malformation. J Thorac Cardiovasc Surg 62:825, 1971.

13. Bharati S, Lev M: The conduction system in double outlet right ventricle with subpulmonic ventricular septal defect and related hearts (the Taussig-Bing group). Circulation 54:459, 1976.

14. Rubay J, Lecompte Y, Batisse A, et al: Anatomic repair of anomalies of ventriculo-arterial connection (REV). Eur J Cardiothorac Surg 2:305, 1988.

15. Vouhe PR, Tamisier D, Leca F, et al: Transposition of the great arteries, ventricular septal defect, and pulmonary outflow tract obstruction: Rastelli or Lecompte procedure? J Thorac Cardiovasc Surg 103:428, 1992.

16. Sakata R, Lecompte Y, Batisse A, et al: Anatomic repair of anomalies of ventriculoarterial connection associated with ventricular septal defect. I. Criteria of surgical decision. J Thorac Cardiovasc Surg 95:90, 1988.

17. Kirklin JW, Barratt-Boyes BG: Double outlet right ventricle. In Kirklin JW, Barratt-Boyes BG (eds): Cardiac Surgery, 2nd ed. New York, Churchill Livingstone, 1993, p 1469.

18. Mason DT, Morrow AG, Elkins RC, Friedman WF: Origin of both great vessels from the right ventricle associated with severe obstruction to left ventricular outflow. Am J Cardiol 24:118, 1969.

19. Lavoie R, Sestier F, Gilbert G, et al: Double outlet right ventricle with left ventricular outflow tract obstruction due to small ventricular septal defect. Am Heart J 82:290, 1971.

20. Sondheimer HM, Freedom RM, Olley PM: Double outlet right ventricle: Clinical spectrum and prognosis. Am J Cardiol 37:709, 1977.

CHAPTER 27

CONGENITALLY CORRECTED TRANSPOSITION OF THE GREAT ARTERIES

ROBERT M. FREEDOM

Congenitally corrected transposition of the great arteries does not convey specific information about the cardiac malformation so designated, and the juxtaposition of *congenitally* and *corrected* is an oxymoron and is mostly unjustified in the consideration of this particularly complex disorder.[1,2] The concept of congenitally corrected transposition of the great arteries is predicated on the perception that the effect of transposition of the great arteries is corrected by inversion of the ventricles.[3-6] But as pointed out by Van Praagh and Warnes amongst others, congenitally corrected transposition of the great arteries is only rarely, if ever, corrected.[1,2,7,8] (See Chapters 19 and 20.)

In its simplest and connection analysis, congenitally corrected transposition is characterized by so-called double discordance, with the morphologically right atrium receiving the superior and inferior caval veins, and the coronary sinus connected to the morphologically left ventricle by the mitral valve (Figs. 27-1 and 27-2). The morphologically left atrium, receiving the pulmonary veins, is connected to the morphologically right ventricle by a tricuspid valve. Thus, the atrioventricular connections are discordant. In addition, the ventriculoarterial connection is also discordant with the transposed pulmonary artery originating from the morphologically left ventricle and the aorta from the morphologically right ventricle (see Figs. 27-1 and 27-2). The mitral valve is in fibrous continuity, or nearly so, with the pulmonary valve, while the subaortic infundibulum is well expanded, preventing continuity between aortic and tricuspid valves.[9-27] The mitral valve does not have septal attachments, but the tricuspid valve does (see Fig. 27-1). In the classic expression of this disorder, and in atrial situs solitus, the aorta is leftward and anterior relative to the rightward and inferior pulmonary valve. At one point in the fascinating history of the nosology of congenital heart disease, a leftward and anterior aorta was considered diagnostic of, or at least consistent with, the diagnosis of congenitally corrected transposition, but this is now known to be incorrect (Fig. 27-3).[28-32] Indeed, these so-called loop rule exceptions were quite important to the development and application of a connections approach.[33-51] A wide variety of congenitally malformed hearts have a levopositioned aorta, but the connections are not invariably that of double discordance.[33-51] In some patients with a levopositioned aorta, the atrioventricular and ventriculoarterial connections are concordant; in others, the atrioventricular connection is concordant, but the ventriculoarterial connection is discordant. Finally, there is the rare patient in whom the atrioventricular connection is discordant, but the ventriculoarterial connection is concordant.[52-66]

PREVALENCE

Bjarke and Kidd and Keith, using data from the Hospital for Sick Children in Toronto, identified among 10,535 patients with congenital heart disease 101 with congenitally corrected transposition of the great arteries, thus giving a prevalence of 0.95%, but these data included patients with a univentricular atrioventricular connection.[67,68] Excluding these patients would reduce the prevalence to 0.57%. The Baltimore-Washington Infant Study identified 47 patients with corrected transposition of the great arteries from 4390 infants surveyed from 1981 to 1989.[69] Data provided by Fyler addressing patients seen at the Boston Children's Hospital revealed that over a 15-year period to 1987, 89 patients with corrected transposition of the great arteries were seen, or 0.6% of those with congenital heart disease.[70] The New England Regional Infant Cardiac Program identified only 16 infants with corrected transposition of the great arteries.[71] Data from the Baltimore-Washington Infant Study indicated that the diagnosis of congenitally corrected transposition of the great arteries was made in more than 93% of patients by 3 months of age.[69] The mean birth weight for this cohort was 3080 g, with 15% having a birth weight below 2501 g and 7.5% below 1501 g. Seventeen and one half percent had a gestational age less than 37 weeks and 7.5% less than 35 weeks. Major chromosomal anomalies were not identified in the 47 patients seen in the Baltimore-Washington Infant Study, but identifiable syndromes were established in 11 (23.4%).

SEGMENTAL ANALYSIS

The heart with congenitally corrected transposition is usually left sided, but in about 30 to 40% of patients the heart is right sided or midline.* Atrial situs solitus is identified in about 80%, with atrial situs inversus in

---

*References 9, 10, 12–17, 22, 27, 57.

375

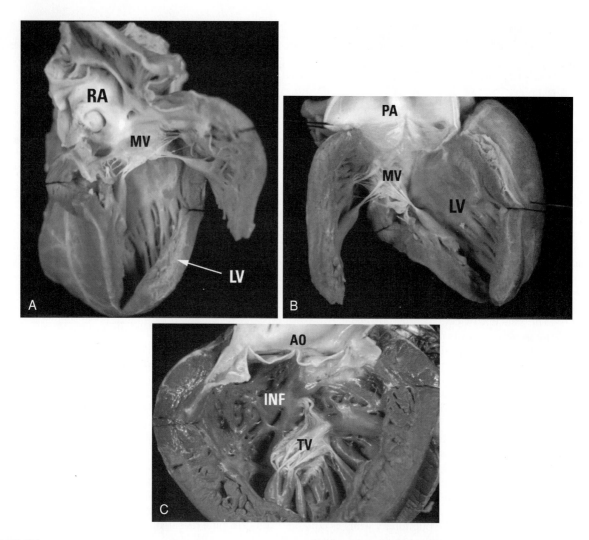

FIGURE 27–1

Internal anatomy of a heart with discordant atrioventricular and ventriculoarterial connections. *A,* Internal view of the right atrium (RA) and the morphologically left ventricle (LV). The atrioventricular junction is guarded by a morphologically mitral valve (MV). *B,* Internal view of a morphologically LV shows the discordantly connected and transposed pulmonary artery (PA). Note the pulmonary-mitral fibrous continuity indicative of the resorption of the subpulmonary conus or its ventriculoinfundibular fold component. *C,* Internal view of the morphologically right ventricle. The internal organization of the left-sided morphologically right ventricle conforms to an L-ventricular loop. The discordantly connected aorta (AO) is supported by a well-defined subaortic infundibulum (INF). TV = tricuspid valve. (*A–C* from Freedom RM, Mawson JB, Yoo SJ, Benson LN [eds]: Congenital Heart Disease: Textbook of Angiocardiography. Armonk, NY, Futura, 1997, pp 1017–1117.)

20%. In those patients with incompletely lateralized atria, one cannot define the atrioventricular connection as discordant.

MORPHOLOGY

Although the ventricles in hearts with corrected transposition of the great arteries may be considered inverted, they are not in a mirror image of a normal heart.[12,14,15] As pointed out by Losekoot and colleagues, this is in large part a consequence of the arterial outflows being parallel to each other, remembering that in the normal heart the outflow tracts cross.[14,22] The ventricles in hearts with solitus atria and atrioventricular discordance have a side-by-side topography with the morphologically left ventricle to

the right of the relatively left-sided morphologically right ventricle (Fig. 27–4). Such hearts may also exhibit supero-inferior disposition of the ventricular masses.[72–88] The internal organization of the morphologically right ventricle in hearts with solitus atria conforms to a left-hand pattern in contrast to the right-hand pattern of the right ventricle when the atrioventricular connections are concordant.[14–17,23–25,51] However, the spatial relationship between the ventricles does not predict the type of atrioventricular connection. Rarely the pattern of internal ventricular organization is nonharmonious with the type of atrioventricular connection.[35–42] Thus, in these unusual hearts, despite an L-ventricular loop in terms of internal organization, the atrioventricular connection is concordant. The connections approach to the definition of congenitally corrected transposition of the great arteries as

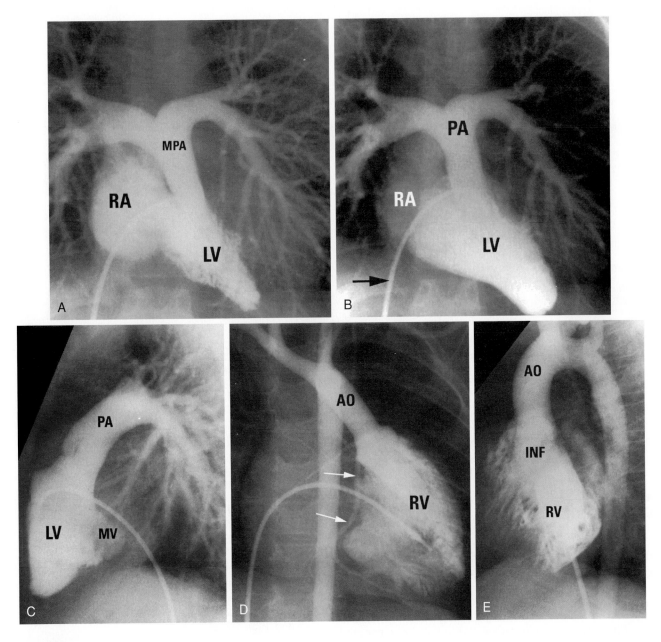

FIGURE 27–2

Angiographic demonstration of discordant atrioventricular and ventriculoarterial connections in a patient with atrial situs solitus and levocardia. *A,* Frontal projection of the morphologically right atrium (RA) showing the connection to the morphologically left ventricle (LV), which supports the discordantly connected main pulmonary artery (MPA). *B,* Selective injection into the LV in the frontal projection shows the medially positioned discordantly connected pulmonary trunk. *C,* The left ventricular injection via the mitral valve (MV) in the lateral projection shows the discordantly connected pulmonary artery (PA). *D, E,* Frontal and lateral right ventriculogram shows the discordantly connected aorta (AO) supported by a well-defined subaortic infundibulum (INF). RV = right ventricle.

that condition characterized by discordant atrioventricular and ventriculoarterial connections does not consider the infundibular anatomy of this condition. The leftward subaortic infundibulum is well expanded, whereas there has been resorption, or nearly so, of the subpulmonary infundibulum. Thus, in the patient with the typical expression of congenitally corrected transposition of the great arteries, the infundibular anatomy is similar, if not identical, to the infundibular anatomy of the heart with the most common form of complete transposition of the great arter-

ies (atrioventricular concordance and ventriculoarterial discordance).

RELATIONSHIP BETWEEN THE GREAT ARTERIES

Usually the aorta is anterior and to the left of the pulmonary trunk in the classic expression of congenitally corrected transposition of the great arteries, but this spatial relationship is not pathognomonic for this condition (see Figs. 27–1 to 27–3). Indeed, this spatial relationship be-

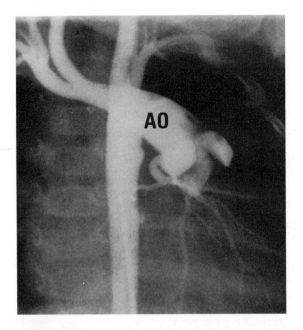

FIGURE 27–3

The levopositioned aorta (AO) was once considered diagnostic of an L-ventricular loop and L-transposition of the great arteries. It is now clear that many hearts with a levopositioned aorta have concordant atrioventricular connections and a wide variety of ventriculoarterial connections.

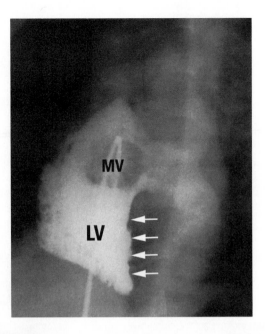

FIGURE 27–4

The disposition of the interventricular septum is usually more vertically or horizontally disposed when the atrioventricular connection is discordant. This frontal left ventriculogram, via the mitral valve (MV), shows the ventricular septum (*arrows*). LV = left ventricle.

tween the great arteries can be seen in a variety of congenitally malformed hearts as discussed earlier in this chapter (Table 27–1).[33–51]

CORONARY ARTERIES

The coronary arteries originate from the facing sinuses of the aortic valve. In patients with atrial situs solitus and congenitally corrected transposition of the great arteries, the coronary arteries show a mirror-image distribution.° The right-sided coronary artery has the pattern of a morphologically left coronary artery, with the main coronary artery bifurcating into circumflex and anterior descending branches, whereas the left-sided coronary artery runs in the left atrioventricular groove and gives rise to infundibular and marginal branches. The coronary artery anatomy in patients with double discordance has assumed more im-

°References 9–12, 14–17, 27, 51, 89–93.

portance since the introduction of the double-switch procedure (see later).

THE VENTRICULOARTERIAL CONNECTION IN HEARTS WITH ATRIOVENTRICULAR DISCORDANCE

These hearts, despite the diversity of ventriculoarterial connection, are unified in many aspects by the implications of the atrioventricular connection and malformations attendant to the discordant atrioventricular connection (Fig. 27–5 and Table 27–2).

COMMONLY ASSOCIATED CARDIAC ANOMALIES

Hearts exhibiting a double discordance are rarely corrected. Indeed, most individuals with atrioventricular and ventriculoarterial discordance have one or more of the following commonly associated cardiac anomalies shown in Table 27–3.

TABLE 27–1

DIFFERENTIAL DIAGNOSIS OF A LEVOPOSITIONED AORTA

Double discordance
Anatomically corrected malposition of the great arteries
Complete transposition of the great arteries with a levopositioned aorta
Double-outlet right ventricle° with a levopositioned aorta
Double-outlet left ventricle° with a levopositioned aorta
Superior-inferior ventricles° with a levopositioned aorta
Crossed or twisted atrioventricular connections

°With concordant atrioventricular connections.

TABLE 27–2

VENTRICULOARTERIAL CONNECTIONS IN HEARTS WITH A DISCORDANT ATRIOVENTRICULAR CONNECTION

Discordant ventriculoarterial connection
Double-outlet right ventricle
Concordant ventriculoarterial connection
Double-outlet left ventricle
Single-outlet aorta°

°Usually from morphologically right ventricle.

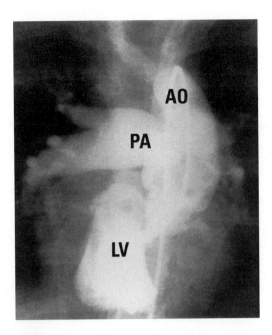

FIGURE 27–5

Double-outlet right ventricle in a patient with atrioventricular discordance. This frontal left ventriculogram demonstrates that both great arteries originate predominately above the right ventricle. AO = aorta; LV = left ventricle; PA = pulmonary artery.

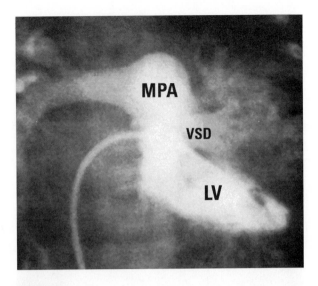

FIGURE 27–6

The ventricular septal defect (VSD) may occupy any position but is usually perimembranous. This frontal left ventriculogram shows the perimembranous ventricular septal defect. MPA = main pulmonary artery; LV = left ventricle.

Indeed, these anomalies are so common in hearts with atrioventricular discordance that they should be considered part of the malformation complex.

Ventricular Septal Defect

A ventricular septal defect is the most common associated malformation in congenitally corrected transposition of the great arteries, having an incidence in clinical material between 60 to 70%, and nearly 80% in autopsy material.* The most common ventricular septal defect is perimembranous and tends to be subpulmonary (Fig. 27–6). The ventricular septal defect is usually large, reflecting in part the malalignment between the atrial septum and the ventricular septum, which is characteristic of hearts exhibiting atrioventricular and ventriculoarterial discordance. The resulting left-to-right shunt is important. The ventricular septal defect may be subarterial and roofed by the semilunar valves. This is uncommon in the Western world, but not uncommon at all in the East.[95] The ventricular septal defect can indeed occupy any position. In the presence of a straddling and overriding tricuspid valve, the ventricular

septal defect involves the inlet portion of the ventricular septum, which is malaligned to the left side from the atrial septum and crux cordis, whereas in that rare situation in which the mitral valve straddles, the ventricular septal defect involves the anterior portion of the ventricular septum. A Swiss-cheese interventricular septum with many ventricular septal defects is uncommon in hearts with atrioventricular and ventriculoarterial discordance.

Pulmonary Outflow Tract Obstruction

Pulmonary outflow tract obstruction is identified in 30 to 50% of patients with corrected transposition of the great arteries and atrial situs solitus.* Such pulmonary outflow tract obstruction uncommonly occurs in isolation at the valve or infundibular level (Fig. 27–7), but it is more typically associated with a large ventricular septal defect (Fig. 27–8). In about one third of these patients with ventricular septal defect and pulmonary outflow tract obstruction, abnormalities of the morphologically tricuspid valve are also seen (Table 27–4).

*References 7–17, 27, 51, 70, 92, 94–102.

*References 9–17, 27, 51, 70, 94–97.

TABLE 27–3

CARDIAC ANOMALIES COMMONLY FOUND IN HEARTS WITH DOUBLE DISCORDANCE

Ventricular septal defect
Left ventricular (pulmonary) outflow tract obstruction
Systemic (tricuspid) atrioventricular valve displacement or dysplasia
Abnormal atrioventricular conduction tissue

TABLE 27–4

MECHANISMS OF LEFT VENTRICULAR OUTFLOW TRACT (PULMONARY) OBSTRUCTION IN DISCORDANT ATRIOVENTRICULAR AND VENTRICULOARTERIAL CONNECTIONS

Potential for left ventricular outflow tract obstruction because of wedging of outflow tract between inverted mitral and tricuspid valves
Infundibular and valvar pulmonary stenosis
Tissue tags derived from intact or perforated membranous septum, inverted tricuspid valve, or pulmonary valve
Blood cysts attached to the pulmonary valve
Subpulmonary tag originating from both sides of the ventricular septum

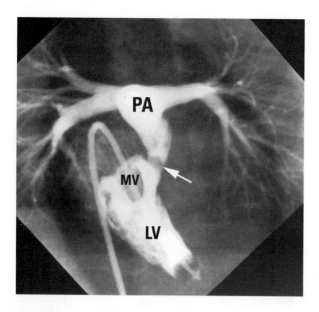

Left ventricular outflow tract obstruction in a patient with atrioventricular and ventriculoarterial discordance and an intact ventricular septum. This frontal left ventriculogram via the mitral valve (MV) demonstrates the subpulmonary left ventricular outflow tract obstruction *(arrow)*. PA = pulmonary artery; LV = left ventricle.

The left ventricular outflow tract obstruction is usually complex and muscular, which reflects wedging of the subpulmonary outflow tract between the infundibular septum and the ventricular free wall, with contributions from the right-sided ventriculoinfundibular fold (see Fig. 27–8). In those patients with a muscular tunnel form of left ventric-

ular outflow tract obstruction, the subpulmonary infundibulum is well developed, and thus bilateral muscular infundibula are present. Fibrous tissue derived from the membranous septum may also contribute to left ventricular outflow tract obstruction, and this may be wholly resectable.[100–102] Tissue tags derived from the tricuspid, mitral, or pulmonary valve itself may obstruct flow into the pulmonary trunk. Blood cysts may also participate in subpulmonary obstruction.[99] Single-outlet aorta with pulmonary atresia is well-recognized with atrioventricular discordance.

Lesions of the Morphologically Tricuspid Valve

Abnormalities of the morphologically tricuspid valve are intrinsic to hearts exhibiting congenitally corrected transposition of the great arteries° (Figs. 27–9 and 27–10). Although at the autopsy table, about 90% of hearts exhibit some abnormality of the morphologically tricuspid valve, considerably fewer demonstrate a functional disturbance during life. The most common and important underlying pathology is dysplasia of the tricuspid valve, with or without displacement of the septal or posterior leaflets of the tricuspid valve° (see Fig. 27–9). Indeed, hearts with double discordance rarely demonstrate the degree of displacement of the systemic atrioventricular (tricuspid) valve as seen in the most severe expression of Ebstein anomaly in the heart with concordant connections. In addition, the anterior leaflet of the left-sided tricuspid valve is rarely as sail-like as its concordant cousin. Some hearts with congenitally corrected transposition of the great arteries ex-

---

°References 1, 2, 7–10, 12–17, 22, 27, 51, 70, 92, 96, 97, 103–112.

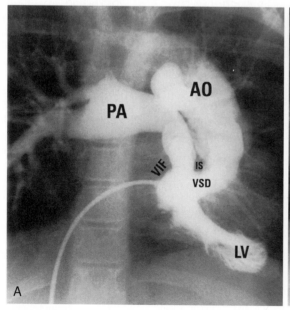
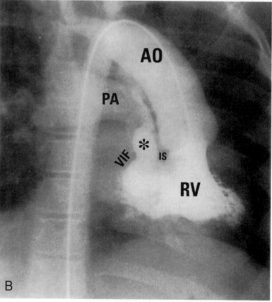

Left ventricular outflow tract obstruction and a ventricular septal defect (VSD) in a patient with atrioventricular and ventriculoarterial discordance. *A,* The frontal left ventriculogram profiles the VSD. The left ventricle (LV) is inferior to the superiorly positioned morphologically right ventricle. The subpulmonary and left ventricular outflow tract is wedged between the infundibular septum (IS) medially and the ventriculoinfundibular fold (VIF) laterally. *B,* Frontal injection into the somewhat small superiorly positioned right ventricle (RV) shows the diffusely narrow left ventricular outflow tract *(asterisk)*. AO = aorta; PA = pulmonary artery.

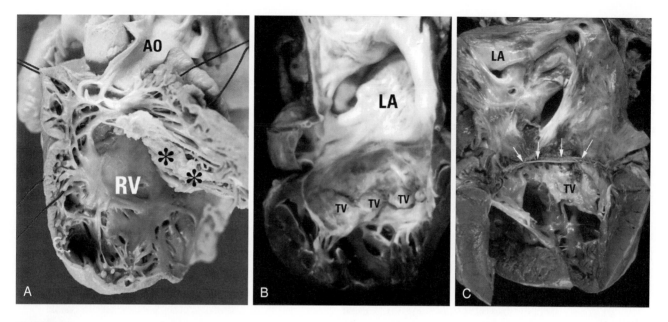

FIGURE 27–9

Various appearances of the morphologically tricuspid valve (TV) in the patient with atrioventricular and ventriculoarterial discordance. *A,* Profound dysplasia of the tricuspid valve *(asterisks)* in a patient with intact ventricular septum, clinically florid tricuspid regurgitation, and interruption of the aortic arch (AO). *B,* Displacement and dysplasia of the tricuspid valve. *C,* Unsuccessful annuloplasty *(arrows)* in a patient with a complex form of atrioventricular and ventriculoarterial discordance and a severely dysplastic TV. LA = left atrium; RV = right ventricle.

hibit an unguarded tricuspid orifice, whereas in others the tricuspid valve straddles and overrides a muscular inlet ventricular septal defect.[113,114] A stenotic, Ebstein-like tricuspid valve, dividing the morphologically right ventricle, has also been described.[115]

Specialized Conduction Tissue

Intrinsic to hearts exhibiting atrioventricular discordance is a particularly unique and fragile specialized conduction system.* It is the unusual disposition of the conduction tissue that predisposes patients with atrioventricular discordance to progressive and spontaneous third-degree heart block. The sinus node is normally positioned in these hearts, but the atrioventricular conduction tissue is grossly abnormal. The abnormal disposition has been elegantly reviewed by Losekoot, Anderson, and others.[116–125] In brief, the basic anatomy dictates that the regular atrioventricular node, located at the apex of the triangle of Koch, cannot give origin to a penetrating atrioventricular conduction bundle. Thus, an anomalous second atrioventricular node is present, located beneath the opening of the right atrial appendage at the lateral margin of the area between pulmonary valve and mitral valve continuity. This anteriorly positioned node gives rise to the atrioventricular bundle that comes to lie immediately underneath the pulmonary valve leaflets.[116–119] The nonbranching bundle has a superficial course underneath the right anterior facing leaflet of the pulmonary valve and descends for some distance before it branches. Rarely, as in the report by Kurosawa and colleagues of a patient with congenitally corrected transposition of the great arteries, large perimembranous ventric-

ular septal defect, and straddling mitral valve, there is a regularly positioned posterior node and bundle.[120]

Other Associated Cardiac Anomalies

Hearts with double discordance have been identified with a wide range of abnormalities of the systemic and pulmonary veins, atrioventricular septal defect, straddling and overriding tricuspid or mitral valves, hypoplasia of the morphologically right or left ventricle, subdivision of the left atrium from either a classic cor triatriatum or a supravalvar-stenosing tricuspid ring, real or functional aortic atresia, subaortic stenosis, aortic coarctation, aortic arch atresia, or aortic interruption* (Fig. 27–11).

Ventricular Hypoplasia

Hypoplasia of either the morphologically left or right ventricle has been well described in patients with atrioventricular and ventriculoarterial discordance, although data from our institution would suggest that hypoplasia of the morphologically left ventricle is less common† (see Fig. 27–8). In those patients with left ventricular hypoplasia, one should certainly scrutinize the form and function of the mitral valve, as stenosis, straddling, and overriding of the mitral valve have been amply recorded.[120,137–139] Severe displacement of the tricuspid valve reduces the functional component of the morphologically right ventricle, and similarly a straddling and overriding tricuspid valve may jeopardize the form, function, and size of the morphologically right ventricle.

---

*References 1, 2, 7–9, 13–17, 51, 70, 90–98, 116–125.

*References 1, 2, 7–17, 26, 27, 51, 70, 72–77, 96, 97, 106–113, 125–145.

†References 16, 51, 129, 130, 133, 134.

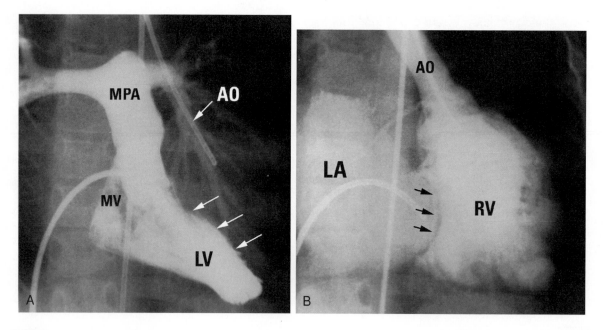

FIGURE 27–10

Severe systemic or tricuspid regurgitation in a child with atrioventricular and ventriculoarterial discordance and an intact ventricular septum. The frontal left ventriculogram shows the discordantly connected main pulmonary trunk (MPA), the ventricular septum *(small white arrows)*, and the course of the retrograde arterial catheter; note the levopositioned aorta (AO). *B*, Retrograde right ventriculogram demonstrates severe tricuspid regurgitation into a much enlarged left atrium (LA); the *small black arrows* indicate the thickened tricuspid valve. MV = mitral valve; LV = left ventricle; RV = right ventricle.

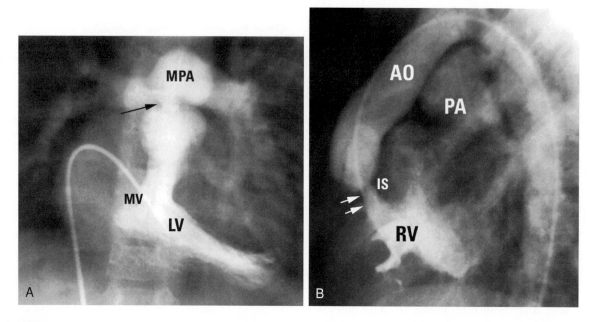

FIGURE 27–11

Severe systemic outflow tract obstruction in a female patient with atrioventricular and ventriculoarterial discordance and a once large ventricular septal defect (VSD) treated elsewhere with palliative pulmonary artery banding. The VSD became restrictive, and the patient developed severe systemic outflow tract obstruction. She underwent successfully a double-switch procedure with a Mustard atrial switch, arterial switch, right ventricular outflow tract patch, and a bidirectional cavopulmonary connection. *A*, The frontal left ventriculogram shows the banded *(arrow)* main pulmonary trunk. *B*, The retrograde lateral right ventriculogram demonstrates the severe and tunnel form *(arrows)* systemic outflow tract obstruction. MPA = main pulmonary artery; MV = mitral valve; LV = left ventricle; AO = aorta; PA = pulmonary artery; IS = infundibular septum; RV = right ventricle.

Systemic Ventricular Outflow Tract Obstruction

The morphologic bases for subaortic stenosis in hearts with double discordance are diverse but may be related to os infundibular stenosis (see Fig. 27–11), a divided right ventricle, strategically disposed tissue tags, or some combination of these.*

Aortic Atresia

Aortic atresia in the setting of double discordance is uncommon, but both functional and anatomic aortic atresia have been described. The one feature common to those patients with either functional or organic aortic atresia is severe systemic (tricuspid) atrioventricular valve regurgitation and a disadvantaged morphologically right ventricle, analogous to the pathogenesis of organic or functional pulmonary atresia in the patient with concordant connections and florid tricuspid regurgitation.[106–112]

Coarctation of the Aorta: Arch Atresia and Interruption of the Aortic Arch

All expressions of an obstructed aortic arch have been recorded in patients with atrioventricular and ventriculoarterial discordance.† Many of these patients have an associated ventricular septal defect with or without significant tricuspid regurgitation. Some years ago, my colleagues and I reported a neonate with interruption of the aortic arch and terribly severe tricuspid regurgitation but no ventricular septal defect or aortopulmonary window; it was likely the severe systemic atrioventricular regurgitation reduced flow to the fourth aortic arch.[146]

CLINICAL FEATURES

Patients with congenitally corrected transposition of the great arteries in isolation should be asymptomatic. Symptoms usually reflect the associated malformations.‡ Thus, individuals with corrected transposition of the great arteries may come to attention because of (1) bradycardia (with or without heart failure), reflecting a high-degree atrioventricular block; (2) tachydysrhythmia; (3) cyanosis, reflecting inadequate pulmonary blood flow (usually indicative of a ventricular septal defect and severe pulmonary outflow tract obstruction); and (4) congestive heart failure. Congestive heart failure may reflect a cardiac dysrhythmia, but more likely heralds structural malformations including a large ventricular septal defect; dysplasia or displacement of the left-sided morphologically tricuspid valve; obstructive anomalies of the aortic arch; functional or organic aortic atresia; or combinations of these anomalies (Table 27–5). Although an older child may be referred to a pediatric cardiologist for evaluation of a loud second heart sound (and thus the clinical suspicion of pulmonary artery hypertension), this is uncommon in a young infant. Rather, a neonate presents for one of the reasons mentioned in Table 27–5. The physical examination only occasionally suggests the possibility of atrioventricular and ventriculoarterial discordance. Clearly the presence of, for example, mitral regurgitation in a neonate or young infant or child should raise the consideration of corrected transposition of the great arteries and a regurgitant systemic atrioventricular valve.

In some neonates with congenitally corrected transposition of the great arteries, regurgitation of the systemic atrioventricular valve may be massive, and such patients may have such profound cardiomegaly that they are clinically considered to have classic Ebstein anomaly of the tricuspid valve (with concordant atrioventricular and ventriculoarterial connections).[51] Organic or functional aortic atresia has been described in these patients and common to them all is a terribly disorganized and deficient morphologically tricuspid valve and an extremely thinned, morphologically right ventricle.

Huhta and colleagues[147] have addressed the natural history of patients with congenitally corrected transposition of the great arteries. The Mayo Clinic reviewed the long-term follow-up of 107 patients seen during a 30-year period (1951 to 1981). The only variable that correlated with decreased survival rate was left atrioventricular valve insufficiency. The survival rate from the date of the Mayo Clinic diagnosis was 70% at 5 years and 64% at 10 years. Clearly this is a biased series because of the unique referral pattern of the Mayo Clinic. The mean age at the Mayo Clinic diagnosis was 12.7 years, ranging from birth to 56 years.

FUNCTION OF THE MORPHOLOGICALLY RIGHT (SYSTEMIC) VENTRICLE

In the conventional operative management of certain forms of congenital heart disease, the morphologically right ventricle must function as the systemic ventricle.[148] And thus the following question has been asked so often in this situation: Can the morphologically right ventricle continue to function for a normal lifetime as the systemic ventricle? All centers have instances of late right ventricular failure after an atrial switch procedure for transposition of the great arteries, a right ventricular failure after the first-stage Norwood operation for hypoplastic left-sided heart syndrome, a bidirectional cavopulmonary connection, or a chronic heart failure after a Fontan operation for a univentricular heart of right ventricular type. A number of studies have addressed right ventricular function in these types of cardiac malformations, and concerns about the morphologically right ventricle after atrial switch surgery have led many centers in the past decade to adopt anatomic repair (arterial repair with coronary transfer) as the procedure of

TABLE 27–5
MODES OF PRESENTATION OF PATIENTS WITH ATRIOVENTRICULAR AND VENTRICULOARTERIAL DISCORDANCE (CORRECTED TRANSPOSITION OF THE GREAT ARTERIES)

Loud second heart sound suggestive of pulmonary hypertension
High-degree atrioventricular block
Heart failure
Cyanosis
Heart murmur
Tachydysrhythmia

---

*References 15, 16, 51, 106–112, 127, 131, 132, 145.
†References 15, 16, 51, 106–112, 127, 131, 132, 145.
‡References 7, 8, 10, 13–17, 51, 58, 70, 82.

choice for transposition of the great arteries. A number of case reports have been published addressing survival to the fifth, sixth, seventh, and eighth decades of life in the individual with uncomplicated congenitally corrected transposition of the great arteries, and these instances have been used to argue that the morphologically right ventricle can function at systemic afterload for many decades.[2,7,8,149–154] Beyond these anecdotal reports, however, Benson and colleagues[155] and others have addressed the function of the morphologically right ventricle using many modes of assessment.[130,156,157] These studies, for the most part, indicate that the morphologically right ventricle can function as normally as the systemic ventricle. My colleagues and I have marshalled evidence based on radionuclide assessment of ventricular function supporting preservation of right ventricular integrity.[155] A similar conclusion based on a different method was reached by Dimas and colleagues.[156] Yet, data from Peterson and colleagues[157] suggest that systemic ventricular ejection fraction does not increase from rest to exercise, indicative of an abnormal exercise response. The issue has not been completely resolved, although at rest, systolic function of the systemic morphologically right ventricle may be reasonably well preserved. Relatively few data on morphologically right ventricular diastolic function are available.

Assessment of right ventricular function is clearly important in these patients. In some patients, progressive systemic atrioventricular valve regurgitation may occur after repair of ventricular septal defect with or without left ventricular outflow tract obstruction.* In this clinical situation, the function of the morphologically right ventricle is often depressed, and thus the atrioventricular valve regurgitation reflects a failing right ventricle and annular dilatation, or it has severe atrioventricular valve regurgitation that has impacted on ventricular function. It may be difficult, if not impossible, in some of these clinical situations to sort out the "chicken from the egg" phenomenon.

DIFFERENTIAL DIAGNOSIS

The differential diagnosis is broad, and for babies in severe heart failure, this includes isolated ventricular septal defect, single- or double-inlet ventricle malformation, tricuspid atresia with increased pulmonary blood flow, double-outlet right ventricle with subaortic ventricular septal defect, and other conditions. When cyanosis and reduced pulmonary blood flow are observed, the differential diagnosis of tetralogy of Fallot is appropriate to consider.

DIAGNOSTIC TECHNIQUES

ELECTROCARDIOGRAPHY

The salient electrocardiographic features have received considerable attention.[9–11,13,16,17,51,70] In an individual with normal atrial situs and discordant atrioventricular and ventriculoarterial connections who is free from significant intracardiac associated malformations, the direction of the frontal P wave axis is normal and therefore positive in leads I, II, III, aVL, and aVF, but negative in aVR. Clearly the position of the heart with the thorax does not influence the P wave vector or axis.

The electrical activation of the ventricles in the normal heart begins in the interventricular septum and is directed from left to right and in a slightly anterior direction as well. This initial activation is responsible for the normal pattern of q waves in the precordial leads: a qR pattern in V_6 and an Rs in V_1. The absence of q waves in the left precordial leads is seldom observed in normal children, but 25% of normal neonates may not demonstrate a q wave in V_6 (see Table 27–3).

In corrected transposition of the great arteries, the interventricular septum is more or less sagittal and is oriented from left posterior to right anterior. With ventricular inversion, both its surfaces and ventricular bundle branches are inverted, and thus the sequence of initial activation is oriented from right to left and usually in a more superior and anterior direction. This results in a reversal of the normal q wave pattern in the precordial leads: q waves are present in the right precordial leads but are absent in the left precordial leads (see Table 27–3). This pattern of reversal is less commonly appreciated when the heart is right sided or when there are confounding associated lesions producing pressure or volume overload (Table 27–6).

CHEST RADIOGRAPHY

The plain chest radiographic findings of patients with congenitally corrected transposition have been extensively reviewed. There is no single feature diagnostic of this condition.* Even though a conspicuous levopositioned aorta may suggest this diagnosis, a levopositioned aorta is not diagnostic of double discordance.

ECHOCARDIOGRAPHY

As in the echocardiographic analysis of any complex heart malformation, atrial situs should be defined as situs solitus or inversus by identifying the spatial relationship of the abdominal aorta and the inferior vena cava. The connections of the systemic and pulmonary veins should be traced to their appropriate atria. This is achieved most readily from a subcostal four-chamber view with superior and inferior angulation to identify the superior and inferior vena cava, and a straight four-chamber view to visualize the pul-

---

*References 9–11, 13, 16, 17, 51, 58, 70, 169.

TABLE 27–6

CAUSES OF A qR PATTERN IN THE RIGHT PRECORDIAL LEADS OF THE ELECTROCARDIOGRAM

Ventricular inversion
Hypoplastic left-sided heart syndrome
Total anomalous pulmonary venous connection
Transposition of the great arteries
Double-outlet ventricle

---

*References 2, 8, 9, 15, 16, 51, 70, 94–98, 130, 155–157.

monary arteries. After the identification of the pulmonary and systemic venous atria, the connections of the atria to the ventricular mass should be identified through the use of a subcostal four-chamber view.[16, 17, 51, 170–174] The striking finding is the vertical, rather than oblique, orientation of the interventricular septum and its malalignment with the interatrial septum. This combination of findings is almost unique for corrected transposition and should alert the examiner to the diagnosis. If the echocardiographer has been performing a sequential examination, this added clue is unnecessary, because it would be obvious that the pulmonary venous atrium corrects with a left-sided (in levocardia) morphologically right ventricle and the systemic venous atrium with a right-sided morphologically left ventricle. The morphology of the ventricles can be identified by their difference in trabecular pattern, which is usually evident even in the neonate or through the identification of the atrioventricular valves. The morphologic right ventricle appears heavily trabeculated and has a moderator band visible at the apex, whereas the left ventricle has a smooth septal surface, and the septum is convex toward the left ventricle. The morphology of the ventricles can also be determined through their corresponding atrioventricular valves. The mitral valve has a typical fish-mouth appearance in the subcostal short-axis view, whereas the tricuspid valve has a clover-leaf configuration with septal attachments. After the identification of the atrioventricular connection, the transducer should be angled superiorly toward the outflow areas of the heart. The pulmonary artery, which is wedged between the atrioventricular valves, originates from the morphologic left ventricle, and the aorta, which is supported by a muscular infundibulum, originates above the morphologically right ventricle. There are ample descriptions of the echocardiographic features of the ventricular septal defect, left ventricular outflow tract obstruction, and form and function of the morphologically tricuspid valve in patients with double discordance.

CARDIAC CATHETERIZATION AND ANGIOCARDIOGRAPHY

The anatomic diagnosis of double discordance should be made before cardiac catheterization, and thus hemodynamic and angiocardiographic data must answer specific questions. The hemodynamics are not specific for corrected transposition of the great arteries but rather reflect the associated intracardiac malformations and cardiac output. Thus, in the absence of pulmonary parenchymal disease, arterial desaturation of a significant degree reflects intracardiac right-to-left ventricular shunting with the anatomic matrix of pulmonary outflow tract obstruction and ventricular septal defect (i.e., tetralogy-like hemodynamics). A large left-to-right shunt at the pulmonary level most likely reflects shunting at the ventricular level, with additional contributions from shunting through an atrial septal defect or stretched foramen ovale, or at the ductal level.

Systemic pressures in the morphologically left ventricle and pulmonary trunk may reflect the presence of a large ventricular septal defect in isolation, a large ventricular septal defect with associated insufficiency of the sys-

temic atrioventricular valve, or severe insufficiency of the systemic atrioventricular valve. An obstructive anomaly of the aortic arch may complicate any of these situations. Systemic pressures in both the morphologically left and the morphologically right ventricles may be defined in those patients with massive insufficiency of the systemic atrioventricular valve and functional or organic aortic atresia.[110]

Angiocardiography performed in both ventricles in frontal and lateral or axial projections confirms the atrioventricular and ventriculoarterial discordance.* The presence or absence of a ventricular septal defect and any morphologic basis for pulmonary outflow tract obstruction are readily defined by axial angiocardiography.

Aortic root angiography should define the integrity of the transverse aortic arch and isthmus, exclude the presence of coarctation of the aorta, define the typical origin and distribution of the coronary arteries, and demonstrate the presence and severity of aortic incompetence.[90, 91, 182–186]

CHANGE IN FORM AND FUNCTION OF HEARTS WITH DOUBLE DISCORDANCE

Hearts with atrioventricular and ventriculoarterial discordance should be expected to demonstrate progressive left ventricular outflow tract obstruction (assuming the substrate exists for this condition); progressive incompetence of the systemic atrioventricular valve; progressive atrioventricular block, culminating in complete or third-degree atrioventricular block; and deterioration in right ventricular function. The observation that progressive deterioration in right ventricular function or tricuspid regurgitation is not necessarily related to operative intervention has led to a re-evaluation of surgical strategies.

SURGICAL CONSIDERATIONS

Historically, operation in patients with double discordance in the setting of a biventricular heart has addressed the associated conditions.† In those with a large left-to-right shunt and congestive heart failure, the ventricular septal defect was closed, with the sutures placed on the right ventricular septal side, a consideration of de Leval and colleagues[124] to reduce the operative incidence of complete heart block. Patients with a large ventricular septal defect and left ventricular outflow tract obstruction required ventricular septal defect closure and a conduit interposed between the morphologically left ventricle and the pulmonary trunk. Some patients either in isolation or with other surgical maneuvers also required attention to the systemic atrioventricular valve, usually tricuspid valvuloplasty or replacement. But despite seemingly successful operations, some patients developed progressive and worsening systemic atrioventricular valve regurgitation, progressive failure of the systemic right ventricle, or both.

---

*References 14–17, 51, 70, 140, 175–184.
†References 7, 8, 13–17, 51, 70, 94–97, 128, 129, 153, 158–168, 187.

These clinical realities led Ilbawi and colleagues[159] to conceive and perform a double-switch operation in two patients. The operation consisted of both a venous switch and a ventricular switch (Rastelli-type) operation. This operation uses the morphologically left ventricle as the systemic pumping chamber, thereby minimizing long-term failure of the morphologically right ventricle. It also allows closure of the defect from the right ventricular side of the septum, thus decreasing the prevalence of complete atrioventricular block. Because the morphologically left ventricle now becomes the systemic ventricle, the tricuspid valve no longer serves as the systemic atrioventricular valve and therefore decreases the chance of postoperative and progressive atrioventricular valve regurgitation. Others have now combined a venous switch of the Mustard or Senning type with a classic arterial switch procedure in the operative strategy for patients with a double discordance[160–168] (see Fig. 27–11). Although these operations potentially have certain benefits for the patient with double discordance, they are not without complications (Table 27–7). For patients undergoing both the venous switch and classic arterial switch procedures, one could expect all the complications of the atrial switch procedures (see Table 27–7) and those of the arterial switch procedure (Table 27–8).

MEDICAL CONSIDERATIONS

For those patients identified to be in sinus rhythm, yearly or more frequent scalar electrocardiograms and Holter ambulatory recordings are absolutely essential.[1, 2, 7, 8, 13–17, 51] When these patients are old enough to exercise, usually older than 6 years, a yearly graded exercise test to assess atrioventricular conduction in response to exercise is recommended. In addition, radionuclide evaluation of the function of the morphologically right ventricle may be helpful in the determination of the timing of intervention.[182]

ADULTS WITH CONGENITALLY CORRECTED TRANSPOSITION OF THE GREAT ARTERIES

Connelly and colleagues[153] have reviewed the course of 52 adults (all older than 18 years) with congenitally corrected transposition of the great arteries seen at the Toronto Con-

---

TABLE 27–7

COMPLICATIONS OF THE ATRIAL SWITCH AND VENTRICULAR SWITCH OPERATIONS

Complications of the Atrial Switch Procedure

  Damage to sinoatrial node or artery
  Baffle complications, including superior or inferior limb or pulmonary venous obstruction; baffle leaks

Complications of the Ventricular Switch Operation

  Restrictive ventricular septal defect producing systemic outflow obstruction
  Aortic incompetence
  Problems related to the right ventricle–pulmonary artery conduit

---

TABLE 27–8

COMPLICATIONS OF THE ARTERIAL SWITCH OPERATION

  Pulmonary outflow and arterial obstruction
  Supra-aortic obstruction
  Aortic incompetence
  Myocardial ischemia
  Late coronary arterial obstruction

---

genital Cardiac Centre for Adults from 1985 to 1996. About 25% died during the study period.[153] Many had undergone prior palliative or definitive repair. Left ventricle-to-pulmonary artery conduit replacement was frequent. Twelve (23%) developed third-degree atrioventricular block at the time of definitive repair, and nine patients developed progressive atrioventricular block unrelated to operation; supraventricular rhythm disturbances developed in 15 patients. Progressive systemic atrioventricular regurgitation developed in 10 patients and endocarditis in 6 patients.

My colleagues and I have reviewed the results of surgery in 124 patients with atrioventricular discordance seen from 1957 to 1997 in our institution.[167] The ventriculoarterial connection was discordant in 88% and concordant in 6%; double-outlet right ventricle was seen in 5% and double-outlet left ventricle in 0.8%. The initial operative mortality rate was only 7%, but 15 years after repair, the survival rate was only 50%, reflecting primarily progressive systemic atrioventricular valve regurgitation, deterioration of the function of the morphologically right ventricle, and reoperation to replace a left ventricle to pulmonary artery conduit. Indeed, in many patients progressive systemic atrioventricular valve regurgitation and deterioration of the function of the morphologically right ventricle occurred after primary repair of the associated lesions (namely, ventricular septal defect and left ventricular outflow tract obstruction). Similar findings have been published by Lundstrum and colleagues[8] reviewing patients from the Great Ormond Street Hospital for Sick Children and the National Heart Hospital, London. The experience with a double-switch procedure is really in its infancy. Only time and a larger cohort of patients surviving a double-switch procedure may demonstrate the efficacy of this operation, providing information about long-term risks and benefits.

ISOLATED ATRIOVENTRICULAR DISCORDANCE

Isolated atrioventricular discordance is quite uncommon,[63–66] and when this occurs without major other malformations, the single discordance produces transposition physiology. Because the aorta originates from the morphologically left ventricle and the pulmonary trunk from the morphologically right ventricle, the great arteries are not transposed. The most commonly associated abnormalities include hypoplasia of the morphologically right ventricle, a ventricular septal defect, and displacement or dysplasia of the tricuspid valve. Although some patients may be candidates for the Mustard or Senning operation, others require a one ventricle approach.[60–62, 66]

REFERENCES

1. Van Praagh R: What is congenitally corrected transposition? N Engl J Med 282:1097, 1970.
2. Warnes CA: Congenitally corrected transposition: The uncorrected misnomer. J Am Coll Cardiol 27:1244, 1996.
3. Von Rokitansky C: Die Defecte der Scheidewande des Herzens. Wien, Wilhelm Braumuller, 1875.
4. Monckeberg JG: Zur Entwicklungsgeschichte des Atrioventrikularsystems. Verh Dtsch Ges Pathol 16:228, 1913.
5. Uher V: Zur Pathologie des Reisleitungssystems bei kongenitalen Herzanomalien. Frankfurter Z Pathol 49:347, 1936.
6. Harris JS, Farber S: Transposition of the great cardiac vessels, with special reference to phylogenetic theory of Spitzer. Arch Pathol 28:427, 1939.
7. Presbitero P, Somerville J, Rabajoli F, et al: Corrected transposition of the great arteries without associated defects in adult patients: Clinical profile and follow up. Br Heart J 74:57, 1995.
8. Lundstrom U, Bull C, Wyse RK, Somerville J: The natural and "unnatural" history of congenitally corrected transposition. Am J Cardiol 65:1222, 1990.
9. Schiebler GL, Edwards JE, Burchell HB, et al: Congenital corrected transposition of the great vessels: A study of 35 cases. Pediatrics 27:851, 1961.
10. Anderson RC, Lillehei CW, Lester RG: Corrected transposition of the great vessels of the heart. Pediatrics 20:626, 1957.
11. Cardell BS: Corrected transposition of the great vessels. Br Heart J 18:186, 1956.
12. Edwards JE, Carey LS, Neufeld HN, Lester RG: Congenital Heart Disease: Correlation of Pathologic Anatomy and Angiocardiography. Philadelphia, WB Saunders, 1965, pp 492–511.
13. Friedberg DZ, Nadas AS: Clinical profile of patients with congenital corrected transposition of the great arteries. A study of 60 cases. N Engl J Med 282:1053, 1970.
14. Losekoot TG, Anderson RH, Becker AE, et al: Congenitally Corrected Transposition. Edinburgh, Churchill Livingstone, 1983, pp 3–190.
15. Kirklin JW, Barratt-Boyes BG: Cardiac Surgery, 2nd ed. New York, Churchill Livingstone, 1993, pp 1263–1300.
16. Freedom RM, Dyck JD: Congenitally corrected transposition of the great arteries. In Emmanouilides GC, Allen HD, Riemenschneider TA, Gutgesell HP (eds): Moss and Adams' Heart Disease in Infants, Children, and Adolescents, Including the Fetus and Young Adult. Baltimore, Williams & Wilkins, 1995, pp 1225–1246.
17. Mullins CE: Ventricular Inversion. In Garson A Jr, Bricker JT, McNamera DG (eds): The Science and Practice of Pediatric Cardiology. Philadelphia, Lea & Febiger, 1990, pp 1233–1245.
18. Macartney FJ, Shinebourne EA, Anderson RH: Connexions, relations, discordance, and distorsions. Br Heart J 38:323, 1976.
19. Shinebourne EA, Macartney FJ, Anderson RH: Sequential chamber localisation—logical approach to diagnosis in congenital heart disease. Br Heart J 38:327, 1976.
20. Anderson RH, Yen Ho S: Sequential segmental analysis: Description and categorization for the millenium. Cardiol Young 7:98, 1997.
21. Losekoot TG, Becker AE: Discordant atrioventricular connexion and congenitally corrected transposition. In Anderson RH, Macartney FJ, Shinebourne EA, Tynan M (eds): Paediatric Cardiology. Edinburgh, Churchill Livingstone, 1987, pp 867–884.
22. Losekoot TG: Conditions with atrioventricular discordance: Clinical investigations. In Anderson RH, Shinebourne EA (eds): Paediatric Cardiology. Edinburgh, Churchill Livingstone, 1978, pp 198–206.
23. Van Praagh R, Weinberg PM, Calder AL, et al: The transposition complexes: How many are there? In Davila JC (ed): The Second Henry Ford Hospital International Symposium on Cardiac Surgery. New York, Appleton-Century-Crofts, 1977, pp 207–213.
24. Van Praagh R: Anatomic variations in transposition of the great arteries. In Takahashi M, Wells WJ, Lindesmith GG (eds): Challenges in the Treatment of Congenital Cardiac Anomalies. Mt. Kisco, NY, Futura, 1986, pp 107–135.
25. Van Praagh R, Layton WM, Van Praagh S: The morphogenesis of normal and abnormal relationships between the great arteries and the ventricles: Pathologic and experimental data. In Van Praagh R, Takao A (eds): Etiology and Morphogenesis of Congenital Heart Disease. Mt. Kisco, NY, Futura, 1980, pp 271–316.
26. Dadez E, Sidi D, Villain E, et al: Double discordance with ventricular septal defect and pulmonary artery hypertension. A study of 21 cases. [Doubles discordances avec communication interventriculaire et hypertension arterielle pulmonaire. Etude de 21 cas.] Arch Mal Coeur Vaiss 83:621, 1990.
27. Allwork SP, Bentall HH, Becker AE: Congenitally corrected transposition of the great arteries. Morphologic study of 32 cases. Am J Cardiol 38:910, 1976.
28. Van Praagh R: The segmental approach to diagnosis in congenital heart disease. Birth Defects Orig Artic Ser 8:4, 1972.
29. Van Praagh R: Diagnosis of complex congenital heart disease: Morphologic-anatomic method and terminology. Cardiovasc Intervent Radiol 7:115, 1984.
30. Van Praagh R, Ongley PA, Swan HJC: Anatomic types of single or common ventricle in man. Morphologic and geometric aspects of sixty autopsied cases. Am J Cardiol 13:367, 1964.
31. Van Praagh R, Van Praagh S, Vlad P, Keith JD: Anatomic types of congenital dextrocardia. Diagnostic and embryologic implications. Am J Cardiol 13:510, 1964.
32. Van Praagh R, Van Praagh S, Vlad P, Keith JD: Diagnosis of the anatomic types of congenital dextrocardia. Am J Cardiol 15:234, 1965.
33. Otero Coto E, Quero Jimenez M, Cabrera A, et al: Aortic levopositions without ventricular inversion. Eur J Cardiol 8:523, 1978.
34. Carr I, Tynan MJ, Aberdeen E, et al: Predictive accuracy of the loop rule in 109 children with classical complete transposition of the great arteries (Abstract). Circulation 38(suppl 5):52, 1968.
35. Anderson RH, Shinebourne EA, Gerlis LM: Criss-cross atrioventricular relationships producing paradoxical atrioventricular concordance or discordance. Their significance to nomenclature of congenital heart disease. Circulation 50:176, 1974.
36. Weinberg PM, Van Praagh R, Wagner HR, Cuaso CC: New form of criss-cross atrioventricular relation: An expanded view of the meaning of D- and L-loops (Abstract 139). Proceedings of the World Congress of Paediatric Cardiology, 1980.
37. Seo JW, Choe GY, Chi JG: An unusual ventricular loop associated with right juxtaposition of the atrial appendages. Int J Cardiol 25:219, 1989.
38. Anderson RH, Smith A, Wilkinson JL: Disharmony between atrioventricular connections and segmental combinations: Unusual variants of "crisscross" hearts. J Am Coll Cardiol 10:1274, 1987.
39. Geva T, Sanders SP, Ayres NA, et al: Two-dimensional echocardiographic anatomy of atrioventricular alignment discordance with situs concordance. Am Heart J 125:459, 1993.
40. Seo J-W, Yoo S-J, Yen Ho S, et al: Further morphological observations on hearts with twisted atrioventricular connections (criss-cross hearts). Cardiovasc Pathol 1:211, 1992.
41. Van Praagh R: When concordant or discordant atrioventricular alignments predict the ventricular situs wrongly. I. Solitus atria, concordant alignments, and L-loop ventricles. II. Solitus atria, discordant alignments, and D-loop ventricles. J Am Coll Cardiol 10:1278, 1987.
42. Anderson RH, Yen Ho S: Editorial note: Segmental interconnexions versus topological congruency in complex congenital malformations. Int J Cardiol 25:229, 1989.
43. Anderson RH, Arnold RB, Jones RS: D-bulboventricular loop with L-transposition in situs inversus. Circulation 46:193, 1972.
44. Freedom RM, Harrington DP, White RI Jr: The differential diagnosis of levo-transposed or malposed aorta. An angiocardiographic study. Circulation 50:1040, 1974.
45. Van Praagh R, Perez-Trevino C, Reynolds JL: Double outlet right ventricle S, D, L with subaortic ventricular septal defect and pulmonary stenosis. Am J Cardiol 35:42, 1975.
46. Van Praagh R, Durnin R, Jockin H, et al: Anatomically corrected malposition of the great arteries (S,D,L). Circulation 51:20, 1975.
47. Anderson RH, Becker AE, Losekoot TG, Gerlis LM: Anatomically corrected malposition of great arteries. Br Heart J 37:993, 1975.
48. Melhuish BPP, Van Praagh R: Juxtaposition of the atrial appendages. A sign of severe cyanotic congenital heart disease. Br Heart J 30:269, 1968.
49. Freedom RM, Harrington DP: Anatomically corrected malposition of the great arteries: Report of two cases, one with congenital asplenia, frequent association with juxtaposition of atrial appendages. Br Heart J 36:207, 1974.

50. Freedom RM: Double-outlet left ventricle; isolated atrioventricular discordance; anatomically corrected malposition of the great arteries; and syndrome of juxtaposition of the atrial appendages. *In* Freedom RM, Benson LN, Smallhorn JF (eds): Neonatal Heart Disease. London, Springer-Verlag, 1992, pp 561–569.

51. Freedom RM, Benson LN: Congenitally corrected transposition of the great arteries. *In* Freedom RM, Benson LN, Smallhorn JF (eds): Neonatal Heart Disease. London, Springer-Verlag, 1992, pp 523–542.

52. Van Praagh R, Van Praagh S: Isolated ventricular inversion. Am J Cardiol 17:395, 1966.

53. Abbott ME, Beattie WW: Rare cardiac anomaly. Am J Dis Child 22:508, 1921.

54. Anderson RH, Wilkinson JL: Isolated ventricular inversion with situs solitus. Br Heart J 37:1202, 1975.

55. Espino-Vela J, De La Cruz MV, Munoz-Castellanos L, et al: Ventricular inversion without transposition of the great vessels in situs inversus. Br Heart J 32:292, 1970.

56. Ostermeyer J, Bircks W, Krain A, et al: Isolated atrioventricular discordance. J Thorac Cardiovasc Surg 86:926, 1983.

57. Quero-Jimenez M, Raposo-Sonnenfeld I: Isolated ventricular inversion with situs solitus. Br Heart J 37:293, 1975.

58. Tandon R, Heineman RP, Edwards JE: Ventricular inversion with normally connected great vessels in situs solitus (atrioventricular discordance with ventriculoarterial concordance). Pediatr Cardiol 7:107, 1986.

59. Tandon R, Moller JH, Edwards JE: Ventricular inversion associated with normally related great vessels. Chest 67:98, 1975.

60. Arciprete P, Macartney FJ, De Leval M, Stark J: Mustard's operation for patients with ventriculoarterial concordance: Report of two cases and a cautionary tale. Br Heart J 53:443, 1985.

61. Leijala MA, Lincoln CR, Shinebourne EA, Nellen M: A rare congenital cardiac malformation with situs inversus and discordant atrioventricular and concordant ventriculoarterial connections: Diagnosis and surgical treatment. Am Heart J 101:355, 1981.

62. Ranjit MS, Wilkinson JL, Mee RB: Discordant atrioventricular connexion with concordant ventriculo-arterial connexion (so-called "isolated ventricular inversion") with usual atrial arrangement (situs solitus). Int J Cardiol 31:114, 1991.

63. Sklansky MS, Lucas VW, Kashani IA, Rothman A: Atrioventricular situs concordance with atrioventricular alignment discordance: Fetal and neonatal echocardiographic findings. Am J Cardiol 76:202, 1995.

64. Pasquini L, Sanders SP, Parness I, et al: Echocardiographic and anatomic findings in atrioventricular discordance with ventriculoarterial concordance. Am J Cardiol 62:1256, 1988.

65. Snider AR, Enderlein MA, Teitel DF, et al: Isolated ventricular inversion: Two-dimensional echocardiographic findings and a review of the literature. Pediatr Cardiol 5:27, 1984.

66. Kothari SS, Kartha CC, Venkitachalam CG, et al: Discordant atrioventricular connection and concordant ventriculoarterial connection in situs inversus: Isolated ventricular noninversion. Pediatr Cardiol 12:126, 1991.

67. Bjarke BB, Kidd BSL: Congenitally corrected transposition of the great arteries. A clinical study of 101 cases. Acta Paediatr Scand 65:153, 1976.

68. Keith JD: Prevalence, incidence, and epidemiology. *In* Keith JD, Rowe RD, Vlad P (eds): Heart Disease in Infancy and Childhood. New York, Macmillan, 1978, pp 3–13.

69. Ferencz C, Rubin JD, McCarter RJ, et al: Congenital heart disease: Prevalence at livebirth. The Baltimore-Washington Infant Study. Am J Epidemiol 121:31, 1985.

70. Fyler DC: Nadas' Pediatric Cardiology. Boston, Mosby–Year Book, 1992, pp 701–708.

71. Fyler DC: Report of the New England Regional Infant Cardiac Program. Pediatrics 65(suppl):376, 1980.

72. Van Praagh S, LaCorte M, Fellows KE, et al: Superoinferior ventricles: Anatomic and angiocardiographic findings in ten postmortem cases. *In* Van Praagh R, Takao A (eds): Etiology and Morphogenesis of Congenital Heart Disease. Mt. Kisco, NY, Futura, 1980, pp 317–378.

73. Freedom RM: Supero-inferior ventricles, criss-cross atrioventricular connections, and the straddling atrioventricular valve. *In* Freedom RM, Benson LN, Smallhorn JF (eds): Neonatal Heart Disease. London, Springer-Verlag, 1992, pp 667–678.

74. Freedom RM: Supero-inferior ventricle and criss-cross atrioventricular connections: An analysis of the myth and mystery. *In* Belloli GP, Squarcia U (eds): Pediatric Cardiology and Cardiosurgery. Modern Problems in Paediatrics. Basel, Karger, 1983, pp 48–62.

75. Anderson RH: Criss-cross hearts revisited. Pediatr Cardiol 3:305, 1982.

76. Freedom RM, Culham G, Rowe RD: The criss-cross and superoinferior ventricular heart: An angiocardiographic study. Am J Cardiol 42:620, 1978.

77. Kinsley RH, McGoon DC, Danielson GK: Corrected transposition of the great arteries. Associated ventricular rotation. Circulation 49:574, 1974.

78. Robinson PJ, Kumping V, Macartney FJ: Cross-sectional echocardiographic correlation in criss-cross hearts. Br Heart J 54:61, 1985.

79. Galinanes M, Chartrand C, Van Doesburg NH, et al: Surgical repair of superoinferior ventricles: Experience with three patients. Ann Thorac Surg 40:353, 1985.

80. Guthaner D, Higgins CB, Silverman JF, et al: An unusual form of the transposition complex. Uncorrected levo-transposition with horizontal ventricular septum: Report of two cases. Circulation 53:190, 1976.

81. Schneeweiss A, Shem-Tov A, Neufeld HN: Coronary arterial pattern in superoinferior ventricular heart. Implications on significance of morphogenesis of this anomaly. Br Heart J 46:559, 1981.

82. Chiu IS, Wang JK, Wu MH: Unusual coronary artery pattern in a criss-cross heart. Int J Cardiol 47:127, 1994.

83. Yamagishi M, Imai Y, Kurosawa H, et al: Superoinferior ventricular heart with situs inversus, levo-loop and dextro-malposition (I,L,D), and double-outlet right ventricle: A case report. J Thorac Cardiovasc Surg 91:633, 1986.

84. Symons JC, Shinebourne EA, Joseph MC, et al: Criss-cross heart with congenitally corrected transposition: Report of a case with d-transposed aorta and ventricular preexcitation. Eur J Cardiol 5:493, 1977.

85. Tadavarthy SM, Formanek A, Castaneda-Zuniga W, et al: The three types of criss cross heart: A simple rotational anomaly. Br J Radiol 54:736, 1981.

86. Ando M, Takao A, Yutani C, et al: What is cardiac looping? Consideration based on morphologic data. *In* Nora JJ, Takao A (eds): Congenital Heart Disease: Causes and Processes. Mt. Kisco, NY, Futura, 1984, pp 553–577.

87. Alday LE, Juaneda E: Superoinferior ventricles with criss-cross atrioventricular connections and intact ventricular septum. Pediatr Cardiol 14:238, 1993.

88. Fontes VF, Malta de Souza JA, Pontes SC Jr: Criss-cross heart with intact ventricular septum. Int J Cardiol 26:382, 1990.

89. Anderson RH, Becker AE: Coronary arterial patterns: A guide to identification of congenital heart disease. *In* Becker AE, Losekoot G, Marcelletti C, Anderson RH (eds): Paediatric Cardiology. Edinburgh, Churchill Livingstone, 1981, pp 251–262.

90. Schwartz HA, Wagner PI: Corrected transposition of the great vessels in a 55-year-old woman; Diagnosis by coronary angiography. Chest 66:190, 1974.

91. Shea PM, Lutz JF, Vieweg WVR, et al: Selective coronary arteriography in congenitally corrected transposition of the great arteries. Am J Cardiol 44:1201, 1979.

92. Becker AE, Anderson RH: Pathology of Congenital Heart Disease. London, Butterworth, 1981, pp 225–240.

93. Neufeld HN, Schneeweiss A: Coronary Artery Disease in Infants and Children. Philadelphia, Lea & Febiger, 1983, p 189.

94. Marcelletti C, Maloney JD, Ritter DG, et al: Corrected transposition and ventricular septal defect: Surgical experience. Ann Surg 191:751, 1980.

95. Okamura K, Konno S: Two types of ventricular septal defect in corrected transposition of the great arteries: Reference to surgical approaches. Am Heart J 85:483, 1973.

96. Williams WG, Suri R, Shindo G, et al: Repair of major intracardiac anomalies associated with atrioventricular discordance. Ann Thor Surg 31:527, 1981.

97. Cohen DM, Freedom RM, Williams WG: Congenitally corrected transposition of the great arteries. *In* Cowgill LD (ed): Cardiac Surgery: Cyanotic Congenital Heart Disease. Philadelphia, Hanley & Belfus, 1989, pp 225–240.

98. Anderson RH, Becker AE, Gerlis LM: The pulmonary outflow tract in classical corrected transposition. J Thorac Cardiovasc Surg 65:747, 1975.

99. Bliddal J, Christensen N, Efsen F: Intracardiac blood cyst causing subpulmonary stenosis in congenitally corrected transposition. Eur J Cardiol 5:17, 1977.

100. Krongrad E, Ellis K, Steeg CN, et al: Subpulmonary obstruction in congenitally corrected transposition of the great arteries due to ventricular membranous septal aneurysms. Circulation 54:679, 1976.

101. Lindenau KF, Olthoff D, Bock K: Accessory valve cusp as a cause of outflow tract obstruction in atrio-ventricular and ventriculo-arterial discordance. Thorac Cardiovasc Surg 36:37, 1988.

102. O'Sullivan JJ, Farrell DJ, Hunter AS: Subpulmonary tag originating from both sides of the ventricular septum in congenitally corrected transposition. Cardiol Young 3:82, 1993.

103. Jaffe RB: Systemic atrioventricular valve regurgitation in corrected transposition of the great vessels. Angiographic differentiation of operable and nonoperable valve deformities. Circulation 37:395, 1976.

104. Anderson KR, Danielson GK, McGoon DW, Lie JT: Ebstein's anomaly of the left-sided tricuspid valve. Pathological anatomy of the valvular malformation. Circulation 58:87, 1978.

105. Horvath P, Szufladowicz M, de Leval MR, et al: Tricuspid valve abnormalities in patients with atrioventricular discordance: Surgical implications. Ann Thorac Surg 57:941, 1994.

106. Brenner JI, Bharati S, Winn WC Jr, Lev M: Absent tricuspid valve with aortic atresia in mixed levocardia (Atria situs solitus, L-loop). A hitherto undescribed entity. Circulation 57:836, 1978.

107. Celermajer DS, Seamus C, Deanfield JE, Sullivan ID: Congenitally corrected transposition and Ebstein's anomaly of the systemic atrioventricular valve: Association with aortic arch obstruction. J Am Coll Cardiol 18:1056, 1991.

108. Deanfield JE, Anderson RH, Macartney FJ: Aortic atresia with corrected transposition of the great arteries (atrioventricular and ventriculoarterial discordance). Br Heart J 46:683, 1981.

109. Matsukawa T, Yoshii S, Miyamura H, Eguchi S: Aortic atresia with Ebstein's and Uhl's anomaly in corrected transposition of the great arteries: Clinicopathologic findings. Jpn Circ J 49:325, 1985.

110. Muster AJ, Idriss FS, Bharati S, et al: Functional aortic valve atresia in transposition of the great arteries. J Am Coll Cardiol 6:630, 1985.

111. Chan KC, Da Costa P, Dickinson DF: Functional aortic atresia in congenitally corrected transposition. Int J Cardiol 25:237, 1989.

112. Craig BG, Smallhorn JF, Rowe RD, et al: Severe obstruction to systemic blood flow in congenitally corrected transposition (discordant atrioventricular and ventriculo-arterial connexions): An analysis of 14 patients. Int J Cardiol 11:209, 1986.

113. Becker AE, Ho SY, Caruso G, et al: Straddling right atrioventricular valves in atrioventricular discordance. Circulation 61:1133, 1980.

114. Rice MJ, Seward JB, Edwards WD, et al: Straddling atrioventricular valve: Two-dimensional echocardiographic diagnosis, classification and surgical implications. Am J Cardiol 55:506, 1985.

115. Schenk M, Gerlis LM, Somerville J: Clinicopathologic correlation—A case of complex congenitally corrected transposition. Cardiol Young 4:238, 1994.

116. Anderson RH, Arnold R, Wilkinson JL: The conducting system in congenitally corrected transposition. Lancet 1:1286, 1973.

117. Anderson RH, Becker AE, Arnold R, Wilkinson JL: The conducting tissues in congenitally corrected transposition. Circulation 50:911, 1974.

118. Kurosawa H, Becker AE: Atrioventricular Conduction in Congenital Heart Disease. London, Springer-Verlag, 1987, pp 225–252.

119. Bharati S, Lev M, Kirklin JW: Cardiac Surgery and the Conduction System. Mt. Kisco, NY, Futura, 1992, pp 123–127.

120. Kurosawa H, Imai Y, Becker AE: Congenitally corrected transposition with normally positioned atria, straddling mitral valve, and isolated posterior atrioventricular node and bundle. J Thorac Cardiovasc Surg 99:312, 1990.

121. Bharati S, Rosen K, Steinfeld L, et al: The anatomic substrate for preexcitation in corrected transposition. Circulation 62:831, 1980.

122. Gillette PC, Busch U, Mullins CE, McNamara DG: Electrophysiologic studies in patients with ventricular inversion and 'corrected transposition'. Circulation 60:939, 1979.

123. Stewart S, Manning J, Siegel L: Automated identification of cardiac conduction tissue in L-TGA and Ebstein's anomaly. Ann Thorac Surg 23:215, 1977.

124. de Leval MR, Bastons P, Stark J, et al: Surgical technique to reduce the risks of heart block following closure of ventricular septal defect in atrioventricular discordance. J Thorac Cardiovasc Surg 78:515, 1979.

125. Ritter M, Schneider J, Schmidin D, Jenni R: Supravalvular tricuspid ring and Ebstein's anomaly in corrected transposition. Am J Cardiol 70:1635, 1992.

126. Chesler E, Beck W, Barnard CN, Schrire V: Supravalvular stenosing ring of the left atrium associated with corrected transposition of the great vessels. Am J Cardiol 31:84, 1973.

127. Cottrell AJ, Holden MP, Hunter S: Interrupted aortic arch type A associated with congenitally corrected transposition of great arteries and ventricular septal defect. Successful direct aortic anastomosis and pulmonary artery banding in an infant. Br Heart J 46:671, 1981.

128. Danielson GK, Tabry IF, Ritter DG, Maloney JD: Successful repair of double-outlet right ventricle, complete atrioventricular canal, and atrioventricular discordance associated with dextrocardia and pulmonary stenosis. J Thorac Cardiovasc Surg 76:710, 1978.

129. Erath HG Jr, Graham TP Jr, Hammon JW Jr, Smith CW: Hypoplasia of the systemic ventricle in congenitally corrected transposition of the great arteries. Preoperative documentation and possible implications of operation. J Thorac Cardiovasc Surg 79:770, 1980.

130. Graham TP Jr, Parrish MD, Boucek RJ Jr, et al: Assessment of ventricular size and function in congenitally corrected transposition of the great arteries. Am J Cardiol 51:244, 1983.

131. Marino B, Sanders SP, Parness IA, Colan SD: Obstruction of right ventricular inflow and outflow in corrected transposition of the great arteries (S,L,L): Two-dimensional echocardiographic diagnosis. J Am Coll Cardiol 8:407, 1986.

132. Ross-Ascuitto NT, Ascuitto RJ, Kopf GS, et al: Discrete subaortic stenosis in a patient with corrected transposition of the great arteries. Pediatr Cardiol 8:147, 1987.

133. Shimizu T, Ando M, Takao A: Pulmonary atresia with intact ventricular septum and corrected transposition of the great arteries. Br Heart J 45:471, 1981.

134. Steeg CN, Ellis K, Bransilver B, Gersony WM: Pulmonary atresia and intact ventricular septum complicating corrected transposition of great vessels. Am Heart J 82:382, 1971.

135. Symons JC, Shinebourne EA, Joseph MC, et al: Criss-cross heart with congenitally corrected transposition; report of a case with d-transposed aorta and ventricular pre-excitation. Eur J Cardiol 5:493, 1977.

136. Tabry IF, McGoon DC, Danielson GK, et al: Surgical management of double-outlet right ventricle associated with atrioventricular discordance. J Thorac Cardiovasc Surg 76:336, 1978.

137. Gerlis LM, Wilson N, Dickinson DF. Abnormalities of the mitral valve in congenitally corrected transposition (discordant atrioventricular and ventriculoarterial connections). Br Heart J 55:475, 1986.

138. Zahn EM, Smallhorn JF, Freedom RM: Congenitally corrected transposition of the great arteries with hypoplasia of the morphologically left ventricle in the setting of situs inversus. Int J Cardiol 36:9, 1992.

139. Garrick ML, Ettedgui JA, Neches WH: Corrected transposition presenting as aortic stenosis in an infant. Int J Cardiol 20:287, 1988.

140. Battistessa S, Soto B: Double outlet right ventricle with discordant atrioventricular connexion: An angiographic analysis of 19 cases. Int J Cardiol 27:253, 1990.

141. Penny DJ, Somerville J, Redington AN: Echo-cardiographic demonstration of important abnormalities of the mitral valve in congenitally corrected transposition. Br Heart J 68:498, 1992.

142. Attie F, Cerda J, Richheimer R, et al: Congenitally corrected transposition with mirror-image atrial arrangement. Int J Cardiol 14:169, 1987.

143. Marino B, Ballerini L, Soro A: Ventricular inversion with truncus arteriosus. Chest 98:239, 1990.

144. Gladman G, Casey F, Adatia I: Supravalvar stenosing tricuspid ring in congenitally corrected transposition. Cardiol Young 6:174, 1996.

145. Miche E, Mannebach H, Boyunovic N, et al: Right ventricular outflow obstruction due to accessory tricuspid valve tissue in corrected transposition of the great arteries with ventricular septal defect. Z Kardiol 80:468, 1991.

146. Freedom RM, Dische MR, Rowe RD: Pathologic anatomy of subaortic stenosis and atresia in the first year of life. Am J Cardiol 39:1035, 1977.

147. Huhta JC, Danielson GK, Ritter DG, Ilstrup DM: Survival in atrioventricular discordance. Pediatr Cardiol 6:57, 1985.

148. McGrath LB, Kirklin JW, Blackstone EH, et al: Death and other events after cardiac repair in discordant atrioventricular connection. J Thorac Cardiovasc Surg 90:711, 1985.

149. Benchimol A, Tio S, Sundararajan V: Congenital corrected transposition of the great vessels in a 58-year-old man. Chest 59:634, 1971.

150. Lieberson AD, Schumacher RR, Childress RH, Genovese PD: Corrected transposition of the great vessels in a 73-year-old man. Circulation 39:96, 1969.

151. Melero-Pita A, Alonso-Pardo F, Bardaji-Mayor JL, Higueras J: Corrected transposition of the great arteries. N Engl J Med 334:866, 1996.

152. Ikeda U, Furuse M, Suzuki O, et al: Long-term survival in aged patients with corrected transposition of the great arteries. Chest 101:1382, 1992.

153. Connelly MS, Liu PP, Williams WG, et al: Congenitally corrected transposition of the great arteries in the adult. Functional status and complications. J Am Coll Cardiol 27:1238, 1996.

154. Ikeda U, Kimura K, Suzuki O, et al: Long-term survival in "corrected transposition." Lancet 337:180, 1991.

155. Benson LN, Burns R, Schwaiger M, et al: Radionuclide angiographic evaluation of ventricular function in isolated congenitally corrected transposition of the great arteries. Am J Cardiol 58:319, 1986.

156. Dimas AP, Moodie DS, Sterba R, Gill CC: Long-term function of the morphologic right ventricle in adult patients with corrected transposition of the great arteries. Am Heart J 118:526, 1989.

157. Peterson RJ, Franch RH, Fajman WA, Jones RH: Comparison of cardiac function in surgically corrected and congenitally corrected transposition of the great arteries. J Thorac Cardiovasc Surg 96:227, 1988.

158. Lamberti JJ, Jensen TS, Grehl TM, et al: Late reoperation for systemic atrio-ventricular valve regurgitation after repair of congenital heart defects. Ann Thorac Surg 47:517, 1989.

159. Ilbawi MN, DeLeon SY, Backer CL, et al: An alternative approach to the surgical management of physiologically corrected transposition with ventricular septal defect and pulmonary stenosis or atresia. J Thorac Cardiovasc Surg 100:410, 1990.

160. Di Donato RM, Wernovsky G, Jonas RA, et al: Corrected transposition in situs inversus. Biventricular repair of associated cardiac anomalies. Circulation 84(suppl III):193, 1991.

161. Di Donato R, Troconis CJ, Marino B, et al: Combined Mustard and Rastelli operations. An alternative approach for repair of associated anomalies in congenitally corrected transposition in situs inversus [I,D,D]. J Thorac Cardiovasc Surg 104:1246, 1992.

162. Stumper O, Wright JG, De Giovanni JV, et al: Combined atrial and arterial switch procedure for congenital corrected transposition with ventricular septal defect. Br Heart J 73:479, 1995.

163. Imai Y, Sawatari K, Hoshino S, et al: Ventricular function after anatomic repair in patients with atrioventricular discordance. J Thorac Cardiovasc Surg 107:1272, 1994.

164. Sano T, Riesenfeld T, Karl TR, Wilkinson JL: Intermediate-term outcome after intracardiac repair of associated cardiac defects in patients with atrioventricular and ventriculoarterial discordance. Circulation 92 (suppl II):272, 1995.

165. Yamagishi Y, Imai Y, Hoshino S, et al: Anatomic correction of atrioventricular discordance. J Thorac Cardiovasc Surg 105:1067, 1993.

166. Yagihara T, Kishimoto H, Isobe F, et al: Double switch operation in cardiac anomalies with atrioventricular and ventriculoarterial discordance. J Thorac Cardiovasc Surg 107:351, 1994.

167. Yeh T Jr, Connelly MS, Coles JG, et al: Atrioventricular discordance: Results of repair in 127 patients. J Thorac Cardiovasc Surg 117:1190, 1999.

168. Delius RE, Stark J: Combined Rastelli and atrial switch procedure: Anatomic and physiologic correction of discordant atrioventricular connection associated with ventricular septal defect and left ventricular outflow tract obstruction. Eur J Cardiothorac Surg 10:551, 1996.

169. Carey LS, Ruttenberg HD: Roentgenographic features of congenital corrected transposition of the great vessels. AJR Am J Roentgenol 92:623, 1964.

170. Carminati M, Valsecchi O, Borghi A, et al: Cross-sectional echocardiographic study of criss-cross hearts and superoinferior ventricles. Am J Cardiol 59:114, 1987.

171. Sutherland GR, Smallhorn JF, Anderson RH, et al: Atrioventricular discordance. Cross-sectional echocardiographic–morphological correlative study. Br Heart J 50:8, 1983.

172. Hagler DJ, Tajik AJ, Seward JB, et al: Atrioventricular and ventriculoarterial discordance. Wide angle two dimensional assessment of ventricular morphology. Mayo Clin Proc 56:591, 1989.

173. Silverman NH, Gerlis LM, Horowitz ES, et al: Pathologic elucidation of the echocardiographic features of Ebstein's malformation of the morphologically tricuspid valve in discordant atrioventricular connections. Am J Cardiol 76:1277, 1995.

174. de Albuquerque TA, Rigby ML, Anderson RH, et al: The spectrum of atrioventricular discordance. A clinical study. Br Heart J 51:498, 1984.

175. Attie F, Soni J, Ovseyevita J, et al: Angiographic studies of atrioventricular discordance. Circulation 62:407, 1980.

176. Soto B, Bargeron LM, Bream PR, Elliott LP: Conditions with atrioventricular discordance—Angiographic study. *In* Anderson RH, Shinebourne EA (eds): Paediatric Cardiology, 1977. Edinburgh, Churchill Livingstone, 1978, pp 207–223.

177. Freedom RM: Axial angiocardiography in the critically ill infant. Indications and contraindications. Cardiol Clin 1:387, 1983.

178. Yoo S-J, Choi Y-H: Angiocardiograms in Congenital Heart Disease. Teaching File of Sejong Heart Institute. Oxford, Oxford Medical Publications, 1991, pp 256–260.

179. Soto B, Pacifico AD: Angiocardiography in Congenital Heart Malformations. Mt. Kisco, NY, Futura, 1990, pp 239–271.

180. Freedom RM, Culham JAG, Moes CAF: Angiocardiography of Congenital Heart Disease. New York, Macmillan, 1984, pp 536–554.

181. Shem-Tov A, Deutsch V, Yahini JH, et al: Corrected transposition of the great arteries. A modified approach to the clinical diagnosis in 30 cases. Am J Cardiol 27:99, 1971.

182. Jennings HSI, Primm RK, Parrish MD, et al: Coronary arterial revascularization in an adult with congenitally corrected transposition. Am Heart J 108:598, 1984.

183. Dabizzi RP, Baarletta G, Caprioli G, et al: Coronary artery anatomy in corrected transposition of the great arteries. J Am Coll Cardiol 12:486, 1988.

184. Freedom RM, Mawson JB, Yoo SJ, Benson LN (eds): Congenital Heart Disease: Textbook of Angiocardiography. Armonk, NY, Futura, 1997, pp 1017–1117.

185. Folliguet TA, Laborde F, Mace L, et al: Aortic insufficiency associated with complex cardiac anomalies. Cardiol Young 5:125, 1995.

186. Capelli H, Ross D, Somerville J: Aortic regurgitation in tetrad of Fallot and pulmonary atresia. Am J Cardiol 49:1979, 1982.

187. Szufladowicz M, Horvath P, de Leval M, et al: Intracardiac repair of lesions associated with atrioventricular discordance. Eur J Cardiothorac Surg 10:443, 1996.

CHAPTER 28

TETRALOGY OF FALLOT AND PULMONARY ATRESIA WITH VENTRICULAR SEPTAL DEFECT

THOMAS P. DOYLE   ANN KAVANAUGH-McHUGH   THOMAS P. GRAHAM

HISTORICAL PERSPECTIVE

In her description of tetralogy of Fallot in 1947, Dr. Helen Taussig relates that more than 100 years before Fallot's report, clear descriptions of this abnormality were published by Peacock in 1866.[1] Indeed, Peacock's report[2] of a patient accredited to 1783 stated, "a child was always dark colored and had presented unusual symptoms of malformation of the heart since shortly after birth and was markedly thin. He was liable to paroxysms and difficulty in breathing, but could arrest them by lying down on the carpet when they were coming on." In 1888, Fallot[3] published a detailed description of three adults with marked cyanosis, harsh systolic murmur, and autopsy findings typical of tetralogy of Fallot. The diagnosis was made premortem in the third patient and later verified at autopsy. He predicted that this cardiac lesion would be encountered with a frequency of probably 75% in older patients with congenital cyanosis. The malformation that he described and that was subsequently given his name consisted of stenosis of the pulmonary artery, intraventricular communication, deviation to the right of the origin of the aorta, and concentric hypertrophy of the right ventricle. In addition, he commented on the unimportance of a patent foreman ovale because previously it was believed to be an important cause of cyanosis.[4]

No treatment for this abnormality was known until the landmark publication by Blalock and Taussig in 1945,[5] in which an aortic-to-pulmonary shunt was successfully introduced in three patients with marked relief of cyanosis. This remarkable achievement opened the way for successful palliation of many patients with cyanotic congenital heart disease.

Subsequently, direct repair of tetralogy was first accomplished by Lillehei and associates[6] using controlled cross-circulation in 1954. With the advent of the successful use of the mechanical pump oxygenator,[7] repair was accomplished in the 1950s[8] and now is performed successfully around the world, even in young infants.

ANATOMY

The embryologic abnormality that gives rise to the constellation of findings found in tetralogy of Fallot is unclear (see Chapter 1). A number of alternative explanations have

been proposed, including abnormalities of bulbotruncal rotation and conotruncal septation, or possibly hypoplasia of the infundibular septum. However, what is clear is that anatomically there is anterior and cephalad deviation of the infundibular septum with resultant encroachment on the right ventricular outflow tract, aortic override, and malaligned ventricular septal defect (VSD). The right ventricular hypertrophy is thought to be secondary to the large VSD and pulmonary outflow obstruction.

RIGHT VENTRICULAR OUTFLOW TRACT OBSTRUCTION

The hallmark of the right ventricular outflow tract obstruction in tetralogy of Fallot is infundibular stenosis (Fig. 28–1). This is the result of a number of factors, the most important of which is the anterior cephalad deviation of the infundibular septum. Outlet obstruction is further aggravated by hypertrophy of the outlet septum, the anterior limb of the septomarginal trabeculation, and the anterior muscle bands.

The right ventricular outflow tract obstruction is not limited to the infundibular region. In the majority of patients, the pulmonary valve is stenotic. The pulmonary valve annulus itself can be hypoplastic. In addition, supravalvar obstruction may be present at the level of the sinotubular ridge. The pulmonary arteries can be diffusely small or may have focal areas of narrowing, most commonly at the bifurcation of the main pulmonary artery, but sometimes further distally in the branch pulmonary arteries. A common area for obstruction is in the proximal left pulmonary artery at the juxtaductal or juxtaligamental site (Fig. 28–2). Delineation of the sites of right ventricular outflow tract obstruction is important for planning repair.

VENTRICULAR SEPTAL DEFECT

The VSD in patients with tetralogy of Fallot is large, usually unrestrictive, and subaortic (Fig. 28–3). In most patients the VSD is perimembranous, with the central fibrous body forming the inferior border and the conduction system running within this region. In approximately 20% of patients a muscular rim along the inferior border of the defect indicates that the defect has extended into the muscular septum. Although the majority of patients have a single large defect, additional VSDs may be found in the muscular septum.

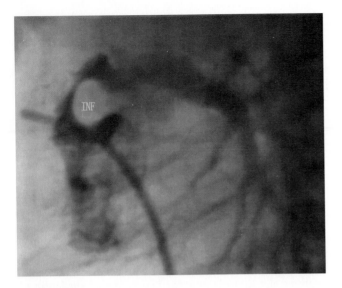

FIGURE 28–1

Lateral projection of a right ventriculogram in a newborn infant with severe infundibular stenosis. The hypertrophied infundibulum (INF) encroaches on the right ventricular outflow tract and causes severe subvalvar stenosis.

AORTIC OVERRIDE

The degree of aortic override can vary considerably in tetralogy of Fallot and to some extent is limited only by the distinction between tetralogy of Fallot and double outlet right ventricle. If the diagnosis of tetralogy of Fallot versus double outlet right ventricle is defined by mitral/aortic valve fibrous continuity,[9] an override of 15 to 95% has been

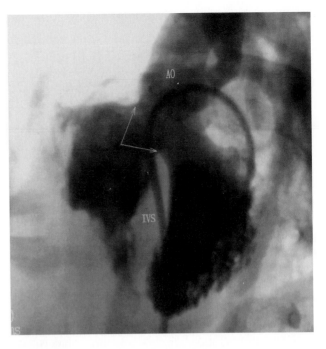

FIGURE 28–3

Left ventriculogram performed in a long axial oblique projection. The aorta (AO) overrides the interventricular septum (IVS), resulting in a large, malaligned ventricular septal defect *(arrows)*.

reported. If one, however, defines double outlet right ventricle as a lesion where greater than 50% of the aorta arises from the right ventricle, one arbitrarily limits the degree of aortic override possible in tetralogy of Fallot.

ASSOCIATED ANATOMIC FEATURES

A variety of anatomic features are frequently associated with tetralogy of Fallot and can have considerable clinical and therapeutic implications. Atrial communications are quite frequent and usually are located at the fossa ovalis as either a patent foramen ovale or rarely a true secundum atrial septal defect. Approximately 25% of patients have a right-sided aortic arch that can alter the approach to a palliative shunt. Abnormalities of the coronary arteries, such as the left anterior descending coronary artery arising from the right coronary artery, occur in about 4% of patients (Fig. 28–4). This anomaly is exceedingly important to recognize, as the left anterior descending coronary then crosses the right ventricular outflow tract, and failure to identify this vessel can result in its inadvertent transection during a right ventriculotomy. Occasionally significant systemic-to-pulmonary collaterals may be present that require occlusion before or at the time of surgery.

TETRALOGY OF FALLOT WITH ABSENT PULMONARY VALVE

Tetralogy of Fallot with absent pulmonary valve is a condition affecting a subgroup of patients without a functioning pulmonary valve. The pulmonary annulus is usually small with vestigial valve leaflets, resulting in some degree of pulmonary stenosis and severe pulmonary insufficiency. The

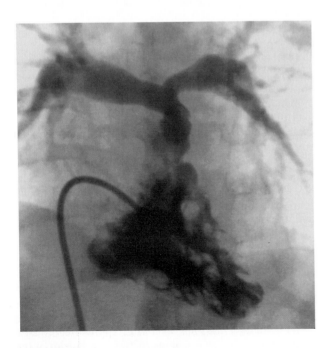

FIGURE 28–2

Right ventriculogram of an 8-month-old infant with tetralogy of Fallot. The camera is angled cranially and left anterior obliquely. Multiple levels of right ventricular outflow obstruction include subvalvar, valvar, supravalvar, and proximal left pulmonary artery.

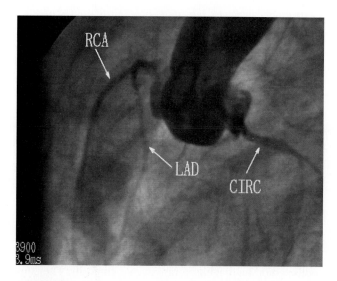

FIGURE 28–4

Aortogram in a long axial oblique/cranial projection. The left anterior descending (LAD) coronary artery can be seen arising from the proximal right coronary artery (RCA) with a course that traverses the right ventricular outflow tract. CIRC = circumflex coronary artery.

anatomic hallmark of this lesion is aneurysmal dilatation of the main and branch pulmonary arteries, particularly the right, which commonly results in bronchial compression and airway compromise that can be life-threatening. The embryologic abnormality that results in this lesion is unclear, but it is interesting that many of these patients do not have a ductus arteriosus. Absence of the ductus arteriosus may alter flow characteristics in the pulmonary arteries and cause subsequent pulmonary artery dilatation.

PULMONARY ATRESIA WITH VENTRICULAR SEPTAL DEFECT

Pulmonary atresia and VSD can be considered at the most severe end of the spectrum of tetralogy of Fallot. The intracardiac anatomy is virtually identical to classic tetralogy of Fallot with a large outlet VSD, an overriding aorta, normal or near-normal size right and left ventricles, and normal atrioventricular valves. The pulmonary artery anatomy is much more variable. In the least complex form of pulmonary atresia, a main pulmonary artery is supplied by the ductus arteriosus, and varying degrees of discontinuity occur between the right ventricular outflow tract and the main pulmonary artery. There can be only a short segment of virtually membranous pulmonary atresia with near-normal main pulmonary artery or there can be only a fibrous strand from the right ventricular outflow tract to the confluence of right and left pulmonary arteries. In contrast to this subset, many patients have either a partial ductal pulmonary blood supply associated with multiple aorticopulmonary collateral arteries (MAPCAs) or a pulmonary artery supply solely from MAPCAs. These MAPCAs arise usually from the descending thoracic aorta, but occasionally from the innominate or subclavian arteries or the upper part of the aortic arch; rarely they can arise from the abdominal aorta. MAPCAs can supply multiple bronchopulmonary segments in either a unifocal manner or a multifocal distribution of pulmonary blood flow to different segments by the ductally supplied right or left pulmonary arteries and the MAPCAs. In addition, MAPCAs may have connections to true central pulmonary arteries. Whether the blood supply to the lung is from the true pulmonary arteries or MAPCAs, the intrapulmonary arteries are usually normal. The difficulty in management increases markedly with the severity of hypoplasia of the central pulmonary arteries and with the MAPCAs supplying various bronchopulmonary segments.

INCIDENCE

Tetralogy of Fallot occurs approximately 3 to 5 times per 10,000 live births (see Chapter 18) and is among the three or four most common cardiac lesions requiring cardiac catheterization or operation in the first year of life.[10–12] It is slightly more common in males than females and is associated with chromosomal abnormalities in approximately 11% of patients, nonchromosomal syndrome complexes in about 8%, and problems of other major organs in approximately 16% (Table 28–1). Reports have indicated that an abnormality of chromosome 22 may be present in 20 to 30% of patients with tetralogy of Fallot. This same chromosome is involved with DiGeorge's syndrome and abnormalities considered previously as the velocardiofacial syndrome (Shprintzen's syndrome).

The recurrence risk for tetralogy of Fallot in families with one affected child is probably between 2 and 5%. For mothers who have tetralogy of Fallot the transmission risk for congenital heart disease in offspring is probably between 5 and 10%; for fathers with tetralogy of Fallot, transmission risk is 5% or less.[13]

NATURAL HISTORY

Fallot's prediction[3] that about 75% of older cyanotic children would have tetralogy of Fallot was true before the ad-

TABLE 28–1

CONDITIONS ASSOCIATED WITH TETRALOGY OF FALLOT

SYNDROMES
   Trisomy 21 (Down)
   Velocardiofacial (Shprintzen's)
   CATCH-22
   Goldenhar's
   Thrombocytopenia absent radius
   CHARGE
   VATER/VACTERL
   Fetal alcohol
   Pierre Robin

ASSOCIATED ORGAN ABNORMALITIES
   Tracheoesophageal fistula
   Imperforate anus
   Hydrocephalus
   Omphalocele

CATCH-22 = Cardiac defects, Abnormal facies, Thymic hypoplasia, Cleft palate, Hypocalcemia, and abnormality of chromosome 22; CHARGE = Coloboma, Heart disease, Atresia choanae, Retarded growth and development, Genital abnormalities, Ear anomalies; VATER = Vertebral defects, Anal atresia, Tracheoesophageal fistula, Renal defects, and Radial upper arm dysplasia; VACTERL = VATER + Cardiac and Limb anomalies.

vent of cardiac surgery. This lesion has the best untreated outcome of any cyanotic malformation, although the median age at death in different series has ranged from age 4 to 12 years.[14,15] Only about 10% of untreated patients live more than 20 years,[16–18] and they have neither pulmonary atresia nor absent pulmonary valves. Less than 5% survive to age 40 years.[19] Most of the long-term survivors had only mild cyanosis, although they are still at risk of many of the complications of chronic cyanotic heart disease (see Chapter 63). In addition, ventricular tachycardia occurs with increasing frequency as they age.[20]

About half of the patients with tetralogy of Fallot and absent pulmonary valve die before 1 year of age,[21] mainly because of airway complications. The remainder continue to be mildly cyanotic for 5 to 20 years but die prematurely because of right ventricular failure caused by volume overload.

About half of the patients with pulmonary atresia and a VSD die before 1 year of age.[21] Most of the others die usually before 10 years of age.

PHYSICAL EXAMINATION AND CLINICAL PRESENTATION

The clinical presentation with tetralogy of Fallot depends primarily on the degree of right ventricular outflow tract obstruction. Presentation can range from a profoundly cyanotic newborn with ductus-dependent pulmonary circulation, to an asymptomatic child with adequate pulmonary flow presenting for evaluation of a murmur. Because of this wide spectrum of presentation, the physical findings vary between individuals. Relatively few of these children are cyanotic at birth, but most become cyanotic by 3 months of age.

Inspection most often reveals an apparently healthy infant or child, although major extracardiac anomalies, such as hypospadias, cleft lip and palate, pectus carinatum, and other bony abnormalities, can be seen.[22] Cyanosis is present to varying degrees and can be best appreciated in the mucous membranes or nail beds. The degree of cyanosis depends not only on the amount of right-to-left intracardiac shunting, but also on the hemoglobin concentration. To appreciate cyanosis, there must be approximately 3 to 5 g/dl of desaturated hemoglobin in arterial blood; this quantity is easier to achieve at higher hemoglobin concentrations. Therefore, a relatively polycythemic neonate may appear more cyanotic shortly after birth than at a few months of age during the period of normal postnatal physiologic anemia.

The level of cyanosis in a given individual varies with activity. Exercise increases the level of cyanosis, primarily as a result of the decreased systemic vascular resistance that normally occurs with exercise and a resultant increase in right-to-left shunting. Additionally, the accentuated inotropic state may aggravate pulmonary outflow obstruction and further contribute to cyanosis.

Older children with unrepaired tetralogy of Fallot often squat. This position is thought to improve systemic saturation by increasing the systemic vascular resistance by kinking the large arterial vessels in the legs. The increased systemic resistance shifts the biventricular output such that

more blood flow enters the lungs across the pulmonary outflow obstruction.

Tetralogy spells or *hypercyanotic spells* are periods of severe cyanosis associated with hyperpnea, tachypnea, and agitation that can result in coma. They may occur without warning but have also been associated with activities such as crying, eating, and defecating. These spells occur more commonly in the mornings, during the summer months, and during intercurrent illnesses. The episodes are usually self-limited and last between 15 and 30 minutes, but they can be prolonged. The hypoxemia can be severe enough to result in altered mental status and even death. The physiologic basis for these episodes remains obscure, although a number of hypotheses have been proposed, including increased infundibular contractility, peripheral vasodilatation, hyperventilation, and stimulation of right ventricular mechanoreceptors.[23] A child admitted with one of these spells should be diagnosed rapidly and clinically. The combination of hyperpnea, deep cyanosis, and normal air entry into lung fields (thus excluding a foreign body in the airways) is pathognomonic. Some infants have minor spells with inconsolable irritability and only a slight increase in cyanosis. They are often erroneously diagnosed as having colic.

Clubbing of the fingers and toes develops in patients with chronic cyanosis. Although usually seen in older patients, it can develop in infancy. With restoration of normal systemic oxygen saturation after complete repair, clubbing resolves.

In a preoperative patient, the jugular venous pulsations are usually normal, although difficult to evaluate in infants. The right ventricle remains relatively compliant with normal or only mildly elevated filling pressures, and significant tricuspid regurgitation is uncommon. Thus the *a* and *v* waves in the jugular pulse are usually normal.

The peripheral pulses are usually normal, and accentuated pulses should suggest a large patent ductus arteriosus or significant aorticopulmonary collateral arteries. The precordial impulse can be normal, but usually a right ventricular parasternal lift can be appreciated. Hepatomegaly is unusual.

Auscultation reveals a normal first sound and a single second sound, which is loudest at the midleft sternal border because of the wide, dextroposed aorta. With significant right ventricular outflow tract obstruction and low pulmonary arterial pressures, the pulmonary component of the second heart sound is usually inaudible. Occasionally, if the outflow tract obstruction is not severe, splitting of the second heart sound can be appreciated. Third and fourth heart sounds are uncommon. An early systolic ejection click can be heard at the left mid-to-upper sternal border caused by the dilated ascending aorta and the increased systemic blood flow.

The murmur in patients with unrepaired tetralogy of Fallot is generated by the right ventricular outflow obstruction. The VSD is large and unrestrictive, and the right-to-left shunt does not produce a murmur. The murmur is classically described as a low-pitched, systolic crescendo/decrescendo ejection murmur best heard at the left mid-to-upper sternal border with radiation to the back. However, it is not uncommon for the murmur to resemble that of an isolated VSD with a pansystolic, plateau quality, best heard at the left mid-to-lower sternal border. In these patients, one needs to rely on other physical findings such as cyanosis or a single second heart sound to suspect the diagnosis of tetralogy of Fallot. In an acyanotic neonate, the murmur caused by the left-to-right shunt across the VSD is difficult to separate from the murmur of infundibular stenosis, and it is easy to misdiagnose the infant as having a small VSD. The distinction can be made clinically in most infants; a neonate with tetralogy will have a forceful right ventricular lift and usually a loud second heart sound, best heard at the midleft sternal border.

Unlike pulmonary valve stenosis with an intact ventricular septum in which the intensity and length of the murmur increase with increasing obstruction, the murmur in tetralogy of Fallot diminishes with worsening obstruction. This is because the intensity of the murmur is related not only to the degree of obstruction, but also to the amount of flow across the obstruction. In tetralogy of Fallot, as the right ventricular outflow tract obstruction progresses, the right ventricular systolic output is preferentially shunted across the VSD and into the systemic circulation. The flow across the right ventricular outflow tract is reduced, resulting in a softer murmur. This phenomenon is best demonstrated by a tetralogy spell, during which the outflow obstruction can become so severe that the murmur becomes inaudible while the patient becomes progressively more cyanotic.

Diastolic murmurs are rarely heard in an unoperated patient with tetralogy of Fallot. A continuous murmur in the left infraclavicular region suggests a patent ductus arteriosus. Very rarely a right-sided ductus arteriosus results in a continuous murmur in the right infraclavicular region. Continuous murmurs heard in the posterior lung fields raise concern about significant aorticopulmonary collaterals. The presence of an early diastolic murmur along the left sternal border is one of the hallmark findings in tetralogy of Fallot with absent pulmonary valve.

The physical examination in a postoperative patient depends on the type of procedure performed. Palliation with a systemic shunt produces a continuous murmur similar to a patent ductus arteriosus. Appreciation of this murmur in the immediate postoperative period may be difficult because of a ventilator or other competing noises. In this situation, auscultating while the bell of the stethoscope is briefly applied to the end of the endotracheal tube often allows appreciation of the murmur because of the proximity of the shunt to the bronchi.

After complete repair of tetralogy of Fallot a variety of physical findings can be found. On inspection, cyanosis should be absent and clubbing should resolve with time. If tricuspid regurgitation has developed, a prominent v wave can be appreciated in the jugular pulsations. Depending on the degree of pulmonary insufficiency and residual outflow tract obstruction, one can palpate a right ventricular parasternal lift. On auscultation, the first heart sound remains normal. The second heart sound frequently remains single. When, however, the pulmonary valve is partially or completely intact, the second heart sound can split normally with respiration or, if there is right bundle branch block, is widely split. It varies with respiration, but the split persists during expiration. Frequently an ejection systolic murmur is present at the left mid-to-upper sternal border

from mild residual right ventricular outflow obstruction. A more intense ejection murmur should raise concern about more significant obstruction. During follow-up, long systolic ejection murmurs that are best appreciated at the left upper sternal border or in either the axilla or the back indicate branch pulmonary artery stenosis and usually warrant further investigation. A blowing, pansystolic murmur from a small residual VSD or tricuspid regurgitation may be heard at the left lower sternal border. A low-pitched delayed diastolic decrescendo murmur at the midleft sternal border is common and results from pulmonary insufficiency caused by relief of the right ventricular outflow obstruction. This diastolic murmur should be differentiated from the high-pitched early diastolic decrescendo murmur at the left sternal border generated from aortic insufficiency. This latter murmur is not expected unless patients have had long-standing pulmonary atresia with a dilated aortic root, and it also warrants further evaluation. Most patients with satisfactory surgical results have soft systolic/diastolic to-and-fro murmurs of mild pulmonary stenosis and regurgitation along the mid-to-upper left sternal border.

ABSENT PULMONARY VALVE

Tetralogy of Fallot with absent pulmonary valve occurs in a small, distinct subpopulation of patients with a unique presentation. This condition is characterized by severe dilatation of the pulmonary arteries with mild pulmonary stenosis and severe pulmonary insufficiency. The dilated pulmonary arteries can compress the bronchi and result in life-threatening airway compromise as early as the immediate newborn period. Standard airway support, such as endotracheal intubation and mechanical ventilation, can be only partially effective. Positioning the infants prone is known to improve airway compromise by removing bronchial compression and can be a life-saving maneuver.

Alternatively, if these infants do not have significant airway compromise, they are more apt to develop congestive heart failure as their right ventricular outflow obstruction is less severe and left-to-right shunting with pulmonary overcirculation is possible. These infants may be intensely cyanotic at birth, but then after a few days, as pulmonary vascular resistance decreases and pulmonary blood flow increases, cyanosis is often mild or absent. On palpation, a prominent precordial impulse with a right ventricular lift is common, and a thrill may be present. Hepatomegaly can accompany other signs of congestive heart failure. On auscultation, the first heart sound is normal, and the second heart sound is single. Third or fourth sounds can be heard. There is a characteristic prominent systolic/diastolic to-and-fro murmur ("sawing wood" murmur) heard along the left sternal border. The systolic component is an ejection quality murmur generated by the pulmonary stenosis, and the diastolic component is a low-pitched decrescendo murmur generated from the severe pulmonary insufficiency.

Postoperatively these patients may still have significant airway compromise. Depending on the type of repair, physical findings on cardiac examination will often not be significantly different from other patients with tetralogy of Fallot.

PULMONARY ATRESIA WITH VENTRICULAR SEPTAL DEFECT

In the neonate with pulmonary atresia and VSD, auscultation reveals a single second heart sound and usually a soft continuous murmur of a ductus or MAPCA. Occasionally, patients have no audible murmur, and, conversely, patients can have loud continuous murmurs and bounding pulses in rare situations in which pulmonary blood flow is unrestrictive and congestive heart failure can ensue.

Patients with a balanced degree of pulmonary flow and soft murmurs may escape detection in the neonatal period and be recognized only as their cyanosis becomes apparent, or physical examination becomes significant in terms of murmur or prominent precordial ventricular impulse.

DIAGNOSIS

The acyanotic neonate needs to be distinguished from an infant with a simple VSD (see earlier). The cyanotic infant needs to be distinguished from infants with other forms of cyanotic heart disease with pulmonic stenosis, including double outlet right ventricle, transposition of the great arteries and a VSD, single ventricle, and tricuspid atresia with normally related great vessels. Each of these has distinctive echocardiographic features. Tricuspid atresia has a characteristic electrocardiogram, and all these entities are much less common than tetralogy of Fallot.

The diagnosis of tetralogy of Fallot is aided by use of electrocardiography and chest radiography. The electrocardiogram is quite useful because it always shows right ventricular hypertrophy. In addition, right atrial enlargement and right-axis deviation are also usually present. Biventricular hypertrophy can be seen in patients who have so-called pink tetralogy with increased pulmonary blood flow. In a neonate, the first or only sign of right ventricular hypertrophy can be an upright T wave in lead V_1 or V_4R after 3 days of age. As the child gets older, typical signs of right ventricular hypertrophy are present with leads V_1 and V_4R showing a tall R wave and small S wave, an rR′

pattern or a QR pattern. Figure 28–5 shows the electrocardiogram of a 6-month-old infant with tetralogy of Fallot.

The chest radiograph of the typical patient shows normal visceroatrial situs, a tilted-up apex, a concave main pulmonary artery segment, and normal to decreased pulmonary vascularity. The heart is usually not enlarged (see Fig. 10–12). A right-sided aortic arch can be identified in approximately 25% of patients with tetralogy of Fallot.

Patients with tetralogy of Fallot and absent pulmonary valve usually have large hearts and markedly enlarged main, right, and left pulmonary arteries. Frequently lung hyperinflation and tracheobronchial compression occur (see Fig. 10–13).

The electrocardiogram and chest radiograph in patients with pulmonary atresia and VSD are usually virtually identical to those found in patients with tetralogy of Fallot. The rare patient with increased pulmonary blood flow caused by a large ductus or a large collateral can show an enlarged heart with increased vascularity and hyperinflated lung fields.

ECHOCARDIOGRAPHY

Two-dimensional echocardiography and Doppler echocardiography are invaluable in the diagnosis of tetralogy of Fallot, both prenatally and postnatally. Tetralogy of Fallot has been diagnosed as early as 14 weeks' gestation using transvaginal ultrasound.[24] This lesion, however, continues to evolve through midgestation and late gestation,[25–27] and serial studies of the embryo and fetus with tetralogy of Fallot are essential in preparing families for the postnatal course of these infants. Early in gestation, the large malalignment perimembranous VSD and aortic override can be seen. Anterior deviation of the conal septum is also apparent. By midgestation, there is considerable variation in the size of the main pulmonary artery, which may be normal or hypoplastic. The branch pulmonary arteries are usually of normal size. In the second half of pregnancy, patients with more severe forms of tetralogy of Fallot demonstrate abnormal growth of the main and branch pulmonary arteries, resulting in progressive hypoplasia, and even in

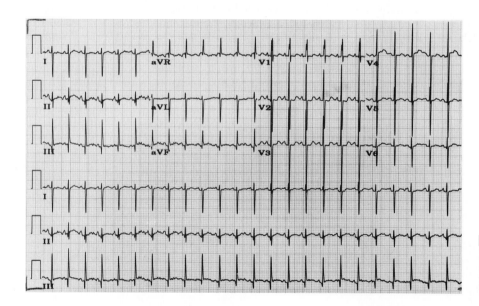

FIGURE 28–5

Electrocardiogram from a 6-month-old infant. The upright T wave in V_1 with the prominent S wave in V_6 indicates right ventricular hypertrophy.

loss of anterograde flow. The aorta may be normal or increased in size during midgestation, with an increased rate of growth when compared with normal controls, resulting in the large ascending aorta characteristic of this lesion.

The likelihood of prenatal detection of tetralogy of Fallot during ultrasound screening depends on both the severity of the defect and the experience of the ultrasonographer. Although the malaligned VSD should be seen in the four-chamber view during obstetric screening (Fig. 28–6), this lesion has been missed during screening examinations that rely on this view alone. Visualization of the outflow tract views can increase the likelihood of prenatal diagnosis of tetralogy of Fallot, although fetuses with milder forms of this anomaly have relatively normal outflow tract views at midgestation. In large prenatal echocardiographic series using multiple imaging planes for comprehensive evaluation, tetralogy of Fallot is one of the more commonly diagnosed lesions, accounting for between 4 and 28% of identified congenital cardiac anomalies. The subset of fetuses with tetralogy of Fallot with absent pulmonary valve are disproportionately represented in prenatal series, almost certainly because the dilated right ventricle and pulmonary arterial tree that characterize this lesion result in their more frequent identification.

During prenatal echocardiographic examination, the characteristic VSD can be demonstrated in the long-axis, sagittal, and four-chamber views. Doppler interrogation of the VSD should be included to rule out the rare restrictive VSD. Short-axis and sagittal views can be used to delineate the right ventricular outflow tract and main and branch pulmonary arteries. Although Doppler interrogation of the right ventricular outflow tract is important in the assessment of the severity of obstruction postnatally, flow velocities in the parallel fetal circulation are usually in the normal range.[28, 29] Doppler interrogation and Doppler color flow mapping can, however, readily demonstrate the to-and-fro flow pattern seen in fetuses with absent pulmonary valve. Sagittal imaging planes also allow examination of the ductus arteriosus and aortic arch. Fetuses with more severe right ventricular outflow tract obstruction have retrograde ductal flow in utero.[30] Other evidence of the severe right ventricular outflow tract obstruction includes significant hypoplasia of the main and branch pulmonary arteries and poor growth of the pulmonary arterial tree during the course of serial examinations.

As with all prenatal diagnoses of congenital heart disease, fetuses with tetralogy of Fallot should undergo assessment of fetal karyotype and comprehensive ultrasound examination to rule out extracardiac anomalies. Families should be counseled regarding the in utero evaluation of this lesion and the need for serial evaluations. All fetuses with the prenatal diagnosis of tetralogy for Fallot should be delivered at a tertiary care center with appropriate support staff for the evaluation and treatment of these infants.

Postnatally, complete echocardiographic evaluation of the infant with tetralogy of Fallot must include examination of all aspects of anatomy important to management. At many institutions, echocardiography is the primary method of evaluation before operation, with cardiac catheterization reserved for those patients with specific unresolved questions after echocardiographic examination. Elements of anatomy that must be assessed include the anatomic type and boundaries of the VSD, the presence or absence of multiple VSDs, the severity and level of right ventricular outflow tract obstruction, the anatomy of the pulmonary arteries, the anatomy of the aortic arch, the course of the coronary arterial tree, and the presence of associated abnormalities.

The large VSD most commonly seen in this lesion can be imaged in multiple views. The relationship among the aorta, the mitral valve, and the large VSD can be seen in the long-axis view (Fig. 28–7). The fibrous continuity between the mitral and aortic valves can be demonstrated, and the degree of aortic override can be assessed. The relationship between the defect and the tricuspid valve can be seen in the parasternal short-axis view, in which the potential for extension into the supracristal region can also be assessed. The apical four-chamber view demonstrates the continuity among the tricuspid, aortic, and mitral valves and also allows assessment of the degree of aortic override. Caudal angulation of the transducer can be used to examine the degree of posterior extension of the defect.

The subcostal right oblique view is perhaps the most useful view to evaluate the VSD (Fig. 28–8). Here, the relationship between the tricuspid and aortic valves in infants with a perimembranous defect is well seen. When the defect is present, a ridge of muscular tissue can be seen separating the tricuspid and aortic valves in this view. Extension of the defect into the supracristal region can also be demonstrated. In the rare instances of obstruction of the VSD, the subcostal coronal view allows demonstration

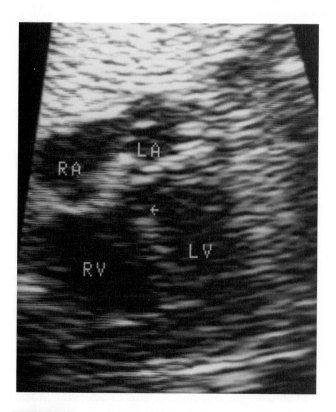

FIGURE 28–6

Echocardiogram showing a four-chamber image of a fetus with tetralogy of Fallot at 32 weeks' gestation, demonstrating large ventricular septal defect *(arrow)*. LA = left atrium; LV = left ventricle; RA = right atrium; RV = right ventricle.

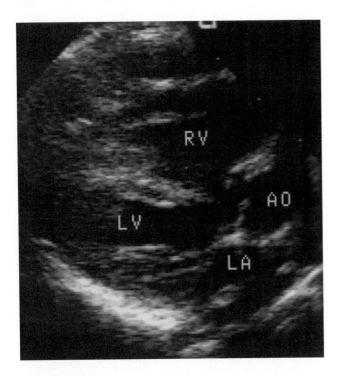

Echocardiogram showing a parasternal long-axis view of an infant with tetralogy of Fallot, demonstrating a large perimembranous ventricular septal defect, aortic override, and mitral/aortic valve fibrous continuity. AO = aorta; LA = left atrium; LV = left ventricle; RV = right ventricle.

of the abnormal or accessory tricuspid valve tissue obstructing the defect and of possible attachments to the infundibular septum.[31,32] This abnormal tricuspid valve tissue can also be imaged in parasternal axis views.

The levels of right ventricular outflow tract obstruction are best assessed in the parasternal short-axis and subcostal

views. The prominent bands of the crista supraventricularis can be seen intruding on the infundibular region in the subcostal coronal view. In the parasternal short-axis and subcostal sagittal views, the anterior and superior deviation of the infundibular septum can be appreciated, and the abnormal pulmonary valve can be seen (Figs. 28–9 and 28–10). Measurements of the pulmonary valve annulus are important in assessing the need for transannular patch.

The parasternal short-axis view allows evaluation of the pulmonary artery confluence and proximal branch pulmonary arteries; the suprasternal notch short- and long-axis views also allow verification of the confluent nature of the pulmonary arteries and visualization of the branch pulmonary arteries more distally. When the pulmonary arteries are not confluent, alternative sources of blood supply can be identified from these views. Assessment of the size and symmetry of the branch pulmonary arteries is important in both the decision regarding the appropriateness of primary repair and the need for patch augmentation of the proximal pulmonary arteries at the time of operation. Despite the multiple levels of right ventricular outflow tract obstruction and the elongated nature of the infundibular obstruction, predicted outflow tract gradients using the modified Bernoulli equation compare favorably with catheterization data,[33] allowing verification of the usually low pulmonary arterial pressure.

These same views can be used to assess the right ventricular outflow tract in infants with tetralogy of Fallot and absent pulmonary valve. In these infants, the infundibular obstruction may not be as severe, although there is significant obstruction at the small pulmonary annulus and, in some patients, by dysplastic valvar tissue. There is marked dilatation of the proximal main and branch pulmonary arteries, and Doppler interrogation demonstrates the severe pulmonary insufficiency that characterizes this lesion.

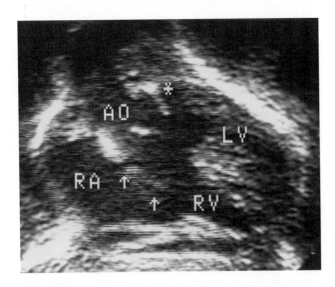

Echocardiogram showing a subcostal right oblique view in a neonate demonstrating large ventricular septal defect, overriding aorta, tricuspid/aortic valve fibrous continuity, and anterior deviation of the infundibular septum (°). *Arrows* identify tricuspid valve leaflet. AO = aorta; LV = left ventricle; RA = right atrium; RV = right ventricle.

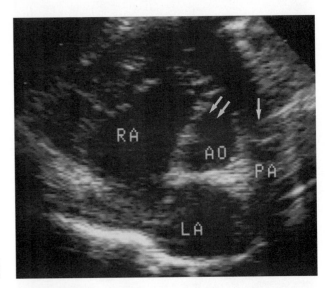

Echocardiogram showing a diastolic frame from parasternal short-axis view of a 3-week-old infant with tetralogy of Fallot. Tricuspid valve leaflets partially obscure ventricular septal defect (*double arrows*). Anterior deviation of the infundibular septum and small pulmonary annulus (*single arrow*) are demonstrated. AO = aorta; LA = left atrium; PA = pulmonary artery; RA = right atrium.

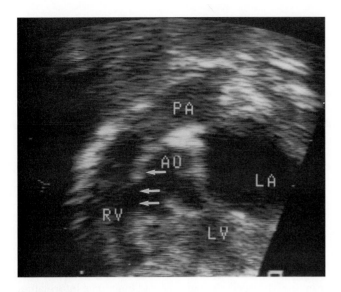

FIGURE 28–10

Echocardiogram demonstrating a subcostal sagittal image from an infant with tetralogy of Fallot and a large ventricular septal defect *(double arrows)* with aortic override and anterior deviation of the infundibular septum *(single arrow)*. AO = aorta; LA = left atrium; LV = left ventricle; PA = pulmonary artery; RV = right ventricle.

Several authors have described the echocardiographic evaluation of coronary artery anatomy in this lesion.[34–36] Echocardiographic evaluation must demonstrate that no major coronary arteries cross the right ventricular outflow tract (Fig. 28–11). The origin and course of the left and

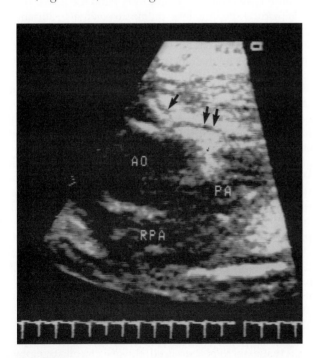

FIGURE 28–11

Echocardiogram showing a parasternal short-axis view with counterclockwise rotation from a neonate with tetralogy of Fallot, demonstrating the right coronary artery *(single arrow)* originating from the right coronary orifice and giving rise to the left anterior descending coronary artery, which crosses the pulmonary outflow tract anteriorly *(double arrows)*. AO = aorta, PA = pulmonary artery; RPA = right pulmonary artery.

right coronary arteries can be traced in multiple views, although the parasternal long- and short-axis views may be the most helpful. Any concerns regarding abnormal coronary anatomy should be verified angiographically.

Aortic arch anatomy can be demonstrated by echocardiography using suprasternal long- and short-axis views, first to determine the relationship between the trachea and the arch, and then to define the branching pattern. Doppler color flow mapping can be used to exclude the presence of a ductus arteriosus or of prominent aorticopulmonary collaterals.

Complete echocardiographic evaluation must also rule out associated anomalies important in planning the surgical approach to this lesion. Two-dimensional imaging and color flow mapping in multiple planes must be used to identify an associated atrial septal defect and additional VSDs. Abnormalities of pulmonary and systemic venous connection must be delineated, and rare left-sided lesions, such as mitral valve abnormalities and subaortic obstruction, must also be identified.

Postoperative studies must define residual septal defects and the degree and level of residual outflow tract obstruction. Care should be taken to carry examination of the branch pulmonary arteries distally to identify branch stenosis at the sites of previous shunts or at the juxtaductal site. Patients after transannular patch repair usually have significant pulmonary insufficiency, which can be assessed either by comparing the width of the regurgitant jet to the annulus[37] or by assessing how far distally the regurgitant jet can be traced beyond the annulus.[38] Although pulmonary insufficiency is generally well tolerated, assessment of right ventricular size and wall motion, as well as tricuspid valve function, should be part of all postoperative echocardiographic studies.

Patients with pulmonary atresia and VSD, as discussed earlier, have similar intracardiac anatomy to patients with classic tetralogy of Fallot. In the absence of anterograde flow from the right ventricle to the pulmonary artery, careful echocardiographic study of the central pulmonary arteries is necessary. The goals of the echocardiographic study are to define the intracardiac anatomy; evaluate ventricular function; evaluate valvar regurgitation; evaluate coronary origins; define the presence or absence of central pulmonary arteries; measure the size of the main, right, and left pulmonary arteries; define the presence or absence of either a left or right ductus arteriosus; and define as many MAPCAs, with their site of origin and proximal distribution to right or left lungs, as possible. These studies can be difficult and time-consuming, with the need for extensive use of color flow mapping. A reasonable road map should be obtained before the necessary cardiac catheterization procedures. Intracardiac anatomy should be defined completely so that contrast media can be conserved at catheterization for comprehensive delineation of pulmonary artery origin, distribution, and anatomy.

MEDICAL MANAGEMENT

The medical management of the tetralogy patient depends on the clinical presentation. The cyanotic neonate who is ductus dependent should be stabilized with prostaglandin

E_1. Further evaluation by cardiac catheterization may be necessary if complete repair is planned or if palliation with balloon valvuloplasty is attempted. If initial palliation is planned with a systemic-to-pulmonary artery shunt, catheterization may be unnecessary at that time, as long as the pulmonary artery anatomy is outlined clearly by noninvasive studies.

In an asymptomatic infant with adequate pulmonary flow and systemic saturation, no initial therapy may be necessary. The infant can be followed as an outpatient with close attention to growth, symptoms, and systemic saturation. If the child develops significant cyanosis or reaches an appropriate size or age, repair can be performed on an elective basis. The development of tetralogy spells is an indication for early intervention.

Medical management of hypercyanotic spells is directed toward improving pulmonary blood flow. Parents should be educated to try and comfort the child while placing him or her in the knee/chest position to increase systemic afterload and force more blood flow across the pulmonary outflow tract. In a hospital setting, the patient's airway and breathing should be assessed, the knee/chest position should be assumed, and 100% oxygen should be given. Sedation with morphine sulfate (0.1 mg/kg) can be given intravenously (IV), or intramuscularly (IM) should an intravenous line not be available; the exact mechanism by which morphine helps is unclear. Acidosis may develop and should be treated with bicarbonate. An intravenous fluid bolus (5–10 ml/kg) of saline or lactated Ringer's solution ensures adequate right ventricular filling, which is thought to improve pulmonary flow. Should these measures fail, intravenous β-blockade with propranolol or esmolol slows the heart rate and improves filling, while decreasing catecholamine stimulation and contractility. Systemic afterload can be increased with α-agonists in an effort to force more blood flow through the right ventricular outflow tract. Continuous infusion of phenylephrine at a rate of 0.5 to 5.0 μg/kg/min has been successful. The effects on blood pressure and symptoms should be monitored. The effect of the medication is enhanced by the fluid administration as described earlier. In fact, some authorities use vasopressors as the first line of treatment. β-Adrenergic agonists are absolutely contraindicated. Finally, should all measures fail, general anesthesia can reverse the episode or prepare the patient for an emergency aorticopulmonary shunt if hypoxemia persists.

In patients with chronic hypoxemia, oral therapy with propranolol (0.5–1 mg/kg qid) can be beneficial in improving saturations and reducing the risk of hypercyanotic spells. These patients are also at risk for thromboembolic complications, a risk that is highest in patients with coexisting iron deficiency anemia. Close monitoring of both hemoglobin concentration and mean corpuscular volume is necessary. These patients should have an elevated hemoglobin at baseline, and a normal hemoglobin value may actually represent a relative anemia. Iron deficiency anemia should be treated with supplemental iron.

Whether an infant or young child undergoes initial palliation or complete repair depends on the institution. In the past, the approach was to try and delay complete repair until later childhood. In the mid-1990s, successful complete repair in early infancy and even the immediate neonatal period has been demonstrated.[39–41] Elective primary repair is usually performed at 6 to 18 months of age.

There are a wide variety of reasons why initial palliation before complete repair might be deemed necessary. These include problems such as small patient size, left anterior descending coronary arising from the right coronary artery, hypoplastic pulmonary arteries, or unresponsive hypercyanotic spell. This palliation previously meant a systemic-to-pulmonary artery shunt. In the mid-1990s, however, adequate palliation has been demonstrated with percutaneous pulmonary valvuloplasty (see later).[42, 43]

CARDIAC CATHETERIZATION

Many institutions continue to perform cardiac catheterization as part of the routine preoperative assessment of the patient with tetralogy of Fallot. Although echocardiography can provide excellent anatomic and functional information, angiography continues to prove useful in delineating certain anatomic details, such as coronary artery distribution, distal branch pulmonary artery anatomy, additional ventricular septal defects, and aorticopulmonary collateral vessels.

The catheterization is most commonly performed from a femoral approach where both arterial and venous access is obtained. The left side of the heart can often be reached via an atrial communication so that most of the hemodynamic measurements can be performed with the venous catheter. Pressures and oxygen saturations should be obtained in the superior vena cava, both ventricles, both atria (if there is an atrial communication), and the aorta. If left atrial saturations are low, pulmonary venous saturations should be obtained. Systemic left and right systolic pressures should be expected, and any variation from this requires further investigation. Ventricular end-diastolic and atrial pressures are often normal or only mildly elevated. A wide systemic pulse pressure should suggest a patent ductus arteriosus or large systemic to pulmonary artery collateral vessels. Saturations usually demonstrate some right-to-left shunting, which can be at both the atrial and ventricular levels. Evidence of left-to-right shunting may also be found if the pulmonary arteries are entered. Whether to cross the right ventricular outflow tract in a patient who is being prepared for elective repair depends on the operator. The benefit is that pulmonary artery pressures and saturations can be obtained; pulmonary flow, pulmonary resistance, and left-to-right shunting can be calculated. Additionally, branch pulmonary artery stenosis may be further examined, although this may be difficult to assess in the face of significant proximal obstruction. The benefits must be weighed against the risks, which include arrhythmia, perforation, and hypercyanotic spells, associated with trying to cross the stenotic outflow tract.

Angiography should be guided by the anatomic questions that need to be answered. Biplane cineangiography is needed, and the angiograms that provide the most important information for a particular patient should be performed first. This ensures adequate contrast availability, should multiple angiograms of a particular structure be necessary.

With multiple levels of obstruction to pulmonary flow, including infundibular, valvar, supravalvar, and branch pulmonary artery, an injection of contrast material into the right ventricle is often indicated (see Fig. 28–2). To visualize the branch pulmonary arteries and their bifurcation better, it is helpful to angle the anteroposterior (AP) camera about 30 degrees cranially with a small amount of left anterior oblique (LAO) rotation. The cranial angulation prevents overlap of the outflow tract onto the pulmonary artery bifurcation. The LAO rotation of the camera improves evaluation of the proximal left pulmonary artery, which may be difficult to see in straight AP projection. Keeping the lateral camera in a straight lateral (90 degrees LAO) projection usually provides excellent imaging of the right ventricular outflow tract and allows evaluation of the infundibular, valvar, and supravalvar areas. Additionally, right-to-left shunting across the VSD may be seen in this view.

Evaluation of the coronary arteries and aorta can often be accomplished with a single injection of contrast material into the ascending aorta. The catheter should be positioned close to the aortic valve to ensure adequate visualization of the coronary arteries. Camera positioning should be tailored to delineate the proximal coronary artery origins and distribution. A variety of camera angles have proved useful, and some authors have even advocated selective coronary angiography, although this has risk in small infants and children. We have found that an injection with the AP camera in 30 degrees right anterior oblique (RAO) and the lateral camera in 70 degrees LAO and 20 degrees cranial (long axial oblique) positions usually results in adequate delineation of the coronary distribution (see Fig. 28–4). Should a particular view not demonstrate the coronary anatomy adequately, the operator should be prepared to try alternative views. The ascending aortic injection also provides information about the aortic arch (right sided or left sided), brachiocephalic vessels (distribution and size), and the presence of a ductus arteriosus and collateral vessels. Embolization of collateral vessels can be performed if deemed necessary.

An injection of contrast material into the left ventricle provides useful information about the VSDs; degree of aortic override; and, if there is any significant left-to-right shunting, the right ventricular outflow tract obstruction. This is often best accomplished with the AP camera in a 30 degrees RAO projection and the lateral camera in a long axial oblique projection.

Postoperative catheterization is usually reserved for patients with residual abnormalities, such as intracardiac shunting, right ventricular outflow tract obstruction, significant pulmonary insufficiency, or branch pulmonary artery stenosis. The goal may be purely diagnostic but is often therapeutic. The refinement of balloon angioplasty and percutaneous stenting techniques have proved invaluable in the management of patients with residual obstruction that may be difficult or impossible to repair surgically (Fig. 28–12).

Patients with pulmonary atresia and VSD present a difficult challenge for both diagnostic and interventional catheterization. Preoperative catheterization must attempt to delineate all sources of pulmonary blood flow and identify the number of bronchopulmonary segments supplied by central pulmonary arteries and by MAPCAs. Ascertaining whether dual blood supply is present is also a goal, in addition to determining the severity of stenoses of central pul-

monary arteries and MAPCAs. Various techniques to obtain these data include balloon occlusion aortography at various levels in the descending aorta (Fig. 28–13), selective injection of MAPCAs or ductus (Figs. 28–14 and 28–15), and pulmonary vein wedge angiography (Fig. 28–16).

Postoperative catheterizations are necessary to assess the patency of shunts or unifocalization procedures that have been carried out, the growth of central pulmonary arteries, the distribution of flow to various bronchopulmonary segments, the presence of stenoses, and the presence of unifocal or dual blood supply from central pulmonary arteries and MAPCAs to various bronchopulmonary segments. Balloon dilatation of stenotic arteries and stenting of vessels are a major part of the reconstructive process for these patients. In addition, some patients need coil occlusion of redundant collaterals or MAPCAs to prevent pulmonary overcirculation.

SURGICAL REPAIR

The report of the Blalock-Taussig (BT) shunt in 1945 opened the door to palliation of patients with tetralogy of Fallot.[5] This technique, often referred to as a *classic BT shunt*, involves anastomosing the subclavian artery to the ipsilateral pulmonary artery to improve pulmonary blood flow. The anastomosis is usually performed on the side opposite the aortic arch because of the greater mobility of the subclavian artery provided by the innominate artery. A more recent modification of the original technique involves placement of an interposition tube graft, usually of GoreTex, between the subclavian artery and the ipsilateral pulmonary artery. This procedure is often referred to as a *modified BT shunt* and can be performed from the subclavian artery, the innominate artery, or the ascending or descending aorta. Other methods of palliation, such as a direct anastomosis of the left pulmonary artery to the descending aorta (Potts' shunt) or of the right pulmonary artery to the ascending aorta (Waterston's shunt), have for the most part been abandoned because of the frequent development of pulmonary vascular disease resulting from excessive pulmonary flow and pressure, and distortion of the pulmonary arteries.

The BT shunt provides excellent palliation, and it was not until 1954 that complete intracardiac repair, with closure of the VSD and relief of the right ventricular outflow obstruction, was demonstrated by Lillehei and colleagues.[6] Although there have been tremendous advances in cardiothoracic surgery and extracorporeal circulation since that time, the standard technique for repair of tetralogy of Fallot has remained relatively unchanged except for minor variations among institutions.[21]

Most commonly a vertical incision is made in the right ventricular outflow tract through which both the outflow tract obstruction and the VSD can be repaired. When a coronary artery crosses the right ventricular outflow tract, a horizontal incision in the outflow tract or a transatrial/pulmonary arterial approach may be preferred. The VSD is closed with artificial patch material, with care taken to avoid injury to the aortic valve leaflets as well as the conduction system, which usually runs along the left posteroinferior margin of the VSD.

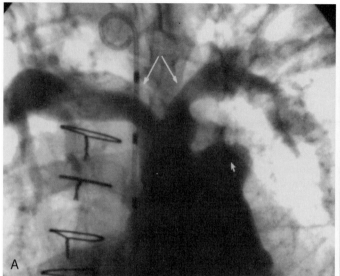

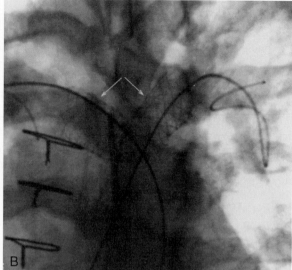

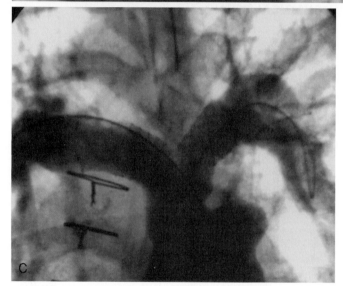

FIGURE 28–12

Three angiograms taken from a 22-year-old patient after complete repair in childhood with residual branch pulmonary artery stenosis and right ventricular hypertension. *A*, The bilateral branch stenosis is well visualized *(long arrows)*. A small diverticulum of the right ventricular outflow tract *(short arrow)* is demonstrated. A marker pigtail catheter is positioned in the right-sided aorta for calibration purposes. *B*, Bilateral stents have been placed *(arrows)*. *C*, Angiography demonstrated relief of proximal pulmonary artery stenosis.

Right ventricular outflow tract obstruction can be at multiple levels. Subvalvar obstruction caused by infundibular tissue and hypertrophied muscle bundles is resected. The pulmonary valve is inspected and is often stenotic; valvotomy is performed as necessary to provide adequate unobstructed flow. If the pulmonary annulus is small, it may be necessary to extend the ventriculotomy incision across the pulmonary annulus so that when the ventriculotomy is closed by a patch there is a widely patent outflow tract and annulus. The drawback to the transannular patch is that it often results in significant pulmonary insufficiency. If there is further supravalvar or branch pulmonary artery stenosis, an incision can be extended along the pulmonary trunk and into the proximal branch pulmonary arteries to allow patch augmentation. If present, an atrial septal defect should be closed, unless there is reason to believe that right ventricular systolic or diastolic dysfunction or residual right ventricular outflow tract obstruction is present. If so, a patent foramen ovale should be left to enhance systemic output from right-to-left atrial shunting in the early postoperative period.

Advances in the surgical approach of a patient with tetralogy of Fallot include early complete repair in infancy and repair through a transatrial approach (see section on future directions).

The surgical approach to the patient with tetralogy of Fallot and absent pulmonary valve is less clear, particularly in the patient with significant respiratory compromise. Arguments have been made both for initial palliation to control the pulmonary blood flow and insufficiency and for initial complete repair. We favor early complete repair for symptomatic infants with pulmonary arterial plication.

Patients with pulmonary atresia and VSD represent a more difficult surgical challenge. Patients with prominent central pulmonary arteries supplied by a ductus with distribution of normal or near-normal branching patterns to the majority of bronchopulmonary segments, and without significant MAPCAs, can have a repair similar to a standard tetralogy of Fallot patient with either an outflow tract patch or a conduit and VSD closure. Unfortunately, a large number of patients have hypoplastic or absent central pulmonary arteries either with MAPCAs supplying the major-

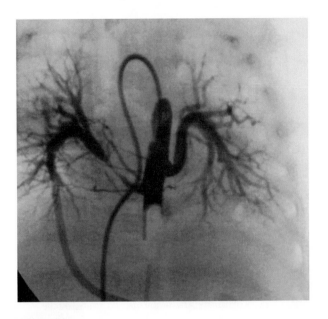

FIGURE 28–13

Balloon occlusion angiogram in the descending aorta. Berman's angiographic catheter has been passed from the right ventricle anterograde into the ascending aorta and positioned in the descending aorta. The balloon has been inflated to prevent runoff into the distal aorta during the injection. Dense opacification of the descending aorta with a large unobstructed collateral to the left lung and a severely stenotic collateral to the right lung can be seen.

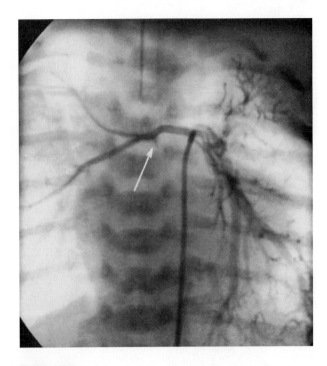

FIGURE 28–14

Selective injection of a major aorticopulmonary collateral vessel. A 4 French right coronary catheter is engaged to the ostium of a single collateral vessel arising from the midthoracic aorta, and contrast agent is injected by hand. Opacification of a well-developed lower left pulmonary artery is demonstrated. In addition, one can clearly see the sea gull appearance of the extremely hypoplastic true or native pulmonary arteries *(arrow)*.

ity of bronchopulmonary segments alone or with a dual blood supply from MAPCAs and central pulmonary arteries. In these, a major goal of the initial operation has been to enlarge central pulmonary arteries by establishing continuity from the right ventricle to the main pulmonary artery or to the confluence of the right and left pulmonary arteries, or by implementing a central shunt to provide growth of these arteries, such that an eventual repair could be performed. When central pulmonary arteries provide blood flow to only a limited number of bronchopulmonary segments, however, unifocalization procedures must be performed so that central pulmonary arteries can be connected to the majority of the bronchopulmonary segments. This may require unifocalization procedures in which shunts are performed to each lung with separate operations in which MAPCAs are divided from the aorta and connected together, with the shunt then providing all the blood flow to the ipsilateral lung. If possible, these unifocalized vessels are connected to a central right or left pulmonary artery. If no central pulmonary arteries are present, the eventual goal is to connect the unifocalized pulmonary arteries in the right and left hila using a central graft that can then be connected to the right ventricle with a valved or nonvalved conduit or homograft. Although this series of operations has been reported since the late 1980s, success has been variable, and many patients have not had adequate growth of pulmonary arteries to undergo repair.[44–49]

Hanley and associates have advocated early repair using extensive mobilization of MAPCAs and central pulmonary arteries with preferred time of operation from 3 to 6 months of age.[50] Small central arteries are enlarged considerably with the use of homograft material, and in the majority of patients, connection is made to the right ventri-

cle with a valved or nonvalved containing graft. If enough bronchopulmonary segments have been connected and the augmented pulmonary arteries appear to be of reasonable size, the VSD can be closed. These authors have described a procedure for help in the decision about closure of the VSD. Immediately after pulmonary artery surgery, the heart/lung pump is used to direct a normal cardiac index through the lungs before the decision is made regarding VSD closure. If the pulmonary arterial pressure has not risen markedly during this procedure, the VSD is closed. With this procedure the authors have been able to achieve complete repair in the majority of infants.[51] This approach has great advantages and we hope can be repeated in other centers. Dobell and associates[52] from Montreal have described successful application of the one-stage repair in four infants ages 2 weeks to 9 months. Despite successful unifocalization and reparative procedures, these patients frequently have multiple stenoses in the surgically created anastomoses and in the native MAPCAs and pulmonary arteries. They require postoperative catheterization and frequently balloon dilatation or stent placement to achieve satisfactory right ventricular pressures.

POSTOPERATIVE PROBLEMS AND LONG-TERM OUTLOOK

Problems that can occur postoperatively include both hemodynamic abnormalities and arrhythmias, which are listed in Table 28–2.

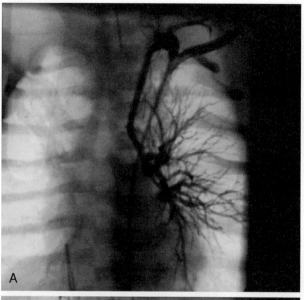

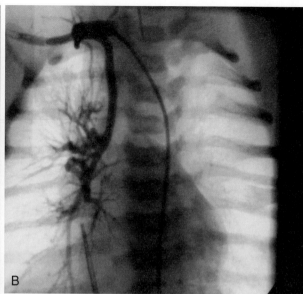

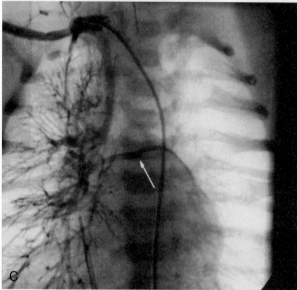

Collateral vessels arising from the brachiocephalic vessels. Selective hand injections are performed in the subclavian arteries. *A*, A small but well-developed left pulmonary artery is supplied by a collateral from the left subclavian artery. *B*, A well-developed right pulmonary artery is supplied by a collateral vessel arising from the right subclavian artery. *C*, As the contrast agent passes further into the right pulmonary artery, the hypoplastic true or native pulmonary arteries can be seen with the typical sea gull appearance *(arrow)*.

TABLE 28–2

POSTOPERATIVE PROBLEMS

RESIDUAL HEMODYNAMIC PROBLEMS
Ventricular septal defect
Right ventricular outflow tract obstruction
Pulmonary valvar and/or annular stenosis
Supravalvar pulmonary artery stenosis
Pulmonary artery branch stenosis
Pulmonary regurgitation
Tricuspid regurgitation
Right ventricular dysfunction
Right ventricular outflow tract aneurysm
Left ventricular dysfunction
Pulmonary hypertension

ARRHYTHMIA AND CONDUCTION DISTURBANCE
Supraventricular tachycardia
Ventricular tachycardia
Complete heart block

Congestive heart failure, extremely rare before surgery, is so common after complete repair that it should not be regarded as a complication. It seems to be due to an acute postoperative decrease in right ventricular compliance, possibly related to injury from oxygen free radicals during reperfusion after cardiopulmonary bypass. After a few weeks of routine treatment for heart failure, it is usually possible to stop all medication.

Residual VSD is uncommon with current surgical techniques. Because preoperatively the left ventricle is normal or slightly small in size without significant ventricular hypertrophy, congestive heart failure frequently supervenes if a significant ventricular defect is present early postoperatively. If there is a question of a significant VSD, cardiac catheterization can be needed to clarify the degree of the shunt and to determine if reoperation is required. Echocardiography is quite useful to detect left-to-right ventricular shunting but, in the presence of a surgical patch, the estima-

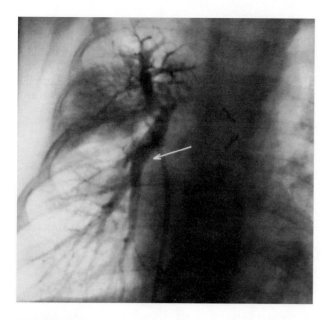

FIGURE 28–16

Pulmonary vein wedge angiogram. No arterial supply could be identified to the right lung in this child after an initial right unifocalization. A wedge catheter has been positioned in the right upper pulmonary vein. The balloon is inflated to occlude flow. Contrast agent is slowly injected retrograde into the capillary bed and then followed rapidly with a saline flush. The right pulmonary artery (*arrow*) is easily seen and densely filled, indicating that it is patent but not being supplied with anterograde flow.

tion of the size of the defect and the degree of shunting is difficult. Most residual VSDs are small and important only in terms of the potential for infective endocarditis.

Residual right ventricular outflow tract obstruction, valvar stenosis, annular stenosis, and supravalvar main pulmonary arterial obstruction can occur, particularly when transannular patching is avoided. The site and severity of obstruction can usually be determined echocardiographically, and balloon valvuloplasty may be useful when there is valvar obstruction. If there is a moderate or severe residual supravalvar, annular, or infundibular stenosis, reoperation is usually required.

Pulmonary artery branch stenosis is relatively common postoperatively and usually occurs in the left pulmonary artery at the site of prior ductus insertion, or at the site of a previous shunt. Fortunately these conditions can now be treated with a high degree of success by using transcatheter balloon arterioplasty with or without the use of stents (see Fig. 28–12).

Tricuspid regurgitation is relatively rare. It usually occurs with moderate to severe right ventricular dilatation secondary to pulmonary regurgitation and/or right ventricular dysfunction. When operation is required for pulmonary valve replacement or correction of residual outflow obstruction, tricuspid valve annuloplasty can be a useful adjunctive procedure.

Pulmonary regurgitation commonly accompanies tetralogy of Fallot repair because of the frequent need for transannular patching for adequate relief of right ventricular outflow tract obstruction. Pulmonary regurgitation is usually well tolerated when pulmonary arterial and right

ventricular pressures are low. If any degree of pulmonary hypertension or pulmonary artery stenosis is present, pulmonary regurgitation is enhanced and right ventricular dilatation is more significant.

The natural history of isolated congenital pulmonary valve incompetence has been reviewed. The development of cardiovascular symptoms increases with age, reaching 20% after 40 years and 48% after 50 years, in patients without associated pulmonary stenosis, pulmonary hypertension, or a right ventriculotomy.[53] If right ventricular dysfunction develops in a high percentage of patients with otherwise normal hearts by age 50 years, postoperative patients with prominent pulmonary regurgitation will almost certainly have similar problems with increasing age.

Exercise performance after tetralogy repair has been found to be less than normal by many investigators, and the degree of impairment is usually directly related to the amount of pulmonary regurgitation in the absence of residual obstruction to right ventricular outflow.[54–57] Right ventricular dysfunction, as assessed by ventricular size and ejection fraction, has often been found in patients with more severe pulmonary insufficiency. These patients also have larger transannular patches and right ventriculotomies, factors that can also depress ventricular function.[58,59] Pulmonary valve replacement usually decreases right ventricular size, increases ejection fraction, and improves exercise capacity.[60–62] However, right ventricular dysfunction[63] and chronotropic impairment of unknown origin[64] also contribute to diminished exercise tolerance.

The decision as to when to perform pulmonary valve replacement for pulmonary regurgitation is difficult. Patients with progressive right ventricular enlargement, decreased exercise tolerance documented with exercise testing, or early signs of right ventricular dysfunction should have the valve replaced, preferably at the earliest time when these signs or symptoms occur. There is usually a modest decrease in heart size after operation and often resolution of symptoms and ventricular ectopy. There have been several reports indicating favorable results with pulmonary valve replacement,[60–62] with an earlier operation associated with better results.

Most right ventricular aneurysms are usually not true aneurysms but simply prominent outflow patches that were too large to begin with. These patches are akinetic, can contribute to right ventricular dysfunction, and should be resected and retailored when reoperation is required.

Arrhythmias can be a significant postoperative problem. There has been a history of late sudden death in as many as 5% of patients on long-term follow-up.[65–71] This incidence appears to be declining with earlier age at operation. Patients who appear to be most at risk for ventricular tachyarrhythmia and sudden death have right ventricular dilatation, right ventricular dysfunction, right ventricular pressure overload, QRS prolongation of 180 msec,[72] and an older age at the time of repair.

Both supraventricular tachycardia and ventricular tachycardia can occur in these patients. Because most patients have right bundle branch postoperatively, they have wide complex tachycardia, and it may be difficult to determine whether the rhythm is ventricular or supraventricular in origin. Patients with documented arrhythmia with symptoms should undergo electrophysiologic studies and concurrent hemodynamic evaluation by electrophysiologists experienced in congenital heart disease. Supraventricular tachycardia and ventricular tachycardia may coexist in these patients. When either type of tachycardia is documented, radiofrequency ablation may be curative, or patients may be treated with an antitachycardia device.

Most postoperative patients lead normal or near-normal lives. Patients who have excellent results with normal to near-normal heart size, and no residual significant hemodynamic lesions, can engage in high-level recreational or sports activities.[73] Like all patients with residual abnormalities after surgery, these patients need prophylaxis against infective endocarditis. Nevertheless, in the absence of a residual VSD, in one series[74] only 1.3% of patients followed for up to 30 years developed infective endocarditis.

Long-term outcome after repair of tetralogy of Fallot has been reported to be very good for most patients, with a 32-year actuarial survival reported as 86% compared with an expected rate of 96% for one group[75] and a 20-year actuarial survival of 84% by another group.[76] These survival rates are for some of the earliest patients receiving repair, and survival after successful early repair with more current techniques would be predicted to be improved over these values.

Complete heart block is now a rare postoperative complication, but patients with a history of syncope or excessive fatigue should have this diagnosis considered. Most patients need yearly follow-up, and any patient with signs of significant arrhythmia, exercise intolerance, or syncope should have urgent referral and evaluation by a physician well trained and experienced in the care of patients with congenital heart disease.

Occasionally an older patient with unoperated tetralogy of Fallot presents. The decision about corrective surgery is often difficult. If the patient is symptomatic, surgery has a relatively low in-hospital mortality and provides significant benefits.[77] Nevertheless, these patients probably have permanent right ventricular damage,[21] and problems with ventricular arrhythmias may not be abolished. If the patient is asymptomatic, the expected survival rate at that age must be considered when making a decision about an operation.

FUTURE DIRECTIONS

Although surgical repair has been available for tetralogy of Fallot since 1954, advances continue to be made in the care of these patients. A number of new approaches are being evaluated and may alter the routine care of tetralogy of Fallot in the future. These include repair in early infancy, repair through the right atrium with avoidance of a ventriculotomy, and preoperative percutaneous balloon valvuloplasty.

The timing of surgical repair of tetralogy of Fallot varies among institutions. In many centers, complete repair is delayed for as long as possible. This approach may include performing a palliative systemic shunt to allow for further growth of the child and/or the pulmonary arteries. The problem with this approach is the need for two operations and the possibility for pulmonary artery distortion with growth after the shunt. A number of institutions have reported excellent results for complete repair in the first few months of life.[39, 40, 78] This early approach is thought to provide a number of benefits, including avoidance of chronic cyanosis, prevention of severe hypertrophy and fibrosis of the right ventricle, and encouragement of normal development of the pulmonary bed. One concern raised with such an early approach has been the possible increase in the number of children who require a transannular patch with subsequent pulmonary insufficiency. Chronic significant pulmonary insufficiency can lead to right ventricular dysfunction. Only long-term follow-up studies will help to clarify whether early repair will decrease the risk of right ventricular dysfunction. We favor elective repair between the age of 6 and 18 months and early repair in symptomatic infants who have reached approximately 2.5 to 3 kg in body weight.

A second innovation has been the repair of tetralogy of Fallot through a transatrial/transpulmonary arterial approach to avoid a significant right ventriculotomy.[79] With this approach the subvalvar obstruction is resected, and the VSD is closed through the right atrium and the tricuspid valve. Further relief of right ventricular outflow obstruction (valvar, supravalvar, branch pulmonary arteries) can be performed through the pulmonary artery. A limited transannular patch can be employed if the pulmonary annulus is too small. This approach offers the benefit of minimizing the right ventricular incision and potentially reducing the possibility of ventricular dysfunction and ventricular arrhythmias that can complicate postoperative recovery. One drawback is that it is difficult to perform in early infancy, and some patients may require a palliative procedure to delay repair until an optimum weight is achieved. As with neonatal repair, only through long-term follow-up studies can the effect on postoperative arrhythmias and ventricular function be clarified.

A third area that has shown promise in the care of patients with tetralogy of Fallot is the use of percutaneous balloon pulmonary valvuloplasty. This procedure has become the standard of care for congenital pulmonary valve stenosis, but it has shown promise in the palliation of some infants with tetralogy of Fallot.[80] By relieving obstruction at the level of the pulmonary valve, it is potentially possible to improve systemic saturation and delay surgical repair or avoid surgical palliation. There is also early evidence that valvuloplasty may improve pulmonary artery growth and increase pulmonary valve annulus. Improvement in pulmonary arterial size may reduce the risk of complete repair, and increasing pulmonary valve annulus size may reduce the number of children requiring transannular patch repair. Further studies are necessary to verify these benefits.

Finally, a few attempts have been made to use lasers or radiofrequency energy to open an atretic pulmonary valve and enable communication with the pulmonary arteries.

REFERENCES

1. Taussig HB: Congenital Malformations of the Heart. New York, Commonwealth Fund, 1945, p 109.
2. Peacock TB: On Malformations of the Heart, etc. With Original Cases and Illustrations, 2nd ed. London, Churchill, 1866.

3. Fallot E: Contribution a l'anatomie pathologique de la maladie bleu (cyanose cardiaque). Marseille-Med 25:418, 1888.

4. Rashkind WJ: Congenital Heart Disease. New York, John Wiley & Sons, 1982, pp 167–175.

5. Blalock A, Taussig HB: Surgical treatment of malformations of the heart: In which there is pulmonary stenosis or pulmonary atresia. Am J Med 128:189, 1945.

6. Lillehei CW, Cohen M, Warden M, Varco RL: The direct vision intracardiac correction of congenital anomalies by controlled cross circulation: Results in 32 patients with ventricular septal defects, tetralogy of Fallot, and atrioventricularis communis defects. Surgery 38:11, 1955.

7. Gibbon JH Jr: Applications of a mechanical heart and lung apparatus to cardiac surgery. Minn Med 37:171, 1954..

8. Kirklin JW, Dushane JW, Patrick RT, et al: Intracardiac surgery with the aid of a mechanical pump-oxygenator system (Gibbon Type): Report of eight cases. Proc Staff Mayo Clin 30:201, 1955.

9. Anderson RH, Allwork SP, Ho SY, et al: Surgical anatomy of tetralogy of Fallot. J Thorac Cardiovasc Surg 81:887, 1981.

10. Fyler DC, Buckley LP, Hellenbrand WE, et al: Report of the New England Regional Cardiac Program. Pediatrics 65(suppl):375, 1980.

11. Mitchell SC, Korones SB, Berendes HW: Congenital heart disease in 56,109 births. Incidence and natural history. Circulation 43:323, 1971.

12. Perry LW, Neill CA, Ferencz ZC, et al: Infants with congenital heart disease: The cases. In Ferencz C, Rubin JD, Loffredo CA, Magee CH (eds): Epidemiology of Congenital Heart Disease: The Baltimore-Washington Infant Heart Study in 1981–1989. Mount Kisco, New York, Futura, 1993.

13. Whittemore R, Wells JA, Castelsague X: A second generation study of 427 probands with congenital heart disease and their 837 children. J Am Coll Cardiol 23:459, 1994.

14. Samánek M: Children with congenital heart disease: Probability of natural survival. Pediatr Cardiol 13:152, 1992.

15. Hoffman JIE: Reflections on the past, present and future of pediatric cardiology. Cardiol Young 4:208, 1994.

16. Rowe RD, Vlad P, Keith JD: Experiences with 180 cases of tetralogy of Fallot in infants and children. Can Med Assoc J 73:23, 1955.

17. Rygg IH, Olesen K, Boesen I: The life history of tetralogy of Fallot. Dan Med Bull 18(suppl 2):25, 1971.

18. Child JS, Perloff JK: Natural survival patterns. A narrowing base. In Perloff JK, Child JS (eds): Congenital Heart Disease in Adults. Philadelphia, WB Saunders, 1991, pp 21–59.

19. Bertranou EG, Blackstone EH, Hazelrig JB, et al: Life expectancy without surgery in tetralogy of Fallot. Am J Cardiol 42:458, 1978.

20. Deanfield JE, McKenna WJ, Presbitero P, et al: Ventricular arrhythmia in unrepaired tetralogy of Fallot: Relation to age, timing of repair and haemodynamic status. Br Heart J 52:77, 1984.

21. Kirklin JW, Barratt-Boyes BG: Ventricular septal defect and pulmonic stenosis or atresia. In Kirklin JW, Barratt-Boyes BG (eds): Cardiac Surgery. New York, Churchill Livingstone, 1993, p 861.

22. Kramer J, Majewski F, Trampisch HJ, et al: Malformation patterns in children with congenital heart disease. Am J Dis Child 141:789, 1987.

23. Kothari SS: Mechanism of cyanotic spells in tetralogy of Fallot—the missing link? Int J Cardiol 37:1, 1992.

24. Achiron R, Weissman A, Rotstein Z, et al: Transvaginal echocardiographic examination of the fetal heart between 13 and 15 weeks' gestation in a low risk population. J Ultrasound Med 13:783, 1994.

25. Allan LD, Sharland GK: Prognosis in fetal tetralogy of Fallot. Pediatr Cardiol 13:1, 1992.

26. Rice M, McDonald RW, Reller MD: Progressive pulmonary stenosis in the fetus: Two case reports. Am J Perinatol 10:424, 1993.

27. Hornberger LK, Sanders SP, Sahn DJ, et al: In utero pulmonary artery and aortic growth and potential for progression of pulmonary outflow tract obstruction in tetralogy of Fallot. J Am Coll Cardiol 25:739, 1995.

28. Shenker L, Reek KL, Marx GR, et al: Fetal cardiac Doppler flow studies in prenatal diagnosis of heart disease. Am J Obstet Gynecol 158:1267, 1988.

29. Gembruch U, Weintraub Z, Bald R, et al: Flow analysis in the pulmonary trunk in fetuses with tetralogy of Fallot by color Doppler flow mapping: Two case reports. Eur J Obstet Gynecol Reprod Biol 27:481, 1996.

30. Berning RA, Silverman NH, Villegas M, et al: Reversed shunting across the ductus arteriosus or atrial septum in utero heralds severe congenital heart disease. J Am Coll Cardiol 27:481, 1996.

31. Musewe NN, Smallhorn JF, Moes CAF, et al: Echocardiographic evaluation of obstructive mechanism of tetralogy of Fallot with restrictive ventricular septal defect. Am J Cardiol 51:664, 1988.

32. Flanagan MF, Foran RB, Van Praagh R, et al: Tetralogy of Fallot with obstruction of the ventricular septal defect. Spectrum of echocardiographic findings. J Am Coll Cardiol 11:386, 1988.

33. Houston AB, Simpson IA, Sheldon CD, et al: Doppler ultrasound in the estimation of the severity of pulmonary infundibular stenosis in infants and children. Br Heart J 55:381, 1986.

34. Berry JM, Einzig S, Krabill KA, Bass JL: Evaluation of coronary artery anatomy in patients with tetralogy of Fallot by two-dimensional echocardiography. Circulation 78:149, 1988.

35. Caldwell RL, Ensing GJ: Coronary artery abnormalities in children. J Am Soc Echocardiogr 2:259, 1989.

36. Jureidini SB, Appleton RS, Nouri S: Detection of coronary artery abnormalities in tetralogy of Fallot by two-dimensional echocardiography. J Am Coll Cardiol 14:960, 1989.

37. Bigras JL, Boutin C, McCrindle BW, Rebeyka IM: Short term effect of monocuspid valves on pulmonary insufficiency and clinical outcome after surgical repair of tetralogy of Fallot. J Thorac Cardiovasc Surg 112:33, 1996.

38. Joffe H, Georgakopoulos D, Celermajar DS, et al: Late ventricular arrhythmia is rare after early repair of tetralogy of Fallot. J Am Coll Cardiol 23:1146, 1994.

39. Reddy VM, Liddicoat JR, McElhinney DB, et al: Routine primary repair of tetralogy of Fallot in neonates and infants less than three months of age. Ann Thorac Surg 60:S592, 1995.

40. Sousa Uva M, Chardigny C, Galetti L, et al: Surgery for tetralogy of Fallot at less than six months of age. Is palliation "old-fashioned"? Eur J Cardiothorac Surg 9:453, 1995.

41. Hennein HA, Mosca RS, Urcelay G, et al: Intermediate results after complete repair of tetralogy of Fallot in neonates. J Thorac Cardiovasc Surg 109:332, 1995.

42. Kreutzer J, Perry SB, Jonas RA, et al: Tetralogy of Fallot with diminutive pulmonary arteries: Preoperative pulmonary valve dilation and transcatheter rehabilitation of pulmonary arteries. J Am Coll Cardiol 27:1741, 1996.

43. Sluysmans T, Neven B, Rubay J, et al: Early balloon dilatation of the pulmonary valve in infants with tetralogy of Fallot. Risks and benefits. Circulation 91:1506, 1995.

44. Sullivan ID, Wren C, Stark J, et al: Surgical unifocalization in pulmonary atresia and ventricular septal defect. A realistic goal? Circulation 78(suppl):III5, 1988.

45. Puga FJ, Leoni FE, Julsrud PR, Mair DD: Complete repair of pulmonary atresia, ventricular septal defect and severe peripheral arborization abnormalities of the central pulmonary arteries: Experience with preliminary unifocalization procedures in 38 patients. J Thorac Cardiovasc Surg 98:1018, 1989.

46. Sawatari K, Imai Y, Kurosawa H, et al: Staged operation for pulmonary atresia and ventricular septal defect with major aortopulmonary collateral arteries: New technique for complete unifocalization. J Thorac Cardiovasc Surg 98:738, 1989.

47. Iyer KS, Mee RBB: Staged repair of pulmonary atresia with ventricular septal defect and major systemic to pulmonary artery collaterals. Ann Thorac Surg 51:65, 1991.

48. Marelli AJ, Perloff JK, Child JS, Laks H: Pulmonary atresia with ventricular septal defect in adults. Circulation 89:243, 1994.

49. Yagihara T, Yamamoto F, Nichigaki K, et al: Unifocalization for pulmonary atresia with ventricular septal defect and major aortopulmonary collateral arteries. J Thorac Cardiovasc Surg 112:392, 1996.

50. Reddy VM, Liddicoat JR, Hanley FL: Midline one-stage complete unifocalization and repair of pulmonary atresia with ventricular septal defect and major aortopulmonary collaterals. J Thorac Cardiovasc Surg 109:832, 1995.

51. Reddy VM, Petrossian E, McElhinney DB, et al: One stage complete unifocalization in infants: When should the ventricular septal defect be closed? J Thorac Cardiovasc Surg 113:858, 1997.

52. Tchervenkov CI, Salasidis G, Cecere R, et al: One-stage midline unifocalization followed by complete repair for complex heart disease with major aortopulmonary collaterals. J Thorac Cardiovasc Surg 114:727, 1997.

53. Shimazaki Y, Blackstone EH, Kirklin JW: The natural history of isolated congenital pulmonary valve incompetence. Thorac Cardiovasc Surg 32:257, 1984.

54. Wessel HV, Cunningham WJ, Paul MH, et al: Exercise performance in tetralogy of Fallot after intracardiac repair. J Thorac Cardiovasc Surg 80:582, 1980.

55. Marx GR, Hicks RW, Allen HD, Goldberg SJ: Noninvasive assessment of hemodynamic responses to exercise in pulmonary regurgitation after operations to correct pulmonary outflow obstruction. Am J Cardiol 61:595, 1988.

56. Rowe SA, Zahka KG, Manolio TA, et al: Lung function and pulmonary regurgitation limit exercise capacity in postoperative tetralogy of Fallot. J Am Coll Cardiol 17:461, 1991.

57. Carvalho JS, Shinebourne EA, Buest C, et al: Exercise capacity after complete repair of tetralogy of Fallot: Deleterious effects of residual pulmonary regurgitation. Br Heart J 67:470, 1992.

58. Graham TP Jr, Cordell D, Atwood GF, et al: Right ventricular volume characteristics before and after palliative and reparative operation for tetralogy of Fallot. Circulation 54:417, 1976.

59. Bove EL, Byrum CJ, Thomas FD, et al: The influence of pulmonary insufficiency in ventricular function following repair of tetralogy of Fallot. Cardiovasc Surg 85:691, 1983.

60. Bove EL, Kavey RW, Byrum CJ, et al: Improved right ventricular function following late pulmonary valve replacement for residual pulmonary insufficiency or stenosis. J Thorac Cardiovasc Surg 90:50, 1985.

61. Ilbawi MN, Idriss FS, DeLeon SG, et al: Long-term results of porcine valve insertion for pulmonary regurgitation following repair of tetralogy of Fallot. Ann Thorac Surg 41:478, 1986.

62. Finck SJ, Puga FJ, Danielson EK: Pulmonary valve insertion during reoperation for tetralogy of Fallot. Ann Thorac Surg 45:610, 1988.

63. Vetter HO, Reichart B, Seidel P, et al: Noninvasive assessment of right and left ventricular volumes 11 to 24 years after corrective surgery on patients with tetralogy of Fallot. Eur J Cardiothorac Surg 4:24, 1990.

64. Perrault H, Drblik SP, Montigny M, et al: Comparison of cardiovascular adjustments to exercise in adolescents 8 to 15 years after correction of tetralogy of Fallot, ventricular septal defect, or atrial septal defect. Am J Cardiol 64:213, 1989.

65. Marin-Garcia J, Moller JH: Sudden death after operative repair of tetralogy of Fallot. Br Heart J 39:1380, 1977.

66. Webb-Kavey RE, Blackmon MS, Sondheimer HM: Incidence and severity of chronic ventricular dysrhythmia after repair of tetralogy of Fallot. Am Heart J 103:342, 1982.

67. Deanfield JE, Ho S-Y, Anderson RH, et al: Late sudden death after repair of tetralogy of Fallot: A clinicopathologic study. Circulation 67:626, 1983.

68. Garson A Jr, Randall DC, Gillette DE, et al: Prevention of sudden death after repair of tetralogy of Fallot: Treatment of ventricular arrhythmias. J Am Coll Cardiol 6:221, 1985.

69. Zhao HZ, Miller G, Reitz BA, Shumway NE: Surgical repair of tetralogy of Fallot: Long term follow-up with particular emphasis on late death and reoperation. J Thorac Cardiovasc Surg 89:204, 1985.

70. Jonsson H, Ivert T, Lars-Ake B, Jonasson R: Late sudden deaths after repair of tetralogy of Fallot. Scand J Thorac Cardiovasc Surg 29:131, 1995.

71. Dietl CA, Cazzaniga ME, Dubner SJ, et al: Life-threatening arrhythmias and RV dysfunction after surgical repair of tetralogy of Fallot. Comparison between transventricular and transatrial approaches. Circulation 90(5 pt 2):II7, 1994.

72. Gatzoulis MA, Till JA, Somerville J, Redington AN: Mechanoelectrical interaction in tetralogy of Fallot. Circulation 92:231, 1995.

73. Graham TP Jr, Bricker JT, James FW, Strong WB: 26th Bethesda Conference: Recommendations for determining eligibility for competition in athletes with cardiovascular abnormalities. Task Force 1: Congenital heart disease. J Am Coll Cardiol 24:867, 1994.

74. Morris CD, Reller MD, Menashe VD: Thirty-year incidence of infective endocarditis after surgery for congenital heart defect. JAMA 279:599, 1998.

75. Murphy JG, Gersh BJ, Mair DD, et al: Long-term outcome in patients undergoing surgical repair of tetralogy of Fallot. N Engl J Med 329:593, 1993.

76. Jonsson H, Ivert T: Survival and clinical results up to 26 years after repair of tetralogy of Fallot. Scand J Thorac Cardiovasc Surg 29:43, 1995.

77. Park I-S, Leachman RD, Cooley DA: Total correction of tetralogy of Fallot in adults: Surgical results and long-term follow-up. Tex Heart Inst J 14:160, 1987.

78. Sousa Uva M, Lacour-Gayet F, Komiya T, et al: Surgery for tetralogy of Fallot at less than six months of age. J Thorac Cardiovasc Surg 107:1291, 1994.

79. Karl TR, Sano S, Porniviliwan S, Mee RBB: Tetralogy of Fallot: Favorable outcome of nonneonatal transatrial, transpulmonary repair. Ann Thorac Surg 54:903, 1992.

80. Sreeram NA, Saleem M, Jackson M, et al: Results of balloon pulmonary valvuloplasty as a palliative procedure in tetralogy of Fallot. J Am Coll Cardiol 18:159, 1991.

CHAPTER 29
TOTAL ANOMALOUS PULMONARY VENOUS CONNECTION

FERNANDO EIMBCKE   GABRIELA ENRÍQUEZ   OSCAR GÓMEZ   RAÚL ZILLERUELO

Total anomalous pulmonary venous connection (TAPVC) can be defined as the failure of connection between the pulmonary veins and their normal site of connection, the left atrium. The pulmonary veins drain into the right atrium, either directly or through tributary veins.

This lesion makes up 1 to 3% of congenital heart disease but is represented more in series of neonates and infants, because many die during the first month after birth.[1,2] The sex distribution is balanced except for the infracardiac form, which predominates in male infants.[3,4] In our series, we have found a significant predominance of TAPVC in patients of a lower income group.

EMBRYOLOGY

TAPVC has a common origin with all the anomalies of the venous connection, both pulmonary and systemic, because it occurs during the embryonic stage of development in which both systems are interconnected and the pulmonary venous system has no direct communication with the heart. In early stages of development, the lungs of the embryo are surrounded by a vascular mesh, called the *splanchnic plexus,* which drains indirectly to the heart through the umbilicovitelline and cardinal venous systems. In a later stage, part of the splanchnic plexus becomes the pulmonary vascular bed and connects to the left atrium through an evagination of the posterior wall of this chamber. This evagination becomes the common pulmonary vein and receives the four pulmonary veins. The initial connections with the umbilicovitelline and cardinal venous systems progressively involute, and the common pulmonary vein becomes incorporated into the posterior wall of the left atrium.

Most anomalies of the pulmonary veins derive from alterations in the development of the common pulmonary vein. TAPVC results from early atresia of the common pulmonary vein when connections between the splanchnic plexus and the cardinal or umbilicovitelline system still exist. These primitive connections grow, widen, and form the collector trunk of the different forms of TAPVC (Fig. 29–1).[4–9]

PATHOLOGY

In TAPVC, all pulmonary veins eventually drain into the right atrium, either directly or through one of the venae cavae, the portal vein, or the coronary sinus. This malformation often occurs in normal infants who have no other significant cardiac anomalies.[10] An interatrial communication or patent foramen ovale is obligatory to allow survival, so mixed blood can pass through this opening into the chambers of the left side of the heart. Another minor association is with patent ductus arteriosus. Because of low systemic blood flow, there may sometimes be variable hypoplasia of the left-sided cardiac chambers. On occasion, TAPVC coexists with other complex cardiac anomalies, such as single ventricle, complete atrioventricular canal, truncus arteriosus, tetralogy of Fallot, and anomalous systemic venous connection.[11–13] A high proportion of these associations have either the asplenia syndrome or the polysplenia syndrome.[14,15]

The most frequently used classification of TAPVC is with respect to the site of connection of the pulmonary veins into the systemic circulation:

Site of Connection	% of TAPVC
Supracardiac	40–59
Cardiac	25–30
Infracardiac	10–20
Mixed	6–8

In the supracardiac form, pulmonary veins connect through a left vertical vein into the right superior vena cava or azygos vein. In the cardiac form, the pulmonary veins connect to the right atrium, either directly and independently or more often through the coronary sinus. In the infracardiac form, the pulmonary veins join a common vein that descends anterior to the esophagus, crosses the diaphragm, and enters usually the portal vein, but occasionally the ductus venosus, inferior vena cava, or suprahepatic veins. In mixed TAPVC, different combinations of these forms can be found (Fig. 29–2).

A feature of great prognostic importance is obstruction to pulmonary venous return. Obstruction almost always exists in the infracardiac form and is responsible for the short natural survival of these neonates. It is due, in part, to the long venous connecting vein; but the main cause is that when the ductus venosus closes, all the pulmonary venous blood must pass through the high-resistance sinusoids of the liver to reach the right atrium. Obstruction occurs less frequently in supracardiac forms and results from intrinsic stenosis at the connection of the systemic vein with the common pulmonary venous channel or from extrinsic compression, when the vertical vein passes between the left pulmonary artery and the left main stem bronchus (hemodynamic vise). Obstruction in TAPVC to the coronary

409

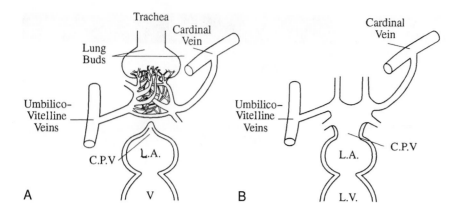

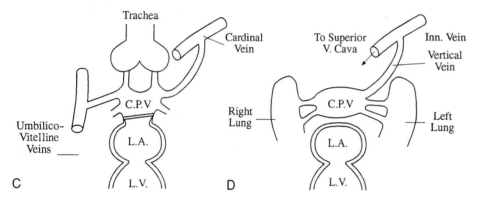

FIGURE 29-1

Embryologic development of TAPVC. *A, B,* Normal evolution with connection of the left atrium to the common pulmonary vein. *C, D,* Atresia of the connection between the common pulmonary vein and the left atrium with persistence of the connections to the umbilicovitelline or cardinal vein. C.P.V. = common pulmonary vein; L.A. = left atrium; L.V. = left ventricle.

sinus is rare.[16] Another site of obstruction can be the interatrial septum from a restrictive atrial septal defect (ASD).[17] Pulmonary vascular disease may develop as early as 4 months of age. Regardless of the site of obstruction, intrapulmonary arterial and vein wall thickness is increased, depending on the duration and severity of the obstruction. In infants with the infracardiac type of return, obstruction and vascular abnormalities are frequently present at or soon after birth, indicating intrauterine change. The common pulmonary venous channel is sometimes obstructed by fibrous tissue at birth. Pulmonary hypertension subsides after repair in almost all patients, and the pulmonary vascular changes apparently regress. Children with the infracardiac type may occasionally have intrinsically small extrapulmonary veins, and pulmonary hypertension may then persist despite adequate reconstruction.

HEMODYNAMICS

The total venous return, both systemic and pulmonary, enters the right atrium, where mixture occurs after the addition of coronary sinus blood. From the right atrium, this mixture is distributed into both systemic and pulmonary circuits: into the right ventricle and to the pulmonary artery, through the atrial communication into the left atrium, and through the left ventricle into the aorta. The amount of flow to each circuit depends partly on the size of the interatrial septal defect, usually nonrestrictive, and mostly on the vasculature resistances of the two circuits.

After the neonatal period, pulmonary vascular resistance is normally much less than systemic. Therefore, pulmonary blood flow may be 3 to 5 times greater than systemic flow. Consequently, there is a high saturation of the mixed blood, around 90%, which is approximately equal in each circuit. This oxygen saturation may change completely if resistance to pulmonary blood flow is high from either pulmonary venous obstruction or arteriolar vasoconstriction. If there is obstructive return, pulmonary venous hypertension is transmitted to the capillary bed. This may produce pulmonary edema if the pressure exceeds the oncotic plasma pressure. A reflex mechanism can sometimes produce pulmonary arteriolar vasoconstriction causing pulmonary hypertension, reduction of pulmonary blood flow, and subsequent lowering of the proportion of oxygenated blood in the mixed blood in the right atrium. Another compensatory mechanism occurs in a neonate with coexistent patent ductus arteriosus, in which pulmonary hypertension is partially relieved through the ductus and the right-to-left shunt increases systemic flow (see Fig. 29–14B).

CLINICAL PRESENTATION

The spectrum of clinical manifestations varies. At one extreme are symptomatic neonates with virtually no response to medical management and a short survival without an emergency operation, as is the rule in nearly all obstructive TAPVC. At the other extreme are the rare patients who are completely asymptomatic and whose clinical picture resembles an ASD. Most of the nonobstructive patients present with congestive heart failure during the first or second year of life. Nevertheless, even these asymptomatic patients can have an unpredictable course, becoming critically ill and dying in a few hours. Therefore, our policy for this malformation is urgent operative treatment, if possible as soon as the diagnosis has been confirmed.[18]

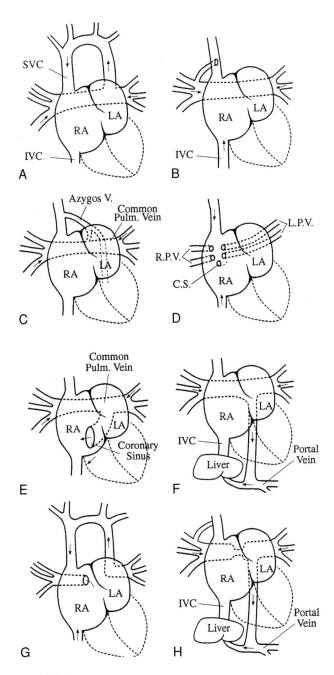

FIGURE 29–2

Types of TAPVC. *A,* Supracardiac, into vertical vein. *B,* Supracardiac, into superior vena cava. *C,* Supracardiac, into azygos vein. *D,* Cardiac, into right atrium. *E,* Cardiac, into coronary sinus. *F,* Infracardiac, into the portal vein. *G,* Mixed: left pulmonary veins (supracardiac) and the right pulmonary veins connect directly to the right atrium (cardiac). *H,* Mixed: right pulmonary veins are predominantly supracardiac into the superior vena cava, and left pulmonary veins drain predominantly infracardiac (portal vein). Both venous systems are interconnected. C.S. = coronary sinus; IVC = inferior vena cava; LA = left atrium; L.P.V. = left pulmonary vein; RA = right atrium; R.P.V. = right pulmonary vein; SVC = superior vena cava.

DIAGNOSIS

Prompt diagnosis depends on the suspicion of a cardiac problem and the immediate transfer of the patient to a cardiac center where the definitive diagnosis can be made. The clinical picture varies significantly, depending on whether obstruction to pulmonary venous return exists. Nevertheless, features of cardiac failure are common in those with and without obstruction.

OBSTRUCTIVE TAPVC

When obstruction of pulmonary venous return exists, the predominant symptom is cyanosis from the first days of life. Tachypnea is common, sometimes as paroxysmal episodes with gasping and intercostal retractions. The symptoms suggest pulmonary edema. Deterioration rapidly progresses, and few neonates survive the first month of life.[15] Sometimes, when the ductus arteriosus persists, the clinical picture can be mistaken for persistence of the fetal pattern of circulation, as part of the blood in the pulmonary trunk flows through the ductus into the aorta, thereby avoiding the pulmonary congestion.

Physical Examination

The neonate usually appears critically ill and shows variable cyanosis, marked tachypnea and retractions, and hepatomegaly. Peripheral pulses are weak. On auscultation, there may be no murmur. The first heart sound is accentuated in the midprecordium and often followed by an ejection click. The second heart sound may be single and loud or narrowly split with an accentuated pulmonary component denoting severe pulmonary hypertension. Exceptionally, a left parasternal venous hum may be present in relation to the site of obstruction in the left vertical vein. Fine rales can be present at both lung bases as an expression of pulmonary edema.

Electrocardiography

Right-axis deviation of the QRS, right atrial enlargement, and marked right ventricular hypertrophy with qR complexes over the right precordium and rS over the left precordium are the most frequent features.

Chest Radiography

The radiographic features of obstructive TAPVC are similar to those of other malformations, such as mitral atresia, with obstruction to pulmonary venous return leading to pulmonary edema. Cardiac size is normal or only slightly enlarged because of right-sided chamber enlargement. Pulmonary vasculature may be passively increased with a reticular pattern throughout both lung fields. With a concomitant ductus arteriosus, the lung pattern resembles that of persistent fetal circulation with peripheral hypovascularity.

Laboratory Study

The oxygen content of arterial blood (PaO_2) is often quite low and shows only little increase during a hyperoxia test. It rarely rises above 100 mm Hg.

Differential Diagnosis

In the differential diagnosis, pulmonary conditions (such as respiratory distress syndrome and persistent fetal circulation) and cardiac causes (such as mitral atresia, hypoplasia of the left side of the heart, aortic coarctation, and complete transposition) must be considered. The cardiac causes are not problems, inasmuch as they lead to a cardiologic referral and the correct diagnosis. The more serious error is the misdiagnosis as pulmonary disease or pulmonary hypertension, thereby delaying operative treatment. This is a common error because there are no characteristic murmurs, and the signs of right ventricular enlargement and the chest radiograph can easily be misinterpreted as lung disease.

NONOBSTRUCTIVE TAPVC

The clinical presentation is different from that of obstructive forms. In general, these patients are not so critically ill, and they may even be asymptomatic during the neonatal period. Diagnosis is often made during the second month of life because heart failure develops after the reduction in pulmonary vascular resistance and the increase in pulmonary blood flow. Even infants who are initially asymptomatic may deteriorate suddenly; approximately 80% die during the first year of life.[15,19]

The symptoms are similar to those with a high-flow interatrial septal defect. There are repeated respiratory infections with subsequent malnutrition and failure to thrive. After 2 months of age, cardiac failure becomes more severe and is manifested by irritability, sweating, tachycardia, tachypnea, hepatomegaly, and feeding problems. Even though these infants have some degree of unsaturation, they seldom show clinical cyanosis; the high pulmonary flow maintains an arterial saturation above 85%. Cyanosis can appear with bronchopneumonia or atelectasis or as a result of organic pulmonary hypertension or polycythemia. The cardiac examination is also similar to that in large ASD: prominent precordial impulse due to a diastolic overloaded right ventricle. On auscultation, there is an accentuated first sound in the midprecordium, sometimes followed by an ejection click, and a fixed split second sound with an increased pulmonary component. A third sound is also frequent. A grade 2–3/6 systolic ejection murmur is present in the pulmonary area and often radiates to the back. A diastolic flow murmur in the tricuspid area is also common. On occasion, a continuous murmur of a patent ductus can be heard.

Electrocardiography

The electrocardiogram resembles an ASD and shows right bundle branch block with a greater degree of right ventricular hypertrophy (rR or qR in V_3R and V_1). There is also often a tall, peaked P wave reflecting right atrial enlargement.

Chest Radiography

The chest radiograph shows cardiomegaly with right chamber enlargement, a prominent pulmonary artery segment, and increase of the pulmonary blood flow. There is no interstitial edema or left atrial enlargement. In older infants and children with TAPVC to the vertical vein, it is possible to see the typical figure-of-eight or snowman produced by the dilatation of the vertical vein or common trunk and the right superior vena cava (see Fig. 10–18).

Magnetic resonance imaging can contribute to the diagnosis of TAPVC.[20,21]

Laboratory Study

Arterial blood gas analyses show a slightly diminished PaO_2. Arterial saturation is between 85 and 90%, which increases to unexpectedly high values with the hyperoxia test because of markedly elevated pulmonary flow.

Echocardiography

Echocardiography is the most useful method in the diagnosis of TAPVC and has almost completely eliminated the need for cardiac catheterization. M-mode and two-dimensional echocardiography[22] and Doppler assessment are able to demonstrate not only the lack of connection between the pulmonary veins and the left atrium to the actual site of connection but also any obstruction to the pulmonary venous flow. The presence of associated structural anomalies can be recognized,[23,24] and the size of the ASD, the size and function of the ventricles, the direction of shunts, and the magnitude of pulmonary hypertension can be assessed. M-mode echocardiography is useful in evaluating the hemodynamic consequences of the anomaly, as expressed by signs of right ventricular volume overload (increase of the anteroposterior diastolic diameter of the right ventricle, paradoxical movement of the interventricular septum) and the indirect signs of pulmonary hypertension (right ventricular hypertrophy, right-sided systolic intervals greater than 0.30, and pulmonary valve excursion with premature closure) (Fig. 29–3).

Two-dimensional echocardiography allows the identification of the pulmonary veins and the pulmonary venous confluence (Fig. 29–4). From a subcostal approach, the ASD is imaged and its size measured.[25] From the parasternal long and short axis together with apical four-chamber views, cardiac morphology can be assessed together with the hemodynamic effects and associated anomalies.

Color Doppler imaging simplifies the identification of the pulmonary veins, the pulmonary confluence, and the connecting vessels. Aliasing makes points of obstruction to venous flow evident.[26] Finally, tricuspid regurgitation can be quantitatively and qualitatively assessed, as can the right-to-left shunt through the patent foramen ovale. Pulsed Doppler interrogation confirms the presence of obstruction by an increase in flow velocity (Fig. 29–5).

Continuous-wave Doppler imaging is frequently needed to measure the peak flow velocities in the obstructive common pulmonary channel and to assess the degree of pulmonary hypertension at the tricuspid level. If there is tricuspid regurgitation, the systolic pressure within the right ventricle can be quantified from the Bernoulli equation:

$$RV = 4V^2 + RA$$

where RV is the systolic pressure in the right ventricle, V is the peak velocity of the flow through the obstruction, and RA is the pressure in the right atrium.

SUPRACARDIAC TAPVC[27,28]

The pulmonary confluence is identified by subcostal and apical four-chamber views, angulating the transducer to

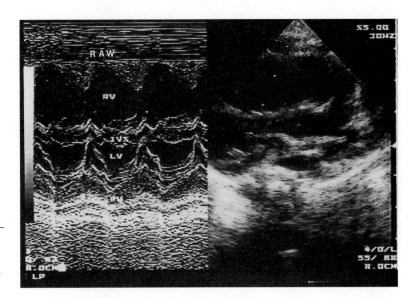

TAPVC, M-mode and 2-dimensional echocardiography recording at the level of the mitral valve. The anterior wall (RAW) is hypertrophic. The right ventricle (RV) is enlarged, and the interventricular septum (IVS) has paradoxical motion. LV = left ventricle.

show the four pulmonary veins. The common pulmonary vein can usually be followed from the suprasternal and subcostal approach and the left parasternal short-axis view (Fig. 29–6). Color Doppler imaging allows determination of whether the common pulmonary vessel reaches the superior vena cava through the azygos vein or through a vertical vein–innominate vein pathway.

CARDIAC TAPVC[27, 28]

CORONARY SINUS TYPE. In this form of TAPVC, the pulmonary veins connect to the coronary sinus either directly or through a small collecting vessel. The latter, an uncommon type, may present with obstruction at the level of the common collecting vessel.

The dilated coronary sinus is easily seen in the parasternal long- and short-axis views. The way in which pulmonary veins and the coronary sinus are connected can be assessed through the subcostal approach (Fig. 29–7).

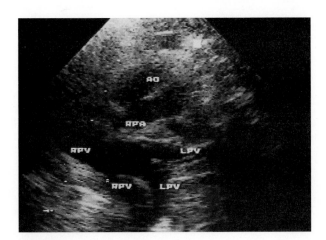

TAPVC, echocardiogram. Suprasternal view demonstrates the left (LPV) and right (RPV) pulmonary veins, the right pulmonary artery (RPA) in long axis, and the aorta (AO) in cross-section.

RIGHT ATRIAL TYPE. Direct cardiac drainage into the right atrium is also seen with suprasternal and subcostal views; with color Doppler imaging, the site of entrance can be assessed (Fig. 29–8).

INFRACARDIAC TAPVC[29, 30]

In this type of TAPVC, the common pulmonary vessel drains into the portal-suprahepatic system (Fig. 29–9 [see also Color Plates]). Characteristically, a transverse view below the diaphragm shows three vascular structures: the normal aorta, the inferior vena cava, and the common pulmonary vein. This pattern is easy for even a noncardiologist to recognize. The pulmonary vein confluence can be imaged from the epigastrium. From this point, slight rotation of the transducer toward the inferior vena cava brings the connecting vessel into view, and the precise site of connection can be identified. This type of connection is almost always obstructive at the entry site into the portal system. We have studied three patients with infracardiac TAPVC directly draining into the inferior vena cava, which is an unusual subtype of TAPVC; none was obstructive (Fig. 29–10 [see Color Plates]).

MIXED TYPE OF TAPVC

This form can easily be missed if there is not an active and thorough search to exclude it. Every possible site of anomalous connection must be investigated carefully. We have had patients in whom some pulmonary veins connect into the coronary sinus while others connect into the superior vena cava with no connection between the respective veins. However, we have also encountered this arrangement in which the systems were interconnected.

ASSOCIATED ANOMALIES

Even though many different anomalies have been described in association with TAPVC, the most common are patent ductus arteriosus and ventricular septal defect. A ductus arteriosus is identified through the suprasternal and parasternal short-axis approach; depending on the degree of pulmonary hypertension, the shunt may be left-to-right

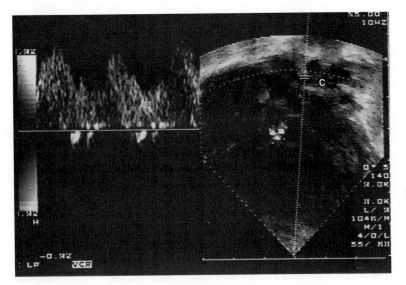

FIGURE 29–5

TAPVC, nonobstructive type. Pulsed Doppler echocardiography recording from the common pulmonary vein (C) of an infant with TAPVC shows venous pattern of flow throughout systole and diastole. The peak velocities of the venous flow signals are low, suggesting no obstruction to forward flow.

or right-to-left. The flow velocity can give an estimation of the magnitude of pulmonary hypertension. To exclude a ventricular septal defect may be difficult in the setting of severe pulmonary hypertension, which is present in many patients. In this circumstance, color Doppler imaging is not useful. Therefore, two-dimensional examination needs to be complete and meticulous, with special emphasis on studying the interventricular septum. Parasternal long- and short-axis views together with apical and subcostal four-chamber views are necessary if a complete diagnosis is to be made.

Ventricular volumes must be assessed, because small left ventricle chambers can be associated with a worse outcome after operation. The morphology and size of the valve rings must be evaluated, particularly those of the mitral and aortic valves, because the amount of flow is increased after correction.[31] They may be functionally normal in the preoperative period and stenotic afterward.

TRANSESOPHAGEAL ECHOCARDIOGRAPHY

Because transthoracic echocardiography provides the necessary anatomic and functional information required for decision-making, we have found no place for transesophageal echocardiography in this particular cardiac anomaly.[32] We use it only as an intraoperative procedure at the surgeon's request.

POSTOPERATIVE EVALUATION

Postoperatively, the return to normal of the signs of right ventricular volume overload and pulmonary hypertension must be ascertained. When these changes do not occur, pulmonary venous obstruction must be excluded. This can be at the level of the left atrium–pulmonary venous confluence anastomosis or within the pulmonary veins.

The size of the anastomotic communication must be assessed as well as the pattern and velocity of the flow within the pulmonary veins and in the left atrium. The most frequent complication is stenosis of the pulmonary veins. In these patients, thin pulmonary veins are seen (1 to 2 mm in

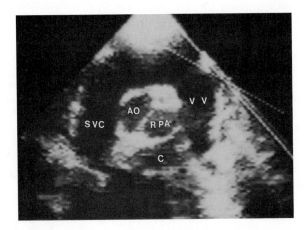

FIGURE 29–6

TAPVC, supracardiac to vertical vein. Echocardiogram in suprasternal view, coronal cut, shows the vertical vein (VV) ascending left to the aorta (AO) and joining the innominate vein, which drains into the superior vena cava (SVC). The pulmonary confluence (C) can be seen underneath the aorta and right pulmonary artery (RPA).

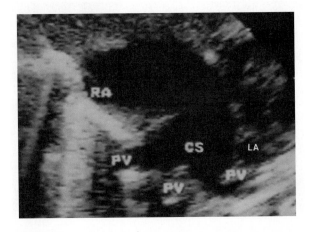

FIGURE 29–7

TAPVC, cardiac to coronary sinus. Echocardiogram in subcostal view shows three pulmonary veins (PV) draining into the coronary sinus (CS) between the left (LA) and right atrium (RA).

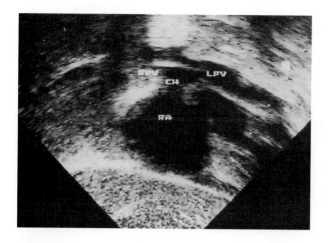

FIGURE 29–8

TAPVC, cardiac to right atrium. Echocardiogram in subcostal view shows left (LPV) and right (RPV) pulmonary veins, the confluence (CH), and the connection to the right atrium (RA).

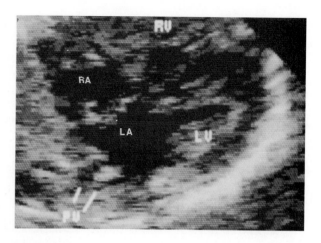

FIGURE 29–11

TAPVC, postoperative pulmonary vein stenosis. Echocardiogram in subcostal view of an infant with surgically corrected TAPVC shows narrowed pulmonary veins (PV). Left ventricle (LV), right ventricle (RV), left atrium (LA), and right atrium (RA) are also identified.

diameter) with turbulent flow. With color Doppler imaging, different flow jets enter the left atrium at different sites and with different peak velocities (Fig. 29–11). When stenosis of the anastomotic communication is present, an image similar to cor triatriatum can be seen with two-dimensional echocardiography. The pulmonary veins are dilated, have a low velocity, and connect to the left atrium through a small communication. At this site, an acceleration of the flow is found.

Cardiac Catheterization and Cineangiocardiography

Before the development of echocardiography, cardiac catheterization and angiography were the most useful

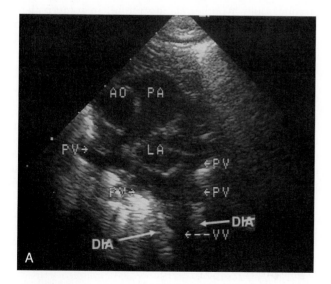

FIGURE 29–9

Infracardiac TAPVC below the diaphragm. *A*, The four pulmonary veins (PV) can be seen to join a venous confluence (VV) that passes caudad through the diaphragm (DIA). *B*, See Color Figure 29–9*B*. AO = aorta; LA = left atrium; PA = pulmonary artery. (*A, B* courtesy of Dr. Norman H. Silverman.)

methods in the final diagnosis of most cardiac malformations including TAPVC. Currently, they are rarely needed; two-dimensional color Doppler echocardiography can provide virtually all the information required to minimize the risk during operation.

In exploration with the catheter, it is possible to enter the anomalous pulmonary veins or their common collecting trunk. This is more frequent in the supracardiac type or some cardiac types. It is also possible to catheterize the left-sided cardiac chambers through the interatrial septal defect or patent foramen ovale. Catheterization of the pulmonary artery is also important for selective cineangiography.

Blood samples taken from the different chambers demonstrate an increase in oxygen saturation at the site where the pulmonary veins connect to the systemic venous system. Complete mixture of systemic and pulmonary venous blood occurs in the right atrium. The oxygen saturation of this mixture is more or less the same in each cardiac chamber and in both great arteries. Its value depends on the relationship between pulmonary and systemic blood flows. In the obstructive TAPVC and with high pulmonary vascular resistance, the pulmonary flow is limited. Consequently, the oxygen saturation of the mixture is lower. In nonobstructive types, pulmonary blood flow may be 3 to 5 times the systemic flow, and the oxygen saturation of the mixture is therefore high (88 to 90%).

Pulmonary hypertension of variable degree is frequently present in infants. It is always present in obstructive forms of TAPVC, in which it reaches systemic levels. Left atrial pressure is normal, and usually no pressure gradient exists between right and left atrium. A gradient greater than 2 mm Hg in favor of the right atrium indicates a restrictive interatrial communication. In some of these patients, atrial septostomy can provide transient improvement, but this procedure should never delay surgical correction.[17, 33, 34]

An obvious complement to catheterization is selective cineangiocardiography. This provides the most accurate in-

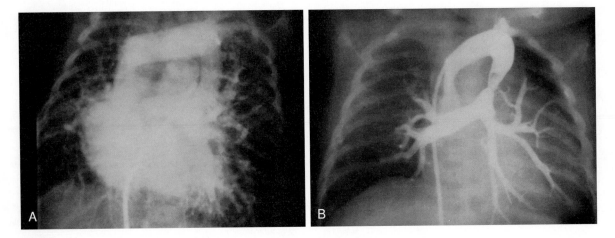

FIGURE 29–12

TAPVC, cineangiography. *A,* Supracardiac connection to vertical vein. *B,* Obstruction in the junction between the common pulmonary vein and the vertical vein.

formation about the site of connection and the existence of obstruction. Selective injection into the common pulmonary vein has the advantage of less dilution of contrast media and consequently better visualization; however, it does not detect mixed types of TAPVC and is impracticable in infracardiac types. Injection into the pulmonary arterial trunk obviates these problems but has the disadvantage of dilution because of high volume of pulmonary blood flow in nonobstructive types. In obstructive TAPVC, one has to program a longer recirculation period because of the slow pulmonary venous return (Figs. 29–12 to 29–14).

PROGNOSIS

TAPVC has an ominous outcome without operation. More than 80% of patients die in the first year of life and a small proportion survive into adult life.[14,34] An especially poor prognosis exists in neonates with obstructive TAPVC, who seldom survive the first month of life without operation. If

they survive an operation and have no residual pulmonary hypertension or venous obstruction, the long-term prognosis is excellent and similar to that for ASD. Long-term postoperative follow-up is recommended to detect late arrhythmias.

TREATMENT

The only effective treatment for this malformation is a cardiac operation as soon as the diagnosis is defined by echocardiography, especially in obstructive forms. Medical treatment is appropriate during the transfer to a cardiac surgical unit and in the hours before planned operation so the patient is in the best possible condition. Ventilatory support, diuretics, and correction of acidosis, hypoglycemia, and hypothermia are useful. In some patients with pulmonary hypertension, prostaglandin E_1 can increase systemic flow by keeping the ductus arteriosus open. In infracardiac TAPVC, prostaglandins may be helpful in maintaining the ductus venosus open.

OPERATIVE TECHNIQUE

The corrective operation is performed with use of cardiopulmonary bypass under hypothermia at 20 to 22°C. Induced circulatory arrest is currently not a routine procedure; if necessary, it is maintained only briefly. Cannulas are placed in the aorta and the caval veins, and catheters are inserted in the radial or femoral artery and jugular vein.[35–37]

The ductus arteriosus is ligated to decompress the lungs and prevent air embolism. When the patient's temperature has reached 25°C, the aorta is clamped and a potassium-rich cardioplegic solution with 4% blood at 4°C is infused at high pressure.

Specific operative correction is carried out according to the anatomic type as explained in the following.

Supracardiac TAPVC

The right pulmonary veins are dissected until the common pulmonary venous confluence is identified, and an incision

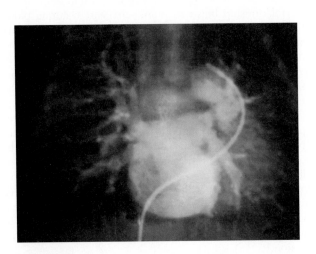

FIGURE 29–13

TAPVC, cineangiography. Cardiac connection to coronary sinus.

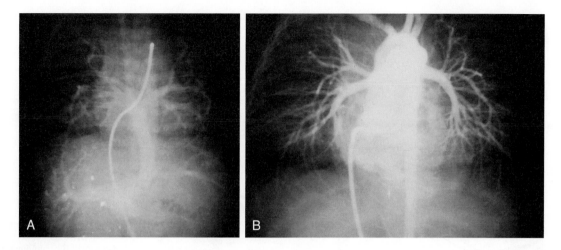

TAPVC, cineangiography. A, Infracardiac drainage to the portal vein. B, Same patient as in A. Because of severe pulmonary hypertension, contrast media enters the descending aorta from the pulmonary artery through a patent ductus arteriosus.

is made to decompress the lungs. The atria are retracted toward the left, and a transverse incision is made in the posterior wall of the left atrium. Both incisions are then sutured in a way that will not induce stenosis. Next, the interatrial communication is closed through a right atriotomy. The patient is warmed, and the bypass is discontinued.

The vertical vein is ligated near its confluence with the innominate vein, a maneuver usually well tolerated by the patient (Fig. 29–15).

Cardiac TAPVC

TO THE CORONARY SINUS. The roof of the coronary sinus is resected, and the orifice of the coronary sinus and the ASD are made confluent. The interatrial communication thus formed is closed with a pericardial or Dacron patch, leaving the pulmonary veins and coronary sinus to drain together into the left atrium. During resection and suturing, damage to the atrioventricular node must be avoided (Fig. 29–16).

TO THE RIGHT ATRIUM. Part of the atrial wall is resected until a wide communication between the pulmonary veins and the atrium is obtained. A patch is then placed to redirect the veins and septate the atria.

Infracardiac TAPVC

The heart is dislocated up and leftward, and the pulmonary venous confluence and pulmonary veins are dissected. The connecting vein is divided near the diaphragm, and a longitudinal incision is performed.[38,39] Some surgeons do not ligate the common vein. A similar incision is made in the left atrium, and a laterolateral anastomosis is performed (Fig. 29–17).

TAPVC, supracardiac type: details of operative approach. Anastomosis is made between the pulmonary veins and the left atrium. LA = left atrium; LPV = left pulmonary vein; RA = right atrium; RPV = right pulmonary vein; VV = vertical vein; SVC = superior vena cava; IVC = inferior vena cava.

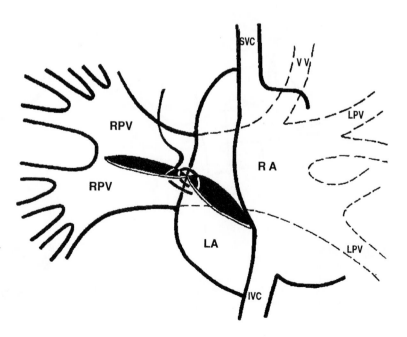

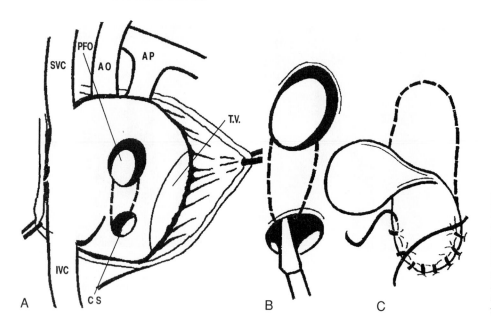

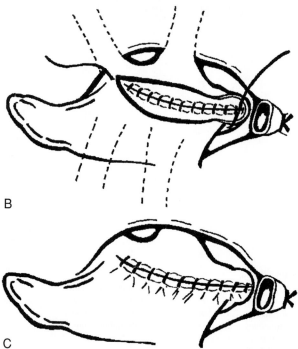

FIGURE 29–16

TAPVC, coronary sinus type: details of operative approach. *A,* Anterior. *B,* Incisions made between coronary sinus (CS) and patent foramen ovale (PFO). *C,* Closure of the common orifice with a patch. AP = pulmonary artery; AO = aorta; IVC = inferior vena cava; SVC = superior vena cava; T.V. = tricuspid valve.

AFTER OPERATION

The patient is left with lines in the left atrium, in the radial or femoral artery, and in the pulmonary artery, the last to monitor possible crises of pulmonary hypertension. Pacemaker wires are also placed in the right atrium and right ventricle.[40]

The operative experience with TAPVC at our center dates to the early 1960s. Since then, more than 200 operative repairs for TAPVC have been performed at the Hospital Calvo MacKenna in Santiago, Chile. In a review from January 1994 to June 1996, 61 patients with TAPVC were operated on.[41] The mean age at operation was 74 days (range, 1 day to 8.9 years), and 26 patients (42%) underwent surgery before 30 days of life. Fourteen cases (22%) were obstructive, and of these, 90% were of the infracardiac forms.

Early mortality in seven (11.4%) was due to pulmonary hypertension, low cardiac output, venous obstruction, bronchopulmonary dysplasia, and sepsis. The late mortality in four (6.5%) was due to pulmonary venous obstruction and pulmonary complications.[16, 42–46]

POSTOPERATIVE PROBLEMS

PULMONARY HYPERTENSION

Pulmonary hypertension is relatively frequent and can be lethal if not properly managed. It must be prevented by us-

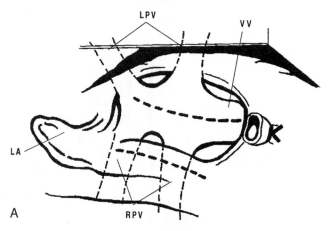

FIGURE 29–17

TAPVC, infracardiac type: details of operative approach. *A,* Incisions are made in the left atrium (LA) and common pulmonary venous chamber. Vertical vein (VV) is ligated. *B,* Anastomosis between the common pulmonary vein and the left atrium. LPV = left pulmonary vein; RPV = right pulmonary vein. *C,* Atrium closed.

ing phenoxybenzamine during bypass, avoiding excessive direct tracheal stimuli, and using adequate sedation and muscle paralysis. The use of prostacyclin and, recently, nitric oxide has been helpful.

PULMONARY EDEMA

Pulmonary edema may represent a continuation of a preoperative problem if the pulmonary veins are stenotic or if the left atrium and ventricle are small. It also occurs if the surgical anastomosis is stenotic, which may be complicated by scar tissue stenosis of the neighboring pulmonary veins. The use of diuretics is required, as is management of the ventilator at high positive end-expiratory pressures.

When the left-sided heart chambers are small, the interatrial communication or the connecting vein may be left patent at the end of the operation. When the pulmonary venous–left atrial anastomosis is stenotic, reoperation to enlarge it is necessary. If there is pulmonary vein hypoplasia or stenosis (5 to 10% of our patients), attempts at surgical enlargement or balloon catheter dilatation are frustrating and usually result in greater stenosis. Stents have been used with limited success.

On occasion, stricture or narrowing of the suture line in the site of anastomosis to the left atrium can occur later (4 to 8 months) and is progressive, with reappearance of signs of pulmonary congestion. The treatment is surgical by resection of the narrowed zone. Results are good when the pulmonary veins are uninvolved.[42] Late results are excellent in most patients, especially if the operation is done early enough to avoid pulmonary vascular obstructive disease. If pulmonary vein obstruction is absent, it can be considered corrective surgery, and the prognosis is as good as in ASD repair.[18]

REFERENCES

1. Byard RW, Moore L: Total anomalous venous drainage and sudden death in infancy. Forensic Sci Int 51:197, 1991.
2. Cabezuelo G, Frontera P: Mortalidad y supervivencia en el DVPAT. Rev Esp Cardiol 43:93, 1990.
3. Fyler DC: Nadas Pediatric Cardiology. Philadelphia, Hanley & Belfus, 1992.
4. Adams FH, Emmanouilides GC, Riemenschneider TA: Moss' Heart Disease in Infants, Children and Adolescents, 4th ed. Baltimore, Williams & Wilkins, 1989, p 839.
5. Lucas RV Jr, Woolfrey BF, Anderson RC, et al: Atresia of the common pulmonary vein. Pediatrics 29:729, 1962.
6. Lucas RV Jr, Anderson RC, Amplatz K, et al: Congenital causes of pulmonary venous obstruction. Pediatr Clin North Am 10:781, 1963.
7. Neill CA: Development of pulmonary veins, with reference to the embryology of anomalies of pulmonary venous return. Pediatrics 18:80, 1956.
8. Darling RC, Rothney WB, Craig JM: Total pulmonary venous drainage into the right side of the heart. Lab Invest 6:44, 1957.
9. Freedom RM, Culham JAG, Moes CAF: Angiocardiography of Congenital Heart Disease. New York, Macmillan, 1984.
10. Delisle G, Ando M, Calder AL, et al: Total anomalous pulmonary venous connection. Report of 93 autopsied cases with emphasis on diagnostic and surgical considerations. Am Heart J 91:99, 1976.
11. Abbattista AD, Marino B, Jovio FS, Marceletti C: Complete atrioventricular canal and total anomalous pulmonary venous drainage: A rare association. J Thorac Cardiovasc Surg 107:1536, 1994.
12. Gerlis LM, Fiddler GI, Pearse RG: Total anomalous venous drainage associated with tetralogy of Fallot: Report of a case. Pediatr Cardiol 4:293, 1983.
13. Gutierrez J, Perez de Leon J, De Marco E, et al: Tetralogy of Fallot associated with total anomalous venous drainage. Pediatr Cardiol 4:293, 1983.
14. Heinemman MK, Hanley FL, VanPraagh S, et al: Total anomalous venous drainage in newborns with visceral heterotaxy. Am Thorac Surg 57:81, 1994.
15. James CL, Keeling JW, Smith NM, Byard RW: Total anomalous pulmonary venous drainage associated with fatal outcome in infancy and early childhood: An autopsy study of 52 cases. Pediatr Pathol 14:665, 1994.
16. Jonas RA, Smolinsky A, Mayer JE, Castaneda AR: Obstructed pulmonary venous drainage with total anomalous pulmonary venous connection to the coronary sinus. Am J Cardiol 59:431, 1987.
17. Ali-Khan M, Brichet J, Mullins C, et al: Blade atrial septostomy: Experience with the first 50 procedures. Cathet Cardiovasc Diagn 23:257, 1991.
18. Galloway AC, Campbell DN, Clarke DR: The value of early repair for total anomalous pulmonary venous drainage. Pediatr Cardiol 6:77, 1985.
19. Long WA: Fetal and Neonatal Cardiology. Philadelphia, WB Saunders, 1990.
20. Kastler B, Livolsi A, Germain P, et al: Contribution of MRI in supracardiac total anomalous pulmonary venous drainage. Pediatr Radiol 22:262, 1992.
21. Hsu YH, Chien CT, Hwang M, Chin IS: Magnetic resonance imaging of total anomalous pulmonary venous drainage. Am Heart J 121:1560, 1991.
22. Huhta JC, Gutgesell HP, Nihill MR: Cross sectional echocardiographic diagnosis of total anomalous pulmonary connection. Br Heart J 53:525, 1985.
23. Anderson RH, Becker AE, Freedom RM, et al: Sequential segmental analysis of congenital heart disease. Pediatr Cardiol 5:281, 1984.
24. Silverman NH, Hunter S, Anderson RH, et al: Anatomical basis of cross sectional echocardiography. Br Heart J 50:421, 1983.
25. Shub C, Dimopdelos IN, Seward JB, et al: Sensitivity of two dimensional echocardiography in the direct visualization of atrial septal defect utilizing the subcostal approach: Experience with 154 patients. J Am Coll Cardiol 2:127, 1983.
26. Sreeramo N, Walsh K: Diagnosis of total anomalous pulmonary venous drainage by Doppler color flow imaging. J Am Coll Cardiol 19:577, 1992.
27. Silverman NH: Pediatric Echocardiography. Baltimore, Williams & Wilkins, 1993.
28. Snider RA: Echocardiography in Pediatric Heart Disease. Chicago, Year Book, 1990.
29. Garcia C, Savio A, Arista O, et al: Two-dimensional and color-coded Doppler echocardiography in the diagnosis of infradiaphragmatic total anomalous pulmonary venous connection to the portal venous system. Rev Esp Cardiol 44:66, 1991.
30. Wang JK, Lue HC, Wu MH, et al: Obstructed total anomalous pulmonary venous connection. Pediatr Cardiol 14:28, 1993.
31. Siewers RD: Total anomalous pulmonary venous drainage and mitral atresia (Letter; comment). Pediatr Cardiol 15:252, 1994.
32. Frommelt PC, Stuth EA: Transesophageal echocardiography in total anomalous pulmonary venous drainage: Hypotension caused by compression of the pulmonary venous confluence during probe passage. J Am Soc Echocardiogr 7:652, 1994.
33. Mullins CE, el Said GM, Neches WH, et al: Balloon atrial septostomy for total anomalous pulmonary venous return. Br Heart J 35:752, 1973.
34. Keith JD, Rowe RD, Vlad P: Heart Disease in Infancy and Childhood, 3rd ed. New York, Macmillan, 1984.
35. Kirklin J, Barratt-Boyes B: Cardiac Surgery, Vol 1, 2nd ed. New York, Churchill Livingstone, 1993.
36. Stark J, de Leval M: Surgery for Congenital Heart Defects, 2nd ed. Philadelphia, WB Saunders, 1994.
37. Castaneda A, Jonas R, Mayer J, et al: Cardiac Surgery of the Neonate and Infant. Philadelphia, WB Saunders, 1994.
38. Sano S, Brawn WJ, Mee RB: Total anomalous pulmonary venous drainage. J Thorac Cardiovasc Surg 97:886, 1989.
39. Long WA, Lawson EE, Harned HS, Henry GW: Infradiaphragmatic total anomalous pulmonary venous drainage: New diagnostic, physiologic, and surgical considerations. Am J Perinatol 1:227, 1984.
40. Wilson WR, Ilbawi MN, De Leon SY, et al: Technical modifications for improved results in total anomalous pulmonary venous drainage. J Thorac Cardiovasc Surg 103:861, 1992.

41. Lopetegui B, Gomez O, Arretz C, et al: Cirugia del drenaje venoso pulmonar anomalo total: Experiencia actual (Abstract). Rev Chil Cardiol Cirug Cardiovasc 15:123, 1996.

42. Schafers HJ, Luhmer I, Oelert H: Pulmonary venous obstruction following repair of total anomalous pulmonary venous drainage. Ann Thorac Surg 43:432, 1987.

43. Oelert H, Schafers HJ, Stegmannt T, et al: Complete correction of total anomalous pulmonary venous drainage: Experience with 53 patients. Ann Thorac Surg 41:392, 1986.

44. Rordam S, Abdelnoor M, Sorland S, Tjonneland S: Factors influencing survival in total anomalous pulmonary venous drainage. Scand J Thorac Cardiovasc Surg 28:55, 1994.

45. Fukushima Y, Onitsuka T, Nakamura K: A simple method for excising pulmonary venous obstruction after repair of total anomalous pulmonary venous drainage. Jpn Circ J 58:805, 1994.

46. van de Wal HJ, Hamilton DI, Godman MJ, et al: Pulmonary venous obstruction following correction for total anomalous pulmonary venous drainage. Eur J Cardiothorac Surg 6:545, 1992.

CHAPTER 30
TRICUSPID ATRESIA

P. SYAMASUNDAR RAO

Tricuspid atresia is a cyanotic cardiac malformation defined as congenital absence or agenesis of the morphologic tricuspid valve.[1,2] It is the third most common cyanotic cardiac anomaly and is the most common cause of cyanosis with left ventricular hypertrophy. The first patient with tricuspid atresia was described by Kreysig in 1817,[3] although the 1812 report by the editors of *London Medical Review*[3] appears to fit the description of tricuspid atresia but without use of the specific term. Some authors[4,5] stated that tricuspid atresia was first described by Kühne in 1906 or Holmes in 1824, but a thorough review by Rashkind[3] suggests that this is not so.

NOMENCLATURE AND CLASSIFICATION

There has been a debate with regard to terminology: tricuspid atresia, univentricular heart, or univentricular atrioventricular connection.[6] On the basis of evidence and arguments presented by Bharati and colleagues,[7–9] Wenink and Ottenkamp,[10] Gessner,[11] and Rao,[6,12] tricuspid atresia is the correct and logical term to describe this well-characterized pathologic and clinical entity and is so used in this chapter.

Tricuspid atresia has been classified on the basis of valve morphology,[13] radiographic appearance of pulmonary vascular markings,[14] and associated cardiac anomalies.[15–17]

CLASSIFICATION BASED ON VALVE MORPHOLOGY

Van Praagh and colleagues[13] proposed a classification based on morphology of the atretic tricuspid valve. This classification was modified and expanded by him and others.[18] The most common is the muscular type, characterized by a dimple or a localized fibrous thickening in the floor of the right atrium at the expected site of the tricuspid valve (Fig. 30–1). The muscular variety constitutes 89% of all tricuspid atresia (Table 30–1). Other types, namely, membranous, valvar, Ebstein, atrioventricular septal defect, and unguarded with muscular shelf, account for the remaining 11% (Table 30–1).[7,13,19–25] The reader is referred to previous publications[18,26] for pathologic, echocardiographic, and angiographic examples of the rare anatomic types.

CLASSIFICATION BASED ON RADIOGRAPHIC PULMONARY VASCULAR MARKINGS

Astley and coworkers[14] classified tricuspid atresia on the basis of pulmonary vascular markings on the chest radiograph: group A, decreased pulmonary vascular markings; and group B, increased pulmonary vascular markings. To this was added a third group by Dick and associates[4]: group C, transition from increased to decreased pulmonary vascular markings. This categorization has clinical value, although more precise noninvasive definition of the problem by echo Doppler studies and pulse oximetry is readily available.

CLASSIFICATION BASED ON ASSOCIATED DEFECTS

Interrelationship of great arteries was used by Kühne[15] in 1906 as a basis for classification, which was expanded later by Edwards and Burchell[16] and popularized by Keith and associates.[17] A variety of other classifications have been proposed.[1,18] To include all variations of great artery anatomy and to maintain uniformity of subgrouping, I proposed a comprehensive yet unified classification[1] that is listed in Table 30–2. The primary grouping is based on great artery relationships: type I, normally related great arteries; type II, D-transposition of great arteries; type III, other malpositions of great arteries, which are subdivided into subtypes 1 through 5 (Table 30–2); and type IV, persistent truncus arteriosus. The major types and subtypes are divided further into subgroup a, pulmonary atresia; subgroup b, pulmonary stenosis or hypoplasia; and subgroup c, normal pulmonary arteries (no pulmonary stenosis). The status of the ventricular septum and the other associated malformations (Table 30–3)[27] should then be stated for each heart.

This unified classification considers all variations in great artery anatomy described thus far, can be expanded if new great artery positional abnormalities are described, and maintains uniformity in subgroups but preserves the basic principles of previous classifications.[15–17] If one wants to follow the terminology of congenital heart disease proposed by Van Praagh,[28] the remaining cardiac segment subsets (i.e., visceroatrial situs and ventricular loop) could be added, and each heart is described by the notations {S,D,S}, {S,D,D}, and {S,D,L} as shown in the schematic drawing depicted in Figure 30–2.

PREVALENCE

The best estimates of the prevalence of tricuspid atresia based on autopsy and clinical series are 2.9% and 1.4% of cardiac malformations, respectively.[29] Assuming a prevalence of congenital heart disease of 0.8% of live births, tricuspid atresia occurs in approximately 1 in 10,000 live

TABLE 30-1

PREVALENCE OF TYPES OF TRICUSPID ATRESIA BASED ON VALVE MORPHOLOGY

Author	Total N	Muscular	Membranous	Valvar	Ebstein	AV Septal Defect	Unguarded with Muscular Shelf
Van Praagh et al,[13] 1971	38	32	3	0	3	0	0
Rao et al,[19] 1973	38	37	0	0	1	0	0
Bharati et al,[7] 1976	172	157	12	0	3	0	0
Anderson et al,[20] 1977	83°	76	4	1	2	0	0
Weinberg,[21] 1980	33	25	4	2	2	0	0
Ando et al,[22] 1980	29	20	8	0	1	0	0
Ottenkamp et al,[23] 1984	34°	29	4	0	1	0	0
Scalia et al,[24] 1984	76°	68	0	3	1	0	4
Rao,[25] 1987	28	27	0	0	0	1	0
Total (%)	531	471 (89)	35 (6.6)	6 (1)	14 (2.6)	1 (0.2)	4 (0.6)

°Number of patients who are common to these three studies cannot be ascertained.

AV = atrioventricular; N = total number of patients.

Adapted from Rao PS: Classification of tricuspid atresia. *In* Rao PS (ed): Tricuspid Atresia, 2nd ed. Mount Kisco, NY, Futura Publishing, 1992, p 59.

births.[29] A slight male preponderance has been suggested for tricuspid atresia,[4,30] but detailed analysis when gender is known[29] did not indicate sex preponderance. However, male preponderance (66% versus 34%) was found in tricuspid atresia patients with transposition of the great arteries (types II and III).[29] Although geographic differences in relative prevalences for aortic coarctation and stenosis have been found, no difference in either geographic prevalence or racial background for tricuspid atresia has been described.[29]

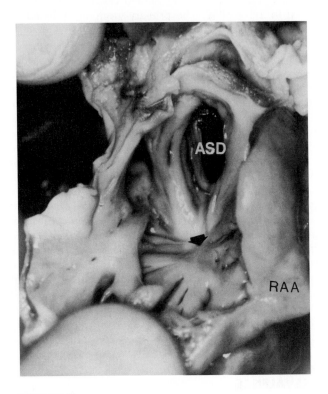

FIGURE 30-1

Muscular type of tricuspid atresia; the right atrium is opened by cutting through the right atrial appendage (RAA). There is a dimple (*arrow*) in the floor of the right atrium with muscle fibers radiating around it. Atrial septal defect (ASD) is shown. (From Rao PS, Levy JM, Nikicicz E, Gilbert-Barness EF: Tricuspid atresia: Association with persistent truncus arteriosus. Am Heart J 122:829–835, 1991.)

PATHOLOGIC ANATOMY

The pathology of this lesion is best described by reviewing variations in the morphology of the atretic tricuspid valve. In the most common muscular type (see Fig. 30–1), no valve material can be identified by either gross or microscopic examination.[17] In the membranous type, the atrioventricular portion of the membranous septum forms the floor of the right atrium at the expected location of the tricuspid valve.[7,13,22] An unusually high incidence of absent pulmonary valve leaflets occurs with this type of tricuspid atresia.[18] In the valvar type, the minute valve cusps are fused.[17,20,21] The Ebstein type, with fusion of the tricuspid valve leaflets (which had been displaced downward and plastered onto the right ventricular wall), is rare.[7,13,19] In the rare atrioventricular septal defect, the valve leaflet of the common atrioventricular valve seals off the only entrance into the right ventricle.[25,31] The final form, in which the right atrioventricular junction is unguarded but the inlet component of the morphologic right ventricle is separated from its outlet by a muscular shelf,[24] is also rare.

The right atrium is usually enlarged and its wall thick and hypertrophied. The interatrial communication, necessary for survival, is usually a stretched patent foramen ovale, sometimes an ostium secundum atrial septal defect, and occasionally an ostium primum atrial septal defect. Rarely, the interatrial communication is obstructive and may form an aneurysm of the fossa ovalis. The left atrium may be enlarged, especially if the pulmonary blood flow is increased. The mitral valve is morphologically normal; the mitral orifice is large and occasionally incompetent. The left ventricle is clearly a morphologic left ventricle with only occasional abnormalities[7]; however, it is enlarged and hypertrophied. In contrast, the right ventricle is small and hypoplastic; even the largest of the right ventricles in patients with a large ventricular septal defect (VSD) or transposition of the great arteries is smaller than normal. Right ventricular size is determined by the anatomic type of tricuspid atresia. In patients with pulmonary atresia and normally related great arteries, the right ventricle may be extremely small and escape detection. However, in most patients, it is a true right ventricle[7,8] consisting of a sharply

TABLE 30–2

A UNIFIED CLASSIFICATION OF TRICUSPID ATRESIA

Type I	Normally related great arteries	
Type II	D-Transposition of the great arteries	
Type III	Malpositions of the great arteries other than D-transposition	
	Subtype 1	L-Transposition of the great arteries
	Subtype 2	Double-outlet right ventricle
	Subtype 3	Double-outlet left ventricle
	Subtype 4	D-Malposition of the great arteries (anatomically corrected malposition)
	Subtype 5	L-Malposition of the great arteries (anatomically corrected malposition)
Type IV	Persistent truncus arteriosus	

Each type and subtype are divided:
Subgroup a   Pulmonary atresia
Subgroup b   Pulmonary stenosis or hypoplasia
Subgroup c   Normal pulmonary arteries (no pulmonary stenosis)

From Rao PS: A unified classification for tricuspid atresia. Am Heart J 99:799–804, 1980.

demarcated infundibulum with septal and parietal bands and a trabeculated sinus portion that communicates with the left ventricle through a VSD. The inflow region of the right ventricle, by definition, is absent, although papillary muscles may be present rarely.

The relative position of the great vessels varies. Most have either normally related great arteries (type I) or D-transposed great arteries (type II), but a few have other positional anomalies of the great arteries (type III) or truncus arteriosus (type IV).

Pulmonary outflow tract obstruction is common in type I tricuspid atresia. The pulmonary valve may be atretic (subgroup a), and either a patent ductus arteriosus or aortopulmonary collateral vessels supply the lungs. A stenotic pulmonary outflow tract (subgroup b) is more common. The stenosis is either subvalvar or valvar in patients with

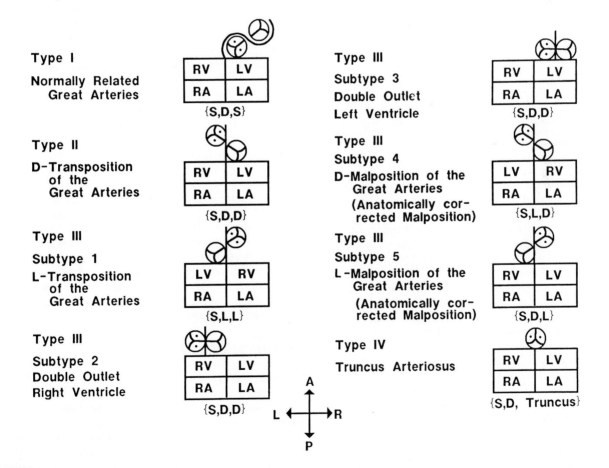

FIGURE 30–2

Representation of segmental subsets of tricuspid atresia with the heart in the left side of the chest. Only commonly described types are depicted. Each type can occur with dextrocardia and atrial inversion. Both double-outlet right ventricle and double-outlet left ventricle can occur with {S, D, L} and {S, L, L}. A = anterior; {–,D,–} = D-loop; {–,–,D} = D-transposition; {–, L, –} = L-loop; {–, –, L} = L-transposition; LA = left atrium; LV = left ventricle; P = posterior; R = right; RA = right atrium; RV = right ventricle; {S, –, –} = situs solitus; {–, –, S} = solitus normal great arteries. (From Rao PS: Classification of tricuspid atresia. *In* Rao PS [ed]: Tricuspid Atresia, 2nd ed. Mount Kisco, NY, Futura Publishing, 1992, p 59.)

ASSOCIATED CARDIAC ANOMALIES IN TRICUSPID ATRESIA

Anomalies that form the basis of classification
 D-Transposition of the great arteries
 L-Transposition of the great arteries
 Double-outlet right ventricle
 Double-outlet left ventricle
 Other malpositions of the great arteries
 Truncus arteriosus

Anomalies that may need attention before or at the time of palliative or total surgical correction
 Absent pulmonary valve
 Aneurysm of the atrial septum
 Anomalous origin of the coronary arteries from the pulmonary artery
 Anomalous origin of the left subclavian artery
 Anomalous origin of the right subclavian artery
 Aortopulmonary fistula
 Coarctation of the aorta
 Common atrium
 Cor triatriatum dexter
 Coronary sinus septal defect
 Double aortic arch
 Double-outlet left atrium
 Hemitruncus
 Hypoplastic ascending aorta and aortic atresia
 Ostium primum atrial septal defect
 Parchment right ventricle
 Patent ductus arteriosus
 Persistent left superior vena cava
 Right aortic arch
 Subaortic stenosis
 Total anomalous pulmonary venous connection
 Tubular hypoplasia of the aortic arch
 Valvar aortic stenosis

Others
 Juxtaposition of the atrial appendages
 Anomalous entry of coronary sinus into the left atrium

From Rao PS, Covitz W, Chopra PS: Principles of palliative management of patients with tricuspid atresia. *In* Rao PS (ed): Tricuspid Atresia, 2nd ed. Mount Kisco, NY, Futura Publishing, 1992, p 297.

transposition of the great arteries, whereas in patients with normally related great arteries, obstruction occurs at the VSD level.[32–38] In a few patients, subvalvar pulmonary stenosis, a narrow outflow tract of the hypoplastic right ventricle, and rarely valvar pulmonary stenosis may be responsible for the pulmonary outflow obstruction. A normal pulmonary outflow tract (subgroup c) without stenosis may be present, although less commonly than those with stenosis. The ascending aorta is normal or enlarged.

The VSD may be large, small, or nonexistent, or multiple VSDs may be present. The VSD may be conoventricular or perimembranous (located inferior to the septal band), show conal septal malalignment (located between the anterosuperior and posteroinferior limbs of the septal band), be muscular (located inferiorly compared with the two previous types), or be of the atrioventricular canal type.[39] Muscular VSDs are most common.[32,33] Furthermore, most VSDs are restrictive, producing subpulmonic stenosis in patients with normally related great arteries and mimicking subaortic obstruction in patients with transposed great arteries.[32–38]

About 30% of tricuspid atresia patients have associated anomalies (see Table 30–3). Significant among these are persistent left superior vena cava and aortic coarctation, the latter more frequent in type II patients.

PATHOPHYSIOLOGY

PRENATAL CIRCULATION

In tricuspid atresia, unlike in normal hearts (see Chapter 4), both vena caval streams are shunted across the foramen ovale into the left atrium and left ventricle. Therefore, the arterial PO_2 is the same in all parts of the body. Whether a higher PO_2 in blood passing to lungs influences the pulmonary arteriolar smooth muscle development is unknown.[40] The lower than normal PO_2 to the brain and upper part of the body does not seem to impair development, at least as observed clinically.

The pulmonary blood flow in type I (normally related great arteries) patients with intact ventricular septum or pulmonary atresia (type Ia) and type II (transposition of the great arteries) patients with pulmonary atresia (type IIa) must be supplied entirely through the ductus arteriosus. Because the ductus carries only the pulmonary blood flow, representing 8 to 10% of combined ventricular output in contrast to 66% in the normal fetus,[40] the ductus arteriosus is smaller than normal. This fact and the acute angulation of the ductus at its aortic origin because of reversal of direction of ductal flow may render the ductus less responsive to the usual postnatal stimuli.[40]

In type I patients with VSD, the amount of blood flow from the left ventricle through the VSD into the right ventricle, pulmonary artery, and ductus arteriosus compared with the quantity of blood flow retrograde from the aorta through the ductus arteriosus varies with size of the VSD. The larger the VSD, the greater is the amount of anterograde ductal flow.

In type I patients with either a small or no VSD, most of the left ventricular blood is ejected into the aorta to the entire body and the placenta. Thus, the aortic isthmus carries a larger proportion of ventricular output than normal; this presumably explains the rarity of coarctation of the aorta in tricuspid atresia without transposition of the great arteries. In type II (transposition) without significant pulmonary stenosis, because the VSD is usually smaller than the pulmonary valve annulus,[41] a larger proportion of blood traverses the pulmonary artery and ductus arteriosus anterograde. Therefore, the isthmic blood flow is less, thus accounting for the high incidence of coarctation of the aorta and aortic arch anomalies in patients with tricuspid atresia and transposition.[40,41]

POSTNATAL CIRCULATION

An obligatory right-to-left shunt occurs at the atrial level in most types and subtypes (exception: type III, subtypes 1 and 4; see Fig. 30–2) of tricuspid atresia. Consequently, the systemic and coronary venous blood mixes with pulmonary venous blood in the left atrium. This mixed pulmonary, coronary, and systemic venous blood enters the left ventricle. In type III, subtypes 1 and 4, because of ventricular inversion, the occluded morphologic tricuspid valve is left-sided and the pathophysiology is that of mitral atresia with left-to-right shunting of pulmonary venous blood.

In type I (normally related great arteries) patients with a VSD, a ventricular left-to-right shunt occurs, thus perfusing the lungs. If the ventricular septum is intact, the pulmonary circulation is derived from a patent ductus arteriosus or through bronchopulmonary or persistent aortopulmonary collateral vessels. The aortic blood flow is derived directly from the left ventricle.

In type II (with D-transposition of the great arteries), the pulmonary circulation is directly supplied from the left ventricle. The systemic circulation is supplied through the VSD and the right ventricle. In other type III and type IV patients, the systemic and pulmonary blood flows are determined by the size of the VSD and other associated anomalies.

OTHER PHYSIOLOGIC PRINCIPLES

Arterial Desaturation

Because of complete admixture of the systemic, coronary, and pulmonary venous returns in the left atrium and left ventricle, systemic arterial desaturation is always present. The oxygen saturation is proportional to the magnitude of the pulmonary blood flow.[41,42] The pulmonary-to-systemic blood flow ratio (Qp/Qs), which represents the pulmonary blood flow, has a curvilinear relationship with the arterial oxygen saturation (Fig. 30–3). A Qp/Qs of 1.5 to 2.5 appears to produce an adequate oxygen saturation.[42]

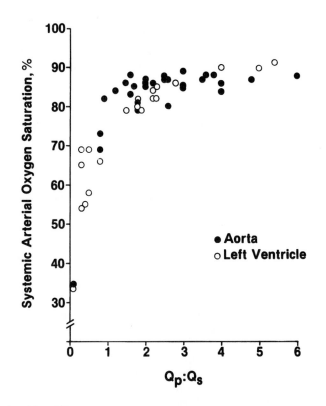

FIGURE 30–3

Systemic arterial saturation of left ventricle or aorta is plotted against the pulmonary-to-systemic blood flow ratio (Qp/Qs). Both type I and type II are included. There is a curvilinear relationship between the two variables. At low Qp/Qs levels, a slight increase in Qp/Qs produces a large increase in systemic oxygen saturation; and at higher Qp/Qs, further increase produces a large increase in systemic oxygen saturation. The ideal Qp/Qs appears to be between 1.5 and 2.5, giving oxygen saturations in the low 80s. Aortic saturations are marked as *solid circles,* LV saturations as *open circles.* (From Rao PS: Cardiac catheterization in tricuspid atresia. *In* Rao PS [ed]: Tricuspid Atresia. Mount Kisco, NY, Futura Publishing, 1982, p 153.)

Pulmonary Blood Flow

The magnitude of pulmonary blood flow is the major determinant of clinical features in tricuspid atresia. An infant with markedly decreased pulmonary blood flow presents early in the neonatal period with severe cyanosis, hypoxemia, and acidosis. An infant with markedly increased pulmonary flow does not have significant cyanosis but usually presents with signs of heart failure. Patients with decreased pulmonary flow usually belong to type I (normally related great arteries), and those with increased pulmonary blood flow are usually type II (transposition of the great arteries) and occasionally type Ic.

The quantity of pulmonary blood flow depends on the degree of obstruction to the pulmonary outflow tract and patency of the ductus arteriosus. The pulmonary outflow obstruction is either valvar or subvalvar in type II patients and valvar, subvalvar, or at VSD level in type I patients. In my experience, I have found the obstruction most commonly at the VSD level.[32–36] If the VSD is large and nonrestrictive and the pulmonary valve nonstenotic, the pulmonary flow is inversely proportional to the pulmonary-to-systemic vascular resistance ratio.

Left Ventricular Volume Overloading

Because the entire systemic, coronary, and pulmonary circulations are supplied by the left ventricle, it has to eject a greater than normal volume. This volume overloading is further increased if the Qp/Qs is increased, because of either minimal obstruction to pulmonary blood flow or a large surgical shunt, and may lead to heart failure. Normal left ventricular function is critical for a successful Fontan-type procedure. Left ventricular function tends to decrease with increasing age, Qp/Qs, and arterial desaturation.[43–45]

Size of the Interatrial Communication

The interatrial communication is usually a patent foramen ovale. Because the entire systemic venous return must pass through the patent foramen ovale, it is not surprising to find interatrial obstruction, although in few patients with tricuspid atresia is this clinically significant.[4] The right-to-left shunt occurs in late atrial diastole with augmentation during atrial systole (*a* wave).[46] A mean atrial pressure gradient greater than 5 mm Hg is usually associated with interatrial obstruction. Tall *a* waves in the right atrial pressure trace also indicate interatrial obstruction.

Changing Hemodynamics

With growth and development, several changes occur in patients with tricuspid atresia. Closure of the ductus arteriosus in the early neonatal period may result in severe hypoxemia. The size of the interatrial communication may diminish either in absolute terms or relative to the volume of the systemic venous return and cause systemic venous congestion. Atrial septostomy may be required.

A VSD is necessary to maintain adequate intracardiac shunting essential for survival of the patient; these types of VSDs are named physiologically advantageous VSDs.[33–36] Intermittent functional[36] and complete or partial anatomic[32,35,37,38,47] closure of the VSD has been reported. Intermittent functional closure of a VSD is likely to produce cyanotic spells in tricuspid atresia. The causes of such functional closure are not clearly delineated but are likely to be similar to those suspected in tetralogy of Fallot.[36, 47] Complete or partial anatomic closure in type I patients produces progressive cyanosis, increasing polycythemia, or disappearance of the heart murmur, requiring an operation earlier than planned. In type II patients, partial closure of the VSD results in subaortic, systemic outflow obstruction; complete VSD closures have not been reported in these patients.

The prevalence of VSD closure in tricuspid atresia is difficult to estimate. The best estimates, based on my data[32, 33, 47] and those of Sauer and Hall,[38] are 38 to 44%, which is similar to that of spontaneous closure of an isolated VSD.[48, 49] The ages at which the VSD closures take place vary, starting before 1 year to 20 years with a median of 1.3 years.[47] Thus, a higher proportion of VSD closure occurs in early life, as has been found with an isolated VSD. Several mechanisms of closure have been observed; the most common is progressive muscular encroachment of the margins of VSD with subsequent fibrosis and covering by endocardial proliferation. The factors initiating closure of VSD are not known. After an extensive review of this subject,[34, 47, 50] I concluded that there is a great natural tendency for a VSD to close spontaneously whether it is isolated or a part of a more complex cardiac anomaly. The reason for this tendency remains unclear.

CLINICAL FEATURES

Nearly half of the patients with tricuspid atresia present with symptoms on the first day after birth, and 80% have symptoms by 1 month of age.[4, 51] Two modes of clinical presentation are recognized: decreased pulmonary blood flow and increased pulmonary blood flow.

Infants with pulmonary oligemia present with symptoms of hypoxemia within the first few days of life; the more severe the pulmonary oligemia, the earlier the clinical presentation. These hypoxemic infants are cyanotic and develop hyperpnea and acidosis if the pulmonary blood flow is markedly decreased. Most are type Ib. Patients with pulmonary atresia (subgroup a) irrespective of the major type also present with early cyanosis, especially as the ductus begins to close. Hypoxic spells are uncommon in a neonate, although they can occur later in infancy. Physical examination reveals central cyanosis, tachypnea or hyperpnea, normal pulses, a prominent *a* wave in the jugular venous pulse (if there is significant interatrial obstruction), and normal hepatic size. Presystolic hepatic pulsations may be felt if severe interatrial obstruction exists. The precordium is quiet, and no thrills are usually felt. The second heart sound is single. A soft holosystolic murmur suggestive of a VSD may be heard at the left lower or midsternal border. Diastole is clear. In patients with associated pulmonary atresia, no murmurs are usually heard, except occasionally the continuous murmur of a patent ductus arteriosus. Signs of congestive heart failure are notably absent.

Infants with pulmonary plethora usually present with signs of heart failure within the first few weeks of life, although an occasional infant may present within the first week of life.[52] They are only minimally cyanotic but present with dyspnea, fatigue, difficulty in feeding, and perspiration. Recurrent respiratory tract infection and failure to thrive are other modes of presentation. Most of these patients belong to type IIc, although a small number may be of type Ic. The association of coarctation of the aorta with type II patients may result in early cardiac failure. Examination reveals tachypnea, tachycardia, decreased femoral pulses (with coarctation of the aorta but without a large patent ductus arteriosus), minimal cyanosis, prominent neck vein pulsations, and hepatomegaly. Prominent *a* waves in jugular veins or presystolic hepatic pulsations may be observed with interatrial obstruction. The precordial impulses are increased and hyperdynamic. The second heart sound may be single or split. A loud holosystolic murmur of a VSD is usually heard at the left lower sternal border. A loud third sound or an apical mid-diastolic murmur is often heard. Signs of congestive cardiac failure are usually present.

Issues related to long-standing cyanosis, such as clubbing, polycythemia, relative anemia, cerebrovascular accident, brain abscess, coagulation problems, and hyperuricemia, are similar to those for any other cyanotic cardiac malformation[53] (see Chapter 63). The risk for development of endocarditis resembles that observed in other cardiac abnormalities.

Patients with tricuspid atresia are particularly prone to atrial arrhythmias; atrial fibrillation is more common, occurring in older children and adolescents with long-standing cyanosis, systemic-to-pulmonary arterial shunt, and left ventricular volume overloading.

NONINVASIVE EVALUATION

CHEST RADIOGRAPHY

Radiographic features depend on the total pulmonary blood flow. In patients with decreased pulmonary flow (most infants fall into this category), cardiac size is either normal or mildly enlarged; whereas in those with increased pulmonary blood flow, moderate to severe cardiomegaly is present. A variety of cardiac configurations have been described in the literature: "characteristic" tricuspid atresia appearance,[54] *coeur en sabot* configuration,[55] and egg-shaped,[56] bell-shaped,[57] and square[14] heart, but in my and others' experience,[56] no consistent pattern diagnostic of tricuspid atresia is found. There may be concavity in the region of the pulmonary artery segment in patients with pulmonary oligemia and a small pulmonary artery. The right atrial shadow may be prominent.

A right aortic arch is present in 8% of patients with tricuspid atresia[56] and is less common than in tetralogy of Fallot (25%) and truncus arteriosus (40%). An unusual contour of the left cardiac border suggestive of L-transposition may be seen in association with or confused with tricuspid atresia.[58]

The greatest use of the chest radiograph is its ability to categorize neonates into those with decreased pulmonary vascular markings and those with increased pulmonary vascular markings. Often, this is all that is necessary to make a correct diagnosis once a history, physical examination, and electrocardiogram have been obtained.[58]

ELECTROCARDIOGRAPHY

The electrocardiogram is virtually diagnostic of tricuspid atresia in the presence of cyanosis. The characteristic features are right atrial hypertrophy; an abnormal, superiorly oriented major QRS vector (so-called left axis deviation) in the frontal plane; left ventricular hypertrophy; and diminished right ventricular forces (Fig. 30–4).

Right atrial hypertrophy, manifested by tall, peaked P waves exceeding 2.5 mm in amplitude, may be present in three fourths of the patients with tricuspid atresia.[59] A double-peak, spike-and-dome configuration of the P wave, referred to as P tricuspidale, may be present.[59] The first taller peak is contributed by the right atrial depolarization, and the second smaller peak is presumed to be due to left atrial depolarization.[60] Irrespective of the configuration, the P wave duration is prolonged, perhaps owing to right atrial enlargement.

An abnormal, superiorly oriented major QRS vector (ASV), more popularly called left axis deviation, between 0 and −90 degrees in the frontal plane is present in most patients with tricuspid atresia (Fig. 30–5). ASV is present in more than 80% of patients with type I anatomy (normally related great arteries), but less than 50% of patients with type II and type III anatomy show such a typical electrocardiographic pattern. Normal (0 to +90 degrees) or right axis deviation is present in a minority of patients, most of them with type II or type III anatomy. The mechanism of ASV has not been clearly delineated; postulated mechanisms include destructive lesions in the left anterior bundle, fibrosis of left bundle branch, abnormal distribution of the conduction system (unusually long right bundle branch

and origin of left bundle branch close to the nodal–His bundle junction), small right ventricle, large left ventricle, and others.[60] More recently, ventricular activation data from my group[60,61] suggested that this characteristic QRS pattern in tricuspid atresia is produced by interaction of several factors, the most important being right-to-left phase asynchrony of ventricular activation, right-to-left ventricular disproportion, and the asymmetric distribution of the left ventricular mass favoring the superior wall.[60,61]

Regardless of the frontal plane mean QRS vector, electrocardiographic left ventricular hypertrophy is present in most patients, manifested by increased (beyond the 95th percentile) S waves in right chest leads and R waves in left chest leads or by adult progression of the QRS in the chest leads in the neonates and infants. ST-T wave changes suggestive of left ventricular strain are present in half of patients.[59] Left ventricular hypertrophy is due to left ventricular volume overload as well as lack of opposition to the left ventricular forces by the hypoplastic right ventricle. Biventricular hypertrophy may occasionally be present, and most of these patients have type II or type III anatomy with an adequately sized right ventricle.[60]

Diminished R waves in right chest leads and S waves in left chest leads are related to right ventricular hypoplasia.

Electrocardiographic features of rare types of tricuspid atresia are reviewed elsewhere.[60]

ECHO DOPPLER STUDIES

M-mode echocardiographic features include an enlarged left atrium (usually proportional to the magnitude of pulmonary blood flow), a dilated left ventricle with normal or decreased

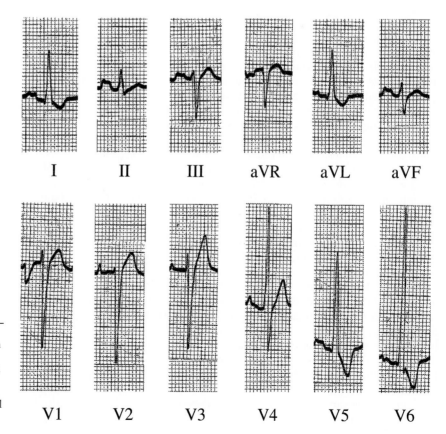

FIGURE 30–4

Electrocardiogram highly suggestive of tricuspid atresia: abnormal, superiorly oriented mean QRS vector in the frontal plane (−45 degrees, left axis deviation), left ventricular hypertrophy, and diminished anterior (R waves in leads V_1 and V_2) and rightward (S waves in leads V_5 and V_6) forces. Prominent P waves appear in several leads.

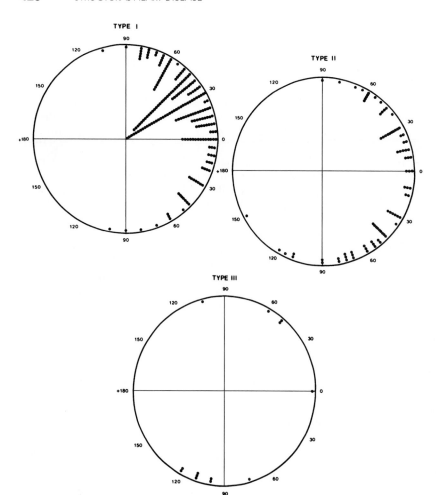

FIGURE 30–5

Frontal plane mean QRS vector in 308 patients, plotted according to anatomic type of tricuspid atresia. Most type I patients have an abnormally superior vector, also called left axis deviation. In type II, only half of the patients have an abnormally superior vector. In type III (subtype a), most have an inferiorly oriented frontal plane vector. (From Rao PS, Kulungara RJ, Boineau JP, Moore HV: Electro-vectorcardiographic features of tricuspid atresia. *In* Rao PS [ed]: Tricuspid Atresia, 2nd ed. Mount Kisco, NY, Futura Publishing, 1992, p 141.)

left ventricular shortening fraction, a large mitral valve in continuity with the posterior semilunar valve, and a small right ventricle.[58, 62] The pulmonary valve may or may not be recorded. The tricuspid valve is conspicuously absent.[58]

Two-dimensional echocardiography, apart from showing an enlarged right atrium, left atrium, and left ventricle and a small right ventricle, demonstrates the atretic tricuspid valve directly. In the most common muscular type, a dense band of echoes is seen at the site where the tricuspid valve should be,[58, 63] and the anterior leaflet of the detectable atrioventricular valve is attached to the left side of the interatrial septum (Fig. 30–6). The anatomy is best demonstrated in the apical and subcostal four-chamber views. A persistent left superior vena cava, when present, can usually be identified emptying into the coronary sinus, as can the entries of the superior and inferior venae cavae into the right atrium. Atrial and ventricular septal defects can also be demonstrated by two-dimensional echocardiography. Semilunar valves can be identified as pulmonic or aortic by following the great vessel until the bifurcation of the pulmonary artery or arch of the aorta is seen; this will help decide whether there is associated transposition of the great arteries. Coarctation of the aorta, often seen in type II patients, may be shown in the suprasternal notch view.

Contrast echocardiography with two-dimensional imaging clearly demonstrates sequential opacification of the right atrium, the left atrium, the left ventricle, and then the right ventricle, although this is unnecessary for diagnosis.

Doppler echocardiography is helpful in demonstrating shunts and the degree of pulmonary stenosis. Right-to-left shunting across the atrial septum can be visualized by placing the pulsed Doppler sample volume on either side of the atrial defect (Fig. 30–7) and by color flow mapping. Most right-to-left shunting occurs during atrial systole. Left-to-right shunting, although transient, can be demonstrated by Doppler study during atrial diastole, secondary to instantaneous pressure differences across the atrial septum.[46] High-flow velocity across the VSD (Fig. 30–7) can be demonstrated in type Ib tricuspid atresia; the higher the velocity, the smaller the defect. Color-guided continuous-wave Doppler, with use of the modified Bernoulli equation, is useful in quantitating the left-to-right ventricular pressure difference, thereby estimating the size of the VSD. Interrogating the right ventricular outflow tract may be useful in demonstrating subvalvar or valvar pulmonic stenosis. Careful interrogation of Doppler velocities across the VSD in type II patients is important to demonstrate subaortic (at the VSD level) obstruction. Similarly, Doppler evaluation of the descending aorta is useful in demonstrating aortic coarctation.

M-mode, two-dimensional, Doppler (pulsed, continuous-wave, and color), and, when indicated, contrast

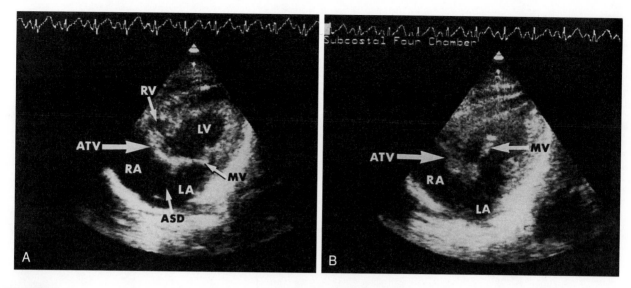

FIGURE 30–6

Subcostal four-chamber two-dimensional echocardiogram of a neonate with tricuspid atresia. *A,* Enlarged left ventricle (LV), small right ventricle (RV), and a dense band of echoes (ATV) are shown at the site where the tricuspid valve echo should be. Atrial (ASD) and ventricular septal defects and the mitral valve (MV) are visualized. *B,* Attachment of anterior leaflet of detectable atrioventricular valve to left side of atrial septum. LA = left atrium; RA = right atrium. (*A, B* from Rao PS: Tricuspid atresia. *In* Long WA [ed]: Fetal and Neonatal Cardiology. Philadelphia, WB Saunders, 1990, p 525.)

echocardiography are useful in delineating most anatomic and physiologic issues related to tricuspid atresia.

OTHER LABORATORY STUDIES

Pulse oximetry is readily available in the outpatient setting for noninvasive measurement of oxygen saturation. Hemoglobin level and hematocrit along with red blood indices should be routinely obtained to assess the degree of polycythemia and hypoxemia and to identify relative iron deficiency anemia.[53]

CARDIAC CATHETERIZATION AND SELECTIVE CINEANGIOGRAPHY

The diagnosis of tricuspid atresia based on clinical, electrocardiographic, and echocardiographic features is relatively simple, and cardiac catheterization with selective cineangiography rarely, if ever, is essential for arriving at the diagnosis.[42] Both anatomic and physiologic definition of the cardiac anomaly can often be achieved by echo Doppler studies. Cardiac catheterization should be performed only if sufficient data needed for management are unavailable from echo Doppler and other noninvasive studies. Catheterization is generally recommended before operative correction to provide the surgeon with accurate anatomic detail. Specific information on the pulmonary artery anatomy, size, and pressures and left ventricular function is necessary before a Fontan-type procedure. Assessment of Choussat's hemodynamic and angiographic parameters[64] (Table 30–4) should be undertaken, although exceptions to some criteria can be made.

CATHETER INSERTION AND COURSE

The percutaneous femoral venous route is used for catheterization.[42,65] The right ventricle cannot be directly entered from the right atrium because of atresia of the tricuspid valve, but the catheter can easily be advanced into the left atrium across the patent foramen ovale and from there into the left ventricle through the mitral valve. With the availability of balloon-tipped catheters and a variety of guide wires, it is usually possible to catheterize the right ventricle (through the VSD), pulmonary artery, and aorta. However, in a sick neonate, the procedure may be terminated after left ventricular angiography because further manipulation of the catheter may produce an arrhythmia or precipitate a hypercyanotic spell. In infants with clinical evidence of aortic coarctation (type II patients), retrograde femoral arterial catheterization may be necessary if left ventricular angiography does not clearly define the problem.

OXYGEN SATURATION

Systemic venous oxygen saturation is decreased in proportion to systemic arterial desaturation and severity of congestive heart failure. Because of obligatory right-to-left shunting across the patent foramen ovale, a left-to-right shunt is ordinarily not detected. However, an increase in right atrial oxygen saturation may be attributed to transient reversal of instantaneous pressure differences between the atria.[46]

The pulmonary venous oxygen saturations are usually normal, with a lower left atrial oxygen saturation reflecting

TABLE 30–4

CHOUSSAT CRITERIA

Normal vena caval connections
Normal right atrial volume
Mean pulmonary artery pressure ≤ 15 mm Hg
Pulmonary vascular resistance ≤ 4 units/m^2
Pulmonary artery to aortic root diameter ratio ≥ 0.75
Normal left ventricular function
Competent mitral valve
Undistorted pulmonary arteries

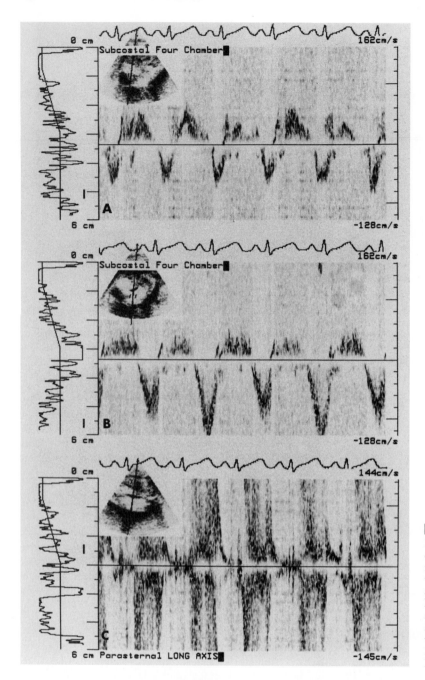

FIGURE 30–7

Pulsed Doppler echocardiography in a subcostal four-chamber view demonstrating left-to-right (*A*) and right-to-left (*B*) shunting across the atrial communication. The right-to-left shunt is expected in tricuspid atresia, but the left-to-right shunt is unexpected and has been explained on the basis of instantaneous pressure differences between atria. *C,* Doppler study shows left-to-right shunting across the ventricular septal defect. (*A–C* from Rao PS: Tricuspid atresia. *In* Long WA [ed]: Fetal and Neonatal Cardiology. Philadelphia, WB Saunders, 1990, p 525.)

the atrial right-to-left shunt. Left ventricular oxygen saturation is also diminished and represents better admixture than that in the left atrium. The oxygen saturations in the left atrium, left ventricle, right ventricle, pulmonary artery, and aorta are similar. Systemic arterial desaturation is always present and is a function of the pulmonary-to-systemic flow ratio (Qp/Qs).

The vena caval, left atrial, and left ventricular oxygen saturations are generally lower in type I than in type II patients, presumably related to greater preponderance of pulmonary oligemia in type I patients.[42]

PRESSURES

The mean right atrial pressure is mildly increased, similar to or slightly higher than that in the left atrium. The right

atrial *a* waves are prominent. A mean atrial pressure difference greater than 5 mm Hg and giant *a* wave in the right atrial pressure trace indicate interatrial obstruction. When the left ventricular end-diastolic pressure is markedly elevated, lack of pressure difference across the atrial septum does not exclude interatrial obstruction.[42]

Mean left atrial and left ventricular end-diastolic pressures are usually normal but increase with increasing Qp/Qs and decreasing left ventricular function. The left atrial *v* waves are lower than *a* waves in patients with decreased pulmonary blood flow. As the pulmonary flow increases, the *v* waves become taller.

The left ventricular peak systolic pressure is usually normal but may be elevated with aortic coarctation or subaortic stenosis. Aortic peak systolic pressure is normal unless there is associated aortic coarctation. Aortic diastolic pressure may be low because of diastolic runoff, secondary to an operatively placed aortopulmonary shunt. In a type II (transposition) patient, careful pressure pullback across the aortic and subaortic region should be performed. A peak pressure gradient between the ventricles indicates subaortic obstruction secondary to a small VSD.[32,33]

The right ventricular peak systolic pressure is usually proportional to the size of the VSD in type I patients; the larger the VSD, the higher is the pressure. The pressure is occasionally high in the face of a small VSD because of right ventricular outflow tract stenosis. The right ventricular pressure is at systemic level in type II patients.

Every attempt should be made to catheterize the pulmonary artery[42] because of the importance of measuring pulmonary artery pressure[64] in evaluating tricuspid atresia patients for corrective operation. When all methods fail, pulmonary venous wedge pressure should be measured to estimate the pulmonary artery pressure.[66] The pulmonary artery pressures are usually normal in type I patients, although they may be high in type Ic patients with a large VSD. In type II patients with transposition, the pulmonary artery pressure depends on the degree of subvalvar and valvar pulmonary stenosis or the effectiveness of an operatively placed pulmonary artery band.

CALCULATED VARIABLES

Pulmonary and systemic blood flows and vascular resistances and shunts may be calculated by the Fick principle, with either assumed or measured oxygen consumption. The principles and methods of calculation are detailed elsewhere.[40,42] Of these, the Qp/Qs and pulmonary vascular resistance are most important. The Qp/Qs is diminished in type I and type II patients with pulmonary atresia and in type Ib patients with a small VSD. It may be markedly increased in type I patients with a large VSD (type Ic) and most type II patients.

In most patients with tricuspid atresia, pulmonary vascular resistance is normal because of pulmonary outflow tract obstruction. In type Ic patients with a large VSD, type IIc patients without pulmonary stenosis, and patients with a large systemic–pulmonary artery shunt, the pulmonary resistance may be elevated.

Another calculated variable described by Mair and associates,[67] the preoperative catheterization index, recognizes the importance of pulmonary vascular resistance and left ventricular diastolic function. This index may be calculated as

$$Rp + \frac{LVEDP}{PI + SI}$$

where Rp is pulmonary vascular resistance (units/m²), LVEDP is left ventricular end-diastolic pressure (mm Hg), and PI and SI are pulmonary and systemic flow indices (L/min/m²).

An index of 4 or less is associated with lower early and total mortality after a Fontan operation than is an index above 4. This is a useful index, although with some limitations.[67]

ANGIOGRAPHY

The absence of direct anatomic continuity between the right atrium and the morphologic right ventricle is the hallmark of the angiographic features of tricuspid atresia. Selective superior vena caval or right atrial angiograms reveal successive opacification of the left atrium and left ventricle without immediate opacification of the right ventricle (Fig. 30–8); this "typical sequence of tricuspid atresia" is con-

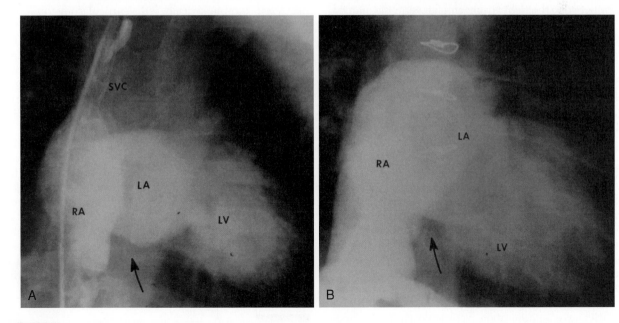

FIGURE 30–8

Cineangiograms from (A) superior vena cava (SVC) and (B) right atrium (RA) in frontal projection from two patients. There is sequential opacification of the left atrium (LA) and left ventricle (LV) without opacification of the right ventricle. The nonopacified right ventricular "window" (arrows) is formed by the RA on the right, the LA superiorly, and the LV on the left. This is a classic appearance of the muscular variety of tricuspid atresia. (From Rao PS: Tricuspid atresia: Anatomy, imaging, and natural history. In Braunwald E [ed]: Atlas of Heart Diseases, Vol XII. Philadelphia, Current Medicine, 1997, p 14.1.)

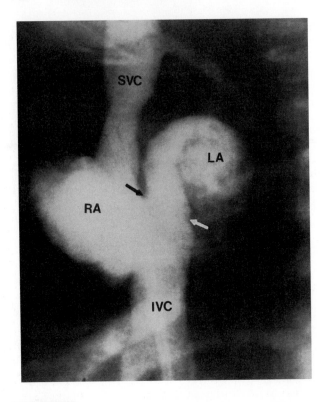

Selective superior vena caval (SVC) angiogram in a four-chamber (hepatoclavicular) projection reveals no opacification of the right ventricle and typical, onionskin appearance of the interatrial communication (arrows). Contrast material streams into the roof of the left atrium (LA). IVC = inferior vena cava; RA = right atrium. (From Schwartz DC, Rao PS: Angiography in tricuspid atresia. In Rao PS [ed]: Tricuspid Atresia, 2nd ed. Mount Kisco, NY, Futura Publishing, 1992, p 233.)

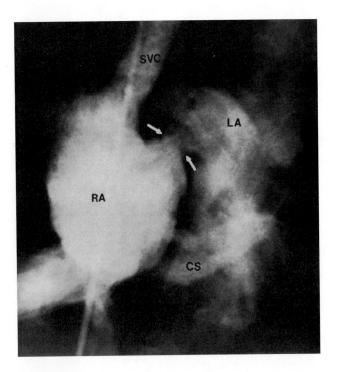

Selective superior vena caval (SVC) injection in four-chamber projection (hepatoclavicular) shows tricuspid atresia and filling of the left atrium (LA) through a restrictive atrial septal defect (arrows). There is retrograde filling of the coronary sinus (CS). RA = right atrium. (From Schwartz DC, Rao PS: Angiography in tricuspid atresia. In Rao PS [ed]: Tricuspid Atresia, 2nd ed. Mount Kisco, NY, Futura Publishing, 1992, p 233.)

sidered a characteristic sign of tricuspid atresia. The negative shadow between the right atrium and left ventricle, named the right ventricular window, corresponds to failure of early filling of the right ventricle (Fig. 30–8). These features are best demonstrated in the posteroanterior view. The size and location of the atrial septal defect are optimally shown in hepatoclavicular or lateral views and may produce the so-called onionskin or waterfall appearance (Fig. 30–9).

Reflux of the contrast material into the venae cavae and hepatic veins is seen normally after right atrial angiography. Dense opacification of the coronary sinus (Fig. 30–10) suggests interatrial obstruction. The size of the right atrium and the location and size of the right atrial appendage should also be evaluated. For example, left-sided juxtaposition of the atrial appendages (Fig. 30–11) occurs more frequently in tricuspid atresia, especially when it is associated with transposition of the great arteries. Finally, different morphologic types of atretic tricuspid valves may be recognized.[18, 26, 68]

Once tricuspid atresia is demonstrated, it is important to define the ventricular anatomy, type and size of the interventricular communication, ventriculoarterial connections, pulmonary artery anatomy, and associated abnormalities. Left innominate vein angiography to demonstrate a persistent left superior vena cava and bridging innominate vein should also be performed; such information is useful in considering bidirectional Glenn and Fontan operations.

Selective left ventricular angiography reveals finely trabeculated, morphologically left ventricular anatomy. The origin and relative positions of the great arteries (Figs. 30–12 and 30–13), the size and location of the VSDs, the presence of mitral insufficiency, and the size of the right ventricle can be demonstrated. I initially perform left ventricular angiography in frontal and lateral views. Angiography is performed in additional views, such as left anterior oblique, hepatoclavicular, or long axial oblique, depending on the structures that need greater definition. Special attention should be paid in evaluating subaortic obstruction at the VSD level in patients with transposition.[32, 33] Quantitative measurements of the size and function of the left ventricle[43–45] should also be undertaken. Selective injections into the right ventricle, aorta, and pulmonary artery provide greater definition of these structures. Particular attention should be paid to define sources of pulmonary blood flow and pulmonary artery anatomy. Selective angiography with the catheter positioned proximal to or in the previously created shunts is also useful in evaluating the pulmonary arteries and, of course, the shunt itself.

DIFFERENTIAL DIAGNOSIS

Differential diagnosis differs with the mode of presentation (Table 30–5).

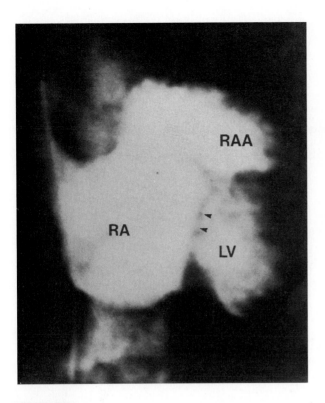

FIGURE 30–11

Selective superior vena caval injection in the right anterior oblique projection shows the right atrial appendage (RAA) juxtaposed leftward. There is an imperforate tricuspid valve *(arrowheads)*. LV = left ventricle; RA = right atrium. (From Schwartz DC, Rao PS: Angiography in tricuspid atresia. *In* Rao PS [ed]: Tricuspid Atresia, 2nd ed. Mount Kisco, NY, Futura Publishing, 1992, p 233.)

DECREASED PULMONARY BLOOD FLOW

Causes of cyanosis with decreased pulmonary blood flow are listed in Table 30–5. The electrocardiogram is most useful in the differential diagnosis (Fig. 30–14).[69] Echocardiography and cineangiography may occasionally be necessary for confirming the diagnosis, especially in complex defects.

INCREASED PULMONARY BLOOD FLOW

The differential diagnostic considerations are also listed in Table 30–5. Although the characteristic electrocardiographic pattern (abnormal, superior vector or left axis deviation) of tricuspid atresia is helpful, it is not always present in tricuspid atresia with transposition. Furthermore, some of the conditions listed in Table 30–5 also have a similar displacement of the mean frontal plane vector. Often, echocardiograms and angiocardiograms are necessary for final diagnosis.

TREATMENT

Physiologically "corrective" operations for tricuspid atresia[70, 71] and their modifications are usually performed in patients older than 2 years. Most patients present with symptoms as neonates and should be effectively palliated to enable them to reach the age at which correction can be undertaken. The objective of the management plan, apart from providing symptomatic relief and increased survival rate, should be to preserve, protect, and restore structure (good-sized and undistorted pulmonary arteries) and function (normal pulmonary artery pressure and preserved left ventricular function) to normal such that a corrective procedure can be performed later. With this objective in mind, the management plan is discussed under the following headings: (1) medical management at the time of initial presentation, (2) palliative treatment of specific physiologic abnormalities, (3) medical management after palliative operation, (4) physiologically corrective operation, and (5) follow-up after corrective operation.

MEDICAL MANAGEMENT AT THE TIME OF PRESENTATION

In infants with low arterial PO_2 and oxygen saturation and with ductus-dependent pulmonary blood flow, the ductus should be kept open by intravenous administration of prostaglandin E_1 (PGE_1).[72] The ductal dilatation increases pulmonary blood flow, thereby improving oxygenation and

TABLE 30–5

DIFFERENTIAL DIAGNOSIS OF TRICUSPID ATRESIA IN THE NEONATE

DECREASED PULMONARY BLOOD FLOW

Tetralogy of Fallot including pulmonary atresia with ventricular septal defect
Pulmonary atresia or severe stenosis with intact ventricular septum
Tricuspid atresia
Complex cardiac anomalies with severe pulmonary stenosis or atresia including D-transposition with ventricular septal defect; L-transposition with ventricular septal defect; single ventricle, double-outlet right ventricle, and asplenia syndrome

INCREASED PULMONARY BLOOD FLOW

D-Transposition of the great arteries with large ventricular septal defect
Coarctation of the aorta with ventricular septal defect
Multiple left-to-right shunts (ventricular septal defect, common atrioventricular canal, and patent ductus arteriosus)
Single ventricle, double-outlet right ventricle, and other complex cardiac defects without pulmonic stenosis
Total anomalous pulmonary venous connection without obstruction
Hypoplastic left heart syndrome
Truncus arteriosus

Modified from Rao PS: Tricuspid atresia. *In* Long WA (ed): Fetal and Neonatal Cardiology. Philadelphia, WB Saunders, 1990, p 535.

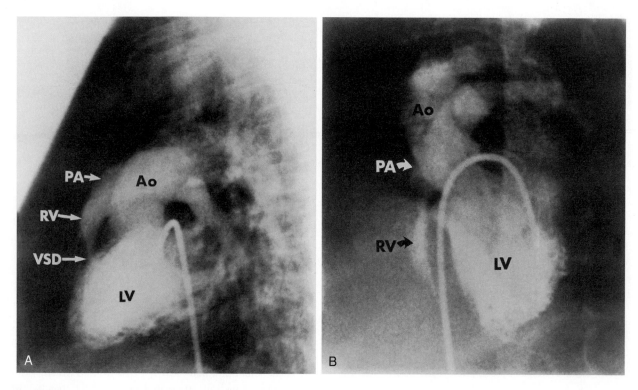

FIGURE 30–12

Selective left ventricular (LV) cineangiograms in lateral (*A*) and four-chamber (*B*) views demonstrate normal position of aorta (Ao) and pulmonary artery (PA). Ventricular septal defect (VSD) is seen with visualization of right ventricle (RV). (*A, B* from Rao PS: Other tricuspid valve anomalies. *In* Long WA [ed]: Fetal and Neonatal Cardiology. Philadelphia, WB Saunders, 1990, p 541.)

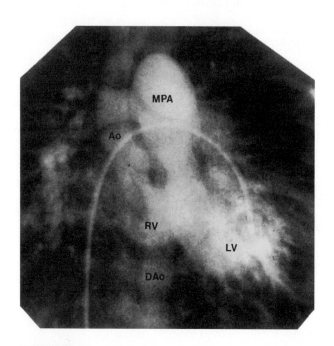

FIGURE 30–13

Selective left ventriculogram in frontal view in infant with type II tricuspid atresia shows transposition of the great arteries. Ao = aorta; DAo = descending aorta; LV = left ventricle; MPA = main pulmonary artery; RV = right ventricle. (From Schwartz DC, Rao PS: Angiography in tricuspid atresia. *In* Rao PS [ed]: Tricuspid Atresia, 2nd ed. Mount Kisco, NY, Futura Publishing, 1992, p 233.)

reversing the metabolic acidosis so that further diagnostic studies and other interventions can be performed with relative safety. I usually begin with a dose of 0.05 μg/kg/min and reduce the rate of infusion, provided that the desired oxygen tension levels are maintained; this has been most helpful in reducing the occurrence and severity of some of the drug's bothersome side effects, namely, apnea and hyperpyrexia. The PGE$_1$ infusion rate may be increased if Po$_2$ does not increase.

An occasional infant who presents with signs of congestive heart failure (more common in type II patients) should be treated with routine anticongestive measures. Patients with associated severe coarctation of the aorta may also be helped with PGE$_1$ infusion; this time, the ductal dilatation improves systemic perfusion. This is followed by relief of aortic obstruction by operation or balloon angioplasty.[73]

PALLIATIVE TREATMENT OF SPECIFIC PHYSIOLOGIC ABNORMALITIES

The type of palliation undertaken depends largely on the hemodynamic abnormality produced by the basic lesion and associated cardiac anomalies. These may be broadly grouped[27] into decreased pulmonary blood flow, increased pulmonary blood flow, and intracardiac obstruction.

Decreased Pulmonary Blood Flow

Since the description of subclavian artery–ipsilateral pulmonary artery anastomosis in 1945 by Blalock and Taussig,[74] several other types of procedures have been devised to improve the pulmonary blood flow. Systemic–pulmonary

DIFFERENTIAL DIAGNOSIS OF INFANTS WITH
CYANOSIS AND DECREASED PULMONARY BLOOD FLOW

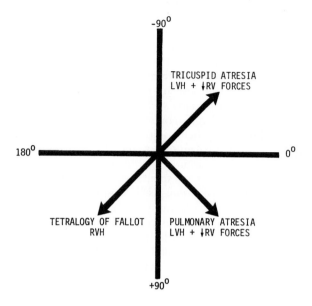

ECG-FRONTAL PLANE MEAN QRS VECTOR ("AXIS")

FIGURE 30-14

Use of electrocardiographic mean QRS vector ("axis") in frontal plane in a differential diagnosis of a cyanotic neonate with decreased pulmonary blood flow. Associated ventricular hypertrophy patterns and decreased right ventricular (RV) forces are also helpful (see text for details). LVH = left ventricular hypertrophy; RVH = right ventricular hypertrophy. (From Rao PS: Management of the neonate with suspected serious heart disease. King Faisal Specialist Hosp Med J 4:213, 1984.)

artery shunts are most commonly used in palliating pulmonary oligemia. Because of the problems associated with the central shunts, most surgeons prefer a modified Blalock-Taussig shunt with a Gore-Tex graft interposed between the subclavian artery and the ipsilateral pulmonary artery,[75] although distortion of the pulmonary artery sometimes created by the shunt may be a problem later.

Enlargement of the VSD or resection of the right ventricular outflow tract stenosis has been suggested by Annecchino and coworkers[76] to augment the pulmonary blood flow. This ingenious approach attacks the site of obstruction rather than bypassing it. However, it requires cardiopulmonary bypass and may not be feasible or necessary in the neonatal period.[27, 76] Stenting the arterial duct, because of limited experience,[77] is not currently an initial therapeutic choice. Rarely, the predominant obstruction may be at the pulmonary valve level, and in such patients, balloon pulmonary valvuloplasty[78] may augment pulmonary blood flow.

In summary, despite the availability of many palliative procedures to increase pulmonary blood flow, some produce serious complications that prevent a successful Fontan-Kreutzer procedure subsequently. The Blalock-Taussig anastomosis or one of its modified versions is the preferred procedure with the least number of long-term complications, but at the same time it preserves suitable anatomy for subsequent corrective procedures and there-

fore is recommended as the procedure of choice for palliation of tricuspid atresia patients with decreased pulmonary blood flow.

Increased Pulmonary Blood Flow
Infants with a moderate increase in pulmonary blood flow do not have any significant symptoms and are less cyanotic than the pulmonary oligemic patients. Markedly increased pulmonary blood flow as in type Ic and type IIc patients, however, can produce congestive heart failure.

In type I patients, aggressive anticongestive measures should be promptly instituted. In the natural history, the VSD becomes smaller, and patients with pulmonary plethora will, in due course, develop pulmonary oligemia requiring a palliative shunt. Right ventricular outflow tract obstruction may also develop, with resultant decrease in pulmonary blood flow. Therefore, pulmonary artery banding should not be performed initially in this group of patients. If optimal anticongestive therapy does not produce adequate relief of symptoms after a time,[27] pulmonary artery banding should be considered. In those who did not have pulmonary artery banding performed, careful follow-up studies with periodic assessment of pulmonary artery pressure and timely intervention are necessary to prevent pulmonary vascular obstructive disease.

In type II patients, banding of the pulmonary artery should be performed once the infant is stabilized with anticongestive therapy. If there is associated coarctation of the aorta, or aortic arch interruption or hypoplasia, adequate relief of the aortic obstruction should be provided concurrently with pulmonary artery banding, and a patent ductus arteriosus should be ligated. The importance of PGE_1 administration in the control of congestive heart failure has already been alluded to. Although I advocate balloon dilatation angioplasty of the coarctation[73] in these complicated lesions, there is no unanimity of opinion among cardiologists and surgeons on this issue.

Intracardiac Obstruction
Intracardiac obstruction can occur at two different levels: patent foramen ovale and VSD.

INTERATRIAL OBSTRUCTION
The interatrial defect should be big enough to accommodate the egress of the entire systemic venous return. A mean atrial pressure difference of 5 mm Hg or more with prominent *a* waves (15 to 20 mm Hg) in the right atrium is generally considered to represent obstruction of the interatrial septum.[27] It may be necessary to relieve the obstruction by balloon atrial septostomy[79]; if that is unsuccessful, by blade atrial septostomy[80, 81]; and rarely by operative atrial septostomy. Significant interatrial obstruction requiring atrial septostomy in the neonate is unusual, although this can be a significant problem later in infancy.[32, 81]

INTERVENTRICULAR OBSTRUCTION
Spontaneous closure of the VSD can occur, causing severe pulmonary oligemia in type I patients and subaortic obstruction in type II patients. Functional and anatomic closures have been reported in patients with normally related great arteries.[33, 36] In functional closure, cyanotic spells similar to those observed in tetralogy of Fallot[36] may occur, and

the management is similar, namely, knee-chest position, humidified oxygen, and morphine sulfate (0.1 mg/kg). If the spells are not averted, β blockers (propranolol or esmolol) or intravenous vasopressors (methoxamine or phenylephrine) may be given to increase systolic blood pressure by 10 to 20%. Correction of metabolic acidosis or anemia, if present, should also be considered. If there is no improvement, immediate operative palliation may be necessary. If the infant improves, correction by a Fontan-type procedure or palliation by a systemic–pulmonary artery shunt or a bidirectional Glenn operation may be performed subsequently.

In partial or complete anatomic closure of the VSD, pulmonary oligemia with consequent hypoxemia and polycythemia ensues. Augmentation of the pulmonary blood flow is indicated and can be accomplished by several methods (see earlier). If the age and size of the patient or cardiac anatomy and hemodynamics are unsuitable for performing a modified Fontan operation, a systemic–pulmonary artery shunt should be undertaken. A classic Glenn procedure should not be performed because if the VSD closes completely, the left pulmonary artery will be without flow (Fig. 30–15), which may result in thrombosis or underdevelopment of the left pulmonary artery. In addition, long-term complications of the Glenn operation,[47] particularly development of pulmonary arteriovenous fistulae, are of concern. Central aortopulmonary shunts should be avoided because they tend to raise pulmonary artery pressure and resistance, frequently kinking or distorting the pulmonary arteries. Thus, a Blalock-Taussig type of shunt (classic or modified [Gore-Tex] Blalock-Taussig) or a bidirectional Glenn procedure is preferable. In younger infants, I prefer a Blalock-Taussig shunt; in older infants and children, I recommend a bidirectional Glenn procedure preparatory to a modified Fontan operation.

Partial spontaneous closure of the VSD in type II patients causes subaortic obstruction,[32, 33, 47] which should be relieved or bypassed lest the resultant left ventricular hypertrophy pose increased risk at the time of the Fontan procedure.[82] The obstruction must be tackled at the time of either a bidirectional Glenn or a modified Fontan operation. Resection of the conal muscular septum,[83, 84] thus enlarging the VSD, is a direct approach, although concern for development of heart block and spontaneous closure of the surgically produced VSD remains.[47] Alternatively, the VSD, right ventricle, and aortic valve may be bypassed by anastomosis of the proximal stump of the divided pulmonary artery to the ascending aorta (Damus-Kaye-Stansel) at the time of the Fontan (or bidirectional Glenn) operation. However, there are limited data from which to draw conclusions of superiority of one method over the other.

MEDICAL MANAGEMENT AFTER A PALLIATIVE OPERATION

Problems encountered with tricuspid atresia patients are similar to those found in other types of cyanotic cardiac malformations. Appropriate monitoring for and treatment of relative anemia, polycythemia, and coagulopathy should be undertaken. Hyperuricemia, gout, and uric acid nephropathy can develop in adolescents and adults with long-standing cyanosis and polycythemia and should be prevented by timely palliative or corrective operative therapy. If prevention is unfeasible, periodic measurement of uric acid levels and treatment with allopurinol (if the uric acid level is above 8 mg/100 ml) may have to be instituted. The risks for development of a cerebrovascular accident or brain abscess are similar to those seen with other cyanotic anomalies, and appropriate consultation and treatment are indicated. Antibiotic prophylaxis before any bacteremia-producing procedures or surgery is indicated, as is routine immunization plus consideration for polyvalent pneumococcal vaccine or influenza vaccine.

CORRECTIVE SURGERY

Since the original descriptions by Fontan[70] and Kreutzer[71] of physiologically corrective operations for tricuspid atresia, many modifications of these procedures have been suggested.[85, 86] The Fontan operation was based on the concept of using the right atrium as a pump. As originally described, it consists of superior vena cava–right pulmonary artery (Glenn) shunt, anastomosis of the proximal end of the divided right pulmonary artery to the right atrium directly or by means of an aortic homograft, closure of the atrial defect, insertion of a pulmonary valve homograft into the inferior vena caval orifice, and ligation of the main pulmonary artery, thus bypassing the right ventricle completely. Kreutzer's concept was that the right atrium may not function as a pump and that the left ventricle is the only suction pump in the system. His original

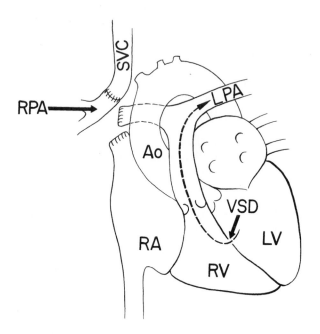

FIGURE 30–15

Drawing of classical Glenn procedure in the presence of a spontaneously closing (closed) ventricular septal defect (VSD). If the VSD closes after a superior vena cava (SVC)–right pulmonary artery (RPA) shunt (Glenn), the left pulmonary artery (LPA) is isolated without anterograde perfusion, which in turn may result in hypoplasia or thrombus formation. Ao = aorta; LV = left ventricle; RA = right atrium; RV = right ventricle. (From Rao PS: Further observations on the spontaneous closure of physiologically advantageous ventricular septal defects in tricuspid atresia: Surgical implications. Reprinted with permission from the Society of Thoracic Surgeons [The Annals of Thoracic Surgery, 1983, Volume 35, Pages 121–131].)

operation consisted of direct anastomosis of the right atrial appendage with the pulmonary artery or through a pulmonary homograft. The atrial septal defect is closed, but neither a Glenn procedure nor prosthetic valve insertion into the inferior vena cava is performed. These procedures were subsequently modified by these and other workers,[86] and there is consensus that there is no need for a classic Glenn anastomosis or a valve at the inferior vena cava–right atrial junction.[85, 86] At the time of extensive review of the literature several years ago,[85, 86] my colleague and I determined that there were four major types of commonly used Fontan-Kreutzer operations: right atrium–pulmonary artery anastomosis with and without valved conduit, and right atrium–right ventricular connection with and without a valved conduit. On the basis of this review, we concluded that direct atriopulmonary anastomosis (without a valved conduit) was the best procedure for tricuspid atresia patients with normally related great arteries and a small right ventricle (≤30% normal) and those with transposed great arteries. On the other hand, a right atrial–right ventricular valved conduit (preferably homograft) anastomosis was better for patients with normally related great arteries and a good-sized right ventricle (>30% of normal, with a trabecular component of the right ventricle).

At the time of our review, we observed several emerging concepts to increase success rate in high-risk patients. On the basis of hydrodynamic studies, de Leval and colleagues[87] concluded that the right atrium has no efficient pump function; pulsations in nonvalved circulation generate turbulence with consequent decrease in net flow; and energy losses occur in the nonpulsatile chambers, corners, and obstructions. They devised and performed total cavopulmonary diversion in which the upper end of the divided superior vena cava is anastomosed end to side with the superior aspect of the undivided right pulmonary artery, and the inferior vena caval blood is directed through an intra-atrial tunnel into the cardiac end of the superior vena cava, which in turn is connected to the undersurface of the right pulmonary artery. The advantages of this procedure are technical simplicity, maintenance of low right atrial and coronary sinus pressure, and reduction in risk of formation of atrial thrombus. Further experimental studies by Sharma and associates[88] suggested that complete or minimal offset between the orifices of the superior vena caval connection may decrease energy losses.

The criteria outlined by Choussat and associates[64] have been modified or exceeded by many groups of workers. These factors, when present, would make the Fontan-Kreutzer operation a high-risk procedure and should be identified at the time of preoperative evaluation. They include elevated pulmonary artery pressure (mean pressure, ≥18 mm Hg) or resistance (≥4 Wood units/m^2), distorted or small (McGoon ratio of 1.8 or less) pulmonary arteries, poor left ventricular function (end-diastolic pressure above 12 mm Hg), significant mitral regurgitation, subaortic obstruction, and severe left ventricular hypertrophy. With one or more of these risk factors, physiologically corrective procedures of the Fontan type may carry significant risk. For these patients, two sets of alternative approaches may be considered: bidirectional cavopulmonary anastomosis and fenestrated Fontan.

In the bidirectional Glenn procedure, the upper end of the divided superior vena cava is anastomosed end to side to the superior aspect of the undivided right pulmonary artery, thus diverting the superior vena caval blood into both right and left pulmonary arteries.[89, 90] Preoperative evaluation should specifically exclude a persistent left superior vena cava because it may divert blood away from the pulmonary arteries. There are hemodynamic advantages associated with the bidirectional Glenn, including improved effective pulmonary flow, reduced total pulmonary flow, and less left ventricular volume overloading. Another advantage is that this procedure preserves pulmonary artery continuity, thus paving the way for a subsequent Fontan-Kreutzer operation. Although some authorities[91] suggest that an additional source of pulmonary blood flow is needed to achieve adequate systemic arterial saturation, and indeed some patients were hypoxemic,[92] I believe that appropriate preoperative selection of patients and adequate relief of pulmonary arterial obstruction during operation circumvent this problem. During preoperative catheterization, the effective pulmonary flow index[42] should be calculated. If it is more than one third of the cardiac index, the bidirectional cavopulmonary anastomosis is not likely to improve systemic arterial oxygen saturation. Also, patients with significant elevation of pulmonary vascular resistance (>3.0 units) are not candidates for this procedure. Calculation of pulmonary vascular resistance after administration of oxygen to ensure that the resistance is less than 3 units should be undertaken. The bidirectional Glenn shunt should be followed later by a lateral tunnel or an extracardiac conduit to divert the inferior vena caval blood into the pulmonary circuit.

In high-risk Fontan-Kreutzer patients, leaving open a small atrial septal defect to allow decompression of the right atrium in the immediate postoperative period with a plan to close the defect later has been used by some workers.[93-95] The atrial defect is closed by a preplaced suture or by transcatheter techniques. Significant improvement in postoperative pleural effusions, systemic venous congestion, and low cardiac output and possibly shorter hospitalization have been the beneficial effects of the fenestration, but at the expense of mild systemic arterial hypoxemia. Although the fenestrated Fontan was originally conceived for high-risk patients, it is now being performed by many surgeons for patients in categories of modest and even low risk.

In summary, operations that divide the pulmonary and systemic venous returns are feasible for most patients with tricuspid atresia. The age (and weight) of the patient and anatomic and physiologic substrate determine the type of palliative and corrective procedures. In neonates and young infants (<6 months), a Blalock-Taussig (classic or modified, Gore-Tex) shunt is the procedure of choice. Between 6 months and 1 year of age, a modified Blalock-Taussig shunt and a bidirectional Glenn procedure are the procedures of choice. Between 1 and 2 years of age, a bidirectional Glenn procedure is used unless there is a contraindication. Beyond 2 years of age, total cavopulmonary anastomosis with or without fenestration, depending on the risk factors, may be performed. In patients with transposition of the great arteries, early pulmonary artery banding, treatment of aortic obstruction, and relieving or bypassing subaortic obstruction should also be incorporated into the treatment plan.

FOLLOW-UP AFTER CORRECTIVE OPERATION

Close follow-up after correction is indicated. Some patients need continued inotropic and diuretic therapy. Afterload reduction with an angiotensin-converting enzyme inhibitor is generally recommended to augment left ventricular outflow with consequent improvement in pulmonary flow, although controlled studies substantiating this principle have not been undertaken. Because of the potential for development of thrombi in the right atrium, anticoagulants are routinely used by most cardiologists. I recommend platelet-inhibiting doses of aspirin; others advocate warfarin anticoagulation.

Most patients do well after operation (Fig. 30–16).[96] However, several problems have been observed after corrective surgery: arrhythmia, obstructed pulmonary outflow pathways, persistent shunts, and systemic venous congestion including protein-losing enteropathy. Supraventricular arrhythmias (atrial flutter or fibrillation, paroxysmal supraventricular tachycardia) are common and should be treated with appropriate pharmacologic therapy. In a patient without adequate control, electrophysiologic study and surgical or transcatheter ablation may be indicated.[97] Revision of the Fontan pathway to a cavopulmonary con-

nection with elimination of the enlarged right atrium has been considered an alternative solution. Sick sinus node syndrome and atrioventricular block occur in some children and may require pacemaker therapy. Ventricular arrhythmia is less frequent.

Symptoms and signs indicative of obstruction to Fontan pathways should be promptly investigated. Poor echo windows make noninvasive evaluation difficult, and catheterization and angiography may be necessary. Obstructive lesions, if identified, should be treated with balloon angioplasty, stenting, or even operation, as indicated.

A persistent shunt may be secondary to intentional fenestration of the atrial septum or a residual atrial septal defect. If significant hypoxemia is present, the residual shunt should be closed, preferably by a transcatheter device.[94,98] Test occlusion of the defect is advisable to ensure that adequate cardiac output is maintained after occlusion.

Recurrent pleural effusion, liver dysfunction, and protein-losing enteropathy have occurred in a small number of patients. Protein-losing enteropathy carries a high (75%) mortality.[99] The cause of protein-losing enteropathy is unknown but appears to be related to loss of protein in the bowel by lymphatic distention secondary to increased systemic venous pressure, although this can occur in patients with reasonably "normal" pressures for the Fontan procedure. Symptoms usually appear 6 months after the Fontan-Kreutzer procedure or later and include diarrhea,

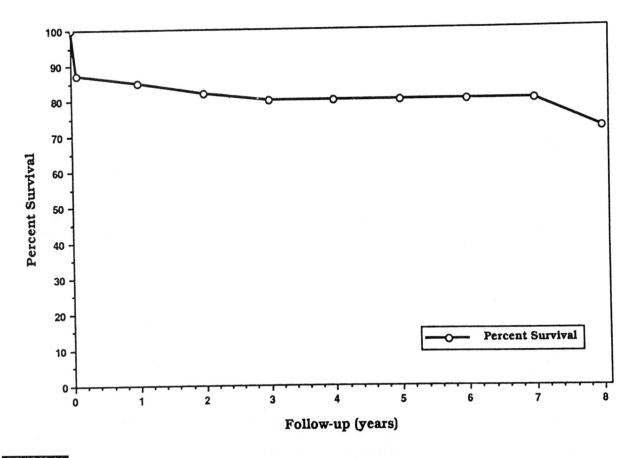

FIGURE 30–16

Actuarial survival of 100 tricuspid atresia patients undergoing a Fontan operation at the Hospital for Sick Children, Toronto, between 1975 and 1989. More than 70% survive 5 years after operation. (From Freedom RM, Gow R, Caspi J, et al: The Fontan procedure for patients with tricuspid atresia: Long-term follow-up. *In* Rao PS [ed]: Tricuspid Atresia, 2nd ed. Mount Kisco, NY, Futura Publishing, 1992, p 377.)

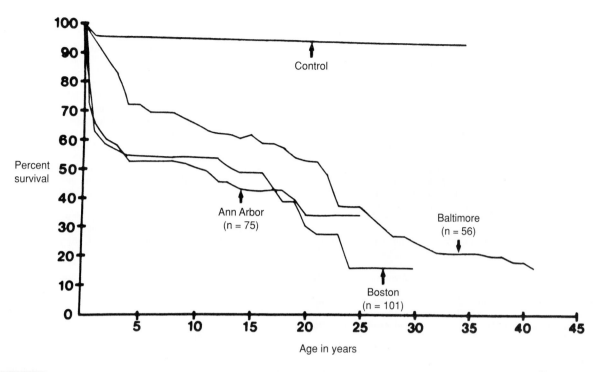

Actuarial survival curves from three series compiled by Dick and Rosenthal[51] show a high initial mortality in the first year of life, a plateau between the first year and the middle of the second decade of life, and a second bout of mortality from the middle of the second decade onward, presumably related to impaired left ventricular function. (From Dick M, Rosenthal A: The clinical profile of tricuspid atresia. *In* Rao PS [ed]: Tricuspid Atresia. Mount Kisco, NY, Futura Publishing, 1982, p 83.)

edema, ascites, and pleural effusion. Significant hypoalbuminemia and increased α_1-antitrypsin in the stool are present. Evidence for obstruction of the Fontan-Kreutzer pathway must be scrutinized and, if found, relieved. Medium-chain triglyceride diet and parenteral albumin supplementation may be supportive. Some workers have used prednisone,[100] with favorable effect, although the experience with this mode of therapy is limited. So, too, is experience with high-molecular-weight heparin. Because protein-losing enteropathy appears to be a fatal complication of the Fontan procedure, aggressive management is suggested. Reduction of right atrial pressure by creation of an atrial septal defect (Brockenbrough's puncture plus static dilatation of the atrial septum[101]) should be considered. Cardiac transplantation is another option that should be considered. However, most patients do well after the Fontan-Kreutzer procedure.

PROGNOSIS

The prognosis for neonates and infants with tricuspid atresia without treatment is poor; only 10 to 20% may survive their first birthday.[4,52] Actuarial survivals from three centers are shown in Figure 30–17. Normalization of the pulmonary blood flow by an aortopulmonary shunt in patients with decreased pulmonary blood flow and by banding of the pulmonary artery in patients with pulmonary plethora has markedly improved the survival. If one carefully examines the survival curves, however, there is still considerable early mortality, which may be related to hypoxemia, car-

diac failure, surgical intervention, or a combination thereof. Recent improvements in early identification and neonatal care, including availability of PGE_1, noninvasive diagnoses, anesthesia, and surgical techniques, may decrease the initial mortality. After the first year of life, survival curves are stable and reach a plateau (Fig. 30–17). A second drop in survival[4] begins at about 15 years of age with continued decline in survival rates. This late mortality is likely to be favorably affected by the physiologically corrective procedures. The advantage of Fontan-Kreutzer procedures, namely, decreasing or eliminating hypoxemia and ventricular volume overloading, may improve the survival rate (see Fig. 30–16) even after accounting for initial and late mortality of the operative procedure. The potential for improved prognosis exists, and therefore each patient with tricuspid atresia should be offered aggressive medical and operative therapy.

REFERENCES

1. Rao PS: A unified classification for tricuspid atresia. Am Heart J 99:799, 1980.
2. Rao PS: Terminology: Tricuspid atresia or univentricular heart? *In* Rao PS (ed): Tricuspid Atresia. Mount Kisco, NY, Futura Publishing, 1982, p 3.
3. Rashkind WJ: Tricuspid atresia: A historical review. Pediatr Cardiol 2:85, 1982.
4. Dick M, Fyler DC, Nadas AS: Tricuspid atresia: Clinical course in 101 patients. Am J Cardiol 36:327, 1975.
5. Rosenthal A, Dick M II: Tricuspid atresia. *In* Adams FH, Emmanouilides GC (eds): Moss' Heart Disease in Infants, Children, and Adolescents, 3rd ed. Baltimore, Williams & Wilkins, 1983, p 271.

6. Rao PS: Is the term "tricuspid atresia" appropriate? (Editorial) Am J Cardiol 66:1251, 1990.

7. Bharati S, McAllister HA Jr, Tatooles CJ, et al: Anatomic variations in underdeveloped right ventricle related to tricuspid atresia and stenosis. J Thorac Cardiovasc Surg 72:383, 1976.

8. Bharati S, Lev M: The concept of tricuspid atresia complex as distinct from that of the single ventricle complex. Pediatr Cardiol 1:57, 1979.

9. Bharati S, Lev M: Reply. Pediatr Cardiol 1:165, 1979/80.

10. Wenink ACG, Ottenkamp J: Tricuspid atresia: Microscopic findings in relation to "absence" of atrioventricular connection. Int J Cardiol 16:57, 1987.

11. Gessner IH: Embryology of atrioventricular valve formation and embryogenesis of tricuspid atresia. In Rao PS (ed): Tricuspid Atresia. Mount Kisco, NY, Futura Publishing, 1982, p 25.

12. Rao PS: Terminology: Is tricuspid atresia the correct term to use? In Rao PS (ed): Tricuspid Atresia, 2nd ed. Mount Kisco, NY, Futura Publishing, 1992, p 3.

13. Van Praagh R, Ando M, Dungan WT: Anatomic types of tricuspid atresia: Clinical and developmental implications (Abstract). Circulation 44(suppl II):115, 1971.

14. Astley R, Oldham JS, Parson C: Congenital tricuspid atresia. Br Heart J 15:287, 1953.

15. Kühne M: Über zwei Falle kongenitaler Atresie des Ostium Venosum Dextrum. Jahrb Kinderh 63:235, 1906.

16. Edwards JE, Burchell HB: Congenital tricuspid atresia: A classification. Med Clin North Am 33:1117, 1949.

17. Keith JD, Rowe RD, Vlad P: Tricuspid atresia. In Heart Disease in Infancy and Childhood. New York, Macmillian, 1958, p 434.

18. Rao PS: Classification of tricuspid atresia. In Rao PS (ed): Tricuspid Atresia, 2nd ed. Mount Kisco, NY, Futura Publishing, 1992, p 59.

19. Rao PS, Jue KL, Isabel-Jones J, et al: Ebstein's malformation of the tricuspid valve with atresia: Differentiation from isolated tricuspid atresia. Am J Cardiol 32:1004, 1973.

20. Anderson RH, Wilkinson JL, Gerlis LM, et al: Atresia of the right atrioventricular orifice. Br Heart J 39:414, 1977.

21. Weinberg PM: Anatomy of tricuspid atresia and its relevance to current forms of surgical therapy. Ann Thorac Surg 29:306, 1980.

22. Ando M, Santomi G, Takao A: Atresia of tricuspid and mitral orifice: Anatomic spectrum and morphogenetic hypothesis. In Van Praagh R, Takao A (eds): Etiology and Morphogenesis of Congenital Heart Disease. Mount Kisco, NY, Futura Publishing, 1980, p 421.

23. Ottenkamp J, Wenink AGG, Rohmer J, et al: Tricuspid atresia with overriding imperforate tricuspid membrane: An anatomic variant. Int J Cardiol 6:599, 1984.

24. Scalia D, Russo P, Anderson RH, et al: The surgical anatomy of the heart with no direct communication between the right atrium and the ventricular mass—so called tricuspid atresia. J Thorac Cardiovasc Surg 87:743, 1984.

25. Rao PS: Atrioventricular canal mimicking tricuspid atresia: Echocardiographic and angiographic features. Br Heart J 58:409, 1987.

26. Rao PS: Tricuspid atresia: Anatomy, imaging, and natural history. In Braunwald E (ed): Atlas of Heart Diseases, Vol XII. Philadelphia, Current Medicine, 1997, p 14.1.

27. Rao PS, Covitz W, Chopra PS: Principles of palliative management of patients with tricuspid atresia. In Rao PS (ed): Tricuspid Atresia, 2nd ed. Mount Kisco, NY, Futura Publishing, 1992, p 297.

28. Van Praagh R: Terminology of congenital heart disease: Glossary and commentary. Circulation 56:139, 1977.

29. Rao PS: Demographic features of tricuspid atresia. In Rao PS (ed): Tricuspid Atresia, 2nd ed. Mount Kisco, NY, Futura Publishing, 1992, p 23.

30. Taussig HB, Keinonen R, Momberger N, et al: Long-term observations of the Blalock-Taussig operation. IV. Tricuspid atresia. John Hopkins Med J 132:135, 1973.

31. Van Praagh R: Discussion after paper by Vlad P: Pulmonary atresia with intact ventricular septum. In Barrett-Boyes BG, Neutze JM, Harris EA (eds): Heart Disease in Infancy: Diagnosis and Surgical Treatment. London, Churchill Livingstone, 1973, p 236.

32. Rao PS: Natural history of the ventricular septal defect in tricuspid atresia and its surgical implications. Br Heart J 39:276, 1977.

33. Rao PS: Further observations on the spontaneous closure of physiologically advantageous ventricular septal defects in tricuspid atresia: Surgical implications. Ann Thorac Surg 35:121, 1983.

34. Rao PS: Physiologically advantageous ventricular septal defects (Letter). Pediatr Cardiol 4:59, 1983.

35. Rao PS, Sissman NJ: Spontaneous closure of physiologically advantageous ventricular septal defects. Circulation 43:83, 1971.

36. Rao PS, Linde LM, Liebman J, Perrin E: Functional closure of physiologically advantageous ventricular septal defects: Observations in three cases with tricuspid atresia. Am J Dis Child 127:36, 1974.

37. Gallaher ME, Fyler DC: Observations on the changing hemodynamics in tricuspid atresia without transposition of the great vessels. Circulation 35:381, 1967.

38. Sauer U, Hall D: Spontaneous closure or critical decrease in size of the ventricular septal defect in tricuspid atresia with normally connected great arteries: Surgical implications. Herz 5:369, 1980.

39. Weinberg PM: Pathologic anatomy of tricuspid atresia. In Rao PS (ed): Tricuspid Atresia. Mount Kisco, NY, Futura Publishing, 1982, p 49.

40. Rudolph AM: Tricuspid atresia with hypoplastic right ventricle. In Congenital Disease of the Heart. Chicago, Year Book, 1974, p 429.

41. Marcano BA, Riemenschnieder TA, Ruttenburg HD, et al: Tricuspid atresia with increased pulmonary blood flow: An analysis of 13 cases. Circulation 40:399, 1965.

42. Rao PS: Cardiac catheterization in tricuspid atresia. In Rao PS (ed): Tricuspid Atresia. Mount Kisco, NY, Futura Publishing, 1982, p 153.

43. LaCorte MA, Dick M, Scheer G, et al: Left ventricular function in tricuspid atresia. Circulation 52:996, 1975.

44. Graham TP, Erath HJG Jr, Boucek RJ, Boerth RC: Left ventricular function in cyanotic congenital heart disease. Am J Cardiol 45:1231, 1980.

45. Rao PS, Alpert BS, Covitz W: Left ventricular function in tricuspid atresia. In Rao PS (ed): Tricuspid Atresia, 2nd ed. Mount Kisco, NY, Futura Publishing, 1992, p 247.

46. Rao PS: Left-to-right shunting in tricuspid atresia. Br Heart J 49:345, 1983.

47. Rao PS: Natural history of ventricular septal defects in tricuspid atresia. In Rao PS (ed): Tricuspid Atresia, 2nd ed. Mount Kisco, NY, Futura Publishing, 1992, p 261.

48. Bloomfield DK: The natural history of ventricular septal defects in patients surviving infancy. Circulation 29:914, 1964.

49. Hoffman JIE, Rudolph AM: The natural history of ventricular septal defects in infancy. Am J Cardiol 16:634, 1965.

50. Rao PS: Subaortic obstruction after pulmonary artery banding in patients with tricuspid atresia and double-inlet left ventricle and ventriculoarterial discordance (Letter). J Am Coll Cardiol 66:406, 1991.

51. Dick M, Rosenthal A: The clinical profile of tricuspid atresia. In Rao PS (ed): Tricuspid Atresia. Mount Kisco, NY, Futura Publishing, 1982, p 83.

52. Rowe RD, Freedom RM, Mehrizi A, Bloom KR: The Neonate with Congenital Heart Disease, 2nd ed. Major Problems in Clinical Pediatrics, Vol 5. Philadelphia, WB Saunders, 1981, pp 456–479.

53. Rao PS: Pathophysiologic consequences of cyanotic heart disease. Indian J Pediatr 50:479, 1983.

54. Taussig HB: The clinical and pathologic findings in congenital malformations of the heart due to defective development of the right ventricle associated with tricuspid atresia or hypoplasia. Bull Hopkins Hosp 59:435, 1936.

55. Wittenborg MH, Neuhauser EBD, Sprunt WH: Roentgenographic findings of congenital tricuspid atresia with hypoplasia of the right ventricle. Am J Roentgenol 64:712, 1951.

56. Vlad P: Tricuspid atresia. In Keith JD, Rowe RD, Vlad P (eds): Heart Disease in Infancy and Childhood, 3rd ed. New York, Macmillan, 1977, p 518.

57. Elster SK: Congenital atresia of pulmonary and tricuspid valves. Am J Dis Child 79:692, 1950.

58. Covitz W, Rao PS: Noninvasive evaluation of patients with tricuspid atresia (roentgenography, echocardiography and nuclear angiography). In Rao PS (ed): Tricuspid Atresia, 2nd ed. Mount Kisco, NY, Futura Publishing, 1992, p 165.

59. Gamboa R, Gersony WM, Nadas AS: The electrocardiogram in tricuspid atresia and pulmonary atresia with intact ventricular septum. Circulation 34:24, 1986.

60. Rao PS, Kulungara RJ, Boineau JP, Moore HV: Electrovectorcardiographic features of tricuspid atresia. In Rao PS (ed): Tricuspid Atresia, 2nd ed. Mount Kisco, NY, Futura Publishing, 1992, p 141.

61. Kulungara RJ, Boineau JP, Moore HV, Rao PS: Ventricular activation and genesis of QRS in tricuspid atresia (Abstract). Circulation 64:IV-225, 1981.

62. Seward JB, Tajik AJ, Hagler DJ, Ritter DG: Echocardiographic spectrum of tricuspid atresia. Mayo Clin Proc 53:100, 1978.

63. Beppu S, Nimura Y, Tamai M, et al: Two-dimensional echocardiography in the diagnosis of tricuspid atresia: Differentiation from other hypoplastic right heart syndromes and common atrioventricular canal. Br Heart J 40:1174, 1978.

64. Choussat A, Fontan F, Besse P, et al: Selection criteria for Fontan procedure. *In* Anderson RH, Shinebourne EA (eds): Paediatric Cardiology 1977. Edinburgh, Churchill Livingstone, 1978, p 559.

65. Rao PS: The femoral route for cardiac catheterization of infants and children. Chest 63:239, 1973.

66. Rao PS, Sissman NJ: The relationship of pulmonary venous wedge to pulmonary arterial pressures. Circulation 44:565, 1971.

67. Mair DD, Hagler DJ, Puga FJ, et al: Fontan operation in 176 patients with tricuspid atresia: Results and a proposed new index for patient selection. Circulation 82(suppl IV):164, 1990.

68. Schwartz DC, Rao PS: Angiography in tricuspid atresia. *In* Rao PS (ed): Tricuspid Atresia, 2nd ed. Mount Kisco, NY, Futura Publishing, 1992, p 223.

69. Rao PS: Management of the neonate with suspected serious heart disease. King Faisal Specialist Hosp J 4:209, 1984.

70. Fontan F, Baudet E: Surgical repair of tricuspid atresia. Thorax 26:240, 1971.

71. Kreutzer G, Bono H, Galindez E, et al: Una operacion para la correccion de la atresia tricuspidea. Ninth Argentinean Congress of Cardiology, Buenos Aires, Argentina, Oct. 31–Nov. 6, 1971.

72. Freed MD, Heymann MA, Lewis AB, et al: Prostaglandin E_1 in the infants with ductus arteriosus dependent congenital heart disease: The US experience. Circulation 64:899, 1981.

73. Rao PS, Thapar MK, Galal O, Wilson AD: Follow-up results of balloon angioplasty of native coarctation in neonates and infants. Am Heart J 120:1310, 1990.

74. Blalock A, Taussig HB: The surgical treatment of malformations of the heart in which there is pulmonary stenosis or pulmonary atresia. JAMA 128:189, 1945.

75. DeLeval M, McKay R, Jones M, et al: Modified Blalock-Taussig shunt: Use of subclavian orifice as a flow regulator in prosthetic systemic-pulmonary artery shunts. J Thorac Cardiovasc Surg 18:112, 1981.

76. Annecchino FP, Fontan F, Chauve A, et al: An operation for the correction of tricuspid atresia. Ann Thorac Surg 29:317, 1979.

77. Gibbs JL, Rothman MT, Rees MR, et al: Stenting of arterial duct: A new approach to palliation of pulmonary atresia. Br Heart J 67:240, 1992.

78. McCredie RM, Lee CL, Swinburn MJ, et al: Balloon dilatation pulmonary valvuloplasty in pulmonary stenosis. Aust N Z J Med 16:20, 1986.

79. Rashkind WJ, Waldhausen JA, Miller WW, et al: Palliative treatment of tricuspid atresia: Combined balloon atrial septostomy and surgical alteration of pulmonary blood flow. J Thorac Cardiovasc Surg 57:812, 1969.

80. Park SC, Neches WH, Zuberbuhler JR, et al: Clinical use of blade atrial septostomy. Circulation 58:600, 1978.

81. Rao PS: Transcatheter blade atrial septostomy. Cathet Cardiovasc Diagn 10:335, 1984.

82. Salim M, Muster AJ, Paul MH, et al: Relation between preoperative left ventricular muscle mass and outcome of the Fontan procedure in patients with tricuspid atresia. J Am Coll Cardiol 14:75, 1989.

83. Ottenkamp J, Wenink ACG, Quaegebeur JM, et al: Tricuspid atresia: Morphology of the outlet chamber with special emphasis on surgical implications. J Thorac Cardiovasc Surg 89:597, 1985.

84. Smolinsky A, Castaneda AR, Van Praagh R: Infundibular septal resection: Surgical anatomy of the superior approach. J Thorac Cardiovasc Surg 95:486, 1988.

85. Chopra PS, Rao PS: Corrective surgery for tricuspid atresia: Which modifications of Fontan-Kreutzer procedure should be used? A review. Am Heart J 123:758, 1992.

86. Rao PS, Chopra PS: Modifications of Fontan-Kreutzer procedure for tricuspid atresia: Can a choice be made? *In* Rao PS (ed): Tricuspid Atresia, 2nd ed. Mount Kisco, NY, Futura Publishing, 1992, p 361.

87. de Leval MR, Kilner P, Gewilling M, et al: Total cavopulmonary connection: A logical alternative to atriopulmonary connection for complex Fontan operation. J Thorac Cardiovasc Surg 96:682, 1988.

88. Sharma S, Goudy S, Walker P, et al: In vitro flow experiments for determination of optimal geometry of total cavopulmonary connection for surgical repair of children with functional single ventricle. J Am Coll Cardiol 27:1264, 1996.

89. Haller JA, Adkins JC, Worthington M, et al: Experimental studies on permanent bypass of the right heart. Surgery 59:1128, 1966.

90. Hopkins RA, Armstrong SE, Serwer GA, et al: Physiologic rationale for a bidirectional cavopulmonary shunt: A versatile complement to the Fontan principle. J Thorac Cardiovasc Surg 90:391, 1985.

91. Schaff HV, Danielson GK: Corrective surgery for tricuspid atresia. *In* Rao PS (ed): Tricuspid Atresia, 2nd ed. Mount Kisco, NY, Futura Publishing, 1992, p 341.

92. Bridges ND, Jonas RA, Mayer JE, et al: Bidirectional cavopulmonary anastomosis as interim palliation for high-risk Fontan candidates: Early results. Circulation 82(suppl IV):170, 1990.

93. Billingsley AM, Laks H, Boyce SM, et al: Definitive repair in some patients with pulmonary atresia with intact ventricular septum. J Thorac Cardiovasc Surg 97:746, 1989.

94. Bridges ND, Lock JE, Castaneda AR: Baffle fenestration with subsequent transcatheter closure: Modification of the Fontan operation for patients with increased risk. Circulation 82:1681, 1990.

95. Laks H, Pearl JM, Haas GS, et al: Partial Fontan advantages of an adjustable interatrial communication. Ann Thorac Surg 52:1084, 1991.

96. Freedom RM, Gow R, Caspi J, et al: The Fontan procedure for patients with tricuspid atresia: Long-term follow-up. *In* Rao PS (ed): Tricuspid Atresia, 2nd ed. Mount Kisco, NY, Futura Publishing, 1992, p 377.

97. Gandhi SK, Bromberg BI, Schuessler RB, et al: Characterization and surgical ablation of atrial flutter after classic Fontan repair in acute canine model. Ann Thorac Surg 61:1666, 1996.

98. Rao PS, Chandar JS, Sideris EB: Role of inverted buttoned device in transcatheter occlusion of atrial septal defect or patent foramen ovale with right-to-left shunting associated with complex congenital cardiac anomalies. Am J Cardiol 80:914, 1997.

99. Hill DJ, Feldt RH, Porter C, et al: Protein losing enteropathy after Fontan operation: A preliminary report (Abstract). Circulation 80(suppl II):490, 1989.

100. Rothman A, Synder J: Protein-losing enteropathy following Fontan operation: Resolution with prednisone therapy. Am Heart J 121:618, 1991.

101. Rao PS: Static balloon dilatation of the atrial septum (Editorial). Am Heart J 125:1824, 1993.

CHAPTER 31
PULMONARY ATRESIA AND INTACT VENTRICULAR SEPTUM

ROBERT M. FREEDOM

Pulmonary atresia and intact ventricular septum is both an uncommon and a peculiar condition, and for many patients afflicted with this anomaly, it is the nature of the disordered coronary circulation that defines the surgical algorithm and outcomes.[1–48] There is tremendous heterogeneity for those hearts designated as having pulmonary atresia and intact ventricular septum. At one end of the continuum are hearts that are truly gigantic, virtually filling the thoracic cavity and often associated with some degree of pulmonary hypoplasia.[1,2,6] Patients with this form of pulmonary atresia and intact ventricular septum have a severely disordered tricuspid valve with massive regurgitation and a profoundly thinned and dysfunctional right ventricle. The coronary artery circulation in this constellation is usually normal. At the other end of the spectrum are those patients with a diminutive, but profoundly hypertensive, right ventricle. Both the right ventricular free wall and septum are hypertrophied, and many of these ventricles are seemingly unipartite, that is, composed only of an inlet component. Although some argue that all three components of the right ventricle are represented but obliterated by hypertrophy, it reflects at least in part the pattern of isometric contraction. The tricuspid valve in these patients is obstructive,[1,2,11] and in this setting, there is likely to be a disordered coronary artery circulation.[1–3,13,14,19,20,32]

MORPHOGENESIS

Kutsche and Van Mierop[49] analyzed a number of morphologic factors, including the diameter of the pulmonary trunk, the morphology of the pulmonary valve, and the morphology and topography of the ductus arteriosus. Their study suggested that pulmonary atresia and ventricular septal defect occur early in cardiac morphogenesis, at or shortly after partitioning of the truncoconal part of the heart but before partitioning of the ventricular septum. They further suggest that pulmonary atresia and intact ventricular septum probably occurs after cardiac septation, speculating that this disorder might reflect a prenatal inflammatory disease rather than a true congenital malformation. Their conclusions of the timing of the maturational arrest may be correct for those patients with pulmonary atresia; intact ventricular septum; and a nearly normal-sized right ventricle, with an imperforate tricuspid pulmonary valve whose commissures are well formed but completely fused. Indeed, there is evidence based on serial

fetal echocardiographic studies that pulmonary atresia may be acquired in some patients, and these hearts tend to have a better developed right ventricle.[50–55] However, there are few data to support an inflammatory process, as infant histopathologic studies have not provided conclusive evidence of acute or subacute inflammation. Furthermore, those hearts with a diminutive right ventricle and ventriculocoronary artery connections likely represent an earlier insult than those with a well-formed right ventricle and a tricuspid-fused imperforate valve, although clearly this is still a postseptational disturbance.

PREVALENCE

Pulmonary atresia and intact ventricular septum accounts for only about 3% of neonates with serious congenital heart disease.[56–58] The more recently completed Baltimore-Washington Infant Study found the prevalence for pulmonary atresia and intact ventricular septum as 0.083 per 1000 live births.[59] This lesion accounts for 0.71% of all patients seen with congenital heart disease at the Toronto Hospital for Sick Children. This disorder ranks third among cyanotic neonates with congenital heart disease after transposition of the great arteries and pulmonary atresia and ventricular septal defect.[56] In other surveys, it may be a little less frequent than truncus arteriosus or single ventricle. There are a few reports of familial aggregation of this disorder,[60] but my colleagues and I have not identified siblings with this disorder among more than 170 families with one affected child seen in our institution. Fetal echocardiography provides a unique window to study the later phases of the fetal heart development and to define specific types of heart predisposed to fetal death.[50–55] There is increasing evidence that fetuses with florid tricuspid regurgitation may develop right-sided heart failure with pleural and pericardial effusions, ascites, and pulmonary hypoplasia; in addition, they may die in utero. Thus, fetal loss might be expected in a specific subset of patients with pulmonary atresia, intact ventricular septum, extremely severe tricuspid regurgitation, and a low-pressure right ventricle.[50–55]

NATURE OF PULMONARY ATRESIA

Pulmonary atresia reflects an imperforate pulmonary valve with a variable expression of leaflet and commissural for-

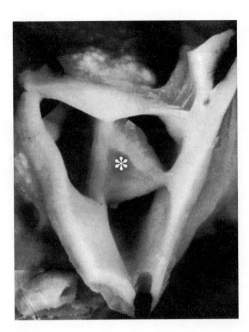

FIGURE 31–1

Morphology of imperforate *(asterisk)* pulmonary valve with well formed, but completely fused, commissures. (From Freedom RM, Mawson JB, Yoo S-J, Benson LN [eds]: Congenital Heart Disease: Textbook of Angiocardiography. Armonk, NY, Futura, 1997, pp 617–662.)

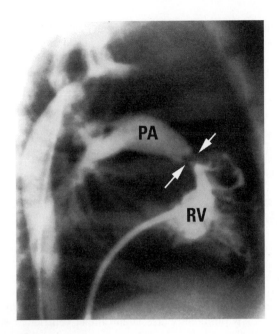

FIGURE 31–2

Double-catheter technique in a newborn with pulmonary atresia and intact ventricular septum demonstrates a short segment *(arrows)* of infundibular atresia. PA = pulmonary artery; RV = right ventricle. (From Freedom RM, Mawson JB, Yoo S-J, Benson LN [eds]: Congenital Heart Disease: Textbook of Angiocardiography. Armonk, NY, Futura, 1997, pp 617–662.)

mation (Fig. 31–1). The morphologic bases for pulmonary atresia in this disorder have been well studied.* Braunlin and colleagues[61] have correlated the type of imperforate pulmonary valve with the nature of the right ventricle and its infundibulum. In patients with a well-formed subpulmonary infundibulum, the imperforate pulmonary valve usually exhibits three semilunar cusps with complete fusion of the commissures, forming a fused imperforate plate. In those patients with an extremely diminutive right ventricle and a severely narrowed or atretic infundibulum, the pulmonary valve is quite primitive. The muscular nature of the infundibulum has received both morphologic and clinicoangiocardiographic attention, and the nature of those right ventricular muscle bundles contributing to the infundibular atresia has been described (Fig. 31–2).[62–63] With radiofrequency or laser interruption of the membranous and muscular forms of pulmonary atresia, these observations have perhaps gained more clinical relevance.[64–70]

PULMONARY CIRCULATION

The pulmonary arteries are almost always confluent in patients with pulmonary atresia and intact ventricular septum.† The pulmonary circulation in the overwhelming majority is maintained by a left-sided patent arterial duct; rarely, it is supplied by large direct aortopulmonary collaterals. There is usually a main pulmonary trunk in continuity with the atretic pulmonary valve. This observation is germane to consideration of catheter intervention in this

disorder. Although left pulmonary artery stenosis at the site of ductal insertion has been observed in these patients,[72–75] my colleagues and I believe that occurs less frequently than in patients with pulmonary atresia and ventricular septal defect (Fig. 31–3). Marino and colleagues[75] have provided data indicating that the arterial duct in patients with pulmonary atresia and intact ventricular septum constricts earlier than the arterial duct in patients with

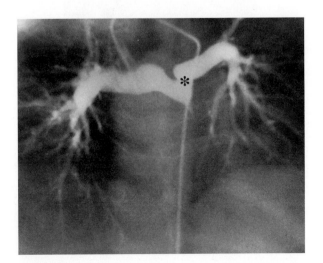

FIGURE 31–3

A patient with pulmonary atresia and intact ventricular septum palliated with a right-sided modified Blalock-Taussig shunt. Note the mildly narrowed *(asterisk)* proximal left pulmonary artery. (From Freedom RM, Mawson JB, Yoo S-J, Benson LN [eds]: Congenital Heart Disease: Textbook of Angiocardiography. Armonk, NY, Futura, 1997, pp 617–662.)

*References 1, 2, 4, 5, 7, 12, 61–63.
†References 1, 2, 4, 5, 7–10, 13, 71–76.

pulmonary atresia and ventricular septal defect. Rarely, the pulmonary arteries in pulmonary atresia and intact ventricular septum are nonconfluent, each supported by its arterial duct.[2, 8] Major aortopulmonary collaterals originating from the descending thoracic aorta have also been described as the source of pulmonary blood flow in these patients.[9, 10] A pulmonary sling has been observed in patients with pulmonary atresia and intact ventricular septum.[76] Isolated distal ductal origin of the left pulmonary artery has not been observed in our large experience of these patients.

SEGMENTAL ANALYSIS

The atrial situs is normal or solitus, the atrioventricular and ventriculoarterial connections are concordant, and the heart is left sided in more than 98% of hearts exhibiting pulmonary atresia and intact ventricular septum.[1, 2, 4, 5, 77–79] Dextrocardia with solitus atria is infrequent, as is pulmonary atresia and intact ventricular septum with discordant atrioventricular and ventriculoarterial connections.[77–79] The aortic arch is usually left sided.

TRICUSPID VALVE

The inlet of the right ventricle with its tricuspid valve is usually quite abnormal and disordered (Figs. 31–4 and 31–5).* The tricuspid valve in some patients with this dis-

---

*References 1–7, 11–18, 32, 45, 80–86.

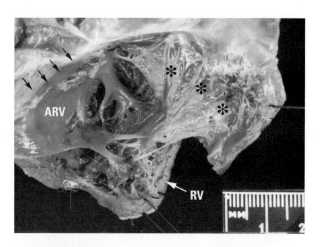

FIGURE 31–5

A severely dysplastic and displaced tricuspid valve promoting severe tricuspid regurgitation. The *black arrows* note that portion of the atrioventricular junction that is virtually unguarded. The dysplastic tricuspid valve tissue is noted by the *asterisks*. ARV = atrialized right ventricle; RV = right ventricle. (From Freedom RM, Mawson JB, Yoo S-J, Benson LN [eds]: Congenital Heart Disease: Textbook of Angiocardiography. Armonk, NY, Futura, 1997, pp 617–662.)

order is severely stenotic (Fig. 31–6; see Fig. 31–4), but in others the tricuspid valve is massively regurgitant, with a dilated annulus, at times virtually unguarded and devoid of valvar tissue (see Fig. 31–5). In those patients with the most stenotic tricuspid valve, the annulus is obstructive and muscularized. All components of the valve apparatus are abnormal with a thickened free-valve margin; thickened, shortened, and attenuated chordae tendineae; and abnormal papillary muscles, including a parachute config-

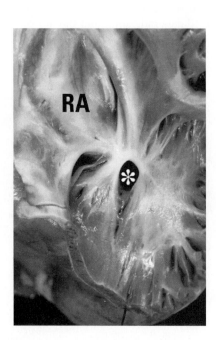

FIGURE 31–4

View of a stenotic tricuspid orifice *(asterisk)* in a patient with pulmonary atresia and intact ventricular septum. RA = right atrium. (From Freedom RM, Mawson JB, Yoo S-J, Benson LN [eds]: Congenital Heart Disease: Textbook of Angiocardiography. Armonk, NY, Futura, 1997, pp 617–662.)

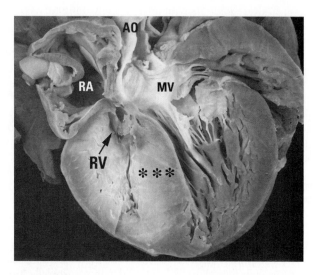

FIGURE 31–6

A diminutive right ventricular cavity with severe hypertrophy of the ventricular septum *(asterisks)* and free wall in a patient with pulmonary atresia and intact ventricular septum. This is the type of right ventricle (RV) in which one would expect ventriculocoronary connections. AO = aorta; MV = mitral valve; RA = right atrium. (From Freedom RM, Mawson JB, Yoo S-J, Benson LN [eds]: Congenital Heart Disease: Textbook of Angiocardiography. Armonk, NY, Futura, 1997, pp 617–662.)

uration (see Figs. 31–4 and 31–6).[1–5,7,11–16] The massively regurgitant tricuspid valve shows a dilated annulus and demonstrates displacement, dysplasia, or both; a portion of the annulus may be unguarded (see Fig. 31–5).* Ebstein anomaly of the tricuspid valve has been found in about 10% of autopsied patients with pulmonary atresia and intact ventricular septum. Displacement without dysplasia is virtually unknown in patients with Ebstein anomaly complicating pulmonary atresia and intact ventricular septum. An obstructive form of Ebstein valve has been observed in some patients with pulmonary atresia and intact ventricular septum.[1,2,6,11,15,86]

The tricuspid Z value has been advocated as a measure of the normalized tricuspid valve diameter.[32] This is the diameter of the tricuspid valve normalized to body surface area and based on the data of Rowlatt and colleagues.[87] The more negative the Z value of the tricuspid valve, the smaller and more obstructive the tricuspid valve; the larger the Z value of the tricuspid valve, the larger the tricuspid valve diameter, and the more severe the regurgitation. The Z value is highly correlated with right ventricular cavity size; the more negative the Z value, the smaller the right ventricle.[32] This correlation was highly significant with ventriculocoronary connections as well. The infundibular diameter has been suggested a better predictor of right ventriculocoronary artery communications than the Z value of the tricuspid valve.[88]

There are some implicit assumptions about the application of the Z score in the determination and application of any surgical algorithm. First, the tricuspid orifice may be elliptical. Second, does the tricuspid annulus adequately represent the tricuspid valve orifice at leaflet level? Most

---

*References 1, 2, 4, 5, 7, 14–18, 45, 80–85.

likely not. The morphologic study of the tricuspid valve carried out here in 1978 indicated that the tricuspid valve annulus did not invariably reflect leaflet-orifice size.[11]

RIGHT VENTRICLE

Numerous classifications or categorizations of the right ventricle have been made in this disorder, including attempts to quantitate its volume. These classifications have evolved from a qualitative assessment of cavity size (from small to extremely large), to a semimorphologic characterization of the ventricle in terms of its morphologic components (inlet, apical trabecular, and outlet zones), to semiquantitative assessment of the inlet-outlet dimensions.[1,19,34–36,89–94] Right ventricular volume determinations have also been reported, but the measurements are complicated by the marked myocardial hypertrophy that attenuates the apical trabecula and infundibulum.[91] The right ventricle in some of these patients is quite underdeveloped, seemingly formed only of an inlet portion (see Fig. 31–6). In others, the right ventricle has an inlet and trabecular portion, and still in others, the right ventricle is represented by inlet, apical trabecular, and infundibular components (Fig. 31–7). The proportion of these components in any given patient may vary considerably, and muscular hypertrophy and overgrowth may obviate recognition of the trabecular and outlet portions of the right ventricle. Thus, in some patients, all three components are clearly recognizable, but the right ventricle is still extremely small, the Z value of the tricuspid valve ranging from −2.5 to −4.5. In contrast, there are those patients with massive tricuspid regurgitation, a Z value of +4.0 to +5.0, a very much enlarged right ventricle, and very well-expanded inlet, trabecular, and infundibular components.

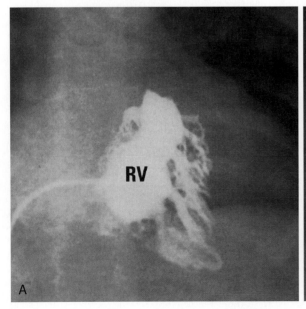
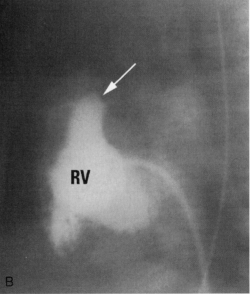

FIGURE 31–7

A nearly normal-sized right ventricle (RV) with an imperforate pulmonary valve and no ventriculocoronary connections. The tricuspid Z value is 0.5. Frontal (*A*) and lateral (*B*) right ventriculogram. The *arrow* in *B* points out the imperforate pulmonary valve. (*A, B* from Freedom RM, Mawson JB, Yoo S-J, Benson LN [eds]: Congenital Heart Disease: Textbook of Angiocardiography. Armonk, NY, Futura, 1997, pp 617–662.)

CORONARY CIRCULATION

Our understanding of the coronary artery circulation in patients with pulmonary atresia and intact ventricular septum has had profound effect on operative management and outcome (Fig. 31–8).* Communications between the cavity of the right ventricle and myocardial sinusoids are an important aspect of this disorder (Figs. 31–9 to 31–12). Data published from the Congenital Heart Surgeons Study indicated that of the 145 patients in whom this information was available (of a total of 171 neonates enrolled in the study), ventriculocoronary connections were observed in 45% of these patients,[32] and 9% were wholly right ventricular dependent. Our own data are similar.† In the United Kingdom National Collaborative study of pulmonary atresia and intact ventricular septum, of 140 patients identified since 1991, the coronary arteries were considered normal in 58%, and minor and major coronary artery fistulae were identified in 15 and 17%, respectively.[130] Ten patients were recognized as having coronary artery stenosis. The median tricuspid Z value for this cohort of patients was 1.6.

Beginning in the early 1960s,[99,111] extensive literature documented the vast array of changes in the coronary arteries in patients with pulmonary atresia and intact ventricular septum.‡ The histopathologic alterations of those

---

*References 1–3, 12–14, 19–21, 26, 30, 32, 39, 41, 46, 47, 48, 79, 95–136.

†References 1–3, 13, 14, 19, 20, 27, 105, 107, 119.

‡References 1–3, 12–14, 79, 100, 104–110, 116, 120, 128, 134.

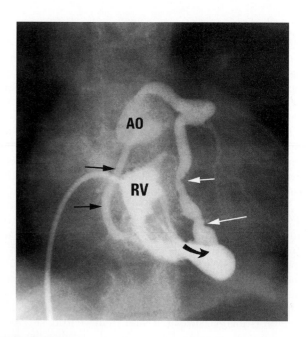

FIGURE 31-9

Ventriculocoronary connections between a diminutive right ventricle and both coronary arteries. Frontal right ventriculogram demonstrates opacification of both right and left coronary arteries. The *curved black arrow* notes the ventriculocoronary connection. The right coronary artery *(black arrows)* is also opacified and shows minimal luminal irregularities. The left anterior descending coronary artery shows multiple levels of stenosis *(white arrows)*. AO = aorta; RV = right ventricle. (From Freedom RM, Mawson JB, Yoo S-J, Benson LN [eds]: Congenital Heart Disease: Textbook of Angiocardiography. Armonk, NY, Futura, 1997, pp 617–662.)

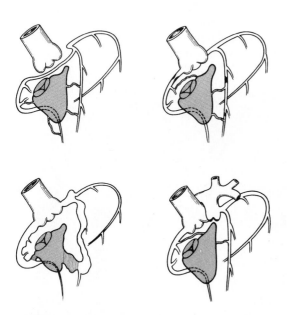

FIGURE 31-8

These diagrams show various types of right ventricular–dependent coronary circulations in pulmonary atresia and intact ventricular septum. *Upper left,* Absent connections between coronary arteries and aorta. *Upper right,* Multiple connections with proximal right coronary artery narrowing and left anterior descending interruption. *Bottom left,* Severe ectasia of both right and left coronary arteries with coronary-cameral fistulae. *Bottom right,* Multiple ventriculocoronary connections with origin of left coronary artery from pulmonary artery. (From Freedom RM, Mawson JB, Yoo S-J, Benson LN [eds]: Congenital Heart Disease: Textbook of Angiocardiography. Armonk, NY, Futura, 1997, pp 617–662.)

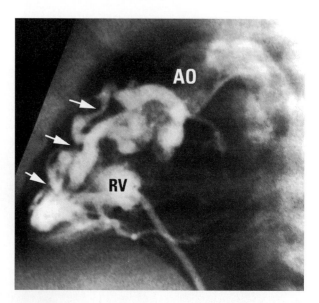

FIGURE 31-10

Multiple levels of coronary artery stenosis and interruption *(arrows)* in this newborn with a right ventricular–dependent coronary circulation is shown by this lateral right ventriculogram. AO = aorta; RV = right ventricle. (From Freedom RM, Mawson JB, Yoo S-J, Benson LN [eds]: Congenital Heart Disease: Textbook of Angiocardiography. Armonk, NY, Futura, 1997, pp 617–662.)

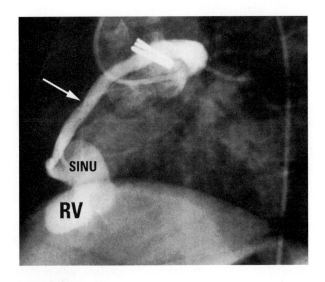

FIGURE 31–11

A ventriculocoronary connection with a distal coronary artery interruption. The *arrow* shows the coronary artery. SINU = sinusoid; RV = right ventricle. (From Freedom RM, Mawson JB, Yoo S-J, Benson LN [eds]: Congenital Heart Disease: Textbook of Angiocardiography. Armonk, NY, Futura, 1997, pp 617–662.)

coronary arteries participating in the ventriculocoronary communications are not characterized by inflammation as once thought but by myointimal hyperplasia with a rich background of glycosaminoglycans (Fig. 31–13). There is a wide spectrum of histopathologic lesions of both the extramural and intramural coronary arteries.° These lesions

range from mild degrees of intimal and medial thickening, in which a continuous internal elastic lamina and normal lumen are present at a loss of normal arterial wall morphology, with replacement of the arterial wall by fibrocellular tissue containing irregular, nonorganized elastin strands and severe stenosis or obliteration of the arterial lumen. Some have designated these changes *fibroelastosis* of the coronary arteries,[116] but it is clear that the emphasis should be placed on myointimal hyperplasia. Staining for glycosaminoglycans shows the prominence of ground substance formation by the activated smooth muscle cells, rather than the reduplicated elastica and collagen characteristic of fibroelastosis. The pathologic process results in profound distortion of the normal architecture, eventuating in endothelial irregularity, stenosis, or interruption.° These coronary arterial changes occur only in patients with ventriculocoronary connections, and by inference, with a hypertensive right ventricle. They have not been observed in those patients with a massively enlarged heart, free tricuspid regurgitation, and a thinned right ventricle incapable of generating systemic pressure. Indeed, ventriculocoronary connections and the thin-walled, low-pressure right ventricle are mutually exclusive (Fig. 31–14). My colleagues and I have speculated that the pathogenesis of these arterial lesions depends on the repeated and sustained injury to the coronary arterial intima from high-pressure right ventricular systolic turbulent blood flow mediated by the presence of the ventriculocoronary connections. Intramural or extramural coronary arteries remote from the ventriculocoronary connections do not demonstrate these arterial lesions; neither do hearts *not* exhibiting ventriculocoronary connections. These lesions

---

°References 1–3, 12–14, 79, 100, 104–110, 116, 120, 128, 134.

°References 1–3, 13, 14, 105, 106, 109, 110, 120, 134.

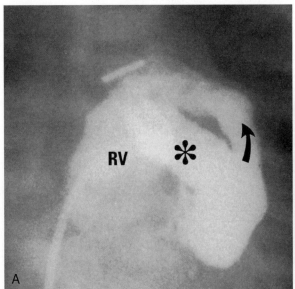

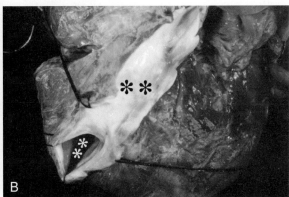

FIGURE 31–12

A massive ventriculocoronary connection mediated by a huge connection. *A,* The injection of contrast material into the right ventricle (RV) fills via the large connection *(asterisk)* to the dilated and ectatic anterior descending coronary artery *(arrow). B,* This postmortem specimen shows the hugely dilated left anterior descending coronary artery *(black asterisks)* and the site of its communication *(white asterisks)* with the right ventricle. (*A, B* from Freedom RM, Mawson JB, Yoo S-J, Benson LN [eds]: Congenital Heart Disease: Textbook of Angiocardiography. Armonk, NY, Futura, 1997, pp 617–662.)

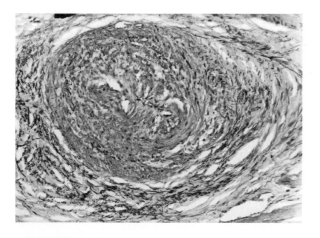

FIGURE 31–13

A cross-section of the anterior descending coronary artery demonstrates virtual luminal occlusion by the process of myointimal hyperplasia in this neonate with, in retrospect, a right ventricular–dependent coronary circulation. (From Freedom RM, Mawson JB, Yoo S-J, Benson LN [eds]: Congenital Heart Disease: Textbook of Angiocardiography. Armonk, NY, Futura, 1997, pp 617–662.)

have been found in fetal hearts with pulmonary atresia and intact ventricular septum and in hearts of immediate newborn infants. The capillary distribution in the ventricles of hearts with pulmonary atresia and intact ventricular septum has been studied by Oosthoek and colleagues.[137] Disarray and other disturbances of capillaries and myocytes were found in hearts with a hypoplastic right ventricle and ventriculocoronary connections. They found that these changes were more extensive when coronary artery interruptions were present. These abnormalities of the coro-

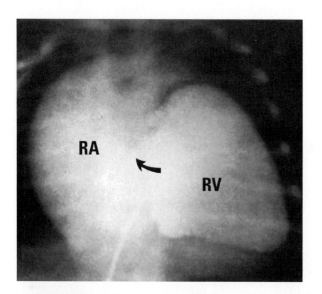

FIGURE 31–14

Massive tricuspid regurgitation (arrow) is shown by this frontal right ventriculogram. The right atrium (RA) is severely dilated. This patient had a right ventricle (RV)/left ventricle pressure ratio less than 1.0, and ventriculocoronary connections in this setting are virtually unknown. (From Freedom RM, Mawson JB, Yoo S-J, Benson LN [eds]: Congenital Heart Disease: Textbook of Angiocardiography. Armonk, NY, Futura, 1997, pp 617–662.)

nary arteries are far more common in those neonates with the smallest tricuspid valve and, by inference, the most underdeveloped right ventricle. However, ventriculocoronary connections have been noted in the right ventricle of normal dimension, or nearly so.[138]

The abnormalities of coronary origin and distribution in patients with pulmonary atresia and intact ventricular septum embrace the same spectrum of those abnormalities as seen in patients with an otherwise normal heart, including abnormalities of origin, epicardial course, and number. A single coronary artery may originate from the aorta or, rarely, the pulmonary trunk. However, a number of congenital and acquired conditions of the coronary circulation, specific to pulmonary atresia and intact ventricular septum, affect surgical management. These include absence of proximal aortocoronary connection between one or both coronary arteries, coronary arterial stenosis or interruption, or a so-called coronary-cameral fistula with a major fistula between right or left coronary artery and the right ventricle.°

RIGHT VENTRICULAR–DEPENDENT CORONARY ARTERY CIRCULATION (See Table 31–1)

Surgical outcomes are determined at least in part by the involvement of the coronary arteries (see Figs. 30–8 to 30–13).† An important concept is that of a right ventricular–dependent coronary artery circulation.‡ In the normal circulation, the aortic diastolic pressure is the driving pressure for coronary blood flow, and those factors reducing aortic diastolic pressure or shortening diastole comprise coronary blood flow. Ventriculocoronary artery connections may promote coronary artery stenosis and interruption, and aortic diastolic pressure may not be sufficient to drive coronary blood flow when there are obstructive lesions within the coronary circulation.§ These babies are ill, tachycardiac, often on prostaglandin, and palliated with a systemic-to-pulmonary artery shunt to augment pulmonary blood flow. As a result, they often have a low aortic diastolic pressure. In such patients, retrograde coronary blood flow from the hypertensive right ventricle, occurring during systole and passing through the ventriculocoronary connections, may be necessary for myocardial perfusion. This process may lead to further coronary arterial distortions. Interference with blood flow into the right ventricle or reduction of right ventricular systolic pressure when the coronary circulation is right ventricular dependent could result in myocardial ischemia, infarction, and death. Multivariable analysis from the Congenital Heart Surgeons Study[32] showed that a small diameter of the tricuspid valve; a coronary circulation that was severely right ventricular dependent; birth weight; and the date and type of initial surgical procedures were risk factors for time-related death. Our data on the deleterious effects of ven-

°References 1–3, 12, 30, 48, 95–114, 117–125, 128–130, 133, 134.
†References 1–3, 12–14, 19–21, 26, 30, 32, 39, 41, 46–48, 79, 95–136.
‡References 1, 2, 103, 105–107, 120, 128, 129, 146.
§References 1–3, 12–14, 19–21, 26, 30, 32, 39, 41, 46–48, 79, 95–136.

TABLE 31–1

CORONARY ARTERY ANOMALIES CONTRIBUTING TO A RIGHT VENTRICULAR–DEPENDENT CORONARY CIRCULATION

Absent proximal aortocoronary connection
Coronary artery interruption or stenosis
Coronary-cameral fistula

triculocoronary connections and a right ventricular–dependent coronary circulation are similar. Giglia and colleagues from the Children's Hospital in Boston came to similar conclusions: "These results support our current hypothesis that coronary artery anatomy and not RV or TV hypoplasia predicts which patients with PA-IVS will do well after early RV decompensation."[129] Mair and colleagues[138] presented a patient with a normal-sized right ventricle and proximal interruption of the left anterior descending coronary artery placed on a Fontan track because of the right ventricular–dependent coronary circulation. Laks and colleagues,[121] De Leval,[123] and others have constructed an aortic-to–right ventricular shunt in patients with pulmonary atresia, an intact ventricular septum, and a right ventricular–dependent coronary circulation to reverse myocardial ischemia.[30, 122] Those patients with a massive coronary artery–cameral (right ventricular) fistula are also right ventricular dependent. If the right ventricular systolic pressure is reduced, such patients develop a fatal steal, rapidly leading to coronary artery insufficiency, and myocardial ischemia or infarction.

Data from a number of institutions indicates that those morphologic and physiologic variables most correlated with a poor outcome are a small diameter of the tricuspid valve, a coronary circulation that is severely right ventricular dependent, and a right ventricular/left ventricular pressure ratio less than 1.[19,20,27,32] This last factor is consistent with a globally disadvantaged right ventricle; the right ventricle is usually thinned, and there is quite severe tricuspid regurgitation. The functional disturbance of severe tricuspid regurgitation correlates with Ebstein abnormality of the tricuspid valve or severe tricuspid valve dysplasia. Rarely, the tricuspid valve may be unguarded or nearly so.

MYOCARDIAL ABNORMALITIES

The myocardium of patients with pulmonary atresia and intact ventricular septum demonstrates a wide range of abnormalities[*] that include frank ischemia, fibrosis, infarction and myocardial rupture. Akiba and Becker[147] suggest that disease of the left ventricle might be the limiting factor for long-lasting successful operation intervention. They found in the hearts of the eight patients that they studied, signs of acute myocardial ischemia and a volume density of interfiber collagen that reached high normal levels in hearts of five patients but exceeded twice the standard deviation of normal in the hearts of the other three patients. The subendocardium showed higher levels of interfiber

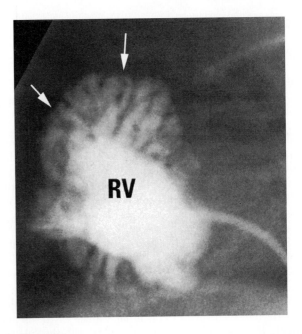

FIGURE 31–15

The angiocardiographic appearance of spongy myocardium (*arrows*) is demonstrated by this lateral right ventriculogram. RV = right ventricle. (From Freedom RM, Mawson JB, Yoo S-J, Benson LN [eds]: Congenital Heart Disease: Textbook of Angiocardiography. Armonk, NY, Futura, 1997, pp 617–662.)

collagen than the subepicardium. They suggest that the high levels of endomysial collagen are consistent with chronic ischemia in relation to left ventricular hypertrophy and that these abnormalities may render the left ventricle less able to cope with a volume load. As a result, the left ventricle might be the limiting factor for long-lasting successful surgical intervention. These observations are consistent with the findings in another form of hypoplastic right ventricle, tricuspid atresia, in that the myocardium is more fibrotic than in normal hearts. Other abnormalities include myocardial disarray, the so-called spongy myocardium appearances (Fig. 31–15), and ventricular endocardial fibroelastosis. There is a reasonably consistent inverse relationship between ventricular endocardial fibroelastosis and extensive ventriculocoronary communications[*]; dense *sugar-coating* right ventricular endocardial sclerosis is uncommon with extensive vasculocoronary communications. Conversely, dense sugar-coating left ventricular endocardial sclerosis is common in those patients with a hypoplastic left-sided heart syndrome, but a perforate mitral valve in which ventriculocoronary connections are less frequent and their pathology less extreme. There is certainly ample clinical and morphologic evidence that the left ventricle in patients with pulmonary atresia and intact ventricular septum is abnormally hypertrophied and noncompliant. The right ventricular myocardium may be particularly thinned in those babies with severe tricuspid regurgitation.

---

[*]References 1, 2, 12, 13, 16, 79, 80, 84, 105, 106, 115, 131–134, 137, 140–147.

[*]References 1, 2, 12, 13, 16, 79, 80, 84, 105, 106, 115, 131–134, 137, 140–147.

FURTHER CHARACTERIZATION OF HEARTS WITH PULMONARY ATRESIA AND INTACT VENTRICULAR SEPTUM

The heart may be only mildly enlarged, due to right atrial enlargement or in patients with extreme tricuspid regurgitation, or tremendously enlarged, with a hugely dilated right atrium occupying much of the right hemithorax[1,2,4,5,80] and compressing the lungs, which may be hypoplastic. Right atrial hypertrophy and dilatation are influenced by restriction of atrial enlargement and the severity of tricuspid regurgitation. When the heart is only mildly enlarged, the course of the anterior descending coronary artery in the anterior interventricular sulcus outlines a smaller than normal right ventricle.

Significant abnormalities of the coronary artery circulation may be present from just external inspection of the heart. The coronary arteries may be obviously thickened and nodular; rarely, the coronary arteries may be seen originating from the pulmonary trunk.[119] So-called dimples may be observed on the epicardial surface of the heart, usually, but not exclusively, in association with the subepicardial coronary arteries. Such dimples may be considered the external stigmata of ventriculocoronary connections and may indicate the site of such connections.

GREAT VEINS, ATRIAL SEPTUM, CORONARY SINUS, AND VENOUS VALVES

The superior and inferior caval veins usually terminate normally in the right atrium. Kauffman and Anderson[111] in 1963 demonstrated the relationship between persistent right venous valve, ventriculocoronary connections, and pulmonary atresia and intact ventricular septum. The coronary sinus usually terminates in the right atrium, although stenosis and atresia of the coronary sinus ostium have been observed, with decompression through an unroofed coronary sinus–left atrial fenestration.[1,2,149,150]

Because of the obligatory right-to-left shunt at the atrial level, with rare exception there is either an ovale foramen defect or a true secundum atrial septal defect. Premature closure of the ovale foramen has been observed in this disorder, usually with fetal death. Rarely, if the interatrial septum is intact or nearly so, alternative pathways for systemic venous return have been recognized, including coronary sinus–left atrial fenestration. The septum primum may assume aneurysmal proportions in those patients with a restrictive atrial septal defect, and herniation through the mitral valve has been observed.[151–153]

The left atrium usually receives the pulmonary veins in a normal fashion, although one or more pulmonary veins may connect anomalously to the systemic circulation. Akiba and Becker[147] found that the hearts of four of eight patients in their study showed short and almost dysplastic chords of the mitral valve, and one patient's heart exhibited a small central cleft of the anterior mitral leaflet. The left ventricle may exhibit variable degrees of hypertrophy, especially in those patients surviving past infancy. A convexity of the outlet portion of the interventricular septum occurs in those patients with a small and hypertensive right ventricle (Fig. 31–16).[1,2,7,153,154] My colleagues and I confirmed this finding. This subaortic bulge has not been observed to promote left ventricular outflow tract obstruction before the Fontan operation. However, we have observed severe left ventricular outflow tract obstruction resulting in

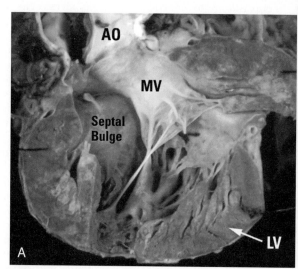

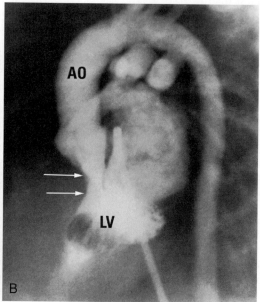

FIGURE 31–16

A, Convex septal bulge in a patient with a small and hypertensive right ventricle. This septal bulge produces the substrate for left ventricular outflow tract obstruction after volume-reducing surgery such as bidirectional cavopulmonary connection or Fontan-type procedure. *B,* Left long axial oblique left ventriculogram demonstrates the convex septal bulge *(arrows)* promoting dynamic left ventricular outflow tract obstruction. AO = aorta; MV = mitral valve; LV = left ventricle. (*A, B* from Freedom RM, Mawson JB, Yoo S-J, Benson LN [eds]: Congenital Heart Disease: Textbook of Angiocardiography. Armonk, NY, Futura, 1997, pp 617–662.)

death, occurring after the Fontan operation when there is an unfavorable change in the ratio between left ventricular mass and end-diastolic volume.[154] Aortic valve stenosis has also been well described in patients with pulmonary atresia and intact ventricular septum, including the neonate with critical aortic stenosis or the somewhat older child with severe aortic valve stenosis.[1, 2, 155] The aortic arch is usually left sided, and we are unaware of the coexistence of pulmonary atresia, intact ventricular septum, and a thoracic coarctation. Coarctation would not be expected to occur because in the fetus with pulmonary atresia, total cardiac output passes through the ascending and transverse aorta, which are wider than normal.

CLINICAL PRESENTATION

Patients with pulmonary atresia and intact ventricular septum have a duct-dependent right ventricular circulation, and thus cyanosis, which increases abruptly after birth, is coincidental with functional and anatomic closure of the arterial duct.[1, 2, 21, 56] Most neonates with pulmonary atresia and intact ventricular septum have an underdeveloped right ventricle—a small tricuspid valve that is both stenotic and often mildly regurgitant. Thus, cardiac examination demonstrates a mild left ventricular lift; a single second heart sound; a soft, blowing pansystolic murmur of tricuspid regurgitation at the lower left sternal border; and, at times, a soft continuous murmur is audible under the left clavicle. Systolic ejection clicks are uncommon. Unless the atrial septum is terribly restrictive and the cardiac output frankly reduced, the caliber of the arterial pulses is normal. In neonates with massive tricuspid regurgitation, the cardiac findings are considerably different. The left side of the chest may be bulging, even in a neonate; the precordium

TABLE 31-2
DIFFERENTIAL RADIOGRAPHIC DIAGNOSIS OF PULMONARY ATRESIA AND INTACT VENTRICULAR SEPTUM
Critical pulmonary stenosis
Tetralogy of Fallot
Pulmonary atresia with ventricular septal defect
Tricuspid and pulmonary atresia
Double inlet ventricle and pulmonary atresia
Hearts with right atrial isomerism and pulmonary atresia

may be rocking; and a systolic thrill is frequently present, accompanying the loud pansystolic murmur. Heart failure is often conspicuous. Because of such gigantic hearts, the lungs may be hypoplastic, and severe respiratory difficulties may be present. In those infants with severe congestive heart failure or a severely restrictive atrial septal defect, the liver is conspicuously enlarged.

DIFFERENTIAL DIAGNOSIS

The differential diagnosis of a cyanotic neonate with oligemic lungs, a soft systolic murmur, and only mild cardiac enlargement is fairly extensive (Table 31–2).

LABORATORY TECHNIQUES

CHEST RADIOGRAPHY

The chest radiograph tends to show mild to moderate cardiac enlargement, some bulging of the right atrium, a left-sided aortic arch, and hypovascular lungs (Fig. 31–17). Some of the largest hearts seen in a neonate occur with

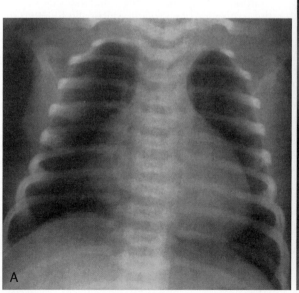
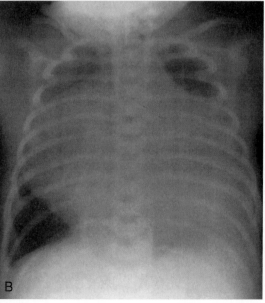

FIGURE 31–17

Chest radiographs from two patients with pulmonary atresia and intact ventricular septum. *A,* This patient had an extremely small and hypertensive right ventricle with a tricuspid Z value of −4.5. *B,* This patient had massive tricuspid regurgitation and a right ventricle/left ventricle pressure ratio less than 1.0.

pulmonary atresia and intact ventricular septum (see Fig. 31–17*B*).[1,2,21,56] Such neonates have massive tricuspid regurgitation. There is a wide spectrum of conditions that produces such massive cardiomegaly in the neonates including functional or organic pulmonary atresia, functional or organic aortic atresia, or intrapericardial teratoma and a large pericardial effusion.

ELECTROCARDIOGRAPHY

The patient with the usual expression of this disorder, a small and hypertensive right ventricle, demonstrates a normal sinus rhythm, a frontal QRS axis from +30 to +90 degrees, a paucity of RV forces with an rS in the right precordial leads (V_4R and V_1) and a pure R wave in the left precordial leads (Fig. 31–18). Right atrial enlargement with tall, peaked P waves is common. ST-T wave changes are not uncommon even in a neonate, and these may progress.[1,2,21,56]

ECHOCARDIOGRAPHY

Identification of ventriculocoronary connections is one of the weakest areas of echocardiography, and recognition is possible only in those with large communications. My colleagues and I have been unable to identify in neonates coronary stenosis or interruption with echo Doppler imaging. As a result of this limitation, we consider angiocardiography essential in neonates with severe hypoplasia of the right ventricle in whom a high incidence of ventriculocoronary artery connections is to be expected. This is not to underestimate the importance of this noninvasive technique as a primary diagnostic tool in those neonates with this lesion. Echocardiography enables the cardiologist to plan the invasive investigation in this subset of patients.[156–162]

The status of the interatrial septum is important because the obligatory right-to-left shunt maintains cardiac

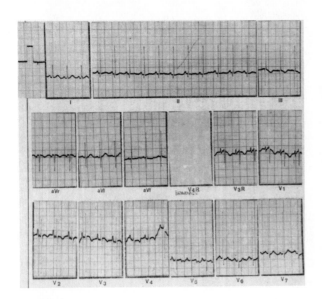

FIGURE 31–18

Electrocardiogram from a patient with pulmonary atresia and intact ventricular septum shows a frontal QRS axis of positive 60%, left ventricular hypertrophy, and right atrial enlargement.

output. The interatrial communication is readily assessed by the subcostal approach with a combination of imaging and Doppler interrogation. Next, the size and morphology of the tricuspid valve are addressed, paying particular attention to the issue of patency. It may be difficult to detect forward flow across an extremely stenotic tricuspid valve into the right ventricle; patency is best determined by identifying tricuspid regurgitation. In the absence of Doppler detection of tricuspid regurgitation, the question of patency cannot always be resolved. Right ventricular size, which usually corresponds with the dimension of tricuspid annulus, can be imaged by a combination of subcostal and precordial views. Absolute volume measurements are of limited value due to the technical limitations of this technique. Although pulmonary infundibular and valve atresia are readily recognized, it may be difficult to distinguish isolated valve atresia from extremely severe stenosis. The size of the right ventricle is not helpful in making this differentiation. Even with the application of Doppler echocardiography, this issue remains a problem, as ductal flow can potentially mask a small jet of forward flow. Pulmonary artery size is best assessed from the suprasternal view, as is the patency of the ductus arteriosus and the laterality and branching pattern of the aortic arch.

It is important to distinguish anatomic from functional pulmonary atresia. In the former, the pulmonary valve is atretic, whereas in the latter, the lack of forward flow is due to poor right ventricular function in the face of high pulmonary artery pressure. Functional pulmonary atresia usually occurs in the setting of Ebstein malformation of the tricuspid valve or with other abnormalities promoting extreme tricuspid regurgitation. Occasionally, transient myocardial ischemia and papillary muscle dysfunction in a stressed neonate provokes functional pulmonary atresia. The patient with Uhl's anomaly or great deficiency in the right ventricular myocardium may also present with functional pulmonary atresia. In general, the pulmonary valve is morphologically normal but functionally closed because of the association of poor right ventricular function and severe tricuspid valve regurgitation. Occasionally, anatomic valve atresia may be present in this setting, hence the importance of being able to differentiate the two entities. With Doppler echocardiography, it is possible to do this by detecting systolic regurgitation of the pulmonary valve, which is caused by a jetting effect of the patent ductus arteriosus against the valve. This is not observed with anatomic pulmonary valve atresia. Another technique is through the use of Doppler echocardiography during positive pressure ventilation, which transiently results in opening of the pulmonary valve and forward Doppler flow.[157,160,161]

HEMODYNAMICS AND ANGIOCARDIOGRAPHY

There are some who suggest that a full hemodynamic and angiocardiographic investigation is not required for the surgical management of the neonate with pulmonary atresia and intact ventricular septum.[184] My colleagues and I take strong issue with this approach, at least for the patient with echocardiographic evidence of a small and hypertensive right ventricle. Rarely, coronary artery interruption can occur in a patient with a normal-sized right ventricle. It is our institutional policy that the coronary artery circu-

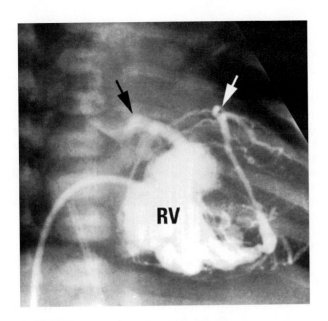

FIGURE 31–19

A newborn with pulmonary atresia and intact ventricular septum and a right ventricular dependent–coronary circulation. The frontal right ventriculogram shows opacification of an ectatic right coronary artery *(black arrow)*. The left coronary artery *(white arrow)* densely opacifies, but there is not reflux of contrast material into the aortic root, indicative of lack of a proximal aortic left coronary artery connection. RV = right ventricle.

lation be evaluated in all patients with elevated right ventricular systolic pressure.[138,163] Although one can recognize large ventriculocoronary connections echocardiographically,[189] this technique does not allow for the recognition of coronary artery stenosis or interruption.[120,134]

The hemodynamic evaluation of the patient with the hypertensive right ventricle establishes right ventricular systolic pressure at or above systemic levels.[1,2,56] Unless the atrial septal defect is significantly obstructive, atrial mean pressures are similar, or the right atrial mean pressure is somewhat higher than the left. Almost always, there is an *a* wave pressure gradient between the right and left atria. When dealing with the patient with massive cardiac enlargement, right ventricular systolic pressure may be substantially less than systemic. These are the patients that raise the possibility that the obstruction to pulmonary blood flow reflects functional pulmonary atresia rather than anatomic pulmonary atresia.

The angiocardiographic investigation of the patient with the hypertensive right ventricle requires right ventricular angiocardiography in frontal and lateral projections* (Fig. 31–19; see Figs. 31–2, 31–3, 31–7, 31–9 to 31–12, and 31–14 to 31–17). Because it may be difficult to enter the small right ventricle using the umbilical venous approach, access through the femoral vein is preferred. Right ventricular angiography is essential, not only to image the form and function of the right ventricle, but also to define any ventriculocoronary artery connections.[8–11,16] Excellent imaging of the coronary circulation in these patients can be achieved with a flow-directed angiocardiographic catheter

advanced from the venous side of the heart to the left atrium, the left ventricle, and the ascending aorta.[1,2,139] Then, using a balloon occlusion technique, contrast agent is directed into the coronary arteries. With release of the balloon, adequate opacification of the aortic arch, brachiocephalic arteries, and pulmonary arteries is achieved as well. We have also been able to perform anterograde selective coronary arteriography from the inferior vena cava, right atrium, left atrium, left ventricle, and ascending aorta. In patients with dense opacification of one or both coronary arteries from the right ventricle, it is important to define coronary arterial stenosis or interruption and to ascertain that each coronary artery has its appropriate proximal aortic connection.[8–11,16] When the coronary arteries densely opacify from the right ventriculogram, one expects subsequent opacification of the aortic root and ascending aorta. When retrograde flow from the coronary artery to the aortic root is not observed, lack of a proximal aortocoronary connection must be excluded. This can usually be accomplished with dense opacification of the aortic root.

BALLOON ATRIAL SEPTOSTOMY

The role of balloon atrial septostomy remains controversial.[38] My colleagues and I advocate septostomy in those patients who unequivocally require a one ventricle repair. In addition, we perform a septostomy when the atrial septum is restrictive and when we have concerns about tricuspid valve and right ventricular size. Obviously, the management algorithm for each patient needs to be individualized. One must balance the consideration of ventricular underfilling and thus reduction of the potential for right ventricular growth vs. the concern that cardiac output after right ventricular outflow tract rehabilitation could be jeopardized by a restrictive ovale foramen in the setting of a noncompliant right ventricle.

CONCEPT OF FUNCTIONAL VS. ORGANIC PULMONARY ATRESIA

A neonate with massive tricuspid regurgitation has a greatly enlarged right atrial and ventricular cavity, and catheter manipulation may provoke atrial tachycardia or flutter. The purpose of any investigation is to exclude functional pulmonary atresia. The concept of functional pulmonary atresia implies an anatomically normal pulmonary infundibulum and valve,[79–82,157,160,161] but with massive tricuspid regurgitation preventing the right ventricle from developing sufficient systolic pressure to open the pulmonary valve in the presence of a relatively muscularized pulmonary vascular bed. Before the routine application of cross-sectional echocardiographic and Doppler imaging, we advocated the role of prostaglandin-enhanced retrograde aortography to demonstrate pulmonary regurgitation, thus defining the atresia as functional.[80] Some patients with functional pulmonary atresia and massive tricuspid insufficiency show resolution and spontaneous improvement. Fetal tricuspid regurgitation may mimic pulmonary atresia and intact ventricular septum.

_____

*References 1, 2, 13–16, 28, 29, 56, 63, 79, 80, 105, 106, 164.

MEDICAL MANAGEMENT

The mainstay of medical management is the administration of prostaglandin E_1 to promote ductal patency.[1,2,56,165,166] In the small preterm infant, prolonged intravenous use or oral administration may permit growth of the infant before operative intervention. Prompt administration of an E-type prostaglandin is important whether the atresia is considered functional or anatomic.

There has been ongoing debate as to the histopathologic effect of prostanoids on the arterial duct.[167–170] Hemorrhage and lacerations have been found in the arterial duct after prostanoid administration, but similar changes have been observed in the closing duct in the absence of prostanoid therapy. Cortical hyperostosis is a well-known complication of prolonged prostanoid administration. In addition, gastric outlet obstruction reflecting antral mucosal hyperplasia is a complication of prolonged prostaglandin administration.[171]

OPERATIVE MANAGEMENT

Our operative experience with pulmonary atresia and intact ventricular septum from 1965 to 1987 has been reviewed.[19,20,27,57] Actuarial survival was only $24.7 \pm 6\%$ at 13 years postoperatively, despite (or perhaps because of) a wide range of procedures. Multivariate analysis indicated that ventriculocoronary connections ($P = .037$), a decreased ratio between right ventricular and left ventricular pressure at the initial cardiac catheterization ($P = .007$), and lower weight at initial operation ($P = .001$) were incremental factors for postoperative death. Of 346 neonates with pulmonary atresia and intact ventricular septum from 32 centers, 41% died before a biventricular, a one ventricle, or a one and a half ventricle repair.[172] Among our patients with severe stenosis or interruption of the left anterior descending coronary artery and thus what we now know to be a right ventricular–dependent coronary circulation, right ventricular outflow tract reconstruction or thromboexclusion of the right ventricle proved uniformly lethal. Indeed, those procedures unmasking a right ventricular–dependent coronary circulation include any procedure reducing right ventricular pressure or thromboexclusion of the right ventricle, which prevents blood from entering the coronary circulation from the right ventricle. Operative results have improved, and when data are stratified by date of operation, the improvement may reflect better understanding of the role of a disordered coronary artery circulation.[19–21,27,57,128,129]

One of the most egregious groups of patients with pulmonary atresia and intact ventricular septum are those with a decreased ratio between right and left ventricular systolic pressure at the initial cardiac catheterization. All have severe tricuspid regurgitation, with most having Ebstein malformation of the tricuspid valve (in itself an additional risk factor in the overall experience, $P = .01$). Many of these neonates die without an operation. Tricuspid valve replacement or annuloplasty has also been attempted in some neonates, but with no survivors at our institution. Starnes and colleagues' novel approach[45] of conversion of these patients from pulmonary atresia and intact ventricular septum to tricuspid and pulmonary atresia with closure of the tricuspid valve and plication of the aneurysmal right atrium may salvage some of these infants.

In the Congenital Heart Surgeons collaborative study, the outcomes of 171 neonates with pulmonary atresia and intact ventricular septum enrolled between January 1, 1987, and January 1, 1991, were evaluated.[32] Survival was 81% at 1 month after the initial surgical intervention and 64% at 4 years. In this study, a systemic-to-pulmonary artery anastomosis with valvotomy or transannular patch was the most commonly performed initial procedure. The risk-adjusted survival rate was the highest after isolated valvotomy, surgical valvotomy with a concomitant systemic-to-pulmonary artery shunt, or transannular patch with a concomitant shunt.

There are many surgical approaches to a neonate with pulmonary atresia and intact ventricular septum. Some with a normal-sized or nearly normal-sized right ventricle are managed with a pulmonary valvulotomy, either by surgery or by catheter techniques, but maintaining the prostaglandin infusion until there is unequivocally good forward pulmonary blood flow. There may initially be a decrease in right ventricular volume after decompression by valvotomy. Despite what appears to be a ventricle of acceptable size, an altered compliance may still eventuate in a shunt. Some surgeons perform an outflow tract patch in these neonates, especially those with a reasonably developed right ventricle. Many of these neonates at some point require a shunt.[32] In neonates with a small ventricle, but with an obvious infundibulum, a pulmonary valvulotomy and a systemic-to-pulmonary artery anastomosis to maintain pulmonary blood flow are usually performed.

Most neonates with pulmonary atresia and intact ventricular septum treated in my unit have a globally disadvantaged unipartite or bipartite right ventricle and ventriculocoronary connections. Many of these patients are never candidates for a biventricular repair. For those considered for a one ventricle repair, the immediate treatment includes a balloon atrial septostomy, followed by a systemic-to-pulmonary artery anastomosis. These patients are converted to a bidirectional cavopulmonary connection from 3 to 6 months of age, addressing any distortion of the right pulmonary artery from the shunt or ductal-induced left pulmonary artery stenosis at that time, with completion of the Fontan procedure from 12 to 24 months of age. In some patients with a vulnerable coronary circulation, simultaneous patency of the arterial duct and surgical shunt may, because of a low diastolic aortic pressure, result in acute left ventricular failure. The long-term outcome for these patients is predicated on preserving the myocardium and pulmonary vascular bed for the Fontan operation. In those patients with ventriculocoronary connections but without a right ventricular–dependent circulation, we consider thromboexclusion of the right ventricle within one to three months after the initial palliation.[45,46,48] The impact of myocardial sinusoids and ventriculocoronary artery connections on ventricular compliance and function clearly affects on some of these patients' ultimate suitability for the Fontan operation.[132,173]

The results of the Fontan procedure for patients with pulmonary atresia and intact ventricular septum are good, and a number with a right ventricular–dependent coronary circulation have successfully undergone a Fontan-type operation.[138,174,175] The long-term fate of the disordered coronary circulation and the impact on the left ventricular myocardium are unclear, but these patients require life-long surveillance for evidence of progressive myocardial ischemia, left ventricular dysfunction, and malignant ventricular dysrhythmia. We have not identified functional left ventricular outflow tract obstruction in a neonate before or after a systemic-to-pulmonary artery anastomosis; however, we have observed mild pressure gradients across the left ventricular outflow tract after a ventricular unloading procedure from either the bidirectional cavopulmonary connection or the Fontan procedure. Indeed, one patient died after a Fontan procedure from severe left ventricular outflow tract obstruction.[154] This form of left ventricular outflow tract obstruction is treated with volume for the low cardiac output but not with inotropes or other modes that could exaggerate the left ventricular outflow tract obstruction. In addition to a one ventricle or a Fontan approach, there is also increasing experience with a one and a half ventricle repair using a bidirectional cavopulmonary connection to unload the borderline or frankly small right ventricle.[176,177]

Finally, there is substantial evidence that right ventricular growth may occur after initial pulmonary outflow tract decompression in some patients.* In some patients, despite adequate relief of the right ventricular outflow tract obstruction, right ventricular growth may not be optimum. Some of these patients may be candidates for a one and a half ventricle repair, complemented with a bidirectional

---

*References 13, 14, 25, 26, 32–35, 38, 39, 43, 94.

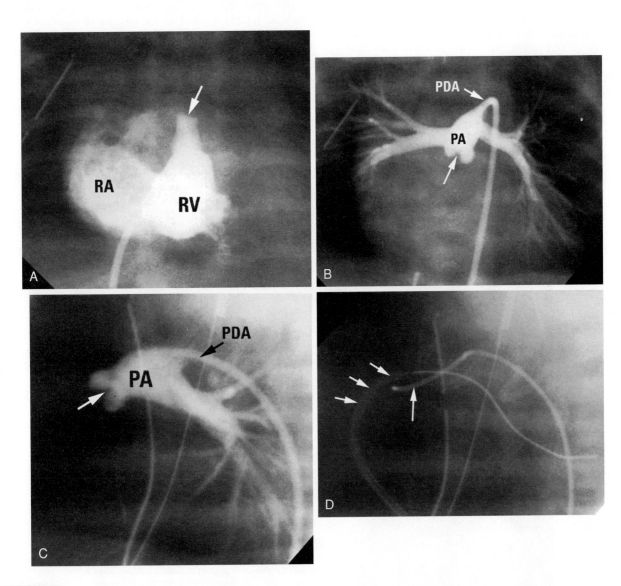

FIGURE 31–20

Catheter-based therapy for pulmonary atresia and intact ventricular septum using radiofrequency-assisted perforation of the atretic pulmonary valve. *A,* Cranially tilted frontal right ventriculogram shows atresia *(arrow)* of the pulmonary valve. Frontal *(B)* and lateral *(C)* pulmonary angiogram shows an imperforate pulmonary valve. *D,* The Judkins right coronary artery catheter is introduced anterograde from the femoral vein to the right ventricular (RV) outlet *(three arrows).* After an application of radiofrequency energy to the atretic valve, a wire has been advanced into the pulmonary artery (PA). The pulmonary valve sinus has been marked by a wire introduced retrograde through the ductus arteriosus *(single arrow).*

Illustration continued on following page

cavopulmonary connection. The preservation of the pulmonary artery anatomy, the functional volumetric capacity of the right ventricle, and the form and function of the tricuspid valve should allow determination of whether any particular patient should be considered a candidate for a biventricular repair or an atriopulmonary bypass. The fabric for many of the patients with pulmonary atresia and intact ventricular septum is clouded by a peculiar coronary artery circulation that may affect the myocardium before or after birth. Cardiac replacement may provide salvation for some of these patients in the neonatal period and beyond.

CATHETER MANAGEMENT OF PULMONARY ATRESIA AND INTACT VENTRICULAR SEPTUM

Surgical algorithms of the management of neonates with this condition have focused on the probability of achieving either a biventricular or a one ventricle repair. In neonates with a right ventricle able to sustain most, if not all, of the systemic venous return, my colleagues and I advocate establishing continuity between the right ventricle and the main pulmonary artery segment using radiofrequency ablation.[76–82] The ideal patient has a tripartite right ventricle

of nearly normal size, with valvar pulmonary atresia and a well-developed pulmonary arterial circulation. Mechanical or thermal transcatheter perforation of the atretic pulmonary valve with subsequent balloon dilatation has been suggested as an alternative to operation in selected patients. Mechanical perforation of the atretic pulmonary valve has been achieved but has the disadvantage of a relatively uncontrolled perforation. Thermal energy applied to the tip of a small wire has allowed more controlled perforation of the atretic valve tissue and has been accomplished in several patients with good results in short-term follow-up. This technique was first reported using excimer laser energy as the energy source.[64–70, 178, 179] However, laser therapy carries the disadvantages of increased risk to staff, the requirement for protective eyewear, limited portability, and considerable capital expense in the setting of an uncommon defect. Radiofrequency energy that can safely achieve well-defined lesions of coagulation necrosis is now widely applied in the treatment of many cardiac dysrhythmias. Utilization of this energy to perforate atretic valve tissue has the advantages of being considerably less expensive, more portable, and less hazardous to staff. The initial results of radiofrequency-assisted perforation of the atretic pulmonary valve have been encouraging

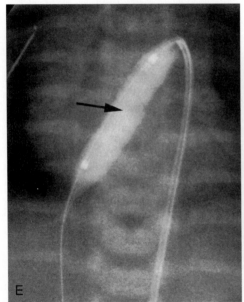

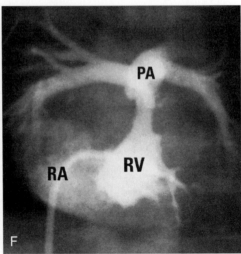

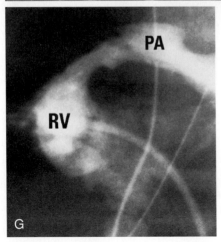

FIGURE 31–20 Continued

E, The wire is advanced from the RV, through the PDA, and into the descending aorta to allow a balloon (*black arrow*) to be introduced across the perforated pulmonary valve for valvotomy. *F, G,* After valvotomy right ventricle–pulmonary artery continuity is clearly established with improvement in tricuspid incompetence. PDA = patent ductus arteriosus; RA = right atrium. (*A–G* from Freedom RM, Mawson JB, Yoo S-J, Benson LN [eds]: Congenital Heart Disease: Textbook of Angiocardiography. Armonk, NY, Futura, 1997, pp 617–662.)

(Fig. 31–20); however, the current literature is confined to early results in small series due to the relative infrequency of the condition.[64–70,178,179] The technique has been applied recently in the setting of longer segment muscular pulmonary atresia. Although initial application is likely to focus on patients destined for a biventricular circulation, application as a technique to decompress the right ventricle in an effort to improve long-term results for those patients on track for a total cavopulmonary connection remains a tantalizing possibility. Such decompression may serve to reduce the potential for left ventricular outflow tract obstruction imposed by the interventricular septum displaced by the hypertensive right ventricle. Decompression may also result in regression of fistulous connections, and improved aortocoronary myocardial perfusion may decrease the incidence of late coronary artery luminal abnormalities associated with high shear stress on the vessels imposed on by the high velocity systolic ventriculocoronary flow, perhaps reducing the incidence of ventricular wall notion abnormalities. Further studies must focus on issues of safety and efficacy. Although a percutaneous approach may avoid or delay the use of cardiopulmonary bypass in the neonatal period, it remains to be seen if it results in a decrease in neonatal or long-term morbidity or mortality.

REFERENCES

1. Freedom RM, Smallhorn JF, Burrows PE: Pulmonary atresia and intact ventricular septum. *In* Freedom RM, Benson LN, Smallhorn JF (eds): Neonatal Heart Disease. London, Springer-Verlag, 1992, pp 285–307.
2. Freedom RM, Mawson JB, Yoo S-J, Benson LN: Congenital Heart Disease: Textbook of Angiocardiography. Armonk, NY, Futura, 1997.
3. Freedom RM: How can something so small cause so much grief? Some thoughts about the underdeveloped right ventricle in pulmonary atresia and intact ventricular septum. J Am Coll Cardiol 19:1038, 1992.
4. Elliott LP, Adams P Jr, Edwards JE: Pulmonary atresia with intact ventricular septum. Br Heart J 25:489, 1963.
5. Van Praagh R, Ando M, Van Praagh S, et al: Pulmonary atresia: Anatomic considerations. *In* Kidd BSL, Rowe RO (eds): The Child With Congenital Heart Disease After Surgery. Mt. Kisco, NY, Futura, 1976, pp 103–135.
6. Bharati S, McAllister HAJ, Chiemmongkoltip P, Lev M: Congenital pulmonary atresia with tricuspid insufficiency: Morphologic study. Am J Cardiol 40:70, 1977.
7. Zuberbuhler JR, Anderson RH: Morphological variations in pulmonary atresia with intact ventricular septum. Br Heart J 41:281, 1979.
8. Milanesi O, Daliento L, Thiene G: Solitary aorta with bilateral ductal origin of non-confluent pulmonary arteries in pulmonary atresia with intact ventricular septum. Int J Cardiol 29:90, 1990.
9. Luciani GB, Swilley S, Starnes VA: Pulmonary atresia, intact ventricular septum, and major aortopulmonary collaterals: Morphogenetic and surgical implications. J Thorac Cardiovasc Surg 110:853, 1995.
10. Mildner RJ, Kiraly L, Sreenam N: Pulmonary atresia, "intact ventricular septum," and aortopulmonary collateral arteries. Heart 77:173, 1997.
11. Freedom RM, Dische MR, Rowe RD: The tricuspid valve in pulmonary atresia and intact ventricular septum. Arch Pathol Lab Med 102:28, 1978.
12. Anderson RH, Anderson C, Zuberbuhler JR: Further morphologic studies on hearts with pulmonary atresia and intact ventricular septum. Cardiol Young 1:105, 1991.
13. Freedom RM, Wilson G, Trusler GA, et al: Pulmonary atresia and intact ventricular septum. A review of the anatomy, myocardium, and factors influencing right ventricular growth and guidelines for surgical intervention. Scand J Thorac Cardiovasc Surg 17:1, 1983.
14. Freedom RM, Wilson GJ: The anatomic substrate of pulmonary atresia and intact ventricular septum. *In* the Third Clinical Conference on Congenital Heart Disease. Obstructive Lesions of the Right Heart. Baltimore, University Park Press, 1984, pp 217–255.
15. Freedom RM, Perrin D: The tricuspid valve: Morphologic considerations. *In* Freedom RM: Pulmonary Atresia and Intact Ventricular Septum. Mt. Kisco, NY, Futura, 1989, pp 37–52.
16. Freedom RM, Perrin D: The right ventricle: Morphologic considerations. *In* Freedom RM: Pulmonary Atresia and Intact Ventricular Septum. Mt. Kisco, NY, Futura, 1989, pp 53–74.
17. Kanjuh VI, Stevenson JE, Amplatz K, Edwards JE: Congenitally unguarded tricuspid orifice with coexistent pulmonary atresia. Circulation 30:911, 1964.
18. Stellin G, Santini F, Thiene G, et al: Pulmonary atresia, intact ventricular septum, and Ebstein anomaly of the tricuspid valve. J Thorac Cardiovasc Surg 106:255, 1993.
19. Coles JG, Freedom RM, Lightfoot NE, et al: Long-term results in neonates with pulmonary atresia and intact ventricular septum. Ann Thorac Surg 47:213, 1989.
20. Lightfoot NE, Coles JG, Dasmahapatra HK, et al: Analysis of survival in patients with pulmonary atresia and intact ventricular septum treated surgically. Int J Cardiol 24:159, 1989.
21. Fyler DC: Nadas' Pediatric Cardiology. Boston, Mosby–Year Book, 1992, pp 557–576.
22. Alboliras ET, Julsrud PR, Danielson GK, et al: Definitive operation for pulmonary atresia with intact ventricular septum. Results in twenty patients. J Thorac Cardiovasc Surg 93:454, 1987.
23. Amodeo A, Keeton BR, Sutherland GR, Monro JL: Pulmonary atresia with intact ventricular septum: Is neonatal repair advisable? Eur J Cardiothorac Surg 5:17, 1991.
24. Battistessa SA, Jackson M, Hamilton DI, et al: Staged surgical management of pulmonary atresia with intact ventricular septum. Cardiol Young 2:395, 1992.
25. Billingsley AM, Laks H, Boyce SW, et al: Definitive repair in patients with pulmonary atresia and intact ventricular septum. J Thorac Cardiovasc Surg 97:746, 1989.
26. Bull C, Kostelka M, Sorensen K, de Leval M: Outcome measures for the neonatal management of pulmonary atresia with intact ventricular septum. J Thorac Cardiovasc Surg 107:359, 1994.
27. Coles J, Williams WG, Trusler GA, et al: Surgical considerations and outcome. *In* Freedom RM (ed): Pulmonary Atresia and Intact Ventricular Septum. Mt. Kisco, New York, Futura, 1989, pp 249–257.
28. De Leval M, Bull C, Hopkins R, et al: Decision making in the definitive repair of the heart with a small right ventricle. Circulation 72(suppl II):52, 1985.
29. De Leval M, Bull C, Stark J, et al: Pulmonary atresia and intact ventricular septum: Surgical management based on a revised classification. Circulation 66:272, 1982.
30. Freeman JE, DeLeon SY, Lai S, et al: Right ventricle-to-aorta conduit in pulmonary atresia with intact ventricular septum and coronary sinusoids. Ann Thorac Surg 56:1393, 1993.
31. Giannico S: Successful balloon avulsion of tricuspid valve in a neonate with pulmonary atresia and intact ventricular septum. J Thorac Cardiovasc Surg 96:488, 1988.
32. Hanley FL, Sade RM, Blackstone EH, et al: Outcomes in neonatal pulmonary atresia with intact ventricular septum. J Thorac Cardiovasc Surg 105:406, 1993.
33. Joshi SV, Brawn WJ, Mee RBB: Pulmonary atresia with intact ventricular septum. J Thorac Cardiovasc Surg 91:192, 1986.
34. Lewis AB, Wells W, Lindesmith GG: Evaluation and surgical treatment of pulmonary atresia and intact ventricular septum in infancy. Circulation 67:1318, 1983.
35. Lewis AB, Wells W, Lindesmith GG: Right ventricular growth potential in neonates with pulmonary atresia and intact ventricular septum. J Thorac Cardiovasc Surg 91:835, 1986.
36. Mainwaring RD, Lamberti JJ: Pulmonary atresia with intact ventricular septum. Surgical approach based on ventricular size and coronary anatomy. J Thorac Cardiovasc Surg 106:733, 1993.
37. McCaffrey FM, Leatherbury L, Moore HV: Pulmonary atresia and intact ventricular septum. Definitive repair in the neonatal period. J Thorac Cardiovasc Surg 102:617, 1991.
38. Milliken JC, Laks H, Hellenbrand H, et al: Early and late results in the treatment of patients with pulmonary atresia and intact ventricular septum. Circulation 72(suppl II):61, 1985.
39. Niederhuser U, Bauer EP, von Segesser LK, et al: Pulmonary atresia and intact ventricular septum: Results and predictive factors of surgical treatment. Thorac Cardiovasc Surg 40:130, 1992.

40. Pawade A, Capuani A, Penny DJ, et al: Pulmonary atresia with intact ventricular septum: Surgical management based on right ventricular infundibulum. J Card Surg 8:371, 1993.

41. Pawade A, Karl T: Management strategy in neonates presenting with pulmonary atresia with intact ventricular septum. Curr Opin Pediatr 6:600, 1994.

42. Ruttenberg HD, Veasy LG, McGough E: Tricuspid valve removal for pulmonic atresia, intact ventricular septum and right ventricular coronary fistulae. Circulation 72(suppl):260, 1985.

43. Schmidt KG, Cloez J-L, Silverman NH: Changes of right ventricular size and function after valvotomy for pulmonary atresia or critical pulmonary stenosis and intact ventricular septum. J Am Coll Cardiol 19:1032, 1992.

44. Squitieri C, Di Carlo D, Giannico S, et al: Tricuspid valve avulsion or excision for right ventricular decompression in pulmonary atresia with intact ventricular septum. J Thorac Cardiovasc Surg 97:779, 1989.

45. Starnes VA, Pitlick PT, Bernstein D, et al: Ebstein's anomaly appearing in the neonate. A new surgical approach. J Thorac Cardiovasc Surg 101:1082, 1991.

46. Waldman JD, Lamberti JJ, Mathewson JW, George L: Surgical closure of the tricuspid valve for pulmonary atresia, intact ventricular septum, and right ventricle to coronary artery communications. Pediatr Cardiol 5:221, 1984.

47. Waldman JD, Karp RB, Lamberti JJ, et al: Tricuspid valve closure in pulmonary atresia and important RV-to-coronary artery connections. Ann Thorac Surg 59:933, 1995.

48. Williams WG, Burrows P, Freedom RM, et al: Thromboexclusion of the right ventricle in a subset of children with pulmonary atresia and intact ventricular septum. J Thorac Cardiovasc Surg 101:222, 1991.

49. Kutsche LM, Van Mierop LHS: Pulmonary atresia with and without ventricular septal defect: A different etiology and pathogenesis for the atresia in the 2 types? Am J Cardiol 51:932, 1983.

50. Hornberger LK, Sahn DJ, Kleinman CS, et al: Tricuspid valve disease with significant tricuspid insufficiency in the fetus: Diagnosis and outcome. J Am Coll Cardiol 17:167, 1991.

51. Roberson DA, Silverman NH: Ebstein's anomaly: Echocardiographic and clinical features in the fetus and neonate. J Am Coll Cardiol 14:1300, 1989.

52. Lang D, Oberhoffer R, Cook A, et al: Pathologic spectrum of malformations of the tricuspid valve in prenatal and neonatal life. J Am Coll Cardiol 17:1161, 1991.

53. Allan LD, Crawford DC, Tynan MJ: Pulmonary atresia in prenatal life. J Am Coll Cardiol 8:1131, 1986.

54. Allan LD, Cook A: Pulmonary atresia with intact ventricular septum in the fetus. Cardiol Young 2:367, 1992.

55. Hornberger LK, Benacerraf BR, Bromley BS, et al: Prenatal detection of severe right ventricular outflow tract obstruction: Pulmonary stenosis and pulmonary atresia. J Ultrasound Med 13:743, 1994.

56. Rowe RD, Freedom RM, Mehrizi A: The Neonate with Congenital Heart Disease. Philadelphia, WB Saunders, 1981.

57. Freedom RM (ed): Pulmonary Atresia and Intact Ventricular Septum. Mt. Kisco, NY, Futura, 1989.

58. Fyler DC: Report of the New England Regional Infant Cardiac Program. Pediatrics 65(suppl):376, 1980.

59. Ferencz C, Rubin JD, McCarter RJ, et al: Congenital heart disease: Prevalence at livebirth. The Baltimore-Washington Infant Study. Am J Epidemiol 121:31, 1985.

60. Chitayat D, McIntosh N, Fouron J-C: Pulmonary atresia with intact ventricular septum and hypoplastic right heart in sibs: A single gene disorder? Am J Med Genet 42:304, 1992.

61. Braunlin EA, Formanek AG, Moller JH, Edwards JE: Angiopathological appearances of pulmonary valve in pulmonary atresia with intact ventricular septum. Interpretation of nature of right ventricle from pulmonary angiography. Br Heart J 47:281, 1982.

62. Arom KV, Edwards JE: Relationship between right ventricular muscle bundles and pulmonary valve. Significance in pulmonary atresia with intact ventricular septum. Circulation 54(suppl 3):79, 1976.

63. Freedom RM, White RI Jr, Ho CS, et al: Evaluation of patients with pulmonary atresia and intact ventricular septum by double catheter technique. Am J Cardiol 33:892, 1974.

64. Parsons JM, Rees MR, Gibbs JL: Percutaneous laser valvotomy with balloon dilatation of the pulmonary valve as primary treatment for pulmonary atresia. Br Heart J 66:36, 1991.

65. Latson LA: Nonsurgical treatment of a neonate with pulmonary atresia and intact ventricular septum by transcatheter puncture and balloon dilation of the atretic valve membrane. Am J Cardiol 68:277, 1991.

66. Rosenthal E, Qureshi SA, Chen KC, et al: Radiofrequency-assisted balloon dilatation in patients with pulmonary valve atresia and an intact ventricular septum. Br Heart J 69:347, 1993.

67. Justo RN, Nykanen DG, Williams WG, et al: Transcatheter perforation of the right ventricular outflow tract as initial therapy for pulmonary atresia and intact ventricular septum in the newborn. Cath Cardiovasc Diagn 40:408, 1997.

68. Gibbs JL, Blackburn ME, Uzan O, et al: Laser valvotomy with balloon valvuloplasty for pulmonary atresia with intact ventricular septum: Five years' experience. Heart 77:225, 1997.

69. Qureshi SA, Rosenthal E, Tynan M, et al: Transcatheter laser assisted pulmonic valve dilatation in pulmonic valve atresia. Am J Cardiol 67:428, 1991.

70. Hausdorf G, Schultze-Neick I, Lange PE: Radiofrequency-assisted "reconstruction" of the right ventricular outflow tract in muscular pulmonary atresia with ventricular septal defect. Br Heart J 69:343, 1993.

71. Freedom RM, Rabinovitch M: The angiography of the pulmonary circulation in patients with pulmonary atresia and ventricular septal defect. *In* Tucker BL, Lindesmith GC, Takahashi M (eds): Obstructive Lesions of the Right Heart. Baltimore, University Park Press, 1984, pp 191–216.

72. Burrows PE, Freedom RM, Rabinovitch M, Moes CAF: The investigation of abnormal pulmonary arteries in congenital heart disease. Radiol Clin North Am 23:689, 1985.

73. Momma K, Takao A, Ando M, et al: Juxtaductal left pulmonary artery obstruction in pulmonary atresia. Br Heart J 55:39, 1986.

74. Elzenga NJ, Gittenberger-de Groot AC: The ductus arteriosus and stenoses of the pulmonary arteries in pulmonary atresia. Int J Cardiol 11:195, 1986.

75. Marino B, Guccione P, Carotti A, et al: Ductus arteriosus in pulmonary atresia with and without ventricular septal defect. Scand J Thorac Cardiovasc Surg 26:93, 1992.

76. Zenati M, del Nonno F, Marino B, di Carlo DC: Pulmonary atresia and intact ventricular septum associated with pulmonary artery sling (Letter). J Thorac Cardiovasc Surg 104:1755, 1992.

77. Steeg CN, Ellis K, Bransilver B, Gersony W: Pulmonary atresia and intact ventricular septum complicating corrected transposition of the great vessels. Am Heart J 82:382, 1971.

78. Shimizu T, Ando M, Takao A: Pulmonary atresia with intact ventricular septum and corrected transposition of the great arteries. Br Heart J 45:471, 1981.

79. Freedom RM, Culham JAG, Moes CAF: Angiocardiography of Congenital Heart Disease. New York, Macmillan, 1984.

80. Freedom RM, Culham G, Moes F, et al: Differentiation of functional and structural pulmonary atresia: Role of aortography. Am J Cardiol 41:914, 1978.

81. Haworth SG, Shinebourne EA, Miller GAH: Right-to-left interatrial shunting with normal right ventricular pressure. A puzzling haemodynamic picture associated with some rare congenital malformations of the right ventricle and tricuspid valve. Br Heart J 37:386, 1975.

82. Schrire V, Sutin GJ, Barnard CN: Organic and functional pulmonary atresia with intact ventricular septum. Am J Cardiol 8:100, 1961.

83. Becker AE, Becker MJ, Edwards JE: Pathologic spectrum of dysplasia of the tricuspid valve: Features in common with Ebstein's malformation. Arch Pathol 91:167, 1971.

84. Anderson RH, Silverman NH, Zuberbuhler JR: Congenitally unguarded tricuspid orifice: Its differentiation from Ebstein's malformation in association with pulmonary atresia and intact ventricular septum. Pediatr Cardiol 11:86, 1990.

85. Berman WJ, Whitman V, Stanger P, Rudolph AM: Congenital tricuspid incompetence simulating pulmonary atresia with intact ventricular septum: A report of two cases. Am Heart J 96:655, 1978.

86. Huhta JC, Edwards WD, Tajik AJ, et al: Pulmonary atresia with intact ventricular septum, Ebstein's anomaly of the hypoplastic tricuspid valve, and double-chamber right ventricle. Mayo Clin Proc 57:515, 1982.

87. Rowlatt JF, Rimoldi MJA, Lev M: The quantitative anatomy of the normal child's heart. Pediatr Clin North Am 10:499, 1963.

88. Drant SE, Allada V, Williams RG: Infundibular diameter predicts the presence of right ventricular-dependent coronary communica-

tions in pulmonary atresia and intact ventricular septum (Abstract). J Am Coll Cardiol 25(suppl):104A, 1995.

89. Davignon AL, Greenwold WE, DuShane JW, Edwards JE: Congenital pulmonary atresia with intact ventricular septum. Clinicopathologic correlation of two anatomic types. Am Heart J 62:591, 1961.

90. Bull C, De Leval M, Mercanti C, et al: Pulmonary atresia and intact ventricular septum: A revised classification. Circulation 66:266, 1982.

91. Patel R, Freedom RM, Moes CAF, et al: Right ventricular volume determinations in 18 patients with pulmonary atresia and intact ventricular septum. Analysis of factors influencing right ventricular growth. Circulation 61:428, 1980.

92. Giglia TM, Jenkins KJ, Matitiau A, et al: Influence of right heart size on outcome in pulmonary atresia with intact ventricular septum. Circulation 88(pt 1):2248, 1993.

93. Freedom RM, Finlay CD: Right ventricular growth potential in patients with pulmonary atresia and intact ventricular septum. In Freedom RM (ed): Pulmonary Atresia and Intact Ventricular Septum. Mt. Kisco, NY, Futura, 1989, pp 239–247.

94. Graham TP Jr, Bender HW, Atwood GF, et al: Increase in right ventricular volume following valvulotomy for pulmonary atresia or stenosis with intact ventricular septum. Circulation 50(suppl II):69, 1974.

95. Grant RT: An unusual anomaly of the coronary vessels in the malformed heart of a child. Heart 13:273, 1926.

96. Anselmi G, Munoz S, Blanco P, et al: Anomalous coronary artery connecting with the right ventricle associated with pulmonary stenosis and atrial septal defect. Am Heart J 62:406, 1961.

97. Williams RR, Kent GBJ, Edwards JE: Anomalous cardiac blood vessel communicating with the right ventricle. Arch Pathol 52:480, 1951.

98. Guidici C, Becu L: Cardio-aortic fistula through anomalous coronary arteries. Br Heart J 22:729, 1960.

99. Lauer RM, Fink HP, Petry EL, et al: Angiographic demonstration of intramyocardial sinusoids in pulmonary-valve atresia with intact ventricular septum and hypoplastic right ventricle. N Engl J Med 271:68, 1964.

100. MacMahon HE, Dickinson PCT: Occlusive fibroelastosis of coronary arteries in the newborn. Circulation 35:3, 1967.

101. Cornell SH: Myocardial sinusoids in pulmonary valvular atresia. Radiology 86:421, 1966.

102. Finegold MJ, Klein KM: Anastomotic coronary vessels in hypoplasia of the right ventricle. Am Heart J 82:678, 1971.

103. Freedom RM, Harrington DP: Contribution of intra-myocardial sinusoids in pulmonary atresia and intact ventricular septum to a right-sided circular shunt. Br Heart J 36:1061, 1974.

104. Calder AL, Co EE, Sage MD: Coronary arterial abnormalities in pulmonary atresia with intact ventricular septum. Am J Cardiol 59:437, 1987.

105. Freedom RM, Benson L, Wilson GJ: The coronary circulation and myocardium in pulmonary and aortic atresia with an intact ventricular septum. In Marcelletti C, Anderson RH, Becker AE, et al (eds): Paediatric Cardiology, Vol 6. Edinburgh, Churchill Livingstone, 1986, pp 78–96.

106. Freedom RM, Benson LN, Trusler GA: Pulmonary atresia and intact ventricular septum: A consideration of the coronary circulation and ventriculo-coronary connections. Ann Cardiac Surg 38, 1989.

107. Gittenberger-De Groot AC, Sauer U, Bindl L, et al: Competition of coronary arteries and ventriculo-coronary arterial communications in pulmonary atresia with intact ventricular septum. Int J Cardiol 18:243, 1988.

108. Kasznica J, Ursell PC, Blanc WA, Gersony WM: Abnormalities of the coronary circulation in pulmonary atresia and intact ventricular septum. Am Heart J 114:1415, 1987.

109. O'Connor WN, Cottrill CM, Johnson GL, et al: Pulmonary atresia with intact ventricular septum and ventriculocoronary communications: Surgical significance. Circulation 65:805, 1982.

110. O'Connor WN, Stahr BJ, Cottrill CM, et al: Ventriculocoronary connections in hypoplastic right heart syndrome: Autopsy serial section study of six cases. J Am Coll Cardiol 11:1061, 1988.

111. Kauffman SL, Anderson DH: Persistent venous valves, maldevelopment of the right heart, and coronary artery-ventricular communications. Am Heart J 66:664, 1963.

112. Hamazaki M: Congenital coronary arterio-ventricular fistulae, associated with absence of proximal coronary artery from aorta. Jpn Heart J 23:271, 1982.

113. Ho SY, De S Carvalho J, Sheffield E: Anomalous origin of single coronary artery in association with pulmonary atresia. Int J Cardiol 20:125, 1988.

114. Lenox CC, Briner J: Absent proximal coronary arteries associated with pulmonic atresia. Am J Cardiol 30:666, 1972.

115. Oppenheimer EH, Esterly JR: Some aspects of cardiac pathology in infancy and childhood. II. Unusual coronary endarteritis with congenital cardiac malformations. Bull Johns Hopkins Hosp 19:343, 1966.

116. Sauer U, Bindl L, Pilossoff V, et al: Pulmonary atresia with intact ventricular septum and right ventricle-coronary artery fistulae: Selection of patients for surgery. In Doyle EE, Engle MA, Gersony WM, et al (eds): Pediatric Cardiology. New York, Springer-Verlag, 1986, pp 566–578.

117. Sissman NJ, Abrams HL: Bidirectional shunting in a coronary artery-right ventricular fistula associated with pulmonary atresia and an intact ventricular septum. Circulation 32:582, 1965.

118. Ueda K, Saito A, Nakano H, Hamazaki Y: Absence of proximal coronary arteries associated with pulmonary atresia. Am Heart J 106:596, 1983.

119. Gerlis LM, Yen Ho S, Milo S: Three anomalies of the coronary arteries co-existing in a case of pulmonary atresia with intact ventricular septum. Int J Cardiol 29:93, 1990.

120. Wilson GJ, Freedom RM, Koike K, Perrin D: The Coronary Arteries: Anatomy and Histopathology. In Freedom RM (ed): Pulmonary Atresia and Intact Ventricular Septum. Mt. Kisco, NY, Futura, 1989, pp 75–88.

121. Laks H, Gates RN, Grant PW, et al: Aortic to right ventricular shunt for pulmonary atresia and intact ventricular septum. J Thorac Cardiovasc Surg 59:342, 1995.

122. Freeman JE, DeLeon SY, Lai S, et al: Right ventricle-to-aorta conduit in pulmonary atresia with intact ventricular septum and coronary sinusoids. Ann Thorac Surg 56:1393, 1993.

123. De Leval M: Myocardial perfusion in congenital heart disease: Surgical implications. In Marcelletti C, Anderson RH, Becker AE, et al (eds): Paediatric Cardiology, Vol 6. New York, Churchill Livingstone, 1986, pp 97–107.

124. Blackman MS, Schneider B, Sondheimer HM: Absent proximal left main coronary artery in association with pulmonary atresia. Br Heart J 46:449, 1981.

125. Garcia OL, Gelband H, Tamer DF, Fojaco RM: Exclusive origin of both coronary arteries from a hypoplastic right ventricle complicating an extreme tetralogy of Fallot: Lethal myocardial infarction following a palliative shunt. Am Heart J 115:198, 1988.

126. Rigby ML, Salgado M, Silva C: Determinants for outcome of hypoplastic right ventricle with duct-dependent pulmonary blood flow presenting in the neonatal period. Cardiol Young 2:377, 1992.

127. Van der Wal HJCM, Smith A, Becker AE, et al: Morphology of pulmonary atresia with intact ventricular septum in patients dying after operation. Ann Thorac Surg 50:98, 1990.

128. Gentles TL, Colan SD, Giglia TM, et al: Right ventricular decompression and left ventricular function in pulmonary atresia with intact ventricular septum. The influence of less extensive coronary anomalies. Circulation 88(pt 2):183, 1993.

129. Giglia TM, Mandell VS, Connor AR, et al: Diagnosis and management of right ventricular-dependent coronary circulation in pulmonary atresia with intact ventricular septum. Circulation 86:1516, 1992.

130. Daubeney PEF, Delany DJ, Slavik Z, et al: Pulmonary atresia with intact ventricular septum: Range of morphology in a population based study. Circulation 92(suppl I):1, 1995.

131. Fyfe DA, Edwards WD, Driscoll DJ: Myocardial ischaemia in patients with pulmonary atresia and intact ventricular septum. J Am Coll Cardiol 8:402, 1986.

132. Hausdorf G, Gravinghoff L, Keck EW: Effects of persisting myocardial sinusoids on left ventricular performance in pulmonary atresia with intact ventricular septum. Eur Heart J 8:291, 1987.

133. Hubbard JF, Girod DA, Caldwell RL, et al: Right ventricular infarction with cardiac rupture in an infant with pulmonary atresia with intact ventricular septum. J Am Coll Cardiol 2:363, 1983.

134. Koike K, Perrin D, Wilson GJ, Freedom RM: Myocardial ischemia and coronary arterial involvement in newborn babies less than one week old with pulmonary atresia and intact ventricular septum. In Freedom RM (ed): Pulmonary Atresia and Intact Ventricular Septum. Mt. Kisco, NY, Futura, 1989, pp 101–108.

135. Akagi T, Benson LN, Williams WG, et al: Ventriculo-coronary arterial connections in pulmonary atresia with intact ventricular septum,

and their influences on ventricular performance and clinical course. Am J Cardiol 72:586, 1993.

136. Dyamenali U, Hanna B, Sharratt GP: Pulmonary atresia with intact ventricular septum: Management of the coronary arterial anomalies. Cardiol Young 7:80, 1997.

137. Oosthoek PW, Moorman AFM, Sauer U, Gittenberger-de Groot AC: Capillary distribution in the ventricles of hearts with pulmonary atresia and intact ventricular septum. Circulation 91:1790, 1995.

138. Mair D, Danielson GK, Puga FJ: The Fontan procedure for pulmonary atresia and intact ventricular septum (PA and IVS): Operative and late results (Abstract). J Am Coll Cardiol 25(suppl):37A, 1995.

139. Burrows PE, Freedom RM, Benson LN, Moes CAF: Coronary angiography of pulmonary atresia, hypoplastic right ventricle, and ventriculocoronary communications. AJR Am J Roentgenol 154:789, 1990.

140. Arcilla RA, Gasul BM: Congenital aplasia or marked hypoplasia of the myocardium of the right ventricle (Uhl's anomaly). J Pediatr 58:381, 1961.

141. Bryan C, Oppenheimer EH: Ventricular endocardial fibroelastosis. Basis for its presence or absence in cases of pulmonic and aortic atresia. Arch Pathol 87:82, 1969.

142. Bulkley BH, D'Amico B, Taylor AL: Extensive myocardial fiber disarray in aortic and pulmonary atresia: Relevance to hypertrophic cardiomyopathy. Circulation 67:191, 1983.

143. Cote M, Davignon A, Fouron J-C: Congenital hypoplasia of right ventricular myocardium (Uhl's anomaly) associated with pulmonary atresia in a newborn. Am J Cardiol 31:658, 1973.

144. Dusek J, Ostadal B, Duskova M: Postnatal persistence of spongy myocardium with embryonic blood supply. Arch Pathol 99:312, 1975.

145. Essed CE, Klein HW, Krediet P, Vorst EJ: Coronary and endocardial fibroelastosis of the ventricles in the hypoplastic left and right heart syndromes. Virchows Arch Pathol Anat Histol 368:87, 1975.

146. Freedom RM, Wilson GJ: Endomyocardial abnormalities. In Freedom RM (ed): Pulmonary Atresia and Intact Ventricular Septum. Mt. Kisco, NY, Futura, 1989, pp 89–99.

147. Akiba T, Becker AE: Disease of the left ventricle in pulmonary atresia with intact ventricular septum. The limiting factor for long-lasting successful surgical intervention. J Thorac Cardiovasc Surg 108:1, 1994.

148. Ho SY, Jackson M, Kilpatrick L, et al: Fibrous matrix of ventricular myocardium in tricuspid atresia compared with normal heart. A quantitative analysis. Circulation 94:1642, 1996.

149. Freedom RM, Culham JAG, Rowe RD: Left atrial to coronary sinus fenestration. (Partially unroofed coronary sinus.) Morphological and angiocardiographic observations. Br Heart J 46:63, 1981.

150. Rose AG, Beckman CB, Edwards JE: Communication between coronary sinus and left atrium. Br Heart J 36:182, 1974.

151. Sahn DJ, Allen HD, Anderson R, Goldberg SJ: Echocardiographic diagnosis of atrial septal aneurysm in an infant with hypoplastic right heart syndrome. Chest 73:227, 1978.

152. Casta A: Atrial septal aneurysm herniation across the mitral valve orifice in pulmonary atresia. Am Heart J 115:1136, 1988.

153. Freedom RM: General morphologic considerations. In Freedom RM (ed): Pulmonary Atresia and Intact Ventricular Septum. Mt. Kisco, NY, Futura, 1989, pp 17–36.

154. Razzouk AJ, Freedom RM, Cohen AJ, et al: The recognition, identification of morphological substrate, and treatment of subaortic stenosis after a Fontan operation: An analysis of 12 patients. J Thorac Cardiovasc Surg 104:938, 1992.

155. Patel RG, Freedom RM, Bloom KR, Rowe RD: Truncal or aortic valve stenosis in functionally single arterial trunk. Am J Cardiol 42:800, 1978.

156. Hanseus K, Bjorkhem G, Lundstrom NR, Laurin S: Cross-sectional echocardiographic measurements of right ventricular size and growth in patients with pulmonary atresia and intact ventricular septum. Pediatr Cardiol 12:135, 1991.

157. Musewe N, Smallhorn JF: Echocardiographic evaluation of pulmonary atresia with intact ventricular septum. In Freedom RM (ed): Pulmonary Atresia and Intact Ventricular Septum. Mt. Kisco, NY, Futura, 1989, pp 133–155.

158. Isaaz K, Cloez JL, Danchin N, et al: Assessment of right ventricular outflow tract in children by two-dimensional echocardiography using a new subcostal view. Am J Cardiol 56:539, 1985.

159. Marino B, Franceschini E, Ballerini L, et al: Anatomical-echocardiographic correlations in pulmonary atresia with intact ventricular septum. Use of subcostal cross-sectional views. Int J Cardiol 11:103, 1986.

160. Smallhorn JF, Izukawa T, Benson L, Freedom RM: Noninvasive recognition of functional pulmonary atresia by echocardiography. Am J Cardiol 54:925, 1984.

161. Silberbach GM, Ferrara B, Berry JM, et al: Diagnosis of functional pulmonary atresia using hyperventilation and Doppler ultrasound. Am J Cardiol 59:709, 1987.

162. Sanders SP, Parness IA, Colan SD: Recognition of abnormal connections of coronary arteries with the use of color flow mapping. J Am Coll Cardiol 13:922, 1989.

163. Mair DD, Julsrud PR, Puga FJ, Danielson GK: The Fontan procedure for pulmonary atresia with intact ventricular septum: Operative and late results. J Am Coll Cardiol 29:1359, 1997.

164. Freedom RM: Angiocardiography of the right ventricle. In Freedom RM (ed): Pulmonary atresia and intact ventricular septum. Mt. Kisco, NY, Futura, 1989, pp 163–206.

165. Olley PM, Coceani F, Bodach E: E-type prostaglandins: A new emergency therapy for certain cyanotic congenital heart malformations. Circulation 53:728, 1976.

166. Haworth SG, Sauer U, Buhlmeyer K: Effect of prostaglandin E1 on pulmonary circulation in pulmonary atresia. A quantitative morphometric study. Br Heart J 43:306, 1980.

167. Calder AL, Kirker JA, Neutze JM, Starling MB: Pathology of the ductus arteriosus treated with prostaglandins: Comparison with untreated cases. Pediatr Cardiol 5:85, 1984.

168. Cole RB, Abman S, Aziz KU, et al: Prolonged prostaglandin E1 infusion: Histologic effects on the patent ductus arteriosus. Pediatrics 67:816, 1981.

169. Park I-S, Nihill MR, Titus JL: Morphologic features of the ductus arteriosus after prostaglandin E1 administration for ductus-dependent congenital heart defects. J Am Coll Cardiol 1:471, 1983.

170. Silver MM, Freedom RM, Silver MD, Olley PM: The morphology of the human newborn ductus arteriosus. Hum Pathol 12:1123, 1981.

171. Peled N, Dagan O, Babyn P, et al: Gastric-outlet obstruction induced by prostaglandin therapy in neonates. N Engl J Med 327:505, 1992.

172. Blackstone EH, Kirklin JW, Hanley FE: What proportion of neonates with pulmonary atresia and intact ventricular septum reach definitive repair? Circulation 94(suppl1):1, 1996.

173. Sideris EB, Olley PM, Spooner E, et al: Left ventricular function and compliance in pulmonary atresia with intact ventricular septum. J Thorac Cardiovasc Surg 84:192, 1982.

174. Najm H, Williams WG, Coles JG, et al: Pulmonary atresia with intact ventricular septum: Results of the Fontan procedure. Circulation 92(suppl 1):1, 1995.

175. Najm H, Williams WG, Coles JG, et al: Pulmonary atresia with intact ventricular septum: Results of the Fontan procedure. Ann Thorac Surg 63:669, 1997.

176. Gentles TL, Keane JF, Jonas RA, et al: Surgical alternatives to the Fontan procedure incorporating a hypoplastic right ventricle. Circulation 90(pt 2):1, 1994.

177. Van Arsdell GS, Williams WG, Maser CM, et al: Superior vena cava to pulmonary artery anastomosis: An adjunct to biventricular repair. J Thorac Cardiovasc Surg 112:1143, 1996.

178. Rosenthal E, Qureshi SA, Kakadekar AP, et al: Technique of percutaneous laser assisted valve dilatation for valvar atresia in congenital heart disease. Br Heart J 69:556, 1993.

179. Redington AN, Cullen S, Rigby ML: Laser or radiofrequency pulmonary valvotomy in neonates with pulmonary atresia and intact ventricular septum—description of a new method avoiding arterial catheterization. Cardiol Young 2:387, 1992.

CHAPTER 32
EBSTEIN ANOMALY OF THE TRICUSPID VALVE

SUSAN G. MACLELLAN-TOBERT   ROBERT H. FELDT

Ebstein anomaly is a rare but well-recognized congenital cardiac anomaly that involves abnormal development of the tricuspid valve and the underlying myocardium. Cardinal anatomic features of Ebstein anomaly include a downward displacement of the septal and posterior leaflets along with a nondisplaced, redundant sail-like anterior leaflet. Thus, the functional tricuspid annulus is displaced downward, resulting in "atrialization" of the right ventricle. An atrial septal defect is commonly present.

This congenital abnormality was first reported by Wilhelm Ebstein in Poland in 1864 after postmortem examination of a 19-year-old laborer who presented with shortness of breath and palpitations.[1] The young man had significant cyanosis and prominent jugular venous pulsations. Dr. Ebstein described severe malformation of the tricuspid valve associated with absence of the thebesian valve and presence of a patent foramen ovale. He published his anatomic findings and details of the associated cardiac murmurs.[2] It was not until 1927 when Alfred Arnstein published the 14th case report that this anomaly was termed *Ebsteinsche Krankheit* (Ebstein disease).[3]

EPIDEMIOLOGY AND GENETICS

Ebstein anomaly is rare, constituting less than 1% of all cardiac malformations and reported in 1 of 1000 autopsies of patients with a congenital cardiac anomaly.[4] The incidence in the general population has been reported to be 1 in 210,000 live births.[5] The New England Regional Infant Cardiac Program reported 13 infants with Ebstein anomaly of 2251 infants (0.5%).[6] Males and females appear to be equally affected.[7,8] Most instances are sporadic, although familial examples have been reported.[9,10] Some authors suggest that there is a basis for inheritance. One large study reporting the outcome of pregnancy in 72 parents with Ebstein anomaly found the incidence of a cardiac anomaly to be 6% (5 of 83) in the offspring of women with Ebstein anomaly and approximately 1% (1 of 75) in the offspring of men.[11] The incidence of Ebstein anomaly in offspring was 0.6% (1 of 158). Other reports have implicated lithium as a possible etiologic agent.[12]

EMBRYOLOGY

During fetal development, the tricuspid valve leaflets and chordae tendineae are formed from the inner surface of the right ventricle by a process known as delamination.[13]

This process involves undermining of the inlet zone of the right ventricle such that the leaflets are lifted off the endocardial surface as they form. The anterior leaflet develops first at the junction of the inlet and trabecular zones. The posterior and septal leaflets develop later at 3 to 4 months of gestation. In Ebstein anomaly, the posterior and septal leaflets insert lower into the ventricle at the junction of the inlet and trabecular zones, suggesting an arrest in the process of delamination. In this region where delamination has failed to occur, the endocardium appears fibrous and thickened. In some patients, the posterior and septal leaflets are absent. Furthermore, the anterior leaflet may contribute to the formation of a membrane covering the tricuspid orifice and making it imperforate or stenotic. Severe tricuspid regurgitation in fetal life results in increased flow across the foramen ovale. The foramen ovale may be enlarged with redundancy of the valve of the fossa ovalis, or an atrial septal defect may be present.

ANATOMY

Displacement of the septal and posterior leaflets of the tricuspid valve is a diagnostic feature of Ebstein anomaly.[14] The septal leaflet normally inserts into the right ventricular myocardium just below the point of septal insertion of the mitral valve. Thus, in Ebstein anomaly, there is an accentuation of the normal downward displacement of the tricuspid valve. The septal and posterior leaflets are variable in size, often thickened, and adherent to the underlying myocardium. In severe displacement, the leaflet tissue and tricuspid orifice move into the region of the right ventricular outflow tract, leaving a large "atrialized" portion of right ventricle above the orifice. The anterior leaflet is generally large and redundant. This sail-like leaflet may also be fenestrated but is not typically displaced into the right ventricle. All the leaflets may be tethered extensively to the underlying myocardium, thus contributing to immobility of the leaflets and to tricuspid regurgitation. Approximately 10% of hearts with Ebstein anomaly have an imperforate tricuspid valve.

Left ventricular dysfunction occurs in patients with Ebstein anomaly.[15,16] Paradoxical septal motion, bowing of the septum leftward, and enlargement of the right side of the heart contribute to a decreased left ventricular cavity size and sometimes to mitral valve prolapse.[17] The left ventricle takes on a banana shape, both in gross appearance and echocardiographically. Left-sided Ebstein anomaly has been described in patients with atrioventricular and ventriculoarterial discordance (congenitally corrected transposition).[18] The posterior and septal leaflets are displaced, but the anterior leaflet tends to be less redundant. Furthermore, right ventricular dilatation is less prominent.

The right atrium, atrioventricular junction, and right ventricle tend to be dilated secondary to volume overload, and there is thinning of the atrialized portion of the right ventricle accompanied by variable ventricular dysfunction. A patent foramen ovale or secundum atrial septal defect is present in as many as 90% of patients.[14] Associated anomalies are rare, with pulmonary stenosis or atresia found in a small percentage of patients. A ventricular septal defect may occasionally be present. Coronary artery anatomy is generally normal except in the presence of an aneurysmal, severely dilated right ventricle, when the right coronary artery may be displaced superiorly.

Conduction tissue abnormalities have been reported. The sinoatrial node and the proximal part of the atrioventricular conduction tissue are normally positioned. Abnormalities of the right bundle branch have been reported. It may be located superficially in the atrialized ventricle, fan out in a similar fashion to the left bundle, or be encased in dense fibroelastic tissue. Accessory conduction pathways have also been described giving rise to a pattern of preexcitation on the electrocardiogram.[19]

PATHOPHYSIOLOGY

A broad spectrum of pathophysiologic findings exists in patients with Ebstein anomaly. The degree of tricuspid regurgitation or stenosis, presence or absence of an atrial communication, factors predisposing to arrhythmias, and degree of right or left ventricular dysfunction all contribute to the pathophysiologic changes found in these patients. The age at presentation of the patient, be it in the fetus or adult, adds an additional dimension to the spectrum of pathophysiologic findings.

Prenatal diagnosis of Ebstein anomaly can be made by fetal echocardiography. In general, the degree of right-sided heart enlargement is a predictor of outcome. Severe right-sided enlargement and hydrops fetalis may be a manifestation of a failing right ventricle. Furthermore, significant cardiomegaly can contribute to the development of pulmonary hypoplasia. The hemodynamic features of Ebstein anomaly in a fetus are dynamic and change with time. For instance, the development of other anomalies, such as pulmonary stenosis or atresia, may be due to impaired forward flow from the right ventricle. Immediately after birth, the infant with Ebstein anomaly may be severely cyanotic.[20] The combination of elevated pulmonary resistance and tricuspid regurgitation can lead to right-to-left shunting at the atrial level, and cyanosis may persist until the pulmonary resistance falls.

In a child or adult, decreased flow into the right ventricle and pulmonary circulation persists in the presence of significant tricuspid regurgitation or, rarely, stenosis. A large volume of blood remains in the right atrium and contributes to atrial distention. During atrial contraction, the atrialized portion of the right ventricle may balloon aneurysmally, acting as a reservoir for blood. With an atrial septal defect or patent foramen ovale, right-to-left shunt-

ing results in cyanosis. Reduced compliance of the right ventricle impairs filling during diastole and contributes to shunting at the atrial level. Each pathophysiologic feature ultimately contributes to the functional capacity of the patient.

In general, the primary focus in patients with Ebstein anomaly has been on the right side of the heart. There have, however, been increasing reports of left-sided abnormalities, involving left ventricular size, shape, and function, that are important. Bowing of the interventricular septum leftward in patients with severe right-sided enlargement compresses the left ventricle and impairs filling.[15,16,18,21] Radionuclide scans and cineangiography have shown impaired left ventricular function at rest in patients who have not had operative repair. With exercise, the ability of the left ventricle to increase end-diastolic volume may be impaired.

CLINICAL FEATURES

HISTORY

Ebstein anomaly may present at any age. In one series at the Mayo Clinic, the mean age at diagnosis was 14.1 years; one patient presented at 79 years of age.[8,22] If the tricuspid valve abnormality is severe, patients present in the fetal or neonatal period. Although some patients are asymptomatic, most exhibit easy fatigability, dyspnea, cyanosis, or palpitations.[7,8] In cyanotic patients, symptoms are exacerbated with exercise. Patients without an atrial shunt have fewer symptoms and fairly normal exercise tolerance. Palpitations may be due to premature atrial or ventricular extrasystoles or tachyarrhythmias. Syncope may be an indication of atrial arrhythmias, because one third of patients have atrial fibrillation or flutter, probably related to right atrial enlargement. A rapid ventricular response in patients with an accessory pathway has led to sudden death. Chest pain is an occasional symptom and is generally sharp or stabbing in nature. Angina-like pain has been reported.

PHYSICAL FINDINGS

Growth and development are generally normal. Cyanosis is not always a presenting sign. Cyanosis and digital clubbing occur in patients with associated right-to-left shunt. Patients may have an unusual facial coloration, described as violaceous hue, flushed, florid, red-cheeked, or malar flush. These patients usually have associated mild polycythemia. A precordial bulge or asymmetry of the precordium is a frequent finding secondary to dilatation of the right-sided heart chambers. Arterial and venous pulsations are usually normal, even with tricuspid insufficiency. The jugular venous pulsations may not have the large V wave because of poor transmission of the venous pulse wave into a dilated, compliant right atrium. An overactive precordium is rarely found.

In general, it is on auscultation that one is first alerted to the diagnosis of Ebstein anomaly. On occasion, the heart sounds are soft, but usually they are of normal intensity. The first heart sound is widely split with an increased second component because of increased excursion of the anterior leaflet and subsequent delayed closure of the abnormal tricuspid valve. The second heart sound is also widely and persistently split owing to late closure of the pulmonic valve, believed to be due to right bundle branch block. Ventricular filling sounds (S_3 or S_4, or both) are common and contribute to the multiplicity of heart sounds with a cadence quality. A holosystolic murmur (grade 2 to 4/6) is heard along the left sternal border and is a manisfestation of tricuspid regurgitation. Frequently, in the same location, diastolic murmurs of low intensity are found and result from anterograde flow across the tricuspid valve. Murmurs vary with respiration, increasing with inspiration.[23]

LABORATORY INVESTIGATIONS

CHEST RADIOGRAPHY

Cardiac size varies, ranging from nearly normal to extreme cardiomegaly. In most patients, the globular heart and narrow base give the cardiac silhouette a balloon shape, similar to that in patients with pericardial effusion (Fig. 32–1). In cyanotic patients, a dilated heart with a narrow base and nearly normal great artery shadows should lead to a diagnosis of Ebstein anomaly. In general, the dilated right atrium and atrialized right ventricle are responsible for the enlarged cardiac shadow.[23] In the lateral projection, the right atrium fills the entire retrosternal space. However, in a neonate, the heart may have a normal size and shape, confusing the diagnosis. The pulmonary vascularity is typically normal except with pulmonary stenosis or significant right-to-left shunt, when the vascularity is decreased. The

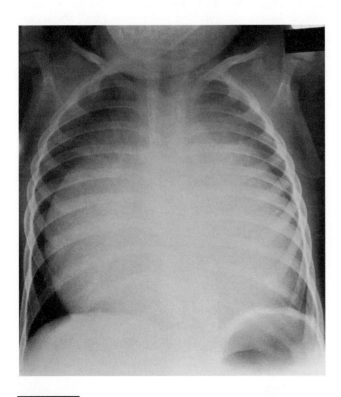

FIGURE 32–1

Chest radiograph of a 2-year-old girl with Ebstein anomaly. Massive cardiomegaly with a cardiothoracic ratio of 0.96.

change in cardiac size can be dramatic after operative repair.

ELECTROCARDIOGRAPHY

The electrocardiogram is usually abnormal, helping to confirm the clinical diagnosis.[8] Sinus rhythm is generally present, although atrioventricular dissociation or atrial fibrillation is occasionally found. Thirty percent to 50% of patients meet the criteria for right atrial enlargement; a large proportion have "Himalayan" P waves.[8] Most patients exhibit right bundle branch block, and many have low-voltage QS complexes in the right precordial leads (Fig. 32–2). Right ventricular hypertrophy and right axis deviation are less common.

Pre-excitation has been reported in 4 to 26% of patients and is due to accessory atrioventricular connections.[8,24] Patients can have a normal PR interval because of delayed conduction through a dilated right atrium. On occasion, the pattern is intermittent, detected only during 24-hour ambulatory monitoring or during exercise electrocardiograms.[25–27] If left axis deviation coexists, an accessory nodoventricular connection or Mahaim fiber should be considered.[28]

Arrhythmias in patients with unrepaired Ebstein anomaly are common. At the Mayo Clinic, 41 of 52 patients (79%) with Ebstein anomaly before operation had documented arrhythmias, history of palpitations, presyncope, or syncope.[29] Paroxysmal supraventricular tachycardia, atrial fibrillation or flutter, and ventricular arrhythmias (premature ventricular complexes or nonsustained ventricular tachycardia) were the most common. Review of 167 patients before and after repair revealed a reduction in arrhythmias from 61% preoperatively to 44% postoperatively (Porter CJ: Personal communication). Early postoperative arrhythmias including supraventricular and ventricular arrhythmias are associated with increased risk of sudden death.

ECHOCARDIOGRAPHY

Angiography was the primary means by which Ebstein anomaly was confirmed until the 1980s. Before the development of two-dimensional echocardiography, the diagnosis of Ebstein anomaly by use of M-mode imaging was limited. The echocardiographic M-mode features of Ebstein anomaly include an enlarged right ventricle, increased amplitude and velocity of the anterior tricuspid leaflet, paradoxical septal motion, and delayed closure of the anterior tricuspid valve leaflet.[30] The most reliable M-mode criterion was thought to be the relationship of mitral valve closure to tricuspid valve closure. The tricuspid valve normally closes within 30 to 50 milliseconds after the mitral valve. If the tricuspid valve closure is more than 50 milliseconds after the mitral valve closure, the diagnosis of Ebstein anomaly should be strongly considered.[31,32] This finding was eventually found to be variable and dependent on the transducer's position. Abnormal activation of the right ventricle (i.e., right bundle branch block) is not responsible for the prolonged mitral-tricuspid closure interval.[33]

With the advent of two-dimensional echocardiography, the diagnosis of Ebstein anomaly became easier. By 1984, two-dimensional imaging was comprehensive enough that

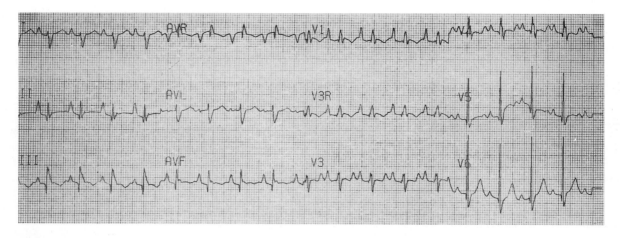

Electrocardiogram of a 15-year-old boy with Ebstein anomaly. Prominent P wave, prolonged atrioventricular conduction, and delay in right ventricular conduction. (From Driscoll DJ, Fuster V, Danielson GK: Ebstein's anomaly of the tricuspid valve. *In* Giuliani ER, Gersh BJ, McGoon MD, et al [eds]: Mayo Clinic Practice of Cardiology, 3rd ed. St. Louis, Mosby, 1996, p 1601. By permission of Mayo Foundation.)

angiography no longer played an integral role in the diagnosis of Ebstein anomaly.[34–36] The single most diagnostic feature is downward displacement of the septal leaflet of the tricuspid valve (virtually all patients); normally, the septal leaflet of the tricuspid valve inserts on the ventricular septum slightly below the insertion of the mitral valve (Fig. 32–3). In patients with Ebstein anomaly, this normal displacement is exaggerated. A "displacement index," which is the distance between septal mitral and septal tricuspid leaflet insertion, can be measured and indexed to body surface area. A value of greater than 8 mm/m² reliably identifies patients with Ebstein anomaly.[37] Others have reported that the "critical difference" for discrimination is greater than 15 mm in children (<14 years old) and greater than 20 mm in adults.[38] Other features consistent with the diagnosis include excessive elongation and displacement of the anterior leaflet (uncommon), leaflet tethering to the underlying myocardium or absence of septal or posterior tricuspid leaflets, and enlargement of the tricuspid valve annulus. Further supporting evidence includes right atrial and ventricular volume overload with paradoxical ventricular septal motion; aneurysmal dilatation of the right ventricular outflow tract and thin, dysfunctional right ventricular myocardium; an atrial septal defect; fenestration of the tricuspid leaflets; and variable tricuspid valve regurgitation.[30,37] Associated anomalies include ventricular septal defects and pulmonary stenosis. Doppler study and color flow assessment aid in determining hemodynamic alterations, such as valve regurgitation and intracardiac shunting. By use of two-dimensional echocardiographic techniques, both the functional and anatomic severity of the malformation of the tricuspid valve should be determined. Anatomic severity and functional severity are not necessarily related. For example, a patient may have a severe anatomic form of Ebstein anomaly with mild functional disease. Both aspects of severity play an important role in determining functional status, prognosis, and reparability of the tricuspid valve.[30,37,39,40]

Echocardiography is also important intraoperatively and postoperatively in assessing adequacy of tricuspid valve repair or replacement.[41] Intraoperative echocardiography can assess prosthetic valve function, detect change in right and left ventricular function, and exclude significant residual right-to-left atrial shunting. Color flow imaging can assess the degree of residual tricuspid regurgitation after valve plication. Similarly, postoperative echocardiography is important to assess the adequacy of repair and exclude postoperative complications. Complications include pericardial or pleural effusion, mediastinal hematoma, and intracardiac thrombus. The degree of residual tricuspid regurgitation or tricuspid stenosis should be determined. Ventricular function and regional wall abnormalities should be assessed. Rarely, right coronary artery flow is

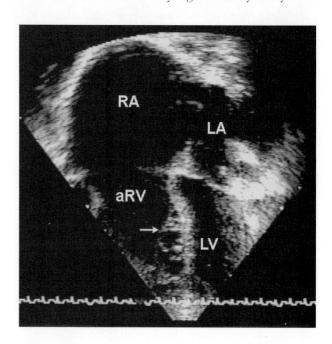

Echocardiogram, apical four-chamber view. Tricuspid valve leaflets (*arrow*) are displaced into the right ventricle. LA = left atrium; LV = left ventricle; RA = right atrium; aRV = atrialized right ventricle.

compromised because of the proximity of the right coronary artery to the plicated portion of the atrialized right ventricle.

Echocardiography can be used to diagnose Ebstein anomaly in the fetus.[42] Characteristics associated with early neonatal mortality include marked right-sided heart enlargement, severe tethering of the anterior tricuspid leaflet tissue, left ventricular compression, and associated lesions such as pulmonary atresia. Pulmonary hypoplasia is secondary to severe cardiomegaly and hydrops with pleural and pericardial effusions. Detection of arrhythmias, such as supraventricular tachycardia, at the time of fetal echocardiography is important, because rhythm disturbances contribute to the development of hydrops.

EXERCISE TESTING

Exercise testing has become part of our routine evaluation of patients with Ebstein anomaly. Decreasing exercise tolerance may be used to determine the optimal time for operative repair. In general, the degree of exercise intolerance correlates with functional capacity.[43–45] Patients with a functionally mild anomaly can have normal or nearly normal exercise capacity. Severely affected patients or those with significant shunt exhibit marked reduction in maximal oxygen uptake and cumulative exercise time.

Maximal oxygen uptake correlates with both rest and exercise systemic arterial saturation in preoperative patients. In a patient with an atrial septal defect, right-to-left shunting is a strong stimulus for increased minute ventilation and a ventilatory equivalent for oxygen; thus, these patients exhibit excessive ventilation at rest and during exercise, and maximal aerobic power might be limited by ventilation as well as by cardiac mechanisms. Operative repair often improves exercise tolerance and maximal oxygen uptake. Exercise often brings out ventricular preexcitation or ectopy.

CARDIAC CATHETERIZATION

Cardiac catheterization plays a limited part in evaluating patients with Ebstein anomaly. Interventional catheterization techniques in patients with associated lesions, such as pulmonary stenosis, and electrophysiologic study of patients with arrhythmias have an ongoing role in management of patients.

Hemodynamic features of the patient with Ebstein anomaly include moderate elevation of the right atrial pressure, most often with a dominant V wave and steep Y descent. If the right atrium is massively dilated, right atrial pressure may be normal in spite of severe tricuspid regurgitation. Right ventricular pressures are usually normal, but the end-diastolic pressure may be elevated in some. The pulmonary artery pressure is generally normal, but it may be decreased in those with severe tricuspid regurgitation and a right-to-left shunt. A right-to-left shunt can be demonstrated by intracardiac dye dilution curves from the inferior or superior vena cava by showing early-appearing dye at the systemic arterial sampling site. Of historical significance is a technique of simultaneous recording of the intracavitary pressure and intracardiac electrogram tracing. When a catheter with an end-hole and an electrode at

the tip was positioned in the atrialized portion of the right ventricle, the pressure tracing recorded was atrial, but the electrogram showed ventricular activity.

ANGIOCARDIOGRAPHY

Right ventricular angiocardiography is usually diagnostic of Ebstein anomaly, except in the mildest forms. In the frontal plane, injection of contrast medium in the right ventricle demonstrates a large sail-like anterior tricuspid leaflet, tricuspid regurgitation, and frequently a distinct notch at the inferior cardiac border to the left of the spine (Fig. 32–4). The notch is the site of abnormal attachment of the displaced anterior leaflet. A "trilobed" appearance results from outlining by contrast medium of the enlarged right atrium, the atrialized ventricle, and the outflow portion of the functional ventricle. Lastly, associated anomalies can be demonstrated by angiocardiography.

In a cyanotic neonate with Ebstein anomaly, injection of contrast medium into the right ventricle may show tricuspid regurgitation and little or no flow of contrast medium into the pulmonary artery, suggesting anatomic obstruction of the right ventricular outflow tract. The same finding occurs in the absence of anatomic obstruction if the pulmonary resistance is elevated. Patency of the right ventricular outflow tract should be established by other techniques, such as catheter advancement through a patent pulmonary valve or injection of contrast medium in the ductus arteriosus to show contrast medium filling the main pulmonary artery and regurgitating into the right ventricle.

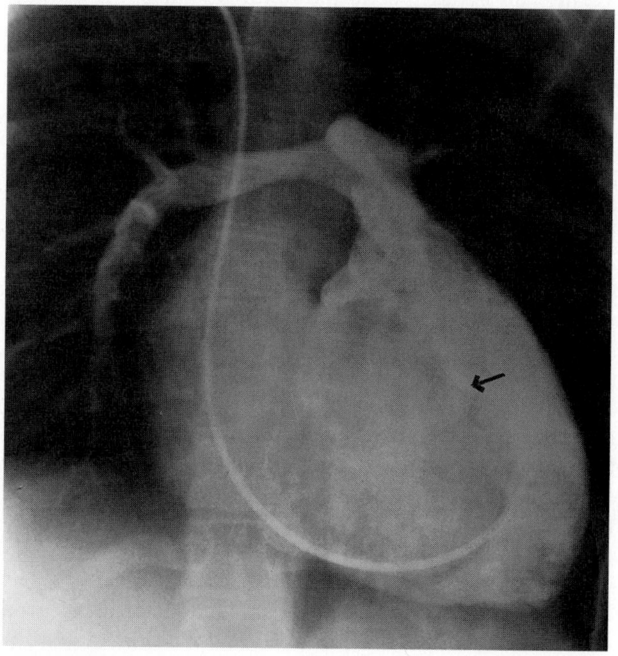

FIGURE 32–4

Right ventriculogram, anteroposterior view, of a 21-year-old woman. Large sail-like anterior leaflet *(arrow)* is displaced well to the left of the spine. Severe tricuspid incompetence is evident. (From Giuliani ER, Fuster V, Brandenburg RO, Mair DD: Ebstein's anomaly: The clinical features and natural history of Ebstein's anomaly of the tricuspid valve. Mayo Clin Proc 54:163, 1979. By permission of Mayo Foundation.)

ELECTROPHYSIOLOGIC STUDY

Electrophysiologic evaluation of patients with Ebstein anomaly has been performed with increasing frequency because of the common occurrence of tachyarrhythmias or symptoms compatible with tachyarrhythmias. Frequently, patients are evaluated just before radiofrequency ablation therapy for the arrhythmia. In 25 patients with Ebstein anomaly who underwent electrophysiologic testing,[46, 47] the mechanisms of arrhythmia included orthodromic reciprocating tachycardia (15), both orthodromic and antidromic reciprocating tachycardia (4), inducible atrial flutter/fibrillation (7), atrioventricular nodal re-entry (2), and ventricular tachycardia (1). Another large series of patients with Ebstein anomaly and pre-excitation who underwent surgical ablation of an accessory pathway was reported by Smith and coworkers.[48] All patients had orthodromic reciprocating tachycardia; but one patient was also thought to have antidromic reciprocating tachycardia, three were believed to have an additional accessory nodoventricular or fasciculoventricular pathway, and one had inducible ventricular tachycardia.

TREATMENT

A wide spectrum of severity exists among patients with Ebstein anomaly; thus, it is difficult to narrow the recommendations for treatment. Patients with a mild functional status do well for years without intervention. A fetus who is significantly affected may die before birth. The neonate presenting with cyanosis can best be managed by supportive and conservative means until the pulmonary resistance falls. At times, nitric oxide therapy may be beneficial in those infants most severely distressed. For the older infant or child with severe disease and clinical deterioration, surgical intervention must be considered.

Because of the success of operative treatment of certain patients with Ebstein anomaly, selection criteria have been defined.[49] At the Mayo Clinic, operation is recommended for patients in the following categories: patients in New York Heart Association (NYHA) class III or class IV; patients in NYHA class I or class II but with a cardiothoracic ratio on a plain chest film of 0.65 or greater; patients with significant cyanosis and polycythemia (an arterial saturation of 80 or less with a hemoglobin level of 16 g/dl or higher); patients who have had a paradoxical embolus, even if they are still in NYHA class I or class II; and patients who have an accessory atrioventricular pathway with medically uncontrolled reciprocating tachycardia. Indications for operation in a neonate with severe congestive cardiac failure or cyanosis are less clear and must be individualized after careful discussion.

The operative approach to Ebstein anomaly has evolved during the past four decades. In the 1950s, systemic–pulmonary artery anastomoses were created to increase pulmonary blood flow, but poor results were achieved. Improved outcomes were obtained with the Glenn shunt, a superior vena cava–pulmonary artery connection.[50] In 1958, Hunter and Lillehei[51] tried repositioning the septal and posterior tricuspid valve leaflets, but this had no apparent success. In 1962, Barnard and Schrire[52] success-fully replaced the tricuspid valve with a prosthesis; this patient was still alive and doing well 19 years after operation.[53] Reconstruction of the tricuspid valve was attempted in 1969 by Hardy and Roe.[54] At present, three approaches are available for repair of Ebstein anomaly: replacement of the valve[9, 55–57] with either a mechanical or "biologic" prosthesis, reconstruction of the valve,[54, 58–61] or both replacement and reconstruction.[62]

From the pioneering efforts of these other surgeons, Danielson and colleagues[63] developed a "plastic" repair based on construction of a monocusp valve by use of the enlarged anterior leaflet of the tricuspid valve. A bicuspid or tricuspid repair can occasionally be performed if there is adequate posterior and septal leaflet tissue. The results of this type of repair have been excellent. Between April 1972 and February 1991, 189 patients with Ebstein anomaly underwent repair; 58% (110 patients) had a plastic repair consisting of plication of the free wall of the atrialized portion of the right ventricle, posterior tricuspid annuloplasty, right reduction atrioplasty, and excision of the attenuated atrial septum with patch closure of the atrial septum in patients with an associated atrial septal defect.[64] Tricuspid valve replacement was performed in 36.5% (69 patients). Porcine bioprostheses were used in 50 patients, and 19 received mechanical prostheses. Twenty-eight patients who had accessory conduction pathways underwent intraoperative mapping of the pathways and successful surgical ablation as part of the operative treatment. Within 30 days of operation, 12 deaths (6%) occurred, 4 of which were related to arrhythmia. There have been 10 late deaths, 4 being sudden and presumably due to arrhythmias. Reoperation was required in four patients (3.4%) 1.4 to 14 years after initial repair. Follow-up of 151 of the 177 operative survivors revealed that 92.9% were in NYHA functional class I or class II.

Radiofrequency current catheter ablation techniques have been employed in patients with Ebstein anomaly who have atrioventricular re-entrant tachycardia associated with an accessory pathway. In a study by Cappato and coworkers,[65] multiple accessory pathways were present in 52% of patients (11 of 21). The presence of multiple pathways and abnormal activation potentials in the atrialized right ventricle adversely influenced ablation. The success rate of ablation in this group of patients was 76% (16 of 21 patients) compared with a 95% success rate for patients with isolated right-sided accessory pathways. A 25% risk of recurrence of tachycardia was noted during follow-up.

NATURAL HISTORY

The natural history of Ebstein anomaly was first reviewed by Watson[66] in 1974. This international cooperative study described 505 patients collected from 61 centers in 28 countries. Thirty-five were younger than 1 year, 403 were between 1 and 25 years, and 67 were older than 25 years. Seventy-two percent of the infants were in heart failure. Growth and development during infancy were either average or good in 81% of the older patients. Seventy-one percent of the patients aged 1 to 25 years and 60% of those older than 25 years had little or no disability and were classified as NYHA class I or class II. Of the total group, 15%

died of natural causes, and 54% who had operative treatment of Ebstein anomaly died. After an initial high mortality from congestive heart failure in the first few months of life, the mortality stabilized uniformly in those older than 1 year, at an average of 13%.

More recently, Celermajer and associates[67] described 220 patients with Ebstein anomaly presenting from fetus to adulthood. The median age at time of presentation was younger than 1 year, emphasizing the role fetal echocardiography now plays in early diagnosis. Early mortality was due to heart failure and pulmonary hypoplasia secondary to cardiomegaly. Associated cardiac anomalies were more common in infants who presented early; however, neonates with isolated Ebstein anomaly showed spontaneous improvement as the pulmonary vascular resistance decreased. In childhood, Ebstein anomaly tended to present with a cardiac murmur discovered incidentally. One major problem in an older child and adult is development of arrhythmias and late hemodynamic deterioration possibly due to increased right-to-left shunting at the atrial level, right-sided heart failure, or progressive left-sided heart dysfunction.

There have been reports of women with mild Ebstein anomaly becoming pregnant and delivering healthy term infants.[68,69] Others, however, have reported fetal deaths and prematurity in mothers who had more significant Ebstein anomaly.[70–72] After operative repair, some women have had uncomplicated and successful pregnancies.[49] Connolly and Warnes[11] reported the outcome of pregnancy in 72 patients with Ebstein anomaly. Pregnancy seemed well tolerated but was associated with an increased risk of prematurity, fetal loss, and congenital heart disease in the offspring. The miscarriage and fetal loss rates were 18%, slightly higher than the expected rate of 10 to 15%. The mean birth weight of infants born to cyanotic women is significantly lower than that of infants born to acyanotic women. No significant maternal complications or death occurred in this series, suggesting that pregnancy in patients with Ebstein anomaly is well tolerated. Maternal arrhythmia and cyanosis, however, warrant close observation during pregnancy.

REFERENCES

1. Mann RJ, Lie JT: The life story of Wilhelm Ebstein (1836–1912) and his almost overlooked description of a congenital heart disease. Mayo Clin Proc 54:197, 1979.
2. Ebstein W: Über einen sehr seltenen Fall von Insufficienz der Valvula tricuspidalis, bedingt durch eine angeborene hochgradige Missbildung derselben. Arch Anat Physiol Wissensch Med 238, 1866.
3. Arnstein A: Eine seltene Missbildung der Trikuspidalklappe ("Ebsteinsche Krankheit"). Virchows Arch Pathol Anat Physiol 266:247, 1927.
4. Abbott MES: Atlas of Congenital Cardiac Disease. New York, American Heart Association, 1936, p 36.
5. Keith JD, Rowe RD, Vlad P: Heart Disease in Infancy and Childhood. New York, Macmillan, 1958, p 314.
6. Report of New England Regional Infant Cardiac Program. Pediatrics 65(suppl):375, 1980.
7. Bialostozky D, Horwitz S, Espino-Vela J: Ebstein's malformation of the tricuspid valve: A review of 65 cases. Am J Cardiol 29:826, 1972.
8. Giuliani ER, Fuster V, Brandenburg RO, Mair DD: Ebstein's anomaly: The clinical features and natural history of Ebstein's anomaly of the tricuspid valve. Mayo Clin Proc 54:163, 1979.
9. Emanuel R, O'Brien K, Ng R: Ebstein's anomaly: Genetic study of 26 families. Br Heart J 38:5, 1976.
10. Rosenmann A, Arad I, Simcha A, Schaap T: Familial Ebstein's anomaly. J Med Genet 13:532, 1976.
11. Connolly HM, Warnes CA: Ebstein's anomaly: Outcome of pregnancy. J Am Coll Cardiol 23:1194, 1994.
12. Nora JJ, Nora AH, Toews WH: Lithium, Ebstein's anomaly, and other congenital heart defects (Letter). Lancet 2:594, 1974.
13. Van Mierop LHS, Gessner IH: Pathogenetic mechanisms in congenital cardiovascular malformations. Prog Cardiovasc Dis 15:67, 1972.
14. Anderson KR, Zuberbuhler JR, Anderson RH, et al: Morphologic spectrum of Ebstein's anomaly of the heart: A review. Mayo Clin Proc 54:174, 1979.
15. Monibi AA, Neches WH, Lennox CC, et al: Left ventricular anomalies associated with Ebstein's malformation of the tricuspid valve. Circulation 57:303, 1978.
16. Benson LN, Child JS, Schwiger M, et al: Left ventricular geometry and function in adults with Ebstein's anomaly of the tricuspid valve. Circulation 75:353, 1987.
17. Anderson KR, Danielson GK, McGoon DC, Lie JT: Ebstein's anomaly of the left-sided tricuspid valve: Pathological anatomy of the valvular malformation. Circulation 58(suppl I):87, 1978.
18. Hurwitz RA: Left ventricular function in infants and children with symptomatic Ebstein's anomaly. Am J Cardiol 73:716, 1994.
19. Lev ML, Gibson S, Miller RA: Ebstein's disease with Wolff-Parkinson-White syndrome: Report of a case with a histopathologic study of possible conduction pathways. Am Heart J 49:724, 1955.
20. Celermajer DS, Cullen S, Sullivan ID, et al: Outcome in neonates with Ebstein's anomaly. J Am Coll Cardiol 19:1041, 1985.
21. Ng R, Somerville J, Ross D: Ebstein's anomaly: Late results of surgical correction. Eur J Cardiol 9:39, 1979.
22. Seward JB, Tajik AJ, Feist DJ, Smith HC: Ebstein's anomaly in an 85-year-old man. Mayo Clin Proc 54:193, 1979.
23. Perloff JK: The Clinical Recognition of Congenital Heart Disease. Philadelphia, WB Saunders, 1987, p 239.
24. Soulié P, Heulin A, Pauly-Laubry C, Degeorges M: Maladie d'Ebstein: Étude clinique et évolation (à propos de 40 observations dont 9 chirurgicales). Arch Mal Coeur Vaiss 63:615, 1970.
25. Schiebler GL, Adams P Jr, Anderson RC: The Wolff-Parkinson-White syndrome in infants and children: A review and a report of 28 cases. Pediatrics 28:585, 1959.
26. Friedman S, Wells CRE, Amiri S: The transient nature of Wolff-Parkinson-White anomaly in childhood, J Pediatr 74:296, 1969.
27. Klein GJ, Gulamhusein SS: Intermittent preexcitation in the Wolff-Parkinson-White syndrome. Am J Cardiol 52:292, 1983.
28. Follath F, Hallidie-Smith KA: Unusual electrocardiographic changes in Ebstein's anomaly. Br Heart J 34:513, 1972.
29. Oh JK, Holmes DR Jr, Hayes DL, et al: Cardiac arrhythmias in patients with surgical repair of Ebstein's anomaly. J Am Coll Cardiol 6:1351, 1985.
30. Seward JB: Ebstein's anomaly: Ultrasound imaging and hemodynamic evaluation. Echocardiography 10:641, 1993.
31. Farooki ZQ, Henry JG, Green EW: Echocardiographic spectrum of Ebstein's anomaly of the tricuspid valve. Circulation 53:63, 1976.
32. Milner S, Meyer RA, Venables AW, et al: Mitral and tricuspid valve closure in congenital heart disease. Circulation 53:513, 1976.
33. Tajik AJ, Gau GT, Giuliani ER, et al: Echocardiogram in Ebstein's anomaly with Wolff-Parkinson-White preexcitation syndrome, type B. Circulation 47:813, 1973.
34. Matsumoto M, Matsuo H, Nagata S, et al: Visualization of Ebstein's anomaly of the tricuspid valve by two-dimensional and standard echocardiography. Circulation 53:69, 1976.
35. Hirschklau MJ, Sahn DJ, Hagan AD, et al: Cross-sectional echocardiographic features of Ebstein's anomaly of the tricuspid valve. Am J Cardiol 40:400, 1977.
36. Ports TA, Silverman NH, Schiller NB: Two-dimensional echocardiographic assessment of Ebstein's anomaly. Circulation 58:336, 1978.
37. Shiina A, Seward JB, Edwards WD, et al: Two-dimensional echocardiographic spectrum of Ebstein's anomaly: Detailed anatomic assessment. J Am Coll Cardiol 3:356, 1984.
38. Gussenhoven EJ, Stewart PA, Becker AE, et al: "Offsetting" of the septal tricuspid leaflet in normal hearts and in hearts with Ebstein's anomaly: Anatomic and echographic correlation. Am J Cardiol 54:172, 1984.

39. Shiina A, Seward JB, Tajik AJ, et al: Two-dimensional echocardiographic-surgical correlation in Ebstein's anomaly: Preoperative determination of patients requiring tricuspid valve plication vs replacement. Circulation 68:534, 1983.
40. Gussenhoven WJ, de Villeneuve VH, Hugenholtz, PG, et al: The role of echocardiography in assessing the functional class of the patient with Ebstein's anomaly. Eur Heart J 5:490, 1984.
41. Hagler DJ: Echocardiographic assessment of Ebstein's anomaly. Prog Pediatr Cardiol 2:28, 1993.
42. Roberson DA, Silverman NH: Ebstein's anomaly: Echocardiographic and clinical features in the fetus and neonate. J Am Coll Cardiol 14:1300, 1989.
43. Barber G, Danielson GK, Heise CT, Driscoll DJ: Cardiorespiratory response to exercise in Ebstein's anomaly. Am J Cardiol 56:509, 1985.
44. Driscoll DJ, Mottram CD, Danielson GK: Spectrum of exercise intolerance in 45 patients with Ebstein's anomaly and observations on exercise tolerance in 11 patients after surgical repair. J Am Coll Cardiol 11:831, 1988.
45. MacLellan-Tobert SG, Driscoll DJ, Mottram CD, et al: Exercise tolerance in patients with Ebstein's anomaly. J Am Coll Cardiol 29:1615, 1997.
46. Olson TM, Porter CJ: Electrocardiographic and electrophysiologic findings in Ebstein's anomaly, pathophysiology, diagnosis and management. Prog Pediatr Cardiol 2:38, 1993.
47. Olson TM, Porter CJ, Danielson GK: Surgical treatment of Ebstein's anomaly and preexcitation. Pacing Clin Electrophysiol 14:645, 1991.
48. Smith WM, Gallagher JJ, Kerr CR, et al: The electrophysiologic basis and management of symptomatic recurrent tachycardia in patients with Ebstein's anomaly of the tricuspid valve. Am J Cardiol 49:1223, 1982.
49. Mair DD, Seward JB, Driscoll DJ, Danielson GK: Surgical repair of Ebstein's anomaly: Selection of patients and early and late operative results. Circulation 72(suppl 2):II-70, 1985.
50. Glenn WWL, Browne M, Whittemore R: Circulatory bypass of the right side of the heart: Cavapulmonary artery shunt—indications and results (report of a collected series of 537 cases). In Cassels DE (ed): The Heart and Circulation in the Newborn and Infant. New York, Grune & Stratton, 1966, pp 345–357.
51. Hunter SW, Lillehei CW: Ebstein's malformation of the tricuspid valve: Study of a case together with suggestion of a new form of surgical therapy. Dis Chest 33:297, 1958.
52. Barnard CN, Schrire V: Surgical correction of Ebstein's malformation with prosthetic tricuspid valve. Surgery 54:302, 1963.
53. Charles RG, Barnard CN, Beck W: Tricuspid valve replacement for Ebstein's anomaly: A 19 year review of the first case. Br Heart J 46:578, 1981.
54. Hardy KL, Roe BB: Ebstein's anomaly: Further experience with definitive repair. J Thorac Cardiovasc Surg 58:553, 1969.
55. Barbero-Marcial M, Verginall, G, Awad M, et al: Surgical treatment of Ebstein's anomaly: Early and late results in twenty patients subjected to valve replacement. J Thorac Cardiovasc Surg 78:416, 1979.
56. Bove EL, Kirsh MM: Valve replacement for Ebstein's anomaly of the tricuspid valve. J Thorac Cardiovasc Surg 78:229, 1979.
57. Melo J, Saylam A, Knight R, Starr A: Long-term results after surgical correction of Ebstein's anomaly: Report of two cases. J Thorac Cardiovasc Surg 78:233, 1979.
58. Danielson GK, Fuster V: Surgical repair of Ebstein's anomaly. Ann Surg 196:499, 1982.
59. Schmidt-Habelmann P, Meisner H, Struck E, Sebening F: Results of valvuloplasty for Ebstein's anomaly. J Thorac Cardiovasc Surg 29:155, 1981.
60. Carpentier A: A new reconstructive operation for Ebstein's anomaly of the tricuspid valve. J Thorac Cardiovasc Surg 96:92, 1988.
61. Quaegebeur JM: Surgery for Ebstein's anomaly: The clinical and echocardiographic evaluation of a new technique. J Am Coll Cardiol 17:722, 1991.
62. Timmis HH, Hardy JD, Watson DG: The surgical management of Ebstein's anomaly: The combined use of tricuspid valve replacement, atrioventricular plication, and atrioplasty. J Thorac Cardiovasc Surg 53:385, 1967.
63. Danielson GK, Maloney JD, Devloo RAE: Surgical repair of Ebstein's anomaly. Mayo Clin Proc 54:185, 1979.
64. Danielson GK: Operative treatment for Ebstein's anomaly. J Thorac Cardiovasc Surg 104:1195, 1992.
65. Cappato R, Schluter M, Weiss C, et al: Radiofrequency current catheter ablation of accessory atrioventricular pathways in Ebstein's anomaly. Circulation 94:376, 1996.
66. Watson H: Natural history of Ebstein's anomaly of tricuspid valve in childhood and adolescence: An international co-operative study of 505 cases. Br Heart J 36:417, 1974.
67. Celermajer DS, Bull C, Till JA, et al: Ebstein's anomaly: Presentation from fetus to adult. J Am Coll Cardiol 23:170, 1994.
68. Littler WA: Successful pregnancy in a patient with Ebstein's anomaly. Br Heart J 32:711, 1970.
69. Waickman LA, Skorton DJ, Varnex MW, et al: Ebstein's anomaly and pregnancy. Am J Cardiol 53:357, 1984.
70. Copeland WE, Wooley CF, Ryan JM, et al: Pregnancy and congenital heart disease. Am J Obstet Gynecol 86:107, 1963.
71. Whittemore R, Hobbins JC, Engle MA: Pregnancy and its outcome in women with and without surgical treatment of congenital heart disease. Am J Cardiol 50:641, 1982.
72. Donnelly JE, Brown JM, Radford DJ: Pregnancy outcome and Ebstein's anomaly. Br Heart J 66:368, 1991.

CHAPTER 33
UNIVENTRICULAR HEART

EDUARDO A. KREUTZER   JACQUELINE KREUTZER   GUILLERMO O. KREUTZER

The univentricular heart,[1] single ventricle or "common" ventricle,[2,3] accounts for up to 2% of congenital cardiac defects,[4] predominating in males by a factor of 1.5 to 2.[2,5] For many years, the definition of a univentricular heart has been disputed by various authors (Table 33–1),[1,3,6,7] differing in terminology and characterization criteria. In 1964, Van Praagh[2] defined single ventricle as the absence of the sinus portion of a ventricular chamber, excluding tricuspid and mitral atresia. On the contrary, Anderson and colleagues[1] and Shinebourne and coworkers,[8] basing their definition on the anatomy of the atrioventricular valves[9] and the atrioventricular connections,[8,10] included hearts with one valve and more than 50% of the second valve, or more than 75% of a common atrioventricular valve, entering one ventricle.[8,9] They therefore included as univentricular hearts the single ventricle, the double-inlet ventricle with overriding atrioventricular valve of more than 50%, the unbalanced common atrioventricular canal,[11] tricuspid atresia, and mitral atresia.[8,9] Because most of these hearts have two ventricles, although one is rudimentary or hypoplastic, single ventricle seemed an inappropriate term. Therefore, the term *univentricular atrioventricular connection*[12] was proposed when two atrioventricular valves (double inlet), one common atrioventricular valve (common inlet), and one single atrioventricular valve (single inlet) are connected completely or in their greater component to a certain ventricle (Fig. 33–1). The second or additional ventricular chamber can be a hypoplastic ventricle when it has an inlet portion (less than 50% of an atrioventricular valve or less than 25% of a common atrioventricular valve), including the overriding atrioventricular valves, or a rudimentary chamber in its absence. When the rudimentary chamber is superior, it is morphologically a right ventricle (thick trabecular component); when it is posteroinferior, it is morphologically a left ventricle (fine trabeculated component).

A univentricular heart can be classified morphologically[13] as follows (Fig. 33–2; see Fig. 33–1):

I. Single ventricle, with two subtypes
   A. Single left ventricle, due to agenesis of the right ventricular inlet
   B. Single right ventricle, due to agenesis of the left ventricular inlet
II. Unbalanced ventricles with a dominant ventricular chamber, which can have either
   A. Dominant left ventricle (hypoplastic right ventricular inlet) or
   B. Dominant right ventricle (hypoplastic left ventricular inlet)

Unbalanced ventricles have more than 1.5 atrioventricular valve rings or more than 75% of a common atrioventricular valve ring aligned to a dominant right or left ventricle; the other atrioventricular valve or portion of it is aligned with a hypoplastic right or left ventricle.

EMBRYOLOGY

Comparative morphologic studies[14] suggest that single ventricle in humans does not represent an evolutionary phylogenetic regression of the human heart toward the single ventricle present in amphibian, fish, and lower reptiles but rather results from defective cardiac ontogenesis. Once cardiac looping is complete, the internal structure of the heart still consists of a single convoluted tube including atria, ventricle, bulbus cordis, and truncus arteriosus. The morphologically left ventricle is known to be derived from the ventricle of the bulboventricular loop.[14] By Streeter's stages XI to XV, the atrioventricular canal of the embryo opens entirely in the left ventricle. Thus, common inlet and double-inlet left ventricle are potentially present in human development and may represent an arrest at this stage.

The morphologic aspects of the embryogenesis of single ventricle are still controversial.[1,7,13,15] According to Van Praagh and colleagues,[13] in single left ventricle, there is agenesis of the right ventricular inlet; the right ventricle fails to evaginate from the ventricle of the bulboventricular loop, and the ventricular septum shifts toward the side of the absent right ventricle (anterior and to the right in a D-loop, anterior and to the left in an L-loop). As the ventricular septum moves beneath the infundibulum, it can create the picture of an infundibular outlet chamber. In a single or dominant right ventricle, the absent or poorly developed left ventricle makes the ventricular septum shift posteriorly and to the left in a ventricular D-loop or posteriorly and to the right in an L-loop. In these anomalies, the location of the ventricular septum away from the infundibulum generally prevents the development of an infundibular outlet chamber.

Others have suggested that double-inlet left or right ventricle results from an abnormal shift of the atrioventricular canal septum by either growth failure or excessive rightward shift. Thus, some examples of straddling atrioventricular valve can be explained as a lesser degree of abnormal positioning of the atrioventricular canal relative to the ventricular chamber.[1,7,15] (See Chapter 1.)

TABLE 33–1		
UNIVENTRICULAR HEART		
Reference	With Rudimentary Outlet Chamber	Without Rudimentary Outlet Chamber
Van Praagh[2] (1964)	Single ventricle type A	Single ventricle types B, C, and D
Lev[3] (1969)	Single or primitive ventricle	Common ventricle
De la Cruz[6,7] (1968, 1973)	Double-inlet left ventricle Double-inlet right ventricle	Common ventricle
Anderson[1] (1976)	Univentricular heart with rudimentary outlet chamber	Univentricular heart without rudimentary outlet chamber
Van Praagh[13] (1979)	Single ventricle type A	Single ventricle type B

PATHOLOGIC ANATOMY

An anatomicoclinical classification of univentricular hearts according to their atrioventricular connection is shown in Figure 33–2.

On the basis of a segmental approach to diagnosis,[8,10] a pathologic study described 22 hearts with univentricular atrioventricular connection from a total of 196 congenital heart defects[16]; of the 22, 6 were single ventricles, 6 were unbalanced ventricles (4 with dominant right ventricle and 2 with dominant left ventricle), 5 had classic tricuspid atresia, and 5 had mitral atresia.

Tricuspid atresia constitutes a typical anatomicoclinical entity among the hypoplastic right ventricles. Similarly, mitral atresia belongs to the hypoplastic left heart syndromes. In both entities, the atrial septum is aligned normally to the interventricular septum at the level of the crux of the heart. This feature allows their echocardiographic characterization. Mitral and tricuspid atresia are not considered in this chapter (see Chapters 30 and 38).

I: SINGLE VENTRICLE, WITH DOUBLE INLET OR WITH COMMON INLET

On the basis of a pathologic study of 60 hearts, single ventricle was classified by Van Praagh and colleagues[2] into four types (Fig. 33–3):

- Type A, single morphologically left ventricle, characterized by numerous fine apical trabeculations, oblique in orientation. The papillary muscles originate from the ventricular free wall, into which two atrioventricular valves drain. An infundibular outlet chamber of superior position is separated from the ventricle by the bulboventricular septum and connected to it by the bulboventricular foramen.
- Type B, single morphologically right ventricle, characterized by thick, few, coarse, and straight apical trabeculations, with septal band and moderator band extending to the papillary muscle of the conus; the atria drain through one or two atrioventricular valves.
- Type C, common ventricle, with severe deficiency of the interventricular septum.
- Type D, undetermined ventricle (diagnosed as neither left nor right ventricle).

With use of the segmental approach, single ventricle was classified according to its arterial relationships (Table 33–2): I, normal or solitus; II, D-aorta anterior; III, L-aorta anterior; IV, L-aorta posterior (inversus). In addition, the ventricular loop was differentiated as dextro (D) or levo (L), according to the ventricular situs. The atrioventricular connections, the ventriculoarterial relationships (transposition, double outlet, or single outlet), and the presence or absence of obstruction at the pulmonary or aortic level were also determined.

The original type C[2] is not currently considered a form of single ventricle because of having two well-developed ventricles with absent or extremely hypoplastic interventricular septum.[13] Type D is considered to be a single right ventricle not adequately identified.[13]

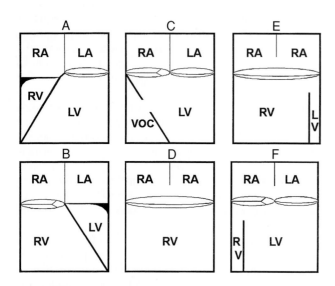

FIGURE 33–1

Schematic classification of univentricular atrioventricular connection. Atretic atrioventricular connection: tricuspid atresia *(A)* and mitral atresia *(B)*. Single ventricle: single left ventricle IA with rudimentary bulboventricular outflow chamber in anterosuperior position (right ventricle) *(C)*; single right ventricle with common atrioventricular valve and atrial dextroisomerism *(D)*. Unbalanced ventricles: dominant right ventricle with hypoplasia of the left ventricle, common atrioventricular valve, and atrial dextroisomerism *(E)*; dominant left ventricle with hypoplastic right ventricular inlet *(F)*. RA = right atrium; LA = left atrium; LV = left ventricle; VOC = ventricular outlet chamber; RV = right ventricle.

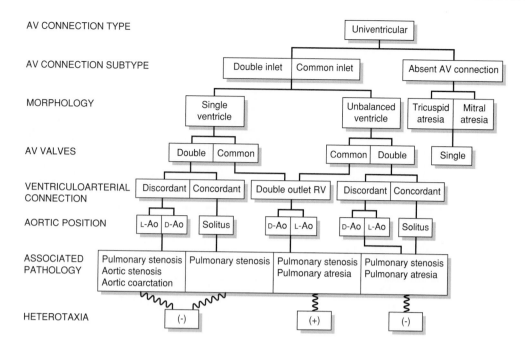

FIGURE 33–2

An anatomicoclinical classification of univentricular hearts according to their atrioventricular (AV) connection. RV = right ventricle; Ao = aorta.

IA: SINGLE LEFT VENTRICLE

Single left ventricle (Fig. 33–4) accounts for 80% of single ventricles,[2,13,17] 90% of which have an infundibular outlet chamber and discordant ventriculoarterial connections (transposition). Ventricular L-loop with L-transposition and left outlet chamber occurs in 55% of patients; ventricular D-loop with D-transposition and right-sided infundibular outlet chamber is less common (35%) (Fig. 33–4A). The remaining 10% have concordant ventriculoarterial connec-

TABLE 33–2

SEGMENTAL ANALYSIS IN SINGLE VENTRICLE
AND UNBALANCED VENTRICLES

Visceral and atrial situs	Solitus
	Inversus
	Heterotaxia
Cardiac position	Levocardia
	Dextrocardia
	Mesocardia
Atrioventricular connection	Double ventricle
	Common inlet
Ventricular morphology	Single ventricle
	Unbalanced ventricle
Ventriculoarterial connection	Discordant
	Concordant
	Double outlet
	Single outlet
Great arteries relationships	Solitus
	Inversus
	D-Aorta
	L-Aorta

tion with right-sided infundibular outlet chamber and normally related great arteries (Holmes heart[18]).

The bulboventricular foramen is restrictive in 40% of the patients with discordant ventriculoarterial connection and subaortic stenosis and in 90% of those with concordant ventriculoarterial connections (Holmes heart), causing subpulmonary stenosis. Coarctation of the aorta is associated in 15% of the patients with type IA and coexists with subaortic stenosis. Pulmonary stenosis or atresia occurs in 40% of patients.

There are usually two atrioventricular valves, right and left sided. The valve in contact with the bulboventricular septum is anatomically a tricuspid valve, and that related to the free wall of the ventricle without attachments to the septum is anatomically a mitral valve. Fibrous continuity commonly exists between the atrioventricular valves and the posterior semilunar valve. The atrioventricular valves appear "normal" in 70% of the patients but can be dysplastic with significant insufficiency (15%), more frequently of the left-sided valve. In 15% of patients, the atrioventricular valves are stenotic or even imperforate, particularly the right one.

When the infundibular outlet chamber is left sided and the ventriculoarterial connection is discordant (type IA III), the left coronary artery is usually dominant.[17] Close to its origin in the posterior and leftward aortic cusp, the left coronary gives origin to a left delimiting artery that outlines the left bulboventricular septal groove. The right coronary originates in the right aortic sinus and runs in the right atrioventricular groove, giving origin to the right delimiting artery and two to six parallel delimiting arteries that cross the anterior surface of the heart, at the site of ventriculotomy for a ventricular septation procedure. When the infundibular chamber is right sided and the ven-

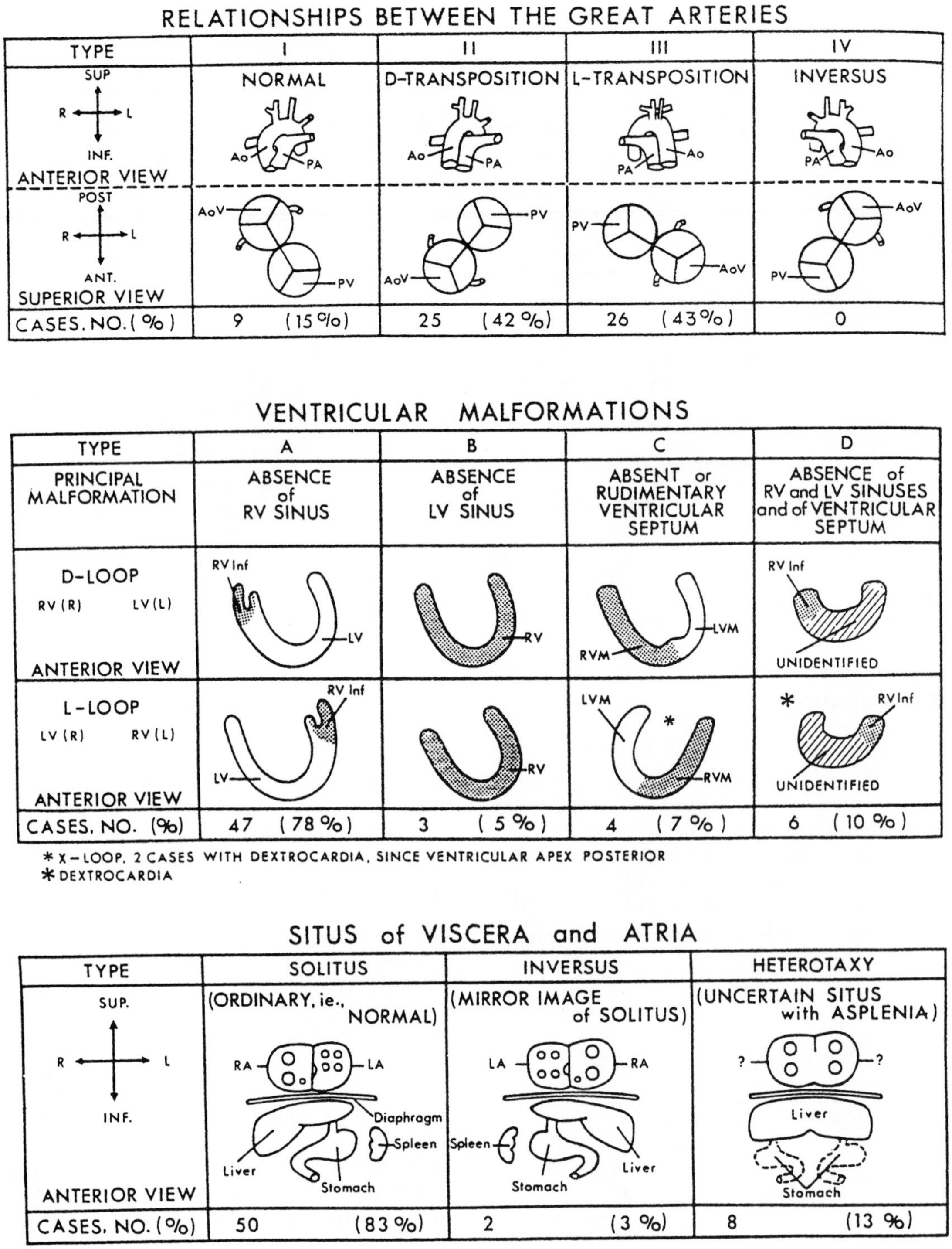

RELATIONSHIPS BETWEEN THE GREAT ARTERIES

TYPE	I	II	III	IV
ANTERIOR VIEW SUP / R—L / INF.	NORMAL	D-TRANSPOSITION	L-TRANSPOSITION	INVERSUS
SUPERIOR VIEW POST / R—L / ANT.				
CASES. NO. (%)	9 (15%)	25 (42%)	26 (43%)	0

VENTRICULAR MALFORMATIONS

TYPE	A	B	C	D
PRINCIPAL MALFORMATION	ABSENCE of RV SINUS	ABSENCE of LV SINUS	ABSENT or RUDIMENTARY VENTRICULAR SEPTUM	ABSENCE of RV and LV SINUSES and of VENTRICULAR SEPTUM
D-LOOP RV (R) LV (L) ANTERIOR VIEW				UNIDENTIFIED
L-LOOP LV (R) RV (L) ANTERIOR VIEW				UNIDENTIFIED
CASES. NO. (%)	47 (78%)	3 (5%)	4 (7%)	6 (10%)

✱ X—LOOP, 2 CASES WITH DEXTROCARDIA, SINCE VENTRICULAR APEX POSTERIOR
✱ DEXTROCARDIA

SITUS of VISCERA and ATRIA

TYPE	SOLITUS	INVERSUS	HETEROTAXY
ANTERIOR VIEW SUP. / R—L / INF.	(ORDINARY, ie., NORMAL)	(MIRROR IMAGE of SOLITUS)	(UNCERTAIN SITUS with ASPLENIA)
CASES. NO. (%)	50 (83%)	2 (3%)	8 (13%)

FIGURE 33–3

Classification of hearts with single ventricle. AoV = aortic valve; Ao = aorta; PA = pulmonary artery; PV = pulmonary valve; RV = right ventricle; LV = left ventricle; Inf = infundibulum; RVM = right ventricular mass; LVM = left ventricular mass; RA = right atrium; LA = left atrium. (Reprinted from *American Journal of Cardiology*, Volume 13, Van Praagh R, Ongley PA, Swan HJC, Anatomic types of single or common ventricle in man. Morphologic and geometric aspects of 60 necropsied cases, Pages 367–386, Copyright 1964, with permission from Excerpta Medica Inc.)

triculoarterial connection is concordant, the delimiting arteries also course around the hypoplastic infundibular chamber.

In double-inlet single ventricle, the conduction system is characterized by an accessory atrioventricular anterolateral node[19,20] localized in the floor of the right atrium, at the acute anterolateral margin of the right atrioventricular ring. Through a nonbranching long bundle, it penetrates the ring, reaches the right parietal wall of the ventricle, and passes toward the rudimentary outlet chamber, following its right edge. If the infundibular outlet chamber is left sided, the bundle crosses the outflow tract of the main chamber anteriorly toward the outlet chamber, immediately anterior and in proximity to the ring of the posterior great artery. If the outlet chamber is right sided, it crosses at the inferior and right edge of the bulboventricular foramen (Fig. 33–5).

The location of the sinoatrial node depends on the atrial situs, which is solitus in most patients, rarely ambiguous, and inversus in 1%.[21]

IB: SINGLE RIGHT VENTRICLE

A single right ventricle is present in 20% of patients with single ventricles.[2,13,22] This includes examples of double-outlet single right ventricle with or without subaortic or bilateral conus, with anterior aorta (subaortic conus) or side-by-side great vessels.

More than 90% of the patients have associated pulmonary stenosis or atresia. Among other associated anomalies are common atrioventricular valve, ambiguous atrial situs,[23,24] ostium primum atrial septal defect or common atrium, double-outlet right ventricle, anomalies of systemic venous return (interrupted inferior vena cava with azygos continuation in patients with polysplenia), inferior vena cava ipsilateral to the descending aorta (in patients with asplenia), double superior venae cavae, unroofed coronary sinus, and anomalous pulmonary venous connec-

tions of the extracardiac variety (asplenia) or at cardiac level (polysplenia) (see Fig. 33–2).[24]

II: UNBALANCED VENTRICLES

We exclude in this chapter the overriding atrioventricular valves, when the overriding into the contralateral ventricle is less than 50% of an atrioventricular valve or less than 75% of a common atrioventricular valve.[25] An unbalanced ventricle with either a dominant left ventricle[5] or hypoplasia of the left ventricular inlet (IIB) (see Figs. 33–1, 33–2, and 33–4) differs from a single ventricle[2,5] in that it has two ventricular inlet portions,[26] resulting in an unbalanced biventricular heart. One ventricle is hypoplastic or secondary, and the other is dominant or major. There can be two atrioventricular valves; a common atrioventricular valve[27]; or a single patent valve with an imperforate second atrioventricular valve, aligned to both ventricles, although predominantly to the dominant one.

Malalignment between the interventricular septum and the atrial septum, with an abnormal atrioventricular septal angle between 30 and 90 degrees (normal 10 degrees), has been described.[28]

Among patients with unbalanced ventricles, 60%[5] have an unbalanced common atrioventricular valve[11] with either a dominant right ventricle (type IIB, 71%; see Fig. 33–4B) or, less frequently, a dominant left ventricle (type IIA, 29%).[29] They are commonly associated with hetero-

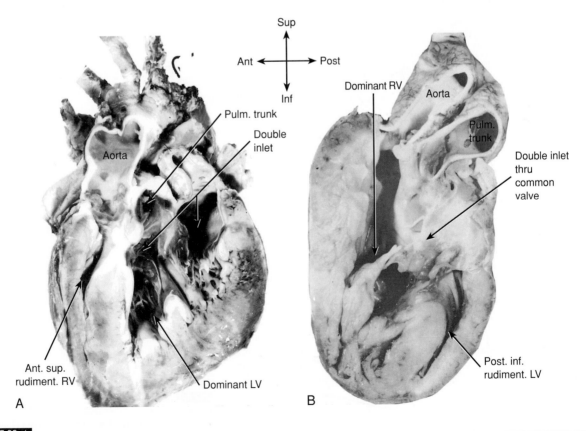

FIGURE 33–4

Parasternal long-axis sections showing the anteroposterior position of the ventricular outlet chamber in single left ventricle IA (*A*) and the posteroinferior position of the hypoplastic left ventricle in unbalanced ventricles with dominant right ventricle IIB (*B*). RV = right ventricle; LV = left ventricle; Sup = superior; Ant = anterior; Post = posterior; Inf = inferior. (*A, B* from Barra Rossi M, Ho SY, Anderson RH: Double-inlet ventricle and its relationships to heart with straddling and overriding atrioventricular valves. Rev Latina Cardiol Cirugia Cardiovasc Infant 3:171, 1986.)

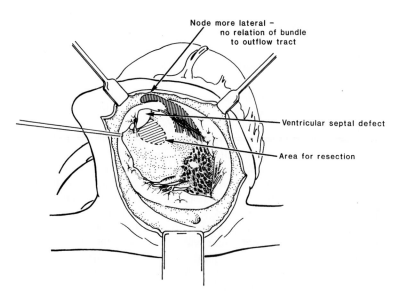

Node more lateral –
no relation of bundle
to outflow tract

Ventricular septal defect

Area for resection

A   Right sided rudimentary right ventricle

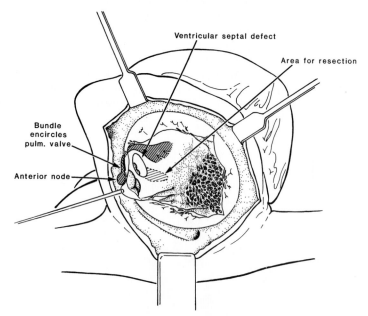

Ventricular septal defect

Area for resection

Bundle
encircles
pulm. valve

Anterior node

B   Left sided rudimentary right ventricle

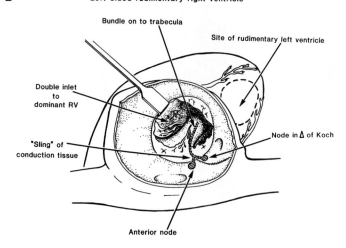

Bundle on to trabecula

Site of rudimentary left ventricle

Double inlet
to
dominant RV

Node in Δ of Koch

"Sling" of
conduction tissue

Anterior node

Right sided rudimentary left ventricle
(left hand ventricular topology)

C

FIGURE 33–5

Diagrams illustrating the conduction system in single left ventricle with right and left ventricular outlet chamber (*A, B*) and in unbalanced ventricle with dominant left ventricle (*C*). (*A, C* from Barra Rossi M, Ho SY, Anderson RH: Double-inlet ventricle and its relationships to heart with straddling and overriding atrioventricular valves. Rev Latina Cardiol Cirugia Cardiovasc Infant 13:171, 1986.)

taxia, often asplenia syndrome, and a large ostium primum atrial septal defect or a common atrium[23, 24] and other associated anomalies (see Table 33–2), such as double-outlet right ventricle and pulmonary stenosis or atresia.

Thirty percent of the patients with unbalanced ventricles have a dominant left ventricle (type IIA) with conoventricular septal defect extending into the inlet septum. The atrioventricular valves are at the same level[5] with overriding of more than 50% of the tricuspid valve and insertion into an anomalous papillary muscle from the free wall of the left ventricle (Fig. 33–6). The remaining 5 to 10% have a dominant right ventricle (type IIB) with overriding and straddling of the anterosuperior portion of the anterior leaflet of the mitral valve. The anterior mitral valve leaflet, commonly with a cleft, inserts on the anterior papillary muscle of the right ventricle through an anterior ventricular septal defect secondary to malalignment of the conal and anterior muscular septum.

When there are two atrioventricular valves, the ventriculoarterial connection is commonly discordant (70% of patients)[26] and occasionally associated with superoinferior ventricles. Double-outlet right ventricle occurs in a few patients. Rarely, the ventriculoarterial connection is concordant. In an unbalanced ventricle, the atrioventricular valves are commonly abnormal.[5] There may be a dysplastic tricuspid valve with insufficiency, a cleft or stenotic mitral valve, or a common atrioventricular valve. The last is common in patients with heterotaxia and unbalanced common atrioventricular valve into a dominant right ventricle.[24–26, 28, 29]

Heterotaxia is common in patients with unbalanced ventricle (60%) and rare in patients with single ventricle (10%). When present, more commonly it is associated with a single right ventricle.[5, 24, 29]

HEMODYNAMICS

Hemodynamic patterns in patients with a univentricular heart[30–34] depend mostly on the presence or absence of obstruction to outflow into either the aorta or pulmonary artery, the morphology and function of the single or dominant ventricle, the type of atrioventricular connection, and the function of the atrioventricular valves.

PULMONARY BLOOD FLOW. Patients without pulmonary stenosis[34] have increased pulmonary blood flow ($Qp/Qs \geq 3$) and signs of congestive heart failure that appear during the first weeks of life. Systemic oxygen saturations approximate 90% without significant clinical cyanosis. When Qp/Qs approaches 2, their cyanosis becomes mild, with oxygen saturation reaching 85%. These patients are generally well compensated hemodynamically. Patients with moderate pulmonary stenosis and Qp/Qs approaching 1 have cyanosis with oxygen saturations close to 80%. When there is severe pulmonary stenosis and Qp/Qs is less than 1, their cyanosis may become extreme with saturations of 60 to 70% or less.

Patients with coexistent pulmonary atresia present in the newborn period when the patent ductus closes spontaneously, as in other ductus-dependent lesions.

MORPHOLOGIC AND FUNCTIONAL ASPECTS OF THE SINGLE VENTRICLE. When the single or dominant ventricle is anatomically a left ventricle, ventricular dysfunction is rare, even with volume or pressure overload or chronic systemic hypoxemia. When the single or dominant ventricle is anatomically a right ventricle, it may perform adequately initially; but with volume and pressure overload, it may

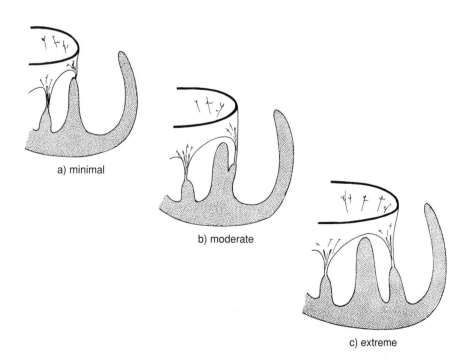

a) minimal

b) moderate

c) extreme

FIGURE 33–6

Diagram illustrating the three grades of straddling of one atrioventricular valve. (From Barra Rossi M, Ho SY, Anderson RH: Double-inlet ventricle and its relationships to heart with straddling and overriding atrioventricular valves. Rev Latina Cardiol Cirugia Cardiovasc Infant 13:171, 1986.)

evolve into a dilated myopathy because of mismatch between the ventricular mass and volume. This occurs commonly in association with progressive atrioventricular valve insufficiency.[35] The clinical scenario resembles that in other patients with a systemic right ventricle, such as those with corrected transposition or transposition of the great arteries after the Senning or Mustard procedure. Abnormal and dysplastic atrioventricular valves can also be insufficient, even without pressure or volume overload.

Rarely, a stenotic or imperforate atrioventricular valve is associated with a restrictive atrial septal defect, causing pulmonary edema early in life and requiring emergency intervention to allow left atrial decompression and adequate mixing.

SUBAORTIC OBSTRUCTION. In single ventricle type IA II or IA III, subaortic obstruction is typically due to a progressive and relative decrease of the size of the bulboventricular foramen.[31] It can also occur acutely after a sudden decrease of preload and ventricular volume when a partial right-sided heart bypass operation is performed (bidirectional Glenn), in patients after pulmonary artery banding,[32,36] or when preload normalizes in patients after total right-sided heart bypass operation.[36] Associated arch obstruction in patients with subaortic stenosis can be severe. If there is severe arch hypoplasia, patients are ductus dependent and present similarly to neonates with hypoplastic left heart syndrome.

NATURAL HISTORY

Most patients with single ventricle develop symptoms during the first weeks or months of life. Those with increased pulmonary blood flow show signs of congestive heart failure and pulmonary hypertension, whereas those with decreased pulmonary blood flow and pulmonary stenosis present with cyanosis. Without treatment by operation, death occurs in infancy in 64% of these patients; more than half die during the neonatal period.[37]

Patients with increased pulmonary blood flow[33] develop permanent pulmonary hypertensive vascular changes after the first year of life. This leads to a decrease in the Qp/Qs ratio and compensation of their congestive heart failure, followed by progressive chronic cyanosis.

Among adult survivors without surgical intervention, three quarters have pulmonary stenosis of moderate degree, and the remaining 25% have pulmonary hypertension with various levels of hypertensive pulmonary arteriopathy.[38,39] Most of the survivors have congestive heart failure and are classified as New York Heart Association class II. They typically have a single left ventricle with two well-functioning atrioventricular valves, situs solitus, nonrestrictive subaortic bulboventricular foramen, and sinus rhythm. Complete heart block develops in 20% of these patients, requiring a pacemaker.[39]

Progressive insufficiency of the atrioventricular valves is poorly tolerated in patients with univentricular heart, especially in the presence of a single or dominant right ventricle.[35]

Single ventricle can be classified into types A and C, according to the presence or absence of a rudimentary outlet

chamber.[33,34] Patients with type C have a poor prognosis, with 50% mortality 4 years after diagnosis, compared with a 50% mortality at 14 years after diagnosis for patients with type A. The cause of death in patients with type A can be congestive heart failure (20%), arrhythmia (20%), or sudden death (10%).[39] Patients with unbalanced ventricles have an even worse prognosis owing to the frequent association with heterotaxia,[25] higher incidence and severity of their pulmonary stenosis, dominant right ventricle, and insufficiency of the atrioventricular valves that can predispose to the development of ventricular dysfunction.[35]

HISTORY AND PHYSICAL EXAMINATION

The presentation of patients with univentricular heart differs according to associated lesions, particularly pulmonary or aortic stenosis. Pulmonary stenosis occurs in 60% of the patients, who develop clinical manifestations similar to those of patients with tetralogy of Fallot with or without pulmonary atresia. Rarely, the pulmonary stenosis is mild, and the patient may be acyanotic.

The remaining 40% of patients present similarly to those with an unrestrictive ventricular septal defect with increased pulmonary blood flow and pulmonary hypertension. In these patients, congestive heart failure occurs early in life.

PULMONARY STENOSIS AND LIMITED PULMONARY BLOOD FLOW. In these patients, cyanosis tends to be moderate to severe; clubbing is evident in older patients. Patients rarely have thoracic deformities. The precordium is commonly normoactive. There may be a left superior parasternal lift in patients with coexistent L-transposition. The peripheral pulses are usually normal. There is a systolic ejection murmur, the intensity and duration of which correlate directly with the amount of pulmonary blood flow and inversely with the severity of the pulmonary stenosis and level of cyanosis. The absence of a systolic ejection murmur suggests severe pulmonary stenosis or atresia. A continuous murmur from a patent ductus arteriosus or a collateral may be heard in the pulmonary areas. The second heart sound is commonly loud and single (aortic component), particularly in patients with L-transposition.

NO PULMONARY STENOSIS AND INCREASED PULMONARY BLOOD FLOW. These patients present with dyspnea, retractions, and poor weight gain secondary to congestive heart failure. Cyanosis in infancy is minimal or absent. They more commonly have thoracic deformities and a hyperdynamic precordium.

A soft systolic ejection murmur in the midprecordium with radiation to the axilla and the back represents relative pulmonary stenosis. The second heart sound is loud and single. An S_3 gallop and a mitral mid-diastolic rumble can be heard in the apex. When a systolic thrill appears at the base and suprasternal notch, subaortic stenosis secondary to a restrictive bulboventricular foramen in types A III and A II should be suspected. On auscultation in such patients, there is a harsh loud systolic ejection murmur at the base and midprecordium with radiation to the neck. If coarctation of aorta is present, the peripheral pulses are diminished or absent in the legs.

More severe pulmonary edema and congestion than could be accounted for by the amount of pulmonary blood flow or ventricular dysfunction suggest either severe stenosis or imperforation of the left atrioventricular valve with restrictive atrial septal defect or anomalous pulmonary venous connections with obstruction, particularly in patients with asplenia.

ELECTROCARDIOGRAPHY

Patients with single left ventricle, leftward bulboventricular outlet chamber, and ventricular L-loop (type IA III) have an inverted initial activation with q waves in the right precordial leads (qRS or qR in V_1) and no q waves in the left precordial leads (RS in V_6). Their QRS axis in the frontal plane is inferior and rightward, simulating left posterior hemiblock with clockwise loop[21] and qR in II, III, and aVF (Fig. 33–7A). With time, complete atrioventricular block may develop.[33] Patients with single left ventricle with rightward outflow chamber and ventricular D-loop (types IA II or IA I)[40–42] have electrocardiograms similar to those of patients with tricuspid atresia, although generally without left anterior hemiblock. The right precordial leads show an rS in V_1. There are tall R waves in the left precordial leads consistent with left ventricular hypertrophy, with or without septal depolarization q waves (qR or R in V_6, due to abnormal initial activation directed anteriorly and to the left) (Fig. 33–7B). In the frontal plane, the QRS axis is often in the left inferior quadrant.

Patients with single right ventricle (type IB) have signs of right ventricular hypertrophy in the right precordial leads with R, qR, or rsR′. The QRS axis is superior in the frontal plane with a counterclockwise loop. Rarely, the electrocardiogram may show rS waves in all the precordial leads. Patients with unbalanced ventricles commonly have a left anterior hemiblock pattern with signs of left ventricular hypertrophy when the left ventricle is dominant (type IIA). If there is a dominant right ventricle (IIB), the electrocardiogram most commonly shows right ventricular hypertrophy (Fig. 33–8).

Patients with heterotaxia and asplenia syndrome or dextroisomerism can have two sinus nodes, and those with polysplenia or levoisomerism may lack a sinus node and have a low atrial rhythm. However, the sinus node can coincide with the anatomic atrial situs in the majority of patients with asplenia.[29] Congenital complete atrioventricular block in fetal life is associated with levoisomerism and a poor prognosis.[43]

CHEST RADIOGRAPHY AND OTHER IMAGING STUDIES

Patients can be characterized by chest radiography[4, 44–46] as follows:

- *Patients with pulmonary stenosis,* normal cardiac size, and diminished pulmonary vascular markings; or

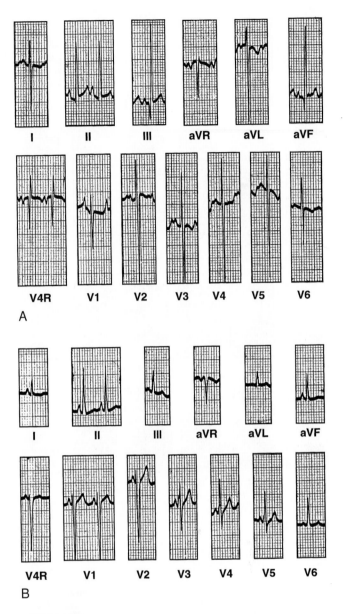

FIGURE 33–7

Electrocardiograms in patients with single left ventricle without pulmonary stenosis. *A,* Type IA III, 28 days old, with QRS axis of 105 degrees and counterclockwise loop, QR in V_4R, and no q waves in left precordial leads. *B,* Type IA II, 45 days old, with QRS axis of 45 degrees, rS in V_1, and R in V_6.

- *Patients without pulmonary stenosis,* severe cardiomegaly (cardiothoracic ratio >65%), and increased pulmonary vascular markings due to either high flow or pulmonary venous congestion (pulmonary venocapillary hypertension secondary to congestive heart failure).

An atypical chest x-ray finding may be the first indication of a complex cardiac anomaly, such as a univentricular heart, in a patient who shows clinical signs consistent with either an unrestrictive ventricular septal defect or tetralogy of Fallot (Fig. 33–9).

Patients with single ventricle typically have a cardiac silhouette with abnormal mediastinal densities, suggesting abnormal position and orientation of the great ves-

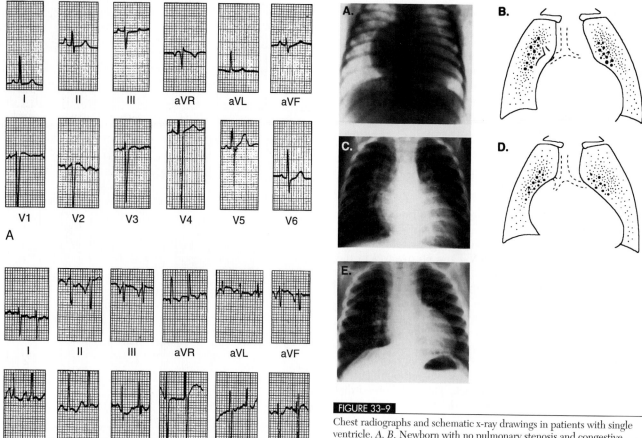

FIGURE 33–8

Electrocardiograms from patients with unbalanced ventricles. *A*, Type IIA with pulmonary stenosis: left anterior hemiblock and absent right ventricular forces in a 2-year-old patient with a double-inlet dominant left ventricle. *B*, Type IIB with pulmonary stenosis: low atrial rhythm, left anterior hemiblock, and right ventricular hypertrophy in a 1-month-old patient with polysplenia with interrupted inferior vena cava and common atrioventricular canal with a dominant right ventricle.

FIGURE 33–9

Chest radiographs and schematic x-ray drawings in patients with single ventricle. *A, B,* Newborn with no pulmonary stenosis and congestive heart failure; L-transposition. *C, D,* Infant with no pulmonary stenosis and congestive heart failure; D-transposition. *E,* A 3-year-old child with pulmonary stenosis and L-transposition.

sels.[4, 44–46] Patients with normally related great arteries often show a "triad of densities" at the superior mediastinum on chest radiography. In the frontal view, these include the ascending aorta, the transverse aortic arch and proximal descending aorta, and the pulmonary trunk.[46] The lack of ascending aorta on the right and its presence on the left can indicate L-transposition (see Fig. 33–9). A narrow superior mediastinum is commonly seen in patients with D-transposition. The left border of the heart can appear abbreviated because of a bulge in the upper third due to an inverted ventricular outlet chamber. Such a notch indicates the edge of the rudimentary outflow chamber located leftward and superior.[46] A left anterior oblique projection demonstrating a hypoplastic right ventricle, with enlargement of the left ventricle, supports the diagnosis of single left ventricle with outflow chamber.

An unbalanced complete atrioventricular canal is suspected on chest radiography in patients with associated abdominal and cardiac malpositions, such as dextrocardia or mesocardia, suggesting heterotaxia. In these patients, dextroisomerism is more common; cardiac anatomy reveals an unbalanced canal with dominant right ventricle and double-outlet right ventricle, with absent or hypoplastic left ventricle.

The development of progressive cardiomegaly in an older patient suggests the onset of dilated myopathy. Signs of pulmonary venous hypertension out of proportion to the amount of pulmonary blood flow can be observed when there is insufficiency or stenosis of the left atrioventricular valve with a restrictive atrial septal defect or when there is anomalous pulmonary venous return with obstruction, most likely in patients with asplenia.

More recently,[47, 48] magnetic resonance imaging with the SPAMM (spatial modulation of magnetization) technique has allowed the study of right ventricular regional wall motion and strain analysis in patients at different stages of bypass of the venous ventricle. With this method, it is possible to compare ventricular mechanics of patients with a single ventricle with those in patients with a systemic right ventricle after a Senning procedure and to study ventriculoventricular interactions. In both groups, there were abnormalities in regional myocardial strain, twisting motion, and regional radial motion. In patients with a univentricular right heart, the lack of ventriculoventricular interaction determined by inferior wall paradoxical systolic wall motion is different from that observed in patients with a Senning operation, in whom paradoxical septal motion occurs.

The abnormalities in ventricular mechanics and geometry secondary to stress, strain, and regional twist in univentricular hearts with a right ventricular anatomy are similar to those in hearts with a left ventricular anatomy.[47] Such changes in ventricular mechanics generate a regional increase in oxygen consumption, which may play a role in the development of ventricular dysfunction.

In addition, magnetic resonance imaging may be useful for defining anatomy before and after a total right-sided heart bypass operation (Fig. 33–10).

ECHOCARDIOGRAPHY

Two-dimensional echocardiography allows sequential determination of thoracoabdominal situs, atrioventricular and ventriculoarterial alignments and connections, morphology and function of the single ventricle or dominant ventricle and atrioventricular valves, position of the infundibular outlet chamber and size of the bulboventricular foramen, and associated cardiac defects.

The thoracoabdominal situs is determined from a subxiphoid window, in a transverse view at the level of the 12th thoracic vertebral space, by analyzing the location of the inferior vena cava and the descending aorta relative to the spine. A second superior vena cava and communicating vein can be investigated from a high parasternal view. From an apical four-chamber view, scanning from posterior to anterior, the atrioventricular connection is demonstrated.[5, 49–53] Patients with a single ventricle can have either two atrioventricular valves positioned at the same

level (Fig. 33–11)[5] or, rarely, one common atrioventricular valve aligned to the only ventricular chamber. In a short-axis view, the morphologic aspects of each valve can be analyzed, including the number of leaflets and their attachments and relationship to each other. In addition, the position of the infundibular outlet chamber can be determined; it is always superior in patients with single left ventricle. The morphologic character of the ventricle can also be diagnosed by echocardiography, by finding either left ventricular thin trabeculations or right ventricular thick trabeculations and moderator band.

From parasternal long-axis, subxiphoid long-axis, and oblique views, the ventriculoarterial relationship is identified. Patients with single left ventricle usually have a posterior pulmonary artery and an anterior aorta arising from the infundibular outlet chamber. In patients with a Holmes heart, the pulmonary artery is anterior and aligned to the infundibular outlet chamber. The aorta is posterior, aligned to the single left ventricle, and has fibrous continuity with the atrioventricular valve.

From these projections, the size of the bulboventricular foramen is determined[51] by the ellipse formula

$$\frac{\pi D_1 D_2}{4} \text{ per m}^2$$

A measurement of less than 2 cm²/m² is consistent with a restrictive bulboventricular foramen. Although the gradient may be underestimated by continuous-wave Doppler study, color Doppler examination may localize the site of turbulent flow and the highest gradient. If the Doppler gradient is more than 1.5 m/sec, the bulboventricular foramen is considered to be restrictive.[51]

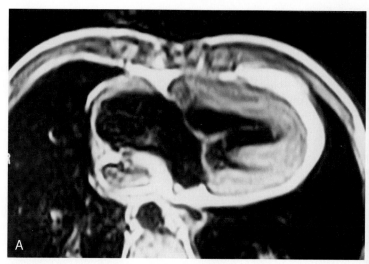
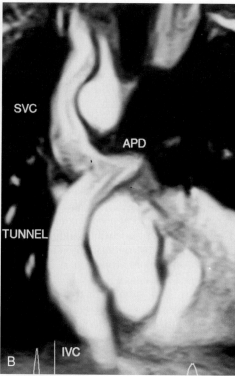

FIGURE 33–10

A, Transverse image obtained by magnetic resonance in a patient with unbalanced ventricles (IIB) with a common atrioventricular canal and right ventricular dominance of more than 75% of the common atrioventricular valve aligned with the right ventricle. Note the hypoplastic posterior left ventricle. *B*, Cine magnetic resonance imaging in a coronal plane of a total cavopulmonary anastomosis through a right-sided intra-atrial lateral tunnel showing widely patent anastomoses. Note direct anastomosis of the superior vena cava (SVC) to the right pulmonary artery (APD) and anastomosis of the inferior vena cava (IVC) to the right pulmonary artery through the intra-atrial tunnel (TUNNEL).

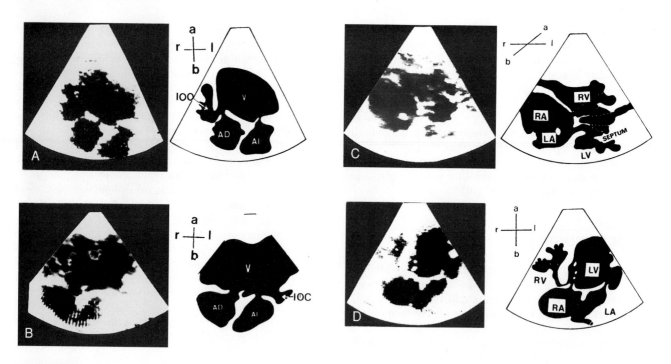

FIGURE 33–11

Echocardiographic views obtained in apical four-chamber view in patients with single left ventricle (*A, B*) and in patients with unbalanced ventricles (*C, D*). *A,* The atrioventricular valves are level, with the annuli at the same plane, aligned with the left ventricle; note the malalignment between inter-atrial and interventricular septum and the right-sided infundibular outlet chamber. *B,* Similar to *A* but with a left-sided infundibular outlet chamber. *C,* Common atrioventricular canal with dominant right ventricle (IIB) and common atrium (atrial dextroisomerism) with common atrioventricular valve aligned almost exclusively with the right ventricle. Note the marked malalignment of the interventricular septum resulting in a hypoplastic left ventri-cle. *D,* Double-inlet unbalanced ventricle with dominant left ventricle (IIA), both atrioventricular valve annuli at the same level, marked malalignment of the interventricular septum, and more than 50% of the tricuspid valve and all the mitral valve aligned to the left ventricle. AD/RA = right atrium; AI/LA = left atrium; V = single ventricle; IOC = infundibular outlet chamber; a = anterior; b = posterior; r = right; l = left; RV = right ventricle; LV = left ventricle. (*A–D* from Binello MM, Roman MI, Granja M, et al: Diferenciacion ecocardiográfica (2-D) de la conexión auriculoventricular en el corazón univentricular, doble entrada ventricular y cabalgamiento auriculoventricular. Implicacias quirurgicas. Rev Latina Cardiol Cirurgia Cardio-vasc Infant 1:25, 1985.)

The morphologic features of the ventricular septal de-fect in patients with unbalanced ventricles and dominant left ventricle (type IIA) can be determined from an apical four-chamber view. Conoventricular septal defects extend to the inlet septum when there is additional malalignment of the ventricular septum to the atrial septum. In such pa-tients, the atrioventricular valve and more than 50% of the second one or more than 75% of a common atrioventricu-lar valve are aligned to the left ventricle (see Fig. 33–11). Patients with dominant right ventricle (type IIB) and com-mon atrioventricular valve also have a primum atrial septal defect.

An unbalanced common atrioventricular canal is best diagnosed from an apical four-chamber view. From a parasternal short-axis view, a small component of the atrio-ventricular valve ring is identified aligned to a hypoplastic left ventricle. A double-outlet right ventricle can be diag-nosed from a subxiphoid projection.

The maximal instantaneous gradients at aortic, subaor-tic, pulmonary, and subpulmonary levels are examined with continuous-wave Doppler study. The function of the atrioventricular valves is examined by color Doppler study.

TRANSESOPHAGEAL ECHOCARDIOGRAPHY. This is particularly indicated for patients with poor echocardio-graphic windows, although patients with adequate trans-

thoracic echocardiogram may also benefit from this diag-nostic tool. A high horizontal plane allows anatomic determination of the atrial appendages and atrioventricu-lar connections. A transgastric short-axis view allows verifi-cation of the atrioventricular connections and gradients across the ventricular outflow tracts.

CATHETERIZATION AND ANGIOGRAPHY

DIAGNOSTIC CARDIAC CATHETERIZATION

Cardiac catheterization and angiography in patients with single ventricle[33,54,55] or unbalanced ventricles[56,57] pro-vide anatomic and hemodynamic information necessary for management. Diagnostic anatomic data, which corrob-orate the results of noninvasive diagnostic tests, include the following:

1. Atrial situs.
2. Systemic venous connections (an additional supe-rior vena cava, innominate vein, site of entry of the inferior vena cava and hepatic veins, interrupted inferior vena cava with azygos continuation).
3. Pulmonary venous connections.
4. Atrioventricular valves and connections.[57] These can be recognized by cineangiocardiography, through

demonstration of anterograde flow through the atrioventricular valves during atrial injection or, more commonly, ventricular injection (unopacified blood). Valvar morphology can be determined by trapping of contrast material underneath the valve leaflet, by delineating the valve ring, or from the configuration of the closed valve after ventricular opacification or as a curved or lineal tangential defect if the valve is stenotic. A large valve annulus suggests either single or common atrioventricular valve, whereas when it is small, a hypoplastic or stenotic valve is likely. The relationship of the atrioventricular valves to the semilunar valves and degree of development of the conal septum (mitral to aortic continuity rules out subaortic conus) are delineated by a ventriculogram. A gooseneck deformity in a left ventriculogram is seen in patients with atrioventricular septal defect.[57]

5. Morphologic aspects of the single or dominant ventricle, infundibular outlet chamber, and hypoplastic rudimentary ventricle. A left ventriculogram in four-chamber view demonstrates the absence of the posterior ventricular septum in single left ventricle (type IA) (Fig. 33–12) or a malaligned interventricular posterior septum in unbalanced ventricles with a dominant left ventricle (type IIA) (Fig. 33–13).

6. Pulmonary or systemic obstruction (restrictive bulboventricular foramen, stenotic pulmonary or aortic valve).

7. Ventriculoarterial alignments and connections.

8. Anatomy of the pulmonary arteries (size of central pulmonary arteries, Nakata index[58] and McGoon ratio,[59] arborization abnormalities and branch pulmonary artery

stenosis, washing out of contrast medium by competing flow from aortopulmonary collaterals, pulmonary transit time, and arteriovenous fistulae).

9. Aortic arch anatomy, branching abnormalities, and any aortopulmonary collaterals.

10. Ventricular function (ejection fraction) and ventricular geometry (mass/volume relationship).

After any surgical procedure, a diagnostic cardiac catheterization should be performed to rule out sequelae from prior operations, such as acquired pulmonary artery stenosis at the site of previous shunt or pulmonary artery banding, pulmonary arteriovenous fistulae in patients with partial right ventricular bypass (classic Glenn, bidirectional Glenn, or Kawashima operation),[60] cavocaval or cavoportal[61] decompressing venous collaterals after partial right-sided heart bypass, sources of right-to-left shunt after a total right-sided heart bypass through fenestration, interatrial communications,[62] and baffle leaks or left-to-right shunts by aortopulmonary collaterals.[63]

A complete hemodynamic study is essential in all patients with univentricular heart before a partial or total right-sided heart bypass operation. It is necessary to use two pressure transducers to record the transpulmonary gradient accurately by simultaneous recording of pulmonary artery and pulmonary venous, left atrial or left ventricular end-diastolic pressures. Oxygen consumption should be measured in all patients. The patient should ideally be sedated but breathing spontaneously, without acidosis to avoid an elevation of the estimated pulmonary vascular resistance. Two sets of hemodynamic data should be collected and be consistent. Because major management decisions depend on the hemodynamic data, these should be collected with the utmost precision and accuracy. As a

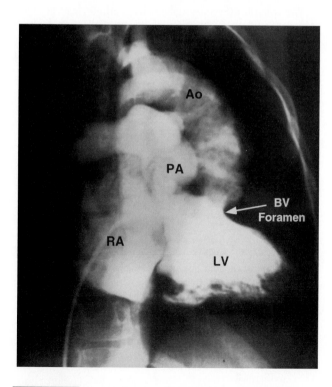

FIGURE 33–12

Angiocardiogram in the frontal plane in a patient with single left ventricle (LV) and L-transposition (IA I). PA = pulmonary trunk; Ao = aorta; RA = right atrium; BV = bulboventricular. (From Elliot LP, Schiebler GH: The X-Ray Diagnosis of Congenital Heart Disease in Infants, Children and Adults. Springfield, IL, Charles C Thomas, 1979. Courtesy of Charles C Thomas, Publisher, Ltd., Springfield, Illinois.)

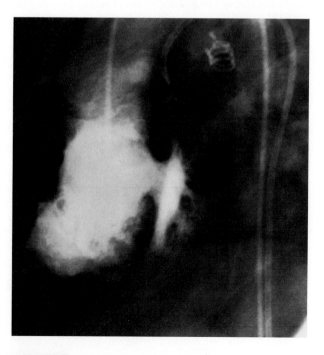

FIGURE 33–13

Angiocardiogram in a patient with unbalanced common atrioventricular canal and dominant right ventricle. There is double-outlet right ventricle and a hypoplastic posteroinferior left ventricle. Lateral view.

result, pulmonary arterial pressure, pulmonary vascular resistance, Qp/Qs ratio, and functional data evaluating ventricular mechanics (ventricular end-diastolic pressure, preload, and afterload) will be determined and calculated.

INTERVENTIONAL CARDIAC CATHETERIZATION

Patients with univentricular heart may require a transcatheter intervention early in their course and before the initial palliative surgical procedure if they have a restrictive atrial septal defect and left atrial outlet atresia or stenosis. Transcatheter creation of a new atrial septal defect with septostomy and balloon septoplasty may allow left atrial decompression and significant preoperative hemodynamic improvement, with reduction in the pulmonary venous congestion and pulmonary vascular resistance. Ductus-dependent patients awaiting cardiac transplantation have been managed by some with stent placement in the ductus arteriosus. The high risk of vessel damage and technical difficulties of this procedure, however, significantly limit its use and indications.

Patients with severe pulmonary stenosis or atresia may have pulmonary arteries that are inadequate to allow future partial or total right-sided heart bypass. Transcatheter pulmonary artery rehabilitation through serial balloon dilatation procedures may be the only option for these patients to become candidates for a right-sided heart bypass procedure, because they are otherwise not good heart transplant candidates.

If a source of potentially detrimental postoperative right-to-left or left-to-right shunting is identified during cardiac catheterization, transcatheter closure is indicated.[64] Examples are a small persistent left superior vena cava draining to the coronary sinus (in the absence of coronary sinus ostia stenosis or atresia), other potential decompressing venous connections (particularly in patients with heterotaxia), and aortopulmonary collaterals.

After a partial or total right-sided heart bypass operation, interventional cardiac catheterization plays a significant role in optimizing hemodynamics and is particularly indicated in symptomatic patients. Many abnormalities are amenable to treatment by transcatheter techniques (Table 33–3). Sometimes, emergency cardiac catheterization in the immediate postoperative period is required in a severely compromised patient to create a new or augment the prior baffle fenestration,[65] to close a baffle leak, or to balloon dilate a stenotic vessel.

At other times, interventions are performed later in the postoperative period. Interventions can be for a coexistent cardiac abnormality. Examples are coil embolization of a small persistent left superior vena cava or aortopulmonary collaterals,[63, 64] balloon dilatation of congenital peripheral pulmonary artery stenosis, and rarely pulmonary valvotomy or balloon dilatation of a native coarctation in selected high-risk surgical patients. Interventions may be performed on postoperative abnormalities,[64–67] such as branch pulmonary artery balloon dilatation or stent placement at a prior shunt insertion site, coil embolization of a patent aortopulmonary shunt and acquired aortopulmonary collaterals after prior thoracotomy, transcatheter closure of residual anterograde flow through the pulmonary valve, coil embolization of decompressing venous collaterals, transcatheter closure of fenestration or baffle leaks, and balloon dilatation of postoperative coarctation (Table 33–4; see also Table 33–3).

The role of interventional cardiac catheterization as adjunct to operation in the management of these patients is clearly illustrated by transcatheter closure of a surgically created baffle fenestration after a total right-sided heart bypass procedure.[66, 67] In such patients, a complete hemo-

---

TABLE 33–3		
"ABNORMALITIES" IN THE TOTAL RIGHT-SIDED HEART BYPASS CIRCULATION		
Obstructions	Ventricular pressure overload	Cardiac: outflow tract obstruction, aortic valve stenosis
		Systemic arterial: arch obstructions, systemic hypertension
	Systemic venous pressure overload	Systemic venous: baffle stenosis
		Pulmonary arterial: branch pulmonary artery stenosis, high pulmonary vascular resistance
		Pulmonary venous: stenosis of pulmonary veins (intrinsic or extrinsic by compression)
Shunts	*Right-to-left shunt* Cyanosis	Cardiac: fenestration, interatrial communications, decompressing veins to left atrium
		Systemic venous: decompressing venous collaterals
		Pulmonary arterial: arteriovenous malformations
	Left-to-right shunt Ventricular volume overload	Cardiac: residual anterograde flow into main pulmonary artery, patch leak in atriopulmonary anastomosis with tricuspid valve patch
		Systemic arterial: aortopulmonary collaterals, residual patent ductus arteriosus or surgical grafts
Pump failure or dysfunction		Cardiomyopathy causing systolic or diastolic dysfunction, arrhythmias, atrioventricular valve insufficiency

TABLE 33–4

SUGGESTED SEQUENTIAL STEPS FOR TRANSCATHETER
FENESTRATION CLOSURE

1	Determine RA or PA and AO saturations and pressures at baseline.
2	Test balloon occlusion for 10 minutes.
3	Determine RA or PA and AO saturations and pressures during balloon occlusion of the fenestration (after 10 minutes).
4	If RA pressures > 16 mm Hg and CI decreases to <2 L/min/m², the fenestration is left open. If RA pressure < 16 mm Hg and CI > 2 L/min/m², the fenestration may be closed.

AO = aorta; CI = cardiac index; PA = pulmonary artery; RA = right atrium.

dynamic study is performed, including test balloon occlusion of the fenestration. If this is well tolerated (see Table 33–4), transcatheter closure is indicated.

MANAGEMENT

In patients with two functioning ventricles, a right ventricle allows an increase in the cardiac output with exercise without increasing systemic venous and ventricular end-diastolic pressures.[68] Ventricular septation developed 165 million years ago, when the right ventricle appeared in reptiles and birds to allow adaptation to air breathing, aerobic exercise, and flying.[69] Patients with univentricular circulation lack this important mechanism of adaptation to aerobic exercise.

The initial objective in the management of patients with univentricular hearts is to protect the pulmonary vasculature and ventricular function, keeping pulmonary artery pressures low while allowing adequate systemic oxygen saturation (≥80%). Early in life, this can be achieved by either a pulmonary artery banding or a Blalock-Taussig shunt (Table 33–5).

Three different types of "corrective" operations have been proposed for these patients. Theoretically, ventricular septation[70] would be ideal, although it is possible only if there are two normal atrioventricular valves with adequate distribution of papillary muscles and attachments to allow repartitioning. The technical difficulties and high early and late mortality have significantly restricted ventricular septation to rare patients with both ideal anatomy and major risk factors that contraindicate a right-sided heart bypass procedure. Ventricular septation has been performed in patients with univentricular heart type IA III, normal atrioventricular valves, nonrestrictive bulboventricular foramen, no prior palliative operations, chronic cyanosis, and severe polycythemia. An additional requirement is a diastolic ventricular volume of 250% larger than that estimated for a normal left ventricle.[70] This procedure is also possible in patients with common ventricle (type C of Van Praagh and colleagues[2]) because there are two well-developed ventricles with markedly deficient interventricular septum.

As a second option, some patients with univentricular heart may undergo cardiac transplantation. The most commonly used surgical approach to manage these patients, however, is to perform a partial or total right-sided heart bypass.

SURGICAL MANAGEMENT

Initial Palliative Surgery
Patients with severe pulmonary stenosis or pulmonary atresia presenting in the neonatal period with marked hypoxia (PO₂ < 30 mm Hg) require prostaglandin E₁ to increase pulmonary blood flow through a patent ductus, until an aortopulmonary shunt is performed. Similarly, those with aortic arch hypoplasia or severe coarctation require prostaglandin infusion until arch reconstruction is performed.

TABLE 33–5

MANAGEMENT ALGORITHM FOR PATIENTS WITH UNIVENTRICULAR HEART

Age	Qp↑		Qp↓	
<3 mo	No AS, subAS (adequate BVF area), and no PS:	AS or subAS and arch hypoplasia:	No AS, subAS, or arch hypoplasia:	AS, subAS, and arch hypoplasia:
	PA banding ± coarctation repair	BT shunt + Stansel ± arch repair	BT shunt	BT shunt + Stansel ± arch repair
	Cardiac catheterization			
>3 mo <2 yr	Pulsatile or nonpulsatile bidirectional Glenn (±takedown of Blalock-Taussig shunt) ±Stansel ±BVF resection ±Plasty of the atrioventricular valve ±Pulmonary artery branch plasty			
	Cardiac catheterization			
>2 yr*	Total right-sided heart bypass (±fenestration)			

Qp↑ = increased pulmonary blood flow; Qp↓ = diminished pulmonary blood flow; AS = aortic stenosis; subAS = subaortic stenosis; BVF = bulboventricular foramen; PA = pulmonary artery; PS = pulmonary stenosis; BT shunt = modified Blalock-Taussig shunt. Stansel = Damus-Kaye-Stansel operation.
*According to institutional preferences, this age may be variable. At the Hospital de Niños of Buenos Aires, the timing of the total right-sided heart bypass tends to be postponed until 4 or 5 years of age according to the patient's saturations.

Neonates with increased pulmonary blood flow, elevated pulmonary artery pressures, and congestive cardiac failure need specific manipulation of the pulmonary vascular resistance by the intensivist to maintain an adequate preoperative Qp/Qs ratio, allowing sufficient systemic perfusion while reducing pulmonary blood flow.[34,71] This may be achieved either by use of a closed hood,[72] to increase inspired PCO_2 and pulmonary vascular resistance, or by hypoventilation using mechanical ventilation, sedation, and paralysis. In some patients, this is accompanied by a low inspired FIO_2 (<21%). Supplemental oxygen and hyperventilation should be avoided, as should any factor that could lower the pulmonary vascular resistance. Once patients are hemodynamically compensated, an initial palliative operation is performed (see Table 33–5). When pulmonary artery banding is indicated, this is achieved leaving a luminal diameter of 21 mm + 1 mm/kg of body weight.[73] The intraoperative distal pulmonary artery pressure measurement should be about 50% of the systemic pressure. If the oxygen saturation drops below 80% or the patient develops bradycardia in the operating room, the band should be made looser. If the banding is unsuitable because of either marked cyanosis (PO_2 of <30 mm Hg) or persistent high pulmonary blood flow (oxygen saturation of >85%, or high pulmonary venous flow velocity by echocardiography of >0.7 m/sec and transmitral flow of E >1 m/sec), a second procedure to revise the banding is indicated.

The early operative mortality for the initial palliative procedures in neonates is 17%.[71] If an aortopulmonary shunt is performed after the neonatal period, the mortality is significantly lower. The early operative mortality in a neonate varies, depending on the severity of the patient's condition and associated cardiac malformations; it ranges from 8 to 47%[71] in those neonates who require additional surgical procedures, such as aortic arch reconstruction or procedures to relieve subaortic stenosis.

After pulmonary artery banding, the reduction in the ventricular volume can decrease the size of the bulboventricular foramen, and subaortic stenosis may develop. This occurs in up to 73% of the patients with transposition,[74] for whom pulmonary artery banding should be avoided whenever there is a risk for development of subaortic stenosis.

In the intermediate and long-term follow-up of patients after the initial palliative procedure, ventricular dysfunction may become significant.[75] The increase in preload relative to the ventricular volumes at end of systole and diastole (2.5 to 3 times normal) causes a reduction in the long-axis/short-axis relationship (normal, 1.9 to 1), so that the ventricle becomes rounder, with increase in the end-systolic stress (afterload) and reduction of ventricular function, mass/volume relationship, and ventricular contractility.[75]

Second-Stage Palliative Surgery: Partial Right-Sided Heart Bypass

A partial right-sided heart bypass can be performed by a right cavopulmonary anastomosis, as proposed by Glenn[76] in 1958 and Bakulev and Kolesnikov.[77] This concept was extended by Hopkins and coworkers[78] in 1985 to a bidirectional cavopulmonary connection.

This operation can be performed with standby cardiopulmonary bypass, except when other intracardiac procedures are performed concomitantly, for example, atrioventricular valvuloplasty, augmentation of the bulboventricular foramen, Damus-Kaye-Stansel procedure (Fig. 33–14), or branch pulmonary arterioplasty.

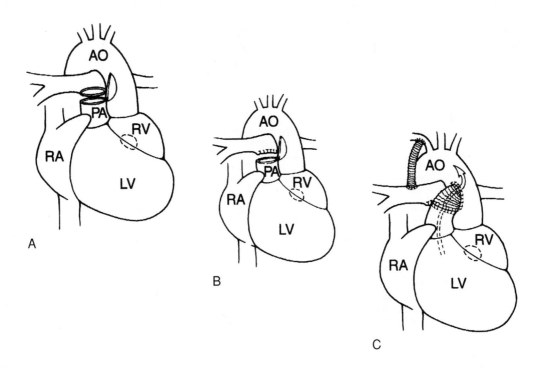

FIGURE 33–14

Damus-Kaye-Stansel anastomosis for single ventricle and subaortic stenosis. *A*, The pulmonary artery (PA) is transected proximal to the bifurcation. An appropriately positioned and sized incision is made in the ascending aorta (AO). *B*, The distal end of the pulmonary artery is oversewn, and the proximal end of the pulmonary artery is anastomosed to the opening in the aorta. *C*, An appropriately shaped hood (Dacron tube, pericardium, allograft, or Gore-Tex) is added to the anastomosis. A systemic–pulmonary artery shunt has been completed. RV = right ventricle; RA = right atrium; LV = left ventricle. (*A–C* from Park MK: Pediatric Cardiology for Practitioners, 3rd ed. St. Louis, Mosby, 1996, p 234.)

TABLE 33–6

RISK FACTORS FOR A TOTAL RIGHT-SIDED HEART BYPASS OPERATION: PROPOSED INCREMENTAL RISK SCALE

Risk Factor	No Incremental Risk	Moderate Increase in Risk	High Risk
Age	<2 yr°	<1.5 yr	<1 yr
Mean PA pressure	<15 mm Hg	≥15 < 18 mm Hg	≥18 mm Hg
McGoon index†	>2.4	>1.8 < 2.4	<1.8
Pulmonary vascular resistance (PVR)	<2 Wood units	>2 < 3 Wood units	>3 Wood units
Transpulmonary gradient	<6 mm Hg	>6 < 12 mm Hg	>12 mm Hg
Ventricular end-diastolic pressure (VEDP)	<10 mm Hg	>10 < 14 mm Hg	>14 mm Hg
Ejection fraction	>60	45–60	<45
AV valve insufficiency	None or mild	Moderate	Severe
Heterotaxia	No heterotaxia	Polysplenia	Asplenia
History of PA banding	No PA banding	Yes	PA band associated with branch PA stenosis
Mayo Clinic index‡	<2	2–4	>4
Nakata index§	>250	250–200	<200
PA stenosis	None	Mild to moderate	Severe
Restrictive BVF	No restriction	Mild (<30 mm Hg)	Moderate to severe (>30 mm Hg)
Left AV valve	Normal	Stenosis	Atresia valve

AV = atrioventricular; BVF = bulboventricular foramen; PA = pulmonary artery.
°According to institutional preferences, this age may be variable. At the Hospital de Niños of Buenos Aires, the cutoff age between low and moderate risk is considered 4 years.
†McGoon index: RPA (mm) + LPA (mm) / descending aorta at the diaphragm (mm).
‡Mayo Clinic index: PVR (Wood units) + VEDP (mm Hg) / Qp (L/min/m²) + Qs (L/min/m²).
§Nakata index: RPA + LPA (mm²/m²).

To optimize pulmonary blood flow distribution, the cavopulmonary anastomosis should be placed as centrally as possible. An end-to-side anastomosis is performed with readsorbable suture, interrupted in four quadrants. The azygos vein and, when present, the hemiazygos are always divided.

Pulsatility can be allowed by leaving anterograde flow across a restrictive open pulmonary outflow tract or a patent modified Blalock shunt, predominantly perfusing the contralateral lung.[79] When anterograde flow is retained, a pulmonary artery band is adjusted over a 3-mm Hegar bougie to control the amount of pulmonary blood flow.

Pulmonary artery branch plasty can be performed with untreated autologous pericardium. In patients who require pulmonary plasty, it is preferable to leave a source of pulsatility. To correct a restrictive bulboventricular foramen, a Damus-Kaye-Stansel procedure or a partial resection of the bulboventricular foramen may be performed (see Fig. 33–14). Atrioventricular valve insufficiency is a difficult problem and is considered to be a significant risk factor, probably because of its association with ventricular dysfunction. When two atrioventricular valves are present and one of them is normal in size and function, closure of the incompetent one may be considered. A valve ring annuloplasty can be performed in the remaining atrioventricular valve to avoid its dilatation secondary to ventricular enlargement. If there is an insufficient single or common atrioventricular valve, an attempt at valvoplasty or even valve replacement may be undertaken.

In patients with both right and left superior venae cavae and no significant communicating vein, the cavopulmonary anastomosis should be performed bilaterally. Around 3 months of age, after cardiac catheterization and angiocardiography to identify risk factors for right-sided heart bypass (Table 33–6), a bidirectional cavopulmonary anastomosis is performed. Severe high-risk factors, such as Nakata index below 120 mm²/m², severe ventricular dysfunction, and severe peripheral pulmonary artery stenosis with distal hypoplasia, contraindicate the operation.

After partial right-sided heart bypass, there is a more efficient pulmonary blood flow, as the Qp becomes effective blood flow (Qe), allowing adequate systemic oxygen saturation (80 to 85%) and a reduction in preload and atrial filling pressures.[80] An aortopulmonary shunt, which requires a Qp/Qs ratio greater than 2 to keep oxygen saturation above 80%, is replaced by a hemodynamically advantageous system that allows adequate saturations with a Qp/Qs ratio less than 1, with no recirculation of blood,[81] while reducing the ventricular volume load and preserving ventricular function.[82, 83] A long-standing ventricular volume overload in patients with aortopulmonary shunts can lead to dilated myopathy and ventricular dysfunction,[35, 84] particularly in those patients with single right ventricle and atrioventricular valve insufficiency. The change in ventricular geometry after a bidirectional Glenn anastomosis (decrease in ventricular volume and increase in the ventricular mass/volume ratio) results in an immediate 25% reduction in the area of the bulboventricular foramen.[85] This frequently produces subaortic stenosis in patients with transposition.[74] Similarly, after a total right-sided heart bypass,[85] such change in ventricular geometry causes a 40% reduction in the bulboventricular foramen size.

A bidirectional Glenn anastomosis is pulsatile when there is additional pulmonary blood flow from a shunt or anterograde flow across the pulmonary valve. In these, the systemic oxygen saturation tends to be higher, but at the expense of some ventricular volume overload and higher pulmonary artery pressures. A pulsatile bidirectional Glenn anastomosis is particularly indicated for patients with small or stenotic pulmonary arteries, in whom a simultaneous pulmonary arterioplasty is performed. If there is significant atrioventricular valve insufficiency and depressed ventricular function, or if the intraoperative superior vena caval pressure is higher than 14 mm Hg, any source of pulsatility should be eliminated.

The technique described by Kawashima[86] can be employed in patients with heterotaxia, interrupted inferior vena cava, and azygos or hemiazygos continuation. After the operation, all systemic venous return, except for the hepatic veins, is directed to the pulmonary arteries. This should be considered a partial right-sided heart bypass operation, because the hepatic venous flow is still excluded from the pulmonary circulation.

RESULTS OF PARTIAL RIGHT-SIDED HEART BYPASS (Table 33–7)
LUNG PERFUSION SCAN. The distribution of pulmonary blood flow after a cavopulmonary connection is preferentially to the ipsilateral pulmonary artery.[87,88] At lung scintigraphy, with upper extremity intravenous isotope injection, both the pulsatile and nonpulsatile bidirectional Glenn procedures show dominant perfusion of the ipsilateral pulmonary artery, and this is reproduced during exercise. With time, this distribution could lead to relative hypoplasia of the contralateral pulmonary artery.[89] Other late complications after a bidirectional Glenn anastomosis include the development of pulmonary arteriovenous microfistulae,[60,90] 50 to 100 μm in diameter, particularly in the lower lobes, which are the best perfused areas. The lack of hepatic flow in the pulmonary circulation has been postulated in their pathogenesis.[60] An additional source of pulmonary blood flow providing pulsatility as well as blood flow that has passed through the liver may prevent the development of these fistulae. In addition, a larger amount of pulmonary blood flow and the pulsatility may play a role in pulmonary arterial growth.[82,91,92] Thus, when possible, a pulsatile bidirectional Glenn anastomosis is preferred[79] with use of a controlled source of pulmonary blood flow, keeping the pulmonary artery mean pressure below 14 mm Hg and a pulsatility amplitude less than 5 mm Hg higher than the mean pulmonary artery pressure.

DOPPLER FLOW DYNAMICS. The echocardiographic evaluation of superior vena cava and pulmonary artery flow dynamics in a bidirectional Glenn procedure demonstrates[88,93] continuous laminar flow of low velocity (<0.5 m/sec) (Fig. 33–15). If there is an additional source of pulsatile flow, there may be in the contralateral pulmonary artery a low or moderate velocity (1 m/sec), continuous flow (aortopulmonary shunt), or systolic flow (anterograde flow through the pulmonary valve). In these patients, Doppler evaluation of the superior vena cava may identify (see Fig. 33–15) continuous venous flow (hypopulsatile bidirectional Glenn), a reduction in the systolic flow (pulsatile bidirectional Glenn), or retrograde flow during systole (hyperpulsatile bidirectional Glenn) (Table 33–8).

RIGHT-TO-LEFT SHUNTS (VENOUS COLLATERALS, ARTERIOVENOUS FISTULAE). The progression in cyanosis in patients after a bidirectional Glenn procedure can be explained by the patient's growth, because the contribution of the head and neck vessels to the total cardiac output diminishes with time.[94] Other common sources of right-to-left shunts, such as decompressing venous collaterals,[95,96] particularly in patients with a bidirectional Glenn anastomosis and history of high pulmonary artery pressure, should be excluded. The reported incidence of decompressing venous collaterals ranges from 13%[90] to 75%.[97]

Contrast echocardiography[90] with fast injection of saline or dextrose solution (3 to 6 ml) in an upper extremity may show rapid filling of the pulmonary veins that suggests pulmonary arteriovenous fistulae but cannot rule out decompressing venous collaterals to the pulmonary veins (Table 33–9). An abnormality in the upper extremity contrast echocardiogram occurs in 15%[97] to 60%[90] of these patients. Arteriovenous fistulae can be suspected from a typical radiographic reticular image in the lower lobes, extending to the periphery. After the Kawashima operation,[86,98] there is evidence of a right-to-left shunt with oxygen saturations of around 90% initially, with progressive cyanosis attributed to the development of arteriovenous fistulae in the lungs.[60,90,98] The progressive right-to-left shunt may result from decompressing venous collaterals, in particular anomalous cavoportal connections,[99] which become more prominent with time. In these patients, transcatheter coil embolization may be therapeutic.

The Doppler evaluation of the lower pulmonary venous flow during inspiration demonstrates continuous flow (>0.5 m/sec) that markedly decreases in expiration (see Fig. 33–15), probably because of collapse of the microfis-

TABLE 33–7

INSTITUTIONAL EXPERIENCE WITH PARTIAL RIGHT-SIDED HEART BYPASS PROCEDURES PERFORMED AT CHILDREN'S HOSPITAL IN BUENOS AIRES

Procedure	No. of Patients	Mortality Early	Late
Classic Glenn	10	0	0
Bidirectional Glenn	90	6	2
Kawashima	3	1	0
Total	103	7	2

TABLE 33–8

FLOW DYNAMICS BY TRANSTHORACIC TWO-DIMENSIONAL ECHO DOPPLER IN BIDIRECTIONAL CAVOPULMONARY CONNECTION

Flow	Superior Vena Cava	Pulmonary Artery (PA)
Nonpulsatile	Continuous <0.5 m/sec ↑ Inspiration	Continuous <0.5 m/sec ↑ Inspiration
Pulsatile	Continuous, decreasing in systole <0.5 m/sec ↑ Inspiration	Rt PA: continuous, <0.5 m/sec, ↑ inspiration Lt PA: pulsatile, >0.5 m/sec
Hyperpulsatile	Retrograde during systole Anterograde during diastole ↑ Inspiration	Rt PA: continuous Lt PA: hyperpulsatile, >1 m/sec

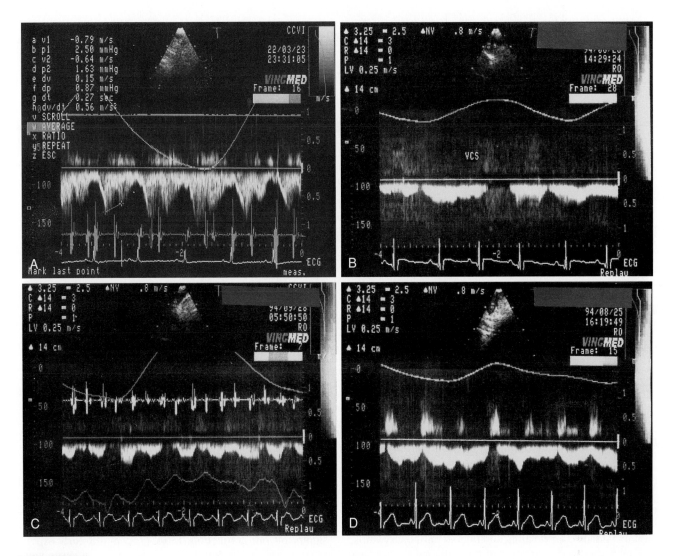

FIGURE 33–15

Two-dimensional Doppler flow dynamics in superior vena cava. *A,* Normal, anterograde biphasic with increase at early inspiration. *B,* Nonpulsatile bidirectional cavopulmonary anastomosis, with continuous flow and inspiratory increase in velocity. *C,* Pulsatile bidirectional cavopulmonary anastomosis, anterograde flow with systolic slowing. *D,* Hyperpulsatile bidirectional cavopulmonary anastomosis, with retrograde systolic flow in superior vena cava.

TABLE 33–9

CONTRAST ECHOCARDIOGRAPHY IN THE RIGHT-SIDED HEART BYPASS

Measure	Procedure						Total No. or Average
	BDGS	PBC	Glenn	Kawashima	APA	TCPC	
No. of patients	29	10	2	2	10	1	54
Age (yr; median)	8.9	14.5	14.8	13	15.2	14.8	12.3
Postoperative period (yr; median)	2.8	2.9	6.6	3.2	7.4	4.7	4.5
PAVMs	4	0	1	1	0	0	6
Venous collaterals	26	3	1	2	0	0	32
Contrast in LA	22	1	0	2	2	0	27

BDGS = bidirectional Glenn shunt with additional pulmonary blood flow; PBC = partial biventricular correction; Glenn = classic Glenn; Kawashima = Kawashima operation or total cavopulmonary shunt in presence of interrupted inferior vena cava and azygos continuation to the superior vena cava; APA = atriopulmonary anastomosis; TCPC = total cavopulmonary connection; PAVMs = pulmonary arteriovenous malformations or fistulae (by contrast echocardiography); venous collaterals = presence of decompressing venous collaterals from superior vena cava to the inferior vena cava; contrast in LA = contrast in the left atrium indicating atrial level right-to-left shunt.

Data from Kreutzer EA, Narkisian G, Vazquez H, et al: Contrast echocardiography in by-passing of the right ventricle. Ultrasound Med Biol 23(suppl 1):S10, 1997.

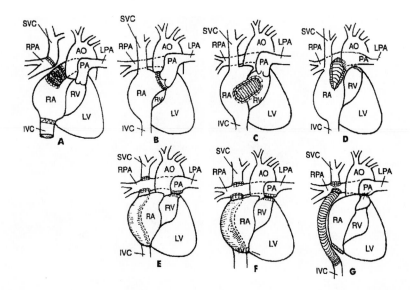

FIGURE 33–16

Modifications of the total right-sided heart bypass operation. *A,* The original Fontan procedure (Fontan and Baudet[106]): an end-to-end anastomosis of the RPA to SVC, an end-to-end anastomosis of the right atrial appendage to proximal end of the RPA by an aortic valved homograft, closure of atrial septal defect, insertion of a pulmonary valve homograft into the IVC, and ligation of the main pulmonary artery. *B,* Total right-sided heart bypass (Kreutzer and coworkers[107]): anastomosis of right atrial appendage to the main pulmonary artery with its intact pulmonary valve (excised from the RV) after closing the atrial and ventricular septal defects. A Glenn operation was not performed, and no IVC valve was used. *C,* Bjork and colleagues[109] anastomosed the right atrial appendage directly to the RV outflow tract if the pulmonary valve was normal, using a roof of pericardium to avoid a synthetic tube graft. *D,* The posterior anastomosis of the RA to the PA (Kreutzer and coworkers[110]). *E, F,* Separate anastomosis of the divided SVC to the RPA; insertion of an IVC to SVC intra-atrial baffle (total cavopulmonary connection) with *(F)* and without *(E)* fenestration. *G,* Extracardiac conduit between the IVC and the RPA and a bidirectional Glenn operation. RPA = right pulmonary artery; SVC = superior vena cava; AO = aorta; PA = pulmonary artery; LPA = left pulmonary artery; RV = right ventricle; RA = right atrium; IVC = inferior vena cava; LV = left ventricle. (*A–G* modified from Park MK: Pediatric Cardiology for Practitioners, 3rd ed. St. Louis, Mosby, 1996, p 217.)

tulae by increase in intrathoracic pressure. Diagnosis of pulmonary arteriovenous fistulae is confirmed by cardiac catheterization. Pulmonary angiograms demonstrate dilated terminal arteries, absent capillary phase, early pulmonary venous opacification, and dilated pulmonary veins. Oximetry reveals desaturation of the pulmonary veins that is not corrected with administration of oxygen. There are few therapeutic options for patients with pulmonary arteriovenous malformations. A brachial or axillary arteriovenous fistula can be performed to increase the pulmonary blood flow and allow blood from the liver to be incorporated in the pulmonary circulation.[100, 101] Regression after liver transplantation in patients with liver disease[102] and after complete right-sided heart bypass[103] supports the hypothesis that pulmonary arteriovenous fistulae can be reversible with incorporation of hepatic blood flow.

EXERCISE CAPACITY. Patients with partial right-sided heart bypass, either pulsatile or not,[104] have markedly depressed exercise capacity (48% of the estimated functional capacity) directly related to the level of systemic desaturation.[104] The chronotropic response is normal, as it is in cyanotic congenital heart defects.[105] Exercise stress testing in these patients demonstrates that even when the systemic saturation is adequate at rest (>85%), marked desaturation (<70%) develops during the study.

Definitive Palliative Surgery: Total Right-Sided Heart Bypass

A total or complete right-sided heart bypass directs all systemic venous return to the pulmonary arteries in the absence of a ventricular pump. The operation was first performed by Fontan in 1971.[106] Shortly thereafter and unaware of Fontan's reported experience, a total right-sided heart bypass was performed in Argentina,[107] considering the right atrium a compliant chamber without any significant pump function. Thus, even in our early experience, valves in the inferior or superior venae cavae were avoided. What is now known as a fenestrated Fontan procedure[67, 108] was first performed in Argentina in 1971 by leaving a residual 6-mm atrial level communication to serve as a pop-off valve. Multiple modifications of the initial Fontan procedure have been proposed and performed (Fig. 33–16):

- Anterior atriopulmonary connections, as reported by Fontan and Baudet,[106] Kreutzer and colleagues,[107] and Bjork and coworkers[109]
- Posterior atriopulmonary connections[110, 111]
- Lateral intra-atrial tunnel[112–115]
- Central tunnel[116, 117]
- Extracardiac tunnel[118, 119]

Each surgical option has advantages and disadvantages. Unfortunately, the late results of each procedure suggest that having a total right-sided heart bypass operation has major adverse consequences.

Authors have differed in the timing of this procedure. There are no studies designed to answer the question of the optimal age for the operation. When, after a partial right-sided heart bypass, systemic oxygen saturation decreases below 80% or the hematocrit rises above 55%, a total right-sided heart bypass should be considered, irrespective of age. Adult patients with single ventricle can undergo total right-sided heart bypass with low morbidity and mortality.[120] After a total bypass, even when it is performed on ideal patients, the clinical status may deteriorate with time, in spite of a Qp/Qs ratio of 1. This observation reinforces the belief in the palliative nature of the procedure. The common long-term complications that follow total right-sided heart bypass operations make one reconsider the approach to timing of this palliative surgery, thereby differing from the criteria used in the repair of other cardiac malformations, in which "early intervention is always advisable." Furthermore, the complications of pregnancy in patients after a total right-sided heart bypass should be considered in committing a female child to it. Limited experience has demonstrated only 45% incidence of live births among 33 pregnancies.[121]

A total right-sided heart bypass normalizes oximetry, eliminates shunts, abolishes the risk of brain abscess, and establishes a series circulation but with a single systemic ventricular pump. Three primary factors are determinants of the total right-sided heart bypass hemodynamics: pulmonary vascular resistance, pulmonary vascular compliance, and left ventricular function. The pulmonary artery index has been demonstrated to correlate poorly with the pulmonary vascular resistance but well with pulmonary vascular compliance. The relationship between pulmonary artery index (PAI), resistance, and compliance is expressed by the formula

$$PAI = Qp \times \text{pulmonary compliance} \\ \times \text{pulmonary resistance}$$

When the normal values for each parameter are taken into account, the result[122] is

$$330 \text{ mm}^2/\text{m}^2 = 3\text{–}4 \text{ L/min/m}^2 \\ \times 40\text{–}55 \text{ ml}^2/\text{m}^2 \cdot \text{mm Hg} \times 2 \text{ U/m}^2$$

In the long-term follow-up of patients with total right-sided heart bypass,[123–133] poor results have been reported from those with heterotaxia, low age at operation, weight less than 15 kg, elevated pulmonary artery pressure, atrioventricular valve dysfunction, and right atrial pressure above 20 mm Hg or left atrial pressure above 10 mm Hg in the early postoperative period. Survival for this group was 60% at 10 years of follow-up. In an attempt to predict the early and late prognosis, a Fontan index was defined as PVR + VEDP/Qs + Qp, where PVR is pulmonary vascular resistance and VEDP is ventricular end-diastolic pressure.[126, 127, 132] Ideally, this should be less than 2. Some

suggest that surgery should be contraindicated when a Fontan index of more than 4 is identified.

After cardiac catheterization and cineangiography for determination of risk factors for a total right-sided heart bypass (Table 33–10; see also Table 33–6), patients undergo either a total cavopulmonary anastomosis[81, 112] with lateral intra-atrial tunnel or extracardiac conduit or a cavoatriopulmonary anastomosis,[116, 117] all of which may or may not be fenestrated.[66, 108] The cavoatriopulmonary surgical modification protects the sinus node and coronary sinus under low pressure[134] and permits homogeneous distribution of pulmonary blood flow, because it includes a mixing chamber similar to that in an atriopulmonary anastomosis.[87]

Associated cardiac malformations increase risks factors for a total right-sided heart bypass (see Table 33–6) and demand technical modifications.

A staged approach for performing a total right-sided heart bypass has allowed a significant reduction in morbidity[135] by avoiding a sudden change in ventricular geometry. After a total right-sided heart bypass performed directly, without a prior staging partial bypass procedure, there is a 100% reduction in the ventricular chamber volume and an increase in both ventricular wall thickness and mass/volume ratio,[136, 137] which leads to diastolic ventricular dysfunction early in the postoperative period.[137]

An atriocavopulmonary anastomosis (central tunnel) (Fig. 33–17),[116, 117] with or without prosthetic material, has

TABLE 33–10
CHOUSSAT'S CRITERIA
Age 4–15 yr
Sinus rhythm
Normal drainage of caval veins
Normal volume of right atrium
Mean PA pressure ≤ 15 mm Hg
Pulmonary resistance < 4 U/m²
Ratio PA/Ao ≥ 0.75
Normal ventricular function
No mitral insufficiency
No impairing effect of shunt

PA = pulmonary artery; Ao = aorta.

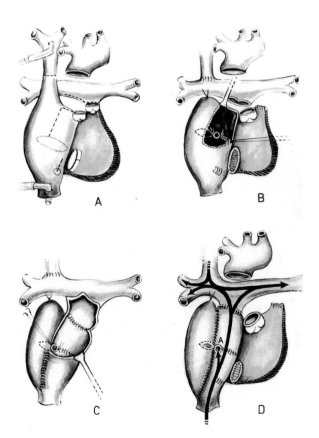

FIGURE 33–17

Surgical technique (*A* through *D*) for the central cavoatriopulmonary anastomosis with autologous material. (*A–D* from Kreutzer C, Schlichter AJ, Kreutzer CO: Cavo-atriopulmonary anastomosis via a non-prosthetic medial tunnel. J Card Surg 12:37, 1997.)

become an acceptable technique for performing a total right-sided heart bypass. This is achieved by creating an intra-atrial tunnel made of autologous tissue, using the patient's own atrial wall, reducing the size of the atrial chamber and thus decreasing atrial afterload. In addition, a bidirectional cavopulmonary anastomosis is performed. The inferior vena cava is connected through this tunnel to the main pulmonary artery trunk and branches, similar to performing an atriopulmonary anastomosis. The advantages of this central tunnel technique[117] are exclusion of the sinus node and coronary sinus from higher pressure,[134] growth potential, absence of suture lines in the proximity of the sinus node and nodal artery, avoidance of the use of prosthetic material, and theoretical allowance of equal bilateral distribution of inferior vena cava blood flow to both lungs. The extracardiac conduit technique[118] shares some advantages with the central tunnel technique, such as the absence of suture lines in the atrium, although it uses prosthetic material, lacks growth potential, and usually causes preferential distribution of inferior vena caval blood flow to the ipsilateral pulmonary artery. The postoperative electrocardiogram in these patients shows small-amplitude P waves in the right precordial leads, suggesting low right atrial wall stress. The flow dynamics by Doppler evaluation demonstrate presystolic pulsatility in the inferior vena cava.

After atriopulmonary connection, late failures are common (Table 33–11),[123] even in patients with ideal preoperative condition according to Choussat's criteria (see Table 33–10).[129] Experience has demonstrated that these criteria should be regarded as only a guide, because the absence of one or more of these factors should not be considered an absolute contraindication to surgery. Some authors believe that to undergo a total right-sided heart bypass procedure, a patient should have a Nakata index[58] of 250 mm²/m² (normal, 330 mm²/m²), or not less than 188 mm²/m²,[130] or a McGoon ratio above 1.8[123] or pulmonary artery branches measuring more than 80% of the normal.[131]

Some patients with two or more high-risk factors for a total right-sided heart bypass, particularly when there is ventricular dysfunction, may benefit from a cardiac transplantation if an experienced transplant team is available.

RESULTS AFTER TOTAL RIGHT-SIDED HEART BYPASS OPERATION

Because of the high incidence of complications reported after a total bypass operation (see Table 33–11), this procedure should be performed only in the patients who strictly meet all the requirements (see Table 33–6). The onset of chronic congestive heart failure in patients who did not fol-

low all the low-risk criteria causes us to select only good candidates for total right-sided heart bypass operations. Patients with high-risk factors who do not comply with all requirements may do better with a pulsatile partial right-sided heart bypass and a systemic-to-pulmonary artery shunt as a source of additional pulmonary blood flow.

No technique of performing a total right-sided heart bypass is ideal. As long-term follow-up becomes available, more complications and disadvantages are identified in association with techniques that are no longer routinely used. Limited follow-up is available of patients with the more recent modifications. Currently, we prefer to use either a central tunnel through a cavoatriopulmonary anastomosis (see Fig. 33–17) or an extracardiac conduit.[118,119] When the left-sided atrioventricular valve is abnormal, a central tunnel as proposed by Kawashima[98] or an extracardiac conduit[118] should be considered. Midterm results after extracardiac conduit are favorable, particularly on the incidence of atrial arrhythmias.[131]

EXERCISE CAPACITY. Patients with total right-sided heart bypass have mildly diminished functional capacity[104] by ergometry to about 79% of estimated capacity. They have mild desaturation and subnormal chronotropic response.[138–142] Cardiac output does not increase normally[138–140]; this results in part from reduced pulmonary blood flow and impaired chronotropic and contractile responses to exercise.[141] Minute ventilation and the ventilatory equivalent for oxygen and carbon dioxide remain above normal.[142] In addition, arrhythmias are more frequent with exercise than at rest.[138]

LUNG PERFUSION SCAN. After total cavopulmonary anastomosis, preferential blood flow distribution to the lung ipsilateral to the cavopulmonary connection is commonly observed (Table 33–12).[87,88,143] Certain technical modifications allow a more homogeneous distribution of blood flow that may have an impact on pulmonary arterial growth.

DOPPLER FLOW DYNAMICS. Hemodynamic failure after total right-sided heart bypass can be detected by Doppler echocardiographic analysis of flow dynamics (Table 33–13; Figs. 33–18 to 33–20).[88]

Among causes or manifestations of failure after a total right-sided heart bypass procedure are the following.

1. *Transpulmonary gradient.* The flow dynamics after a total right-sided heart bypass depends on the pressure gradient between the right atrium and the left atrium or transpulmonary gradient. This gradient should ideally not exceed 6 mm Hg. Failure after a total right-sided heart bypass may be secondary to a rise in the transpulmonary gradient with time. Various factors may contribute to this increase, such as deficient pulmonary arterial growth (Nakata index getting smaller with time)[144,145] or chronic pulmonary microthromboembolism or macrothromboembolism.[146,147] In these patients, oral anticoagulants should be routinely prescribed.

2. *Giant right atrium.* Another long-term complication after total right-sided heart bypass of the atriopulmonary anastomosis variety is the development of a giant right

---

TABLE 33–11

INSTITUTIONAL EXPERIENCE WITH TOTAL RIGHT-SIDED HEART BYPASS PROCEDURES PERFORMED AT CHILDREN'S HOSPITAL IN BUENOS AIRES

Diagnosis	No. of Patients	Mortality Early	Late
Left univentricular heart (IA, IIA)	62	6 (9.8%)	6
Right univentricular heart (IB, IIB)	18	2 (11%)	2

TABLE 33–12

CHARACTERISTICS OF VARIOUS SURGICAL TECHNIQUES FOR TOTAL RIGHT-SIDED HEART BYPASS

Total Bypass	Energy Loss	Pulmonary Blood Flow Distribution	Incidence of Arrhythmias	Prosthetic Material	Limitation
Atriopulmonary anastomosis	High	Homogeneous to both lungs	Late; atrial flutter most common	No	—
Lateral tunnel	Not significant	80% ipsilateral lung to tunnel anastomosis, 20% contralateral lung	Early sinus node dysfunction more common	Yes	—
Extracardiac tunnel	Not significant	80% ipsilateral lung to tunnel anastomosis, 20% contralateral lung	?	Yes	—
Autologous extracardiac tunnel	Not significant	Homogeneous to both lungs	?	No	Only in L-aorta
Central tunnel	Not significant	Homogeneous to both lungs	?	Yes	—
Autologous central tunnel	Not significant	Homogeneous to both lungs	?	No	Normal left AV valve and coronary sinus

atrium. These patients commonly have associated atrial arrhythmias and thromboembolic complications, and they may develop compression of the right pulmonary veins by the posterior wall of the right atrium, which further increases the transpulmonary gradient. They benefit from conversion to a lateral tunnel connection[148, 149] to increase their functional capacity and release compression of the right pulmonary veins.

3. *Right-to-left shunts.* In some patients, failure after a total right-sided heart bypass is characterized by cyanosis.

Right-to-left shunting can result from a baffle leak, fenestration, and decompressing venous collaterals to pulmonary veins or to cardiac veins. Small interatrial communications can develop and cause cyanosis in the long-term follow-up, particularly in patients with atriopulmonary connections.[150] To date, there have been no reports of pulmonary arteriovenous fistulae in patients with atriopulmonary connections or total cavopulmonary shunts with homogeneous distribution of hepatic venous blood flow to both lungs.

TABLE 33–13

FLOW DYNAMICS BY TRANSTHORACIC TWO-DIMENSIONAL ECHO DOPPLER IN ATRIOPULMONARY ANASTOMOSIS

Flow	"Normal" Function	Dysfunctional
Inferior vena cava	Anterograde biphasic S/D <0.5 m/sec ↑ Inspiration	Anterograde in inspiration Retrograde in expiration
Pulmonary artery	Anterograde triphasic S/D with PS exacerbation =0.5 m/sec ↑ Inspiration	Anterograde in inspiration <0.5 m/sec Retrograde in expiration
Pulmonary veins	Anterograde biphasic D > S <0.6 m/sec ↑ Inspiration	Anterograde diastolic >1 m/sec ↑ Inspiration
Mitral valve	E > A < 0.6 m/sec ↑ Inspiration	Restrictive E ≥1 m/sec ↑ Inspiration Gradient VP–MV

A = late diastolic filling; E = early diastolic filling; VP = pulmonary veins; MV = mitral valve; PS = presystolic; S = systolic; D = diastolic.

4. *Thromboembolism.* Patients with atriopulmonary anastomosis can develop atrial flutter and chronic thromboembolism.[146,147] The incidence of thromboembolic complications seems to be independent of the type of connection used for total right-sided heart bypass (3.9%).[146] Systemic embolism can also occur after a total right-sided heart bypass, particularly in those patients with a remaining source of right-to-left shunting (fenestration). Such patients should continue to receive at least aspirin or a combination of platelet antiaggregant agents.

5. *Arrhythmias.* In patients with total cavopulmonary anastomosis, the prevalence of sinus node dysfunction is significant (37%).[151,152] This may occur from direct damage to the artery of the sinus node or to the node itself. Si-

nus node dysfunction can also occur after atriopulmonary connection (12%) and is particularly frequent after bidirectional Glenn or hemi-Fontan procedures.[152]

Arrhythmias may occur in the early postoperative period, particularly in patients with high-risk factors and poor postoperative hemodynamics. Among these, atrial arrhythmias, junctional ectopic tachycardia, and even ventricular arrhythmias may develop.[153] Junctional ectopic tachycardia can occur in the immediate postoperative period after total right-sided heart bypass,[154] particularly in patients younger than 3 years, and has a poor prognosis.

Supraventricular tachycardia seems to be less frequent in patients with total cavopulmonary connection

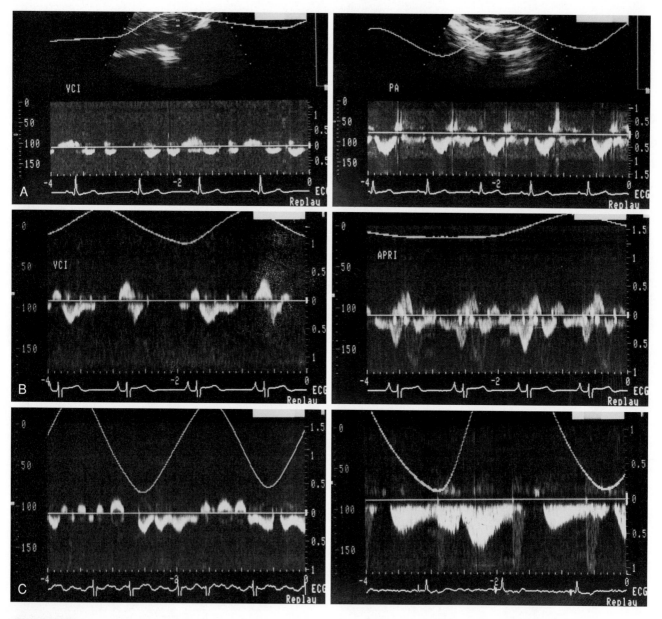

FIGURE 33–18

Echocardiographic flow dynamics by two-dimensional Doppler evaluation at inferior vena cava *(left)* and pulmonary artery *(right)* in normal *(A)*, atriopulmonary anastomosis *(B)*, and failure after atriopulmonary anastomosis *(C)*. Note that the flow in the pulmonary artery in *B* is triphasic systolic-diastolic, with presystolic exacerbation, of low velocity, and increased in inspiration. In *C*, there is atrial flutter and the flows in the inferior vena cava and pulmonary artery are retrograde in expiration.

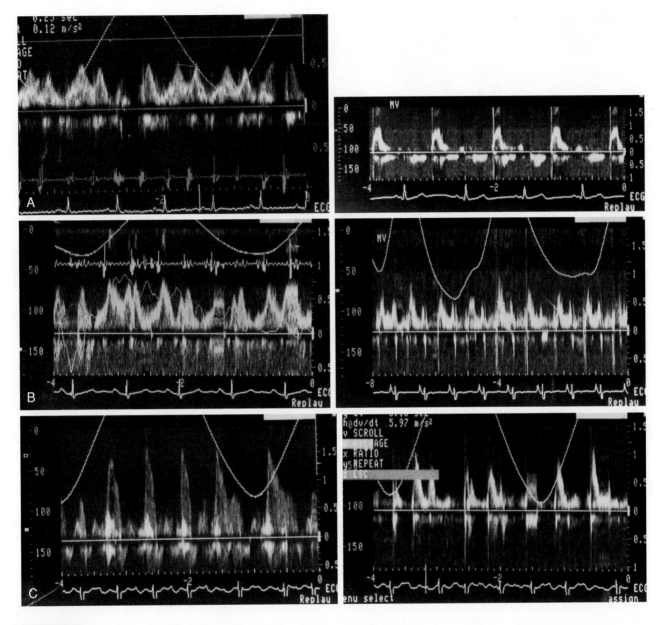

Flow dynamics by two-dimensional Doppler echocardiography at pulmonary veins *(left)* and mitral valve *(right)* in normal *(A)*, atriopulmonary anastomosis *(B)*, and late failure after atriopulmonary anastomosis *(C)*. The pulmonary venous flow in *B* is triphasic anterograde (protodiastolic, telediastolic, and protosystolic), with increase in velocity during inspiration, same as the transmitral flow. In *C*, there are high velocities recorded in pulmonary veins (1.5 m/sec) with a monophasic protodiastolic flow, differing from the transmitral flow velocity (0.7 to 1 m/sec). Atrial flutter is present.

than in those with atriopulmonary connection, although the follow-up periods are not comparable.[154]

6. *Protein-losing enteropathy.* This serious complication of chronic venous hypertension occurs in up to 11% of the patients.[127] They present with hypoproteinemia, hypoalbuminemia, chronic edema, pleural effusions, ascites, pericardial effusions, and increase of fecal α_1-antitrypsin. Clearance of α_1-antitrypsin is currently the best method of evaluating protein-losing enteropathy. Various management options have been considered for such patients, including steroid treatment, low-molecular-weight heparin, fenestration creation, heart transplantation, and Fontan takedown.

Another rare manifestation of failure after a total right-sided heart bypass has been chyloptysis and expectoration of bronchial casts.[155]

Clinical failure after a total right-sided heart bypass is managed according to the specific hemodynamic abnormality or manifestation of failure. Anticongestive medications, afterload-reducing agents, and oral anticoagulants are universally used. Cardiac catheterization and potential transcatheter interventions should always be performed. Invasive evaluation of arrhythmias with possible ablation, in addition to medical management, may be beneficial.[156] Some patients have improved after conversion from one form of total bypass to another with more favorable hemo-

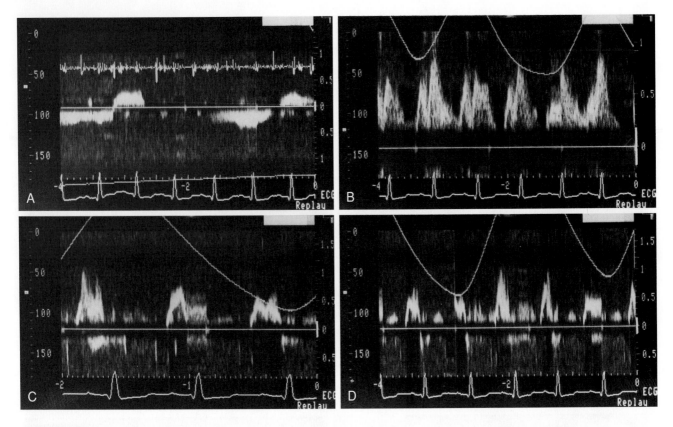

FIGURE 33–20

Two-dimensional Doppler flow dynamics in a patient with total cavopulmonary anastomosis. The flow in the inferior vena cava (IVC) is continuous (A), of low velocity, anterograde in inspiration, and retrograde with Valsalva or forced expiration. The flow in the pulmonary veins (B) is biphasic anterograde: diastolic and protodiastolic. The transmitral flow (C, D) markedly increases with inspiration.

dynamics.[149, 157] Other patients can only be either taken down to a partial right-sided heart bypass or referred for cardiac transplantation.

PROGNOSIS

When managed surgically, patients with single ventricle and low pulmonary blood flow who undergo an aortopulmonary shunt in the newborn period have an immediate mortality of 17%.[71] Among survivors with an aortopulmonary shunt, Taussig[158] reported 72% survival at 10 years of age and 50% at 20 years.

Patients with increased pulmonary blood flow who undergo pulmonary artery banding in the newborn period have an initial mortality of 8%. The mortality increases up to 47%[71] in those patients who require concomitant operation of aortic coarctation or subaortic stenosis. When pulmonary artery banding is performed during the first 6 months of life, the mortality is low.[74]

On follow-up, three quarters of patients with single ventricle type A II or A III will require subaortic stenosis repair at a mean age of 8 months.[74]

A Damus-Kaye-Stansel operation or a subaortic resection associated with a bidirectional cavopulmonary anastomosis or total cavopulmonary anastomosis has been reported to carry a mortality of 19%.[74] After the initial palliative procedure (shunt or banding), the second opera-

tion or partial right-sided heart bypass (bidirectional Glenn procedure) has low mortality (4%). The total right-sided heart bypass has a mortality of about 11%.[81]

Critical risk factors for a total right-sided heart bypass procedure,[58, 129–131] which may influence long-term outcome, include (1) pulmonary vascular resistance or transpulmonary gradient; (2) systolic ventricular function (ejection and shortening fraction), ventricular mechanics (contractility, preload, and afterload), and diastolic ventricular function (ventricular filling indices, pulmonary venous flow by Doppler); and (3) atrioventricular valve function.

Multiple modifications of the original Fontan procedure have evolved over time, and early mortality and morbidity after a total right-sided heart bypass have improved. There continues, however, to be progressive attrition at long-term follow-up, and this does not seem to relate to procedural variables.[133]

A common hemodynamic mechanism of failure after an atriopulmonary anastomosis is that of progressive atrial dilatation and higher venous pressure, which cause more atrial dilatation and progressive increase in systolic venous pressures,[132] rise in the atrial afterload, and electromechanical dissociation. In addition, the turbulent flow causes a loss of energy. All this predisposes to the development of atrial arrhythmias, such as atrial flutter.[153]

The subnormal growth of the pulmonary arteries or the reduction in their size after total right-sided heart bypass[144, 145] and the higher morbidity and mortality for patients of younger age[123, 133] suggest that early operation for total right-sided heart bypass may not be as beneficial as it is for other anomalies. Assuming that pulmonary arterial growth after total right-sided heart bypass is abnormal, a Nakata index of 330 mm²/m² in a patient with a body surface area of 1 m² would allow adequate pulmonary artery size at the end of the growth curve (Nakata index >200 mm²/m²), even in the absence of any pulmonary artery growth. A pulsatile bidirectional Glenn procedure may be the ideal intermediate palliative surgery, and it allows better pulmonary artery growth. Despite the disadvantages of progression of cyanosis by development of decompressing venous collaterals and a higher volume load to the single ventricle compared with a nonpulsatile bidirectional Glenn procedure, it may be the optimal approach for many patients who are not optimal candidates for a total right-sided heart bypass.

REFERENCES

1. Anderson RH, Becker AE, Wilkinson JL, Gerlis LM: The morphogenesis of univentricular heart. Br Heart J 38:558, 1976.
2. Van Praagh R, Ongley P, Swan H: Anatomic types of single or common ventricle in man: Morphologic and geometric aspects of 60 necropsied cases. Am J Cardiol 13:367, 1964.
3. Lev M, Libertson RR, Kirkpatric KJ, et al: Single (primitive) ventricle. Circulation 39:577, 1969.
4. Kreutzer E, Flores J, Viegas C, et al: Radiología Cardiovascular en Pediatría. Buenos Aires, Editorial Médica Panamericana, 1982.
5. Binello M, Roman MI, Granja M, et al: Diferenciación ecocardiográfica (2-D) de la conexión auriculoventricular en el corazón univentricular, doble entrada ventricular y cabalgamiento auriculoventricular. Implicancias quirúrgicas. Rev Latina Cardiol Cirugia Cardiovasc Infant 1:25, 1985.
6. De la Cruz MV, Miller VL: Double inlet left ventricle: Two pathological specimens with comments on the embryology and on its relation to single ventricle. Circulation 37:249, 1968.
7. Muñoz Castellanos L, De la Cruz MV, Cieslinski A: Double-inlet right ventricle: Two pathological specimens with comments on embryology. Br Heart J 35:292, 1973.
8. Shinebourne EA, Macartney FJ, Anderson RH: Sequential chamber localization—Logical approach to diagnostics in congenital heart disease. Br Heart J 38:327, 1976.
9. Anderson RH, Becker A, Freedom R, et al: Analysis of the atrioventricular junction—connections, relations and ventricular morphology. In Godman MJ (ed): Paediatric Cardiology, Vol 4. New York, Churchill Livingstone, 1981, p 169.
10. Van Praagh R: The segmental approach to diagnosis in congenital heart disease. Birth Defects Orig Artic Ser 8(5):4, 1972.
11. Bharati S, Lev M: The spectrum of common atrioventricular orifice (canal). Am Heart J 86:553, 1973.
12. Anderson RH, Macartney FJ, Tynan M, et al: Univentricular atrioventricular connection, the single ventricle trap unsprung. Pediatr Cardiol 4:273, 1983.
13. Van Praagh R, Plett JA, Van Praagh S: Single ventricle pathology, embryology, terminology and classification. Hertz 4:113, 1979.
14. Lyons GE: Vertebrate heart development. Curr Opin Genet Dev 6:454, 1996.
15. Van Mierop LHS: Embryology of the univentricular heart. Hertz 4:78, 1979.
16. Viegas C, Kreutzer EA: Estudio anatomico de 196 corazones con cardiopatias congenitas aplicando el analisis segmentario secuencial. In Kreutzer EA (ed): Cardiología y Cirugía Cardiovascular Infantil. Buenos Aires, Doyma Arg. Buenos Aires, 1993, p 152.
17. Keeton BR, Lie JT, Mc Goon DC, et al: Anatomy of coronary arteries in univentricular heart and its surgical implications. Am J Cardiol 43:569, 1979.
18. Holmes AF: Case of malformation of the heart. Trans Med Chir Soc Edinb 1:252, 1824.
19. Anderson RH, Arnold R, Thapar MK, et al: Cardiac specialized tissues in heart with an apparently single ventricular chamber (double inlet left ventricle). Am J Cardiol 33:95, 1974.
20. Davies MJ, Anderson RH, Becker AE: Atrioventricular conduction tissues in congenital heart disease. In Davies MJ, Anderson RH, Becker AE (eds): The Conduction System of the Heart. London, Butterworth-Heinemann, 1983, p 135.
21. Van Praagh R, Van Praagh S, Vlad P, Keith JD: Diagnosis of the anatomic types of single or common ventricle. Am J Cardiol 15:345, 1965.
22. Quero Jimenez M, Anderson RH, Tynan M, et al: Summation of anatomic patterns of atrioventricular and ventriculo-arterial connections. In Godman MJ (ed): Paediatric Cardiology, Vol 4. Edinburgh, Churchill Livingstone, 1981, p 211.
23. Van Mierop LHS, Gessner IH, Schiebler GL: Asplenia and polysplenia syndromes. Birth Defects Orig Articl Ser 8(5):36, 1972.
24. Uemura H, Ho S, Devine W, Anderson RH: Analysis of visceral heterotaxy according to splenic status, appendage morphology or both. Am J Cardiol 76:846, 1995.
25. Milo S, Ho SY, Macartney FJ, et al: Straddling and overriding atrioventricular valves, morphology and classification. Am J Cardiol 44:1122, 1979.
26. Liberthson R, Paul M, Muster A, et al: Straddling and displaced atrioventricular orifices and valves with primitive ventricles. Circulation 43:213, 1971.
27. Barra Rossi M, Ho SY, Anderson RH: Double-inlet ventricle and its relationships to hearts with straddling and overriding atrioventricular valves. Rev Latina Cardiol Cirugia Cardiovasc Infant 2:171, 1986.
28. Van Praagh R: The importance of ventriculoatrial malalignment in anomalies of the atrioventricular valves, illustrated by "mitral atresia" and congenital mitral stenosis with large left ventricle. In Doyle EF, Engle MA, Gersony W, et al (eds): Paediatric Cardiology. New York, Springer-Verlag, 1986, p 901.
29. Van Praagh S, Santini F, Sanders SP: Cardiac malpositions with special emphasis on visceral heterotaxy (asplenia and polysplenia syndromes). In Fyler DC (ed): Nadas' Paediatric Cardiology. Philadelphia, Hanley & Belfus, 1992, p 589.
30. Rahimtoola SH, Ongley P, Swan HJC: The hemodynamics of common (or single) ventricle. Circulation 34:14, 1966.
31. Somerville J, Becu L, Ross D: Common ventricle with acquired subaortic obstruction. Am J Cardiol 34:206, 1974.
32. Freedom RM, Sondheimer H, Dische R, Rowe RD: Development of "subaortic stenosis" after pulmonary arterial banding for common ventricle. Am J Cardiol 39:78, 1977.
33. Ritter DG, Seward JB, Moodie D, et al: Univentricular heart (common ventricle): Preoperative diagnosis, hemodynamic, angiocardiographic and echocardiographic features. Hertz 4:198, 1979.
34. Wernovsky G, Chang AC, Wessel AL: Intensive care. In Emmanouilides GC, Allen H, Riemenschneider TA, Gutgesell HP (eds): Moss and Adams' Heart Disease in Infants, Children and Adolescents: Including the Fetus and Young Adult, 5th ed. Baltimore, Williams & Wilkins, 1995, p 398.
35. Sano T, Ogawa M, Taniguchi K, et al: Assessment of ventricular contractile state and function in patients with univentricular heart. Circulation 79:1247, 1989.
36. Rychik KJ, Jacobs M, Norwood W: Acute changes in left ventricular geometry after volume reduction operation. Am Thorac Surg 60:1267, 1995.
37. Kidd BSL: Single ventricle. In Keith JD, Rowe RD, Vlad P (eds): Heart Disease in Infancy and Childhood, 3rd ed. New York, Macmillan, 1978, p 405.
38. Moodie DS, Ritter DG, Tajik AJ, et al: Long-term follow-up in the non-operated univentricular heart. Am J Cardiol 53:1124, 1984.
39. Ammash NM, Warnes CA: Survival into adulthood of patients with unoperated single ventricle. Am J Cardiol 77:542, 1996.
40. Elliot LP, Ruttenberg HD, Elliot RS, Anderson RC: Vectorial analysis of the electrocardiogram in common ventricle. Br Heart J 26:302, 1964.
41. Quero-Jimenez M, Casanova Gomez M, Castro C, et al: Electrocardiographic finding in single ventricle and related conditions. Am Heart J 86:449, 1973.
42. Guller B, Mair D, Ritter D, Smith R: Frank vectocardiogram in common ventricle: Correlation with anatomic finding. Am Heart J 90:290, 1975.

43. Phoon CK, Villegas M, Ursell P, Silverman NH: Left atrial isomerism detected in fetal life. Am J Cardiol 77:1083, 1996.

44. Carey L, Ruttenberg H: Roentgenographic features of common ventricle with inversion of the infundibulum. Corrected transposition with rudimentary left ventricle. AJR Am J Roentgenol 92:652, 1964.

45. Elliot LP, Gedgadus E: The roentgenologic findings in common ventricle with transposition of the great vessels. Radiology 82:850, 1964.

46. Elliot LP, Schiebler GH: The X-Ray Diagnosis of Congenital Heart Disease in Infants, Children and Adults. Springfield, IL, Charles C Thomas, 1979, p 282.

47. Fogel MA, Weinberg PM, Fellows KE, Hoffman EA: A study in ventricular-ventricular interaction. Single right ventricle compared with systemic right ventricles in a dual-chamber circulation. Circulation 92:219, 1995.

48. Fogel MA, Gupta KB, Weinberg PM, Hoffman EA: Regional wall motion and strain analysis across stages of Fontan reconstruction by magnetic resonance tagging. Am J Physiol 269:H1132, 1995.

49. Shiraishi H, Silverman NH: Echocardiographic spectrum of double inlet ventricle: Evaluation of the interventricular communication. J Am Coll Cardiol 15:1401, 1990.

50. Bevilacqua M, Sanders SP, Van Praagh S, et al: Double inlet single left ventricle: Echocardiographic anatomy with emphasis on the morphology of the atrioventricular valves and ventricular septal defect. J Am Coll Cardiol 18:559, 1991.

51. Matitau A, Geva T, Colan SD, et al: Bulboventricular foramen size in infants with double inlet left ventricle or tricuspid atresia with transposed great arteries: Influence on mitral palliative operation and rate of growth. J Am Coll Cardiol 19:142, 1992.

52. Rigby ML, Anderson RH, Gibson D, et al: Two dimensional echocardiographic categorisation of the univentricular heart. Ventricular morphology, type, and mode of atrioventricular connection. Br Heart J 46:603, 1981.

53. Smallhorn JF, Tommasini G, Macartney FJ: Detection and assessment of straddling and overriding atrioventricular valves by two dimensional echocardiography. Br Heart J 46:254, 1981.

54. Soto B, Pacifico AD, Di Sciascio G: Univentricular heart: An angiographic study. Am J Cardiol 49:787, 1982.

55. Soto B, Bertranou EG, Bream PR, et al: Angiographic study of univentricular heart of right ventricular type. Circulation 60:1325, 1979.

56. Soto B, Ceballos R, Nath PH, et al: Overriding atrioventricular valves. An angiographic-anatomical correlate. Int J Cardiol 9:327, 1985.

57. Ellis K: Angiocardiography in complex congenital heart disease: Single ventricle, double-inlet, double outlet, and transposition. In Davila JC (ed): Second Henry Ford Hospital International Symposium on Cardiac Surgery. Norwalk, CT, Appleton-Century-Crofts, 1977, p 220.

58. Nakata S, Yasuharu T, Kurosawa H, et al: A new method for quantitative standardization of cross sectional areas of the pulmonary arteries in congenital heart disease with decreased pulmonary blood flow. J Thorac Cardiovasc Surg 88:610, 1984.

59. Piehler MJ, Danielson GK, McGoon DC, et al: Management of pulmonary atresia with ventricular septal defect and hypoplastic pulmonary arteries. J Thorac Cardiovasc Surg 80:552, 1980.

60. Srivastava D, Preminger T, Lock J, et al: Hepatic venous blood and the development of pulmonary arteriovenous malformations in congenital heart disease. Circulation 92:1217, 1995.

61. Stumper O, Wright J, Sadiq M, De Giovani JV: Late systemic desaturation after total cavopulmonary shunt operations. Br Heart J 74:282, 1995.

62. Hsu H, Nykanen D, Williams W, et al: Right to left interatrial communications after the modified Fontan procedure: Identification and management with transcatheter occlusion. Br Heart J 74:548, 1995.

63. Treidman JK, Bridges N, Mayer JE, Lock JE: Prevalence and risk factors for aortopulmonary collateral after Fontan and bidirectional Glenn procedures. J Am Coll Cardiol 92:1021, 1993.

64. Kreutzer J: Interventional cardiac catheterization in patients with Fontan circulation. Rev Argent Cardiol 64:379, 1996.

65. Kreutzer J, Lock JE, Jonas RA, Keane JF: Transcatheter fenestration dilation and/or creation in postoperative Fontan patients. Am J Cardiol 79:228, 1997.

66. Bridges ND, Lock JE, Castaneda AR: Baffle fenestration with subsequent transcatheter closure. Circulation 82:1681, 1990.

67. Bridges ND, Lock JE, Mayer JE, et al: Cardiac catheterization and test occlusion of the interatrial communication after the fenestrated Fontan operation. J Am Coll Cardiol 25:1712, 1995.

68. Fully S, Zieske H, Levy M: The essential function of the right ventricle. Am Heart J 107:404, 1984.

69. Colbert EH: El Libro de los Dinosaurios. Buenos Aires, Eudeba, 1979, p 35.

70. Imai Y, Hoshino S, Koh Y, et al: Ventricular septation procedure for univentricular connection of left ventricular type. Semin Thorac Cardiovasc Surg 6:48, 1994.

71. Mayer JE: Initial management of the single ventricle patient. Semin Thorac Cardiovasc Surg 6:2, 1994.

72. Kreutzer C, Kreutzer EA, Varon RF, et al: Preoperative management of congestive heart failure in neonates: The closed hood. Int J Cardiol 60:139, 1997.

73. Trusler GA, Mustard WT: A method of banding the pulmonary artery for large isolated ventricular septal defect with and without transposition of the great arteries. Ann Thorac Surg 13:351, 1972.

74. Jensen RA, Williams RG, Laks H, et al: Usefulness of banding of the pulmonary trunk with single ventricle. Physiology at risk for subaortic obstruction. Am J Cardiol 77:1089, 1996.

75. Sluysmans T, Sanders S, Van der Velde M, et al: Natural history and patterns of recovery of contractile function in single left ventricle after Fontan operation. Circulation 86:1753, 1992.

76. Glenn WWL: Circulatory bypass of the right heart: II. Shunt between superior vena cava and distal right pulmonary artery. Report of a clinical application. N Engl J Med 259:117, 1958.

77. Bakulev AN, Kolesnikov SA: Anastomosis of superior vena cava and pulmonary artery in surgical treatment of certain congenital defects of the heart. J Thorac Surg 37:693, 1959.

78. Hopkins RA, Armstrong BE, Serwer GA, et al: Physiological rationale for a bidirectional cavopulmonary shunt: A versatile complement to the Fontan principle. J Thorac Cardiovasc Surg 90:391, 1985.

79. Kobayashi J, Matsuda H, Nakano S, et al: Hemodynamic effects of bidirectional cavopulmonary shunt with pulsatile pulmonary flow. Circulation 84(suppl III):219, 1991.

80. Salim MA, Case C, Sade RM, et al: Pulmonary/systemic flow ratio in children after cavopulmonary anastomosis. J Am Coll Cardiol 25:735, 1995.

81. Jonas RA: Indications and timing for the bidirectional Glenn shunt versus the fenestrated Fontan circulation. J Thorac Cardiovasc Surg 108:522, 1998.

82. Uemura H, Yagihara T, Kawashima Y, et al: Use of bidirectional Glenn procedure in the presence of forward flow from the ventricle to the pulmonary arteries. Circulation 92(suppl II):II-228, 1995.

83. Fogel M, Weinberg P, Chin AJ, et al: Late ventricular geometry and performance changes of functional single ventricle throughout staged Fontan reconstruction assessed by magnetic resonance imaging. J Am Coll Cardiol 28:212, 1996.

84. Kuroda O, Sano T, Matsuda H, et al: Analysis of the effects of the Blalock-Taussig shunt on ventricular function and prognosis in patient with single ventricle. Circulation 76(suppl III):III-24, 1987.

85. Donofrio MT, Jacobs ML, Norwood WI: Early changes in ventricular septal defect size in the single ventricle after volume unloading surgery. J Am Coll Cardiol 23(suppl A):105A, 1994.

86. Kawashima Y, Kitamura S, Matsuda H, et al: Total cavopulmonary shunt operations in complex cardiac anomalies. J Thorac Cardiovasc Surg 87:74, 1984.

87. Kreutzer EA, Quilindro AH, Barber B, et al: Study of pulmonary perfusion using scintigraphy in total or partial bypass of the right ventricle at rest and with exertion. J Am Coll Cardiol 25(suppl A):305A, 1995.

88. Kreutzer EA, Quilindro AH, Roman MI, et al: Distribución y dinámica del flujo pulmonar en los diferentes by pass de ventriculo derecho. Rev Argent Cardiol 63:565, 1995.

89. Mendelson AM, Bove EL, Lupinetti FM, et al: Central pulmonary artery growth patterns after the bidirectional Glenn procedure. J Thorac Cardiovasc Surg 107:1284, 1994.

90. Bernstein HS, Brook MM, Silverman NH, Bristow J: Development of pulmonary arteriovenous fistulae in children after cavopulmonary shunt. Circulation 92(suppl II):II-309, 1995.

91. Slavik Z, Salmon A, Daubeney P, et al: Do central pulmonary arteries grow following bidirectional superior cavopulmonary anastomosis? J Am Coll Cardiol 25(suppl A):304A, 1995.

92. Miyaji K, Shimada M, Sekiguchi A, et al: Usefulness of pulsatile bidirectional cavopulmonary shunt in high-risk Fontan patients. Ann Thorac Surg 65:845, 1996.

93. Salzer-Muhar V, Marx M, Ties M, et al: Doppler flow profiles in the right and left pulmonary artery in children with congenital heart disease and a bidirectional cavopulmonary shunt. Pediatr Cardiol 15:302, 1994.

94. Gross G, Jonas R, Castaneda AR, et al: Maturational and hemodynamic factors predictive of increased cyanosis after bidirectional cavopulmonary anastomosis. Am J Cardiol 74:705, 1994.

95. Koff GH, Laks H, Stansel H, et al: Thirty year follow-up of superior vena cava pulmonary artery (Glenn) shunt. J Thorac Cardiovasc Surg 100:662, 1990.

96. Magee AG, McCrindle BW, Benson L, et al: Systemic venous collaterals after the bidirectional cavopulmonary anastomosis. Prevalence and risk factors. Circulation 92(suppl I):I-126, 1995.

97. Kreutzer EA, Narkizian G, Vazquez H, et al: Contrast echocardiography in bypassing of the right ventricle. Ultrasound Med Biol 23(suppl):S10, 1997.

98. Kawashima Y, Matsuki O, Yagihara T, Matsuda H: Total cavopulmonary shunt operation. Semin Thorac Cardiovasc Surg 6:17, 1994.

99. Stumper O, Wright SG, Sadig M, De Giovanni JV: Late systemic desaturation after total cavopulmonary shunt operations. Br Heart J 74:282, 1995.

100. Mitchell IM, Goh DW, Abrams LD: Creation of brachial artery–basilic vein fistula. A supplement to the cavopulmonary shunt. J Thorac Cardiovasc Surg 98:214, 1989.

101. Magee A, Sim E, Benson LN, et al: Augmentation of pulmonary blood flow with an axillary arteriovenous fistula after a cavopulmonary shunt. J Thorac Cardiovasc Surg 111:176, 1996.

102. Lacroix J, Blanchard H, de Viele de Goyet J, et al: Reversal of cirrhosis-related pulmonary shunting in two children by orthotopic liver transplantation. Transplantation 53:1135, 1992.

103. Brodie Knight W, Mee RBB: A cure for pulmonary arteriovenous fistulas? Ann Thorac Surg 59:999, 1995.

104. Abella I, Torres I, Leveroni A, et al: Ergometría en el bypass total vs bypass parcial del ventrículo derecho. Rev Argent Cardiol 64:517, 1996.

105. Sietsema KE, Cooper D, Perloff JK, et al: Dynamic of oxygen uptake during exercise in adults with cyanotic congenital heart disease. Circulation 73:1137, 1986.

106. Fontan F, Baudet E: Surgical repair of tricuspid atresia. Thorax 26:240, 1971.

107. Kreutzer G, Galindez E, Bono H, et al: An operation for the correction of the tricuspid atresia. J Thorac Cardiovasc Surg 66:613, 1973.

108. Billingsley AM, Laks H, Boyce SW, et al: Definitive repair in patients with pulmonary atresia and intact ventricular septum. J Thorac Cardiovasc Surg 97:746, 1989.

109. Bjork VO, Olin CL, Bjarke BB, Thoren CA: Right atrial–right ventricular anastomosis for correction of tricuspid atresia. J Thorac Cardiovasc Surg 77:452, 1979.

110. Kreutzer GO, Vargas FJ, Schlichter AJ, et al: Atriopulmonary anastomosis. J Thorac Cardiovasc Surg 83:427, 1982.

111. Kreutzer GO, Allaria A, Schlister A, et al: A comparative long-term follow-up of the results of anterior and posterior approaches in bypassing the rudimentary right ventricle in patients with tricuspid atresia. Int J Cardiol 19:167, 1988.

112. deLeval MR, Kliner P, Gewilling M, Bull C: Total cavopulmonary connection; a logical alternative to atriopulmonary connection for complex Fontan operations. Experimental studies and early clinical experience. J Thorac Cardiovasc Surg 3:91, 1988.

113. Puga JF, Chiavarelli M, Hagler DJ: Modification of the Fontan operation applicable to patients with left atrioventricular valve atresia or single atrioventricular valve. Circulation 76:1153, 1987.

114. Vargas FJ, Mayer JE, Jonas RA, Castaneda AR: Anomalous systemic and pulmonary venous connection in conjunction with atriopulmonary anastomosis (Fontan-Kreutzer). Technical considerations. J Thorac Cardiovasc Surg 83:523, 1987.

115. Jonas RA, Castañeda AR: Modified Fontan procedure: Atrial baffle and systemic venous to pulmonary artery anastomotic techniques. J Card Surg 3:91, 1988.

116. Uemura H, Yagihara T, Kawashima Y, et al: What factors affect ventricular performance after a Fontan-type operation? J Thorac Cardiovasc Surg 110:405, 1995.

117. Kreutzer C, Schlichter AJ, Kreutzer GO: Cavoatriopulmonary anastomosis via a nonprosthetic medial tunnel. J Card Surg 12:37, 1997.

118. Marcelletti C, Corno A, Giannico S, Marino B: Inferior vena cava pulmonary artery extracardiac conduit: A new form of right heart bypass. J Thorac Cardiovasc Surg 100:228, 1990.

119. Gundry SR, Razzouk AJ, del Rio MS, et al: The optimal Fontan connection: A growing extracardiac lateral tunnel with pedicled pericardium. J Thorac Cardiovasc Surg 114:552, 1997.

120. Gates RN, Laks H, Drinkwater DC Jr, et al: The Fontan procedure in adults. Ann Thorac Surg 63:1085, 1997.

121. Canobbio MM, Mair DD, Van der Velde M, Koos BJ: Pregnancy outcomes after the Fontan repair. J Am Coll Cardiol 28:763, 1996.

122. Senzaki H, Isoda T, Ishizawa A, Hishi T: Reconsideration of criteria for the Fontan operation. Influence of pulmonary artery size on postoperative hemodynamics of the Fontan operation. Circulation 89:1196, 1994.

123. Fontan F, Kirklin JW, Fernandez G, et al: Outcome after a "perfect" Fontan operation. Circulation 81:1520, 1990.

124. Humes RA, Porter CJ, Mair D, et al: Intermediate follow-up and predicted survival after the modified Fontan procedure for tricuspid atresia and double-inlet ventricle. Circulation 76(suppl 3):67, 1987.

125. Driscoll DJ, Offord KP, Feldt RH, et al: Five to fifteen year follow-up after Fontan operation. Circulation 85:469, 1992.

126. Mair DD, Hagler DJ, Julsrud PR, et al: Early and late results of the modified Fontan procedure for double-inlet left ventricle. The Mayo Clinic experience. J Am Coll Cardiol 18:1727, 1991.

127. Feldt RH, Driscoll DJ, Offord KP, et al: Protein-losing enteropathy after the Fontan operation. J Thorac Cardiovasc Surg 112:672, 1996.

128. Moore JW, Kirby WC, Madden W, Gaiber NS: Development of pulmonary arteriovenous malformations after modified Fontan operation. J Thorac Cardiovasc Surg 98:1045, 1989.

129. Choussat A, Fontan F, Besse P, et al: Selection criteria for Fontan's procedure. In Anderson RH, Shinebourne EA (eds): Pediatric Cardiology 1977. Edinburgh, Churchill Livingstone, 1978, p 559.

130. Fontan F, Fernandez G, Costa F, et al: The size of the pulmonary arteries and the results of the Fontan operation. J Thorac Cardiovasc Surg 98:711, 1989.

131. Amadeo A, Galletti L, Marianeschi S, et al: Extracardiac Fontan operation for complex cardiac anomalies: Seven years' experience. J Thorac Cardiovasc Surg 114:1020, 1997.

132. Knott-Craig CJ, Danielson GK, Schaff HV, et al: The modified Fontan operation. An analysis of risk factors for early postoperative death or takedown in 702 consecutive patients from one institution. J Thorac Cardiovasc Surg 109:1237, 1995.

133. Gentles TL, Mayer JE, Gauvreau K, et al: Fontan operation in five hundred consecutive patients: Factors influencing early and late outcome. J Thorac Cardiovasc Surg 114:376, 1997.

134. Miura T, Hiramatsu T, Forbess JM, Mayer JE: Effects of elevated coronary sinus pressure on coronary blood flow and left ventricular function. Implications after the Fontan operation. Circulation 92(suppl II):II-298, 1995.

135. Castaneda A: From Glenn to Fontan. A continuing evolution. Circulation 86(suppl II):II-80, 1992.

136. Mayer JE, Bridges N, Lock JE, et al: Factors associated with marked reduction in mortality for Fontan operations in patients with single ventricle. J Thorac Cardiovasc Surg 103:444, 1992.

137. Gewillig M, Daenen W, Aubert A, Van der Hauwaert L: Abolishment of chronic volume overload. Implications for diastolic function of the systemic ventricle immediately after Fontan repair. Circulation 86(suppl):II-93, 1992.

138. Driscoll D, Danielson G, Puga F, et al: Exercise tolerance and cardiorespiratory response to exercise after the Fontan operation for tricuspid atresia or functional single ventricle. J Am Coll Cardiol 7:1087, 1986.

139. Zellers T, Driscoll D, Mottram C, et al: Exercise tolerance and cardiorespiratory response to exercise before and after the Fontan operation. Mayo Clin Proc 64:1489, 1989.

140. Ben Schachar G, Fuhrman B, Wang Y, et al: Rest and exercise dynamics after the Fontan procedure. Circulation 65:1043, 1982.

141. Gewillig MH, Lundstrom UR, Bull C, et al: Exercise responses in patients with congenital heart disease after Fontan repair: Patterns and determinants of performance. J Am Coll Cardiol 15:1424, 1990.

142. Grant G, Mansell A, Garfano R, et al: Cardiorespiratory response to exercise after the Fontan procedure for tricuspid atresia. Pediatr Res 24:1, 1988.

143. Lardo AC, Webber S, del Nido PJ, et al: Does the right lung receive preferential blood flow in Fontan repair? Comparison of total cavopulmonary and atriopulmonary connections: An in vitro study. Circulation 92(suppl I):I-579, 1995.

144. Siggfusson G, Webber S, Myers JL, et al: Growth of pulmonary arteries following Fontan operation: Influence of age and type of connection. Circulation 92(suppl I):I-55, 1995.

145. Buheitel G, Hofbeck M, Tenbrink V, et al: Changes in pulmonary artery size before and after total cavopulmonary connection. Heart 78:488, 1997.

146. Rosenthal D, Friedman A, Kleinman CH, et al: Thromboembolic complications after Fontan operations. Circulation 92(suppl II):II-287, 1995.

147. Day RW, Boyer RS, Tait VF, Ruttenberg HD: Factors associated with stroke following the Fontan procedure. Pediatr Cardiol 16:270, 1995.

148. Brestcker M, Myers J, Cyran SE: Conversion of modified Fontan-Kreutzer connection to total cavopulmonary connection. Result in improved exercise tolerance and quality of life. Circulation 92(suppl I):I-55, 1995.

149. Kreutzer J, Keane JF, Lock JE, et al: Conversion of modified Fontan procedure to lateral atrial tunnel cavopulmonary anastomosis. J Thorac Cardiovasc Surg 111:1169, 1996.

150. Hsu H, Nykanen DG, Williams WG, et al: Right to left interatrial communications after the modified Fontan procedure: Identification and management with transcatheter occlusion. Br Heart J 74:548, 1995.

151. Kavey RW, Gaum W, Byrum CJ, et al: Loss of sinus rhythm after total cavopulmonary connection. Circulation 92(suppl II):II-304, 1994.

152. Manning PB, Mayer JE, Wernovsky G, et al: Staged operation to Fontan increases the incidence of sinoatrial node dysfunction. J Thorac Cardiovasc Surg 112:833, 1996.

153. Gelatt M, Hamilton RM, McCrindle BW, et al: Risk factors for atrial tachyarrhythmias after the Fontan operation. J Am Coll Cardiol 24:1735, 1994.

154. Cecchini F, Johnsrude CL, Perry JC, Friedman RA: Effect of age and surgical technique on symptomatic arrhythmias after the Fontan procedure. Am J Cardiol 76:386, 1995.

155. Robotin MC, Edis BD, Weintraub RG, et al: Heart transplantation for chyloptysis after Fontan operation. Ann Thorac Surg 59:1570, 1995.

156. Treidman JK, Saul PS, Wendling SN, Walsh EP: Radiofrequency ablation of intraatrial reentrant tachycardia after surgical palliation of congenital heart disease. Circulation 91:707, 1995.

157. Kao JM, Alejos JC, Grant PW, et al: Conversion of atriopulmonary to cavopulmonary anastomosis in management of late arrhythmias and atrial thrombosis. Ann Thorac Surg 58:1510, 1994.

158. Taussig HB: Long-time observations on the Blalock-Taussig operation. Single ventricle (with apex to the left). Johns Hopkins Med J 139:69, 1976.

CHAPTER 34
PERSISTENT TRUNCUS ARTERIOSUS

J. F. N. TAYLOR

The term *truncus arteriosus* denotes a single arterial trunk that arises from the heart and is the common origin of the systemic, pulmonary, and coronary circulations. The original description is attributed to Wilson in 1798.[1]

Truncus arteriosus accounts for 2% of congenital cardiac abnormalities (see Chapter 18). Its frequency is constant throughout the reported series from the Western world.[2–4]

EMBRYOLOGY

The cephalad segment of the straight primitive cardiac tube is designated the truncus arteriosus, a single structure that begins at the outlet of the ultimate heart at the level of the semilunar valve. This segment then divides into two separate major arterial outlets, one to the systemic circulation and one to the developing pulmonary circulation. There remains debate as to whether this septation is created by ingrowth of the two ridges that develop in a spiral, so that in joining the normal way the pulmonary trunk twists around the aortic root, or whether this spiral is formed as a consequence of the looping of the primitive ventricle and subsequent differential growth of neural crest–derived tissue.[1,5] In either event, failure of this process takes place at the 4- to 5-mm embryonic stage (4- to 5-week embryo), at the same time that the outlet ventricular septum is developing, and there will be mutual interaction between these developments.[6]

There is an association with an absent thymus, immunodeficiency, and hypocalcemia that became known as the DiGeorge syndrome,[7] although not all the features are universally present (see Chapter 2). The degree of immunodeficiency is one of the more variable features; thus, the term partial DiGeorge syndrome[8] came to be used. Coincidentally, other workers, notably Takao and colleagues,[9] described a typical abnormal facies seen with many conotruncal malformations including truncus arteriosus. This feature, but with variable expression of severity of the cardiac defect,[10] was familial and suggested an inheritance pattern following mendelian lines. A genetic basis for the disease entity was postulated[11] and confirmed by identification of a deletion on the long arm of chromosome 22 (designated 22q11) by Scambler and colleagues.[12] The deletion may involve a long segment of the long arm or there may be different microdeletions, thus demonstrating a basis for a varied clinical picture incorporating some or all of a series of characteristics. These were defined by Wilson and coworkers[13] as conofacial anomaly, absent thymus, hypocalcemia, and heart defect, embodied in the acronym CATCH-22. There is overlap with other syndromes involving cardiac malformation, such as the velocardiofacial syndrome (Shprintzen's syndrome),[10] and there is wider family grouping around individuals with or without these features (see Chapter 2). There is some experimental evidence in dogs to support this theory.[14]

Much attention has been given to the role played by migrating neural crest tissue in the developing cardiac tube and the cellular contribution to the development of the ridges described before.[15–23] The teratogenic effects of cytotoxic agents in producing this defect seem to be related to this specific effect on migration of the neural crest tissue.[24–27] There is experimental evidence to support the link between an identifiable gene defect (microdeletion), its effect on a particular cell type and its migration (the neural crest), and the ultimate expression of one or more developmental abnormalities (specifically in context, truncus arteriosus).

CLASSIFICATION

It is usual to classify truncus arteriosus in relation to the origin of the pulmonary circulation from the arterial trunk.[28–34] A single pulmonary artery arising posteriorly and to the left of the trunk immediately above the semilunar valve, which then branches after a variable length into right and left pulmonary arteries, is type I. From the bifurcation of the pulmonary artery, a ductus arteriosus may connect to the descending thoracic aorta.[29,34] If the orifices of the two pulmonary arteries arise separately from the arterial trunk, although close together and still just above the semilunar valve, this is designated type II. It can be difficult to distinguish a true type II lesion from a type I with a short common pulmonary trunk (Fig. 34–1). Type III is the designation when the two pulmonary arteries have separate origins either distinctly separated from each other or displaced cranially from the semilunar valves but still proximal to the origin of the brachiocephalic arteries.

Two other terms have been used but in fact describe particular types of pulmonary atresia with ventricular septal defect. These are pseudotruncus, in which an unrestricted ductus arteriosus supplies confluent right and left pulmonary arteries, and the so-called type IV truncus, in which the blood supply to the lungs arises from the descending thoracic aorta, from arteries that are major aortopulmonary communicating arteries. In both these variants, examination of the right ventricle demonstrates an

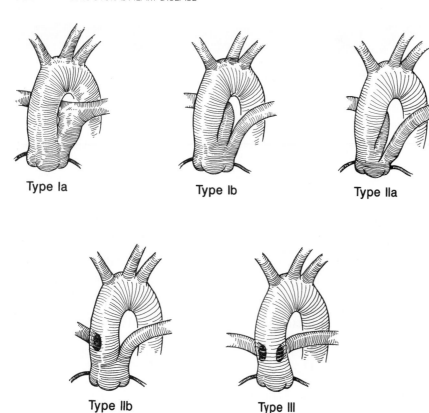

Type Ia

Type Ib

Type IIa

Type IIb

Type III

FIGURE 34–1

Truncus arteriosus—illustration of types. It may be difficult to distinguish type Ib from type IIa by imaging studies.

infundibular portion, albeit hypoplastic and atretic. The pathologic differences between truncus arteriosus and pulmonary atresia have been documented.[35]

PATHOLOGIC ANATOMY

The single arterial trunk usually arises from a heart with two ventricles communicating with each other by a nonrestrictive ventricular septal defect immediately below the semilunar valve that guards the orifice of the arterial trunk. A right-sided arch occurs in a third,[28–30] interruption of the aortic arch is common (11 to 19%),[28–30] there is no ductus arteriosus or ligamentum arteriosum in at least half of the subjects,[28–30] and an anomaly of the pulmonary venous connection is not unusual.[32] One pulmonary artery is occasionally absent.[28–36]

The atrial arrangement is usual for situs solitus with concordant atrioventricular relationships and two equal-sized ventricles. The right ventricle is hypertrophied and without an outflow portion; thus, there is no infundibular septum. Although this describes most instances of truncus arteriosus, a wide variety of univentricular and biventricular connections, with and without two distinct ventricular components or ventricular septal defect, have been described.[37–45] A number of abnormal coronary artery arrangements have also been described[34, 46–50] and need to be identified in any preoperative investigation. The intrapulmonary arterial circulation is normal; occasionally the pulmonary venous connection is abnormal.

The most important associated extracardiac malformations are anomalies of the aortic arch, which may be simply right-sided with a right descending thoracic aorta, or the arch may be interrupted whether it is left- or right-sided.[28–30] As with interruption of the aortic arch in the usual situation (i.e., with only a malalignment ventricular septal defect), the arch may be interrupted as depicted in Figure 34–2. The exact arrangement has no influence on presentation given the presence of interruption, although the palpability of individual pulses may vary on detailed clinical examination (see later).

HEMODYNAMICS

The increased volume load in the left ventricle is derived not only from the increased pulmonary blood flow but also from regurgitation of the truncal valve. To this may be added an increased resistance to outflow if the truncal valve is also stenotic. The combined effects of these changes increase the end-diastolic volume and the end-diastolic pressure; there will be left atrial enlargement, pulmonary venous distention, and raised left atrial pressure.

Pulmonary blood flow comes directly from the systemic circulation and is restricted only by the size of the pulmonary arteries (especially in types II and III), which varies from individual to individual, and by the pulmonary arteriolar resistance. This falls after birth, but often faster than when pulmonary blood flow is enhanced solely by a communication at the ventricular level; thus, even with a competent truncal valve, the effect of increased pulmonary blood flow and distention of the left ventricle leads to respiratory embarrassment, difficulty in feeding, excessive diaphoresis, and poor weight gain before the end of the

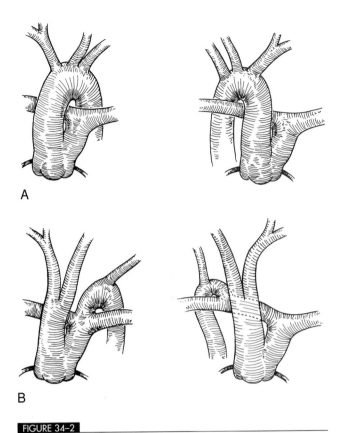

FIGURE 34–2

Truncus arteriosus. *A*, Type I with left aortic arch (*left*) and with right aortic arch (*right*). *B*, Type I with interruption of aortic arch between ipsilateral carotid and subclavian arteries (type B). Left aortic arch (*left*) and right aortic arch (*right*).

neonatal period. If the truncal valve is abnormal, these effects are demonstrated earlier, even before pulmonary vascular resistance falls.[32] Thus, the more severe the truncal valve malformation, the earlier the clinical presentation in cardiac failure, which may occur within a day or two of birth.

Without a major truncal valve abnormality, the hemodynamic changes follow a pattern dictated by the pulmonary vascular response. The pulmonary vascular resistance falls early and then in some patients may rise markedly before 3 months of age.[51,52] In others, the slow and inexorable progressive change of typical advancing pulmonary vascular disease is delayed until after 1 or 2 years of age, with falling pulmonary blood flow and increasing cyanosis. Pulmonary vascular resistance is almost always at the systemic level and no longer capable of reversal before the end of the first decade, and survival beyond the second decade is unlikely.

The truncal valve is rarely totally competent, and with the passage of time, the degree of incompetence increases. This comes from the progressive increase in diameter of the truncal root (as occurs with the aortic root in longstanding pulmonary atresia with ventricular septal defect or tetralogy of Fallot), precluding appropriate apposition of the valve leaflets, plus an increase in combined systemic and pulmonary resistance.

There is only one exit from the right ventricle, that is, through the ventricular septal defect directly through the truncal valve as it overlies the septal defect. The ventricu-

lar septal defect is only rarely restrictive. The right ventricular volume partially reflects the changes in left ventricular volume with increasing pulmonary flow but is also affected directly by the regurgitant flow from an incompetent truncal valve. Right ventricular performance is thus affected in both the short and long term more directly by truncal valve performance than by pulmonary blood flow.

The common origin of systemic, coronary, and pulmonary circulations results in common mixing, systemic and pulmonary venous returns becoming admixed at the level of the ventricular septal defect and the orifice of the truncal valve itself. The level of saturation in blood reaching the periphery depends on the relative volumes of saturated blood (from the pulmonary venous return) and of desaturated blood from the body. Pulmonary venous return is likely to exceed systemic flow because the pulmonary vascular resistance is usually lower than systemic, and restriction of pulmonary blood flow by anatomic narrowing of the pulmonary arteries is rare.

Thus, as pulmonary vascular resistance falls in the neonatal period, pulmonary blood flow increases, the arterial saturation rises, and cardiac failure supervenes. Rarely, pulmonary blood flow is restricted by an anatomic narrowing at the origins of the pulmonary arteries or by hypoplasia of the main branches themselves; cyanosis is then significant and remains severe. (In a common mixing lesion, such as common atrium, effective single-ventricle chamber, and truncus arteriosus, equal pulmonary and systemic blood flow usually gives an arterial saturation in the low 80s, whereas if the pulmonary-to-systemic flow ratio exceeds 3, arterial saturation will be in the mid-90s, assuming a near-normal systemic flow.)

After the neonatal fall in pulmonary vascular resistance and in the absence of significant truncal valve regurgitation, the hemodynamic situation remains stable, with an oxygen saturation in the 80s for many months. However, once pulmonary vascular resistance starts to rise, it continues to rise inexorably. This is associated with clinical improvement as the lower pulmonary blood flow diminishes cardiac output; systemic flow increases but at first with little change in saturation. Ultimately, arterial saturation falls significantly as pulmonary vascular resistance continues to rise. In the face of the total increase in vascular resistance, the truncal valve may become regurgitant or progressively more so. The clinical course becomes common to all lesions leading to progressive pulmonary vascular disease.

The coexistence of interrupted aortic arch influences the hemodynamic changes described before, particularly the rapidity with which obstructive pulmonary vascular change takes place such that the whole natural history may be experienced within 2 years. It is likely that the early features of cardiac failure will be pronounced.

NATURAL HISTORY

Many infants with truncus arteriosus present in cardiac failure during the first 2 weeks. Such early development of cardiac failure with an interventricular communication before the pulmonary vascular resistance falls from its neonatal level, implies that there is a valve lesion also present and should suggest this diagnosis. The other common lesion that shares the same early history is a complete atrioventricular septal defect with regurgitant common atrioventricular orifice. Early death, often unexpected, is not rare.[53]

The cardiac failure, although severe, may not progress for several weeks, but eventually an increasing volume load to the heart from the increasing pulmonary flow as the vascular resistance falls may exacerbate the clinical signs. Weight gain remains inadequate, and the infant appears marasmic. Survival will be prejudiced further by a severe lower respiratory tract infection. Eighty-five percent of untreated children die before 1 year of age.[54]

With a competent nonrestrictive truncal valve, the infant may thrive initially. By 3 months, weight gain may have slowed, although height increase remains unchecked. The degree of cyanosis is usually so mild as to be unnoticed except by an experienced observer, but there are signs of mild cardiac failure, and the overactive precordial impulse persists for at least 2 years. Thereafter, in the absence of treatment, the child's general condition may improve with better growth. Cyanosis is recognized by this time but still mild. This improvement is a consequence of the progressive rise in resistance from pulmonary vascular obstructive disease, limiting pulmonary blood flow and thus the volume of the left-to-right shunt.

Pulmonary flow has fallen to equal systemic blood flow toward the end of the first decade and thereafter, as the teenage years progress, falls below it. Cyanosis increases, and effort tolerance and stamina that had previously increased in early childhood now fall again; increased fatigability and lassitude rather than breathlessness become factors limiting effort tolerance.

Toward the end of the second decade, pulmonary vascular obstructive disease becomes so severe that cyanosis and poor stamina result in a limited existence. A degree of breathlessness, now from hypoxemia, may develop on minimal effort, and the extremities may be cold from inadequate cardiac output.

Survival into the third decade is unusual, death resulting from hemoptysis, intrapulmonary arterial thrombotic events, or ventricular (predominantly right) failure. Sudden death, that is to say an event without significant change in general status in the antecedent weeks, is not uncommon. This is frequently from cardiac standstill, although tachyarrhythmias and ventricular fibrillation are recognized terminal events.

CLINICAL HISTORY AND PHYSICAL EXAMINATION

Although fetal echocardiography may suggest a congenital cardiac lesion or even be diagnostic (see Chapter 12), recognition of the cardiac anomaly usually occurs within the first week of life because of cyanosis and cardiac failure, which can become severe within the first 10 days, responding little to conventional anti-failure regimens. A murmur, detected at the immediate routine postnatal examination, also leads to recognition of the abnormality. An abnormal facies is present in some, although the incidence depends on the diligence with which the particular features of the "conotruncal facies"[55] are sought, and similar features may be recognized in retrospect in other family members.

Cyanosis is moderate and changes little in the early months. From 6 weeks onward, digital clubbing is recognizable and, although progressive, does not reach the extreme degree encountered in long-standing untreated tetralogy of Fallot and other lesions with restricted pulmonary blood flow. Growth rate is slow, and in common with many lesions with an excessive pulmonary blood flow, there is air trapping in the lungs leading to increased anteroposterior and lateral diameters of the chest with mild to moderate subcostal and intercostal recession.

There is easy palpability of the peripheral pulses, sometimes of bounding quality. The precordial impulse is hyperdynamic and suggests enlargement of both ventricles, with displacement of the apex beat toward the axilla. There may be a systolic thrill, occasionally a diastolic thrill, appreciated at the apex. There is a prominent ejection click, often palpable; care should be taken to identify its timing relative to the first sound rather than to confuse it with an accentuated delayed pulmonary component to the second sound. There is universally a long ejection systolic murmur and frequently an immediate diastolic murmur after the single second component of the heart sound. From the lower left sternal border to the apex, the third sound and mid-diastolic rumble are appreciated.

The chest is sometimes deformed, the transverse and anteroposterior diameters being increased with a prominent sternum (so-called pigeon chest deformity in common with all lesions producing a large left-to-right shunt). In young infants, the respiratory rate is increased, and subcostal and intercostal recession is evident. Without a concomitant respiratory tract infection, there are no other abnormal signs other than the appreciation in some infants that air entry to the left base is significantly reduced; because of the lobar collapse, fine crepitations are heard on inspiration, even in the absence of infection. The liver is palpable below the right costal margin; occasionally, the spleen tip is palpable as well. Abdominal examination otherwise does not differ from normal.

Two signs suggest that the aortic arch is, in addition, interrupted. Neither is pathognomonic. The first is a degree of cardiac failure out of proportion to the signs of truncal valve malformation (stenosis or regurgitation). The second is an appreciation that the carotid pulsation is less than the leg pulsation. (If the arch is interrupted, the ascending aorta may be significantly underdeveloped; it is always smaller than the normal ascending aorta. Preferential flow is thus to the pulmonary trunk and lower half of the body through a persistent ductus arteriosus. Differential cyanosis is not detectable because there is mixing proximal to the ascending aorta.)

As pulmonary vascular resistance rises with advancing age, the clinical features in the older child (or young adult) differ significantly from those described in infancy and childhood. General physical development remains marginally affected, particularly in a lean build relative to a mildly compromised stature. Cyanosis, however, is marked, with severe digital clubbing. Although arterial pulse volume tends to be normal, the venous pressure in the neck has a prominent *a* wave. The precordial impulse is characterized by a sustained left parasternal heave, indicating predominantly right ventricular hypertrophy, and there is little displacement of the apex beat. The heart sounds differ little, with a prominent ejection click and single component to the second sound. The systolic murmur, however, is short, midsystolic, or even absent. The immediate diastolic murmur is more definite, high pitched, and decrescendo, rarely passing beyond middiastole. Although a third sound may be heard, there is no mid-diastolic murmur.

Ultimately, pulmonary vascular disease progresses to a stage at which fatigability is such as to limit activities to the house, cyanosis is extreme, and peripheral circulatory failure results in cold extremities. Three events determine the final outcome: uncontrollable hemoptysis after one or more lesser episodes; congestive cardiac failure with florid ascites and peripheral edema, accompanied by painful hepatic enlargement and central chest pain ("right ventricular angina"); and sudden death. The last, however, is not always completely unheralded; it may be preceded by one or two syncopal episodes or by an unrelated intercurrent illness. Such an evolution of the natural history is now unlikely.

ELECTROCARDIOGRAPHY

There are no electrocardiographic features specific to persistent truncus arteriosus. Electrocardiograms recorded during the first week of life may have normal precordial voltages or show the moderate excess of right ventricular activity common to many other cardiac lesions at this age. With advancing age (about 3 months), virtually all patients show the features of biventricular enlargement, the signs of left ventricular hypertrophy exceeding those of right ventricular hypertrophy but without prominent Q waves in the left precordial leads. The mean frontal QRS axis tends to lie in the arc from +30 to +120; P waves are prominent but not abnormally large, and the ST segment and T waves are normal in the absence of digoxin administration (Fig. 34–3). There are no special features that help to identify the severe truncal valve malformation, a right aortic arch, or interruption of the aortic arch.

CHEST RADIOGRAPHY AND OTHER IMAGING TECHNIQUES

THE PLAIN CHEST RADIOGRAPH (see Chapter 10)

The cardiac silhouette lies in the usual position but is enlarged with a contour associated with left ventricular enlargement, the apex lying on or below the level of the left dome of the diaphragm. Left atrial enlargement may be evident from splaying of the bronchi, and the right atrial border is usually prominent. A right-sided aortic arch may be identified by the characteristic indentation on the right margin of the tracheal shadow.

Pulmonary plethora is prominent, the enlarged pulmonary arterial markings being evident well into the pe-

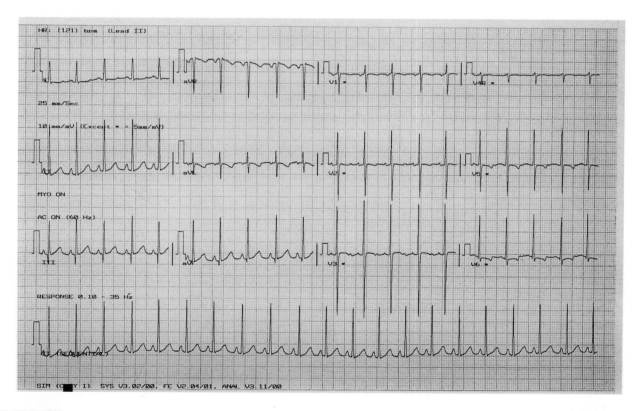

FIGURE 34–3

Electrocardiogram from an infant with truncus arteriosus showing the dominant left ventricular forces. The T wave inversion in lateral chest leads may be a digoxin effect.

riphery of the lung fields. An element of pulmonary venous congestion is often in evidence, and when there is failure with fluid overload, the interlobar and interlobular fissures are prominent, with blurring of the two costophrenic angles. The central right and left pulmonary arteries are usually enlarged, irrespective of whether they have taken a single type I or separate type II or type III origin from the common trunk; however, their origin and immediate course toward each lung lie more cephalad than normally arising pulmonary arteries. As a consequence, the hilar shadows in persistent truncus arteriosus are more cephalad than normal, and this may allow distinction from an isolated ventricular septal defect.

As a consequence of enlargement of the central pulmonary arteries and the left atrium and ventricle, there may be bronchial compression and collapse of certain bronchopulmonary segments. The most common are collapse of the left lower lobe (bronchial compression between the main left pulmonary artery and the left atrium plus direct compression from the enlarged left ventricle) and right middle lobe collapse and consolidation from compression of the bronchi at the point of bifurcation within the hilum where the enlarged pulmonary artery branches take origin. Infective changes may be widespread and in fact related to bronchial compression.

Progressive pulmonary vascular obstructive disease may be inferred from the plain radiograph by the second decade. The central pulmonary arteries remain enlarged, but there is progressive diminution in the size of the peripheral pulmonary arteries to produce the radiographic appearance of "pruning." Compared with similar changes due to isolated ventricular septal defect (often a decade later), the transverse cardiac diameter does not change and remains enlarged. Left basal collapse tends to remain. The changes of pulmonary vascular disease are more evident if the ductus arteriosus remains patent, with or without in-terruption of the arch. If it is not interrupted, because the ascending aortic components are smaller than normal, there may be little mediastinal shadowing to the right of the trachea; similarly, in a right aortic arch, the more prominent mediastinal shadow is on the right.

MAGNETIC RESONANCE IMAGING

Magnetic resonance images can be superior to echocardiograms or angiocardiograms in defining the abnormal origins of the pulmonary arteries from the common trunk. Sufficient information may also be available to define the anatomy of the ventricular septal defect.[56]

Conventional techniques will become fast enough to supplant more costly spin-echo techniques,[57,58] which had sufficiently rapid acquisition times to be useful in the younger infant.

ECHOCARDIOGRAPHY

A ventricular septal defect will be shown in the outlet position, Doppler color flow interrogation showing bidirectional flow. Careful interrogation will exclude additional smaller defects. The ventricular septal defect lies under the single semilunar valve, with the single outlet coming predominantly from one or other ventricle rather than equally above the two ventricles. There is no outlet septum or other outlet anterior to the great artery overlying the ventricular septal defect (Fig. 34–4A).[59]

Careful inspection of the cross-sectional image may determine the number of sinuses (usually three, although it may be two, four, or six) and demonstrate morphology and limitation of cusp movements. Doppler interrogation may reveal an increased velocity to suggest stenosis or may show regurgitation (Fig. 34–4B; see Color Plates).

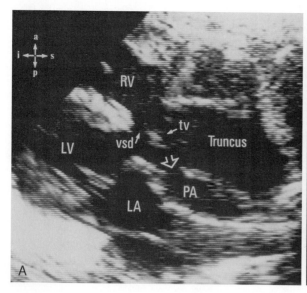
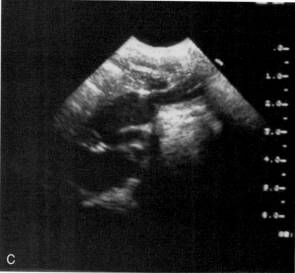

FIGURE 34–4

Truncus arteriosus, cross-sectional echocardiograms. *A,* Parasternal long-axis view of typical type I truncus. LA = left atrium; LV = left ventricle; PA = pulmonary artery; RV = right ventricle; tv = truncal valve; vsd = ventricular septal defect. *B,* See Color Figure 34–4B. *C,* The pulmonary artery arises from behind and to the left of the truncus. The first branch of the aorta bifurcates, that is, it is the brachiocephalic artery lying to the left, indicating a right aortic arch.

One pulmonary artery can usually be defined arising from the posterior and leftward aspect of the common trunk, but it can be difficult to define the origin of the other (usually right) pulmonary artery, unless it is remote (i.e., type III). It is also difficult to establish continuity between the two pulmonary arteries and thus correctly differentiate a type I from a type II origin.

High parasternal views, both left and right, together with suprasternal notch and infraclavicular views, may be necessary to define the arch anatomy correctly; not only should a left arch be distinguished from the right (Fig. 34–4C), but a patent ductus on the side of the arch should be identified. If a ductus appears to be present, it is necessary to establish whether there is also a true aortic arch; otherwise, an interruption may be overlooked. Clues to interruption are a smaller dimension of the ascending aortic component than of the apparent arch (i.e., ductus) and descending aorta and a simple bifurcation of the ascending aorta into the two carotids. Interruption of the arch associated with truncus arteriosus is usually immediately distal to the origin of the left carotid artery, and both subclavian arteries may arise from the descending thoracic aorta just below ductal insertion. Thus, one of the subclavian arteries (depending on the side of the descending thoracic aorta) passes behind the esophagus.

Possibly the most difficult echocardiographic distinction to make is interruption of a right aortic arch from a right-sided ductus with right arch and descending thoracic aorta. Recognition that the thymus is absent may help in evaluating the potential presence of the DiGeorge syndrome.[60] Persistent truncus arteriosus can be identified echocardiographically during fetal life.[61,62]

The usual questions that remain after a carefully conducted echocardiogram are the site of origin and course of the second pulmonary artery and the integrity of the aortic arch.

CARDIAC CATHETERIZATION AND ANGIOGRAPHY

HEMODYNAMIC ASSESSMENT

Hemodynamic investigation and invasive imaging, if undertaken, should confirm the diagnosis, add to the detail of information available concerning an individual patient, and exclude additional lesions likely to influence management.[63] It should be complete in its own right, with no assumption made from the previous clinical and echocardiographic findings.

There is typically a bidirectional shunt, the left-to-right component of which is at the ventricular level, although the right-to-left component may not be defined until the great arterial sample is analyzed. The oxygen saturation in the ascending aorta may differ significantly from that in the pulmonary artery even though both arise from the common trunk. The respective ventricular outputs do not mix above the single semilunar valve, and the less saturated right ventricular outflow blood passes preferentially to the pulmonary artery. The pulmonary artery saturation cannot be assumed from any sample of aortic origin. To do so results in erroneous calculation of pulmonary blood flow (too high) and pulmonary vascular resistance (too low).

In small infants particularly, when the pulmonary blood flow is high, a left-to-right shunt may be detected at atrial level, the high pulmonary venous return being associated with a "stretched" foramen ovale, although a true (secundum) atrial septal defect may be present.[28] This must be distinguished from anomalous pulmonary venous connection by judicious catheter probing and angiography.

It is not possible to rely on catheter passage alone (either anterograde or retrograde) to distinguish the additional presence of a ductus arteriosus with or without aortic interruption. With aortic interruption, however, the pulmonary artery saturation is identical to the descending aortic saturation, but the ascending aortic value may be higher.

The ventricular systolic pressures are equal, although the end-diastolic pressure may be higher on the left. A critically important pressure difference is that between the ventricles and the common trunk or ascending aorta. A systolic pressure difference in excess of 10 mm Hg (ignoring any ventricular pressure overshoot) implies a restrictive semilunar valve but may on occasion be associated with an excessive "runoff" into the pulmonary circulation if the pulmonary vascular resistance is low.

Pulmonary artery pressure (ideally, both right and left) must be recorded separately from the truncal/ascending aortic pressure because, even with a free communication, a lower pulmonary vascular resistance results in appreciable difference in perfusion pressure of pulmonary and systemic vascular beds. This is not so if the ductus remains widely patent, when truncal, ascending aortic, pulmonary arterial, and descending aortic pressures are the same. If the arch is interrupted, there may be a narrower pulse pressure in the ascending aortic component and its immediate branches.

In following the catheter's passage between ascending aortic and descending aortic components in truncus arteriosus, it may be difficult to be certain whether the aortic arch has been followed or the catheter passed through the ductus arteriosus; careful differential angiography may be required for definitive delineation. Distinction of right or left descending thoracic aorta is easy, and identifying the position of the ascending aorta is relatively easy, but the most difficult differentiation is between a right-sided ductus with interruption and an intact right arch.

With an older child particularly, accurate collection of pressure and saturation data is mandatory if a representative measurement of pulmonary vascular resistance is to be made. This also demands a reliable method of assessing oxygen uptake if the Fick principle[63] is to be used as the basis of calculation. These factors may become crucial in assessing indication for operation.

ANGIOGRAPHY

Although all aspects of the central circulation should be identified angiographically,[63] the left ventricular angiogram and an angiogram taken by injecting contrast medium immediately above the single semilunar valve are two basic requirements. The most useful projections for the left ventricular angiograms are the long-axis view[64] and the lateral. These two views define the margins of the ventricular septal defect and the origin of the great artery relative to the outlet of the two ventricles. They may also indicate the morphology of the semilunar valves (thickened leaflets, doming, possibly number of sinuses) and delineate the site of origin from the common trunk of at least one pulmonary artery; this is the main trunk of type I and the left pulmonary artery in type II and possibly type III. It is difficult to differentiate a type I origin from a type II if the common pulmonary segment between the truncus and bifurcation is extremely short; it may be little more than a diverticulum from the apex of which the right and left pulmonary arteries arise. This is usually classified as type II surgically. The long-axis view, because it profiles the length of the interventricular septum, excludes additional, often unsuspected ventricular septal defects.

It is not possible to define one or two projections that invariably yield all requisite information, but at least two if not four orthogonal views may be required. These may be supplemented by more specifically sited injections in the pulmonary component of the trunk or the ascending aortic component proximal to the expected commencement of the arch (Fig. 34–5).

A right ventricular injection documents the size of the ventricular chamber and confirms its only outlet to the common trunk by way of the ventricular septal defect. The absence of a true infundibular region to the ventricle will be demonstrated and the commitment of the single semilunar valve to one or other ventricle emphasized, although sole origin from either ventricle is rare.

Because the pulmonary circulation is defined from all these injection sites, at least one angiographic series should be allowed to run until the ventricles reopacify. This permits delineation of the pulmonary venous return and the integrity of the atrial septum. Limited angio-

graphic exploration may be required to document atrial situs, cavoatrial connection, and a left superior vena cava.

A complete study permits differentiation of types I, II, and III as distinct from bilateral ductal origin of pulmonary arteries and pulmonary atresia with ventricular septal defect; so-called pseudotruncus; unilateral ascending aortic origin of one pulmonary artery, the other from a ductus or major aortopulmonary communicating artery; aortic valve atresia with aortopulmonary window; pulmonary valve atresia with aortopulmonary window; and a large aortopulmonary window alone, with or without patency of the ductus arteriosus.[65] Origin of the single great artery from one ventricle with hypoplasia or absence of the other may be seen occasionally.

MANAGEMENT

MEDICAL MANAGEMENT

Medical treatment is not the definitive management for this condition but is useful in optimizing the patient's cardiac and nutritional state and maintaining stability before an operation is undertaken (see Chapter 54).

Because of the frequent association of the DiGeorge syndrome (partial or complete), specific additional measures may be necessary to correct the associated hypocalcemia (calcium and magnesium supplements) and to take account of the thymus-based immune deficiency. This includes treatment of and subsequent prophylaxis against pneumococcal and streptococcal infections, and avoidance of immunization procedures with live vaccines. As a precaution, operative intervention in infancy, often on an urgent basis, should use only irradiated blood products

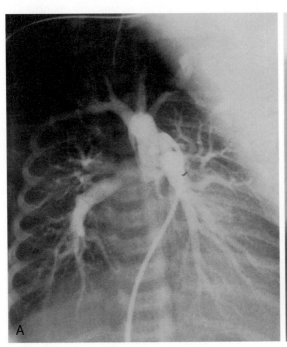 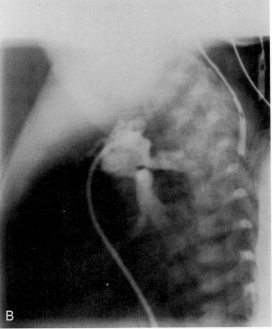

FIGURE 34–5

Angiograms after truncal root injections. *A*, Type I truncus, anteroposterior projection. *B*, Type IIb truncus, lateral projection showing separate origins of the two pulmonary arteries, each with a constriction at its origin. Note also the unusual origin of the right coronary artery.

because there may be insufficient time to assess the infant's immune status accurately.

OPERATIVE MANAGEMENT

Because many infants present early in life with severe cardiac failure, the earliest attempts to improve survival at this age came from banding of the pulmonary arteries, the common origin in type I, otherwise the individual arteries themselves. Although there was some success in reducing early mortality,[66] the procedure was difficult to perform adequately and did not address the fundamental hemodynamic problem. As primary repair of a variety of severe lesions in infancy became feasible, it seemed appropriate to include this lesion among those suitable for early repair.[51,67] The results in early infancy depend on the status of the semilunar valve, particularly its competence.[33,68] The level of pulmonary vascular resistance becomes the determinant in later (8 years or beyond) rather than earlier (around 2 years) childhood. Pulmonary vascular resistance is likely to be normal or nearly normal in infants and young children presenting with severe cardiac failure. Elevation of pulmonary vascular resistance to levels deemed inappropriate for attempted complete repair are unlikely to be met before 2 years of age. Thereafter, the level of resistance tends to increase with age so that few teenagers with this lesion will have a resistance value within the "operable" range. On the basis of a calculation of pulmonary vascular resistance using pulmonary blood flow measurements derived by the Fick principle in a spontaneously ventilating subject with a normal carbon dioxide level, a normal pulmonary vein oxygen saturation, and a normal systemic arterial acid-base status, a value of 8 units/m^2 (640 dyne · sec/cm^5) is deemed the upper limit for safe operative intervention with a good chance of significant long-term improvement. A value of 10 units/m^2 (800 dyne · sec/cm^5) or above raises the immediate operative risks to unacceptable levels with little chance of long-term improvement if survival ensues. The gray area between these limits (8 to 10 units/m^2) demands careful assessment of all the individual factors involved, including competence of the semilunar valve and ventricular performance, but more particularly with respect to age and the sequelae of severe lower respiratory tract infections.[32,35,36,69]

OPERATIVE TECHNIQUES

Operative repair of truncus arteriosus, originally achieved in 1968,[70] comprises three major steps: (1) separation of the pulmonary artery or arteries from the truncus and repair of the aortic defects thus created, (2) closure of the ventricular septal defect, and (3) establishment of continuity between the right ventricle and pulmonary artery or arteries. In addition, it may be necessary to repair the truncal valve or to undertake repair of an aortic arch interruption. Thus, deep hypothermia with periods of circulatory arrest may be needed; otherwise, the cardiopulmonary bypass procedure follows conventional lines, including infusing cardioplegic solution (directly into the coronary ostia if the truncal valve is incompetent) and ultrafiltration as bypass is terminated.[71,72]

Repair of the defects in the aortic wall after removal of the pulmonary arteries may be by direct suture or by patch

closure. The ventricular septal defect is always closed with a patch, and if the defect extends into the perimembranous region, the conducting system may be at risk of damage from any suture placed near the tricuspid valve. The patch should allow free passage of the left ventricular output to the aorta and provide a buttress on which to support the extracardiac conduit.

Whether the conduit should contain a valve, particularly when primary repair is undertaken in early infancy, remains contentious. Homograft valve material is superior to heterograft,[73,74] and the mode of preparation of homograft material affects the durability,[75] but the use of valveless conduits in the primary repair may improve the time to replacement by avoiding unnecessary obstruction by degenerative change in the valve itself.[76,77]

FOLLOW-UP AND LONGER TERM MANAGEMENT

After successful primary repair, the outcome depends on three factors: the continued adequate function of the conduit, the competence of the original truncal (now aortic) valve, and the pulmonary vascular resistance. In the mid term, the dominant problem lies with the function of the conduit.

Malfunction of the conduit in this lesion follows from three often interrelated facets.[78] With growth, the conduit becomes too small, and given otherwise good function in a conduit placed in infancy, it becomes restrictive around a mean age of 8 years, with right ventricular systolic pressure approaching systemic artery systolic pressure. In addition, the conduit may malfunction by degeneration and calcification, leading to earlier severe obstruction.[79] Calcification in the wall alone has no hemodynamic consequence, but this process may affect the leaflets of the valve within the conduit, producing a rigid ring-like obstruction, or the leaflets may degenerate completely, and a regurgitant volume load is added to the work of a ventricle with an already restricted outlet. Finally, the position of the conduit within the chest may lead to its obstruction if its anterior wall is against the sternum, which thus limits its free anterior displacement by a heart enlarging with growth. The obstruction may be enhanced by angulation at the level of the proximal anastomosis and by muscular hypertrophy. As a separate problem, constricting peripheral pulmonary arterial lesions may develop, particularly at the site of the distal conduit anastomosis. These lesions may develop in isolation, when relief by balloon dilatation or stent placement is appropriate, or at least be part of a complex right ventricular outflow obstruction necessitating reoperation.

The original semilunar valve, if competent at the time of initial operation, is likely to remain so at least into the long term (in excess of 10 years), although it may ultimately become increasingly regurgitant. Obviously, if the valve is regurgitant at the time of original repair, progressive increase in severity will lead to the need for intervention at about the same time as conduit replacement. Adequate repair of the native valve is not feasible in most patients, so prosthetic valve replacement is preferred.

If the original operation was undertaken before 2 years of age, it is likely that the pulmonary vascular resistance was normal, and the probability for the long term is that it will remain within or near normal limits and does not become a factor limiting long-term survival. The more severely elevated the pulmonary vascular resistance at the time of primary repair, the more likely it is to be a determinant of outcome and of duration of survival.[68,80] The degree of elevation may remain stable for a decade or so, but there will be a final inexorable climb. More difficult to evaluate is the progression of pulmonary vascular disease if there is a significant degree of obstruction to right ventricular outflow at conduit level. This leads to a more profound load on the right ventricle under conditions of exercise, even if the resting gradient is not severe. The adverse hemodynamic effects are not solely borne by the right ventricle, but the long-term left ventricular performance is affected by the duration and magnitude of the original volume load before primary repair and the severity and duration of semilunar valve regurgitation. As yet, there are no long-term studies (longer than 20 years) of patients with truncus arteriosus who underwent repair as young infants.

PROGNOSIS

The prognosis for untreated truncus arteriosus is poor. Death in early infancy from cardiac failure is common,[28,51,52] with further fall in survival during childhood from cardiac failure and pulmonary infection. A few who survive succumb to pulmonary vascular disease in the teenage years,[81] although individual survival to middle age is documented.[82–84]

Early surgical management, namely, primary repair, even with associated aortic arch interruption, now carries a good chance of survival, at least initially.[80,85–92]

With judicious operative intervention, the prognosis, however, is certainly good in the short term; most enjoy a symptom-free childhood free from medication. Inevitably, there is a morbidity associated with the unavoidable conduit change. The relative importance thereafter of right ventricular outflow obstruction, pulmonary vascular obstructive disease, aortic (original truncal) valve function, and ventricular performance has been discussed before.

At the time of leaving full-time education and passing into adult life, counseling to the patient should have covered the prospects for sustained employment, genetic counseling, marriage, childbearing and upbringing, personal life, and health insurance as well as preventive health advice (exercise, eating habits, alcohol, drugs, smoking).[93,94]

REFERENCES

1. Van Mierop LHS, Patterson DF, Schnarr WR: Pathogenesis of persistent truncus arteriosus in light of observations made in a dog embryo with the anomaly. Am J Cardiol 41:755, 1978.
2. Dickinson DF, Arnold R, Wilkinson JL: Congenital heart disease among 160,480 liveborn children in Liverpool 1960 to 1969. Br Heart J 46:55, 1981.
3. Grabitz RG, Joffres MR, Collins-Nakai RL: Congenital heart disease: Incidence in the first year of life. Am J Epidemiol 128:381, 1988.
4. Samanek M, Slavik Z, Zborilova B, et al: Prevalence, treatment, and outcome of heart disease in live-born children: A prospective analysis of 91,823 live-born children. Pediatr Cardiol 10:205, 1989.
5. de la Cruz MV, Pio da Rocha J: An ontogenetic theory for the explanation of congenital malformations involving the truncus and conus. Am Heart J 51:782, 1956.
6. Bartelings MM, Gittenberger-de Groot AC: Morphogenetic considerations on congenital malformations of the outflow tract. Part I: Common arterial trunk and tetralogy of Fallot. Int J Cardiol 32:213, 1991.
7. DiGeorge AM: Discussions on the new concept of the cellular basis of immunity. J Pediatr 67:907, 1965.
8. Conley ME, Beckwith JB, Mancer JFK, Tenckhoff L: The spectrum of the DiGeorge syndrome. J Pediatr 94:883, 1979.
9. Takao A, Ando M, Cho K, et al: Etiological categorization of common congenital heart disease. In Van Praagh R, Takao A (eds): Etiology and Morphogenesis of Congenital Heart Disease. New York, Futura Publishing, 1980, p 253.
10. Shprintzen RJ, Goldberg RB, Young D, Wolford L: The velo-cardio-facial syndrome: A clinical and genetic analysis. Pediatrics 67:161, 1981.
11. De la Chapelle A, Herva R, Koivisto M, Aula P: A deletion in chromosome 22 can cause DiGeorge syndrome. Hum Genet 57:253, 1981.
12. Scambler PJ, Kelly D, Linsay E, et al: Velo-cardio-facial syndrome associated with chromosome 22 deletions encompassing the DiGeorge locus. Lancet 339:1138, 1992.
13. Wilson DJ, Burn J, Scambler P, Goodship J: DiGeorge syndrome: Part of CATCH 22. J Med Genet 30:852, 1993.
14. Patterson DF, Pexieder T, Schnarr WR, et al: A single major gene defect underlying cardiac conotruncal malformations interferes with myocardial growth during embryonic development: Studies in the CTD line of keeshond dogs. Am J Hum Genet 52:388, 1993.
15. Besson WT, Kirby ML, Van Mierop LHS, Teabeaut JR: Effects of the size of lesions of the cardiac neural crest at various embryonic ages on incidence and type of cardiac defects. Circulation 73:360, 1986.
16. Van Mierop LHS, Kutsche LM: Cardiovascular anomalies in DiGeorge syndrome and importance of neural crest as a possible pathogenetic factor. Am J Cardiol 58:133, 1986.
17. Kirby ML: Cardiac morphogenesis—recent research advances. Pediatr Res 21:219, 1987.
18. Nishibatake M, Kirby ML, Van Mierop LHS: Pathogenesis of persistent truncus arteriosus and dextroposed aorta in the chick embryo after neural crest ablation. Circulation 75:255, 1987.
19. Franz T: Persistent truncus arteriosus in the Splotch mutant mouse. Anat Embryol (Berl) 180:457, 1989.
20. Kirby ML: Plasticity and predetermination of mesencephalic and trunk neural crest transplanted into the region of the cardiac neural crest. Dev Biol 134:402, 1989.
21. Leatherbury L, Gauldin HE, Waldo K, Kirby ML: Microcinephotography of the developing heart in neural crest–ablated chick embryos. Circulation 81:1047, 1990.
22. Tomita H, Connuck DM, Leatherbury L, Kirby ML: Relation of early hemodynamic changes to final cardiac phenotype and survival after neural crest ablation in chick embryos. Circulation 84:1289, 1991.
23. Kirby ML, Kumiski DH, Myers T, et al: Backtransplantation of chick cardiac neural crest cells cultured in LIF rescues heart development. Dev Dyn 198:296, 1993.
24. Nishibatake M, Kargas SA, Bruyere HJ, Gilbert EF: Cardiovascular malformations induced by bromodeoxyuridine in the chick embryo. Teratology 36:125, 1987.
25. Miyagawa S, Kirby ML: Pathogenesis of persistent truncus arteriosus induced by nimustine hydrochloride in chick embryos. Teratology 39:287, 1989.
26. Tasaka H, Takenaka H, Okamoto N, et al: Abnormal development of cardiovascular systems in rat embryos treated with bisdiamine. Teratology 43:191, 1991.
27. Okishima T, Takamura K, Matsuoka Y, et al: Cardiovascular anomalies in chick embryos produced by bis-diamine in demethylsulfoxide. Teratology 45:155, 1992.
28. Van Praagh R, Van Praagh S: The anatomy of common aorticopulmonary trunk (truncus arteriosus communis) and its embryologic implications. A study of 57 necropsy cases. Am J Cardiol 16:406, 1965.
29. Calder L, Van Praagh R, Van Praagh S, et al: Truncus arteriosus communis: Clinical, angiographic and pathologic findings in 100 patients. Am Heart J 92:23, 1976.

30. Crupi G, Macartney FJ, Anderson RH: Persistent truncus arteriosus: A study of 66 autopsy cases with special reference to definition and morphogenesis. Am J Cardiol 40:569, 1977.

31. Butto F, Lucas RV, Edwards JE: Persistent truncus arteriosus: Pathologic anatomy in 54 cases. Pediatr Cardiol 17:95, 1986.

32. Mair DD, Ritter DG, Davis GD, et al: Selection of patients with truncus arteriosus for surgical correction: Anatomic and hemodynamic considerations. Circulation 49:144, 1974.

33. Gelband H, Van Meter S, Gersony WM: Truncal valve abnormalities in infants with persistent truncus arteriosus: A clinicopathologic study. Circulation 45:397, 1972.

34. Collett RW, Edwards JE: Persistent truncus arteriosus: A classification according to anatomic type. Surg Clin North Am 29:1245, 1949.

35. Fyfe DA, Driscoll DJ, Di Donato RM, et al: Truncus arteriosus with single pulmonary artery: Influence of pulmonary vascular obstructive disease on early and late operative results. J Am Coll Cardiol 5:1168, 1985.

36. Mair DD, Ritter DG, Danielson GK, et al: Truncus arteriosus with unilateral absence of a pulmonary artery. Criteria for operability and surgical results. Circulation 55:641, 1977.

37. Schofield DE, Anderson RH: Common arterial trunk with pulmonary atresia. Int J Cardiol 20:290, 1988.

38. Rosenquist GC, Bharati S, McAllister HA, Lev M: Truncus arteriosus communis: Truncal valve anomalies associated with small conal or truncal septal defects. Am J Cardiol 37:410, 1976.

39. Carr I, Bharati S, Kusnoor VS, Lev M: Truncus arteriosus communis with intact ventricular septum. Br Heart J 42:97, 1979.

40. Shapiro SR, Ruckman RN, Kapur S, et al: Single ventricle with truncus arteriosus in siblings. Am Heart J 102:456, 1981.

41. Alves PM, Ferrari AH: Common arterial trunk arising exclusively from the right ventricle with hypoplastic left ventricle and intact ventricular septum. Int J Cardiol 16:99, 1987.

42. Shaddy RE, McGough EC: Successful diagnosis and surgical treatment of single ventricle, truncus arteriosus. Ann Thorac Surg 48:298, 1989.

43. Rao PS, Levy JM, Nikicicz E, Gilbert-Barness EF: Tricuspid atresia: Association with persistent truncus arteriosus. Am Heart J 122:829, 1991.

44. Rice MJ, Andrilenas K, Rellar MD, McDonald RW: Truncus arteriosus associated with mitral atresia and a hypoplastic left ventricle. Pediatr Cardiol 12:128, 1991.

45. Zeevi B, Dembo L, Berant M: Rare variant of truncus arteriosus with intact ventricular septum and hypoplastic right ventricle. Br Heart J 68:214, 1992.

46. Shrivastava S, Edwards JE: Coronary arterial origin in persistent truncus arteriosus. Circulation 55:551, 1977.

47. Anderson KR, McGoon DC, Lie JT: Surgical significance of the coronary arterial anatomy in truncus arteriosus communis. Am J Cardiol 41:76, 1978.

48. Mair DD, Edwards WD, Julsrud PR, et al: Truncus arteriosus. In Emmanouilides GC, Riemenschneider TA, Allen HD, Gutgesell HP (eds): Moss and Adams Heart Disease in Infants, Children and Adolescents. Baltimore, Williams & Wilkins, 1995, p 1026.

49. de la Cruz MV, Cayre R, Angelini P, et al: Coronary arteries in truncus arteriosus. Am J Cardiol 66:1482, 1990.

50. Lenox CC, Debich DE, Zuberbuhler JR: The role of coronary artery abnormalities in the prognosis of truncus arteriosus. J Thorac Cardiovasc Surg 104:1728, 1992.

51. Ebert PA, Turley K, Stanger P, et al: Surgical treatment of truncus arteriosus in the first 6 months of life. Ann Surg 200:451, 1984.

52. Juaneda E, Haworth SG: Pulmonary vascular disease in children with truncus arteriosus. Am J Cardiol 54:1314, 1984.

53. Abu-Harb M, Hey E, Wren C: Death in infancy from unrecognised congenital heart disease. Arch Dis Child 71:3, 1994.

54. Stanger P: Truncus arteriosus. In Moller JH, Neal WM (eds): Fetal, Neonatal and Infant Heart Disease. Norwalk, CT, Appleton & Lange, 1990, p 587.

55. Bell RA, Arensman FW, Flannery DB, et al: Facial dysmorphologic and skeletal cephalometric findings associated with conotruncal cardiac anomalies. Pediatr Dent 12:152, 1990.

56. Donnelly LF, Higgins CB: MR imaging of cono-truncal abnormalities. Am J Roentgenol 166:925, 1996.

57. Chrispin A, Small P, Rutter N, et al: Transectional echo planar imaging of the heart in cyanotic congenital heart disease. Pediatr Radiol 16:293, 1986.

58. Chrispin A, Small P, Rutter N, et al: Echo planar imaging of normal and abnormal connections of the heart and great arteries. Pediatr Radiol 16:289, 1986.

59. Sullivan ID, Gooch VM: Echocardiography. In Stark J, de Leval MR (eds): Surgery for Congenital Heart Defects, 2nd ed. Philadelphia, WB Saunders, 1994, p 59.

60. Yeager SB, Sanders SP: Echocardiographic identification of thymic tissue in neonates with congenital heart disease. Am Heart J 129:837, 1995.

61. Achiron R, Glaser J, Gelernter I, et al: Extended fetal echocardiographic examination for detecting cardiac malformations in low risk pregnancies. Br Med J 304:671, 1992.

62. Achiron R, Rotstein Z, Lipitz S, et al: First-trimester diagnosis of fetal congenital heart disease by transvaginal ultrasonography. Obstet Gynecol 84:69, 1994.

63. Taylor JFN: Investigation. In Stark J, de Leval MR (eds): Surgery for Congenital Heart Defects, 2nd ed. Philadelphia, WB Saunders, 1994, p 37.

64. Fellows KE, Keane JF, Freed MD: Angled views in cine-angiography of congenital heart disease. Circulation 56:485, 1977.

65. Yoshizato T, Julsrud PR: Truncus arteriosus revisited: An angiographic demonstration. Pediatr Cardiol 11:36, 1990.

66. Singh AK, de Leval MR, Pincott JR, Stark J: Pulmonary artery banding for truncus arteriosus in the first year of life. Circulation 54(suppl III):17, 1976.

67. Stark J, Gandhi D, de Leval M, et al: Surgical treatment of persistent truncus arteriosus in the first year of life. Br Heart J 40:1280, 1978.

68. de Leval M, McGoon D, Wallace RB, et al: Management of truncal valvular regurgitation. Ann Surg 180:427, 1974.

69. Marcelletti C, McGoon DC, Danielson GK, et al: Early and late results of surgical repair of truncus arteriosus. Circulation 55:636, 1977.

70. McGoon DC, Rastelli GC, Ongley PA: An operation for the correction of truncus arteriosus. JAMA 205:69, 1968.

71. de Leval MR: In Stark J, de Leval M (eds): Surgery for Congenital Heart Defects. New York, Grune & Stratton, 1983, p 417.

72. Elliott MJ: Ultrafiltration and modified ultrafiltration in pediatric open heart operations. Ann Thorac Surg 56:1518, 1993.

73. Almeida RS, Wyse RKH, de Leval MR, et al: Long-term results of homograft valves in extracardiac conduits. Eur J Cardiothorac Surg 3:488, 1989.

74. Reddy VM, Rajasinghe HA, McElhinney DB, Hanley FL: Performance of right ventricle to pulmonary artery conduits after repair of truncus arteriosus: A comparison of Dacron-housed porcine valves and cryopreserved allografts. Semin Thorac Cardiovasc Surg 7:133, 1995.

75. Stark J, Weller P, Leanage R, et al: Late results of surgical treatment of transposition of the great arteries. Adv Cardiol 27:254, 1988.

76. Spicer RL, Behrendt D, Crowley DC, et al: Repair of truncus arteriosus in neonates with the use of a valveless conduit. Circulation 70(suppl I):I-26, 1984.

77. Behrendt DM, Dick M: Truncus repair with a valveless conduit in neonates. J Thorac Cardiovasc Surg 110:1148, 1995.

78. Taylor JFN: Investigation before reoperations for congenital heart disease. In Stark J, Pacifico AD (eds): Reoperations in Cardiac Surgery. New York, Springer-Verlag, 1989, p 3.

79. Bull C, Macartney FJ, Horvath P, et al: Evaluation of long term results of homograft and heterograft valves in extracardiac conduits. J Thorac Cardiovasc Surg 94:12, 1987.

80. Hanley FL, Heinemann MK, Jonas RA, et al: Repair of truncus arteriosus in the neonate. J Thorac Cardiovasc Surg 105:1047, 1993.

81. Fuster V, Mair DD, Ritter DG, McGoon DC: Truncus arteriosus with pulmonary vascular obstructive disease: Medical vs surgical management (Abstract). Am J Cardiol 45:450, 1980.

82. Hicken P, Evans D, Heath D: Persistent truncus arteriosus with survival to the age of 38 years. Br Heart J 28:284, 1966.

83. Silverman JJ, Scheenesson GP: Persistent truncus arteriosus in a 43 year old man. Am J Cardiol 17:94, 1966.

84. Wilton NC, Traber KB, Deschner LS: Anaesthetic management for caesarean section in a patient with uncorrected truncus arteriosus. Br J Anaesth 62:434, 1989.

85. Parenzan L, Crupi G, Alfieri O, et al: Surgical repair of persistent truncus arteriosus in infancy. J Thorac Cardiovasc Surg 28:18, 1980.

86. Musumeci F, Piccoli GP, Dickinson DF, Hamilton DI: Surgical experience with persistent truncus arteriosus in symptomatic infants under 1 year of age. Br Heart J 46:179, 1981.

87. Sano S, Brawn WJ, Mee RB: Repair of truncus arteriosus and interrupted aortic arch. J Card Surg 5:157, 1990.

88. Pearl JM, Laks H, Drinkwater DC, et al: Repair of truncus arteriosus in infancy. Ann Thorac Surg 52:780, 1991.

89. Turley K: Current method of repair of truncus arteriosus. J Card Surg 7:1, 1992.

90. Bove EL, Lupinetti FM, Pridjian A, et al: Results of a policy of primary repair of truncus arteriosus in the neonate. J Thorac Cardiovasc Surg 105:1057, 1993.

91. Slavik Z, Keeton BR, Salmon AP, et al: Persistent truncus arteriosus operated during infancy: Long-term follow up. Pediatr Cardiol 15:112, 1994.

92. Lacour-Gayet F, Serraf A, Komiya T, et al: Truncus arteriosus repair: Influence of techniques of right ventricular outflow tract reconstruction. J Thorac Cardiovasc Surg 111:849, 1996.

93. Mitchell JH, Haskell WH, Raven PB: Classification of sports. 26th Bethesda Conference: Recommendations for determining eligibility for competition in athletes with cardiovascular disease. J Am Coll Cardiol 24:864, 1994.

94. Thorne S, Deanfield JE: Long term outlook in treated congenital heart disease. Arch Dis Child 75:6, 1996.

CHAPTER 35
AORTIC STENOSIS

JOHN M. NEUTZE A. LOUISE CALDER THOMAS L. GENTLES NIGEL J. WILSON

In this chapter, we discuss left ventricular outflow obstruction, including fixed obstruction at the valve, supravalve, and subvalve levels, and hypertrophic cardiomyopathy. Obstruction associated with complex anomalies, such as double-inlet ventricles and transposition, is not included.

AORTIC VALVE STENOSIS

Some 60 to 75% of left ventricular outflow tract obstructions occur at valve level. The prevalence is commonly quoted as about 1%, although there are variations in estimates related largely to the population sampled.[1] The pattern of occurrence of aortic valve stenosis usually fits a multifactorial origin, and it is about four times more common in males as in females. The risk of recurrence in the next generation is reported as 8% from mothers and 3.8% from fathers,[2] although higher figures have been quoted. The most commonly associated lesions are coarctation of the aorta and patent ductus arteriosus.

PATHOLOGIC ANATOMY

The aortic valve develops by cavitation of three tubercles, two situated on the distal edge of the truncal swellings that divide the primitive truncus and the third on the free wall opposite. Failure of separation and cavitation of these tubercles leads to stenosis. In a necropsy series of 62 stenotic aortic valves in our department (stillborn to 81 years, median 13 days), the valve was unicommissural in more than 50% (Table 35–1). A commissure is the site where contiguous leaflets meet the aortic wall. The number of leaflets is determined by the number of commissures, a unicommissural valve having one leaflet (Fig. 35–1A). Additional raphes and partially formed sinuses may lead to confusion about the number of leaflets.

Bicommissural Aortic Valves
The most common congenital heart defect is a bicommissural aortic valve. In 100 necropsies with bicommissural aortic valves (stillborn to 69 years, median 1 month), the deficient or absent commissure was intercoronary in 57 (Table 35–2). In patients with this anatomy and normally related great arteries, the functional commissures were right anterior and left posterior (Fig. 35–1B), although there may be some variation in the degree of obliquity.[3] When the right noncoronary or the left noncoronary commissure was deficient, the commissures were left anterior and right posterior (Fig. 35–1C). In most subjects, the

combined leaflet was larger than the single leaflet. If a raphe could not be identified, the valve was classified as indeterminate when the coronary arteries arose from separate sinuses (Table 35–2).

In utero, the fetus is generally untroubled by aortic stenosis and the left ventricle usually maintains a normal output. In severe disease, however, left ventricular filling becomes restricted, thus minimizing atrial right-to-left shunt and increasing right ventricular contribution to systemic flow through the ductus. This redistribution of flow can result in hypoplasia of the ascending aorta and arch and heightens the risk of coarctation of the aorta. The whole left ventricular apparatus including the mitral valve may be hypoplastic.

HEMODYNAMICS

Important left ventricular hypertrophy is primarily a postnatal problem. The stimulus for hypertrophy is peak myocardial force, which can be quantified as wall stress, and it is directly proportional to ventricular systolic pressure and chamber size and inversely proportional to chamber thickness. Peak wall stress acts as a servomechanism, increasing as left ventricular obstruction increases and normalizing as the myocardium hypertrophies.[4] Thus, in stable aortic stenosis, left ventricular mass is increased, and peak systolic wall stress is normal.[4]

Except for the neonate with critical aortic stenosis, ventricular systolic dysfunction is rarely a problem during childhood. In fact, "function," as measured by fractional shortening or ejection fraction or by velocity of fiber shortening, is frequently enhanced. Left ventricular function is inversely related to end-systolic wall stress,[5] and several investigators have demonstrated that the hyperdynamic systolic function seen in patients with congenital aortic stenosis is a result of reduced end-systolic wall stress rather than an expression of enhanced myocardial contractility (Fig. 35–2).[4] End-systolic wall stress is reduced because end-systolic wall thickness is increased, and end-systolic pressure (i.e., pressure at the time of aortic valve closure) is normal (Fig. 35–3).[5]

With exercise to a level that approximately doubles the cardiac output (e.g., jogging), much of the increased output results from an increase in heart rate, but some associated increase in stroke volume and reduction in ejection time increase the outflow gradient. Higher exercise levels demand a progressively increasing stroke volume with a sharp increase in gradient, the change being proportional to the square of the increase in flow velocity. Concomitant

TABLE 35–1

AORTIC VALVE STENOSIS: GREEN LANE HOSPITAL

	Tricommissural	Bicommissural	Unicommissural	Total
Isolated	4 (11%)	9 (25%)	23 (64%)	36
Coarctation, mitral stenosis	3 (21%)	5 (36%)	6 (43%)	14
Major associated anomalies	2 (17%)	6 (50%)	4 (33%)	12
Total	9 (15%)	20 (32%)	33 (53%)	62

TABLE 35–2

BICOMMISSURAL AORTIC VALVES: GREEN LANE HOSPITAL

Deficient or Absent Commissure	No.	Associated Defects			
		Coarctation or Interrupted Aortic Arch	Aortic Stenosis: Valvar or Subvalvar	Transposition or Malposition of the Great Arteries	Associated Bicommissural Pulmonary Valve
Right-left, intercoronary	57	35 (76%)	22 (71%)	8 (53%)	3 (25%)
Right coronary–noncoronary	18	4 (9%)	4 (13%)		3 (25%)
Left coronary–noncoronary	14	4 (9%)	5 (16%)	3 (20%)	2 (17%)
Indeterminate	11	3 (6%)		4 (27%)	4 (33%)
Total	100	46	31	15	12

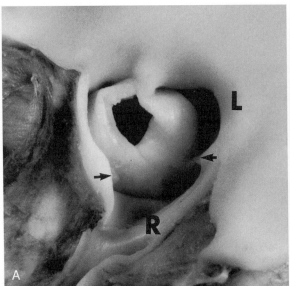

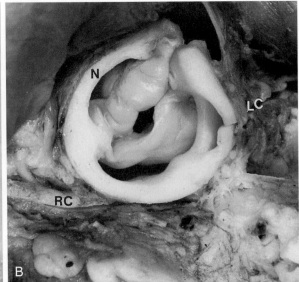

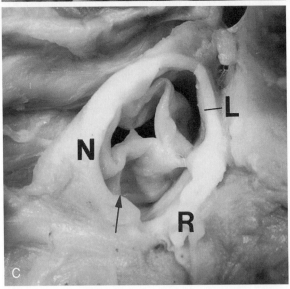

FIGURE 35–1

Superior views of three aortic valves. *A,* Unicommissural, stenotic, and hypoplastic valve from an 8-day-old girl. The only commissure present is between the left (L) and noncoronary sinuses. Two rudimentary commissures are represented by raphes only *(arrows).* The leaflet is thickened and domed. R = opened right coronary artery. *B,* Bicommissural stenotic aortic valve from a 4-month-old boy. The intercoronary commissure is absent or deficient. The leaflets are thickened, domed, and mildly fused at the right noncoronary commissure. LC = left coronary artery; N = noncoronary sinus; RC = right coronary artery. *C,* Bicommissural aortic valve from a 2-day-old boy due to deficiency of the commissure *(arrow)* between the right coronary and noncoronary leaflets. L = left aortic sinus; N = noncoronary sinus; R = right aortic sinus. Note the different position of the commissures and leaflets compared with *B.* (*B* and *C* modified from Kirklin JW, Barratt-Boyes BG: Congenital aortic stenosis. *In* Cardiac Surgery, 2nd ed. New York, Churchill Livingstone, 1993, p 1195.)

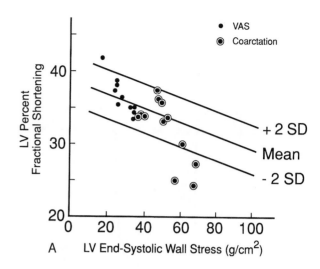

FIGURE 35–2

Relationship between fractional shortening and left ventricular (LV) end-systolic wall stress (A) and rate-corrected velocity of shortening and LV end-systolic wall stress (B). Enhanced ventricular function in patients with aortic stenosis is related to low end-systolic wall stress. Lower indices, related to higher end-systolic wall stress, are shown in subjects with coarctation. In all but three of these patients, however, contractility is within the normal range. VAS = valvar aortic stenosis. (From Borow KM, Colan SD, Neumann A: Altered left ventricular mechanics in patients with valvular aortic stenosis and coarctation of the aorta: Effects on systolic performance and late outcome. Circulation 72[3]:515–522, 1985.)

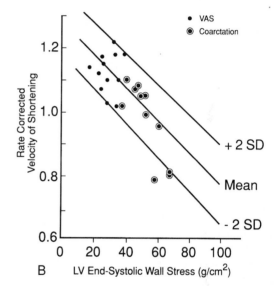

reduced filling time restricts coronary blood flow, particularly in the subendocardial region where flow is almost entirely diastolic in a hypertrophied chamber. An estimate of potential coronary flow can be made from the area between the aortic and left ventricular pressures in diastole, the diastolic pressure time index (DPTI) (Fig. 35–4).[6] Similarly, an estimate of left ventricular oxygen requirement can be obtained from the area under the ventricular pressure curve during ejection, the systolic pressure time index (SPTI). In the absence of coronary disease, the ratio

FIGURE 35–3

Illustration of the mechanism of reduced end-systolic stress in aortic stenosis (AS). Although left ventricular (LV) peak pressure is elevated (left), the pressure at end systole is normal. Hypertrophy takes place until peak stress is normalized, resulting in "excess" hypertrophy at end systole relative to end-systolic pressure. Consequently, end-systolic stress (ESS) is low compared with normal values (right). AP = aortic pressure. (From Colan SD: Noninvasive assessment of myocardial mechanisms—a review of analysis of stress-shortening and stress-velocity. Cardiol Young 2:1, 1992.)

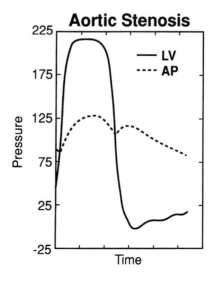

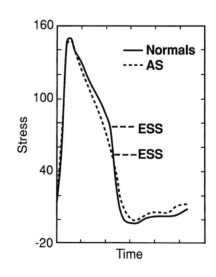

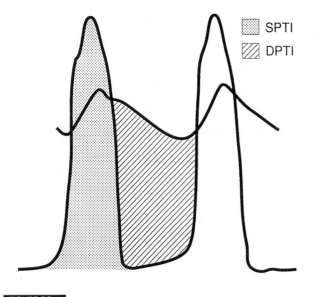

SPTI
DPTI

Illustration of left ventricular and aortic pressures in a patient with aortic stenosis showing the diastolic pressure time index (DPTI) and systolic pressure time index (SPTI). The ratio DPTI/SPTI gives a measure of the oxygen supply/demand ratio (see text). (From Vincent WR, Buckberg GD, Hoffman JI: Left ventricular subendocardial ischemia in severe valvar and supravalvar aortic stenosis: A common mechanism. Circulation 49[2]:326–333, 1974.)

DPTI/SPTI gives a measure of the oxygen supply/demand ratio. Patients with an aortic valve area less than 0.7 cm^2/m^2 and a heart rate of 100 per minute have a ratio DPTI × arterial oxygen content (g/dl)/SPTI below 10, consistent with subendocardial ischemia.[7] With exercise-induced tachycardia, diastolic filling time is reduced even more than systolic ejection time, and myocardial oxygen delivery is decreased just as systolic work is increasing markedly. Electrocardiographic ST depression appears consistently in left ventricular leads with exercise in patients with a resting left ventricular aortic catheter gradient of around 50 mm Hg.[8] With time, myocardial damage and subendocardial fibrosis develop. The limits of exercise tolerance may be heralded by presyncope or, in extreme instances, present with sudden death. A ventricular arrhythmia may be the trigger, especially in a ventricle with dilatation and fibrosis. The discovery of left ventricular baroreceptors in dogs[9] led to speculation that such receptors could also contribute to syncope in aortic stenosis. Stress or exercise that raises left ventricular systolic pressure might stimulate the receptors, producing vasodilatation that could reduce coronary flow to a critical level, triggering a precipitous drop in left ventricular output.

Left ventricular diastolic function may be impaired even when systolic function is well preserved.[10] As left ventricular hypertrophy progresses, elastic recoil and ventricular relaxation rate are reduced, so that passive chamber stiffness increases and active relaxation becomes impaired. In time, these functions are further affected by the development of fibrosis.

NATURAL HISTORY

Natural history very much depends on the severity of obstruction at birth. About 10% of patients presenting in childhood develop congestive heart failure in the first year of life, two thirds in the first 2 months.[11] Those with extreme stenosis and a small left ventricle develop failure, often with a shock-like syndrome as the ductus closes. In a small group with severe but not extreme stenosis, breathlessness and failure to thrive present during a period of months. In an era before treatment was possible, Campbell[12] reported a death rate of 23% in patients presenting in the first year. By contrast, annual mortality in those surviving the first year was 1.2% for the next two decades. Looking at the whole group of patients, about 60% survived until age 30 years and 40% until age 40 years.[12, 13]

Patients with signs of trivial aortic stenosis may show minimal progression for half a lifetime. From the late 30s onward, thickening and eventually calcification of leaflets and commissures become more common, but the rate of progression is individual and difficult to predict. In a Liverpool study (31% observed for 15 years), 17 of 39 patients presenting with trivial aortic stenosis progressed to a mild grade, the remainder staying trivial.[14] In our study of 218 patients presenting after 1 year of age with mild or greater aortic stenosis, we found that 55% initially graded as mild retained this grade after 18 years, and 42% initially graded as moderate retained this grade after 15 years (Fig. 35–5). Only two unexpected deaths occurred in this study, both patients having been lost to follow-up for some years. This was in the pre-echocardiographic era, when assessment relied primarily on clinical findings with selective catheterization.[15]

The Second Natural History Study of congenital heart defects[16] presented a long-term follow-up of 432 subjects recruited after 2 years of age in the years 1958 to 1969. Compared with a predicted 96% survival in an age-matched normal population, 25-year survival of study patients was 92.5% for those with an initial catheter gradient less than 50 mm Hg and 81% in those with an initial gradient of 50 mm Hg or above. In 217 patients under medical observation, there were 6 sudden deaths, 3 deaths from other cardiac causes, and 8 noncardiac deaths. In 240 patients observed after operation, there were 12 perioperative deaths, 19 sudden deaths, 4 deaths from other cardiac causes, and 5 noncardiac deaths. Surgical intervention is palliative. As expected, the timing of operation depended on the severity of stenosis at the time of recruitment (Fig. 35–6). In subjects with full information, about 40% receiving medical treatment initially required operation, and almost 40% of those needed a second operation.

Many other studies have examined the progressive nature of aortic valve stenosis. The risk of serious arrhythmias and sudden death rises once the catheter gradient exceeds 50 mm Hg.[16] Once congestive heart failure has developed, life expectancy is about 2 years. Deciding on the appropriate time of intervention is a key factor in management.

HISTORY AND PHYSICAL EXAMINATION

Although a typical ejection murmur may be heard at birth in an infant with moderate aortic stenosis, the murmur is often minimal when obstruction is extreme. Systemic circulation is sustained until the ductus narrows, when a shock-like state may develop in a matter of hours. Dyspnea becomes marked, pulses are almost impalpable, the liver

Mild A.S.

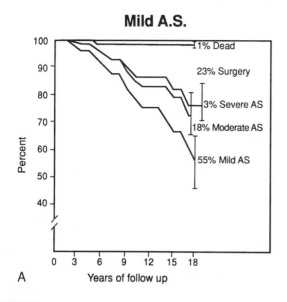

A   Years of follow up

Moderate A.S.

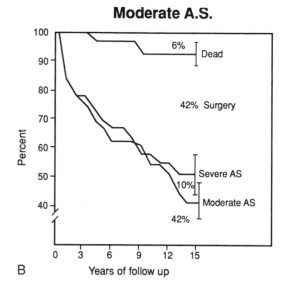

B   Years of follow up

A, Cumulative actuarial curves of 153 patients presenting with mild aortic stenosis. The actuarial curves are plotted to the point where the smallest subgroup has 10 members at risk, and bars show 1 SE at this point. Mean age at presentation, 6.5 years (1 to 25 years); mean follow-up, 8.8 years (1 to 26 years). *B,* Cumulative actuarial curves of 54 patients presenting with moderate aortic stenosis. Mean age at presentation, 11.8 years (1 to 25 years); mean follow-up, 8.5 years (1 to 24 years). (From Hossack KF, Neutze JM, Lowe JB, Barratt-Boyes BG: Congenital valvar aortic stenosis. Natural history and assessment for operation. Br Heart J 43:561, 1980.)

enlarges rapidly, there is a modest ejection murmur with a prominent gallop, and acidosis develops rapidly. The picture may be indistinguishable from that of aortic atresia. With an intermediate presentation, signs of low output, tachypnea, and other evidence of failure develop more gradually. Infants with mild or moderate stenosis have signs similar to those of older children.

Beyond 1 year, most patients with mild aortic stenosis (Doppler gradient around 30 to 40 mm Hg or catheter gra-

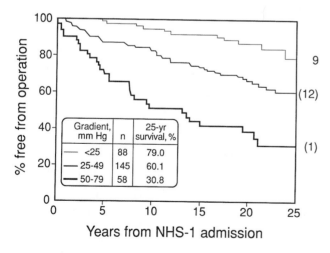

Gradient, mm Hg	n	25-yr survival, %
<25	88	79.0
25-49	145	60.1
50-79	58	30.8

Years from NHS-1 admission

Second Natural History Study: aortic stenosis. Kaplan-Meier curves of percentage free from operation for aortic stenosis of 235 subjects with full information. All were at least 2 years of age when admitted to the first Natural History Study (NHS-1). Numbers in parentheses indicate the number of patients remaining under observation at 25 years. Gradient denotes catheterization left ventricular aortic pressure difference at recruitment. (From Keane JF, Driscoll DJ, Gersony WM, et al: Second natural history study of congenital heart defects. Results of treatment of patients with aortic valve stenosis. Circulation 87[2 suppl]:I16–27, 1993.)

dient of 25 to 30 mm Hg) have no cardiac symptoms, and 95% show normal growth and development.[17] In general, convincing cardiac symptoms are rare in patients with moderate stenosis (Doppler gradients up to approximately 70 mm Hg or catheter gradients of 55 mm Hg), although as this level is approached, a lack of competitive stamina is sometimes evident. Specific inquiry does not always establish the significance of a symptom. For example, fatigability has been reported in 15% of children with catheter gradients below 25 mm Hg and in only 30% of children with severe stenosis.[18] Angina is rare, not reported in patients with a catheter gradient below 25 mm Hg but described in 9% with moderate to severe stenosis.[18] In the same study, syncope occurred in only 9% of patients with a catheter gradient above 80 mm Hg.

In children, the typical signs of mild aortic stenosis include normal venous pressure and a pulse that is normal or slightly jerky. There is a long ejection systolic murmur radiating to the suprasternal notch and usually associated with a thrill, and the second heart sound varies normally with respiration. The intensity and length of the murmur correlate poorly with severity of stenosis; but as the severity increases, the frequency of the murmur rises. With moderate obstruction, the venous A wave becomes prominent over the years, illustrating the effect of left-sided hypertrophy on right ventricular filling. The signs most reliably related to moderate obstruction are not the intensity of the murmur but a reduction in pulse pressure and the respiratory variation in splitting of the second heart sound.[15] Variation in output makes it difficult to ascribe a figure to an unusually narrowed pulse pressure, but subjective assessment of a large artery (usually the brachial artery) is surprisingly consistent between observers. Gradual prolongation of left ventricular systole with progressive overload narrows the inspiratory gap between aortic and pulmonary closure. Eventually a stage may be reached

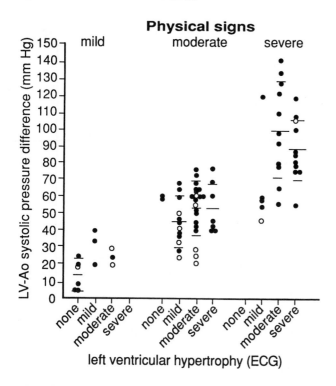

Physical signs

Relation between physical signs, electrocardiographic assessment, and left ventricular–aortic (LV-AO) pressure difference at catheterization; 79 studies in 65 patients. Patients were judged to have mild, moderate, or severe stenosis on clinical signs. Note the failure of the electrocardiogram (ECG) to discriminate between moderate and severe obstruction. *Open circles* denote patients with some aortic regurgitation. (From Hossack KF, Neutze JM, Lowe JB, Barratt-Boyes BG: Congenital valvar aortic stenosis. Natural history and assessment for operation. Br Heart J 43:561, 1980.)

when splitting is detected only on expiration, but this finding is rarely present in children. The presence of either a small pulse pressure or minimal splitting of the second heart sound provides strong evidence of a moderate obstruction (Fig. 35–7).[15] A systolic click is recorded in 60 to 90% of children but may be intermittent.[17, 19] It is usually heard best between the fourth left interspace and the apex. As stenosis increases, the click comes closer to the first heart sound and eventually may be inaudible. A fourth heart sound is usually a sign of long-term ventricular pressure overload and is uncommon in young children unless obstruction is severe. The early diastolic murmur of aortic regurgitation has been recorded in 15 to 25% of pediatric patients.[15, 19] Regurgitation is usually minor, but it is occasionally an important component of the hemodynamic disturbance.

ELECTROCARDIOGRAPHY AND EXERCISE TESTING

Electrocardiographic demonstration of left ventricular hypertrophy depends on chamber size as well as wall thickness. In the first month of life, right ventricular dominance is usual regardless of the severity of aortic stenosis, but left ventricular dominance and frank hypertrophy become manifest in three quarters of older infants with important aortic stenosis and good left ventricular volume.[11] Shift of the frontal plane axis to the left is usually slow but useful when present. Increased posterolateral voltages are also useful, but the association with left ventricular hypertrophy is weak. For example, an R wave in V_6 greater than 30 mm or beyond 2 SD from the mean for age occurs in 40% of patients with a gradient above 25 mm compared with 68% in patients with a gradient above 80 mm. We prefer simply to regard the sum of the voltages of the S wave in V_2 and the R wave in V_6 of 40 mm as carrying an approximately 70% probability of left ventricular hypertrophy at any age.[20] In the absence of myocardial or pericardial disease, ST or T wave depression is virtually diagnostic of important hypertrophy. Although customarily looked for in lateral chest leads, such depression frequently appears first in the inferior leads.

Exercise stress testing adds some further information. ST depression greater than 1 mm for more than 0.08 second after the J point is generally recognized as a pointer to subendocardial ischemia and, in the present context, to important left ventricular overload. Although initially thought to provide a reliable indication of a resting gradient above 50 mm Hg, subsequent reports showed a false-positive rate up to 40% in patients with gradients as low as 30 mm Hg.[21]

The electrocardiogram therefore contributes to assessment but does not reliably predict a gradient or exclude important hypertrophy. Exercise adds a dimension and has a significant role in assessing symptoms when there is uncertainty about their significance. Undue dyspnea, chest pain, dizziness, arrhythmias, or failure to develop a normal rise in blood pressure all point to limited capacity of the left ventricle to increase its output and to a significant increase in risk. We reserve exercise testing for answering specific questions about risks or management.

CHEST RADIOGRAPHY

Almost all infants with severe aortic stenosis show cardiomegaly, particularly marked in those younger than 1 month with congestive heart failure.[11] Pulmonary venous congestion is evident in those with frank failure, but the lung fields may be surprisingly clear in older infants despite persistent tachypnea and an important lesion. On the other hand, critical neonatal aortic stenosis is often accompanied by a large left-to-right atrial shunt that causes pulmonary plethora. Normal heart size has been reported in 90% of children with catheter gradients below 65 mm Hg,[18] although left ventricular hypertrophy may be suspected because of a prominent posterior displacement of the cardiac outline. Radiologic enlargement of the heart always suggests cardiac dilatation from failure or an additional lesion. Poststenotic dilatation of the ascending aorta is rare before 5 to 6 years of age but is seen in more than 50% of adults.

ECHOCARDIOGRAPHY

The development of echo Doppler techniques transformed assessment and monitoring of aortic stenosis. Excellent images are usually obtained in the pediatric age group, although sedation may be required in younger patients to achieve all the detail required. Provided that full

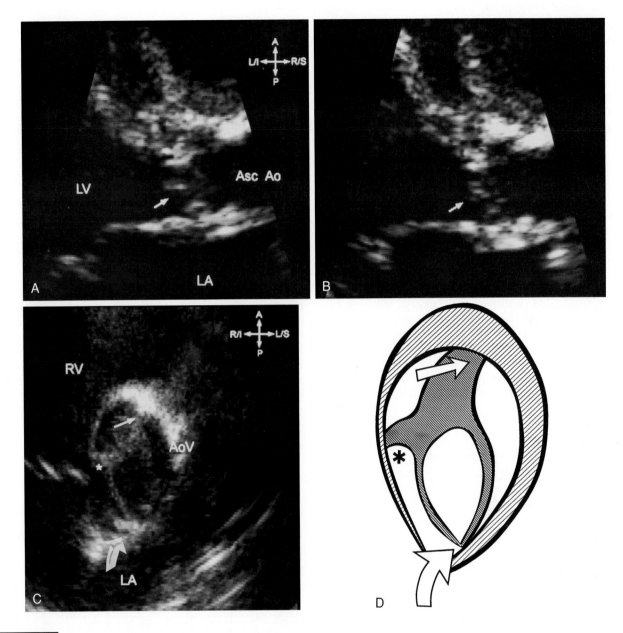

Parasternal long-axis views in systole *(A)* and diastole *(B)*. Note the thickened leaflets with minimal movement *(arrows)* (Doppler gradient 120 mm Hg). *C,* Parasternal short-axis view in systole in a different patient. The view is angulated to show each leaflet, and the right lower aortic margin is not visible. There is major fusion of the right and left leaflets *(arrow)* and lesser fusion between the right and noncoronary leaflets *(asterisk)*. Because the leaflets do not meet the aortic wall at either site, the valve should strictly speaking be labeled unicommissural. (The commissure is marked by the *curved arrow* in both *C* and *D*.) Nevertheless, some separation of leaflets might be expected with balloon or surgical valvuloplasty at each site of leaflet fusion. *D,* Line drawing of *C*. A = anterior; AoV = aortic valve; Asc Ao = ascending aorta; LA = left atrium; L/I = left and inferior; L/S = left and superior; LV = left ventricle; P = posterior; R/I = right and inferior; R/S = right and superior; RV = right ventricle.

anatomic and hemodynamic information can be recorded, diagnostic catheterization is now rarely required.[22] Comprehensive systematic imaging is required to assess the lesion, quantitate left ventricular function, and demonstrate or exclude other anomalies. Two-dimensional images of the aortic valve are obtained from subcostal, apical, and parasternal long-axis and short-axis positions. Long-axis views allow assessment of leaflet thickening and display limitations of movement with doming of the valve in systole (Fig. 35–8*A, B*). Imaging in the parasternal short-axis plane usually allows visualization of leaflet anatomy,

establishing the orientation of the opening plane and allowing judgment of leaflet numbers and structure. A valve that appears to be tricommissural in diastole (even though somewhat distorted) is frequently shown in systole to be essentially bicommissural but with a raphe in the fused leaflet. Some degree of fusion is frequently also shown at one of the two commissures; if marked, this can effectively produce a unicommissural valve (Fig. 35–8*C, D*).

Detailed two-dimensional and M-mode measurements are required to measure the aortic annulus and septal and free wall thickness, to make observations of papillary muscle anatomy and bulk, to record chamber dimensions, and to assess ventricular function. All figures are compared with normal values.

Assessment of the adequacy of the left ventricle and aortic arch is particularly important in critical aortic stenosis of the newborn. Highly echogenic endocardium suggests endocardial fibroelastosis, particularly when regional movement is restricted. The size and function of the mitral valve, left ventricular volume, and the anatomy of the left ventricular outflow and aortic arch may render effective left ventricular function impossible even if valve opening can be achieved.

Pulsed, continuous-wave, and color Doppler interrogations are pivotal in assessing the site and severity of obstruction and associated lesions.[23–25] Assessment can be based on the left ventricular aortic gradient with use of the modified Bernoulli equation[26] or the valve area according to the continuity equation.[27] The reliability of the simplified Bernoulli equation, pressure gradient = 4 × peak velocity[2], has been confirmed. This records the peak instantaneous (P-I) gradient, which is generally significantly higher than the peak to peak (P-P) gradient recorded at cardiac catheterization.[28] Part of the difference can be explained by variations in sedation and inherent damping in catheter systems, but most is due to the inherent difference in the phase of the pressure pulses recorded. This is

well shown in Figure 35–9 with catheter pressure recordings. Taking two patients with similar P-P gradients, both the P-I and mean gradients are much greater in a patient with a higher pulse pressure, a finding associated with a lesser degree of stenosis and augmented by aortic regurgitation. There is thus no consistent correction factor to allow comparison between catheter P-P and echocardiographic P-I measurements, although the catheter figure is commonly about 80% of the echo figure in patients with critical stenosis. On the other hand, mean velocity as measured by the echocardiogram is usually much closer to the catheter figure.[23, 29, 30]

With echo Doppler, valve area is derived from a direct application of the continuity equation:

$$\text{valve area} = A\ (\text{LVOT}) \times V\ (\text{LVOT})/V\ (\text{AV})$$

where A is area, LVOT is left ventricular outflow tract, V is mean velocity, and AV is aortic valve. The left ventricular outflow tract is measured 2 to 3 mm below the aortic valve in infants and 5 to 10 mm below the valve in teenagers. Meticulous alignment of the Doppler signal is essential. Because the left ventricular outflow tract and the aorta share the same ejection volume, measurement is valid in the presence of aortic regurgitation.

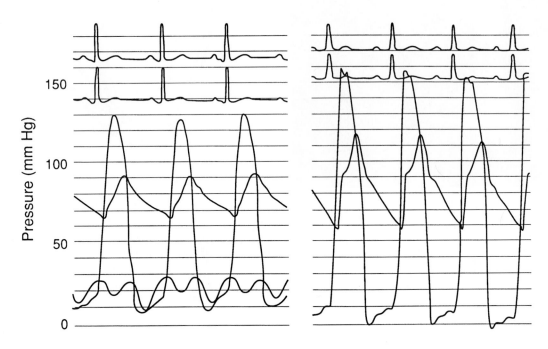

FIGURE 35–9

Pressure tracings from two children with valvar aortic stenosis and equal peak to peak systolic gradients of approximately 40 mm Hg. The larger aortic pulse pressure explains the greater mean and peak instantaneous gradients of the patient in the right panel:

	P-P Gradient	Pulse Pressure	Mean Gradient	P-I Gradient
Patient 1	38	28	28	45
Patient 2	40	62	42	67

P-I gradient = peak instantaneous gradient, equivalent to a Doppler gradient; P-P gradient = peak to peak gradient. Pressures were obtained from digitized simultaneous tracings. (Reprinted from American Journal of Cardiology, Volume 69, Beekman RH, Rocchini AP, Gillon JH, Mancini GB, Hemodynamic determinants of the peak systolic left ventricular–aortic pressure gradient in children with valvar aortic stenosis, Pages 813–815, Copyright 1992, with permission from Excerpta Medica Inc.)

CARDIAC CATHETERIZATION

Previously the routine technique for establishing the severity of aortic stenosis, diagnostic catheterization is now restricted to those rare patients in whom doubt about the severity of stenosis remains despite echocardiography or in whom it has been impossible to exclude a specific associated anomaly. Right-sided and left-sided heart catheterizations are then usually required with cardiac output measurements by Fick, dye dilution, or thermodilution methods.

Some units prefer the trans-septal technique to enter the left ventricle, often the Mullins long trans-septal sheath technique.[31] Most units, however, make limited use of trans-septal puncture techniques and routinely use the femoral artery approach for both diagnostic and treatment steps. Simultaneous pressures in left ventricle and ascending aorta provide optimal pressure data. Femoral arterial pressures can be misleading because of variable peripheral amplification of peak systolic pressure. Alternatively, sequential recordings in the aorta and left ventricle may be judged adequate. Retrograde entry to the left ventricle can be difficult, and it is then best approached by defining the left ventricular aortic jet on biplane cineangiography and positioning an appropriately shaped catheter in the ejection stream. When centrally positioned, the catheter is deflected at one moment to one sinus and then to the other, but well-timed catheter movements usually achieve left ventricular entry.

In borderline situations, pressure measurements must be accompanied by cardiac output measurement, and valve area can be calculated from the Gorlin formula[32] or some modification.[33] The Gorlin formula is

$$\text{cardiac output} = \text{ejection time (seconds/minute)} / 44.3 \times \sqrt{\text{mean systolic gradient}}$$

This formula assumes that 100% of the pressure drop across the aortic valve produces flow, and this is not always true, particularly at low flows. Wide discrepancies have been noted between valve areas calculated from the Gorlin formula and actual measured areas,[34] with questionable increases during exercise[35] and dubious measurements at low flows.[36] An in vitro model showed that the estimate from the Gorlin formula of a known area increased directly with increasing flow, so that substantial errors are to be expected at both low and high flows.[37] Further, at a critical point, small errors become important—an area of 0.6 cm^2/m^2 is on the margin of the severe range, and an area of 0.8 cm^2/m^2 is in the mild to moderate range. The formula remains the basis for comparisons with other methods, but it is by no means a true "gold standard."

Although best views of the whole left ventricular outflow are usually achieved with left ventricular injections using cranial tilt of the left anterior oblique view, straight oblique views (usually about 60 degrees left anterior oblique and 30 degrees right anterior oblique) profile the aortic annulus well and facilitate balloon valvuloplasty. Typical appearances with aortography are shown for the various forms of stenosis in Figure 35–10.

We use a convention that aortic regurgitation is mild if opacification of the left ventricle does not equal that of the aorta, moderate if opacification is equalized after three cycles, and severe if it is equalized in less than three cycles.[38,39] In our hands, this has proved more satisfactory than the method of calculating the regurgitant volume by subtracting net forward flow measured by the Fick method from angiographically determined forward flow.[40] Satisfactory correlation with echocardiographic assessment has been shown using the Brandt convention.[41]

COMPARISONS BETWEEN CATHETERIZATION AND DOPPLER ASSESSMENTS

Earlier studies in adults[29,30,42] showed that catheter P-P gradients averaged about 80% of Doppler P-I gradients with reasonable correlation but moderate scatter. Interestingly, Doppler P-I gradients in these studies averaged only a little above 80% of catheterization P-I gradients, partly because of difficulty in aligning Doppler signals in some studies; this is probably a lesser problem in the pediatric age group. The study by Currie and associates,[30] the only one that included simultaneous echocardiographic and catheter studies, showed excellent correlation between simultaneous catheter and echo P-I gradients and illustrated very well the variation to be expected when these studies are carried out at different times (Fig. 35–11).

Assessments of mean gradients by echo Doppler and catheterization are much closer, catheter figures ranging from 2 to 4 mm Hg on average higher than echo. Mean pressures therefore have appeal on both theoretical and practical grounds, but mean levels requiring intervention have not been securely established. For example, in an adult population judged to need operation because valve area was less than 0.75 cm^2, all patients had a mean gradient greater than 30 mm Hg, more than half greater than 50 mm Hg.[43] In a pediatric population, by contrast, 11 patients with a mean gradient in the range of 17 to 27 mm Hg were judged to need operation.[23] More information is required to establish boundaries with confidence.

Correlations between Doppler and catheterization measurements of valve area have been reasonable in adult patients although there is considerable scatter and different studies have derived varying regression equations.[29] Assessment of valve area is mandatory in patients with significant aortic regurgitation and desirable in patients with borderline gradients associated with unfavorable clinical features. Minor errors in dimension measurements can lead to substantial errors in area assessment.

To summarize, technically good simultaneous catheterization and Doppler assessments of P-I and mean gradients give excellent correlation; toward the critical end of the spectrum, P-P measurements are about 80% of P-I measurements; technically satisfactory Doppler assessment of aortic valve area appears at least as reliable as catheter assessment. Further, a Doppler P-I gradient of 90 to 100 mm Hg (equivalent to a P-P catheter gradient of more than 75 mm Hg) or a valve area of 0.5 cm^2/m^2 usually justifies early intervention; a Doppler P-I gradient of 70 mm Hg (equivalent to a P-P gradient of about 55 mm Hg) or an area less than 0.7 cm^2/m^2 justifies intervention in the presence of other unfavorable features. Intervention may be judged appropriate in patients with a catheter or Doppler mean gradient of 30 mm Hg, but a level of 50 mm

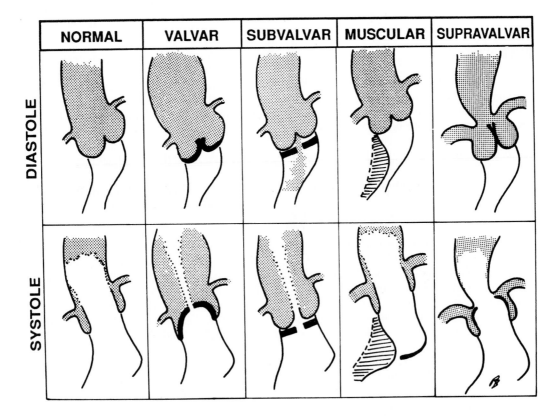

NORMAL	VALVAR	SUBVALVAR	MUSCULAR	SUPRAVALVAR

DIASTOLE

SYSTOLE

FIGURE 35–10

Aortography in various types of aortic stenosis compared with normal. In a normal aortic valve, the opening of the leaflets allows full-width bolus of contrast medium to pass through. In aortic valvar stenosis, the thickened, domed, fused leaflets restrict the bolus of contrast material, seen as a jet, which may be asymmetric. With subvalvar fixed or membranous stenosis, there is a jet of contrast material without doming of the leaflets. With hypertrophic cardiomyopathy (muscular), the aortic valve may appear normal. Septal hypertrophy and systolic anterior motion of the anterior leaflet of the mitral valve are also seen in the diagram. In supravalvar stenosis, the narrowing is above the top of the sinuses; the aortic leaflets may form a dome because of leaflet adherence to the supravalvar ridge. The coronary arteries are dilated. (From Brandt PW, O'Brien KP, Glancy DL: Cardiac catheterization. 3. Angiocardiography. Australas Radiol 14:398–408, 1970.)

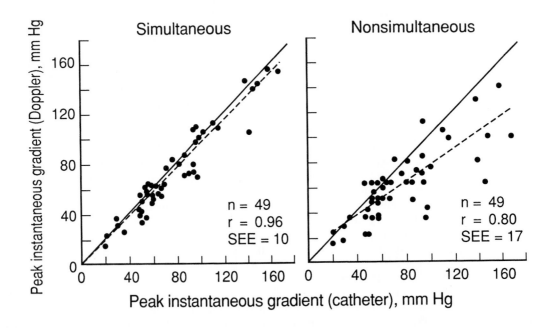

FIGURE 35–11

Simultaneous *(left)* and nonsimultaneous *(right)* Doppler and catheterization measurements of peak instantaneous gradients in patients with aortic stenosis. The Doppler spectral envelope and left ventricular and aortic catheterization gradients were digitized at 10-millisecond intervals to obtain these measurements. The excellent correlation with simultaneous recordings compared with the wider scatter in sequential recordings. *Dotted lines* denote regression lines; *solid lines* denote lines of identity. (From Currie PJ, Hagler DJ, Seward JB, et al: Instantaneous pressure gradient: A simultaneous Doppler and dual catheter correlative study. Reprinted with permission from the American College of Cardiology [Journal of the American College of Cardiology, 1986, Volume 7, Pages 800–806].)

Hg is more common in older patients. These variations should not be surprising in view of the relationship between cardiac output and outflow gradient. Hemodynamic measurements contribute only part of the decision process.

TREATMENT

Natural history studies of aortic stenosis include patients in whom the diagnosis is clear-cut. In addition, there is a large group of children whose only sign is a modest systolic murmur that radiates to the neck more than expected with the ubiquitous functional murmurs of young children. All that is required in this situation is the advice that there could be a trivial flaw in the aortic valve, with a recommendation for endocarditis precautions and a later check. Echocardiography rarely plays a useful role in this situation in infancy, because it cannot exclude a trivial anomaly of the valve. By 4 or 5 years of age, echocardiographic confirmation or exclusion may be desirable when signs are suggestive of an aortic valve anomaly.

MANAGEMENT OF INFANTS YOUNGER THAN 1 YEAR

Infants presenting with severe failure in the neonatal period pose the most formidable problem. An apparently well baby can become critically ill in a matter of hours, the common differential diagnosis being overwhelming sepsis. This situation has been triggered by ductus constriction, and immediate treatment is an infusion of prostaglandin E. Although usually successful, systemic vasodilatation may be a problem if ductus flow is only partly restored,[44] and moderate inotropic support, usually with dopamine, is often needed. Intubation and positive-pressure ventilation are frequently required. The patient having been stabilized, treatment is then decided primarily by echocardiography. With a widely patent ductus and a low output, the gradient may be in the 20s in the presence of extreme stenosis. Morphology of the valve and ventricle then dictates management.

Effective treatment may be impossible for a valve with a small annulus and poorly formed myxomatous leaflets. A small left ventricle greatly increases the risk of intervention,[45] especially with endocardial fibroelastosis,[46] small mitral annulus,[44] or infarction of papillary muscles with mitral regurgitation.[47] Pointers to a high likelihood of a poor outcome with intervention are an end-diastolic volume less than 20 ml/m^2, left ventricular inflow dimension (aortic annulus to apex) less than 25 mm, aortic annulus less than 5 mm, and mitral annulus less than 9 mm.[48,49] A single factor does not always provide a reliable prediction of outcome, however, because multiple factors appear to interact even if they are above the recognized borderline.

An equation correctly predicted outcome in almost 90% of patients, a discriminating score less than −0.35 predicting death (Fig. 35–12)[50]:

$$score = 14.0 \, (BSA) + 0.943 \, (AOi) + 4.78 \, (LAR)$$
$$+ \, 0.157 \, (MVAi) - 12.03$$

where BSA is body surface area, AOi and MVAi are aortic sinus dimension and mitral valve area indexed to body sur-

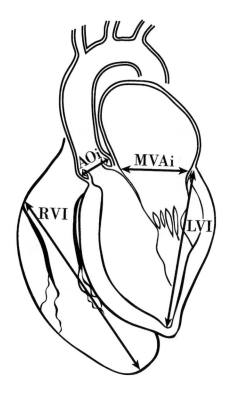

FIGURE 35–12

Measurements used in patients to predict outcome from aortic valvotomy in neonates.[50] See text. In this example, LAR is LVI/RVI.

face area, and LAR is the ratio of the long axis of the left ventricle (from the plane of the mitral valve annulus to the apex of the ventricle) to the long axis of the heart (apical four-chamber view of the distance from the crux of the heart to the apical endocardium, either left or right ventricle, whichever forms the apex of the heart). Infants with a score below the critical level have a better outlook with a Norwood approach[51] than with valvotomy. In this situation, the ascending aorta is often small, and the papillary muscle structure of the mitral valve is single or hypoplastic with short chordae tendineae. Meticulous interrogation of the aortic arch is required to assess associated hypoplasia and coarctation.

Operation

Survival rates as high as 90% and as low as 10% have been recorded with surgery in neonates.[52] Differences in these earlier studies are probably related more to anatomy than to technique. The Second Natural History Study[16] in patients recruited in the years 1958 to 1969 presents a sobering picture of surgery in infants. Of 21 documented patients, 13 underwent surgery in the first year, of whom 7 died within 2 days and 3 of the remaining 6 required reoperation. Of eight medically managed patients, five required an operation beyond 1 year. When the overall dimensions discussed before are adequate, acceptable medium-term results are now possible with severe aortic stenosis even if left ventricular function is significantly impaired. In infants with good left ventricular function, immediate intervention is not mandatory even if the obstruction is severe. Postponement of operation under careful observation may lower the risk further.

Balloon Valvuloplasty

In early experience of balloon aortic valvuloplasty (BAV) in infancy, survival of about 50% was achieved.[53] Zeevi compared outcomes of a sequential series of 16 operations and 16 BAVs in similar groups of infants. After follow-up for 18 months, there were seven deaths (or staging for the Norwood operation) in each group. In surgical patients with adequate documentation, death occurred in each of 3 with a hypoplastic left ventricle and in 3 of 10 with normal left ventricular size. Corresponding figures for the BAV group were 5 of 6 and 2 of 10, respectively. In the collaborative Valvuloplasty and Angioplasty of Congenital Anomalies (VACA) Registry, 4 of the 5 deaths among 204 patients occurred in infants younger than 1 month, as did all 3 life-threatening arrhythmias.[54] In a series of 80 patients, Sholler and colleagues[55] reported 3 early deaths among 12 neonates but none in 68 older patients. Potential complications include major hemorrhage from the femoral or central arteries, avulsion of part of an aortic leaflet, and perforation of the mitral valve or left ventricle. Permanent loss of the femoral pulse occurs in about 10% of infants younger than 1 year. Although complications are much higher in a neonate, results appear comparable with those of operation, and balloon valvuloplasty is now regarded as the first step in management in many centers.

MANAGEMENT OF CHILDREN OLDER THAN 1 YEAR

Operation

Beyond 1 year, operation mortality is less than 2%.[15,56] In most children and teenagers, a valvotomy is practical, using cardiopulmonary bypass. The commissures are incised to mobilize the fused leaflets. Considerable judgment is required to achieve the largest possible opening without compromising leaflet stability and producing important aortic regurgitation that may increase further as time goes by.

As already noted, intermediate outcome in any patient with aortic stenosis is related to the initial severity of the lesion, and this also applies to postoperative progress. Survival after surgical valvotomy is around 95% at 5 years, 85% at 15 years, and 75% at 25 years.[52,56] Valvotomy provides no protection against infectious endocarditis, and the specter of sudden death is not abolished. In earlier studies, mild or moderate aortic regurgitation was reported in 10 to 28% of patients after surgical valvotomy. This may progress with time and it may be underestimated on clinical examination. In the Second Natural History Study, moderate or severe aortic regurgitation was diagnosed at follow-up of medical patients in 8% clinically and 24% by echocardiography; in the operatively treated group, the corresponding figures were 12% and 30%. Continued monitoring of patients is required to detect changes in valve and ventricular function. The need for reoperation begins 4 to 5 years after the first procedure, and almost 40% of patients require a second operation by 25 years.[16,56]

Balloon Valvuloplasty

The role of balloon valvuloplasty has been assessed in the light of this experience, and in the shorter follow-up period since the first reports of the early 1980s,[57] results appear comparable to operation. Because valvuloplasty is less traumatic and cheaper and does not cause mediastinal scarring, it is now usually the first intervention. A typical operative outcome achieves a P-P reduction in gradient at catheterization from 70 mm Hg or higher to 25 to 40 mm Hg.[58,59] In reported catheterization assessments after BAV, gradients on average have fallen from 70 mm Hg or higher to 30 mm Hg.[54,55,57] With both techniques, there is of course a considerable range of residual gradients. In the VACA study,[54] 192 of 204 patients showed some benefit.

Principles of valvuloplasty have been established and apply in all age groups. In 16 lambs, Helgason and colleagues[60] defined the safe limits of balloon size for BAV. In three with no balloon inflations and six in which the balloon/aortic annulus ratio (BAR) was 0.9 to 1.1, there was no damage to the left ventricular outflow. In seven animals in which the BAR was 1.2 to 1.5, ventricular tachycardia and ST depression were common, and two animals developed aortic regurgitation. Tears, hematomas, or both were found in the aortic valve (three), mitral leaflets (four), and interventricular septum (four). Clinical experience confirms that increasing the BAR beyond 1 increases the risk of aortic regurgitation without improving the level of dilatation (Fig. 35–13).[54,55]

Annulus size should be measured both at echocardiography and on aortography because definition of the true boundaries is sometimes difficult. A caliber check of the inflated balloon is useful because the inflated diameter is sometimes smaller than specified. Catheterization from the femoral artery is usual. A carotid approach has been used when access is difficult, and a cutdown carotid approach has been used in some centers in neonates. An approach from the umbilical artery has also been advocated in neonates but does not allow free manipulation. Others have recommended anterograde passage of the balloon catheter. This may be achieved by trans-septal entry to the left atrium and ventricle, placement of a sheath with a J loop pointing toward the aortic valve, anterograde passage of a balloon-type catheter to the aorta, and either capture of the wire through a femoral puncture to allow a venous arterial loop[61] or simply placing the wire in descending aorta.[62] In most patients, however, retrograde entry can be achieved by placing an appropriately curved catheter above the aperture in the valve and passing a small-gauge soft-tip wire to the left ventricle. An appropriate curve for the catheter can be made by amputating a pigtail catheter at a selected point. The aperture through the valve is often posterior, and the catheter can be placed in the jet stream with reference to the aortogram. Echocardiography has been used in some units. After the ventricle has been entered, placement of an extra-stiff wire with the soft tip curled in the left ventricle provides stability for the balloon. Balloon placement must be accurate, relying initially on landmarks identified by the aortogram. The balloon should have a BAR of 0.9 to 1. Firm control of the catheter shaft is required to avoid displacement either to left ventricle or aorta. A mobile balloon probably increases the risk of an unsatisfactory valvotomy and significant aortic regurgitation. A recent trial of adenosine (0.125–0.55 mg/kg) to produce temporary asystole could point the way to improved outcomes.[63] Full dilatation should be maintained for about 5 seconds, and unless there is a prompt return of heart rate and blood pressure, the balloon should be withdrawn to the aorta between dilatations. No benefit has

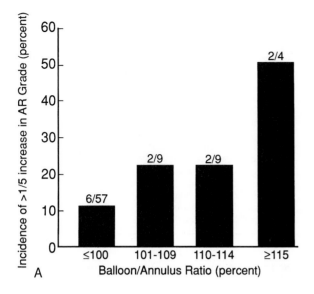

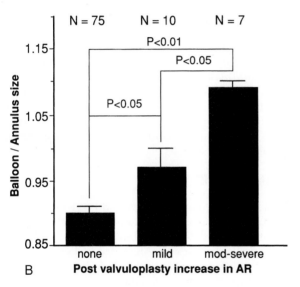

Relation between the diameter of the valvuloplasty balloon/aortic annulus ratio and the development of aortic regurgitation (AR). (*A* from Sholler GF, Keane JF, Perry SB, et al: Balloon dilation of congenital aortic valve stenosis. Results and influence of technical and morphological features on outcome. Circulation 78[2]:351–360, 1988. *B* reprinted from American Journal of Cardiology, Volume 65, Rocchini AP, Beekman RH, Ben Shachar G, et al: Balloon aortic valvuloplasty: Results of the Valvuloplasty and Angioplasty of Congenital Anomalies Registry, Pages 784–789, Copyright 1990, with permission from Excerpta Medica Inc.)

been demonstrated in repeating the dilatation once the waist has been eliminated, but we carry out at least one further dilatation to observe the constrictive pattern on re-inflation. In neonates with a myxomatous valve, there may be little if any waist even with the first inflation.

A trivial increase in aortic regurgitation has been reported in 14% of patients, moderate or severe regurgitation in 4%.[54,55] The risk appeared greater with a unicuspid valve but otherwise was not appreciably higher in infants. Permanent pulse loss occurred in 5 to 10% of patients, the risk being higher in infants. Improvement in balloons allowing smaller catheter size has reduced this risk, but initial pulse

reduction is common. If it is persistent, intravenous heparin should be given at 4 hours and fibrinolysis at 24 hours. Rarely, surgical thrombectomy may be required. Transient left bundle branch block, complete atrioventricular block, and ventricular ectopics may occur, although ventricular tachycardia requiring cardioversion is rare beyond 1 year of age. Insertion of a pacing wire, or at least providing venous access for pacing, is recommended before balloon insertion. Life-threatening complications are extremely uncommon beyond early infancy, and the risk of death at intervention is probably about 1%. Early operation has been required in 5% of patients, about half of these because of failure to cross the valve or otherwise achieve adequate dilatation, and the other half because of complications. Again, the risk is lower beyond the early infant period.

Some units have advocated the use of two balloons with a combined area (not diameter) giving a BAR of 0.9 to 1. Better results have been suggested with this technique by some[64] but not confirmed by others.[55] Satisfactory BAV has been demonstrated in patients who have had previous surgical valvotomy[65,66] and in younger adults with noncalcified valves.[67] Although long-term follow-up is awaited, BAV has been established as the preferred technique, and repeated BAV should be possible in many patients during the first three or four decades of life, postponing the need for aortic valve replacement.

PROGNOSIS

Long-term prognosis will always be less good in those presenting at a young age with a severe lesion. Continued supervision will help preserve left ventricular function and minimize the risk both of sudden death and of heart failure. Most patients requiring intervention as a child or young adult will, however, ultimately need valve replacement. Long-term survival after replacement has been around 75% at 5 years, 60% at 10 years, and 40% at 15 years,[68] but most series included many patients with impaired left ventricular function. All interventional steps in aortic stenosis must be regarded as palliative. Nevertheless, with meticulous care and precautions against the ever-present risk of endocarditis, many patients can approach a normal life span with a satisfactory lifestyle.

FUTURE DIRECTIONS

Despite the interesting report of attempted antenatal BAV,[69] it is difficult to envisage intrauterine interventions early enough to alter the infant's outcome substantially, and severe neonatal aortic stenosis is likely to remain a formidable problem. In older children, endoscopic and laser techniques could make it possible to develop a surgical approach with modestly invasive techniques. The success of BAV is intriguing, however. The inflated balloon often appears to provide a nearly optimal result, perhaps by producing just enough local stress to open the appropriate commissure without damaging adjacent tissues. Indeed, balloon valvotomy has been recommended at an open chest, nonbypass operation.[70] Continued improvement in balloon technology, together with careful recording of pressure, time, and diameter of dilatation to fit the anatomy, should gradually increase success rates. Continu-

TABLE 35–3

TYPES OF PATIENTS WITH SUPRAVALVAR AORTIC STENOSIS (N = 43) AND ASSOCIATED CARDIAC LESIONS: GREEN LANE HOSPITAL

Williams' syndrome (n = 20)
  8 branch pulmonary stenosis
  1 pulmonary valve stenosis
  1 dysplastic aortic and pulmonary valves

Familial (n = 8)
  6 unusual facies:
    5 branch pulmonary stenosis
  2 normal facies:
    no associated congenital heart defects

Down syndrome (n = 1)
  No other associated congenital heart defects

Sporadic (n = 14)
  Congenital cardiac defects
    3 coarctation
    2 mitral valve stenosis
    2 bicommissural aortic valve
    1 asplenia syndrome
    1 prolapsed mitral valve
    1 ventricular septal defect
    1 pulmonary valve stenosis
    6 without associated congenital heart defects
  Acquired cardiac defects
    1 calcific aortic valve stenosis
    1 rheumatic heart disease
    1 bacterial endocarditis

ous improvement in prosthetic and tissue valves could certainly improve long-term outcome in patients who frequently require valve replacement in the first half of their natural life span. The potential of the Ross procedure,[71] replacing the aortic valve with the patient's own pulmonary valve and inserting an allograft in the pulmonary area, may lead to its wider application in young children.

SUPRAVALVAR AORTIC STENOSIS

Supravalvar aortic stenosis is the least common type of aortic stenosis or left ventricular outflow obstruction. In a report of 104 patients, supravalvar aortic stenosis was found in 6% in contrast to 71% valvar and 23% subvalvar aortic stenosis.[72] Supravalvar aortic stenosis occurs in at least three types of patients: in association with Williams' syndrome,[73] in autosomal dominant familial disease,[74] and sporadically. Most instances of Williams' syndrome occur spontaneously although occasional familial instances have been reported, suggesting a possible autosomal dominant inheritance.[75] The autosomal dominant, nonsyndromic, familial type has usually been described with normal facies and intelligence; however, we have seen two families with unusual facies and low intelligence (Table 35–3) and one patient with Down syndrome. In a series of 81 patients,[76] nearly 50% had Williams' syndrome, 22% were familial, 25% were sporadic, 2% had Noonan's syndrome, and one had rubella, in contrast to combined surgical series,[77,78] in which 29% had Williams' syndrome, 8% were familial, and 63% were sporadic.

GENETIC BASIS FOR SUPRAVALVAR AORTIC STENOSIS

Mutations in the elastin gene of chromosome 7 have been seen in families with supravalvar aortic stenosis, whereas submicroscopic deletions of chromosome 7q11.23 are associated with Williams' syndrome (Table 35–4).[79] These deletions of the elastin gene are detectable by fluorescent in situ hybridization and are found in 90% of patients with classical features of Williams' syndrome.[80] Reduction of the elastin content of the media, abnormalities in the internal elastic lamina, or abnormalities of the elastic fibers may lead to the vascular anomalies seen in patients with supravalvar aortic stenosis.[79]

WILLIAMS' SYNDROME

In 1961, Williams, Barratt-Boyes, and Lowe described the triad of supravalvar aortic stenosis, mental subnormality, and unusual facial features (Table 35–5),[73] and subsequently, similar findings were reported by Beuren and colleagues.[81] Earlier reports suggested an association with idiopathic hypercalcemia of infancy. This appears less common now,[82,83] but serum calcium levels should be checked in infants with symptoms suggesting hypercalcemia (vomiting, constipation, irritability; Table 35–6).[84]

The characteristic facial features (Fig. 35–14), general somatic abnormalities, and cardiovascular defects are listed in Tables 35–5 to 35–8. The typical facial features may not be obvious at birth but become more characteristic with time.[84] Supravalvar aortic stenosis has been reported in 37 to 73% of patients with Williams' syndrome[82,84,85] (Tables 35–7 and 35–8).

TABLE 35–4

MOLECULAR GENETICS OF SUPRAVALVAR AORTIC STENOSIS AND WILLIAMS' SYNDROME

Clinical Disorder	Mode of Inheritance	Chromosome	Gene	Associated Mutations	Genetic Testing	Mechanism
Supravalvar aortic stenosis	Autosomal dominant	7q11.23	Elastin	Intragenic deletion and translocation	Linkage and mutational analyses	Probable reduction in elastin content during development
Williams' syndrome	Sporadic	7q11.23	Elastin and adjacent genes	De novo deletion (complete)	Fluorescent in situ hybridization	Probable contiguous gene disorder

From Keating MT: Genetic approaches to cardiovascular disease. Supravalvular aortic stenosis, Williams syndrome, and long-QT syndrome. Circulation 92(1):142–147, 1995.

TABLE 35–5

FACIAL FEATURES IN WILLIAMS' SYNDROME

Large mouth, prominent lips in 89%[82]
Hypoplastic teeth with malocclusion in 85%[84]
Medial flare to eyebrows in 81%[82]
Anteverted nostrils in 74%[82]
Flat nasal bridge, full tip of nose in 68%[82]
Stellate iris in 72%[82]
Short palpebral fissures in 58%[82]
Supraorbital fullness in 56%[82]
Long philtrum in 56%[82]
Ocular hypotelorism in 53%[82]
Strabismus in 35%[82]

TABLE 35–6

WILLIAMS' SYNDROME—GENERAL FEATURES

Dysmorphic facial appearance (see Table 35–5)
Mental retardation, IQ average 58, range 20–106,[84] mild to severe
    learning difficulties
Characteristic learning profile: poor visual-motor integration, good
    language skills, poor motor skills
Attention deficit disorder in 84%[84]
Failure to thrive in 81%[84]
Congenital heart defects in 79%[84] and vascular changes involving aorta,
    pulmonary, renal, and coronary arteries
Hoarse voice in 78%[82]
Early feeding difficulties in 71%[84]
Hypersocial personality, gregarious, engaging personalities in 67%[82]
Infantile hypercalcemia in 4/6,[84] 0/8[82]
Hypertension in 8%[97] to 82%[95]
Hallux valgus in 78% with small curved fifth digit in 42%[82]
Vomiting, constipation in 40%[84]
Pectus excavatum in 39%[82]
Intrauterine growth retardation
Inguinal or umbilical hernia in 14%[84]
Joint abnormalities—contractures or limitations in 5%[84]

TABLE 35–7

CONGENITAL HEART DEFECTS IN WILLIAMS' SYNDROME

Supravalvar aortic stenosis in 37–73%[82, 84]
Peripheral pulmonary stenosis in 3–39%[85, 97]
Coronary artery anomalies in 6%[85]
Prolapse of mitral valve in 1–15%[85, 97]
Bicommissural aortic valve in 11%[97]
Aortic valve stenosis
Ventricular septal defects in 1.6%[97]
Coarctation of aortic isthmus in 1%[85]
Anomalous left pulmonary artery

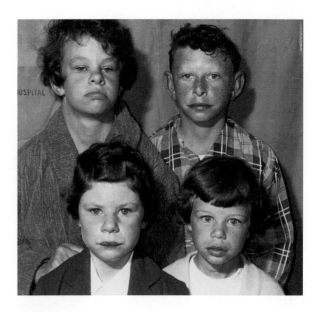

FIGURE 35–14

Photograph of the first four patients reported with supravalvar aortic stenosis and the characteristic facial features of Williams' syndrome. (From Williams JCP, Barratt-Boyes BG, Lowe JB: Supravalvular aortic stenosis. Circulation 24:1311–1318, 1961.)

dysplasia,[86, 87] may be completely or only partially circumferential. The stenosis is a localized, hourglass deformity in about 80% of patients and more diffuse in 20% (Fig. 35–16).[72, 77, 78, 88] In most patients, the proximal ascending aorta is mildly narrowed or at least smaller than normal (Fig. 35–16*B*). In the more severe diffuse type, the narrowing may extend around the aortic arch and involve the brachiocephalic arteries (Fig. 35–16*C*).[72, 77, 78, 88]

The aortic valve leaflets are frequently abnormal.[72] Bicommissural aortic valves have been reported in about 26%.[77, 78] The free edges of the aortic valve leaflets may be partially or completely adherent to the wall of the aorta at the site of the medial thickening, sometimes obstructing coronary arterial flow. Restriction of coronary arterial flow can also be produced by stenosis of the origin of the coronary artery, which may be narrowed at or just distal to the ostium, as found in 20 of 33 patients described by Peterson and coworkers.[72] Thickening of the wall encroaches on the lumen. On histologic examination, coronary arterial wall dysplasia (disorganization) involves all three layers, not just the media, with varying degrees of intimal hyperplasia, fibrosis, and disorganization; disruption and loss of internal elastic lamina with indistinct intimal medial junctions; medial hypertrophy and dysplasia; and adventitial fibroelastosis.[87] Other coronary arteries may be dilated and tortuous (Fig. 35–16*C*).

PATHOLOGIC ANATOMY

Supravalvar stenosis is produced by thickening of the wall of the ascending aorta in the region of the sinotubular ridge, at the top of the commissures (Fig. 35–15). The thickening, which is produced by medial hypertrophy and

TABLE 35–8

CARDIOVASCULAR LESIONS IN WILLIAMS' SYNDROME (N = 25): GREEN LANE HOSPITAL

Supravalvar aortic stenosis (n = 20)	Without supravalvar aortic stenosis (n = 5)
8 branch pulmonary stenosis	3 no heart disease
1 pulmonary valvar stenosis	1 branch pulmonary stenosis
1 dysplastic aortic and pulmonary valves	1 ventricular septal defect, anomalous left pulmonary artery

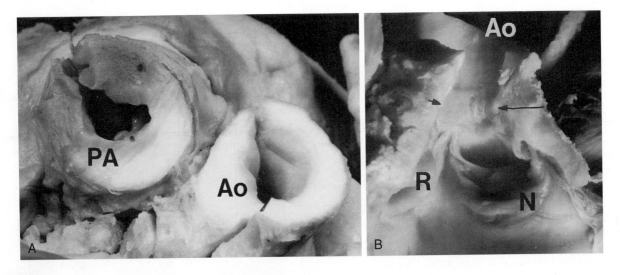

FIGURE 35-15

Heart specimen of 5-month-old girl with supravalvar aortic and pulmonary stenoses and generalized arteriopathy involving coronary arteries as well as brachiocephalic arteries. *A*, Superior view of transected, thick-walled great arteries, viewed from behind. The aorta (Ao) measured 2 mm in thickness, the main pulmonary artery (PA) 3 mm. *B*, Opened left ventricular outflow to aorta (Ao). The supravalvar ridge *(arrows)*, which is seen superior to the right (R) and noncoronary (N) aortic valve leaflets, produced further thickening of the wall and narrowed the lumen to 4 mm.

Associated cardiac lesions are common, particularly branch and peripheral pulmonary arterial stenoses (Fig. 35–17).[72,89] Pulmonary arterial branch stenoses are found more frequently in patients with the familial type of supravalvar aortic stenosis or with Williams' syndrome. The right and left pulmonary arterial branches are usually diffusely hypoplastic, but discrete stenosis may occur, usually of more peripheral branch origins (Fig. 35–17). Additional associated cardiac lesions are listed in Table 35–9. The most severely affected infants often have significant right- and left-sided obstruction with generalized arteriopathy[90] in addition to mitral valve prolapse, with dysplasia of aortic, pulmonary, and mitral valves.[91]

HEMODYNAMICS

The hemodynamic findings are similar to those of aortic valvar stenosis, but the gradient is found in the proximal ascending aorta. Thus, the systolic pressure that perfuses coronary arteries is elevated, although the diastolic coronary pressure is normal. Coronary arterial anomalies may lead to important limitation of subendocardial coronary flow in addition to that imposed by left ventricular hypertrophy. The jet through the supravalvar narrowing passes more distally, often hugging the aortic wall (Coanda effect), with the right brachial pressure greater than the left.[92,93] In patients with associated pulmonary valve or branch stenoses, right-sided heart pressures are elevated.

NATURAL HISTORY

The natural history is affected by the associated cardiovascular and other lesions. Isolated supravalvar aortic stenosis does not appear to require an operation in infancy. Neonates who underwent an operation also had severe associated lesions.[77] Other described patients have been older than age 1 year,[77,78,88] the mean age at operation in two large series being 12 years.[77,78] The severity of the

supravalvar aortic stenosis may progress with time,[88,94,95] although one patient showed reduction in severity of obstruction.[75] Wren and colleagues[88] found an increase in the degree of supravalvar aortic stenosis produced by failure of normal growth of the region in about 80% of their patients, being most rapid in the younger patients. By contrast, the stenoses of peripheral pulmonary arterial branches may spontaneously improve.[88,94] Right ventricular systolic pressure decreased in about 80% of those with peripheral pulmonary arterial stenosis,[88,94] and diffusely hypoplastic pulmonary arteries increased in size on cineangiograms.[85,88,94]

There is a significant incidence of bacterial endocarditis or mycotic aneurysms of the aorta. Sudden death is not uncommon, for example, in 3 of 104 patients,[95] and is probably related to coronary arterial lesions. Coronary arterial stenoses were found in more than 70% of patients with Williams' syndrome who died suddenly.[96] Severe biventricular outflow tract obstruction may also predispose individuals to sudden death.[96]

HISTORY, PHYSICAL EXAMINATION, CHEST RADIOGRAPHY, AND ELECTROCARDIOGRAPHY

Symptoms are similar to those of aortic valvar stenosis, although many young patients are asymptomatic and the age at presentation is usually older.[84] The male preponderance seen in other types of aortic stenosis is not found in supravalvar aortic stenosis, particularly in patients with Williams' syndrome, for which the female/male ratio is 1.2:1.[84,85,97] Apart from associated syndromes, the clinical features are also similar to those of aortic valve stenosis except that the systolic murmur is along the upper right sternal border, and there is no click. The murmur may radiate superiorly with or without a palpable thrill in the suprasternal notch. Systemic hypertension is frequent, noticed in 50% in a series of 104 patients.[95] Asymmetric

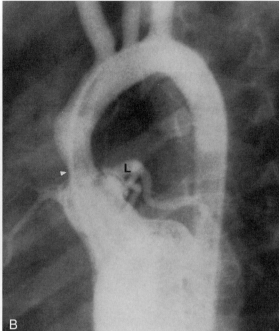

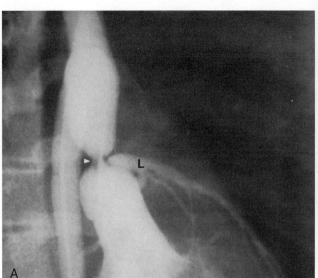

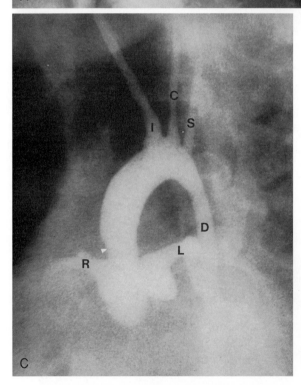

FIGURE 35–16

Frames from cineangiograms in three patients with supravalvar aortic stenosis and dilatation of aortic valve ring and sinuses. *A,* Injection in left ventricle in right anterior oblique projection in a 15-year-old girl with severe stenosis *(arrowhead)* above the aortic valve. The diameter measured 5 mm compared with 26 mm across the aortic sinus. The left coronary artery (L) is dilated. *B,* Left ventricular injection in left anterior oblique projection in a 7-year-old boy with moderate supravalvar stenosis *(arrowhead),* diameter 6 mm. The ascending aorta is mildly hypoplastic, diameter 12 mm. The aortic valve leaflets are thickened and domed, and adherence of the left leaflet obstructed flow into the dilated left coronary artery (L). *C,* Aortogram in left anterior oblique projection in a 14-year-old girl with the diffuse type of supravalvar aortic stenosis. The right (R) and left (L) coronary arteries are dilated. The descending thoracic aorta (D) is diffusely hypoplastic, diameter 5 mm compared with 22 mm across the aortic sinuses, 9 mm above the aortic valve *(arrowhead),* and 17 mm in the ascending aorta. The brachiocephalic arteries are also hypoplastic. C = left common carotid; I = innominate artery; S = left subclavian artery. Compare size of these arteries with *B.*

blood pressures have been noted, with pressure in the right arm usually higher.[92, 93] Electrocardiograms are similar to those in aortic valvar stenosis except that additional right ventricular hypertrophy may be found when there is significant associated pulmonary branch stenosis. Chest films do not usually show dilatation of the ascending aorta.

ECHOCARDIOGRAPHY

The diagnosis of supravalvar aortic stenosis can be made noninvasively by two-dimensional echocardiography.[74] Imaging from the parasternal and suprasternal windows can identify the type and localize the site of obstruction, although on occasion it may not be possible to image the entire length of the ascending aorta. In patients with an hourglass deformity or with diffuse hypoplasia of the ascending aorta, the diameter of the proximal ascending aorta is less than that of the aortic annulus (Fig. 35–18). This is in contrast to normal subjects, in whom the diameter of the annulus is similar to, or slightly less than, the diameter of the proximal ascending aorta. Two-dimensional echocardiography can also define the morphology of the aortic valve, identifying leaflet thickening and tethering. Careful imaging may demonstrate coronary ostial abnormalities, al-

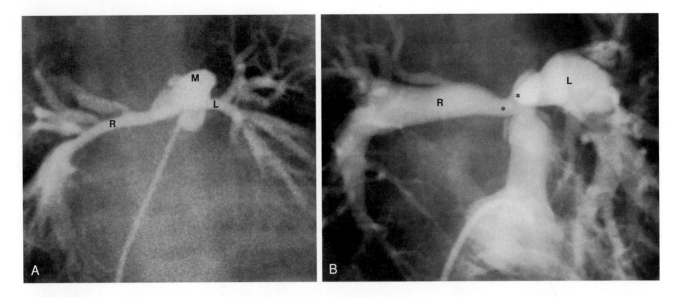

Frames from cineangiocardiograms in two patients with pulmonary arterial branch or origin stenoses. *A*, Injection in main pulmonary artery (M) in anteroposterior view in a 2-year-old boy. There is diffuse hypoplasia of right (R) and left (L) pulmonary arteries and localized stenoses of the origins of the right upper and middle lobe branches. *B*, Right ventricular injection in right anterior oblique view in a 10-month-old boy. The pulmonary valve leaflets are thickened, domed, and tethered. There is supravalvar pulmonary stenosis and moderate stenoses of proximal right (R) and left (L) pulmonary arteries *(asterisks)*. The origin of the right upper lobe branch is mildly stenosed.

though intermittent coronary artery obstruction by tethered aortic valve leaflets may be difficult to diagnose.

The gradient across the obstruction can be estimated by two-dimensional image-guided pulsed and continuous-wave Doppler from the apical and suprasternal windows. Repeated examinations will document progression of obstruction. Serial obstruction (at the valve and the supravalvar level) may result in an overestimation of the gradient, whereas the modified Bernoulli equation may underestimate the gradient when there is long-segment stenosis.[98] Echocardiography may also identify branch pulmonary artery stenosis and elevated right ventricular pressure.

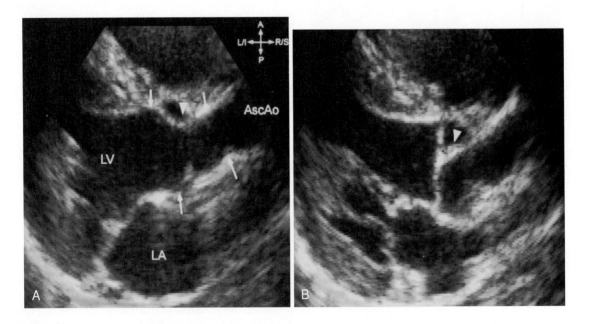

Two-dimensional echocardiogram, parasternal long-axis image. *A*, In systole, the right coronary leaflet *(arrowhead)* is tethered to the supra-aortic ridge *(right arrows)*. The diameter of the aortic annulus *(left arrows)* is larger than the supra-aortic region. *B*, In diastole, there is persistent adherence of the leaflet *(arrowhead)* to the supra-aortic ridge. A = anterior; AscAo = ascending aorta; LA = left atrium; L/I = left and inferior; LV = left ventricle; P = posterior; R/S = right and superior.

TABLE 35–9

ASSOCIATED CARDIOVASCULAR DEFECTS IN SUPRAVALVAR AORTIC STENOSIS

Peripheral pulmonary arterial branch stenosis in 24–68%[72, 77, 78]
Dilated coronary arteries in 24%[77, 78]
Coronary artery stenosis in 24%[78]
Bicuspid aortic valve in 26%[77, 78]
Aortic valve stenosis in 23%[77, 78]
Aortic arch branch stenosis in 6–21%[72, 77, 78]
Subaortic stenosis in 11%[77, 78]
Mitral stenosis in 9%[78]
Pulmonary stenosis—valvar, subvalvar, or both in 7.5%[78]
Coarctation in 7%[77, 78]
Ventricular septal defect in 2.6%[77, 78]
Patent ductus arteriosus in 2.6%[77, 78]
Mitral regurgitation in 2%[77]

CARDIAC CATHETERIZATION AND CINEANGIOGRAPHY

In patients considered for an operation, cardiac catheterization is required to assess coronary and pulmonary arterial anomalies and to confirm the gradient that is detected above the aortic valve (Fig. 35–19). The flow pattern through the stenotic region is different from that in patients with subvalvar or valvar stenoses (see Fig. 35–10).[99] Cineangiocardiograms may show a discrete hourglass narrowing or diffuse hypoplasia of the aorta and sometimes stenosis of the branches. Stenosis of the origins of the coronary arteries may be demonstrated (see Fig. 35–16). Most patients with discrete stenosis show some hypoplasia of the proximal ascending aorta.

Patients with peripheral pulmonary arterial stenoses often have associated diffuse hypoplasia of the branch pulmonary arteries (see Fig. 35–17). There may be discrete stenosis, more often of peripheral branches. Stenotic lesions may be displayed with magnetic resonance imaging rather than cineangiography, provided that coronary artery detail is adequate in small patients.[100]

MANAGEMENT

Management of supravalvar stenosis depends on severity. If the stenosis is mild, no treatment is required.[95] Once the diagnosis is made, serial echocardiography is required to detect progression before important left ventricular hypertrophy or coronary arterial stenoses develop, particularly in younger patients.[94] If the supravalvar aortic stenosis is associated with generalized arteriopathy involving the coronary arteries and polyvalvar disease, no surgical correction may be feasible except possible cardiac transplantation; if peripheral pulmonary arteries are severely hypoplastic and stenosed, heart and lung transplantation may be required if it is considered practicable. Although balloon dilatation of stenotic supravalvar aortic lesions has been performed with some success, benefit is likely to be limited except in localized lesions.[101] Stent treatment has been reported.[102]

Patients who have symptoms or left ventricular strain pattern on electrocardiography or have gradients of 50 mm Hg at cardiac catheterization or 75 mm Hg at echocardiography require an operation.[76] A variety of procedures have been used for the localized type, usually tear-shaped or pantaloon-shaped patches, excision of the stenosing ring

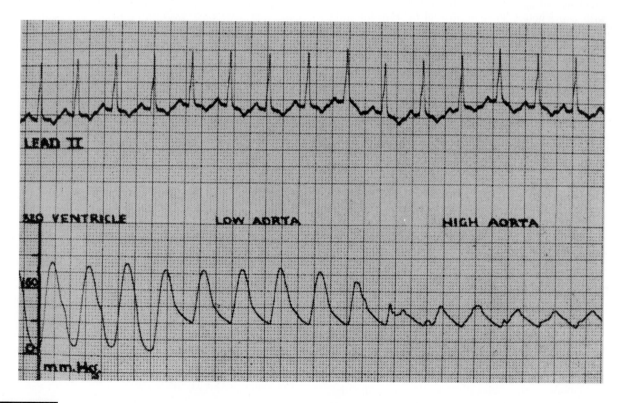

FIGURE 35–19

Withdrawal pressure tracing from left ventricle to ascending aorta in a patient with supravalvar aortic stenosis to show the pressure gradient within the ascending aorta. (From Williams JCP, Barratt-Boyes BG, Lowe JB: Supravalvular aortic stenosis. Circulation 24:1311–1318, 1961.)

below commissures, or extended aortoplasty.[77,78] Aortic valve regurgitation may develop after operation or balloon dilatation. For the diffuse type, various procedures have been tried, including extended patch aortoplasty with apicoaortic conduits, extensive endarterectomy, and conduit from ascending to descending aorta with side branches to stenotic arch vessels. Coronary arterial lesions may require treatment.

Early operative intervention is recommended to minimize development of coronary obstruction, to allow regression of left ventricular hypertrophy, and to prevent progressive ventricular dysfunction.[78]

Strict antibiotic prophylaxis is required in patients with supravalvar aortic stenosis.

PROGNOSIS

The actuarial survival data of Kececioglu and associates[95] in 104 patients with Williams' syndrome and supravalvar aortic stenosis show a decline to 90% at age 18 years and then remain stable. The causes of death in 10 patients were perioperative in 2, during attempted balloon angioplasty for severe peripheral pulmonary stenosis in 1, sudden in 3, and noncardiac in 4. The event-free curve fell to 46% at 21 years of age; surgery (29 patients), reoperation, residual aortic gradients above 50 mm Hg, and bacterial endocarditis were considered events. In 81 patients with supravalvar aortic stenosis (including 40 patients with Williams' syndrome), Kitchiner and colleagues[76] found that survival gradually decreased with time to 71% 17 years after presentation. Long-term survival was related to younger age or severity of aortic stenosis at presentation, with a predicted 30-year survival of 95% for mild stenosis, 73% for moderate stenosis, and 12% for severe stenosis.

Two large operative series have been reported.[77,78] Sharma and coworkers[77] reported 8 early deaths (11%) in 73 patients and 4 late deaths (6%), the latter all due to bacterial endocarditis. The important determinants of death were preoperative functional class 3 or 4, diffuse type of supravalvar aortic stenosis, and associated congenital cardiac lesions. van Son and colleagues[78] reported an operative mortality of 2 among 13 patients with the diffuse type of stenosis, but none of 67 patients with the localized form. Survival, excluding operative mortality, was 94% at 10 years and 91% at 20 years; all patients were in functional class 1 or 2. The only independent predictor for late death was associated aortic valve disease, which was also a risk for late reoperation.

FUTURE DIRECTIONS

More detailed delineation of the anomalies of the elastin gene may allow differentiation between types of autosomal dominant families. Intravascular ultrasound imaging may enable a more rational approach to therapeutic interventions.[103] Intra-arterial interventions might be conceivable in some patients with localized thickening. Keating[79] has suggested that once the pathogenic mechanisms underlying supravalvar aortic stenosis are understood, medical therapy to arrest progression of lesions might be possible.

FIXED SUBAORTIC STENOSIS

Fixed subaortic stenosis is responsible for up to 20% of left ventricular outflow obstruction requiring intervention.[19,104] It affects males more frequently than females,[19,104–106] is rarely seen in infancy, and tends to progress.[107–109] Other cardiac anomalies are present in about two thirds of patients. The most frequent of these are ventricular septal defect, patent ductus arteriosus, coarctation of the aorta, anomalies of the aortic and mitral valves, and double-chambered right ventricle.[108–110]

PATHOLOGY

There are a number of different entities, the most common of which are fibromuscular or membranous subaortic stenosis and tunnel-type subaortic stenosis (Table 35–10). Fibromuscular and membranous subaortic stenosis have been differentiated on the basis of angiographic appearance and the site of obstruction: membranous subaortic stenosis (type I) consists of a thin membrane obstructing the left ventricular outflow tract. This membrane does not involve the aortic or mitral valve. Conversely, with fibromuscular subaortic stenosis (type II), there is a wider fibromuscular ridge 3 to 4 mm proximal to the aortic valve that may involve the anterior leaflet of the mitral valve (Fig. 35–20).[111] The abnormal fibromuscular ridge varies in length, thickness, and shape.[112] It may be crescentic, extending across the anterior portion of the left ventricular outflow tract, or it may be circumferential and extend onto the anterior leaflet of the mitral valve.[111–113] The histologic appearance is variable with irregularly oriented acellular dense collagen fibers, sparse fibroblasts, a smooth muscle cell layer, amounts of elastic tissue, and occasionally areas of myocytes with an associated capillary network.[113,114] The extreme form, tunnel-type subaortic stenosis, with an elongated, narrow, and often convoluted subaortic outflow tract, is usually associated with other left ventricular anomalies including the Shone complex (supramitral ring, parachute mitral valve, subaortic stenosis, and coarctation of the aorta).[115]

In reality, the pathologic anatomy of fixed subaortic stenosis is highly variable, and the differentiation between

TABLE 35–10

CLASSIFICATION OF FIXED SUBAORTIC STENOSIS

Anomalies of the left ventricular outflow tract
    Discrete membranous or fibromuscular subaortic stenosis
    Tunnel-type subaortic stenosis
Mitral valve anomalies
    Anomalous attachments of mitral valve chordae or papillary muscles
    Accessory mitral valve tissue
    Mitral valve prostheses
Cardiac tumors
Complex cardiac anomalies
    Atrioventricular septal defects°
    Single ventricle with rudimentary outflow chamber°
    Conoventricular septal defects°

°Discussed elsewhere.

Adapted from Edwards JE: Pathology of left ventricular outflow tract obstruction. Circulation 31:586–599, 1965.

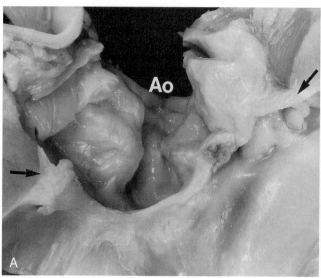

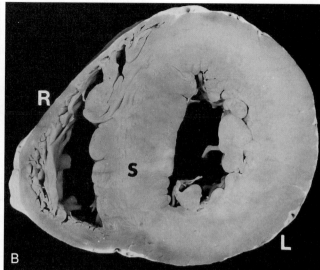

Heart specimen from an 18-year-old man with fibrous subaortic stenosis who died suddenly. *A*, Opened left ventricular outflow to aorta (Ao) to show the ridge *(between arrows)* below the aortic valve leaflets. *B*, A transverse section of the myocardium demonstrates concentric left ventricular hypertrophy. L = left ventricle; R = right ventricle; S = ventricular septum.

membranous and fibromuscular stenosis is often difficult. Membranous and fibromuscular subaortic stenosis represent a spectrum of disease; a membrane is frequently associated with a fibromuscular ridge and, less commonly, with a diffusely narrowed left ventricular outflow tract.[116] When obstruction is significant, there may be considerable left ventricular hypertrophy, especially involving the septum, that may further contribute to left ventricular outflow tract obstruction. Thus, the obstruction is rarely discrete[117] and often involves some length of the left ventricular outflow tract. It may also involve the mitral valve and frequently extends onto the aortic valve.

Aortic valve anomalies are common. The valve may be bicommissural or tricommissural, and valvar aortic stenosis is not uncommon.[104, 106, 109, 111] More frequently, there is leaflet thickening in the absence of stenosis. Aortic regurgitation is seen in 40 to 60% and may be a result of leaflet trauma from the high-velocity subaortic jet.[118] Aortic valve deformation and dysfunction may also be secondary to extension of the fibromuscular subaortic ridge onto the valve itself.[111, 112] Feigl and coworkers[112] described involvement of at least one cusp of the aortic valve in 16 of 18 postmortem specimens and speculated that this is the mechanism of aortic valve damage and aortic regurgitation in some patients.

Other forms of left ventricular outflow tract obstruction are uncommon. Rarely, accessory tissue related to the mitral valve apparatus or myocardial tumors may obstruct the left ventricular outflow tract.[119] Hypertrophic cardiomyopathy with obstruction is discussed separately.

PATHOGENESIS

The etiology of subaortic stenosis is uncertain. Almost all instances are sporadic with no apparent genetic or environmental predilection. Nevertheless, an autosomal pattern of transmission has been documented in Newfoundland dogs,[120] and in humans there have been occasional reports of occurrence in siblings.[121] Because it is rare in infancy, fixed subaortic stenosis is often considered an acquired disease. However, a number of reports provide evidence that it may be a secondary response to a congenital abnormality of left ventricular outflow tract morphometry and geometry.[122–124]

Rosenquist and colleagues[122] demonstrated increased mitral aortic separation in cardiac specimens with isolated subaortic stenosis. They speculated that this could alter the angle of ejection of blood from the left ventricle and cause abnormal in utero accumulation of embryonic cells that could eventually differentiate into fibroelastic tissue. Two-dimensional echocardiography has allowed detailed observation of cardiac anatomy before the development of subaortic obstruction. Kleinert and Geva[123] observed increased mitral-aortic separation, a steeper aortoseptal angle, and exaggerated aortic override in patients with fixed subaortic stenosis (Fig. 35–21). There were similar anomalies in a group of 23 patients with ventricular septal defect, double-chambered right ventricle, or coarctation of the aorta who *subsequently* developed subaortic stenosis. Although there was some overlap between patients and control subjects with each of these measurements, those with a coarctation, a ventricular septal defect, or both were likely to develop subaortic stenosis if the aortoseptal angle was 135 degrees or less or mitral aortic separation was 4 mm or more (negative predictive value of 90%, positive predictive value of 84%).[123] Using Doppler color flow mapping, Gewillig and colleagues[124] demonstrated areas of turbulent flow originating proximal to the site of subaortic ridge resection in postoperative patients. The turbulence appeared to arise from a more proximal ridge of

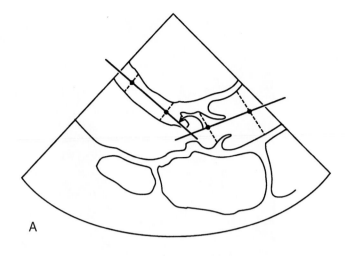

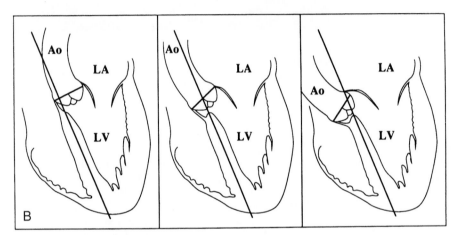

FIGURE 35–21

A, Diagrammatic presentation of an echocardiographic parasternal long-axis view in a patient with fixed subaortic stenosis demonstrating measurement of the aortoseptal angle, that is, the angle between the long axis of the aortic root and proximal ascending aorta and the midline of the interventricular septum. *B,* Diagrammatic representation of an echocardiographic five-chamber view illustrating the criteria used to grade the degree of aortic override: *left,* normal; *center,* mild override; *right,* marked override. Ao = ascending aorta; LA = left atrium; LV = left ventricle. (*A, B* modified from Kleinert S, Geva T: Echocardiographic morphometry and geometry of the left ventricular outflow tract in fixed subaortic stenosis. Reprinted with permission from the American College of Cardiology [Journal of the American College of Cardiology, 1993, Volume 22, Pages 1501–1508].)

muscle in the left ventricle or be caused by misalignment of the muscular and membranous septum. The authors speculated that left ventricular outflow tract flow disturbances caused by these minor "downstream" anomalies might lead to cellular proliferation. Although these studies provide clues to the development and progression of this complex disease, an underlying etiologic mechanism is yet to be defined.

NATURAL HISTORY

Subaortic stenosis is rare in infancy, is commonly diagnosed in childhood, and tends to progress. Although there have been occasional reports of subaortic stenosis presenting in the neonatal period,[123, 125] a postmortem study of 99 infant hearts (≤1 year) with subaortic stenosis or atresia included only 3 with isolated subaortic stenosis. The remainder had complex associated intracardiac anomalies, including ventricular septal defect and interrupted aortic arch, transposition complexes, and various forms of "single ventricle."[125] The median age at the time of diagnosis of isolated subaortic stenosis is between 5 and 9 years in most series, with a trend toward earlier diagnosis since the advent of two-dimensional echocardiography.[105, 106, 109, 110] Progression of stenosis is well documented (Fig. 35–22)[104–107, 109, 126] but is not universal.[106, 107] For example, important progression of the subaortic gradient was seen in 76% in one series; age at diagnosis was younger, and progression was particularly rapid in those with tunnel-type subaortic stenosis.[107] Progression is often asso-

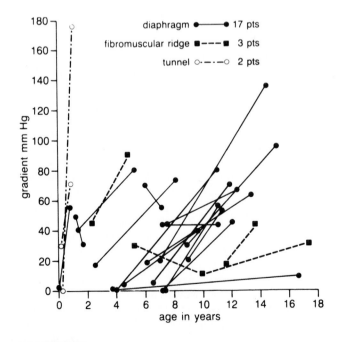

FIGURE 35–22

Graph depicting serial change in left ventricular outflow tract gradient among 22 patients with the three pathologic forms of discrete subaortic stenosis (diaphragm denotes "membranous" subaortic stenosis). (Reprinted from International Journal of Cardiology, Volume 8, Freedom RM, Pelech A, Brand A, et al: The progressive nature of subaortic stenosis in congenital heart disease, Pages 137–148, Copyright 1985, with permission from Elsevier Science.)

ciated with further narrowing of membranous or fibromuscular obstruction, but it may also be related to septal hypertrophy or development of more diffuse elongation and narrowing of the left ventricular outflow tract.[110] Data from the presurgical era are sparse, but untreated there is a significant risk of death, either sudden or with congestive heart failure, when subaortic stenosis is severe.[104,106,108]

Fixed subaortic stenosis can develop in patients with an isolated ventricular septal defect, coarctation, or other intracardiac lesions some time after repair or spontaneous closure.[109,123,127] Leichter and coworkers[127] documented 35 patients in whom subaortic stenosis was not present at the initial catheterization but developed subsequently. Sixteen of these patients had serial hemodynamic data. In this selected group, the left ventricular outflow tract gradient increased from near zero to a mean of 58 mm Hg during a mean interval of approximately 5 years. Subaortic stenosis also occurs in association with double-chambered right ventricle, and several reports have stressed the importance of thoroughly examining the left ventricular outflow tract in patients with this lesion.[128,129]

AORTIC REGURGITATION.   Aortic regurgitation is common, is usually hemodynamically insignificant in childhood, tends to be progressive,[106,109,126] and is related to the degree of left ventricular outflow tract obstruction.[106,126] de Vries and colleagues[106] reported regurgitation in 30% of patients at the time of diagnosis, increasing to 54% during a mean follow-up interval of 3.7 years. Regurgitation is more common in those with high gradients, supporting the concept of progressive damage to the aortic valve by the high-velocity left ventricular outflow tract jet. In contrast to children, adult patients with fixed subaortic stenosis have a high incidence of significant aortic regurgi-

tation and frequently require aortic valve replacement at the time of surgical intervention.[118]

ENDOCARDITIS.   Fixed subaortic regurgitation is associated with a high risk of endocarditis,[108,109] which occurs at a rate up to 19.3 per 1000 patient-years.[109] The risk appears to increase with increasing gradient and with aortic regurgitation.[109] Endocarditis may involve the subaortic area, the aortic valve, or an associated lesion (Fig. 35–23).

CLINICAL FINDINGS

Symptoms and signs vary, depending on the severity of obstruction, the presence and severity of aortic regurgitation, and associated lesions. The child with isolated fixed subaortic stenosis is frequently asymptomatic, although fatigue, dyspnea, chest discomfort, and syncope with exertion may be present when obstruction is severe.[104,111,113,116] Congestive heart failure is uncommon unless it is precipitated by an associated lesion.[105] With severe subaortic stenosis, findings commonly include a thrusting apical impulse, a palpable thrill, and a grade 4 or louder ejection systolic murmur that peaks in late systole and radiates to the carotid arteries. The aortic component of the second heart sound is frequently soft.[111] An early diastolic murmur indicates aortic regurgitation. The systolic thrill and the intensity of the murmur are related to the severity of obstruction, so that the only physical sign of mild subaortic stenosis is often a soft systolic ejection murmur heard at the mid left sternal edge, radiating toward the base of the heart and to the neck. Differentiation from a pulmonary flow murmur, a vibratory murmur, or a small ventricular septal defect may be difficult.[104,105] The clue to clinical diagnosis may be a systolic murmur increasing in intensity or a new murmur appearing in the patient with a

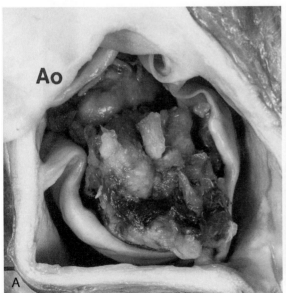
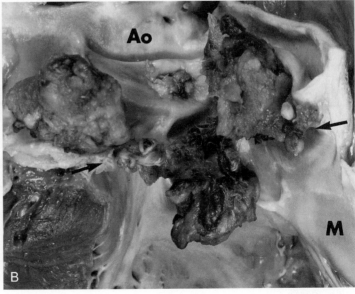

FIGURE 35–23

Specimen from a patient with bacterial endocarditis and a large vegetation attached to the subaortic membrane. *A*, Superior view of the aortic valve demonstrating masses protruding into the aorta (Ao). *B*, Opened left ventricular outflow to aorta (Ao). Masses are attached both superiorly and inferiorly to a subaortic membrane (between arrows). M = anterior leaflet of the mitral valve.

known small ventricular septal defect or a previously repaired cardiac lesion. Peripheral pulses may be normal even when obstruction is severe.[111] Clinical differentiation from valvar aortic stenosis is usually not possible; the systolic murmur is similar in both lesions, and an ejection click, heard in some patients with subaortic stenosis, may not be present in older children with valvar aortic stenosis.[111]

The chest radiograph is frequently normal. There may be left atrial enlargement. Mild cardiomegaly is not uncommon,[116] but important cardiomegaly is unusual and suggests significant aortic regurgitation or a large left-to-right shunt.[113] Dilatation of the ascending aorta occurs in 20 to 30% of patients.[111,113]

The electrocardiogram may demonstrate left ventricular hypertrophy with or without ST depression and T wave changes. There is some correlation between the degree of obstruction and electrocardiographic changes,[106,113] and progressive left ventricular outflow tract obstruction may be reflected in progressive increases in left precordial voltages and T wave changes.[104] However, as with valvar aortic stenosis, the electrocardiogram cannot be relied on to assess severity or progression; some patients with a significant gradient have a normal electrocardiogram.[19,106,111,113]

ECHOCARDIOGRAPHY

Echocardiography is the preferred technique for the diagnosis and serial assessment of fixed subaortic stenosis and for the delineation of associated lesions (Fig. 35–24). Diagnosis can be made at an early stage, and serial follow-up will establish the rate of progression.[130,131] M-mode echocardiography is useful in assessing left ventricular function and measuring chamber thickness; the mechanism and severity of obstruction are assessed by two-dimensional imaging and by pulsed, color, and continuous-wave Doppler echocardiography. M-mode findings of systolic aortic valve flutter and early valve closure[132] may be a clue to the diagnosis when two-dimensional image quality is poor. Two-dimensional imaging can detect small irregularities in the left ventricular outflow tract that may subsequently cause more significant obstruction[105,107] and may prove useful in predicting the development of subaortic stenosis in high-risk individuals.[123] Careful imaging can characterize the morphology of the subaortic obstruction and detect abnormal aortic valve thickening[110,133] with greater accuracy than angiography[134] (Fig. 35–24 and 35–25). Color Doppler mapping can demonstrate the presence and degree of aortic regurgitation. The gradient across the left ventricular outflow tract can be serially assessed by pulsed and continuous-wave Doppler, assisting the evaluation of patients during follow-up and after intervention.[105,110,126] In older patients with suboptimal transthoracic image quality, transesophageal echocardiography may be necessary to differentiate fixed subaortic stenosis from valvar aortic stenosis or idiopathic hypertrophic cardiomyopathy.[135]

CARDIAC CATHETERIZATION

An operation can usually be undertaken in patients without prior cardiac catheterization when there is echocardiographic evidence of severe obstruction and significant left ventricular hypertrophy. Nevertheless, some patients require cardiac catheterization to confirm the left ventricular outflow tract gradient and, if echocardiographic images are suboptimal, to assess the degree of aortic regurgitation and

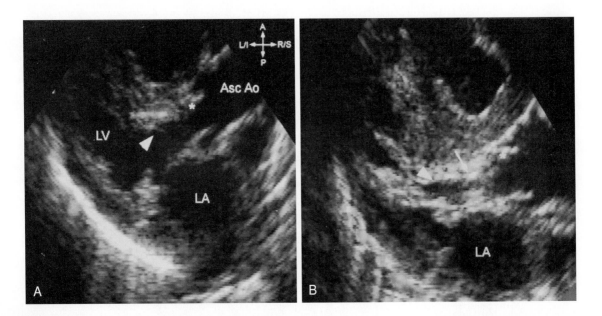

FIGURE 35–24

Two-dimensional echocardiographic images during systole from the parasternal long-axis window in an infant with tunnel-type subaortic stenosis. *A,* At 2 weeks of age, there is mild narrowing of the left ventricular outflow tract. There is also irregularity *(arrowhead)* on the septal surface of the left ventricular outflow tract, which is elongated and mildly narrowed. There is also mild hypoplasia of the aortic annulus *(asterisk).* *B,* The same infant at 9 months of age. There is severe tunnel-type subaortic stenosis with marked narrowing of the left ventricular outflow tract proximally *(arrowhead)* and an area of severe stenosis *(arrow)* immediately below the aortic valve *(asterisk).* A = anterior; Asc Ao = ascending aorta; LA = left atrium; L/I = left and inferior; LV = left ventricle; P = posterior; R/S = right and superior.

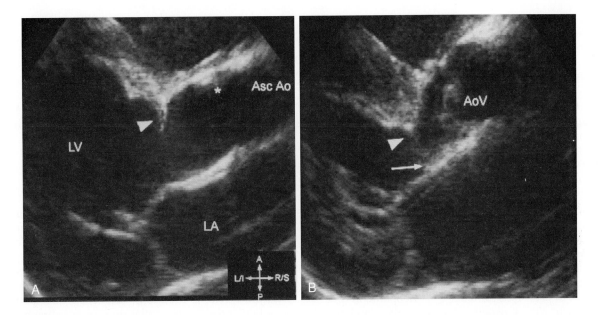

Two-dimensional images from the parasternal long-axis window in a 10-year-old boy with discrete subaortic stenosis. In systole *(A)*, a fibromuscular ridge can be seen arising from the septum *(arrowhead)* below the aortic annulus *(asterisk)*; and in diastole *(B)*, an irregular ridge can be seen arising from the posterior wall of the left ventricular outflow tract and anterior leaflet of the mitral valve *(arrow)*. A = anterior; AoV = aortic valve; Asc Ao = ascending aorta; LA = left atrium; L/I = left and inferior; LV = left ventricle; P = posterior; R/S = right and superior.

identify associated lesions. Careful withdrawal of an end-hole catheter from the body of the left ventricle to the ascending aorta may document the gradient at a single site or at multiple levels within the left ventricular outflow tract. This may not be possible when the obstruction is adjacent to the aortic valve or in the severely narrowed outflow tract

where catheter manipulation provokes ventricular ectopy. Biplane axial left ventricular angiography with cranial angulation in either the left anterior oblique or lateral projection is required to visualize the left ventricular outflow tract (Fig. 35–26). On occasion, membranous obstruction is not well defined.[134] An aortogram should be undertaken

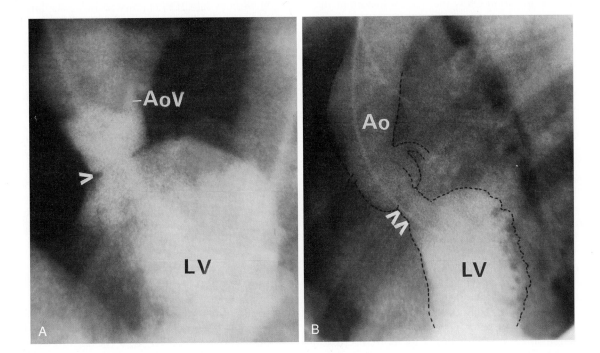

Left ventricular (LV) cineangiograms in the left anterior oblique projection with cranial angulation in two patients with subaortic stenosis. *A*, A thin ridge *(arrowhead)* is seen a few millimeters below the aortic valve (AoV). *B*, A thicker fibromuscular stenosis *(arrowheads)* extends close to the aortic valve. Ao = ascending aorta. (*A, B* modified from Kirklin JW, Barratt-Boyes BG: Congenital aortic stenosis. *In* Cardiac Surgery, 2nd ed. New York, Churchill Livingstone, 1993, p 1195.)

to grade aortic regurgitation, and when this is present, the subaortic obstruction area may be better visualized from the aortic injection than from the ventriculogram.

INTERVENTION

Operative techniques include excision of the membrane or fibromuscular ridge and blunt enucleation. Some advocate myectomy as a routine.[136] Tunnel-type stenosis is best dealt with by variations of the Konno procedure, whereby the left ventricular outflow tract is enlarged by extensive aortoventriculoplasty with or without aortic root replacement.[137,138] The operative mortality after excision or enucleation is low, and complete heart block is infrequent, but there is a significant rate of restenosis, the cause of which is unclear. Some consider it to be related to scar formation from the initial operation,[139] but others consider it to be secondary to the proliferation of abnormal residual tissue,[136] to the persistence of abnormal outflow tract geometry,[113] or to persistent turbulence.[124] Reoperation is necessary in 7 to 25% of patients at a mean follow-up interval of 4 to 5 years,[106,109,139] and the event-free survival has been reported at about 65% at 10 years.[108]

The palliative nature of operative intervention has led several centers to consider transcatheter balloon dilatation as treatment for subaortic stenosis.[133,140] de Lezo and coinvestigators[133] demonstrated a 70% overall reduction in gradient in 33 patients who underwent dilatation of membranous subaortic stenosis. Seven of these patients developed restenosis at a mean follow-up interval of almost 3 years. Further experience and longitudinal study are necessary to determine the role of this form of intervention in the treatment of subaortic stenosis, but long-term benefit is yet to be demonstrated.

Whether an operation alters the natural history of the development and progression of aortic regurgitation is unclear. The retrospective, uncontrolled nature of available reports and the heterogeneity of the lesion, together with its unpredictable natural history, probably account for this uncertainty. Several series report progression of aortic regurgitation despite operation.[109,141] However, some with similar postoperative follow-up demonstrate little change,[142] and others have concluded that early operation decreases the incidence of aortic regurgitation at late follow-up.[126] Endocarditis can occur after operation, but the risk is probably reduced when there has been gradient relief and there is no aortic regurgitation or associated lesion.[109] Late sudden death has been reported after adequate relief of the left ventricular outflow tract obstruction.[109]

The indications for intervention in fixed subaortic stenosis are controversial. Factors complicating decision-making include the unpredictable pattern of progression of obstruction, the likelihood of progression of aortic regurgitation over time, and the high frequency of restenosis after an operation. An increased incidence of residual stenosis in patients with high preoperative gradients[126] and the association of aortic regurgitation with more severe obstruction[126] have led some to advocate excision or enucleation with peak to peak catheter gradients in the region of 25 to 30 mm Hg[142] or mean Doppler-derived or catheter-measured gradients of 30 mm Hg.[126] Others rec-

ommend intervention when the gradient is higher, or when there is progression of obstruction or regurgitation, on the basis that some with mild or moderate gradients remain stable for many years and that the risk of restenosis is high.[106] Our current practice is to operate when the Doppler-derived peak gradient reaches 50 mm Hg or when there is mild or more aortic regurgitation. We observe patients with lesser degrees of obstruction at regular intervals with serial echocardiography.

FUTURE DIRECTIONS

Recent advances in the three-dimensional reconstruction of echocardiographic and magnetic resonance images may provide further insight into the etiology of fixed subaortic stenosis. These techniques may also demonstrate left ventricular outflow tract abnormalities associated with postoperative recurrence, leading to modifications of surgical technique. In addition, further longitudinal evaluation may clarify the role of routine myectomy in association with resection of the fibromuscular ridge or membrane.

HYPERTROPHIC CARDIOMYOPATHY

Hypertrophic cardiomyopathy (HCM) is a heterogeneous, usually familial disorder of heart muscle sarcomere[143–145] characterized by a hypertrophied, nondilated left ventricle. Missense mutations of genes for contractile protein on chromosome 14 and other chromosome loci are responsible for the condition.[143,144,146–151] Histologic and morphologic abnormalities produce a disorder of relaxation and sometimes outflow obstruction, but overt clinical manifestations may not present for decades. The earliest reports of HCM were by late 19th century pathologists, but Teare is attributed with characterizing the condition in 1958,[152] Brock's surgical case report appearing only months earlier. More than 70 terms have been used to describe HCM, emphasizing different aspects such as the site and asymmetry of left ventricular hypertrophy, left ventricular outflow obstruction, and the familial nature of the disease. By the 1980s, the term *hypertrophic cardiomyopathy* was favored,[153] although it remains clinically useful to refer to obstructive or nonobstructive HCM. Knowledge of HCM has evolved with the development of the investigative techniques available to cardiology.[154] The true prevalence of HCM is unknown in children because many patients are asymptomatic. Prevalence estimates in adults are 0.1 to 0.2% of the general population.[155] Conditions with left ventricular hypertrophy found in childhood that should not be regarded as HCM are listed in Table 35–11.

THE GENETIC BASIS OF HYPERTROPHIC CARDIOMYOPATHY

The mode of inheritance in HCM is autosomal dominant with variable penetrance. Teare's original report identified the familial nature of HCM.[152] Echocardiography suggested that HCM is familial in 50% of patients,[156,157] but genetic testing of large kindreds has proved more sensitive than echocardiography in identifying patients.[158–160] In 1989, the β-myosin heavy chain (β-MHC) gene was identi-

TABLE 35–11

CONDITIONS WITH LEFT VENTRICULAR HYPERTROPHY NOT
REGARDED AS HYPERTROPHIC CARDIOMYOPATHY

All secondary cardiomyopathies causing left ventricular hypertrophy
Infants of diabetic mothers
Glycogen storage diseases
Gigantism and acromegaly
Myocardial iron deposition (e.g., β-thalassemia)
Athlete's heart

fied as the candidate gene for HCM at chromosome locus 14q1.[146] To date, more than 40 missense mutations in the β-MHC gene have been reported worldwide in families with HCM.[143,147,148,161] Other abnormal genes identified are those for α-tropomyosin on chromosome 15q2,[149] troponin T on chromosome 1q3,[150] and myosin-binding protein C on chromosome 11p11.2.[144,151] In addition, linkage to a fragile site on chromosomes 16 and 18 has been reported without identification of the responsible genes.[148] Mutations of the two myosin light chain genes have been reported in a rare form of HCM.[162] To date, abnormal β-MHC, troponin T, α-tropomyosin, and myosin-binding protein C genes account for approximately 30%, 15%, 3%, and 10% of HCM families, respectively, with the responsible gene for the remainder unknown. It is likely that HCM will ultimately prove to be familial. Certainly HCM should always be regarded as a genetic disorder even though it may not exhibit familial inheritance.[148] Sporadic mutations accounting for some isolated instances support the concept that the β-MHC gene is highly mutagenic. Disease expression varies with gene abnormalities—there is more nonpenetrance with mutations of α-tropomyosin and troponin T than with β-MHC.

Studies have begun to unravel the connection between the genetic and histologic abnormalities and identify the primary defect initiated by the mutations.[148] In vitro studies indicate that mutated proteins have defective contractile function leading to compensatory hypertrophy.[163] This hypothesis received support in a mouse HCM model with sarcomere disarray that progressed to compensatory hypertrophy with abnormalities of systolic and diastolic function.[145] There are at least 1000 genes responsible for cardiac growth, possibly explaining the variations in degrees of hypertrophy in the same family with the same mutant gene. These findings go some way to explain the apparent paradox of impaired contractile proteins at molecular level and apparently excessive contractility at the clinical level.

Metabolic abnormalities, rather than contractile protein abnormalities, may also cause HCM. In most instances, it is not known whether there is an etiologic relationship.[164]

PATHOLOGIC ANATOMY

Before the era of two-dimensional echocardiography, asymmetric septal hypertrophy was regarded as the gross anatomic marker of HCM.[165] Although the hypertrophy is characteristically asymmetric and maximal in the cephalad portion of the ventricular septum, it may be apical, midventricular, or concentric (Figs. 35–27 and 35–28). Moreover, degrees of asymmetric septal hypertrophy vary, confined to the basal third or even extending to the apex. Hypertrophy may be diffuse, involving the left ventricular free wall as well as the septum (Fig. 35–27B)[165] or it may be mild and segmental.[166] The patterns of hypertrophy were so diverse in a study that the authors concluded that there is no characteristic pattern of hypertrophy in HCM.[166] Cardiac mass may be three times greater than

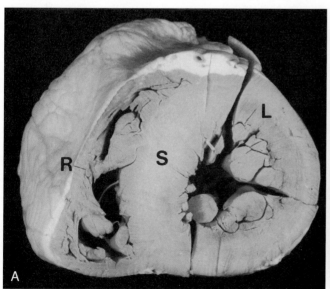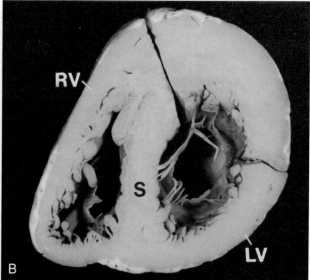

FIGURE 35–27

Heart specimens from patients with hypertrophic cardiomyopathy. *A,* Transverse view in a 23-year-old man with prominent hypertrophy of the ventricular septum (S) that measured 23 mm in thickness compared with a left ventricular (L) wall thickness of 18 mm, exclusive of trabeculations and papillary muscles. R = right ventricle. *B,* Transverse view from a 15-year-old boy who died suddenly, with the dominant hypertrophy superiorly measuring about 30 mm in thickness compared with 16 mm laterally and 12 mm inferiorly. The ventricular septum (S) measured 12 mm. LV = left ventricle; RV = right ventricle.

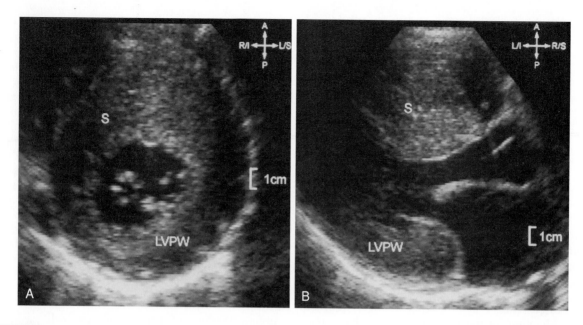

Two-dimensional echocardiogram of a 15-year-old with left ventricular hypertrophy. *A,* Parasternal short-axis image with the dominant hypertrophy anteriorly and in the free wall of the left ventricle. *B,* Parasternal long-axis image showing typical septal hypertrophy. A = anterior; L/I = left and inferior; L/S = left and superior; LVPW = left ventricular posterior wall; P = posterior; R/I = right and inferior; R/S = right and superior; S = septum.

normal. Molecular studies, although confirming that hypertrophy is compensatory, have yet to explain the asymmetric rather than concentric hypertrophy.[161] Maron and colleagues,[167] using serial echocardiography, showed the progressive development of left ventricular hypertrophy through childhood and adolescence, usually complete by 18 years. Septal hypertrophy may reach 50 mm in diameter. Individuals with asymmetric septal hypertrophy often have a subaortic gradient (obstructive HCM) caused by anterior systolic motion of the anterior leaflet of the mitral valve and its apposition with the bulging septum. Right ventricular hypertrophy also occurs in HCM, more frequently recognized in children[153] and often severe in infants,[168] sited in the right ventricular outflow tract or midventricle.

The histologic hallmark of HCM is extensive myocardial fiber disarray interspersed with a variable amount of loose connective tissue (Fig. 35–29). The myocardial cells are disorganized, lying at perpendicular or oblique angles to each other rather than showing the usual parallel arrangement. The cells are hypertrophied, with an increased transverse diameter, and have intercellular connections. Within the myocardial cells, the myofibrils also show disarray. Myocardial disarray occurs on average in 35% of the septum and 24% of the left ventricular free wall.[169] Myocardial disarray is not pathognomonic for

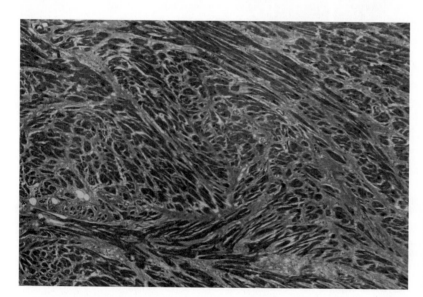

Histology of hypertrophic cardiomyopathy, photomicrograph of ventricular septum (magnification ×200). The cardiac muscle cells are hypertrophied and show disarray. There is an increased amount of connective tissue interspersed between muscle cells.

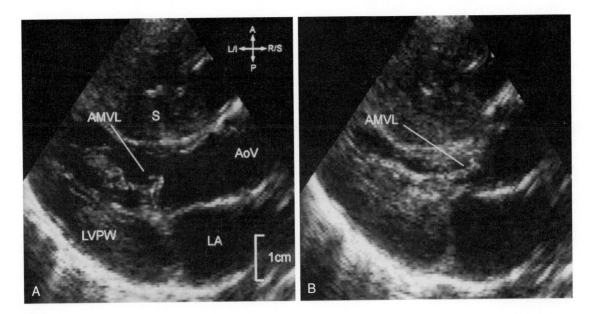

FIGURE 35–30

Echocardiographic systolic anterior motion of the mitral valve. *A,* Two-dimensional echocardiogram showing the anterior mitral valve leaflet in early systole beginning to move anteriorly. *B,* By midsystole, there is anterior mitral valve leaflet–septum contact. *C,* See Color Figure 35–30C. A = anterior; AMVL = anterior mitral valve leaflet; AoV = aortic valve; LA = left atrium; L/I = left and inferior; LVOT = left ventricular outflow tract; LVPW = left ventricular posterior wall; P = posterior; R/S = right and superior; S = septum.

HCM because small foci of disorganized myocardial cells occur in other forms of congenital and acquired heart disease. There is no specific histochemical marker for HCM. Myocardial disarray may occur without increased myocardial mass in some kindreds.[170]

The mitral valve is often closer to the septum than usual, crowded by the septum in diastole and pulled closer to the septum in systole. The increased length and greater area of anterior and posterior leaflets may allow interleaflet coaptation in the body rather than at the leaflet tips. The distal free segment or tip of the anterior leaflet moves anteriorly and superiorly (systolic anterior motion of the mitral valve) (Fig. 35–30 [see also Color Plates]) with varying degrees of septal contact, subaortic obstruction, and mitral valve regurgitation. Fibrous plaques on the ventricular septum and fibrous thickening of the anterior leaflet of the mitral valve are found at the point of septum–mitral leaflet contact. Structural mitral valve abnormalities including increased size of either leaflet or absent chordae tendineae with insertion of the papillary muscle directly into the anterior mitral leaflet have been reported in one fifth to two thirds of patients,[153,171,172] allowing an alternative mechanism for mitral regurgitation.

The intramural coronary arteries show increased intimal and medial thickening, causing luminal narrowing. The left anterior descending artery and septal perforating arteries may become occluded in systole. Other postulated mechanisms for myocardial ischemia include microvascular spasm, decreased coronary perfusion pressure, reduced coronary vasodilator response, and myocardial bridging.[153,173,174] Wigle[153,175] has emphasized the cycle of the effect of decreased coronary filling and myocardial ischemia with impaired diastolic relaxation in HCM.

PATHOPHYSIOLOGY

Diastolic Function

The primary pathophysiologic disturbance of HCM is a disorder of diastolic relaxation. There is a decrease in rate and volume of early rapid filling and a compensatory increase in atrial filling.[153] Ventricular relaxation as well as ventricular contraction is load dependent,[176] and abnormal diastolic function occurs whether or not there is left ventricular outflow obstruction. Decreased compliance (increased chamber stiffness) also occurs in HCM because of increased muscle mass and increased muscle fibrosis. Ventricular volumes are decreased. Diastolic dysfunction is invariably present in HCM and can usually be demonstrated in most patients with M-mode and echo Doppler, nuclear, angiographic, and hemodynamic techniques.[177,178] Diastolic dysfunction may contribute to dyspnea and ischemic symptoms, but correlation between symptoms[179] and the degree of hypertrophy[180] is low.

Systolic Function and Left Ventricular Outflow Tract Obstruction

HCM produces an increase in left ventricular ejection fraction and rate of early ejection[181] without an increase in contractility. Systolic anterior motion of the mitral valve occurs in early systole and peaks in midsystole with or without contact with the septum, and the leaflet moves abruptly posteriorly at the end of systole.[182] In general, patients with obstruction have a narrowed left ventricular outflow tract dimension, the anterior basal septum is significantly hypertrophied, and the mitral valve is positioned anteriorly closer to the septum than normal.[183] Those without obstruction have a wider left ventricular outflow tract, there is less septal hypertrophy, and the mitral valve is positioned more normally. The left ventricular outflow tract gradient occurs because of early and prolonged septum–anterior mitral leaflet contact; the greater the contact, the greater the obstruction and the greater the mitral regurgitation.[171,182] When the septum–mitral leaflet contact occurs in midsystole, a larger proportion of left ventricular emptying has already occurred and there is minimal obstruction.

There is debate whether systolic anterior motion is due to a Venturi effect that pulls the mitral leaflets toward the septum or whether it is due to flow drag.[154] Transesophageal echocardiography has demonstrated that by midsystole, the septal contact of the anterior mitral leaflet has created a funnel-shaped gap between the leaflets.[171] This allows posteriorly directed mitral regurgitation (Fig. 35–31). There is thus an eject-obstruct-leak sequence in subaortic obstructive HCM.[153,171,175] Patients with HCM occasionally have massive midventricular hypertrophy, and gradient occurs at this level.[153]

Despite high early systolic flow, left ventricular ejection time is increased as obstruction increases and aortic flow decreases; little blood remains in the ventricle at end systole. The subaortic gradient in HCM shows spontaneous variability, and characteristic techniques at the bedside demonstrate this. The evidence that the subaortic gradient is obstructive and clinically important, and that its relief improves symptoms, is now convincing.[154,184–187] Earlier, some investigators attributed pressure gradients to the phenomenon of cavity obliteration whereby part of the ventricle completely empties in systole,[188] producing catheter entrapment. Although this sometimes happens, true mechanical impedance to left ventricular ejection has been clearly established.[153,171,184]

A small proportion of patients show measurable deterioration of systolic function with ventricular dilatation, decreased shortening fraction by echocardiography,[189] and eventually wall thinning. Myocardial fibrosis is implicated.[153] This dilated end-stage phase is associated with worsening of symptoms and onset of heart failure[154] but is rarely seen in childhood.

NATURAL HISTORY, SUDDEN DEATH, AND PROGNOSIS

Prognosis is significantly affected by age and mode of presentation. Mortality for HCM is twice as high in children as in adults.[190,191] McKenna's 1981 natural history study of HCM in childhood is still useful as a guide to survival based on the diagnosis of HCM by clinical findings (Fig. 35–32).[191] Presentation with symptoms in infancy has an extremely poor prognosis; many die of congestive heart failure. Infantile HCM is more likely to be caused by a metabolic abnormality than by sarcomeric protein abnormalities. Even infants who present with only a heart murmur have a 50% mortality by 1 year,[192,193] and another 25% will succumb later. However, the remaining 25% may have a benign course.[194] Beyond a year, presentation in congestive failure is unusual, but the patients are at risk of sudden death. During childhood, septal hypertrophy rapidly increases with somatic growth (Fig. 35–33).[167] By age 15 to 18 years, hypertrophy will have developed in most patients and is thus detectable, at least by echocardiography. Although the degree of left ventricular hypertrophy does not correlate with poorer prognosis, mortality in childhood is probably worse with left ventricular outflow tract obstruction.[194] In adults, the degree of left ventricular hypertrophy contributes to the degree of subaortic obstruction, heart failure, and arrhythmias.[165] However, the correlation of clinical outcomes and the degree of left ventricular hypertrophy is poor, as witnessed by pedigrees with sudden arrhythmic death and minimal or no left ventricular hypertrophy.[195] Of interest is a mild form of HCM

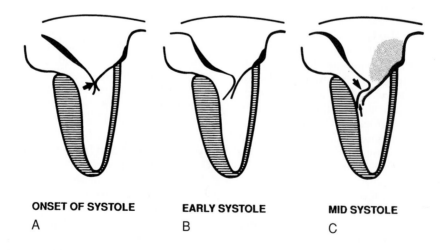

ONSET OF SYSTOLE

A

EARLY SYSTOLE

B

MID SYSTOLE

C

FIGURE 35–31

Septum-leaflet contact and mitral regurgitation. Line diagram of a transesophageal echocardiogram (horizontal plane) demonstrating the anterior and basal motion of the anterior mitral leaflet to produce septum–anterior mitral valve leaflet contact and failure of leaflet coaptation in midsystole. At the onset of systole (A), the coaptation point (arrow) is in the body of the anterior and posterior leaflets. During early systole (B) and midsystole (C), there is anterior and basal movement of the residual length of the anterior mitral leaflet (thick arrow), with septal contact and failure of leaflet coaptation (thin arrow), with consequent mitral regurgitation directed posteriorly into the left atrium (stippled area). (A–C from Grigg LE, Wigle ED, Williams WG, et al: Transesophageal Doppler echocardiography in obstructive hypertrophic cardiomyopathy: Clarification of pathophysiology and importance in intraoperative decision making. Reprinted with permission from the American College of Cardiology [Journal of the American College of Cardiology, 1992, Volume 42, Pages 42–52].)

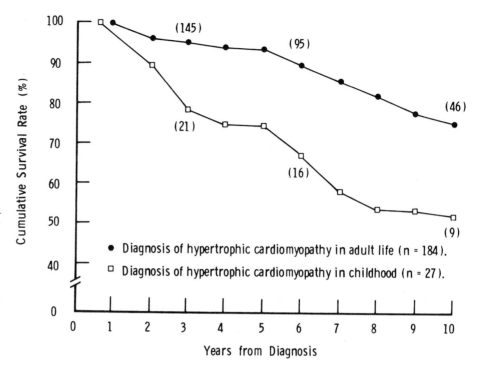

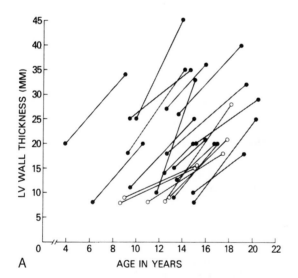

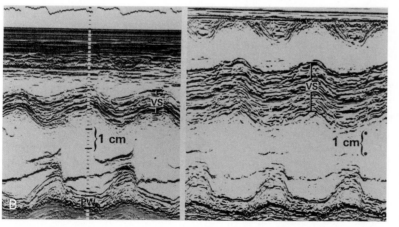

FIGURE 35–33

A, Development and progression of left ventricular hypertrophy in hypertrophic cardiomyopathy, changes in left ventricular (LV) wall thickness in 22 children. Each patient is represented by the left ventricular segment that showed the greatest change in wall thickness. *Open symbols* denote five patients who had a family history of hypertrophic cardiomyopathy but no evidence of hypertrophy in any segment of the left ventricle at the initial evaluation. *B,* Development of marked hypertrophy in the anterior basal ventricular septum. M-mode echocardiograms were obtained at the same cross-sectional level in a girl with a family history of hypertrophic cardiomyopathy. At age 11 years, the anterior ventricular septal (VS) thickness was at the upper limit of normal (10 mm); at age 15 years, it had markedly increased (to 33 mm), and the image is typical of hypertrophic cardiomyopathy. PW = posterior left ventricular free wall. Calibration marks are 1 cm apart. (*A, B* adapted with permission from Maron BJ, Spirito P, Wesley Y, Arce J: Development and progression of left ventricular hypertrophy in children with hypertrophic cardiomyopathy. N Engl J Med 315:610–614, 1986. Copyright © 1986 Massachusetts Medical Society. All rights reserved.)

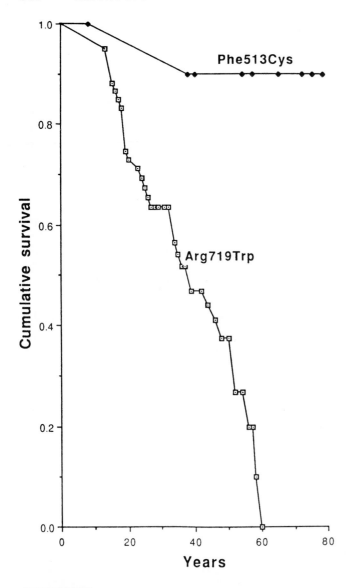

FIGURE 35–34

Genetic survival. Kaplan-Meier product limit curves for the survival of individuals bearing the Arg719Trp or Phe513Cys mutation. Data from four unrelated families with the Arg719Trp mutation are combined because no differences were detected between these families. A significant difference ($P < .001$) in life expectancy was observed in individuals with the Arg719Trp compared with the Phe513Cys mutation. (From Anan R, Greve G, Thierfelder L, et al: Prognostic implications of novel β cardiac myosin heavy chain gene mutations that cause familial hypertrophic cardiomyopathy. J Clin Invest 93:280, 1994.)

presenting in the sixth to eighth decades with a benign prognosis unless it is associated with hypertension.[196]

Evidence is emerging of different prognoses for different point mutations, and this may prove to be the most powerful prognostic predictor.[158,175,197,198] For example, the "charge" change mutations of 403 Arg→Gln and 606 Val→Met on the β-MHC have high penetrance and a high incidence of sudden death, whereas 908 Leu→Val and 256 Gly→Glu mutations have low disease penetrance and a benign prognosis (Fig. 35–34).[158,197] Sudden death and end-stage heart failure have occurred in the same kindred, reflecting the diverse expression of HCM and inexact genotype-phenotype correlations,[158] which limits genetic

predictions of outcome. Studies do not show any clear racial or sex prevalence differences,[155] as expected for an autosomal dominant condition. There is evidence that race may alter the phenotype of the same missense mutation[143,199] and that black individuals with HCM are more at risk of sudden cardiac death.[199,200]

SUDDEN DEATH. HCM is the most common cause of sudden death during exercise in the young.[170,200] Earlier data on sudden death, derived from adult HCM tertiary-center cohorts, estimated a rate of 2 to 4% per year, but population-based adult estimates are 0.1 to 0.7% per year.[196,201] Estimates of sudden death for children are up to 6% per year,[194,202] derived from tertiary-care centers. The most common age for sudden death is 12 to 35 years.[192] Predictive variables for sudden death in children with HCM have not been defined except for those with a malignant family history of sudden death[191] and recurrent syncope.[203]

Even in adults, hemodynamic predictors for sudden death, including the degree of left ventricular outflow obstruction, are inconsistent or unreliable.[191,192,204] Two independent studies in 1981 showed that symptomatic and asymptomatic nonsustained ventricular tachycardia on Holter monitoring was associated with an approximate 8% incidence of sudden death.[205,206] Later, Fananapazir and colleagues[204] demonstrated that only those in whom nonsustained ventricular tachycardia was associated with impaired consciousness or those with inducible sustained ventricular tachycardia at electrophysiologic study were at high risk of sudden death. Signal-averaged electrocardiography has not defined those at high risk of sudden death. In a retrospective study in adults, increased QT dispersion was associated with ventricular arrhythmia. Neither the corrected QT interval nor QT dispersion has been shown to predict ventricular arrhythmias and cardiac arrest in children.[207] Sudden death often occurs shortly after rather than during exercise.[192,208] McKenna and coinvestigators demonstrated abnormal blood pressure responses during exercise in a third of HCM patients.[206] Others postulated that the greater than normal drop in systemic vascular resistance, often without accompanying symptoms, may be the initiating mechanism of sudden death.[209] However, sudden death also occurs without exercise or with minimal exertion. Supraventricular arrhythmias are associated with death in adults,[210] and prognosis is improved with antiarrhythmic treatment,[211] but there are no comparable data for children.

Sudden death due to arrhythmia may occur in patients without obstruction, histologic areas of myocyte disarray, myocyte replacement fibrosis, or interstitial fibrosis providing arrhythmogenic foci. An alternative explanation is that myocardial ischemia plays a primary role in cardiac arrest and syncope. Dilsizian and colleagues[212] studied 23 patients aged 6 to 23 years deemed at high risk for sudden death by exercise thallium scintigraphy, Holter monitoring, cardiac catheterization, and an electrophysiologic study. All 15 patients who had syncope or cardiac arrest had evidence of myocardial ischemia, but sustained ventricular tachycardia was induced in only 4 of these patients. Three of the eight patients with a family history of sudden death had myocardial ischemia, and ventricular tachycardia was not induced in any of them. After a mean 2-year follow-up, four further episodes of cardiac arrest or syncope occurred in those with myocardial ischemia, not those with inducible ventricular tachycardia. Interestingly, three of these four patients had discontinued verapamil.

In summary, infants and children with symptoms of HCM have a poor prognosis. The main risk in infants is congestive heart failure. The main risk in older children and adolescents is sudden death, for which there are no proven predictive risk factors other than recurrent syncope, a family history of sudden death, or a malignant genotype. Variation of clinical expression in HCM makes prediction of prognosis difficult, but genetic markers may provide further insight. No treatment modality has to date been shown to alter the natural history of HCM, but promising strategies are emerging.

CLINICAL FINDINGS

Clinical manifestations of HCM are diverse, varying from a benign asymptomatic course to heart failure and sudden death. In infants who present with congestive heart failure, the diagnosis may be initially missed when both right- and left-sided obstruction is present. Beyond infancy, most children are asymptomatic and are diagnosed because of a systolic heart murmur or referred as a relative of an index patient. Others have variable symptoms, often compatible with aortic stenosis, even in the absence of obstruction. These include exertional dyspnea or fatigue, chest pain, dizziness, syncope, and palpitations. Chest pains may be anginal or atypical, aching, and prolonged. Symptoms are more frequent and severe in obstructive HCM.[153]

The physical signs are extremely variable but relate more closely to the hemodynamic state than do symptoms. There is often a prominent A wave in the jugular venous pulse related to diastolic dysfunction or right ventricular obstruction. Without obstruction, other findings may be entirely normal or consist of a systolic murmur, typical of an innocent flow murmur. With outflow obstruction, the pulses are jerky, the brisk initial upstroke is interrupted in midsystole as rapid ventricular ejection is impeded, and ejection is completed more slowly. The left ventricular impulse may be double in patients with obstruction and triple with a palpable fourth heart sound. The first heart sound is normal, the second often normally split but, as in aortic stenosis, narrow and even paradoxical with significant obstruction. Third and fourth heart sounds are more frequently present with phonocardiography than on auscultation. The murmur of obstruction is ejection, midsystolic, and radiates widely but not prominently to the carotids, unlike in aortic stenosis. The murmur is louder with greater degrees of obstruction. At the apex, the murmur may be ejection, or holosystolic with mitral regurgitation. The murmur is increased by maneuvers that increase systolic anterior motion of the mitral valve, such as standing or the Valsalva maneuver (decreased preload and afterload), amyl nitrite (decreased afterload), and isoproterenol (increased contractility). Conversely, the murmur is decreased by a volume load (increased preload), by squatting or a handgrip (increased afterload), or by verapamil and disopyramide (decreased contractility). An apical mid-diastolic murmur may be associated with mitral regurgitation or impaired ventricular diastolic function.

ELECTROCARDIOGRAPHIC FINDINGS IN HYPERTROPHIC CARDIOMYOPATHY

Normal electrocardiogram
Left ventricular hypertrophy
Q waves of pseudoinfarction
Right ventricular hypertrophy (in infancy)
Right or left bundle branch block
Giant negative T waves V_4 through V_6 in apical hypertrophic cardiomyopathy
Left, right, or left and right atrial hypertrophy
Nonspecific ST changes

ELECTROCARDIOGRAPHY

Most index patients have an abnormal electrocardiogram, but up to 25% of non–index patients diagnosed by M-mode echocardiography have a normal electrocardiogram.[156] There is a diverse range of electrocardiographic abnormalities (Table 35–12). The electrocardiogram may be abnormal when the echocardiogram is normal.[213] Subtle electrocardiographic changes without overt left ventricular hypertrophy may be detectable in childhood as left ventricular hypertrophy is developing.[167] Electrophysiologic study is indicated for patients with nonsustained ventricular tachycardia,[204] but the predictive accuracy of inducible arrhythmias for prediction of sudden death has not been prospectively assessed.[214]

RADIOGRAPHY AND OTHER IMAGING

Most infants with hypertrophic cardiomyopathy have radiographic cardiomegaly.[192] In older children and adults, the heart size on chest radiography is often normal, even with significant left ventricular hypertrophy.[156] Pulmonary vascular markings will be abnormal if there is heart failure. Thus, except for infants, the chest film is of limited value in asymptomatic patients and unhelpful as a screening method for HCM.

Radionuclide studies can be useful in assessing systolic and diastolic function.[215] Thallium scans can demonstrate the extent and distribution of left ventricular hypertrophy and detect regional perfusion abnormalities in assessment of patients with and without chest pain.[212] Positron emission tomography is an alternative method to detect evidence of myocardial ischemia.[216] Magnetic resonance imaging may be helpful if apical hypertrophic cardiomyopathy is suspected by electrocardiography but not demonstrated by echocardiography.[217]

ECHOCARDIOGRAPHY

An M-mode,[156, 157] two-dimensional,[98, 166] and echo Doppler[157, 165, 171] study is the most useful investigation for the diagnosis and evaluation of systolic and diastolic function in HCM. It should still be complementary to genetic testing for screening family members of index patients and is indispensable for serial evaluation and evaluation of treatment. Two-dimensional echocardiography defines the type and degree of left ventricular hypertrophy.[98, 166] Individuals with classical HCM have asymmetric septal hypertrophy, with an M-mode ratio of thickness of basal ventricular septum to posterior left ventricular wall of 1.3:1 or greater. In children, causes of hypertrophy other than HCM have led to the recommendation by some of a ratio of 1.5:1 as evidence of HCM. Septal and posterior wall diagnosis of hypertrophy should be based on comparison with normal data indexed for body surface area. Systolic anterior motion of the mitral valve, characteristically shown by M-mode imaging, is even better shown by real-time, two-dimensional echocardiography. Maron and Epstein reported the specificity of asymmetric septal hypertrophy and systolic anterior motion for HCM to be 90% and 97%, respectively.[184] Although systolic anterior motion usually indicates a diagnosis of HCM (high sensitivity), its absence does not exclude HCM (low specificity). Systolic notching may be seen on the aortic valve as ejection is impeded.

Pulsed Doppler mapping of the left ventricular outflow tract shows different patterns of acceleration at different sites, maximal just beyond the mitral valve–septal coaptation point. Continuous-wave and color Doppler imaging estimates the severity of the subaortic gradient, demonstrates midventricular obstruction, and grades the degree of mitral regurgitation. Provocation maneuvers can be used in cooperative children to elicit systolic anterior motion. The size of the left atrium and left ventricular cavity, morphology of the mitral valve, and degree of right ventricular obstruction should be examined. Transesophageal echocardiography can elegantly show the interrelationship of septal hypertrophy and systolic anterior motion, obstruction and mitral regurgitation, and changes after surgical septal reduction.[171]

Athlete's heart can usually be differentiated easily from HCM by echocardiography; left ventricular wall thickness does not usually exceed 15 mm, there is regression of hypertrophy after a short period without training, and left ventricular end-diastolic dimension is usually greater than 55 mm.[218]

CATHETERIZATION AND ANGIOGRAPHY

Echocardiography has replaced routine cardiac catheterization, because left ventricular hypertrophy, systolic gradient, and degree of mitral regurgitation are usually well shown by echocardiography. However, invasive studies may better clarify systolic and diastolic function. Characteristic hemodynamic features of HCM include elevated left ventricular end-diastolic pressure, gradients more proximal to the aortic valve than in non-HCM subaortic stenosis, a left ventricular outflow tract pressure trace showing a midsystolic dip and a secondary elevation in late systole with a similar systolic contour in the aortic pressure pulse (Fig. 35–35), failure of a postectopic beat to exceed the preceding beat (Brockenbrough's phenomenon) (Fig. 35–35), and isoproterenol-induced or isoproterenol-enhanced obstruction (Fig. 35–36). Right-sided heart studies clarify the site and extent of right ventricular outflow tract obstruction.

Cineangiography with injections in the left ventricle may show the hypertrophy of the septum and papillary muscles. In systole, there is abnormal complete emptying often with obliteration of the mid, interpapillary, or apical regions. The abnormal shape may be seen in the right anterior oblique projection. Systolic anterior motion of the

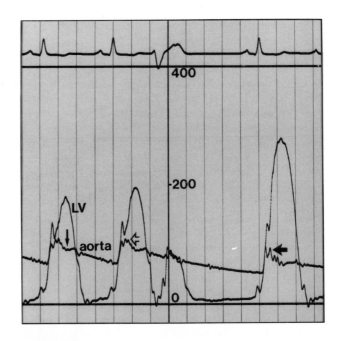

FIGURE 35–35

Simultaneous left ventricular (LV) and aortic pressure tracing in hypertrophic cardiomyopathy. Note the spike and dome LV pressure trace, the midsystolic dip (*vertical arrow*) in the aortic trace, and the left ventricular outflow tract pressure gradient (first two complexes). After an ectopic beat, the gradient is increased but the aortic pressure fails to exceed that of the preceding beats (*horizontal arrows*).

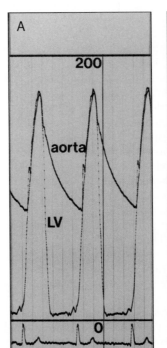
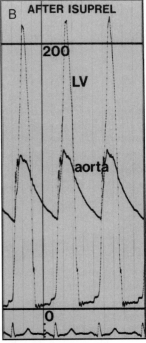

FIGURE 35–36

Induction of a left ventricular (LV) outflow tract gradient in an adult patient with hypertrophic cardiomyopathy. At rest, there is no gradient (*A*); with isoproterenol, a significant gradient is induced (*B*).

anterior leaflet of the mitral valve and the closeness of the mitral leaflet to the ventricular septum are seen in the lateral view. The degree of mitral regurgitation can also be assessed.

MANAGEMENT

HCM has a variety of presentations and as such should never be far from the physician's mind in patients with heart murmurs and especially those with syncope. The diagnosis should be considered in children with unexplained left ventricular hypertrophy after congenital disease and systemic hypertension are excluded. Limitations of diagnosis based on the presence of left ventricular hypertrophy do not allow for patients who have inherited a gene for HCM but have not developed hypertrophy.[199] At the time of diagnosis, investigations should include 24-hour Holter monitoring, an exercise test with measurement of maximal oxygen consumption, and detailed clinical and echocardiographic evaluation. Some investigators have emphasized the pivotal role of stress thallium studies in their algorithm of management.[212] Patients with a history of syncope and those found to have nonsustained ventricular tachycardia should have electrophysiologic testing.[204, 214] The diverse genetic and clinical features of HCM render guidelines for management difficult.[203] However, an attempt to stratify all patients for risk of sudden death should be undertaken.

Symptomatic Hypertrophic Cardiomyopathy

β-Blockers have been the conventional therapy for symptomatic children,[173, 174] their effect being mediated through reduced heart rate with prolongation of diastole and by reduced left ventricular contractility. Noncardioselective β-blockers such as propranolol should be used. Initial recommended dosage of propranolol is 2.0 mg/kg/day, but dosage may need to be 1.5 to 2.0 mg/kg per dose three times a day to achieve adequate β-blockade in children. Because β-blockers have no effect on the degree of left ventricular hypertrophy or sudden death,[192] they should be regarded as symptomatic treatment only.

There is extensive experience with verapamil for HCM in adults,[154, 219] which can be tried for symptomatic children whose β-blockade fails.[220] Verapamil improves diastolic filling as well as decreases systolic gradients, so it could be regarded as more physiologic treatment than β-blockers for HCM. It is uncertain whether verapamil reduces sudden death in adults. In some patients, excessive vasodilatation may worsen obstruction and cause death,[221] and extreme care is needed in any patient with obstruction and in infants.[222] It is contraindicated for those with conduction disturbances without a pacemaker. Nifedipine has been used in infants, but its more potent vasodilatory properties should contraindicate its use in patients with obstructive HCM.[153] Disopyramide has been used extensively in adults by the Toronto group[154] on the basis of its negative inotropic and antiarrhythmic effect, and it could be of benefit in children on its own or in conjunction with β-blockers.[203] Digoxin, other inotropes, and angiotensin-converting enzyme inhibitors are contraindicated in HCM because they worsen obstruction, but they have a role in end-stage dilated thin-walled HCM[154] or where there is impaired left ventricular function.[173, 174] Diuretics are rel-

atively contraindicated because of their reduction in preload[154, 173, 174] but can be used judiciously in the symptomatic infant with heart failure.

SURGICAL METHODS. Surgery is the most effective form of treatment of symptomatic obstructive HCM, usually producing a satisfactory reduction in gradient and reducing or abolishing symptoms.[185–187] Surgical techniques (myotomy or myectomy) through differing approaches (aortic, aortic–left ventricular approach, modified Konno) have evolved. Currently, we favor myectomy through the aortic valve approach. The myectomy needs to be extended beyond the point of the anterior mitral valve–septum contact, widening the left ventricular outflow tract, reducing or abolishing the subaortic obstruction, and reducing mitral regurgitation.[171, 186] Earlier reported mortality was 5 to 7%, but it would currently be expected to be less than 3%.[185–187] There was 1 death in a pediatric cohort of 17 patients commencing in the 1960s.[223] Complications include inadequate myectomy and hence inadequate relief of symptoms, perforation of the ventricular septum, and complete heart block. Approximately 10% of patients have a recurrence of symptoms despite an adequate myectomy. Surgery may not reduce the risk of sudden death late postoperatively, so that continued close medical follow-up is important. It remains unproven whether operation is indicated for asymptomatic patients with a marked gradient.[203] Mitral valve replacement may occasionally be indicated in patients with severe mitral regurgitation and intrinsic abnormalities of the mitral valve.[172] It has been shown that alcohol injected into the left anterior descending coronary septal perforating arteries can produce septal infarction and relief of subaortic obstruction,[224] but further trials with longer follow-up are needed to establish the role of this technique.

PACEMAKER THERAPY. There has been enthusiasm for dual-chamber (DDD) pacing for adult HCM patients by some groups,[225] first reported in 1975. DDD pacing decreases subaortic obstruction by RV apical pacing, but the exact mechanism of gradient reduction is not certain, and the degree of gradient reduction is less than with surgery.[203] Atrioventricular delay must be optimal, and if the intrinsic PR interval is short, either β-blockers or atrioventricular nodal ablation is required for pacing to be effective.[154] Symptoms are improved in many patients, but results from a randomized, double-blind, crossover study indicate a significant placebo effect on symptoms.[226] Currently, the role and efficacy of DDD pacing are keenly debated.[227, 228] It would seem prudent for some of these issues to be resolved in adult patients and a limited number of pediatric centers[229] with longer follow-up before the widespread use of pacing in asymptomatic children is recommended.

ARRHYTHMIA TREATMENT. Amiodarone was previously recommended for treatment of any patient with nonsustained ventricular tachycardia.[230] More recent modifications are to treat only those with associated impaired consciousness,[204] or those with sustained ventricular tachycardia at electrophysiologic study,[214] and those with at least 10 beat runs of ventricular tachycardia.[203] Although it is rare in young children, adolescents have shown nonsustained ventricular tachycardia in 16 to 18% of two cohorts of more than 30 patients.[231,232] However, the absence of ventricular arrhythmia does not indicate a low risk of sudden death in children[231] as it does for adults.[205,206] Inducible ventricular tachycardia should be treated by myectomy, amiodarone, both, or an implantable cardiac defibrillator.[212] Atrial fibrillation, uncommon in childhood, may cause deterioration and cardiac failure and should be treated with amiodarone.[231] Amiodarone, or myectomy for those with obstruction to reduce left atrial size, is the treatment most likely to achieve sinus rhythm.

Asymptomatic Hypertrophic Cardiomyopathy

There is no proven therapy for asymptomatic individuals, and β-blockers are now no longer routinely recommended.[212,214] Spirito and coauthors[203] argue that those with massive left ventricular hypertrophy and those with marked outflow tract gradients could reasonably be given prophylactic drug treatment. Evidence of myocardial ischemia should be sought by stress thallium scintigraphy and treated by verapamil.[212] Supportive treatment for the asymptomatic child should include prophylaxis for infectious endocarditis because of the mitral valve abnormalities and avoidance of intense sports training and competition. Individuals with a history of exercise-induced syncope or a malignant family history or genotype should avoid all strenuous exercise. Conversely, those considered at low risk for sudden death require little or no restriction with regard to recreational sports.[203] Family members of index patients should be screened for HCM by an electrocardiogram and echocardiogram. The role of genetic testing is still evolving, but it is unhelpful in individuals without a positive family history, whereas those from large kindreds of HCM are more likely to have the abnormal gene identified. A potential negative effect of genetic testing is the psychological burden for those identified with an HCM gene with incomplete penetrance who may never develop the clinical disease.[199] Similarly, children identified with HCM by mass screening with use of echocardiography may represent a mild form of the disease.[233]

Prenatal diagnosis is possible in the first trimester by chorionic villous biopsy using linkage analysis for a fetus with a large HCM kindred. Prenatal diagnosis of HCM by fetal echocardiography has been reported.[234] The range of septal thickness for fetuses with HCM has not been defined, but many presumably will not develop hypertrophy in utero. Fetal left ventricular hypertrophy may also result from placental insufficiency and maternal exposure to steroids or dopamine.

FUTURE DIRECTIONS

Small numbers of children per center, genetic variables, and duration of follow-up limit the evaluation of medical, surgical, and pacemaker modalities to improve the natural history of HCM. The prevention of sudden death remains an important challenge, and the efficacy of amiodarone and implantable defibrillators for children in particular needs clarification. Gene therapy for HCM provides the most exciting challenge.

REFERENCES

1. Beppu S, Suzuki S, Matsuda H, et al: Rapidity of progression of aortic stenosis in patients with congenital bicuspid aortic valves. Am J Cardiol 71:322, 1993.
2. Nora JJ: From generational studies to a multilevel genetic-environmental interaction (Editorial; Comment), J Am Coll Cardiol 23:1468, 1994.
3. Roberts WC: The congenitally bicuspid aortic valve. A study of 85 autopsy cases. Am J Cardiol 26:72, 1970.
4. Borow KM, Colan SD, Neumann A: Altered left ventricular mechanics in patients with valvular aortic stenosis and coarctation of the aorta: Effects on systolic performance and late outcome. Circulation 72:515, 1985.
5. Colan SD: Noninvasive assessment of myocardial mechanisms—a review of analysis of stress-shortening and stress-velocity. Cardiol Young 2:1, 1992.
6. Vincent WR, Buckberg GD, Hoffman JI: Left ventricular subendocardial ischemia in severe valvar and supravalvar aortic stenosis: A common mechanism. Circulation 49:326, 1974.
7. Lewis AB, Heymann MA, Stanger P, et al: Evaluation of subendocardial ischemia in valvar aortic stenosis in children. Circulation 49:978, 1974.
8. Kveselis DA, Rocchini AP, Rosenthal A, et al: Hemodynamic determinants of exercise-induced ST-segment depression in children with valvar aortic stenosis. Am J Cardiol 55:1133, 1985.
9. Mark AL, Abboud FM, Schmid PG, Heistad DD: Reflex vascular responses to left ventricular outflow obstruction and activation of ventricular baroreceptors in dogs. J Clin Invest 52:1147, 1973.
10. Villari B, Hess OM, Kaufmann P, et al: Effect of aortic valve stenosis (pressure overload) and regurgitation (volume overload) on left ventricular systolic and diastolic function. Am J Cardiol 69:927, 1992.
11. Hastreiter AR, Oshima M, Miller RA: Congenital aortic stenosis syndrome in infancy. Circulation 28:1084, 1963.
12. Campbell M: The natural history of congenital aortic stenosis. Br Heart J 30:514, 1968.
13. Frank S, Johnson A, Ross J Jr: Natural history of valvular aortic stenosis. Br Heart J 35:41, 1973.
14. Kitchiner D, Jackson M, Walsh K, et al: The progression of mild congenital aortic valve stenosis from childhood into adult life. Int J Cardiol 42:217, 1993.
15. Hossack KF, Neutze JM, Lowe JB, Barratt-Boyes BG: Congenital valvar aortic stenosis. Natural history and assessment for operation. Br Heart J 43:561, 1980.
16. Keane JF, Driscoll DJ, Gersony WM, et al: Second natural history study of congenital heart defects. Results of treatment of patients with aortic valvar stenosis. Circulation 87(suppl 1):1–16, 1993.
17. Cohen LS, Friedman WF, Braunwald E: Natural history of mild congenital aortic stenosis elucidated by serial hemodynamic studies. Am J Cardiol 30:1, 1972.
18. Ellison RC, Wagner HR, Weidman WH, Miettinen OS: Congenital valvular aortic stenosis: Clinical detection of small pressure gradient. Prepared for the joint study on the natural history of congenital heart defects. Am J Cardiol 37:757, 1976.
19. Braunwald E, Goldblatt A, Aygen MM, et al: Congenital aortic stenosis. I: Clinical and hemodynamic findings in 100 patients. II: Surgical treatment and the results of operation. Circulation 27:426, 1963.
20. Keith JD, Rowe RD, Vlad P: Electrocardiography. In Heart Disease in Infancy and Childhood, 2nd ed. New York, Macmillan, 1967, p 39.
21. James FW, Schwartz DC, Kaplan S, Spilkin SP: Exercise electrocardiogram, blood pressure, and working capacity in young patients with valvular or discrete subvalvular aortic stenosis. Am J Cardiol 50:769, 1982.
22. Krabill KA, Ring WS, Foker JE, et al: Echocardiographic versus cardiac catheterization diagnosis of infants with congenital heart disease requiring cardiac surgery. Am J Cardiol 60:351, 1987.
23. Bengur AR, Snider AR, Serwer GA, et al: Usefulness of the Doppler mean gradient in evaluation of children with aortic valve stenosis and comparison to gradient at catheterization. Am J Cardiol 64:756, 1989.

24. Bengur AR, Snider AR, Meliones JN, Vermilion RP: Doppler evaluation of aortic valve area in children with aortic stenosis. J Am Coll Cardiol 18:1499, 1991.

25. Nishimura RA, Pieroni DR, Bierman FZ, et al: Second natural history study of congenital heart defects. Aortic stenosis: Echocardiography. Circulation 87(suppl):I66, 1993.

26. Hatle L, Angelsen BA, Tromsdal A: Noninvasive assessment of aortic stenosis by Doppler ultrasound. Br Heart J 43:284, 1980.

27. Skjaerpe T, Hegrenaes L, Hatle L: Noninvasive estimation of valve area in patients with aortic stenosis by Doppler ultrasound and two-dimensional echocardiography. Circulation 72:810, 1985.

28. Beekman RH, Rocchini AP, Gillon JH, Mancini GB: Hemodynamic determinants of the peak systolic left ventricular–aortic pressure gradient in children with valvar aortic stenosis. Am J Cardiol 69:813, 1992.

29. Otto CM, Pearlman AS, Comess KA, et al: Determination of the stenotic aortic valve area in adults using Doppler echocardiography. J Am Coll Cardiol 7:509, 1986.

30. Currie PJ, Hagler DJ, Seward JB, et al: Instantaneous pressure gradient: A simultaneous Doppler and dual catheter correlative study. J Am Coll Cardiol 7:800, 1986.

31. Duff DF, Mullins CE: Transseptal left heart catheterization in infants and children. Cathet Cardiovasc Diagn 4:213, 1978.

32. Gorlin R, McMillan IKR, Medd WE, et al: Dynamics of the circulation in aortic valvular disease. Am J Med 18:855, 1955.

33. Bache RJ, Jorgensen CR, Wang Y: Simplified estimation of aortic valve area. Br Heart J 34:408, 1972.

34. Ubago JL, Figueroa A, Colman T, et al: Hemodynamic factors that affect calculated orifice areas in the mitral Hancock xenograft valve. Circulation 61:388, 1980.

35. Bache RJ, Wang Y, Jorgensen CR: Hemodynamic effects of exercise in isolated valvular aortic stenosis. Circulation 44:1003, 1971.

36. Richter HS: Mitral valve area: Measurement soon after catheterization. Circulation 28:451, 1963.

37. Cannon SR, Richards KL, Crawford M: Hydraulic estimation of stenotic orifice area: A correction of the Gorlin formula. Circulation 71:1170, 1985.

38. Hunt D, Baxley WA, Kennedy JW, et al: Quantitative evaluation of cineaortography in the assessment of aortic regurgitation. Am J Cardiol 31:696, 1973.

39. Brandt PWT, Roche AHG, Barratt-Boyes BG, Lowe JB: Radiology of homograft aortic valves. Thorax 24:129, 1969.

40. Kennedy JW, Twiss RD, Blackmon JR, Dodge HT: Quantitative angiocardiography. III. Relationships of left ventricular pressure, volume, and mass in aortic valve disease. Circulation 38:838, 1968.

41. Jaffe WM, Coverdale HA, Roche AHG, et al: Doppler echocardiography in the assessment of the homograft aortic valve. Am J Cardiol 63:1466, 1989.

42. Oh JK, Taliercio CP, Holmes DR Jr, et al: Prediction of the severity of aortic stenosis by Doppler aortic valve area determination: Prospective Doppler-catheterization correlation in 100 patients. J Am Coll Cardiol 11:1227, 1988.

43. Yeager M, Yock PG, Popp RL: Comparison of Doppler-derived pressure gradient to that determined at cardiac catheterization in adults with aortic valve stenosis: Implications for management. Am J Cardiol 57:644, 1986.

44. Pelech AN, Dyck JD, Trusler GA, et al: Critical aortic stenosis. Survival and management. J Thorac Cardiovasc Surg 94:510, 1987.

45. Kugler JD, Campbell E, Vargo TA, et al: Results of aortic valvotomy in infants with isolated aortic valvular stenosis. J Thorac Cardiovasc Surg 78:553, 1979.

46. Mocellin R, Sauer U, Simon B, et al: Reduced left ventricular size and endocardial fibroelastosis as correlates of mortality in newborns and young infants with severe aortic valve stenosis. Pediatr Cardiol 4:265, 1983.

47. Moller JH, Nakib A, Edwards JE: Infarction of papillary muscles and mitral insufficiency associated with congenital aortic stenosis. Circulation 34:87, 1966.

48. Parsons MK, Moreau GA, Graham TP Jr, et al: Echocardiographic estimation of critical left ventricular size in infants with isolated aortic valve stenosis. J Am Coll Cardiol 18:1049, 1991.

49. Leung MP, McKay R, Smith A, et al: Critical aortic stenosis in early infancy. Anatomic and echocardiographic substrates of successful open valvotomy. J Thorac Cardiovasc Surg 101:526, 1991.

50. Rhodes LA, Colan SD, Perry SB, et al: Predictors of survival in neonates with critical aortic stenosis. Circulation 84:2325, 1991.

51. Rychik J, Murdison KA, Chin AJ, Norwood WI: Surgical management of severe aortic outflow obstruction in lesions other than the hypoplastic left heart syndrome: Use of a pulmonary artery to aorta anastomosis. J Am Coll Cardiol 18:809, 1991.

52. Keane JF, Bernhard WF, Nadas AS: Aortic stenosis surgery in infancy. Circulation 52:1138, 1975.

53. Zeevi B, Keane JF, Castaneda AR, et al: Neonatal critical valvar aortic stenosis. A comparison of surgical and balloon dilation therapy. Circulation 80:831, 1989.

54. Rocchini AP, Beekman RH, Ben Shachar G, et al: Balloon aortic valvuloplasty: Results of the Valvuloplasty and Angioplasty of Congenital Anomalies Registry. Am J Cardiol 65:784, 1990.

55. Sholler GF, Keane JF, Perry SB, et al: Balloon dilation of congenital aortic valve stenosis. Results and influence of technical and morphological features on outcome. Circulation 78:351, 1988.

56. Hsieh KS, Keane JF, Nadas AS, et al: Long-term follow-up of valvotomy before 1968 for congenital aortic stenosis. Am J Cardiol 58:338, 1986.

57. Lababidi Z, Wu JR, Walls JT: Percutaneous balloon aortic valvuloplasty: Results in 23 patients. Am J Cardiol 53:194, 1984.

58. Fisher RD, Mason DT, Morrow AG: Results of operative treatment in congenital aortic stenosis: Pre- and postoperative hemodynamic evaluations. J Thorac Cardiovasc Surg 59:218, 1970.

59. Wagner HR, Ellison RC, Keane JF, et al: Clinical course in aortic stenosis. Circulation 56:I-47, 1977.

60. Helgason H, Keane JF, Fellows KE, et al: Balloon dilation of the aortic valve: Studies in normal lambs and in children with aortic stenosis. J Am Coll Cardiol 9:816, 1987.

61. Hosking MC, Benson LN, Freedom RM: A femoral vein–femoral artery loop technique for aortic dilatation in children. Cathet Cardiovasc Diagn 23:253, 1991.

62. Hausdorf G, Schneider M, Schirmer KR, et al: Anterograde balloon valvuloplasty of aortic stenosis in children. Am J Cardiol 71:460, 1993.

63. De Giovanni JV, Edgar RA, Cranston A: Adenosine induced transient cardiac standstill in catheter interventional procedures for congenital heart disease. Heart 80:330,1998.

64. Nihill MR, O'Laughlin MP, Mullins CE: Aortic balloon valvuloplasty in congenital aortic stenosis. Proceedings of the World Congress of Pediatric Cardiology, Bangkok. New York, Excerpta Medica, 1989.

65. Meliones JN, Beekman RH, Rocchini AP, Lacina SJ: Balloon valvuloplasty for recurrent aortic stenosis after surgical valvotomy in childhood: Immediate and follow-up studies. J Am Coll Cardiol 13:1106, 1989.

66. Sreeram N, Kitchiner D, Williams D, Jackson M: Balloon dilatation of the aortic valve after previous surgical valvotomy: Immediate and follow up results. Br Heart J 71:558, 1994.

67. Rosenfeld HM, Landzberg MJ, Perry SB, et al: Balloon aortic valvuloplasty in the young adult with congenital aortic stenosis. Am J Cardiol 73:1112, 1994.

68. Kirklin JW, Barratt-Boyes BG: Congenital aortic stenosis. In Cardiac Surgery, 2nd ed. New York, Churchill Livingstone, 1993, p 1195.

69. Allan LD, Maxwell DJ, Carminati M, Tynan MJ: Survival after fetal aortic balloon valvoplasty. Ultrasound Obstet Gynecol 5:90, 1995.

70. Neish SR, O'Laughlin MP, Nihill MR, et al: Intraoperative balloon valvuloplasty for critical aortic valvular stenosis in neonates. Am J Cardiol 68:807, 1991.

71. Gula G, Wain WH, Ross DN: Ten years' experience with pulmonary autograft replacements for aortic valve disease. Ann Thorac Surg 28:392, 1979.

72. Peterson TA, Todd DB, Edwards JE: Supravalvular aortic stenosis. J Thorac Cardiovasc Surg 50:734, 1965.

73. Williams JCP, Barratt-Boyes BG, Lowe JB: Supravalvular aortic stenosis. Circulation 24:1311, 1961.

74. Ensing GJ, Schmidt MA, Hagler DJ, et al: Spectrum of findings in a family with nonsyndromic autosomal dominant supravalvular aortic stenosis: A Doppler echocardiographic study. J Am Coll Cardiol 13:413, 1989.

75. Geggel RL: Supravalvar aortic stenosis: Discordance in monozygotic twins and reduction in severity of obstruction during childhood. Pediatr Cardiol 13:170, 1992.

76. Kitchiner D, Jackson M, Walsh K, et al: Prognosis of supravalve aortic stenosis in 81 patients in Liverpool (1960–1993). Heart 75:396, 1996.

77. Sharma BK, Fujiwara H, Hallman GL, et al: Supravalvar aortic stenosis: A 29-year review of surgical experience. Ann Thorac Surg 51:1031, 1991.

78. van Son JA, Danielson GK, Puga FJ, et al: Supravalvular aortic stenosis. Long-term results of surgical treatment. J Thorac Cardiovasc Surg 107:103, 1994.

79. Keating MT: Genetic approaches to cardiovascular disease: Supravalvular aortic stenosis, Williams syndrome, and long-QT syndrome. Circulation 92:142, 1995.

80. Nickerson E, Greenberg F, Keating MT, et al: Deletions of the elastin gene at 7q11.23 occur in approximately 90% of patients with Williams syndrome. Am J Hum Genet 56:1156, 1995.

81. Beuren AJ, Schulze C, Eberle P, et al: The syndrome of supravalvular aortic stenosis, peripheral pulmonary stenosis, mental retardation and similar facial appearance. Am J Cardiol 13:471, 1964.

82. Jones KL, Smith DW: The Williams elfin facies syndrome. A new perspective. J Pediatr 86:718, 1975.

83. Jones KL: Williams syndrome: An historical perspective of its evolution, natural history, and etiology. Am J Med Genet Suppl 6:89, 1990.

84. Morris CA, Demsey SA, Leonard CO, et al: Natural history of Williams syndrome: Physical characteristics. J Pediatr 113:318, 1988.

85. Zalzstein E, Moes CA, Musewe NN, Freedom RM: Spectrum of cardiovascular anomalies in Williams-Beuren syndrome. Pediatr Cardiol 12:219, 1991.

86. O'Connor WN, Davis JB Jr, Geissler R, et al: Supravalvular aortic stenosis. Clinical and pathologic observations in six patients. Arch Pathol Lab Med 109:179, 1985.

87. van Son JA, Edwards WD, Danielson GK: Pathology of coronary arteries, myocardium, and great arteries in supravalvular aortic stenosis: Report of five cases with implications for surgical treatment. J Thorac Cardiovasc Surg 108:21, 1994.

88. Wren C, Oslizlok P, Bull C: Natural history of supravalvular aortic stenosis and pulmonary artery stenosis. J Am Coll Cardiol 15:1625, 1990.

89. Garcia RE, Friedman WF, Kaback MM, Rowe RD: Idiopathic hypercalcemia and supravalvar aortic stenosis: Documentation of a new syndrome. N Engl J Med 271:117, 1964.

90. McDonald AH, Gerlis LM, Somerville J: Familial arteriopathy with associated pulmonary and systemic arterial stenoses. Br Heart J 31:375, 1969.

91. Blieden LC, Lucas RV Jr, Carter JB, et al: A developmental complex including supravalvular stenosis of the aorta and pulmonary trunk. Circulation 49:585, 1974.

92. French JW, Guntheroth WG: An explanation of asymmetric upper extremity blood pressures in supravalvular aortic stenosis: The Coanda effect. Circulation 42:31, 1970.

93. Goldstein RE, Epstein SE: Mechanism of elevated innominate artery pressures in supravalvular aortic stenosis. Circulation 42:23, 1970.

94. Giddins NG, Finley JP, Nanton MA, Roy DL: The natural course of supravalvar aortic stenosis and peripheral pulmonary artery stenosis in Williams's syndrome. Br Heart J 62:315, 1989.

95. Kececioglu D, Kotthoff S, Vogt J: Williams-Beuren syndrome: A 30-year follow-up of natural and postoperative course. Eur Heart J 14:1458, 1993.

96. Bird LM, Billman GF, Lacro RV, et al: Sudden death in Williams syndrome: Report of ten cases. J Pediatr 129:926, 1996.

97. Hallidie-Smith KA, Karas S: Cardiac anomalies in Williams-Beuren syndrome. Arch Dis Child 63:809, 1988.

98. Snider AR, Serwer GA: Abnormalities of ventricular outflow. *In* Echocardiography in Pediatric Heart Disease. Chicago, Year Book Medical Publishers, 1990, p 231.

99. Brandt PWT: Cineangiography in congenital lesions of the aortic valve. Proceedings of the VII Asian-Pacific Congress of Cardiology. Bangkok, Bangkok Medical Publishers, 1979, p 61.

100. Boxer RA, Fishman MC, LaCorte MA, et al: Diagnosis and postoperative evaluation of supravalvular aortic stenosis by magnetic resonance imaging. Am J Cardiol 58:367, 1986.

101. Pinto RJ, Loya Y, Bhagwat A, Sharma S: Balloon dilatation of supravalvular aortic stenosis: A report of two cases. Int J Cardiol 46:179, 1994.

102. DeLezo JS, Pan M, Romero M, et al: Tailored stent treatment for severe supravalvular aortic stenosis. Am J Cardiol 78:1081, 1996.

103. Rein AJ, Preminger TJ, Perry SB, et al: Generalized arteriopathy in Williams syndrome: An intravascular ultrasound study. J Am Coll Cardiol 21:1727, 1993.

104. Newfeld EA, Muster AJ, Paul MH, et al: Discrete subvalvular aortic stenosis in childhood. Study of 51 patients. Am J Cardiol 38:53, 1976.

105. Frommelt MA, Snider AR, Bove EL, Lupinetti FM: Echocardiographic assessment of subvalvular aortic stenosis before and after operation. J Am Coll Cardiol 19:1018, 1992.

106. de Vries AG, Hess J, Witsenburg M, et al: Management of fixed subaortic stenosis: A retrospective study of 57 cases. J Am Coll Cardiol 19:1013, 1992.

107. Freedom RM, Pelech A, Brand A, et al: The progressive nature of subaortic stenosis in congenital heart disease. Int J Cardiol 8:137, 1985.

108. Vogt J, Dische R, Rupprath G, et al: Fixed subaortic stenosis: An acquired secondary obstruction? A twenty-seven year experience with 168 patients. Thorac Cardiovasc Surg 37:199, 1989.

109. Wright GB, Keane JF, Nadas AS, et al: Fixed subaortic stenosis in the young: Medical and surgical course in 83 patients. Am J Cardiol 52:830, 1983.

110. Choi JY, Sullivan ID: Fixed subaortic stenosis: Anatomical spectrum and nature of progression. Br Heart J 65:280, 1991.

111. Kelly DT, Wulfsberg E, Rowe RD: Discrete subaortic stenosis. Circulation 46:309, 1972.

112. Feigl A, Feigl D, Lucas RV, Edwards JE: Involvement of the aortic valve cusps in discrete subaortic stenosis. Pediatr Cardiol 5:185, 1984.

113. Somerville J, Stone S, Ross D: Fate of patients with fixed subaortic stenosis after surgical removal. Br Heart J 43:629, 1980.

114. Ferrans VJ, Muna WFT, Jones M, Roberts WC: Ultrastructure of the fibrous ring in patients with discrete subaortic stenosis. Lab Invest 39:30, 1978.

115. Shone JD, Sellers RD, Anderson RC, et al: The developmental complex of "parachute mitral valve," supravalvular ring of left atrium, subaortic stenosis, and coarctation of the aorta. Am J Cardiol 11:714, 1963.

116. Maron BJ, Redwood DR, Roberts WC, et al: Tunnel subaortic stenosis. Left ventricular outflow tract obstruction produced by fibromuscular narrowing. Circulation 54:404, 1976.

117. Somerville J: Fixed subaortic stenosis—a frequently misunderstood lesion. Int J Cardiol 8:145, 1985.

118. Sung C, Price EC, Cooley DA: Discrete subaortic stenosis in adults. Am J Cardiol 42:283, 1978.

119. Edwards JE: Pathology of left ventricular outflow tract obstruction. Circulation 31:586, 1965.

120. Pyle RL, Patterson DF, Chacko S: The genetics and pathology of discrete subaortic stenosis in the Newfoundland dog. Am Heart J 92:324, 1976.

121. Diglio MC, Giannotti A, Marino B, et al: Discrete membranous subaortic stenosis in siblings. Eur J Pediatr 152:622, 1993.

122. Rosenquist GC, Clark EB, McAllister HA, et al: Increased mitral-aortic separation in discrete subaortic stenosis. Circulation 60:70, 1997.

123. Kleinert S, Geva T: Echocardiographic morphometry and geometry of the left ventricular outflow tract in fixed aortic stenosis. J Am Coll Cardiol 22:1501, 1993.

124. Gewillig M, Daenen W, Dumoulin M, van der Hauwaert L: Rheologic genesis of discrete subvalvular aortic stenosis: A Doppler echocardiographic study. J Am Coll Cardiol 19:818, 1992.

125. Freedom RM, Dische RM, Rowe RD: Pathological anatomy of subaortic stenosis and atresia in the first year of life. Am J Cardiol 39:1035, 1977.

126. Coleman DM, Smallhorn JF, McCrindle BW, et al: Postoperative follow-up of fibromuscular subaortic stenosis. J Am Coll Cardiol 24:1558, 1994.

127. Leichter DA, Sullivan I, Gersony WM: "Acquired" discrete subvalvar aortic stenosis: Natural history and hemodynamics. J Am Coll Cardiol 14:1539, 1989.

128. Baumstark A, Fellows KE, Rosenthal A: Combined double chambered right ventricle and discrete subaortic stenosis. Circulation 57:299, 1978.

129. Vogel M, Smallhorn JF, Freedom RM, et al: An echocardiographic study of the association of ventricular septal defect and right ventricular muscle bundles with a fixed subaortic abnormality. Am J Cardiol 61:857, 1988.

130. Berry TE, Aziz KU, Paul MH: Echocardiographic assessment of discrete subaortic stenosis in childhood. Am J Cardiol 43:957, 1979.

131. Weyman AE, Feigenbaum H, Hurwitz RA, et al: Cross-sectional echocardiography in evaluating patients with discrete subaortic stenosis. Am J Cardiol 37:358, 1976.

132. ten Cate FJ, Van Dorp WG, Hugenholtz PG, Roelandt J: Fixed subaortic stenosis. Value of echocardiography for diagnosis and differentiation between various types. Br Heart J 41:159, 1979.

133. Suarez de Lezo J, Pan M, Medina A, et al: Immediate and follow-up results of transluminal balloon dilation for discrete subaortic stenosis. J Am Coll Cardiol 18:1309, 1991.

134. Wilcox WD, Seward JB, Hagler DJ, et al: Discrete subaortic stenosis: Two-dimensional echocardiographic features with angiographic and surgical correlation. Mayo Clin Proc 55:425, 1980.

135. Essop MR, Skudicky D, Sareli P: Diagnostic value of transesophageal versus transthoracic echocardiography in discrete subaortic stenosis. Am J Cardiol 70:962, 1992.

136. Lupinetti FM, Pridjian AK, Callow LB, et al: Optimum treatment of discrete subaortic stenosis. Ann Thorac Surg 54:467, 1992.

137. Reddy VM, Rajasinghe HA, Teitel DF, et al: Aortoventriculoplasty with the pulmonary autograft: the "Ross-Konno" procedure. J Thorac Cardiovasc Surg 111:158, 1996.

138. Bjornstad PG, Rastan H, Keutel J, et al: Aortoventriculoplasty for tunnel subaortic stenosis and other obstructions of the left ventricular outflow tract: Clinical and hemodynamic results. Circulation 60:59, 1979.

139. Stewart JR, Merrill WH, Hammon JW, et al: Reappraisal of localized resection for subvalvar aortic stenosis. Ann Thorac Surg 50:197, 1990.

140. Lababidi Z, Weinhaus L, Stoeckle H, Walls JT: Transluminal balloon dilatation for discrete subaortic stenosis. Am J Cardiol 59:423, 1987.

141. Binet JP, Losay J, Demontoux S, et al: Subvalvular aortic stenosis: Long-term surgical results. Thorac Cardiovasc Surg 31:96, 1983.

142. Rizzoli G, Tiso E, Mazzucco A, et al: Discrete subaortic stenosis: Operative age and gradient as predictors of late aortic valve incompetence. J Thorac Cardiovasc Surg 106:95, 1993.

143. Watkins H, Rosenzweig A, Hwang DS, et al: Characteristics and prognostic implications of myosin missense mutations in familial hypertrophic cardiomyopathy. N Engl J Med 326:1108, 1992.

144. Watkins H, Conner D, Thierfelder L, et al: Mutations in the cardiac myosin binding protein-C gene on chromosome 11 cause familial hypertrophic cardiomyopathy. Nat Genet 11:434, 1995.

145. Geisterfer Lowrance AA, Christe M, Conner DA, et al: A mouse model of familial hypertrophic cardiomyopathy. Science 272:731, 1996.

146. Jarcho JA, McKenna W, Pare JAP, et al: Mapping a gene for familial hypertrophic cardiomyopathy to chromosome 14q1. N Engl J Med 321:1372, 1989.

147. Dausse E, Komajda M, Fetler L, et al: Familial hypertrophic cardiomyopathy: Microsatellite haplotyping and identification of a hot spot for mutations in the β-myosin heavy chain gene. J Clin Invest 92:2807, 1993.

148. Marian AJ, Roberts R: Recent advances in the molecular genetics of hypertrophic cardiomyopathy. Circulation 92:1336, 1995.

149. Thierfelder L, MacRae C, Watkins H, et al: A familial hypertrophic cardiomyopathy locus maps to chromosome 15q2. Proc Natl Acad Sci U S A 90:6270, 1993.

150. Watkins H, MacRae C, Thierfelder L, et al: A disease locus for familial hypertrophic cardiomyopathy maps to chromosome 1q3. Nat Genet 3:333, 1993.

151. Carrier L, Hengstenberg C, Beckmann JS, et al: Mapping of a novel gene for familial hypertrophic cardiomyopathy to chromosome 11. Nat Genet 4:311, 1993.

152. Teare RD: Asymmetrical hypertrophy of the heart in young adults. Br Heart J 20:1, 1958.

153. Wigle ED, Sasson Z, Henderson MA, et al: Hypertrophic cardiomyopathy: The importance of the site and the extent of hypertrophy: A review. Prog Cardiovasc Dis 28:1, 1985.

154. Wigle ED, Rakowski H, Kimball BP, Williams WG: Hypertrophic cardiomyopathy: Clinical spectrum and treatment. Circulation 92:1680, 1995.

155. Maron BJ, Gardin JM, Flack JM, et al: Prevalence of hypertrophic cardiomyopathy in a general population of young adults: Echocardiographic analysis of 4111 subjects in the CARDIA Study. Circulation 92:785, 1995.

156. Greaves SC, Roche AHG, Neutze JM, et al: Inheritance of hypertrophic cardiomyopathy: A cross sectional and M mode echocardiographic study of 50 families. Br Heart J 58:259, 1987.

157. Maron BJ, Nichols PF, Pickle LW, et al: Patterns of inheritance in hypertrophic cardiomyopathy: Assessment by M-mode and two-dimensional echocardiography. Am J Cardiol 53:1087, 1984.

158. Fananapazir L, Epstein ND: Genotype-phenotype correlations in hypertrophic cardiomyopathy: Insights provided by comparisons of kindreds with distinct and identical β-myosin heavy chain gene mutations. Circulation 89:22, 1994.

159. Anan R, Greve G, Thierfelder L, et al: Prognostic implications of novel β cardiac myosin heavy chain gene mutations that cause familial hypertrophic cardiomyopathy. J Clin Invest 93:280, 1994.

160. Solomon SD, Wolff S, Watkins H, et al: Left ventricular hypertrophy and morphology in familial hypertrophic cardiomyopathy associated with mutations of the beta-myosin heavy chain gene. J Am Coll Cardiol 22:498, 1993.

161. Schwartz K, Carrier L, Guicheney P, Komajda M: Molecular basis of familial cardiomyopathies. Circulation 91:532, 1995.

162. Poetter K, Jiang H, Hassanzadeh S, et al: Mutations in either the essential or regulatory light chains of myosin are associated with a rare myopathy in human heart and skeletal muscle. Nat Genet 13:63, 1996.

163. Yu QT, Ifegwu J, Marian AJ, et al: Hypertrophic cardiomyopathy mutation is expressed in messenger RNA of skeletal as well as cardiac muscle [published errata appear in Circulation 87:1775, 1993 and 87:2070, 1993]. Circulation 87:406, 1993.

164. Schwartz ML, Cox GF, Lin AE, et al: Clinical approach to genetic cardiomyopathy in children. Circulation 94:2021, 1996.

165. Maron BJ, Gottdiener JS, Epstein SE: Patterns and significance of distribution of left ventricular hypertrophy in hypertrophic cardiomyopathy: A wide angle, two dimensional echocardiographic study of 125 patients. Am J Cardiol 48:418, 1981.

166. Klues HG, Schiffers A, Maron BJ: Phenotypic spectrum and patterns of left ventricular hypertrophy in hypertrophic cardiomyopathy: Morphologic observations and significance as assessed by two-dimensional echocardiography in 600 patients. J Am Coll Cardiol 26:1699, 1995.

167. Maron BJ, Spirito P, Wesley Y, Arce J: Development and progression of left ventricular hypertrophy in children with hypertrophic cardiomyopathy. N Engl J Med 315:610, 1986.

168. Maron BJ, Tajik AJ, Ruttenberg HD, et al: Hypertrophic cardiomyopathy in infants: Clinical features and natural history. Circulation 65:7, 1982.

169. Maron BJ, Anan TJ, Roberts WC: Quantitative analysis of the distribution of cardiac muscle cell disorganization in the left ventricular wall of patients with hypertrophic cardiomyopathy. Circulation 63:882, 1981.

170. Maron BJ, Fananapazir L: Sudden cardiac death in hypertrophic cardiomyopathy. Circulation 85:I-57, 1992.

171. Grigg LE, Wigle ED, Williams WG, et al: Transesophageal Doppler echocardiography in obstructive hypertrophic cardiomyopathy: Clarification of pathophysiology and importance in intraoperative decision making. J Am Coll Cardiol 20:42, 1992.

172. Klues HG, Maron BJ, Dollar AL, Roberts WC: Diversity of structural mitral valve alterations in hypertrophic cardiomyopathy. Circulation 85:1651, 1992.

173. Maron BJ, Bonow RO, Cannon RO 3d, et al: Hypertrophic cardiomyopathy: Interrelations of clinical manifestations, pathophysiology, and therapy (1). N Engl J Med 316:780, 1987.

174. Maron BJ, Bonow RO, Cannon RO 3d, et al: Hypertrophic cardiomyopathy: Interrelations of clinical manifestations, pathophysiology, and therapy (2). N Engl J Med 316:844, 1987.

175. Wigle ED: Hypertrophic cardiomyopathy. In Willerson JT, Cohn JN (eds): Cardiovascular Medicine. New York, Churchill Livingstone, 1995, p 852.

176. Brutsaert DL, Rademakers FE, Sys SU: Triple control of relaxation: Implications in cardiac disease. Circulation 69:190, 1984.

177. Maron BJ, Spirito P, Green KJ, et al: Noninvasive assessment of left ventricular diastolic function by pulsed Doppler echocardiography in patients with hypertrophic cardiomyopathy. J Am Coll Cardiol 10:733, 1987.

178. Shaffer EM, Rocchini AP, Spicer RL, et al: Effects of verapamil on left ventricular diastolic filling in children with hypertrophic cardiomyopathy. Am J Cardiol 61:413, 1988.

179. Nihoyannopoulos P, Karatasakis G, Frenneaux M, et al: Diastolic function in hypertrophic cardiomyopathy: Relation to exercise capacity. J Am Coll Cardiol 19:536, 1992.

180. Spirito P, Maron BJ: Relation between extent of left ventricular hypertrophy and diastolic filling abnormalities in hypertrophic cardiomyopathy. J Am Coll Cardiol 15:808, 1990.

181. Murgo JP, Alter BR, Dorethy JF, et al: Dynamics of left ventricular ejection in obstructive and nonobstructive hypertrophic cardiomyopathy. J Clin Invest 66:1369, 1980.

182. Pollick C, Rakowski H, Wigle ED: Muscular subaortic stenosis: The quantitative relationship between systolic anterior motion and the pressure gradient. Circulation 69:43, 1984.

183. Panza JA, Maris TJ, Maron BJ: Development and determinants of dynamic obstruction to left ventricular outflow in young patients with hypertrophic cardiomyopathy. Circulation 85:1398, 1992.

184. Maron BJ, Epstein SE: Clinical significance and therapeutic implications of the left ventricular outflow tract pressure gradient in hypertrophic cardiomyopathy. Am J Cardiol 58:1093, 1986.

185. Schulte HD, Bircks WH, Loesse B, et al: Prognosis of patients with hypertrophic obstructive cardiomyopathy after transaortic myectomy: Late results up to twenty-five years. J Thorac Cardiovasc Surg 106:709, 1993.

186. Williams WG, Wigle ED, Rakowski H, et al: Results of surgery for hypertrophic obstructive cardiomyopathy. Circulation 76(suppl V):V-104, 1987.

187. Kirklin JW, Barratt-Boyes BG: Hypertrophic obstructive cardiomyopathy. In Cardiac Surgery, 2nd ed. New York, Churchill Livingstone, 1993, p 1239.

188. Criley JM, Lewis KB, White RI, et al: Pressure gradients without obstruction: A new concept of "hypertrophic subaortic stenosis." Circulation 32:881, 1965.

189. Seiler C, Jenni R, Vassalli G, et al: Left ventricular chamber dilatation in hypertrophic cardiomyopathy: Related variables and prognosis in patients with medical and surgical therapy. Br Heart J 74:508, 1995.

190. Koga Y, Itaya K, Toshima H: Prognosis in hypertrophic cardiomyopathy. Am Heart J 108:351, 1984.

191. McKenna W, Deanfield J, Faruqui A, et al: Prognosis in hypertrophic cardiomyopathy: Role of age and clinical, electrocardiographic and hemodynamic features. Am J Cardiol 47:532, 1981.

192. Maron BJ, Roberts WC, Epstein SE: Sudden death in hypertrophic cardiomyopathy: A profile of 78 patients. Circulation 65:1388, 1982.

193. Schaffer MS, Freedom RM, Rowe RD: Hypertrophic cardiomyopathy presenting before 2 years of age in 13 patients. Pediatr Cardiol 4:113, 1983.

194. Maron BJ, Henry WL, Clark CE, et al: Asymmetric septal hypertrophy in childhood. Circulation 53:9, 1976.

195. Maron BJ, Kragel AH, Roberts WC: Sudden death in hypertrophic cardiomyopathy with normal left ventricular mass. Br Heart J 63:308, 1990.

196. Cannan CR, Reeder GS, Bailey KR, et al: Natural history of hypertrophic cardiomyopathy: A population-based study, 1976 through 1990. Circulation 92:2488, 1995.

197. Epstein ND, Cohn GM, Cyran F, Fananapazir L: Differences in clinical expression of hypertrophic cardiomyopathy associated with two distinct mutations in the β-myosin heavy chain gene. A $908^{Leu \to Val}$ mutation and a $403^{Arg \to Gln}$ mutation. Circulation 86:345, 1992.

198. Marian AJ, Mares A Jr, Kelly DP, et al: Sudden cardiac death in hypertrophic cardiomyopathy: Variability in phenotypic expression of beta-myosin heavy chain mutations. Eur Heart J 16:368, 1995.

199. Fananapazir L, Epstein ND: Prevalence of hypertrophic cardiomyopathy and limitations of screening methods. Circulation 92:700, 1995.

200. Maron BJ, Shirani J, Poliac LC, et al: Sudden death in young competitive athletes: Clinical, demographic, and pathological profiles. JAMA 276:199, 1996.

201. Cecchi F, Olivotto I, Montereggi A, et al: Hypertrophic cardiomyopathy in Tuscany: Clinical course and outcome in an unselected regional population. J Am Coll Cardiol 26:1529, 1995.

202. Maron BJ, Epstein SE: Hypertrophic cardiomyopathy. Recent observations regarding the specificity of three hallmarks of the disease: asymmetric septal hypertrophy, septal disorganization and systolic anterior motion of the anterior mitral leaflet. Am J Cardiol 45:141, 1980.

203. Spirito P, Seidman CE, McKenna WJ, Maron BJ: The management of hypertrophic cardiomyopathy (Review). N Engl J Med 336:775, 1997.

204. Fananapazir L, Chang AC, Epstein SE, McAreavey D: Prognostic determinants in hypertrophic cardiomyopathy: Prospective evaluation of a therapeutic strategy based on clinical, Holter, hemodynamic, and electrophysiological findings. Circulation 86:730, 1992.

205. Maron BJ, Savage DD, Wolfson JK, Epstein SE: Prognostic significance of 24 hour ambulatory electrocardiographic monitoring in patients with hypertrophic cardiomyopathy: A prospective study. Am J Cardiol 48:252, 1981.

206. McKenna WJ, England D, Doi YL, et al: Arrhythmia in hypertrophic cardiomyopathy. I: Influence on prognosis. Br Heart J 46:168, 1981.

207. Martin AB, Garson A Jr, Perry JC: Prolonged QT interval in hypertrophic and dilated cardiomyopathy in children. Am Heart J 127:64, 1994.

208. Maron BJ: New observations on the interrelation of dynamic subaortic obstruction and exercise in hypertrophic cardiomyopathy (Editorial). J Am Coll Cardiol 19:534, 1992.

209. Frenneaux MP, Counihan PJ, Caforio AL, et al: Abnormal blood pressure response during exercise in hypertrophic cardiomyopathy. Circulation 82:1995, 1990.

210. Krikler DM, Davies MJ, Rowland E, et al: Sudden death in hypertrophic cardiomyopathy: Associated accessory atrioventricular pathways. Br Heart J 43:245, 1980.

211. Canedo MI, Frank MJ, Abdulla AM: Rhythm disturbances in hypertrophic cardiomyopathy: Prevalence, relation to symptoms and management. Am J Cardiol 45:848, 1980.

212. Dilsizian V, Bonow RO, Epstein SE, Fananapazir L: Myocardial ischemia detected by thallium scintigraphy is frequently related to cardiac arrest and syncope in young patients with hypertrophic cardiomyopathy. J Am Coll Cardiol 22:796, 1993.

213. Ryan MP, Cleland JG, French JA, et al: The standard electrocardiogram as a screening test for hypertrophic cardiomyopathy. Am J Cardiol 76:689, 1995.

214. McKenna WJ, Sadoul N, Slade AKB, Saumarez RC: The prognostic significance of nonsustained ventricular tachycardia in hypertrophic cardiomyopathy. Circulation 90:3115, 1994.

215. Bonow RO, Frederick TM, Bacharach SL, et al: Atrial systole and left ventricular filling in hypertrophic cardiomyopathy: Effect of verapamil. Am J Cardiol 51:1386, 1983.

216. Nienaber CA, Gambhir SS, Mody FV, et al: Regional myocardial blood flow and glucose utilization in symptomatic patients with hypertrophic cardiomyopathy. Circulation 87:1580, 1993.

217. Higgins CB, Byrd BFI, Stark D, et al: Magnetic resonance imaging in hypertrophic cardiomyopathy. Am J Cardiol 55:1121, 1985.

218. Pelliccia A, Maron BJ, Spataro A, et al: The upper limit of physiologic cardiac hypertrophy in highly trained elite athletes. N Engl J Med 324:295, 1991.

219. Bonow RO, Dilsizian V, Rosing DR, et al: Verapamil-induced improvement in left ventricular diastolic filling and increased exercise tolerance in patients with hypertrophic cardiomyopathy: Short- and long-term effects. Circulation 72:853, 1985.

220. Spicer RL, Rocchini AP, Crowley DC, Rosenthal A: Chronic verapamil therapy in pediatric and young adult patients with hypertrophic cardiomyopathy. Am J Cardiol 53:1614, 1984.

221. Epstein SE, Rosing DR: Verapamil: Its potential for causing serious complications in patients with hypertrophic cardiomyopathy. Circulation 64:437, 1981.

222. Garson A Jr: Medicolegal problems in the management of cardiac arrhythmias in children. Pediatrics 79:84, 1987.

223. Stone CD, McIntosh CL, Hennein HA, et al: Operative treatment of pediatric obstructive hypertrophic cardiomyopathy: A 26-year experience. Ann Thorac Surg 56:1308, 1993.

224. Gleichmann U, Seggewiss H, Faber L, et al: Catheter treatment of hypertrophic obstructive cardiomyopathy. Dtsch Med Wochenschr 121:679, 1996.

225. Fananapazir L, Cannon ROI, Tripodi D, Panza JA: Impact of dual-chamber permanent pacing in patients with obstructive hypertrophic cardiomyopathy with symptoms refractory to verapamil and beta-adrenergic blocker therapy. Circulation 85:2149, 1992.

226. Nishimura RA, Trusty JM, Hayes DL, et al: Dual-chamber pacing for hypertrophic obstructive cardiomyopathy: A randomized, double-blind, crossover study. J Am Coll Cardiol 29:435, 1997.

227. Fananapazir L, Epstein ND, Curiel RV, et al: Long-term results of dual-chamber (DDD) pacing in obstructive hypertrophic cardiomyopathy: Evidence for progressive symptomatic and hemodynamic improvement and reduction of left ventricular hypertrophy. Circulation 90:2731, 1994.
228. Spirito P, McKenna WJ, Schultheiss H-P: DDD pacing in obstructive HCM (Letter). Circulation 92:1670, 1995.
229. Rishi F, Hulse JE, Auld DO, et al: Effects of dual-chamber pacing for pediatric patients with hypertrophic obstructive cardiomyopathy. J Am Coll Cardiol 29:734, 1997.
230. McKenna WJ, Oakley CM, Krikler DM, Goodwin JF: Improved survival with amiodarone in patients with hypertrophic cardiomyopathy and ventricular tachycardia. Br Heart J 53:412, 1985.
231. McKenna WJ, Franklin RC, Nihoyannopoulos P, et al: Arrhythmia and prognosis in infants, children and adolescents with hypertrophic cardiomyopathy. J Am Coll Cardiol 11:147, 1988.
232. Muller G, Ulmer HE, Hagel KJ, Wolf D: Cardiac dysrhythmias in children with idiopathic dilated or hypertrophic cardiomyopathy. Pediatr Cardiol 16:56, 1995.
233. Ino T, Okubo M, Nishimoto K, et al: Clinicopathologic characteristics of hypertrophic cardiomyopathy detected during mass screening for heart disease. Pediatr Cardiol 17:295, 1996.
234. Stewart PA, Buis Liem T, Verwey RA, Wladimiroff JW: Prenatal ultrasonic diagnosis of familial asymmetric septal hypertrophy. Prenat Diagn 6:249, 1986.

CHAPTER 36
PULMONIC STENOSIS

LEONARD C. BLIEDEN   MICAEL BERANT   BENJAMIN ZEEVI

Pulmonic stenosis with an intact ventricular septum obstructs right ventricular flow. This obstruction may occur within the ventricle, at the valve itself, or in the pulmonary arteries. The obstruction may be solitary or occur at multiple levels. As an isolated lesion, pulmonic stenosis accounts for approximately 10% of cardiac malformations. In association with other lesions, the incidence may be as high as 25 to 30% of congenital heart disease.

VALVAR PULMONIC STENOSIS

This is a common lesion that may occur sporadically or recur in families (up to 3% of siblings also have pulmonic stenosis).[1] It may occur in the Noonan syndrome,[2,3] the LEOPARD syndrome, or neurofibromatosis.

PATHOLOGY

Pulmonic stenosis may occur in a tricuspid, bicuspid, or dysplastic pulmonic valve. In the most common and classic form, there are three cusps with fusion of the commissures. As a result, the valve becomes dome shaped and projects into the pulmonary trunk.[4] Sometimes the valve is bicuspid. The stenotic valve usually has a central orifice, but the orifice is occasionally eccentric. The valve cusps are usually thin, but they can be thickened and may even be calcified.

As a result of the obstruction, generalized right ventricular hypertrophy occurs. This may be more marked in the infundibular region, where dynamic obstruction may develop. The right atrium may become dilated if the stenosis is severe and compliance of the right ventricle decreased. The wall of the right atrium may thicken, and the foramen ovale may dilate.

The pulmonary artery shows poststenotic dilatation, which may extend into one of the branches and is almost always present after infancy. The left pulmonary artery is usually dilated as the "jet" through the stenotic orifice is directed toward the left pulmonary artery. There is no correlation between severity of the obstruction and the degree of poststenotic dilatation; mild stenosis, for example, may be associated with marked poststenotic dilatation. Although poststenotic dilatation may differentiate classic valvar stenosis from dysplastic valve stenosis, it may occur in a dysplastic valve, although the incidence is lower than that in patients with classic pulmonic stenosis.

An important pathologic subgroup (having clinical and therapeutic implications) is that of the dysplastic valve.[2,3] This valve consists of three thickened, immobile cusps with little, if any, commissural fusion. The cusps are composed of disorganized myxomatous tissue. The valve annulus is usually narrow, and the supravalvar area of the pulmonary trunk is also hypoplastic.

ETIOLOGY

The pathologic process has been ascribed to an abnormality in the development of the distal bulbus cordis.[5] The cause is unclear. A genetic cause is likely, considering the numerous familial and isolated syndromic examples.

PHYSIOLOGY

Regardless of the features of the pulmonary valve, the physiologic effects depend on the degree of stenosis. As the size of the valve orifice narrows, right systolic ventricular pressure increases (roughly as a squared function) to maintain the cardiac output. Right ventricular hypertrophy develops, the severity of which depends on the level of the right ventricular systolic pressure. If the obstruction is severe, significant hypertrophy is present. The trabeculations of the ventricle are increased. In severe stenoses, the right ventricular cavity is decreased in size.

In severe stenosis with suprasystemic right ventricular systolic pressure and especially if it is long-standing (rare in the modern era and in developed countries), myocardial ischemia may occur and lead to myocardial fibrosis and eventually congestive cardiac failure.[6] We have observed one infant—with severe right ventricular hypertrophy from pulmonic stenosis—who developed fatal right ventricular infarction after becoming ill with a respiratory infection that caused moderate hypoxemia, enough to upset the delicate supply-demand equilibrium of the hypertrophied right ventricle. Rudolph[7] has made a significant contribution to our understanding of fetal and neonatal factors contributing to the physiology in such patients. An essential difference in the response of the very young to afterload is hyperplasia in addition to hypertrophy of myocardial fibers. In the neonatal response to afterload, the number of capillaries is increased. This provides the capacity to produce extremely high systolic ventricular pressures. The stroke volume is usually maintained by the hypertrophied muscle, although after a period of sustained elevated pressure, cardiac failure may occur if the ventricle dilates. Cardiac output is usually maintained.

Pulmonary blood flow is decreased and cyanosis is present when right-to-left shunting occurs at the atrial level in association with right ventricular fibrosis (and decreased compliance), right ventricular failure, or decreased size of the right ventricle (due to hypertrophy, which also causes decreased compliance). Hypoplasia of the right ventricle, a separate entity, may simulate the last condition.[8]

CLINICAL HISTORY

In these patients, intelligence is usually normal. Most patients are asymptomatic, even if the stenosis is severe. Currently, most patients undergo treatment to relieve the stenosis before symptoms appear (certainly those beyond the neonatal period). In infancy, symptoms are rare. Patients with critical stenosis may be in congestive heart failure or be cyanotic because of a right-to-left shunt at the atrial level.

Symptoms include dyspnea and fatigue on effort. Even in severe stenosis, marked symptoms are unusual because the right ventricle maintains cardiac output for long periods before decompensation. Rarely, chest pain, syncope, and even sudden death may occur during exercise in patients with severe stenosis.

Cyanosis is rare in childhood but possibly occurs in older, untreated patients, as right ventricular compliance decreases and shunting occurs through a patent foramen ovale.

PHYSICAL EXAMINATION

The general appearance is usually normal. In many patients, however, there is a "moon-like" face, or prominent frontal bossing. Growth and development are usually normal, regardless of the degree of the stenosis. Facial as well as other features may be specific in the Noonan syndrome,[2,3] the LEOPARD syndrome, and neurofibromatosis. In the first two conditions, there are triangular facies, ptosis, and hypertelorism. In syndromic patients (e.g., those with the Noonan and LEOPARD syndromes), both growth and development may be subnormal (often below the 10th percentile).

Cardiac findings depend on the severity of the obstruction. Signs of congestive cardiac failure are usually present only in severe stenosis during infancy. The peripheral pulse and systemic blood pressure are normal. The jugular venous pulse may be altered in severe stenosis, with the *a* wave being prominent. A right ventricular heave may be found, depending on the degree of right ventricular hypertrophy. A systolic thrill at the second and third left intercostal spaces is common; it does not parallel severity of the lesion and is often present in mild to moderate stenosis.

Auscultation is particularly accurate in predicting severity of the lesion, probably more so than in any other congenital lesion.[9,10] The first heart sound is usually normal. An early ejection systolic click is a typical and often identifying feature of classic pulmonic valvar stenosis. It does not occur in subvalvar or supravalvar stenosis. The click becomes louder during expiration and softer in inspiration. In expiration, the right atrial contractile force decreases so that the pulmonary valve is in a relatively closed position when the right ventricle contracts; therefore, its systolic excursion is

increased, and the ejection sound is louder. The ejection sound is heard with mild or moderate stenosis but is absent in patients with severe stenosis or a dysplastic valve.

A systolic ejection murmur is heard best at the upper left sternal border. It may be transmitted throughout the precordium and importantly to the left upper back. In general, louder murmurs indicate more severe stenosis, but the distinction is imperfect.

The length and peak of the murmur vary with the severity of stenosis, which obviously determines the length of contraction. In patients with mild stenosis, the murmur is relatively short, and the peak does not occur beyond midsystole. In moderate stenosis, the peak occurs later, and the murmur may end at or slightly beyond the aortic component of the second heart sound. With severe stenosis, the peak occurs even later in systole, and the murmur ends beyond the aortic component of the second sound. With increasing severity of stenosis, the frequency of the murmur increases as well.

The degree of splitting of the second heart sound varies with severity. In mild stenosis, the split is normal, and the pulmonic component is clearly audible. The degree of splitting increases with increasing severity and the pulmonic component becomes softer in severe stenosis so that the duration of the split may be 0.12 to 0.14 second and the pulmonic component soft or inaudible. In addition, if it is audible, the split may be almost unchanging because of a fixed right ventricular volume. A fourth heart sound may be heard in patients with severe stenosis. In infants with severe stenosis, an additional systolic murmur that increases with inspiration, indicative of tricuspid insufficiency, may be audible.

ELECTROCARDIOGRAPHY

The electrocardiogram reflects the degree of severity accurately, probably more than in any other cardiac malformation.[11] The electrocardiographic changes are right atrial enlargement, right-axis deviation, and right ventricular hypertrophy. In mild valvar stenosis, the electrocardiogram is often normal, with only mild right-axis deviation and often an rSR' or rR' pattern in lead V_1. In moderate stenosis, the electrocardiogram is abnormal in more than 90% of patients. Right-axis deviation may be present (usually between 90 and 130 degrees mean frontal axis). On occasion, right atrial enlargement is found. An rR' or RS complex is usually present in lead V_1. In severe stenosis, an abnormal P wave is found. The mean frontal axis varies from +100 to +170 degrees. In lead V_1, a pure R wave or RS or QR pattern may be present. The T waves may remain negative but often become upright in severe stenosis. Beyond infancy, the height of the R wave in V_1 has correlated roughly with pressure in the right ventricle. Two formulae have been suggested:

$$R(V_1) \times 3 + 49 \text{ mm Hg}$$
$$= \text{right ventricular systolic pressure} \quad (1)$$

$$R(V_1) \times 5 = \text{right ventricular systolic pressure} \quad (2)$$

An R wave above 30 mV in lead V_1 correlates with severe stenosis. Although the electrocardiogram may be normal in aortic stenosis, even in severe stenosis, this is extremely rare in pulmonic stenosis.

In patients with a dysplastic valve (usually those with Noonan's syndrome), the electrocardiogram is atypical with a left anterior hemiblock and counterclockwise QRS frontal plane loop. The mean frontal QRS axis is superiorly directed, and deep S waves are present in the precordium, regardless of the level of systolic pressure in the right ventricle. If there is an associated hypertrophic cardiomyopathy, left ventricular hypertrophy may be present.

ARRHYTHMIA

Arrhythmias are rare in pulmonic stenosis. Supraventricular arrhythmia may occur in an untreated patient with severe stenosis, and ventricular arrhythmias may occur in the older untreated patients, especially during exercise.

RADIOGRAPHY

Radiographic features are much less reliable than physical findings and electrocardiographic features in assessing the severity of the lesion. Cardiac size is usually normal. Poststenotic dilatation of the main and often the left pulmonary artery is present and causes the appearance of a prominent pulmonary artery segment on the posteroanterior chest radiograph. The prominence of the pulmonary artery does not correlate with the degree of stenosis, and although dysplastic valves may have little or no poststenotic dilatation, this is certainly not a general rule.[12] In addition, it is not uncommon for a normal adolescent to be referred for evaluation of possible congenital heart disease because of a prominent pulmonary artery segment on the chest radiograph.

ECHOCARDIOGRAPHY

The abnormal pulmonary valve can be visualized on a parasternal short-axis view at the level of the great arteries. The valve may also be evaluated (Fig. 36–1) from a subxiphoid short-axis view. The valve domes during systole, appearing as a convex line of varying thickness at the pulmonary annulus. The pulmonary trunk is dilated (poststenotic dilatation). Color Doppler imaging shows the direction of the jet through the valve, and continuous-wave Doppler imaging allows assessment of the severity of the stenosis (see Fig. 36–1). The peak instantaneous systolic gradient across the valve may be calculated by the simplified Bernoulli equation ($\Delta P = 4 \times V_{max}^2$). A gradient up to 40 mm Hg is considered mild, 40 to 70 mm Hg is considered moderate, and exceeding 70 mm Hg is severe. The right ventricular systolic pressure is increased according to the severity of the pulmonic stenosis. The severity of stenosis may be assessed qualitatively by the degree of thickening of the right ventricular wall or by the presence or absence of systolic flattening of the intraventricular septum on a short-axis view. If the systolic pressure in the right ventricle is less than systemic, the left ventricle appears round at end systole, and the septum is convex toward the right ventricular cavity. Flattening of the septum appears at higher right ventricular systolic pressures; the septum appears straight when the right ventricular systolic pressure reaches systemic level and may show convexity toward the left ventricular cavity at suprasystemic right ventricular systolic pressures. If there is tricuspid regurgitation, the right ventricular systolic pressure may be assessed quantitatively by applying the simplified Bernoulli equation to the regurgitation jet. The right ventricular systolic pressure equals the peak systolic gradient of this jet in addition to the right atrial pressure (usually 5 to 10 mm

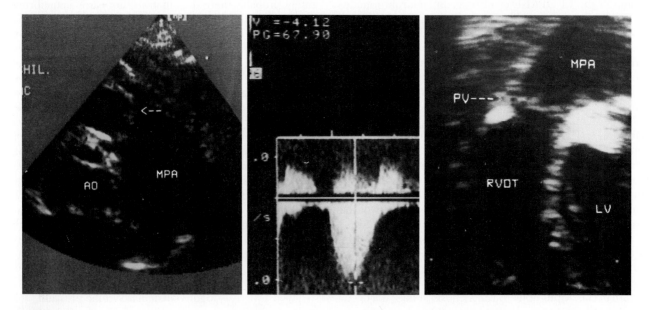

FIGURE 36–1

Echocardiogram in a parasternal short-axis view (*left*) and a subcostal sagittal view (*right*) of the ventricular outflow, doming pulmonary valve, and dilated pulmonary trunk. Continuous-wave Doppler imaging yields a peak instantaneous gradient of 68 mm Hg (*center*). AO = aorta; LV = left ventricle; MPA = main pulmonary artery; PV = pulmonary valve; RVOT = right ventricular outflow tract.

Hg). This pressure may be compared with the systemic blood pressure measured by the blood pressure cuff.

In infants with severe valvar pulmonic stenosis, a right-to-left shunt across the foramen ovale may be demonstrated by color Doppler or contrast-enhanced echocardiography. In these infants, some hypoplasia of the right ventricular cavity may be present, and this decreases the compliance of the ventricle and enhances the right-to-left shunt. Bowing of the atrial septum from right to left may be seen in the presence of a right-to-left shunt at the atrial level because of the increased right atrial pressure. In a dysplastic pulmonary valve, the leaflets are markedly thickened and move poorly. This may be accompanied by hypoplasia of the pulmonary valve annulus and narrowing of the pulmonary trunk.

CARDIAC CATHETERIZATION

Cardiac catheterization is principally performed for balloon valvoplasty. In most patients, oxygen saturation data do not demonstrate an intracardiac shunt, although the combination of pulmonic stenosis and a secundum atrial septal defect is common. In patients with severe obstruction and associated intracardiac communication, a right-to-left shunt through a foramen ovale may be detected.

The severity of the stenosis is determined by the peak systolic pressure gradient across the pulmonary valve and the systolic pressure ratio of the right ventricle to the aorta or the left ventricle. Carefully obtained withdrawal pressure tracings from the pulmonary artery to the right ventricle, using an end-hole catheter, provide information concerning the site and severity of the stenosis.

When the resting right ventricular systolic pressure is less than 50 mm Hg or the gradient is less than 30 mm Hg, the stenosis is characterized as mild. In moderate valvar pulmonic stenosis, the right ventricular systolic pressure may equal that of the aorta or the gradient may be between 30 and 50 mm Hg. In severe obstruction, the resting right ventricular pressure is suprasystemic, and the gradient exceeds 50 mm Hg. (Note that the gradients measured at catheterization are usually less than those measured by Doppler echocardiography.) The pulmonary valve area may be calculated by use of the Gorlin formula and is normally about 2 cm^2/m^2. Because cardiac output is usually normal, even in severe stenosis, the valve area is only rarely calculated. The most important hemodynamic factor that influences the systolic pressure gradient is the heart rate.

The end-diastolic pressure in the right ventricle may be normal, but when there is severe obstruction or right ventricular dysfunction, it may be elevated. Tall right atrial *a* waves are usually present in severe pulmonic stenosis, particularly when there is only a small interatrial communication. Tall right atrial *v* waves are present when moderately severe tricuspid insufficiency is associated. In severe stenosis, there is obliteration of the pulsatile configuration of the pulmonary artery pressure tracing. Associated infundibular stenosis may be present, especially in severe stenosis, and may be suspected from the withdrawal pressure tracing. When multiple obstructions are in close proximity, this technique may be inadequate to identify each of them. A double-pressure balloon catheter capable of measuring pressures through closely spaced ports allows accurate simultaneous measurement of pressure gradients across the pulmonary valve and in the subvalvar area.

ANGIOGRAPHY

Right ventriculograms in the anteroposterior and lateral projections with a 25-degree cranial tilt provide information about the right ventricular size and function, the presence or absence of associated infundibular stenosis, and the pulmonary valve.

The right ventricular size is usually normal although there can be moderate to severe right ventricular hypoplasia, especially in neonates. The typical stenotic valve is thickened and domes during systole. The annulus is usually normal but may be hypoplastic in neonates or infants and in those with severe valvar pulmonic stenosis. Poststenotic dilatation of the pulmonary trunk and left pulmonary artery is usually seen. In a dysplastic valve, the leaflets are thickened and relatively immobile. The main pulmonary artery and the annulus may be moderately hypoplastic. There may be poststenotic dilatation of the pulmonary trunk, although this is less marked than in classic valvar stenosis.

In patients with severe valvar pulmonic stenosis, diffuse narrowing of the right ventricular outflow tract due to hypertrophy may be seen during middle to late systole, but this narrowing disappears during diastole.

NATURAL HISTORY

The Natural History Study produced important information.[13] In most patients, the probability of survival is similar to that of the general population, and they are asymptomatic. In postoperative patients, reoperation is rarely necessary.

Patients with pressure gradients below 25 mm Hg did not experience an increase in gradient with time. If the gradient was above 50 mm Hg, valvotomy was deemed necessary. The management of patients with a gradient between 40 and 49 mm Hg was controversial. (The introduction of balloon valvoplasty has altered this approach and is discussed later.) There were 22 deaths, 19 in the surgically managed patients and 3 in the medically managed patients.[13] In the medical group, two of the three deaths were noncardiac related, and the third death was a result of ventricular fibrillation during catheterization. In the surgical group, 12 of 19 patients died of cardiac-related causes, including 8 perioperative deaths. Morbidity after admission to the study was uncommon but was significant in the individual patients, related to such conditions as bacterial endocarditis, brain abscess, syncope, congestive cardiac failure, stroke, and pacemaker implantation.

EXERCISE TOLERANCE

In general, exercise tolerance is good and may be normal and equal to that of peer groups. In patients with severe stenosis or in those operated on late and in whom fibrosis may have developed, exercise tolerance may be decreased.[14]

BACTERIAL ENDOCARDITIS

The incidence of bacterial endocarditis in patients with pulmonic stenosis is low. In spite of the low incidence, endocarditis prophylaxis is warranted.

TREATMENT

Patients with mild valvar pulmonic stenosis do not require intervention. They should be treated as normal children and should not be restricted in physical activity.[15–17] An indication for treatment in infants, children, and adolescents, with or without symptoms, is a transvalvar gradient above 40 mm Hg in the absence of fixed subpulmonary obstruction or additional lesions that need operative interventions. Most patients are asymptomatic, including most patients with severe obstruction.[17–20] The successful relief of obstruction has been associated with improved clinical outcome.[19, 21] Severe valvar pulmonic stenosis leads to symptoms and signs of right-sided heart failure, especially in long-standing obstruction in adults.[21, 22]

Infants

Asymptomatic infants with severe valvar pulmonic stenosis should be treated electively, usually around the age of 9 to 12 months. Balloon valvoplasty may be performed earlier if the lesion is extremely severe. The rationale for intervention has included the relief of symptoms, the prevention of secondary changes in the right ventricle and pulmonary artery, and the prevention of progression to more severe obstruction.[17–19] The successful relief of obstruction improves clinical outcome.[19, 21]

Neonates

In contrast to older infants and children, critical pulmonic stenosis in neonates requires emergency treatment to reduce the mortality rate that exists in the absence of intervention.[19, 23, 24] Treatment, when necessary, consists of valvotomy or valvoplasty. Valvotomy has been used for more than 4 decades but has been replaced by valvoplasty by catheter techniques.

Surgical Valvotomy

Surgical valvotomy may be performed by an open or closed technique, although almost all are performed under direct vision.[25] The approach is through the pulmonary artery, and valvotomy is performed. With a dysplastic pulmonary valve, the same approach is used. Balloon valvoplasty is attempted; should this fail because of either the thickened leaflets or the supravalvar stenosis, operative treatment is necessary. Valvotomy alone does not usually suffice, and valvectomy, partial or total, may be necessary. Enlargement of the annulus and patch enlargement of the pulmonary trunk may also be necessary.

The results of the surgical valvotomy on nondysplastic valves are excellent. Mortality should be minimal, although in the Natural History Study, 3.4% of patients undergoing operations died of cardiac-related causes. These included 8 of 12 perioperative deaths, 1 sudden death, and 1 death each attributed to myocardial infarction, congestive heart failure, and cardiomyopathy. Subsequently, $96 \pm 1.2\%$ of patients remained free of reoperation for 10 years.

After an operation, some degree of pulmonary insufficiency may be present. This is usually minor and clinically insignificant. Rarely, the insufficiency needs valve replacement. Associated infundibular hypertrophy, which occurs in severe stenosis and is probably secondary or functional, poses a special situation. Occasionally, infundibular obstruction does not regress after valvotomy, or the obstruction increases postoperatively. Death has been reported from the so-called suicidal right ventricle. Significant subvalvar obstruction recurring immediately after valvotomy may require treatment with a β-blocker. If there is no response, resection may be necessary. In most patients, however, the secondary obstruction decreases and resolves with time.

Balloon Valvuloplasty

Balloon valvoplasty has become the treatment of choice for patients with valvar pulmonic stenosis of any age and with any valve morphology.[26–58] The procedure of balloon valvoplasty is not technically difficult.[27, 37, 39, 49, 50]

After hemodynamic measurements of the right ventricle/aortic pressure ratio and the transvalvar gradient, accurate measurements of the diameter of the valve annulus are obtained from posterior-anterior and lateral angiocardiograms. An extra stiff exchange guide wire is positioned in a distal pulmonary artery. With the wire carefully fixed in place, the prepared balloon dilatation catheter is advanced over the wire until the valve lies exactly halfway along the length of the balloon. When a single balloon is used, the balloon diameter should be 50 to 60% greater than the diameter of the pulmonary valve annulus. The balloon is inflated to its *prescribed pressure;* observations are made first for the development of a circumferential indentation (or "waist") in the balloon, and then for the disappearance of this waist as the balloon reaches maximal pressure. The balloon is then rapidly deflated, with the entire cycle of inflation and deflation taking no more than 10 to 15 seconds. The inflation-deflation process is repeated with the balloon repositioned slightly forward or backward between each inflation.

For a larger valve annulus, a double-balloon technique was developed. For this technique, a second exchange wire is introduced from the opposite femoral vein, and the second balloon is passed over this wire to a position side by side with the first balloon across the pulmonary valve. When two balloons are used, the combined diameters of the two balloons should be at least 1.6 to 1.8 times the actual diameter of the valve annulus. The two balloons are inflated and deflated simultaneously. Several added advantages to the double-balloon technique immediately become apparent. The two balloons inflate and deflate faster than a single larger balloon. This, coupled with the persistent "lumen" through the valve between the two inflated balloons, results in much less effect on the systemic arterial pressure at maximal inflation than with a single balloon. Even in smaller valves, the relatively smooth contour of the two much lower profile balloons results in less trauma to the vessels at the site of introduction. Because of these advantages, the double-balloon technique has been adapted for most pulmonary valve dilatations even if a single adequate-sized balloon is available.

The goal of the pulmonary valve dilatation is to "ablate" or destroy the pulmonary valve with the balloons, with little concern about the low-pressure pulmonary regurgitation created. When properly performed, the gradient across the valve should be reduced to less than 10 to 15 mm Hg. Often, particularly in patients with more severe stenosis, dynamic subvalvar right ventricular outflow tract obstruction is associated. Once the valvar obstruction is relieved, the subvalvar gradient becomes manifest, and angiographically the subvalvar area narrows markedly. This reaction was recognized long ago by the surgeons as the "suicide right ventricle" after operative relief of valvar stenosis. Fortunately, in the catheterization laboratory, without the trauma of operation and cardiopulmonary bypass, this is a nonfatal reaction, and the stenosis regresses with time if the valvar stenosis has been adequately relieved.

Some dysplastic pulmonary valves cannot be dilated adequately. Unless there are extreme degrees of these echocardiographic and angiocardiographic features, the valve may be mildly dysplastic and possible to dilate. An attempt should be made to dilate these valves when significant stenosis is present.

Although operation for valvar pulmonary stenosis is considered simple and low risk, catheter dilatation of the pulmonary valve in experienced hands is effective, is virtually risk free, and has associated minimal discomfort or morbidity. Balloon dilatation of the pulmonary valve has become the standard treatment for pulmonary valvar stenosis.

The safety and efficacy of balloon valvoplasty of a stenotic pulmonary valve in infants, children, adolescents, and adults have been confirmed by numerous studies.[27-58] Acute and long-term results are excellent with reduction of valve gradient in most patients to a hemodynamically insignificant level (Fig. 36–2). In comparison with valvotomy, balloon valvoplasty provides equivalent long-term gradient relief with less valvar insufficiency.[35]

Follow-up data for 533 patients from 22 institutions up to 7 years after an initial balloon valvoplasty[59] demonstrated that 23% of patients had a suboptimal outcome because of either a residual peak systolic gradient at or above 36 mm Hg or further treatment of pulmonic stenosis by repeated balloon pulmonary valvoplasty or surgical valvotomy. Significant independent predictors of suboptimal long-term outcome are an earlier year of the initial valvoplasty, a small valve hinge point diameter, and a higher immediate residual gradient. A small ratio of balloon-to-valve hinge point diameter significantly predicted suboptimal outcome for patients with valves morphologically classified as either typical or complex (primarily postsurgical valvotomy) but not for patients with dysplastic or combined morphologic features (dysplasia with commissural fusion). The patient's age, Noonan's syndrome or associated cardiac lesions, pre–balloon valvoplasty gradient, and use of the double-balloon technique did not independently predict follow-up outcome.[47] Other investigators[60] found that intervention in patients with a systolic gradient between 40 and 60 mm Hg achieved a lower long-term gradient and fewer late symptoms.

Data from the Valvuloplasty and Angioplasty of Congenital Anomalies (VACA) Registry study[59] suggest that the significant residual gradients are usually located at the infundibular level and that the higher the degree of obstruction before valvoplasty, the higher the infundibular gradient immediately after balloon pulmonary valvoplasty. Regression of infundibular hypertrophy has been associated with resolution of residual gradient in many patients.[32, 57, 58, 61-63]

Results of balloon pulmonary valvoplasty for patients with a dysplastic pulmonary valve are variable and may depend on the relative contribution to the degree of obstruc-

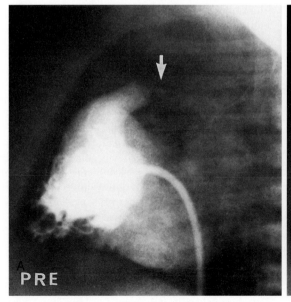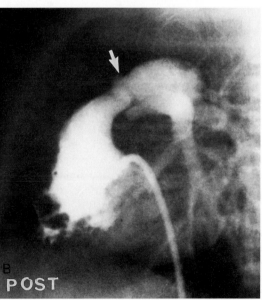

FIGURE 36–2

Right ventriculogram in a lateral projection showing severe valvar pulmonic stenosis. *A,* Before balloon valvoplasty. *Arrow* shows severe obstruction with minimal passage of contrast medium across the valve. *B,* After balloon valvoplasty. *Arrow* shows valve with good filling of pulmonary arteries.

tion made by the thickened and immobile leaflets, the nodular tissue in the leaflet, the sinuses, and the commissural fusion, all of which may form a continuum with typical pulmonic stenosis. Because the degree of valve fusion is difficult to define, in the absence of a hypoplastic annulus (<75% of that predicted for age and body surface area) and perhaps the finding of a dilated pulmonary trunk, balloon valvoplasty should be attempted.[32,34,64–69] Although undersized balloons may be associated with a poor acute result, the use of oversized balloons increases the risk of valve disruption, outflow tract damage, and vascular complications.[70] Unsuccessful results were generally due to inability to cross the valve, especially in neonates.

Few major complications occur beyond the neonatal period. In the VACA Registry,[59] among 822 children, there were only five major complications (0.6%), including two deaths, one cardiac perforation with tamponade, and two new occurrences of tricuspid insufficiency. These complications were observed in infants and neonates. Other complications are complete heart block,[71,72] transient prolongation of the QTc interval,[73] right-sided endocarditis,[74] and transient pulmonary hypertension.[75] Transient systemic hypotension and arrhythmias can occur during the dilatation process.[76–78] A long-term success rate of 86% was noted, confirming the long-term effectiveness of balloon pulmonary valvoplasty.[34,79] Electrocardiographic evidence of regression of right ventricular hypertrophy provides further confirmation of the success of this intervention in relieving the excessive pressure load imposed on the right ventricle.[33] At follow-up, most patients show echocardiographic evidence of pulmonary insufficiency, although this is usually trivial to mild.[32,34,52]

Acute and midterm results have been as good in neonates as in older patients. Successful dilatation occurs in up to 95% of neonates.[79–95] In some neonates, the smaller and noncompliant right ventricle may be inadequate for maintaining a normal pulmonary blood flow. Prolonged prostaglandin infusion for up to 3 weeks gives time for the right ventricular compliance to increase after regression of its hypertrophy. If cyanosis persists (oxygen saturation <80%) after 3 weeks of prostaglandin infusion, a systemic-to-pulmonary artery shunt should be placed.

Complications are more common in neonates than in older patients, with a mortality rate of 3%, major complications 3.5%, and minor complications 15%.[32,78–89] On longer follow-up, about 10 to 15% of patients need reintervention,[78–89] either repeated balloon dilatation or surgery for either infundibular stenosis or a dysplastic valve. Morphologic follow-up studies have confirmed that the valve matures from its dysplastic appearance, and the annulus and right ventricular cavity grow.[94] The results compare favorably with operation.[95] Thus, we currently consider balloon valvoplasty the treatment of choice in neonates with isolated critical valvar pulmonic stenosis, regardless of mild right ventricular hypoplasia or valve morphology.

With this experience, balloon valvoplasty of the pulmonary valve has similarly been applied as a palliative approach in children with complex forms of cyanotic heart disease, especially in tetralogy of Fallot.[96–100] This approach is effective in improving pulmonary blood flow and oxygen saturation. The pulmonary annulus and pulmonary

arteries grow.[96,101–105] The experience in adults confirms the technical simplicity and hemodynamic improvement seen in the pediatric age groups.[22,63,101–111]

PERIPHERAL PULMONIC STENOSIS

Peripheral pulmonic stenosis (PPS) may occur at a single site or, more commonly, at multiple sites of obstruction. The stenosis may be present at any level above the pulmonary valve and may involve one or many pulmonary artery branches. In a simplified classification,[112] four types of obstruction were described: (1) stenosis of the pulmonary trunk, (2) bifurcation stenosis extending into the right or left pulmonary arteries (or both), (3) multiple peripheral pulmonary artery stenoses, and (4) stenoses of both the pulmonary trunk and peripheral arteries. PPS may be sporadic or familial; it may occur as an isolated lesion (40%) or in combination with other cardiac lesions (60%). These associated lesions include valvar pulmonic stenosis, atrial septal defect, ventricular septal defect, and patent ductus arteriosus; about 20% of patients with tetralogy of Fallot have associated PPS. Other complex-associated lesions include mitral obstruction and transposition of the great arteries.

Another important association is with supravalvar aortic stenosis.[113] We believe this association is more common than is usually recognized, and it should be carefully evaluated in all patients with PPS. The combination is classically present in the Williams syndrome. It is also present as the central feature of a developmental complex that includes supravalvar stenosis of the aorta and pulmonary trunk, dysplasia of valves, and stenosis of ostia of coronary arteries and branches of the aortic arch.[114] In this complex, histologic examination of the aorta and major pulmonary arteries showed two patterns that may alternate from segment to segment in a given patient. One pattern is of a mosaic orientation of medial elements, and the other pattern is of thickening of the media that appears to have an excess number of units of elastic and intervening layers.

Other syndromes that have PPS as an important feature include the rubella, Alagille, Keutel,[115] cutis laxa, Noonan, and Ehlers-Danlos syndromes.

Functional or *physiologic* PPS is a relatively common feature in both premature and full-term neonates. The stenosis, evidenced by the typical murmur and a small gradient (echo Doppler), is mild. With time, these arteries grow, and the murmur usually disappears within a few months and almost invariably is gone by the first birthday.

In premature infants, closure of the ductus arteriosus has been proposed as the determining factor in the occurrence of PPS. Gradients not present after birth in preterm infants may appear after ductal closure.

HEMODYNAMICS

The hemodynamics resembles valvar pulmonic stenosis. Proximal to the obstruction, the systolic pressure is elevated, and distally, it is normal or low. Thus, depending on the degree of obstruction, the systolic pressure is elevated in the right ventricle and also in the pulmonary artery proximal to the obstruction. The diastolic pressure is low and equal in the pulmonary artery both proximal and distal to the obstruction, so that the pressure tracing in the proximal pulmonary artery resembles the right ventricular pressure contour, although the diastolic pressure is not zero.

As a result of the elevated pressure, right ventricular hypertrophy develops, and the right atrium may also enlarge. The degree of obstruction varies from mild to severe. The severity does not usually change with time. In some patients, especially with the Williams syndrome, a decrease in gradient may occur.

CLINICAL FEATURES

The general appearance is either normal or that of the associated syndrome involved with possible typical facial features of the Noonan, rubella, Williams, or Alagille syndromes. Growth and development are normal in most patients or possibly delayed in the syndromes. Most patients are asymptomatic. With severe obstruction, fatigue or dyspnea on exertion is usually present. Signs of congestive cardiac failure are rare. Decreased compliance of the right ventricle may be associated with a right-to-left shunt at the atrial level and cyanosis. In mild to moderate stenosis, no thrills or heaves are palpable; with severe obstruction, a right ventricular heave may be palpable.

The first heart sound is normal. The second sound is split, the width intensifying with the increasing severity of the stenosis. No ejection click is present. Typically, the murmur is absent or soft over the precordium. It is heard below both clavicles. Of particular importance is the wide distribution of the murmur over the back and axillae; this is often the clinical clue to diagnosis. With multiple PPS or an associated left-to-right shunt, a continuous murmur may be present and widely distributed over the precordium, back, and axillae. Its intensity varies, depending on the degree of stenosis.

ELECTROCARDIOGRAPHY

The electrocardiographic features are similar to those of valvar pulmonic stenosis. They vary from normal to those of severe right ventricular hypertrophy and even "strain" pattern.

RADIOLOGIC FEATURES

Pulmonary vasculature is usually normal regardless of severity, although decreased vasculature may be present in severe stenosis. The main pulmonary artery segment is not prominent (as opposed to valvar stenosis). In severe unilateral stenosis, a difference may be seen between the two lung fields. Often with marked differences of stenosis in the two lungs, no significant differences in vasculature may be evident.

Radioisotope studies[116,117] are useful in determining the degree of perfusion to each lobe and are a more reliable indicator of the relative stenoses (Fig. 36–3).

ECHOCARDIOGRAPHY

Narrowing of the pulmonary artery branches may be present in either diffuse or discrete forms. The proximal right

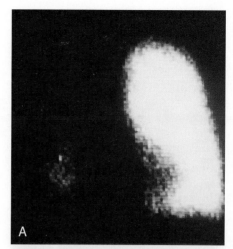

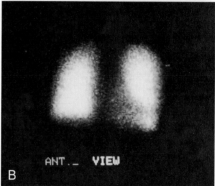

FIGURE 36–3

Pulmonary scintigram of peripheral right pulmonary artery stenosis. *A*, Markedly decreased perfusion of right lung before dilatation. *B*, Markedly improved perfusion of right lung after balloon dilatation of right pulmonary artery.

and left pulmonary arteries may be imaged from the suprasternal, high parasternal short-axis, or subxiphoid view (Fig. 36–4). Flow into the narrow pulmonary artery branches is anterograde throughout the cardiac cycle, and this causes a characteristic systolic-diastolic high-velocity flow on Doppler study. The systolic Doppler gradient across a long obstruction is unreliable, but the severity of the narrowing may be assessed by the right ventricular systolic pressure.

CARDIAC CATHETERIZATION

Cardiac catheterization is important to confirm the diagnosis of PPS and may sometimes be an important therapeutic modality with balloon angioplasty and endovascular stent implantation. The indications for cardiac catheterization are symptoms or noninvasive evidence of right ventricular hypertension (>80% systemic pressure) and assessment after surgical repair (e.g., after repair of tetralogy of Fallot or the Fontan operation).

Carefully obtained withdrawal pressure tracings from the distal branches demonstrate systolic pressure gradients across the narrowest segment of the arteries. Systolic pressure gradients more than 10 mm Hg are considered abnormal. With unilateral stenosis, a pressure gradient is usually

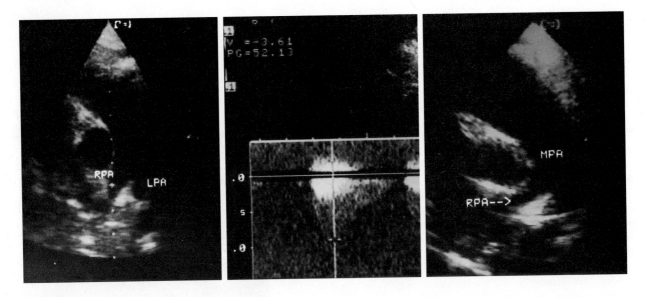

FIGURE 36–4

Echocardiogram showing peripheral stenosis of the pulmonary artery. *Left,* Parasternal short-axis view shows a normal-sized pulmonary trunk and small origin of its major branches. *Middle,* Doppler recording shows a jet peaking in systole to 52 mm Hg but extending throughout diastole. *Right,* Small right pulmonary artery is obtained with a clockwise rotation of the transducer. LPA = left pulmonary artery; MPA = main pulmonary artery; RPA = right pulmonary artery.

present across the narrowed segment, with the proximal pulmonary artery pressure being elevated. Sometimes, pressure is elevated in the contralateral pulmonary artery as well. The pressure tracing proximal to the obstruction has a contour similar to that of the right ventricle in length and time up to the dicrotic notch; it also has a wide pulse pressure that becomes more pronounced with increasing severity of the obstruction. Unlike a ventricular pressure tracing, diastolic pressure is not near zero.

ANGIOGRAPHY

Selective angiography is important to define the exact location, extent, and distribution of the lesions in each pulmonary artery. The right pulmonary artery is best seen in the anteroposterior view and the left pulmonary artery in the left anterior oblique view with cranial angulation. Demonstration of stenosis in the main pulmonary artery and the origin of both left and right pulmonary arteries requires cranial angulation. Aortography should be performed to exclude the presence of frequently associated systemic arterial stenosis.

TREATMENT

Mild or moderate unilateral or bilateral PPS does not usually require treatment. The indications for treatment of severe PPS include the following: cardiovascular symptoms, such as exercise intolerance, dyspnea, cyanosis, or signs of right-sided heart failure; near-systemic (or higher) right ventricular pressure; markedly decreased flow to affected lung segments, as assessed by radionuclide scans; hypertension in the unobstructed pulmonary artery; and documented stenosis in distal pulmonary arteries not easily accessible by an approach as a surgical prelude to definitive repair of a coexistent cardiac anomaly.[118, 119]

An operation performed to directly relieve pulmonary artery stenosis has been found to be difficult and often ineffective with a success rate of approximately 30%.[120–122] In the surgical approach, a pericardial or Dacron ellipsoid patch is used to widen the lumen of the vessel. Furthermore, the surgical approach is confined to a small group of patients with well-localized stenosis of the pulmonary trunk or bifurcation of the origins of the main branch pulmonary arteries. The intraparenchymal pulmonary arteries are surgically inaccessible. For patients with multiple PPS or hypoplastic pulmonary arteries, there is no surgical alternative; therefore, the interventional options such as balloon angioplasty and endovascular stent placement have been developed.

Successful angioplasty results in longitudinal or oblique intimal tears, medial disruption, and, in some patients, transmedial tears, with organization of intramural hemorrhage and scar formation as the mode of healing.[123, 124] Pseudoendothelialization is complete in 3 to 6 weeks; areas of mural thinning within the scar may predispose to aneurysm formation. After angioplasty, perivascular fibrosis may reinforce the outer vessel wall, but several months must pass to allow complete tissue granulation and healing of transmedial tears induced by catheter intervention.[124, 125] The techniques are described in detail in Chapter 13.

Balloon dilatation is usually well tolerated and should be considered an initial form of intervention (Fig. 36–5). Acute technical success is judged by the modified criteria of the Boston group[118] and includes at least two of the following criteria: an increase in vessel diameter of more than 50% of the predilatation diameter, an increase of more than 20% in the relative blood flow to the affected lung, and a decrease to less than 60% of the systolic right ventricular/aortic pressure ratio. Balloon angioplasty for PPS has been effective with use of these criteria in 50 to 60% of the patients.[118, 119] Restenosis occurs in 15 to 20% of patients[118, 119] and a long-term favorable result is achieved in 35 to 50% of patients[119, 126] by the following criteria: resolution of the stenosis and avoidance of surgical

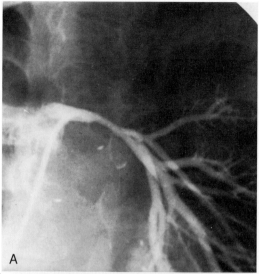

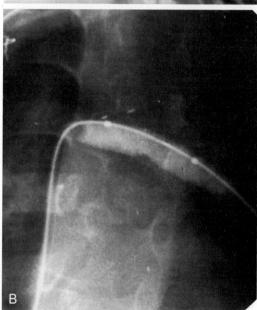

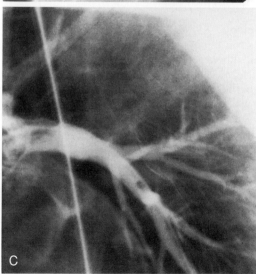

FIGURE 36-5

Peripheral stenosis of left pulmonary artery. *A,* Right ventriculogram shows narrow left pulmonary artery. *B,* Inflated balloon in proximal left pulmonary artery. *C,* Angiogram shows successfully dilated left pulmonary artery.

intervention; optimization of future surgical intervention, judged by one of two standards: (1) pulmonary artery anatomy or pressure suitable for surgical repair in patients with pulmonary artery anatomy or pressure that was previously considered a contraindication for surgical repair or (2) obviation of the need for surgical intervention in the areas of balloon angioplasty during the succeeding surgical repairs and reduction of the systolic right ventricular/aortic pressure ratio to less than 60%.[127,128] Lung perfusion scintigraphy is a relatively easy noninvasive method for accurate determination of relative pulmonary blood flows,[116,117] allowing the clinician to plan and follow up transcatheter interventions in the pulmonary arteries.[118,119,126,127] Clinicians must, however, be aware of the anatomic or technical limitations of the scanning results; "washout" effect from additional blood supply to the lung can cause inaccuracy of the scan.

Significant complications may follow percutaneous balloon angioplasty of PPS.[125–129] These complications include a mortality rate of about 1 to 2%, usually from exsanguination from a ruptured pulmonary artery during dilatation; other complications include hemoptysis, transient pulmonary edema, clotted iliac veins, pulmonary artery aneurysm, cyanosis, and hypotension. Late death may also occur from aneurysm rupture.*

Even after a technically successful procedure, these patients require careful serial evaluation and may need follow-up cardiac catheterization to evaluate accurately the midterm and long-term results of the angioplasty procedure. Patients who develop aneurysms should be observed even more closely because the prognosis of these aneurysms remains unknown.

ENDOVASCULAR STENTS

The incidence of recurrent narrowing after balloon angioplasty (about 17%) could be related to the elastic recoil of the pulmonary artery wall. The efficacy of endovascular stents[132–135] to relieve such obstructions and the safety of implantation have been demonstrated with a success rate above 96% (Fig. 36–6).

Major complications are few but include death from fatal pulmonary artery embolism and embolization of incorrectly placed stents.[136–139] Minor complications include occlusion of side branches,[136,139] longitudinal break of the stent during redilatation, acute thrombosis of the pulmonary artery distal to the stent that resolves after thrombolytic therapy, and balloon rupture during expansion.[133]

SUBVALVAR STENOSIS

Two main types of obstruction may occur within the right ventricle.

ISOLATED INFUNDIBULAR STENOSIS

This rare condition consists of narrowing of the infundibulum. The narrowing is fibromuscular in type.

*References 118, 119, 125, 127, 130, 131.

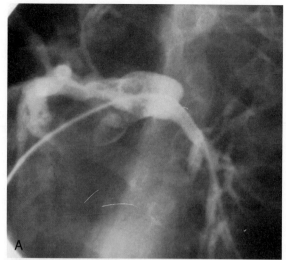

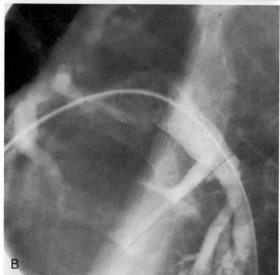

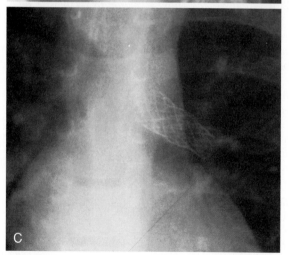

FIGURE 36–6

Peripheral pulmonary artery stenosis. *A,* Pulmonary arteriogram shows stenosis of left pulmonary artery. *B,* Dilated left pulmonary artery with stent. *C,* Chest radiograph shows stent in position in left pulmonary artery.

Physiology

The hemodynamics resembles that of other right-sided obstructions with a gradient being present within the right ventricle, causing hypertrophy of the proximal chamber. Clinically, the general features are similar to valvar stenosis. The features of right ventricular hypertrophy depend on severity of obstruction. The murmur is systolic ejection and heard along the left sternal border or in the pulmonary area. In severe stenosis, cyanosis develops from a right-to-left shunt at the atrial level.

The absence of an ejection click and the often lower position of the murmur help in the differentiation from valvar stenosis. The murmur is often harsher than in valvar stenosis. The second sound is usually narrowly split. The electrocardiogram is nondiagnostic, depending on the degree of right ventricular hypertrophy. The chest radiograph shows normal cardiac size. No dilatation of pulmonary arteries is present; the pulmonary vasculature is usually normal. The apex may be elevated in severe stenosis.

Echocardiography

An infundibular subpulmonic obstruction may be present transiently after relief of valvar pulmonic stenosis. A characteristic Doppler jet with a concave downstroke is indicative of a dynamic subvalvar narrowing (Fig. 36–7). When a fixed obstruction is present, the jet has a regular, convex downstroke.

Natural History

The degree of obstruction tends to increase with age.

Treatment

Treatment is surgical with good results.

ANOMALOUS MUSCLE BUNDLES

The other form of stenosis within the right ventricle is anomalous muscle bundles.

Physiology

In this condition, muscle bundles divide the ventricle into two chambers (hence, the synonym *two-chambered right ventricle*).[140] The muscle bundles pass from the septal wall close to the base of the anterior papillary muscle to the anterior wall of the right ventricle. A ventricular septal defect is present in most patients, although in some, the muscle bundles may functionally close the septal defect. In addition, a discrete membranous subaortic membrane completes a triad of commonly associated pathologic findings.

The severity of right ventricular obstruction often progresses (as may the coexistent subaortic stenosis). Clinically, the patients are usually asymptomatic. The position of the ventricular septal defect may occasionally affect the clinical picture. If the septal defect is situated above the muscle bundles, a left-to-right shunt may predominate and even lead to heart failure. However, right-to-left shunting may be present only occasionally when the septal defect is below the muscle bundles.

The most striking clinical feature is a long, usually harsh, ejection systolic murmur heard along the left sternal

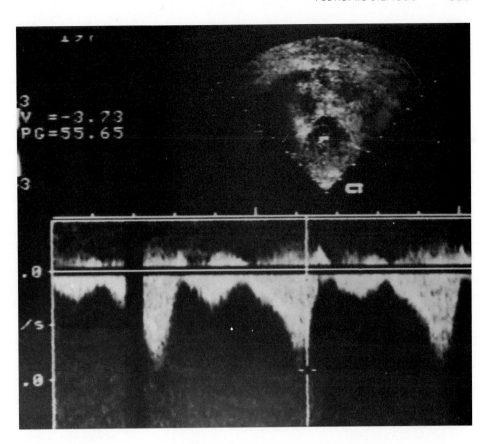

FIGURE 36-7
Echocardiogram of a dynamic subvalvar pulmonic stenosis. Doppler recording shows concave downstrike typical of dynamic nature.

border, possibly radiating to the pulmonary area. A thrill is often present. The heart sounds are usually normal. A systolic click is not audible. The electrocardiogram shows different degrees of right ventricular hypertrophy, depending on severity of the obstruction. The radiographic features are nonspecific.

Echocardiography
On echocardiography, the muscle bundle may be well imaged from a subxiphoid short-axis or a right anterior oblique view, which can be obtained by counterclockwise rotation of the transducer. The severity of the obstruction may be assessed by continuous-wave Doppler imaging.

Cardiac Catheterization
Usually no evidence of shunt is found. On occasion, left-to-right or right-to-left shunting may be present. A pressure gradient is measured by catheter withdrawal.

Angiocardiography
The muscle bundles are characteristically demonstrated by filling defects in the right ventricle. The left-to-right or right-to-left shunt may also be demonstrated.

Treatment
When indicated by the severity of the gradient, treatment is surgical with removal of the muscle bundles. A characteristic dimple is the surgical landmark of the muscle bundle attachment to the right ventricular free wall. The associated ventricular septal defect is closed, and the subaortic membrane is excised.

RARE CAUSES OF RIGHT VENTRICULAR OBSTRUCTION

Rare additional causes of right ventricular obstruction include the following:

- Pouch-like structures in the right ventricle, such as the "windsock" lesion.
- Tumors in the right ventricle—rhabdomyoma.
- Prolapse of right aortic cusp through a ventricular septal defect.
- Sinus of Valsalva aneurysm, which may prolapse into the right ventricular outflow region.[141]

IDIOPATHIC DILATATION OF THE PULMONARY ARTERY

Although it may seem incongruous to include this entity, we do so because we believe it may represent an extremely mild form of valvar pulmonic stenosis associated with marked dilatation of the pulmonary trunk. Because the obstruction is mild, secondary hemodynamic effects are not evident.

The patients are always asymptomatic and usually examined because of a murmur or finding on the chest radiograph. Clinical findings may be those of mild pulmonic stenosis: systolic ejection click, normal first and second heart sounds, and a soft systolic ejection murmur at the upper left sternal border; a soft diastolic murmur of pulmonary insufficiency may occasionally be audible. Electrocardiography is normal; the chest radiograph shows a dilated pulmonary artery. Echocardiography shows a small pulmonic valve gradient, with occasional insufficiency and a greatly dilated pulmonary artery.

REFERENCES

1. Driscoll DJ, Michels VJ, Gersony WM, Hayes CT: Occurrence risk for congenital heart defect in relatives of patients with aortic stenosis, pulmonary stenosis or ventricular septal defect. Circulation 87(suppl 1):114, 1993.
2. Rodriquez-Fernandez HL, Char F, Kelly AT, Rowe RD: The dysplastic pulmonary valve and neonatal syndrome. Circulation 98(suppl II):45, 1972.
3. Koretzky ED, Moller JH, Korns ME, et al: Congenital pulmonary stenosis resulting from dysplasia of the valve. Circulation 40:43, 1969.
4. Edwards JE: Congenital malformations of the heart and great vessels. In Gould SE (ed): Pathology of the Heart. Springfield, IL, Charles C Thomas, 1960, pp 391–397.
5. Campbell M: Factors in the aetiology of pulmonary stenosis. Br Heart J 24:625, 1962.
6. Francioso RA, Blanc WA: Myocardial infarct in infants and children. I. A necropsy study in infants and children. J Pediatr 73:309, 1968.
7. Rudolph AM: Congenital Diseases of the Heart. Chicago, Year Book, 1974.
8. Raghib G, Amplatz K, Moller JH, et al: Hypoplasia of right ventricle and of tricuspid valve. Am Heart J 70:806, 1965.
9. Leatham A, Weitzman D: Auscultatory and phonocardiographic signs of pulmonic stenosis. Br Heart J 19:303, 1957.
10. Vogelpoel L, Schrire V: Auscultatory and phonocardiographic assessment of pulmonary stenosis with intact ventricular septum. Circulation 22:55, 1960.
11. Bassingthwaighte JB, Parkin TW, Dushane JW, et al: The electrocardiographic and hemodynamic findings in pulmonary stenosis with intact ventricular septum. Circulation 28:893, 1963.
12. Schneeweiss A, Shem-tov A, Blieden LC, et al: Diagnostic angiographic criteria in pulmonic stenosis due to dysplastic pulmonary valve. Am Heart J 106:761, 1983.
13. Hayes CJ, Gersony WM, Driscoll DJ, et al: Results of treatment of patients with pulmonary valve stenosis. Circulation 87(suppl I):28, 1993.
14. Driscoll DF, Wolfe RR, Gersony WM, Hayes CJ: Cardiorespiratory response to exercise of patients with aortic stenosis, pulmonary stenosis and ventricular septal defect. Circulation 87(suppl I):102, 1993.
15. Wennevold A, Jacobsen JR: Natural history of valvular pulmonary stenosis in children below the age of two years: Long-term follow-up with serial heart catheterization. Eur J Cardiol 83:371, 1978.
16. Hayes CJ, Gersony WM, Driscoll DJ: Second natural history study of congenital heart defects: Results of treatment of patients with pulmonary valvar stenosis. Circulation 87(suppl I):28, 1993.
17. Mody MR: The natural history of uncomplicated valvular pulmonic stenosis. Am Heart J 90:317, 1975.
18. Tinker J, Howitt G, Markman P, Wade EG: The natural history of isolated pulmonary stenosis. Br Heart J 27:151, 1965.
19. Nugent EW, Freedom RM, Nora JJ, et al: Clinical course in pulmonary stenosis. Circulation 56(suppl I):38, 1977.
20. Johnson LW, Grossman W, Dalen JE, Dexter L: Pulmonic stenosis in the adult. Long-term follow-up results. N Engl J Med 287:1159, 1972.
21. Engle MA, Ito T, Goldberg HP: The fate of the patient with pulmonic stenosis. Circulation 30:554, 1964.
22. Shrivastava S, Kumar K, Dev V, et al: Pulmonary balloon valvotomy for severe valvular pulmonic stenosis with congestive heart failure beyond infancy. Cathet Cardiovasc Diagn 28:137, 1993.
23. Gersony WM, Bernard WF, Nadas AS, Gross RE: Diagnosis and surgical treatment of infants with critical pulmonary outflow obstruction. Circulation 35:767, 1967.
24. Freed MD, Rosenthal A, Bernhard WF, et al: Critical pulmonary stenosis with a diminutive right ventricle in neonates. Circulation 48:875, 1973.
25. Gersony WM, Bernhard WF, Nadas AS, Gross RE: Diagnosis and surgical treatment of pulmonic stenosis. Circulation 13:765, 1967.

26. Kan SJ, White RI Jr, Mitchell SE, Gardner TJ: Percutaneous balloon valvuloplasty: A new method for treating congenital pulmonary valve stenosis. N Engl J Med 307:540, 1982.
27. Lock JE, Keane JF, Fellows KE: Diagnostic and Interventional Catheterization in Congenital Heart Disease. Boston, Martinus Nijhoff, 1987.
28. Rao PS (ed): Cardiac interventions in the pediatric patient. J Invas Cardiol 8:278, 1996.
29. Benson LN, Smallhorn JS, Freedom RM, et al: Pulmonary valve morphology after balloon dilation of pulmonary valve stenosis. Cathet Cardiovasc Diagn 11:161, 1985.
30. Lababidi Z, Wu JR: Percutaneous balloon pulmonary valvuloplasty. Am J Cardiol 52:560, 1983.
31. Walls JT, Lababidi Z, Curtis JJ, Silver D: Assessment of percutaneous balloon pulmonary and aortic valvuloplasty. J Thorac Cardiovasc Surg 88:352, 1984.
32. Stanger P, Cassidy SC, Girod DA, et al: Balloon pulmonary valvuloplasty: Results of the Valvuloplasty and Angioplasty of Congenital Anomalies Registry. Am J Cardiol 65:775, 1990.
33. Kan JS, White RI, Mitchel SE, et al: Percutaneous transluminal balloon valvuloplasty for pulmonary valve stenosis. Circulation 69:554, 1984.
34. McCrindle B, Kan SJ: Long-term results after balloon pulmonary valvuloplasty. Circulation 83:1915, 1991.
35. O'Connor BK, Beekman RH, Lindauer A, Rocchini A: Intermediate-term outcome after pulmonary balloon valvuloplasty. Comparison with a matched surgical control group. J Am Coll Cardiol 20:169, 1992.
36. Witsenburg M, Talsma M, Rohmer J, Hess J: Balloon valvuloplasty for valvular pulmonary stenosis in children over 6 months of age: Initial results and long-term follow up. Eur Heart J 14:1657, 1993.
37. Elliott JM, Tuzcu EM: Recent developments in balloon valvuloplasty techniques. Curr Opin Cardiol 10:128, 1995.
38. Ettedgui JA, Ho SY, Tynan M, et al: The pathology of balloon pulmonary valvuloplasty. Int J Cardiol 16:285, 1987.
39. Lau KW, Hung JS: Controversies in percutaneous balloon pulmonary valvuloplasty: Timing, patient selection and technique. J Heart Valve Dis 2:321, 1993.
40. Ali Khan MA, al-Yousef S, Moore JW, Sawyer W: Results of repeat percutaneous balloon valvuloplasty for pulmonary valvar stenosis. Am Heart J 120:878, 1990.
41. Rao PS: Balloon pulmonary valvuloplasty: A review. Clin Cardiol 12:55, 1989.
42. Miller GA: Balloon valvuloplasty and angioplasty in congenital heart disease. Br Heart J 54:285, 1985.
43. Sullivan ID, Robinson PJ, Macartney FJ, et al: Percutaneous balloon valvuloplasty for pulmonary valve stenosis in infants and children. Br Heart J 54:435, 1985.
44. Hwang B, Chen LY, Lu JH, Meng CC: A quantitative analysis of the structure of right ventricle–pulmonary artery junction for balloon pulmonary valvuloplasty in children. Angiology 46:383, 1995.
45. Jaing TL, Hwang B, Lu JH, et al: Percutaneous balloon valvuloplasty in severe pulmonary valvular stenosis. Angiology 46:503, 1995.
46. Medina A, Bethencourt A, Olalla E, et al: Intraoperative balloon valvuloplasty in pulmonary valve stenosis. Cardiovasc Intervent Radiol 12:199, 1989.
47. Melgares R, Prieto JA, Azpitarte J: Success determining factors in percutaneous transluminal balloon valvuloplasty of pulmonary valve stenosis. Eur Heart J 12:15, 1991.
48. Cazzaniga M, Vagnola O, Aldayl O, et al: Balloon pulmonary valvuloplasty in infants: A quantitative analysis of pulmonary valve-anulus-trunk structure. J Am Coll Cardiol 20:345, 1992.
49. Fedderly RT, Beekman RH III: Balloon valvuloplasty for pulmonary valvuloplasty. J Intervent Cardiol 8:451, 1995.
50. Rao PS: Balloon pulmonary valvuloplasty for isolated pulmonic stenosis. In Rao PS (ed): Transcatheter Therapy in Pediatric Cardiology. New York, Wiley-Liss, 1993, p 59.
51. Burrows PE, Benson LN, Smallhorn JF, et al: Angiographic features associated with percutaneous balloon valvotomy for pulmonary valve stenosis. Cardiovasc Intervent Radiol 11:111, 1988.
52. Masura J, Burch M, Deanfield JE, Sullivan ID: Five-year follow-up after balloon pulmonary valvuloplasty. J Am Coll Cardiol 21:132, 1993.
53. Schmaltz AA, Bein G, Gravinghoff L, et al: Balloon valvuloplasty of pulmonary stenosis in infants and children—co-operative study of

the German Society of Pediatric Cardiology. Eur Heart J 10:967, 1989.

54. Rocchini AP, Kveselis DA, Crowley D, et al: Percutaneous balloon valvuloplasty for treatment of congenital pulmonary valvular stenosis in children. J Am Coll Cardiol 3:1005, 1984.

55. Tynan M, Baker EJ, Rohmer J, et al: Percutaneous balloon pulmonary valvuloplasty. Br Heart J 53:520, 1985.

56. Rao PS, Fawzy ME, Solymar L, Mardini MK: Long-term results of balloon pulmonary valvuloplasty of valvar pulmonic stenosis. Am Heart J 115:1291, 1988.

57. Mullins CE, Ludomirsky A, O'Laughlin MP, et al: Balloon valvuloplasty for pulmonic valve stenosis. Two-year follow-up: Hemodynamic and Doppler evaluation. Cathet Cardiovasc Diagn 14:76, 1988.

58. Fontes VF, Sousa EMR, Esteves CA, et al: Pulmonary valvoplasty—experience of 100 cases. Int J Cardiol 21:335, 1988.

59. McCrindle BW: Independent predictors of long-term results after balloon pulmonary valvuloplasty. Valvuloplasty and Angioplasty of Congenital Anomalies (VACA) Registry investigators. Circulation 89:1751, 1994.

60. Mendelson AM, Banerjee A, Meyer RA, Schwarz DC: Predictors of successful pulmonary balloon valvuloplasty: 10-year experience. Cathet Cardiovasc Diagn 39:236, 1996.

61. Ben-Shachar G, Cohen MH, Sivakof MC: Development of infundibular obstruction after percutaneous pulmonary balloon valvuloplasty. J Am Coll Cardiol 11:161, 1985.

62. Nakanishi T, Tsuji T, Nakazawa M, Momma K: Configurations of right ventricular pressure curves and infundibular stenosis after balloon pulmonary valvuloplasty. Cardiol Young 5:44, 1995.

63. Fawzy ME, Galal O, Dunn B, et al: Regression of infundibular pulmonary stenosis after successful balloon pulmonary valvuloplasty in adults. Cathet Cardiovasc Diagn 21:77, 1990.

64. Musewe NN, Robertson MA, Benson LN, et al: The dysplastic pulmonary valve: Echographic features and results of balloon dilatation. Br Heart J 57:364, 1987.

65. Ballerini L, Mullins CE, Cifarelli A, et al: Percutaneous balloon valvuloplasty of pulmonary valve stenosis, dysplasia, and residual stenosis after surgical valvotomy for pulmonary atresia with intact ventricular septum: Long-term results. Cathet Cardiovasc Diagn 19:165, 1990.

66. David SW, Goussous YM, Harbi N, et al: Management of typical and dysplastic pulmonic stenosis, uncomplicated or associated with complex intracardiac defects, in juveniles and adults: Use of percutaneous balloon pulmonary valvuloplasty with eight-month hemodynamic follow-up. Cathet Cardiovasc Diagn 12:105, 1993.

67. Rao PS: Balloon dilatation in infants and children with dysplastic pulmonary valves: Short-term and intermediate-term results. Am Heart J 116:1168, 1988.

68. Marantz PM, Huhta JC, Mullins CE, et al: Results of balloon valvuloplasty in typical and dysplastic pulmonary valve stenosis: Doppler and echocardiographic follow-up. Am J Coll Cardiol 12:476, 1988.

69. DiSessa TG, Alpert BS, Chase NA, et al: Balloon valvuloplasty in children with dysplastic pulmonary valves. Am J Cardiol 66:405, 1987.

70. Ring JC, Kulik TJ, Burke BA, Lock JE: Morphologic changes induced by dilation of the pulmonary valve anulus with overlarge balloons in normal newborn lambs. Am J Cardiol 55:210, 1984.

71. Lo RNS, Lau KC, Leung MP: Complete heart block after balloon dilatation for congenital pulmonary stenosis. Br Heart J 59:384, 1988.

72. Steinberg C, Levin AR, Engle MA: Transient complete heart block following percutaneous balloon pulmonary valvuloplasty: Treatment with systemic corticosteroids. Pediatr Cardiol 13:181, 1992.

73. Martin GR, Stanger P: Transient prolongation of the QTc interval after balloon valvuloplasty and angioplasty in children. Am J Cardiol 58:1233, 1986.

74. Kalra GS, Wander GS, Anand IS: Right sided endocarditis after balloon dilatation of the pulmonary valve. Br Heart J 63:368, 1990.

75. Bhagwat AG, Loya YS, Sharma S: Transient pulmonary hypertension following pulmonary balloon valvuloplasty. Am Heart J 123:1397, 1992.

76. Rao PS, Solymar L: Electrocardiographic changes following balloon dilatation of valvar pulmonic stenosis. J Intervent Cardiol 1:189, 1988.

77. Kveselis DA, Rocchini AP, Snider AR, et al: Results of balloon valvuloplasty in the treatment of congenital valvar pulmonary stenosis in children. Am J Cardiol 56:527, 1985.

78. Lloyd TR, Donnerstein RL: Rapid T-wave normalization after balloon pulmonary valvuloplasty in children. Am J Cardiol 64:399, 1989.

79. Zeevi B, Keane JF, Fellows KE, Lock JE: Balloon dilation of critical pulmonary stenosis in the first week of life. J Am Coll Cardiol 11:821, 1988.

80. Caspi J, Coles J, Benson L, et al: Management of neonatal critical pulmonary stenosis in the balloon valvotomy era. Ann Thorac Surg 49:273, 1990.

81. Ali Khan MA, al-Yousef S, Huhta JC, et al: Critical pulmonary valve stenosis in patients less than 1 year of age: Treatment with percutaneous gradational balloon pulmonary valvuloplasty. Am Heart J 117:1008, 1989.

82. Ladusans EJ, Qureshi SA, Parson JM, et al: Balloon dilation of critical stenosis of the pulmonary valve in neonates. Br Heart J 64:362, 1990.

83. Gournay V, Piechaud JF, Delogu A, et al: Balloon valvotomy for critical stenosis or atresia of pulmonary valve in newborns. J Am Coll Cardiol 26:1725, 1995.

84. Santoro G, Formigari R, Di Carlo D, et al: Midterm outcome after pulmonary balloon valvuloplasty in patients younger than one year of age. Am J Cardiol 75:637, 1995.

85. Fedderly RT, Lloyd TR, Mendelsohn AM, Beekman RH: Determinants of successful balloon valvotomy in infants with critical pulmonary stenosis or membranous pulmonary atresia with intact ventricular septum. J Am Coll Cardiol 25:460, 1995.

86. Talsma M, Wittenburg M, Rohmer J, Hess J: Determinants for outcome of balloon valvuloplasty for severe pulmonary stenosis in neonates and infants up to six months of age. Am J Cardiol 71:1246, 1997.

87. Colli AM, Perry SB, Lock JE, Keane JF: Balloon dilation of critical pulmonary stenosis in the first month of life. Cathet Cardiovasc Diagn 34:23, 1995.

88. Gildein HP, Kleinert S, Goh TH, Wilkinson JL: Treatment of critical pulmonary valve stenosis by balloon dilatation in the neonate. Am Heart J 131:1007, 1996.

89. Rao PS: Balloon valvuloplasty in the neonate with critical pulmonary stenosis (Editorial). J Am Coll Cardiol 27:479, 1996.

90. Burzynski JB, Kveselis DA, Byrum CJ, et al: Modified technique for balloon valvuloplasty of critical pulmonary stenosis in the newborn. J Am Coll Cardiol 19:947, 1994.

91. Weber HS, Cyran SE, Gleason MM, et al: Critical pulmonary valve stenosis in the neonate: A technique to facilitate balloon dilatation Am J Cardiol 73:310, 1994.

92. Latson L, Cheatham J, Froemming S, Kugler J: Transductal guidewire "rail" for balloon valvuloplasty in neonates with isolated critical pulmonary valve stenosis or atresia. Am J Cardiol 73:713, 1994.

93. Zellers TM, Moake L, Wright J: Use of the Terumo SP catheter system for crossing the pulmonary valve in infants with critical pulmonary valve stenosis. Am J Cardiol 76:1082, 1995.

94. Tabatabaei H, Boutin C, Nykanen DG, et al: Morphologic and hemodynamic consequences after percutaneous balloon valvotomy for neonatal pulmonary stenosis: Medium-term results. J Am Coll Cardiol 27:473, 1996.

95. Hanley FL, Sade RM, Freedom RM, et al: Outcomes in critically ill neonates with pulmonary stenosis and intact ventricular septum. A multi-institutional study. J Am Coll Cardiol 22:183, 1993.

96. Rao PS, Brais M: Balloon pulmonary valvuloplasty for congenital cyanotic heart defects. Am Heart J 115:1105, 1988.

97. Rao PS, Wilson AD, Thapar MK, Brais M: Balloon pulmonary valvuloplasty in the management of cyanotic congenital heart defects. Cathet Cardiovasc Diagn 25:16, 1992.

98. Boucek MM, Webster HE, Orsmond GS, Ruttenberg HD: Balloon pulmonary valvotomy: Palliation for cyanotic heart disease. Am Heart J 115:318, 1988.

99. Qureshi SA, Kirk CR, Lamb RK, et al: Balloon dilatation of the pulmonary valve in the first year of life in patients with tetralogy of Fallot: A preliminary study. Br Heart J 60:232, 1988.

100. Sreeram N, Saleem M, Jackson M, et al: Results of balloon pulmonary valvuloplasty as a palliative procedure in tetralogy of Fallot. J Am Coll Cardiol 18:159, 1991.

101. Parsons JM, Ladusans EJ, Qureshi SA: Growth of the pulmonary artery after neonatal balloon dilatation of the right ventricular outflow tract in an infant with the tetralogy of Fallot and atrioventricular septal defect. Br Heart J 62:65, 1989.

102. Battistessa SA, Robles A, Jackson M, et al: Operative findings after percutaneous pulmonary balloon dilatation of the right ventricular outflow tract in tetralogy of Fallot. Br Heart J 64:321, 1990.

103. Sluysmans T, Neven B, Rubay J, et al: Early balloon dilatation of the pulmonary valve in infants with tetralogy of Fallot. Risks and benefits. Circulation 91:1506, 1995.

104. Stumper O, Piechaud JF, Bonhoeffer P, et al: Pulmonary balloon valvuloplasty in the palliation of complex cyanotic congenital heart disease. Heart 76:364, 1996.

105. Kreutzer J, Perry SB, Jonas RA, et al: Tetralogy of Fallot with diminutive pulmonary arteries: Preoperative pulmonary valve dilation and transcatheter rehabilitation of pulmonary arteries. J Am Coll Cardiol 27:1741, 1996.

106. Kaul UA, Singh B, Tyagi S, et al: Long-term results after balloon pulmonary valvuloplasty in adults. Am Heart J 126:1152, 1993.

107. Lau KWE, Hung JS, Wu JJ, et al: Pulmonary valvuloplasty in adults using the Inoue balloon catheter. Cathet Cardiovasc Diagn 29:99, 1993.

108. Fawzy ME, Mercer EN, Dunn B: Late results of pulmonary balloon valvuloplasty in adults using double balloon techniques. J Intervent Cardiol 1:35, 1988.

109. Sherman W, Hershman R, Alexopoulos D, et al: Pulmonic balloon valvuloplasty in adults. Am Heart J 119:187, 1990.

110. Herrmann HC, Hill JA, Krol J, et al: Effectiveness of percutaneous balloon valvuloplasty in adults with pulmonic valve stenosis. Am J Cardiol 68:1111, 1991.

111. Chen CR, Cheng TO, Huang T, et al: Percutaneous balloon valvuloplasty for pulmonic stenosis in adolescents and adults. N Engl J Med 335:21, 1996.

112. Gay BB, Franch RH, Shuford WH, Rogers JV: Roentgenologic features of simple and multiple coarctations of the pulmonary artery and its branches. AJR Am J Roentgenol 90:599, 1963.

113. Bourassa MG, Campeau L: Combined supravalvar aortic and pulmonic stenosis. Circulation 28:572, 1963.

114. Blieden LC, Lucas RV Jr, Miller JB, et al: A developmental complex including supravalvar stenosis of the aorta and pulmonary trunk. Circulation 49:585, 1974.

115. Keutel J, Jorgensen G, Gabriel R: A new autosomal recessive syndrome: Peripheral pulmonic stenosis, brachytelephalangism, neural hearing loss and abnormal cartilage calcification/ossifications. Birth Defects Orig Artic Ser 8:60, 1995.

116. Raj BL, Sakowitz M, Golfarm R, et al: Lung-scan abnormalities in pulmonary artery branch stenosis. J Nucl Med 21:495, 1980.

117. Tamir A, Melloul M, Berant M, et al: Lung perfusion scans in patients with congenital heart defects. J Am Coll Cardiol 19:382, 1991.

118. Rothman A, Perry JB, Keane JF, Lock JE: Early results and follow-up of balloon angioplasty for branch pulmonary artery stenosis. J Am Coll Cardiol 15:1109, 1990.

119. Hosking MCK, Thomaidis A, Hamilton R, et al: Clinical impact of balloon angioplasty for branch pulmonary artery stenosis. Am J Cardiol 69:1467, 1992.

120. Cohn LH, Sanders JHT, Collins JJ-N: Surgical treatment of congenital unilateral pulmonary arterial stenosis with contralateral pulmonary hypertension. Am J Cardiol 38:257, 1976.

121. McGoon DC, Kincaid OW: Stenosis of branch of the pulmonary arteries: Surgical repairs. Med Clin North Am 48:1083, 1976.

122. Gill CC, Moodie DS, McGoon DC: Staged surgical management of pulmonary atresia with diminutive pulmonary arteries. J Thorac Cardiovasc Surg 73:436, 1997.

123. Lock JE, Niemi T, Einzig S, et al: Transvenous angioplasty of experimental branch pulmonary artery stenosis in newborn lambs. Circulation 64:886, 1981.

124. Edwards BS, Lucas RV, Lock JE, Edwards JE: Morphologic changes in the pulmonary arteries after percutaneous balloon angioplasty for pulmonary arterial stenosis. Circulation 71:195, 1985.

125. Fellows KE, Radke W, Keane JE: Acute complications of catheter therapy for congenital heart disease Am J Cardiol 60:679, 1987.

126. Kan JS, Marvin WJ, Bass JL, et al: Balloon angioplasty–branch pulmonary artery stenosis: Results from the Valvuloplasty and Angioplasty of Congenital Anomalies Registry. Am J Cardiol 65:798, 1990.

127. Zeevi B, Berant M, Blieden LC: Midterm clinical impact versus procedural success of balloon angioplasty for pulmonary artery stenosis. Pediatr Cardiol 18:101, 1997.

128. Fuster V, McGoon DC, Kennedy MA, et al: Long term evaluation (12–22 years) of open heart surgery for tetralogy of Fallot. Am J Cardiol 40:635, 1980.

129. Saxena A, Fong W, Ogilvie BC, Keeton BR: Use of balloon dilatation to treat supravalvar pulmonary stenosis developing after anatomical correction for complete transposition. Br Heart J 64:151, 1990.

130. Zeevi B, Berant M, Blieden LC: Late death from aneurysm rupture following balloon angioplasty for branch pulmonary artery stenosis. Cathet Cardiovasc Diagn 39:284, 1996.

131. Arnold LW, Keane JF, Kan JS, et al: Transient unilateral pulmonary edema after successful balloon dilation of peripheral pulmonary artery stenosis. Am J Cardiol 62:327, 1988.

132. Mullins CE, O'Laughlin MP, Dick M III, et al: Implantation of balloon-expandable intravascular grafts by catheterization in pulmonary arteries and systemic veins. Circulation 77:188, 1988.

133. O'Laughlin MP, Perry SB, Lock JE, Mullins CE: Use of endovascular stents in congenital heart disease. Circulation 83:1923, 1991.

134. Benson LN, Hamilton F, Dasmahaptra H, et al: Percutaneous implantation of a balloon-expandable endoprosthesis for pulmonary artery stenosis: An experimental study. J Am Coll Cardiol 18:1303, 1991.

135. Mendelson AM, Bove EL, Lupinetti FM, et al: Intraoperative and percutaneous stenting of congenital pulmonary artery and vein stenosis. Circulation 88(pt 2):210, 1993.

136. Fogelman R, Nykanen D, Smallhorn JF, et al: Endovascular stents in the pulmonary circulation. Clinical impact on management of medium-term follow-up. Circulation 92:881, 1995.

137. Hatai Y, Nykanen D, Williams WG, et al: The clinical impact of percutaneous balloon expandable endovascular stents in the management of early postoperative vascular obstruction. Cardiol Young 6:48, 1996.

138. Moore JW, Spicer RL, Perry JC, et al: Percutaneous use of stents to correct pulmonary artery stenosis in young children after cavopulmonary anastomosis. Am Heart J 130:1245, 1995.

139. Hijazi ZM, Al-Fadzey F, Geggel RL, et al: Stent implantation for relief of pulmonary artery stenosis: Immediate and short-term results. Cathet Cardiovasc Diagn 36:16, 1996.

140. Rowland TW, Rosenthal A, Castaneda AR: Double-chamber right ventricle: Experience with 17 cases. Am Heart J 89:445, 1975.

141. Chesler E, Korns ME, Edwards JE: Anomalies of the tricuspid valve, including pouches, resembling aneurysms of the membranous ventricular septum. Am J Cardiol 21:661, 1968.

CHAPTER 37
COARCTATION OF THE AORTA AND INTERRUPTED AORTIC ARCH

ALBERT P. ROCCHINI

COARCTATION OF THE AORTA

Coarctation of the aorta is the seventh or eighth most common form of congenital cardiovascular disease.[1] The prevalence of coarctation of the aorta is significantly higher for white males (6.52 per 10,000 live births) than for white females (3.17 per 10,000 live births). In contrast, coarctation is significantly less common in black males and females, and there is no significant difference between the two sexes (2.64 per 10,000 live black male births versus 1.69 per 10,000 live black female births).[2]

Coarctation of the aorta usually occurs in a sporadic fashion; however, genetic factors occasionally play an important role, for example, Turner's syndrome. Cardiovascular abnormalities and coarctation of the aorta are present in up to 36% of girls with Turner's syndrome.[3] There are reports of monozygotic twins concordant for coarctation,[4] and there are a number of families in which coarctation has occurred in more than one family member.[5]

PATHOLOGY AND EMBRYOLOGY

Pathology

The anatomist Johann Meckel in 1750 first described coarctation of the aorta.[6] Coarctation of the aorta is a narrowing of the aortic lumen that causes an obstruction to blood flow. Most coarctations are congenital and are usually discovered in infancy; however, some coarctations can be acquired, such as in Takayasu's arteritis or after surgical procedures such as the arterial switch procedure of complete transposition.[7] The coarctation is typically localized in the thoracic aorta just distal to the origin of the left subclavian artery and opposite the ductus (or ligamentum) arteriosus. The narrowing may be discrete, or there may be a diffusely narrowed segment. When the narrowing is diffuse, the aortic isthmus is involved and the coarctation is usually associated with other cardiac malformations, such as a ventricular septal defect, atrioventricular septal defect, or double-outlet right ventricle. In the older literature, coarctation of the aorta was divided into two types: preductal or infantile and postductal or adult. The term *juxtaductal* is currently used because it more clearly describes the pathologic anatomy. The coarctation is usually related anatomically to an abnormality in the media of the aortic wall that gives rise to a posterior "ridge-like" infolding (Fig. 37–1).[8] This *posterior shelf* can be clearly observed echocardiographically and an-giographically and is an important anatomic landmark for making the diagnosis of coarctation. Dilatation of the left subclavian artery and intercostal arteries often occurs, and the right subclavian artery originates below the coarctation in approximately 5% of the patients.[8] Rarely, a coarctation may occur in other locations, such as the aortic arch or descending thoracic or abdominal aorta (Fig. 37–2). Renal and mesenteric artery involvement frequently occurs with abdominal coarctation.[9]

On histologic examination, the posterior shelf is composed of infolding of medial tissue that eccentrically narrows the aortic lumen. In addition, intimal thickening is usually present. Distal to the obstruction, the aorta is usually dilated (poststenotic dilatation), and the aortic wall in this area is histologically associated with intimal proliferation and medial and elastic tissue disruption. Infective endarteritis may occur in this location (Fig. 37–3).

The terms *simple* and *complex* are used to describe coarctations that are either isolated (with or without a patent ductus) or associated with other cardiac malformations. Of infants with coarctation who present in congestive heart failure, 40% have simple coarctation and 60% have complex coarctation.[6] The most frequently coexisting cardiac abnormalities consist of ventricular septal defect (either isolated or multiple), aortic stenosis (valvar or subvalvar), and mitral valve anomalies (supravalvar ring, dysplasia of mitral leaflets, and "parachute" mitral valve). The combination of coarctation of the aorta, subaortic stenosis, and mitral stenosis is known as Shone's syndrome.[10] Other cardiac lesions commonly associated with coarctation include double-outlet right ventricle, especially Taussig-Bing anomaly (Fig. 37–4); tricuspid atresia, especially with D-transposition of the great arteries; D-transposition of the great arteries with an inlet ventricular septal defect and right ventricular hypoplasia; atrioventricular septal defect; hypoplastic left heart syndrome; double-inlet left ventricle; and L-transposition of the great arteries.

As a result of aortic obstruction, there is a progressive development of collateral blood flow around the coarcted segment (Fig. 37–5). The collaterals develop mainly from the subclavian artery and its branches through the internal mammary, intercostal, musculophrenic, transverse cervical, scapular, lateral thoracic, superior epigastric, and spinal arteries.[11] These dilated and tortuous collateral arteries erode the lower margins of the ribs in older children and produce the characteristic chest x-ray appearance of "rib notching."

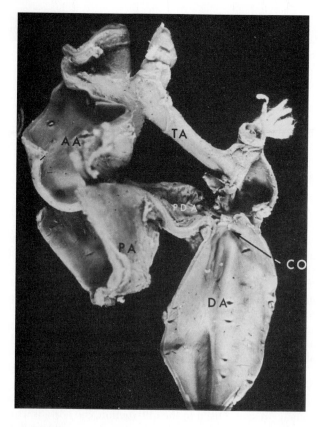

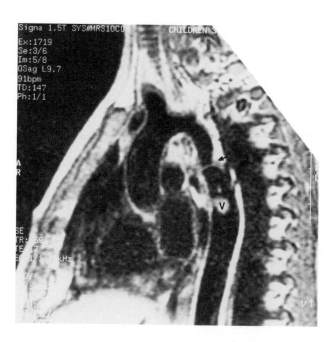

FIGURE 37-3

A magnetic resonance image of a 12-year-old boy with coarctation of the aorta endocarditis. The coarctation is seen on this sagittal section as a white linear line *(arrow).* Distal to the coarctation is a circular vegetation (V). There are also collateral vessels that enter into the descending aorta, suggesting a rich collateral circulation.

FIGURE 37-1

A pathologic specimen of the ascending aorta, descending aorta, and pulmonary artery in a patient with coarctation of the aorta. The ascending aorta (AA) gives rise to a hypoplastic transverse aorta (TA). The patent ductus arteriosus (PDA) enters opposite the coarctation (CO). A prominent posterior shelf *(arrow)* is seen. Large ostia of the intercostal arteries suggest a generous collateral system. PA = pulmonary artery; DA = descending aorta.

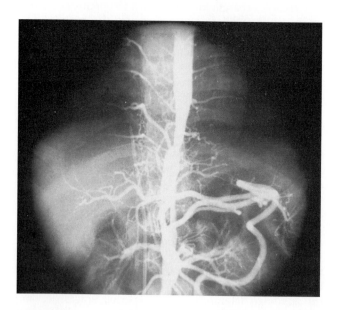

FIGURE 37-2

Abdominal aortic angiogram demonstrates coarctation of the abdominal aorta beginning just proximal to the celiac axis. Dilated splenic and mesenteric arteries provide collateral circulation.

Other vascular anomalies can also be associated with coarctation of the aorta, including berry aneurysms of the circle of Willis,[12, 13] anomalous right subclavian artery arising distal to the coarctation, and coronary artery anomalies. Musculoskeletal (including the late development of scoliosis in boys), gastrointestinal, genitourinary, and respiratory system developmental anomalies also occur in individuals with coarctation of the aorta.[14, 15]

Pseudocoarctation is a "kinking or buckling" of the aorta that results in an x-ray picture similar to coarctation of the aorta. However, in pseudocoarctation, unlike in coarctation, there is little or no obstruction to blood flow. Although pseudocoarctation is usually a benign lesion, there is a tendency in some patients for dilatation and aneurysm formation to develop just distal to the pseudocoarctation.[16]

Embryology

The embryonic origin of coarctation has not been completely defined. The two theories that have been proposed to explain the development of coarctation are an intrinsic defect in the development of the aortic wall and an abnormality of fetal hemodynamics. Coarctation can develop as the result of an intrinsic defect in media of the aortic arch. In mice, a deficiency of endothelin-1 has been associated with the development of tubular hypoplasia of the aortic arch, aberrant right subclavian artery, ventricular septal defect, abnormalities of the left ventricular outflow tract, and interrupted aortic arch.[17] Anomalous fibroductal tissue that circumferentially surrounds the aorta has been demonstrated to occur at a greater frequency in individuals with coarctation than is observed in the general population.[18] Contraction and fibrosis of this tissue at the time of ductal closure pulls the coarctation shelf toward the con-

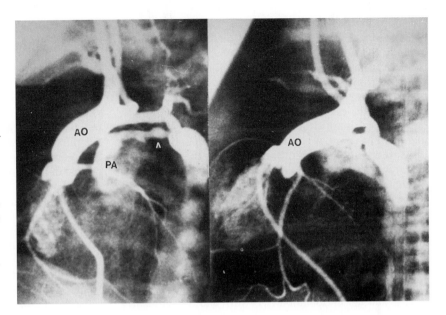

FIGURE 37-4

An angiogram from a patient with double-outlet right ventricle (Taussig-Bing type) and coarctation of the aorta. The angiogram was performed in the left anterior oblique projection. The aorta (AO) is anterior to the pulmonary artery (PA), and there is subaortic and pulmonary conus. The transverse aortic arch and isthmus are hypoplastic, and a patent ductus arteriosus (*arrow*) is also evident. (Adapted from Muster A: Angiographic anatomy of aortic coarctation: A classification based on the associated morphology of the aortic arch. *In* Mavroudis C, Backer C [eds]: Cardiac Surgery: State of the Art Reviews. Philadelphia, Hanley & Belfus, 1993, pp 24–45.)

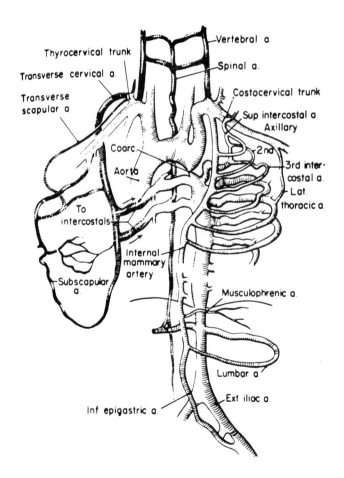

FIGURE 37-5

Collateral circulation associated with coarctation is depicted. On the right side of the figure, the anterior collateral system can be seen to arise from the internal mammary artery. The left side of the figure demonstrates that the posterior system arises from the posterior branches of the subclavian artery. (From Moller JH, Amplatz K, Edwards JE: Congenital Heart Disease for the Universities Associated for Research and Education in Pathology Incorporated. Kalamazoo, MI, The Upjohn Corporation, 1971, pp 1–3.)

tralateral wall, causing constriction of the aorta and obstruction to blood flow.

Rudolph and coworkers[19] have suggested that abnormal fetal hemodynamics may also promote the development of coarctation of the aorta. The region between the left subclavian artery and the ductus arteriosus, the aortic isthmus, receives less than 10% of the combined ventricular output in the normal fetus and is therefore smaller in diameter than either the ascending or descending aorta. Any associated cardiac lesions that reduce left ventricular output could cause reduced blood flow through the aortic isthmus, thus promoting underdevelopment of this portion of the aortic arch and leading to the development of coarctation. Consistent with this hypothesis are the high association of coarctation with a ventricular septal defect that is the result of posterior malalignment of the conal septum and the fact that coarctation does not exist in individuals with pulmonary atresia. The hemodynamic theory alone does not explain, however, the pathogenesis of isolated coarctation of the aorta.

HEMODYNAMICS

Obstruction in the aortic arch results in a selective elevation in pressure and resistance in the upper extremity arterial vessels and ultimately in an increase in left ventricular work. In a neonate with coarctation, closure of the ductus results in an acute increase in left ventricular afterload and the development of left ventricular failure. In infants with milder degrees of coarctation, the left ventricle ultimately adapts to the increase in afterload, and heart failure does not occur. The cardiovascular system has four compensatory mechanisms to respond to the increased systemic afterload produced by coarctation of the aorta. The first and most important compensatory mechanism is left ventricular hypertrophy. Myocardial hypertrophy is the major adaptive mechanism that enables the left ventricle to develop increased systolic pressure yet still maintain a normal or nearly normal left ventricular wall stress.[20] The second mechanism, the Frank-Starling mechanism, is used in individuals with coarctation who develop severe congestive heart failure. With heart failure, the left ventricular end-diastolic volume and pressure increase, and to a point, this increase in preload sustains a nearly normal cardiac output. The third mechanism for cardiovascular compensation in children with coarctation of the aorta is activation of the sympathetic nervous system, a short-term (hours to days) compensatory mechanism. Sympathetic activation increases myocardial contractility and increases systemic pressure that helps maintain perfusion of the descending aorta and the abdominal organs. The fourth and final mechanism to compensate for the increased systemic afterload is the development of a collateral circulation to bypass the aortic obstruction. As the child develops a collateral circulation, systemic arterial pressure and afterload are reduced and blood supply improves to the abdominal organs such as the liver, gastrointestinal tract, and kidneys. Lack of blood flow to the descending aorta leads to ischemia of abdominal organs and the lower extremities (i.e., resulting in metabolic acidosis and renal insufficiency).

Associated cardiovascular lesions aggravate the hemodynamic burden associated with coarctation. A coarctation and the concomitant increase in systemic afterload increase both the amount of left-to-right shunting that results from defects in the atrial and ventricular septum and the amount of mitral regurgitation that occurs in atrioventricular septal defects and other congenital anomalies of the mitral valve. In coexistent aortic stenosis, the addition of coarctation further increases both left ventricular afterload and myocardial oxygen demand.

NATURAL HISTORY

Untreated coarctation of the aorta significantly impairs long-term survival; death frequently occurs within the fourth to fifth decade of life. Campbell[21] reported that of all individuals with an unrepaired coarctation of the aorta who survive the first 2 years of life, 25% die before they reach 20 years, more than 50% before they reach 30 to 31 years, 75% before they reach 43 years, and 90% before 55 years of age. Causes of death in individuals with unrepaired coarctation of the aorta include congestive heart failure, aortic rupture, bacterial endocarditis, and intracranial hemorrhage. With use of autopsy data, the incidence of death due to an intracranial hemorrhage was 11.5%. Campbell and Baylis[22] reported that both intracranial hemorrhage and ruptured aorta occurred in children and young adults who did not have exceptionally high blood pressures. Even in the 1990s, ruptured cerebral aneurysms occur in patients with unrepaired coarctation of the aorta.[13] Campbell[21] has estimated the risk of endocarditis in unrepaired coarctation of the aorta to be 1.3% per year, but this was largely before antibiotic prophylaxis was recommended.

HISTORY AND PHYSICAL EXAMINATION

Clinical Features

Most individuals with coarctation are asymptomatic. If symptoms are present, they are usually nonspecific and relate either to the result of upper extremity hypertension (headaches or frequent nosebleeds) or to reduced blood supply to the lower extremities (exercise-induced claudication).

In infancy, coarctation can be associated with congestive heart failure. Although heart failure can develop any time during the first 6 months of life, it typically develops during the first 6 weeks of life. If heart failure develops after 6 months of age, a cause other than isolated coarctation of the aorta needs to be sought. In infants with complex coarctation, such as coarctation with a large ventricular septal defect, heart failure usually develops within the first 2 weeks of life. These infants are usually discharged from the hospital and then present with an acute onset of tachypnea, tachycardia, and pallor. If these neonates are not immediately diagnosed and correctly treated, shock, acidosis, and death can rapidly occur. In fact, a neonate presenting in shock is more likely to have a critical coarctation (or aortic stenosis) than sepsis or a metabolic disorder that is often erroneously diagnosed. Other infants with coarctation may have a more chronic presentation of congestive heart failure. These infants have a history from birth of dyspnea and diaphoresis with feedings, but failure to thrive is usually what causes them to seek medical attention.

Physical Findings

The hallmarks of coarctation of the aorta are absent or diminished femoral pulses and a difference in systolic blood pressure between the arms and legs. Hypertension is usually noted in the upper extremities; however, in young infants in severe congestive failure, generalized hypotension is usually present. Systolic and mean pressures are elevated in the upper extremities, whereas diastolic pressure is usually similar in the upper and lower extremities (Fig. 37–6). Because the left subclavian artery is frequently involved with the coarcted segment and is hypoplastic, the right arm is the preferred location for measurement of upper extremity blood pressure. However, in three situations, almost no blood pressure gradient or pulse difference will be found on physical examination in an individual with coarctation of the aorta:

1. In an infant with coarctation, the right ventricle may be perfusing the lower part of the body through an unrestrictive patent ductus arteriosus, thus virtually eliminating a pressure difference between the arms and legs.

2. When the left ventricle is severely dysfunctional, blood pressures throughout the body are severely low, and therefore blood pressure differences may not be detectable.

3. A small number of individuals have an aberrant right subclavian artery that arises below the coarctation; thus, it is impossible to measure a blood pressure difference between upper and lower extremities.

The precordial examination usually includes a prominent left ventricular impulse, a heave. With isolated coarctation, a systolic thrill is uncommon; however, with complex coarctation, a systolic thrill, due to the other associated cardiovascular anomalies, is the rule. The first heart sound is normal. Because a bicuspid aortic valve and aortic stenosis frequently coexist in patients with coarctation of the aorta, a systolic ejection click is frequently present.

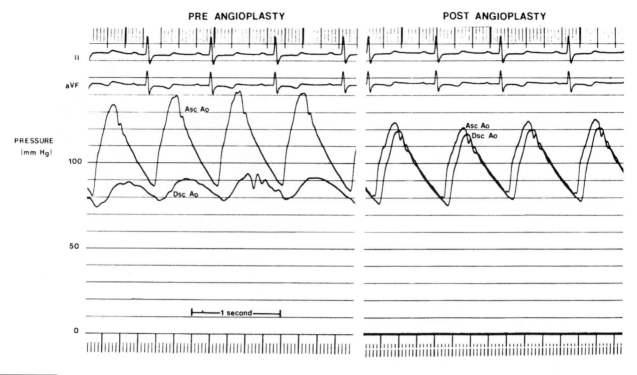

FIGURE 37-6

A pressure tracing before and after balloon angioplasty in a 13-year-old boy with coarctation of the aorta. Before angioplasty, there is a systolic gradient of 50 mm Hg from the ascending aorta (Asc Ao) to the descending aorta (Dsc Ao). The descending aorta has a reduced pulse pressure and a delayed upstroke. After angioplasty, the systolic gradient is approximately 5 mm Hg, and both the pulse pressure and upstroke in the descending aorta have become normal.

The second heart sound is usually normal; however, in an infant with congestive heart failure and pulmonary hypertension, the second heart sound is usually narrowly split with increased intensity of the pulmonary component. A grade 2–3/6 systolic ejection murmur is usually present. The systolic murmur is heard well along the left sternal border and is maximal in intensity in the left subscapular region. If a prominent subscapular murmur is not heard and the child has a blood pressure difference between arms and legs, an abdominal coarctation should be considered. Other systolic murmurs associated with aortic stenosis, mitral regurgitation, or a ventricular septal defect also occur in patients with coarctation. In older children with unrepaired coarctation, continuous murmurs, usually due to collateral blood flow, can be heard over the back and chest. Collateral pulsation can often be felt, especially over the scapular margins. Apical diastolic murmurs, usually of mitral origin, are frequently heard. Finally, neonates with congestive heart failure usually have a gallop and significant hepatomegaly.

Ing and coworkers[23] reviewed the medical records of 50 consecutive patients older than 1 year who had surgical repair of coarctation of the aorta. The most consistent clinical findings associated with coarctation were a cardiac murmur and a systolic blood pressure gradient between the arms and legs of greater than 10 mm Hg. Coarctation would have been missed in 82% of children if absent lower extremity pulses were required as a diagnostic feature. The most discouraging finding in Ing's study was that the timing of, reason for, and source of referral for coarctation compared with data from the previous decade[24] indicated no improvement in early detection of coarctation by pediatricians.

A coarctation is rarely located in the abdominal aorta. The physical examination in abdominal coarctation differs from that of thoracic coarctation in the following ways: abdominal coarctation occurs predominantly in girls; it is associated with a loud murmur in the abdomen, not the chest; it is frequently associated with stenoses of other abdominal arteries (mesenteric, hepatic, and renal); and it is usually associated with more severe elevation in diastolic blood pressure.

ELECTROCARDIOGRAM

The electrocardiogram varies according to the patient's age. In infants, right ventricular hypertrophy is the rule[25]; however, by the second to third year of life, a left ventricular hypertrophy pattern may gradually emerge. In addition, a number of patients with isolated coarctation of the aorta have a normal electrocardiogram. In the neonate or infant with congestive heart failure and coarctation of the aorta, right ventricular hypertrophy is always encountered. The right ventricular hypertrophy reflects the increased in utero volume load that the right ventricle faces, pulmonary hypertension, and the fact that the descending aorta may be perfused by a large patent ductus arteriosus. In a neonate with associated cardiac failure, the T waves are inverted in the left precordial leads. If an infant or neonate with suspected coarctation has an electrocardiogram that demonstrates left rather than right ventricular hypertrophy, the infant is likely to have coexisting severe aortic stenosis.

CHEST FILM

In a neonate, the chest film shows severe cardiomegaly and increased pulmonary vascular markings (consistent with pulmonary edema). In an older child, the typical radiologic features of coarctation are a "3" sign consisting of the ascending aortic knob and the poststenotic dilatation that is usually present. (On barium swallow examination, the 3 turns into an E, which is composed of the indentation on the esophagus by the ascending and poststenotic aorta [Fig. 37–7].) Above 5 years of age, rib notching may be noted (Fig. 37–8). The rib notching is most prominent in the apical ribs; if prominent notching of the lower ribs is present, the diagnosis of an abdominal coarctation should be considered.

ECHOCARDIOGRAPHIC FEATURES

The two-dimensional echo Doppler has replaced cardiac catheterization as the primary diagnostic tool for coarctation of the aorta. The echocardiogram is also useful in delineating other associated cardiac lesions, such as aortic stenosis, mitral valve abnormalities, and ventricular septal defects. Table 37–1 outlines the various echocardiographic views used to image the entire aortic arch. The echocardiographic assessment of coarctation of the aorta should include the sidedness of the aortic arch, the anatomy of each of the aortic arch segments (ascending aorta, transverse aortic arch, isthmus, and descending aorta), the presence or absence of the ductus arteriosus, and a Doppler examination (Fig. 37–9).

A number of investigators have reported excellent sensitivity of two-dimensional echocardiographic Doppler in the assessment of coarctation of the aorta.[26–33] Doppler features that are characteristic of coarctation include progressive increase in systolic flow velocity, development of continuous anterograde flow in diastole, and flow accelera-

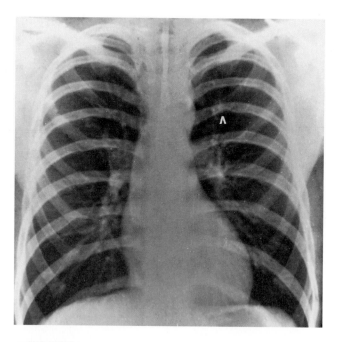

FIGURE 37–8

A chest film from an 8-year-old boy with coarctation of the aorta is depicted. Marked rib notching (*arrow*) is present bilaterally. Rib notching of the upper ribs is classically observed in individuals with thoracic coarctation; coarctation of the abdominal aorta usually results in notching of the lower ribs.

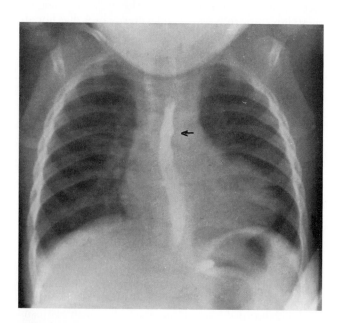

FIGURE 37–7

A chest film with barium in the esophagus from a child with coarctation of the aorta is depicted. The heart is mildly enlarged; the esophagus, indented from the coarctation, demonstrates the "E" sign (*arrow*).

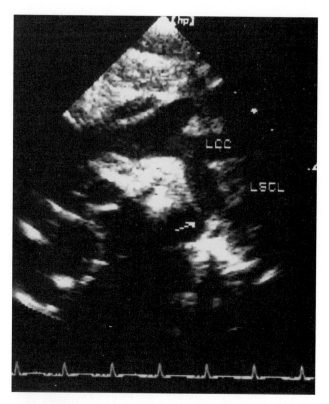

FIGURE 37–9

Echocardiogram. Suprasternal view of a coarctation of the aorta reveals increased distance between the left common carotid and the left subclavian artery. The arrow indicates the coarctation site. LCC = left common carotid; LSCL = left subclavian artery. (Courtesy of Dr. Nina Gotteiner and Kaliope Berdusis.)

TABLE 37–1

ECHOCARDIOGRAPHIC VIEWS FOR VISUALIZATION OF THE AORTIC ARCH

View	Portions of Aortic Arch Visualized
PARASTERNAL VIEWS	
Standard left	Aortic root and proximal ascending aorta
High left "ductus view"	Aortic isthmus, ductus, and descending aorta
Right subclavian	Ascending aorta
SUPRASTERNAL NOTCH VIEWS	
Short axis	Ascending aorta
Long axis	Ascending and transverse arch, isthmus, part of the descending aorta and branching pattern of arch vessels
SUBCOSTAL VIEWS	
Short axis	Abdominal aorta and in infants, sometimes the entire ascending and descending aorta

tion with a long first alias—and sometimes a second or third alias—throughout most of systole in the area proximal to coarctation (Fig. 37–10). Doppler estimates of the gradient across the coarctation correlate poorly with catheter-measured peak systolic gradients owing to difficulties in accurately measuring proximal velocity, increased viscous resistance associated with small orifice diameters, and multiple areas of aortic arch obstruction (tubular hypoplasia of the transverse aortic arch and isthmus). Other difficulties in echocardiographic diagnosis of aortic coarctation include false-negative diagnosis of coarctation when isthmic hypoplasia is associated with a widely patent ductus arteriosus that obscures the discrete coarctation, false-negative diagnosis when a suprasternal notch long-axis view alone is used and the posterior shelf of the coarctation cannot be visualized because the isthmus is parallel to the ultrasound beam, and false-positive diagnosis of coarctation if the normal anterior shelf associated with the entry of the ductus into the aorta is mistaken for a coarctation. Because imaging the region of the coarctation can deceive even the most expert echocardiographers, it is essential to evaluate the acceleration of flow above and below the region of the coarctation. Any significant obstruction makes acceleration much lower in the distal than in the proximal aorta, similar to the acceleration of pressure shown in Figure 37–6.

Echocardiographic studies are also useful for the prenatal diagnosis of coarctation[34, 35] (see Chapter 12). Severe coarctation is usually associated with hypoplasia of the left-sided heart structures. Quantitative hypoplasia of the aortic isthmus and transverse aortic arch is the most reliable finding associated with a correct prenatal diagnosis of coarctation. Milder forms of coarctation have a normal early fetal echocardiogram, which therefore makes an early prenatal diagnosis impossible. In late pregnancy, it may be impossible to exclude coarctation categorically because in the normal fetus, the right-sided heart structures may appear larger than those of the left side. Although a combination of echocardiographic features, such as a left-to-right shunt across the foramen ovale,

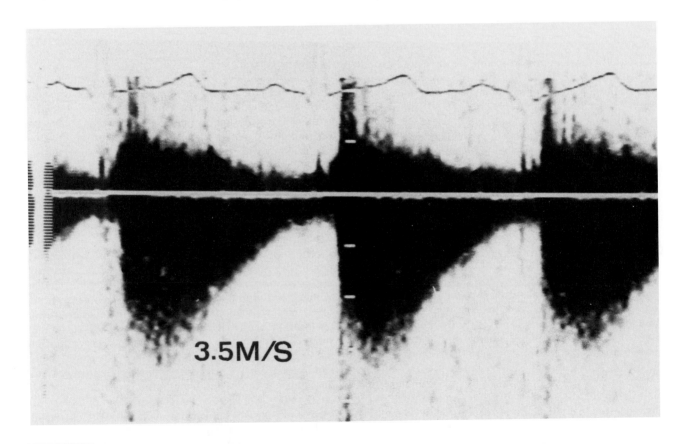

3.5M/S

FIGURE 37–10

Echocardiogram. Continuous-wave Doppler tracing across the site of coarctation measures a maximal systolic gradient of 3.5 m/sec with diastolic continuation of flow. (Courtesy of Dr. Nina Gotteiner and Kaliope Berdusis.)

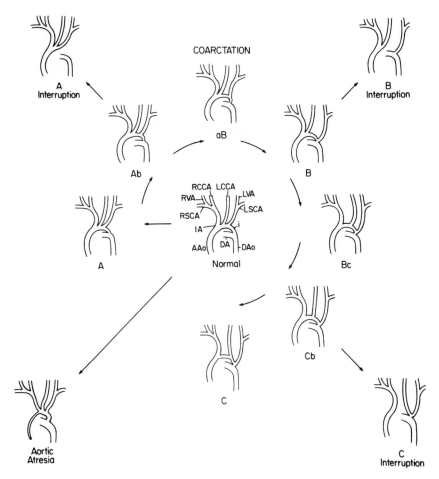

COARCTATION

A Interruption

B Interruption

Ab

aB

B

RCCA LCCA
RVA — LVA
RSCA — LSCA
IA — i
AAo — DA — DAo
Normal

A

Bc

Cb

C

Aortic Atresia

C Interruption

FIGURE 37–11

Classification of coarctation based on the configuration of the aortic arch as proposed by Dr. A. S. Muster. Muster has speculated that the variety of arch configurations found in association with coarctation of the aorta is indicative of the close developmental relationship between coarctation and interruption of the aortic arch. He believes that the differences in arch involvement may be purely quantitative; thus, according to Muster, coarctation and interrupted arches can be similarly classified. RCCA = right common carotid artery; LCCA = left common carotid artery; LVA = left vertebral artery; LSCA = left subclavian artery; RVA = right vertebral artery; RSCA = right subclavian artery; DAo = descending aorta; DA = ductus arteriosus; AAo = ascending aorta; IA = innominate artery; i = isthmus. (Adapted from Muster A: Angiographic anatomy of aortic coarctation: A classification based on the associated morphology of the aortic arch. *In* Mavroudis C, Backer C [eds]: Cardiac Surgery: State of the Art Reviews. Philadelphia, Hanley & Belfus, 1993, pp 23–45.)

a small left ventricle or aortic arch, or associated cardiac lesions, can correctly diagnose coarctation in the fetus, none of these features either alone or in combination can always clearly distinguish between real and false-positive coarctations.[34,35]

Noninvasive assessment of coarctation can also be made by computed tomography, cine computed tomography, magnetic resonance imaging, and cine magnetic resonance imaging (see Fig. 37–3). The major limitations of these other noninvasive tests are their cost and the fact that the patient needs to be absolutely still for a prolonged time.

CARDIAC CATHETERIZATION AND ANGIOGRAPHY

The place of cardiac catheterization in the management of coarctation of the aorta has greatly changed. With the advent of echocardiography, catheterization is now performed only because the cardiac anatomy or pathophysiologic process cannot be adequately delineated by the echocardiogram or for treatment of the coarctation with the use of balloon angioplasty.

Considering the embryology of the aortic arches[36] and the existing classification of arch interruption,[37] Muster[38] has suggested that coarctation of the aorta can be similarly classified (Fig. 37–11). By use of this angiographic classification, a coarctation that occurs in the isthmus is type A (Fig. 37–12); in the distal arch, type B (Fig. 37–13); and in the proximal aorta, type C.

MANAGEMENT

Management of a patient with coarctation of the aorta must be individualized. In an asymptomatic individual without hypertension, in whom a coarctation is detected on routine examination, repair of the coarctation, either surgically or with use of interventional catheterization, is not recommended before 18 to 24 months of age. For an infant with hypertension but without congestive heart failure, repair is recommended if the hypertension is severe, greater than the 95th percentile for age and sex,[39] or if significant left ventricular hypertrophy is documented echocardiographically.

The initial management of a neonate or infant with coarctation who presents in congestive heart failure consists of stabilization with intravenous inotropes (dopamine or dobutamine) and diuretics. Most critically ill neonates require mechanical ventilation. For neonates younger than 2 weeks, an infusion of prostaglandin E_1 (0.05 to 0.1 µg/kg/min) should be tried to open a closed or closing ductus arteriosus. Side effects of prostaglandin include fever, seizures, apnea, and hypotension if a responsive ductus is not present.[40] Acidosis, hypoglycemia, and hypothermia are frequently present in critically ill neonates and require prompt therapy. After a brief period of stabilization, all infants with coarctation and congestive heart failure require correction.

In the past, there was controversy regarding the management for an infant with congestive heart failure and simple coarctation of the aorta. For infants with congestive

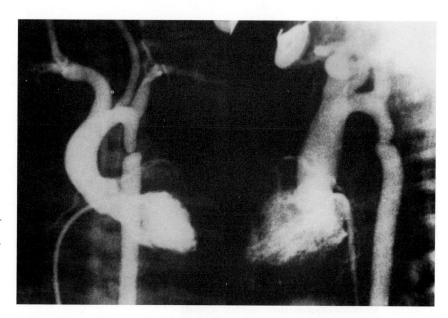

FIGURE 37–12

Left ventriculogram demonstrates the anterior-posterior (*left*) and lateral (*right*) projections of a child with coarctation of the aorta. According to the scheme proposed by Muster, this patient has type A coarctation (a discrete coarctation located at the site of the ductus with mild hypoplasia of the isthmus).

heart failure and a simple coarctation (with or without a patent ductus), the New England Regional Infant Cardiac Program reported a 31% first-year mortality with operative treatment compared with 43% with medical management.[14] However, since 1980, the surgical mortality for simple coarctation has progressively declined. From 1979 to 1993 at Children's Memorial Hospital, Chicago, 96 infants with simple coarctation and congestive heart failure underwent repair without early deaths.[41] On the basis of this experience, I and others believe that all infants with simple coarctation and congestive heart failure should have surgical repair.

Infants with complex coarctation of the aorta require urgent repair. Controversy exists regarding the timing and the type of correction of both the coarctation and, if present, the other major cardiovascular anomalies. The most common type of complex coarctation of the aorta is with an associated ventricular septal defect. In infants with a ventricular septal defect and coarctation, our approach at the Children's Memorial Hospital, Chicago, is to repair the coarctation and ventricular septal defect at the same operative setting, provided that the ventricular septal defect is large. From 1979 through 1996, 32 infants with coarctation and a ventricular septal defect have undergone primary repair with an operative mortality of less than 10%.[41] Other approaches to such patients include repair of coarctation and pulmonary artery band or repair of coarctation with subsequent repair of the ventricular septal defect a few weeks after coarctation repair.

For children (age 2 years or older) with coarctation but without congestive heart failure, elective repair of the coarctation could consist of either surgical repair or balloon angioplasty. For either of these modalities, treatment can safely be undertaken with minimal risk of mortality or morbidity. Minich and colleagues[42] suggested that an appropriate treatment strategy for children (age 2 years or older) with native discrete coarctation of the aorta but without congestive heart failure is the initial use of balloon angioplasty if coarctation anatomy is suitable (i.e., short segment and no arch hypoplasia), followed by operative repair if the angioplasty proved to be unsuccessful.

Finally, there are rare individuals who have a mild coarctation with a systolic arm-leg gradient of less than 20 mm Hg and no upper extremity hypertension. In these individuals, no intervention, either operative or balloon angioplasty, may be necessary. However, they need to be carefully observed because increasing aortic obstruction can occur, and these individuals are at risk for the development of endarteritis.

Operative Repair
RESECTION AND END-TO-END ANASTOMOSES

The first successful operative repair of coarctation of the aorta was reported in 1945 by Craaford and Nylin.[43] A similar report was made in that same year by Gross and Hufnagel.[44] Both reports described resection of the coarctation with primary end-to-end anastomosis (Fig. 37–14A). The first successful surgical repair of coarctation of the aorta in a neonate was reported in 1952 by Kirklin and coworkers.[45]

Resection with end-to-end anastomosis is classically performed through a left posterior lateral thoracotomy. Extensive mobilization of the aorta from the left subclavian artery past the ductus arteriosus to the descending aorta is required along with ductus division and ligation. Although attempts are made to spare dilated collateral intercostal arteries, it is often necessary to sacrifice the first and rarely the second pair of intercostal arteries. Adequate repair is achieved only when the entire segment of narrowing is resected and a tension-free anastomosis is created. Early repairs used silk suture in a continuous running fashion, both anteriorly and posteriorly; however, these repairs were associated with a high incidence of restenosis.[46] Currently, most surgeons advocate a continuous suture posteriorly and an interrupted layer anteriorly. The choice of suture material is either nonabsorbable polypropylene or absorbable polydioxanone.[47–49] Resection with end-to-end anastomosis is advantageous in that it theoretically removes all abnormal ductal and coarctation tissue while avoiding the use of prosthetic material. Extensive dissection is required, and a tension-free anastomosis is occasionally impossible, especially in young infants with com-

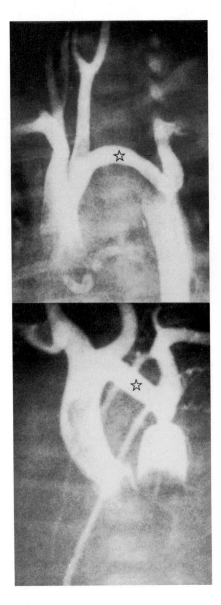

FIGURE 37–13

Angiograms of Muster's type B coarctation of the aorta. The aortic isthmus is absent, and the coarctation develops at the junction of the fourth arch, left subclavian artery, dorsal aorta, and ductus. The long and narrow transverse arch is hypoplastic (*stars*). (Adapted from Muster A: Angiographic anatomy of aortic coarctation: A classification based on the associated morphology of the aortic arch. *In* Mavroudis C, Backer C [eds]: Cardiac Surgery: State of the Art Reviews. Philadelphia, Hanley & Belfus, 1993, pp 23–45.)

plex coarctation of the aorta, so an alternative method of repair is frequently required. The potential for growth of the circumferential anastomosis is controversial, although reports of interrupted suture techniques and use of monofilament suture suggested that there is adequate potential for growth.[48,49]

PROSTHETIC PATCH AORTOPLASTY
The prosthetic patch aortoplasty was first introduced in 1957 by Vosschulte[50] (see Fig. 37–14B). This repair uses a longitudinal incision through the coarctation with extension both distally and proximally. An elliptical prosthetic patch made of either Dacron or polytetrafluoroethylene is

then sutured in place, longitudinally along the aortotomy edges. The major advantage of the prosthetic patch aortoplasty versus the classic end-to-end technique is avoidance of both an extensive dissection and a prolonged operative time. The initial enthusiasm for this technique has diminished because of the development of late aneurysms on the posterior aortic wall opposite the patch, especially a Dacron patch.[51–56]

Two theories have been proposed to explain the prevalence of aneurysm formation. One is that excision of the posterior coarctation membrane weakens the posterior aortic wall and predisposes to late aneurysm formation.[54,55] The other theory contends that aneurysm formation is secondary to altered hemodynamics arising from the difference in tensile strength between the prosthetic patch and the posterior aortic wall.[57,58] Because of the incidence of aneurysms after prosthetic patch aortoplasty, this operative technique has fallen out of favor, although it still is a valuable option in selected circumstances.

INTERPOSITION GRAFTS
The use of a prosthetic or homograft interposition graft to repair coarctation of the aorta was first described by Morris and coworkers[59] (see Fig. 37–14C). Interposition grafts are currently used only for older individuals with an associated aneurysm or in selective instances of recoarctation when resection and end-to-end anastomosis cannot be accomplished. The major disadvantages with interposition grafts are their predisposition to potential infection and aneurysm formation and their lack of growth potential.

SUBCLAVIAN FLAP AORTOPLASTY
The subclavian flap aortoplasty was introduced in 1966 by Waldhausen and Nahrwold[60] (see Fig. 37–14D). The operation consists of mobilizing, ligating, and dividing the subclavian artery; making a longitudinal incision across the coarctation; and opening the subclavian artery along its anterior surface, then folding it down and anastomosing it to the edge of the aortotomy. The subclavian flap aortoplasty has been widely used in repair procedures for infants and young children. The major appeal of the subclavian flap has been its simplicity, and the lack of extensive aortic dissection results in a decreased aortic cross-clamp time. Other advantages include the avoidance of prosthetic patch material, hemostasis control, and increasing growth potential for the anastomosis. Disadvantages of this procedure have been complications associated with sacrificing the major vascular supply to the left upper extremity,[61,62] the occurrence of aneurysms,[63,64] and the belief that inadequate resection of ductus tissue could result in an unacceptably high recurrence of coarctation.[65–67]

EXTENDED END-TO-END ANASTOMOSIS
The extended end-to-end repair is the newest of the surgical options for coarctation of the aorta (see Fig. 37–14E). It was introduced in 1984 by Lansman and associates[68] and later revised by Zannini and coworkers[69] and Elliott.[70] The operative approach in the extended end-to-end anastomosis is similar to that of a classic resection and end-to-end technique; however, proximally a long incision is made on the inferior surface of the arch (frequently requiring temporary occlusion of the left subclavian artery and left

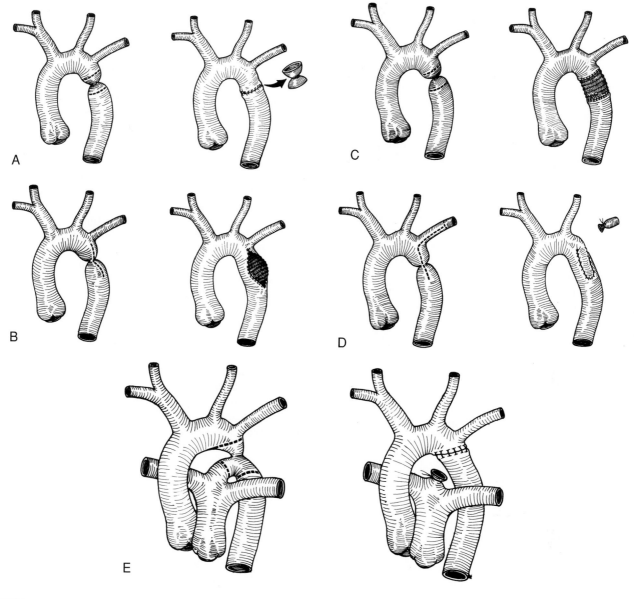

Types of surgical repair of coarctation of the aorta. *A*, Resection with primary end-to-end anastomosis. *B*, Prosthetic patch angioplasty. *C*, Prosthetic interposition graft. *D*, Subclavian flap aortoplasty. *E*, Resection with extended end-to-end repair.

carotid artery and part of the right innominate artery), and the distal aorta is then brought up and sutured to this incision. The most obvious advantages to this technique are the excision of all potentially abnormal aortic tissue and, by extending the proximal incision across the isthmus and transverse aortic arch, correction of the distal arch hypoplasia. The disadvantages of the extended end-to-end anastomosis are similar to those of the end-to-end repair; most specifically, this technique requires extensive dissection and sacrificing of many intercostal collaterals. A tension-free anastomosis is necessary, and occasionally this is technically difficult to achieve.

EARLY COMPLICATIONS AFTER SURGICAL REPAIR

The major operative complications include hemorrhage, paradoxical hypertension, stroke, paraplegia, and damage to adjacent structures. The most common early postopera-

tive complication after surgical correction of coarctation of the aorta is paradoxical hypertension.[71,72] In a review of the first 274 patients operated on at the University of Minnesota between 1948 and 1976, paradoxical or persistent postoperative hypertension occurred in 85 (34%) of the patients.[73] Post-coarctation hypertension has been shown to be due to transection of the aorta and damage to sympathetic afferent or efferent nerves.[74] During the initial phase, the hypertension is initiated through activation of the sympathetic nervous system with a marked increase in systemic catecholamine secretion. During the second phase, the catecholamine hyperactivity activates the renin-angiotensin-aldosterone system, ultimately leading to sustained hypertension and fluid retention. If untreated, the hypertension can result in post-coarctation syndrome. Post-coarctation syndrome is due to acute inflammatory changes in the mesenteric arteries (possibly due to overdistention of the thin-walled arteries below the obstruction that have not previously been exposed to a normal pulse pressure) that can result in intestinal ischemia, necrosis, and even death. Symptoms of post-coarctation syndrome consist of severe abdominal pain, distention, and tenderness, and there may also be fever.[71] Paradoxical hypertension can be prevented if β-blockers are administered before surgery,[75] or it can be treated early in the postoperative course by the intravenous administration of β-blockers, converting enzyme inhibitors, or nitroprusside.

The second most common complication after coarctation repair in the Minnesota series was bleeding. This occurred in seven patients (3%). Bleeding after coarctation repair is usually due to a postoperative coagulopathy. Turner's syndrome is associated with an increased incidence of hemorrhage because of abnormal tissue fragility.[76] Another factor predisposing to hemorrhage is extensive tension along the suture line, especially if the patient has severe paradoxical hypertension.

Another important complication associated with coarctation repair is infection. This occurred in seven patients (3%) in the Minnesota series and was due to *Staphylococcus epidermidis*. All of the infections occurred early in the series before the use of prophylactic antistaphylococcal agents.

Stroke and paraplegia are complications after coarctation repair, but their occurrence is rare. In our series from Minnesota, spinal cord paralysis, probably due to anterior spinal artery syndrome, occurred in two patients (1%). In other reported series, paraplegia has been reported to occur in 0.4% of patients.[77] Brewer and colleagues[77] demonstrated that neither sacrificing intercostal arteries nor aortic cross-clamp time was related to the occurrence of spinal cord injuries. In Brewer's report, predisposing factors included poor collaterals, anomalous origin of the right subclavian artery, and prolonged distal hypotension. In an attempt to prevent spinal cord paraplegia, most surgeons try to maintain distal aortic pressure above 50 mm Hg. If the distal aortic pressure does fall below this critical range, pharmacologic attempts (such as the use of isoproterenol and metaraminol) should be undertaken to raise the pressure. If pharmacologic measures are ineffective in preventing the hypotension, surgical procedures should be used, such as a Gott shunt or femoral bypass with a distal pump oxygenator.[78] Other means for monitoring potential spinal cord injury include the intraoperative monitoring of somatosensory evoked potentials.[79, 80] Loss of these somatosensory evoked potentials indicates that additional pharmacologic or operative intervention should be done to improve distal aortic perfusion.

Finally, damage to adjacent structures can also occur during surgical repair of coarctation. This most often involves injury to the phrenic nerve, resulting in diaphragmatic paralysis; injury to the recurrent laryngeal nerve; damage to the sympathetic trunk, resulting in Horner's syndrome; and, rarely, the development of chylothorax due to injury of the thoracic duct.

The mortality for coarctation repair is low. In the Minnesota series,[73] of 274 patients operated on between 1948 and 1976, the operative mortality for all patients was only 7%. With prostaglandin therapy and appropriate medical stabilization, the mortality rate has been significantly reduced. Since 1989 at the Children's Memorial Hospital of Chicago, we have had no operative deaths for individuals, regardless of age, with isolated coarctation of the aorta.

Primary coarctation repair in adults has a higher risk. The aorta above and below the coarctation is atheromatous and friable, and there are often large, thin-walled intercostal aneurysms.

Balloon Angioplasty as Treatment

Percutaneous balloon angioplasty is an alternative therapy for both native and recurrent coarctation of the aorta. Angioplasty in the treatment of coarctation dates to 1979 when Sos and coworkers[81] reported the successful balloon dilatation of aortic coarctation in postmortem neonates. Lock and coworkers[82, 83] in 1982, using an experimental model, demonstrated that balloon dilatation could successfully treat coarctation. After Lock's experimental work, numerous investigators have used balloon angioplasty to treat coarctation of the aorta.[84–92]

TECHNIQUE FOR PERFORMING ANGIOPLASTY FOR COARCTATION

Angioplasty is usually performed in older children; therefore, if possible, both femoral arteries are cannulated percutaneously, and the patient is then heparinized. The coarctation is crossed retrograde, and simultaneous recording of ascending and descending aorta pressure is made. Angiography of the arch is performed in the left anterior oblique and lateral projections. The diameter of the coarctation site and the aorta proximal to the coarctation is measured by use of either a video freeze frame or digital imaging. Correction for magnification should be made with either a calibrated marker catheter positioned in the superior vena cava or other calibration devices. An angioplasty catheter is chosen whose balloon diameter is approximately equal to or slightly larger than the diameter of the aortic isthmus. The deflated balloon is advanced over an exchange guide wire until the balloon is positioned across the coarctation; the balloon is inflated by hand until the indentation produced on the balloon by the coarctation disappears. The angioplasty catheter is then removed, and an angiographic catheter is exchanged over a guide wire.

Angioplasty enlarges the area of coarctation by splitting the coarctation shelf. The tears in the coarctation shelf extend through the aortic wall intima and into the media. If these tears extend through the media, an acute dissection or aortic perforation can occur. Perforation can be avoided by using the proper size angioplasty balloon and by never advancing a catheter through a freshly dilated aorta unless it is guided by a wire (Fig. 37–15).

EARLY COMPLICATIONS AFTER BALLOON ANGIOPLASTY

Early complications after angioplasty are uncommon and include hemorrhage, femoral artery damage, and possible cerebrovascular accidents. Tynan and colleagues[84] reported the results of the Valvuloplasty and Angioplasty of Congenital Anomalies Registry. Among 140 patients who had balloon angioplasty of coarctation of the aorta, complications occurred in 24 (17%) of the patients. There was only one death. The most common complication in Tynan's

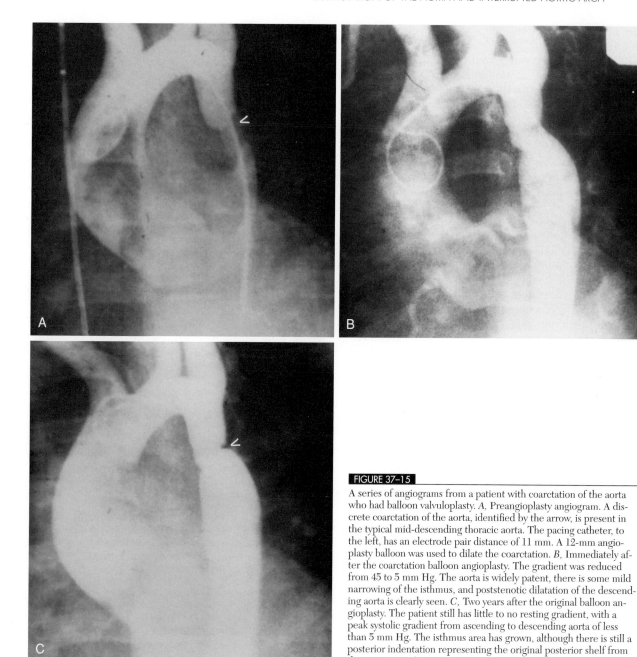

FIGURE 37–15

A series of angiograms from a patient with coarctation of the aorta who had balloon valvuloplasty. *A,* Preangioplasty angiogram. A discrete coarctation of the aorta, identified by the arrow, is present in the typical mid-descending thoracic aorta. The pacing catheter, to the left, has an electrode pair distance of 11 mm. A 12-mm angioplasty balloon was used to dilate the coarctation. *B,* Immediately after the coarctation balloon angioplasty. The gradient was reduced from 45 to 5 mm Hg. The aorta is widely patent, there is some mild narrowing of the isthmus, and poststenotic dilatation of the descending aorta is clearly seen. *C,* Two years after the original balloon angioplasty. The patient still has little to no resting gradient, with a peak systolic gradient from ascending to descending aorta of less than 5 mm Hg. The isthmus area has grown, although there is still a posterior indentation representing the original posterior shelf from the coarctation *(arrow).*

series was femoral artery injury in 14 (10%): in six patients, there was dissection of the femoral artery; in one patient, femoral artery thrombosis severe enough to require operative intervention occurred; and the remaining seven patients had transient loss of femoral artery pulses that responded to 12 hours of intravenous heparin. Prolonged bleeding at the puncture site requiring transfusion or the administration of fresh frozen plasma occurred in 2 of the 140 patients, and one patient had a cerebrovascular accident. Unlike with operative repair, paradoxical hypertension after angioplasty was uncommon.

PROGNOSIS

The long-term outcome after repair of coarctation of the aorta, whether by operation or angioplasty, can be divided

into two major categories: recoarctation of the aorta and long-term survivability.

Recoarctation

Operative repair of coarctation of the aorta in children older than 3 years is associated with excellent long-term relief of the coarctation gradient. Beekman and co-workers[93] demonstrated that patients who had undergone coarctation of the aorta repair after 3 years of age experienced less than a 3% incidence of recoarctation. The length of follow-up in Beekman's study was 1 to 10 years. Likewise, in a long-term follow-up project performed at the University of Minnesota,[73] when patients were followed up for more than 20 to 25 years, the incidence of recoarctation was less than 3% in patients operated on after 5 years of age. In patients operated on in infancy, the incidence of recoarctation after operative repair is much higher. In Beekman's study, the incidence of recoarctation was 30 to 40% when patients younger than 3 years were treated with end-to-end anastomosis. Similar incidences of recoarctation are seen with the patch angioplasty and with subclavian artery aortoplasty. Van Heurn and coworkers[67] evaluated the results of coarctation repair of 151 patients younger than 3 months at the time of repair and who were treated between 1985 and 1990. The actuarial freedom from recoarctation after 4 years of follow-up was 57% (confidence limits, 28 to 78%) after subclavian flap repair, 77% (confidence limits, 60 to 87%) after classic end-to-end anastomosis, and 83% (confidence limits, 66 to 92%) after extended end-to-end anastomosis. Merrill and coworkers[66] reported their results of coarctation repair in 139 infants younger than 1 month who underwent repair between 1970 and 1993. Restenosis requiring reoperation or balloon dilatation developed in 28% of the children at 5 years after operation. For patients observed longer than 5 years, the recurrence of coarctation was higher in those who had undergone subclavian flap repair than in those who had undergone end-to-end repair. Kappetein and coworkers[46] evaluated 109 patients (younger than 3 years) with isolated coarctation repaired between 1953 and 1988. They found that if the coarctation anastomosis was repaired by use of a polypropylene suture material, the incidence of recoarctation was significantly reduced.

On the basis of a review of the surgical literature, if repair of coarctation is performed after infancy, there is excellent long-term relief with a low incidence of restenosis; if surgical repair is performed during the first 3 months of life, recoarctation is common, occurring in 30 to 40% of individuals, and the type of surgical repair can affect the incidence of recoarctation. The highest rates of recoarctation are seen in the classic end-to-end anastomosis, followed by the subclavian flap and patch aortoplasty; early results of the new extended end-to-end anastomosis suggest that it may be the best surgical procedure.

It is difficult to compare the efficacy of angioplasty with surgical correction of coarctation, because angioplasty has been performed as therapy for coarctation of the aorta only since the mid-1980s. A number of important pieces of information regarding the use of angioplasty to treat coarctation of the aorta are unknown. Numerous investigators have demonstrated that although angioplasty of native coarctation of the aorta can successfully relieve gradients in patients, regardless of age, the incidence of recoarctation in children younger than 1 year appears to be much higher in the angioplasty-treated group than in the surgical group. Rao and coworkers[94] reported on the immediate results of balloon angioplasty to treat native coarctation of the aorta in 16 infants aged 3 days to 12 months. The patients were observed for 36 ± 18 months after angioplasty, and 5 of 16 infants (31%) had evidence of significant recoarctation that required either repeated angioplasty or operation. Rao compared the results of angioplasty with those of operation and found that mortality rates with angioplasty appeared to be less, but recoarctation rates were slightly higher. More recently, Johnson and colleagues[95] in a literature review compared the treatment of coarctation of the aorta in infancy by surgical repair (n = 1189 patients) with that by balloon angioplasty (n = 57 patients).

This review demonstrated that balloon angioplasty and surgery had similar early mortality rates but that the recoarctation rates were significantly higher in the balloon-treated group, averaging 57% compared with 14% for the operation.

Thus, from the current data, angioplasty does not offer an advantage over operation in the neonatal period. For children older than 1 year, the recurrence rates after angioplasty are much lower. Fletcher and coworkers[96] reported their follow-up (up to 117 months) of 102 patients who underwent balloon angioplasty for treatment of native coarctation of the aorta. Their results demonstrated that immediate success with balloon angioplasty was achieved in 93 patients (91%); 71 of the 93 patients remained asymptomatic and normotensive with insignificant arm-to-leg blood pressure gradients. Twenty-one patients (22%) with initial successful treatment developed an increase in gradient during the follow-up, requiring a repeated intervention. Most patients, however, were infants younger than 7 months, and for those children older than 7 months, the incidence of recoarctation was only 10%. Similarly, Mendelsohn and associates[97] reported their long-term results after balloon angioplasty in children with native coarctation of the aorta. Of 59 patients who underwent balloon angioplasty for native coarctation of the aorta, effective gradient relief was achieved in 41. Restenosis occurred in 6 of these patients, in 3 of 5 who were infants and in only 3 of 41 who were older than 1 year. These authors concluded that balloon angioplasty provided effective relief of coarctation of the aorta in older children but not in neonates.

Shaddy and coworkers[98] compared angioplasty and surgery for unrepaired coarctation of the aorta. In a randomized study of 36 patients, 20 randomized to angioplasty and 16 to operation, no statistical difference in the incidence of restenosis was found between the angioplasty and the surgical groups. There was, however, a tendency toward angioplasty's having more restenosis than surgery did.

Finally, Kaine and coworkers[99] using echocardiographic analysis of the aortic arch, determined predictors of outcome of balloon angioplasty for native coarctation of the aorta. The predictors of an unsuccessful angioplasty outcome were younger age (<7 months); a patent ductus arteriosus; and an aortic isthmus diameter, distal transverse arch diameter, and aortic valve annulus less than 2 SD below population norms. Thus, on the basis of current available literature, it appears that in selected patients, angioplasty offers results similar to those of surgery. The important criteria for selection of patients for balloon angioplasty of native coarctation are that children should be older than 1 year and without arch hypoplasia.

Before 1983, reoperation was the accepted treatment of recoarctation.[93, 100–102] Operation, however, did not always abolish the residual obstruction. In a series of 26 patients operated on for recoarctation, there was a residual mean aortic gradient of 15 mm Hg after reoperation.[101] The mortality for recoarctation of the aorta has been reported to be between 3 and 33%.[93, 100–102] The operative morbidity after reoperation for coarctation of the aorta has included spinal cord damage, cerebrovascular events, pulmonary collapse or infection, wound sepsis, and endocarditis.[93, 100–102] After early reports suggesting that balloon angioplasty is an effective alternative to operation with a low incidence of complications, balloon angioplasty has replaced surgery as the preferred method of treating recoarctation of the aorta in many centers.[85, 103, 104]

Balloon angioplasty of recurrent coarctation of the aorta is performed like that previously described for native coarctation. In very young infants or in patients who have previously undergone a stage I Norwood procedure, either a transvenous anterograde or intraoperative approach may be preferable.[105, 106]

Acute efficacy for the use of balloon angioplasty to treat recurrent coarctation of the aorta was established from a multicenter prospective study.[107] This series reported the acute results of 200 patients aged 1 month to 26 years (mean, 7 years) who underwent angioplasty of recurrent coarctation of the aorta 45 days to 20 years (mean, 5.4 years) after the operation to repair coarctation of the aorta. For the entire group, the peak systolic pressure gradient across the coarctation site was decreased by angioplasty from 42 ± 20 to 13 ± 12 mm Hg (mean $\pm$ SD, $P < .0001$). Overall, 149 of the 200 patients (74.8%) had a good or excellent result (residual coarctation gradient of less than 20 mm Hg). In this series, the hemodynamic adequacy of angioplasty was not correlated with the type of previous operative procedure, the ratio of balloon diameter to aortic diameter both proximal and distal to the coarctation site, the inflation pressure of the angioplasty balloon, age at initial surgery, or the time interval between surgery and angioplasty. The only variable that appeared to relate to angioplasty success was age at the time of angioplasty, in that the average age of the patients who had a residual gradient of less than 10 mm Hg was significantly less than that of patients who had a residual gradient of 11 mm Hg or more ($P < .025$). Similar results have been reported in other smaller series.[19–27]

In this series, there were five deaths (2.5%) directly associated with balloon angioplasty for recoarctation of the aorta.[107] Two of the deaths were believed to be the result of sudden and unexpected arrhythmias occurring 6 and 14 hours after the procedure. In both patients, necropsy showed no rupture at the angioplasty site and no anatomic explanation for the arrhythmias. The other deaths were related to left ventricular failure 36 hours after the angioplasty, acute cerebral edema after a cerebrovascular accident that occurred at the time of the procedure, and acute aortic rupture at the time of balloon inflation. Acute intimal dissection occurred in three other patients; one required immediate surgical repair, and two others were small and required no surgical intervention. Balloon angioplasty of recoarctation has a higher risk of acute aortic rupture than when angioplasty is used in a patient with native coarctation. The higher incidence of aortic rupture in patients with recoarctation is related to both the need to use higher balloon inflation pressures and the types of operative repair. Patients with recoarctation after repair with a prosthetic patch have the highest risk of aortic rupture after balloon angioplasty. Joyce and McGrath[108] reported rupture of the aortic wall and pseudoaneurysm formation after balloon angioplasty of a previous Gore-Tex patch angioplasty. In this patient, the aortic wall ruptured at the anastomosis between a previously placed Gore-Tex patch and native aortic wall.

Nonlethal neurologic complications occurred in three patients. These were occlusion of the right middle cerebral artery and acute hemiplegia, transient hemianopia 12 hours after the angioplasty, and transient headache and visual complaints.

In all reported series, femoral artery injury is the most frequently cited complication. In one series, 17 of 200 patients (8.5%) developed femoral artery complications.[107] These included 11 femoral artery thromboses, and another six patients had transient loss of femoral artery pulse. Eight of these patients required surgical thrombectomy, two resolved with streptokinase therapy, three resolved with heparin therapy, and four resolved spontaneously. Cooper and associates[109] reported femoral artery injury in 8 of 44 (18%). At follow-up, 3 of 44 (7%) had angiographic confirmation of superficial femoral artery occlusion. Saul and coworkers[110] reported femoral artery occlusion in 5 of 27 (19%) of their patients. On the basis of these reports and others,[86, 94] the two factors most frequently associated with femoral artery injury after balloon angioplasty of recoarctation of the aorta are the patient's size (90% of all reported femoral artery injuries occurred in children who weighed less the 12 kg at the time of angioplasty) and the angioplasty balloon's rupture.

In most centers, follow-up cardiac catheterization is not performed routinely in all patients after angioplasty for treatment of recoarctation of the aorta. There are a limited number of reports on the long-term follow-up of patients who have had angioplasty of recoarctation of the aorta.[86–88, 94, 109–112] Of the 76 patients for whom follow-up data are available, 12 of 76 (16%) had significant residual stenosis or restenosis at follow-up. In 7 of 12, repeated balloon angioplasty was used to treat the residual obstruction. In the other 64 patients, the gradient relief persisted, and further improvement in gradient reduction occurred in many patients over time. On the basis of follow-up magnetic resonance images, Soulen and colleagues[112] speculated that the progressive improvement in coarctation gradient was related to an increase in size of the aorta at the angioplasty site. At follow-up, aneurysms of the aorta at the site of the angioplasty occurred in 5 of the 76 patients (7%). However, because not all of the 76 patients in these studies underwent angiography at follow-up evaluation, the true incidence of late aneurysms after angioplasty for recoarctation of the aorta is unknown.

In summary, regardless of whether recoarctation occurred after surgical correction or after balloon angioplasty, percutaneous balloon angioplasty is currently considered to be the treatment of choice for aortic recoarctation.

Long-Term Survival

The long-term survival of patients treated for coarctation is less than the general population's. There are several long-term studies of survivors of coarctation repair.[113–119] These studies, although retrospective, have shown that individuals with repaired coarctation of the aorta do not have a normal survival and that they suffer from significant cardiovascular problems, including ischemic heart disease, cerebral hemorrhage, development of aortic aneurysms, and late development of hypertension. At the University of Minnesota, we recently had the opportunity to evaluate the long-term results of 254 survivors of coarctation repair performed between 1948 and 1976[73]; follow-up data were obtainable on all but two of these patients. During this time, of the 252 long-term survivors, there were 45 deaths. A survival analysis revealed that 87% of the patients were alive at 10 years, 82% at 20 years, 74% at 30 years, and 75% at 40 years. Of the 45 postoperative deaths, the mean age at death was 34.4 years ± 22.1 years. Survival was significantly related to age at the time of original coarctation repair, in that for individuals operated on before 14 years of age, the 30-year survival rate was 81%, whereas for those patients operated on after 14 years of age, the 30-year survival rate was only 62%. The most common causes of death included coronary artery disease (10 patients); a second cardiac operation, usually for coexistent aortic valve disease (8); sudden death, presumed due to an arrhythmia or coronary artery disease (7); a ruptured aortic aneurysm (6); cardiomyopathy (3); endocarditis (1); and miscellaneous causes in the remaining 10 patients including cerebrovascular accident, motor vehicle accidents, and other noncardiac causes of death. On the basis of this study and other retrospective analysis, survival, despite successful repair of coarctation of the aorta, is not normal.

One of the most common medical problems in patients who have had successful repair of coarctation is systemic hypertension. In the series from Minnesota,[73] 48% of the patients had high blood pressure (>140/90) at 10 years after repair, 55% at 20 years, 60% at 30 years, and 74% at 40 years. The most important predictor of late hypertension was age at operation, with those individuals operated on after 9 years of age having the highest incidence of hypertension. Sigurdardottir and Helgason[120] documented that exercise-induced hypertension is more common in patients with coarctation operated on after the first year of life. The exact mechanism for late systemic hypertension after coarctation repair still remains unclear. Potential causes of late hypertension relate to mild residual obstruction and abnormalities of compliance of the proximal or distal vascular beds. Parrish and colleagues[121] used ambulatory blood pressure monitoring to demonstrate that the degree of systolic blood pressure lability directly correlates with mild residual aortic obstruction. Johnson and coworkers[122] have documented abnormal peripheral flow kinetics in patients with successfully repaired coarctation of the aorta. They observed that compared with control subjects, surgically corrected coarctation patients experienced a greater degree of exercise-induced femoral artery vasodilatation but had an impaired lower limb blood flow in response to strenuous dynamic exercise. They speculated that alterations in peripheral vascular flow could result from exaggerated flow turbulence in the descending aorta distal to the site of coarctation correction because of loss of elasticity of the aorta either at or below the site of the resection. Gardiner and coworkers[123] demonstrated that in individuals with successfully repaired coarctation of the aorta, arterial dilatation capacity is reduced in the precoarctation vascular bed. These investigators suggested that this may be a significant contributor to long-term systemic hypertension. Beekman and coworkers[124] have previously demonstrated altered carotid baroreceptor function in post-coarctation patients. Gidding and colleagues[125] have shown abnormal vasoreactivity to catecholamines in the upper extremities compared with the lower extremities. Thus, despite successful repair of coarctation of the aorta, alterations in structure and function of the vascular bed seem to persist and may contribute to late systemic hypertension.

Exercise testing in patients after repair of coarctation of the aorta can be useful in assessing the etiology of residual or recurrent hypertension after presumedly successful repair. Abnormally increased blood pressure response to exercise can occur in patients with and without significant recoarctation of the aorta.

Recoarctation of the aorta and residual coarctation are the most common causes of exercise-induced hypertension in this group of patients. Investigators have reported abnormally high systolic blood pressure at peak exercise in patients after successful coarctation repair.[126] Other investigators have reported exercise-induced systolic blood pressure greater than 200 mm Hg with arm-to-leg blood pressure gradients of greater than 15 mm Hg at rest and greater than 35 mm Hg with exercise in patients with significant recoarctation of the aorta (ratio of aortic diameter at coarctation site to aortic diameter at diaphragm was less than 0.4).[127] Many patients with rest- or exercise-induced hypertension have no significant hemodynamic evidence of residual coarctation.[126, 128] In addition, investigators have demonstrated that the absence of a resting arm-to-leg blood pressure gradient does not exclude significant residual or recurrent coarctation.[129]

Exercise testing can provide valuable objective data in the assessment of patients after repair of coarctation of the aorta. The following general statements are helpful in the assessment of patients after coarctation repair[130]:

1. The presence of normal upper extremity systolic blood pressure response to exercise with lack of significant arm-to-leg blood pressure gradient at rest is consistent with adequate repair of coarctation of the aorta.

2. Systolic hypertension, whether at rest or with exercise, can occur in the absence of significant residual or recurrent coarctation of the aorta.

3. Significant coarctation can be present despite normal upper extremity blood pressure at rest.

4. Postexercise arm-to-leg blood pressure gradients must be evaluated with caution owing to technical difficulties in their acquisition and variable rate in the decrease of blood pressure after exercise in patients with coarctation.

Aneurysms of the aorta frequently occur in patients who have had successful repair of coarctation. These aneurysms occur in both the ascending and descending aorta and whether the coarctation has been treated by operation or angioplasty. Kaemmerer and associates[131] used magnetic resonance imaging to assess the long-term results of 25 patients who had coarctation repair. An aneurysm of the ascending aorta was observed in four patients and an aneurysm of the descending aorta was found in three patients. Each individual with an ascending aortic aneurysm had a bicuspid aortic valve. In our study,[73] aortic root dilatation was documented by magnetic resonance imaging in 27 of the 85 patients who had magnetic resonance imaging. The most common findings associated with aortic root dilatation were older age at operation and a bicuspid aortic valve. In this study, six patients had rupture of

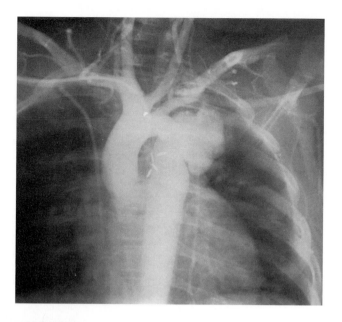

Angiogram, left anterior oblique projection, from a patient who had a patch angioplasty. A large aneurysm has developed at the site of the patch angioplasty.

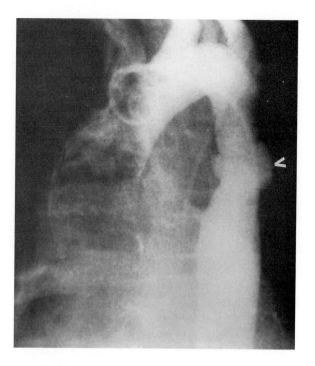

Angiogram, left anterior oblique projection, from a patient who had balloon angioplasty of a native coarctation. The arrow denotes the small circumferential aneurysm at the site of the coarctation angioplasty.

an ascending aortic aneurysm as a cause of late death. Aneurysms of the descending aorta occur with all types of coarctation surgical repair; however, the use of synthetic patch aortoplasty is the most common surgical procedure associated with aneurysms (Fig. 37–16). In a prospective study of 29 children who had Dacron patch angioplasty repair of coarctation, Bromberg and colleagues[52] found that 7 of the 29 (24%) had an aortic aneurysm. These investigators also documented that a chest film provided a sensitive screening test for detecting an aneurysm after correction of coarctation. In a study by Knyshov and coworkers,[56] of 891 long-term survivors of coarctation repair, aneurysms were documented to occur in 48 (5.4%) of all the patients who underwent repair. Aneurysms occurred with a repair using a synthetic patch aortoplasty in 43 of 48, with an end-to-end anastomosis in 4 of 48, and after coarctectomy and placement of a prosthetic graft in 1 of 48. Kino and coworkers[64] as well as Martin and coworkers[63] have reported late aneurysms associated with coarctation repair by use of a subclavian flap angioplasty.

Although the exact mechanisms responsible for aneurysm formation after surgical repair are unknown, Bogaert and coworkers[132] suggested that aneurysm formation at the repair site is directly related to hypoplasia of the transverse arch. These investigators believe that dynamic phenomena, such as flow acceleration and turbulence, originating in a narrow transverse arch may contribute to aneurysm formation at the repair site. McGiffin and associates[58] described a mathematical model for determining aortic wall stress. This model is useful in understanding why aneurysms may occur after surgical repair. The model predicts that the major variable affecting aortic wall stress after coarctation repair is patch geometry. If the patch is allowed to balloon, the wall stress increases out of proportion to the increase in aortic diameter. This model also predicts that aortic wall stress is concentrated opposite the

patch site, the site at which aneurysms are known to occur. Extending McGiffin's observation, one could assume that regardless of cause (the result of surgery, balloon angioplasty, or genetics), alterations in the elasticity of the aorta wall would be expected to be associated with increasing incidences of aneurysms. Aneurysms also follow balloon angioplasty,[89–91, 109, 133] and in fact, the late development of aortic aneurysms after angioplasty has made many cardiologists hesitant to perform angioplasty in patients with native coarctation (Fig. 37–17). On the basis of a review of multiple follow-up studies on balloon angioplasty,[89–91, 96–98, 109, 133] the incidence of aneurysms of the aorta after balloon angioplasty is approximately 6%. It is impossible to determine which patient will develop aneurysms after balloon angioplasty. Rothman and colleagues[134] described the use of intraluminal ultrasound imaging during balloon angioplasty of experimentally created coarctations in dogs and found that this technology permitted a more accurate anatomic visualization of the coarcted segment and also helped to determine the risk factors for development of aneurysms after balloon angioplasty. On the basis of subsequent studies in humans, these investigators have reported a high incidence of intimal tears (Fig. 37–18) and dissections immediately after balloon angioplasty.[135, 136] However, they have also documented that even significant intimal tears are not necessarily associated with aneurysm formation at follow-up.

Coronary artery disease seems to be accelerated in patients who have had coarctation of the aorta. In long-term follow-up studies,[113–119] early cardiac death from coronary artery disease has been observed in post-coarctation patients. Although the etiology of this accelerated atherosclerotic heart disease is unknown, a number of factors proba-

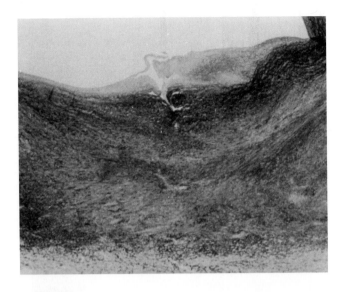

FIGURE 37–18

A photomicrograph of a coarctation that was surgically removed. The patient had a previous unsuccessful balloon angioplasty 6 weeks before the surgery. A small intimal flap can be noted with intimal hyperplasia and a tear in the aortic wall that extends midway into the aortic media.

bly play a role. Hypertension, as already discussed, is a known risk factor for the development of coronary artery disease. There must be factors other than hypertension, because even considering the higher incidence of hypertension, the incidence of coronary artery disease is much higher than one would expect. Some individuals with coarctation in the aorta are known to have altered structure and function of both the coronary and other systemic arteries. Chen and coworkers[137] described severe atherosclerosis and calcification in internal mammary arteries of two patients with previous coarctation repair who required coronary artery bypass surgery.

FUTURE DIRECTIONS

Although coarctation of the aorta appears to be a simple lesion that should be corrected with surgical repair, we now know that many individuals with coarctation of the aorta still present major diagnostic and therapeutic dilemmas. Cardiologists must determine the factor or factors that need to be modified to improve the longevity of individuals with coarctation of the aorta. This undoubtedly will include a better understanding of blood pressure regulation and coronary biology. The second major area of advancement will probably come with the repair of coarctation of the aorta in neonates. Currently, the extended end-to-end anastomosis technique offers great promise in reducing the incidence of restenosis in these individuals. In the future, there may also be catheter-based technologies that will be useful in these patients. Suarez de Lezo and coworkers[138] have reported on the use of balloon expandable stents for repair of severe coarctation of the aorta. Balloon expandable stents are also a nonsurgical therapeutic alternative in selected individuals with native or recurrent coarctation of the aorta.[139–141] The balloon expandable stent eliminates some of the limitations of balloon angioplasty in individuals with recurrent stenosis due to either vessel recoil or long tubular narrowing. Stents can be especially useful in individuals with Takayasu's arteritis who have diffuse long-segment aortic obstruction.[142] Because the stents are rigid and will not increase in size as a child grows, most cardiologists have reserved the use of aortic stents to fully or near-fully grown individuals. As with balloon angioplasty, aortic aneuryms can occur after placement of a balloon expandable stent.[143] Currently, most cardiologists consider the use of balloon expandable stents to treat coarctation as an investigational technique.

INTERRUPTED AORTIC ARCH

Interrupted aortic arch differs from coarctation of the aorta in that the continuity between the descending and ascending aorta is absent. Interrupted aortic arch is a rare anomaly that accounts for less that 1.5% of all congenital heart disease.[144]

PATHOLOGY AND EMBRYOLOGY

On the basis of the site of the interruption, Celoria and Patton[37] anatomically divided interrupted aortic arch into three types: type A, distal to the left subclavian artery; type B, between the left subclavian artery and the left common carotid artery; and type C, between the left common carotid and innominate arteries (Fig. 37–19). Types A and B have been further subdivided according to whether the right subclavian artery arises anomalously from the descending aorta, designated type A2 or type B2. The most common type of interrupted aortic arch is type B, and type C is the rarest.[37, 145, 146] Interrupted aortic arch is almost always associated with other intracardiac anomalies, the most common being a ventricular septal defect. Of 105 patients described by Moller and Edwards,[145] ventricular septal defect was present in 98, and in 58 of these, the ventricular septal defect was the only malformation. Other cardiac vascular malformations can coexist, but there have been no reports describing interrupted aortic arch associated with pulmonary atresia. The most common extracardiac anomaly associated with interrupted aortic arch is DiGeorge's syndrome, chromosomally localized to a microdeletion in the long arm of chromosome 22.[147, 148] DiGeorge's syndrome occurs in at least 15% of the patients with interrupted aortic arch (always type B).

In the past, the most widely accepted theory on the embryologic basis of interrupted aortic arch was that intracardiac malformations altered fetal hemodynamics, causing faulty development of the aortic arch. Thus, the magnitude of blood flow through the fetal arch would be critically important to both its enlargement and its evolution.[149, 150] However, with the recent understanding that microdeletions of the long arm of chromosome 22 are present in many patients with interrupted aortic arch, one has to question the importance of this hemodynamic theory. Type C interruption, between the right and left carotid arteries, and the rare patient of Pillsbury and coworkers,[151] who did not have any intracardiac malformation, also suggest that morphogenic factors other than anterograde aortic blood flow must be involved.

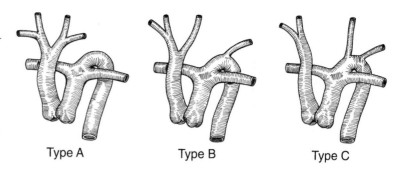

FIGURE 37–19

Three types of aortic arch interruption are classified as by Celoria and Patton[37]: type A interruption, distal to the left subclavian artery; type B interruption, between the left common carotid and left subclavian arteries; and type C interruption, between the innominate and left carotid arteries. (From Beekman R, Rocchini A: Coarctation of the aorta and interruption of the aortic arch. *In* Moller J, Neal W [eds]: Fetal, Neonatal, and Infant Cardiac Disease. Norwalk, CT, Appleton & Lange, 1990, pp 497–521. Reproduced with permission of The McGraw-Hill Companies.)

Type A   Type B   Type C

HEMODYNAMICS

In most types of interrupted aortic arch, flow to the descending aorta depends on a patent ductus arteriosus. As the ductus closes, perfusion to the lower part of the body and kidneys becomes inadequate. Urine output and renal function become impaired, and metabolic acidosis ultimately develops. In addition, as the ductus constricts, blood flow is redirected through the pulmonary circulation, resulting in left-sided volume and pressure overload that ultimately leads to rapid, progressive biventricular failure. Without treatment of interrupted aortic arch, the median age of death is 4 to 10 days.[144]

HISTORY AND PHYSICAL EXAMINATION

Patients with interrupted aortic arch have symptoms, usually severe, soon after birth. In a group of 50 infants observed at the Children's Memorial Medical Center between 1951 and 1996, all patients presented in severe congestive heart failure during the first 10 days of life.

The physical findings depend on the size of the ductus arteriosus and the severity of intracardiac malformations. The neonate always has tachypnea, tachycardia, and hepatomegaly and usually has rales. Precordial activity is always increased, the second sound is accentuated, and there is a loud systolic murmur usually present along the left sternal border. In all of our patients, a gallop and mid-diastolic rumble were also heard.

Femoral pulses are usually weak, and there is almost always a blood pressure difference between upper and lower extremities. The difference in pulse character can be helpful in differentiating on physical examination the type of interrupted aortic arch. In type C interrupted arch, absent femoral and left carotid pulses and a normal right carotid pulse are found; type B interruption may have abnormal left subclavian and femoral pulses, yet normal right and left carotid pulses. If the ductus is widely patent, there is little difference in upper and lower extremity pulses and pressures.

In individuals who have normally related great arteries, differential cyanosis between the upper and lower parts of the body may be noted (a pink head and blue abdomen), but this is usually not striking because of massive intracardiac left-to-right shunting. In patients with double-outlet right ventricle or D-transposition, the upper part of the body may be cyanotic while the lower part of the body is acyanotic, resulting in reversed differential cyanosis. Although these differences in oxygen saturation may not be detected by physical examination alone, they can frequently be detected with the use of pulse oximetry.

Peripheral edema, although rare among infants in congestive heart failure, is occasionally noted with interrupted aortic arch and is one of the few cardiac malformations associated with edema. Infants should be closely examined for features of DiGeorge's syndrome; the facial characteristics include hypertelorism, antimongoloid slant of the eyes, shortened philtrum, low-set ears and notched pinna, and micrognathia.

ELECTROCARDIOGRAM AND CHEST FILM

The electrocardiogram is usually not diagnostic with interrupted aortic arch and its pattern is usually dependent on associated anomalies. As with most types of congenital heart disease, there is usually right-axis deviation and right ventricular hypertrophy. Likewise, the chest film is also nondiagnostic and resembles the features of complex coarctation of the aorta with a large heart and increased pulmonary vascular markings.

ECHOCARDIOGRAPHIC FEATURES

Much of the discussion about echocardiograms for coarctation of the aorta also applies for patients with interrupted aortic arch. The suprasternal arch long-axis view is usually best to visualize the interruption of the arch.[27, 152, 153] In the most common type of interrupted aortic arch, type B, the ascending aorta can be seen to terminate in the left carotid artery, and the ductus arteriosus continues into the descending aorta. There is no evidence of an aortic arch linking the descending and ascending portions of the aorta. The two-dimensional echocardiogram and Doppler study can also be used to evaluate other intracardiac anomalies.

One of the most important abnormalities associated with interrupted aortic arch is left ventricular outflow tract obstruction. Left ventricular outflow tract obstruction occurs in more than 50% of children with interrupted aortic arch but is seldom recognized preoperatively. Geva and coworkers[154] demonstrated that preoperative echocardiographic predictors of left ventricular outflow tract obstruction can be useful in determining the surgical approach for patients with interrupted aortic arch. They analyzed the preoperative and postoperative echocardiograms in 37 infants and classified predictors of left ventricular outflow tract obstruction after repair. They found that the cross-sectional area of the left ventricular outflow tract was significantly smaller in patients who developed subaortic obstruction. Left ventricular outflow tract and aortic valve diameters and aortic valve areas did not predict postoperative left ventricular outflow tract obstruction. They found that a left ventricular outflow tract area that was less than $0.7 \text{ cm}^2/\text{m}^2$ was a sensitive predictor of left ventricular outflow tract obstruction. Arch anatomy was also an important predictor of postoperative left ventricular outflow tract obstruction, because type B interruptions had a much higher incidence of outflow tract obstruction than type A had, and an aberrant subclavian artery was also a strong predictor of left ventricular outflow tract obstruction.

CARDIAC CATHETERIZATION AND ANGIOGRAPHY

In the past, cardiac catheterization was used to diagnose interrupted aortic arch. With the important information that can now be obtained by two-dimensional echocardiography, catheterization is rarely performed, even in critically ill infants with interrupted aortic arch (Figs. 37–20 to 37–22). When catheterization is performed, it is usually to answer questions that have not been clearly resolved by the two-dimensional echocardiogram. The current indications for cardiac catheterization are to help delineate exact arch anatomy and to document the presence or hemodynamic significance of other intracardiac abnormalities.

If a catheterization is performed and the ventricular injection does not precisely delineate the arch anatomy, an ascending aortic injection is indicated. The ascending aorta can usually be entered from the left ventricle with the aid of a tip deflector or torque control soft guide wire. The presence of the characteristic "V" sign, that is, an ascending aorta that ends in the right common carotid arteries and left common carotid on the left ventricular injection, should alert the cardiologist to the diagnosis of type B interruption.

MANAGEMENT

The initial principles of management of interrupted aortic arch are identical to those of coarctation of the aorta,

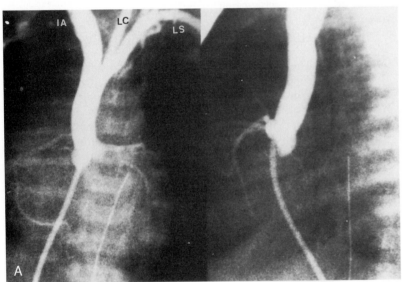

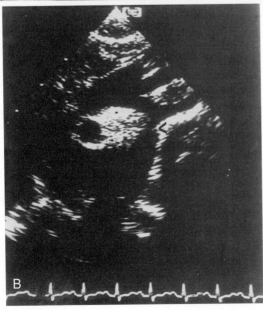

FIGURE 37–20

Interrupted aortic arch, type A. *A,* Anterior-posterior *(left)* and lateral *(right)* projections of an aortic angiogram. Left subclavian (LS), left carotid (LC), and innominate (IA) arteries arise from the ascending aorta. *B,* Echocardiogram, suprasternal view, with an interrupted arch just distal to the left subclavian artery *(arrow)*. (Courtesy of Dr. Nina Gotteiner and Kaliope Berdusis.)

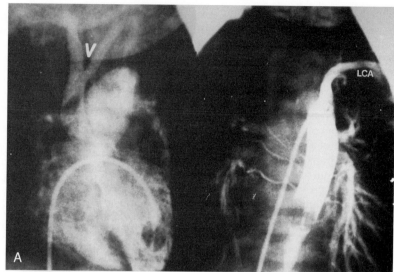

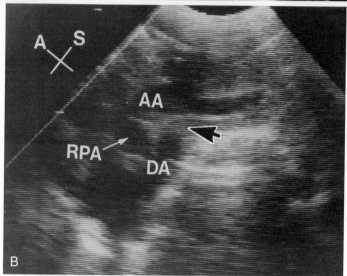

FIGURE 37–21

Interrupted aortic arch, type B. A, Left ventricular angiogram demonstrates a large left ventricle and ventricular septal defect that give rise to the ascending aorta, and the descending aorta arises from the ductus. The ascending aorta forms the typical "V" sign by ending in the right common carotid and left common carotid arteries. The panel on the right demonstrates a descending aortogram. The descending aorta is supplied by the ductus arteriosus, and the left subclavian artery (LCA) can be seen to arise from the descending aorta. B, Two-dimensional echocardiogram (suprasternal notch long-axis view). The ascending aorta (AA) terminates in the left carotid artery. There is no evidence (arrow) of an aortic arch linking the ascending and descending aorta (DA). A = anterior; RPA = right pulmonary artery; S = superior. Courtesy of Dr. A. Rebecca Snider. (From Beekman R, Rocchini A: Coarctation of the aorta and interruption of the aortic arch. In Moller J, Neal W [eds]: Fetal, Neonatal, and Infant Cardiac Disease. Norwalk, CT, Appleton & Lange, 1990, pp 497–521. Reproduced with permission of The McGraw-Hill Companies.)

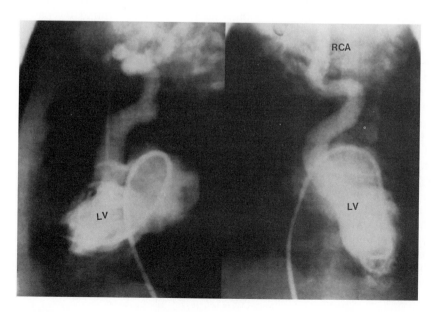

FIGURE 37–22

Interrupted aortic arch, type C. Left ventricular angiogram (LV) demonstrates filling of the ascending aorta, which ends with the right subclavian and right common carotid (RCA) arteries. The ventricular septum is intact, and a large patent ductus, not shown, supplies the descending aorta. (Adapted from Muster A: Angiographic anatomy of aortic coarctation: A classification based on the associated morphology of the aortic arch. In Mavroudis C, Backer C [eds]: Cardiac Surgery: State of the Art Reviews. Philadelphia, Hanley & Belfus, 1993, pp 23–45.)

namely, to stabilize the patient with the use of prostaglandin and inotropes. In all critically ill neonates in whom interrupted aortic arch is suspected, prostaglandin E₁ therapy should be given in an attempt to either dilate the ductus or maintain ductus patency. In a multicenter study,[155] prostaglandin infusion was beneficial in more than 75% of the infants with interrupted aortic arch. This study observed improved femoral pulses, peripheral infusion, increased urine output, and correction of the acidosis. As in coarctation of the aorta, the beneficial effects of prostaglandin E₁ in patients with interrupted aortic arch are less dependent on the age of the neonate, and it does take longer for improvement of ductal flow to occur. In addition to prostaglandin E₁ therapy, cardiac failure needs to be treated with inotropes (such as dopamine and dobutamine) and diuretics. Acidosis needs to be corrected aggressively with bicarbonate. A high inspired concentration of oxygen is not recommended because an elevated PO_2 tends to reduce pulmonary vascular resistance and increases systemic vascular resistance, thus altering the blood flow distribution such that more blood is directed to the pulmonary circulation and less blood to the systemic circulation. Blood calcium levels need to be routinely checked because the number of infants with DiGeorge's syndrome can approach 30% or greater. Finally, if DiGeorge's syndrome is suspected on the basis of facial features or absence of a thymus, only irradiated blood should be used for transfusion.

Once the infant has been successfully stabilized and the diagnosis is confirmed, operative therapy should be attempted. The first successful repair of interrupted aortic arch was in 1957 by Merrill and colleagues,[156] who divided the ductus and performed an end-to-side anastomosis between the descending and ascending aorta in the 3½-year-old child. Two ventricular septal defects were subsequently closed 4 years later. The goals of surgery are establishment of continuity between the ascending and descending aorta and correction of the intracardiac anomalies. These goals can be achieved either primarily or in different stages of repair. The ideal method of surgical management for interrupted aortic arch still remains controversial. Palliative operations were commonly used in the past but are less frequently employed now (Fig. 37–23). Noncorrective procedures include application of a pulmonary artery band and establishment of continuity between the ascending and descending aorta with a synthetic conduit. The change from palliated to primary repair is best illustrated in a paper by Menahem and coworkers.[157] From 1979 through 1984, 17 infants were treated; a single-stage repair was used in 2 of the 17, and a two-stage repair with initial reconstruction of the arch and pulmonary artery banding was used in the remaining 15. The surgical mortality with use of a predominantly two-stage repair was 65%. In the next 5 years, 1984 through 1988, 29 infants underwent surgery, and 22 of 29 had a single-stage repair with only three deaths in this group. Other excellent institutions have come to the same conclusion.[158–161] The basic approach to infants with ventricular septal defect and left-sided obstruction is best summarized in a 1994 review by Gersony.[162] He stated that complete repair at the time of diagnosis in the neonate, regardless of whether associated obstructions are present, remains the "gold standard" (Fig. 37–24).

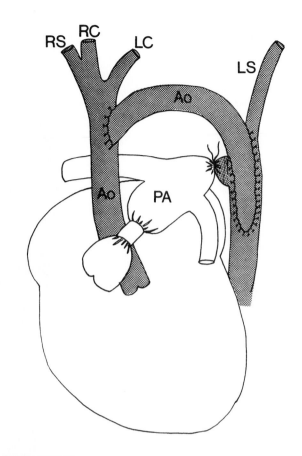

Staged repair of type B interrupted aortic arch with a ventricular septal defect. A large polytetrafluoroethylene conduit is interposed between the ascending and descending aorta (Ao) and the pulmonary artery (PA) is banded. The patent ductus arteriosus is ligated. LC = left carotid artery; LS = left subclavian artery; RC = right carotid artery; RS = right subclavian artery. (From Beekman R, Rocchini A: Coarctation of the aorta and interruption of the aortic arch. *In* Moller J, Neal W [eds]: Fetal, Neonatal, and Infant Cardiac Disease. Norwalk, CT, Appleton & Lange, 1990, pp 497–521. Reproduced with permission of The McGraw-Hill Companies.)

Currently, the most challenging and controversial aspect in the treatment of patients with interrupted aortic arch and ventricular septal defect is the management of severe left ventricular outflow tract obstruction. During the past 3 years, several new procedures have been advocated for this group of patients. Starnes and coworkers[163] reported the use of aortic root replacement with pulmonary autografts in children with complex obstructive lesions of the left side of the heart. Three of the eight patients described in this series had interrupted aortic arch with ventricular septal defect and subaortic stenosis. The surgical technique advocated by Starnes included replacement of the aortic root with a pulmonary autograft, combined with incision of the conal septum to relieve subaortic stenosis and a pulmonary homograft placed in the right ventricular outflow tract. Reddy and coworkers[164] described a similar procedure for treating patients with complex left ventricular outflow tract obstruction. Other approaches for severe left ventricular outflow tract obstruction associated with interrupted arch and ventricular septal defect have included transplantation, as reported by Razzouk and coworkers,[165] and the Norwood procedure, as reported by Jacobs and coworkers.[166] In 1993, Bove and coworkers[167] reported their results of man-

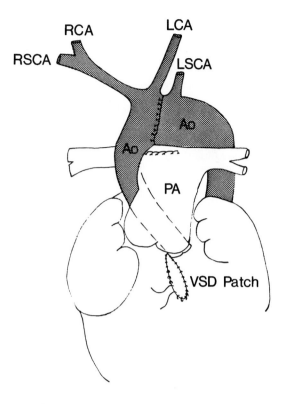

FIGURE 37–24

Repair of type B interrupted aortic arch and ventricular septal defect (VSD). The ventricular septal defect is patched through the right atrium. End-to-side anastomosis of the ascending and descending aorta (Ao) is performed with running sutures. The pulmonary artery (PA) is repaired. LCA = left carotid artery; LSCA = left subclavian artery; RCA = right carotid artery; RSCA = right subclavian artery. (From Beekman R, Rocchini A: Coarctation of the aorta and interruption of the aortic arch. *In* Moller J, Neal W [eds]: Fetal, Neonatal, and Infant Cardiac Disease. Norwalk, CT, Appleton & Lange, 1990, pp 497–521. Reproduced with permission of The McGraw-Hill Companies.)

agement of severe subaortic stenosis and aortic arch obstructions in the neonate. Their approach was through the right atrium to remove part of the superior margin of the ventricular septal defect up to the aortic annulus. The resulting enlarged ventricular septal defect was then closed with a patch to widen the subaortic area. Of seven patients who were treated in this fashion, there was only one operative death. In 1996, Starnes and coworkers[163] suggested a one-stage repair of interrupted aortic arch with subaortic stenosis by a new approach, which did not include resection of the conal septum; rather, the ventricular septal defect patch was placed on the left side of the septum to deflect the conal septum anteriorly and away from the subaortic area. They reported their results in nine neonates treated in this fashion with no early or late deaths in the mean follow-up of 12 months. At follow-up, they reported that no patient had subaortic obstruction.

In patients with complex intracardiac anomalies and interrupted aortic arch, the general principles should be that if two ventricles are present, a biventricular repair should be undertaken during the neonatal period. This would hold, for example, with children with truncus arteriosus and interrupted aortic arch or double-outlet right ventricle and interrupted aortic arch. Management of the child with a functional single ventricle and an interrupted arch pre-

sents a much more challenging problem. There is frequently an important obstruction within the single ventricle often in the form of an obstructive bulboventricular foramen. This obstruction must be bypassed by use of a pulmonary-aortic anastomosis, such as the Damus-Kaye-Stansel procedure or the Norwood procedure, or it must be relieved by resection of the bulboventricular foramen. Because the ultimate corrective procedure involves the use of a Fontan-type repair, it is therefore mandatory to preserve ventricular function without leaving any significant outflow tract obstruction.

PROGNOSIS

The outcome of operation for interrupted aortic arch was clearly defined in a multi-institutional study of the Congenital Heart Surgeons Society.[161] In this study, 183 neonates with interrupted arch and ventricular septal defect entered a multi-institutional study between 1987 and 1989. Nine died before repair was accomplished. For the remaining 74, survival at 1 month and 1, 3, and 4 years after repair was 73%, 65%, 63%, and 63%, respectively. The risk factors for death were low birth weight and younger age at repair, interrupted aortic arch type B, outlet and trabecular ventricular septal defect, small size of ventricular septum, and subaortic narrowing. The cardiac center at which the operation was performed was also thought to be a risk factor in two centers and possibly in two others. Procedural risk factors for death after repair were repair without concomitant procedures in patients with other important levels of obstruction on the left side of the heart and aorta, a Damus-Kaye-Stansel anastomosis, and a subaortic myotomy or myomectomy in the face of subaortic narrowing. The Congenital Heart Surgeons Society study also concluded that a one-stage repair, plus ascending aortic arch augmentation, had the highest predicted time-related survival.

FUTURE DIRECTIONS

In the future, major advances will be made into our understanding of the genetic basis of interrupted aortic arch. Although we know that interrupted aortic arch type B is frequently associated with the DiGeorge deletion on chromosome 22, not all children with interrupted arch have this genetic defect. Once we understand all of the genetic causes of interrupted aortic arch, preventive strategies might then be initiated to reduce the incidence of this complex lesion.

The management of children with complex intracardiac anomalies and interrupted aortic arch is currently challenging and difficult. In the future, new surgical procedures will need to be developed to improve both the short-term and long-term outcome for these children.

REFERENCES

1. Keith J: Coarctation of the aorta. *In* Keith J, Rowe R, Vlad P (eds): Heart Disease in Infancy and Children. New York, Macmillan, 1978, pp 736–760.
2. Storch T, Mannick E: Epidemiology of congenital heart disease in Louisiana: An association between race and sex and the prevalence of specific cardiac malformations. Teratology 46:271, 1992.

3. Ravela H, Stephenson LW, Freidman S: Coarctation resection in children with Turner's syndrome. J Thorac Cardiovasc Surg 80:427, 1980.

4. Sehester J: Coarctation of the aorta in monozygotic twins. Br Heart J 47:619, 1882.

5. Beekman R, Robinow M: Coarctation of the aorta inherited as an autosomal dominant trait. Am J Cardiol 56:818, 1985.

6. Beekman R, Rocchini A: Coarctation of the aorta and interruption of the aortic arch. In Moller J, Neal W (eds): Fetal, Neonatal, and Infant Cardiac Disease. Norwalk, CT, Appleton & Lange, 1990, p 497.

7. Mulder H, Kaan G, Nijveld A, et al: Coarctation developing after arterial switch repair for transposition of the great arteries. Ann Thorac Surg 58:227, 1994.

8. Edwards J, Christensen N, Clagett O: Pathologic considerations in coarctation of the aorta. Mayo Clin Proc 23:324, 1948.

9. Graham M, Zelenock G, Erlandson E, Stanley J: Abdominal aortic coarctation and segmental hypoplasia. Surgery 86:519, 1979.

10. Shone J, Seller R, Anderson R: The developmental complex of "parachute mitral valve," supravalvar ring of left atrium, subaortic stenosis and coarctation of the aorta. Am J Cardiol 11:714, 1963.

11. Blankl H: Coarctation of the aorta. In Blankl H (ed): Congenital Malformations of the Heart and Great Vessels: Synopsis of Pathology, Embryology, and Natural History. Baltimore, Urban & Schwarzenberg, 1977, p 45.

12. Hobes H, Steinfeld L, Blumenthal S: Congenital cerebral aneurysms and coarctation of the aorta. Arch Paediatr 76:28, 1959.

13. Serizawa T, Satoh A, Miyata A, et al: Ruptured cerebral aneurysm associated with coarctation of the aorta—report of two cases. Neurol Med Chir (Tokyo) 32:342, 1992.

14. Fyler D, Buckley L, Hellenbrand W: Report of the New England Regional Infant Cardiac Program. Pediatrics 65:432, 1980.

15. Greenwood R, Rosenthal A, Parisi L: Extracardiac abnormalities in infants with congenital heart disease. Pediatrics 55:485, 1975.

16. Perloff J: Coarctation of the aorta. In Perloff J (ed): The clinical recognition of congenital heart disease. Philadelphia, WB Saunders, 1978, pp 126–153.

17. Kurihara Y, Kurihara H, Oda H, et al: Aortic arch malformations and ventricular septal defect in mice deficient in endothelin-1. J Clinic Invest 96:293, 1995.

18. Russell G, Berry P, Watterson K: Patterns of ductal tissue in coarctation in the first three months of life. J Thorac Cardiovasc Surg 102:596, 1991.

19. Rudolph A, Heymann M, Spitznas U: Hemodynamic considerations in the development of narrowing of the aorta. Am J Cardiol 30:514, 1972.

20. Graham T, Lewis B, Jarmakani M: Left ventricular volume and mass quantification in children with left ventricular pressure overload. Circulation 41:203, 1970.

21. Campbell M: Natural history of coarctation of the aorta. Br Heart J 32:633, 1970.

22. Campbell M, Baylis J: The course and prognosis of coarctation of the aorta. Br Heart J 18:475, 1956.

23. Ing F, Starc T, Griffiths S, Gersony W: Early diagnosis of coarctation of the aorta in children: A continuing dilemma. Pediatrics 98:378, 1996.

24. Stafford M, Griffiths S, Gersony W: Coarctation of the aorta: A study in delayed detection. Pediatrics 69:159, 1982.

25. Sinha S, Kardatzke M, Cole R, Paul M: Coarctation of the aorta in infancy. Circulation 40:385, 1969.

26. Sahn D, Allen H, McDonald G, Goldberg S: Real-time cross-sectional echocardiographic diagnosis of coarctation of the aorta: A prospective study of echocardiographic-angiographic correlations. Circulation 56:762, 1977.

27. Snider AR, Silverman N: Suprasternal notch echocardiography: A two-dimensional technique for evaluation of congenital heart disease. Circulation 63:165, 1981.

28. Hatle L, Angelsen B: Doppler Ultrasound in Cardiology. Philadelphia, Lea & Febiger, 1985.

29. Huhta J, Gutgesell H, Latson L, Huffines F: Two-dimensional echocardiographic assessment of the aorta in infants and children with congenital heart disease. Circulation 70:417, 1984.

30. Smallhorn J, Huhta J, Adams P: Cross-sectional echocardiographic assessment of coarctation in the sick neonate and infant. Br Heart J 50:349, 1983.

31. Snider RA, Serwer G: Quantitative echocardiographic exam. In Snider AR, Serwer G (eds): Echocardiography in Pediatric Heart Disease. Chicago, Year Book Medical Publishers, 1990, p 78.

32. Carvalho J, Remington A, Shinebourne E: Continuous wave Doppler echocardiography and coarctation of the aorta: Gradients and flow pattern in the assessment of severity. Br Heart J 64:133, 1990.

33. Simpson I, Sahn D, Valdes-Cruz L: Color Doppler flow mapping in patients with coarctation of the aorta: New observations and improved evaluations with color flow diameter and proximal acceleration as predictors of severity. Circulation 77:736, 1988.

34. Sharland G, Chan K, Allan L: Coarctation of the aorta: Difficulties in prenatal diagnosis. Br Heart J 71:70, 1994.

35. Hornberger L, Sahn D, Kleinman C, et al: Antenatal diagnosis of coarctation of the aorta: A multicenter experience. J Am Coll Cardiol 23:2417, 1994.

36. Barry A: The aortic arch derivatives in the human adult. Anat Rec 111:221, 1951.

37. Celoria G, Patton R: Congenital absence of the aortic arch. Am Heart J 58:407, 1959.

38. Muster A: Angiographic anatomy of aortic coarctation: A classification based on the associated morphology of the aortic arch. In Mavroudis C, Backer C (eds): Cardiac Surgery: State of the Art Reviews. Philadelphia, Hanley & Belfus, 1993, p 23.

39. Task Force on Blood Pressure in Children: Report of the Second Task Force on Blood Pressure Control in Children—1987. Pediatrics 79:1, 1987.

40. Lewis A, Freed M, Heymann M, et al: Side effects of therapy with prostaglandin E$_1$ in infants with critical congenital heart disease. Circulation 64:893, 1981.

41. Backer C, Paape K, Zales V, et al: Coarctation of the aorta. Repair with polytetrafluoroethylene patch aortoplasty. Circulation 92(suppl):II-132, 1995.

42. Minich L, Beekman R, Rocchini A, et al: Surgical repair is safe and effective after unsuccessful balloon angioplasty of native coarctation of the aorta. J Am Coll Cardiol 19:389, 1992.

43. Craaford C, Nylin G: Congenital coarctation of the aorta and its surgical management. J Thorac Surg 14:347, 1945.

44. Gross R, Hufnagel C: Coarctation of the aorta: Experimental studies regarding its surgical correction. N Engl J Med 233:287, 1945.

45. Kirklin J, Burchell H, Pugh D, et al: Surgical treatment of coarctation of the aorta in a ten week old infant: Report of a case. Circulation 6:411, 1952.

46. Kappetein A, Zwinderman A, Bogers A, et al: More than thirty-five years of coarctation repair. An unexpected high relapse rate. J Thorac Cardiovasc Surg 107:87, 1994.

47. Messmer B, Minale C, Muhler E: Surgical correction of coarctation in early infancy: Does surgical technique influence the results? Ann Thorac Surg 52:594, 1991.

48. Arenas J, Myers J, Gleason M, et al: End-to-end repair of aortic coarctation using absorbable polydioxanone suture. Ann Thorac Surg 51:413, 1991.

49. Myers J, Campbell D, Waldhausen J: The use of absorbable monofilament polydioxanone suture in pediatric cardiovascular operations. J Thorac Cardiovasc Surg 92:771, 1986.

50. Vosschulte K: Surgical correction of coarctation of the aorta by an "isthmus-plastic" operation. Thorax 16:338, 1961.

51. Bergdahl L, Ljungqvist A: Long-term results after repair of coarctation of the aorta by patch grafting. J Thorac Cardiovasc Surg 80:177, 1980.

52. Bromberg B, Beekman RH, Rocchini A, et al: Aortic aneurysm after patch aortoplasty repair of coarctation: A prospective analysis of prevalence, screening tests and risks. J Am Coll Cardiol 14:734, 1989.

53. Clarkson P, Brandt P, Barratt-Boyes B, et al: Prosthetic repair of coarctation of the aorta with particular reference to Dacron onlay patch grafts and late aneurysm formation. Am J Cardiol 56:342, 1985.

54. Heikkinen L, Sariola H, Salo J, et al: Morphological and histopathological aspects of aneurysms after patch aortoplasty for coarctation. Ann Thorac Surg 50:946, 1990.

55. DeSanto A, Bills R, King H: Pathogenesis of aneurysm formation opposite prosthetic patches used for coarctation repair. J Thorac Cardiovasc Surg 94:720, 1987.

56. Knyshov G, Sitar L, Glagola M, Atamanyuk M: Aortic aneurysms at the site of the repair of coarctation of the aorta: A review of 48 patients. Ann Thorac Surg 61:935, 1996.
57. Rheuban K, Gutgesell H, Carpenter M, Jedeiken R: Aortic aneurysm after patch angioplasty for aortic isthmic coarctation in childhood. Am J Cardiol 58:178, 1986.
58. McGiffin D, McGiffin P, Galbraith A, Cross R: Aortic wall stress profile after repair of coarctation of the aorta: Is it related to subsequent true aneurysm formation? J Thorac Cardiovasc Surg 104:924, 1992.
59. Morris G, Cooley D, DeBakey M, Crawford R: Coarctation of the aorta with particular emphasis upon improved technique of surgical repair. J Thorac Cardiovasc Surg 40:705, 1960.
60. Waldhausen J, Nahrwold D: Repair of coarctation of the aorta with a subclavian flap. J Thorac Cardiovasc Surg 51:532, 1966.
61. Van Son J, Van Asten W, Van Lier H, et al: Detrimental sequelae on the hemodynamics of the upper left limb after subclavian flap angioplasty in infancy. Circulation 81:996, 1990.
62. Van Son J, Daniels O, Vincent J, et al: Appraisal of resection and end-to-end anastomosis for repair of coarctation of the aorta in infancy: Preference for resection. Ann Thorac Surg 48:496, 1989.
63. Martin M, Beekman R, Rocchini A, et al: Aortic aneurysms after subclavian angioplasty repair of coarctation of the aorta. Am J Cardiol 61:951, 1988.
64. Kino K, Sano S, Sugawara E, et al: Late aneurysm after subclavian flap aortoplasty for coarctation of the aorta. Ann Thorac Surg 61:1262, 1996.
65. Beekman R, Rocchini A, Behrendt D, et al: Long-term outcome for repair of coarctation in infancy: Subclavian angioplasty does not reduce the need for reoperation. J Am Coll Cardiol 8:1406, 1986.
66. Merrill W, Hoff S, Stewart J, et al: Operative risk factors and durability of repair of coarctation of the aorta in the neonate. Ann Thorac Surg 58:399, 1994.
67. Van Heurn L, Wong C, Spiegelhalter D, et al: Surgical treatment of aortic coarctation in infants younger than three months: 1985 to 1990. Success of extended end-to-end arch aortoplasty. J Thorac Cardiovasc Surg 107:74, 1994.
68. Lansman S, Shapiro A, Schiller M, et al: Extended aortic arch anastomoses for repair of coarctation in infancy. Circulation 74:136, 1986.
69. Zannini L, Lecompte Y, Galli R: Aortic coarctation with arch hypoplasia: A new surgical technique. G Ital Cardiol 15:1045, 1985.
70. Elliott M: Coarctation of the aorta with arch hypoplasia: Improvements on a new technique. Ann Thorac Surg 44:321, 1987.
71. Sealy W, Harris J, Young W: Paradoxical hypertension following resection of coarctation of the aorta. Surgery 42:135, 1957.
72. Rocchini A, Rosenthal A, Barger A, et al: Pathogenesis of paradoxical hypertension after coarctation resection. Circulation 54:382, 1976.
73. Salazar O, Steinberger J, Carpenter B, et al: Predictors of hypertension in long term survivors of repaired coarctation of the aorta. J Am Coll Cardiol 27(suppl A):35A, 1996.
74. Choy M, Rocchini A, Beekman R, et al: Paradoxical hypertension after repair of coarctation of the aorta in children: Balloon angioplasty versus surgical repair. Circulation 75:1186, 1987.
75. Gidding S, Rocchini A, Beekman R, et al: Therapeutic effect of propanolol on paradoxical hypertension after repair of coarctation. N Engl J Med 312:1224, 1985.
76. Brandt B, Heintz S, Rose E: Repair of coarctation of the aorta in children with Turner's syndrome. Pediatr Cardiol 5:175, 1984.
77. Brewer L, Fosberg R, Mulder G: Spinal cord complications following surgery for coarctation of the aorta. J Thorac Cardiovasc Surg 64:368, 1972.
78. Moreno N, de Campo T, Kaiser G: Technical and pharmacologic management of distal hypotension during repair of coarctation of the aorta. J Thorac Cardiovasc Surg 80:182, 1980.
79. Pollock J, Jamieson M, McWilliams R: Somatosensory evoked potentials in the detection of spinal cord ischemia in aortic coarctation repair. Ann Thorac Surg 41:251, 1986.
80. Dasmahapatra H, Coles J, Taylor M: Identification of risk factors for spinal cord ischemia by the use of monitoring of somatosensory evoked potentials during coarctation repair. Circulation 76:14, 1987.
81. Sos T, Sniderman K, Rettek-Sos B, et al: Percutaneous transluminal dilatation of coarctation of thoracic aorta post mortem. Lancet 2:970, 1979.
82. Lock J, Castaneda-Zuniga W, Bass J, et al: Balloon dilatation of excised aortic coarctation. Radiology 143:689, 1982.
83. Lock J, Niemi T, Burke B, et al: Transcutaneous angioplasty of experimental aortic coarctation. Circulation 66:1280, 1982.
84. Tynan M, Finley J, Fontes V, et al: Balloon angioplasty for the treatment of native coarctation: Results of Valvuloplasty and Angioplasty of Congenital Anomalies Registry. Am J Cardiol 65:790, 1990.
85. Beekman R, Rocchini AP: Transcatheter treatment of congenital heart disease. Prog Cardiovasc Dis 32:1, 1989.
86. Allen HD, Marx G, Ovitt T, Goldberg S: Balloon dilatation angioplasty for coarctation of the aorta. Am J Cardiol 57:828, 1986.
87. Lock J, Bass J, Amplatz K, et al: Balloon dilation angioplasty of aortic coarctations in infants and children. Circulation 68:109, 1983.
88. Lababidi Z, Daskalopoulos D, Stoeckle H: Transluminal balloon coarctation angioplasty: Experience with 27 patients. Am J Cardiol 54:1288, 1984.
89. Wren C, Peart J, Bain H, Hunter S: Balloon dilatation of unoperated coarctation: Immediate results and one year follow-up. Br Heart J 58:369, 1987.
90. Morrow W, Vick G, Nihill M, et al: Balloon dilation of unoperated coarctation of the aorta: Short and intermediate term results. J Am Coll Cardiol 11:133, 1988.
91. Beekman R, Rocchini A, Dick M, et al: Percutaneous balloon angioplasty for native coarctation of the aorta. J Am Coll Cardiol 10:1078, 1987.
92. Rao P: Balloon angioplasty of native coarctations. Am J Cardiol 66:1401, 1990.
93. Beekman R, Rocchini A, Behrendt D, Rosenthal A: Reoperation for coarctation of the aorta. Am J Cardiol 48:1108, 1981.
94. Rao P, Mohinder K, Galal O, Wilson A: Follow-up results of balloon angioplasty of native coarctation in neonates and infants. Am Heart J 120:1310, 1990.
95. Johnson M, Canter C, Strauss A, Spray T: Repair of coarctation of the aorta in infancy: Comparison of surgical and balloon angioplasty. Am Heart J 125:464, 1993.
96. Fletcher S, Nihill M, Grifka R, et al: Balloon angioplasty of native coarctation of the aorta: Midterm follow-up and prognostic factors. J Am Coll Cardiol 25:730, 1995.
97. Mendelsohn A, Lloyd T, Crowley D, et al: Late follow-up of balloon angioplasty in children with a native coarctation of the aorta. Am J Cardiol 74:696, 1994.
98. Shaddy R, Boucek M, Sturtevant J, et al: Comparison of angioplasty and surgery for unoperated coarctation of the aorta. Circulation 87:793, 1993.
99. Kaine S, Smith EO, Mott A, et al: Quantitative echocardiographic analysis of the aortic arch predicts outcome of balloon angioplasty of native coarctation of the aorta. Circulation 94:1056, 1996.
100. Cerilli J, Lauridsen P: Reoperation for coarctation of the aorta. Acta Chir Scand 129:391, 1965.
101. Pollack P, Freed M, Castenada A, Norwood W: Reoperation for isthmic coarctation of the aorta: Follow-up of 26 patients. Am J Cardiol 51:1690, 1983.
102. Kirklin J, Barratt-Boyes B: Coarctation of the aorta and aortic arch interruption. In Kirklin J, Barratt-Boyes B (eds): Cardiac Surgery: Morphology, Diagnostic Criteria, Natural History, Techniques, Results and Indications. New York, John Wiley & Sons, 1986, p 1030.
103. Kan J, White R, Mitchell S, et al: Treatment of restenosis of coarctation by percutaneous transluminal angioplasty. Circulation 68:1087, 1983.
104. Lock J, Keane J, Fellows K: The use of catheter intervention procedures for congenital heart disease. J Am Coll Cardiol 7:1420, 1986.
105. Beekman R, Meliones J, Riggs T, Rocchini A: Antegrade transvenous balloon angioplasty of recurrent coarctation in infancy. J Intervent Cardiol 1:137, 1988.
106. Murphy J, Sands BL, Norwood, WI: Intraoperative balloon angioplasty of aortic coarctation in infants with hypoplastic left heart syndrome. Am J Cardiol 59:949, 1987.
107. Hellenbrand W, Allen H, Golinko R, et al: Balloon angioplasty for aortic recoarctation: Results of Valvuloplasty and Angioplasty of Congenital Anomalies Registry. Am J Cardiol 65:793, 1990.
108. Joyce D, McGrath L: Pseudo-aneurysm formation following balloon angioplasty for recurrent coarctation of the aorta. Cathet Cardiovasc Diagn 20:133, 1990.
109. Cooper R, Ritter S, Golinko R: Balloon dilation angioplasty: Nonsurgical management of coarctation of the aorta. Circulation 70:903, 1984.

110. Saul J, Keane J, Fellows K, Lock J: Balloon dilation angioplasty of postoperative aortic obstruction. Am J Cardiol 59:943, 1987.

111. Lorber A, Ettedgui J, Baker E, et al: Balloon angioplasty for re-coarctation following the subclavian flap operation. Int J Cardiol 10:57, 1986.

112. Soulen R, Kan J, Mitchell S, White RJ: Evaluation of balloon angioplasty of coarctation restenosis by magnetic resonance imaging. Am J Cardiol 60:343, 1987.

113. Clarckson P, Nicholson M, Barratt-Boyes B, et al: Results after repair of coarctation of the aorta beyond infancy. A 10 to 28 year follow-up with particular reference to late systemic hypertension. Am J Cardiol 51:1481, 1983.

114. Cohen M, Fuster V, Steele P, et al: Coarctation of the aorta. Long-term follow-up and prediction of outcome after surgical correction. Circulation 80:840, 1989.

115. Koller M, Rothlin M, Senning A: Coarctation of the aorta: Review of 362 operated patients. Long term follow-up and assessment of prognostic variables. Eur Heart J 8:670, 1987.

116. Marrion B, Humphries J, Rowe R, Mellits E: Prognosis of surgically corrected coarctation of the aorta. A 20 year postoperative appraisal. Circulation 47:119, 1973.

117. Presbitero P, Demaire D, Perinetto E, et al: Long term results (15–30 years) of surgical repair of aortic coarctation. Br Heart J 57:462, 1987.

118. Sorland S, Rostad H, Forfang K, Abyholm G: Coarctation of the aorta. A follow-up study after surgical treatment in infancy and childhood. Acta Paediatr Scand 69:113, 1980.

119. Stewart A, Ahmed R, Travill C, Newman C: Coarctation of the aorta life and health 20–44 years after surgical repair. Br Heart J 69:65, 1993.

120. Sigurdardottir L, Helgason H: Exercise-induced hypertension after corrective surgery for coarctation of the aorta. Pediatr Cardiol 17:301, 1996.

121. Parrish M, Torres E, Peshock R, Fixler D: Ambulatory blood pressure in patients with occult recurrent coarctation of the aorta. Pediatr Cardiol 16:166, 1995.

122. Johnson D, Bonnin P, Perrault H, et al: Peripheral blood flow responses to exercise after successful correction of coarctation of the aorta. J Am Coll Cardiol 26:1719, 1995.

123. Gardiner H, Celermajer D, Sorensen K, et al: Arterial reactivity is significantly impaired in normotensive young adults after successful repair of aortic coarctation in childhood. Circulation 89:1745, 1994.

124. Beekman R, Katz B, Moorehead-Steffens C, Rocchini A: Altered baroreceptor function in children with systolic hypertension after coarctation repair. Am J Cardiol 52:112, 1983.

125. Gidding S, Rocchini A, Moorehead C, et al: Increased forearm vascular reactivity in patients with hypertension after repair of coarctation. Circulation 71:495, 1985.

126. Freed M, Rocchini A, Rosenthal A, et al: Exercise-induced hypertension after surgical repair of coarctation of the aorta. Am J Cardiol 43:253, 1979.

127. Markel H, Rocchini A, Beekman R, et al: Exercise-induced hypertension after repair of coarctation of the aorta: Arm versus leg exercise. J Am Coll Cardiol 8:165, 1986.

128. Pelech AN, Kartodihardjo W, Balfe JA, et al: Exercise in children before and after coarctectomy: Hemodynamic, echocardiographic, and biochemical assessment. Am Heart J 112:1263, 1986.

129. Waldman J, Goodman A, Tumeau A, et al: Coarctation of the aorta: Noninvasive physiological assessment in infants and children before and after operation. J Thorac Cardiovasc Surg 80:187, 1980.

130. Driscoll DJ: Diagnostic use of exercise testing in pediatric cardiology: The noninvasive approach. In Bar-Or MD (ed): Advances in Pediatric Sport Sciences, Vol III: Biological Issues. Champaign, IL, 1989, p 223.

131. Kaemmerer H, Theissen P, Konig U, et al: Follow-up using magnetic resonance imaging in adult patients after surgery for aortic coarctation. J Thorac Cardiovasc Surg 41:107, 1993.

132. Bogaert J, Gewillig M, Rademakers F, et al: Transverse arch hypoplasia predisposes to aneurysm formation at the repair site after patch angioplasty for coarctation of the aorta. J Am Coll Cardiol 26:521, 1995.

133. Marvin W, Mahoney L, Lauer R: Pathologic sequelae of balloon dilation angioplasty for unoperated coarctation of the aorta in children (Abstract). J Am Coll Cardiol 7:117, 1986.

134. Rothman A, Ricou F, Weitraub R, et al: Intraluminal ultrasound imaging through a balloon dilation catheter in an animal model of coarctation of the aorta. Circulation 85:2291, 1992.

135. Degoff C, Rice M, Reller M, et al: Intravascular ultrasound can assist angiographic assessment of coarctation of the aorta. Am Heart J 128:836, 1994.

136. Sohn S, Rothman A, Shiota T, et al: Acute and follow-up intravascular ultrasound findings after balloon dilation of coarctation of the aorta. Circulation 90:340, 1994.

137. Chen R, Reul G, Cooley D: Severe internal mammary artery atherosclerosis after correction of coarctation of the aorta. Ann Thorac Surg 59:1228, 1995.

138. Suarez de Lezo J, Pan M, Romero M, et al: Balloon-expandable stent repair of severe coarctation of the aorta. Am Heart J 129:1002, 1995.

139. Ebeid MR, Prieto LR, Latson LA: Use of balloon-expandable stents for coarctation of the aorta: Initial results and intermediate-term follow-up. J Am Coll Cardiol 30:1853, 1997.

140. Ovaert C, Benson LN, Nykanen D, Freedom RM: Transcatheter treatment of coarctation of the aorta: A review. Pediatr Cardiol 19:27, 1998.

141. Bulbul ZR, Bruckheimer E, Love JC, et al: Implantation of balloon-expandable stents for coarctation of the aorta: Implantation data and short-term results. Cathet Cardiovasc Diagn 39:36, 1996.

142. D'Souza SJ, Tsai WS, Silver MM, et al: Diagnosis and management of stenotic aorto-arteriopathy in childhood. J Pediatr 132:1016, 1998.

143. Fletcher SE, Cheatham JP, Froeming S: Aortic aneurysm following primary balloon angioplasty and secondary endovascular stent placement in the treatment of native coarctation of the aorta. Cathet Cardiovasc Diagn 44:45, 1998.

144. Collins-Nakai R, Dick M, Parisi-Buckley L, et al: Interrupted aortic arch in infancy. J Pediatr 88:959, 1976.

145. Moller J, Edwards J: Interruption of aortic arch. Anatomic patterns and associated cardiac malformations. Am J Roentgenol 95:557, 1967.

146. Van Praagh R, Bernhard W, Rosenthal A, et al: Interrupted aortic arch surgical treatment. Am J Cardiol 27:200, 1971.

147. Momma K, Kondo C, Matsuoka R, Takao A: Cardiac anomalies associated with a chromosome 22q11 deletion in patients with conotruncal anomaly face syndrome. Am J Cardiol 78:591, 1996.

148. Puder K, Humes R, Gold R, et al: The genetic implication for preceding generations of the prenatal diagnosis of interrupted aortic arch in association with unsuspected DiGeorge anomaly. Am J Obstet Gynecol 173:239, 1995.

149. Congdon E, Wang H: The mechanical processes concerned in the formation of the differing types of aortic arches of the chick and the divergent early development of the pulmonary arches. Am J Anat 37:499, 1926.

150. Jaffee O: The development of the arterial outflow tract in the duck embryo heart. Anat Rec 158:35, 1967.

151. Pillsbury R, Lower R, Shumway N: Atresia of the aortic arch. Circulation 30:749, 1964.

152. Silverman N, Snider A: Two-Dimensional Echocardiography in Congenital Heart Disease. Norwalk, CT, Appleton-Century-Crofts, 1982.

153. Smallhorn J, Anderson R, Macartney F: Cross-sectional echocardiographic recognition of interruption of aortic arch between left carotid and subclavian arteries. Br Heart J 48:229, 1982.

154. Geva T, Hornberger L, Sanders S, et al: Echocardiographic predictors of left ventricular outflow tract obstruction after repair of interrupted aortic arch. J Am Coll Cardiol 22:1953, 1993.

155. Freed M, Heymann M, Lewis A, et al: Prostaglandin E$_1$ in infants with ductus arteriosus–dependent congenital heart disease. Circulation 64:899, 1981.

156. Merrill D, Webster C, Samson P: Congenital absence of the aortic isthmus. J Thorac Cardiovasc Surg 33:311, 1957.

157. Menahem S, Rahayoe A, Brawn W, Mee R: Interrupted aortic arch in infancy: A 10-year experience. Pediatr Cardiol 13:214, 1992.

158. Luciani G, Ackerman R, Chang A, et al: One-stage repair of interrupted aortic arch, ventricular septal defect and subaortic obstruction in the neonate: A novel approach. J Thorac Cardiovasc Surg 111:348, 1996.

159. Jacobs M, Chin A, Rychik J, et al: Interrupted aortic arch. Impact of

subaortic stenosis on management and outcome. Circulation 92(suppl):II-128, 1995.

160. Sandhu S, Beekman R, Mosca R, Bove E: Single-stage repair of aortic arch obstruction and associated intracardiac defects in the neonate. Am J Cardiol 75:370, 1995.

161. Jonas R, Quaegebeur J, Kirklin J, et al: Outcomes in patients with interrupted aortic arch and ventricular septal defect. A multi-institutional study. Congenital Heart Surgeons Society. J Thorac Cardiovasc Surg 107:1099, 1994.

162. Gersony W: Ventricular septal defect and left sided obstructive lesions in infants. Curr Opin Pediatr 6:596, 1994.

163. Starnes V, Luciani G, Wells W, et al: Aortic root replacement with the pulmonary autograft in children with complex left heart obstruction. Ann Thorac Surg 62:442, 1996.

164. Reddy V, Rajasinghe H, Teitel D, et al: Aortoventriculoplasty with the pulmonary autograft: The "Ross-Konno" procedure. J Thorac Cardiovasc Surg 111:158, 1996.

165. Razzouk A, Chinnock R, Gundry S, et al: Transplantation as a primary treatment for hypoplastic left heart syndrome: Intermediate-term results. Ann Thorac Surg 62:1, 1996.

166. Jacobs M, Rychik J, Murphy J, et al: Results of Norwood's operation for lesions other than hypoplastic left heart syndrome. J Thorac Cardiovasc Surg 110:1555, 1995.

167. Bove E, Minich L, Pridjian A, et al: The management of severe subaortic stenosis, ventricular septal defect, and aortic arch obstruction in the neonate. J Thorac Cardiovasc Surg 105:289, 1993.

CHAPTER 38
HYPOPLASTIC LEFT HEART SYNDROME

AMNON ROSENTHAL

Each year, approximately 1000 infants with hypoplastic left heart syndrome are born in the United States. The prevalence is estimated at 0.162 to 0.267 per 1000 live births.[1] Hypoplastic left heart syndrome is the fourth most common congenital cardiac lesion presenting within the first year of life. Preceding it in frequency are ventricular septal defect, transposition of the great arteries, and tetralogy of Fallot in that order. In many major pediatric cardiac centers, hypoplastic left heart syndrome is the most frequent diagnostic category resulting in hospitalization, cardiac catheterization, and surgery. Infants with hypoplastic left heart syndrome are usually full term; they have a normal birth weight and few significant extracardiac malformations. Two thirds of the reported cases occur in male infants. Prematurity and small for gestational age at birth are observed in 5.5%. Noncardiac malformations are uncommon (12%), and serious or major malformations are rare (2.3%).[1] Hypoplastic left heart syndrome has been observed in siblings. Autosomal recessive and multifactorial inheritance have both been postulated. The recurrence rate in siblings is estimated at 0.5% for hypoplastic left heart syndrome and 2.2% for all other cardiac malformations. A predilection for bicuspid aortic valve in first-degree relatives has also been noted. In addition to Turner's syndrome, other chromosome abnormalities have been reported, including duplication of the short arm of chromosome 12 and a rare case of trisomy 18, 4q− and 4p−.

The pathologic anatomy was first described in 1952 by Lev[2] as a constellation of lesions with hypoplasia of the left ventricle associated with obstruction or atresia of both the left ventricular inflow and outflow tracts (Table 38–1). In 1958, Noonan and Nadas[3] coined the phrase hypoplastic left heart syndrome and described the pathophysiologic features and implications of the lesion. The epidemiology was well outlined by the New England Regional Infant Cardiac Program, initiated by Fyler in 1968.[1] The ability to make a precise diagnosis by echocardiography and the subsequent introduction of prostaglandin E_1 to maintain patency of the ductus arteriosus in the mid to late 1970s prepared the way for the staged surgical reconstructive procedures as well as for cardiac transplantation. The first successful reconstructive procedure, performed by Norwood in 1980,[4] involved connecting the right ventricle to the systemic circulation by the main pulmonary artery and restricting pulmonary blood flow by the creation of an aortopulmonary shunt. A second or intermediate stage, modeled after the operation proposed by Glenn in 1958,[5] was subsequently performed, with the creation of a superior vena cava–pulmonary artery connection and elimination of

the aortopulmonary artery shunt. At a third stage, the entire systemic venous flow is connected to the pulmonary artery by the Fontan and Baudet procedure introduced in 1971 for treatment of tricuspid atresia.[6] There have subsequently been numerous modifications of the initial reconstructive (Norwood's), bidirectional Glenn's, and Fontan's procedures. The alternative operative procedure for hypoplastic left heart, cardiac transplantation, was first performed by Yacoub in London in 1984, and the first successful transplantation was performed by Bailey in Loma Linda in 1985.[7]

Before the introduction of the Norwood reconstructive procedure and cardiac transplantation, infants with hypoplastic left heart syndrome, with rare exception, died within the first month of life. Prognosis and survival have dramatically improved in the past two decades.

PATHOLOGIC ANATOMY

The hypoplastic left heart syndrome is a continuum of congenital heart anomalies characterized by underdevelopment of the aorta, aortic valve, left ventricle, mitral valve, and left atrium. The major morphologic features of the syndrome are outlined in Table 38–2. Although these features represent the classic hypoplastic left heart syndrome, there are a number of anatomic variations and additional defects, including atrioventricular septal defect, double-outlet right ventricle, and atrioventricular discordance; approximately 5% of infants have structural abnormalities of the pulmonary or tricuspid valves, pulmonary arteries, or pulmonary venous connection. There is a small group of patients (approximately 5 to 7%) with aortic atresia and a normal-sized left ventricle. These usually have a ventricular septal defect, and some may benefit from a biventricular repair. The multiple variations in the anatomic features are well described by Freedom and Nykanen.[8]

Juxtaductal coarctation of the aorta occurs in most patients (70%) with hypoplastic left heart syndrome. Aortic arch interruption coexisting with aortic atresia is rare. Blood flow in this last malformation is usually provided to the ascending aorta by an aortopulmonary window or a right-sided patent ductus arteriosus. Coronary artery size and distribution in infants with hypoplastic left heart syndrome are usually normal. Ventricular coronary connections may also occur in the subepicardial coronary vessels. Overall heart size is large, left ventricular cavity and ascending aorta are diminutive, and left atrium is small. The right atrium, right ventricle, and pulmonary artery are en-

TABLE 38–1
_____
HYPOPLASTIC LEFT HEART SYNDROME: HISTORICAL LANDMARKS

Date	Landmark	Originator
1952	Pathologic anatomy	M. Lev
1958	Hypoplastic left heart syndrome (HLHS)	J. Noonan and A.S. Nadas
1968	New England Regional Infant Program	D. Fyler
1970s	Introduction of prostaglandin E_1	Upjohn Company
1980	Norwood procedure and staged approach	W. Norwood
1984	First cardiac transplant for HLHS	M. Yacoub
1985	First successful cardiac transplant for HLHS	L. Bailey

larged. The morphologic right ventricle is hypertrophied and dilated, and the pulmonary valve is usually normal. A patent foramen ovale is commonly present; there is a secundum atrial septal defect in a few, and ostium primum atrial septal defect occurs in a rare infant. In some infants, premature closure of the foramen ovale occurs in utero. The myocardium is usually normal. Endocardial fibroelastosis of the left ventricle may also be present. When complete closure of the foramen ovale and mitral atresia are present, pulmonary venous return may be through a left atrial to coronary sinus window or a levocardinal vein connecting the left atrium or pulmonary vein to the brachiocephalic vein.

PATHOPHYSIOLOGY

The cardiac structural defects associated with the hypoplastic left heart syndrome may be variable, but the accompanying pathophysiologic changes are similar. There is an obligatory left-to-right shunt at the atrial level; the right ventricle supplies both the pulmonary blood flow and, through the patent ductus arteriosus, the systemic blood flow. Because the mitral valve is atretic or stenotic and the left ventricle is hypoplastic and nonfunctional, the pulmonary venous return must enter the right atrium. It reaches the right atrium through a stretched patent foramen ovale. In the right atrium, the oxygenated pulmonary venous blood mixes with the systemic venous return, and the mixed blood then flows into the right ventricle. From the right ventricle, the blood is delivered to the pulmonary circulation; systemic blood flow is maintained through the ductus arteriosus. The brachiocephalic vessels and coronary arteries are perfused through retrograde flow from the ductus into the transverse aortic arch and hypoplastic ascending aorta (Fig. 38–1).

TABLE 38–2
_____
MAJOR MORPHOLOGIC FEATURES OF THE HYPOPLASTIC LEFT HEART SYNDROME

Aortic atresia or stenosis
Hypoplasia of ascending aorta
Coarctation of the aorta
Mitral stenosis or atresia
Left ventricular hypoplasia
Patent ductus arteriosus
Restrictive foramen ovale

After birth, the physiologic changes that result in serious hemodynamic consequences and complications are due to three major factors: gradual decrease in pulmonary vascular resistance, spontaneous constriction of the ductus arteriosus, and inadequate interatrial communication. One or more of these factors may occur in any one patient. The gradual decrease in pulmonary vascular resistance in the first few days of life leads to progressive increase in pulmonary blood flow, which in turn leads to improved systemic arterial oxygen saturation but also results in diminution of systemic blood flow, lower perfusion pressure, and volume overload of the right ventricle. The increased pulmonary blood flow is also accompanied by pulmonary congestion and an increase in left atrial and pulmonary venous pressure. A restrictive interatrial communication and usually a small and poorly compliant left atrium lead to further elevation in left atrial and venous pressure. Because the systemic and coronary circulations are totally dependent on maintaining flow through the ductus, its constriction in the first few days of life leads to progressively poor systemic perfusion, tissue hypoxemia, and metabolic acidosis, eventually resulting in vascular shock and death. The coronary blood flow is dependent on the perfusion pressure in the aortic arch and the size of the ascending aorta. Various compensatory mechanisms, including redistribution of blood away from the less vital organs such as the gastrointestinal tract, kidney, and muscles, temporarily result in maintenance of nearly normal arterial pressure and coronary perfusion.

The pulmonary and systemic blood flows in infants with hypoplastic left heart syndrome are determined by the ratio of the pulmonary-to-systemic vascular resistances. When the ductus arteriosus remains patent, the majority of infants are able to maintain a precarious balance between the pulmonary and systemic resistance, resulting in appropriate pulmonary and systemic perfusion. However, in some infants, excessive reduction of the pulmonary-to-systemic vascular resistance ratio will lead to marked pulmonary hyperperfusion with the development of increasing congestive heart failure, relatively adequate systemic arterial oxygen saturation, but gradually progressive diminution of peripheral perfusion. Less often, the presence of a higher pulmonary-to-systemic vascular resistance ratio will lead to diminished pulmonary blood flow. This situation may occur when pulmonary arteriolar resistance remains high in infants with persistent fetal circulation or in the presence of severe restriction of the interatrial septum. The consequence is severe hypoxemia resulting in progressive tissue hypoxia, leading to metabolic acidosis and death. The significance of the interaction between the pulmonary and systemic resistance in determining pulmonary and systemic blood flow as well as systemic arterial oxygen saturation is crucial to the understanding of the clinical presentation of these infants and the preoperative and postoperative ventilatory and pharmacologic management.[9]

CLINICAL MANIFESTATIONS

There are no adverse effects on circulatory hemodynamics in the fetus with hypoplastic left heart syndrome because

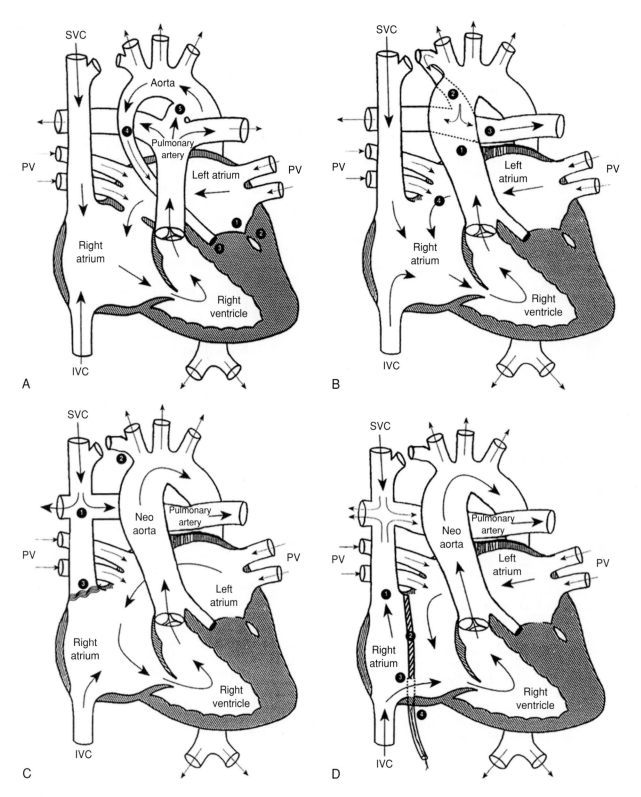

FIGURE 38–1

Circulation pattern in the infant with hypoplastic left heart syndrome, before surgery (*A*) and after each stage of the reconstructive surgical procedure (*B* to *D*). *A,* Hypoplastic left heart syndrome. 1, Atretic mitral valve. 2, Hypoplastic left ventricle. 3, Atretic aortic valve. 4, Hypoplastic ascending aorta. 5, Patent ductus arteriosus. IVC = inferior vena cava; PV = pulmonary veins; SVC = superior vena cava. *B,* The Norwood Procedure. 1, Neoaorta, constructed from the main pulmonary artery and the hypoplastic ascending aorta. 2, Modified Blalock-Taussig shunt. 3, Pulmonary artery. 4, Large atrial septal defect. *C,* The hemi-Fontan (bidirectional Glenn) procedure. 1, Anastomosis of superior vena cava to right pulmonary artery. 2, Ligated modified Blalock-Taussig shunt. 3, Patch closure of superior vena cava to right atrial junction. *D,* The fenestrated Fontan procedure. 1, Removed superior vena cava to right atrial patch. 2, Right atrial pulmonary baffle. 3, Fenestration in the baffle. 4, Snare employed for delayed fenestration closure.

oxygenation is provided through the placenta and the right ventricle pumps blood to the systemic circulation through the ductus arteriosus. At birth, therefore, the infant tends to be well developed, without circulatory symptoms and with normal Apgar scores. However, symptoms may appear soon after birth and usually within the first few days. Clinical presentation in the neonate may occur in one of three ways: respiratory distress, shock, or cyanosis. Respiratory distress with tachypnea and mild cyanosis usually begins in the second or third day of life. Here, the ductus arteriosus is open; there is large pulmonary blood flow and an adequate atrial opening to allow the obligatory left-to-right shunt. The infant is in congestive heart failure. Presentation in shock occurs with constriction of the ductus arteriosus, resulting in hypotension, poor peripheral perfusion, and severe metabolic acidosis. The least common presentation is that of severe cyanosis, usually occurring on day 1 of life. The cyanosis results from premature closure of the foramen ovale, inadequate atrial septal defect, or persistence of pulmonary artery hypertension of the newborn. The high pulmonary vascular resistance and associated low pulmonary blood flow diminish oxygenated blood returning to the right ventricle. All of these presentations constitute a cardiac emergency and require prompt therapy.

The most frequent presentation of infants with hypoplastic left heart syndrome is between day 1 and day 3, occasionally as late as a week of age, with respiratory symptoms including tachypnea, dyspnea, and mild duskiness. These respiratory symptoms are due to progressive increase in pulmonary blood flow and pulmonary congestion that result from the gradual decrease in pulmonary vascular resistance during the first week of life. The duskiness is the result of mild hypoxemia associated with admixture of the pulmonary and systemic blood flows at the atrial level and hence into the right ventricle, ductus arteriosus, and systemic circulation. The congestive heart failure tends to be progressive, and as the ductus arteriosus starts to constrict, there is diminished peripheral perfusion. Physical examination discloses marked tachypnea, tachycardia, a gallop rhythm, and hepatomegaly. Right ventricular impulse is hyperdynamic at the xiphoid and left parasternal area, and the second heart sound is single. There is often a low-intensity systolic ejection murmur audible at the bases and back bilaterally due to physiologic peripheral pulmonary stenosis, accentuated by the increased pulmonary blood flow. An additional regurgitant systolic murmur may be heard at the left lower sternal border if tricuspid regurgitation is present. A mid-diastolic rumble is unusual. The peripheral pulses are diminished throughout because of a narrow pulse pressure associated with a diminished stroke volume. There is poor capillary filling and mottling of the skin. Cyanosis is often not apparent because hypoxemia is relatively mild and may be masked by the simultaneous presence of neonatal icterus. An arterial blood gas sample obtained in room air usually has a PaO_2 of approximately 45 to 60 mm Hg, with normal or moderately decreased $PaCO_2$ of 30 to 35 mm Hg and low pH as a result of moderate metabolic acidosis. When the infant is breathing 100% oxygen, the PaO_2 may rise to 100 mm Hg or greater. Systemic arterial oxygen saturation measured by pulse volume oximeter may be in the mid to high 80s or low 90s and

is similar in all four extremities. The second most frequent presentation, usually occurring after discharge from the hospital and on arrival in the emergency department, is vascular collapse often mistaken for septic shock. The cardiovascular collapse results from marked constriction of the ductus arteriosus or progressive congestive failure associated with increased pulmonary blood flow, right ventricular volume overload, and diminished peripheral perfusion. Vascular collapse often occurs during or after the second or third day and results in poor systemic, renal, cerebral, and coronary perfusion. There is profound myocardial dysfunction, metabolic acidosis, and anuria. Seizures may also occur. The physical findings on examination are those of shock and severe cardiac failure. There is mild cyanosis and no heart murmur. Arterial blood gas analysis discloses a low pH (often less than 7.1), low bicarbonate concentration, and mild to moderate diminution of arterial PaO_2 to perhaps 30 to 45 mm Hg. With persistent poor perfusion and increasing metabolic acidosis, there may be associated hypoglycemia, hypocalcemia, and hyperkalemia and subsequently the development of disseminated intravascular coagulopathy.

The least common presentation, severe cyanosis, occurs within the first day of life and is associated with marked diminution in pulmonary blood flow due to obstruction of the interatrial communication or persistence of high pulmonary vascular resistance. Because the diagnosis can readily be made in the fetus, some of the physiologic changes observed postnatally, such as with premature closure of the foramen ovale, may be anticipated before delivery. On physical examination, there is profound cyanosis, tachypnea, tachycardia, single second heart sound, and no murmur. Arterial blood gas measurement discloses a low PaO_2, usually less than 25 mm Hg, with no significant change on the administration of oxygen. On chest x-ray examination, the heart may be normal or minimally enlarged. There is evidence of pulmonary venous congestion in the case of a restrictive foramen ovale or diminution in pulmonary blood flow in the presence of persistent pulmonary artery hypertension of the neonate. Urgent precise anatomic and physiologic diagnosis with appropriate therapy directed at enlarging the interatrial communication and reducing pulmonary vascular resistance is necessary.

DIAGNOSIS

PRENATAL DIAGNOSIS

A prenatal diagnosis of the hypoplastic left heart may be made by fetal echocardiography as early as 16 weeks of gestation. It is often suspected during a screening procedure when an ultrasound examination is performed for obstetric reasons or when there is a family history of congenital heart disease or other chromosome abnormalities. The prenatal diagnosis has led to a greater understanding of the etiology of the malformation and the ability to plan for care and provide counseling to the family. In some instances, prenatal diagnosis leads to the termination of pregnancy and thus reduction in the postnatal prevalence of hypoplastic left heart syndrome. Sequential observations of serial prenatal echocardiograms in fetuses with hypoplastic left heart syndrome have disclosed nearly 40% with chromosome abnormalities and extracardiac defects and the natural progression of hypoplasia or atresia of left ventricular structures. Longitudinal studies have shown progression of a dilated and dysfunctional left ventricle to ventricular and aortic root hypoplasia, and aortic valve or mitral valve to critical stenosis or atresia.

POSTNATAL DIAGNOSIS

Early postnatal detection of infants with hypoplastic left heart syndrome may be difficult because overt symptoms and signs may not occur before early discharge from the hospital at a day or two of age. Routine measurement of systemic arterial oxygen saturation by pulse volume oximeter may provide the first clue to the presence of underlying heart disease. An arterial oxygen saturation in the high 80s or low 90s should raise suspicion that an underlying cardiac disease may be present and lead to further assessment. The chest radiograph may be normal immediately after birth but within 1 day usually discloses cardiomegaly and an increase in both active and passive pulmonary plethora. In infants with a restrictive interatrial communication, there is usually a pattern of pulmonary edema; in those with persistent fetal circulation of the newborn, there is a diminution of pulmonary blood flow. While the infant is receiving prostaglandin E_1 and awaiting a palliative Norwood procedure or cardiac transplantation, progressive pulmonary plethora and cardiomegaly are usually observed. After the Norwood procedure, the heart generally diminishes in size, although some cardiomegaly persists, and blood flow is generally normal or slightly diminished. There is often prominence of the newly constructed neoaorta. The electrocardiogram in the newborn with hypoplastic left heart is usually similar to that of a normal newborn and is thus not helpful in establishing a diagnosis. Subsequent electrocardiographic changes are related to hypoplasia of the left ventricle and right ventricular volume and pressure overload. These changes may include right atrial hypertrophy, right ventricular hypertrophy, and progressive diminution in left ventricular electromotive forces with absence of a Q wave in the left precordial leads and a pure R or QR in lead V_1. The subsequent development of right ventricular myocardial ischemic ST-T wave changes may appear. Conduction disturbances and Wolff-Parkinson-White patterns are rare.

ECHOCARDIOGRAPHY

A definitive diagnosis is made by two-dimensional echocardiography and Doppler study (Fig. 38–2). The characteristic echocardiographic features of the hypoplastic left heart syndrome include (1) marked hypoplasia of the left ventricle, (2) hypoplasia of the ascending aorta and transverse arch with or without associated discrete coarctation, (3) atresia or marked hypoplasia of the mitral valve, and (4) right ventricular enlargement. To assess the needs for further medical, catheter interventional, or operative procedure, it is essential to define clearly the various anatomic cardiac structures and functional abnormalities. Special attention should be given to the interatrial communication, patency and flow through the ductus arteriosus, pulmonary venous connections, pulmonary valve morphology, presence and severity of tricuspid regurgitation, and right ventricular function.

CARDIAC CATHETERIZATION

Cardiac catheterization is rarely necessary to establish the diagnosis. However, cardiac catheterization may be useful

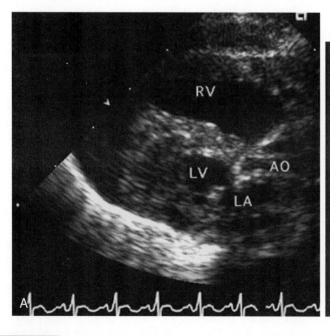 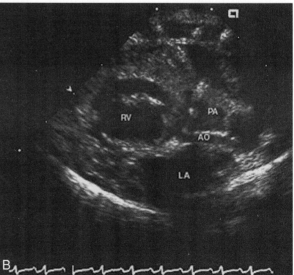

FIGURE 38–2

Aortic atresia. Echocardiograms, long-axis view. *A,* Hypoplastic left ventricle (LV) and ascending aorta (AO); dilated right ventricle (RV). *B,* Absent left ventricle; hypoplastic ascending aorta (AO) and dilated right ventricle (RV). LA = left atrium; PA = pulmonary artery. (Echocardiograms provided by Norman Silverman, MD.)

in delineating complex anomalies of the pulmonary venous connections, identifying associated abnormalities of the pulmonary arteries, and resolving uncertainties with respect to the severity of left-sided obstruction or hypoplasia. Angiography may be useful in the infant with critical aortic stenosis and a small but not diminutive left ventricle if biventricular repair is contemplated. Interventional cardiac catheterization, with performance of an atrial septostomy or blade septectomy, may be necessary for urgent relief of severe interatrial obstruction. Cardiac catheterization may be performed postoperatively to assess hemodynamics, patency of an aortopulmonary shunt, or deformity of the pulmonary artery or other confounding anatomic features. Cardiac catheterization and angiography are also currently performed in evaluating the anatomic and hemodynamic changes after the initial stage of construction surgery (Norwood's operation), just before the second-stage hemi-Fontan (or a bidirectional Glenn) and before the third-stage Fontan procedure.

In the infant with hypoplastic left heart syndrome, blood oxygen saturations disclose an obligatory left-to-right shunt at the atrial level with usually complete mixing at the right atrium and therefore similar oxygen saturations in the right ventricle, pulmonary artery, and aorta. Systemic arterial oxygen saturation is only mildly decreased unless there is markedly diminished pulmonary blood flow associated with increased pulmonary vascular resistance, restrictive interatrial communication, severe pulmonary congestion, or inadequate ventilation. Right ventricular and main pulmonary artery pressures are equal to or greater than systemic arterial pressure. A higher pressure in the right side of the heart than the systemic arterial pressure occurs when there is constriction of the ductus arteriosus. Left atrial pressure may be the same as or higher than right atrial pressure, depending on the adequacy of the interatrial communication. Hemodynamic

study and angiography (Fig. 38–3) are performed while prostaglandin E_1 is infused. Access at cardiac catheterization is best achieved through the femoral artery and vein, although umbilical artery access may be useful for monitoring systemic pressure and blood gas. Manipulation of the catheter into the aortic arch or ascending aorta or through the ductus arteriosus may significantly compromise the coronary and systemic circulation. Catheter interventional study is best done in institutions where appropriate surgical procedures for these infants are performed.

Echocardiography in conjunction with cardiac catheterization and angiography are essential for complete functional and anatomic assessment after the initial Norwood procedure. Before performance of the hemi-Fontan or bidirectional Glenn procedure at age 4 to 6 months, cardiac catheterization is done for assessment of any stenoses, hypoplasia, or deformity of the pulmonary arteries; for direct or indirect (by pulmonary vein wedge) measurement of pulmonary artery pressures; and for assessment of the presence of recurrent coarctation of the aorta and, if necessary, balloon dilatation of the aortic obstruction. Echocardiography is most helpful in assessment of right ventricular and tricuspid valve function as well as the adequacy of the interatrial communication, any functional abnormality of the pulmonary valve, and presence of a left superior vena cava. If a right and left superior vena cava are present, and there is no bridging innominate vein, a bilateral bidirectional caval-pulmonary connection may need to be established. Imaging of the venous anatomy is also well delineated by angiography at cardiac catheterization. Before physiologic repair by the Fontan procedure or one of its modifications, at approximately 18 to 30 months of age, cardiac hemodynamic and angiographic studies are obtained to determine pulmonary artery pressure, any possible deformity or obstruction of the pulmonary arteries, tricuspid valve competency, and right ventricular function.

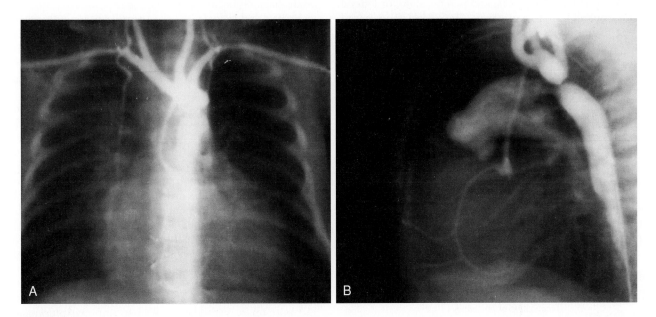

FIGURE 38–3

Aortic atresia. Aortogram, anteroposterior (A) and lateral (B). A very hypoplastic ascending aorta gives rise to the right coronary artery. Isolated coarctation with filling of the main and branch pulmonary arteries through a patent arterial duct is seen.

The presence of major systemic venous collaterals that may be associated with obstruction of the cavopulmonary connection or the presence of large aortopulmonary collaterals, particularly from the internal mammary arteries, may require therapy. The systemic venous collaterals may steal or direct blood away from the lungs. Aortopulmonary collaterals result in increased pulmonary blood flow and subsequent right ventricular volume overload as well as pulmonary congestion. Large collaterals are occluded at the time of cardiac catheterization by the use of metal coils or other devices.

TREATMENT

The management of infants with hypoplastic left heart continues to vary among different physicians, institutions, and countries. Overall management options are shown in Table 38–3. If the diagnosis is made in the early prenatal period, termination of pregnancy may be an acceptable option to some families and is certainly the preferred option in many European countries. Once the infant is born, some parents may elect to provide supportive care only. This decision is highly individualized and dependent on the family, physician, and available services for care of these patients. It used to be much more prevalent in the United States in the past than it is today. Most often, all options are discussed with the family, and the recommendation, in the majority of centers, is staged palliative reconstructive surgery. Cardiac transplantation is the initial and primary option in some centers, but it obviously cannot be used for all infants with this disease, because there are not enough heart donors available. Cardiac transplantation also remains an option in the future for any of the children who have had staged palliative reconstructive procedures. The ethical and economic dilemmas in infants with hypoplastic left heart syndrome are societal issues in which families, physicians, insurers, and private, state, or federal institutions all need to participate. The ethical issues raised in the management of these infants include the cost and potential benefits of treatment in an era of limited resources, potential distress and suffering of the infant and family associated with multiple reconstructive and invasive procedures (or heart transplantation), and uncertain long-term prognosis. Recognizing the rarity of serious noncardiac abnormalities among infants with hypoplastic left heart syndrome and having witnessed the incredible progress made in management and outcome in the last 20 years, I recommend, with few exceptions, the staged palliative reconstructive surgical approach.

After the establishment of a diagnosis by echocardiography and Doppler study, the major initial steps in the management of an infant with hypoplastic left heart syndrome and otherwise uncomplicated course include maintenance

TABLE 38–3

MANAGEMENT OPTIONS IN HYPOPLASTIC LEFT HEART SYNDROME

Termination of pregnancy
Supportive care only
Staged palliative reconstruction
Cardiac transplantation

of ductal patency by prostaglandin E_1 and the performance of the Norwood procedure within the first 3 weeks of life.[4, 10, 11] Cardiac catheterization and a superior vena cava–to–pulmonary artery anastomosis (a bidirectional Glenn or hemi-Fontan operation) is then performed at approximately 6 months of age. Repeated cardiac catheterization and a fenestrated cavopulmonary tunnel (a modified Fontan) procedure are carried out at 18 to 24 months of age; and finally, if appropriate, closure of the fenestration at cardiac catheterization is done 6 to 12 months later.

NEONATAL MANAGEMENT

Immediate medical therapy in infants with hypoplastic left heart is designed to maintain patency of the ductus arteriosus with intravenous prostaglandin E_1 infusion in preparation for surgery. In the infant with increased pulmonary blood flow and congestive heart failure, pharmacologic and ventilatory management is designed to maintain a pulmonary-to-systemic flow ratio as near to 1 as possible.[12] Additional pharmacologic therapy includes use of digoxin to improve right ventricular contractility, diuretics to decrease pulmonary edema, and low-dose dopamine or dobutamine (3 to 5 μg/kg/min) to improve cardiac output and renal perfusion. High doses of inotropic agents are avoided because of the resultant increase in systemic vascular resistance and thus enhancement of pulmonary blood flow with simultaneous decrease in systemic perfusion. Infants with a large pulmonary blood flow or those presenting in shock require intubation, mechanical ventilation, neuromuscular blockade to reduce pulmonary blood flow, and at the same time correction of the metabolic acidosis by intravenous administration of sodium bicarbonate or tromethamine.[12] Decrease in the partial pressure of inspired oxygen by mixing oxygen with room air or an increase in inspired carbon dioxide may be used to cause increased pulmonary vasoconstriction and an appropriate balance between systemic and pulmonary vascular resistance and flow. In the infants presenting with severe cyanosis due to persistent pulmonary artery hypertension of the newborn, a reduction in pulmonary vascular resistance and improved pulmonary blood flow may be accomplished by increased inspired oxygen inhalation and alkalization. When the severe cyanosis is associated with a markedly restrictive or absent atrial communication, in addition to the hyperventilation and supplemental oxygen, urgent intervention is required to relieve the interatrial obstruction. This can be performed by balloon septostomy or blade septostomy at cardiac catheterization or atrial septectomy at surgery. The option of intervention at the cardiac catheterization, the surgical septectomy, or the early Norwood procedure depends on the initial severity of the interatrial obstruction, the cardiac anatomy, and the experience and availability of the medical or surgical team. In patients with severe cyanosis due to persistent high pulmonary vascular resistance, in addition to increasing inspired oxygen and hyperventilation (designed to achieve a pH of 7.5 to 7.6), intravascular volume may be augmented and pulmonary vasodilators used to improve pulmonary blood flow.[12] Blood transfusions may be required to maintain the appropriate oxygen-carrying capacity to maximize oxygen delivery.

THE NORWOOD OPERATION

The first stage in the three-stage reconstructive surgical palliation is the Norwood operation (see Fig. 38–1B).[4] This procedure is designed for the following:

    1. To provide unobstructed systemic blood flow to the ascending and descending aorta by dividing the main pulmonary artery and creating an anastomosis between the proximal main pulmonary artery trunk and the ascending aorta. Patch augmentation is generally required in enlarging the ascending aorta and extending it across the arch and the coarctation.

    2. To provide a measured pulmonary blood flow by creating an aortic-to-pulmonary artery anastomosis. This is usually carried out with an interposed Gore-Tex 3.5-mm graft between the right subclavian and right pulmonary arteries. Various modifications may be used, depending on the anatomy and infant's size.

    3. To create a large interatrial communication by performing a generous atrial septectomy.

The first-stage palliation by the Norwood procedure leads to hemodynamic parameters similar to those that existed preoperatively, with pulmonary blood flow and systemic blood flow closely related to the ratio of pulmonary-to-systemic vascular resistance. In the immediate postoperative period, there is commonly pulmonary vasoconstriction with moderate to severe hypoxemia that usually resolves with appropriate ventilatory support and maintenance of normal acid-base balance and oxygen-carrying capacity. Persistent elevation of pulmonary vascular resistance and inadequate pulmonary blood flow may require increasing concentration of inspired oxygen, hyperventilation with alkalization, and sometimes the use of nitric oxide as a selective pulmonary vasodilator. The infants are sedated with a continuous infusion of fentanyl because of its ability to reduce lability in pulmonary vascular resistance in the postoperative period and its suppression of hormonal stress response to cardiac surgery. Intravenous infusion of morphine is used for sedation and analgesia. Patients are weaned from the ventilator when hemodynamic parameters are stable, respiratory effort is adequate, and edema or pulmonary congestion has significantly decreased. Parenteral alimentation is started on the second postoperative day, particularly in those with significant preoperative risk factors and at risk for necrotizing enterocolitis. In the less seriously ill infants, early feedings are initiated by nasogastric tube and subsequently given orally. Digoxin and diuretic therapy are often started before discharge from the hospital, and angiotensin-converting enzyme inhibitors are occasionally required to decrease right ventricular workload and improve pulmonary blood flow. A small dose (20 mg/day) of aspirin is administered as an anticoagulant. During the immediate postoperative period, parameters monitored include central venous pressure, arterial blood pressure, heart rate and rhythm, systemic arterial oxygen saturation, and core temperature. Atrial and ventricular epicardial pacemaker leads are placed intraoperatively to permit more accurate analysis as well as therapy of any immediate postoperative arrhythmias or conduction disturbance. The importance of a well-trained staff and a designated pediatric cardiac intensive care unit cannot be overemphasized as essential for optimal outcome of infants with hypoplastic left heart syndrome.

THE HEMI-FONTAN OPERATION

The second reconstructive operation is a hemi-Fontan procedure, which is performed at approximately 4 to 6 months of age (see Fig. 38–1C). In this operation, the superior vena cava blood flow is directed to the pulmonary arteries, and the connection between the superior vena cava and right atrium is closed with the placement of a patch. At the same time, the aortopulmonary shunt is closed. Systemic venous blood from the head and arms now perfuses the lungs to provide oxygenated blood, which then returns to the left atrium and through the atrial septal defect into the right atrium. After mixing with all the unoxygenated blood from the inferior vena cava, it is then pumped by the right ventricle into the aorta. The advantages of this operation are that it removes the right ventricular volume overload from the prior aortopulmonary shunt, tends to protect the pulmonary vascular bed from the subsequent development of pulmonary artery hypertension, and increases the diastolic systemic arterial blood pressure by removing the parallel pulmonary vascular resistance circuit. The hemi-Fontan procedure allows remodeling of right ventricular geometry, reducing stress while normalizing the mass-to-volume ratio of the chamber. It is also during this stage that other associated cardiac problems are corrected, such as tricuspid valve repair for tricuspid regurgitation, pulmonary angioplasty for any pulmonary artery deformity or stenosis, and, if necessary, further enlargement of a restrictive interatrial defect.[11] The performance of an intermediate bidirectional Glenn or hemi-Fontan before the Fontan procedure has resulted in significant improvement in survival and decrease in postoperative complications after the Fontan procedure. It is also better tolerated in younger infants than the Fontan procedure and obviates the need for long-term right ventricular volume overload through a persistent shunt or the need for multiple shunt revisions in cases of inadequate pulmonary blood flow. Immediate postoperative management includes weaning of low-dose inotrope support during 48 to 72 hours, discontinuation of fentanyl infusion and neuromuscular blockade within 12 to 24 hours, and extubation in 2 to 3 days after surgery. Diuresis is often necessary within approximately 24 hours. Postoperative complications, such as right ventricular dysfunction, persistent tricuspid regurgitation, rhythm disturbances, and more rarely superior vena cava obstruction or thrombosis, may require further therapy.

THE FONTAN OPERATION

The third stage of the physiologic repair is the fenestrated Fontan procedure. This is performed at approximately 1.5 to 2 years of age (see Fig. 38–1D). It involves removal of the previously placed patch at the entrance of the superior vena cava to the right atrium, with creation of a cavopulmonary tunnel with a separation between the oxygenated and unoxygenated blood in the right atrium so that blood from the inferior vena cava as well as from the superior vena cava flows directly into the pulmonary arteries. A small fenestration or hole is left in the medial patch of the tunnel wall. The fenestration may be created in a variety of ways: by a punched lesion of approximately 4 mm; by multiple smaller punched lesions; or with a snare around it, which is left buried subcutaneously in the abdominal wall. The fenestration is designed to allow gradual accommodation for the increased venous flow, decompression of the tunnel should systemic venous pressure rise excessively, and reduction in the frequency and severity of postoperative pleural effusions and other complications. The fenestration may diminish in size or close spontaneously with time, or it may be closed at cardiac catheterization some 6 to 12 months after surgery. If a snare is used, it is tightened, tied, and buried in the subcutaneous tissue of the abdomen. A punched-out lesion may be closed with the use of an occluding device. Immediate postoperative management is designed to maintain adequate pulmonary blood flow by hyperoxygenation, hyperventilation, and the development of mild respiratory and metabolic alkalosis. Transpulmonary pressure gradient is monitored from a central venous line and a line placed in the "left" atrial chamber. Elevation in the transpulmonary gradient may be the result of increased pulmonary vascular resistance or anatomic obstruction. Persistent postoperative pulmonary effusions may require prolonged pleural drainage and adequate fluid replacement therapy. Some of those patients will eventually need ligation of the thoracic duct or pleurodesis.

Extracorporeal membrane oxygenation is occasionally used in the postoperative infant with hypoplastic left heart and is limited to patients with myocardial dysfunction that is likely to be reversible, unexplained increase in pulmonary vascular resistance, or acute respiratory disease.

CARDIAC TRANSPLANTATION

Cardiac transplantation is the preferred surgical treatment for infants with hypoplastic left heart syndrome in a number of major cardiac centers.[13] Heart replacement allows more normal cardiac physiology. Infants with hypoplastic left heart syndrome who are waiting for a transplant organ are maintained with prostaglandin E_1 until a donor heart is available. In some, ductal patency is accomplished by stent placement; others may require atrial septostomy or septectomy while awaiting transplantation. The shortage of donor organs results in an approximately 25% mortality rate before availability of a donor heart.[13] After appropriate procurement of the donor organ and preparation of the recipient with an intravenous infusion of cyclosporine, cardiac transplantation is performed with use of profound hypothermic circulatory arrest. Immediate postoperative management generally includes inotropic and ventilatory support for a few days. Oversized grafts may require delayed sternal closure, and early associated postoperative hypertension and cerebral edema may require vigorous diuresis and blood pressure control. Renal failure with associated general edema may be treated effectively with peritoneal dialysis. The immunosuppression that began when the donor was identified is then maintained by use of a variety of medications including cyclosporine, a steroid, and azathioprine. The patients continue immunosuppressive therapy for life and are closely monitored for rejection, superimposed infections, and other complications. Although

the overall results from transplantation are similar to those of the three-stage physiologic repair, one may expect an increasing number of recipients with hypoplastic left heart as well as other malformations and a decreasing number of donors, in part because of the implementation of infant car safety laws. The need for chronic immunosuppressive therapy, associated renal dysfunction, hypertension, and the risk of lymphoproliferative disease as well as graft coronary vasculopathy remain major limitations for the long-term survival of these infants.

PROGNOSIS, RESIDUA, AND SEQUELAE

Surgical treatment has dramatically altered the prognosis and natural history of infants born with hypoplastic left heart syndrome. Without treatment, 95% of infants with hypoplastic left heart syndrome die within the first month of life, and 97.2% are dead within 1 year.[9] The average age at death is 4.5 days. A rare patient whose ductus arteriosus remains patent, with well-balanced pulmonary and systemic vascular resistance, may survive to mid-childhood or adolescence. The oldest known survivor without surgery was 24 years old. The introduction of reconstructive staged palliative surgery and cardiac transplantation has markedly improved prognosis. The 5-year survival rates for staged reconstructive palliative surgery and cardiac transplantation are virtually identical.[13,14] With staged reconstruction, 1-year survival of all patients with hypoplastic left heart at my institution is 63 ± 5%, and 5-year survival is 58 ± 4%. In patients operated on at standard risk, 1-year survival is 80 ± 5%; at 5 years, it is 73 ± 5%.[14] Standard risk group includes patients without major serious associated cardiac anomalies or prematurity, those who undergo repair before 1 month of age; it excludes those with severe pulmonary venous obstruction. Comparison to primary therapy with cardiac transplantation discloses a 1-year survival of 62% (including those who died before they could undergo transplantation) and a 5-year survival of 58%. The corresponding survival for transplant recipients is 83% at 1 year and 75% at 5 years.[13] The overall mortality for the Norwood procedure is 15% in standard risk patients and 22% in altered risk patients. The mortality for the bidirectional Glenn procedure for all patients is approximately 3%; for the Fontan procedure, it is 10% and more recently 5%.

Although the improvement in survival has been dramatic during the past two decades, morbidity remains significant. Complications, residua, and sequelae persist after the reconstructive surgery. After the initial palliative Norwood procedure, a number of problems persist and others develop (Table 38–4). Persistent hypoxemia is invariably present and is expected because pulmonary blood flow is supplied by an aortopulmonary shunt and most of the systemic venous return is not oxygenated. The hypoxemia may be progressive owing to inadequate shunt size associated with the infant's growth, pulmonary artery obstruction, diminution in the size of the atrial defect, or development of relative anemia. Congestive heart failure is usually the result of a large aortopulmonary shunt, right ventricular dysfunction, tricuspid regurgitation, or significant residual neoaortic coarctation. The atrial septum may be-

TABLE 38–4

RESIDUA AND SEQUELAE AFTER THE NORWOOD PROCEDURE

Hypoxemia
Congestive heart failure
Restrictive atrial septal defect
Pulmonary hypoplasia or stenosis
Right ventricular dysfunction
Tricuspid regurgitation
Coarctation of the aorta
Tracheobronchial obstruction
Sudden unexplained death

come restrictive or inadequate despite initial surgical septectomy, resulting in the development of increasing cyanosis or pulmonary edema. Pulmonary hypoplasia or stenosis may be the consequence of obstruction at the site of shunt placement into the pulmonary artery. Right ventricular dysfunction, present preoperatively or developing in the perioperative period, is a major and not infrequent problem. Tricuspid regurgitation may be due to right ventricular dilatation or be associated with inherent abnormalities of the tricuspid valve. Residual coarctation or subsequent stenosis at the site of neoaortic reconstruction can be relieved by balloon dilatation or further surgery. Tracheobronchial obstruction is rare and is usually due to extrinsic pressure by a large neoaorta on the tracheobronchial tree. Perhaps the most baffling and serious complication is sudden unexpected death, which may occur while the infant is in the hospital or shortly after discharge, after the Norwood procedure in an infant who is hemodynamically stable and seems to be doing well. There is usually bradycardia followed by hypotension and the inability to resuscitate the infant. The etiology remains unclear; it may be related to extensive denervation of autonomic fibers that occurs during surgical reconstruction of the neoaorta or be due to sudden changes in coronary blood flow.

Because the systemic circulation is dependent on the right ventricle, the maintenance of normal right ventricular function is essential. The factors that affect right ventricular function before and subsequent to the various staged procedures are outlined in Table 38–5. After the Norwood procedure, there is clearly right ventricular pressure overload, because the right ventricle is the systemic ventricle and there is additional volume overload from the aortopulmonary shunt. Both these factors lead to increased right ventricular stress and increased workload and myocardial demand for oxygen. The pressure overload

TABLE 38–5

FACTORS LEADING TO RIGHT VENTRICULAR DYSFUNCTION

Right ventricular pressure overload
Right ventricular volume overload
Decreased systemic flow
Decreased diastolic aortic pressure
Decreased resting coronary flow
Decreased myocardial oxygen delivery
Increased collagen in myocardium or endocardium
Tricuspid regurgitation
Associated right-sided heart abnormalities
Absence of ventricle-ventricle interaction

may be aggravated by such factors as residual coarctation and volume overload complicated by residual tricuspid regurgitation. If the aortopulmonary shunt is large, there may be decrease in systemic blood flow and perfusion with low diastolic pressure, which may in turn lead to diminished coronary blood flow and may further decrease myocardial oxygen delivery when it is coupled with low oxygen saturation or anemia. Positron emission tomography has shown a significant decrease in absolute myocardial blood flow in infants after the Norwood procedure at rest and after the administration of adenosine.[15] The reason for the decrease in coronary blood flow is unclear, but it may be due to lower diastolic pressure or relative disproportionate increased steal to the small left ventricle or perhaps coronary abnormalities. The ischemia and hypertrophy of the right ventricle may in turn lead to increased collagen deposition,[16] which further decreases myocardial function. Associated right-sided heart abnormalities, such as tricuspid malformations, bicuspid pulmonary valve, or coronary artery fistula or stenoses, may also lead to poor myocardial performance. Others have postulated that the left ventricle is necessary for the systemic right ventricle to function normally. The left ventricle augments right ventricular function and affects the biomechanics in such a way as to reduce the stress and dyskinesis.[17]

The second-stage bidirectional Glenn or hemi-Fontan procedure is advantageous in that it removes ventricular volume overload, normalizes ventricular mass-to-volume ratio, protects the pulmonary vascular bed from increased flow or elevation in pressure, and increases systemic diastolic blood pressure. Postoperative complications are infrequent, and the infant's overall cardiovascular status improves because many of the adverse residua after the Norwood procedure (such as persistent or developing neocoarctation of the aorta, pulmonary artery stenosis, and tricuspid regurgitations) are repaired. Residua or sequelae after the hemi-Fontan procedure include hypoxemia; occasionally congestive heart failure, particularly if there is persistent right ventricular dysfunction or tricuspid incompetence; and rarely thromboses of the superior vena cava or pulmonary arteries. Marked increase in superior vena cava pressure may lead to the development of hydrocephalus. Other potential complications, common to all of the staged procedures, include chylothorax, diaphragmatic paralysis, and vocal cord paralysis.

The long-term residua and sequelae of the Fontan procedure or one of its modifications for hypoplastic left heart syndrome are shown in Table 38–6. Rhythm and conduction disturbances are often accompanied by symptoms and may be life-threatening. Atrial tachyarrhythmias and sick sinus syndrome increase in frequency with advancing age and require close monitoring, pharmacologic therapy, and not infrequently interventional or surgical therapy. Resistant atrial flutter may require conversion of a classic Fontan to a cavopulmonary tunnel or extracardiac conduit or performance of the maze procedure alone or combined with epicardial pacemaker implementation. Protein-losing enteropathy develops in approximately 4 to 13% of patients who have had a Fontan procedure for univentricular heart and often presents with abdominal pain, diarrhea, or peripheral edema. It occurs on the average of approximately 3 years after the Fontan procedure with the devel-

TABLE 38-6

LONG-TERM RESIDUA AND SEQUELAE OF THE FONTAN PROCEDURE OR ONE OF ITS MODIFICATIONS

Right-sided obstruction to flow
  Persistent pulmonary artery hypoplasia or stenosis
  Narrow anastomosis (direct, conduit, or cavopulmonary baffle)
  Pulmonary artery or conduit thrombosis
  Pulmonary vascular obstructive disease (? microemboli)
Intracardiac and extracardiac shunts
  Right-to-left through
    Interatrial leak, baffle, fenestration
    Intrapulmonary shunts through arteriovenous fistulae
    Systemic venous–to–pulmonary venous channel
  Left-to-right through
    Large or extensive aortopulmonary collaterals
    Incomplete ligation of aortopulmonary shunt
Systemic venous hypertension
  Liver dysfunction
  Protein-losing enteropathy
  Portal hypertension
    Esophageal varices
    Hypersplenism
  Varicose veins
Right ventricular dysfunction
  Tricuspid regurgitation
Rhythm and conduction disturbances
  Atrial tachyarrhythmia or bradycardia (20%)
  Ventricular ectopy
  Complete heart block
Miscellaneous
  Infective endocarditis
  Neurodevelopmental abnormalities

opment of albuminemia, malnutrition, and a compromised immune state. The loss of albumin leads to depletion in intravascular volume, and when it is coupled with a higher central venous pressure, it predisposes the patients to thromboses and cerebrovascular accidents. The diagnosis can be made by low serum albumin concentrations, fecal α_1-antitrypsin assay, histopathologic examination, and a variety of other studies. Protein-losing enteropathy in these patients is difficult to treat. The multiplicity of available treatments suggests that none is fully effective. Diet alone and periodic albumin replacement may be effective in mild or early cases. Steroids may lead to transient remission in some patients, but the enteropathy often recurs when the steroids are tapered or discontinued because of their side effects. Fenestration of the atrial septum with reduction in systemic venous pressure is helpful in perhaps half the patients but at the price of significant increase in cyanosis and frequent return of the enteropathy a few years later. Other operative approaches, such as small bowel resection or diversion of the hepatic veins to the systemic circulation, have also been proposed. Cardiac transplantation has been curative in all but a few cases. Subcutaneous heparin injection[18] has been effective in many patients by eliminating symptoms and maintaining a satisfactory albumin level. It is postulated that heparin acts by stabilizing the cell-matrix interaction at the capillary level or intestinal mucosa, resulting in decreased leakage of albumin across it. The patient may have a recurrence while receiving heparin therapy with progressive increase in central venous pressure or in the presence of severe intercurrent infection.

Neurodevelopmental abnormalities are one of the greatest long-term concerns in children with hypoplastic left heart. The potential risks for the developmental abnormalities are multiple because both cyanosis and congestive heart failure are known to lead to developmental delay; the infants undergo three major operations in early childhood, including the requirement for circulatory arrest, which has been shown to predispose to developmental delay. An additional contributing factor is the association of the lesion with other acquired or congenital structural abnormalities of the central nervous system. Reported associated congenital malformations include agenesis of the corpus callosum, holoprosencephaly, microcephaly, Arnold-Chiari malformation, and immature cortical mantle. Some of the acquired central nervous system abnormalities noted on magnetic resonance imaging or postmortem studies have included periventricular leukomalacia, brain stem or cerebral necrosis, intracranial hemorrhage, and evidence of cerebral ischemia or infarction. More recent developmental studies of patients with hypoplastic left heart syndrome at my institution[19] at age 3 to 8 years have disclosed neurodevelopment in the normal range. Tests using the Wechsler Preschool and Primary Scale of Intelligence–Revised disclosed a mean verbal score of 103.2 (range, 68 to 109), mean performance score of 97.8 (range, 62 to 127), and mean overall score of 97.9 (range, 62 to 131). For all tests, the normal range is 90 to 109. Verbal scores tended to be higher than performance scores in these children. It would seem that most Fontan survivors demonstrate normal intelligence and verbal and communication skills that are significantly and consistently better than performance and motor skills. When patients who have had the Fontan operation for hypoplastic left heart syndrome are compared with those undergoing the procedure for other lesions, the hypoplastic left heart patients are within the normal range but tend to have somewhat lower scores than do patients being operated on for other cardiac abnormalities.

FUTURE DIRECTIONS

Much has been accomplished in helping infants born with this malformation and their families in the past two decades. However, many unresolved issues remain. Few children have reached adulthood, and the long-term outcome achieved by staged reconstruction or cardiac transplantation therefore needs to be elucidated. Some questions require further exploration. What is the etiology of the unexplained death in some infants after the Norwood procedure? Can some of the intermediate procedures currently being performed, such as multiple cardiac catheterizations, hemi-Fontan, or baffle fenestration, be eliminated or modified and how? We need to assess the quality of life 20 to 30 years after operation and how long the systemic right ventricle will continue to function well. Can cardiac transplantation be made preferable to reconstructive surgery, particularly if more donor hearts become available? Perhaps most important, can the malformation be prevented or growth of the left ventricle chamber be enhanced in the fetus?

REFERENCES

1. Fyler DC: Report of the New England regional infant cardiac program. Pediatrics 65(suppl 1):437, 1980.
2. Lev M: Pathologic anatomy and interrelationship of hypoplasia of the aortic tract complexes. Lab Invest 1:61, 1952.
3. Noonan JA, Nadas AS: The hypoplastic left heart syndrome. Pediatr Clin North Am 5:1029, 1958.
4. Norwood WI, Kirklin JK, Sanders SP: Hypoplastic left heart syndrome. Experience with palliative surgery. Am J Cardiol 45:87, 1980.
5. Glenn WWL: Circulatory by-pass of the right side of the heart, IV. Shunt between superior vena cava and distal right pulmonary artery—report of clinical application. N Engl J Med 259:117, 1958.
6. Fontan F, Baudet E: Surgical repair of tricuspid atresia. Thorax 26:240, 1971.
7. Bailey L, Conception W, Shattuck H, Huang C: Method of heart transplantation for treatment of hypoplastic left heart syndrome. J Thorac Cardiovasc Surg 92:1, 1986.
8. Freedom RM, Nykanen D: Hypoplastic left heart syndrome: Pathologic considerations of aortic atresia and variations on the theme. Prog Pediatr Cardiol 5:3, 1966.
9. Rosenthal A: Physiology, diagnosis and clinical profile of the hypoplastic left heart syndrome. Prog Pediatr Cardiol 5:19, 1996.
10. Iannettoni MD, Bove EL, Mosca RS, et al: Improving results with first-stage palliation for hypoplastic left heart syndrome. J Thorac Cardiovasc Surg 107:934, 1994.
11. Bove EL, Mosca RS: Surgical repair of the hypoplastic left heart syndrome. Prog Pediatr Cardiol 5:23, 1966.
12. Charpie JR, Kulik TJ: Pre- and post-operative management of infants with hypoplastic left heart syndrome. Prog Pediatr Cardiol 5:49, 1996.
13. Razzouk AJ, Chinnock RE, Gundry SR, Bailey LL: Cardiac transplantation for infants with hypoplastic left heart syndrome. Prog Pediatr Cardiol 5:37, 1966.
14. Lloyd TR: Prognosis of the hypoplastic heart syndrome. Prog Pediatr Cardiol 5:57, 1996.
15. Donnelly JP, Raffel DM, Shulkin BL, et al: Resting coronary flow and coronary flow reserve in human infants following repair or palliation for congenital heart defects or measured by positron emission tomography. J Thorac Cardiovasc Surg 115:103, 1998.
16. Schwartz SN, Gordon D, Mosca RS, et al: Collagen content in normal pressure and pressure-volume overloaded developing human hearts. Am J Cardiol 77:734, 1996.
17. Fogel MA, Weinberg PM, Chein AJ, et al: Late ventricular geometry and performance changes of functional single ventricle throughout staged Fontan reconstruction assessed by magnetic resonance imaging. J Am Coll Cardiol 28:212, 1996.
18. Donnelly JP, Rosenthal A, Castle VP, Holmes RD: Reversal of protein losing enteropathy with heparin therapy in three patients with univentricular hearts and Fontan palliation. J Pediatr 130:474, 1997.
19. Goldberg CS, Schwartz EM, Brunberg JA, et al: Neurodevelopmental outcome of children following the Fontan procedure. Circulation 96:I-300, 1997.

CHAPTER 39
CORONARY ARTERIAL ABNORMALITIES AND CONGENITAL ANOMALIES OF THE AORTIC ROOT

JULIEN I. E. HOFFMAN

CORONARY VASCULAR ANOMALIES

Coronary vascular anomalies discussed in this chapter include

- Ectopic aortic origin of coronary arteries, either isolated or associated with congenital heart disease (Table 39–1)
- Anomalous connection of a coronary artery to main or peripheral pulmonary arteries (Table 39–1)
- Miscellaneous coronary arterial abnormalities (Table 39–2)

Chapter 42 discusses fistulae between coronary arteries and cardiac chambers, pulmonary arteries, or other vessels and anomalies of the coronary venous system.

INCIDENCE
Isolated coronary vascular anomalies (excluding innocuous variants) have been found in 0.3 to 1.3% of autopsies at all ages,[1] 0.5% of pediatric autopsies,[2] and about 0.3 to 1.3% of angiograms for possible myocardial ischemia.[3–5] They may cause disability and death in an unknown proportion of people; however, their similar prevalence in autopsy and clinical studies argues that most are important. In congenital heart disease, different coronary vascular anomalies that may be important only during surgery are common.

EMBRYOLOGY
The primitive myocardium has sinusoids that develop into the intramural vessels. These join a network of subepicardial vessels, which in turn join endothelial buds that emerge from the sinuses of Valsalva of both aorta and main pulmonary artery.[6] The regulation of this organization is not known, but it is easy to see how anomalous connections could be established to structures that in the early embryo are only a few micrometers away from the correct site.

ANATOMY
This is described in many texts and summarized by Hoffman.[7,8] The important factor in all primates is that the right coronary artery normally supplies part of the left ventricle.

PHYSIOLOGY
This is summarized in Chapter 6.

ECTOPIC AORTIC ORIGIN OF ONE OR MORE CORONARY ARTERIES

Innocuous Anomalies
About 1% of people have separate orifices for the left anterior descending and left circumflex coronary arteries, and 50% have a separate conus branch from the right sinus of Valsalva (Fig. 39–1). Sometimes coronary orifices arise high above the correct sinuses, above the supravalvar ridge. None of these variants appears to be clinically important unless it affects the conduct of percutaneous transluminal coronary angioplasty.

Serious or Potentially Serious Anomalies
STENOSIS OR ATRESIA OF A CORONARY OSTIUM. Bilateral coronary atresia is rare and occurs mainly with coexistent pulmonary or aortic atresia. In this circumstance, the distal coronary branches are perfused retrograde from the ventricles by sinusoids.

Stenosis or atresia of the ostium or first few millimeters of the left main coronary artery is rare.[9–11] The more distal branches are normal and supplied by multiple collaterals from the right coronary artery. Patients may present from 3 months to 60 years of age with sudden death, angina pectoris, myocardial infarction, or congestive heart failure. If they present in childhood, signs of anterolateral ischemia or infarction of the left ventricle make one suspect anomalous origin of the left coronary artery from the pulmonary artery, a suspicion supported when echocardiography or cineangiography fails to show the left coronary artery arising from the aorta and when attempts made to catheterize the left main coronary artery from the aorta fail. The distinction between these two entities is that with atresia, no flow enters the pulmonary artery from the left coronary artery by Doppler echocardiography or cineangiography studies; in particular, failure to fill the anomalous left coronary artery during a pulmonary angiogram favors the diagnosis of atresia.

Like an atretic left coronary artery, a single right coronary artery shows a large right main coronary artery and no left main coronary artery arising from the aorta or pulmonary artery. However, by angiography, the atretic coronary artery anomaly shows collaterals from the right coronary artery entering large major branches of the left coronary artery, whereas in a single right coronary artery, blood flows through progressively smaller arteries as it passes toward the periphery.[11]

TABLE 39–1

CLASSIFICATION OF CORONARY ARTERIAL CONGENITAL ANOMALIES

Coronary Arterial Anomaly	Prevalence per Million Population
ECTOPIC ORIGIN FROM AORTA	
Innocuous anomalies	
Separate orifice for conal branch of RCA	500,000 (50%)
Separate orifices for LAD, LC	10,000 (1%)
Potentially serious anomalies	
Stenosis or atresia of coronary ostium	
Abnormal orifice or intramural course from normal SV	
Origin from wrong SV	
LMCA from RSV	1,070
RCA from LSV	170
LAD, LC, or both from RSV	300
Single CA	450
Miscellaneous anomalies	
ECTOPIC ORIGIN FROM MPA OR PPA	
All CA from MPA	
LMCA from MPA	80
RCA from MPA	20
LAD from MPA	8
LC from MPA or PPA	

SV = sinus of Valsalva; LMCA = left main coronary artery; RSV = right sinus of Valsalva; RCA = right coronary artery; LSV = left sinus of Valsalva; LAD = left anterior descending coronary artery; LC = left circumflex coronary artery; CA = coronary artery; MPA = main pulmonary artery; PPA = peripheral branch pulmonary artery.

TABLE 39–2

MISCELLANEOUS CORONARY ARTERIAL DISEASES

Calcific arteriopathy of infancy
Myocardial infarction
Coronary arterial aneurysms
Myocardial bridges

There are several reports of successful coronary artery bypass grafting, either with the saphenous vein[12] or with the internal mammary artery, for atresia of the left coronary artery.[9–11, 13]

ORIGIN OF A CORONARY ARTERY FROM THE APPROPRIATE SINUS OF VALSALVA, BUT WITH AN ABNORMAL ORIFICE OR INTRAMURAL COURSE. The coronary arterial orifice is normally round, and the artery emerges radially with a short intramural course. In some autopsies in patients who died suddenly, and in a few patients at operation, a coronary artery, usually the right, has a long intramural aortic course and emerges tangentially (Fig. 39–2). The ostium of the artery tends to be slit-like and may be partly covered by a valve-like ridge.[14, 15] Most of these patients have been adults, but the abnormality has occurred in children.[16]

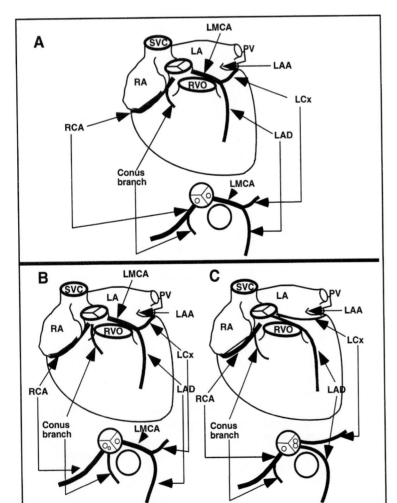

FIGURE 39–1

Normal and innocuous variations, seen in an exploded frontal view *(above)* and diagrammatically from above *(below)*. *A,* Normal main right and left coronary arteries. *B,* Separate origin of conus branch of right coronary artery. *C,* Separate origins of left circumflex and left anterior descending coronary arteries. SVC = superior vena cava; LA = left atrium; LMCA = left main coronary artery; PV = pulmonary vein; LAA = left atrial appendage; RVO = right ventricular outflow tract; RA = right atrium; RCA = right coronary artery; LCx = left circumflex coronary artery; LAD = left anterior descending coronary artery.

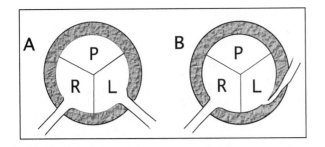

FIGURE 39-2

Diagram of origins of right and left coronary arteries. *A*, Normal radial course, with short intramural portion. *B*, Left main coronary artery arises tangentially, has a long intramural course, and may be narrowed at its initial portion. The orifice (not shown) is slit-like and often covered by a flap. P = posterior sinus; R = right sinus; L = left sinus.

ABNORMAL ORIGIN OF ONE CORONARY ARTERY OR A BRANCH FROM THE WRONG SINUS OF VALSALVA

Left Main Coronary Artery From Right Sinus of Valsalva. This is common.[3, 4, 17, 18] Four patterns are found.[19–21] The most common pattern is the septal type; the left main artery has an intramyocardial course through the ventricular septum along the floor of the right ventricular outflow tract, then reaches the surface and divides into circumflex and anterior descending branches (Fig. 39–3*A*). Second is the posterior type, in which a long left main coronary artery passes behind the aorta and pulmonary artery before dividing into its two branches (Fig. 39–3*B*). Third is the anterior type, in which the left coronary artery runs on the anterior surface of the right ventricle almost like a nor-

mal conus branch and divides at about the midseptum into its two main branches (Fig. 39–3*C*). These three patterns are usually harmless in the absence of coronary atheroma. The fourth pattern, however, is more sinister. The left main coronary artery courses obliquely through the aortic wall and then runs between the aorta and the main pulmonary artery before it bifurcates (Fig. 39–3*D*). Its aortic origin may be slit-like and covered by a flap. Roberts[17] described 43 necropsy reports with this lesion: 9 deaths were due to other factors, and 26 of the remaining 34 died before 20 years of age. Herrmann and colleagues[22] and Duran and associates[23] described 10 infants who had died with ectopic coronary arterial origins. Three had ectopic left coronary arteries from the right aortic sinus; one had a septal course, one had a posterior course, and one was interarterial.

Right Coronary Artery From Left Sinus of Valsalva. This accounts for about one third of all major coronary arterial anomalies.[3, 4, 17, 18] The artery leaves the left sinus of Valsalva and passes between the aorta and the right ventricular outflow tract to reach the atrioventricular groove, after which it is distributed normally (Fig. 39–4). The orifice is often slit-like, and the proximal portion of the artery is angulated.[24–26] There are many reports of myocardial ischemia, infarction, deaths, and near deaths with this lesion.[27] Most deaths occur in teenagers or young adults, but seven neonates and infants have died with this anomaly.[22, 23]

Origin of Left Anterior Descending, Left Circumflex, or Both Arteries From the Right Sinus of Valsalva or Right Coronary Artery. A left circumflex coronary artery coming from the right coronary artery or right sinus of Valsalva is

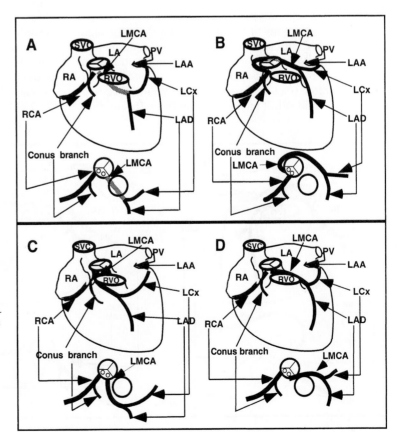

FIGURE 39-3

Left main coronary artery from right sinus of Valsalva, seen in an exploded frontal view *(above)* and diagrammatically from above *(below)*. *A*, Intramural septal course. *B*, Posterior course. *C*, Anterior course. *D*, Interarterial course. SVC = superior vena cava; LA = left atrium; LMCA = left main coronary artery; PV = pulmonary vein; LAA = left atrial appendage; RVO = right ventricular outflow tract; RA = right atrium; RCA = right coronary artery; LCx = left circumflex coronary artery; LAD = left anterior descending coronary artery.

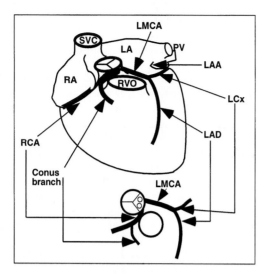

Right coronary artery from left sinus of Valsalva, seen in an exploded frontal view *(above)* and diagrammatically from above *(below)*. SVC = superior vena cava; LA = left atrium; LMCA = left main coronary artery; PV = pulmonary vein; LAA = left atrial appendage; RVO = right ventricular outflow tract; RA = right atrium; RCA = right coronary artery; LCx = left circumflex coronary artery; LAD = left anterior descending coronary artery.

common.[3, 4, 17, 18] The circumflex artery runs posteriorly around the aorta and then travels in the atrioventricular sulcus (Fig. 39–5A). This anomaly is usually benign (but see Piovesana and coworkers[28]) except that it may be liable to premature atherosclerosis,[18] and it can be compressed if both aortic and mitral prosthetic fixation rings are implanted.[29]

The left anterior descending coronary artery can originate in the right sinus of Valsalva or from the right main coronary artery. This anomaly is rare in the absence of congenital heart disease[3,4,17,18] but is common in tetralogy of Fallot. The artery usually passes in front of the right ventricular outflow tract or through the interventricular septum, but occasionally it passes between the aorta and right ventricular outflow tract (Fig. 39–5B). Should there be atheroma near the beginning of the common arterial trunk, most of the heart will become ischemic, so that the lesion is the equivalent of a left main coronary arterial stenosis.[30]

On occasion, both the left circumflex and the left anterior descending arteries arise by separate orifices from the right sinus of Valsalva. These arteries take posterior and anterior courses, respectively, as described in the two preceding paragraphs, and produce no pathologic changes except as noted before.

Single Coronary Artery.   Single coronary arteries represent about 5 to 20% of major coronary arterial anomalies. They may be isolated but are often associated with transposition of the great vessels, tetralogy of Fallot, truncus arteriosus, coronary cameral fistulae, and bicuspid aortic valves.[3, 4, 17, 18, 31–34] The anomaly comes usually from failure of the vascular anlage to make the correct connections to the sinuses of Valsalva, so that the single artery combines the branches of the right and left coronary systems.

There are many classifications of these anomalies, the best known being those by Ogden and by Lipton and their colleagues[31,33] and a variant by Shirani and Roberts.[34] There is a single ostium in the right or the left sinus of Valsalva. The single main artery arising from this ostium may form a left coronary artery that divides into left anterior and left circumflex arteries, the latter continuing past the crux to form the right coronary artery (type L1 of Lipton or IB of Shirani and Roberts) (Fig. 39–6), or it may form a right coronary artery that is normally distributed but continues beyond the crux of the heart to form the left circumflex and anterior coronary arteries (type R1 of Lipton, IIA of Shirani and Roberts; Fig. 39–7). Alternatively, the single artery branches early into typical right and left coronary arteries; each of these patterns is further subdivided according to whether the transverse branch passes anterior to the pulmonary artery (R2a and L2a, or IB_1 and IIB_1), between the great arteries (R2b and L2b, or IB_2 and IIB_2), posterior to the aorta (R2p and L2p, or IB_4 and IIB_4), or through the septum (IB_3 and IIB_3) (see Figs. 39–6 and 39–7). Both classifications introduce added groups (3 for

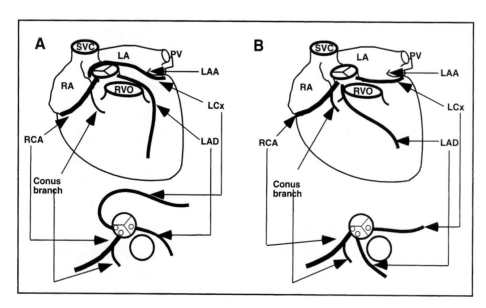

Branch of left coronary artery from right sinus of Valsalva, seen in an exploded frontal view *(above)* and diagrammatically from above *(below)*. *A*, Left circumflex coronary artery from right sinus of Valsalva. *B*, Left anterior descending coronary artery from right sinus of Valsalva. SVC = superior vena cava; LA = left atrium; PV = pulmonary vein; LAA = left atrial appendage; RVO = right ventricular outflow tract; RA = right atrium; RCA = right coronary artery; LCx = left circumflex coronary artery; LAD = left anterior descending coronary artery.

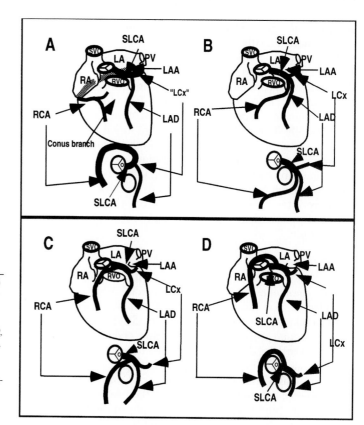

FIGURE 39–6

Single left coronary artery, seen in an exploded frontal view *(above)* and diagrammatically from above *(below)*. *A,* Right coronary artery as continuation of left coronary artery (L1 or IA). *B,* Transverse right coronary artery with anterior course (L2a or IB$_1$). *C,* Transverse right coronary artery with interarterial course (L2b or IB$_2$). *D,* Transverse right coronary artery with posterior course (L2p or IB$_4$). Classifications with L by Lipton and colleagues,[33] with I by Shirani and Roberts.[34] SVC = superior vena cava; LA = left atrium; PV = pulmonary vein; LAA = left atrial appendage; RVO = right ventricular outflow tract; RA = right atrium; RCA = right coronary artery; LCx = left circumflex coronary artery; LAD = left anterior descending coronary artery; SLCA = single left coronary artery.

Lipton, IIC and IID for Shirani and Roberts) in which the branching patterns are not similar to any normal patterns.

A single coronary artery usually produces no symptoms in the absence of severe atheroma (which is more serious when there is only one main artery supplying the whole heart), but a small number of premature deaths or infarctions have been reported with this anomaly.[32, 35] Possibly those variants in which a major branch passes between the

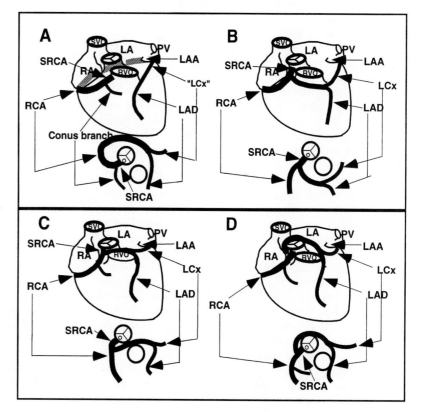

FIGURE 39–7

Single right coronary artery, seen in an exploded frontal view *(above)* and diagrammatically from above *(below)*. *A,* Left coronary artery as continuation of right coronary artery (R1 or IIA). *B,* Transverse left coronary artery with anterior course (R2a or IIB$_1$). *C,* Transverse left coronary artery with interarterial course (R2b or IIB$_2$). *D,* Transverse left coronary artery with posterior course (R2p or IIB$_4$). Classifications with R by Lipton and colleagues,[33] with II by Shirani and Roberts.[34] SVC = superior vena cava; LA = left atrium; PV = pulmonary vein; LAA = left atrial appendage; RVO = right ventricular outflow tract; RA = right atrium; RCA = right coronary artery; LCx = left circumflex coronary artery; LAD = left anterior descending coronary artery; SRCA = single right coronary artery.

aorta and the right ventricular infundibulum are at greatest risk for sudden death.

Miscellaneous Anomalies. Many possible variations of coronary arterial origins have been reported. For example, the right or left coronary arteries may arise from the posterior (noncoronary) sinus of Valsalva.[36] Two circumflex or two left anterior descending coronary arteries can arise from the left sinus of Valsalva, or a large septal branch of the left coronary artery may come from the right sinus of Valsalva. There may be two right coronary arteries. Sometimes one coronary arterial ostium straddles a commissure and arises from two adjacent sinuses of Valsalva. A major coronary artery occasionally comes from a ventricle or atrium. Hypoplastic coronary arteries may cause death in young adults.[37]

PATHOLOGY
About 20% of the autopsies in patients with these coronary arterial anomalies have a subendocardial scar due to episodes of ischemia, and occasionally there is a major myocardial infarct. The suddenness of death in most of these patients prevents infarction from occurring, however, even with total occlusion of the coronary artery. A few subjects had left ventricular hypertrophy, perhaps the result of prolonged subclinical ischemia or an associated cardiomyopathy, but more likely because these subjects were athletes with physiologic work hypertrophy of the left ventricle. Severe atherosclerosis has been observed occasionally in a segment of the abnormal coronary arteries, even in children. In some of the anomalies, the initial few millimeters of artery may actually run in the aortic wall or may be narrowed; occasionally, the whole anomalous artery is hypoplastic. Finally, the anomalous artery may arise tangentially from the aorta, its ostium may be slit-like, and the ostium may be partly covered by a valve-like flap.

MECHANISMS OF DEATH
Death is almost certainly due to myocardial ischemia. The left ventricular myocardium, sometimes hypertrophied, has an enormous demand for oxygen during strenuous exercise. Systolic pressure rises during strenuous exercise, and the sympathetic nervous system is activated. The root of the aorta therefore distends in systole, and there might be excessive contraction of smooth muscle in the aortic wall. If part of the anomalous artery runs in the wall, it may be compressed; and if the artery runs adjacent to the wall, it may be stretched, compressed, or both. Another possible mechanism is that the flap over the ostium may occlude the inflow into the artery at a time when maximal flow is needed. The severe myocardial ischemia that would occur from any of these mechanisms probably produces ventricular fibrillation or electromechanical dissociation. In those with previous episodes of syncope, the severe ischemia might have produced transient ventricular tachycardia or fibrillation,[38] or else sudden impaired ventricular function might have decreased cardiac output catastrophically. It is even possible that ischemia leads to acute ventricular dilatation with abnormal stimulation of cardiac sensory nerve endings that causes vasodepressor syncope, just as it does in the syncope of severe aortic stenosis. In a few adults, ergonovine has provoked spasm and regional ischemia in these anomalous arteries. Why several patients have apparently identical anomalies but survive without ischemia un-

til their 70s and 80s is unknown; it is possible that there is progressive obstruction to the orifice and first part of the artery with aging.

CLINICAL FEATURES
Anomalous coronary arteries may be found during angiography in patients with congenital heart disease or adults with myocardial ischemia. As lesions causing primary problems, they are most often found in autopsies done for sudden death. At times, however, they are detected by imaging studies performed in children and young adults presenting with syncope, chest pain, arrhythmia, or other evidence of myocardial ischemia, including myocardial infarction. These symptoms almost invariably come on during or just after strenuous exercise, and most of the victims have been athletes.

GENERAL FEATURES. Failure to recognize an anomalous coronary arterial branching pattern can lead to erroneous diagnosis of occlusion of a branch when selective coronary arteriography is done or a sinus of Valsalva shows no coronary ostium during an aortic root angiogram. The anomalous artery may be injured if an operation is done near the aortic and pulmonary arterial roots, particularly if the anomalous artery is buried in muscle or concealed in scar tissue from a prior operation. All these sources of error may be prevented if the anomalous coronary artery can be recognized by good aortic root imaging (see later). Finally, some of these anomalous arteries may be subject to premature atherosclerosis (although usually well beyond childhood). This would be particularly dangerous if the obstruction is in the proximal part of a single coronary artery or of the right main coronary artery from which the left anterior descending coronary artery arises.

Apart from these problems, most of these anomalous arteries do not cause myocardial ischemia, particularly if the anomalous branch does not pass between the aorta and the right ventricular infundibulum. Even those that do run between these structures do not always lead to sudden or premature death. However, this anatomic pattern accounts for a large proportion of anginal symptoms and sudden death in children, adolescents, and young adults.

DIAGNOSIS
Any episode of syncope or severe chest pain during or after exercise calls for intensive investigations. Apart from a standard clinical examination, which shows no abnormalities, there should be a resting electrocardiogram to look for ventricular hypertrophy and arrhythmias. An exercise test to evaluate blood pressure response and the electrocardiogram at nearly maximal exercise can be useful, but there is some risk; injection of thallium at peak exercise might reveal ischemic regions. A nearly maximal stress test result has been reported normal, however, in patients who subsequently died suddenly and were found to have an anomalous left main coronary artery.[39-42] Because of this, exertional syncope or prolonged chest pain in a child or young adult warrants careful imaging studies.

IMAGING STUDIES
AORTIC AND CORONARY ANGIOGRAPHY. Ishikawa and Brandt[43] described the classical cineangiographic features of the various types of course taken by a left main

coronary artery arising from the right aortic sinus. This approach was extended to other anomalies by Serota and coworkers,[44] and details of the patterns in single coronary arteries are provided by Lipton and colleagues.[33]

OTHER IMAGING STUDIES. Because classical angiography gives a two-dimensional picture with superimposition of structures in a plane, even biplane studies can be difficult to interpret. Therefore, tomographic or semi-tomographic techniques like echocardiography, ultrafast computed tomography, and magnetic resonance imaging (with or without flow encoding) have been used with increasing success.

An echocardiogram with Doppler interrogation should always be done to exclude intracardiac anomalies and hypertrophic cardiomyopathy, the latter a common cause of syncope and sudden death in the young.[45–47] Because the coronary anomalies affect the origins of the major arteries or their major branches, they should be detectable by echocardiography, although the sensitivity and specificity of this technique have not been evaluated. Those anomalies in which the arteries arise tangentially from the sinuses of Valsalva should be readily detectable. It might be more difficult to trace peripheral coronary branches. On the other hand, there are already several reports in which satisfactory transthoracic echocardiography failed to detect what was later proved to be an anomalous coronary artery. In larger children and adults, transesophageal echocardiography has been more useful diagnostically than has transthoracic echocardiography.[48–50] In about 25% of adults with normal coronary arterial origins, however, it is not possible to visualize the origin of the right coronary artery, so that failure to detect an anomalous origin does not eliminate this possibility.

Magnetic resonance imaging has been shown to have excellent sensitivity and specificity for detecting these anomalies[51, 52]; the anomaly was missed in only 1 of 34 patients. An alternative is computed tomography,[53, 54] but the sensitivity and specificity of this technique, although likely to be good, have not been evaluated.

TREATMENT

If there are symptoms indicating myocardial ischemia and one of the known sinister coronary arterial anomalies is found, it would be prudent to reroute the abnormal artery or to do a coronary arterial bypass graft. Although grafting might be suitable in an older adult, its use in children is less advisable because of doubts about the longevity of these grafts. There are many isolated reports of short-term revascularization or reimplantation. In older patients with atherosclerotic occlusion of the anomalous artery, percutaneous transluminal coronary angioplasty or one of its variants has been used with due regard for the abnormal position of the anomalous artery.[55, 56]

If a patient has one of the more benign anomalies, with or without symptoms, provocative testing with pacing, dobutamine, or ergonovine might help to determine whether the anomaly indeed puts the patient at risk.

Coronary Artery Patterns Associated With Congenital Heart Defects

These are discussed in detail in chapters on the individual lesions. The anomalies of greatest importance for the surgeon are those that cross the right ventricular outflow tract where an incision needs to be made to open up the tract or place a conduit in it[57,58]; lesions commonly affected are tetralogy of Fallot, truncus arteriosus, and pulmonary atresia. Other anomalies of the coronary arteries influence reimplantation of the arteries during an arterial switch procedure.[59]

ECTOPIC ORIGIN OF ONE OR BOTH CORONARY ARTERIES FROM THE MAIN OR PERIPHERAL PULMONARY ARTERIES

All Coronary Arteries From Pulmonary Trunk

Rarely, both right and left coronary arteries come from the pulmonary trunk, or a single coronary artery does; by 1986, only 25 such anomalies had been described. Unless there is a cardiac lesion causing pulmonary hypertension, these children usually do not survive infancy, and survivors are rare even with other lesions.[60–62]

Left Main Coronary Artery From the Pulmonary Trunk

This anomaly has been found in 24 of 23,249 coronary arteriograms done in older children and adults.[3, 4, 41, 63] The first report relating clinical and autopsy findings in a 3-month-old boy was by Bland and coworkers,[64] and the anomaly is often called the Bland-White-Garland syndrome.

PATHOPHYSIOLOGY

In fetal life, this anomaly is probably not harmful; pressures and oxygen saturations are similar in aorta and pulmonary artery. Myocardial perfusion is presumably normal, and there is no stimulus to collateral formation. After birth, however, the pulmonary artery contains desaturated blood at low pressures. Therefore, the left ventricle, with its huge demand for oxygen, is perfused with desaturated blood at low pressures. Collateral vessels between the normal right and abnormal left coronary artery enlarge, and so does the right coronary artery itself. However, unlike the coronary collaterals in coronary arterial stenosis, this collateral flow may be of little use. Blood does enter the left coronary arterial system through the collaterals, but because the left coronary artery is connected to the low-pressure pulmonary artery, the collateral flow tends to pass into the pulmonary artery rather than into the high-resistance myocardial blood vessels (Fig. 39–8). This pulmonary-coronary steal was first demonstrated by Sabiston and colleagues,[65] who observed a large increase in distal left coronary arterial pressure when the origin of that artery was occluded. Subsequently, the left-to-right shunt was demonstrated angiographically.[66, 67] The amount of left-to-right shunting is small in terms of cardiac output but large in terms of coronary flow. The left ventricular myocardial vessels dilate to reduce their resistance and increase flow, but soon coronary vascular reserve becomes exhausted, and myocardial ischemia ensues. At first, ischemia is transient and occurs only with exertion, such as feeding or crying, but further increases in myocardial oxygen demand lead to infarction of the anterolateral left ventricular free wall. This causes congestive heart failure, often made worse by mitral incompetence secondary to a dilated mitral valve ring or infarction of the anterior papillary muscle.[68]

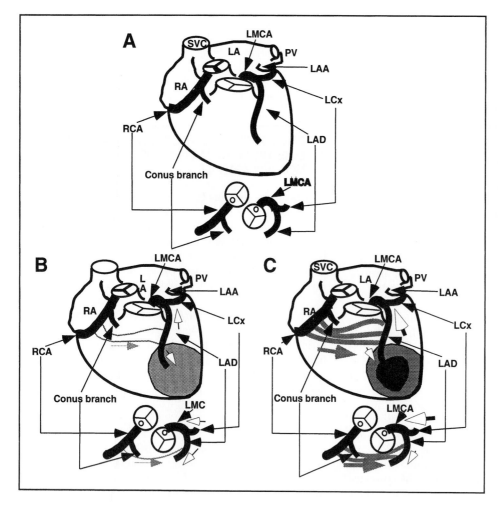

FIGURE 39–8

Left main coronary artery from pulmonary artery, seen in an exploded frontal view *(above)* and diagrammatically from above *(below)*. *A,* In fetus. *B,* In neonate. The light gray apical region indicates the ischemic region. *C,* In older infant. The slightly darker gray apical region indicates worsening ischemia, and the dark central area is the infarct. The gray vessels joining left anterior descending and right coronary arteries are collaterals. The *pale gray arrows* indicate the direction and approximate magnitude of collateral blood flow and its distribution. The *open arrows* indicate the direction and approximate quantity of flow in the proximal and distal left coronary artery. SVC = superior vena cava; LA = left atrium; LMCA = left main coronary artery; PV = pulmonary vein; LAA = left atrial appendage; RA = right atrium; RCA = right coronary artery; LCx = left circumflex coronary artery; LAD = left anterior descending coronary artery.

In about 15% of patients with these anomalies, myocardial blood flow is adequate to sustain myocardial function at rest or even during exercise, and these are the patients who reach adult life.[60]

PATHOLOGY

This anomaly is usually isolated but has been associated with patent ductus arteriosus,[60,69] ventricular septal defect, tetralogy of Fallot, and coarctation of the aorta.[60] If there is pulmonary hypertension, as with a large ventricular septal defect, left ventricular perfusion may be adequate to prevent ischemia. Under these circumstances, closure of the defect with a fall of pulmonary arterial pressure may be catastrophic.[70]

The right coronary artery is greatly dilated, and large collaterals are seen on the surface of the heart. The left coronary artery enters the main pulmonary artery, usually in the left pulmonary sinus, but rarely enters a branch pulmonary artery. It is usually only 2 to 5 mm long before it branches.

In infancy, the hearts are large, and the left ventricle and atrium are dilated and hypertrophied. The anterolateral papillary muscle is atrophic and scarred, and its chordae may be shortened. Sometimes the posterior papillary muscle is similarly affected.[60,71] There may be diffuse endocardial fibroelastosis of the left ventricle, and the anterior mitral valve leaflet is often thickened. Thinning and

scarring of the anterolateral left ventricular wall and apex due to infarction are seen, and there are often mural thrombi.

In adults, the left coronary artery is thin walled, resembling a vein. The heart is usually enlarged, but not as much as in infants, and there is usually no endocardial fibroelastosis. However, there is usually scarring and calcification of the anterolateral papillary muscle and occasionally even of the adjacent left ventricle.[17,72]

CLINICAL FINDINGS

In infancy, the description by Bland and coworkers[64] still pertains. They wrote:

Nothing remarkable was noted about the patient until the tenth week; while nursing from the bottle, the onset of an unusual group of symptoms occurred which consisted of paroxysmal attacks of acute discomfort precipitated by the exertion of nursing. The infant appeared at first to be in obvious distress, as indicated by short expiratory grunts, followed immediately by marked pallor and cold sweat with a general appearance of severe shock. Occasionally, with unusually severe attacks, there appeared to be a transient loss of consciousness. The eructation of gas at times seemed to relieve the discomfort and to shorten the duration of the attack which usually lasted from 5 to 10 minutes, and following which the infant might proceed to nurse without difficulty and remain free of symptoms for several days. . . . It seems probable that in this infant the curious attacks of paroxysmal discomfort . . . were those of angina pectoris. If this is true, it represents the earliest age at which this condition has been recorded.

Some infants present with the signs and symptoms of congestive heart failure. A few children have severe difficulties in infancy and then gradually improve until they are asymptomatic. On the other hand, this anomaly is a rare cause of sudden death in infancy. Older children and adults may be entirely asymptomatic or may have dyspnea, syncope, ventricular arrhythmias, or angina pectoris on effort. Sudden death after exertion has been common.[73] Typical myocardial infarction or congestive heart failure is rare in adults.

On physical examination, there may be signs of congestive heart failure. In infants, the heart is usually enlarged, the left ventricle being the predominant ventricle affected. There may, however, be right ventricular enlargement and loud pulmonic closure if left ventricular failure has caused considerable pulmonary hypertension. The first heart sound may be soft or absent (if there is mitral incompetence), and apical gallop rhythms are common. There may be no murmurs or the murmur of mitral incompetence; at times, a soft continuous murmur is heard at the upper left sternal border that is reminiscent of the murmur of a coronary arteriovenous fistula or a small patent ductus arteriosus.

RADIOLOGIC FINDINGS

These are nonspecific, with marked cardiomegaly, predominantly of the left atrium and ventricle, and pulmonary edema, features similar to those of many forms of cardiomyopathy with which this anomaly is often confused.

Thallium scintigraphy is a useful added investigation that will show reduced uptake in the anterolateral ischemic region.[74, 75] This finding has been seen in some patients with cardiomyopathies.[76]

ELECTROCARDIOGRAPHY

Classically, because there is usually an anterolateral infarct by the time the infant presents for diagnosis, there will be abnormal q waves (≥ 3 mm deep and ≥ 30 milliseconds in duration[77]) in leads I and aV_1 and precordial leads V_4 through V_6. There may also be abnormal R waves or R wave progression in the left precordial leads. Although this pattern is not pathognomonic for this anomaly (it could be seen in myocardial infarcts from other causes or occasionally in various cardiomyopathies), its presence should be sought, and if it is found, the diagnosis of this anomaly should be considered and evaluated by other means. Even in asymptomatic adults, the resting electrocardiogram is abnormal, and abnormal ischemic responses occur with exercise.[72]

ECHOCARDIOGRAPHY

Doppler echocardiography has replaced cardiac catheterization as the standard method of diagnosis.[78–80] The abnormal attachment of the origin of the left coronary artery can be seen, but it must be sought in more than one view to avoid problems due to lateral dropout. The addition of Doppler interrogation is essential, because it will show flow passing from the coronary artery to the great artery instead of from the great artery to the coronary artery. Therefore, even if the attachment of coronary artery to great artery is uncertain, the direction of flow will be informative. The transverse sinus of the pericardium should not be confused with a normal left coronary artery.[81] False-negatives are rare, but one has been described[82]; the correct diagnosis was made in this patient by magnetic resonance imaging, which presumably has higher sensitivity.

The study also shows the large right coronary artery. In addition, the size and function of the cardiac chambers (particularly the left ventricle), regional left ventricular wall motion abnormalities, and mitral regurgitation are shown. There may be increased echogenicity of the papillary muscle and adjacent endocardium due to fibrosis and fibroelastosis.

CARDIAC CATHETERIZATION

This can be used if the results of echocardiography are uncertain but is done much less frequently today than it used to be; deaths due to arrhythmias have occurred during catheterization. An unnecessary cardiac catheterization is better than missing a potentially treatable anomaly, however, especially because failure to diagnose this anomaly usually leads to the diagnosis of idiopathic cardiomyopathy for which no specific treatment other than cardiac transplantation is available.

Symptomatic infants have a low cardiac output, high filling pressures, and usually some pulmonary hypertension. In asymptomatic older patients, cardiac output and pressures are usually normal except perhaps for a slight increase in left ventricular end-diastolic pressure. There may be a left-to-right shunt at the pulmonary arterial level, but because the amount of shunting may be small, its absence does not exclude the diagnosis of this anomaly. Angiography reveals the dilated left ventricle and atrium with dysfunction of the anterolateral left ventricular free wall and shows any mitral regurgitation. Aortic root angiography shows the dilated right coronary artery; and if there are large collaterals, it shows filling of the left coronary artery and passage of contrast material from the left coronary to the main pulmonary artery. Main pulmonary arterial angiography often shows reflux of contrast medium into the origin of the left coronary artery. This anomaly is to be distinguished from the rare anomaly of an atretic left main coronary artery (see earlier).

NATURAL HISTORY

About 87% of children born with this rare anomaly present in infancy,[60] and about 65 to 85% die before 1 year of age from intractable congestive heart failure,[83, 84] usually after 2 months of age. A few of these children have been observed to improve spontaneously.[46] Others never have symptoms, perhaps because they have extensive collaterals and even a restrictive opening between the origin of the left coronary artery and the pulmonary trunk. Nevertheless, even these people are at high risk of sudden death,[73] especially during exercise. Some of these present as adults with angina of effort[72, 85, 86] or with congestive heart failure in association with mitral incompetence.[17, 46] In the past 5 or 6 years, there has been an increased number of reports of adults treated for this anomaly. Operation markedly improves function. Whether an operation is required for an adult with this anomaly but with no evidence of ischemia at rest or on exercise is not known.

TREATMENT

The first effective operation for this anomaly was ligation of the origin of the left coronary artery to prevent the steal.[65] Most children benefit initially from this procedure, especially if they have extensive coronary-to-pulmonary arterial shunting, but late sudden death can occur.[72, 86–88] Ligation is done without cardiopulmonary bypass and is quick, but the circulation cannot be supported if ventricular fibrillation occurs. Furthermore, the origin of the coronary artery occasionally runs in the aortic wall so that ligation is distal to the origin, and collaterals can bypass the ligature and reconstitute the shunt.

Ligation of the origin of the left coronary artery with reconstitution of flow through it by a subclavian arterial or saphenous venous graft has also been successful,[89–93] although clotting or stenosis of the graft has occurred. Late obliterative changes in saphenous vein grafts have occurred.[94] These are potentially serious because by about 3 years after successful saphenous vein grafting for this anomaly, there is usually marked reduction of collaterals from the right coronary artery.[95, 96] Grafts using the internal thoracic artery would possibly have a longer survival.

Surgeons and cardiologists currently favor direct reimplantation of the origin of the left coronary artery into the aorta (with a button of pulmonary artery around the origin)[91, 97–100] or creation of an aortopulmonary window and then fashioning of a tunnel that directs the blood from the aorta to the left coronary ostium.[101–105] There have been few reports of occlusion of either of these nongrafted connections, and a short, wide connection is not likely to become occluded. The longer the follow-up period, the more this approach seems to be better than ligation or bypass grafting.[86, 105–111]

The mortality of surgery in the very sick infant is high, up to 20%, often because of ventricular fibrillation occurring before the sternotomy,[112] so that the less desirable but safer simple ligation procedures (with or without cardiopulmonary bypass) have been recommended for the sickest infants.[112] Reports indicate that satisfactory results can be obtained in good centers with even the sickest infants,[106, 107, 110] although postoperative support with a left ventricular assist device or extracorporeal membrane oxygenation might sometimes be needed.[109]

The late results after operation are usually good, even in adults. The heart becomes smaller, symptoms of congestive heart failure abate, mitral incompetence regresses, and left ventricular shortening fraction improves.* Furthermore, the region of hypoperfusion shown by thallium scans or positron emission tomography may disappear or become smaller, suggesting that some of the ischemic tissue was hibernating and not just scar tissue. Because of the improvement in mitral incompetence, mitral valve repair should not usually be done during the initial operation; it might, however, be required later.[93]

---

*References 87, 101, 106–109, 111, 113.

Right Main Coronary Artery From Pulmonary Trunk

This anomaly is rare. Only 43 reports have appeared in the literature up to 1992.[114]

PATHOLOGY

Myocardial infarction does not occur, and the only grossly abnormal findings are increased size of the left main coronary artery and thinning of the wall of the right coronary artery. The right coronary artery is usually free from atheroma, probably as a result of the low pressure in it.

CLINICAL FINDINGS

Most patients are asymptomatic. Syncope, cardiac arrest, sudden death, angina pectoris (due to coronary steal), and congestive heart failure have been described, however.[17, 114] The youngest patient was 2 months old.[114] There may be a continuous murmur at the left sternal border in some patients.

DIAGNOSIS

The electrocardiogram and chest radiograph are usually normal, and it is left for imaging studies (usually echocardiography or angiography) to demonstrate the abnormal attachment of the right coronary artery to the pulmonary trunk and the retrograde flow from right coronary artery to pulmonary artery.

TREATMENT

Most patients are asymptomatic, and there is no good way to determine which patients are at risk of sudden death without surgical correction of this defect. Nevertheless, most cardiologists recommend operation, especially if there are symptoms or objective evidence of myocardial ischemia. This can be done by reimplanting the right coronary artery into the aortic root.[114–117]

Left Anterior Descending Coronary Artery From Pulmonary Trunk

This is rare; only nine patients have been described by 1992.[17, 118] Apart from a 7-month-old child who died with an anterior myocardial infarct, all the others have been 18 to 55 years old. Five had angina pectoris, one an anterior myocardial infarct, and one mitral regurgitation from papillary muscle dysfunction. Precordial murmurs were common, and most had electrocardiographic evidence of ischemia; radiographs were normal in three and showed cardiomegaly in three. Cardiac catheterization and angiocardiography were diagnostic.

Surgical treatment by ligation of the anomalous artery or its connection to the aorta by a conduit is recommended.[17, 118, 119]

Left Circumflex Coronary Artery From Pulmonary Trunk or Arteries

A few of these anomalies have been reported[17]; in many, the circumflex coronary artery was attached to a branch pulmonary artery rather than to the main pulmonary trunk. All but two have been in children, and all but one child and one adult had other congenital cardiac lesions.[120] One child had ischemic symptoms and was cured after reimplantation of the artery into the aorta.

MISCELLANEOUS CORONARY ARTERIAL DISEASES

The coronary arteries can be involved in many forms of generalized systemic disease, for example, Kawasaki disease, systemic lupus erythematosus, and infantile polyarteritis nodosa. These are not discussed further here, but certain other abnormalities are. (See Chapters 47 and 60.)

Calcific Arteriopathy of Infancy

Arterial calcification of infancy is rare; only 90 patients have been diagnosed before 1975.[121] This disease affects mainly the muscular arteries: coronary arteries in 90% of patients and renal, pancreatic, and splenic arteries in 50% of patients. The internal elastic lamina fragments, and then calcification begins there and extends to the media, where large calcium clumps form and destroy the muscle. Intimal connective tissue proliferation occurs and eventually occludes the lumen. The process probably begins in utero.[122] We do not know whether there is a single cause or several different processes with a common end result.[123] In some patients, similar processes with minimal calcification may or may not be from the same cause.[124]

The patients present with congestive heart failure by about 2 months of age and may have signs of myocardial ischemia and infarction; less often, they have renal failure and hypertension.[125, 126] Diagnosis may be made by palpating hardened superficial arteries in the neck and limbs, by finding calcified arteries on x-ray examination,[124, 127] and sometimes by ophthalmoscopy. Most infants die before 6 months of age, but spontaneous improvement has occurred.[127] Diphosphonates have been used therapeutically, but their effectiveness has not been proved.[128]

Myocardial Infarction

Myocardial infarction in the fetus or neonate is rare.[129, 130] Most of these infarcts are probably due to intrauterine emboli from umbilical, hepatic, or renal veins[129, 130]; some are associated with coronary arteriopathy, a few with severe intrauterine hypoxia and stress,[131] and a few with coagulopathies, but most are of unknown cause. There is occasionally postnatal paradoxical embolism, and there are reports of embolism from material extruded from cardiac catheters, particularly if there have been several changes of guide wires.[132] The risk of coronary embolism may be particularly high in children with cyanotic heart disease. If there is an infarct, it is essential to exclude an anomalous coronary artery arising from the pulmonary artery.

Coronary Aneurysms

These have been found in 1 to 5% of coronary angiograms, the difference depending in part on the definition of an aneurysm.[133, 134] Possible causes are listed in Table 39–3. The most common cause in children is Kawasaki syndrome (see Chapter 47); in adults, it is coronary atherosclerosis. All other causes are rare.

These aneurysms seldom have specific clinical features and are usually found during investigation of other problems. They occasionally appear on x-ray films because of calcification. They are shown best by imaging techniques, usually echocardiography or angiography.

Apart from any problems pertaining to the basic disease, aneurysms may thrombose and cause either coro-

TABLE 39–3
CAUSES OF CORONARY ARTERIAL ANEURYSMS

Congenital[135]
Atherosclerotic[133, 134]
Inflammatory and infectious causes
    Kawasaki syndrome[136]
    Syphilis
    Mycotic
    Infective endocarditis
Trauma, including percutaneous transluminal coronary angioplasty
Connective tissue disorders
    Marfan's syndrome
    Ehlers-Danlos syndrome
Vasculitides
    Takayasu arteritis
    Polyarteritis nodosa
    Scleroderma
    Systemic lupus erythematosus
Miscellaneous
    Osler-Rendu-Weber disease
    Metastatic tumor

nary stenosis or distal coronary embolism, with resulting myocardial ischemia or infarction. Rupture has been described but is rare.[137] Treatment ranges from nothing to antiplatelet medication, thrombolytic agents for acute thrombosis, coronary bypass grafting for occlusive disease, and even excision of the aneurysm.[137]

Myocardial Bridges

The large epicardial coronary arteries run on the surface of the heart, with only their terminal branches penetrating the muscle; but in about 50% of people, part of the epicardial artery dips beneath the epicardial muscle for several millimeters so that there is a muscle bridge over the large artery.[138] These bridges are probably present at birth. Most bridges are on the left anterior descending coronary artery, predominantly its proximal half.[139] Before 20 years of age, the bridges average 14 mm in length, but they are 20 to 30 mm long in older people.[139] In about 75%, the left anterior descending coronary artery runs in the interventricular groove and may be covered by a few superficial bridging muscle fibers; in 25%, the left anterior descending coronary artery deviates toward the right ventricle and runs deep in the ventricular septum, where it is crossed by a bundle of muscle extending from the right ventricular apex to the septal muscle.[139] Most of these bridges are not functionally important, particularly if they are superficial. However, there are documented examples of myocardial ischemia[139, 140] and infarction[141] associated with these bridges, including relief of ischemia after myotomy.[142] Symptoms may occur if the bridge is abnormally long or deep, especially if the right coronary artery is small.[143]

During coronary angiography, a portion of the coronary artery appears to be narrowed in systole but widely patent in diastole, distinguishing it from an anatomically occlusive lesion of the artery.[138, 139, 144]

Because myocardial bridges are so common and do not necessarily indicate present or future coronary arterial disease, the decision about myotomy to relieve anginal symptoms must be made carefully. In addition to a well-defined muscle bridge, there should be ischemia based on lactate production in the regional vein, electrocardiographic changes, or deficient thallium uptake in the region supplied by the artery with the bridge. Ischemia may be due to long, thick bridges that compress the artery and relax unusually slowly so that diastolic filling of the coronary artery beyond the bridge is impaired. Under these circumstances, disappearance of symptoms and of signs of ischemia may follow myotomy. Some patients obtain relief from antianginal therapy with β-adrenergic blockade.[145] Myocardial bridges causing ischemia are rare in children; I have seen them in only a few children with ventricular hypertrophy, particularly hypertrophic cardiomyopathy.

REFERENCES

1. Alexander RW, Griffith GC: Anomalies of the coronary arteries and their clinical significance. Circulation 14:800, 1956.
2. Lipsett J, Cohle SD, Berry PJ, et al: Anomalous coronary arteries: A multicenter pediatric autopsy study. Pediatr Pathol 14:287, 1994.
3. Wilkins CE, Betancourt B, Mathur VS, et al: Coronary artery anomalies: A review of more than 10,000 patients from the Clayton Cardiovascular Laboratories. Tex Heart Inst J 15:166, 1988.
4. Yamanaka O, Hobbs RE: Coronary artery anomalies in 126,595 patients undergoing coronary arteriography. Cathet Cardiovasc Diagn 21:28, 1990.
5. Topaz O, DeMarchena EJ, Perin E, et al: Anomalous coronary arteries: Angiographic findings in 80 patients [see comments]. Int J Cardiol 34:129, 1992.
6. Hutchins GM, Kessler-Hanna A, Moore G: Development of the coronary arteries in the human heart. Circulation 77:1250, 1988.
7. Hoffman JIE: Coronary physiology. In Garfein OB (ed): Current Concepts in Cardiovascular Physiology. New York, Academic Press, 1990, p 290.
8. Hoffman JIE: Congenital anomalies of the coronary vessels and the aortic root. In Emmanouilides GC, Riemenschneider TA, Allen HD, Gutgesell HP (eds): Heart Disease in Infants, Children, and Adolescents: Including the Fetus and Young Adult, Vol 1. Baltimore, Williams & Wilkins, 1995, p 769.
9. Fortune RL, Baron PJ, Fitzgerald JW: Atresia of left main coronary artery. Repair with internal mammary artery by-pass. Cardiovasc Surg 94:150, 1987.
10. Gay F, Vouhé P, Lecompte Y, et al: Atrésie de l'ostium coronaire gauche. Réparation chez un nourrison de deux mois. Arch Mal Coeur Vaiss 82:807, 1989.
11. Bedogni F, Castellani A, La Vecchia L, et al: Atresia of the left main coronary artery: Clinical recognition and surgical treatment. Cathet Cardiovasc Diagn 25:35, 1992.
12. Mullins CE, El-Said G, McNamara DG, et al: Atresia of the left coronary artery ostium: Repair by saphenous vein graft. Circulation 46:989, 1972.
13. Serraf JW: Atresia of left main coronary artery. Repair with internal mammary artery by-pass. Cardiovasc Surg 94:150, 1987.
14. Virmani R, Chun PKC, Goldstein RE, et al: Acute takeoffs of the coronary arteries along the aortic wall and congenital ostial valve-like ridges: Association with sudden death. J Am Coll Cardiol 3:766, 1984.
15. Basso C, Frescura C, Corrado D, et al: Congenital heart disease and sudden death in the young. Hum Pathol 26:1065, 1995.
16. Tuna IC, Bessinger FB, Ophoven JP, Edwards JE: Acute angular origin of left coronary artery from aorta: An unusual cause of left ventricular failure in infancy. Pediatr Cardiol 10:39, 1989.
17. Roberts WC: Major anomalies of coronary arterial origin seen in adulthood. Am Heart J 111:941, 1986.
18. Click RL, Holmes DJ Jr, Vlietstra RE, et al: Anomalous coronary arteries: Location, degree of atherosclerosis and effect on survival—a report from a coronary artery study. J Am Coll Cardiol 13:531, 1989.
19. Kragel AH, Roberts WC: Anomalous origin of either the right or left main coronary artery from the aorta with subsequent coursing between aorta and pulmonary trunk: Analysis of 32 necropsy cases. Am J Cardiol 62:771, 1988.
20. Roberts WC, Shirani J: The four subtypes of anomalous origin of the left main coronary artery from the right aortic sinus (or from the right coronary artery). Am J Cardiol 70:119, 1992.
21. Selig MB, Jafari N: Anomalous origin of the left main coronary artery from the right coronary artery ostium–interarterial subtype: Angiographic definition and surgical treatment. Cathet Cardiovasc Diagn 31:41, 1994.
22. Herrmann MA, Dousa MK, Edwards WD: Sudden infant death with anomalous origin of the left coronary artery. Am J Forensic Med Pathol 13:191, 1992.
23. Duran AC, Angelini A, Frescura C, et al: Anomalous origin of the right coronary artery from the left aortic sinus and sudden infant death. Int J Cardiol 45:147, 1994.
24. Chu E, Cheitlin MD: Diagnostic considerations in patients with suspected coronary artery anomalies. Am Heart J 126:1427, 1993.
25. Ghosh PK, Agarwal SK, Kumar R, et al: Anomalous origin of right coronary artery from left aortic sinus. J Cardiovasc Surg (Torino) 35:65, 1994.
26. Rinaldi RG, Carballido J, Giles R, et al: Right coronary artery with anomalous origin and slit ostium. Ann Thorac Surg 58:828, 1994.
27. Taylor AJ, Rogan KM, Virmani R: Sudden cardiac death associated with isolated congenital coronary artery anomalies. J Am Coll Cardiol 20:640, 1992.
28. Piovesana P, Corrido D, Verlato R, et al: Morbidity associated with anomalous origin of the left circumflex coronary artery from the right aortic sinus. Am J Cardiol 63:762, 1989.
29. Roberts WC, Morrow AG: Compression of anomalous left circumflex coronary arteries by prosthetic valve fixation rings. J Thorac Cardiovasc Surg 57:834, 1969.
30. Roberts WC, Waller BF, Roberts CS: Fatal atherosclerotic narrowing of the right main coronary artery: Origin of the left anterior descending or left circumflex coronary artery from the right (the true "left main equivalent"). Am Heart J 104:863, 1982.
31. Ogden JA: Congenital anomalies of the coronary arteries. Am J Cardiol 25:474, 1970.
32. Sharbaugh AH, White RS: Single coronary artery. Analysis of the anatomic variation, clinical importance, and report of five cases. JAMA 230:243, 1974.
33. Lipton MJ, Barry WH, Obrez I, et al: Isolated single coronary artery: Diagnosis, angiographic classification, and clinical significance. Radiology 130:39, 1979.
34. Shirani J, Roberts WC: Solitary coronary ostium in the aorta in the absence of other major congenital cardiovascular anomalies. J Am Coll Cardiol 21:137, 1993.
35. Liberthson RR, Zaman L, Weyman A, et al: Aberrant origin of the left coronary artery from the proximal right coronary artery: Diagnostic features and pre- and postoperative course. Clin Cardiol 5:377, 1982.
36. Lawson MA, Dailey SM, Soto B: Selective injection of a left coronary artery arising anomalously from the posterior aortic sinus. Cathet Cardiovasc Diagn 30:300, 1993.
37. Zugibe FT, Zugibe FT Jr, Costello JT, Breithaupt MK: Hypoplastic coronary artery disease within the spectrum of sudden unexpected death in young and middle age adults. Am J Forensic Med Pathol 14:276, 1993.
38. Amarasena NL, Pillai RP, Forfar JC: Atypical ventricular tachycardia and syncope with left coronary artery origin from the right coronary sinus. Br Heart J 70:391, 1993.
39. Barth CW III, Roberts WC: Left main coronary artery originating from the right sinus of Valsalva and coursing between the aorta and the pulmonary trunk. J Am Coll Cardiol 7:366, 1986.
40. Cheitlin MD, De Castro CM, McAllister HA: Sudden death as a complication of anomalous left coronary origin from the anterior sinus of Valsalva: A not-so-minor congenital anomaly. Circulation 50:780, 1974.
41. Donaldson RM, Raphael M, Radley-Smith R, et al: Angiographic identification of primary coronary anomalies causing impaired myocardial perfusion. Cathet Cardiovasc Diag 9:237, 1983.
42. Mustafa I, Gula G, Radley-Smith R, et al: Anomalous origin of the left coronary artery from the anterior aortic sinus: A potential cause of sudden death. J Thorac Cardiovasc Surg 82:297, 1981.
43. Ishikawa T, Brandt PWT: Anomalous origin of the left main coronary artery from the right anterior aortic sinus: Angiographic definition of anomalous course. Am J Cardiol 55:770, 1985.
44. Serota H, Barth CW III, Seuc CA, et al: Rapid identification of the course of anomalous coronary arteries in adults: The "dot and eye" method. Am J Cardiol 65:891, 1990.
45. Maron BJ, Roberts WC, McAllister HA, et al: Sudden death in young athletes. Circulation 62:218, 1980.

46. Driscoll DJ, Edwards WD: Sudden unexpected death in children and adolescents. J Am Coll Cardiol 5(suppl B):118B, 1985.

47. Topaz O, Edwards JE: Pathologic features of sudden death in children, adolescents, and young adults. Chest 87:476, 1985.

48. Gaither NS, Rogan KM, Stajduhar K, et al: Anomalous origin and course of coronary arteries in adults: Identification and improved imaging utilizing transesophageal echocardiography. Am Heart J 122:69, 1991.

49. Fernandes F, Alam M, Smith S, Khaja F: The role of transesophageal echocardiography in identifying anomalous coronary arteries. Circulation 88:2532, 1993.

50. Nowak B, Voigtlander T, Kolsch B, et al: Echocardiographic visualization of anomalous left main coronary arteries originating from the right sinus of Valsalva. Int J Cardiol 46:67, 1994.

51. McConnell MV, Ganz P, Selwyn AP, et al: Identification of anomalous coronary arteries and their anatomic course by magnetic resonance coronary angiography. Circulation 92:3158, 1995.

52. Post JC, van Rossum AC, Bronzwaer JG, et al: Magnetic resonance angiography of anomalous coronary arteries. A new gold standard for delineating the proximal course? Circulation 92:3163, 1995.

53. Kaku B, Simizu M, Kajinami K, et al: Ultrafast computed tomography in the diagnosis and evaluation of anomalous origin of the right coronary artery. Jpn Heart J 36:807, 1995.

54. van Straalen MJ, Gijs Mast E, Ernst SM: The value of computed tomography in combination with a percutaneous transluminal coronary angioplasty guide wire for identifying the definite course of an anomalous left anterior descending artery. Int J Cardiol 53:189, 1996.

55. Ilia R: Percutaneous transluminal angioplasty of coronary arteries with anomalous origin. Cathet Cardiovasc Diagn 35:36, 1995.

56. Oral D, Dagalp Z, Pamir G, et al: Percutaneous transluminal coronary angioplasty of anomalous coronary arteries. Case reports. Angiology 47:77, 1996.

57. Driscoll DJ: Congenital coronary artery anomalies. In Garson A Jr, Bricker JT, McNamara DG (eds): The Science and Practice of Pediatric Cardiology. Philadelphia, Lea & Febiger, 1990, p 1453.

58. Fellows KE, Smith J, Keane JF: Preoperative angiography in infants with tetrad of Fallot. Am J Cardiol 47:1279, 1981.

59. Mayer JE Jr, Sanders SP, Jonas RA, et al: Coronary artery pattern and outcome of arterial switch operation for transposition of the great arteries. Circulation 82(suppl IV):139, 1990.

60. Neufeld HN, Schneeweiss A: Coronary Artery Disease in Infants and Children. Philadelphia, Lea & Febiger, 1983.

61. Heifetz SA, Robinowitz M, Mueller KH, Virmani R: Total anomalous origin of the coronary arteries from the pulmonary artery. Pediatr Cardiol 7:11, 1986.

62. Urcelay GE, Iannettoni MD, Lutomirsky A, et al: Origin of both coronary arteries from the pulmonary artery. Circulation 980:2379, 1994.

63. Thomas CS Jr, Campbell WB, Alford WC, et al: Complete repair of anomalous origin of the left coronary artery in the adult. J Thorac Cardiovasc Surg 66:439, 1973.

64. Bland EF, White PD, Garland J: Congenital anomalies of the coronary arteries: Report of an unusual case associated with cardiac hypertrophy. Am Heart J 8:787, 1993.

65. Sabiston DC Jr, Neill CA, Taussig HB: The direction of blood flow in anomalous left coronary artery arising from the pulmonary artery. Circulation 22:591, 1960.

66. Augustsson MN, Gasul BM, Lundquist R: Anomalous origin of the left coronary artery from the pulmonary artery (adult type). Pediatrics 29:274, 1962.

67. Rudolph AM, Gootman NL, Kaplan N, Rohman M: Anomalous left coronary artery arising from the pulmonary artery with large left-to-right shunt in infancy. J Pediatr 63:543, 1963.

68. Foster HJ, Hagstrom J, Ehlers K, Engle MA: Mitral insufficiency due to anomalous origin of the left coronary artery from the pulmonary artery. Pediatrics 34:649, 1964.

69. Ogden JA, Goodyer AVN: Patterns of distribution of the single coronary artery. Yale J Biol Med 43:11, 1970.

70. Rao BNS, Lucas RV Jr, Edwards JE: Anomalous origin of the left coronary artery from the right pulmonary artery associated with ventricular septal defect. Chest 59:616, 1970.

71. Vlodaver Z, Neufeld HN, Edwards JE: Coronary Artery Variations in the Normal Heart and in Congenital Heart Disease. New York, Academic Press, 1975.

72. Moodie DS, Fyfe D, Gill CC, et al: Anomalous origin of the left coronary artery from the pulmonary artery (Bland-White-Garland syndrome) in adult patients. Long term follow-up after surgery. Am Heart J 106:381, 1983.

73. George JM, Knowlan DM: Anomalous origin of the left coronary artery from the pulmonary artery in an adult. N Engl J Med 261:993, 1959.

74. Finley JP, Howman-Giles R, Gilday DL, et al: Thallium-201 myocardial imaging in anomalous left coronary artery arising from the pulmonary artery. Am J Cardiol 42:675, 1978.

75. Rabinovitch M, Rowland T, Castaneda AR, Treves S: Thallium 201 scintigraphy in patients with anomalous origin of the left coronary artery from the main pulmonary artery. J Pediatr 94:244, 1979.

76. Gutgesell HP, Pinsky WW, DePuey EG: Thallium-201 myocardial perfusion imaging in infants and children, value in distinguishing anomalous left coronary artery from congestive cardiomyopathy. Circulation 61:596, 1980.

77. Johnsrude CL, Perry JC, Cecchin F, et al: Differentiating anomalous left main coronary artery originating from the pulmonary artery in infants from myocarditis and dilated cardiomyopathy by electrocardiogram. Am J Cardiol 75:71, 1995.

78. Caldwell RL, Hurwitz RA, Girod DA, et al: Two-dimensional echocardiographic differentiation of anomalous left coronary artery from congestive cardiomyopathy. Am Heart J 106:710, 1983.

79. King DH, Danforth DA, Huhta JC, Gutgesell HP: Noninvasive detection of anomalous origin of the left main coronary artery from the pulmonary trunk by pulsed Doppler echocardiography. Am J Cardiol 55:608, 1985.

80. Schmidt KG, Cooper MJ, Silverman NH, Stanger P: Pulmonary artery origin of the left coronary artery: Diagnosis by two-dimensional echocardiography, pulsed Doppler ultrasound and color flow mapping. J Am Coll Cardiol 11:396, 1988.

81. Robinson PJ, Sullivan ID, Kumpeng V, et al: Anomalous origin of the left coronary artery from the pulmonary trunk. Potential for false negative diagnosis with cross sectional echocardiography. Br Heart J 52:272, 1984.

82. Breuer J, Barth H, Steil E, et al: Anomalous origin of the left coronary artery from the pulmonary artery. Variability of clinical aspects, echocardiography and angiography findings [in German]. Monatsschr Kinderheilkd 140:346, 1992.

83. Keith JD: Anomalous origin of the left coronary artery from the pulmonary artery. Br Heart J 21:149, 1959.

84. Wesselhoeft H, Fawcett JS, Johnson AL: Anomalous origin of the left coronary artery from the pulmonary trunk. Its clinical spectrum, pathology, and pathophysiology, based on a review of 140 cases with seven further cases. Circulation 38:403, 1968.

85. Roche AHG: Anomalous origin of the left coronary artery from the pulmonary artery in the adult. Report of uneventful ligation in two cases. Am J Cardiol 20:561, 1967.

86. Wilson CL, Dlabal PW, McGuire SA: Surgical treatment of anomalous left coronary artery from pulmonary artery. Follow-up in teenagers and adults. Am Heart J 98:440, 1979.

87. Shrivastava S, Castenada AR, Moller JH: Anomalous left coronary artery from pulmonary trunk. Long-term follow-up after ligation. J Thorac Cardiovasc Surg 76:130, 1978.

88. Backer CL, Stout MJ, Zales VR, et al: Anomalous origin of the left coronary artery. A twenty-year review of surgical management. J Thorac Cardiovasc Surg 103:1049, 1992.

89. Cooley DA, Hallman GL, Bloodwell RD: Definitive qualified treatment of anomalous origin of left coronary artery from pulmonary artery. J Thorac Cardiovasc Surg 59:789, 1966.

90. Meyer BW, Stefanik G, Stiles QR, et al: A method of definitive surgical treatment of anomalous origin of left coronary artery—a case report. J Thorac Cardiovasc Surg 56:104, 1968.

91. Neches WH, Mathews RA, Park SC, et al: Anomalous origin of the left coronary artery from the pulmonary artery. A new method of surgical repair. Circulation 50:582, 1974.

92. Stephenson LW, Edmunds LH Jr, Friedman S, et al: Subclavian–left coronary artery anastomosis (Meyer operation) for anomalous origin of the left coronary artery from the pulmonary artery. Circulation 64(suppl II):130, 1981.

93. Bojar RM, Ilbawai MN, De Leon SY, et al: Surgical management of anomalous left coronary artery with mitral insufficiency in infancy: Contribution of echocardiography. Pediatr Cardiol 5:35, 1984.

94. El-Said GM, Ruzyllo MD, Williams RL, et al: Early and late results of saphenous vein graft for anomalous origin of left coronary artery from pulmonary artery. Circulation 48(suppl III):2, 1976.

95. Moodie DS, Gill C, Loop FD, Sheldon WC: Anomalous left main coronary artery originating from the right sinus of Valsalva. Patho-

physiology, angiographic definition and surgical approaches. J Thorac Cardiovasc Surg 80:198, 1980.

96. Donaldson RM, Raphael MJ, Yacoub MH, Ross DN: Hemodynamically significant anomalies of the coronary arteries. Surgical aspects. Thorac Cardiovasc Surg 30:7, 1982.

97. Grace RR, Angelini P, Cooley DA: Aortic implantation of anomalous left coronary artery arising from pulmonary artery. Am J Cardiol 39:608, 1977.

98. Stiles QR: Surgery for anomalous origin of the left coronary artery from the pulmonary artery. In Tucker BL, Lindesmith GG (eds): First Clinical Conference on Congenital Heart Disease. New York, Grune & Stratton, 1979, p 285.

99. Levitsky S, van der Horst RL, Hastreiter AR, Fisher EA: Anomalous left coronary artery in the infant: Recovery of ventricular function following early direct aortic implantation. J Thorac Cardiovasc Surg 79:598, 1980.

100. Laborde F, Marchand M, Leca F, et al: Surgical treatment of anomalous origin of the left coronary artery in infancy and childhood; early and late results in 20 consecutive cases. J Thorac Cardiovasc Surg 82:423, 1981.

101. Arciniegas E, Farooki ZQ, Hakimi M, Green EW: Management of anomalous left coronary artery from the pulmonary artery. Circulation 62(suppl I):180, 1975.

102. Hamilton DI, Ghosh PK, Donnelly RJ: An operation for anomalous origin of the left coronary artery. Br Heart J 41:121, 1979.

103. Takeuchi S, Imamura H, Katsumoto K, et al: New surgical method for repair of anomalous left coronary artery from pulmonary artery. J Thorac Cardiovasc Surg 78:7, 1979.

104. Midgley FM, Watson DC Jr, Scott LP III, et al: Repair of anomalous origin of the left coronary artery in the infant and small child. J Am Coll Cardiol 4:1231, 1984.

105. Laks H, Ardehali A, Grant PW, Allada V: Aortic implantation of anomalous left coronary artery. An improved surgical approach. J Thorac Cardiovasc Surg 109:519, 1995.

106. Vouhé PR, Tamisier D, Sidi D, et al: Anomalous left coronary artery from the pulmonary artery: Results of isolated aortic reimplantation [see comments]. Ann Thorac Surg 54:621, 1992.

107. Dua R, Smith JA, Wilkinson JL, et al: Long-term follow-up after two coronary repairs of anomalous left coronary artery from the pulmonary artery. J Card Surg 8:384, 1993.

108. Wollenek G, Domanig E, Salzer-Muhar U, et al: Anomalous origin of the left coronary artery: A review of surgical management in 13 patients. J Cardiovasc Surg (Torino) 34:399, 1993.

109. Alexi-Meskishvili V, Hetzer R, Weng Y, et al: Anomalous origin of the left coronary artery from the pulmonary artery. Early results with direct aortic reimplantation. J Thorac Cardiovasc Surg 108:354, 1994.

110. Raanani E, Abramov D, Abramov Y, et al: Individual anatomy demands various techniques in correction of an anomalous origin of the left coronary artery in the pulmonary artery. Thorac Cardiovasc Surg 43:99, 1995.

111. Turley K, Szarnicki RJ, Flachsbart KD, et al: Aortic implantation is possible in all cases of anomalous origin of the left coronary artery from the pulmonary artery. Ann Thorac Surg 60:84, 1995.

112. Kirklin JW, Barratt-Boyes BG: Congenital aneurysm of the sinus of Valsalva. In Cardiac Surgery, Vol 1, 2nd ed. New York, John Wiley & Sons, 1993, p 825.

113. Alexi-Meskishvili V, Berger F, Weng Y, et al: Anomalous origin of the left coronary artery from the pulmonary artery in adults. J Card Surg 10:309, 1995.

114. Vairo U, Marino B, De Simone G, Marcelletti C: Early congestive heart failure due to origin of the right coronary artery from the pulmonary artery. Chest 102:1610, 1992.

115. Bregman D, Brennan FJ, Singer A, et al: Anomalous origin of right coronary artery from pulmonary artery. J Thorac Cardiovasc Surg 72:626, 1976.

116. Lerberg DB, Ogden JA, Zuberbuhler JR, Bahnson HT: Anomalous origin of the right coronary artery from the pulmonary artery. Ann Thorac Surg 27:87, 1979.

117. Tinglestad JB, Lower RR, Eldredge WJ: Anomalous origin of the right coronary artery from the main pulmonary artery. Am J Cardiol 30:670, 1972.

118. Fu M, Hung JS, Yeh SJ, Chang CH: Reversal of silent myocardial ischemia by surgery for isolated anomalous origin of the left anterior descending coronary artery from the pulmonary artery. Am Heart J 124:1369, 1992.

119. Tamer DF, Mallon SM, Garcia OL, Wolff GS: Anomalous origin of the left anterior descending coronary artery from the pulmonary artery. Am Heart J 108:341, 1984.

120. Chopra PS, Reed WH, Wilson AD, Rao PS: Delayed presentation of anomalous circumflex coronary artery arising from the pulmonary artery following repair of aortopulmonary window in infancy. Chest 106:1920, 1994.

121. Stolte M, Jurowich B: Arteriopathia calcificans infantum. Basic Res Cardiol 70:305, 1975.

122. Traisman HS, Limperis NM, Traisman AS: Myocardial infarction due to calcification of the arteries in an infant. Am J Dis Child 91:34, 1956.

123. MacMahon HE, Dickinson PCT: Occlusive fibroelastosis of coronary arteries in the newborn. Circulation 35:3, 1967.

124. Witzleben CL: Idiopathic infantile arterial calcification—a misnomer? Am J Cardiol 26:305, 1970.

125. Schiffmann JH, Wessel A, Bruck W, Speer CP: Idiopathic infantile arterial calcinosis. A rare cardiovascular disease of uncertain etiology—case report and review of the literature [in German]. Monatsschr Kinderheilkd 140:27, 1992.

126. Gleason MM, Weber HS, Cyran SE, et al: Idiopathic infantile arterial calcinosis: Intermediate-term survival and cardiac sequelae. Am Heart J 127:691, 1994.

127. Sholler GF, Yu JS, Bale PM, et al: Generalized arterial calcification of infancy: Three case reports, including spontaneous regression with long-term survival. J Pediatr 1105:257, 1984.

128. Thiaville A, Smets A, Clercx A, Perlmutter N: Idiopathic infantile arterial calcification: A surviving patient with renal artery stenosis. Pediatr Radiol 24:506, 1994.

129. Kilbride H, Way GL, Mersenstein GB, Winfield JM: Myocardial infarction in the neonate with normal heart and coronary arteries. Am J Dis Child 134:759, 1980.

130. Bernstein D, Finkbeiner WE, Soifer S, Teitel D: Perinatal myocardial infarction: A case report and review of the literature. Pediatr Cardiol 6:313, 1986.

131. DeMoor MMA, Vosloo SM, Human DG: Myocardial infarction in a neonate with cyanotic congenital heart disease. Pediatr Cardiol 6:219, 1986.

132. Klys HS, Salmon AP, DeGiovanni JV: Paradoxical embolisation of a catheter fragment to a coronary artery in an infant with congenital heart disease. Br Heart J 66:320, 1991.

133. Swaye PS, Fisher LD, Litwin P, et al: Aneurysmal coronary arterial disease. Circulation 67:134, 1983.

134. Robinson FC: Aneurysms of the coronary arteries. Am Heart J 109:129, 1985.

135. Seabra-Gomez R, Somerville J, Ross DN, et al: Congenital coronary artery aneurysms. Br Heart J 36:329, 1974.

136. Kato H, Ichinose E, Yoshioka F, et al: Fate of coronary aneurysms in Kawasaki disease: Serial coronary angiography and long-term follow-up study. Am J Cardiol 49:1758, 1982.

137. Burns CA, Cowley MJ, Wechsler AS, Vetrovec GW: Coronary aneurysms: A case report and review. Cathet Cardiovasc Diagn 27:106, 1992.

138. Angelini P, Trivellato M, Donis J, Leachman RL: Myocardial bridges: A review. Prog Cardiovasc Res 26:75, 1983.

139. Ferreira AG Jr, Trotter SE, König B Jr, et al: Myocardial bridges: Morphological and functional aspects. Br Heart J 66:364, 1991.

140. Hill RC, Chitwood WR Jr, Bashore TM, et al: Coronary flow and regional function before and after supraarterial myotomy for myocardial bridging. Ann Thorac Surg 31:176, 1981.

141. Bestetti RB, Costa RS, Zucolotto S, Olivara JSM: Fatal outcome associated with autopsy proven myocardial bridging of the left anterior descending coronary artery. Eur Heart J 10:573, 1989.

142. Iversen S, Hake U, Mayer E, et al: Surgical treatment of myocardial bridging causing coronary artery obstruction. Scand J Thorac Cardiovasc Surg 26:107, 1992.

143. Morales AR, Romanelli R, Tate LG, et al: Intramural left anterior descending coronary artery: Significance of the depth of the muscular tunnel. Hum Pathol 24:693, 1993.

144. Bezarra AJC, Prates JC, Didio LJC: Incidence and clinical significance of bridges of myocardium over the coronary arteries and their branches. Surg Radiol Anat 9:273, 1987.

145. Schwarz ER, Klues HG, vom Dahl J, et al: Functional, angiographic and intracoronary Doppler flow characteristics in symptomatic patients with myocardial bridging: Effect of short-term intravenous beta-blocker medication. J Am Coll Cardiol 27:1637, 1996.

CHAPTER 40

MALPOSITION OF THE HEART

BRUNO MARINO   PAOLO GUCCIONE   ADRIANO CAROTTI

Malposition of the heart is a nonspecific term used to indicate an abnormal position of the heart within or outside the thorax, without giving information about cardiac structure such as atrial situs, ventricular arrangement, or position of great arteries. This term refers not only to the position of the heart but also to the appropriateness of the position of the heart in the thorax in relation to the situs. *Levocardia* indicates a left-sided heart and is the normal position of the heart in individuals with situs solitus; *dextrocardia* indicates a right-sided heart and is the normal position in individuals with situs inversus; and *mesocardia* is the midline position of the heart in the thorax. *Ectopia cordis* is the classic cardiac malformation in which the heart is outside the thorax.

Cardiac position is embryologically determined by the ventricular loop and by the degree of pivoting of the ventricular portion of the cardiac tube. The embryologic events that result in D–ventricular looping also result in levocardia, whereas events producing L–ventricular looping result in dextrocardia. When there is concordance between the situs and the position of the heart in the thorax (levocardia in a D-loop and dextrocardia in an L-loop), the pivoting of the ventricle has been complete. On the other hand, the pivoting of the heart is incomplete when discordance between the situs and the position of the heart occurs, resulting in malposition. With atrioventricular discordance, either in situs solitus or in situs inversus, the pivoting of the heart is more often incomplete, resulting in varying cardiac positions (levocardia, dextrocardia, mesocardia). The same concept may be applied to cases of asplenia/right isomerism or polysplenia/left isomerism. These conditions preclude a designated situs and therefore a concordant loop. It is not surprising to find a high prevalence of cardiac malposition in situs ambiguus.

The classification of cardiac malposition is not easy, and few discussions have been more controversial than those about the nomenclature of complex cardiac malformations.[1–9] These discussions are valuable in helping us to focus on issues of cardiac anatomy of different types of malformation of the heart. There is general agreement about applying a segmental approach to diagnosis[1, 6, 8] of patients with complex cardiac anomalies and in particular children with malposition of the heart. Because intracardiac anomalies frequently coexist in cardiac malpositions, segmental analysis is essential to understand and describe the sequential anatomy of the heart. Three segments must be considered: (1) atrial situs, (2) ventricular position and connection to the atria, and (3) position of great arteries and connections to the ventricle. In this chapter, the atrial situs is discussed; the second and third segments are discussed in Chapters 19 and 20.

ATRIAL SITUS

The first step to understand the morphology of a heart is the determination of visceroatrial situs. The left-right orientation of the abdominal organs and of the hearts in vertebrates is a nonrandom and highly conserved phenomenon[10, 11] probably controlled by several genes.[12–19] Visceroatrial situs refers to the relationship between the abdominal viscera and the cardiac atria. The three types of visceroatrial situs are *situs solitus* (normal), *situs inversus* (mirror image of normal), and *situs ambiguus* (irregular relationship between viscera and atria).

SITUS SOLITUS

Visceroatrial situs solitus is the usual pattern present in normal subjects and also frequently occurs with malformed hearts.

In situs solitus, the major lobe of the liver, the inferior vena cava, and the anatomic right atrium are on the right side of the body, as is the trilobed lung and the eparterial bronchus. The stomach, the spleen, the descending aorta, and the anatomic left atrium are on the left side of the body, as is the bilobed lung and the hyparterial bronchus.

In individuals with situs solitus, the heart is usually located in the left hemithorax. Cardiac malposition in situs solitus includes dextrocardia and mesocardia.

SITUS INVERSUS

Situs inversus is the mirror image of situs solitus so that the major lobe of the liver, the inferior vena cava, and the anatomic right atrium are on the left side of the body, as is the trilobed lung and the eparterial bronchus. The liver, descending aorta, anatomic left atrium, bilobed lung, and hyparterial bronchus are on the right side of the body.

The characteristic position of the heart in subjects with situs inversus is in the right hemithorax (dextrocardia), but the cardiac mass may also be "malposed" in the left side.

SITUS AMBIGUUS

In any arrangement other than situs solitus or situs inversus, there is random orientation of different organs. This situation is defined as situs ambiguus or *heterotaxia*.[20–31]

Heterotaxia includes all abnormalities of lateralization consisting of anomalous relationships between major organs whose anatomic position becomes unpredictable.

Altered left-right asymmetry (heterotaxia) is often (more than 90% of instances) accompanied by severe cardiac malformations consisting of disarrangement of cardiac chambers, abnormal venous connections, and altered great arterial alignment. It is frequently associated with cardiac malposition such as mesocardia or dextrocardia.

Furthermore, other organs, such as the liver, the spleen, and the intestine, show abnormal morphology and position. In patients with heterotaxia, the genetic message of visceral asymmetry is lost. There is a tendency toward morphologic symmetry of some organs, such as atrial appendages, bronchi, and lungs. This aspect prompted some authors to define these conditions as *atrial isomerism* initially[24,25] and more recently as *isomerism of the atrial appendages*.[27,30,31] On the contrary, other investigators[26,28,29,32] contest this definition, affirming that the concept of isomerism as it relates to the heart has never been biologically proved, is diagnostically difficult to assess, and is surgically irrelevant. However, two forms of situs ambiguus have been defined according to the status of the spleen and the morphology of the atrial appendages, bronchi, and lungs.[21–23]

The first subtype of situs ambiguus is the *asplenia syndrome* with *right isomerism* of atrial appendages. In this type of heterotaxia, the spleen is absent *(asplenia)* and the atrial appendages, bronchi, and lungs tend to be mirror images of each other and to show the anatomic features of the right-sided structures *(right isomerism)*.[24–31]

The second subtype of situs ambiguus is the *polysplenia syndrome* with *left isomerism* of atrial appendages. In this type of heterotaxia, two or more splenic masses *(polysplenia)* are present along the greater curvature of the stomach on the right or left side of the abdomen. The atrial appendages, bronchi, and lungs tend to be mirror images of each other and to show the anatomy of the left-sided structures *(left isomerism)*.[21–26] In patients with heterotaxia (including asplenia/right isomerism and polysplenia/left isomerism), there is no characteristic position of the heart, because it is possible to find the cardiac mass in the left (levocardia) or in the right (dextrocardia) hemithorax or in the intermediate position (mesocardia).[33]

After the diagnosis of visceroatrial situs, the segmental analysis includes the definition of ventricular loop (atrioventricular connections) and conotruncal and great arterial alignment (ventriculoarterial connections).[1,6,8]

Along with the categorization of visceroatrial situs, we can classify cardiac malpositions in three types: cardiac malposition with situs solitus, cardiac malposition with situs inversus, and cardiac malposition with situs ambiguus and heterotaxia.

CARDIAC MALPOSITION WITH SITUS SOLITUS

DEXTROCARDIA

Dextrocardia is the most common type of malposition. Dextrocardia, initially described by Fabricius in 1749,[34] simply means that the heart is predominantly in the right

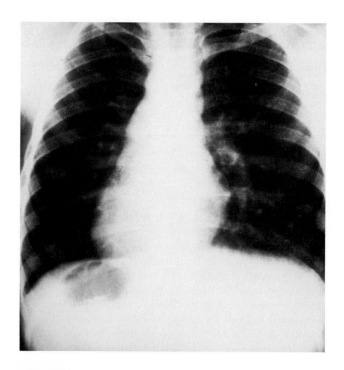

FIGURE 40–1

Dextrocardia, thoracic radiograph in posteroanterior projection. The heart is displaced in the right hemithorax with the apex toward the patient's right.

hemithorax. A wide variety of terms have been proposed in an attempt to fully describe all variants of dextrocardia. Numerous classifications of dextrocardia have been proposed. Terms such as isolated dextrocardia, mirror-image dextrocardia, false dextrocardia, primary or secondary dextrocardia, dextroversion, and dextrorotation represent the attempts to describe and categorize this condition.[35,36] In this chapter, we distinguish dextrocardia and dextroversion. Dextrocardia is the location of the heart in the right thorax with the apex pointing to the right (Fig. 40–1), and it is usually due to anomalous pivoting of the ventricles.[7] Dextroversion is the location of the heart in the right thorax with the apex normally pointed to the patient's left; it occurs in those congenital or acquired lesions that push the heart to the right, such as diaphragmatic hernia and right lung hypoplasia (Fig. 40–2).

Dextrocardia With Situs Solitus

This is the most common type of dextrocardia in reported pathologic series.[3,37] The atrial and ventricular septa are in the same plane as in levocardia with either concordant or discordant atrioventricular connection. In mesocardia and dextrocardia, the incomplete pivoting of the ventricular septum determines a progressively narrower angle between the atrial and ventricular septa.

Dextrocardia With D–Ventricular Loop and Normally Related Great Arteries {S,D,S}

This is the second most frequent type of cardiac condition in dextrocardia; corrected transposition in situs solitus {S,L,L} is the most common one. A wide variety of associated malformations have been described in situs solitus and dextrocardia[3,37]: ventricular septal defect, aortic

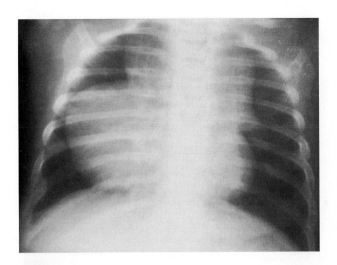

FIGURE 40–2

Dextroversion of the heart, thoracic radiograph in posteroanterior projection. The major part of the heart is displaced in the right hemithorax because of the enormous dilatation of the right atrium (Ebstein malformation). The apex of the heart is pointed toward the patient's left.

coarctation, secundum atrial septal defect, atrioventricular canal, anomalies of the systemic veins, persistent left superior vena cava to the coronary sinus, tricuspid atresia, double-outlet right ventricle, and tetralogy of Fallot.

Dextrocardia with normal atrioventricular and ventriculoarterial relations {S,D,S} is often part of a syndrome[38, 39] usually with midline defects, an association initially described by Cantrell and colleagues.[40] In this syndrome, sporadically associated with trisomy 18,[41] five components are present: midline epigastric abdominal wall defect, often associated with herniation or omphalocele; defect of the lower sternum; deficiency of the anterior diaphragm; defect of the diaphragmatic portion of the pericardium;

and diverticulum of the left or right ventricle. Cardiac malformation often coexists, most frequently tetralogy of Fallot or ventricular septal defect. Although the presentation of Cantrell's syndrome can be variable, one-stage repair of the cardiac defect is usually feasible.[42]

Dextroversion of the Heart

The malposition of a heart with atrioventricular and ventriculoarterial concordance {S,D,S} in the right thorax with the apex normally pointed toward the patient's left is defined as *dextroversion* (see Fig. 40–2). This condition that mimics dextrocardia is generally due to anatomic or functional abnormalities of the lung, diaphragm, or thoracic cage or marked dilatation of the right atrium as in infants with the Ebstein malformation (see Fig. 40–2).

Right lung hypoplasia and dextroversion[43] of the heart are usually associated with congenital lesions, such as renal abnormalities (oligohydramnios), right bronchial tree abnormalities,[44] deformity of the thoracic spine and rib cage, and diaphragmatic hernia. Diaphragmatic hernia is the most common cause of congenital dextroversion. During fetal life when the embryonic heart is looping, as the hernia develops, the heart is displaced, resulting in malposition. The space occupation by the hernia within the thorax can compress the left-sided heart structures and lead to their underdevelopment.

Acquired lesions resulting in dextroversion are left pneumothorax and tumor of the pericardium[45] or of the mediastinum. *Scimitar syndrome* is one well-described[39] condition associated with dextroversion. The scimitar syndrome combines hypoplasia of the right lung, right pulmonary artery, and right bronchus; partial anomalous connection of the right pulmonary veins to the inferior vena cava; and anomalous arterial vessels arising from the descending aorta and directed to the right lung (Figs. 40–3 and 40–4).

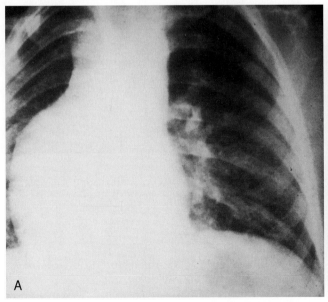
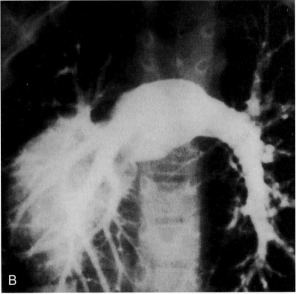

FIGURE 40–3

Dextroversion of the heart, scimitar syndrome. *A*, Thoracic radiograph, heart in right hemithorax. The right hemithorax is smaller than the left because of the right lung hypoplasia. The right hemidiaphragm is elevated. *B*, Pulmonary arteriogram shows hypoplastic vasculature in the right lung.

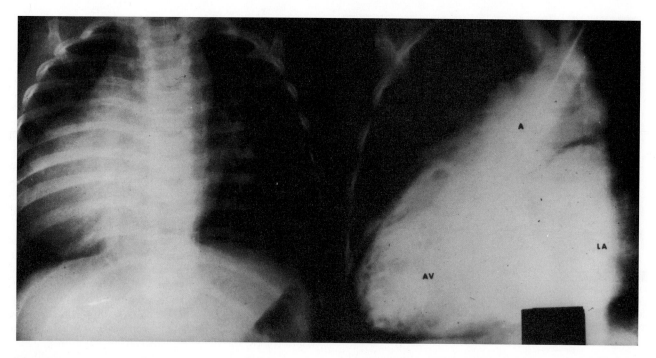

FIGURE 40–4

Dextroversion of situs solitus. *Left,* Heart in right hemithorax. *Right,* Injection in anterior ventricle (AV). Aorta (A) and left atrium (LA) are opacified. The descending aorta is on the left.

Dextrocardia With D–Ventricular Loop and Transposition of the Great Arteries {S,D,D}

Transposition of great arteries occurs in dextrocardia (Fig. 40–5). Complex forms of transposition of great arteries are more common in dextrocardia than in levocardia. In a series, 75% of instances of {S,D,D} and transposition of great arteries had a ventricular septal defect, and 75% had left atrial appendage juxtaposition.[37] Dextrocardia is twice as common in transposition of great arteries with left atrial juxtaposition than in simple transposition of great arteries.[46] Dextrocardia in situs solitus reduces the size of the atrial free wall and may cause difficulties in creating an atrial baffle.[47]

Dextrocardia With D–Ventricular Loop and L-Malposition of the Aorta {S,D,L}

Dextrocardia is frequent in this group of rare cardiac malformations that include double-outlet right ventricle with L-aorta and subaortic ventricular septal defect (dextrocardia, 30%), anatomically corrected malposition of the great arteries (dextrocardia, 30%), and double-outlet left ventricle or crisscross heart (dextrocardia, 25%). Left atrial juxtaposition is frequent in patients with {S,D,D} and dextrocardia (Fig. 40–6).[37, 46]

A peculiar form of dextrocardia with {S,D,L} arrangement is represented by the crisscross heart.[48] In these patients, the right-sided right atrium is connected with the left-sided right ventricle, and the left-sided left atrium is connected to the right-sided left ventricle, so that the atrioventricular valves cross each other. The great arteries are transposed, or both arise from the right ventricle with

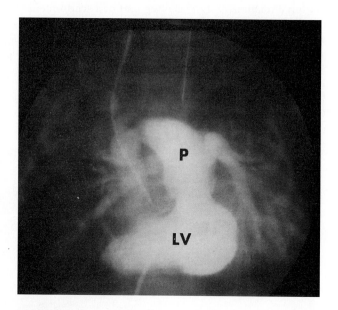

FIGURE 40–5

Left ventricular angiogram in a patient with dextrocardia and {S,D,D} and transposition of the great arteries. The pulmonary artery (P) originates from the left ventricle (LV).

the aorta anterior and left-sided. In crisscross heart, the tricuspid valve and the right ventricle are always anterior and usually hypoplastic. The right ventricle frequently lies in a superior position so that crisscross heart and upstairs-downstairs ventricle (superoinferior ventricle) coexist (Fig. 40–7).[48]

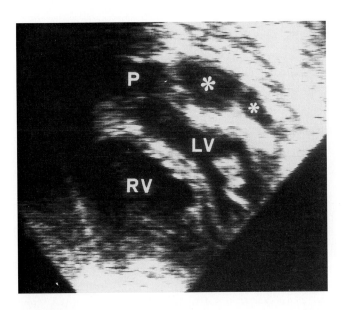

FIGURE 40–6

Two-dimensional echocardiography in subcostal view {S,D,D}, transposition of great arteries, left juxtaposition of the atrial appendages, and dextrocardia. The juxtaposed atrial appendages are indicated by the asterisks. RV = right ventricle; LV = left ventricle; P = pulmonary artery. (From Marino B, Thiene G: Anatomia Ecocardiografia delle Cardiopatie Congenite. Florence, Italy, USES Edizioni Scientifiche, 1990, p 177.)

Dextrocardia With L–Ventricular Loop and Transposition of the Great Arteries or Double-Outlet Right Ventricle {S,L,L}

This condition is characterized by discordant atrioventricular connection (L–ventricular loop) and discordant ventriculoarterial connection with anterior and left-sided aorta (L-aorta) (Fig. 40–8). The morphologic right atrium receives the systemic venous blood and is connected to the morphologic left ventricle through a right-sided mitral valve, and the morphologic left ventricle supports the pulmonary artery. The morphologic left atrium is connected with a left-sided morphologic right ventricle through a left-sided tricuspid valve, and the aorta (supported by a muscular infundibulum) originates from the left-sided morphologic right ventricle. In double-outlet right ventricle with L-loop of the ventricles (atrioventricular discordance), both great arteries arise from the left-sided morphologic right ventricle.

Dextrocardia is associated in about 40% of patients with corrected transposition in situs solitus.[7] The frequently associated anomalies are, singly or in combination, ventricular septal defect, pulmonary outflow tract stenosis, Ebstein-like deformity of the left (tricuspid) atrioventricular valve, double outlet from the morphologic right ventricle (Fig. 40–9), and complete atrioventricular block. Corrected transposition of the great arteries in situs solitus is the most common condition in one pathologic series of dextrocardia.[37] The degree of pivoting of the ventricular septum[7] that is shown by its orientation varies, depending on the presence of dextrocardia or levocardia. In {S,L,L} and dextrocardia, the ventricular septum is oriented in a plane between the coronal and sagittal plane, whereas in levocardia, it is oriented in the sagittal plane. There is no evidence that the associated anomalies of corrected transposition of the great arteries (see Chapter 27) have a different prevalence in dextrocardia or levocardia.

Dextrocardia With L–Ventricular Loop and Inverted Related Great Arteries {S,L,I}

In hearts with situs solitus, atrioventricular discordance and ventriculoarterial concordance, and inverted related great arteries, dextrocardia is common.[37] This rare condition is associated with conotruncal anomalies, often tetralogy of Fallot. Atresia of the right superior vena cava with left superior vena cava connecting to the coronary sinus is

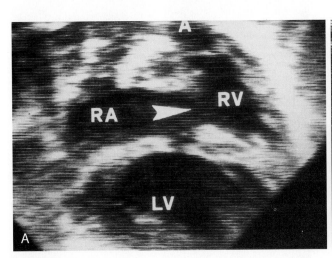
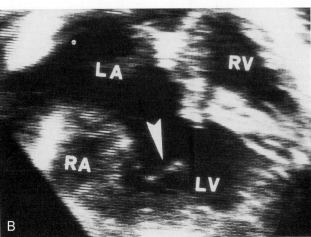

FIGURE 40–7

Two-dimensional echocardiography in an {S,D,L} crisscross heart. *A,* The right atrium (RA) is connected (*arrowhead*) with the left-sided right ventricle (RV), which is anterosuperior and gives rise to the aorta (A). Note the horizontal position of the interventricular septum and the superoinferior position of the ventricles. The right ventricle is hypoplastic. *B,* In a more posterior plane with respect to *A,* the left atrium (LA) is connected (*arrowhead*) with the right-sided left ventricle (LV). Note the inferior position of the left ventricle compared with the right ventricle. (*A, B* from Marino B, Thiene G: Anatomia Ecocardiografia delle Cardiopatie Congenite. Florence, Italy, USES Edizioni Scientifiche, 1990, pp 72–73.)

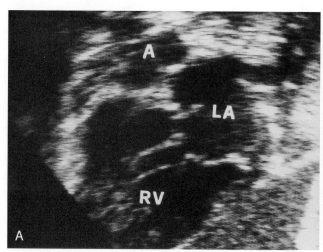

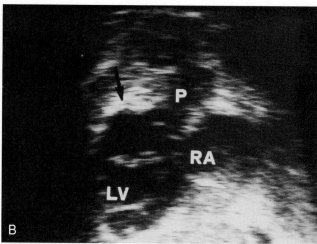

FIGURE 40–8

A, Two-dimensional echocardiography in a patient with {S,L,L}, corrected transposition of great arteries, and dextrocardia. The left atrium (LA) is connected with the left-sided morphologic right ventricle (RV), which gives rise to the aorta (A) supported by a muscular infundibulum. *B,* The right atrium (RA) is connected with the right-sided morphologic left ventricle (LV), which gives rise to the pulmonary artery (P). The *arrow* indicates the left ventricular outflow tract. (*A, B* from Marino B, Thiene G: Anatomia Ecocardiografia delle Cardiopatie Congenite. Florence, Italy, USES Edizioni Scientifiche, 1990, p 60.)

reported in the series of Pasquini and colleagues[49] and has been found in our experience.

CARDIAC MALPOSITION WITH SITUS INVERSUS

Situs inversus with atrioventricular concordance (L–ventricular loop) shows dextrocardia as a frequent feature (Fig. 40–10). As already stated, the cardiac position in the thorax is a function of the ventricular loop and the degree of pivoting. An L–ventricular loop, normal in situs inversus, pivots the heart into the right hemithorax. In situs inversus and dextrocardia, there is alignment between the atrial and the ventricular septa, as in situs solitus and D–ventricular loop. Consequently, malposition of the heart in situs inver-

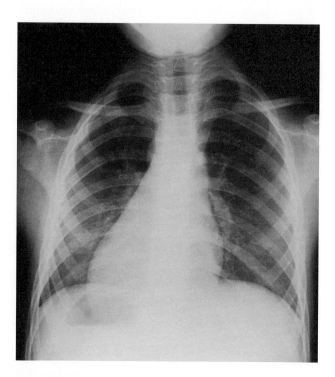

FIGURE 40–9

Left ventricular angiogram in a patient with {S,L,L} and double-outlet right ventricle (RV). The angiogram shows dextrocardia, situs solitus (the catheter is on the right side of the spine and the aorta [A] on the left), atrioventricular discordance (the morphologic left ventricle [LV] is on the right), and double outlet from the left-sided morphologic right ventricle.

FIGURE 40–10

Posteroanterior chest radiograph in a patient with dextrocardia and atrial and visceral situs inversus. The liver shadow is in the left upper quadrant of the abdomen, and the stomach bubble is on the right. The apex of the heart is pointed toward the patient's right.

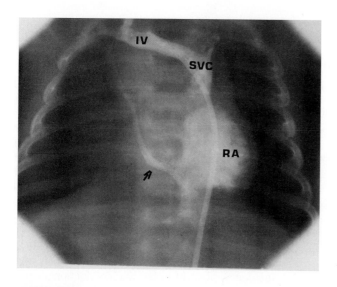

FIGURE 40–11

Angiogram in a patient with situs inversus and levocardia (so-called isolated levocardia). The angiogram demonstrates the innominate vein (IV) and the superior vena cava (SVC) (both on the left) connecting with the left-sided morphologic right atrium (RA). The coronary sinus (*arrow*) drains into the right atrium.

sus should be defined in cases with L–ventricular loop and levocardia.

The expected position of a normal heart in situs inversus, that is, L–ventricular loop and inverted normal related great arteries (also called mirror-image dextrocardia), is in the right thorax. There is no report in the literature of a malposition of such a heart into the left thorax. This condition, situs inversus and levocardia (Fig. 40–11), also called isolated levocardia, is almost always associated with a cardiac malposition. On the other hand, in the chapters about malposition of the heart in situs inversus, they are classically included in the descriptions of the different positions of the heart in the thorax and the patterns of associated defects.[35,36] Thus, we include these conditions, for example, the normal dextrocardia heart in situs inversus, in this chapter, although the fact is they are not truly malpositions.

DEXTROCARDIA

Dextrocardia With L–Ventricular Loop and Inverted Related Great Arteries {I,L,I}

This represents the normal heart in situs inversus. It is characterized by situs inversus (I), L–ventricular loop (L), and inverted, normally related great arteries (I). This condition is not the most common in the pathologic series, but because it might escape clinical detection when there are no associated malformations, its exact incidence is not defined. The commonly associated anomalies are ventricular septal defect, atrial septal defect, tetralogy of Fallot, double-outlet right ventricle, and pulmonary atresia with intact ventricular septum.

KARTAGENER'S SYNDROME. Kartagener first described a group of children and adults with situs inversus, chronic sinusitis, and airway disease.[50] This triad of symptoms with familial occurrence, known as Kartagener's syn-

drome, appears to be primarily due to ciliary dyskinesia. Subsequent clinical studies indicated that infertility was present in males as a result of sperm tail motility disorders.[51] Ciliary action is important in the embryogenesis, probably being a determinant of the situs. Abnormal ciliary motility has been found in patients with left isomerism.[52] In conclusion, in primary ciliary dyskinesia, situs is random, so that individuals with this inheritable condition may have situs inversus (Kartagener's syndrome), situs solitus, or situs ambiguus. Patients with a cardiac anomaly can undergo cardiac surgery successfully.

Dextrocardia With L–Ventricular Loop and Transposition of the Great Arteries {I,L,L}

Associated cardiac anomalies are frequent in this condition and include ventricular septal defect, hypoplastic left ventricle, and pulmonary stenosis with intact ventricular septum.

Dextrocardia With D–Ventricular Loop and Transposition of the Great Arteries {I,D,D}

This is homologous with corrected transposition in situs solitus {S,L,L}. It occurs in about 5 to 8% of all patients with corrected transposition.[53,54] The segmental description of this anomaly is {I,D,D} and consists of situs inversus (I), atrioventricular discordance (ventricular D-loop), and ventriculoarterial discordance (D-transposition of the great arteries). The combination of atrioventricular and ventriculoarterial discordance allows a physiologic circulation pattern. In about 70% of patients, the heart is anomalously in the right thorax; in the remaining 30%, the position of the heart is either mesocardia or levocardia. Corrected transposition in situs inversus is associated with ventricular septal defect in 60 to 100% of patients[53,55,56] and with subvalvar and valvar pulmonary stenosis or pulmonary atresia in 70 to 100% of patients.[53,55,56] The incidence of either spontaneous or operatively related atrioventricular block appears less common than in patients with corrected transposition in situs solitus[57]; this may be due to the more usual location of the conduction tissue in these patients.

DIAGNOSTIC FEATURES OF MALPOSITION OF THE HEART IN SITUS SOLITUS AND INVERSUS

On clinical inspection, the right and left hemithoraces should show symmetric excursion in both levocardia and dextrocardia. A reduced excursion of the right hemithorax may be evident in patients with dextroversion due to right lung hypoplasia, as in scimitar syndrome, or in patients with diaphragmatic hernia; in these, on percussion, reduced movement of the right hemidiaphragm is noted.

The thoracic radiograph is characteristic in determining the position of the heart in the thorax and situs. The apex of the heart points downward and to the left in the normal heart of levocardia, downward and to the right in dextrocardia (see Figs. 40–1, 40–2, and 40–10). In dextroversion, the heart is in the right hemithorax but with the apex pointing toward the left; in this circumstance, there is usually an evident cause of dextroversion, for example, left pneumothorax or diaphragmatic hernia. The situs can usually be determined, considering the position of the abdominal viscera. There are few exceptions corresponding with atrial situs; that is, the anatomic right atrium is almost always on the same side as the main liver mass. The best radiologic guide to abdominal visceral situs is the gastric air bubble. Intrathoracic situs that closely corresponds to atrial situs may be determined by the main bronchial morphology, often evident on the standard or overpenetrated chest radiographs.

The electrocardiogram in many patients allows determination of the situs and the position of the heart in the thorax. The P wave represents the atrial activation. In situs solitus, the mean P wave vector in the frontal plane is approximately +60. It is directed away from the sinus node located in the high right atrium. This results in a positive P wave in leads I, II, and aVF and a negative P wave in lead aVR. In situs inversus, the mean vector of the atrial activation on the frontal plane is +120, because the sinus node in the anatomic right atrium is on the patient's left. The P wave on the horizontal plane proceeds posteroanteriorly in both types of situs but is toward the left (solitus) or right (inversus).

Echocardiography is the best tool for recognizing the cardiac situs and cardiac anatomy. The abdominal aorta and the inferior vena caval relationship, cardiac chamber morphology, and their orientation in space or connections are easily recognizable by echocardiography, allowing a precise identification of the situs, atria, ventricular loop, and great artery relationship.

Cardiac catheterization and angiocardiography are now indicated in the preoperative physiologic assessment and in the evaluation of some anatomic details, such as the anatomy of the branch pulmonary arteries, the coronary artery circulation, or the anatomy of the venae cavae. Intracardiac anatomy is usually better assessed by two-dimensional echocardiography.

SURGICAL TREATMENT

A variety of cardiac lesions can exist in a malpositioned heart. To describe an operative classification of such abnormalities, one can roughly separate hearts amenable to univentricular palliation from those treatable with biventricular repair. Among the latter group, biventricular hearts with atrioventricular and ventriculoarterial concordance or with either ventriculoarterial or double (atrioventricular and ventriculoarterial) discordance constitute the most common anatomic arrangements.

Atrioventricular with ventriculoarterial concordance is usually associated with a D–ventricular loop. A wide variety of cardiac lesions amenable to total repair can coexist, such as isolated atrial septal defect or ventricular septal defect, atrioventricular septal defect, and tetralogy of Fallot.

With anomalies of ventriculoarterial connection associated with ventricular septal defect and balanced ventricles, a biventricular repair can usually be carried out with an intraventricular repair,[58,59] a Rastelli-type procedure[60] or the REV (Reparation Etage Ventriculaire) procedure,[61] or an arterial switch procedure (with the construction of a left ventricle–to–pulmonary orifice tunnel).[58,59]

With combined atrioventricular and ventriculoarterial discordance and balanced ventricles, double-switch procedures can provide anatomic repair of the condition.

Double discordance with left ventricular outflow tract obstruction (pulmonary or subpulmonary stenosis) can be treated by combined Senning-Mustard and Rastelli procedures,[62,63] whereas patients with unrestricted pulmonary blood flow are best treated by combined atrial and arterial switch, provided there is an adequate preoperative left ventricular pressure.[64–66] Double-switch procedures are usually feasible, irrespective of the cardiac malposition or atrial situs; however, because of the posterior location of the atria and the small amount of lateral free atrial wall, if there is apicocaval juxtaposition, the atrial switch is best achieved with a Mustard procedure, using some additional material for augmentation of the atrial volume.[65] With specific reference to abnormalities of the atrial situs, double-switch procedures in patients with situs inversus have been described as more advantageous because of the D-loop arrangements of double discordance in situs inversus with a lower incidence of atrioventricular conduction disturbances compared with L-loop arrangement of hearts in situs solitus.[63]

Isolated ventriculoarterial or, sporadically, atrioventricular discordance can occur in malpositioned hearts. Arterial switch and atrial switch constitute the procedures of choice for such anatomic arrangements.

Scattered reports have also suggested biventricular repair for crisscross heart,[67] a form of positional abnormality of the ventricles often associated with dextrocardia. A right ventricular volume greater than 45% of normal and absence of straddling atrioventricular valves constitute the main requirements for a biventricular repair of crisscross heart,[68] even though the possible recourse to a pulsatile bidirectional cavopulmonary anastomosis has expanded the spectrum of cardiac lesions with right ventricular hypoplasia amenable to biventricular repair (i.e., one-and-a-half ventricle repair).[69]

CARDIAC MALPOSITION WITH SITUS AMBIGUUS

Heterotaxia is one of the most intriguing mysteries in pediatric cardiovascular medicine. The prevalence of this syndrome was estimated to be 1 per 22,000 to 24,000, accounting for 1 to 3% of cardiac malformations[70–72] and for 30% of patients dying with cardiac malposition.[73] Asplenia/right isomerism is more common in males, whereas polysplenia/left isomerism has an equal sex ratio.[23] These syndromes are usually sporadic, but there are several familial occurrences,[14,74] in particular to children born of consanguineous parents. In some instances, there are in the same family heterogeneous laterality defects including situs inversus, asplenia, and polysplenia.[74]

PATHOLOGIC ANATOMY

There are extracardiac and cardiac anomalies common to both asplenia/right isomerism and polysplenia/left isomerism syndromes, but there are particular differences between these two conditions.

1. The abdominal organs are abnormal in shape and position. The liver tends to be symmetric and to occupy a

transverse position across the upper abdomen,[75] and abnormalities of the biliary tract may be found. The gallbladder may be absent or hypoplastic. Malrotation of the bowel and of the midgut loop is present[24] and may cause intestinal obstruction.[21] Adrenal and genitourinary tract anomalies have been described.[23]

Extrahepatic biliary atresia leading to obstructive jaundice[76] has been found in polysplenia/left isomerism. The spleen is absent in asplenia/right isomerism and multiple in polysplenia/left isomerism.

2. The thoracic organs tend to be symmetric.[21–24] In patients with asplenia/right isomerism, there are trilobed bilateral eparterial bronchi; in each lung, the pulmonary artery courses anterior to the main stem bronchus.[23] In patients with polysplenia/left isomerism, there are bilateral bilobed lungs and hyparterial bronchi. In each lung, the pulmonary artery courses over and behind the main stem bronchus.[21] Pulmonary arteriovenous fistulae have been reported in patients with polysplenia/left isomerism.[77] In about 40% of children with asplenia/right isomerism and with polysplenia/left isomerism, cardiac malpositions including mesocardia and dextrocardia are present.

3. Systemic venous connections are frequently anomalous.[21, 23, 78, 79] In more than half of patients with heterotaxia, bilateral superior venae cavae connect to the superior and posterior portion of the respective atria. In these patients, the innominate vein is absent. If a single superior vena cava is present, it is usually opposite to the cardiac apex. In most patients, the coronary sinus is absent.

In patients with asplenia/right isomerism, the inferior vena cava and the abdominal aorta are ipsilateral. They lie together on the right or left side of the spine (Fig. 40–12). The inferior vena cava connects with the right or left side of the atria. In a few of these patients, the hepatic veins connect with the atria separately from the inferior vena

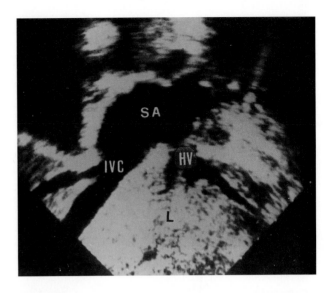

FIGURE 40–13

Two-dimensional echocardiography in subcostal view in a patient with asplenia/right isomerism shows the hepatic veins (HV) connected with the single atrium (SA) separately from the inferior vena cava (IVC). L = liver. (From Marino B, Thiene G: Anatomia Ecocardiografia delle Cardiopatie Congenite. Florence, Italy, USES Edizioni Scientifiche, 1990, p 48.)

cava (Fig. 40–13). Interrupted inferior vena cava is extremely rare in patients with asplenia/right isomerism.

In more than 70% of patients with polysplenia/left isomerism, the infrahepatic portion of the inferior vena cava is interrupted. It connects into the azygos vein and terminates in either the left or right superior vena cava. The hepatic veins connect directly to the left or right side of the floor of the atria. In a few patients, a small inferior vena cava persists on one side of the abdomen connecting to the atria, and an enlarged azygos vein connects to a superior vena cava on the opposite side. In other patients, the inferior vena cava ascends on one side of the abdomen and crosses to the opposite side at the level of the diaphragm to enter the azygos vein.

4. Pulmonary venous connections are often anomalous.[20–23, 29, 31, 78–81] In more than 80% of patients with asplenia/right isomerism, total anomalous pulmonary venous connection is present; in nearly half of these, it is obstructed. The anomalous pulmonary venous connection may be to either a supracardiac or an infradiaphragmatic location.[29–31]

In children with polysplenia/left isomerism, the pulmonary venous connection is into the atria, and an extracardiac total anomalous pulmonary venous connection virtually does not occur. In approximately 40% of these patients, the pulmonary veins from each lung enter the posterior wall of the atria separately on opposite sides of the midline, simulating a partial anomalous pulmonary venous connection.[81]

5. Anomalies at atrial level and of the atrioventricular valves are frequent.[20–23, 29, 31, 78–81] A common atrium with virtually absent atrial septum is present in asplenia/right isomerism. There is usually a narrow band, a remnant of the atrial septum, passing in an anteroposterior direction and crossing the midportion of the atria (Fig. 40–14). Each

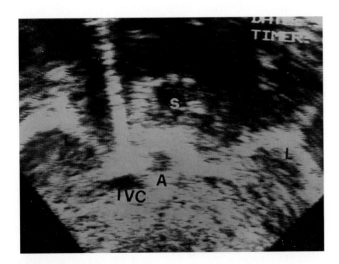

FIGURE 40–12

Two-dimensional echocardiography in abdominal short-axis view in a patient with asplenia/right isomerism. Note the ipsilateral position of the aorta (A) and of the inferior vena cava (IVC) lying together on the right side of the spine (S). The liver (L) presents a symmetric transverse position. (From Marino B, Thiene G: Anatomia Ecocardiografia delle Cardiopatie Congenite. Florence, Italy, USES Edizioni Scientifiche, 1990, p 47.)

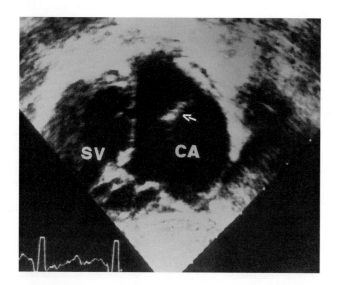

Two-dimensional echocardiography in subcostal view in a patient with asplenia/right isomerism and dextrocardia. In the common atrium (CA), a narrow band (*arrow*) crosses the midportion of the atria. SV = single ventricle. (From Marino B, Thiene G: Anatomia Ecocardiografia delle Cardiopatie Congenite. Florence, Italy, USES Edizioni Scientifiche, 1990, p 49.)

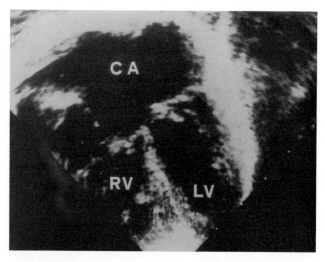

Two-dimensional echocardiography in subcostal four-chamber view in a patient with polysplenia/left isomerism shows common atrium (CA) with biventricular heart, D-loop of the ventricles, and intact ventricular septum. RV = right ventricle; LV = left ventricle. (From Marino B, Thiene G: Anatomia Ecocardiografia delle Cardiopatie Congenite. Florence, Italy, USES Edizioni Scientifiche, 1990, p 69.)

atrial appendage shows a broad-based pyramidal morphology (right isomerism). In children with asplenia/right isomerism, the complete form of atrioventricular septal defect is the rule, with a common atrioventricular valve. The morphology of the common atrioventricular valve in asplenia/right isomerism is different from the one observed in complete atrioventricular canal with situs solitus. In patients with asplenia/right isomerism, the common atrioventricular valve is rudimentary, showing a reduced number of leaflets and papillary muscles, and these muscles appear short and hypoplastic.[82]

A common atrium is also present in patients with polysplenia/left isomerism (Fig. 40–15), but the more frequent atrial pattern in this syndrome is a large ostium primum defect with a partial atrioventricular canal and a cleft of the mitral valve. Malposition of the atrial septum is also frequent in these patients. The septum primum may be displaced either leftward or rightward, depending on whether there is levocardia or dextrocardia, respectively. This displacement is responsible for the apparent partial anomalous pulmonary venous connection.[21, 81] Each atrial appendage is long and narrow, showing the features of a left appendage (left isomerism). This atrial anatomy is similar to that observed in patients with Ellis–van Creveld syndrome.[83]

6. Anomalies at ventricular level are also frequent.° An L-loop of the ventricles occurs in approximately 40% of patients with both asplenia/right isomerism and polysplenia/left isomerism.

A single ventricle of right ventricular type due to malalignment of the atrioventricular canal with a hypoplas-

tic left ventricle is the more frequent pattern at the ventricular level in children with asplenia/right isomerism, but a single left ventricle and a biventricular heart are also represented. Ventricular septal defect is constant in these children.

On the contrary, in patients with polysplenia/left isomerism, a single ventricle is less frequent and the biventricular heart (with D- or L-loop ventricle) is the more common pattern with intact ventricular septum in 20 to 30% (Fig. 40–15).

7. Conotruncal defects and anomalies of the great arteries are usual.° The classic conotruncal pattern in patients with asplenia/right isomerism, which occurs in more than 80% of patients, is double-outlet right ventricle with the aorta in the anterior position surrounded by muscular infundibulum, pulmonary stenosis or atresia, and hypoplasia of the infundibular septum. Transposition of great arteries is also present. The normal relations and alignment of the great arteries are rare. In infants and children with asplenia/right isomerism and pulmonary atresia, there is a prevalence of confluent pulmonary arteries with ductus-dependent pulmonary circulation, sometimes with bilateral ductus arteriosus (Fig. 40–16).[86–88] Moreover, a correlation has been noted between atresia of the pulmonary valve and obstruction of the pulmonary venous connection.[29, 80, 84]

On the contrary, in more than 70% of children with polysplenia/left isomerism, concordant ventriculoarterial connection is present.[79, 85] The great arteries are normally related in patients with D-loop ventricles, or inversely normally related (mirror image) in patients with L-loop ventricles.[85] Double-outlet right ventricle is also present with in-

---

°References 20–23, 29, 31, 78–81, 84, 85.

°References 20–23, 29, 31, 78–81, 84–88.

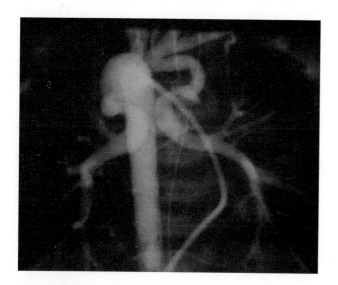

FIGURE 40-16

Angiocardiography with injection into the aorta in a patient with asplenia/right isomerism and pulmonary atresia. Bilateral ductus arteriosus supplies the right and left pulmonary arteries.

fundibular morphology of tetralogy of Fallot, whereas transposition of great arteries is rare. Obstruction of the pulmonary blood flow is present in approximately 30%; one third have pulmonary atresia. Systemic outflow tract obstructions including mitral stenosis, hypoplastic left ventricle, aortic stenosis, and coarctation are present in 25%.

In summary, in patients with asplenia/right isomerism, the cardiac malformations are complex because of an early embryologic abnormality. The classic anatomy includes transverse liver; bilateral trilobed lungs and eparterial bronchi; levocardia, mesocardia, or dextrocardia; bilateral superior venae cavae with absent coronary sinus; inferior vena cava coursing with the abdominal aorta on the same side of the spine connecting to the atria; extracardiac total anomalous venous connection (frequently obstructed); common atrium; right bilateral morphology of the atrial appendages; complete atrioventricular canal malaligned to a dominant right ventricle; D- or L-loop ventricle; double-outlet right ventricle with anterior aorta; and pulmonary stenosis or atresia.

In patients with polysplenia/left isomerism, the pattern of cardiac anomalies is less rudimentary, and they are less complex. The usual morphology includes transverse liver; bilateral bilobed lungs and hyparterial bronchi; levocardia, mesocardia, or dextrocardia; bilateral superior venae cavae; interruption of inferior vena cava with azygos continuation; pulmonary veins draining into the right and left posterior sides of the atria; common atrium or large ostium primum atrial septal defect; left bilateral morphology of the atrial appendages; partial atrioventricular canal; D- or L-loop ventricles with balanced ventricular masses; concordant ventriculoarterial connection; ventricular septal defect (frequent); pulmonary stenosis (possible); and systemic outflow tract obstruction (possible).

Some crossover exists, however, with individuals presenting anatomic patterns of asplenia/right isomerism in the presence of polysplenia/left isomerism, and vice versa.

Moreover, the heart may be completely normal in patients with polysplenia/left isomerism and, exceptionally, in patients with asplenia/right isomerism. An interesting subgroup of patients shows a hypoplastic or rudimentary spleen with many of the features of asplenia/right isomerism but sometimes presenting systemic obstruction.[33]

CLINICAL FEATURES AND DIAGNOSTIC APPROACH

Asplenia/Right Isomerism

The most frequent presentation is in a male neonate with intense cyanosis, respiratory distress, and systolic murmur or no murmur. A right-sided apical impulse, the heart sounds and murmur heard better over the right hemithorax, and the transverse lower hepatic margin are characteristic of this syndrome.

The electrocardiogram is generally abnormal. The P wave axis is directed inferiorly and to the right (90 to 105 degrees) in patients with levocardia and to the left (75 to 90 degrees) in those with dextrocardia.[89] The frontal plane QRS axis is usually directed superiorly because of atrioventricular septal defect.

Clues to the diagnosis of asplenia/right isomerism are often present on the thoracic radiograph, which shows cardiac malposition frequently with mesocardia or dextrocardia and with the cardiac apex discordant with the position of the liver and the stomach. The lower hepatic margin lies horizontally across the upper abdomen, the cardiac size is normal, and either the pulmonary vascular markings are diminished owing to pulmonary stenosis or atresia (Fig. 40–17) or there are signs of pulmonary edema in patients with obstruction of the pulmonary venous connection (Fig. 40–18). Moreover, by use of tomography or the high-

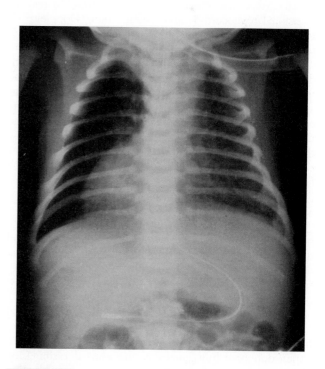

FIGURE 40-17

Chest radiograph in a patient with asplenia/right isomerism shows symmetric liver, dextrocardia, and reduced pulmonary blood flow.

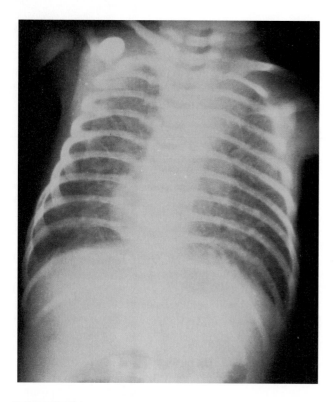

FIGURE 40–18

Chest radiograph in a patient with asplenia/right isomerism shows symmetric liver and mesocardia.

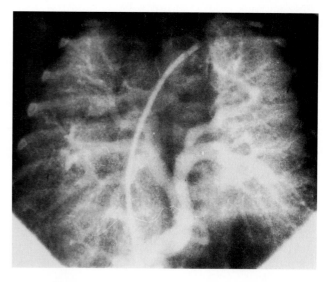

FIGURE 40–19

Angiocardiography in a patient with asplenia/right isomerism shows an obstructed total anomalous pulmonary venous connection. All pulmonary veins empty into an anomalous venous channel that descends below the diaphragm to join the portal vein.

kilovoltage radiographs, it is possible to visualize the bilateral eparterial bronchial position.[90,91]

The precise diagnosis of this syndrome and of the associated cardiac malformation can be established by two-dimensional echocardiography with color Doppler.[92–96] With the short-axis subcostal view, it is possible to visualize the abdominal aorta and the inferior vena cava lying on the same side of the spine (see Fig. 40–13); with a long-axis abdominal cut with the aid of color Doppler, the infracardiac total anomalous pulmonary venous connection can be imaged.[97] Furthermore, two-dimensional echocardiography can directly detect the agenesis of the spleen,[98] but isomerism of the atrial appendages is difficult to diagnose by this method. Common atrium, complete atrioventricular canal,[95] and single ventricle[94] are well imaged with echocardiography (see Fig. 40–14), and the other details of intracardiac anatomy, including the conotruncal morphology, can be defined.

A cardiac malposition (dextrocardia or mesocardia) or horizontal liver on the chest radiograph (heterotaxia) and the echocardiographic recognition of common atrium, complete atrioventricular canal, single ventricle with anterior aorta, and pulmonary stenosis or atresia are the most precise diagnostic signs of asplenia/right isomerism.

The introduction of cine magnetic resonance imaging seems to improve the morphologic diagnosis in these patients.[99] However, because of anatomic complexity and to obtain definitive functional data including determination of pulmonary vascular resistance, preoperative evaluation by means of cardiac catheterization and angiocardiography is still indicated in many of these children.[80] On angiocar-

diography, the aorta and inferior vena cava lie together on the same side of the spine, and this technique is particularly useful to document the anatomy of pulmonary arteries and the pulmonary blood supply in patients with pulmonary atresia.[86,88,100] Moreover, angiocardiography reveals the site of pulmonary venous connection and the presence of pulmonary venous obstruction (Fig. 40–19) although it is masked by the pulmonary stenosis or atresia. Furthermore, angiocardiography in association with color Doppler echocardiography can quantify the degree of atrioventricular valve regurgitation that in neonates, but in particular in older children, can deeply influence the natural history of these patients.[101–103]

Polysplenia/Left Isomerism

The clinical manifestations of these patients are variable and usually appear later compared with those of children with asplenia/right isomerism because the pulmonary obstruction is less severe and the pulmonary veins are not obstructed. Cyanosis is present only in children with pulmonic stenosis or atresia, and most patients show various degrees of congestive heart failure due to left-to-right shunts. Other patients may be asymptomatic.

The electrocardiographic observations in polysplenia/left isomerism demonstrate similar but distinctive findings in respect to asplenia/right isomerism. Because the sinus node is a right atrial structure, hearts with polysplenia/left isomerism are usually characterized by an absent, displaced, or hypoplastic sinus node.[104] A leftward and superiorly directed P wave axis and ectopic atrial rhythm are frequently present.[89] Even the QRS axis is superiorly directed because of the atrioventricular canal. Congenital complete atrioventricular block is occasionally present.[105]

Thoracic radiographs may suggest this syndrome, showing dextrocardia or mesocardia with discordance between the position of the heart and that of the liver and the stomach. Moreover, the absence of an inferior vena caval shadow on the lateral view and the enlargement of the azygos vein consistent with a round density along the upper left or right cardiac border suggest polysplenia/left isomerism.[106] High-kilovoltage chest radiographs may show the symmetric bronchial branching pattern characteristic of left pulmonary isomerism.[90, 91]

Echocardiography is the best tool for the noninvasive diagnosis of intracardiac malformations. Interruption of the inferior vena cava with azygos continuation and the pattern of pulmonary venous connection can be identified,[92, 93] as can the atrial, ventricular, and great artery malformations.[85]

A cardiac malposition (dextrocardia or mesocardia) or horizontal liver on the chest radiograph and the echocardiographic recognition of azygos continuation, partial atrioventricular septal defect, biventricular heart or single ventricle, and normally aligned great arteries (concordant ventriculoarterial connections) are the best diagnostic signs of polysplenia/left isomerism.

Fetal echocardiography can reliably detect heterotaxia.[107] Some authors have demonstrated that the spectrum of fetal cardiac defect in polysplenia/left isomerism seems to be more complex than previously shown in postnatal life.[108] Moreover, echocardiography can identify the presence of multiple spleens.[98]

Cardiac catheterization and angiocardiography are often required for the definitive preoperative anatomic and functional assessment of these patients. Interruption of the inferior vena cava often requires a percutaneous approach from the neck to reach the heart directly and avoid the catheter loop in the azygos vein and superior vena cava.[109] Angiocardiography on a lateral view of a pulmonary arteriogram can demonstrate the superimposed branches of the pulmonary arteries arching posteriorly from the pulmonary trunk, because each has the characteristics of a left pulmonary artery.[110]

NATURAL HISTORY

Asplenia/Right Isomerism

The natural history of asplenia/right isomerism is extremely poor. Mortality has been reported to occur in more than one third of untreated neonates in the first week of life[111] and up to 85% of patients during the first year of life.[22] Hypoxemia related to cardiovascular abnormalities is the predominant cause of death, followed by sepsis due to the increased susceptibility to infections when the spleen is absent.[23, 112]

Polysplenia/Left Isomerism

The natural history of polysplenia/left isomerism has been associated with a 65% mortality rate within the first year of life.[79] Associated cardiac abnormalities constitute the main cause of death, followed by rhythm disturbances[105] and extrahepatic biliary atresia.[113, 114]

MEDICAL MANAGEMENT

Asplenia/Right Isomerism

Patients with asplenia/right isomerism usually develop severe cyanosis with hypoxemia and metabolic acidosis during the first hours after birth. The severe illness of such neonates is almost certainly related to either pulmonary inflow (pulmonary stenosis or atresia) or outflow obstruction (obstructed total anomalous pulmonary venous connection).

Early prostaglandin therapy may improve the oxygen saturation as long as the pulmonary venous system is not obstructed. Otherwise, prostaglandin therapy can either unmask or increase the degree of pulmonary venous obstruction by increasing the total pulmonary blood flow.[101, 115, 116] Patients with infracardiac pulmonary venous connection should be operated on without delay. In the remaining neonates, the degree of pulmonary venous obstruction should be carefully evaluated under prostaglandin infusion[116] to provide the best indication for operation.

Because of the susceptibility to infection of asplenia/right isomerism patients,[112] aggressive perioperative antibiotic prophylaxis may play an important role. Antibiotic prophylaxis against encapsulated bacteria with penicillin or amoxicillin is indicated as a daily requirement. Immunization against pneumococcus is indicated at age 2 years.

Polysplenia/Left Isomerism

Few patients with polysplenia/left isomerism develop severe cyanosis soon after birth. These usually have some anatomic features of asplenia/right isomerism and require the same management as those patients. Vice versa, neonates with polysplenia/left isomerism can become severely symptomatic soon after birth with congestive heart failure and metabolic acidosis because of pulmonary overcirculation associated with systemic obstruction. In most of such patients, severe aortic stenosis or hypoplastic left heart syndrome occurs. Those patients should be managed according to the general criteria for the treatment of hypoplastic left heart syndrome.[117, 118] Rarely, a complete atrioventricular block constitutes the main cause for neonatal symptomatic presentation of polysplenia/left isomerism.[105]

Most patients with polysplenia/left isomerism become symptomatic some months after birth. Clinical manifestations differ according to the underlying lesions. Cyanosis is usually related to pulmonary outflow tract obstruction, even though it has occasionally been associated with pulmonary arteriovenous fistulae occurring early in the natural history.[77] On the other hand, heart failure is usually related to complete atrioventricular septal defect or isolated ventricular septal defect. Patients with common atrium or partial atrioventricular septal defect usually become symptomatic later in life, often in association with cardiac rhythm disturbances.[119, 120]

OPERATIVE TREATMENT

Initial Palliation

ASPLENIA/RIGHT ISOMERISM

The most important goal of the operative treatment of these ill and delicate neonates is palliation to make the patient survive. Indeed, even though extensive palliation with use of cardiopulmonary bypass has been reported as not increasing operative mortality,[121] there is agreement concerning the poor results of complex neonatal approaches to this condition.[110, 111]

As far as neonatal survival is concerned, whenever possible, simple palliation with a reliable, controlled pulmonary blood supply by means of a prosthetic shunt appears to be the best approach to improve the eventual outcome. This can be done only to patients with confluent pulmonary arteries, without juxtaductal pulmonary stenosis, and with unobstructed pulmonary venous connection. In all other neonates, a more extensive palliation with cardiopulmonary bypass must be performed. The choice of a small shunt, even though potentially disadvantageous in terms of early recurrence of cyanosis, carries the advantage of keeping the Qp/Qs ratio within an acceptable range, with beneficial effects on the pulmonary venous connection (inability to unmask potentially obstructive pulmonary venous connections) and on the common atrioventricular valve function.

A complex operative approach to patients with asplenia/right isomerism presenting after the first month of life carries a better chance of survival than does the same type of palliation performed in the neonatal period.[111] Indeed, the goal of the minimal palliation in the neonatal period should be to delay a more extensive approach to the disease (i.e., correction of total anomalous pulmonary venous connection). An early bidirectional cavopulmonary anastomosis[122,123] can replace the systemic-pulmonary shunt as a source of pulmonary blood flow, with beneficial effects on ventricular function and on the atrioventricular valve competence by reducing the volume load to the heart.

On the other hand, if obstructed pulmonary venous connection coexists, neonatal palliation by repair of total anomalous pulmonary venous connection associated with a systemic-pulmonary shunt is mandatory. The need of a concomitant shunt in obstructed total anomalous pulmonary venous connection can initially be underestimated in patients with patent, even though stenotic, pulmonary inflow.

Because the combination of potentially abnormal pulmonary inflow and outflow makes the assessment of pulmonary blood flow unreliable,[102] whenever neonatal repair of obstructed total anomalous pulmonary venous connection is carried out, a concomitant systemic-pulmonary shunt should always be performed to ensure an adequate pulmonary blood supply.[121]

POLYSPLENIA/LEFT ISOMERISM

Patients with early presentation of symptoms usually require an operation with a systemic-pulmonary shunt (pulmonary obstruction), a Norwood-type procedure (hypoplastic left heart syndrome), or a pulmonary artery banding (complete atrioventricular septal defect).

Early palliation, usually advisable in patients with single-ventricle physiology, is frequently required also in patients with two ventricles because of anomalies of systemic and pulmonary venous connection that make atrial partition difficult in small children.

Biventricular Repair

ASPLENIA/RIGHT ISOMERISM

Sporadic examples of biventricular atrioventricular connection can be amenable to complex biventricular repair. Common atrium, balanced complete atrioventricular sep-

tal defect, double-outlet right ventricle, pulmonary stenosis, and total anomalous pulmonary venous connection constitute the usual anatomy of patients treated with biventricular repair described in the literature.[124–126]

POLYSPLENIA/LEFT ISOMERISM

In contrast to asplenia/right isomerism, biventricular atrioventricular connection has been reported to be present in up to 72% of patients with polysplenia/left isomerism, with two separate atrioventricular valves in 43%.[126] Not all of those patients were amenable to biventricular repair because of abnormalities of atrioventricular concordance or systemic and pulmonary venous connections. However, biventricular repair has been reported in up to 30% of patients with polysplenia/left isomerism.[127] The main requirements to achieve a biventricular repair are balanced ventricles and concordant ventriculoarterial connection.[127,128]

In these patients, the operative procedure consists mainly of atrial septation associated with septation of a common atrioventricular valve and ventricular septal closure (complete atrioventricular septal defect), suture of a mitral cleft (partial atrioventricular septal defect), and right ventricular outflow tract reconstruction or ventricular septal defect closure (tetralogy-type double-outlet right ventricle, ventricular septal defect), depending on the coexistent conditions. Atrial septation may require partition with a straight patch, when systemic and pulmonary veins connect into either side of the atrium independently; intra-atrial rerouting with a tailored baffle, to separate the pulmonary veins from systemic veins; or atrial switch, when the pulmonary veins connect into the functional right atrium or more than two systemic veins connect into the functional left atrium.[126] Because of the high incidence of cardiac rhythm disturbances with progressive slowing of the atrial rhythm and occasional occurrence of atrioventricular block,[119,120] the implantation of a permanent pacing device at the time of operation should be preoperatively evaluated by careful Holter monitoring or electrophysiologic study.

Staging Toward Single-Ventricle Repair

ASPLENIA/RIGHT ISOMERISM

Most patients with asplenia/right isomerism undergo staging toward a modified Fontan operation. Key requirements for the staging include an unobstructed pulmonary venous connection into the common atrium and a reduced volume load to the heart, which is achievable both by providing pulmonary blood flow through a bidirectional cavopulmonary anastomosis and by adequate competence of the common atrioventricular valve. There is some controversy concerning the role of the bidirectional cavopulmonary anastomosis in reducing the regurgitation of a common atrioventricular valve.[122]

Right univentricular hearts gain little muscle mass after systemic-pulmonary shunt, compared with left ventricular hearts. Consequently, regurgitation of the common atrioventricular valve in a right univentricular heart, most commonly associated with asplenia/right isomerism, occurs more frequently and earlier.[129] Under such circumstances, the reduction of volume load to the heart is unlikely to improve the competence of a moderately to severely regurgitant common atrioventricular valve. Moreover, moderate to severe regurgitation of the atrioventricular valve has been postulated to constitute a risk factor for early mortality after a bidirectional cavopulmonary anastomosis.[122] Reports have described encouraging results of valvuloplasty or annuloplasty of incompetent common atrioventricular valves in asplenia/right isomerism associated with bidirectional cavopulmonary anastomosis.[130–132] The double reduction of the volume load to the heart obtained by such a combined procedure may decrease the risk after a bidirectional cavopulmonary anastomosis and improve the candidacy for a subsequent Fontan procedure.

POLYSPLENIA/LEFT ISOMERISM

About 70% of cardiac malformations associated with polysplenia/left isomerism do not fulfill the criteria for biventricular repair and require staging toward a Fontan operation by means of a bidirectional cavopulmonary anastomosis. Because of the high incidence of azygos/hemiazygos continuation in polysplenia/left isomerism, the bidirectional cavopulmonary anastomosis under such circumstances becomes an almost total cavopulmonary anastomosis, with only the hepatic and coronary venous blood draining into the functional left atrium.

Since the first description of the Kawashima operation,[133] great attention has been paid to atrioventricular valve function: 75% of patients who received this procedure underwent concomitant replacement of the incompetent common atrioventricular valve. Preliminary enthusiasm for the Kawashima operation, initially considered a sort of definitive palliation for single ventricles with polysplenia/left isomerism, has diminished in subsequent reports[77,134,135] showing an increased occurrence of pulmonary arteriovenous fistulae in this setting early postoperatively compared with the bidirectional cavopulmonary anastomosis performed in patients without polysplenia/left isomerism. The occurrence of pulmonary arteriovenous fistulae in patients with hepatic disease and their regression after improvement in hepatic function[136] or after hepatic transplantation[137] have led investigators to postulate the existence of a labile hepatic factor that prevents precapillary channels of the pulmonary microcirculation from dilating. The exclusion of the hepatic venous blood from the pulmonary circulation by the Kawashima operation, just like the modified Glenn operation, could explain the occurrence of pulmonary arteriovenous fistulae in these patients.

An increased incidence of pulmonary arteriovenous malformations in patients with azygos/hemiazygos continuation and bidirectional cavopulmonary anastomosis could be related to other factors associated with their development, such as polysplenia/left isomerism per se[77,138] or a lesser extent of bronchial collateral flow[139] related to a higher Qp/Qs ratio compared with bidirectional cavopulmonary anastomosis in the absence of azygos/hemiazygos continuation. Complete regression of pulmonary arteriovenous fistulae developed after the Kawashima operation has been reported when the hepatic veins were connected to the confluent pulmonary arteries with an atrial tunnel.[139] Pulmonary arteriovenous fistulae have also been described as increasing early morbidity and mortality after a modified Fontan operation owing to severe arterial desaturation.[140]

Patients with polysplenia/left isomerism who have undergone a bidirectional cavopulmonary anastomosis should be strictly followed-up to assess the early onset of pulmonary arteriovenous fistulae. Contrast echocardiography, even more than transcutaneous pulse oximetry, has proved to be a sensitive and reliable method of assessment.[141]

Single-Ventricle Repair

ASPLENIA/RIGHT ISOMERISM

The final step in the operative treatment of patients with asplenia/right isomerism and single functional ventricle consists of a modified Fontan procedure.[142] Actually, preliminary reports described an increased mortality after the Fontan operation in patients with asplenia/right isomerism, compared with patients with polysplenia/left isomerism. Initial reasons for the difference were unexplained but definitely not related to infectious or septic causes. A prevalence of right ventricular morphology in right isomerism, especially when associated with anomalous pulmonary venous connection, could explain the increased risk. Furthermore, the Fontan operation in patients with heterotaxia syndrome had a significantly higher risk than in patients without this syndrome.[143]

Reports on survival of patients with heterotaxia syndrome undergoing the Fontan procedure fail to identify asplenia/right isomerism alone as a significant risk factor for higher mortality rate. On the other hand, significantly increased mortality occurs in the groups of patients with moderate or severe atrioventricular valve regurgitation, hypoplastic pulmonary arteries, and mean pulmonary artery pressure of 15 mm Hg or higher after 6 months of age.[103] Current literature shows that early mortality after the Fontan operation for heterotaxia patients has decreased dramatically during the past few years, approaching the results obtained in nonisomeric patients.[144,145] Moreover, in recent experience, early mortality after the Fontan operation is similar in asplenia/right isomerism and polysplenia/left isomerism.[145] Improved selection of patients, younger age at operation, and refinements in operative techniques and postoperative management may have had important roles. Perhaps early ventricular volume unloading associated with aggressive treatment of the atrioventricular valve incompetence during the staging toward the Fontan procedure may preserve the single ventricular function to fulfill the requirements for a subsequent corrective, safe Fontan repair.[122,123,130–132,146] Moreover, recent techniques of total cavopulmonary connection,[147,148] with the possible advantages carried by the fenestration,[149,150] may contribute to further improvement of survival of patients with asplenia/right isomerism.

POLYSPLENIA/LEFT ISOMERISM

Completion of the Fontan repair constitutes the final step of the treatment of many patients with left isomerism and single-ventricle physiology.

The current literature reports decreasing early mortality after the Fontan operation for heterotaxia, with the results being similar for asplenia/right isomerism and polysplenia/left isomerism and approaching those obtained in nonisomeric patients.[144,145] Even for polysplenia/left isomerism, the degree of preoperative atrioventricular valve regurgitation constitutes a significant risk factor for higher mortality rate at the time of the Fontan operation.[103] Accurate evaluation and possible treatment of atrioventricular valve incompetence during staging are mandatory to improve the subsequent candidacy of such patients for the Fontan operation.

Cardiac Transplantation

ASPLENIA/RIGHT ISOMERISM AND POLYSPLENIA/LEFT ISOMERISM

Neonatal cardiac transplantation has been advocated by some as a primary therapy for some forms of complex cardiac anomalies, such as those associated with asplenia/right isomerism.[151,152] Apart from the general shortage of adequate donors for small recipients, there is general agreement to reserve cardiac transplantation for patients with asplenia/right isomerism, either already palliated or not, with uncorrectable atrioventricular valve incompetence associated with severe ventricular dysfunction. From this viewpoint, asplenia/right isomerism does not differ from polysplenia/left isomerism or from other cardiac malformations with single-ventricle physiology.[153]

In the peculiar subset of patients with heterotaxia, a few scattered instances of pediatric cardiac transplantation are reported.[153–157] Generally speaking, operative technique can be made extremely difficult by the position of the heart,[158] the abnormalities of systemic and pulmonary venous connections,[153,156–159] the relationship between the great vessels,[160,161] and the effects of previous palliative procedures on the pulmonary arterial tree and on chest adhesions.[155,157–159]

Early results of pediatric cardiac transplantation for cardiac malformations showed a significantly increased early mortality compared with idiopathic cardiomyopathy[162,163] because of major operative procedure–related complications. Current literature describes increasing proportions of positive results with cardiac transplantation in children with cardiac malformations, despite multiple previous cardiac operations.[153,157,159,164,165]

ECTOPIA CORDIS

CLASSIFICATION

Ectopia cordis represents the partial or complete location of the heart outside the thorax. This extremely rare condition occurs in 5.5 to 7.9 per million live births.[166,167] Kanagasuntheran and Verzin[168] divided ectopia cordis into five types: cervical, thoracocervical, thoracic, thoracoabdominal, and abdominal. The cervical form was found only in malformed fetuses; the abdominal form is extremely rare, with only one patient described. Thus, for practical purposes, only two types of ectopia cordis must be considered: the thoracic and the thoracoabdominal forms.

The thoracic type is the classic form of ectopia cordis. In these patients, there is a cleft of the sternum that allows protrusion of the heart outside the thoracic cavity, absence

of the parietal pericardium, cephalic orientation of the cardiac apex, epigastric omphalocele, diastasis recti, and small thoracic cavity. The thoracoabdominal form is a partial form of ectopia cordis that is characterized by partial absence or cleft of the lower sternum, defect of the parietal diaphragmatic pericardium, midline diaphragmatic defect resulting in a free communication between the pericardium and abdominal cavity, and diastasis recti with partial displacement of the ventricular portion of the heart into the epigastrium. Many types of cardiac malformations are associated with ectopia cordis: tetralogy of Fallot, ventricular septal defect, atrioventricular septal defect, common atrium, tricuspid atresia, pulmonary stenosis and atresia, and transposition of the great arteries. There are at least five instances of ectopia cordis without a cardiac anomaly.[37]

Oligohydramnios due to amnion rupture causing compression of the heart during cardiogenesis has been hypothesized as a mechanism of both thoracic and thoracoabdominal ectopia cordis.[169] Despite this mechanical explanation, chromosome abnormalities[166,170,171] and associated anomalies such as cleft lip and palate, cranial anomalies, gastrointestinal and renal anomalies, and pulmonary hypoplasia have been identified in some affected patients.[37,172,173]

TREATMENT

A dismal outcome is generally reported in patients with ectopia cordis,[172,174] mainly because of associated extracardiac and cardiac anomalies.[172–175] The first successful operative treatment of thoracoabdominal ectopia cordis without cardiac and extracardiac anomalies was performed in 1888 by Lannelongue and reported 22 years later.[176] Major extracardiac problems in the treatment of ectopia cordis include external cardiac compression, lung hypoplasia, and large airway obstruction due to distorted vascular anatomy.

The prognosis is particularly poor in patients with the thoracic form of ectopia cordis. In these patients, even though the thoracic cavity may appear normal in size, the liver occupies much of the cavity and precludes placement of the heart in the thorax. Although the outcome for patients with thoracoabdominal ectopia cordis is considered more favorable than that for patients with the thoracic form, the mortality is still high in both groups. The outcome of a large group of children and infants with ectopia cordis and cardiac anomalies treated at Children's Hospital of Boston has been reported by Hornberger and colleagues.[177] This report provides evidence that affected infants and children can survive beyond early infancy and undergo successful repair or definitive palliation of their cardiac anomaly.

THORACOPAGUS CONJOINED TWINS

The most common form of conjoined twins shows a fusion in the midportion of the body, and these children are called thoracopagus twins. These patients represent a rare type of cardiac malposition because the fusion involves the anterior chest region and the heart. Conjoined twins occur in every 50,000 births. Female twins represent more than three fourths of the patients.[178]

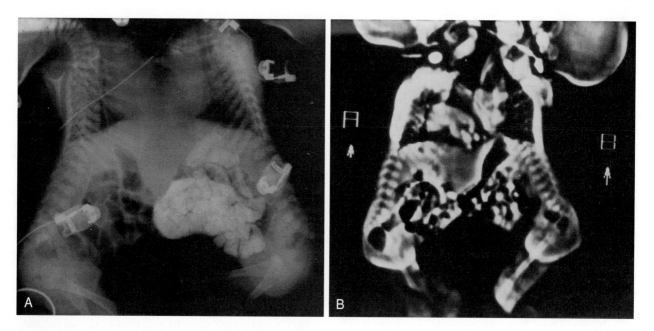

Chest radiograph *(A)* and computed tomographic angiogram *(B)* in thoracopagus twins. Note the conjoined livers and the fusion of the chests (the twin A is right-sided and the twin B is left-sided in the figure).

In thoracopagus twins, the livers are conjoined and the sternum is usually partially or totally absent (Fig. 40–20). The pericardial and pleural cavities may be either separate or common to both children, and the cardiovascular fusion may be classified into three types[179]: common pericardium but separate hearts; fusion at atrial and ventricular levels; and fusion at atrial level only. Simple or, more frequently, complex cardiac malformations may coexist and may be discordant between the children.

Because anomalies of the visceroarterial situs and discordant atrioventricular and ventriculoarterial connections are frequent,[180] the segmental approach to cardiac diagnosis[1, 2, 6, 8] is mandatory in these patients.

At atrial level, the most frequent anomalies are single atrium and large atrial septal defect. Venous channels interposed between the superior venae cavae and connecting the systemic venous drainages of the twins are frequent, as is partial or total anomalous pulmonary venous connection. At ventricular level, the most common anomalies are single ventricle and ventricular septal defect[181]; transposition of the great arteries and double-outlet right ventricle are the most common conotruncal defects. Pulmonary and aortic stenosis or atresia occur frequently, and one twin may show one of these conditions and the opposite twin the other.[182]

The fetal diagnosis can be made by radiography.[183] Prenatal echocardiographic examination details the intracardiac anatomy.[184]

At birth, the diagnosis of separate hearts can be suspected if one twin differs from the other in pulse rate and

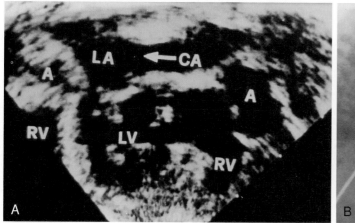

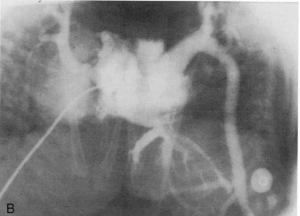

A, Two-dimensional echocardiography in thoracopagus twins. Note the fusion of the cardiac masses at atrial (CA *arrow* to LA) and ventricular (LV, RV) levels. The aorta (A) of the twin A (which is right-sided in the figure) is smaller than the aorta (A) of the twin B (which is left-sided in the figure). CA = common atrium; LA = left atrium; LV = left ventricle; RV = right ventricle. *B,* Angiocardiography in the same thoracopagus twins shows the conjoined hearts.

if they show separate QRS complexes on an electrocardiogram.[183] Echocardiography can diagnose the site and dimension of the heart fusion and the morphology of intracardiac anomalies (Fig. 40–21A).[182] Computed tomographic angiography (Fig. 40–20B)[182, 185] may also be useful for the diagnosis, but cardiac catheterization and angiocardiography, although technically difficult in these patients, are mandatory to assess the feasibility of separation (Fig. 40–21B).[182, 186] Aortography and coronary angiography should be indicated to exclude fusion of the coronary vascular beds at ventricular level. Furthermore, the assessment of electromyocardial continuity should be considered in the preoperative work-up.[187]

Separation of conjoined twins represents an operative challenge[188–195] and is best delayed until the infants are relatively mature (6 to 12 months of age). The assessment of the cardiovascular system is fundamental in planning the operative separation, but the evaluation of the liver, pancreaticobiliary tract, gastrointestinal tract, urinary tract, and central nervous system is also important. Therefore, the operative team must include many specialty consultants and surgeons. Moreover, the use of skin expanders and prosthetic mesh is mandatory to facilitate wound closure.

The moral, ethical, and legal problems of separation of conjoined twins are important aspects in medical and surgical treatment.[194, 195] With conjoined hearts, the possibility of sacrificing one twin, allowing the other to lead a potentially normal life, comes into question.[195] The hospital's ethics committee has been helpful in this respect, but obviously the parents always have the right to refuse surgical separation.

There are no reported long-term instances of separation of twins with conjoined ventricles (one patient survived for 3 months),[194] and there is only a single success when the junction was at atrial level.[189]

REFERENCES

1. Van Praagh R, Van Praagh S, Vlad P, Keith JD: Anatomic types of congenital dextrocardia. Diagnostic and embryologic implications. Am J Cardiol 13:510, 1964.
2. Van Praagh R, Van Praagh S, Vlad P, et al: Diagnosis of anatomic types of congenital dextrocardia. Am J Cardiol 15:234, 1965.
3. Lev M, Liberthson RR, Eckner FA, et al: Pathologic anatomy of dextrocardia and its clinical implications. Circulation 37:979, 1968.
4. Anselmi G, Munoz S, Blanco P, et al: Systematization and clinical study of dextroversion, mirror-image dextrocardia and laevoversion. Br Heart J 34:1085, 1972.
5. Squarcia U, Ritter DG, Kincaid OW: Dextrocardia: Angiocardiographic study and classification. Am J Cardiol 32:965, 1973.
6. Shinebourne EA, Macartney FI, Anderson RH: Sequential chamber localization: The logical approach to diagnosis in congenital heart disease. Br Heart J 38:327, 1976.
7. Stanger P, Rudolph AM, Edwards JE: Cardiac malpositions: An overview based on study of 65 necropsy specimens. Circulation 56:159, 1977.
8. Van Praagh R: Terminology of congenital heart disease. Glossary and commentary. Circulation 56:139, 1977.
9. Calcaterra G, Anderson RH, Lau KC, et al: Dextrocardia—value of segmental analysis in its categorization. Br Heart J 42:497, 1979.
10. Brown NA, Wolpert J: The development of handedness in left/right asymmetry. Development 109:1, 1990.
11. Splitt MP, Burn J, Goodship J: Defects in the determination of left-right isomerism. J Med Genet 33:498, 1996.
12. Wilson GN, Stout JP, Schneider NR, et al: Balanced translocation 12/13 and situs abnormalities. Homology of early pattern formation in man and lower organisms? Am J Med Genet 38:601, 1991.
13. Carmi R, Boughman JA, Rosenbaum KR: Human situs determinant is probably controlled by several different genes. Am J Med Genet 44:246, 1992.
14. Casey B, Devoto M, Jones KL, Ballabio A: Mapping a gene for familial situs abnormalities to human chromosome Xq24-q27.1 Nature 5:403, 1993.
15. Britz-Cunningham S, Shah M, Zuppan C, Fletcher W: Mutations of the connexin43 gap-junction gene in patients with heart malformations and defects of laterality. N Engl J Med 332:1323, 1995.
16. Gebbia M, Towbin JA, Casey B: Failure to detect connexin43 mutations in 38 cases of sporadic and familial heterotaxy. Circulation 94:1909, 1996.
17. Casey B, Cuneo BF, Vitali C, et al: Autosomal dominant transmission of familial laterality defects. Am J Med Genet 61:325, 1996.
18. Marino B, Digilio MC, Giannotti A, et al: Heterotaxia syndromes and 22q11 deletion. J Med Genet 33:1052, 1996.
19. Kato R, Yamada Y, Niikawa N: De novo balanced translocation (6;18) (q21;q21.3) in a patient with heterotaxia. Am J Med Genet 66:184, 1996.
20. Ivemark B: Implication of agenesis of the spleen on the pathogenesis of cono-truncus anomalies in childhood. Acta Paediatr Scand 44 (suppl):1, 1955.
21. Moller JH, Nakib A, Anderson RC, et al: Congenital cardiac disease associated with polysplenia: A developmental complex of bilateral "left-sideness." Circulation 36:789, 1967.
22. Van Mierop LH, Gessner IH, Schiebler GL: Asplenia and polysplenia syndrome. Birth Defects 3:74, 1972.
23. Rose V, Izukawa T, Moes CA: Syndromes of asplenia and polysplenia. A review of cardiac and non-cardiac malformations in 60 cases with special reference to diagnosis and prognosis. Br Heart J 37:840, 1975.
24. Macartney FJ, Zuberbuhler JR, Anderson RH: Morphological considerations pertaining to recognition of atrial isomerism. Consequences for sequential chamber localisation. Br Heart J 44:657, 1980.
25. Sapire DW, Yen Ho S, Anderson RH, Rigby ML: Diagnosis and significance of atrial isomerism. Am J Cardiol 58:342, 1986.
26. Van Praagh R, Van Praagh S: Atrial isomerism on the heterotaxy syndromes with asplenia, or polysplenia, or normally formed spleen: An erroneous concept. Am J Cardiol 66:1504, 1990.
27. Sharma S, Devine W, Anderson RH, Zuberbuhler JR: The determination of atrial arrangement by examination of appendage morphology in 1842 heart specimens. Br Heart J 60:227, 1988.
28. Phoon CK, Neill CA: Asplenia syndrome: Insight into embryology through an analysis of cardiac and extracardiac anomalies. Am J Cardiol 73:581, 1994.
29. Rubino M, Van Praagh S, Kadoba K, et al: Systemic and pulmonary venous connections in visceral heterotaxy with asplenia. J Thorac Cardiovasc Surg 110:641, 1995.
30. Uemura H, Yen Ho S, Devine WA, Anderson RH: Analysis of visceral heterotaxy according to splenic status, appendage morphology, or both. Am J Cardiol 76:846, 1995.
31. Uemura H, Yen Ho S, Devine WA, et al: Atrial appendages in venoatrial connections in hearts from patients with visceral heterotaxy. Ann Thorac Surg 60:561, 1995.
32. Geva T, Vick GW III, Wendt RE, Rokey R: Diagnosis of heterotaxy syndrome. Circulation 91:907, 1995.
33. Frescura C, Marino B, Bosman C, Thiene G: Sindromi asplenica e polisplenica: Malformazioni cardiovascolari ed interpretazioni embriogenetiche. In Progressi in Cardiologia Pediatrica. Trieste, LINT, 1981, p 123.
34. Fabricius, cited by Cleveland M: Situs inversus viscerum: Anatomic study. Arch Surg 13:343, 1926.
35. Nadas AS, Fyler DC: Dextrocardias. In Nadas AS, Fyler DC (eds): Pediatric Cardiology. Philadelphia, WB Saunders, 1972, p 657.
36. Friedberg CK: Dextrocardia. In Friedberg CK (ed): Disease of the Heart. Philadelphia, WB Saunders, 1966, p 1284.
37. Van Praagh R, Weinberg PM, Smith SD, et al: Malpositions of the heart. In Adams FH, Emmanouilides GC, Riemenschneider TA (eds): Heart Disease in Infants, Children, and Adolescents, 4th ed. Baltimore, Williams & Wilkins, 1989, p 530.
38. Stratton RF, Parker MW: Growth hormone deficiency, wormian bones, dextrocardia, brachycamptodactily, and other midline defects. Am J Genet 32:169, 1989.
39. Neil CA, Ferencz C, Sabiston DC, Sheldon H: The familial occurrence of hypoplastic right lung with systemic arterial supply and venous drainage: "Scimitar syndrome." Johns Hopkins Med J 107:1, 1960.

40. Cantrell JR, Haller JA, Ravitch MM: A syndrome of congenital defects involving the abdominal wall, sternum, diaphragm, pericardium and heart. Surg Gynecol Obstet 107:602, 1958.

41. Fox JE, Gloster ES, Mirchandani R: Trisomy 18 with Cantrell pentalogy in a stillborn infant. Am J Med Genet 31:391, 1988.

42. Borges AJ, Hazebroek FW, Hess J: Left and right diverticula, ventricular septal defect and ectopia cordis in a patient with Cantrell's syndrome. Eur J Cardiothorac Surg 7:334, 1993.

43. Husain AN, Hessel RG: Neonatal pulmonary hypoplasia: An autopsy study of 25 cases. Pediatr Pathol 13:475, 1993.

44. Mannes GPM, Van der Jagt EJ, Wouters B, Postmus PE: Dextrocardia? Chest 96:2, 1989.

45. Reddy SCB, Taneja K, Kothari SS, et al: Mediastinal lipoma mimicking dextrocardia and cardiac enlargement: Diagnosis by magnetic resonance imaging. Am Heart J 132:94, 1996.

46. Van Praagh S, O'Sullivan J, Brili S, Van Praagh R: Juxtaposition of the morphological right atrial appendage in solitus and inversus atria: A study of 35 postmortem cases. Am Heart J 132:382, 1996.

47. Wood AE, Freedom RM, Williams WG, Trusler GA: The Mustard procedure in transposition of the great arteries associated with juxtaposition of the atrial appendage with or without dextrocardia. J Thorac Cardiovasc Surg 85:451, 1983.

48. Marino B, Sanders S, Pasquini L, et al: Two-dimensional echocardiographic anatomy in criss-cross heart. Am J Cardiol 58:325, 1986.

49. Pasquini L, Sanders SP, Parness IA, et al: Echocardiographic and anatomic findings in atrioventricular discordance and ventriculoarterial concordance. Am J Cardiol 62:1256, 1988.

50. Kartagener M: Zur Pathogenese der Bronchiektasian: Bronchiektasian bei Situs Viscerum Inversus. Beitr Klin Tuberk 83:489, 1933.

51. Eliasson R, Mossberg B, Cammer P: The immotile cilia syndrome. A congenital abnormality as an etiologic factor in chronic airway infection and male sterility. N Engl J Med 297:1, 1977.

52. Shidlow DV, Katz SM, Turtz MG: Polysplenia and Kartagener syndromes in a sibship: Association with abnormal respiratory cilia. J Pediatr 100:401, 1982.

53. Losekoot TG, Anderson RH, Becker AE, et al: Congenitally Corrected Transposition. New York, Churchill Livingstone, 1983, p 5.

54. McGrath LB, Kirklin JW, Blackstone EH, et al: Death and other events after cardiac repair of discordant atrioventricular connection. J Thorac Cardiovasc Surg 90:711, 1985.

55. Attie F, Cerda J, Richheimer R, et al: Congenitally corrected transposition with mirror image atrial arrangement. Int J Cardiol 14:169, 1987.

56. Di Donato RM, Wernovsky G, Jonas R, et al: Corrected transposition in situs inversus. Biventricular repair of cardiac anomalies. Circulation 62:194, 1989.

57. Hutha JC, Maloney JD, Ritter DJ, et al: Complete atrioventricular block in patient with atrioventricular discordance. Circulation 94:2, 1996.

58. Sakata R, Lecompte Y, Batisse A, et al: Anatomic repair of anomalies of ventriculoarterial connection associated with ventricular septal defect: Criteria of surgical decision. J Thorac Cardiovasc Surg 95:90, 1988.

59. Borromée L, Lecompte Y, Batisse A, et al: Anatomic repair of anomalies of ventriculoarterial connection associated with ventricular septal defect: Clinical results in 50 patients with pulmonary outflow tract obstruction. J Thorac Cardiovasc Surg 95:96, 1988.

60. Rastelli GC: A new approach to "anatomic" repair of transposition of the great arteries. Mayo Clin Proc 44:1, 1969.

61. Lecompte Y, Neveux JY, Leca F, et al: Reconstruction of the pulmonary outflow tract without prosthetic conduit. J Thorac Cardiovasc Surg 84:727, 1982.

62. Ilbawi MN, DeLeon SY, Backer CL, et al: An alternative approach to the surgical management of physiologically corrected transposition with ventricular septal defect and pulmonary stenosis or atresia. J Thorac Cardiovasc Surg 100:410, 1990.

63. Di Donato RM, Troconis CJ, Marino B, et al: Combined Mustard and Rastelli operations: An alternative approach for repair of associated anomalies in congenitally corrected transposition in situs inversus {I,D,D}. J Thorac Cardiovasc Surg 104:1246, 1992.

64. Yamagashi Y, Imai Y, Hoshino S, et al: Anatomic correction of atrioventricular discordance. J Thorac Cardiovasc Surg 105:1067, 1993.

65. Yagihara T, Kishimoto H, Isobe F, et al: Double switch operation in cardiac anomalies with atrioventricular and ventriculoarterial discordance. J Thorac Cardiovasc Surg 107:351, 1994.

66. Imai Y, Sawatari K, Hoshino S, et al: Ventricular function after repair in patients with atrioventricular discordance. J Thorac Cardiovasc Surg 107:1272, 1994.

67. Sato K, Ohara S, Tsukaguchi I, et al: A criss-cross heart with concordant atrioventriculoarterial connections. Circulation 57:396, 1978.

68. Ohtakae S, Shimazaki Y, Kawata H, et al: Surgical management of criss-cross heart in association with complex cardiac anomalies. Cardiol Young 3(suppl 1):58, 1993.

69. Muster AJ, Zales VR, Ilbawi MN, et al: Biventricular repair of hypoplastic right ventricle assisted by pulsatile bidirectional cavopulmonary anastomosis. J Thorac Cardiovasc Surg 105:112, 1993.

70. Webber SA, Sandor GGS, Patterson MWH, et al: Prognosis in asplenia syndrome—a population based review. Cardiol Young 2:129, 1992.

71. Gatrad AR, Read AP, Watson GH: Consanguinity and complex cardiac anomalies with situs ambiguus. Arch Dis Child 59:242, 1984.

72. Rowe RD, Freedom RM, Mehrizi A, Bloom KR: The Neonate With Congenital Heart Disease, 2nd ed. Philadelphia, WB Saunders, 1981, p 484.

73. Van Praagh R, Weinberg PM, Matsuoka R, Van Praagh S: Malpositions of the heart. In Adams FH, Emmanouilides GC (eds): Moss' Heart Disease in Infants, Children, and Adolescents, 3rd ed. Baltimore, Williams & Wilkins, 1983, p 422.

74. Niikawa N, Koshaka S, Mizumoto M, et al: Familial clustering of situs inversus totalis and asplenia and polysplenia syndromes. Am J Med Genet 16:43, 1983.

75. Randall PA, Moller JH, Amplatz K: The spleen and congenital heart disease. Am J Roentgenol 119:551, 1973.

76. Carmi R, Magee CA, Neill CA, Karrer FM: Extrahepatic biliary atresia and associated anomalies: Etiologic heterogeneity suggested by distinctive patterns of associations. Am J Med Genet 45:683, 1993.

77. Amodeo A, Di Donato R, Carotti A, et al: Pulmonary arteriovenous fistulas and polysplenia syndrome. J Thorac Cardiovasc Surg 107:1379, 1994.

78. Ruttenberg HD, Neufeld HN, Lucas RV Jr, et al: Syndrome of congenital heart disease with asplenia. Distinction from other forms of congenital cyanotic cardiac disease. Am J Cardiol 13:387, 1964.

79. Peoples WM, Moller JH, Edwards JE: Polysplenia: A review of 146 cases. Pediatr Cardiol 4:129, 1983.

80. Marino B, Pasquini L: Systemic and venous connection in asplenia syndrome. J Thorac Cardiovasc Surg 111:1109, 1996.

81. Van Praagh S, Carrera ME, Sanders S, et al: Partial or total direct pulmonary venous drainage to right atrium due to malposition of septum primum. Chest 107:1488, 1995.

82. Francalanci P, Marino B, Boldrini R, et al: Morphology of the atrioventricular valve in asplenia syndrome: A peculiar type of atrioventricular canal defect. Cardiovasc Pathol 5:145, 1996.

83. Digilio MC, Marino B, Giannotti A, Dallapiccola B: Single atrium, atrioventricular canal/postaxial hexodactyly indicating Ellis–van Creveld syndrome. Hum Genet 96:251, 1995.

84. Vairo U, Marino B, Parretti di Iulio D, et al: Isomerismo atriale destro con atresia polmonare: Caratteristiche angiocardiografiche e modelli di circolazione polmonare. G Ital Cardiol 21:669, 1991.

85. Vairo U, Marino B, Parretti di Iulio D, et al: Morfologia ventricolo-infundibolare nell'eterotassia viscerale con isomerismo sinistro. Studio eco-angiocardiografico. G Ital Cardiol 21:969, 1991.

86. Marino B, Calabrò R, Gagliardi MG, et al: Patterns of pulmonary arterial anatomy and blood supply in complex congenital heart disease with pulmonary atresia. J Thorac Cardiovasc Surg 4:518, 1987.

87. Formigari R, Vairo U, de Zorzi A, et al: Prevalence of bilateral ductus arteriosus in patients with pulmonic valve atresia and asplenia syndrome. Am J Cardiol 70:1219, 1992.

88. Vitiello R, Moller JH, Marino B, et al: Pulmonary circulation in pulmonary atresia associated with the asplenia cardiac syndrome. J Am Coll Cardiol 20:363, 1992.

89. Blieden LC, Moller JH: Analysis of the P wave in congenital cardiac malformations associated with splenic anomalies. Am Heart J 85:439, 1973.

90. Partridge JB, Scott O, Deverall PB, et al: Visualization and measurement of the main bronchi by tomography as an objective indicator of thoracic situs in congenital heart disease. Circulation 51:188, 1975.

91. Deanfield JE, Leanage R, Stroobant J, et al: Use of high kilovoltage filtered beam radiographs for detection of bronchial situs in infants and young children. Br Heart J 44:577, 1980.

92. Hutha JC, Smallhorn JF, Macartney FJ: Two-dimensional echocardiographic diagnosis of situs. Br Heart J 48:97, 1982.

93. Hutha JC, Hagler DJ, Seward JB, et al: Two-dimensional echocardiographic assessment of cardiac malposition. Am J Cardiol 50:1351, 1982.

94. Smallhorn JS, Tommasini G, Macartney FJ: Two-dimensional echocardiographic assessment of common atrioventricular valves in univentricular hearts. Br Heart J 46:30, 1981.

95. Arisawa J, Morimoto S, Ikezoe J, et al: Cross sectional echocardiographic anatomy of common atrioventricular valve in atrial isomerism. Br Heart J 62:291, 1989.

96. Silverman NH, de Araujo LML: An echocardiographic method for the diagnosis of cardiac situs and malpositions. Echocardiography 4:35, 1987.

97. Van Der Velte ME, Parness IA, Colan SD, et al: Two-dimensional echocardiography in the pre- and postoperative management of totally anomalous pulmonary venous connection. J Am Coll Cardiol 18:1746, 1991.

98. O'Leary PW, Seward JB, Hagler DJ, Tajik J: Echocardiographic documentation of splenic anatomy in complex congenital heart disease. Am J Cardiol 68:1536, 1991.

99. Geva T, Wesley V III, Wendt RE, Rokey R: Role of spin echo and cine magnetic resonance imaging in presurgical planning of heterotaxy syndrome. Comparison with echocardiography and catheterization. Circulation 90:348, 1994.

100. Marino B, Vairo U, Marcelletti C, Calabrò R: Morphology of ductus arteriosus in patients with pulmonary atresia and complex congenital heart disease. Chest 97:766, 1990.

101. Di Donato R, di Carlo D, Squitieri C, et al: Palliation of cardiac malformations associated with right isomerism (asplenia syndrome) in infancy. Ann Thorac Surg 44:35, 1987.

102. DeLeon SY, Gidding SS, Ilbawi MN, et al: Surgical management of infants with complex cardiac anomalies associated with reduced pulmonary blood flow and total anomalous pulmonary venous drainage. Ann Thorac Surg 43:207, 1987.

103. Culbertson CB, George BL, Day RW, et al: Factors influencing survival of patients with heterotaxy syndrome undergoing the Fontan procedure. J Am Coll Cardiol 20:678, 1992.

104. Dickinson DF, Wilkinson JL, Anderson KR, et al: The cardiac conduction system in situs ambiguus. Circulation 59:879, 1979.

105. Garcia OL, Mehta AV, Pickoff AS, et al: Left isomerism and complete atrioventricular block: A report of six cases. Am J Cardiol 48:1103, 1981.

106. Heller RM, Dorst JP, James AE, Rowe RD: A useful sign in the recognition of azygos continuation of the inferior vena cava. Radiology 101:519, 1971.

107. Parness IA, Yeager SB, Sanders SP, et al: Echocardiographic diagnosis of fetal heart defects in mid trimester. Arch Dis Child 63:1137, 1988.

108. Phoon CK, Villegas MD, Ursell PC, Silverman NH: Left atrial isomerism detected in fetal life. Am J Cardiol 77:1083, 1996.

109. Guccione P, Gagliardi MG, Bevilacqua M, et al: Cardiac catheterization through the internal jugular vein in pediatric patients. An alternative to the usual femoral vein access. Chest 101:1512, 1992.

110. Moller JH: Malposition of the heart. In Moller JH, Neal WA (eds): Fetal, Neonatal and Infant Cardiac Disease. Norwalk, CT, Appleton & Lange, 1990, p 755.

111. Sadiq M, Stümper O, De Giovanni JV, et al: Management and outcome of infants and children with right isomerism. Heart 75:314, 1996.

112. Waldman JD, Rosenthal A, Smith AL, et al: Sepsis and congenital asplenia. J Pediatr 90:555, 1977.

113. Chandra RS: Biliary atresia and other structural anomalies in the congenital polysplenia syndrome. J Pediatr 85:649, 1974.

114. Dimmick JE, Bove KE, McAdams AJ: Extrahepatic biliary atresia and the polysplenia syndrome. J Pediatr 86:644, 1975.

115. Gersony WM: Obstruction to pulmonary venous return obscured by decreased pulmonary blood flow. Chest 64:283, 1973.

116. Freedom RM, Olley PM, Coceani F, Rowe RD: The prostaglandin challenge: Test to unmask obstructed total pulmonary venous connections in asplenia syndrome. Br Heart J 40:91, 1978.

117. Norwood WI: Hypoplastic left heart syndrome. Cardiol Clin 7:377, 1989.

118. Jobes DR, Nicolson SC, Steven JM, et al: Carbon dioxide prevents pulmonary overcirculation in hypoplastic left heart syndrome. Ann Thorac Surg 54:150, 1992.

119. Wren C, Macartney FJ, Deanfield JE: Cardiac rhythm in atrial isomerism. Am J Cardiol 59:1156, 1987.

120. Momma K, Takao A, Shibata T: Characteristics and natural history of abnormal atrial rhythms in left isomerism. Am J Cardiol 65:231, 1990.

121. Heinemann MK, Hanley FL, Van Praagh S, et al: Total anomalous pulmonary venous drainage in newborns with visceral heterotaxy. Ann Thorac Surg 57:88, 1994.

122. Albanese SB, Carotti A, Di Donato RM, et al: Bidirectional cavopulmonary anastomosis in patients under two years of age. J Thorac Cardiovasc Surg 104:904, 1992.

123. Chang AC, Hanley FL, Wernovsky G, et al: Early bidirectional cavopulmonary anastomosis shunt in young infants. Postoperative course and early results. Circulation 88:II-149, 1993.

124. Ando F, Shirotani H, Kawai J, et al: Successful total repair of complicated cardiac anomalies with asplenia syndrome. J Thorac Cardiovasc Surg 72:33, 1976.

125. Pacifico AD, Fox LS, Kirklin JW, Bargeron LM Jr: Surgical treatment of atrial isomerism. In Anderson RH, Macartney FJ, Shinebourne EA, Tynan M (eds): Paediatric Cardiology, Vol 5. Edinburgh, Churchill Livingstone, 1983, p 223.

126. Hirooka K, Yagihara T, Kishimoto H, et al: Biventricular repair in cardiac isomerism. Report of seventeen cases. J Thorac Cardiovasc Surg 109:530, 1995.

127. Carotti A, Marino B, Oppido G, Marcelletti C: Biventricular repair in patients with left isomerism. J Thorac Cardiovasc Surg 110:1151, 1995.

128. Di Donato R, Marino B, Carotti A, et al: Biventricular repair in left atrial isomerism (polysplenia syndrome). Circulation 80:II-363, 1989.

129. Kuroda O, Sano T, Matsuda H, et al: Analysis of the effects of Blalock-Taussig shunt on ventricular function and the prognosis in patients with single ventricle. Circulation 76:III-24, 1987.

130. Okita Y, Miki S, Kusuhara K, et al: Annuloplastic reconstruction for common atrioventricular valvular regurgitation in right isomerism. Ann Thorac Surg 47:302, 1989.

131. Tatsuno K, Suzuki K, Kikuchi T, et al: Valvuloplasty for common atrioventricular valve regurgitation in cyanotic heart disease. Ann Thorac Surg 58:154, 1994.

132. Takayama T, Nagata N, Miyairi T, et al: Bridging annuloplasty for common atrioventricular valve regurgitation. Ann Thorac Surg 59:1003, 1995.

133. Kawashima Y, Kitamura S, Matsuda H, et al: Total cavopulmonary shunt operation in complex cardiac anomalies. A new operation. J Thorac Cardiovasc Surg 87:74, 1984.

134. Matsuda H, Kawashima Y, Hirose H, et al: Evaluation of total cavopulmonary shunt operation for single ventricle with common atrioventricular valve and left isomerism. Am J Cardiol 58:180, 1986.

135. Cloutier A, Ash JM, Smallhorn JF, et al: Abnormal distribution of pulmonary blood flow after the Glenn shunt or Fontan procedure: Risk of development of arteriovenous fistulae. Circulation 72:471, 1985.

136. Silverman A, Cooper MD, Moller JH, Good RA: Syndrome of cyanosis, digital clubbing, and hepatic disease in siblings. J Pediatr 72:70, 1968.

137. Krowka MJ, Cortese DA: Hepatopulmonary syndrome: An evolving perspective in the era of liver transplantation. Hepatology 11:138, 1990.

138. Papagiannis J, Kanter RJ, Effman EL, et al: Polysplenia with pulmonary arteriovenous malformations. Pediatr Cardiol 14:127, 1993.

139. Knight WB, Mee RBB: A cure for pulmonary arteriovenous fistulas? Ann Thorac Surg 59:999, 1995.

140. Lamberti JJ, Spicer RL, Waldman JD, et al: The bidirectional cavopulmonary shunt. J Thorac Cardiovasc Surg 100:22, 1990.

141. Bernstein HS, Brook MM, Silverman NH, Bristow J: Development of pulmonary arteriovenous fistulae in children after cavopulmonary shunt. Circulation 92:II-309, 1995.

142. Marcelletti C, Di Donato R, Nijveld A, et al: Right and left isomerism: The cardiac surgeon's view. Ann Thorac Surg 35:400, 1983.

143. Humes RA, Feldt RH, Porter CJ, et al: The modified Fontan operation for asplenia and polysplenia syndromes. J Thorac Cardiovasc Surg 96:212, 1988.

144. Michielon G, Gharagozloo F, Julsrud PR, et al: Modified Fontan operation in the presence of anomalies of systemic and pulmonary venous connections. Circulation 88:II-141, 1993.

145. Cetta F, Feldt RH, O'Leary PW, et al: Improved early morbidity and mortality after Fontan operation: The Mayo Clinic experience, 1987 to 1992. J Am Coll Cardiol 28:480, 1996.

146. Bridges ND, Jonas RA, Mayer JE, et al: Bidirectional cavopulmonary anastomosis as interim palliation for high-risk Fontan candidates. Early results. Circulation 82:IV-170, 1990.

147. de Leval MR, Kilner P, Gewilling M, Bull C: Total cavopulmonary connection: A logical alternative to atriopulmonary connection for complex Fontan operations. J Thorac Cardiovasc Surg 96:682, 1988.

148. Marcelletti C, Corno A, Giannico S, Marino B: Inferior vena cava–pulmonary artery extracardiac conduit: A new form of right heart bypass. J Thorac Cardiovasc Surg 100:228, 1990.

149. Laks H, Pearl JM, Haas GS, et al: Partial Fontan: Advantages of an adjustable interatrial communication. Ann Thorac Surg 52:1084, 1991.

150. Bridges ND, Mayer JE, Lock JE, et al: Effects of baffle fenestration on outcome of the modified Fontan operation. Circulation 86:1762, 1992.

151. Bailey LL, Assaad AN, Trimm RF, et al: Orthotopic transplantation during early infancy as therapy for incurable congenital heart disease. Ann Surg 208:279, 1988.

152. Boucek MM, Mathius CM, Razzouk A, et al: Indications and contraindications for heart transplantation in infancy. J Heart Lung Transplant 12:S154, 1993.

153. Mayer JE, Perry S, O'Brien P, et al: Orthotopic heart transplantation for complex congenital heart disease. J Thorac Cardiovasc Surg 99:484, 1990.

154. Kanter KR, Vincent RN, Miller BE, McFadden C: Heart transplantation in children who have undergone previous heart surgery: Is it safe? J Heart Lung Transplant 12:S218, 1993.

155. Bailey LB: Heart transplantation techniques in complex congenital heart disease. J Heart Lung Transplant 12:S168, 1993.

156. Vouhé PR, Tamisier D, Le Bidois J, et al: Pediatric cardiac transplantation for congenital heart defects: Surgical considerations and results. Ann Thorac Surg 56:1239, 1993.

157. Turrentine MW, Kesler KA, Caldwell R, et al: Cardiac transplantation in infants and children. Ann Thorac Surg 57:546, 1994.

158. Doty DB, Renlund DG, Caputo GR, et al: Cardiac transplantation in situs inversus. J Thorac Cardiovasc Surg 99:493, 1990.

159. Menkis AH, McKenzie FN, Novick RJ, et al: Expanding applicability of transplantation after multiple prior palliative procedures. Ann Thorac Surg 52:722, 1991.

160. Reitz BA, Jamieson SW, Gaudiani VA, et al: Method for cardiac transplantation in corrected transposition. J Cardiovasc Surg 23:293, 1982.

161. Harjula ALJ, Heikkilä LJ, Nieminen MS, et al: Heart transplantation in repaired transposition of the great arteries. Ann Thorac Surg 46:611, 1988.

162. Trento A, Griffith BP, Fricker FJ, et al: Lessons learned in pediatric heart transplantation. Ann Thorac Surg 48:617, 1989.

163. Parness IA, Nadas AS: Cardiac transplantation in children. Pediatr Rev 10:111, 1988.

164. Chartrand C, Guerin R, Kangah M, Stanley P: Pediatric heart transplantation: Surgical considerations for congenital heart diseases. J Heart Transplant 9:608, 1990.

165. Merrill WH, Frist WH, Stewart JR, et al: Heart transplantation in children. Ann Surg 213:393, 1991.

166. Khoury MJ, Cordero JF, Rasmussen S: Ectopia cordis, midline defects and chromosomal abnormalities: An epidemiologic perspective. Am J Med Genet 30:811, 1988.

167. Carmi R, Boughman JA: Pentalogy of Cantrell and associated midline anomalies: A possible midline developmental field. Am J Med Genet 42:90, 1992.

168. Kanagasuntheran R, Verzin JA: Ectopia cordis in man. Thorax 17:159, 1962.

169. Torpin R: Fetal Malformation Caused by Amnion Rupture During Gestation. Springfield, IL, Charles C Thomas, 1968.

170. King CR: Ectopia cordis and chromosomal errors. Pediatrics 66:328, 1980.

171. Soper SP, Roe LR, Hoyme HE, Clemmons JJW: Trisomy 18 with ectopia cordis, omphalocele and ventricular septal defect: Case report. Pediatr Pathol 5:481, 1986.

172. Shambererg RC, Welk KJ: Sternal defect. Pediatr Surg 5:90, 1990.

173. Toyoma WM: Combined congenital defect of the anterior abdominal wall, sternum diaphragm, pericardium and heart: A case report and review of the syndrome. Pediatrics 50:778, 1972.

174. Leca F, Thilbert M, Khoury W, et al: Extrathoracic heart (ectopia cordis): Report of two cases and review of the literature. Int J Cardiol 22:221, 1989.

175. Millhouse RF, Joos HA: Extrathoracic ectopia cordis: Report of cases and review of the literature. Am Heart J 57:470, 1959.

176. Lannelongue OM, in discussion of Kermisson EF: Volumineuse hernie sub-umbilicale avec ectopia cardiaque. Bull Acc Med Paris 63:215, 1910.

177. Hornberger LK, Colan SD, Lock J, et al: Outcome of patients with ectopia cordis and significant intracardiac defect. Circulation 94(suppl):II-32, 1996.

178. Izukawa T, Kidd BS, Moes CA, et al: Assessment of the cardiovascular system in conjoined twins. Am J Dis Child 132:19, 1978.

179. Leachman RD, Latson JR, Kohler CM, et al: Cardiovascular evaluation of conjoined twins. Birth Defects 3:52, 1967.

180. Nichils BL, Blattner RJ, Rudolph AJ: General clinical management of thoracopagus twins. Birth Defects 3:38, 1967.

181. Rossi MB, Burn J, Yen Ho S, et al: Conjoined twins, right atrial isomerism and sequential segmental analysis. Br Heart J 58:518, 1987.

182. Gugliantini P, Marino B: Ecocardiografia, angio-TC e angiocardiografia per valutare la possibilità di separazione di gemelli siamesi. Radiol Med 88:130, 1994.

183. Rudolph AJ, Michael JP, Nichols BL: Obstetric management of conjoined twins. Birth Defects 3:207, 1975.

184. Sanders SP, Chin AJ, Parness IA, et al: Prenatal diagnosis of congenital heart defects in thoracoabdominally conjoined twins. N Engl J Med 313:370, 1985.

185. Rossi P, Bordiuk JM, Golinko RJ: Angiographic evaluation of conjoined twins. Ann Radiol 14:341, 1971.

186. Rossi P, Cozzi F, Iannaccone G: CT for assessing feasibility of separation of thoracopagus twins. J Comput Assist Tomogr 5:574, 1981.

187. Wu MH, Lai YC, Lo HM, et al: Assessment of electromyocardial continuity in conjoined (thoracopagus) twins. Am J Cardiol 69:830, 1992.

188. Simpson JS, Mustard WT, Moes CAF, et al: Emergency separation of thoracopagus twins (conjoined at thorax) in the newborn period: Importance of careful preoperative cardiac evaluation. Surgery 67:697, 1970.

189. Synhorst D, Matlak M, Roan Y: Separation of conjoined thoracopagus twins joined at the right atria. Am J Cardiol 43:662, 1979.

190. Boles ET, Vassy LE: Thoraco-omphalopagus conjoined twins: Successful surgical separation. Surgery 86:485, 1979.

191. Cloutier R, Levasseur L, Copty M, Roy JP: The surgical separation of pygopagus twins. J Pediatr Surg 14:554, 1979.

192. Hoshina H, Tanaba O, Obara H, Iwai S: Thoracopagus conjoined twins: Management of anesthetic induction and postoperative chest wall defect. Anesthesiology 66:424, 1987.

193. Roy M: Anesthesia for separation of conjoined twins. Anesthesia 39:1225, 1984.

194. O'Neill JA, Holcomb GW, Schnaufer L, et al: Surgical experience with thirteen conjoined twins. Ann Surg 208:299, 1988.

195. Annas GJ: Siamese twins: Killing one to save the other. Hastings Cent Rep 17:27, 1987.

MICHAEL L. EPSTEIN

The terms *vascular rings* and *vascular slings* refer to various arrangements of the great arteries, which may lead to symptoms primarily because of their effect on the large airways or esophagus. Although these anomalies may be seen in association with structural cardiac malformations, they often occur in the absence of associated anomalies. Some of them cause marked and even life-threatening respiratory difficulty. Vascular rings, a variety of vascular arrangements that completely encircle the trachea and esophagus, are discussed separately from vascular sling, a less common anomaly that is much more uniform in its anatomic arrangement.

VASCULAR RINGS

Before the variations in pathologic anatomy are considered, it is useful to review the embryologic development of the aortic arch and pulmonary arteries. These vessels develop from persistence or dissolution of all or portions of the six paired aortic arches connecting the truncal aortic sac with the paired dorsal aortae that eventually fuse to form the definitive descending aorta. Although these six paired aortic arches do not exist simultaneously, remnants of the various vessels eventually form the various structures that constitute the final structure of the aortic arch, brachiocephalic arteries, and pulmonary arteries. The development of the various arrangements of vessels resulting in vascular rings can be most easily understood from understanding the hypothetical double aortic arch pattern described by Edwards.[1] In this pattern, the ascending aorta gives rise to two intact aortic arches, which in turn give rise to brachiocephalic arteries on either side before eventually joining posteriorly to continue as the descending aorta, as depicted in a report by Shuford and Sybers[2] (Fig. 41–1). In this theoretical arrangement, a ductus arteriosus is present bilaterally with connection to the ipsilateral pulmonary artery. The resulting patterns of vascular rings can be understood by persistence, narrowing, or loss of certain segments of the hypothetical double aortic arch system.

The definition of a left or a right aortic arch is determined by the main stem bronchus that is crossed by the vessel. This arrangement becomes important in trying to diagnose a vascular ring from various diagnostic studies and is obviously important in planning operative intervention. In a normal aortic arch, the right innominate artery is the first branch arising from the aortic arch, and it divides into the right subclavian and right carotid arteries. The left carotid artery is the second branch, and the left subclavian artery is the final branch. This pattern results from dissolution of the right aortic arch between the right subclavian artery and descending aorta (Fig. 41–1C).

In the section to follow, a number of anomalies are discussed that are considered abnormalities of the fourth embryonic arch. In addition, cervical aortic arch is described, and this is thought to be an abnormality of the third arch (Table 41–1).

DOUBLE AORTIC ARCH

If both right and left aortic arches persist, a double aortic arch is created (Fig. 41–1E, 1G).[3] The trachea and esophagus are encircled by the ascending aorta anteriorly, the two aortic arches laterally, and the descending aorta posteriorly. When the descending aorta lies to the left of the spine, the right aortic arch is usually larger than the left and courses behind the esophagus to join the smaller left arch before continuing as the descending aorta.[2,3] Although less common, the descending aorta may lie to the right of the spine, and then the left aortic arch is usually larger than the right.

With double aortic arch, an innominate artery does not exist. Four major brachiocephalic arteries arise in a relatively symmetric pattern from their respective arches. In a double aortic arch, the ductus arteriosus, which can be on either side, plays no role in the formation of the vascular ring. Although uncommon, atresia of a segment of one of the aortic arches (usually the left arch) may occur. Depending on the location of the atresia, this lesion may be impossible to distinguish from right aortic arch with an anomalous left subclavian artery.[3,4]

RIGHT AORTIC ARCH WITH RETROESOPHAGEAL VESSEL

In this category of vascular ring, the right aortic arch persists. Two variations may occur. In one, an aberrant left subclavian artery passes posterior to the trachea and esophagus (Fig. 41–1B). The ductus arteriosus is almost always left-sided, connecting the aberrant subclavian artery to the ipsilateral pulmonary artery.[2,5] The vascular ring is then formed by the ascending aorta anteriorly, the aortic arch to the right of the trachea and esophagus, the aberrant left subclavian artery posterior to the esophagus, and the ductus arteriosus completing the ring to the left of the esophagus and trachea.

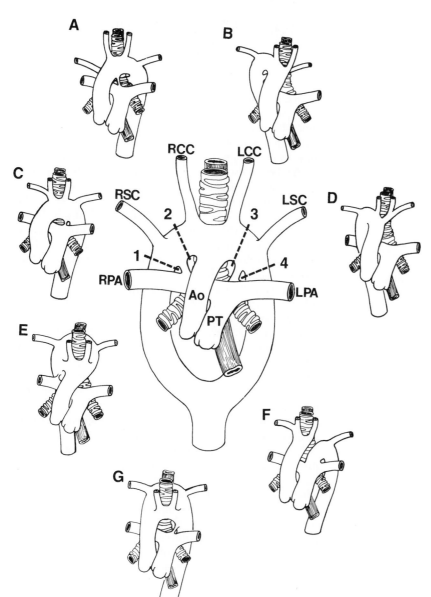

FIGURE 41–1

Hypothetical double aortic arch. During development, interruptions may occur at various sites (1 to 4), which give rise to different anatomic patterns of arch anatomy. If interruption occurs at site 1, a normal left aortic arch forms (C). If interruption occurs at site 4, a right aortic arch with mirror-image branching is formed (D). Interruption at sites 2 and 3 form a left aortic arch with aberrant right subclavian artery (A) or right artery arch with aberrant left subclavian artery (B), respectively. If neither arch is interrupted, double aortic arch with either right descending aorta (E) or left descending aorta (G) results. Two interruptions may occur in the hypothetical double aortic arch, giving rise to interruption of the aortic arch. One example is shown (F) in which the double arches were interrupted at sites 1 and 3, giving rise to interruption of the aorta distal to the left carotid artery.
Ao = aorta; LCC = left common carotid artery; LPA = left pulmonary artery; LSC = left subclavian artery; PT = pulmonary trunk; RCC = right common carotid artery; RPA = right pulmonary artery; RSC = right subclavian artery.

The second variation is created by a right aortic arch and a descending aorta on the left. The ductus arteriosus arises either directly from the descending aorta or from a retroesophageal diverticulum (of Kommerell) connecting to the left pulmonary artery.[6] This vascular ring is formed by the ascending aorta anteriorly and the aortic arch to the right and posterior to the trachea and esophagus. The ring is completed by the ductus arteriosus. This type of vascular ring may be difficult if not impossible to distinguish from a double aortic arch with atresia of one segment of the left-sided arch. Because this malformation does not include an aberrant subclavian artery, the brachiocephalic arteries arise in a "mirror-image" pattern to the normal.

LEFT AORTIC ARCH WITH RETROESOPHAGEAL VESSEL

The most common variant of the hypothetical double arch is left aortic arch with an aberrant right subclavian artery (Fig. 41–1A), the mirror image of the preceding pattern

(Fig. 41–1B).[7] The major difference is that the ductus arteriosus is almost always left-sided so that a vascular ring is not present. This occurs in 0.5% of the population and may indent the esophagus deeply. Rarely does it cause symptoms and require an operation. There are three rare varieties. A right-sided ductus arteriosus may connect the anomalous right subclavian artery to the ipsilateral pulmonary artery, completing a vascular ring.[8] Second, the ductus arteriosus may arise from a diverticulum of Kommerell and connect with the right pulmonary artery. Finally, in patients with left aortic arch and anomalous right subclavian artery, the aorta may descend on the right with a right-sided ductus, thereby creating a vascular ring.[9–11]

CERVICAL AORTIC ARCH

Cervical aortic arch is a rare aortic arch configuration that may cause a vascular ring. This lesion is defined by the aortic arch lying above the level of the clavicle and has been

TABLE 41–1

ANOMALIES OF AORTIC ARCH SYSTEM

ABNORMALITIES OF THIRD AORTIC ARCH SYSTEM

Cervical aortic arch
  Left
  Right

ABNORMALITIES OF FOURTH AORTIC ARCH SYSTEM

No regression
  Double left aortic arch
  Double right aortic arch
One regression
  Left aortic arch
  Left aortic arch with aberrant right subclavian artery
  Left aortic arch with right descending aorta
  Right aortic arch ("mirror" image)
  Right aortic arch with aberrant left subclavian artery
  Right aortic arch with left descending aorta
Two regressions
  Interruption of left aortic arch
    Interruption beyond left subclavian artery (type A)
    Interruption between left carotid and left subclavian arteries
      (type B) with or without aberrant right subclavian artery
    Interruption between carotid arteries (type C)
  Interruption of right aortic arch
    Interruption beyond right subclavian artery (type A)
    Interruption beyond right carotid and right subclavian arteries
      (type B)
    Interruption between carotid arteries (type C)
  Isolation of subclavian artery

ABNORMALITIES OF FIFTH AORTIC ARCH SYSTEM

Persistent fifth arch, "double-lumen aorta"

ABNORMALITIES OF SIXTH AORTIC ARCH SYSTEM

Patent ductus arteriosus
Proximal interruption of sixth aortic arch
  "Absence of a pulmonary artery"
  "Ductal origin of a pulmonary artery"
Pulmonary artery sling

VARIATIONS OF BRACHIOCEPHALIC ARTERIES

Common
  Left carotid arises from innominate artery
  Separate origin of left vertebral artery from aortic arch
  Separate origin of right vertebral artery from aortic arch
  Separate origin of right carotid artery from aortic arch
Less common
  Common arterial trunk with origin of each brachiocephalic artery
  Two arterial trunks, each supplying a carotid and a subclavian artery
  Separate origin of each brachiocephalic artery from aortic arch
  Common origin of right carotid, left carotid, and left subclavian
    arteries
  Common origin of right and left subclavian arteries

postulated to result from abnormal persistence of the second or third primitive aortic arch.[2, 12] A cervical arch can be recognized because five brachiocephalic arteries arise from the arch: external carotid and internal carotid arteries (on side of arch), ipsilateral carotid artery, and two subclavian arteries. The most common variation of this condition is a right aortic arch that begins to descend on the right but crosses behind the esophagus to the left where it descends further. If the ductus arteriosus arises from the descending aorta and communicates with the left pulmonary artery, a vascular ring is created. An even less common variation includes a right aortic arch that continues to descend on the right side but gives rise to an aberrant left subclavian artery. A vascular ring is again created if a ductus arteriosus arises from the left subclavian artery and communicates with the left pulmonary artery. A variety of other vascular

arrangements occur with cervical aortic arch but do not form vascular rings. Even in those arterial arrangements in which a vascular ring is present, symptoms occur in only about half of the patients.[12]

Clinical Features

In patients with a vascular ring, the hemodynamics are generally normal unless structural cardiac anomalies are associated. Symptoms in patients with a vascular ring, if they occur, are almost always caused from compression of the trachea or esophagus.[2, 6, 13] Although dysphagia can occur in unusual instances, the most common symptoms are related to tracheal compression and include stridor, wheezing, and other forms of dyspnea, all of which may become worse with feeding. The age at onset of symptoms and the severity depend on the type of vascular ring. Double aortic arch presents early in life, and infants may have severe respiratory distress. Patients with other forms of vascular ring, such as right aortic arch with anomalous left subclavian artery and left ductus arteriosus, usually present later in life and have milder symptoms.

The natural history of vascular rings depends on the severity of the lesion. In the most severe illness, the respiratory symptoms resulting from vascular rings can be fatal.[14] If the particular anomaly present is unrecognized, patients may have recurrent pneumonia or difficulty eating, especially in swallowing solid foods. If the vascular ring does not cause compression of the trachea or esophagus, a patient has no symptoms at all.

On physical examination, findings relate to airway compression. Infants with a relatively tight vascular ring may have stridor at rest or may develop respiratory distress only when they are agitated on feeding. They often hyperextend the neck. Episodes of cyanosis, apnea, or unconsciousness may occur. In the absence of associated structural heart disease, the cardiac examination is normal. In cervical aortic arch, a pulsatile mass may be noted at the base of the neck, and there may be an associated thrill and systolic murmur at the same location. Diminution or disappearance of the femoral pulses during compression of the mass has been considered pathognomonic of cervical aortic arch.[12]

Any of these patients may have the CATCH-22 (DiGeorge) syndrome, a condition that should be excluded.

Electrocardiography is normal unless there is concomitant structural heart disease. In patients with milder forms of airway obstruction, a mild degree of right ventricular hypertrophy develops during months or years, because of chronic obstructive airway disease.

Radiography of the chest is helpful if not diagnostic of the specific lesions, in most instances. An abnormality of the aortic arch vessels may be suggested by deviation of the trachea. For example, a right-sided aortic arch in a patient with persistent or recurrent respiratory symptoms should suggest the possibility of a vascular ring. The findings on the plain chest radiograph are nonspecific, however. A barium swallow, on the other hand, has proved to be an extremely valuable diagnostic study.[15, 16] In patients suspected of having a vascular ring, both posterior-anterior and lateral views should be obtained, and fluoroscopy might be considered. In patients with a double aortic arch, the posterior-anterior view demonstrates bilateral indenta-

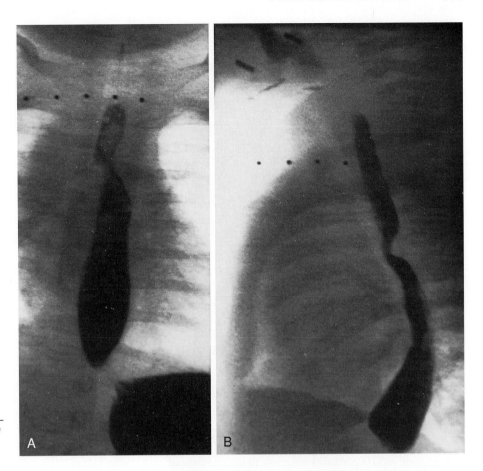

Double aortic arch, posterior-anterior (*A*) and lateral (*B*) chest radiograph and barium esophagogram.

tion on the upper esophagus (Fig. 41–2). The lateral view shows indentation of the esophagus posteriorly. In patients with an aberrant subclavian artery, the frontal view demonstrates an oblique filling defect on the barium column. In a patient with a left aortic arch and an aberrant right subclavian artery, the filling defect courses superiorly and to the right; in patients with a right aortic arch and aberrant left subclavian artery, the filling defect is in the opposite direction.

Two-dimensional echocardiography is a valuable diagnostic tool for patients with suspected vascular ring, especially in patients with double aortic arch.[17–19] This technique has eliminated the need for cardiac catheterization and cineangiography. The most helpful view is obtained from the suprasternal notch or high parasternal locations. The laterality of the aortic arch can be determined not only from the position of the transducer during visualization of the ascending aorta but also by the direction of the first brachiocephalic artery. In the normal patient with a left aortic arch, the initial branch is the innominate artery, which courses to the right and bifurcates into separate carotid and subclavian arteries. If the initial branch from the ascending aorta does not bifurcate, an aberrant subclavian artery should be sought and can often be visualized arising from the descending aorta. Similarly, in a patient with a right aortic arch and mirror-image branching of the brachiocephalic arteries, an opposite pattern can be found. In patients with double aortic arch, two separate aortic arches can be visualized, each giving rise to separate carotid and subclavian arteries (Fig. 41–3). If questions re-

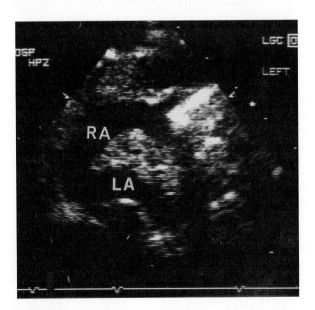

FIGURE 41–3

Double aortic arch, echocardiogram. Double aortic arch recorded from an oblique suprasternal notch position. LA = left-sided arch; RA = right-sided arch.

main, magnetic resonance imaging can be performed. Cardiac catheterization and cineangiography should be undertaken only if more anatomic detail is necessary before operative intervention. Intracardiac hemodynamic

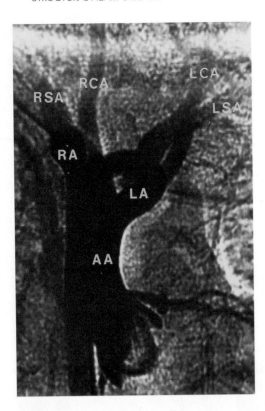

FIGURE 41–4

Double aortic arch, ascending aortogram. As depicted in Figure 41–1, the brachiocephalic arteries arise separately. AA = ascending aorta; LA = left aortic arch; LCA = left carotid artery; LSA = left subclavian artery; RA = right aortic arch; RCA = right carotid artery; RSA = right subclavian artery.

parameters are abnormal only if a cardiac anomaly is associated. Aortography, or left ventriculography in some instances, demonstrates the anatomy (Fig. 41–4). Angulated views should be used because overlying shadows may obscure the anatomy if only the posterior, anterior, and lateral projections are obtained.

Patients presenting with symptoms of respiratory or feeding difficulties shown to be due to a vascular ring should undergo an operation.[20–23] In patients with a double aortic arch, the decision regarding where to divide the arch depends on the specific anatomy. In general, division of the smaller of the two aortic arches is undertaken. Because the right-sided aortic arch is usually the dominant structure, a left thoracotomy is usually chosen.[22] The left (anterior) arch is usually divided distal to the left subclavian artery, which results in the anatomy of a right-sided aortic arch with mirror-image branching of the brachiocephalic arteries. The aortic arch can also be divided between the left carotid and left subclavian arteries. For those patients with an aberrant retroesophageal subclavian artery, surgery is usually performed through a thoracotomy opposite to the side of the aortic arch so that the ductus arteriosus or ligamentum arteriosum can be divided between the retroesophageal subclavian artery and the ipsilateral pulmonary artery. In patients with a cervical aortic arch and associated vascular ring, the operative technique is based on the specific anatomy of the lesion.

In general, the prognosis of these patients depends on the exact anatomy and severity of the vascular ring. If untreated, the symptoms that brought the individual to medical attention persist, and death can occur from pulmonary disease secondary to the compromised airway.[13] If an operation is undertaken, the prognosis for full recovery is excellent. Patients presenting in infancy, who are likely to have a double aortic arch, can be expected to have persistent respiratory symptoms after surgical relief of the vascular ring because of tracheomalacia. In time, the airway compression improves, unless another abnormality involving the trachea, such as complete tracheal rings, coexists.[23–25]

Future directions are likely to be determined only by changes in surgical technique. For example, these lesions may become easily treatable by new thoracoscopic surgical techniques, thereby obviating the need for thoracotomy.

VASCULAR SLINGS

Vascular sling refers to a condition in which the left pulmonary artery arises anomalously from the right pulmonary artery.[26] It is considered an abnormality of the sixth aortic arch system. In this condition, the pulmonary trunk is normal, but rather than bifurcating into the branch pulmonary arteries, it continues as the right pulmonary artery only. The left pulmonary artery then arises as a proximal branch of the right pulmonary artery and passes between the trachea and esophagus, proceeding to the hilum of the left lung posterior to the left main stem bronchus (Fig. 41–5). This anatomic configuration often results in

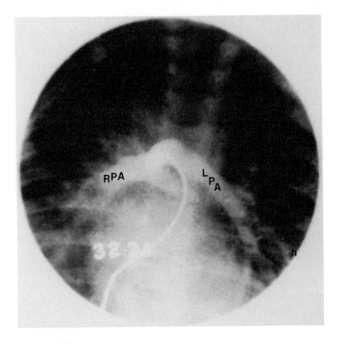

FIGURE 41–5

Pulmonary artery sling. Posterior-anterior projection of a pulmonary arteriogram. Left pulmonary artery (LPA) arises from proximal right pulmonary artery (RPA) and courses leftward between esophagus and trachea to reach hilum of left lung.

compression of the right main stem bronchus and lower trachea, causing airway obstruction with subsequent respiratory distress, the most common presenting symptom.[27,28] Although variations in anatomic features have been described, the anomalous left pulmonary artery is usually the only arterial supply to the left lung. In half of patients, associated cardiac anomalies are present.[28,29] In addition, a variety of malformations of the trachea and bronchi can be present and may be the cause of much of the respiratory problems. The most significant tracheal malformation is complete cartilaginous rings, which may require surgical intervention along with the repair of the cardiac anomaly.[30]

Hemodynamic findings are normal in the absence of associated cardiac malformations. In patients with normal hearts, abnormal hemodynamic findings are secondary to severe obstructive airway disease.

Most patients with a pulmonary artery sling present in infancy with severe respiratory symptoms, often with overinflation of the right lung. Significant morbidity and death can occur without prompt intervention. Even when an operation is undertaken, the mortality rate remains considerable. The presentation of this anomaly may be variable, however, and it may be found incidentally in adolescents and adults.[31,32]

Significant findings on history and physical examination relate either to associated structural heart disease or to respiratory symptoms. In mild forms of pulmonary artery sling, history and physical examination findings are normal. Symptoms of severe respiratory distress or stridor should raise suspicion for this diagnosis.

The chest radiograph may show deviation of the lower end of the trachea toward a leftward and inferior position. There may also be evidence of air trapping in the right lung. The most diagnostic radiographic procedure is a barium swallow. Pulmonary artery sling is the only vascular anomaly that results in anterior indentation of the esophagus (see Fig. 10–22).[26,33,34] Although this finding is almost pathognomonic, other diagnostic modalities can confirm the diagnosis. Echocardiography demonstrates the absence of normal pulmonary artery bifurcation and the anomalous origin of the left pulmonary artery from the proximal right pulmonary artery. Cardiac catheterization and pulmonary artery angiography should be undertaken if an operation is being considered, both to exclude a cardiac abnormality and to demonstrate variations of the blood supply into the left lung.[31,32]

In symptomatic patients, an operation is necessary. The most common operation is division of the left pulmonary artery from the right pulmonary artery with subsequent reimplantation into the pulmonary trunk after transposing the left pulmonary artery anterior to the trachea.[35–37] An alternative has been suggested in which the trachea is transected and moved posterior to the anomalous left pulmonary artery.[38] An operation on the trachea itself is often necessary for those patients who have associated primary airway disease, such as complete cartilaginous rings.

The prognosis for patients with pulmonary artery sling depends, largely, on the degree of airway obstruction at presentation. In patients with severe symptoms, urgent intervention may be necessary in infancy. Milder cases may not require an operation, and this anomaly may occasionally go unrecognized for many years and never require treatment.[32]

MISCELLANEOUS CONDITIONS

Vascular compression of the trachea and esophagus can occur in the absence of a vascular ring. On occasion, an innominate artery compresses the trachea and may need a pexy procedure to move it.

A number of other variations of the origin of the brachiocephalic arteries occur and are listed in Table 41–1.

REFERENCES

1. Edwards JE: "Vascular rings" related to anomalies of the aortic arches. Mod Concepts Cardiovasc Dis 17:19, 1948.
2. Shuford WH, Sybers RG: The Aortic Arch and Its Malformations with Emphasis on the Angiographic Features. Springfield, IL, Charles C Thomas, 1974.
3. Ekstrom G, Sandblom P: Double aortic arch. Acta Chir Scand 102:183, 1952.
4. Griswold HE, Young MD: Double aortic arch: Report of two cases and review of the literature. Pediatrics 4:751, 1949.
5. Knight L, Edwards JE: Right aortic arch: Types and associated cardiac anomalies. Circulation 50:1047, 1974.
6. Kommerell B: Verlagerung des Osophagus durch eine abnorm verlaufende Arteria sublavia dextra (Arteria lusoria). Fortschr Geb Rontgenstr 54:590, 1936.
7. Edwards JE: Malformations of the aortic arch system manifested as "vascular rings." Lab Invest 2:56, 1953.
8. McFaul R, Millard P, Nowicki E: Vascular rings necessitating right thoracotomy. J Thorac Cardiovasc Surg 82:306, 1981.
9. Edwards JE: Retro-esophageal segment of the left aortic arch, right ligamentum arteriosum and right descending aorta causing a congenital vascular ring about the trachea and esophagus. Proc Staff Meet Mayo Clin 23:108, 1948.
10. Park SC, Siewers RD, Neches WH, et al: Left aortic arch with right descending aorta and right ligamentum arteriosum: A rare form of vascular ring. J Thorac Cardiovasc Surg 71:779, 1976.
11. Berman W Jr, Yabek SM, Dillon T, et al: Vascular ring due to left aortic arch and right descending aorta. Circulation 63:458, 1981.
12. Mullins CE, Gillette PC, McNamara DG: The complex of cervical aortic arch. Pediatrics 51:210, 1973.
13. Gross RE, Neuheuser EBD: Compression of the trachea or esophagus by vascular anomalies: Surgical therapy in 40 cases. Pediatrics 7:69, 1951.
14. Wolman IJ: Syndrome of constricting double aortic arch in infancy. J Pediatr 14:527, 1939.
15. Neuheuser EBD: The roentgen diagnosis of double aortic arch and other anomalies of the great vessels. Am J Roentgenol Radium Ther Nucl Med 56:1, 1946.
16. Stewart JR, Kincaid OW, Titus JL: Right aortic arch: Plain film diagnosis and significance. Am J Roentgenol Radium Ther Nucl Med 97:377, 1966.
17. Sahn DJ, Valdes-Cruz LM, Ovitt TW, et al: Two-dimensional echocardiography and intravenous digital video subtraction angiography for diagnosis and evaluation of double aortic arch. Am J Cardiol 50:342, 1982.
18. Celano V, Pieroni DR, Gingell RL, Roland JMA: Two-dimensional echocardiographic recognition of the right aortic arch. Am J Cardiol 51:1507, 1983.
19. Enderlein MA, Silverman NH, Stanger P, Heymann MA: Usefulness of suprasternal notch echocardiography for diagnosis of double aortic arch. Am J Cardiol 57:359, 1986.
20. Gross RE: Surgical relief for tracheal obstruction from a vascular ring. N Engl J Med 233:586, 1945.
21. Wychulis AR, Kincaid OW, Weidman WH, Danielson GK: Congenital vascular rings. Surgical considerations and results of operation. Mayo Clin Proc 46:182, 1971.

22. Arciniegas E, Hakimi M, Hertzler JH, et al: Surgical management of congenital vascular rings. J Thorac Cardiovasc Surg 77:721, 1979.

23. Backer CL, Ilbawi MN, Idriss FS, DeLeon SY: Vascular anomalies causing tracheo-esophageal compression: Review of experience in children. J Thorac Cardiovasc Surg 97:725, 1989.

24. Gross RE: Arterial malformations which cause compression of the trachea or esophagus. Circulation 11:124, 1955.

25. Eklof O, Ekstrom G, Eriksson BO, et al: Arterial anomalies causing compression of the trachea and/or oesophagus. Acta Paediatr Scand 60:81, 1971.

26. Contro S, Miller RA, White H, Potts WJ: Bronchial obstruction due to pulmonary artery anomalies. I: Vascular sling. Circulation 17:418, 1958.

27. Murphy DR, Dunbar FS, MacEwan DW, et al: Tracheobronchial compression due to a vascular sling. Surg Gynecol Obstet 118:572, 1964.

28. Sade RM, Rosenthal A, Fellows K, Castaneda AR: Pulmonary artery sling. J Thorac Cardiovasc Surg 69:333, 1975.

29. Jacobson JH, Morgan BC, Andersen DH, Humphreys GH III: Aberrant left pulmonary artery: A correctable cause of respiratory obstruction. J Thorac Cardiovasc Surg 39:602, 1960.

30. Berdon WE, Baker DH, Wung JT, et al: Complete cartilage-ring tracheal stenosis associated with anomalous left pulmonary artery: The ring-sling complex. Radiology 152:57, 1984.

31. Gumbiner CH, Mullins CE, McNamara DG: Pulmonary artery sling. Am J Cardiol 45:311, 1980.

32. Dupuis C, Vaksmann G, Pernot C, et al: Asymptomatic form of left pulmonary artery sling. Am J Cardiol 61:177, 1988.

33. Capitanio MA, Ramos R, Kirkpatrick JA: Pulmonary sling: Roentgen observations. Am J Roentgen 112:28, 1971.

34. Berdon WE, Baker DH: Vascular anomalies and the infant lung: Rings, slings, and other things. Semin Roentgenol 7:39, 1972.

35. Lenox CC, Crisler C, Zuberbuhler JR, et al: Anomalous left pulmonary artery. Successful management. J Thorac Cardiovasc Surg 77:748, 1979.

36. Koopot R, Nikaidoh H, Idriss FS: Surgical management of anomalous left pulmonary causing tracheobronchial obstruction. J Thorac Cardiovasc Surg 69:239, 1975.

37. Backer CL, Idriss FS, Holinger MD, Mavroudis C: Pulmonary artery sling: Results of surgical repair in infancy. J Thorac Cardiovasc Surg 103:683, 1992.

38. Jonas RA, Spevak PJ, McGill T, Castaneda AR: Pulmonary artery sling: Primary repair by tracheal resection in infancy. J Thorac Cardiovasc Surg 97:548, 1989.

CHAPTER 42
ARTERIOVENOUS FISTULAE AND ALLIED LESIONS

CARLO KALLFELZ

GENERAL ASPECTS

DEFINITION AND CLASSIFICATION

Arteriovenous (AV) fistulae are anomalous vascular connections between arteries and veins by which the capillary bed is partially bypassed. These lesions occur in all regions of the body, in the systemic as well as in the pulmonary circulation. In the heart, the fistulae may enter a cardiac chamber, hence the term *coronary-cameral fistula.* Large fistulae cause congestive heart failure, whereas small fistulae cause only local effects.

The classification proposed by Mulliken and Glowacki,[1] based on clinical appearance, histology, histochemistry, and tissue culture, separates the lesions into two groups: *hemangiomas,* which can proliferate or involute; and *vascular malformations,* which are subdivided according to structure, number, and size of the abnormal vessels (Table 42–1).

PREVALENCE

AV malformations leading to significant hemodynamic alterations are rare, accounting for less than 1% of congenital cardiovascular lesions.[2] Coronary AV or coronary-cameral anomalies constitute 0.2 to 0.4% of all congenital cardiac anomalies.[3,4] They have been found in 0.08 to 0.18% of routine coronary angiograms in adults and make up 8 to 13% of the congenital coronary artery anomalies observed in these studies.[5,6] In a 10-year experience at the Mayo Clinic,[7] mainly with older children and adults, most fistulae occurred in the extremities, about one third were seen within the lungs, and less than 10% were around the neck and face; no cerebral and intra-abdominal AV fistulae were encountered. In the series of Knudson and Alden,[8] however, in 156 patients younger than 6 months, more than 50% (n = 81) were intracranial and almost 40% (n = 61) in the liver, the remainder being in the lungs. These differences of local distribution are due to the age of the patients[9] and the hemodynamic significance at presentation dependent on the site and size of shunting. With the exception of intracranial AV malformations, which show a male preponderance, the lesions affect both sexes equally.

Acquired AV fistulae of the systemic circulation, commonly caused by trauma, play a minor role in childhood. However, following the growing number of invasive vascular procedures, they have increased during the last two decades in the young.

Multiple small intrapulmonary AV shunts may develop in patients with chronic liver disease, mainly cirrhosis,[10,11] and after cavopulmonary (unilateral and bilateral) shunts.[12–15]

Angiomatous anomalies constitute the great majority of vascular lesions, being present in up to 10% of newborns if all vascular birthmarks are included.[16,17] Hemodynamically significant hemangiomas and hemangioendotheliomas present with a high female preponderance.[17] The Rendu-Osler-Weber syndrome (hereditary hemorrhagic telangiectasia) is rare in children. The frequency of the disease is assumed to be 1 in 16,000.[18]

EMBRYOLOGY, GENETICS, AND ETIOLOGY

The vascular system develops between the 5th and 10th weeks of embryonic life, and its abnormalities are probably the result of persistence of primitive vessel connections.[19,20] Capillary endothelial cells may play the most important role in creating the vascular network.[21] Coronary-cameral fistulae may result from persistence of the wide intertrabecular spaces of the primitive myocardium, and coronary-to-pulmonary arterial fistulae probably result from communication between the primitive coronary arteries and the mediastinal plexus of vessels. Not all malformations can be explained by developmental arrest. Some behave like neoplasms,[22] for instance, proliferating hemangiomas and hemangioendotheliomas, and some may show spontaneous involution.

The vascular anomaly is often associated with abnormalities of neighboring tissues, but whether the AV malformation leads to the abnormalities or whether the combined lesion is produced by a common causative factor is uncertain. Typical examples are the grossly deformed hypertrophied extremities in the Klippel-Trénaunay-Weber syndrome. The abnormality is usually obvious at birth but becomes more pronounced as the patients grow. On the other hand, hereditary hemorrhagic telangiectasia, transmitted as an autosomal dominant trait, can be diagnosed only later in life: The vasculature seems to be normal at birth but becomes abnormal with time: a structural weakness leads to a dilatation of the wall of small arteries, arterioles, and capillaries, producing visible telangiectasias (skin and mucous membranes) and progressively growing AV fistulae, particularly involving the liver, the lungs, and the brain.[23,24] McAllister and colleagues[18] demonstrated that the basic molecular abnormality is a defective synthesis of endoglin, a membrane glycoprotein expressed on human endothelial cells. This abnormality leads to poor re-

TABLE 42–1

CLASSIFICATION OF ARTERIOVENOUS LESIONS

Measure	Vascular Malformation	Hemangioma
Present at birth	90%	30%
Tumor-like	–	+
Spontaneous growth	–	+
Female/male	1/1	5/1
Basement membranes of vascular walls	Thin	Thick
Vascular stroma	–	+
Mast cells per high power field	<1	>25
Tissue culture	Almost impossible	Easy
Angiogenesis in vitro	No	Yes
Capillary formation		
Cell culture	No	1–2 mo
Clot culture	No	5 days
Proliferating cell nuclear antigen	?	±
Type IV collagenase	–	+
Vascular endothelial growth factor	?	±
Fibroblast growth factor	–	+
Inhibition of cellular proliferation by interferon alfa	–	+

Modified from Mulliken JB, Young AE (eds): Vascular Birthmarks: Hemangiomas and Malformations. Philadelphia, WB Saunders, 1988, and extended by recent data.

sponse of the cells to transforming growth factor β_1, a potent mediator of vascular remodeling. Deletions in the long arm of chromosome 9 (q33 to q34) have been identified as the underlying cause.

PATHOLOGIC ANATOMY

AV fistulae show four different vascular patterns:

- Large truncal arterial and venous channels called truncal AV fistulae
- Several smaller AV fistulae, directly connecting the arterial to the venous system, named macrofistulae
- Multiple small arteries join to the draining veins by a "nidus" known as a microfistulous malformation, also called a plexiform AV lesion
- Capillary hemangiomas composed of masses of rapidly proliferating endothelial cells and with vascular channels of different size

Examples of truncal AV fistulae are aneurysm of the great vein of Galen and coronary-cameral fistulae. Many peripheral AV malformations belong to the second type, but truncal and macrofistulous lesions are often present in the same angioma. The third category, the microfistulous AV malformation, may be difficult to assess in practice, because there are vague transitions between the second pattern and capillary angiomas. A mixture of histologic features characteristic of both types is often present in one lesion. Because of this, an exact classification of each vascular malformation is sometimes difficult or even impossible. Therefore, it seems appropriate to name all these lesions AV malformations.[17, 24, 25]

The tortuous and dilated arterial vessels may develop aneurysms. On histopathologic examination, the vessel wall is frequently dysplastic, the smooth muscle cells being hypertrophied and disorganized. The internal elastic lamina is fragmented and sometimes missing. The endothelium consists of a flat and single layer of cells and contains a normal number of mast cells. There is no tendency for endothelial proliferation. The structure of the venous walls resembles that of an artery. These anomalous channels are characterized by reactive hyperplasia of the smooth muscle cells and later by degenerative changes such as fibrosis; multiple thrombi, even calcified, are sometimes present.[17, 26]

In infancy and childhood, almost all AV malformations are single or involve a single localized area only. Regions of predilection are brain,[24, 27] thorax,[28] and lungs[7, 29] and the extremities and liver.[8] In older patients, the diffusely disseminated lesions in hereditary hemorrhagic teleangiectasia affect all organs.[18, 23, 24]

Larger AV fistulae may affect the surrounding tissue by their size or by dilatation of the draining veins that compress neighborhood structures; for instance, an intracranial aneurysm may lead to local ischemia and collateral edema in the brain.[24] In addition, a steal phenomenon may play a major role.

In older children or in adults, grossly dilated aneurysms may rupture. The resulting hemorrhage[24, 30] is often life-threatening.

Large AV fistulous malformations rarely develop in the placenta. They lead to a hyperkinetic circulation in the fetus and to considerably enlarged umbilical and central venous and arterial vessels.[31]

PATHOPHYSIOLOGY AND HEMODYNAMICS

The disturbances due to AV malformations and hemangiomas depend mainly on the age of the patient and on

1. The size and region of the (systemic or pulmonic) AV shunt
2. The steal phenomenon
3. Compression or dilatation of adjacent structures
4. Alterations of vascular autoregulation
5. Disturbances in coagulation
6. Hemorrhage due to vessel rupture

The hemodynamic alterations depend on the amount of and direction of blood shunted. Thus, volume overloading is most pronounced in truncal and macrofistulous lesions. In the neonatal period, AV fistulous malformations in the central nervous system and hemangioendotheliomas of the liver are causes of serious congestive heart failure,[8, 9, 32–37] a form of high-output failure. These patients resemble those with a widely open arterial duct leading to a big left-to-right shunt with all its consequences. High pulse pressure and markedly increased flow velocity in the afferent and efferent vessels due to the low resistance in the malformation are constant features. A steal phenomenon accentuated by a loss of arterial autoregulation in the surrounding tissue causes regional hypoperfusion that may provoke collateral edema and even hemorrhage in cerebral lesions. Ischemia has also been documented in tissue surrounding hepatic and pulmonic AV malformations.[38–41]

If the malformation allows a large shunt prenatally, intrauterine congestive heart failure may develop and lead to fetal hydrops. Another serious consequence occurs postnatally. Because of the markedly increased cardiac output, the cardiac workload is elevated and myocardial oxygen consumption increases. The low peripheral resistance due to large AV fistulae causes a low diastolic pressure and diminishes the blood supply to all organs even more.[32] In early infancy, the increased myocardial oxygen requirement caused by the high volume load is met almost entirely by increasing the heart rate, leading to a shortened diastolic filling that adds to myocardial dysfunction and initiates a vicious circle. In a neonate, too, the foramen ovale and the arterial duct are patent, the pulmonary vascular resistance is elevated, and the right ventricle is relatively hypertrophic and less compliant than normal. This hemodynamic pattern together with the low systemic resistance resulting from the AV fistula and the increased systemic venous return leads to a right-to-left shunt through both connections and thus lowers arterial oxygen saturation.

The pathophysiologic features in neonates with large AV fistulous malformations are impressive. In contrast, the hemodynamic alterations in infants and older children and more so in adults are less remarkable because these patients have hemodynamically less significant lesions. The development of significant heart failure is the exception in this age group. Nonetheless, a hemodynamically insignificant AV malformation may lead to serious complications, depending on its location. Examples are intracranial or intraspinal hemorrhage, provoking seizures, and subdural or subarachnoid bleeding, gastrointestinal bleeding, hemoptysis, and others.

NATURAL HISTORY

The lesions allowing a large shunt, such as many of the intracranial, intrahepatic, and intrapulmonary AV fistulae, may cause severe heart failure within the early neonatal period, eventually leading to death if untreated. An additional problem in large hemangiomas is thrombocytopenia as part of the Kasabach-Merritt syndrome,[42] which may lead to profuse bleeding that is difficult to control.

Hemangiomas and hemangioendotheliomas often regress spontaneously. Involution rarely starts before the sixth month of life, except if it is induced by corticosteroids[16, 43–45] or α-interferon. The biologic activity of these vascular tumors may be monitored by measuring the level of the basic fibroblast growth factor in the urine.[46] Thus, the response to therapy can be evaluated.

HISTORY AND PHYSICAL EXAMINATION

Symptoms and signs produced by systemic or pulmonic AV fistulae vary according to their location and size, their hemodynamic significance, and the patient's age at presentation. Neonates with large AV shunts present with a history of irritability, restlessness, poor feeding, breathlessness, pallor, or cyanosis. Rarely, the babies have had intrauterine congestive heart failure as manifested by hydrops at birth. Neonatal congestive heart failure was present in 50% of the patients with hepatic AV malformations in the series of

Knudson and Alden[8] and in more than 90% of the infants with intracranial lesions of the vein of Galen type.[47]

Many young patients present with a hyperkinetic circulatory state causing tachycardia, bounding peripheral pulses, and wide pulse pressures. A systolic or continuous soft murmur can usually be detected over the region affected. The correct diagnosis may be missed initially if there are no distinct external abnormalities, except for general signs of congestive heart failure, and the heart and great vessels seem to be structurally normal although enlarged on echocardiogram. A key to the diagnosis is often the hypercirculatory state that cannot be easily explained except by an arterial runoff. The next step should be careful auscultation of the abdomen, thorax, and skull. A thrill or a murmur often alerts the examiner to the underlying lesion.

If the lesions are hemodynamically less significant, symptoms and signs develop later and are less prominent.

Neurologic symptoms such as headaches, seizures, transitory speech disorders, and local numbness as well as ocular disturbances are common in patients with hereditary hemorrhagic teleangiectasia. Dizziness, vertigo, paresthesia and tinnitus, and even hemiplegia are also reported beyond adolescence.[24] Both sexes are equally affected.

ELECTROCARDIOGRAPHY

The electrocardiogram does not contribute to the diagnosis, because its pattern is nonspecific. However, it might demonstrate changes compatible with myocardial ischemia. In neonates with a large cerebral AV fistula, variable ST segment and T wave changes have been reported[34] in a high percentage. At necropsy, subendocardial myocyte necrosis involving mainly the right ventricle was detected in a large number of these lesions. In the neonate, right axis deviation and right ventricular hypertrophy are common, whereas in older infants and children, left ventricular hypertrophy is found. In most older infants and children with hemodynamically insignificant AV malformations, the electrocardiogram is normal.

RADIOGRAPHIC FEATURES

The size and configuration of the heart are usually normal. In symptomatic infants with large AV shunts, however, the cardiac silhouette is significantly enlarged. In addition to cardiomegaly, both the aorta and pulmonary artery are enlarged, and increased pulmonary markings and sometimes pulmonary edema are noted.

ULTRASONOGRAPHY

Two-dimensional ultrasonography and color Doppler ultrasonography are the most important diagnostic tools. These techniques not only allow a qualitative diagnosis but also give a clear picture of the localization, extent, and hemodynamic significance of the AV malformation. Suspicion of an AV fistulous lesion should arise whenever the aorta and one or more of the big central arteries and, of course, the draining veins are dilated. On echocardiography, the cardiac anatomy is normal, but all the chambers and central vessels involved in the increased blood flow are enlarged.[48]

According to its site, size, and hemodynamic importance, each fistulous malformation produces different but characteristic patterns. These are described later in their respective sections.

ADDITIONAL NONINVASIVE IMAGING TECHNIQUES

Computed tomography (CT) and magnetic resonance imaging (MRI) are by far the best and most reliable imaging techniques for exact localization and demonstration of the extent and nature of AV malformations in all regions of the body. CT using the conventional or the fast spiral technique produces excellent images of the anatomy[49]; MRI allows in addition a biologic classification.[24,50]

The application of contrast material enhances the visibility of vascular structures on CT, thus demonstrating the hypervascularity of the lesions. MRI is in some respects superior to CT; it does not involve radiation, and the vascular nature of the malformation can be demonstrated clearly without additional application of contrast material. High-flow lesions are impressively visualized by T2-weighted spin-echo images that allow distinct differentiation from adjacent soft tissue structures. T1-weighted images are especially useful in showing both the solid tissues (for instance, bones) and the increased blood flow in hemangiomas. The size, shape, and relationship of the lesions to the adjacent structures are even better demonstrated on three-dimensional reconstructions.

Besides being time-consuming and needing general anesthesia in infants and young children, the only disadvantage of these imaging modalities is seen in postinterventional artifacts produced by embolizing agents. Ferromagnetic coils interfere with the imaging process, leading to voiding of the signal flow when CT is used; in addition, they are a contraindication for MRI at least for several months after placement, because of potential migration of the coils induced by the magnetic forces.[24] Therefore, more and more, platinum devices that have no ferromagnetic properties are used for embolization.[51]

CARDIAC CATHETERIZATION AND ANGIOGRAPHY

Up to the 1980s, a complete catheterization was performed in infants and children presenting with a hemodynamically significant AV malformation or an otherwise unexplained vascular anomaly to define its nature. When cardiac failure was present, high oxygen saturations were detected in the draining veins, sometimes only a small percentage lower than on the arterial side. Reliable shunt calculations, however, were impossible, because a correct mixed venous saturation could never be obtained. Nevertheless, there were serious hemodynamic alterations, like a high arterial pulse pressure, a large left-to-right shunt, and pulmonary hypertension, which could be at systemic levels in the neonate.

Whenever an AV malformation has been detected, an angiographic delineation of the lesion is necessary[25,52–58] to assess the risk of complications and to plan the therapeutic strategy. Currently, catheterization and angiography

are undertaken only to perform a therapeutic intervention at the same session, when feasible.

The goal of the angiographic investigation is to outline the origin, number, and size of the afferent arteries; to demonstrate their relationship to the arteries supplying the organ involved; and to assess the treatment that would yield the best results. Because the afferent arteries are often multiple and may originate from different arteries, selective or superselective injections of contrast material in different imaging projections will provide the complete anatomic information needed. Therefore, a biplane angiographic x-ray unit with the ability to produce images in variable axial, sagittal, and coronal angles should be used. Wherever possible, digital subtraction angiography should be used, because even with a lower application of contrast agent, the demonstration of the arterial and venous vessels is clearer and more precise. A few examples of typical angiograms in intracranial, cardiac, intra-abdominal, and peripheral AV lesions are demonstrated in Figures 42–1 to 42–4.

Angiography plays a crucial role in the diagnosis of most intrapulmonary fistulae that are difficult to visualize clearly by other imaging modalities. Angiography is also obligatory in patients with acquired fistulous communications. This applies in particular to patients with systemic venous–to–pulmonary venous shunts after a Glenn procedure or a Fontan-like operation[13,59] or systemic-to-pulmonary shunts, as seen after atrial switch procedures for transposition of the great arteries or after surgical correction of pulmonary atresia with ventricular septal defect. In those patients, arteries from the mediastinum or chest wall may be involved. Angiography is also necessary in a sequestrated lung lobe or segments receiving arterial blood from the abdominal aorta.

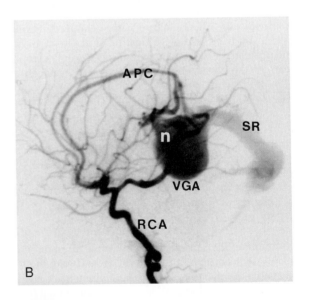

FIGURE 42–1

Vein of Galen aneurysmal malformation of the choroideal type. A, See Color Figure 42–1A. B, Cerebral angiography in a 3-month-old infant with a similar lesion. Lateral view after a right carotid artery (RCA) injection. This vessel gives rise to several fistulous arteries connected to the ectatic vein of Galen (VGA) by a nidus (n). The sinus rectus (SR) drains the VGA. Note the similarity to A. APC = arteria pericallosa.

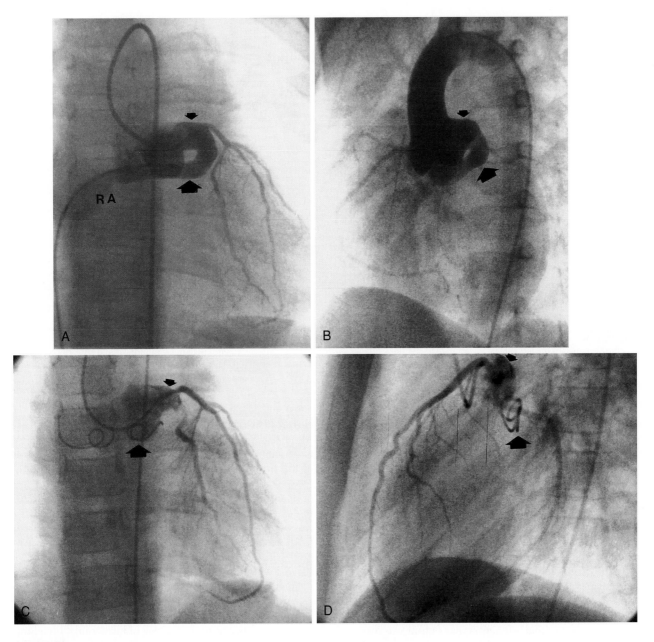

FIGURE 42–2

Coronary AV fistula to the right atrium in a 4-month-old infant with moderate heart failure. Frontal *(A)* and lateral *(B)* left coronary arteriogram. A large fistulous channel artery with a diameter of 5 to 6 mm at its origin *(large arrows)* originates from the left main coronary and runs behind the aortic root to the upper portion of the right atrium (RA). Note the extreme dilatation of the proximal left coronary artery *(small arrows). C, D,* Complete occlusion of the fistula 20 minutes after placement of a Jackson coil *(large arrows).*

MANAGEMENT AND PROGNOSIS

All patients showing signs of congestive heart failure or hemorrhage need urgent diagnostic evaluation. As soon as the true nature and significance of the malformation have been clarified, treatment should be started. In symptomatic neonates and infants with a large intracranial or hepatic AV fistula leading to serious circulatory overload, reducing the amount of shunting is the most important goal. Beyond medical treatment of congestive heart failure, which is rarely successful, surgical or catheter intervention offers better chances for improvement.[24, 60–62] Because the number of patients treated by either method is small, no reliable data on the postinterventional course and prognosis are available.

SPECIFIC REGIONAL FISTULAE

CENTRAL NERVOUS SYSTEM

Pathologic Anatomy

A typical example of a truncal AV fistula is the vein of Galen aneurysm, the result of multiple direct arterial connections to the great cerebral vein. In addition to the grossly increased arterial blood flow, associated obstructive

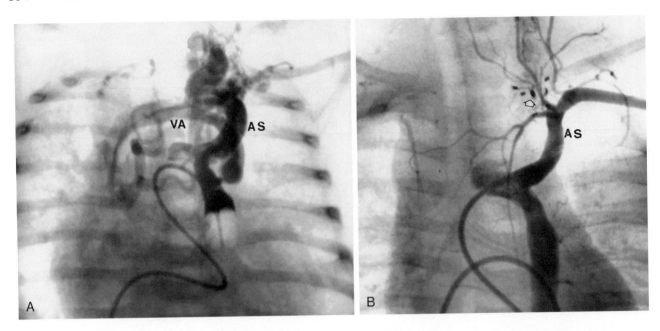

FIGURE 42-3

Large fistula between the left subclavian artery (AS) and the left innominate vein (VA). Arteriographic appearance before (*A*) and after (*B*) occlusion with a Rashkind PDA device (*arrow*). Note the steal phenomenon in the AS before treatment and its normal flow and size afterward. (*A, B,* courtesy of Professor G. Hausdorf, Hanover, Germany.)

anomalies of the draining cerebral sinuses play a significant role in causing aneurysmal dilatation of the vein of Galen. The cerebral arteries involved, mostly the anterior cerebral, the lenticulostriate, and the perforating thalamic, are markedly enlarged and tortuous.[24,32,47,63,64]

Pathophysiology

These infants have features of a huge left-to-right shunt, as described before. In addition, a steal phenomenon accentuated by a loss of arterial autoregulation in the surrounding tissue causes regional hypoperfusion and thus may provoke collateral edema and even hemorrhage in cerebral lesions. Neonates may have findings of coarctation of the aorta from relative hypoplasia of the aortic isthmus because most of the fetal left ventricular output was diverted to the head and the intracranial fistula.

Natural History

About 90% of the symptomatic newborns with a vein of Galen aneurysmal malformation die within the first week of life from intractable congestive heart failure or serious complications such as intracranial bleeding.[34] In the study of Knudson and Alden[8] of 156 infants younger than 6 months, the mortality was 64% when the AV malformation was symptomatic. Spontaneous regression of intracranial fistulous malformations occurs rarely after partial or complete thrombosis. Even if the patients with cerebral lesions survive without invasive treatment, they are prone to later serious complications such as intracranial hemorrhage, seizures, internal hydrocephalus, and mental retardation. Symptomless patients with a hemodynamically insignificant AV malformation face a risk of intracranial bleeding of 2 to 3% per year with a peak in the second and third

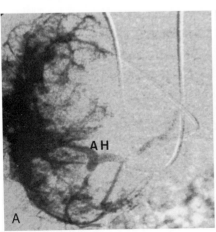
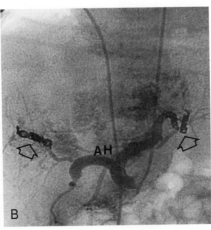

FIGURE 42-4

Hepatic hemangioendothelioma in a neonate. *A,* Large hypervascularized tumor in the right liver lobe. The catheter had been pushed from the venous side through a patent ductus arteriosus down to the hepatic artery (AH). *B,* Selective arteriography and embolization with tungsten coils (*open arrows*) was accomplished by the same route. (*A, B,* courtesy of Professor G. Hausdorf, Hanover, Germany.)

decades.[63,65] If the lesion presents with bleeding as the first sign, a 10% mortality and a 50% risk of neurologic residua are noted.[65,66]

Intracranial AV malformations with hydrocephalus sometimes produce rapid growth of head circumference and prominent, congested-looking skull veins.[64,67]

Radiologic Features

There may be superior mediastinal widening due to a dilated ascending aorta when huge intracranial fistulae are present.[27,48]

Ultrasonography

In a few patients, intracranial AV malformations have been diagnosed antenatally[68] by color flow Doppler ultrasound examination or by MRI.[69]

Intracranial lesions are readily diagnosed as long as an echo window is available, and this often happens even beyond infancy because many patients develop hydrocephalus leading to delayed closure of the anterior fontanelle. Even if this does not occur in older children, however, transcranial color-coded duplex sonography may identify these anomalies, albeit the method is inferior to other imaging modalities, such as CT and MRI.[70] Cerebral ultrasonography allows good delineation of the position and size of the lesion and its relationship to the cerebral structures as well as visualization of the resulting pathologic process, for instance, intraventricular or intracerebral bleeding and hydrocephalus. The dilated vein of Galen appears as a large fluid-filled structure with turbulent flow and thus can be easily differentiated from other echolucent intracranial structures, such as cysts or enlarged ventricles (see Fig. 42–1). Doppler and color Doppler studies often enable the experienced examiner to demonstrate the origin and number of feeding vessels and to estimate the amount of shunt flow.[71–73] However, the first suspicion of a significant intracranial AV malformation usually arises when the ascending aorta, the brachiocephalic arteries, and the draining veins are found to be dilated at echocardiographic screening. In patients with a big intracranial runoff, retrograde diastolic flow in the transverse and descending aorta may be demonstrated, just as in premature infants or neonates with a widely patent ductus arteriosus.[72] Intraspinal and paraspinal lesions usually cannot be detected by this technique, unless they are located in the neck region.

Management

AV malformations of the central nervous system, being the most frequent lesions causing symptoms in the young, have been treated aggressively during the last three decades. The results of surgery, especially in neonates and young infants, were disappointing, with either death or serious brain damage occurring in most of the patients.[32] The poor course of the critically ill neonates has been attributed partly to prenatal or perinatal cerebral tissue damage and concomitant hemorrhage or to uncontrollable heart failure due to the large AV shunt.[47,53] In published series, the outcome of symptomatic newborn infants has not been improved much by embolization of the lesions; there is still a death rate of 30 to 40%, and an additional 30 to 50% of the survivors

show serious residual brain damage.[24,67] Better survival rates of 70 to 100% were reported by Friedman and coworkers[61,74] and Ciricillo and associates,[75] but there was a high percentage of cerebral damage. Considering the even worse prognosis of neonates in heart failure without aggressive treatment, there is, however, no other option than to attempt embolization as early as is feasible. Still, a careful preinterventional assessment is mandatory, because the outcome will be poor in patients with preexisting serious brain damage, leading to either death or severe neurologic sequelae. In those infants, active intervention should be withheld. This applies specifically to neonates with encephalomalacia and perhaps even multiorgan failure.[56] It needs much expertise of the neuroradiologic interventionist and good cooperation and long experience within the group taking care of the newborn with an intracranial AV malformation to decide whether to go ahead and to determine the type of intervention.[24] Whenever the neonatal heart failure is controlled by appropriate medical treatment (digoxin, afterload reduction, diuretics, and sedation) and serious progressive brain damage can be excluded, intervention should be postponed. In a few patients, spontaneous regression early in life may occur, probably because of thrombosis of the vein of Galen.[76] The prognosis is obviously better when the patient has survived the first 3 months[24,68,75,77] and intervention can be done later.[51,67,74,78] Other complications, however, threaten the patient's prognosis. The persistently elevated cerebral venous pressure may cause two major complications:

1. Development of hydrocephalus, due to compression of the aqueduct or the third ventricle, or due to the increased cerebrospinal fluid pressure secondary to the venous hypertension compromising the reabsorption of cerebrospinal fluid[53,68,77,79]

2. Progressive ischemic brain damage, subcortical calcifications, and eventually neurologic deterioration[24,68,77]

In general, the outcome of direct surgical treatment is worse than that of endovascular embolization regardless of the size and location of the intracranial lesion and the age of the patient.[47] Neuroradiologic interventions are preferred, irrespective of the location of the intracranial AV shunt (subdural, subarachnoid, or subpial space).[24,51,80,81] The preferred approach to occlude the lesion or at least to reduce the shunt is transarterial embolization with platinum coils if the feeding vessels are large (>0.5 mm). In more plexiform AV malformations, where multiple small arteries enter the lesion, as in most of the so-called pial AV malformations, in addition to the coils or as the only embolizing agent, acrylic glue or a newer degradable material (Ethibloc) sometimes combined with silk or nylon filaments has been used.[24,51,67,80] Most patients need more than one treatment session for successful complete or almost complete occlusion. A transvenous retrograde approach is feasible but often leads to complete thrombosis of the dilated vein of Galen.[24,67] Stereotactic radiotherapy was applied in the 1980s but resulted in neurologic abnormalities in about 35 to 40% of the patients.[24] This method is today used only as an adjunctive measure to embolization when this is not completely curative.[24,51,67]

CORONARY-CAMERAL AND CORONARY ARTERIOVENOUS FISTULAE

Another common example of the truncal type is the coronary AV fistula,[82–84] 90% of which drain into the right side of the heart, usually the right ventricle, or the pulmonary artery.[85–87] About 60 to 70% of the fistulae arise from the right coronary artery. Bilateral coronary artery communications have been described, 60% of which empty into the pulmonary artery.[88] The fistulous coronary artery may be small or may be dilated and tortuous, and it enters the affected chamber by one or several openings; occasionally, plexiform lesions are seen. Saccular aneurysmal dilatation of the fistula can be seen, but spontaneous rupture is rare.[4,89] Other congenital cardiac lesions can coexist,[4,90] but most coronary artery fistulas are isolated.

Coronary AV fistulae rarely cause congestive heart failure in infancy and childhood.[20,82,84,86] Because the shunt is usually of small to moderate size, most of the patients are asymptomatic for the first 20 to 30 years of life.[83,86] Larger fistulae may cause congestive heart failure, dyspnea, fatigue, angina pectoris due to a coronary steal or accelerated atherosclerosis, or rarely myocardial infarction. They have twice been reported to rupture,[4,89] a surprising rarity because of the massive aneurysmal dilatation of the fistulae that may occur. Small fistulae, usually between a coronary artery and the pulmonary artery, may never increase in size and never cause hemodynamic problems. They may, however, develop infective endocarditis.[90,91] Spontaneous closure of fistulae has been described in four patients,[92,93] possibly as a result of infection.

Clinical Features

In coronary AV fistulae draining into the atria or the right ventricle, the resulting continuous murmur may be mistaken for a patent ductus arteriosus. The murmur is best heard at the midsternal region over the third or fourth intercostal space, however. The murmur often has a louder mid-diastolic than midsystolic component when the fistula enters the right ventricle. In coronary-to-pulmonary artery fistulae, the murmur may be heard at the upper left sternal border, and clinical differentiation from a patent ductus arteriosus is impossible.[87,94] Continuous murmurs, however, are not heard when the fistula drains into the left ventricle, and these fistulae may even be silent.[95,96] If there is a wide pulse pressure with jerky pulses and the diastolic murmur is heard along the left sternal border toward the apex, aortic incompetence may be incorrectly diagnosed.[83,97] Other features are nonspecific: signs of a large left-to-right shunt, congestive heart failure, and occasionally accentuated pulmonary valve closure. In smaller lesions of insignificant hemodynamic importance, particularly when no specific symptoms or signs are present, the clinical diagnosis is difficult or impossible.

Echocardiography

Coronary AV fistulae can be diagnosed fairly easily by echo Doppler study if the examiner is careful.[87,98] The proximal segment of the feeding coronary artery is enlarged, and whenever the arterial runoff is more than trivial, the chamber into which the fistula is draining can be identified by turbulent flow. The transesophageal approach may be helpful in difficult problems.[84]

Management

About 30% of coronary artery fistulae cause congestive heart failure in infancy,[87] and urgent intervention is indicated. Apart from this emergency, a coronary fistula should be closed as soon as the diagnosis has been made.[82,85,87] Long-term experiences of several centers have shown that with increasing age, the risk of endocarditis, congestive heart failure, or myocardial damage becomes more prominent, and the complications of surgical treatment increase.[82,85–87] On the other hand, in a few patients, spontaneous complete obliteration of a coronary fistula has been documented (personal observation).[84] Until recently, surgical interruption of the fistula was the only available therapy. The fistula was ligated near its origin and also near its entrance to the cardiac chamber when multiple fistulae were present. Proximal ligation alone may be followed by reestablishment of the fistula by collaterals that bypass the site of ligation. The operation can be done usually without cardiopulmonary bypass, but it is often necessary to open the cardiac chamber to find and ligate the points of entry. There are risks of surgery in an older patient; myocardial ischemia or infarction, thrombosis of the parent coronary artery, rupture of the fistula, and ventricular fibrillation have all been reported.[4]

Fistulae from the left anterior descending and right coronary arteries to the pulmonary artery have been closed by microparticle embolization.[99] Obviously, nonsurgical closure with particles, coils, or detachable balloons should be reserved for fistulae draining the right side of the circulation. They run the risk of proximal extension of thrombosis and also of recurrence of the fistula through small collaterals not visible at the time of the original investigation.

PERIPHERAL ARTERIOVENOUS FISTULAE

Pathologic Anatomy

When AV malformations affect a limb, generalized overgrowth of bone, muscle, and fat sometimes leads to gross disfiguration.[100,101] Parkes Weber termed this phenomenon hemiangiectatic hypertrophy. In large lesions located in one of the extremities, hypoplasia of the distal part is common, probably secondary to hypoperfusion because of a steal.[102]

Peripheral systemic AV malformations rarely cause congestive heart failure.[103,104] They may be static, may grow larger, or may even involute. When they present in the neonatal period and if they are not large, hemodynamic alterations do not occur and the course tends to be benign. Although life-threatening events are rare in infancy and early childhood, there is a tendency for complications subsequently.

Peripheral angiomatous malformations, particularly in the neck or the extremities, cause circumscribed, often nodular soft swellings that may grow. If the malformation is found in one limb and it is hemodynamically significant, it might be possible to elicit Branham's sign: digital compression of the afferent artery makes the murmur disappear, the mean arterial blood pressure increase, and the heart rate slow.

The clinical diagnosis is fairly easy in patients presenting with externally visible abnormalities indicative of vascular anomalies, such as cutaneous or subcutaneous nontender nodular, soft, compressible, prominent peripheral swellings often identifying themselves by hemangioma-like color and structure. A thrill is often felt on careful palpation. Distended veins in the neighborhood of the malformation becoming larger in their centripetal course are typical.

Radiographic Examination

In peripheral AV malformations involving the limbs, radiographs allow a rough evaluation of the size of the lesion and show the extent of hypertrophy or hypotrophy of bones in the region affected.[105]

Management

This may be done by surgical ligation of the fistula or by various occlusive devices.

PULMONARY ARTERIOVENOUS FISTULAE

Pathologic Anatomy

In the lung, there are either localized anomalies, such as isolated truncal,[106, 107] macrofistulous, or microfistulous pulmonary AV malformations, or diffuse small intrapulmonary shunting vessels that develop mostly beyond childhood in patients suffering from hereditary hemorrhagic teleangiectasia. In chronic liver disease,[10] in portal hypertension, and in patients with severe congenital heart disease late after having had a Glenn or a Fontan procedure,[12, 14, 15, 108] acquired diffuse microfistulous shunts may enlarge. The fistulae vary from small vessels to huge tubular, sometimes multilobulated structures, mostly confined to one lobe or lung. The larger isolated lesions may occupy a whole lobe and tend to be subpleural, usually involving the lower lobes.[26, 109] As the patient grows, degenerative changes may develop in the fistula and lead to vessel rupture with hemoptysis and even hemothorax.[41, 110]

Major aortopulmonary collateral arteries, persisting segmental arterial vessels, arising from the descending aorta and connecting the systemic to the pulmonic circulation in pulmonary atresia, for instance, are also AV fistulae. This also applies to systemic arteries from the abdominal aorta that supply sequestrated lung segments or lobes, as in the scimitar syndrome.

Pathophysiology

In patients with large intrapulmonary AV shunts, a variable amount of the desaturated pulmonary arterial blood is directly diverted to the pulmonary veins, resulting in arterial hypoxemia.[106]

Natural History

The few patients with a large intrapulmonary AV fistula deteriorate rapidly because of progressive heart failure and arterial desaturation. If the lesions are smaller, the immediate danger is low, but with time, an increasing risk of aneurysm formation, rupture, and life-threatening parenchymal or endobronchial bleeding develops. Further potential complications are cerebral abscesses and endocarditis. In the series reported by Sloan and Cooley,[52] 27% of patients died in childhood or adult life, 37% were alive and asymptomatic, 12% were alive but symptomatic, and 24% had died from unrelated causes. If the underlying reason for the intrapulmonary AV shunt is hereditary hemorrhagic telangiectasia, the course is prolonged. Most affected patients become cyanotic only after puberty. In the long term, however, the symptoms progress and complications occur.

Clinical Features

A history of generalized cyanosis, increasing on exercise, is more the exception than the rule in patients with intrapulmonary AV fistula. Although neonates may rarely present with congestive heart failure and cyanosis,[40, 106, 107, 111] most patients present only after 20 years of age.[29, 112] Pulmonary AV fistulae localized in one lobe tend to produce symptoms earlier in life because they are large and present from birth, whereas diffuse small AV connections as part of hereditary hemorrhagic telangiectasia develop with time and therefore may not cause suspicious symptoms until adult life.[110] In a solitary fistula, a soft continuous murmur is usually heard on one side of the back.

Asymptomatic patients are occasionally discovered by a chest x-ray examination showing an abnormal shadow.[110, 113] Others are identified by mucocutaneous telangiectasias becoming more numerous as the patient becomes older. In such patients, epistaxis and bleeding from mouth, lips, and gastrointestinal tract are frequent and recurrent. Dyspnea and fatigue appear later than cyanosis. Hemoptysis is common beyond adolescence but is rare in infants and children. Hemothorax due to rupture of subpleural lesions may manifest as pleural pain.[112, 114] Repeated blood loss may lead to anemia, thus obscuring arterial hypoxemia.[112]

Electrocardiography

Only those with a huge intrapulmonary shunt due to large fistulae or the rare direct communication between pulmonary artery and left atrium[106] may show left axis deviation, left atrial enlargement, and left ventricular hypertrophy.[41]

Radiologic Findings

In patients with intrapulmonary AV malformations, cardiomegaly is seen only with a large shunt, but unilateral or bilateral rounded opacities are apparent in about 50% of the patients.[52, 113] These homogeneous and well-circumscribed lesions are seen in the peripheral lung fields. The afferent and efferent vessels sometimes may be identified as cord-like stalks reaching to the hilum.[29] Intrapulmonary AV fistulae are almost impossible to identify directly, but on careful screening, a suspicion may be confirmed by detection of a much increased pulmonary venous blood flow on one side. In patients with large intrapulmonary shunts, the pulmonary artery branch feeding the lesion will be dilated.

Ultrasonography

In patients with large intrapulmonary shunts, the pulmonary artery branch feeding the lesion is dilated. A more reliable method of diagnosis, however, is contrast echocardiography. Peripherally injected contrast medium quickly passes through the fistulae and appears as small cavitations in the left atrium and ventricle. This phenomenon must be differentiated from an early right-to-left shunt through a patent foramen ovale. Because of its sensitivity, contrast echocardiography is widely used for the evaluation of the immediate result of interventions and for the long-term follow-up of patients with intrapulmonary AV shunts.[41, 115]

Management

Management of patients with pulmonary AV lesions depends on their number, size, structure, and hemodynamic significance. A large solitary fistula confined to one lung and causing arterial hypoxemia should be treated as early and as completely as feasible. Two therapeutic options are available: surgical excision of the segment or lobe affected[109] and transcatheter embolization.[115–117] The less invasive interventional procedure is preferred and generally yields good results with few complications.

Metal coils alone and detachable balloons[116] and metal coils in combination[117] are used. Both methods are equally successful, but coils are preferred. It is crucial to investigate carefully the location, number, and size of the lesions and to deliver the devices as distally as possible to avoid impairment of neighborhood structures. In large communications with a high flow, there exists the risk of systemic embolization. To avoid this potentially serious complication, distal placement of a spider has been advocated with additional coils until the feeding artery is completely blocked.[115] Results of treatment in AV fistulae occurring in one segment or lobe only or in single large communications between pulmonary artery and vein or left atrium[106] are in general excellent, leading to cure in most patients. The prognosis regarding permanent relief of pulmonary AV shunts is guarded when the communications are multiple and located in more than one lobe. These patients tend to form new shunts or to increase previously undetected AV shunts, and after some years, they may present with the same clinical picture.[117] This course is particularly seen in patients with the Rendu-Osler-Weber syndrome, whose prognosis therefore cannot be altered. The management of patients developing intrapulmonary AV fistulae after cavopulmonary anastomosis is still unclear.[15, 108]

HEPATIC ARTERIOVENOUS FISTULAE

Pathophysiology

Extrahepatic or prehepatic AV shunts are caused by arterioportal fistulae that may produce severe portal hypertension, giving rise to symptoms such as ascites and gastrointestinal bleeding from esophageal and intestinal venous collaterals.[20, 58, 118–120] AV shunting lesions within the liver and around the hepatic hilum behave differently, however, owing to their basic tissue structure, hemodynamic effects, consequences on neighborhood structures, and potential either to grow or to regress spontaneously. Most intrahepatic lesions are hemangioendotheliomas, densely vascularized benign tumors, often causing early congestive heart failure. In contrast to fistulous AV malformations of the liver[55] presenting with the same clinical picture, hemangioendotheliomas may undergo spontaneous involution once treatment with steroids, interferon, or partial embolization has been started.[25, 60, 121, 122]

Rydell and Hoffbauer[123] were the first to report the association of juvenile liver cirrhosis and multiple pulmonary AV fistulae. This peculiar combination has been confirmed by others.[124] These AV communications are acquired and therefore are histologically different from the usual congenital lesions. Disappearance of the intrapulmonary right-to-left shunt is reported after liver transplantation.[10] The same unknown pathologic mechanism is probably responsible for the development of intrapulmonary AV fistulae in patients with pulmonary or tricuspid atresia after palliation by cavopulmonary anastomosis (a classic Glenn or bidirectional cavopulmonary anastomosis) or a complete Fontan procedure.[12, 14, 15, 108] Kawata and associates[125] described two patients with left isomerism in whom they observed pulmonary as well as systemic AV fistulae.

Clinical Features

Hepatic hemangioendotheliomas are constantly accompanied by abdominal swelling, often extreme.[126–128] Intra-abdominal AV lesions, in particular hepatic hemangiomas, are associated with cutaneous (raspberry) hemangiomas in 30 to 40%.[8, 126]

Radiologic Features

Dilatation of the descending aorta has been described as a characteristic sign in infants with hepatic AV fistula.[48]

Ultrasonography

In patients with a dilated descending aorta and inferior caval vein, the suspicion of an AV malformation in the lower torso or limbs has to be entertained. Intra-abdominal fistulae, the majority of which are intrahepatic hemangioendotheliomas, and rarer intrahepatic AV malformations or extrahepatic arterioportal fistulae are readily visualized.[120, 128, 129] The sonographic diagnosis and localization of the rare AV fistulae of the bowel, however, are difficult.[53]

Splenic and renal AV malformations are well identified by Doppler ultrasonography.

Cardiac Catheterization and Angiography

Intrahepatic AV shunting lesions need special consideration because of their different vascular structure and variable biologic behavior.[126] Hemangioendotheliomas or infantile hemangiomas consist of highly vascular solid masses, about 60% of which are multiple with associated large afferent and efferent vessels and sponge-like parenchyma. They often receive additional arterial supply from the abdominal wall and from retroperitoneal as well as periportal vessels.[55, 130] In contrast, AV malformations in the liver consist almost entirely of high-flow vascular channels without solid cellular components[55, 130] and are supplied by the hepatic artery only. These lesions may also be multiple. Because it seems impossible to differentiate clearly between both lesions by the noninvasive methods, angiography is necessary. Careful search for all arterial vessels supplying the lesion is needed to plan therapy. In addition to the arterial flow to the lesion, extensive portal vein supply, including direct portal vein–hepatic vein fistulae, has been described,[55, 129] making the therapeutic decision even more difficult and the outcome doubtful.

Management

Hemangioendotheliomas, in general being benign tumors, can grow and regress spontaneously. Therefore, besides surgical ligation of the hepatic artery or resection of the "tumor,"[131,132] medical treatment with steroids[38,131,133] and even cytotoxins has been tried. In a few seriously impaired patients, liver transplantation has been carried out successfully.[55,127] Transcatheter hepatic artery embolization is currently the first choice for treatment. Although the AV shunt decreases, however, the benefit may be temporary, and because of new recruitment of collateral arteries, congestive heart failure may recur.[55,121] In contrast to this evolution, the patient's life is endangered by total hepatic artery occlusion if there is no collateral arterial supply to the organ.[129] Hepatic necrosis or disseminated intravascular coagulation and finally death may result. Liver transplantation is the last therapeutic option in this situation.[121] Long-term administration of interferon alfa-1 or alfa-2a has been effective in accelerating the regression of hepatic angioendotheliomas,[121,126,134] even when they are resistant to steroids. Interferon is an antiangiogenic agent that inhibits endothelial cell proliferation and migration, and it can be used in addition to embolization to treat angiomatous lesions successfully in various other anatomic sites.[117,134]

Intrahepatic AV malformations of the fistulous or angiomatous type often present with the same clinical picture as soon as they allow a large left-to-right shunt. The therapeutic strategy therefore has to be pragmatic: reduction (but no attempt at complete abolition) of the shunt by embolization. Whenever possible, the embolization procedure should be directed to selective or even superselective occlusion of the feeding vessels, avoiding complete blockage of the arterial supply because of its serious consequences.[55] With this strategy, more than one interventional session will be necessary in most patients.[130]

LESIONS RESEMBLING ARTERIOVENOUS FISTULAE

AORTIC–LEFT VENTRICULAR DEFECT (TUNNEL)

This rare lesion connects the aorta and the left ventricle with a tunnel that begins above the right coronary ostium and passes behind the right ventricular infundibulum and through the anterior upper part of the ventricular septum to enter the left ventricle just below the right and left aortic cusps.[135] It is usually short and direct but may be aneurysmal. Some investigators regard this lesion as acquired,[136] but this is unlikely because of its frequent appearance in the immediate neonatal period.

These patients often present in infancy with congestive heart failure and signs resembling marked aortic incompetence: a wide pulse pressure with a low diastolic blood pressure, a hyperactive dilated left ventricle and enlarged left atrium, and a loud to-and-fro murmur at the base. The electrocardiogram shows varying degrees of left ventricular and atrial hypertrophy. The chest radiograph shows variable cardiomegaly and possibly signs of congestive heart failure; but there is a dilated ascending aorta in all patients and a bulge of the enlarged right aortic sinus in

some. Echocardiography with Doppler color flow mapping and aortography separate this lesion from aortic incompetence by the lack of retrograde flow through the aortic valve; from a coronary artery–left ventricular fistula by normal right and left main coronary arteries; from an associated ventricular septal defect by the absence of a left-to-right shunt through the defect; and from a ruptured sinus of Valsalva by the anterior position of the tunnel and an undilated sinus of Valsalva.[137]

Treatment is surgical, but there is a high incidence of aortic incompetence after surgery.[137,138]

ANEURYSMS OF THE SINUS OF VALSALVA

A localized weakness of the wall of a sinus of Valsalva leads to aneurysmal bulging and even rupture. It is distinguished from Marfan's syndrome in which there is diffuse dilatation of all the sinuses that do not rupture. The localized aneurysms are usually congenital, with thinning just above the annulus at the leaflet hinge due to absence of normal elastic and muscular tissue.[139] However, they can follow infective endocarditis, and it may be impossible to decide whether the endocarditis is the cause or the consequence of the aneurysm or associated lesions.

Pathologic Anatomy and Physiology

About 75% of the patients are male. Two thirds of the aneurysms are located in the right aortic sinus, one quarter are in the noncoronary sinus, and the rest are in the left aortic sinus.[140–144] The aneurysms may be isolated or, in about 40%, may be associated with a ventricular septal defect,[142,143,145,146] especially in the outlet septum and when the aneurysm arises from the right sinus. With an associated ventricular septal defect, particularly if it is subpulmonic, there is often prolapse of the aortic valve cusp with aortic incompetence, similar to the association of subpulmonic ventricular septal defect with aortic incompetence without an aneurysm of the sinus of Valsalva. The aortic incompetence tends to progress as the valve prolapses further and becomes fibrous and stiff.[145,147] Coarctation of the aorta, atrial septal defect, tetralogy of Fallot, and patent ductus arteriosus may coexist. Because the aortic root is surrounded by cardiac structures, the aneurysms can rupture into any cardiac chambers, and virtually all combinations of sinus and chamber fistulae have been described. Rupture is most frequently of the right sinus aneurysm into the right ventricle, particularly if there is an outlet ventricular septal defect. The next most frequent site of rupture is into the right atrium from an aneurysm in the noncoronary sinus. Rupture into the pericardium is rare. At operation, most fistulae look like windsocks projecting from the sinus into the chamber of entry, with one or more openings near the end of the windsock.

Unruptured aneurysms may cause symptoms by obstructing the right ventricular outflow tract, distorting the aortic valve and causing aortic incompetence, compressing the left coronary artery and causing myocardial ischemia, or causing conduction disturbances or even complete heart block by compressing the conduction system.[148] Because all complications of these aneurysms depend on their size and because they grow slowly, they seldom present in infancy and early childhood. The mean age at the onset of symptoms due to sudden rupture of the aneurysms was 31 years.[140] Rupture can follow acute chest trauma or severe exertion. If the aneurysm ruptures, the size of the fistula determines how large the shunt will be, and its site of entry into the heart often determines the specific features. Aneurysmal rupture into the left side of the heart does not produce signs of a left-to-right shunt, but rupture into the right side of the heart produces a left-to-right shunt of variable size.

Infective endocarditis is an important complication of smaller fistulae and may occur in 5 to 10% of patients with a congenital aneurysm.[140]

Clinical and Laboratory Features

Before rupture, these aneurysms are diagnosed only accidentally on imaging for other lesions. Rupture may be associated with a tearing pain in the chest or upper abdomen. If a huge shunt develops rapidly, features of congestive heart failure appear almost immediately; with smaller fistulae, it may take several months for heart failure to develop.[140] About 20% of patients are asymptomatic.

With a small fistula, there may be only a continuous murmur like that of a patent ductus arteriosus but with its maximal intensity in the third or fourth intercostal space near the sternal edge or even at the xiphisternum; in a fistula entering the right atrium, the murmur may be maximal to the right of the sternum. With a larger fistula, there is a wide pulse pressure, a collapsing pulse, and left ventricular overactivity. In a right-sided fistula, there is also right ventricular overactivity. A large fistula into the left ventricle may have a to-and-fro murmur and simulate aortic incompetence. On occasion, there is only a diastolic murmur when the fistula enters the left ventricle or the high-pressure right ventricle in a neonate. If a ventricular septal defect is present, especially with infundibular obstruction, the combined murmurs can be confusing.[147]

With a large chronic fistula, the electrocardiogram shows hypertrophy of the appropriate chambers. Signs of myocardial ischemia or conduction defects occur occasionally.

With a large left-to-right shunt, the chest radiograph shows enlargement of the appropriate chambers and pulmonary overcirculation. Evidence of congestive heart failure may be seen. The aortic root is not enlarged, although rarely with aneurysms of the left sinus of Valsalva, there may be a bulge on the left aortic root border.

Two-dimensional echocardiography with Doppler color flow mapping shows the aneurysmal dilatation, even before rupture,[149] and pulsed Doppler studies show the site of drainage of the fistula.[150,151] Transesophageal echocardiography shows features not obtainable by routine transthoracic echocardiography.

Cardiac Catheterization and Angiocardiography

Cardiac catheterization data show the size of any left-to-right shunt, ventricular systolic and diastolic pressures, pulmonary hypertension, and any infundibular obstruction. Associated lesions, including coarctation of the aorta, ventricular septal defect, small patent ductus arteriosus, coronary arteriovenous fistula, and small aortopulmonary window, will be revealed.

High-quality angiography from the left ventricle and the aortic root in the long-axis and frontal views shows the aneurysm, the fistula, associated aortic incompetence, and other lesions.

Management

Congestive heart failure is treated, with emphasis on afterload reduction to minimize runoff through the fistula. Cardiopulmonary bypass is used for definitive therapy. Moderate hypothermia and cardioplegia, including perfusion of the coronary arteries, are recommended.[112] The fistula should be closed from inside the aorta so that the coronary arteries can be avoided and the aortic valve inspected and protected. The other end of the aneurysm is usually approached from within the cavity that it enters, the aneurysms are removed, and the orifices of the aneurysm and an associated ventricular septal defect are closed with patches. If aortic incompetence remains, an attempt may be made to repair the valve or, if that is not possible, to replace it.[152] An unruptured aneurysm should be repaired electively at the time of operation for the other lesions. The hospital mortality for this operation is currently below 5%.[152] Late results are excellent in the absence of aortic valve damage.[143,146]

REFERENCES

1. Mulliken JB, Glowacki J: Hemangiomas and vascular malformations in infants and children: A classification based on endothelial characteristics. Plast Reconstr Surg 69:412, 1982.
2. Musewe NN, Burrows PE, Culham JAG, Freedom RM: Arteriovenous fistulae: A consideration of extracardiac causes of congestive heart failure. In Freedom RM, Benson LN, Smallhorn JF (eds): Neonatal Heart Disease. Berlin, Springer-Verlag, 1992, p 759.
3. McNamara JJ, Gross RE: Congenital coronary artery fistula. Surgery 65:59, 1969.
4. Neufeld HN, Schneeweiss A: Coronary Artery Disease in Infants and Children. Philadelphia, Lea & Febiger, 1983.
5. Wilkins CE, Betancourt B, Mathur VS, et al: Coronary artery anomalies: A review of more than 10,000 patients from the Clayton Cardiovascular Laboratories. Tex Heart Inst J 15:166, 1988.
6. Yamanaka O, Hobbs RE: Coronary artery anomalies in 126,595 patients undergoing coronary arteriography. Cathet Cardiovasc Diagn 21:28, 1990.
7. Gomes MMR, Bernartz PE: Arteriovenous fistulas: A review and ten year experience at the Mayo Clinic. Mayo Clin Proc 45:81, 1970.
8. Knudson RP, Alden ER: Symptomatic arteriovenous malformation in infants less than 6 months of age. Pediatrics 64:238, 1979.
9. Moller JH: Arteriovenous fistula in the neonate. J Am Coll Cardiol 12:1536, 1988.
10. Laberge JM, Brandt ML, Lebecque P, et al: Reversal of cirrhosis-related pulmonary shunting in two children by orthotopic liver transplantation. Transplantation 53:1135, 1992.
11. Toyosaka A, Okamoto E, Okasora T, et al: Outcome of 21 patients with biliary atresia living more than 10 years. J Pediatr Surg 28:1498, 1993.
12. Cloutier A, Ash JM, Smallhorn JF, et al: Abnormal distribution of pulmonary blood flow after the Glenn shunt or Fontan procedure: Risk and development of arteriovenous fistulae. Circulation 72:471, 1985.
13. Leung MP, Benson LN, Smallhorn JF, et al: Abnormal cardiac signs after Fontan type of operation: Indicators of residua and sequelae. Br Heart J 61:52, 1989.
14. Puga JF: Pulmonary arteriovenous malformations after modified Fontan operation. J Thorac Cardiovasc Surg 98:1144, 1989.
15. Bernstein HS, Brook MM, Silverman NH, Bristow J: Development of arteriovenous fistulae in children after cavopulmonary shunt. Circulation 92(suppl II):II-309, 1995.

16. Mulliken JB: Classification of vascular birthmarks. *In* Mulliken JB, Young AE (eds): Vascular Birthmarks: Hemangiomas and Malformations. Philadelphia: WB Saunders, 1988, p 35.

17. Enjolras O, Riche MC, Merland JJ, Escande JP: Management of alarming hemangiomas in infancy: A review of 25 cases. Pediatrics 85:491, 1990.

18. McAllister KA, Grogg KM, Johnson DW: Endoglin, a TGF-β binding protein of endothelial cells, is the gene for hereditary haemorrhagic teleangiectasia type 1. Nat Genet 59:369, 1994.

19. Reid L: Lung growth in health and disease. Br J Dis Chest 78:113, 1984.

20. Young AE: Pathogenesis of vascular malformations. *In* Mulliken JB, Young AE (eds): Vascular Birthmarks: Hemangiomas and Malformations. Philadelphia, WB Saunders, 1988, p 107.

21. Folkman J: Toward a new understanding of vascular proliferative disease in children. Pediatrics 74:850, 1984.

22. Folkman J: How is blood vessel growth regulated in normal and neoplastic tissue? Cancer Res 46:467, 1986.

23. Lande A, Bedford A, Schechter LS: The spectrum of arteriographic findings in Osler-Weber-Rendu disease. Angiology 27:223, 1976.

24. Lasjaunias P: Vascular Diseases in Neonates, Infants and Children. Interventional Neuroradiology Management. Berlin, Springer, 1997.

25. Fellows KE: What is an arteriovenous malformation? Cardiovasc Intervent Radiol 10:53, 1987.

26. Avery JB: Cardiovascular Pathology in Infants and Children. Philadelphia, WB Saunders, 1984.

27. Schauseil-Zipf U, Thun F, Kellermann K, et al: Intracranial arteriovenous malformations and aneurysms in childhood and adolescence. Eur J Pediatr 140:260, 1983.

28. Bopp P, Faidutti B, Fornet PC, et al: Congenital arterio-venous fistula of the internal mammary vessels: Report of a case and review of the literature. J Cardiovasc Surg 18:79, 1977.

29. Dines DE, Seward JB, Bernatz PE: Pulmonary arteriovenous fistulas. Mayo Clin Proc 58:176, 1983.

30. Dehner LP, Ishak KG: Vascular tumors of the liver in infants and children. Arch Pathol 92:101, 1971.

31. Benson DF: Cardiomegaly in a newborn due to placental chorioangioma. Br Med J 262:102, 1961.

32. Holden AM, Fyler DC, Shillito J, et al: Congestive heart failure from intracranial arteriovenous fistula in infancy. Pediatrics 49:30, 1972.

33. McLean RH, Moller JH, Warwick WJ, et al: Multinodular hemangiomatosis of the liver in infancy. Pediatrics 49:563, 1972.

34. Hoffman HJ, Chuang S, Hendrichs EB, et al: Aneurysms of the vein of Galen. J Neurosurg 57:316, 1982.

35. Jedekin R, Rowe RD, Freedom RM, et al: Cerebral arteriovenous malformations in neonates: The role of myocardial ischemia. Pediatr Cardiol 4:29, 1983.

36. Nielsen G: Arteriovenous malformations as a cause of congestive heart failure in the newborn and infant. Eur J Pediatr 142:298, 1984.

37. Pellegrino PA, Milanesi O, Saia OS, Carollo C: Congestive heart failure secondary to cerebral arteriovenous fistula. Childs Nerv Syst 3:141, 1987.

38. Rocchini AP, Rosenthal A, Issenberg HG, et al: Hepatic hemangioendothelioma: Hemodynamic observations and treatment. Pediatrics 57:131, 1976.

39. Nornes H, Grip A: Hemodynamic aspects of cerebral arteriovenous malformations. J Neurosurg 53:456, 1980.

40. Fried R, Amberson JB, O'Loughlin JF, et al: Congenital pulmonary arteriovenous fistula producing pulmonary arterial steal syndrome. Pediatr Cardiol 2:313, 1982.

41. Chilvers ER: Clinical and physiological aspects of pulmonary arteriovenous malformations. Br J Hosp Med 39:188, 1988.

42. Kasabach HH, Merritt KK: Capillary hemangioma with extensive purpura: Report of a case. Am J Dis Child 59:1063, 1940.

43. Brown SH Jr, Neerhout RC, Fonkalsrud EW: Prednisone therapy in the management of large hemangiomas in infants and children. Surgery 71:168, 1972.

44. Bartoshesky LE, Bull M, Feingold M: Corticosteroid treatment of cutaneous hemangiomas: How effective? A report on 24 children. Clin Pediatr (Phila) 17:625, 1978.

45. Enjolras O, Merland JJ: The current management of vascular birthmarks. Pediatr Dermatol 10:311, 1993.

46. Takahashi K, Mulliken JB, Kozakewich HPW, et al: Cellular markers that distinguish the phases of hemangioma during infancy and childhood. J Clin Invest 93:2357, 1994.

47. Johnston JH, Whittle JR, Besser M, Morgan MK: Vein of Galen malformation: Diagnosis and management. Neurosurgery 20:747, 1987.

48. Sapire DW, Casta A, Donner RM, et al: Dilatation of the descending aorta: A radiologic and echocardiographic sign in arterio-venous malformations in neonates and young infants. Am J Cardiol 44:493, 1979.

49. Leblanc R, Ethier R, Little JR: Computerized tomography findings in arteriovenous malformations of the brain. J Neurosurg 51:765, 1979.

50. Meyer JS, Hoffer FA, Barnes PD, Mulliken JB: Biological classification of soft tissue vascular anomalies: MR correlation. AJR Am J Roentgenol 157:559, 1991.

51. Brassel F, Bertram H: Endovaskuläre Therapie bei arteriovenösen Malformationen des Zentralnervensystems im Kindesalter. Monatschr Kinderheilkd 146:38, 1998.

52. Sloan RD, Cooley RD: Congenital pulmonary arteriovenous aneurysm. Am J Roentgenol 70:183, 1953.

53. Meyer CT, Troncale FJ, Galloway S, Sheahan DG: Arteriovenous malformations of the bowel: An analysis of 22 cases and review of the literature. Medicine (Baltimore) 60:36, 1981.

54. Widlus DM, Murray RR, White JR, et al: Congenital arteriovenous malformations. Tailored embolotherapy. Radiology 169:511, 1988.

55. Burrows PE: Variations in the vascular supply to infantile hepatic hemangioendotheliomas. Radiology 181:631, 1991.

56. Lasjaunias P, Hui F, Zerah M, et al: Cerebral arteriovenous malformations in children. Management of 179 consecutive cases and review of the literature. Childs Nerv Syst 11:66, 1995.

57. Rodesch G, Pongpech S, Alvarez H, et al: Spinal cord arteriovenous malformations in a pediatric population. Intervent Neuroradiol 1:29, 1995.

58. Maeda N, Horie Y, Kocla M, et al: Extrahepatic portal obstruction without hepatopetal pathway associated with congenital arterioportal fistula: A case report. Hepatogastroenterology 44:1317, 1997.

59. Clapp S, Morrow WR: Development of superior vena cava to pulmonary vein fistula following modified Fontan operation: Case report of a rare anomaly and embolization therapy. Pediatr Cardiol 19:363, 1998.

60. Burrows PE, Rosenberg HC, Chang HS: Diffuse hepatic hemangiomas: Percutaneous transcatheter embolization with detachable silicone balloons. Radiology 156:85, 1985.

61. Friedman DM, Verma R, Madrid M, et al: Recent improvement in outcome using transcatheter embolization techniques for neonatal aneurysmal malformations of the vein of Galen. Pediatrics 91:583, 1993.

62. Gomes AS, Busattal RW, Baker JD, et al: Congenital arteriovenous malformations. The role of transcatheter embolization. Arch Surg 118:817, 1983.

63. Aicardi J: Cerebrovascular Disorders. London, MacKeith Press, 1992.

64. Cronquist S: Hydrocephalus and congestive heart failure caused by intracranial arteriovenous malformation in infants. J Pediatr 89:343, 1976.

65. Graf CJ, Perret GE, Torner JC: Bleeding from cerebral arteriovenous malformations as part of their natural history. J Neurosurg 58:331, 1983.

66. Perret G, Nishioka H: Report of the cooperative study of intracranial aneurysms. J Neurosurg 25:467, 1966.

67. Borthne A, Carteret M, Baraton J, et al: Vein of Galen vascular malformations in infants: Clinical, radiological and therapeutic aspect. Eur Radiol 7:1252, 1997.

68. Rodesch G, Hui F, Alvarez H, et al: Prognosis of antenatally diagnosed vein of Galen aneurysmal malformations. Childs Nerv Syst 10:79, 1994.

69. Martinez-Lage JF, Garcia Sautos JM, Poza M, Garcia Sanchez F: Prenatal magnetic resonance imaging detection of a vein of Galen aneurysm. Childs Nerv Syst 9:377, 1993.

70. Baumgartner RW, Mattle HP, Aaslid R, Kaps M: Transcranial color-coded duplex sonography in arterial cerebral vascular disease. Cerebrovasc Dis 7:57, 1997.

71. Bertram H, Hoyer PF, Brassel F: Stellenwert der cerebralen Sonographie in der Diagnostik arteriovenöser Malformationen der Vena

Galeni vor und nach Embolisationsbehandlung. *In* Gross-Selbeck G (ed): Aktuelle Neuropädiatrie. Wehr, Germany, Ciba-Geigy, 1995, p 568.

72. Starc TJ, Krongrad E, Bierman FZ: Two-dimensional echocardiography and Doppler findings in cerebral arteriovenous malformation. Am J Cardiol 64:252, 1989.

73. Westra SJ, Curran JG, Duckwiler GR, et al: Pediatric intracranial vascular malformations: Evaluation of treatment results with color Doppler US. Radiology 186:775, 1993.

74. Friedman DM, Madrid M, Berenstein A, et al: Neonatal vein of Galen malformations: Experience in developing a multidisciplinary approach using an embolization treatment protocol. Clin Pediatr 30:621, 1991.

75. Ciricillo SF, Edwards MSB, Schmidt KG, et al: Interventional neuroradiological management of vein of Galen aneurysms. Neurosurgery 27:22, 1990.

76. Hanigan WC, Brady T, Medlock M, Smith EB: Spontaneous regression of giant arteriovenous fistulae during the perinatal period. J Neurosurg 73:954, 1990.

77. Lylyk P, Viñuela T, Dion JE, et al: Therapeutic alternatives for vein of Galen vascular malformations. J Neurosurg 78:438, 1993.

78. Lasjaunias P, Garcia-Monaco R, Rodesch G, et al: Vein of Galen malformation. Endovascular management of 43 cases. Childs Nerv Syst 7:360, 1991.

79. Brunelle F: Arteriovenous malformation of the vein of Galen in children. Pediatr Radiol 27:501, 1997.

80. Halbach VV, Dowd CF, Higashida RT, et al: Endovascular treatment of mural-type vein of Galen malformations. J Neurosurg 89:74, 1998.

81. Verma R, Friedman DM, Madrid M, et al: Recent improvement in outcome using transcatheter embolization techniques for neonatal aneurysmal malformations of the vein of Galen. Pediatrics 91:583, 1993.

82. Davis JT, Allen HD, Wheller JJ, et al: Coronary artery fistula in the pediatric age group: A 19-year institutional experience. Ann Thorac Surg 58:760, 1994.

83. de Nef JJE, Varghese PJ, Losekoot G: Congenital coronary artery fistula. Analysis of 17 cases. Br Heart J 33:857, 1971.

84. Farooki ZQ, Nowlen T, Hakimi M, Pinsky W: Congenital coronary artery fistula: A review of 18 cases with specific emphasis on spontaneous closure. Pediatr Cardiol 14:208, 1993.

85. Kirklin JW, Barratt-Boyes BG (eds): Cardiac Surgery. New York, Churchill Livingstone, 1993, p 1167.

86. Liberthson RR, Sagar K, Berkoben JP, et al: Congenital coronary arteriovenous fistula. Circulation 59:849, 1979.

87. Schumacher G, Roithmaier A, Lorenz HP, et al: Congenital coronary artery fistula in infancy and childhood: Diagnostic and therapeutic aspects. Thorac Cardiovasc Surg 45:287, 1997.

88. Vanselow B, Fallen H, Zimmermann A, et al: Beidseitige Koronarfistel: Eine Fallpräsentation und Übersicht. Z Kardiol 85:214, 1996.

89. Kugelmass AD, Manning WJ, Piana RN, et al: Coronary arteriovenous fistula presenting as congestive heart failure. Cathet Cardiovasc Diagn 26:19, 1992.

90. Ogden JA, Stansel HC: Coronary arterial fistulas terminating in the coronary venous system. J Thorac Cardiovasc Surg 63:172, 1972.

91. Vlodaver Z, Neufeld HN, Edwards JE: Coronary Arterial Variations in the Normal Heart and in Congenital Heart Disease. New York, Academic Press, 1975.

92. Griffiths SP, Ellis K, Hordof AJ: Spontaneous complete closure of a congenital coronary artery fistula. J Am Coll Cardiol 2:1169, 1983.

93. Hackett D, Hallidie-Smith A: Spontaneous closure of a coronary artery fistula. Br Heart J 52:477, 1984.

94. Olearchyk AS, Runk DM, Alavi M, Grosso MA: Congenital bilateral coronary-to-pulmonary artery fistulas. Ann Thorac Surg 64:233, 1997.

95. Vogelbach K-H, Edmiston WA, Stenson RE: Coronary artery–left ventricular communications: A report of two cases and review of the literature. Cathet Cardiovasc Diagn 5:159, 1979.

96. Ahmed S, Haider B, Regan T: Silent left coronary artery–cameral fistula: Probable cause of myocardial ischemia. Am Heart J 104:869, 1982.

97. Dobell ARC, Lony RW: Right coronary–left ventricular fistula, mimicking aortic valve insufficiency in infancy. J Thorac Cardiovasc Surg 82:785, 1981.

98. Fang BR, Chiang CW, Liu FC, et al: Two dimensional and Doppler-echocardiographic features of coronary arteriovenous fistula. J Ultrasound Med 9:39, 1990.

99. Strunk BL, Hieshima GB, Shafton EP: Treatment of congenital coronary arteriovenous malformations with micro-particle embolization. Cathet Cardiovasc Diagn 22:133, 1991.

100. Klippel M, Trénaunay I: Du naevus variqueux et ostéohypertrophique. Arch Gen Med 3:641, 1900.

101. Szilagyi DE, Smith RF, Elliott JP, Hageman JH: Congenital arteriovenous anomalies of the limbs. Arch Surg 111:423, 1976.

102. Malan E, Puglionisi A: Congenital angiodysplasias of the extremities. J Cardiovasc Surg (Torino) 5:87, 1964.

103. Ford EG, Stanley P, Tolo V, Woolley MM: Peripheral congenital arteriovenous fistulae: Observe, operate or obturate? J Pediatr Surg 27:714, 1992.

104. Kuint J, Bilik R, Heyman Z, et al: Congenital aorto-caval fistula in the newborn: A case report. J Pediatr Surg 33:743, 1998.

105. Schobinger RA: Periphere Angiodysplasien. Bern, Verlag H. Huber, 1977.

106. Jimenez M, Fournier A, Chossat A: Pulmonary artery to the left atrium fistula as an unusual cause of cyanosis in the newborn. Pediatr Cardiol 10:216, 1989.

107. Clarke CP, Goh TH, Blackwood A, Venables AW: Massive pulmonary arteriovenous fistula in the newborn. Br Heart J 38:1092, 1976.

108. Srivastava D, Preminger T, Lock JE, et al: Hepatic venous blood and the development of pulmonary arteriovenous malformations in congenital heart disease. Circulation 2:1217, 1995.

109. Kallfelz HC, Borst HG: Solitäre arteriovenöse Lungenfistel im Säuglings- und Kindesalter. Thoraxchirurgie 23:238, 1975.

110. Moyer JH, Glantz G, Brest AN: Pulmonary arteriovenous fistulas. Am J Med 32:417, 1962.

111. Hall RJ, Nelson WP, Blake HA, Geiger JP: Massive pulmonary arteriovenous fistula in the newborn; a correctable form of 'cyanotic heart disease,' an additional cause of cyanosis with left axis deviation. Circulation 31:765, 1965.

112. Hodgson CH, Burchell HB, Good CA, Clagett OT: Hereditary hemorrhagic telangiectasia and pulmonary arteriovenous fistula; survey of a large family. N Engl J Med 261:625, 1959.

113. Steinberg I, Finby N: Roentgen manifestations of pulmonary arteriovenous fistula. Am J Roentgenol 78:234, 1957.

114. Brummelkamp WH: Unusual complication of pulmonary arteriovenous aneurysm: Intrapleural rupture. Dis Chest 39:218, 1961.

115. Hirota S, Matsumoto S, Tomita M, et al: Pulmonary arteriovenous fistula: Long-term results of percutaneous transcatheter embolization with spring coils. Radiat Med 16:17, 1998.

116. Kumar S, Ruttley MI, Fisher DI: Bilateral pulmonary arteriovenous fistulae treated with balloon embolization. Postgrad Med J 62:209, 1986.

117. White CW, Sondheimer HM, Crouch EC, et al: Treatment of pulmonary hemangiomatosis with recombinant interferon alfa-2a. N Engl J Med 320:1197, 1989.

118. Altuntas B, Erden A, Karakurt C, et al: Severe portal hypertension due to congenital hepatoportal arteriovenous fistula associated with intrahepatic portal vein aneurysm. J Clin Ultrasound 26:357, 1998.

119. Billing JS, Jamieson NV: Hepatic arterioportal fistula: A curable cause of portal hypertension in infancy. HPB Surg 10:311, 1997.

120. Vauthey JN, Tomczak RJ, Helmberger T, et al: The arterioportal fistula syndrome: Clinicopathologic features, diagnosis, and therapy. Gastroenterology 113:1390, 1997.

121. Fok TF, Chan MSV, Metreweli C, et al: Hepatic hemangioendothelioma presenting with early heart failure in a newborn: Treatment with hepatic artery embolization and interferon. Acta Paediatr 85:1373, 1996.

122. Peuster M, Windhagen-Mahnert B, Fink C, et al: Interventionelle Therapie eines Hämangioendothelioms der Leber bei einem Neugeborenen über einen venösen Zugang. Z Kardiol 87:832, 1988.

123. Rydell R, Hoffbauer FW: Multiple pulmonary arteriovenous fistulas in juvenile cirrhosis. Am J Med 21:450, 1956.

124. El Gamal M, Stoker JB, Spiers EM, Whitaker W: Cyanosis complicating hepatic cirrhosis: Report of a case due to multiple pulmonary arteriovenous fistulas. Am J Cardiol 25:490, 1970.

125. Kawata H, Kishimoto H, Ikawa S, et al: Pulmonary and systemic arteriovenous fistulas in patients with left isomerism. Cardiol Young 8:290, 1998.

126. Boon LM, Burrows PE, Paltiel HJ, et al: Hepatic vascular anomalies in infancy: A twenty-seven-year experience. J Pediatr 129:346, 1996.

127. Egawa H, Berquist W, Garcia-Kennedy R, et al: Respiratory distress from benign liver tumors: A report of two unusual cases treated with hepatic transplantation. J Pediatr Gastroenterol 19:114, 1994.

128. Iyer CP, Stanley P, Mahour H: Hepatic hemangiomas in infants and children: A review of 30 cases. Am Surg 62:356, 1996.

129. McHugh K, Burrows PE: Infantile hepatic hemangioendotheliomas: Significance of portal venous and systemic collateral arterial supply. J Vasc Interv Radiol 3:337, 1992.

130. Fellows KE, Hoffer FA, Markowith RI, O'Neill JA: Multiple collaterals to hepatic infantile hemangioendotheliomas and arteriovenous malformations: Effect on embolization. Radiology 181:813, 1991.

131. Davenport M, Hansen L, Heaton ND, Howard ER: Hemangioendothelioma of the liver in infants. J Pediatr Surg 30:44, 1995.

132. Samuel M, Spitz L: Infantile hepatic hemangiothelioma: The role of surgery. J Pediatr Surg 30:1425, 1995.

133. Jackson C, Greene HL, O'Neill J, Kirchner S: Hepatic hemangioendothelioma: Angiographic appearance and apparent prednisone responsiveness. Am J Dis Child 131:74, 1977.

134. Ezekowitz RAB, Mulliken JB, Folkman J: Interferon alfa-2a therapy for life-threatening hemangiomas of infancy. N Engl J Med 326:1456, 1992.

135. Levy MJ, Schachner A, Blieden LC: Aortico–left ventricular tunnel. Collective review. J Thorac Cardiovasc Surg 84:102, 1982.

136. Llorens R, Arcas R, Herreros J, et al: Aortico–left ventricular tunnel: A case report and review of the literature. Tex Heart Inst 9:169, 1982.

137. Fripp RR, Werner JC, Whitman V, et al: Pulsed Doppler and two-dimensional echocardiographic findings in aortico–left ventricular tunnel. J Am Coll Cardiol 4:1012, 1984.

138. Serino W, Andrade JL, Ross D, et al: Aorto–left ventricular communication after closure. Late postoperative problems. Br Heart J 49:501, 1983.

139. Edwards JE, Burchell HB: The pathological anatomy of deficiencies between the aortic root and the heart, including aortic sinus aneurysms. Thorax 12:125, 1957.

140. Nowicki ER, Aberdeen E, Friedman S, Rashkind WJ: Congenital left aortic sinus–left ventricle fistula and review of aortocardiac fistulas. Ann Thorac Surg 23:378, 1977.

141. Henze A, Huttunen H, Björk VO: Ruptured sinus of Valsalva aneurysms. Scand J Thorac Cardiovasc Surg 17:249, 1983.

142. Dev V, Goswami KC, Shrivastava S, et al: Echocardiographic diagnosis of aneurysm of the sinus of Valsalva. Am Heart J 126:930, 1993.

143. van Son JA, Danielson GK, Schaff HV, et al: Long-term outcome of surgical repair of ruptured sinus of Valsalva aneurysm. Circulation 90(suppl I):I-20, 1994.

144. van Son JA, Sim EK, Starr A: Morphometric features of ruptured congenital sinus of Valsalva aneurysm: Implication for surgical treatment. J Cardiovasc Surg (Torino) 36:433, 1995.

145. Sakakibara S, Konno S: Congenital aneurysm of the sinus of Valsalva associated with ventricular septal defect. Anatomical aspects. Am Heart J 75:595, 1968.

146. Hamid IA, Jothi M, Rajan S, et al: Transaortic repair of ruptured aneurysm of sinus of Valsalva. Fifteen-year experience. J Thorac Cardiovasc Surg 107:1464, 1994.

147. Taguchi K, Sasaki N, Matasuura Y, Mura R: Surgical correction of aneurysm of the sinus of Valsalva. A report of 45 consecutive patients, including 8 with total replacement of the aortic valve. Am J Cardiol 23:180, 1969.

148. Hoffman JIE: Congenital anomalies of the coronary vessels and the aortic root. In Emmanouilides GC, Riemenschneider TA, Allen HD, Gutgesell HP (eds): Moss and Adams Heart Disease in Infants, Children, and Adolescents: Including the Fetus and Young Adult, Vol 1, 5th ed. Baltimore, Williams & Wilkins, 1995, p 769.

149. Hands ME, Lloyd BJ, Hung J: Cross-sectional echocardiographic diagnosis of unruptured right sinus of Valsalva aneurysm dissecting into the interventricular septum. Int J Cardiol 9:380, 1985.

150. Chiang CW, Lin FC, Fang BR, et al: Doppler and two dimensional echocardiographic features of sinus of Valsalva aneurysm. Am Heart J 116:1283, 1986.

151. Sahasakul Y, Panchavinnin P, Chaithiraphen S, Sakiyalak P: Echocardiographic diagnosis of a ruptured aneurysm of the sinus of Valsalva: Operation without catheterisation in seven patients. Br Heart J 64:195, 1990.

152. Kirklin JW, Barratt-Boyes BG: Congenital aneurysm of the sinus of Valsalva. In Kirklin JW, Barratt-Boyes BG (eds): Cardiac Surgery, Vol 1, 2nd ed. New York, John Wiley & Sons, 1993, p 825.

CHAPTER 43
CARDIAC VALVAR ANOMALIES

JULIA STEINBERGER

In this chapter, abnormalities of the mitral, tricuspid, and pulmonary valves that are not discussed elsewhere in this book are described. Primary abnormalities of these valves are uncommon but can be serious and life-threatening.

MITRAL VALVE AND LEFT ATRIAL ABNORMALITIES

MITRAL VALVE ABNORMALITIES

In the pediatric population, abnormalities of the mitral valve are usually associated with other congenital or acquired anomalies. Isolated mitral valve anomalies are rare in children. The most prevalent mitral valve disease in children worldwide is acquired secondary to rheumatic fever (see Chapter 48), which is now rare in the United States.

CONGENITAL MITRAL STENOSIS

Mitral stenosis and other left atrial obstructive lesions limit diastolic blood flow into the left ventricle. When alterations in left-sided inflow occur early in fetal development (the extreme end of the spectrum), the mitral valve may be hypoplastic or atretic, and the left ventricular cavity small or hypoplastic. At the other end of the spectrum, the left ventricle is fully developed. The degree of obstruction to left ventricular inflow varies.

Pathology

Congenital mitral stenosis results in infancy from several different anatomic states,[1] the most frequent being parachute mitral valve.[2] In this form, only a single left ventricular papillary muscle is present. The chordae tendineae from both mitral valve leaflets insert into this single papillary muscle (Fig. 43–1). The chordae tendineae are short and thickened and restrict movement of the leaflets. The mitral valvar leaflets and commissures are normal. Mitral stenosis results from convergence of the chordae tendineae and narrowing of the interchordal spaces by the thickened and fused chordae tendineae.

Parachute mitral valve is frequently a portion of a developmental complex (Shone) that includes supravalvar mitral stenosis, subaortic stenosis, and coarctation of the aorta. It also occurs in patients with ventricular septal defect or origin of both great vessels from the right ventricle and supracristal ventricular septal defect.[3]

Mitral stenosis also occurs from abnormally large papillary muscles.[1,4] In this condition, also known as mitral ar-

cade, the mitral valvar leaflets are normal. Large bulky papillary muscles are situated immediately beneath the mitral valve and attach to the valvar leaflets by shortened chordae tendineae. The obstruction is basically subvalvar.

Another anatomic cause of mitral stenosis is congenital commissural fusion, and this resembles rheumatic mitral stenosis.[3] The leaflets are thickened and fused, the chordae tendineae are also distorted, and the papillary muscles may be poorly developed.

Double-orifice mitral valve is an unusual congenital anomaly that can be found incidentally at autopsy in association with a number of cardiac malformations. Although mitral valve function is usually normal, both stenosis and insufficiency have been reported with double-orifice mitral valve. Unlike in parachute mitral valve, in double-orifice mitral valve, two papillary muscles are present; there may be multiple small papillary muscles. Two-dimensional echocardiography (Fig. 43–2) can usually delineate three leaflets. The orifices are usually positioned anteriorly and posteriorly. The double orifice must be differentiated from cleft mitral valve in endocardial cushion defect, in which the cleft mitral valve appears as a defect in the anterior leaflet, resulting in a two-sided mitral valve structure. Thickening of the leaflets may be seen in double-orifice mitral valve when stenosis or insufficiency is present.

Mitral stenosis, regardless of anatomic detail, can occur as an isolated lesion or coexist with other conditions.[1,2,5] In this chapter, the isolated form is considered. When mitral stenosis coexists with another lesion, the major clinical features usually resemble those of the associated condition.

The normal mitral valve orifice area in adults is 4 to 6 cm^2. An orifice of 2 cm^2 usually causes mild symptoms, and an orifice of 1 cm^2 causes severe symptoms of mitral stenosis. Normal values in children depend on body surface area.[6] The most commonly used formula for calculating the valve area is based on the work of Gorlin and Gorlin[7] and relies on the principle that the valve area is directly related to the flow rate and inversely related to the velocity of flow and the coefficient of orifice contraction (see Chapter 13).

Hemodynamics

Normally, there is no pressure difference between the left atrium and left ventricle in diastole. With mitral stenosis, left atrial pressure increases and a gradient develops between the left atrium and the left ventricle. The pressure gradient is proportional to the degree of mitral stenosis. Left atrial hypertension is transmitted to the pulmonary veins and pulmonary capillaries, where, if oncotic pressure is exceeded, fluid transudation and pulmonary edema de-

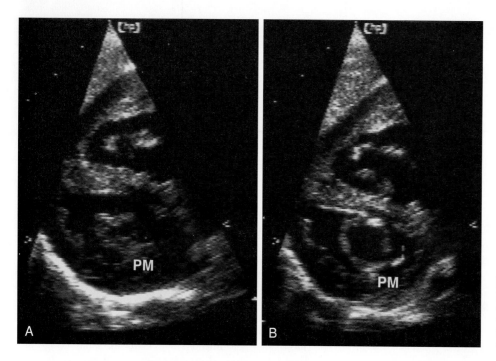

Parachute mitral valve. Short-axis view of the left ventricle. All mitral valve chords insert into a single anterolateral papillary muscle (PM) in systole (A) and diastole (B).

velop. According to Gorlin's formula, small changes in flow across the obstructed valve alter the gradient exponentially. With increasing heart rate, the diastolic filling period is shortened; the available time for mitral flow per minute is shortened, and the necessary pressure gradient is higher. Consequently, patients who are asymptomatic at rest may experience dyspnea and pulmonary edema with activity. The elevated pulmonary venous and capillary pressures can cause reflex pulmonary arteriolar vasoconstriction and pulmonary arterial hypertension.

Clinical Manifestations

The first symptom of mitral stenosis is dyspnea in older children and tachypnea in infants, but symptoms are unusual except in advanced stenosis. Relatively severe mitral stenosis at birth may be surprisingly well tolerated because of secondary persistent pulmonary hypertension. Poor growth is unusual even with maximal obstruction. The usual patient with mitral stenosis has an associated anomaly that attracts attention through symptoms or a murmur. On physical examination, there is an apical low-pitched diastolic rumble. It is present in all patients with rheumatic mitral stenosis but is not always present in patients with congenital mitral stenosis. The murmur is mid-diastolic or presystolic and, in its characteristic form, begins in mid-diastole and is accentuated in presystole. Although an opening snap is rarely noted in congenital mitral stenosis, it is almost invariably present in patients with rheumatic disease. Whether this is related to the difficulty of examining infants with a faster heart rate as opposed to older children with rheumatic heart disease or whether this is inherent in the valve anatomy is unclear. The first heart sound is accentuated in either form. Mitral stenosis may produce an apical diastolic thrill in patients with rheumatic or congenital heart disease. With secondary pulmonary hypertension, there is accentuation of the second heart sound; and sometimes early in diastole, the murmur of pulmonary regurgitation (Graham Steell's murmur) can be heard.

Electrocardiography

With minimal stenosis, the electrocardiogram is normal. With increasing degrees of mitral stenosis, there is increasing evidence of right ventricular hypertrophy and P mitrale.

Double-orifice mitral valve. Short-axis view of the left ventricle with anterior (A) and posterior (P) orifice of the mitral valve.

Chest Radiography

The cardiac silhouette may be enlarged, but the degree of enlargement is minimal and does not approach that seen in patients with mitral regurgitation. The left atrial enlargement is modest compared with that in mitral regurgitation, but it is detectable as a double density and by elevation of the left main bronchus. There may be posterior displacement of the esophagus. In severe obstruction, there is redistribution of the pulmonary blood flow; when the patient is upright, the apical regions are better perfused than they are in normal individuals. Late in the course, Kerley's B lines and pulmonary edema are evident.

Echocardiography

Two-dimensional echocardiography is essential in demonstrating the morphologic and functional details of the mitral valve, such as limited motion of the mitral valve, abnormal tethering of the mitral valve leaflets, a single papillary muscle, and a small valve orifice. Doppler demonstration of a pressure gradient across the valve is helpful in the diagnosis and quantification of mitral stenosis. Any suggestion that the patient has a supravalvar membrane or cor triatriatum (sometimes confused with valvar mitral stenosis) must be diligently pursued because those lesions are readily corrected.

Cardiac Catheterization

With the availability of high precision provided by echo Doppler in the evaluation of mitral stenosis, cardiac catheterization is reserved mostly for balloon valvuloplasty of the mitral valve. Nevertheless, catheterization is advocated by many before a mitral valve operation is undertaken. Direct measurement of left atrial and left ventricular diastolic pressures is made, as well as the best available estimation of blood flow across the valve, and the valve area is calculated. Puncture of the atrial septum to gain access to the left atrium is undertaken, even though the targeted left atrium may not be particularly large. In general, good-quality pressure tracings of the left atrium and left ventricle, which can be overlaid for precise comparison, are obtained.

Angiography with left atrial injection not only usually confirms the echocardiographic findings but provides further confidence in deciding a plan of operative management. A contrast agent with low osmolality should be used when high left atrial pressures are discovered.

Management

Operations for congenital mitral stenosis are often unsatisfactory because valvuloplasty rarely produces sufficient benefit, and valve replacement, even if possible, is undesirable in small children. Additional cardiac malformations may need to be corrected. The mortality is high. The valve annulus is often small, and valve replacement results in some residual obstruction that is likely to become worse as the child grows. Later, as the child grows, replacement with a larger valve is difficult and sometimes impossible. Various solutions, none completely satisfactory, have been suggested. Sometimes the best approach is to excise the mitral valve and insert a prosthesis above the valve ring.[8–12] For these reasons, if possible, operation for congenital mitral stenosis is avoided in infancy and delayed until the child is larger. Only when it is certain that there is no alternative to valve replacement is surgery undertaken, even though it is expected that valvuloplasty might offer a possible solution. Correction of associated anomalies, such as a patent ductus arteriosus or ventricular septal defect, that cause increased mitral valve flow may reduce the transvalvar gradient enough to relieve symptoms.

Rheumatic mitral stenosis is a different problem. In pure form, it is amenable to balloon valvuloplasty[13] or, if necessary, to the full variety of surgical possibilities.

Course

Congenital mitral stenosis tends to remain stable for many years. Often, however, there is concern about pulmonary hypertension that is associated with mitral stenosis. In general, this is reversible with correction of the stenosis. For this reason, only symptoms of tachypnea, significant exercise intolerance, and evidence of pulmonary edema are indications for intervention in children with congenital mitral stenosis.

COR TRIATRIATUM

In this rare cardiac anomaly, the pulmonary veins enter a chamber that communicates with the left atrium through a small orifice. It must be considered in the differential diagnosis of pulmonary venous obstruction because it can be operatively corrected and the results are excellent.

Pathology

Several reviews[14–16] have described the anatomy of cor triatriatum. This anomaly is generally considered to result from faulty incorporation of the common pulmonary vein into the left atrium, so that the pulmonary veins do not directly join the left atrium. Rather, they enter an accessory atrial chamber that communicates through an opening or, occasionally, through several openings with the left atrium proper. The size of the orifice varies.

Marin-Garcia and coworkers[16] classified cor triatriatum into three types: (1) diaphragmatic type, in which a fibromuscular diaphragm divides the left atrium from the accessory chamber, and there is no external evidence of two distinct chambers; (2) hourglass type, in which a constriction is observed externally between the two chambers; and (3) tubular type, which is apparent externally, with a tubular channel joining the chambers receiving the pulmonary veins with the left atrium.

The left atrial appendage arises from the left atrium below the cor triatriatum. This is an important anatomic feature that distinguishes cor triatriatum from mitral stenosis and supravalvar stenosing ring. The fossa ovalis almost always connects between the right atrium and the true left atrium. Partial anomalous pulmonary venous connection can coexist with cor triatriatum.[17–20]

Hemodynamics

The hemodynamics of this condition resembles that of mitral stenosis. Elevated pulmonary venous pressure results from the narrowed orifice in the channel separating the anomalous chamber from the left atrium.

Echocardiography

The membrane crossing the left atrium can be visualized on two-dimensional echocardiography. Documentation that the accessory atrial chamber accepts the pulmonary veins, whereas the distal segment (left atrium) is associated with the foramen ovale and the left atrial appendage, makes the diagnosis. The entry point of each of the pulmonary veins should be identified because of the tendency for anomalous connection in these patients.

The distinction between cor triatriatum and a supravalvar stenosing ring is usually readily apparent. In cor triatriatum, although the membrane may balloon into the mitral valve, the left atrial appendage communicates with the distal compartment, as does the foramen ovale, because they are proximal to the stenosing structure.

The obstructing membrane of cor triatriatum can be imaged in subxiphoid or apical chamber views (Fig. 43–3). Doppler color flow mapping is useful for detecting the orifice in the membrane and for quantitating the obstruction. If tricuspid regurgitation is present, the right ventricular systolic pressure can be estimated from the velocity of the regurgitant jet. Otherwise, the right ventricular systolic pressure can be grossly estimated from the orientation of the ventricular septum.

Cardiac Catheterization

Patients with cor triatriatum may undergo cardiac catheterization because the diagnosis is sufficiently rare that direct physiologic measurements are usually recorded.

Nevertheless, accurate echocardiographic evaluation may eliminate the need for catheterization.

Management

The obstructing membrane of cor triatriatum should be resected if the infant is symptomatic. Asymptomatic patients without significant obstruction are managed expectantly. A membrane of cor triatriatum is often removed during a surgical procedure to repair associated cardiac anomalies. Ordinarily, removal of the obstructing membranes is curative.[21–23]

SUPRAVALVAR STENOSING RING

A supravalvar stenosing ring is situated immediately above the mitral valve leaflets and is distinguished from cor triatriatum because the left atrial appendage communicates with the proximal part of the atrium. It is a rare anomaly, occurring about as frequently as cor triatriatum, but it is almost always associated with other cardiac defects (i.e., the Shone syndrome).

Clinical Manifestations

The clinical features are those of the associated malformations, except in the rare isolated membrane severe enough to cause pulmonary venous hypertension and dyspnea.

Echocardiography

The diagnosis can often be recognized by echocardiography. It is necessary to separate the image of the supravalvar membrane from that of the mitral valve leaflets.[24] Sometimes a thin membrane is adherent to the leaflets and is difficult to distinguish. Apical two- and four-chamber views and the parasternal long-axis view are most useful for imaging the membrane (Fig. 43–4 [see also Color Plates]). The

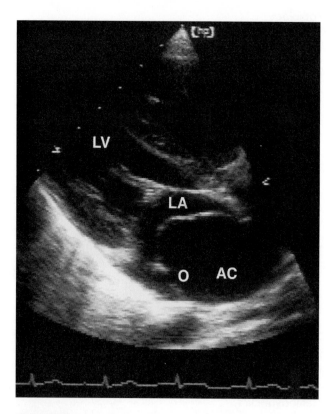

FIGURE 43–3

Cor triatriatum. Parasternal short-axis view. The accessory atrial chamber (AC) receives the pulmonary veins and communicates with the true left atrium (LA) through a small opening (O). LV = left ventricle.

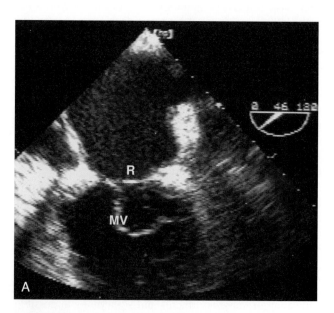

FIGURE 43–4

Supravalvar stenosing ring. A, Transesophageal apical view of the left ventricle and left atrium with the ring (R) situated above the mitral valve (MV) leaflets. B, See Color Figure 43–4B.

membrane is usually at the annulus of the valve, but it may occasionally attach to the leaflet slightly below the annulus. In all patients with evidence of mitral stenosis, a supravalvar membrane should be considered because it is usually a curable lesion,[25] whereas most forms of mitral stenosis are not.

MITRAL VALVE INSUFFICIENCY

In pediatric patients, mitral valve insufficiency usually results from acquired conditions. Mitral insufficiency can develop secondary to myocarditis, congestive or hypertrophic cardiomyopathy, bacterial endocarditis, coronary insufficiency due to myocardial infarction or papillary muscle infarction, connective tissue diseases or storage diseases affecting the cardiac muscle, rupture of the chordae tendineae or papillary muscles, annular dilatation, and chronic rheumatic heart disease or after catheter or surgical procedures that involve the mitral valve.[6, 26] Mitral valve prolapse, often accompanied by mitral regurgitation, is discussed in Chapter 44.

Hemodynamics

During mitral regurgitation, the left ventricle decompresses into the left atrium. Half of the regurgitant volume during systole occurs before the opening of the aortic valve. When the regurgitant volume exceeds the stroke volume, cardiac output decreases in the baseline state. With a normal left ventricle, the ejection fraction or shortening fraction is usually increased; normal or decreased left ventricular function may imply left ventricular cardiomyopathy. The left ventricular wall stress and tension are decreased in mild regurgitation; therefore, the oxygen consumption in the left ventricle is not significantly elevated.[6, 26]

Clinical Manifestations

Symptoms of mitral insufficiency depend on the severity of regurgitation, associated cardiac abnormalities, left ventricular function, pulmonary artery pressure, and the rate of development of the regurgitation. Acute mitral regurgitation of moderate to severe degree, usually due to acquired rupture of the chordae tendineae or destruction of the atrioventricular valve, is poorly tolerated and leads to acute pulmonary edema and respiratory distress. Chronic mitral regurgitation often results in diaphoresis, recurrent respiratory symptoms and infections, exercise intolerance, tachypnea, and in infants failure to thrive.

On cardiovascular examination, there is usually a diffuse left ventricular lift with a palpably enlarged heart. The first heart sound is normal or decreased, and the pulmonary component of the second heart sound may be either normal or increased (pulmonary hypertension). Mitral regurgitation causes an apical high-pitched pansystolic murmur, which must be differentiated by its location and radiation from the murmur of tricuspid insufficiency. The murmur of mitral regurgitation radiates into the axilla and may be associated with a low-pitched diastolic flow rumble or third heart sound when regurgitation is moderate or severe.

Electrocardiography

The electrocardiogram usually shows left atrial enlargement and left ventricular hypertrophy. Atrial fibrillation is uncommon in children.

Chest Radiography

Radiography shows enlargement of the left atrial shadow, splaying of the right and left bronchi, and generalized cardiomegaly with left ventricular enlargement. The pulmonary venous markings may be increased. Pulmonary edema and Kerley's B lines are uncommon in children.

Echocardiography

The appearance, motion, and chordal attachments can be assessed by two-dimensional echocardiography. Systolic left ventricular function is usually normal or increased. The degree of mitral regurgitation can be qualitatively assessed by color flow Doppler mapping. This is generally accomplished by determining the width of the regurgitant volume and the penetration into the left atrium; grades are mild, moderate, and severe. The left atrial pressure can be quantitated in the absence of distal stenosis by computing the difference in the systemic blood pressure and the gradient across the mitral valve, as determined by the regurgitant flow velocity.[27]

Cardiac Catheterization

Isolated mitral insufficiency does not require cardiac catheterization, which is usually undertaken to assess associated lesions. Pulmonary capillary wedge pressure and pulmonary arterial pressure are often mildly elevated, but rarely as high as in mitral stenosis. Abnormally high v waves are typical for significant mitral insufficiency. Angiography of the left ventricle provides additional assessment of the degree of mitral insufficiency.

Course

As opposed to mitral stenosis, which tends to remain stable for many years, "mitral regurgitation begets mitral regurgitation" by causing left atrial enlargement, which further stretches the mitral annulus and worsens the regurgitation. Eventually, left ventricular enlargement and decreasing systolic function develop.

Management

Mild or moderate insufficiency often requires no treatment. Afterload reduction may be of some benefit in children with moderate to severe regurgitation. Indications for cardiac operation include symptomatic mitral regurgitation that is poorly controlled by medical management. Worsening cardiomyopathy or the steady decrease in left ventricular contraction indices over time may also be an indication for mitral valve replacement. The surgical treatment of choice is valvuloplasty or annuloplasty, although mitral valve replacement is frequently necessary.[28, 29]

TRICUSPID VALVE ABNORMALITIES

TRICUSPID VALVE STENOSIS

Congenital tricuspid stenosis is usually associated with other anomalies, most commonly severe pulmonary stenosis or atresia, with secondary hypoplasia of the right ventricle. The tricuspid annulus in this complex is small, but the valve apparatus, although diminutive, is usually normally

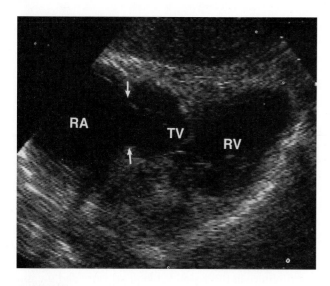

FIGURE 43–5

Tricuspid stenosis. Subcostal view of enlarged right atrium (RA) with hypoplastic tricuspid valve annulus *(arrows)*, doming tricuspid valve leaflets (TV), and hypoplastic right ventricle (RV).

formed (Fig. 43–5). The narrow tricuspid orifice in these patients, therefore, should more properly be referred to as being hypoplastic rather than stenotic, even though a certain degree of commissural fusion coexists in some. Tricuspid valve hypoplasia has also been associated with ventricular septal defect, tetralogy of Fallot, double-outlet right ventricle, single ventricle, and mitral stenosis.[30–32] In all of these, the clinical manifestations are determined by the associated anomalies.

Isolated tricuspid stenosis is rare. Many examples reported in adults are almost certainly acquired, probably secondary to rheumatic valvulitis. Gueron and colleagues[33] commented on the strong predominance of females in this group. Isolated congenital tricuspid stenosis is extremely rare.[34–36] In some patients, there is associated moderate or severe hypoplasia of the right ventricle.[37–42] This combination has a tendency to occur in families.

Clinical Manifestations

The clinical signs and symptoms of isolated congenital tricuspid stenosis resemble those seen in tricuspid atresia, and the two anomalies may be difficult to distinguish even with angiocardiography. Cyanosis is present in both, and in both the electrocardiogram may demonstrate left-axis deviation, right atrial hypertrophy, and left ventricular hypertrophy with absent or reduced QRS voltage in the right precordial leads.

TRICUSPID VALVE INSUFFICIENCY

Tricuspid insufficiency may be related to a variety of cardiac problems and should not in itself be considered a primary diagnosis until various etiologic factors have been excluded. A number of the conditions that lead to tricuspid insufficiency are discussed in other chapters. A classification is given here:

I. Involvement of tricuspid valve as part of another cardiac condition directly involving the tricuspid valve
    A. Ebstein's malformation
    B. Atrioventricular septal defect
    C. Endocarditis
II. Tricuspid insufficiency secondary to a condition affecting the right ventricle
    A. Associated with increased right ventricular systolic pressure
        1. Pulmonary stenosis or atresia with intact ventricular septum
        2. Pulmonary hypertension
    B. Right ventricular dilatation
        1. Cardiomegaly
        2. Premature closure of foramen ovale
        3. Obstructive pulmonary disease
III. Primary abnormalities of the tricuspid valve
    A. Dysplastic tricuspid valve
    B. Papillary muscle dysfunction secondary to asphyxia or metabolic insult (usually transient)

Pathology

Congenital tricuspid valve insufficiency as an isolated anomaly is rare.[43] In most instances, it is associated with severe stenosis or atresia of the right ventricular outflow tract, at either the infundibular or valvar level or both. In some of these, the insufficiency is functional and not due to a tricuspid valve anomaly. In others, some or all of the valve cusps are dysplastic and attached to the right ventricular myocardium by anomalous, short chordae tendineae. The features of tricuspid valve dysplasia have been well described.[44] There is great variation in the severity of the dysplasia from slight nodular thickening of the cusps of an otherwise normal valve apparatus to irregularly thickened, redundant cusps with abnormal chordae tendineae. There may be agenesis of part or even all[45,46] of the tricuspid valve, and in others, the valve is merely represented by a ridge of nodular thickening. Only a few instances of tricuspid valve dysplasia without downward displacement of the valve are without right ventricular outflow obstruction.

Clinical Manifestations

The manifestations of severe congenital tricuspid insufficiency in neonates and infants are remarkably similar.[47–50] They include extreme cardiomegaly, heart failure, cyanosis, a precordial thrill and harsh pansystolic murmur, and decreased second heart sound.

Electrocardiography

Right atrial enlargement is commonly seen. Right-axis deviation is occasionally demonstrated.

Chest Radiography

A massively enlarged heart and diminished vascular pattern of the lungs are seen on radiography. In neonates, the appearance resembles that of severe Ebstein's malformation.

Echocardiography

The mainstay of diagnosis is two-dimensional echocardiography and Doppler interrogation. These studies demonstrate the anatomy of the tricuspid valve, the presence of tricuspid insufficiency, and enlargement of the right-sided cardiac chambers. The right ventricular systolic pressure may be normal or elevated. Apparently in neonates, the free regurgitation across the tricuspid valve makes it impossible for the right ventricle to generate enough pressure to open the pulmonary valve in the presence of the high pulmonary vascular resistance. It is crucial to differentiate this condition from pulmonary atresia, in which the pulmonary valve is not patent (discussed in Chapter 31).

Course

The prognosis of severe congenital tricuspid insufficiency is poor, probably in part because of the high frequency of associated severe pulmonary stenosis or atresia. Surgical replacement of the tricuspid valve in the neonatal period carries high mortality. Patients with milder forms of tricuspid valve dysplasia have a much better prognosis and may be asymptomatic for many years.[48]

A transient form of tricuspid insufficiency in the newborn[51,52] resembles congenital tricuspid insufficiency due to malformed tricuspid valve. With vigorous medical treatment, and often spontaneously, the infant's condition improves. The cardiovascular status eventually becomes normal. All 14 term infants with the syndrome reported by Bucciarelli and colleagues[51] had experienced significant perinatal stress. The two babies who died had histologic evidence of right ventricular anterior papillary muscle necrosis. This, and the commonly seen electrocardiographic and biochemical[53] evidence of myocardial ischemia, led to the view that the syndrome was due to a reversible form of papillary muscle dysfunction.

PULMONARY REGURGITATION

Rarely is pulmonary regurgitation an isolated congenital anomaly. This is usually a benign condition and well tolerated, unless pulmonary hypertension is present. Nevertheless, a study of the natural history of isolated congenital pulmonary valve incompetence[54] showed that even in the absence of associated lesions, symptoms developed in 6% of patients within 20 years and in 29% of patients within 40 years of the angiographic diagnosis of pulmonary regurgitation. Neonates with pulmonary regurgitation or adults who develop pulmonary hypertension from any cause may be extremely symptomatic. It is manifested by an early diastolic, decrescendo murmur that is accidentally discovered during routine auscultation; the main pulmonary artery is large and is sometimes coincidentally recognized on a chest radiograph taken for some other reason. Since the advent of Doppler echocardiography, the incidence of isolated pulmonary regurgitation has risen 10-fold. Most normal individuals have trivial pulmonary regurgitation that can be detected only by this technique.[55] Hence, there is little relation between the incidence of isolated pulmonary regurgitation recognized by auscultation and that recognized by echocardiography.

Pulmonary regurgitation is common after repair of tetralogy of Fallot and is seen occasionally after relief of pulmonary stenosis. In some patients after pulmonary

valvotomy or valvuloplasty, replacement of the valve is required to avoid excessive right ventricular dilatation and dysfunction. Severe, hemodynamically significant pulmonary insufficiency may occur with the absent pulmonary valve syndrome that usually accompanies tetralogy of Fallot. This condition is described in detail in Chapter 28.

REFERENCES

1. Davachi F, Moller JH, Edwards JE: Diseases of the mitral valve in infancy. An anatomic analysis of 55 cases. Circulation 43:565, 1971.
2. Shone JD, Sellers RD, Anderson RC, et al: The developmental complex of "parachute mitral valve," supravalvular ring of left atrium, subaortic stenosis, and coarctation of aorta. Am J Cardiol 11:714, 1963.
3. Zamora R, Moller JH, Edwards JE: Double outlet right ventricle. Anatomic types and associated anomalies. Chest 68:672, 1975.
4. Castaneda AR, Anderson RC, Edwards JE: Congenital mitral stenosis resulting from anomalous arcade and obstructing papillary muscles. Report of correction by use of ball valve prosthesis. Am J Cardiol 24:237, 1969.
5. Van der Horst RL, Hastreiter AR: Congenital mitral stenosis. Am J Cardiol 20:773, 1967.
6. Braunwald E: Heart Disease: A Textbook of Cardiovascular Medicine. Philadelphia, WB Saunders, 1984.
7. Gorlin R, Gorlin SG: Hydraulic formula for calculation of the area of the stenotic, mitral valve, other cardiac valves, and central circulatory shunts. Am Heart J 41:1, 1951.
8. Corno A, Giannico S, Leibovich S, et al: The hypoplastic mitral valve. When should a left atrial–left ventricular extracardiac valved conduit be used? J Thorac Cardiovasc Surg 91:848, 1986.
9. Laks H, Hellenbrand WE, Kleinman C, et al: Left atrial–left ventricular conduit for relief of congenital mitral stenosis in infancy. J Thorac Cardiovasc Surg 80:782, 1980.
10. Lansing AM, Elbl F, Solinger RE, et al: Left atrial–left ventricular bypass for congenital mitral stenosis. Ann Thorac Surg 35:667, 1983.
11. Mazzera E, Corno A, Di Donato R, et al: Surgical bypass of the systemic atrioventricular valve in children by means of a valved conduit. J Thorac Cardiovasc Surg 96:321, 1968.
12. Midgley FM, Perry LW, Potter BM: Conduit bypass of mitral valve: A palliative approach to congenital mitral stenosis. Am J Cardiol 56:493, 1985.
13. Lock JE, Khalilullah M, Shrivastava S, et al: Percutaneous catheter commissurotomy in rheumatic mitral stenosis. N Engl J Med 313:1515, 1985.
14. Van Praagh R, Corsini I: Cor triatriatum: Pathologic anatomy and a consideration of morphogenesis based on 13 postmortem cases and a study of normal development of the pulmonary vein and atrial septum in 83 human embryos. Am Heart J 78:379, 1960.
15. Niwayama G: Cor triatriatum. Am Heart J 59:291, 1960.
16. Marin-Garcia J, Tandon R, Lucas RV Jr, Edwards JE: Cor triatriatum: Study of 20 cases. Am J Cardiol 35:59, 1975.
17. Jennings RB Jr, Innes BJ: Subtotal cor triatriatum with left partial anomalous pulmonary venous return. Successful surgical repair in an infant. J Thorac Cardiovasc Surg 74:461, 1977.
18. Wilson JW, Graham TP, Gehweiler JA, Canent RV: Cor triatriatum with intact subdividing diaphragm and partial anomalous pulmonary venous connection to the proximal left atrial chamber (an unreported type). Pediatrics 47:745, 1971.
19. Shone JD, Anderson RC, Amplatz K, et al: Pulmonary venous obstruction from two separate coexistent anomalies. Subtotal pulmonary venous connection to cor triatriatum and subtotal pulmonary venous connection to left innominate vein. Am J Cardiol 11:525, 1963.
20. Nakib A, Moller JH, Kanjuh VI, Edwards JE: Anomalies of the pulmonary veins. Am J Cardiol 20:77, 1967.
21. Jegier W, Gibbons JE, Wiglesworth FW: Cor triatriatum: Clinical, hemodynamic and pathological studies: Surgical correction in early life. Pediatrics 31:255, 1963.
22. Anderson RC, Varco RL: Cor triatriatum: Successful diagnosis and surgical correction in a three year old girl. Am J Cardiol 7:436, 1961.

23. Perry LW, Scott LP, McClenathan JE: Cor triatriatum: Preoperative diagnosis and successful surgical repair in a small infant. J Pediatr 71:840, 1967.

24. Glaser J, Yakirevich V, Vidne BA: Preoperative echographic diagnosis of supravalvular stenosing ring of the left atrium. Am Heart J 108:169, 1984.

25. Sullivan ID, Robinson PJ, de Leval M, et al: Membranous supravalvular mitral stenosis: A treatable form of congenital heart disease. J Am Coll Cardiol 8:159, 1986.

26. Braunwald E, Ross RS, Morrow AG, Roberts WC: Differential diagnosis of mitral regurgitation in childhood: Clinical pathological conference at the National Institutes of Health. Ann Intern Med 54:1223, 1961.

27. Zile MR, Gaash WH, Carroll JD, Levine HJ: Chronic mitral regurgitation: Predictive value of preoperative echocardiographic indices of left ventricular function and wall stress. J Am Coll Cardiol 3:235, 1984.

28. Roberts WC, Perloff JK: Mitral valvular disease: A clinicopathologic survey of the conditions causing the mitral valve to function abnormally. Ann Intern Med 77:939, 1972.

29. Christakis GT, Kormos RL, Weisel RD, et al: Morbidity and mortality of mitral valve surgery. Circulation 72(suppl II):120, 1985.

30. Gasul BM, Arcilla RA, Lev M: Heart Disease in Children. Diagnosis and Treatment. Philadelphia, JB Lippincott, 1971, p 731.

31. Calleja HB, Hosier DM, Kissane RW: Congenital tricuspid stenosis. The diagnostic valve of cineangiocardiography and hepatic pulse tracing. Am J Cardiol 6:821, 1960.

32. Salazar E, Benavides P, Contreras R, et al: Congenital mitral and tricuspid stenoses. Am J Cardiol 16:758, 1965.

33. Gueron M, Hirsh M, Borman J, et al: Isolated tricuspid valvular stenosis: The pathology and merits of surgical treatment. J Thorac Cardiovasc Surg 63:760, 1972.

34. Bharati S, McAllister HA, Tatooles CJ, et al: Anatomic variations in underdeveloped right ventricle related to tricuspid atresia and stenosis. J Thorac Cardiovasc Surg 72:383, 1976.

35. Lewis T: Congenital tricuspid stenosis. Clin Sci 5:261, 1945.

36. Medd WE, Neufeld HH, Weidman WH, et al: Isolated hypoplasia of the right ventricle and tricuspid valve in siblings. Br Heart J 23:25, 1961.

37. Scheibler GL, Gravenstein JS, Van Mierop LHS: Ebstein's anomaly of the tricuspid valve. Translation of original description with comments. Am J Cardiol 22:867, 1968.

38. Westaby S, Karp RB, Kirklin JW, et al: Surgical treatment in Ebstein's malformation. Ann Thorac Surg 34:388, 1982.

39. Davachi F, McLean RH, Moller JH, et al: Hypoplasia of the right ventricle and tricuspid valve in siblings. J Pediatr 71:869, 1967.

40. Dimich I, Goldfinger P, Steinfeld L, et al: Congenital tricuspid stenosis: Case treated by heterograft replacement of tricuspid valve. Am J Cardiol 31:89, 1973.

41. Medd WE, Kinmonth JB: Congenital tricuspid stenosis: A case treated by open operation. Br Med J 1:598, 1962.

42. Sackner MA, Robinson MJ, Jamison WL, et al: Isolated right ventricular hypoplasia with atrial septal defect or patent foramen ovale. Circulation 24:1388, 1961.

43. Rowe RD, Freedom RM, Mehrizi A: The Neonate with Congenital Heart Disease. Philadelphia, WB Saunders, 1981, p 515.

44. Edwards JE: Pathology of the Heart and Blood Vessels, 3rd ed. Springfield, IL, Charles C Thomas, 1968, p 316.

45. Becker AE, Becker MJ, Edwards JE: Pathologic spectrum of dysplasia of the tricuspid valve. Arch Pathol 91:167, 1971.

46. Kanjuh VI, Stevenson JE, Amplatz K, et al: Congenitally unguarded tricuspid orifice with coexistent pulmonary atresia. Circulation 30:911, 1964.

47. Reisman M, Hipona FA, Bloor CN, et al: Congenital tricuspid incompetence. J Pediatr 66:869, 1965.

48. Barritt DW, Urich H: Congenital tricuspid incompetence. Br Heart J 18:133, 1956.

49. Barr PA, Celermajer JM, Bowdler JS, et al: Severe congenital tricuspid incompetence in the neonate. Circulation 49:962, 1974.

50. Kincaid OW, Swan HJC, Ongley PA, et al: Congenital tricuspid insufficiency: Report of two cases. Mayo Clin Proc 37:640, 1962.

51. Bucciarelli RL, Nelson EM, Egan EA, et al: Transient tricuspid insufficiency of the newborn: A form of myocardial dysfunction in stressed newborns. Pediatrics 59:330, 1977.

52. Freymann R, Kallfelz HC: Transient tricuspid incompetence in a newborn. Eur J Cardiol 2:467, 1975.

53. Nelson RM, Bucciarelli RL, Eitzman DV, et al: Serum creatine phosphokinase MB fraction in newborns with transient tricuspid insufficiency. N Engl J Med 298:146, 1978.

54. Shimazaki Y, Blackstone EH, Kirklin JW: The natural history of isolated congenital pulmonary valve incompetence: Surgical implications. Thorac Cardiovasc Surg 32:257, 1984.

55. Takao S, Miyatake K, Izumi S, et al: Clinical implications of pulmonary regurgitation in healthy individuals: Detection by cross sectional pulsed Doppler echocardiography. Br Heart J 59:542, 1988.

CHAPTER 44
MITRAL VALVE PROLAPSE

RUSSELL V. LUCAS, JR.

Mitral valve prolapse (MVP) is an alteration in mitral valve function. It is not a single entity. MVP has been called by many names that provide insight into our perception of this condition over the years (Table 44–1). No pathognomonic sign, symptom, or feature allows reliable diagnosis of MVP. Diagnostic criteria have changed since the late 1960s, resulting in a variation in the reported prevalence of MVP ranging from more than 40% to less than 1%. Using current diagnostic criteria, MVP has an average prevalence of 4% (2.5% in males and 6% in females). MVP occurs in all ages, from the neonate to the ninth decade, but it is more common in young adults. MVP is more common in young females than in young males (male/female ratio = 1:2), although minimal gender differences are present in infants, young children, and older adults.

ETIOLOGY

MVP can be caused by a large number of cardiac conditions (Table 44–2). Primary MVP occurs in patients without any evidence of underlying cardiac disease and accounts for about 80 to 90% of MVP in the United States. In developing countries, MVP secondary to rheumatic carditis or rheumatic heart disease is estimated to cause about 30% of all MVP.

DIAGNOSTIC CRITERIA

The methods used to observe, define, and diagnose MVP illustrate different facets of the condition and do not always concur in the same patient.

CARDIAC AUSCULTATION

Auscultatory findings in MVP are a midsystolic click, a late-systolic murmur, or both. Currently accepted auscultatory diagnostic criteria allow consistent and reliable identification of MVP. Auscultation does not differentiate between primary or secondary MVP.

NONCONCURRENCE OF DIAGNOSTIC METHODS

The disparities in anatomic, echocardiographic, and auscultatory features in MVP have made absolute diagnosis of MVP difficult. They require evaluation of prior studies extremely carefully to determine precisely what diagnostic criteria were used to identify patients with MVP. Moreover, precise diagnostic criteria must be used in a disciplined manner to define accurately and understand MVP.

PRIMARY MITRAL VALVE PROLAPSE

PATHOLOGIC ANATOMY

This review of pathologic anatomy of MVP is based on general autopsy studies, autopsy studies of specific cardiac diseases, autopsy studies of the complications of MVP, and surgical pathologic studies of resected mitral valves. Death rarely occurs in young patients with primary MVP, so anatomic studies of the mitral valve in young patients with primary MVP are rare.

TABLE 44–1

SYNONYMS OF MITRAL VALVE PROLAPSE

Floppy mitral valve
Myxomatous degeneration of the mitral valve
Billowing mitral valve
Midsystolic click, late-systolic murmur syndrome
Barlow's syndrome
Prolapsing mitral leaflet syndrome
Ballooning mitral cusp syndrome
Redundant cusp syndrome

TABLE 44–2

ETIOLOGY OF MITRAL VALVE PROLAPSE

Primary

Familial
Nonfamilial

Secondary

Genetic (Hereditary)

Part of a clearly defined genetic syndrome, which may include Marfan syndrome, Ehlers-Danlos syndrome, osteogenesis imperfecta, homocystinuria, pseudoxanthoma elasticum, fragile X syndrome, cutis laxa, mucopolysaccharidoses, and others

Acquired

Acute rheumatic carditis
Nonrheumatic carditis
Rheumatic heart disease
Cardiomyopathy
Myocardial ischemia secondary to coronary artery disease
Secondary to papillary muscle dysfunction

Microscopic Anatomy of the Mitral Valve

A normal mitral valve leaflet is composed of the following four layers (Fig. 44–1):

1. Atrialis—a thin layer of collagen and elastic tissue that forms the atrial aspect of the leaflet and is continuous with the endocardium of the left atrium.

2. Spongiosa—delicate myxomatous connective tissue between the atrialis and the fibrosa.

3. Fibrosa—composed of dense layers of collagen and elastic tissue that form the basic support of the leaflet.

4. Ventricularis—a thin layer of collagen and elastic tissue that forms the ventricular surface of the mitral valve leaflet and tends to disappear toward the free end of the leaflet. The ventricularis may be considered part of the fibrosa.

The pathologic features of primary MVP are significant thickening of the spongiosa and spongiosal invasion of the fibrosa.[1] The latter causes focal interruption of the fibrosa and loss of structural integrity of the valve leaflet (see Fig. 44–1). Considerable variation occurs in the amount of spongiosa in the normal mitral valve leaflet. Those patients who have a thickened spongiosa layer that does not invade or interrupt the fibrosa represent a variation of the normal mitral valve anatomy. The histologic diagnosis of primary MVP (floppy mitral valve) cannot be made in the absence of spongiosal invasion and disruption of the fibrosa. The hypertrophied spongiosa contains an excessive amount of acid mucopolysaccharide material, which is not abnormal but simply increased in amount.

Ultrastructural studies of mitral valve leaflets in primary MVP reveal alterations in the fibrosal elements and chordae. The collagen fibers in the fibrosa and chordae are swollen, fragmented, and split. The collagen fibers are also coarsely granular, spiraled, and twisted. Some elastic fibers are fragmented and have cystic spaces. These alterations of ultrastructure may produce focally weak areas in the fibrosa that allow spongiosal penetration and enlargement of the valve leaflet. The chordal changes may allow stretching and elongation of the chordae.

Gross Anatomy of the Mitral Valve

In the normal mitral valve, the larger anterior leaflet is somewhat circular, and the small posterior leaflet is composed of three scallops. Each leaflet has a rough zone toward the free edge of the leaflet and a central clear zone toward the base (Fig. 44–2).

The following features define the gross anatomic diagnosis of MVP (Fig. 44–3)[1]:

1. Interchordal hooding involving both the rough and clear zones of the involved leaflet or leaflets. Leaflet enlargement is usually present.

2. Height of interchordal hooding of 4 mm or greater.

3. Interchordal hooding involving at least one half of the anterior leaflet, two thirds of the posterior leaflet, or both. When lesser degrees of hooding occur, they may represent variations of normal mitral valve anatomy.

Hooding represents bulging or prolapse of the mitral valve into the left atrial cavity. The mitral valve ring is positioned normally; the body of the mitral valve leaflet bulges into the left atrium; the free edges of the mitral valve

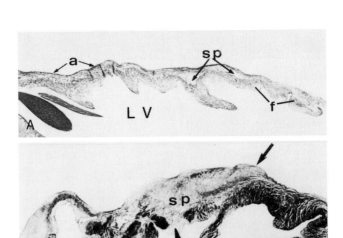
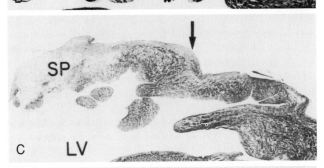
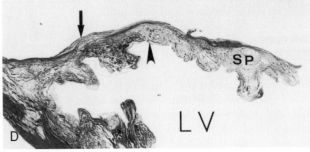

FIGURE 44–1

Photomicrographs of a normal mitral valve and three mitral valves with primary mitral valve prolapse (MVP). *A*, Normal mitral valve. The atrialis (a) is a thin layer of fibrous tissue on the left atrial side of the valve. The central layer is the spongiosa (sp), a layer of loose connective tissue, which is relatively sparse in a normal valve. The inner layer on the left ventricular surface is the fibrosa (f). This layer is composed of collagen and elastic tissue and serves as the skeleton of the valve leaflet. Elastin Van Gieson stain (ELVG) ×75. *B*, Anterolateral scallop of posterior leaflet in a 3-month-old girl with grade II primary MVP. The *arrowhead* on the left ventricular side of the valve demonstrates a distinct break in the fibrosa, which has been eroded by the spongiosa (sp). Several more distal breaks in the fibrosa are produced by spongiosal invasion. Note the fibrous scarring on the atrial surface of the valve *(arrow)*, which is secondary to the mitral valve contacting the left atrial wall during prolapse. Elastic tissue stain ×125. *C*, The central scallop of the posterior leaflet in a 4-year-old girl with grade II primary MVP. The spongiosa (SP) has eroded through the fibrosa at several sites in the distal one third of the leaflet. The *arrow* demonstrates the build-up of fibrous tissue where the prolapsing leaflet strikes the left atrial wall. Elastic tissue stain ×125. *D*, A 73-year-old man with grade II MVP. The spongiosa (sp) has completely eroded the fibrosa from the point of the *arrowhead* to the tip of the valve. The *arrow* demonstrates the build-up of fibrous tissue where the valve leaflet makes contact with the left atrial wall during prolapse. Note how little change is present in the histology of primary MVP between children in their first months and years of life and the elderly. ELVG ×125. LV = left ventricle.

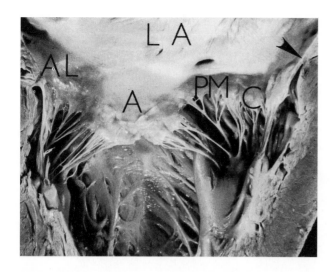

FIGURE 44–2

Normal mitral valve. The left atrium (LA) and left ventricle have been opened. The components of the mitral valve from left to right are a portion of the anterior lateral (AL) scallop of the posterior leaflet, the anterior (A) leaflet, the posteromedial (PM) and central (C) scallops of the posterior leaflet, and a portion of the bisected anterolateral scallop. The peripheral (rough) zone of both leaflets is normally thickened. There is minimal interchordal hooding, which is normal. The central portions of both leaflets are clear. The papillary muscles are normally located, and the chordae tendineae are of normal diameter and length. Note the continuity of the mitral valve fibrosa with the left atrial endocardium at the right (*arrowhead*).

leaflets may coapt normally or may occasionally allow mitral valve regurgitation.

Other specific anatomic findings are the result of different underlying cardiac causes of MVP, secondary effects of MVP, and complications of MVP.

Our definition of severity of MVP was based solely on the degree of interchordal hooding. This was an important proviso. The anatomic features resulting from complications of MVP, such as fibrosis of the atrial and ventricular surfaces of the mitral valve, friction lesions on the left ventricular wall, ruptured chordae tendineae, bacterial endocarditis, anatomic evidence of mitral regurgitation, anatomic evidence of left ventricular failure, and anatomic features of other cardiac causes of MVP, were not considered in our severity definition. The average severity of MVP did not increase in general autopsy studies as patients grew older.[1–3]

The prevalence of MVP in these autopsy studies was 7.4%,[1] 4.5%,[3] and 1%.[2] These prevalence figures are comparable to the current prevalence estimates based on auscultation and echocardiography.

Typical gross and histologic features of primary MVP have been reported in infants as young as 2 months of age, in children, and in adults of all ages.

FIBROELASTIC LESIONS. Fibroelastic lesions on the mitral valve leaflets, on the chordae, or on both regions occur in all patients with MVP (see Figs. 44–1 and 44–3B). These appeared to be related to the stress and tension imposed by the MVP as well as friction between the mitral valve leaflets and the atrial and ventricular surfaces.

THICKENED CHORDAE. Thickened chordae tendineae can be present (see Fig. 44–3B). Thickened chordae

were sometimes associated with friction lesions of the left ventricular wall and were most likely related to the friction of the chordae on the left ventricular wall (see Fig. 44–3C). Thinning and elongation of the chordae occurred in about 25% of MVP patients. We were unable to define any gross or histologic reason for the thinning or elongation of the chordae. It is pertinent that 75% of patients with primary MVP had chordae of normal length and normal thickness.[4] In primary MVP, no commissural fusion or chordal fusion occurs.

LEFT VENTRICULAR FRICTION LESIONS. Left ventricular friction lesions (Salazar lesions) consist of fibrous patches on the left ventricular endocardium, oriented parallel to the contiguous chordae. They appear to be related to friction between the contiguous chordae and the left ventricular wall (see Fig. 44–3B,C). Friction lesions were present in 75% of the patients with MVP in the study of Lucas and Edwards,[1] and in three patients the mitral valve chordae were entrapped in the left ventricular friction lesions, resulting in mitral valve regurgitation.

ASSOCIATED ANATOMIC CONDITIONS. Certain conditions have been reported as having a higher-than-expected frequency in patients with primary MVP.

Floppiness of Other Valves. In one study, 41% of patients with primary MVP had comparable histologic changes in the tricuspid valve.[1] None of the patients had clinically significant complications, and none had evidence of tricuspid valve regurgitation or bacterial endocarditis. Floppy pulmonary valves are occasionally noticed (11%), and floppy aortic valve is rarely present (2%) in patients with MVP.

Secundum Atrial Septal Defect. Mitral valve regurgitation in MVP may lead to left atrial dilatation and stretching of the foramen ovale, which results in a secondary atrial septal defect. Because primary MVP may be present in 2 to 6% of the general population, the finding of a significant number of patients with MVP among a series of secundum atrial septal defects is not surprising and may be explained by chance alone. A fundamental relationship between a secundum atrial septal defect and MVP has not been conclusively demonstrated.

HEMODYNAMICS

Mechanism of Mitral Valve Prolapse

The spongiosal invasion and destruction of the fibrosal integrity cause the mitral valve leaflet to become enlarged and redundant. In early systole, the mitral valve closes completely as the anterior and posterior leaflets coapt. As systole progresses, the left ventricle empties, the left ventricular dimensions decrease, and the papillary muscles and mitral ring attachments of the posterior leaflet move closer to each other. The posterior leaflet is rendered redundant and prolapses into the left atrium. If apposition between the two leaflets is lost, mitral regurgitation occurs. Less often, the anterior leaflet prolapses. Enlargement of the valve leaflets, elongation of the chordae tendineae, and dilatation of the mitral valve ring augment the prolapse process.

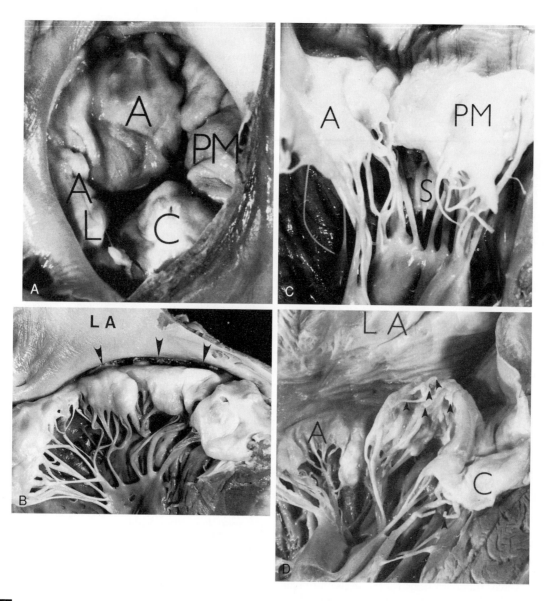

A, Primary mitral valve prolapse (MVP) in a 74-year-old woman who died of metastatic breast cancer. The left atrium has been resected at the atrioventricular groove. The anterior leaflet (A) and the anterior lateral (AL), the central (C), and the posteromedial (PM) scallops of the posterior leaflet are thickened, hooded, and prolapsed into the left atrial cavity. *B,* The left atrium (LA) and left ventricle of the same patient have been opened. There is prominent prolapse of the anterior leaflet *(at left)* and the three scallops of the posterior leaflet *(center* and *right).* A mound of fibrous tissue can be seen along the atrial surface of all the mitral valve leaflets where the leaflets hit the left atrial wall during prolapse (see Fig. 44–1 for the histologic depiction of this fibrous tissue mound). A deep pocket is formed when the valve leaflet strikes the left atrial wall during prolapse. Thrombi sometimes form in the pocket *(arrowheads).* Some chordae are thickened. A left ventricular friction (Salazar) lesion is present under the chordae to the central scallop of the posterior leaflet. *C,* Close-up of the anterior leaflet (A) and posteromedial (PM) scallop of the posterior leaflet in a 69-year-old man who died of a ruptured aneurysm of the descending aorta. He had no features of Marfan syndrome. There is grade II primary MVP. The chordae are thickened. There is a friction (Salazar) lesion (S) on the posterior wall of the ventricle where the chordae rub on the left ventricular wall. The chordae are scarred and thickened. *D,* Ruptured chordae tendineae serving the posteromedial scallop of the posterior leaflet in a 62-year-old man with grade II primary MVP. There are multiple sites of chordal rupture *(arrowheads).* The posteromedial scallop prolapses into the left atrium (LA). The resulting mitral regurgitation has scarred the prolapsing scallop.

These features allow the valve leaflets to "slip" after their initial contact (midsystolic click), thereby prolapsing into the left atrium. In some patients, mitral valve regurgitation occurs after the leaflets slip into the left atrium (late-systolic murmur). In others, the leaflet slippage does not unguard the mitral valve orifice, and no mitral valve regurgitation occurs (no murmur).

Effect of Left Ventricular Volume on Mitral Valve Prolapse

The left ventricular end-diastolic volume influences MVP. Decreased left ventricular end-diastolic volume favors MVP, whereas MVP is less common as left ventricular volume increases. For example, a woman with MVP loses the auscultatory and echocardiographic features of MVP in the third trimester of pregnancy when left ventricular end-diastolic volume is increased. After delivery, left ventricular volume decreases and the findings of MVP return.

Changes of left ventricular volume induced by changes in body position, heart rate, Valsalva's maneuver, and drug infusions result in alterations of diagnostic auscultatory features of MVP.

The effect of left ventricular volume on MVP may be additive to the anatomic abnormalities of the mitral valve leaflet that produce prolapse. However, it is possible that left ventricular volume dynamics could be the sole cause of MVP in patients having anatomically normal mitral valve leaflets.

Mitral Valve Regurgitation

ABSENT OR MILD.   The hemodynamics are normal in patients with uncomplicated primary MVP and absent or mild mitral valve regurgitation. Left ventricular function as measured by angiography or echocardiography is also normal.

CLINICALLY SIGNIFICANT.   Clinically significant mitral valve regurgitation is present in 5 to 20% of patients with primary MVP. Severe mitral regurgitation typically develops in the sixth and seventh decades of life. Mitral valve regurgitation results in dilatation of the left ventricle, left atrial enlargement, dilatation of the mitral valve orifice, apical displacement of the papillary muscles, and stretching and thinning of the chordae tendineae. Left atrial enlargement tends to pull the mitral valve leaflets into the left atrium because the mitral valve fibrosa and the left atrial endocardium are continuous. All of these events result in more mitral valve regurgitation. Thus, mitral valve regurgitation becomes progressively more severe and leads to left ventricular failure.

NATURAL HISTORY

Routine necropsy studies[1,3] indicate that patients with primary MVP have a normal life expectancy (Fig. 44–4). In a study of 119 children followed for an average of 6.9 years, one child developed bacterial endocarditis, and a second had a cerebrovascular accident. All of the rest remained well and without symptoms.[4] In a 9- to 22-year follow-up of 62 adults with MVP,[5] 5 (8%) died at an average age of 67 years. Five (8%) had bacterial endocarditis (one death), two had ruptured chordae (one died and one had valve replacement), and six developed mitral regurgitation but had slight symptoms. Forty-one patients (66%) remained completely asymptomatic.

Most studies suggest that primary MVP rarely produces symptoms in children or young adults. Long-term follow-up of adult patients with MVP indicates that the mortality of patients with MVP was not significantly different from that of age- and sex-matched controls.[6] When symptoms and complications of MVP occur, they are usually in patients older than 60 years.

Complications
MITRAL VALVE REGURGITATION
Minimal or clinically insignificant mitral valve regurgitation appears in many patients with MVP. Mild mitral valve regurgitation appears to increase the risk of bacterial endocarditis and rupture of the chordae. When mitral valve regurgitation is mild, its severity does not appear to progress over time. These patients have a normal life expectancy. In the Framingham study,[7] MVP patients had no evidence of clinically significant mitral valve regurgitation.

Mitral valve regurgitation severe enough to require mitral valve replacement occurs in about 4% of men and 1.5% of women, usually between the ages of 60 and 80 years.[8] Others with MVP die as a result of mitral valve regurgitation. Devereau and associates[8] suggested that 10% of men and 5% of women with MVP develop serious mitral valve regurgitation. Significant mitral valve regurgitation is rarely present before age 60 years in patients with primary MVP. The mean age at death of patients with MVP and significant mitral valve regurgitation was 76 years in one general population autopsy study.[1] In that study, 18% of patients with MVP had evidence of mitral valve regurgita-

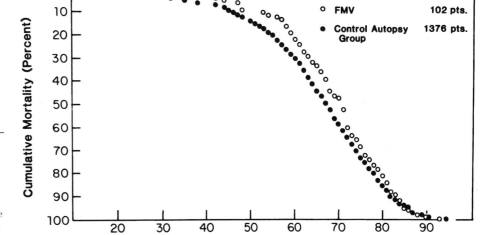

FIGURE 44–4

Cumulative mortality in all patients with MVP and in all patients in the community hospital control autopsy group. The MVP patients live slightly longer than control group patients, but the difference is not statistically significant. Of the 102 MVP patients, 62 were males and 40 were females. FMV = floppy mitral valve. (From Lucas RV Jr, Edwards JE: The floppy mitral valve. Curr Probl Cardiol 7:48, 1982.)

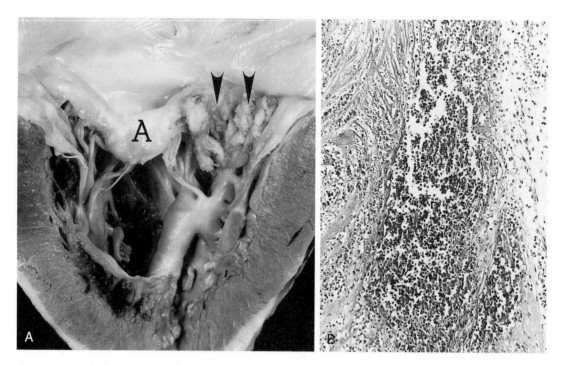

FIGURE 44–5

A, Bacterial endocarditis in a 44-year-old woman with mitral valve prolapse. The infection has destroyed the posteromedial and central scallops of the posterior leaflet of the mitral valve *(arrowheads).* Many of the chordae serving these scallops are ruptured. There was severe mitral valve regurgitation. The left atrium became greatly dilated and death ensued. A = anterior leaflet of mitral valve. *B,* Photomicrograph of the posteromedial scallop depicted in *A.* The colony of cocci has disrupted and partially destroyed the mitral valve tissue. H&E ×150.

tion: dilated mitral valve annulus, left atrial and ventricular dilatation, and jet lesions on the left atrial wall. The basis of the mitral valve regurgitation was primary rupture of the chordae tendineae in seven patients (see Fig. 44–3D), bacterial endocarditis in four patients (Fig. 44–5), chordal enlargement in a friction lesion in three patients, and MVP itself in four patients. In another general autopsy study,[3] virtually all the deaths resulting from mitral valve regurgitation occurred in patients between 60 and 90 years of age.

RUPTURE OF CHORDAE TENDINEAE

The prevalence of primary ruptured chordae in MVP was 7% in one autopsy study[1] and 2% in another study.[3] The posterior leaflet is the usual site of chordal rupture; the anterior leaflet is less commonly affected. The distribution of severity of MVP was identical in those patients with and without ruptured chordae. Chordal rupture occurs late in life (Fig. 44–6). In two autopsy series the mean age at death was 63.5 years[3] and 66 years.[1] The severity of MVP, presence of mitral valve regurgitation, and male gender predispose to ruptured chordae in MVP. Bacterial endocarditis is the underlying cause of about 20% of chordal rupture.[1,3] The mean age at operation in the 66 patients with MVP and ruptured chordae reported by Salomon and colleagues[9] was 58 years. Clinical chordal rupture is a common cause of mitral valve replacement in patients older than 60 years.

BACTERIAL ENDOCARDITIS

Two autopsy series of MVP had a prevalence of bacterial endocarditis of 7%[1] and 6%.[3] Clinical studies confirm that

the occurrence of bacterial endocarditis in patients with MVP is rare in children and more common in adults older than 40 years (see Fig. 44–6).

Studies of patients with bacterial endocarditis revealed that approximately one third of these patients had primary MVP as a predisposing cardiac condition.[10,11] A study suggested a lower prevalence of bacterial endocarditis in pa-

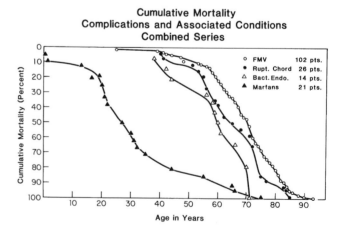

FIGURE 44–6

Cumulative mortality from complications and associated conditions of mitral valve prolapse (MVP). The cumulative mortality of the 102 patients with MVP (see Fig. 44–4) is shown for comparison. The other curves represent the total experience of Lucas and Edwards in the complication or associated condition recorded. FMV = floppy mitral valve. (From Lucas RV Jr, Edwards JE: The floppy mitral valve. Curr Probl Cardiol 7:48, 1982.)

tients with MVP,[12] but the risk of bacterial endocarditis in all patients with MVP is 5 times that of persons without MVP. The presence of a systolic murmur, the patient age older than 45 years, and the male gender all were independently associated with increased prevalence of bacterial endocarditis in patients with MVP.

Bacterial endocarditis has serious consequences. It produces severe mitral valve regurgitation, rupture of the chordae, or both in most patients. Nearly half of the patients die or require mitral valve replacement.[1, 10] The remainder are at high risk of more rapidly progressive mitral valve regurgitation.

SUDDEN UNEXPECTED OR UNEXPLAINED DEATH

Sudden death occurs in patients with primary MVP who have severe mitral valve regurgitation and dysfunction of the right or left ventricle. Sudden death also occurs in patients with secondary MVP due to myocardial ischemia, carditis, or cardiomyopathy. In none of these patients, however, is death unexpected or unexplained, because sudden death is typical in patients with these underlying cardiac diseases.

Sudden death that is truly unexpected and unexplained is rare in patients with MVP. I am aware of no evidence that either implicates or exonerates MVP as the cause of sudden unexpected or unexplained death. In these patients, the anatomic features of MVP are not unusual. The risk of sudden death in a patient with primary MVP without complications or associated cardiac disease is not high enough to warrant prophylactic therapy, and the risk should be minimized to the patient.

FIBRIN DEPOSITS AT THE LEFT ATRIUM–MITRAL VALVE JUNCTION

Fibrin deposits at the junction of the left atrium and mitral valve leaflets were present in 4% of the specimens with MVP in a general autopsy series and in 16% of specimens with MVP referred for study.[1] The fibrin collects in the pocket formed between the left atrium–mitral valve junction and the site of impact of the mitral valve leaflet on the left atrial wall (see Fig. 44–3B).

Fibrin deposits are transient. They either organize or embolize. Transient ischemic attacks have been reported in children and young adults with MVP.[13] Cerebrovascular accidents occur in children[4] and patients younger than 45 years[14] with MVP. Stroke and transient ischemic attacks are rare but real risks in patients of all ages with MVP.

EFFECT OF PREGNANCY ON MITRAL VALVE PROLAPSE

The prevalence of a midsystolic click and a late-systolic murmur is low in pregnant women. Prevalence of MVP defined by echocardiography is also lower in pregnant women than in nonpregnant women. As explained previously, women who have an echocardiographic or auscultatory diagnosis of MVP before pregnancy often lose the features of MVP during pregnancy only to have the features of MVP recur in the postpartum period.[15]

EFFECT OF MITRAL VALVE PROLAPSE ON PREGNANCY

No adverse effects of MVP on pregnancy or delivery have been reported in controlled studies. There is no apparent adverse effect on the fetus.[15]

Antibiotic prophylaxis to prevent bacterial endocarditis is indicated in women with echocardiographically defined MVP, in women with midsystolic click and late-systolic murmur, and in women with midsystolic click alone, at the time of routine and complicated deliveries.

HISTORY AND PHYSICAL FINDINGS

The keys to auscultatory findings are a midsystolic click and a late apical systolic murmur and postural changes in both.

Barlow and associates defined the midsystolic (nonejection) click and late-systolic murmur as cardiac in origin and diagnostic of MVP.[16, 17] The prevalences of the midsystolic (nonejection) click and the late-systolic murmur both peak in the adolescent and young adult years. Prevalence is less in the child younger than 6 years and the adult older than 60 years.[18] The prevalence of these auscultatory features is greater in females than in males. The average prevalence is approximately 4%. Midsystolic click and late-systolic murmurs have been documented in infants 1 to 3 days of age.[19]

Midsystolic (Nonejection) Click

The snapping, midsystolic or late-systolic click or clicks are characteristically variable: variable in the same patient from time to time and variable among different patients. One or more clicks may be present in early, middle, or late systole. They always precede the late-systolic murmur (if present). They are best heard in the left lateral position and are brought out, augmented, or changed in character and location in systole by change of position of the patient.

Late-Systolic Murmur

A late-systolic murmur is rarely louder than grade III and has a crescendo-decrescendo quality. The murmur always extends to the aortic component of the second heart sound, is often best heard in the left lateral position, and may be brought out or accentuated by sitting, leaning forward, squatting, or standing. Auscultation must be performed with the patient in several positions to assess variations in length and loudness of a murmur.

A late-systolic "honk" or "whoop" is rare. It is loud and may be heard by the patient. It is associated with a thrill. It is widely transmitted. A typical late-systolic murmur may become a honk on change of position, usually sitting, standing, or squatting. The honk is associated with the typical MVP features noted on echocardiography. The honk does not appear to alter the prognosis or natural history of MVP.

Effects of Postural Changes and Other Maneuvers on Timing of Click and Murmur

In early systole, the anterior and posterior leaflets of the mitral valve coapt normally. As systole progresses, left ventricular volume decreases. At a certain left ventricular volume, the posterior leaflet and, less often, the anterior leaflet slip or prolapse into the left atrium, producing the click. If the two mitral valve leaflets lose apposition, mitral valve regurgitation occurs (late-systolic murmur).

The volume of the left ventricle at the beginning of systole influences the timing of the midsystolic click and late-systolic murmur.[20] The supine position is the control position for left ventricular volumes. Sitting and standing reduce left ventricular volume at beginning systole. As a result, the click appears progressively earlier and the late-systolic murmur starts earlier and is longer (Fig. 44–7). However, squatting increases left ventricular volume at the beginning of systole. The click appears later in systole, and the murmur appears later and is shorter. The murmur may be significantly louder.

The Valsalva maneuver, tachycardia, and amyl nitrite also reduce left ventricular volume at beginning systole. They result in earlier clicks and longer systolic murmurs. Bradycardia and propranolol increase left ventricular volume at beginning systole and thereby produce later systolic clicks and shorter systolic murmurs.

These changes in "timing" of the midsystolic click are required to identify the click as the result of MVP. Moreover, these positional changes may initiate a click or murmur not otherwise heard.

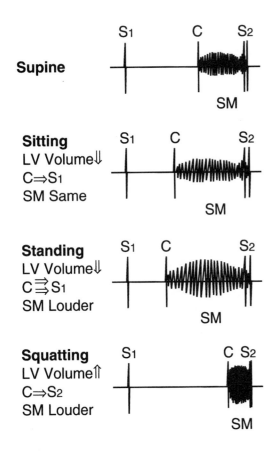

<u>FIGURE 44–7</u>

Effect of body position on the midsystolic click and late-systolic murmur in mitral valve prolapse. I consider the supine position as the control position. Sitting or standing reduces left ventricular end-diastolic volume. As left ventricular volume decreases, mitral valve prolapse is more likely and the click occurs earlier in systole. Squatting increases left ventricular end-diastolic volume. The click moves later in systole and may disappear. Maneuvers that reduce left ventricular volume (Valsalva's, tachycardia, amyl nitrite) result in clicks earlier in systole. Bradycardia and propanolol increase left ventricular volume and produce later systole clicks and shorten late-systolic murmurs. S_1 = first heart sound; C = midsystolic click; S_2 = second heart sound; SM = late-systolic murmur.

Mitral Valve Prolapse Syndrome

A large number of symptoms and signs have been correlated with MVP in past uncontrolled studies. In fact, a constellation of signs and symptoms has been called the mitral valve prolapse syndrome. Controlled studies provide no evidence that this syndrome occurs in adults or in children. Controlled studies in adults[7,8] and in children[21] found no correlation of MVP with symptoms such as chest pain, dyspnea, fatigue, palpitations, dizziness, or anxiety scores.

Skeletal Abnormalities

There appear to be no reliable data supporting increased incidence of skeletal abnormalities in patients with primary MVP as compared with that of the normal population.

Decreased Body Weight, Thinness, Asthenia

Several investigations have confirmed lower body weight in MVP patients compared with that in control groups.[22–24] This relationship holds for both adult men and adult women.

Nine (32%) of 28 patients with anorexia nervosa studied by Meyers and associates[24] had MVP diagnosed by echocardiography compared with a 7% incidence of MVP in the normal weight control groups. Seven of the nine patients with MVP gained to above 80% expected normal weight. In all nine patients, the echocardiographic evidence of MVP disappeared. Two of these patients then lost weight back to their previous severe weight loss state. The echocardiographic evidence of MVP recurred.

Reduced body size is correlated with reduced left ventricular volume, which in turn is correlated with MVP. Confirmation of this hypothesis requires additional study.

DIAGNOSTIC METHODS

Electrocardiography

The electrocardiogram (ECG) in most children and adults with a clinical diagnosis of primary MVP is normal. Many of the reported abnormalities in the ECG are secondary to the cardiac disease producing MVP. Some of the ECG abnormalities reported appear to be coincidental. Other ECG features that are described are variations of normal.

CHARACTERISTIC PATTERN

Pocock and Barlow[25] called attention to a "characteristic" ECG pattern in patients with MVP. This pattern was suggestive of posteroinferior myocardial ischemia. The pattern consisted of small q waves, elevated ST segments, and inverted T waves in leads II, III, and aVF. These changes could be present in two or three of these leads. In a few patients, these changes were also noted in leads V_5 and V_6. These so-called characteristic ECG findings have been described in both children and adults.[22,25,26] The incidence in adults was 9% and in children 48%. Some authors suspect that some of these patients with the characteristic ECG pattern suggestive of posteroinferior myocardial ischemia had underlying acute rheumatic carditis as a cause of the MVP. Others believe that nonrheumatic carditis might have been the underlying cause of MVP. In other studies, the ST and T wave changes have reverted to normal over time. There appears to be no relationship between the presence of the characteristic ECG findings and the severity of MVP or its natural history.[27]

Devereau and associates[8] found an equal incidence (10%) of inferior lead ECG repolarization abnormalities in patients with MVP and in a control group of first-degree relatives and spouses of the MVP patients. They believe that these so-called characteristic ECG abnormalities are not useful in establishing the diagnosis of primary MVP.

PREMATURE VENTRICULAR AND ATRIAL CONTRACTIONS

Unifocal premature ventricular and atrial contractions are commonly noted in the ECGs of patients with MVP. Most of these patients represent coincidental association of MVP with these benign ectopics. Multifocal premature ventricular and atrial contractions that increase in frequency with exercise also occur in patients with MVP.

Nearly 50% of the patients with MVP in the Framingham study[27] had complex or frequent premature ventricular contractions. The incidence of these ectopics was the same in controls. The presence of complex premature ventricular contractions may not be related to, or a result of, primary MVP but may represent an underlying cardiac etiology, such as myocarditis, myopathy, or myocardial ischemia.

ARRHYTHMIAS

Tachyarrhythmias occur in the ECG of patients with MVP. The Framingham study[27] revealed no statistical difference in the incidences of dysrhythmias in the 208 patients with echocardiographically defined MVP and their 2639 controls. Supraventricular tachycardias, atrial flutter, atrial fibrillation, and ventricular tachycardias have been reported.

CONDUCTION DISTURBANCES

First-degree heart block occurs in the ECG of approximately 3% of the patients with MVP.[20] Intraventricular conduction delays (right bundle branch block, left anterior hemiblock), second-degree heart block, and complete heart block are rare. When these occur in patients with MVP, they may be a chance association.[20]

EXERCISE STUDIES

Results of graded exercise on the ECG in patients with MVP have been variable. In numerous reports the incidence of ST depression during exercise in patients with MVP has varied from 0 to 60% of the patients.[4, 25, 26] In these studies, the frequency of development of premature ventricular contractions varied from 0 to 30%. Because in some studies the underlying etiology of MVP was not clearly identified in the exercised patients, the ECG changes could be related to an underlying myocardial disease and not to MVP.

COMMENT

There appears to be no correlation between ECG findings and MVP. No clear relationships between the resting or exercise ECG and the severity of MVP, the etiology of MVP, or the natural history of MVP have been proved. Most of the arrhythmias appear to be a chance coexistence of MVP and the arrhythmia.

The ST segment changes in the characteristic MVP ECG pattern occur in equal frequency in control non-MVP patients.

It is my practice to evaluate the ECG abnormalities as independent variables for all patients with MVP. Arrhythmias should be evaluated and treated in the usual fashion. Ventricular function should also be evaluated and appropriate treatment started if impaired ventricular function underlies the arrhythmia.

The presence of a significant arrhythmia imputes its own prognosis, independent of that of MVP.

Chest Radiography

The chest radiograph in most patients with primary MVP is normal. Those few patients who develop clinically significant mitral valve regurgitation have left ventricular and left atrial enlargement. As mitral valve regurgitation becomes more severe, pulmonary edema, enlargement of the main pulmonary artery segment, and right ventricular hypertrophy also occur. Levy and Savage[22] pointed out that the left atrial enlargement occurs less often in patients with MVP (7.5%) than in control patients without evidence of MVP (11.5%).

The typical age of the patient with MVP who develops ruptured chordae is usually around 60 years. These patients have the sudden onset of mitral valve regurgitation and left ventricular failure. Chest radiography reveals dilatation of the left ventricle, enlargement of the left atrium, and pulmonary edema. The pulmonary artery segment may be enlarged, and the right ventricle may also be dilated.

Echocardiography

The recognition and diagnosis of MVP and the technical improvements in and understanding of echocardiography occurred simultaneously. Initially, the sensitivity and specificity of echocardiography in the diagnosis of MVP were variable.

M-MODE ECHOCARDIOGRAPHY

M-mode echocardiography is not spatially oriented, and the mitral valve leaflets and the plane of the mitral valve annulus cannot be appreciated by the operator. Thus, a minor change in angulation of the M-mode beam might result in the appearance of MVP in a normal individual, on the one hand, or in normal appearance of the mitral valve in a patient who had MVP, on the other hand. Differences in criteria applied to the M-mode echocardiogram resulted in variations in prevalence of MVP defined by this method from 4 to 20%. As more strict diagnostic criteria were applied, the prevalence of prolapse was reduced to approximately 1 to 4%. The M-mode echocardiogram will never be able to define the spatial relationship of the mitral valve leaflets to the mitral valve annulus.[28]

TWO-DIMENSIONAL ECHOCARDIOGRAPHY

The two-dimensional echocardiogram, however, allows the relationship between the mitral valve leaflets and the plane of the mitral valve annulus to be identified. Because the mitral valve annulus is not flat but saddle shaped, slight variations in angulation of the transducer beam may result in erroneous identification of MVP.

Initially, the apical four-chamber view was considered to be the best method of defining MVP (Fig. 44–8). However, the saddle shape of the mitral valve annulus allowed for false-positives to be defined in children.[29]

In a parasternal long-axis view when the mitral valve is imaged in the anteroposterior direction, both leaflets can be well seen. Superior prolapse of the mitral valve leaflets into the left atrium can be defined by this view (see Fig. 44–8). In addition, the mitral valve leaflets may be carefully inspected for myxomatous thickening. Finally, this view allows excellent identification of mitral valve regurgitation by color flow Doppler. M-mode echocardiographic recordings can also clearly indicate prolapse (Fig. 44–9).

DIAGNOSTIC CRITERIA

The echocardiographic criteria for the diagnosis of MVP are not uniform. I believe the following criteria of MVP advanced by Snider and Serwer[30] are the most useful:

Systolic prolapse of one or both of the mitral valve leaflets posterior and superior to the plane of the mitral annulus in at least two echocardiographic views; or prolapse in one echocardiographic view, when associated mitral regurgitation and/or myxomatous enlargement of the mitral valve leaflets are present.

ASSOCIATED CONDITIONS

SEVERE MITRAL VALVE REGURGITATION. In these patients, the echocardiogram reveals a dilated left ventricle and impaired left ventricular function. The left atrium is enlarged. The mitral valve annulus may be significantly dilated. Color flow Doppler evaluation defines significant

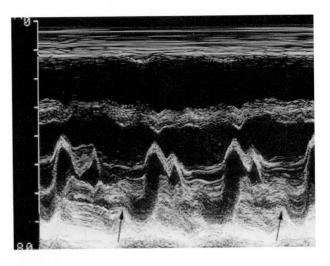

M-mode echocardiogram shows prolapse of the posterior mitral valve leaflet starting at about midsystole (*arrows*). (Courtesy of Dr. Norman H. Silverman.)

mitral valve regurgitation, and right ventricular pressure may be elevated.

RUPTURED CHORDAE TENDINEAE. The subcostal view is excellent to define the detail of the mitral valve and, particularly, ruptured chordae, which can be seen flailing around in the left atrium. Mitral valve regurgitation occurs, and often one valve leaflet or a portion of the leaflet is completely detached from its chordae and prolapses completely into the left atrial cavity.[30]

Cardiac Catheterization and Angiography

Cardiac catheterization and angiography in MVP are primarily of historical interest. These studies are not often performed today in patients with MVP. In the patient with primary MVP, without clinically significant mitral valve regurgitation, the hemodynamics are normal. Left ventricular size and function are normal, and left atrial size is normal.

Cardiac catheterization and angiography are occasionally indicated in a patient with primary MVP and a severe complication, such as mitral valve regurgitation and left ventricular failure, ruptured chordae tendineae, or bacterial endocarditis. Even then, echocardiography is usually sufficient to plan appropriate management, including surgery.

ANGIOGRAPHIC FEATURES

Prolapse of the posterior mitral leaflet and its three scallops is best defined in the right anterior oblique projection. In the 30- to 40-degree right anterior oblique projection, the mitral valve annulus is in the plane of the x-ray beam, and the mitral valve leaflets are superimposed.[31] Prolapse of the posterior leaflet and its scallops can be well seen in this view. However, lesser degrees or greater degrees of obliquity produce a more elliptic view of the annulus. This may result in a false-positive or false-negative diagnosis of MVP.

The anterior leaflet, not well visualized in the right anterior oblique position, may be seen better in the straight

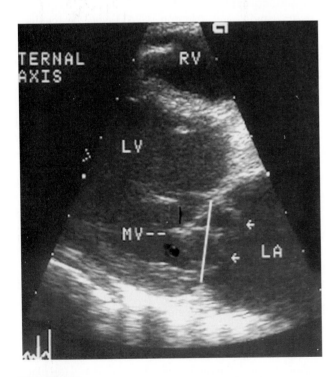

Two-dimensional echocardiogram shows prolapse of both mitral valve leaflets (MV) into the left atrium (LA). The leaflets are seen behind the plane of the mitral valve annulus, indicated by the *straight line*. The *arrows* point to the prolapsed portion of the valve leaflets. RV = right ventricle; LV = left ventricle. (Courtesy of Dr. Norman H. Silverman.)

lateral view in which anterior leaflet prolapse may be defined. Even with several views, the severity of MVP is difficult to estimate using angiography, because the degree of angulation of the view influences the apparent degree of prolapse significantly.[31] Specific angiographic criteria for the diagnosis of MVP have not been systematically or prospectively tested in patients with MVP defined by other methods. Because of this and because MVP can be clinically well defined by auscultation and echocardiography, invasive contrast angiography is rarely used as a diagnostic method in the definition of MVP.[8]

MANAGEMENT AND PROGNOSIS

Management of MVP varies from reassurance to mitral valve replacement. The basis of appropriate management is an accurate and definitive diagnosis. Although there is better agreement today than in the past on the appropriate diagnostic criteria for MVP, there is no generally accepted standard. MVP has no pathognomonic sign or feature to ensure accurate diagnosis.

Diagnostic Criteria

Devereau and associates[8] have defined diagnostic criteria for MVP that are a good start to standardized diagnosis. Widespread agreement and appropriate modification are still required.

My criteria for the diagnosis of MVP are influenced by several publications[8, 20, 28, 30] and are outlined in Table 44–3.

TABLE 44–3

CRITERIA FOR DIAGNOSIS OF MITRAL VALVE PROLAPSE

Auscultation

1. Apical midsystolic click alone
   Moderately high accuracy if typical timing changes are present
2. Midsystolic click and late-systolic murmur
   High accuracy if patient examined in multiple positions and typical timing changes are present
3. Late-systolic murmur alone
   Moderate accuracy if murmur persists to aortic closure sound
4. Holosystolic murmur alone
   Low accuracy

M-Mode Echocardiography

Poor diagnostic value unless confirmed by two-dimensional echocardiography

Two-Dimensional Echocardiography

1. Prolapse of one or both mitral valve leaflets during systole; posterior and superior to the plane of the mitral valve ring; in at least two echocardiographic views
   High accuracy
2. Prolapse in only one echocardiographic view when associated with
   a. Mitral valve regurgitation and/or
   b. Myxomatous thickening of mitral valve leaflet(s)
   High accuracy
3. Prolapse in only one echocardiographic view
   Nondiagnostic

Left Ventricular Angiogram

Angiography rarely used in the clinical diagnosis of primary mitral valve prolapse
Degree of angulation of x-ray beam influences magnitude of prolapse
Severity of prolapse difficult to define
High accuracy requires mitral valve prolapse in two angiographic views

---

The tendency to add up several nondiagnostic features of MVP and conclude that the patient has MVP must be resisted. Much of the past misdiagnosis, disagreement, and confusion is based on this natural and human tendency. For example, the patient who has a midsystolic click that does not change its timing with position, has prolapse in only one plane on echocardiography, has the characteristic ECG findings in leads II, III and aVF, and suffers from chest pain, palpitations, and anxiety does *not* have MVP.

Further Patient Evaluation

Appropriate management requires a further definition of the etiology, clinical severity, and complications of MVP (Table 44–4).

The patient who has only a midsystolic click with appropriate timing changes with position should undergo echocardiography. If the echocardiogram is nondiagnostic of MVP, the patient should be reassured that the click is benign and that his or her life expectancy is normal. Long-term follow-up (every 2 to 3 years) is appropriate. Bacterial endocarditis prophylaxis is recommended.

If the echocardiogram is diagnostic of MVP, the patient has primary MVP. The patient should be reassured that he or she has a normal life expectancy and that complications may occur late in life. Bacterial endocarditis prophylaxis is required and long-term follow-up is necessary. A careful family history will establish if this primary MVP is familial.

The patient with a midsystolic click with typical timing changes and a late-systolic murmur extending to the aortic closure sound has MVP. Echocardiography is not required for the diagnosis of MVP, but it is useful in ruling out one of the secondary causes of MVP. This patient needs reassurance, a careful family history, bacterial endocarditis

---

TABLE 44–4

MANAGEMENT CONSIDERATIONS IN MITRAL VALVE PROLAPSE

Etiology

Primary
  Familial
  Nonfamilial
Secondary
  Marfan syndrome and other connective tissue disorders
  Carditis: rheumatic, nonrheumatic
  Rheumatic heart disease
  Cardiomyopathy
  Ischemic myocardium

Mitral Valve Abnormality

Prolapse—specify leaflets
Leaflet enlargement
Leaflet thickening
Chordal redundancy
Chordal rupture
Mitral ring dilatation

Clinical Severity of Mitral Regurgitation

No mitral regurgitation
Trivial or mild
Moderate to severe

Other Complications

Left ventricular failure
Bacterial endocarditis
Transient ischemic attacks
Significant electrocardiographic abnormality

prophylaxis, and long-term follow-up. Symptoms or complications are rare before the age of 60.

A routine ECG should be obtained with a diagnosis of primary MVP. If it is abnormal, the patient requires a complete evaluation to determine the cause of the ECG changes. ECG findings that are abnormal are not usually caused by MVP.

Identification of one of the genetic syndromes can be done without difficulty. The management and natural history of these patients are determined by the syndrome and are not typical of primary MVP.

Clinical Severity of Mitral Valve Regurgitation

The presence and severity of mitral valve regurgitation in primary MVP are major determinants in its natural history and management.

ABSENCE OF MITRAL VALVE REGURGITATION

These patients have a normal life expectancy. The occurrence of severe mitral valve regurgitation or other complications of MVP is rare. These patients require maximal reassurance as to their "normal" heart and normal life expectancies. Bacterial endocarditis prophylaxis is recommended. Long-term (every 2 to 3 years) follow-up is indicated.

TRIVIAL OR MILD MITRAL VALVE REGURGITATION

These patients have normal cardiac function and appear to have a normal life expectancy. The incidence of clinically significant mitral valve regurgitation is 5% or less and occurs usually in the sixth and seventh decades of life. Bacterial endocarditis prophylaxis is mandatory. These patients need maximal reassurance as to their optimistic natural history. Annual clinical follow-up is indicated.

MODERATE OR SEVERE MITRAL VALVE REGURGITATION

Once the patient with primary MVP develops moderate to severe mitral valve regurgitation, the prognosis worsens. Specific complications of MVP leading to mitral valve regurgitation (e.g., ruptured chordae, entrapped chordae, and bacterial endocarditis) must be identified if present. Appropriate medical management with digitalis, diuretics, and afterload reducers is indicated when left ventricular dilatation or failure occurs.

Mitral valve replacement is indicated when left ventricular function is declining or left ventricular dilatation is increasing. Bacterial endocarditis prophylaxis is mandatory.

Other Complications
LEFT VENTRICULAR FAILURE

Severe mitral valve regurgitation, chordal rupture, and bacterial endocarditis may cause left ventricular failure. Left ventricular failure causes enlargement of the left ventricle, mitral valve ring, and left atrium, as well as causing pulmonary edema and right ventricular failure. Bacterial endocarditis, if present, must be established and treated bacteriologically. Staged valve replacement is usually also required. Bacterial endocarditis occurs in children and young adults but is more common in middle-aged and older patients. Ruptured chordae can be diagnosed by echocardiography. In these patients, left ventricular failure requires mitral valve replacement.

TRANSIENT ISCHEMIC ATTACKS

Transient ischemic attacks (TIAs) and strokes with residual central nervous system findings occur in patients with MVP. These are presumed to be secondary to embolization of the left atrium–mitral valve junction thrombi that are noted on autopsy in about 4% of the patients with MVP. Appropriate management of the patient with primary MVP to prevent the first TIA or stroke is not established. Daily or every-other-day low-dose aspirin therapy seems an appropriate recommendation for the adult with primary MVP.

Once the patient with MVP has had a stroke or TIA, some physicians recommend low-dose aspirin or warfarin (Coumadin). The efficacy of these in preventing subsequent events is not established.

SUDDEN DEATH

Sudden death is an exceedingly rare complication of primary MVP in the absence of left ventricular failure or other life-threatening complications or in the absence of ECG abnormalities. It is a great disservice to the patient with uncomplicated primary MVP to bring up sudden death as a potential complication.

Sudden death is not unexpected in patients with MVP secondary to left ventricular dysfunction and in patients with MVP and left ventricular failure.

SUMMARY

- The greatest enemy of appropriate management of the patient with primary MVP is sloppy diagnosis.
- The diagnosis of primary MVP should be disciplined and based on defined criteria.
- The patient should be given an accurate and complete prognosis based on precise and specific findings.
- Reassurance is the cornerstone of management in more than 90% of patients with primary MVP. You must keep up the reassurance throughout the life of the patient.
- Management of the complications of MVP and of the secondary causes of MVP is well established in medical practice and poses no problem to the informed physician. Controlled studies do not support the existence of the mitral valve prolapse syndrome.

SECONDARY MITRAL VALVE PROLAPSE

MITRAL VALVE PROLAPSE IN GENETIC OR HEREDITARY SYNDROMES

These syndromes are listed in Table 44–2. The histologic and anatomic features in these syndromes are similar to those in primary MVP. They differ from primary MVP by (1) an earlier onset and more severe mitral valve pathology, (2) the typical clinical features characteristic of each of these syndromes, and (3) the natural history dominated by the underlying syndrome.

ACQUIRED MITRAL VALVE PROLAPSE

ACUTE RHEUMATIC CARDITIS. This is a rare cause of MVP in the United States. Prevalence of acute rheumatic carditis as a cause of MVP is as high as 30% in developing countries. Anatomic and histologic features are typical for acute rheumatic carditis.[32] Anatomic and histologic features of primary MVP are not present. Use of the Jones criteria for the diagnosis of acute rheumatic fever allows an appropriate differential diagnosis between primary MVP and MVP secondary to acute rheumatic carditis.

RHEUMATIC HEART DISEASE. Patients with mitral valve regurgitation as a result of well-documented acute rheumatic fever have MVP demonstrated by echocardiography in 30%[33] to 80%.[34] Careful documentation of prior acute rheumatic fever allows an appropriate differential diagnosis.

LEFT VENTRICULAR DYSFUNCTION. MVP has been noted in patients with left ventricular dysfunction due to myocarditis, cardiomyopathy, coronary artery disease, and other causes. Left ventricular dilatation, papillary muscle dysfunction, dilated mitral valve ring, and mitral valve regurgitation are usual. Left ventricular failure may occur, and mitral valve replacement may be recommended.

The clinical features of these acquired cardiac diseases usually allow appropriate differential diagnosis. The histologic and anatomic features of these diseases are diagnostic. The histologic features of primary MVP are not present.

FUTURE DIRECTIONS

DIAGNOSTIC CRITERIA

Understanding of the diagnosis, management, and etiology of MVP requires the identification of diagnostic criteria that are generally accepted by the medical profession. The great variety of diagnostic criteria casts a wide net that catches many patients who do not have MVP. We are truly in the same state of affairs as the medical profession was before the Jones commission report in 1944 outlined the diagnostic criteria for acute rheumatic fever. When the Jones criteria were learned and accepted, our diagnosis, management, and understanding of rheumatic fever were greatly facilitated.

ETIOLOGY OF PRIMARY MVP

Understanding the precise etiology of MVP might establish more exact diagnostic criteria and perhaps identify a pathognomonic sign or laboratory test. One wonders if the hypertrophy of the spongiosa, invasion of fibrosa, and the collagen and elastic fiber changes seen in the valve and chordae are similar in etiology to the changes seen in Marfan syndrome and the other connective tissue diseases. Is there a relationship between the familial occurrence of primary MVP and the genetically related causes of MVP?

Many patients with primary MVP have specific histologic and anatomic abnormalities of the mitral valve leaflets. I believe that another group of patients with anatomically normal mitral valve leaflets have primary MVP solely on the basis of left ventricular volume characteristics. This opinion cannot be supported by the known data. Moreover, both causes of MVP may coexist. Do they

have a different natural history? Which one of them is more likely to be familial in occurrence?

THERAPEUTIC CONSIDERATIONS

A major clinical problem that requires solution is whether a patient with primary MVP needs antithrombotic therapy to prevent the occurrence of fibrin deposits in the left atrium–mitral valve junction to prevent TIAs and strokes in these patients. Moreover, once a TIA or stroke has occurred, is anticoagulant treatment necessary?

REFERENCES

1. Lucas RV Jr, Edwards JE: The floppy mitral valve. Curr Probl Cardiol 7:48, 1982.
2. Pomerance A: Ballooning deformity of atrioventricular valves. Br Heart J 31:343, 1969.
3. Davies MJ, Moore BP, Braimbridge MV: The floppy mitral valve: Study in incidence, pathology and complications in surgical, necroscopy and forensic material. Br Heart J 40:468, 1978.
4. Bissett GS, Schwartz DC, Meyer RA, et al: Clinical spectrum and long-term follow-up of isolated mitral valve prolapse in 119 children. Circulation 62:423, 1980.
5. Allen H, Harris A, Leatham A: Significance and prognosis of an isolated late systolic murmur: A 9- to 22-year follow-up. Br Heart J 36:525, 1974.
6. Nishimura RA, McGoon MD, Shub C, et al: Echocardiographically documented mitral valve prolapse: Long-term follow-up of 237 patients. N Engl J Med 313:1305, 1985.
7. Savage DD, Devereau RB, Garrison RJ, et al: Mitral valve prolapse in the general population. 2. Clinical features: The Framingham study. Am Heart J 106:577, 1983.
8. Devereau RV, Kramer-Fox R, Shear MK, et al: Diagnosis and classification of severity of mitral valve prolapse: Methodologic, biologic, and prognostic considerations. Am Heart J 113:1255, 1987.
9. Salomon NW, Stinson EB, Griepp RB, Shumway NE: Surgical treatment of degenerative mitral regurgitation. Am J Cardiol 38:463, 1976.
10. Nolan CM, Kane JJ, Grunow WA: Infective endocarditis and mitral valve prolapse: A comparison with other types of endocarditis. Arch Intern Med 141:447, 1981.
11. Corrigal D, Bolen J, Hancock EW, et al: Mitral valve prolapse and infective endocarditis. Am J Med 63:215, 1977.
12. MacMahon SW, Roberts JK, Kramer-Fox R, et al: Mitral valve prolapse and infective endocarditis. Am Heart J 113:1291, 1987.
13. Barnett HJM, Jones MW, Boughner DR: Cerebral ischemic events associated with prolapsing mitral valve. Arch Neurol 33:777, 1976.
14. Bogousslavsky J, Hommel M, Stauffer JC, et al: Patent foramen ovale in young stroke patients with mitral valve prolapse. Acta Neurol Scand 89:23, 1994.
15. Rayburn WF: Mitral valve prolapse and pregnancy. In Elkayam W, Gleicher N (eds): Cardiac Problems in Pregnancy. New York, AR Liss, 1990, pp 181–188.
16. Barlow JB, Bosman CK, Pocock WA, Marchand P: Late systolic murmurs and non-ejection ("mid-late") systolic clicks. Br Heart J 30:203, 1968.
17. Pocock WA, Barlow JB: Etiology and electrocardiographic features of the billowing posterior mitral leaflet syndrome. Am J Med 51:731, 1971.
18. McLaren MJ, Hawkins DM, Lachman AS, et al: Non-ejection systolic clicks and mitral systolic murmurs in Black school children of Soweto, Johannesburg. Br Heart J 38:718, 1976.
19. Chandraratna PAN, Vlahovich G, Kong Y, Wilson D: Incidence of mitral valve prolapse in 100 clinically stable newborn girls: An echocardiographic study. Am Heart J 98:312, 1979.
20. Devereau RB, Perloff JK, Reichek N, Josephson ME: Mitral valve prolapse. Circulation 54:3, 1976.
21. Arfken CL, Leachman AS, MacLaren MJ, et al: Mitral valve prolapse: Associations with symptoms and anxiety. Pediatrics 85:311, 1990.

22. Levy D, Savage D: Prevalence and clinical features of mitral valve prolapse. Am Heart J 113:1281, 1987.

23. Devereau RV, Kramer-Fox R: Gender differences in mitral valve prolapse. Cardiovasc Clin 19:243, 1989.

24. Meyers DG, Starke EH, Pearson PH, Wilken MR: Mitral valve prolapse in anorexia nervosa. In Proceedings of the Second International Conference on Eating Disorders. New York, John Wiley & Sons, 1986, p 184.

25. Pocock WA, Barlow JB: Etiology and electrocardiographic feature of the billowing posterior mitral valve leaflet syndrome. Analysis of a further 130 patients with a late systolic murmur or nonejection systolic click. Am J Med 51:731, 1971.

26. Kavey RW, Sondheimer HM, Blockman MS: Detection of dysrhythmia in pediatric patients with mitral valve prolapse. Circulation 62:582, 1980.

27. Savage DD, Levy D, Garrison RT, et al: Mitral valve prolapse in the general population. 3. Dysarrhythmias: The Framingham study. Am Heart J 106:582, 1986.

28. Judd VE: Mitral valve prolapse. In Garson A Jr, Bricker JT, McNamara DG (eds): The Science and Practice of Pediatric Cardiology. Philadelphia, Lea & Febiger, 1990, pp 1973–1986.

29. Warth DC, King ME, Cohen J, et al: Prevalence of mitral valve prolapse in normal children. J Am Coll Cardiol 5:1173, 1985.

30. Snider AR, Serwer G: Echocardiography in Pediatric Heart Disease. St. Louis, Mosby–Year Book, 1990.

31. Amplatz K, Moller JH, Castaneda-Zuniga WR: Radiology of Congenital Heart Disease. New York, Thieme Medical, 1986.

32. Marcus RH, Sardi P, Pocock W, et al: Functional anatomy of severe mitral regurgitation in active rheumatic carditis. Am J Cardiol 63:577, 1989.

33. Wu M, Lue H, Wang J, et al: Implications of mitral valve prolapse in children with rheumatic mitral regurgitation. J Am Coll Cardiol 23:1199, 1994.

34. Lembo NJ, Dell'Italia LJ, Crawford MH, et al: Mitral valve prolapse in patients with prior rheumatic fever. Circulation 79:830, 1988.

CHAPTER 45
CARDIAC PROBLEMS OF ADULTS WITH CONGENITAL HEART DISEASE

JANE SOMERVILLE

The success of cardiac surgery for congenital heart disease not only stimulated the development of the specialty pediatric cardiology but, more important, transformed the prognosis of congenital heart disease. Once, 60 to 70%[1] of those born with congenital heart disease died during infancy, and now 70 to 75% reach adolescence and become adults.[2-5] The management of congenital heart disease has undergone a revolution. It is no longer only the neonate, infant, and child with congenital heart disease who need specialist cardiac medicine and surgery, but also the fetus and the adult. Many pediatric cardiology practices may have to change when the triumphs and disasters in the adult are evaluated. Some of today's practices will not be tomorrow's, as occurs in all branches of evolving medicine.

Thus, a new adult medical population has been created—the grown-up congenital heart (GUCH as known in the United Kingdom, Europe, and Japan)—which includes the adolescents, in transition between childhood and adulthood, and adults. The group has various names according to local sensitivity and geography—for example, ACH (Adult Congenital Hearts), CACH (Canadian version), BACH (Boston)—with various overseeing bodies, such as Working Group on GUCH of the European Society of Cardiology.

The size of this population in most countries is unknown or can only be guessed, unless the country is small and has strong and organized health services, as in Iceland and the Scandinavian countries. Perhaps there are 100,000 to 500,000 GUCH patients in the United States.[3] In the United Kingdom, our estimate of the hospital attending population is about 10,000 to 15,000, with less than 1000 admissions per annum. The number unseen and untreated is not known. Many GUCH patients may not need medical care, and those with a simpler lesion (Table 45–1) lead normal lives, requiring little cardiologic follow-up. The formation of a GUCH Patients' Association in the United Kingdom, separate from the medical profession, has brought many patients into the open; this identification has encouraged them to share and lobby to improve their care. The lack of GUCH statistics results from inaccuracy of hospital diagnostic codes. In addition, because there are few such patients, the number of patients an individual physician sees is limited, and because many have good health, they do not seek medical attention.

WHO ARE THE GUCH PATIENTS, AND WHAT ARE THEIR SPECIFIC PROBLEMS?

1. They are those with minor lesions, such as a small atrial or ventricular septal defect or mild pulmonic stenosis. Other than precautions against infective endocarditis (rare in atrial septal defects and pulmonic stenosis), they need little cardiac care because these conditions are stable throughout life. An exception is the patient with a bicuspid, nonstenotic aortic valve who may do well until middle age and then develop severe calcific aortic stenosis or devastating aortic incompetence.[6,7]

2. They are those with a significant but unoperated lesion, such as a large atrial septal defect, patent ductus arteriosus, univentricular heart, transposition of the great arteries with a ventricular septal defect and pulmonic stenosis, Eisenmenger's syndrome, or tetralogy of Fallot. Many of these are candidates for operative correction of the defect, although some will have a lesion that is uncorrectable because of anatomic features or pulmonary vascular disease.

3. They are those with a prior "reparative" operation who have a residual problem. Long-term follow-up studies[2,4] have shown that most of these patients do well for at least 25 to 30 years, as long as they have no major residua. What happens beyond that period is unknown.

DIFFERENCES BETWEEN AN ADULT AND A CHILD WITH CONGENITAL HEART DISEASE

1. The adult is older and has more and tougher scar tissue in the heart or vessels. These differences probably explain why sustained atrial flutter and fibrillation are much more common in adults than in children. The larger size also makes transthoracic echocardiography more difficult because of the limited available windows, so that transesophageal echocardiography plays a greater role than in children. Even with this modality, the need for deeper penetration restricts the transducers to lower frequencies and thus yields lower resolution.

2. The longer duration of the cardiac malformation means that the cumulative risk of infective endocarditis is greater. It means, too, that the myocardium is subjected to a greater preload or afterload for a longer time, so that dysfunction of atrial or ventricular myocardium is often a major problem in the GUCH patient. Young children with

687

TABLE 45–1

SIMPLE LESIONS FOUND IN GUCH PATIENTS WHO RARELY
NEED MEDICAL HELP AND USUALLY LEAD NORMAL LIVES

> Atrial septal defect (smaller)
> Bicuspid aortic valve and mild aortic valve stenosis°
> Coarctation of the aorta with mild gradient
> Mild pulmonary valve stenosis
> Persistent ductus arteriosus
> Small ventricular septal defect

°Many of these become severely stenotic or incompetent beyond 50 to 60 years of age, in women later than in men.

congenital heart disease who have cardiac failure often have relatively good muscle function but an excessive volume or pressure load. Removal of the load usually restores excellent cardiac function. In contrast, the GUCH patient may have cardiac failure based partially on chronic muscle dysfunction despite a smaller preload or afterload. Relief of the load, although helpful, may not relieve the dysfunction. In addition, the abnormal fibrotic ventricular myocardium may form the substrate for a serious ventricular arrhythmia, just as the abnormal scarred atria are the site of origin of atrial fibrillation and particularly atrial flutter.

3. Female GUCH patients may have specific problems during pregnancy and delivery, and they need special precautions when using contraceptives. Female patients have a different prognosis in certain diseases and face different general problems. Gender as well as the specific form of congenital heart disease should be considered in management.

4. As they age, GUCH patients acquire other diseases, such as coronary artery disease, diabetes mellitus, kidney or liver disease, blood dyscrasias, and pulmonary disease, which occur in greater frequency in older individuals. Systemic hypertension is also acquired, especially when there is a family history of hypertension. It may cause the underlying defect to become symptomatic, particularly in those

with an atrial septal defect or tetralogy of Fallot. These added diseases may greatly affect the outcome of operative or medical management of the cardiac lesion.

5. A number of psychosocial problems need to be considered. The GUCH patient may have difficulty getting work or insurance. Marriage may be deferred or avoided because of the heart disease. Other issues are dealt with later in the chapter.

Organization of professional care for GUCH patients in most countries continues to be difficult because of lack of interest and expertise of adult cardiologists and the understandable concern and vested interests of pediatric cardiologists, who usually lack knowledge of adult medicine and facilities to treat GUCH patients outside a children's hospital. The frequent result is inadequate care for the GUCH patient. The difficulties are further compounded in countries such as the United States and the United Kingdom by insurability and payment mechanisms that make it difficult for the GUCH patient, even if the anomaly is complex, to receive treatment from a center with experience and expertise. There is a tendency in the profession to hold on to the interesting GUCH patient, thereby preventing concentration of these patients in a few centers of excellence.

Pediatric cardiologists need to ensure that their patients are transferred to long-term informed care and identify those GUCH patients who have or will have special problems. Ideally, care of such GUCH patients should be provided by a cardiologist knowledgeable about congenital heart disease, with training in adult medicine and with access to appropriate facilities. Professional recognition of a subspecialty for GUCH within adult cardiology, with the trainee coming from pediatric or adult cardiology with crossover experience, is needed.[8] The GUCH specialist should function in a region, state, or province (depending on population served and geography) at a center that provides the necessary cardiologic, surgical, and support ser-

TABLE 45–2

COMPLEX ANOMALIES/REPAIRS REQUIRING SPECIALIZED CARE*

Aorta–left ventricular fistula	Pulmonary atresia
Atrioventricular septal defects	Pulmonary atresia with intact ventricular septum
Corrected transposition	Total anomalous pulmonary venous drainage
Double-outlet ventricle	Transposition
Ebstein anomaly	Tricuspid atresia
Eisenmenger's syndrome	Truncus arteriosus/hemitruncus
Tetralogy of Fallot	Mitral atresia
One ventricle	Ventricular septal defect
(also called double inlet, double outlet, common,	+ Aortic regurgitation
single, primitive)	+ Subaortic stenosis
	+ Mitral disease
	+ Absent valves
	+ Straddling tricuspid/mitral valve

Other abnormalities of atrioventricular and ventriculoarterial connection not included above, i.e., crisscross heart, isomerism; always complex

ADDITIONAL LESIONS CONSIDERED TO BE COMPLEX WITH PREVIOUS OPERATION BEFORE 12 YEARS OF AGE AND REQUIRING FURTHER SURGERY

Coarctation of the aorta
Left ventricular outflow obstruction (valve, subvalve, supravalve) and regurgitation
Ventricular septal defect with other anomalies
Mitral and tricuspid valve disease (congenital)
Pulmonary valve needing replacement

*These patients should be considered "at risk" or have special risks and needs requiring a specialist cardiologist.

KNOWLEDGE AND SKILLS REQUIRED TO CARE
FOR GUCH PATIENTS

Cardiologist with knowledge of congenital and acquired heart disease
Experience with adolescents
Invasive and interventional catheterization
Cardiac surgery for congenital heart disease
Integrated transplant service*
Arrhythmia management
Echocardiography in congenital heart disease
Fetal echocardiography
Transesophageal echocardiography service
Specialist in hematology, particularly for cyanotic patients
Magnetic resonance imaging
At-risk pregnancy service*
General surgery, plastic surgery, orthopedics, and chest surgery*
Access to specialties: endocrine, dermatology, gynecology, and others*

*Not necessarily on site, but easy to access and close geographically.

vices needed by GUCH patients.[9] Because of the expertise required and the relatively small numbers of patients, GUCH services should be centralized.

Patients with complex anomalies or operative repairs (Table 45–2), about 15% of the GUCH population, require specialized support services led by cardiologists and cardiac surgeons but with access to and close integration with other specialists (Table 45–3). Because many psychosocial difficulties exist in this group, psychological support is necessary and often best managed by available GUCH counselors who are trained in this field. Nurses or mother figures may play prominent roles in giving advice.

The GUCH database at the Royal Brompton Hospital provides statistics based on the work of a specialized GUCH unit with a bias of referral toward the complex and severe. The data serve, however, to show a perspective of current and future complications and the conditions that need ongoing attention. Similar information has been reported by other centers.[3, 10–14]

ORGANIZATION OF A GUCH UNIT

A specialist GUCH unit should be designed to provide inpatient services for adolescents and young adults to 30 years of age with congenital heart disease, congenital syndromes (Marfan's syndrome, muscular dystrophies), primary disorders of rhythm, and cardiomyopathies and exceptionally for the young with rheumatic or traumatic heart disease. Older patients or those with particular requirements can be admitted to contiguous adult cardiology medical and surgical units. Within a GUCH unit, a high-dependence unit for early postoperative patients, intervention, and emergency admission is useful. Other facilities include a five- to seven-bed area with a mobile partition (to separate sexes); an isolation room for septic patients or those with special needs, such as GUCH mothers with babies; a quiet sitting room for patients studying for examinations and for parents; a room for interviewing or counseling patients; and a recreation area and a kitchen, which have been found useful for occupational therapy. Postoperative GUCH patients often return to the GUCH unit or general cardiology unit because of lack of expertise in dealing with congenital heart disease

in the cardiac surgical unit. There are too few patients in most nations for formal specialized training for nurses. This emphasizes the importance of centralization of special GUCH patients into a few supraregional centers. Ideally, a GUCH unit should be formed in relation to an active pediatric cardiac surgical unit.

MAJOR MEDICAL ISSUES

GUCH patients requiring admission to the hospital represent about 7% of the total population cared for by a specialist GUCH unit, and they may be only 2 to 3% of those in a region or province because of the large number of patients with simple or trivial congenital heart disease who never need a cardiologic admission until they acquire degenerative disease. Those with complex problems collect where specialist expertise exists, as demonstrated by the types of lesions in patients admitted to the Royal Brompton Hospital unit in 1 year (Fig. 45–1).

GUCH admissions have predictably increased, which must be considered by those planning a GUCH service. There are more adults than adolescents, a fundamental reason not to consider GUCH care to be an extension of pediatrics. The most common reason for hospital admission is for cardiac catheterization, with increasing needs for therapeutic interventions and assessment for transplantation. Day patient rooms with night stay areas can be used for some of these patients and those needing transesophageal imaging (transesophageal echocardiography) or other investigations, such as computed tomography and magnetic resonance imaging (MRI) studies for patients who travel long distances.

ARRHYTHMIAS

Arrhythmias are a common cardiac reason for admission to the GUCH unit. Arrhythmias alter hemodynamics and ventricular function and always herald clinical deterioration despite optimal therapy. These are usually various forms of atrial or ventricular tachycardias; less frequently, they are disorders with slow heart rates due to complete atrioventricular block or defective sinus node function.

Atrial Flutter
The most common arrhythmia in GUCH patients is atrial flutter. It occurs before operation in the natural history of certain lesions; incidence increases with age in the Ebstein anomaly, atrial or atrioventricular septal defect, tricuspid and mitral atresia, pulmonary atresia (with intact septum—a rare GUCH patient), and univentricular heart (double inlet). It is common after procedures such as the Fontan, the Mustard, and right ventricular reconstruction in tetralogy of Fallot and pulmonary atresia. Atrial flutter occurs early in the postoperative course of atrial septal defect in patients who have had preoperative attacks of atrial flutter and also after pulmonary autograft surgery for aortic valve disease. It can lead to hemodynamic compromise and need urgent cardioversion or rate control by intravenous administration of amiodarone or digoxin in digitalizing doses.

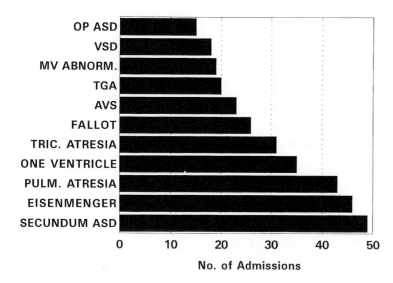

FIGURE 45–1

Basic diagnosis of patients 16 years of age and older with congenital heart disease admitted to the GUCH unit, Royal Brompton Hospital, in 1996. Secundum atrial septal defect is most common, but complex lesions are present in the majority. Abnorm = abnormality; ASD = atrial septal defect; AVS = aortic valve stenosis; MV = mitral valve; OP = ostium primum; PULM = pulmonary; TGA = transposition of the great arteries; TRIC = tricuspid; VSD = ventricular septal defect.

Diagnosis of atrial flutter is not always obvious, and it is missed particularly in patients with an atrial baffle (a Mustard or Senning procedure) or with flat or small P waves. Attention must be paid to all the standard electrocardiographic leads, and the possibility of atrial flutter must be considered in any GUCH patient with new deterioration or tachycardia. Corrected transposition, with and without added defects, can occasionally present to the cardiologist for the first time after the age of 40 years with the onset of atrial flutter or fibrillation that may lead to pulmonary edema. It is usually associated with worsening of left atrioventricular valve regurgitation. In this condition, a previously asymptomatic patient developing dyspnea and with chest pain may end up in a coronary care unit, erroneously diagnosed with a myocardial infarct because of large Q waves in anterior and inferior leads. Those without good bedside skills will not appreciate that the loud second sound in the pulmonary area is really A_2 and that the chest radiograph is atypical, so the corrected transposition remains undiagnosed.

Atrial flutter with a 1:1 response is a cause of sudden death in GUCH patients. Some patients who have been resuscitated after cardiac arrest are given antiarrhythmics for what is perceived to be ventricular arrhythmia, but these agents may have a proarrhythmic effect and unmask the cause as atrial flutter at the next attack.

The principles of treatment of this arrhythmia are the same as for atrial fibrillation:

1. Return to sinus rhythm as soon as possible. Unfortunately, the general cardiologist, to slow the heart rate, may give a medication with negative inotropic effect, or a physician may fail to recognize the reason for symptoms. If the rhythm remains, persistent right atrial hypertension, ascites, liver pain, symptomatic deterioration, and progressive tricuspid regurgitation develop. Drugs such as flecainide and propafenone are used to the detriment of ventricular function; intravenous verapamil can cause cardiac arrest. Loading with intravenous amiodarone can sometimes cause reversion to sinus rhythm, but it can cause severe bradycardia, atrioventricular block, and cardiac failure. Scrutiny of previous data is vital before a therapy is chosen (see Chapter 55).

2. Anticoagulate. In GUCH patients, atrial flutter usually arises from lesions affecting the right atrium, so the danger of systemic embolism is nonexistent unless there is a patent foramen ovale or atrial septal defect. Pulmonary emboli from right atrial thrombi are, however, more common than once thought. Delay while heparin is administered is unnecessary if cardioversion is needed urgently because of hemodynamic compromise. It is usually better, however, to give 24 hours of full heparinization before electrical DC conversion. If the lesion affects the left atrium, as in mitral valve disease or congenitally corrected transposition, either give heparin and do transesophageal echocardiography first to check for thrombi or anticoagulate for 2 to 3 weeks and do transesophageal echocardiography just before cardioversion. In time, and in certain circumstances (as after a Fontan procedure), an atrial thrombus will form because of stasis, sometimes before the atrial flutter occurs; this should not prevent an attempt to cardiovert unless there is evidence that the thrombus is recent. Because atrial flutter is likely to recur and ultimately become atrial fibrillation, long-term anticoagulation should be instituted. If there are contraindications to full anticoagulation, aspirin should be started and maintained instead.

3. Investigate to exclude a hemodynamic basis for the arrhythmia, irrespective of whether sinus rhythm is regained. It may be possible to intervene to prevent further deterioration (e.g., relieve obstruction in Fontan's circulation) or replace a regurgitant or stenotic pulmonary valve or homograft. The onset of atrial flutter is frequently related to right atrial hypertension, distention and scars, tricuspid stenosis, chronic right ventricular obstruction, or pulmonary regurgitation or occurs late after a Mustard or Senning procedure. Less often in GUCH patients, the basic lesion is in the left atrium. It is possible to have atrial flutter in the right atrium and atrial fibrillation in the left atrium at the same time, giving the appearance of atrial "flutter"—flutter/fibrillation.

4. Maintenance therapy to prevent further attacks and diminish their frequency is important. Atrial flutter recurs in 95% of GUCH patients because the anatomic disturbance remains. Disopyramide is poor; sotalol is better but

patients should be observed for lethargy and depression even at a low dose. Amiodarone is the most successful prophylactic but has late side effects, particularly serious thyrotoxicosis that may precipitate the atrial arrhythmia for which it is given. Thyroid ablation may be necessary to continue the amiodarone.

5. Reports show success of radiofrequency ablation in certain conditions, but where it is most needed (e.g., after a Fontan procedure) the circuits are complex and multiple. Thus, this procedure is not yet as successful as claimed by electrophysiologists used to the general cardiologic population.

Atrial Fibrillation

Atrial fibrillation in GUCH patients, also age related, generally has more disastrous long-term effects than does atrial flutter. It may follow periods of paroxysmal atrial flutter or appear de novo, initially in paroxysms, and then become established. It always adds atrioventricular valve regurgitation to ventricular dysfunction and produces deterioration as in atrial flutter. When, however, the ventricle has decreased compliance and is unable to fill, symptomatic deterioration may be greater with atrial flutter, and the atrial pressure waves are higher than with atrial fibrillation. Conversion to sinus rhythm is urgent, but it is less likely to be successful than in atrial flutter, particularly if the arrhythmia has been established for more than 6 months, the hemodynamic parameters are poor, there have been more than three previous attacks, or either atrium is larger than 6 cm. Intensive medical therapy and anticoagulants are mandatory. Atrial fibrillation is part of the natural history of atrial septal defect after age 35 years, becoming permanent in more than 50% after age 50 years, and it is the major cause of deterioration leading to chronic right-sided heart failure with the addition of gross tricuspid regurgitation. Atrial fibrillation is frequent after operation for atrial septal defect in those older than 35 years and has been cited as the reason for not closing an atrial septal defect in adults older than 40 years.[15] The effects of atrial fibrillation, however, are less devastating in patients with closed atrial septal defect than in those with an open atrial septal defect. Thus, this arrhythmia is not a contraindication to recommending surgery in adults.

Atrial fibrillation occurs in all the conditions associated with atrial flutter and may be the first atrial arrhythmia. It always needs prompt treatment, long-term anticoagulants, and attempted cardioversion. If cardioversion fails, as it often does, long-term control of rate with digoxin (not amiodarone) is important, as are long-term anticoagulants and diuretics.

Ventricular Arrhythmias

Ventricular tachycardia after repair of tetralogy of Fallot was the first rapid arrhythmia to attract the attention of investigators because of its dramatic consequences and the assumption that it was a cause of sudden death from ventricular fibrillation and torsades de pointes. As a cause of sudden death, ventricular arrhythmias are probably less frequent than atrial flutter. Ventricular tachycardia occurs late in repaired tetralogy of Fallot and appears sometimes after closure of a ventricular septal defect, aortic valvotomy, or resected subaortic stenosis; it occurs with dilated failed ventricles (right or left), a small ventricular septal defect with severe pulmonary regurgitation, or late after a pulmonary autograft. Sometimes it appears without obvious reason, arising from the left ventricle late after surgical repair of a right-sided lesion, possibly because of ischemic damage during the bypass period, particularly in the years before the mid-1970s. It occurs in unoperated congenital heart anomalies such as univentricular heart (when dilating) and sinisterly with right ventricular dysplasia, in which it heralds impending death.

Repair of tetralogy of Fallot with infundibular resection leaves a scar of variable extent and site in the right ventricular outflow tract. This scar is the main location where a re-entrant circuit can arise. Arrhythmias can also originate from the cardiac apex (or be induced artificially), less often from the free wall. In these patients, there is more fibrosis in the myocardium of both ventricles than is appreciated from simple inspection. Ventricular tachycardia is associated with severe pulmonary regurgitation and wide right bundle branch block (>0.14 second), which has led to postulation of an electromechanical etiology.[16] Patients live, however, through many decades with QRS duration of more than 0.14 second without ventricular tachycardia or sudden death. I doubt the importance of long QRS duration as a lone contributor. In some patients, combined with significant pulmonary regurgitation that causes chronic right ventricular dilatation, the situation resembles dilated cardiomyopathy in terminal failure with progressively widening QRS, in which ventricular tachycardia is frequent, often induced by phasic low serum potassium concentration from diuretic therapy. After repair of tetralogy of Fallot, ventricular tachycardia and sudden unexpected death can occur in patients with narrow QRS and without serious pulmonary regurgitation, although less frequently than with wide QRS. The problem is that a wide QRS (>0.12 second) occurs in at least 80% of these patients, and with increasing age, the QRS duration widens naturally.

Thus, after repair of tetralogy of Fallot, reconstructed pulmonary atresia, or resection of infundibular stenosis, there are two populations with ventricular tachycardia. The first has sudden death, resuscitated or not. The other group has, during many years, recurrent ventricular tachycardia that responds in part to therapy and, although symptomatic and troublesome, is relatively benign as far as survival is concerned.

Patients with disabling symptoms require therapy. Whether treatment is indicated in an asymptomatic patient with short runs of tachycardia (or when the arrhythmia is discovered by investigation or induced by electrophysiologic study) or whether asymptomatic frequent single-focus ventricular ectopics should be treated is debatable. Treatment for sustained ventricular tachycardia is urgent cardioversion. If this is unavailable or contraindicated, procaine, lidocaine, or amiodarone can be tried; flecainide should be avoided because it is dangerously proarrhythmic in this type of heart with an abnormal ventricle.

Ablation of the re-entrant circuit has been successful at operation with cryoablation or with radiofrequency applied at cardiac catheterization. Surgical treatment for major lesions such as pulmonary regurgitation (pulmonary valve replacement) combined with mapping and surgical ablation may abolish these attacks or diminish their frequency; if they recur, they are less harmful. Even without ablation, improving the hemodynamics by replacing the pulmonary valve, closing a residual ventricular septal defect, or removing obstructing lesions improves symptoms and probably the prognosis despite persistence of ventricular tachycardia.

Ventricular tachycardia is a special problem that may need a variety of treatments—drug therapy, automatic internal cardiac defibrillator (AICD) implantation, and even transplantation on occasion. Problems now arise in relation to the need for AICD, from costs and indications. These devices will improve, but currently they are too sensitive, firing frequently and having to be explanted. Added therapy with amiodarone or β blockade may be useful, but β blockade is contraindicated in the dilated failing ventricle for which the AICD may be most needed.

Recurrent and unstoppable ventricular tachycardia with right ventricular dysplasia is a cardiomyopathy that may need emergency transplantation. Such patients must be prepared and ready for such an event despite severe clinical deterioration.

Complete Heart Block

Heart block in a GUCH patient might have been present at birth (congenital) with or without structural congenital heart disease or be secondary to an intrauterine myocarditis. Heart block may also develop at any time in the natural history of certain lesions, such as the Ebstein malformation, atrioventricular septal defect, or corrected transposition of the great arteries, or be acquired after a cardiac operation (Fig. 45–2).

Some GUCH patients have a lifelong need for a pacemaker. This will mean several lead and battery changes during their life span. There may be complex anatomy, difficulty in finding an acceptable threshold, abnormal venous connections and ventricular anatomy, and risks of endocarditis from sepsis. Therefore, an expert in cardiac pacing, preferably one who understands the complexities of anatomy, is mandatory. Identification of a left superior vena cava and other venous anomalies or disturbance of visceral situs is vital before a transvenous pacemaker is placed.

Patients with an anomaly causing a right-to-left shunt present special risks for endocardial pacing. In my experience, they have an increased frequency of infection, so antibiotics should be used for at least 4 to 5 days after pacemaker placement. Also, they have delayed skin healing, so stitches should be left in for about 7 to 10 days. The risk of thromboembolism in the first 6 months after implantation is at least 15%. For this reason, in our unit, all cyanotic GUCH patients with endocardial pacing have long-term anticoagulation. We maintain their international normalized ratio between 2 and 2.5. This has made embolic incidents exceptional, but hemorrhagic problems are frequent (5 to 8% during 5 years) because of difficulty in hemostatic control.

There may be difficulty in finding an adequate electrode position in abnormally placed or formed ventricles. Thresholds tend to be higher in the left ventricle of atrioventricular discordance than in a normally placed right ventricle.

Patients with congenital complete atrioventricular block without associated cardiac lesions were once thought to have an excellent prognosis. Long-term follow-up studies[17] have shown, however, that they may have significant mortality and morbidity. They have unpredictable Stokes-Adams attacks (the first of which can be fatal), may have decreased exercise tolerance because of the low heart rate, and sometimes acquire mitral incompetence. Consideration needs to be given to prophylactic pacing,[17,18] particularly before permanent pacing and if the patient wishes to hold a vocational driving licence. In the United Kingdom, this refers to buses, public service vehicles, and heavy lorries.

ACQUIRED HEART BLOCK IN THE NATURAL HISTORY OF CONGENITAL HEART DISEASE

Patients with a variety of conditions can acquire complete heart block as they age. This includes atrioventricular septal defects of all types, particularly single (common) atrium; corrected transposition of the great arteries, with and without intracardiac lesions; occasionally the Ebstein anomaly; double-inlet ventricle; and defects associated with left isomerism. Complete heart block uncommonly

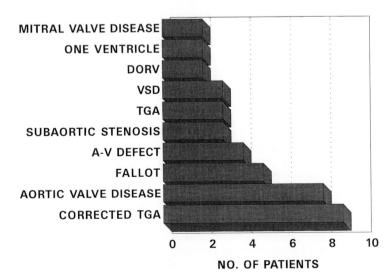

FIGURE 45–2

Basic anomalies that acquired heart block after corrective surgery. Data from the GUCH database, Royal Brompton Hospital. A-V = atrioventricular; DORV = double-outlet right ventricle; TGA = transposition of the great arteries; VSD = ventricular septal defect.

occurs with atrial septal defect, tetralogy of Fallot, and pulmonary valve stenosis and in fact can coexist as a separate congenital abnormality with any congenital cardiovascular condition, including fibroelastosis. Patients with syndromes such as Holt-Oram and allied chromosome defects, ventricular septal defect, or atrial septal defect may have heart block, a long PR interval, or left axis deviation, and/or they may have siblings with congenital heart disease.

POSTOPERATIVE HEART BLOCK

Complete heart block or variable atrioventricular block may develop during cardiac operative repair or subsequently. The likelihood of such an occurrence is greater if there has been transient block soon after operation or prolongation of the PR interval or transient block before operation. Lesions prone to this serious complication include corrected transposition, in which it may occur at any time, even before thoracotomy, and not in relation to the defect closure; closure of a ventricular septal defect, particularly the inlet type; ventricular septal defect with subaortic stenosis; and atrioventricular defects.

The heart block may be intermittent. Ventricular rate varies during the day but usually slows to 20 to 30 beats per minute at night. The block causes syncope, transient giddiness, heart failure particularly if a left-to-right shunt is present, and new chronic fatigue, or it may be asymptomatic. Atrial contraction is needed in most types of structural cardiac abnormalities, and therefore dual chamber pacing is needed in such patients. This is important in patients after an atrial switch, corrected transposition, and complex repairs. Fortunately, complete heart block is rare after Fontan-type surgery, but when it does occur, it poses a difficult pacemaker problem. In this situation, pacing the left ventricle through the coronary sinus is possible; otherwise, pacing must be achieved through the atrial septum or through the epicardium, requiring a thoracotomy. In fact, lack of venous access, tricuspid atresia, and the Fontan procedure are today the main indications for epicardial pacing, which has become uncommon since the 1980s. Epicardial atrial leads remain a problem because of myocardial irritability, lead fractures, rising thresholds, and atrial fibrillation or flutter.

Sinus Node Disease

Sinus node disease is another common reason for placing an artificial pacemaker, either to control extreme bradycardia or to allow the use of drugs that suppress tachycardia without slowing the heart too much in the sick sinus syndrome. Although sinus node disease can occur as an isolated entity, it most often follows atrial surgery, especially atrial switch repair of transposition of the great arteries or total anomalous pulmonary venous connection. By 10 years of age, only 50% of children with atrial switch repairs have sinus rhythm all day, and the percentage is less by the time they reach adult life (see Chapter 25).

INFECTIVE ENDOCARDITIS

Infective endocarditis is the cause for about 8% of admissions to a GUCH unit. Endocarditis occurs in certain anomalies (Fig. 45–3) but not in others (Table 45–4).[19] After operative repair of congenital heart disease, the 25-year cumulative incidence of infective endocarditis is below 2.5% for many major lesions, provided that they have no residual defects (Fig. 45–4).[20] The major exception is after aortic valvotomy, in which the 25-year cumulative incidence of infective endocarditis is above 20%; this predilection for aortic valve infection has been reported previously.[21]

Without operative repair, the abnormal aortic valve (the most common congenital abnormality) is the most frequently affected, followed by small ventricular septal defects, which are also common. The organisms found are the usual, but bizarre organisms may be cultured from patients with a homograft infected at the time of implantation, from patients with unusual occupations (such as sewer workers, fish marketers, and animal handlers), and from patients with long-term lines in intensive care. Predisposing events are dental treatment, including scaling and cleansing, extraction, and fillings; skin infection; genitourinary surgery; and operative abortion. Endocarditis

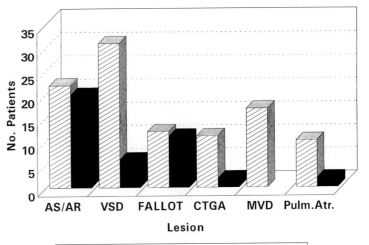

FIGURE 45–3

Infective endocarditis in various congenital lesions before and after surgery in an adolescent and adult population. AR = aortic regurgitation; AS = aortic stenosis; CTGA = corrected transposition of the great arteries; MVD = mitral valve disease: Op. = operation; Pulm.Atr. = pulmonary atresia; Rep. = repair; VSD = ventricular septal defect. (Data from Li W, Somerville J: Infective endocarditis in the grown-up congenital heart (GUCH) population. Eur Heart J 19:166, 1998.)

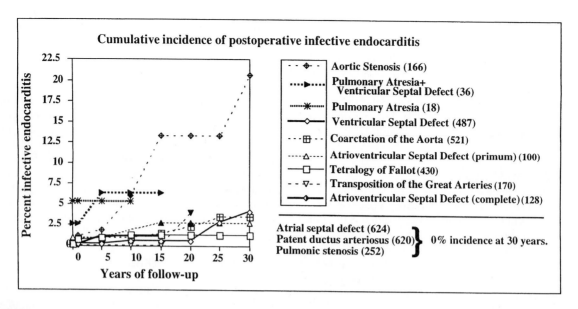

FIGURE 45–4

Cumulative incidence of infective endocarditis in 25 years after operative repair of the most common congenital heart defects. Most of the episodes recorded after repair of ventricular septal defect or tetralogy of Fallot had small residual defects. Parentheses contain numbers of patients in each group. (Data from Morris CD, Reller MD, Menashe VD: Thirty-year incidence of infective endocarditis after surgery for congenital heart defect. JAMA 279:599, 1998.)

has occurred exceptionally after prolonged transesophageal echocardiography,[22] after fitting of an intrauterine coil, and with vaginal delivery. In a cyanotic patient with transposition, deep dental scaling with ultrasonic jets has led to cerebral abscess rather than endocarditis. New dental techniques involving intensive scaling for long periods are not recommended for such patients. I suggest short sessions with antibiotic coverage.

The diagnosis of endocarditis in GUCH patients is too frequently delayed (Fig. 45–5) by poor medical practice, not examining the patients, or not considering the diagnosis. Diagnosis is even later when the right side of the heart is infected, as in small ventricular septal defect or an infected right-sided valve, unless pyogenic organisms are involved and cause dramatic presentations. The incidence of negative blood cultures is high because of the habit of pre-scribing random antibiotics without prior blood tests, blood cultures, or diagnosis. Education of physicians has failed, so patients at risk should be educated to demand blood tests and cultures before taking antibiotics for nonspecific illnesses. Unfortunately, the patient's understanding of his or her own heart disease and the prevention of infective endocarditis is often inadequate.[23,24]

Transesophageal echocardiography has an important role in the management of GUCH patients with endocarditis, particularly because the transthoracic echo window may be poor; furthermore, certain areas are more completely visualized by transesophageal echocardiography. It is useful for diagnosis and assessment of vegetations, aortic root abscess, and atrioventricular valve function and should be part of management unless the routine transthoracic echocardiogram has provided adequate views. If the patient is too toxic because of sepsis, and the site of the infection is known, transesophageal echocardiography should be delayed.

Outcomes of treatment are generally satisfactory, but emergency or elective surgery may be required for uncontrolled sepsis, acute hemodynamic disturbance, or large vegetations. Mortality varies, and in a large series of GUCH patients,[19] death was related to *Staphylococcus aureus* infection, emergency operation, and increasing number of re-operations. Hemoptysis, related to infection of collaterals, shunts, coarctation, or pulmonary artery aneurysms, portends disaster.

The practice of the GUCH unit should involve the cardiac surgeon early in management, particularly if cardiac surgery has already been performed. When the vegetations are large, and if there are pyogenic or fungal organisms, operation should be considered after a short period (1 to 2 weeks) of antibiotics. Some conditions, such as failing single ventricles, Eisenmenger's syndrome with an infected

TABLE 45–4

CONGENITAL HEART LESIONS THAT ARE NOT SUSCEPTIBLE TO BACTERIAL ENDOCARDITIS

Pulmonary valve stenosis and postoperative pulmonary valvotomy
Secundum/sinus venosus atrial septal defect (without mitral valve lesion)
Postoperative closed*
    Ventricular septal defect
    Atrial septal defect
    Ductus arteriosus
Total anomalous pulmonary venous connection
Tetralogy of Fallot, well repaired†
    No shunts
    No aortic regurgitation
    No ventricular septal defect
    No valve grafts
Eisenmenger patients without valve abnormalities†

*Completely closed without left valve lesion.
†Bacterial endocarditis occurs exceptionally.

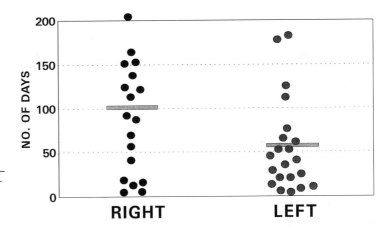

FIGURE 45–5

Time (days) between onset of symptoms and diagnosis of endocarditis in GUCH patients with various anomalies. Delay is greater when emboli go to the lungs (right-sided) compared with the left side. The delay is serious in all types of lesion.

valve, and complex pulmonary atresia, may not be reparable. In these patients, the risk of removing the vegetation alone ("vegetectomy") may have to be taken. In many patients with aortic and mitral valve endocarditis, early surgery can prevent morbidity and mortality.

Infection on Right-Sided Homografts or Xenografts

These can be difficult to diagnose, and the diagnosis must be considered early in patients who have a biologic valve on the right side of the heart (and indeed on the left side) and continue to be unwell after the operation. The infection may be in the valve at the time of implantation of an antibiotic-sterilized valve or acquired during a difficult early postoperative course. This infection may give rise to a florid septic illness, which becomes apparent when the postoperative antibiotics are stopped, or else to a low-grade fever; unusual organisms cause general nonspecific ill health for months or years with "rheumatic" manifestations and fever, formation of shadows in lungs, and even development of aneurysms. Unless the vegetations are large, pulmonary emboli may be too small to be noted. When a fungus attacks a homograft valve, the vegetations are large and obvious, especially when they are mobile. Fungal endocarditis should be the first diagnosis when an acutely painful red eye develops in the postoperative febrile patient or when a pulmonary embolus (so rare now) occurs. *Candida albicans* endocarditis should be treated with amphotericin. If it occurs on a dead homograft, lysozymal preparations may not control fungal infections. Renal function needs assessment. Pulmonary arterial cultures taken from a catheter may provide the organism and the correct diagnosis; considering the diagnosis is the most important step.

New infections late after a right-sided homograft are rare.[25] Vegetations can be difficult to differentiate from calcific lumps and fragments of ruptured cusp.

Small Ventricular Septal Defect

At least 10% of adults with a small ventricular septal defect acquire endocarditis between the ages of 16 and 50 years.[26] This occurs commonly with a subtricuspid ventricular septal defect and is associated with vegetations on the tricuspid valve and/or around the defect. Endocarditis is also found in outflow tract defects with a contiguous prolapsed aortic valve cusp, which as a result may become

more regurgitant, and also affects defects associated with coexistent mitral valve abnormality. The high incidence from the GUCH unit is only in part explained by referral to a specialist unit. Characteristically, the illness starts with nonspecific febrile symptoms (diagnosed as "flu," depending on the season); transient chest pains; and cough diagnosed variously as pleurisy, pneumonia, or recurrent bronchitis, none of which is likely in a young healthy adult. Embolic lesions are often discrete on the chest radiograph, small, round, and missed.

Coarctation of the Aorta: Native and After Repair

Infection is uncommon at the site of the coarctation either before or after operation; if endocarditis occurs, it more often attacks the coexistent abnormal (bicuspid) aortic valve. Emboli from the site of the coarctation pass to the abdomen and legs only; pain in the back may be the first symptom of a false aneurysm or infected intercostal aneurysm. Hemoptysis signals disaster as the pseudoaneurysm bleeds into the left bronchus. Bronchoscopy is dangerous; and although transesophageal echocardiography usually delineates the lesion, unless it is posterior, this investigation causes hypertension *during* intubation and can lead to rupture of both false and true aneurysms. The investigation of choice is magnetic resonance imaging (MRI) and not angiography, which may fail to show the lesion, risks rupture, and can give a false sense of security.

Cyanotic Cardiac Disease

Patients with cyanotic congenital heart disease were not considered susceptible to endocarditis. This is not true; perhaps too few survived to get it, because it is an age-related disease. Of our GUCH patients with endocarditis,[19] 25% were cyanotic, with tetralogy of Fallot being the most common. Operatively created aortopulmonary shunts, stenotic congenital collaterals in complex pulmonary atresia, the tricuspid or mitral valve in a univentricular heart, and the aortic valve in tetralogy of Fallot are the usual sites of infection. Cerebral abscess is probably as common as endocarditis in the cyanotic patient,[27] originating from the same sources. Fortunately, infective endocarditis is rare in the Eisenmenger group of patients but does occur on the tricuspid and aortic (or truncal) valve. Special risks exist in these patients having intravenous therapy, particularly with large neck and subclavian lines, from bubbles of air that lead to unexpected seizures. Careful briefing of nurses administering the antibiotics is essential, and mandatory use of filters requires standing orders. Infective endocarditis is a particularly serious disease in the cyanotic patient because of the risk of cerebral complications.

Staphylococcus epidermidis albus; Coagulase-Negative Staphylococcus

This infection is usually acquired intraoperatively or perioperatively; it may come from the surgeons, infected tissue, or a complicated course in intensive care. Rarely is it acquired de novo unless there is a history of cut skin, particularly on the face and involving the lip or nose. Infection is usually low grade, with a long history of illness, and may take at least 6 months' treatment (oral after intravenous) to be eradicated. In a patient with an aortic valve replaced by an aortic homograft, there had been a nonspecific illness for 5 years since the surgery. On inquiry into the pedigree of the homograft, the donor had had a blood culture positive for *Staphylococcus epidermidis,* as did the patient with the homograft.

HEART FAILURE

Heart failure in GUCH patients occurs in several conditions (Fig. 45–6): as part of the natural history; after aorticopulmonary shunts, particularly in those with "single" right ventricle; and after radical reparative procedures, such as in complex pulmonary atresia, repeated aortic valve surgery, aged Mustard patients, and tetralogy of Fallot shunted for too long a period or with severe pulmonary regurgitation. In patients with Fontan-type operations, ventricular dysfunction develops insidiously after a long period of well-being. Although systolic function appears to be moderately good, the problems stem from diastolic dysfunction that may worsen after relief of obstruction in the preloaded Fontan circulation; these patients are often in trouble soon after reoperation. It is important not to miss postoperative constrictive pericarditis, too often diagnosed as restrictive cardiomyopathy and even referred wrongly for transplantation! Calcification in the pericardium on the lateral chest radiograph or echocardiogram suggests the correct diagnosis.

Atrial flutter and fibrillation frequently herald ventricular dysfunction or result from it. Function worsens precipitously once atrial fibrillation is established because of the addition of atrioventricular regurgitation and reduced forward flow.

The right ventricle as a systemic ventricle does not have the longevity of the left; "single" right ventricles have not lasted beyond 35 years in my experience, irrespective of having had caval shunts, Fontan's procedures, or other systemic–pulmonary artery shunts. Treatment strategies are the same as for any cardiac failure: digoxin, diuretics, angiotensin-converting enzyme (ACE) inhibitors, suppression of arrhythmias, and avoidance of negative inotropic therapy; flecainide is contraindicated. Cyanotic patients become more cyanotic with ACE inhibitors, and these drugs should be used with caution, if at all.

Patients with the Eisenmenger reaction usually do not develop heart failure until after the age of 40 years unless there is a single ventricle (which fails earlier), anemia, intercurrent disease, or fluid-retaining therapy (nonsteroidal anti-inflammatory drugs and steroids). ACE inhibitors improve the heart failure but increase the cyanosis (right-to-left shunt) by lowering the systemic vascular resistance, and they are contraindicated in most circumstances; the possible exception is when there is a failing systemic ventricle with mitral regurgitation, but if they are used, dyspnea increases from hypoxemia. Treatment of systemic hypertension with a β blocker can be helpful; the systemic systolic blood pressure is the same as the pulmonary artery pressure and needs reduction, but not by vasodilatation, which increases cyanosis.

TRANSPLANTATION

Assessment and management of patients for transplantation of heart, lungs, or heart and lung are inevitable and resource-consuming demands on GUCH units. These patients require medical and social support for long waiting periods, but large numbers develop renal and multiorgan dysfunction awaiting donor organs. Transplant evaluation

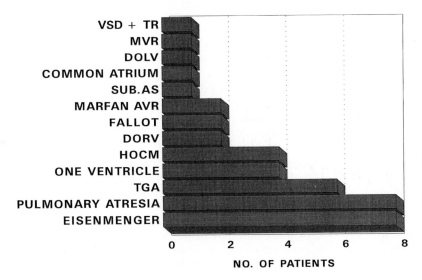

FIGURE 45–6

Congenital cardiac lesions that are associated with right, left, and biventricular congestive heart failure, usually terminal, in adults. AVR = aortic valve replacement; DOLV = double-outlet left ventricle; DORV = double-outlet right ventricle; HOCM = hypertrophic obstructive cardiomyopathy; MVR = mitral valve replacement; SUB.AS = subaortic stenosis; TGA = transposition of the great arteries; TR = tricuspid regurgitation; VSD = ventricular septal defect.

must be available for GUCH patients. Unfortunately, those patients who have had a complex repair or multiple palliative procedures do not have as good an outcome after transplantation as do those with cardiomyopathies or those without a previous operation. Given the donor shortage, there is an unadmitted reluctance to give a precious donor heart to a complex GUCH patient. Top priority category for the transplant is awarded too late to the GUCH patients, who rapidly become untransplantable because of renal dysfunction. A particularly difficult group includes those in a terminal state after Fontan-type surgery, so often cachectic with unrecognized protein-losing enteropathy. They have a high morbidity and mortality from unexpected hyper-rejection and/or sepsis, and the protein-losing enteropathy may not stop after the transplant.[28]

The number of patients needing lung transplantation (single, double, or heart and lung) is increasing; the most frequent claimants are those with Eisenmenger's syndrome, followed by those with progressive pulmonary vascular disease because their defect was closed too late. The rarest group are those with primary pulmonary hypertension and pulmonary venous disease, but these appear to have the best results (Radley-Smith R: Personal communication, 1997).

Eisenmenger patients survive less well after transplantation than do other groups, probably because of their age and their renal dysfunction. They are usually minimally symptomatic before 30 years of age and, with good care, may reach 40 to 50 years. After age 40 years, when symptoms worsen, the results are poor. Currently, there is reluctance to transplant lungs in an older symptomatic patient; lungs go to younger patients with cystic fibrosis. Patients, particularly with cyanotic heart disease and complex pulmonary atresia, are referred for consideration of transplantation when a palliative or reparative operation might be possible. It is vital for GUCH experts to see such patients before consideration for a transplant. Even a palliative operation that defers transplantation helps patients and units in these days of severe donor shortage and rising numbers of potential recipients.

Many technical considerations, such as transposition, abnormal situs, previous surgery and difficulties of connec-

tion, and distorted pulmonary arteries, are involved with transplantation in GUCH patients. These influence not only the actual transplantation but also the harvesting of the hearts, which may need longer segments of great vessels and major veins.

GUCH transplantation can cause more difficulties than occur in other forms of heart and lung disease and thus requires expertise, much counseling, and support to maintain morale and adequate "health."

PULMONARY HYPERTENSION

The Eisenmenger reaction, a term coined by Paul Wood,[29] which complicates various malformations, is the most common form of pulmonary hypertension seen in the GUCH population (Fig. 45–7). Large ventricular septal defect is the most frequent association but is less now because of successful infant cardiac surgery. Another group of patients who need admission are the few with residual pulmonary hypertension that persists and progresses after cardiac surgery in childhood (postoperative pulmonary hypertension). These patients need admission for right-sided heart failure, hemoptysis, extracardiac surgery, and cerebral events.

When significant pulmonary hypertension (50 to 70% of systemic pressure) remains after closure of a large ventricular septal defect in childhood, it can progress unexpectedly and unsuspectedly. This course occurs also in tetralogy of Fallot or double-outlet right ventricle with pulmonary stenosis, when a left-to-right shunt has been left for too long before corrective operation or when the shunt was too large. In a series of postoperative pulmonary hypertension patients treated in the GUCH unit, age at death was earlier than in those with Eisenmenger's syndrome (Fig. 45–8). Pregnancy for these patients is particularly hazardous. Accepting that there might have been selection bias in referral of the worst affected patients, it is possible that there is a population of asymptomatic patients whose modest residual pulmonary hypertension remains constant.

Primary pulmonary hypertension beginning in childhood, manifesting in adolescence or young adulthood, is

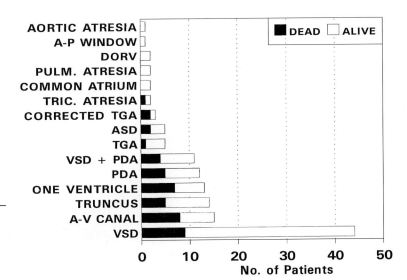

FIGURE 45–7

Lesions associated with the Eisenmenger reaction. A-P = aortopulmonary; ASD = atrial septal defect; A-V = atrioventricular; DORV = double-outlet right ventricle; PDA = persistent ductus arteriosus; PULM. = pulmonary; TGA = transposition of the great arteries; TRIC. = tricuspid; VSD = ventricular septal defect.

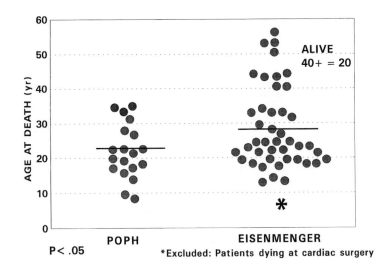

FIGURE 45–8

Age at death of patients with residual pulmonary hypertension after closure of large defects in children 2 years and older compared with age at death of patients with Eisenmenger's syndrome and the same or similar lesions. POPH = postoperative pulmonary hypertension.

more common in female patients and has a poor prognosis once symptoms occur. Sometimes there is a family history, or the disease may be acquired from taking a diet medication; exceptionally, it is secondary to thromboembolism after administration of estrogens, trauma or orthopedic surgery, or long-standing ventriculoatrial shunts for hydrocephalus.

Primary pulmonary venous disease is a rare cause of pulmonary hypertension. It is worsened by pulmonary arteriolar dilatation from calcium blockers and prostacyclin, which lead to pulmonary edema.

Treatment of right-sided heart failure—oxygen, diuretics, digoxin—is ancillary to attempts to lower the pulmonary artery pressure. Sometimes oral diltiazem helps, but it is contraindicated in pulmonary venous disease. Chronic infusion of prostacyclin and even oral prostacyclin may be beneficial, particularly while awaiting lung transplantation. Nitric oxide helps a few. Long-term strategies need further evaluation and development.

Treatment is highly specialized and requires management by a specialist for pulmonary hypertension[30, 31] because the field is changing rapidly. Understanding pulmonary hypertension and its prevention and treatment is a major challenge for pediatric cardiology, but currently, management is better undertaken by specialist pretransplant units, such as that in Columbia University.

DEATH

All deaths are associated with disorders of cardiac rhythm (ventricular fibrillation or asystole), but these may be secondary to other serious catastrophes, such as hemorrhage (ruptured heart, aneurysm, or vessels), blocking of outlets by thrombus, terminal ventricular dilatation, and chemical disorders.[32] Reoperation and related events are the most common primary events leading to death in GUCH patients (Fig. 45–9). The second most frequent cause documented in GUCH patients is sudden unexpected death.[33] Retrospective review at the Royal Brompton Hospital of 80 GUCH patients categorized as having sudden death shows predictors or management omissions that preceded the event in at least 20%. These included arrhythmia in the days or weeks before the event, low or unmeasured electrolyte concentrations in chronically diuresed patients, and unrecognized severe but correctable hemodynamic disorders. Thus, the label of sudden unexpected death may be

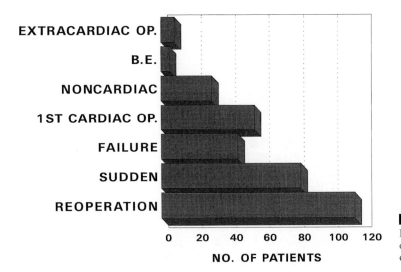

FIGURE 45–9

Primary events involved in deaths of patients in the GUCH database, Royal Brompton Hospital. B.E. = bacterial endocarditis; OP. = operation.

incorrect; the physician may not have anticipated events or managed appropriately.

INVASIVE INVESTIGATION AND INTERVENTION

As noninvasive imaging has improved, the need for diagnostic cardiac catheterizations to diagnose congenital heart disease has diminished. Several forms of imaging, including angiocardiography, are often required for full diagnosis; surprises for the GUCH surgeon increase mortality and morbidity and must be minimized.

Cardiac catheterization and angiography in a GUCH patient pose difficulties. Pediatric cardiologists undoubtedly are the best to perform catheterization, producing good anatomic and physiologic data, whereas adult cardiologists do better with the coronary arteries.

Difficulties with venous access are common; bilateral femoroiliac vein obstruction, even inferior vena caval obstruction, may be present as a result of infant catheterization. Unusual anomalies are encountered, large chambers need large amounts of contrast medium, calcified conduits and valves may be difficult to cross, friable clot may be dislodged from the right atrium (particularly in those with a failed Fontan procedure), and many other hazards have to be overcome.

Cyanotic patients have special risks for catheterization and angiography; dehydration can lead to oliguria and even anuria, and there can be thromboembolic complications during and after the procedure that should be mentioned when consent is obtained for the procedure. Heparin should probably be given for 24 to 48 hours until full mobilization of the patient, because a clot that must form to close the intubated vessels can easily embolize to the brain. Induced arrhythmias (not cardiac arrest) may lead to clinical deterioration after the procedure. Special nursing precautions, care, and experience are needed. All patients should have an intravenous infusion on the day of the procedure and supervised fluid balance for at least 24 hours. If the blood urea concentration rises on the following day, the fluid balance should be supervised until urea concentrations return to precatheterization levels. Renal function, hemoglobin level, and hematocrit must be measured before cardiac catheterization in an adult cyanotic patient. If the hemoglobin level exceeds 18 g/dl, it may be useful at catheterization to hemodilute, removing 500 to 700 ml of whole blood and replacing it with colloid or plasma substitutes (*not* crystalloids, which encourage dehydration).

There is an increasing use of therapeutic interventions to treat residual, new, and native lesions.[34] Patent ductus arteriosus can be successfully closed if it is neither too wide (>1 cm) nor window-like, as can small atrial septal defects and patent foramen ovale; as yet, no device is big enough and safe enough for the standard-sized secundum defect in an adult (1.7 to 2.5 cm). Stents have improved outcomes in pulmonary arterial stenoses, more so in acquired than in native lesions, which may pose danger with dilatation from rupture of the thin-walled vessel distal to the stenosis. In complex pulmonary atresia, stents have been useful in opening collaterals, resulting in improved exercise tolerance and decreased cyanosis.[35] The major effect of intervention in GUCH patients is to reduce the need for reoperation with its own particular risks.

Recoarctation is helped by balloon dilatation, and stenting has further improved results. This can be applied with success to native coarctation, but I remain anxious about aneurysm formation, so that surgical treatment is still preferred unless there are special circumstances. Patients feel considerable pain during balloon dilatation of aortic coarctation. In older patients, the aortic wall may show changes of cystic medial necrosis. This may be the cause of aortic dissection in this disease and also leads to concern about balloon dilatation of the coarctation in adults.

CARDIAC SURGERY

Statistics from a specialized unit show that one in five admissions is for a cardiac operation, a ratio that despite increased numbers of admissions has changed little in our unit for a decade. Catheter interventions have increased and produced a slight decrease in surgery, certainly for simpler lesions. Cardiac surgery is likely to be greater when GUCH surgery is integrated with a pediatric cardiac service with more adolescents and less in a more general regional service with simpler lesions. The big challenge comes more from reoperations, which are more common than first operations, but this varies according to referral patterns and the success of infant surgery. Where there are immigrants or asylum seekers, the incidence of first operations on serious congenital heart disease, particularly the cyanotic forms, increases. In an established specialist unit in a capital city, there are likely to be a larger number of complex, difficult problems that need admission for evaluation and operation.[36,37] The most common reoperations are on the left ventricular outflow tract and changing the conduit and valves in the right ventricular outflow tract.

In some patients, several reoperations are needed during a lifetime, a factor that must be considered and discussed in childhood when the initial valve or conduit is chosen. Patients and parents often have not been warned of the future need and risks, which increase with the number of operations.[37] Reoperating on Fontan-type procedures has a higher mortality and morbidity in GUCH patients than in children with congenital heart disease. When a conduit has been placed between the right atrium and the right ventricle, enlarging the cavity, relief of obstruction is difficult and requires either right atrial–pulmonary artery connection or construction of a new total cavalpulmonary anastomosis.[38] The systemic ventricle may fail after relief of long-standing right atrial obstruction, because when obstruction is relieved, serious diastolic dysfunction appears.

The serious and unexpected problems in adulthood posed by an apparently simple ventricular septal defect with aortic regurgitation in GUCH patients with previous operation deserve special mention. Several operations may be needed on the seriously deformed aortic root, which remains a susceptible site for endocarditis.

GUCH surgery is demanding of all facilities, skills, and resources. It is costly and requires experience not only of the cardiac surgeon and cardiologist, who should work closely with intensivists, but of nursing and junior staff, who need special training. Because reoperation is the most common factor in deaths of GUCH patients, it is the most vulnerable part of the GUCH patients service and demands great expertise. It is unreasonable to nurse these patients in an environment where neither adult cardiac surgical staff nor nurses are familiar with the needs and complexity of congenital heart disease. It highlights the need for specialist units, concentration of patients (who are relatively rare), and experience and expertise with all the available facilities. Operating on and managing the occasional patient with complex congenital heart disease in a regional cardiac unit is a formula for disastrous outcome. The type of cardiac surgery performed is shown in Figure 45–10.

NONCARDIAC SURGERY

Certain patients with complex and advanced congenital heart disease have special risks for commonplace interven-

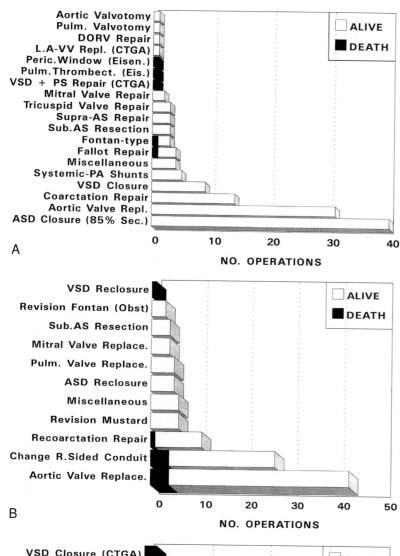

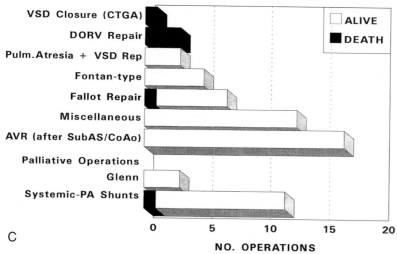

FIGURE 45–10

Type of cardiac surgery performed in the GUCH population, 1991 to 1994, at the Royal Brompton Hospital. *A*, First operations. *B*, Reoperations. *C*, Definitive repair after other cardiovascular surgery and palliative procedures. AS = aortic stenosis; ASD = atrial septal defect; AVR = aortic valve replacement; CoAo = coarctation of the aorta; CTGA = corrected transposition; DORV = double-outlet right ventricle; Eisen./Eis. = Eisenmenger; L.A-VV = left atrioventricular valve; Obst = obstruction; PA = pulmonary artery; Peric. = pericardial; PS = pulmonary stenosis; Pulm. = pulmonary; R. = right; Rep. = repair; Repl./Replace. = replacement; Sec. = secundum; Sub.AS = subaortic stenosis; Thrombect. = thrombectomy; VSD = ventricular septal defect; Supra-AS = supra-aortic stenosis.

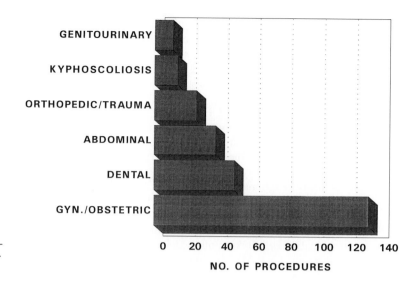

FIGURE 45–11

Type of extracardiac surgery needed by GUCH patients.
Gyn. = gynecologic.

tions and surgery (see Table 45–2). With their underlying cardiac abnormality, they are at higher risk of death and morbidity than those with a normal heart are. Consultation with a trained GUCH cardiologist and a cardiac anesthetist will help to minimize the risks.[39] Particular care must be given to avoid volume overload in those with poor ventricular function and to avoid decreasing systemic blood pressure and sudden changes in circulating volume, including hemorrhage, in those with cyanotic heart disease or pulmonary hypertension.[40]

Some of the commonly required types of noncardiac surgery are shown in Figure 45–11. To these should be added removal of wisdom teeth, which may have to be done in the specialized unit if there are special risks from the heart disease. The GUCH unit in the Royal Brompton Hospital provides this service with visiting dentists, a cardiac anesthetist, and available intensive care or a high-dependency unit when needed.

OUTPATIENT AND OUT-OF-HOSPITAL SERVICE

General

Ninety percent to 95% of the care of the GUCH population is on an outpatient basis; only 5 to 8% need admission. Thus, if a GUCH service cares for 5000 GUCH patients, 250 to 400 will require admission for cardiac problems per annum. This does not include admission for pregnancy and

delivery, general surgery, or trauma. These figures vary according to the type of lesion under surveillance, referrals, and geography. A specialized unit will see a large proportion of the complex and difficult patients. A large proportion of mild and more common lesions are followed in smaller centers outside the larger center; this means that in smaller centers, the GUCH admissions for cardiac needs are likely to be less (i.e., 2 to 4% of their GUCH population) than those of the specialized supraregional (or national) center.

Basic clinical investigative procedures must be available for care of the GUCH outpatient population. A written protocol for investigation of each disease or condition is useful. Communication to referring physicians and the patients by fax and a medical help line with a GUCH NETWORK for advice have meant an increase in secretarial staff and availability.

It is important that a counselor, separate from the physicians, be available for inpatients and outpatients. These patients have many problems in trying to lead normal lives, and many need nonmedical help and advice (Table 45–5). Although they often need psychosocial counseling, full psychiatric syndromes are no higher than in the general population.

GUCH patients need the full range of laboratory and diagnostic studies. Chest radiographs,[41] including a lateral view, are useful and often ignored by clinicians. Inspecting

TABLE 45–5

MEDICAL AND NONMEDICAL PROBLEMS FOR WHICH GUCH PATIENTS CONTACT THE GUCH UNIT, SECRETARIES, COUNSELORS, AND HELP LINE

Adoption	Fitness to fly
Attempted suicide	Housing
Chest scars	Life insurance
Contraception	Marriage
Court appearances/prison sentences	Multiple anxieties
Dangerous hobbies	Organ donation
Dentistry	Pregnancy
Driving license	Psychological problems in relation to heart disease
Education and further education	Risks to offspring
Employment	Social service support
Extracardiac surgery	

chest radiographs should be part of the routine bedside examination, like looking at the electrocardiogram, and should not require a special trip to the radiology department.

Magnetic Resonance Imaging

MRI has a particular value in GUCH patients, especially for assessment of operated and unoperated coarctation of the aorta, right ventricular outflow conduit, Fontan's obstruction, atrial baffle obstruction, and intrathoracic aneurysms.[42–45] It may be of value in acute situations, such as hemoptysis after operations on coarctation of the aorta. It must be interpreted by a consultant experienced with congenital heart disease in adults. MRI obviates the need for diagnostic catheterization or may direct the need for cardiac catheterization or intervention, which can thereby be planned electively. Cine MRI has increased the scope and use of this diagnostic method, as has velocity mapping for conduit obstruction. MRI does not detect calcium and is interfered with by metallic implants.

MRI is a good way to show adherence of the right ventricle to the sternum and dictate extreme caution to the surgeon to be ready with femorofemoral bypass.

Computed Tomography

This technique may be useful in assessing pulmonary artery thrombosis and aneurysm and pulmonary lobar lesions. Its main value is in the evaluation of clinical lung problems, such as infarction, emphysema, and interlobular effusions, and the delineation and localization of a lung opacity. The technique can also be helpful in evaluating dissection of the aorta, showing the pulmonary arteries, displaying calcification, and evaluating complications related to coarctation when the patient cannot undergo MRI.

Transesophageal Echocardiography

This is a routine investigation but is invasive and needs antibiotic coverage if prolonged or traumatic. Although anesthesia may be achieved by midazolam, there are, however, instances when it fails or when hypoxia and suppressed respiratory effort are hazardous. Because the investigations are longer and more complex than in the routine adult cardiac problem, an anesthetist should be present, and when there is concern about hypoxia (Eisenmenger's syndrome) or untoward effects of hypertension (coarctation with aneurysm), a quick general anesthetic may be safer as well as more agreeable to the patient.

Transesophageal echocardiography gives valuable information about the atrial septum, size and site of ventricular septal defects, venous connections, atrial baffle leaks and venous obstruction, ventricular function, dissection of the aorta, isthmus region and aortic root size, left ventricular outflow anomaly, and atrioventricular valve function. As for any procedure in a GUCH patient, dehydration must not occur while the patient is waiting for the procedure. Such patients can recover under observation, staying overnight in the hospital environment if there is any instability.

PREGNANCY AND CONTRACEPTION

Pregnancy produces many physiologic changes that might affect the GUCH patient. Increased blood volume and cardiac output could precipitate cardiac failure; decreased systemic vascular resistance could increase a right-to-left shunt; hypercoagulability and venous stasis in the legs could cause venous thrombosis and perhaps embolism; and the large uterus, by pressing on the diaphragm, decreases total lung capacity and vital capacity.[46–49]

In general, pregnancy is well tolerated by women classified in New York Heart Association (NYHA) categories I and II, but those in NYHA classes III and IV are at significant risk of cardiac failure or death during pregnancy or delivery. To be more specific, those with minimal lesions or adequately corrected congenital heart anomalies have no difficulties during pregnancy. Those with a large left-to-right shunt tolerate the increased blood volume of pregnancy well, and they and their infants usually do well, provided that the mothers do not have pulmonary vascular disease. On the other hand, patients older than 40 years with an atrial septal defect have a tendency toward supraventricular arrhythmias and cardiac failure.[49] Those with an atrial septal defect are also at risk of paradoxical embolism if they develop deep venous thrombosis, and precautions against venous stasis are needed.

Pregnancy is usually well tolerated in those with pulmonic or aortic stenosis, but occasionally the increased cardiac output causes a large increase in ventricular systolic pressure and even cardiac failure.[50,51] In addition, the associated low systemic blood pressure of pregnancy may decrease myocardial blood flow and produce ischemia of the ventricle, particularly the left ventricle.[50] Balloon valvotomy may at times be needed to relieve the obstruction.[52] In coarctation of the aorta, pregnancy increases the risks of aortic dissection or rupture of an aneurysm of the circle of Willis.[49] An increased risk of aortic rupture is noted in patients with Marfan's syndrome.

In the Ebstein anomaly, the inadequate right ventricle does not tolerate the gestational rise in cardiac output. Paroxysmal atrial arrhythmias are common, right-to-left shunting may occur for the first time or increase, and the risks to mother and fetus have been reported to be high.[53] This has not been my experience, in which mothers with the Ebstein anomaly have easily controlled problems and usually deliver normal babies successfully.

Patients with uncorrected cyanotic heart disease have reduced fertility. If they become pregnant, they have a greatly increased risk of spontaneous abortion, premature labor, or delivery of small-for-date infants at term.[54–56] These complications are all substantially reduced if pregnancy follows successful operative correction of the defect.[56,57] This is true even with complex lesions that are corrected by a Fontan type of operation.[58]

Patients with pulmonary hypertension, whether primary or secondary to pulmonary vascular disease (Eisenmenger's syndrome), are at high risk of dying during pregnancy, labor, and delivery.[49,59] The high fixed pulmonary vascular resistance increases the right-to-left shunt when cardiac output rises, thus affecting the fetus. Labor and bearing down increase systemic vascular resistance and so reduce systemic blood flow. Any fall in systemic blood pressure, even transient, can result not only in an increased right-to-left shunt but also in sudden underperfusion of the right ventricular wall with acute heart failure and fatal arrhythmias. Maternal mortality in these lesions is high (but not always[60]), reportedly about 30 to 50% even today. Deaths said to be due to pulmonary embolism are usually not so, in my experience. Eisenmenger patients and those with primary pulmonary hypertension may have fibrinoid destruction of small pulmonary arterioles. Even patients with modest pulmonary hypertension (about 50% of systemic pressure) after closure of cardiac defects are at risk of sudden death in the third stage after delivery or may deteriorate after completion of pregnancy.

Women with congenital heart disease are at risk for infective endocarditis immediately after delivery because of the large raw uterine surface, although the risk appears to be low. Antibiotic prophylaxis is not recommended for uncomplicated deliveries, but it may be needed when the risk of bacterial invasion is increased by premature rupture of the membranes or prolonged labor or if the patient has a prosthetic valve. The risk applies as much to those with a minor lesion as to those with a more significant uncorrected anomaly or with a residual lesion after correction.

Management of Pregnancy

Salt restriction (not diuretics) may help to reduce volume overloading. Adequate rest and avoiding extreme heat reduce cardiac work. Prompt treatment of an infection, especially of the genitourinary tract, and good dental hygiene may reduce the risks of infective endocarditis. Elastic stockings may be needed to minimize the risk of venous thrombosis in the legs.

Particularly difficult problems occur when a pregnant woman is taking anticoagulants for venous thrombosis or a mechanical aortic or mitral valve. Because of this, pregnancy should be undertaken before valve replacement if possible, or else a homograft valve should be used. Aspirin is contraindicated because of its possible effect on the fetal ductus arteriosus and relatively poor anticoagulant properties. Warfarin (Coumadin) is a teratogen, and it also increases fetal wastage substantially.[61] This is mainly related to dosage. Most authorities recommend prescribing the pregnant woman subcutaneous heparin throughout the pregnancy, because heparin does not cross the placenta, but fetal losses remain high,[61] and thromboembolism may not be prevented[62]; regular checking must be done of the adequacy of anticoagulation. Whether anticoagulation with low-molecular-weight heparin or hirudin will improve the outcome in these patients remains to be determined. Currently, our practice is to prescribe warfarin at the lowest dose that will maintain adequate anticoagulation until the last month. Then the patient is admitted to the hospital and given intravenous heparin by pump.

Contraception

Intrauterine devices may be associated with the risk of bacteremia and so should be avoided. Oral contraceptives with low-dose estrogen are not harmful, except in patients at risk of thrombosis (pulmonary hypertension, cyanotic heart disease). A diaphragm, used with a spermicide, is benign, although not always effective. In those women with severe pulmonary hypertension, uncorrectable severe left ventricular outflow tract obstruction, Marfan's syndrome, or poor ventricular function, tubal ligation should be considered.

GENETIC COUNSELING

Genetic counseling should be made available to the GUCH patients, who are at increased risk of having children with congenital heart disease. Although the transmission risk is usually below 10%, it may be increased in certain syndromes.[63] If there is a pregnancy, fetal echocardiography done by an expert in the field should be offered (see Chapter 12).

EXERCISE

Exercise recommendations for GUCH patients obviously depend on their cardiac function. After operative correction of many anomalies, those with no residual defects may undertake any level of exercise. Those with residual defects might need restriction of activity based on recommendations that differ for each lesion and problem.[64, 65] If there are concerns, formal exercise testing to assess how much the patient may safely exercise can be useful.

INSURANCE PROBLEMS AND EMPLOYMENT

Life insurance for patients with congenital heart disease may be obtained for many but not all lesions; depending on the lesion, premiums might be normal or increased.[66–70] The studies cited covered only children, adolescents, and young adults; data for older adults have not been published. Furthermore, the practices of life insurance companies probably differ greatly among countries.

What is of more importance to the GUCH patient is the ability to obtain health insurance. This ability clearly varies with the country and its type of health system. When various forms of managed care are involved, as in the United States, it may be difficult for people with a pre-existing health problem to get health insurance. Furthermore, if there is no national health plan, health insurance is inextricably bound up with employment, because health insurance is often obtained through the employer. Employers may be reluctant to hire people with serious health problems who might need time off work and have high medical costs. In fact, even without consideration of health insurance, employers may be reluctant to hire the GUCH patient.[66, 69] On the other hand, at least one survey[70] found that less than 10% of GUCH patients had difficulty applying for jobs.

Despite all the potential problems of the GUCH patient, many of them do well after their lesions have been corrected, and personal satisfaction and assessment of their well-being have apparently been high.[71, 72]

THE FUTURE

The standard of care for GUCH patients needs to be improved in most countries, an issue becoming increasingly important because of the growing numbers of GUCH patients. A proper system of referral and transfer is needed. Those at risk of difficult problems, the complex and rare anomalies, and those who need reoperations should all be treated in a center where the volume of patients is sufficient for good experience and professional expertise. Too often these patients are held as occasional curiosities in private practices or small centers without appropriate expertise. Managed care and health authorities have made it difficult for the GUCH patient to find and reach the few available experts. Although a few practice optimal care of GUCH patients, many patients fail to receive it, appearing to the specialist only in an emergency or a terminal state. The profession as a whole needs to realize the need to improve care for this special group of patients, an improvement achieved by referring them to a centralized group with appropriate resources and personnel for grown-up congenital heart disease patients—the GUCH patients.

REFERENCES

1. MacMahon B, McKeown T, Record RG: The incidence and life expectation of children with heart disease. Br Heart J 15:121, 1953.
2. Morris C, Menashe VD: 25-Year mortality after surgical repair of congenital heart defect in childhood. A population-based cohort study. JAMA 266:3447, 1991.
3. Perloff JK, Miner PD: Specialized facilities for the comprehensive care of adults with congenital heart disease. In Perloff JK, Child JS (eds): Congenital Heart Disease in Adults. Philadelphia, WB Saunders, 1998, p 9.
4. Moller JH, Anderson RC: Natural history of congenital heart disease. 1000 consecutive children with cardiac malformations with 26–37 year follow-up. Am J Cardiol 70:661, 1992.
5. Immer FF, Haefeli-Bleuer B, Seiler A, et al: Angeborene Herzfehler: Vorkommen und Verlauf wahrend der Schulzeit (8. bis 16. Lebensjahr). Schweiz Med Wochenschr 124:894, 1994.
6. Roberts WC: The congenitally bicuspid aortic valve. A study of 85 autopsy cases. Am J Cardiol 26:26, 1970.
7. Cheitlin MD, Gertz EW, Brundage BH, et al: Rate of progression of severity of valvular aortic stenosis in the adult. Am Heart J 98:689, 1979.
8. Skorton DJ, Cheitlin MD, Freed MD, et al: Training in the care of adult patients with congenital heart disease. J Am Coll Cardiol 25:31, 1995.
9. Connelly MS, Webb GD, Somerville J, et al: Canadian Consensus Conference on Adult Congenital Heart Disease. Can J Cardiol 14:395, 1998.
10. Webb GD, Harrison DA, Connelly MS: Challenges posed by the adult patient with congenital heart disease. Adv Intern Med 41:437, 1996.
11. Dodo H, Perloff JK: Congenital heart disease in adults—collaboration between pediatric and medical cardiologists. Jpn Circ J 60:895, 1996.
12. Findlow D, Doyle E: Congenital heart disease in adults. Br J Anaesth 78:416, 1997.
13. Muhler EG, Franke A, Lepper W, et al: Die Betreuung von Adoleszenten und Erwachsenen mit angeborenem Herzfehler: 3 Jahre Erfahrungen mit einer interdisziplinären Sprechstunde. [The management of adolescents and adults with congenital heart defects: 3 years experience with interdisciplinary consultation.] Z Kardiol 84:532, 1995.
14. Wagdi P, Fluri M, Meier B: Adulte Patienten mit kongenitalen Herzvitien: Berner Zahlen. [Adult patients with congenital heart disease: Berne statistics]. Schweiz Rundsch Med Prax 84:623, 1995.
15. Shah D, Azhar M, Oakley CM: Natural history of atrial septal defect in adults after medical or surgical treatment: A historical perspective study. Br Heart J 71:224, 1994.
16. Gatzoulis MA, Till JA, Somerville J, Redington AN: Mechanoelectrical interaction in tetralogy of Fallot. QRS prolongation relates to right ventricular size and predicts malignant ventricular arrhythmias and sudden death. Circulation 92:231, 1995.
17. Michaelsson M, Jonzon A, Riesenfeld T: Isolated congenital complete atrioventricular block in adult life. A prospective study. Circulation 92:442, 1995.
18. Michaelsson M, Riesenfeld T, Jonzon A: Natural history of congenital complete atrioventricular block. Pacing Clin Electrophysiol 20:2098, 1997.
19. Li W, Somerville J: Infective endocarditis in the grown-up congenital heart (GUCH) population. Eur Heart J 19:166, 1998.
20. Morris CD, Reller MD, Menashe VD: Thirty-year incidence of infective endocarditis after surgery for congenital heart defect. JAMA 279:599, 1998.
21. Gersony WM, Hayes CJ, Driscoll D, et al: Bacterial endocarditis in patients with aortic stenosis, pulmonary stenosis, or ventricular septal defects. Circulation 87(suppl II):21, 1993.
22. Read RC, Finch RG, Donald FE, et al: Infective endocarditis after transesophageal echocardiography. Circulation 87:1426, 1993.
23. Cetta F, Warnes CA: Adults with congenital heart disease: Patient knowledge of endocarditis prophylaxis. Mayo Clin Proc 70:50, 1995.
24. Kantoch MJ, Collins-Nakai RL, Medwid S, et al: Adult patients' knowledge about their congenital heart disease. Can J Cardiol 13:641, 1997.
25. Somerville J, Stone S: Homograft reconstruction of the right ventricular outflow tract: Late results of homograft function. In Anderson RH, Neches WH, Park SC, Zuberbuhler JR (eds): Perspectives in Pediatric Cardiology. Mount Kisco, NY, Futura Publishing, 1988, p 189.
26. Neumayer U, Stone S, Somerville J: Small ventricular septal defects in adults. Eur Heart J 19:1573, 1998.
27. Ammash N, Warnes CA: Cerebrovascular events in adult patients with cyanotic congenital heart disease. J Am Coll Cardiol 28:768, 1996.
28. Mertens L, Hagler DJ, Sauer U, et al: Protein-losing enteropathy after the Fontan operation: An international multicenter study. PLE study group. J Thorac Cardiovasc Surg 115:1063, 1998.
29. Wood P: The Eisenmenger syndrome or pulmonary hypertension with reversed central shunt (The Croonian Lectures). Br Med J 2:701, 755, 1958.
30. Barst RJ, Rubin LJ, McGood MD, et al: Survival in primary pulmonary hypertension with long-term continuous intravenous prostacyclin. Ann Intern Med 121:409, 1994.
31. Barst RJ, Long W, Gersony W: Long-term vasodilator treatment improves survival in children with primary pulmonary hypertension. Cardiol Young 3(suppl 1):89, 1993.
32. Somerville J: Near misses and disasters in the treatment of grown-up congenital heart patients. J R Soc Med 90:124, 1997.
33. Harrison DA, Connelly M, Harris L, et al: Sudden cardiac death in the adult with congenital heart disease. Can J Cardiol 12:1161, 1996.
34. Harrison DA, McLaughlin PR: Interventional cardiology for the adult patient with congenital heart disease: The Toronto Hospital experience. Can J Cardiol 12:965, 1996.
35. Redington AN, Weil J, Somerville J: Self-expanding stents in congenital heart disease. Br Heart J 72:378, 1994.
36. Laks H, Pearl JM: The surgeon's responsibility: Operation and reoperation: The UCLA experience. J Am Coll Cardiol 18:327, 1991.
37. Dore A, Glancy DL, Stone S, et al: Cardiac surgery for grown-up congenital heart patients: Survey of 307 consecutive operations 1991–1994. Am J Cardiol 80:906, 1997.
38. de Leval M, Kilner P, Gewillig M, Bull C: Total cavopulmonary connection: A logical alternative to atriopulmonary connection for complex Fontan operations. J Thorac Cardiovasc Surg 96:682, 1988.
39. Ritchie JL, Cheitlin MD, Eagle KA, et al: Guidelines for perioperative cardiovascular evaluation for noncardiac surgery. Circulation 93:1278, 1996.
40. Perloff JK, Sangwan S: Noncardiac surgery. In Perloff JK, Child JS (eds): Congenital Heart Disease in Adults. Philadelphia, WB Saunders, 1998, p 291.
41. Steiner RM, Gross GW, Flicker S, et al: Congenital heart disease in the adult patient: The value of plain film chest radiology. J Thorac Imaging 10:1, 1995.
42. Hirsch R, Kilner PJ, Connelly MS, et al: Diagnosis in adolescents and adults with congenital heart disease: Prospective assessment of individual and combined roles of magnetic resonance imaging and transesophageal echocardiography. Circulation 90:2937, 1994.
43. Wexler L, Higgins CB, Herfkens RJ: Magnetic resonance imaging in adult congenital heart disease. J Thorac Imaging 9:219, 1994.
44. Wexler L, Higgins CB: The use of magnetic resonance imaging in adult congenital heart disease. Am J Card Imaging 9:15, 1995.
45. Hartnell GG, Meier RA: MR angiography of congenital heart disease in adults. Radiographics 15:781, 1995.
46. Pitkin RM, Perloff JK, Koos BJ, et al: Pregnancy and congenital heart disease. Ann Intern Med 112:445, 1990.

47. Shime J, Mocarski EJM, Hastings D, et al: Congenital heart disease in pregnancy: Short- and long-term implications. Am J Obstet Gynecol 156:313, 1987.

48. Mendelson MA: Congenital heart disease and pregnancy. Clin Perinatol 24:467, 1997.

49. Perloff JK, Koos B: Pregnancy and congenital heart disease: The mother and the fetus. *In* Perloff JK, Child JS (eds): Congenital Heart Disease in Adults. Philadelphia, WB Saunders, 1998, p 144.

50. Easterling TR, Chadwick HS, Otto CM, Bendetti TJ: Aortic stenosis in pregnancy. Obstet Gynecol 72:113, 1988.

51. Presbitero P, Somerville J, Rabajoli F: Pregnancy in patients with congenital heart disease. Schweiz Med Wochenschr 125:311, 1995.

52. Angel JL, Chapman C, Knappel RA, et al: Percutaneous balloon aortic valvuloplasty in pregnancy. Obstet Gynecol 72:438, 1988.

53. Waickman LA, Skorton DJ, Varner MW, et al: Ebstein's anomaly and pregnancy. Am J Cardiol 53:357, 1984.

54. Whittemore R, Hobbins JC, Engle MA: Pregnancy and its outcome in women with and without surgical treatment of congenital heart disease. Am J Cardiol 50:641, 1982.

55. Presbitero P, Somerville J, Stone S, et al: Pregnancy in cyanotic heart disease. Outcome of mother and fetus. Circulation 89:2673, 1994.

56. Neumayer U, Somerville J: Outcome of pregnancies in patients with complex pulmonary atresia. Heart 78:16, 1997.

57. Oliveira TA, Avila WS, Grinberg M: Obstetric and perinatal aspects in patients with congenital heart disease. Rev Paul Med 114:1248, 1996.

58. Canobbio MM, Mair DD, Van der Velde M: Pregnancy outcomes after Fontan repair. J Am Coll Cardiol 28:763, 1996.

59. Bitsch M, Johansen C, Wennevold A, Osler M: Eisenmenger's syndrome and pregnancy. Eur J Obstet Gynecol Reprod Biol 28:69, 1988.

60. Avila WS, Grinberg M, Snitcowsky R, et al: Maternal and fetal outcome in pregnant women with Eisenmenger's syndrome. Eur Heart J 16:460, 1996.

61. Hall JG, Pauli RM, Wilson KM: Maternal and fetal sequelae of anticoagulation during pregnancy. Am J Med 68:122, 1980.

62. Salazar E, Izaguirre R, Verdejo J, et al: Failure of adjusted doses of subcutaneous heparin to prevent thromboembolic phenomena in pregnant patients with mechanical cardiac valves. J Am Coll Cardiol 27:1698, 1996.

63. Burn J: The aetiology of congenital heart disease. *In* Anderson RH, Macartney FJ, Shinebourne EA, Tynan M (eds): Paediatric Cardiology. London, Churchill Livingstone, 1987, p 15.

64. Kaplan S, Perloff JK: Exercise and athletics before and after surgery or interventional catheterization. *In* Perloff JK, Child JS (eds): Congenital Heart Disease in Adults. Philadelphia, WB Saunders, 1998, p 189.

65. Graham TP Jr, Bricker JT, James FW, Strong WB: Task Force 1: Congenital heart disease. 26th Bethesda Conference: Recommendations for determining eligibility for competition in athletes with cardiovascular abnormalities. J Am Coll Cardiol 24:867, 1994.

66. Manning JA: Insurability and employability of young cardiac patients. Cardiovasc Clin 11:117, 1980.

67. Truesdell SC, Skorton DJ, Lauer RM: Life insurance for children with cardiovascular disease. Pediatrics 77:687, 1986.

68. Allen HD, Gersony WM, Taubert KA: Insurability of the adolescent and young adult with congenital heart disease. Circulation 86:703, 1992.

69. Celermajer DS, Deanfield JD: Employment and insurance for young adults with congenital heart disease. Br Heart J 69:539, 1992.

70. Kaemmerer H, Tintner, Konig U, et al: Psychosoziale probleme Jugendlicher und Erwachsener mit angeborenen Herzfehlern [Psychosocial problems of adolescents and adults with congenital heart defects]. Z Kardiol 83:194, 1994.

71. Ferencz C: The quality of life of the adolescent cardiac patient. Postgrad Med 56:67, 1974.

72. Utens EM, Verhulst FC, Erdman RA, et al: Psychosocial functioning of young adults after surgical correction for congenital heart disease in childhood: A follow-up study. J Psychosom Res 38:745, 1994.

SECTION IV
MISCELLANEOUS ACQUIRED DISEASE

CHAPTER 46
PULMONARY HYPERTENSION

SHEILA GLENNIS HAWORTH

Pulmonary hypertension is a common cause of morbidity and mortality. It is a major complicating factor in the management of children with many types of congenital heart disease, preventing intracardiac repair in those with established pulmonary vascular disease. It exists in a primary form and as persistent primary hypertension of the newborn (PPHN) when the pulmonary circulation fails to adapt normally to extrauterine life. In many children with congenital heart disease, the increasing sophistication of surgery and cardiopulmonary bypass make it feasible to carry out a primary intracardiac repair in early infancy and so prevent the development of pulmonary vascular obstructive disease. The emphasis has shifted, therefore, from morphologic studies of established disease to a concern about understanding the early, neonatal origins of pulmonary vascular disease and a need to understand the functional derangements that complicate the postoperative management of these children. Primary pulmonary hypertension is almost always universally fatal in an untreated patient, but genetic studies on the familial form of this disease open up new lines of enquiry into the pathogenesis of this and other forms of pulmonary hypertension. Unlike the situation with pulmonary hypertensive congenital heart disease and primary pulmonary hypertension, it is relatively easy to model PPHN experimentally. Using this approach has taught us much about the cellular and molecular biology of pulmonary hypertension. The principal management of pulmonary hypertension is still limited to timely, effective surgery in patients with congenital heart disease; the use of nitric oxide (NO) to treat postoperative pulmonary hypertension and neonates with persistent pulmonary hypertension; and the indefinite, intravenous administration of prostacyclin in patients with primary pulmonary hypertension. Ultimately, the only "cure" for advanced pulmonary vascular obstructive disease is lung transplantation. Thus, although the outlook during the past few years has improved for many patients with pulmonary hypertension, there is still much work to do.

PULMONARY HYPERTENSION CAUSED BY CONGENITAL HEART DISEASE

A marked, sustained increase in pulmonary arterial pressure and flow leads to pulmonary vascular obstructive disease, which is a major limiting factor in the successful treatment of many children with congenital heart disease. This section is concerned only with severe pulmonary hypertension, generally in the presence of a left-to-right shunt. The rate at which pulmonary vascular disease develops varies according to the type of intracardiac abnormality, and an appreciation of the natural history makes it possible to prevent the development of significant disease by operative intervention in early infancy. As the seeming inevitability of severe pulmonary vascular obstructive disease has receded, so we have become more aware of the functional disturbances in pulmonary vascular reactivity that can prejudice surgical outcome.

In patients who present later in life, predicting the outcome of intracardiac repair with a marked increase in pulmonary vascular resistance calls for fine clinical judgement. Is an early improvement in quality of life worth the risk of reducing long-term survival? For those with irreversible pulmonary vascular disease, medical treatment remains empirical. Therapeutic pulmonary vascular remodeling remains only a theoretical possibility. For the minority of patients offered lung transplantation, the outlook is also unsatisfactory. Transplantation should be offered only when the probability of survival with a satisfactory quality of life is better than that without transplantation.

ASSESSMENT OF THE HYPERTENSIVE PULMONARY CIRCULATION

In children with a left-to-right shunt, the nature of the anatomic abnormality determines the clinical picture, as described in the preceding chapters. But if pulmonary vascular disease is allowed to pursue its natural course, most of the findings become common to all types of congenital heart disease. At the onset, a high pulmonary blood flow is frequently associated with feeding difficulties, failure to thrive, and recurrent respiratory tract infections. Dilated pulmonary arteries compress the main and lobar bronchi in children with and without pulmonary hypertension, leading to the familiar problem of recurrent collapse of different lobes or segments of lung. The respiratory complications of congenital heart disease often constitute an indication for corrective surgery in infancy. After the operation, the deformity of the bronchi may persist for some time and in some patients prolonged compression appears to be associated with bronchomalacia. Cardiac failure may appear to improve as pulmonary vascular resistance increases. Without surgical intervention, the resistance continues to increase until the shunt is bidirectional or reversed. This physiologic situation is known as *Eisenmenger's complex*, defined as pulmonary hypertension at the systemic level due to a high pulmonary vascular resistance (more than 10 Wood units or 800 dyne-sec/cm[5]) and with a reversed shunt at any level.[1,2] Patients have exercise intolerance, central cyanosis, clubbing, and polycythemia, and they can develop hemoptysis in early adult life. Paul Wood described a series of 727 patients with congenital heart disease with a systemic-to-pulmonary connection, of whom 17.5% developed Eisenmenger's complex.[2] (This early study could not have taken into account a substantial, early attrition.) The physical signs include a small or normal volume pulse; a right (or subpulmonary) ventricular lift extending to the pulmonary artery; a loud pulmonary ejection click, followed by a short pulmonary systolic murmur; and a palpable, accentuated pulmonary component of the second heart sound. Eventually, a pulmonary regurgitant murmur and signs of tricuspid incompetence develop.

The chest radiograph is reassuringly plethoric when the resistance is sufficiently low to permit a high blood flow, and it is depressingly evident when pulmonary vascular disease is advanced (Fig. 46–1). Severe obstructive disease in the muscular pulmonary arteries leads to peripheral pruning and a hypertranslucent appearance in association with dilatation of the hilar and proximal vessels. Wedge angiography is not widely used, although it is helpful in demonstrating advanced pulmonary vascular obstructive disease, because it cannot discriminate between less severe degrees of disease when the patient may still be potentially operable. The abnormal pulmonary wedge angiogram is characterized by decreased arborization, reduced background opacification, and delayed venous filling. The arteries may appear tortuous or have segments of dilatation, constriction, or marginal defects suggestive of

obliterative disease. Quantitative wedge angiography represents an attempt to improve the correlation between structure and function.[3] In the normal lung, the pulmonary arteries taper toward the periphery, but the vessels narrow over a shorter distance when pulmonary vascular resistance is elevated. The rate of tapering can be related to the pulmonary arterial pressure and vascular resistance and to the structural changes found at lung biopsy. Abrupt tapering is associated with a resistance greater than 3.5 U/m[2], but further discrimination is difficult.

The pulmonary arterial pressure can be reliably determined noninvasively by Doppler interrogation, but resistance cannot. At cardiac catheterization, the lowest determinations of pulmonary arterial pressure and vascular resistance are conventionally accepted as a guide to outcome. This is based on the premise that if the predominant structural abnormality in the pulmonary circulation is an increase in muscularity, the circulation responds to vasodilator substances. To this end, the patient is usually given 100% oxygen to breathe, with or without prostacyclin.[4] Giving both vasodilator agents together may produce a greater fall in resistance than if either is given alone. Inhalation of NO has come into vogue, because it is a specific pulmonary vasodilator. In those patients with an elevated pulmonary vascular resistance, inhalation of NO lowers resistance and can be more effective than giving a high oxygen concentration. In one study, inhalation of NO at 40 ppm reduced the resistance from a mean of 8.6 to 5.7 U/m[2].[5] When used together, NO and a high oxygen concentration can produce a greater fall in resistance than either used alone.[6] Endothelium-dependent and endothelium-independent vasodilatation can be studied by the sequential infusion of acetylcholine and sodium

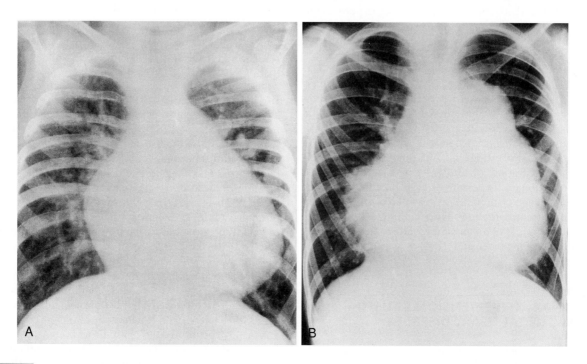

FIGURE 46–1

A, Chest radiograph of a 4-month-old child with a ventricular septal defect and pulmonary hypertension showing an enlarged heart, pulmonary plethora, and prominent pulmonary artery. *B,* Eisenmenger's syndrome, showing dilatation of the pulmonary artery with a marked reduction in pulmonary vascular markings.

nitroprusside.[7] Endothelium-dependent vasodilatation is impaired early in children with pulmonary hypertensive congenital heart disease and a high pulmonary blood flow, but the response to sodium nitroprusside is preserved. Endothelium-independent dilatation is diminished in patients with an elevated pulmonary vascular resistance.[7] With any vasodilator, the release of vasoconstrictor tone lowers pulmonary vascular resistance, increases the magnitude of the left-to-right shunt, and may lower the pulmonary arterial pressure. Failure to achieve this response implies fixed, organic obstruction of the pulmonary circulation. In practice, however, it is often difficult to predict pulmonary vascular structure in this manner, particularly after the first year of life. Children with Down syndrome are particularly difficult to assess because they often suffer from upper airway obstruction, which may contribute to the increased pulmonary vascular resistance determined at cardiac catheterization. The pathologist will then find less pulmonary vascular damage in a lung biopsy than is expected for the increase in pulmonary arterial pressure and resistance.

If a child is deemed inoperable and is likely to be offered a transplant, reassessment should include catheterization. Conventionally, the clinical status determines the necessity for transplantation. In patients with advanced disease, however, survival can be predicted from the product of mean right atrial pressure and pulmonary vascular resistance.[8] The optimal time to offer transplantation is when the expected survival time is less than the expected time of survival after transplantation, bearing in mind the quality of life achieved.

STRUCTURAL DEVELOPMENT OF PULMONARY VASCULAR DISEASE

Children are occasionally born with pulmonary vascular disease, but this is rare. Pulmonary vascular disease usually begins at birth when the vasculature fails to adapt normally to extrauterine life. An increase in pulmonary blood flow with little increase in pressure causes peripheral extension of muscle from differentiating pericytes and intermediate cells in precapillary vessels. Simultaneously, the media of larger arteries increases in thickness as smooth muscle cells hypertrophy and excessive connective tissue is deposited both in the media and adventitia (Fig. 46–2).[9, 10] The normal postnatal increase in contractile myofilaments is accelerated and the myofilament concentration normally present by 6 months is achieved during the first weeks of life. In the endothelial cells, microfilament disarray is seen in early infancy and the cells become partially detached from the basement membrane, although the cell sheet is still continuous. There is abundant evidence of early endothelial dysfunction.

If the pulmonary arterial pressure is allowed to remain elevated, the outer subadventitial layers of smooth muscle cells appear well differentiated. They contain abundant smooth muscle–specific α- and γ-actin; the smooth muscle–specific myosin heavy chain isoforms, SM1 (204 kDa) and SM2 (200 kDa); the contractile regulatory proteins calponin and caldesmon; and cytoskeletal markers of differentiated smooth muscle cells, such as desmin. The innermost smooth muscle cells, however, have a more

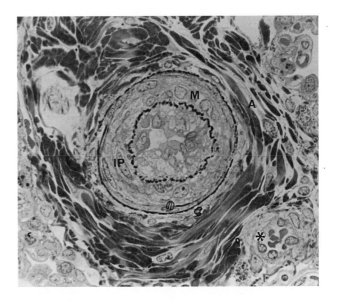

FIGURE 46–2

Photomicrograph of lung tissue from a 5-month-old child with univentricular heart without pulmonary outflow tract obstruction, showing severe medial hypertrophy, intimal proliferation, and a dense adventitia (A) composed of thick bundles of collagen. The *asterisk* denotes a small, normally thin-walled precapillary vessel. IP = intimal proliferation; M = media. Magnification ×553.

synthetic phenotype, cease to express many smooth muscle–specific contractile and cytoskeletal proteins, and appear to migrate through gaps in the internal elastic lamina to produce intimal proliferation. Heightened activity of a proteolytic enzyme, endogenous vascular elastase, is thought to help induce structural remodeling and cause disruption of the internal elastic lamina to facilitate smooth muscle cell migration.[11] The intimal obstruction to flow is strategically placed at the entrance to each respiratory unit (Fig. 46–3).[12] The rate at which these changes occur depends on the type of intracardiac abnormality, and intimal proliferation can develop rapidly in certain abnormalities. In transposition of the great arteries with ventricular septal defect, for example, severe obstructive intimal proliferation increases resistance to flow during the first months of life. In such infants, intimal proliferation is cellular and exuberant, obstructing and even occluding the lumen before there has been sufficient time to achieve neat, circumferential intimal fibrosis, known as the *onionskin picture,* seen in older patients (Fig. 46–4A, B).[13] The veins show a slight increase in wall thickness, commensurate with the increase in pulmonary arterial wall thickness.

As intimal proliferation increases in severity in the small muscular arteries, it narrows the lumen, and the medial thickness of the more peripheral respiratory unit arteries decreases (Fig. 46–4B). The transitory near-normal appearance of the peripheral intra-acinar arteries can be misleading, but it reflects the severity of more proximal obstruction in patients with a high pressure and resistance (Fig. 46–4C). Therefore, to interpret a lung biopsy with confidence, it is important that the biopsy be sufficiently deep to include some of the preacinar and terminal bronchiolar arteries in which intimal proliferation first develops.[12, 14] The appearance of these arteries is crucial to the

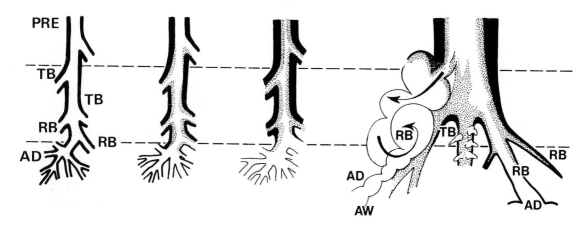

Diagram of the end of four pathways from the preacinar (PRE) and terminal bronchiolar (TB) arteries to the intra-acinar respiratory bronchiolar (RB) and alveolar duct (AD) arteries. Note the alveolar wall (AW), showing the gradual development of intimal proliferation (stippling) associated with a progressive increase in wall thickness of preacinar arteries and a decrease in wall thickness of intra-acinar arteries until dilatation lesions develop. The *upper horizontal interrupted line* indicates the plane of section of satisfactory biopsies, and the *lower interrupted line* illustrates the plane of section of biopsies taken too close to the pleura to sample the distal preacinar vessels and all the intra-acinar vessels.

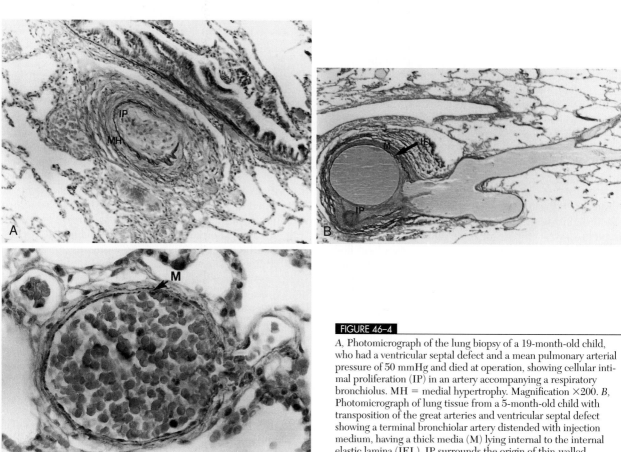

A, Photomicrograph of the lung biopsy of a 19-month-old child, who had a ventricular septal defect and a mean pulmonary arterial pressure of 50 mmHg and died at operation, showing cellular intimal proliferation (IP) in an artery accompanying a respiratory bronchiolus. MH = medial hypertrophy. Magnification ×200. *B,* Photomicrograph of lung tissue from a 5-month-old child with transposition of the great arteries and ventricular septal defect showing a terminal bronchiolar artery distended with injection medium, having a thick media (M) lying internal to the internal elastic lamina (IEL). IP surrounds the origin of thin-walled branches (Miller's elastin counterstained with van Gieson's stain). Magnification ×200. *C,* From the parent artery shown in *A,* a view of a more peripheral vessel accompanying an alveolar duct. Note absence of MH. M = media. Magnification ×595.

evaluation of the intra-acinar arteries beyond. If preacinar arteries are not present in the specimen, a mean percentage medial thickness less than 14% in arteries 50 to 100 μm in diameter, particularly when associated with respiratory unit arteries that are slightly larger than normal for age, is suggestive of predilatation in patients with severe pulmonary hypertension and elevated resistance.[14] This stage in the evolution of pulmonary vascular disease is associated with an increase in mortality and morbidity at, and after, intracardiac repair. The number of intra-acinar arteries is reduced with severe pulmonary hypertension. Ultrastructural examination reveals many occluded vessels.[15] This is an early change and can be seen in young infants with a low resistance. Whether there is also a primary failure of postnatal angiogenesis is unknown.

In children with a sustained, high pulmonary arterial pressure, the obstruction to flow increases with age, and dilatation lesions develop from the walls of small muscular arteries. The smooth muscle cells of the thick-walled arteries continue to synthesize transforming growth factor β (TGFβ), a potent mitogen. The walls of both the original vessels and the dilatation lesions contain smooth muscle–specific contractile proteins and regulatory proteins, but how these vessels function in relation to each other is unknown (Fig. 46–5 [see Color Plates]). The structurally abnormal, dysfunctioning endothelium synthesizes vascular endothelial growth factor (VEGF), even when covering a thick layer of intimal proliferation. The dilatation lesions contain abundant VEGF. In vitro, VEGF induces endothelium-dependent relaxation,[16] and its presence in unobstructed pulmonary arteries and in dilatation lesions may help ensure continued perfusion of the capillary bed. The VEGF colocalizes with TGFβ1 in the endothelium of both the pulmonary arteries and the dilatation lesions. VEGF is a potent angiogenic factor, and TGFβ upregulates its angiogenic activity in vitro.[17] Plexiform lesions accompany or follow the appearance of dilatation lesions, and they also contain abundant VEGF. VEGF is not present, however, in obstructed arteries. The role of VEGF in the pathogenesis of pulmonary vascular disease is unclear, but it may have an angiogenic effect after peripheral pulmonary arterial occlusion. Obstructive intimal proliferative tissue shows intense tenascin expression, which localizes with epidermal growth factor and indices of cell replication.[18] Expression of fibronectin is widespread. These findings are consistent with in vitro studies showing that tenascin modulates epidermal growth factor–dependent neointimal smooth muscle cell proliferation, and fibronectin provides a gradient for migration from the media to the neointima.

When the pulmonary arterial pressure remains elevated after birth, whatever the reason, the structure of the pulmonary trunk retains its fetal appearance and contains long, thick elastin fibers.[19] If pulmonary hypertension develops later in life, the pulmonary trunk becomes thicker because of the deposition of connective tissue and smooth muscle cell hypertrophy in a normally adapted vessel.

CORRELATION BETWEEN STRUCTURE AND FUNCTION

In 1958, Heath and Edwards published their classic papers on the evolution of pulmonary vascular disease.[20–22] They classified pulmonary vascular disease into six grades, in order of increasing severity (Table 46–1). Grades I to III indicate a *low resistance, high reserve,* still a labile pulmonary vascular bed. The pulmonary arterial pressure is high, the pulmonary blood flow is high, and the direction of the shunt is left to right. Grades V and VI indicate a high *resistance, low reserve* pulmonary vascular bed, which is no longer labile because the lumen of many of the arteries is occluded. Pulmonary arterial pressure is higher in patients with these grades than in those with grades I to III pulmonary vascular disease. Flow is low, and the direction of the shunt is predominantly right to left. Grade IV represents a transitional stage. However, although grades I to III reflect a succession of structural changes, grades IV to VI probably do not. Necrotizing arteritis can precede the development of plexiform lesions but is rare in pulmonary hypertensive congenital heart disease. Wagenvoort and Wagenvoort[23] found that none of these advanced lesions carried a more severe prognosis than the others, save for the plexiform lesion.

All the patients with congenital heart disease in the Heath and Edwards study were at least 10 months of age, and most had either an atrial or ventricular septal defect or a patent ductus arteriosus. Our problems now concern patients with more complex types of congenital heart disease, many of whom develop pulmonary vascular obstructive disease during the first months of life. In certain anomalies, exuberant cellular intimal proliferation obstructs and even occludes the lumen of small muscular and terminal bronchiolar arteries, as noted previously, but the Heath and Edwards classification of grade II disease would suggest a less dangerous situation. The Heath and Edwards classification has been, and still is, invaluable in the management of older children and adults with pulmonary hypertension. A more recent classification system concentrates on the early structural changes when medial hypertrophy is developing, before intimal damage appears. It emphasizes the importance of assessing the muscularity, size, and number of vessels in a pulmonary vascular bed that is still developing (Table 46–2).[24] Both classifications are helpful when describing a group of patients, but when evaluating an individual lung biopsy, it is wiser to describe all the abnormalities present, rather than to try to classify them, and then relate the structural findings to the clinical and hemodynamic data. We know too little about the cells that compose the vessel walls and about how the pulmonary circulation functions to make definitive correlations between structure and function, much less growth potential.

TABLE 46–1

THE HEATH AND EDWARDS CLASSIFICATION OF PULMONARY VASCULAR DISEASE (1958)

Grade	Severity
I	Medial hypertrophy
II	Medial hypertrophy with cellular intimal proliferation
III	Progressive fibrous vascular occlusion
IV	Progressive generalized arterial dilatation + complex dilatation lesions
V	Chronic dilatation + dilatation lesions + pulmonary hemosiderosis
VI	Necrotizing arteritis

TABLE 46–2

EARLY DEVELOPMENT OF PULMONARY VASCULAR DISEASE

Grade A

Extension of muscle into smaller and more peripheral arteries than in normal. Extension of muscle may be found alone and is associated with increased pulmonary blood flow without increased pressure.

Grade B

In association with abnormal extension of muscle, the medial muscular coat of the small intra-acinar arteries is thicker than normal; this feature is most effectively recognized on biopsy specimens by analyzing arteries 50–100 μm in diameter. When mild, it is not associated with pulmonary arterial hypertension; when more than twice normal, it invariably is.

Grade C

In association with abnormal extension of muscle and increased thickness of the medial muscular coat, the number of small arteries is reduced.

It is more difficult to relate the structural findings in the pulmonary vasculature to hemodynamic observations and to outcome in young children than it is in older children. Medial hypertrophy is usually associated with a low pulmonary vascular resistance and is potentially reversible. However, in young children the resistance may be elevated, and the children can die in the postoperative period after a technically successful intracardiac repair because the pulmonary arterial pressure is high, either continuously or sporadically (Fig. 46–6). Sporadic increases in pressure are known as *pulmonary hypertensive crises.* Medial hypertrophy, although a potentially reversible lesion, is therefore not necessarily a safe lesion. At the other extreme, extensive dilatation plus the other features of classic grade IV pulmonary vascular disease is invariably associated with a high resistance and a poor prognosis. In practice, most patients fall between the two extremes. As intimal proliferation increases in small muscular arteries, the medial thickness of more peripheral arteries decreases. Resistance is inversely proportional to peripheral arterial

muscularity (Fig. 46–7; see Fig. 46–3). In practice, it is usually possible to predict the structural changes present in the pulmonary vascular bed from the hemodynamic findings, when these findings are considered in conjunction with the age of the patient and the type of intracardiac abnormality. The effect of associated lesions, such as coarctation of the aorta, must also be taken into account, even when they have been repaired earlier. If there is doubt about the likely outcome of surgical repair, an open lung biopsy should clarify the position.

EVOLUTION OF PULMONARY VASCULAR DISEASE IN COMMON TYPES OF CONGENITAL HEART DISEASE

In children with severe pulmonary hypertension, the rate at which pulmonary vascular disease progresses depends on the type of intracardiac abnormality.

Abnormalities Associated With an Increase in Pulmonary Blood Flow

In children with a hypertensive *ventricular septal defect,* the pulmonary vasculature fails to develop normally after birth.[14, 25] With a high pulmonary blood flow, the pulmonary arterial and venous muscularity increases, the muscle extends into more peripheral arteries than normal, and the size and number of intra-acinar arteries are reduced. Occluded alveolar wall arteries are seen with electron microscopic examination, probably secondary to the hyperplasia and hypertrophy of differentiating smooth muscle cells in small, normally thin-walled precapillary segments. Intimal proliferation tends to develop toward the end of the first year, and fibrosis develops during the third year of life. Patients with severe pulmonary hypertension should thus be operated on before the age of 2 years and preferably before the age of 1 year. Intimal abnormalities gradually worsen with age and resistance increases (Fig. 46–8; see Fig. 46–4A, C). Progression is relatively slow in most children with this abnormality, and grade IV pulmonary vascular disease seldom occurs in

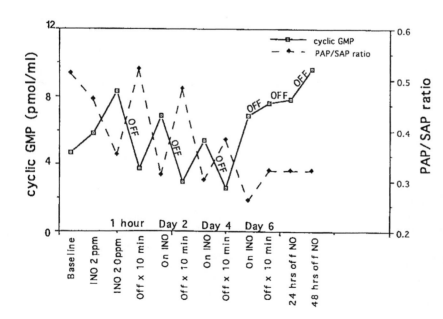

FIGURE 46–6

Concentration of cyclic guanosine monophosphate (GMP) and ratio of pulmonary arterial pressure (PAP) to systemic arterial pressure (SAP), showing the early inverse relationship between the pressure ratio and cyclic GMP concentration during treatment with nitric oxide (NO). INO = inhaled nitric oxide.

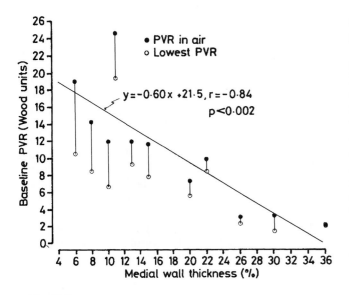

FIGURE 46–7

Medial wall thickness of intra-acinar arteries plotted against pulmonary vascular resistance (PVR), showing baseline PVR and fall in PVR after 100% oxygen and prostacyclin.

young children with a ventricular septal defect. In the minority of children who develop severe obstructive intimal proliferation early, the arteries beyond the intimal obstruction have a relatively normal medial thickness. There is no generalized arterial dilatation or other stigmata of grade IV pulmonary vascular disease, and the pulmonary arteriolar resistance can exceed 6 U · m².[14] In one study, these predilatation features were present in 62% of patients who either died at operation or had postoperative pulmonary hypertension. These observations suggest that a relatively low peripheral pulmonary arterial muscularity in patients with a ventricular septal defect and severe pulmonary hypertension (mean pulmonary arterial pressure > 40 mm Hg after 6 months of age) represents a predilatation phase

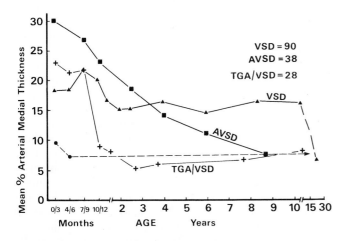

FIGURE 46–8

Mean percentage arterial medial thickness ([2 × medial thickness ÷ external diameter] × 100) in arteries 50 to 100 μm in diameter in 90 children with a ventricular septal defect (VSD), 38 with an atrioventricular septal defect (AVSD), and 28 with transposition of the great arteries and ventricular septal defect (TGA/VSD), shown at different ages.

and that the severity of proximal luminal obstruction may prejudice the outcome of intracardiac repair.

In transposition of the great arteries, patient outcome correlates with the pulmonary arterial pressure.[26] With a large ventricular septal defect, the pulmonary vasculature does not remodel normally after birth, and this failure to remodel marks the onset of rapidly progressive pulmonary vascular obstructive disease[9, 27, 28] (see Figs. 46–4B and 46–8). Intimal proliferation is seen from 2 months of age and is abundant by 5 months of age.[13] As the intimal obstruction increases in severity, the muscularity decreases in more distal vessels. After the patient reaches 7 to 9 months of age, the medial thickness is normal or even less than normal in the distal vessels. These patients have a high resistance and are usually inoperable. A patent ductus arteriosus also leads to the early development of pulmonary vascular disease in children with transposition, and it should have been closed therapeutically, if not spontaneously, by 3 months of age. With an intact ventricular septum, the pulmonary circulation usually adapts normally to extrauterine life. The bronchial circulation is enlarged, making a substantial but unknown contribution to total pulmonary blood flow, probably from birth. An enlarged bronchial circulation can sometimes persist after successful intracardiac repair. Patients are now operated on soon after birth, and nearly all patients with transposition and an intact ventricular septum undergo intracardiac repair with a relatively normal pulmonary vasculature. Rarely, infants who have had an apparently successful arterial switch operation have later developed severe progressive pulmonary vascular disease. In the days before an intracardiac repair could be carried out in early infancy, children developed severe polycythemia and pulmonary thromboembolism, and some showed pulmonary hypertension.

In infants with an *atrioventricular septal defect,* cellular intimal proliferation develops earlier and is more severe than in those with an isolated ventricular septal defect, but it develops more slowly than in those with transposition and ventricular septal defect (see Fig. 46–8). Severe medial hypertrophy and intimal proliferation can be present by 6 or 7 months of age, and intracardiac repair should be carried out in early infancy.[29, 30] Pulmonary vascular structure can be particularly difficult to evaluate in complete atrioventricular defect because of the varying degrees of incompetence of the left atrioventricular valve. When this is severe, the vein walls are abnormally thick, and perivascular connective tissue deposition is excessive, particularly around the capillary bed and small veins.

Pulmonary hypertension rarely develops in children with a *secundum atrial septal defect.* Most children are asymptomatic, but in the exceptional patient who develops cardiac failure, the pulmonary arterial pressure is usually considerably higher than in an older patient in cardiac failure. Such children are generally inoperable.[31] The pulmonary vascular abnormalities in these children resemble those in children with a hypertensive ventricular septal defect. They are unlike those seen in most middle-aged pulmonary hypertensive patients, in whom the preacinar arteries are dilated and usually undergo a modest increase in pulmonary arterial muscularity. The dominant change at the periphery is fibrotic occlusion of the small alveolar duct and the alveolar wall arteries, leading to a reduction in the capacity of the peripheral pulmonary vascular bed. Presentation of an atrial septal defect in infancy has been attributed to a primary abnormality of the pulmonary vasculature, causing persistence of the fetal circulation; the atrial septal defect is incidental. However, the presentation and clinical findings are usually unlike those seen in infants with persistent fetal circulation. The symptoms in infants with an atrial septal defect are attributable to a left-to-right shunt and a high pulmonary blood flow, whereas in persistent fetal circulation blood is shunted right to left through persistent fetal channels.

Thus far, this chapter has addressed the structural features associated with an increase in pulmonary blood flow. In pulmonary venous hypertension, the vein wall thickening and the deposition of connective tissue, particularly around the capillary bed, are more pronounced. Pulmonary arterial medial hypertrophy can be severe, but intimal damage is rare because the children normally present early in infancy, extremely ill.

Abnormalities Causing Pulmonary Venous Obstruction

Total anomalous pulmonary venous connection is an anomaly of early infancy, presenting with cyanosis at or soon after birth when the common pulmonary venous channel becomes obstructed. Only a minority of children survive infancy without surgery, and then the pulmonary venous return is usually cardiac or supradiaphragmatic, and pulmonary blood flow is elevated for some time before obstruction develops. Rarely, infants may present to the pediatrician with a history of episodic collapse, indicative of pulmonary hypertensive crises. Regardless of the site of obstruction, intrapulmonary arterial and vein wall thickness is increased, depending on the duration and severity of the obstruction. In infants with the infradiaphragmatic type of connection, obstruction and vascular abnormalities are frequently present at or soon after birth, indicating intrauterine change.[32] The common pulmonary venous channel is sometimes obstructed by fibrous tissue at birth. Pulmonary hypertension subsides after repair in almost all patients, and the pulmonary vascular changes apparently regress. Children with infradiaphragmatic total anomalous pulmonary venous connection may occasionally have intrinsically small extrapulmonary veins, and pulmonary hypertension may then persist despite adequate reconstruction.[32]

In other cardiac abnormalities causing pulmonary venous obstruction, such as cor triatriatum, congenital mitral stenosis, or stenosis of individual pulmonary veins at their junction with the left atrium, the vascular abnormalities are similar to those in total anomalous pulmonary venous return, but the arterial changes are less prominent. The lymphatic channels are dilated and abnormally thick walled, and the perivascular connective tissue is abnormally dense.

Other Problems

SCIMITAR SYNDROME. Pulmonary hypertension is not usually a feature of the scimitar syndrome in older patients, when the diagnosis is an incidental finding, but it can occur in infants. The scimitar syndrome consists of anomalous pulmonary venous connection of the right lung into the inferior vena cava, hypoplasia of the right lung with dextroposition of the heart, hypoplasia or other malformations of the right pulmonary artery, and anomalous systemic arterial supply to the lower lobe of the right lung from the abdominal aorta or its main branches.[33] In four children presenting between 1 and 5 months of age, microscopic examination showed normal peripheral airway and alveolar development.[34] The pulmonary arterial branching pattern was deficient in three children, and in areas of lung not perfused by the right pulmonary artery, the systemic arteries from the upper abdominal aorta anastomosed with the pulmonary arteries to distribute blood to a dilated capillary bed. Pulmonary arterial medial wall thickness was increased and vein wall morphology was normal. Early correction is recommended, but a report commented that surgical repair abolishes the left-to-right shunt but seldom results in a normal blood flow to the right lung, and postoperative pulmonary venous obstruction is common.[35]

EFFECT OF PALLIATIVE SURGERY ON THE LUNG. In patients with pulmonary hypoperfusion, insertion of a systemic-to-pulmonary artery shunt may lead to pulmonary hypertension. In patients with congenital heart disease associated with pulmonary hypertension, banding the pulmonary trunk may fail to adequately reduce the pulmonary arterial pressure and flow. For many years, a less than perfect result has not impaired the outcome of intracardiac repair in most patients. The introduction of the Fontan circulation and cardiac transplantation, however, has emphasized the need to achieve a structurally normal pulmonary vascular bed or at least one with normal resistance. A moderate increase in pulmonary arterial medial thickness may have little or no effect on the outcome of a repair in which a subpulmonary ventricle exists, such as tetralogy of Fallot, but offers too great an afterload for a transplanted normal, unhypertrophied right ventricle or for the systemic venous pressure when the right ventricle is missing.

MISSING A SUBPULMONARY VENTRICLE. The Fontan procedure provides a physiologic correction for tricuspid atresia and other abnormalities with only one functioning ventricle.[36, 37] The systemic venous blood is channeled into the pulmonary arteries from either the right atrium or the venae cavae. Pulmonary blood flow and survival are dependent on the postoperative gradient between the systemic venous or right atrial pressure and the left atrial pressure. Pulmonary vascular resistance must be low. The pulmonary blood flow may have been abnormally low in patients being assessed for a Fontan procedure, as in tricuspid atresia, or high, as in a univentricular heart without pulmonary stenosis. All such patients will have required palliative surgery. Those patients with a low pulmonary blood flow usually have a systemic-to-pulmonary artery shunt. This procedure provides symptomatic relief; encourages small, thin-walled intrapulmonary arteries to grow normally; and causes a modest increase in pulmonary arterial smooth muscle. The outlook is usually good. By contrast, when the pulmonary blood flow is initially high, arterial medial hypertrophy develops, and the pulmonary artery is banded in early life to prevent the development of obstructive pulmonary vascular disease. Banding reduces pulmonary flow and pressure, but the arterial medial hypertrophy does not usually regress sufficiently to produce a low resistance. Even when the Fontan criteria are fulfilled, muscularity can sometimes be increased. A lung biopsy may be helpful in determining clinical management, but the pathologist must appreciate the peculiar constraints that the lack of a subpulmonary ventricle imposes on the pulmonary vasculature.

FUNCTIONAL MANIFESTATIONS OF PULMONARY VASCULAR DISEASE AND EFFECTS OF CARDIOPULMONARY BYPASS

Pulmonary endothelial dysfunction is present early in the course of pulmonary vascular disease in young children who are potentially operable. The balance between the mechanisms controlling relaxation and contraction is disturbed (Fig. 46–9), and the relaxant response to acetylcholine is impaired.[7] However, the blood nitrite and nitrate concentrations were increased in a group of infants with pulmonary hypertension who were in cardiac failure, suggesting enhanced basal release of NO.[38] Such children have high circulating levels of thrombomodulin, an endothelial cell surface glycoprotein released by injured cells. The thromboxane/prostacyclin ratio is increased, tipping the balance between these two physiologic mediators of vascular tone in favor of vasoconstriction and platelet aggregation.[39] (After successful intracardiac repair, the ratio becomes normal within a year.) The plasma norepinephrine level is increased and increases as pulmonary vascular resistance rises. Impaired endothelium-independent relaxation in response to the NO donor sodium nitroprusside occurs later,[7] usually in association with advanced structural disease.

The diseased pulmonary vasculature is extremely vulnerable to the traumatic effects of cardiopulmonary bypass. Enhanced pulmonary vascular reactivity is a major problem after open heart surgery in children, quickly manifested as pulmonary hypertensive crises. Circulating levels of vasoconstrictor mediators such as endothelin-1,[40,41] catecholamines,[42] and thromboxane increase.[43] The vasodilator response to acetylcholine is attenuated.[44] Nitrate anion levels, reflecting NO release, are not increased,[45,46] and cyclic guanosine monophosphate (cGMP) levels can be reduced. Experimental studies indicate an impairment of NO production.[47] By contrast, the release of prostacyclin is enhanced.[43] The picture is extremely complex, made more so by the fact that the effect of any vasodilator agonist is dependent on the nature of the predominant contractile stimulus. If, as seems likely, cardiopulmonary bypass evokes a generation of many contractile agonists in varying amounts and proportions, a delay in meeting this challenge with intrinsic vasodilator agonists seems likely.

OUTCOME OF INTRACARDIAC REPAIR: FACTORS INFLUENCING EARLY AND LATE RESULTS

The outcome of a satisfactory intracardiac repair is largely determined by the state of the pulmonary vascular bed at the time of repair. In the perioperative period, the problems are associated with endothelium–smooth muscle cell dysfunction. Late outcome is determined by the extent to which the structural abnormalities are reversible.

Pulmonary hypertensive crises are now a well-recognized complication of intracardiac repair. They are particularly associated with the labile pulmonary vascula-

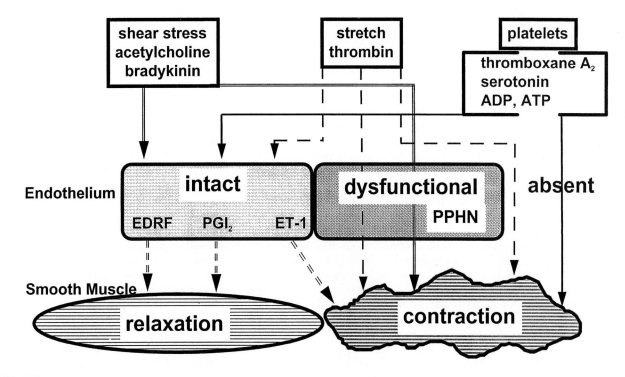

FIGURE 46–9

A diagram showing the shift in balance of vascular tone from relaxation to contraction in the presence of a dysfunctioning endothelium and the effect of exposing denuded smooth muscle cells to plasma and blood products. ADP = adenosine diphosphate; ATP = adenosine triphosphate; EDRF = endothelium-derived relaxing factor; PGI_2 = prostaglandin I_2; PPHN = persistent pulmonary hypertension of the neonate; ET-1 = endothelin-1.

ture of young children with marked pulmonary arterial medial hypertrophy, a potentially reversible state. Pulmonary hypertensive crises are sporadic increases in pulmonary arterial pressure above a normal or elevated baseline. In these cases, the pulmonary arterial pressure normally exceeds the systemic arterial pressure and left atrial return, and then cardiac output falls. Hypoxia is probably the most common identifiable precipitating factor. Crises tend to cluster and can be fatal. Cardiopulmonary bypass is thought to cause further damage to the already traumatized pulmonary endothelium, and excess reactivity is evidence of disturbed control of smooth muscle cell contractility. The ventilatory management of pulmonary hypertension involves manipulating factors that control pulmonary vascular resistance, which include alveolar oxygenation, blood pH, and lung volume. Adequate oxygenation should be maintained with an appropriate fraction of inspired oxygen (FIO_2) and mean airway pressure to achieve a PaO_2 of 10 to 14 kPa. Hypoxia and hypercapnia should be avoided. The ventilation strategy involves maintaining a normal lung volume with optimum positive end expiratory pressure. Lung overdistention or low lung volume results in increased pulmonary vascular resistance. Normocapnia or mild hypocapnia, in addition to systemic alkalosis, should be used to achieve an alkalotic pH (pH 7.45 to 7.5).[48] Volume-preset ventilation is useful to avoid detrimental fluctuations in carbon dioxide and pH. In patients with acute lung injury after cardiopulmonary bypass, high-frequency ventilation may be beneficial. Adequate analgesia and sedation are necessary to avoid severe pulmonary vasoconstriction in response to noxious stimuli such as endotracheal suctioning. Marked hyperventilation and hyperoxia should be avoided as these result in secondary lung injury from barotrauma and oxygen toxicity.[49] But the management of pulmonary hypertensive crises has been transformed by the introduction of NO therapy.[50,51] The dose of NO is titrated against the pulmonary arterial pressure, and the patient is then maintained on the lowest possible dose. A reduction in pulmonary arterial pressure and vascular resistance accompanies an increase in the plasma level of cGMP.[52] It can be difficult to wean some patients off NO, possibly because exogenous NO may depress the release of endogenous cGMP (see Fig. 46–6). This situation may be alleviated by adding a phosphodiesterase inhibitor dipyridamole. The combination of NO and dipyridamole is more effective in reducing pulmonary arterial pressure in adult patients than is NO alone.[53] Rebound pulmonary hypertension can occur after discontinuing NO, but this usually settles after an hour or so,[54] unless there are other compromising factors present. The design and use of systems delivering NO require meticulous care, with monitoring for potentially toxic levels of nitrogen dioxide and for methemoglobin, which may increase as a result of cardiopulmonary bypass.[55] Intravenous prostacyclin was used extensively to control pulmonary vascular resistance postoperatively, before the advent of NO, despite its being nonselective and possibly prejudicing the systemic circulation. Studies, however, show that prostacyclin, when given by inhalation, can be extremely helpful. In adults it has been shown to reduce pulmonary vascular resistance postoperatively in a dose-dependent manner.[56]

After repair, extensive clinical and experimental evidence has shown that pulmonary arterial medial hypertrophy, even with a modest amount of cellular intimal proliferation and fibrosis, is potentially reversible. Complete obliteration of the arterial lumen by intimal proliferation, even when highly cellular, is not usually reversible. Plexiform lesions are regarded as irreversible. It is not entirely certain whether these lesions are irreversible when present in early childhood but, given the severity of obstructive pathology with which they are associated, reversibility seems unlikely. The reduction in small intra-acinar arteries seen particularly in young children with severe pulmonary hypertension is probably not reversible. Normally about half of the intra-acinar arteries and the alveoli that they supply are present at birth, and the remainder form mainly during the first year of life.[57] Hence, it is desirable to operate as early in life as possible to encourage the development of new, normal vessels to help achieve a normal pulmonary arterial pressure and mitigate against the effects of existing obstructive disease.

The age at which intracardiac repair is carried out is the most crucial factor. In 1978, a group of 67 children with different types of intracardiac abnormalities underwent lung biopsy at the time of intracardiac repair, and the structural changes present were related to the mean pulmonary pressure the day after operation, and the mean pressure and vascular resistance determined 1 year later.[24,58] On the day after surgery, patients whose biopsies showed only a modest increase in pulmonary arterial smooth muscle generally had a normal or near-normal pulmonary arterial pressure. Those whose biopsies showed severe arterial medial hypertrophy or a reduction in peripheral arterial number had an increase in pressure, which was greater in those patients who also had intimal proliferation. Those whose lung biopsy showed intimal fibrosis had a higher mean pulmonary arterial pressure of approximately 40 mm Hg or more, regardless of the morphometric findings. One year after surgical repair, however, all those operated on before 9 months of age had a normal pressure, resistance, or both, regardless of the severity of the pulmonary vascular lesions at the time of repair. Of the children surgically repaired after 9 months of age, those who had extension of muscle and an increase in pulmonary arterial smooth muscle had normal hemodynamic findings 1 year later, whereas those with more advanced changes generally did not. This study emphasized the desirability of repairing the abnormalities in early infancy.

Emphasis in clinical management must be on the prevention of pulmonary vascular disease. When the natural history of the cardiac abnormality is that of rapidly progressive pulmonary vascular disease, as in transposition of the great arteries with ventricular septal defect or univentricular heart without pulmonary outflow tract obstruction, the child should undergo either corrective surgery or banding of the pulmonary artery soon after birth. For conditions in which the natural history of pulmonary vascular disease is less aggressive, as in a ventricular septal defect, the abnormality should be corrected before 1 year of age if the pulmonary arterial pressure remains high. In those patients operated on before the age of 1 year, pulmonary vascular resistance usually falls to normal. Surgery soon after the age of 2 years is associated with a fall in resistance but not usually to a normal level. Repairing an intracardiac abnormality in the presence of established pulmonary vascular disease accelerates the progression of disease and the onset of right ventricular failure and death. An early study described a group of children with a ventricular septal defect who underwent intracardiac repair at a mean age of 4.8 years, with a pulmonary vascular resistance more than 25% of the systemic vascular resistance and in excess of 400 dyne = sec $\cdot$ cm^{-5} $\cdot$ m^2.[59] The operative mortality was high, and 18% of those patients surviving the operation died between 1 and 7 years after the operation with Eisenmenger's syndrome, when they were 7 to 16 years old.

LATE FOLLOW-UP OF PATIENTS WITH PULMONARY HYPERTENSION

The clinical features of patients who have been deemed inoperable have been described earlier in this chapter. Treatment is largely empirical. Dipyridamole is given to reduce platelet aggregation but may also have a beneficial vasodilatory effect as a phosphodiesterase inhibitor. Because thrombi become superimposed on the obstructive lesions of pulmonary vascular disease, there is an argument for using anticoagulation in patients with this condition. Venesection with plasma dilution in those with a high hematocrit affords symptomatic relief to some patients and reduces the risk of cerebrovascular accidents. Calcium channel blockers are not used routinely. Long-term oxygen treatment at home gives subjective improvement and can increase survival.[60] Prostacyclin when given by inhalation becomes a selective pulmonary vasodilator and remodeling agent. Given long term, it is hoped that, like intravenous prostacyclin, it could increase survival and retard the progressive obstruction of the pulmonary vascular bed. (For a drug not to have a selective action on the pulmonary vasculature in the presence of a systemic-to-pulmonary communication would be dangerous.) Domiciliary NO is not yet a routine treatment, although NO can be given safely to children breathing spontaneously.[61] Patients with advanced pulmonary vascular obstructive disease, like those with primary pulmonary hypertension, may be unable to increase their NO production on exercise.[62] Chronic administration of L-arginine might be helpful if it could be shown conclusively that these patients have a relative substrate deficiency of NO production.

Finally, the only effective treatment for the very sick patient is transplantation, either a combined heart-lung transplantation or a lung transplantation with intracardiac repair. Conventionally, transplantation is recommended when the patient's condition begins to deteriorate rapidly. However, a more active approach is to be recommended, which includes recatheterization as part of the routine reassessment.[8] Survival has been found to correlate with the product of pulmonary vascular resistance and mean right atrial pressure, a relatively crude evaluation of right ventricular function. Because the results of transplantation are unsatisfactory, transplantation should be considered only when the expected survival time is less than the expected survival after transplantation. We do well to remember how long many of these patients can live with a relatively good quality of life. The average age at death for untreated patients, reported in the 1950s, was 33 years for aortopulmonary and ventricular septal defects and 36 years for atrial defects.[2] The maximum age reached was 65 years for

patients with ventricular and atrial septal defects and 55 years for those with patent ductus arteriosus.

In patients in whom pulmonary hypertension is secondary to left heart failure, it is infinitely preferable to transplant only the heart, for which long-term survival is good. In discriminating between the need for heart rather than heart-lung transplantation, inhalation of NO can be particularly helpful.[63] A study showed that in those patients in whom the mean left atrial pressure was more than 15 mm Hg on NO, the pulmonary vascular resistance decreased to 7.6 U $\cdot$ m^2, a figure thought to be compatible with transplantation of the heart alone. But those patients with a left atrial pressure of less than 15 mm Hg had a minimum pulmonary vascular resistance of 30 U $\cdot$ m^2. In giving NO to patients with left ventricular dysfunction after surgery, the beneficial effect on the pulmonary vasculature must be balanced against the detrimental effect of increasing left ventricular preload.[64]

In patients with postoperative pulmonary hypertension, the management is similar to that outlined previously, with one exception. Because patients with congenital heart disease and a high resistance can survive longer with a defect, rather than without, and because the life expectancy of patients presenting with primary pulmonary hypertension is shorter than in those with Eisenmenger's syndrome, it is logical to restore a defect.[65] When blade atrial septectomy was carried out in a group of patients with primary pulmonary hypertension, in New York Heart Association class IV, the symptoms and signs of right-sided heart failure improved, there was no further syncope, and there was a sustained increase in cardiac index and in survival.[66] Because the procedure carries a significant mortality in very sick patients with either primary or postoperative pulmonary hypertension, the procedure should probably be carried out when it is clear that the pulmonary vascular resistance is, and will remain, high after surgery. Further studies are warranted.

PRIMARY PULMONARY HYPERTENSION

Primary pulmonary hypertension is diagnosed when there is no explanation for the increase in pulmonary arterial pressure. The mean pressure exceeds 25 mm Hg at rest and 30 mm Hg on exercise. There is a progressive increase in right ventricular pressure leading to right-sided heart failure and death. An early study reported a 5-year survival rate of 9% in children and young adults not treated with vasodilator drugs.[67] Long-term vasodilator treatment has markedly improved survival: the 5-year survival rate is 88% in children who present at less than 6 years of age and 25% in older patients. In 1975 a World Health Organization committee defined primary pulmonary hypertension according to morphologic criteria, as being caused by pulmonary arterial obstruction, the most common pathology; pulmonary venoocclusive disease; or thromboembolism. This unsatisfactory definition was revised in 1998. The reclassification includes all forms of severe pulmonary hypertension, including primary pulmonary hypertension. It is based on three features—the anatomic localization of the disease, the presence or absence of associated disease, and the severity of the circulatory disturbance. The incidence of primary pulmonary hypertension is approximately 1 to 2 per million people in Western countries.[68] Women are most frequently affected. The sex incidence (female-to-male ratio) in the adult population is 1.7:1, and although the sex incidence in children had always been thought to be equal, recent studies show that a female preponderance is present from early childhood.[69] Most instances are sporadic but 6% are familial.[70] The disease is inherited in an autosomal dominant manner with incomplete penetrance.[71,72] Familial primary pulmonary hypertension shows gene anticipation, presenting at a younger age in successive generations.[73] Studies have located the gene for familial primary pulmonary hypertension to chromosome 2q31–32.[74]

Patients can present throughout childhood, after a period of apparently normal growth and development. PPHN is excluded from this diagnostic group, although in some young patients with primary pulmonary hypertension, the pulmonary circulation may have failed to grow and to develop normally. In most patients with primary pulmonary hypertension, adults and children, the organization of elastin in the pulmonary trunk indicates that pulmonary hypertension was not present from birth. In general, the disease is similar in adults and children, but there are important differences.

Indian children suffer from a particularly vicious form of primary pulmonary hypertension. The clinical picture is distinctive. The majority of patients present in late adolescence, although they can present as young as 4 years of age. Many patients die within 2 years of diagnosis, a few surviving as young as 10 years. Pulmonary vascular change is described as grade IV to VI, using the Heath and Edwards classification.[20,75] In patients from Sri Lanka, Wallooppillai and Wagenvoort found the picture of plexogenic pulmonary arteriopathy.[23] There is generally no familial incidence, and no evidence of a collagen disorder, coagulation defect, eosinophilia, or thromboembolism.

PATHOLOGY AND PATHOGENESIS

The structural abnormalities in the pulmonary vasculature are similar to those seen in patients with pulmonary hypertension and a left-to-right shunt. At autopsy, most adults have advanced pulmonary vascular obstructive disease with plexiform lesions. This picture is also common in older children and can be seen before 3 years of age. Severe pulmonary arterial medial hypertrophy with marked intimal proliferation almost occluding the lumen can also occur, however, and is seen more commonly in young children. The changes can be so exuberant and rapidly progressive that they obstruct the lumen before intimal fibrosis and plexiform lesions have had time to develop.

The pathogenesis of primary pulmonary hypertension is unknown. The evidence suggests that it is a disease of those with a genetic predisposition to respond adversely to a variety of stimuli, the response initiating the development of pulmonary vascular disease. The clinical and structural findings represent the final common pathway. Likely triggers include drugs, particularly anorexic agents such as fenfluramine, dexfenfluramine, and aminorex[76]; toxins; hypoxia, including high-altitude hypoxia; lung injury; catecholamine-induced increases in sympathetic tone; and autoimmune diseases, such as disseminated lupus erythe-

matosus.[77,78] Intense vasoconstriction is thought to be the common early response to injury. Experimental studies show that, like hypoxia, the anorexic agents that cause primary pulmonary hypertension inhibit potassium current in the smooth muscle cells of pulmonary resistance arteries, causing membrane depolarization and hence vasoconstriction.[79] The association between autoimmune diseases and pulmonary hypertension has long been recognized, including Raynaud's syndrome, which is a systemic vasospastic condition.[80,81] Children, unlike adults, do not show an increased incidence of antinuclear antibodies, but their healthy mothers do, and some children seroconvert when they get older.[69] Most autoimmune diseases are associated with an increase in certain human leukocyte antigen (HLA) class II alleleles, and children with primary pulmonary hypertension have an increased frequency of HLA-DR3, -DR52, and -DQ2.[82] These observations suggest that primary pulmonary hypertension is autoimmune in origin in some children. The endothelium probably plays a crucial role in the pathogenesis of primary pulmonary hypertension, influencing both vasoconstriction and structural remodeling, functions that are inseparable (see Fig. 46–9). Vasoconstrictor agents such as endothelin are also vascular smooth muscle mitogens, whereas vasodilator agents such as prostacyclin and NO can be antiproliferative and antimigratory (Fig. 46–10). Two of the most powerful intrinsic vasodilators are thought to be deficient in patients with primary pulmonary hypertension, namely prostacyclin and NO. The amount of exhaled NO is normal at rest but fails to increase on exercise.[62] Other metabolic indicators of endothelial dysfunction include an excess of circulating thromboxane in relation to prostacyclin, elevated endothelin levels predisposing to vasoconstriction, and coagulation abnormalities that might encourage platelet aggregation.[83,84] The role of platelet aggregation in the pathogenesis of primary pulmonary hypertension is unknown, but elevated fibrinopeptide A levels indicate that thrombosis occurs in situ, and thrombosis is frequently evident in the established disease seen at autopsy.[85] Anticoagulation therapy increases survival.[86] The rationale for giving chronic vasodilator therapy is that a reduction in vasoconstriction not only alleviates symptoms but retards the progression of vascular disease from medial hypertrophy to plexogenic arteriopathy. This is particularly so for chronic intravenous prostacyclin therapy.

CLINICAL FEATURES

Symptoms vary and are age related. Young children fail to thrive, whereas others appear remarkably normal but tire easily and are said to be "very good children." Young children can also present with syncope, sometimes fatally. Older children, like adults, have exertional dyspnea and may have chest pain. Evaluation includes exclusion of other causes of pulmonary hypertension and screening other siblings for the familial form of the disease. Chronic thromboembolic disease must be excluded because it could be amenable to thromboendarterectomy. Therefore, ventilation-perfusion scintigraphy and, if necessary, pulmonary angiography are carried out. Echocardiography, radionuclide angiography and magnetic resonance imaging, pulmonary function and exercise testing, and continu-

Shear stress
Hypoxia
Cytokines

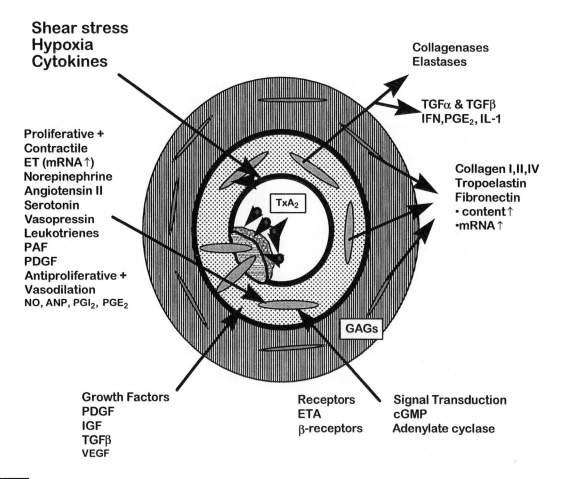

Proliferative +
Contractile
ET (mRNA↑)
Norepinephrine
Angiotensin II
Serotonin
Vasopressin
Leukotrienes
PAF
PDGF
Antiproliferative +
Vasodilation
NO, ANP, PGI₂, PGE₂

Collagenases
Elastases

TGFα & TGFβ
IFN,PGE₂, IL-1

Collagen I,II,IV
Tropoelastin
Fibronectin
• content↑
•mRNA ↑

TxA₂

GAGs

Growth Factors
PDGF
IGF
TGFβ
VEGF

Receptors
ETA
β-receptors

Signal Transduction
cGMP
Adenylate cyclase

FIGURE 46–10

A diagram showing the factors influencing vessel wall remodeling and the interaction between proliferative and contractile agonists, and between antiproliferative and vasodilator agonists. ET = endothelin; PAF = platelet-activating factor; PDGF = platelet-derived growth factor; NO = nitric oxide; ANP = atrial natriuretic peptide; PG = prostaglandin; IGF = insulin-like growth factor; TGF = transforming growth factor; VEGF = vascular endothelial growth factor; TxA₂ = thromboxane A₂; GAGs = glycosaminoglycans; ETA = endothelin type A receptor; IFN = interferon; IL = interleukin; cGMP = cyclic guanosine monophosphate.

ous measurement of oxygen saturation during sleep are all noninvasive tests that are important not only in diagnosis but also in monitoring the progression of disease and the effect of treatment. Echocardiography generally reveals dilated right-sided heart chambers with posterior bowing of the ventricular septum and, in the absence of a small atrial communication, the atrial septum. Doppler interrogation detects tricuspid and pulmonary insufficiency, and the velocity of the regurgitant jets gives an estimate of the pulmonary systolic and diastolic pressures. Lung function testing can demonstrate small airway obstruction, and according to Mikkilineni and coworkers,[87] the degree of obstruction correlates with the degree of symptoms and hemodynamic findings.[87,88] On exercise testing, an exercise capacity of less than 10% of the predicted value indicates an increased risk of developing complications during cardiac catheterization.[88] Conversely, a capacity of more than 75% of the predicted value may identify a subgroup likely to respond well to vasodilator therapy. Some children with primary pulmonary hypertension have immunoglobulin deficiency. They may have a low level of antithrombin III, protein S, or protein C, which may be genetic in origin or result from a consumption coagulopathy.[89]

At cardiac catheterization, the pulmonary arterial pressure, vascular resistance, and cardiac index are higher in children than in adults presenting with primary pulmonary hypertension, and in one study measured 70 ± 15 mm Hg, 28.1 ± 18.1mm Hg/L/min/m², and 4.3 L/min/m², respectively.[69] Catheterization is extremely hazardous in these patients, and adequate sedation, optimal ventilation, and meticulous attention to acid-base status and blood loss are mandatory. Taking an open lung biopsy is also not without risk, but when the clinical picture is uncertain, a biopsy can be invaluable in excluding other pathologies before embarking on long-term therapy.

TREATMENT

Treatment for primary pulmonary hypertension is treatment for life. The therapeutic regimen has to be tailored to meet the needs of each individual and adjusted when required according to changes in clinical and hemodynamic status. Optimizing the management of these patients markedly improves quality of life and survival. Conventional treatment consists of giving anticoagulants and oral vasodilator therapy, usually a calcium channel blocker.

Warfarin rather than aspirin or dipyridamole is recommended to prevent thrombosis in situ. But only 40% of children showed a clinical and hemodynamic improvement and lived longer when treated with oral vasodilator therapy.[90] Studies have shown that long-term intravenous prostacyclin therapy is more effective.[67,91,92]

The most important determinants of survival are age and the acute response to prostacyclin. A study by Barst and colleagues[67] reported a 5-year survival rate of 88% in children of less than 6 years of age, as compared with 25% for older children.[93] In a later study of children who responded satisfactorily to acute prostacyclin at catheterization, the 5-year survival rate was 86%, as compared with 33% for nonresponders.[67] The response to an acute vasodilator drug at cardiac catheterization is used to assess the desirability of using chronic vasodilator therapy. In children with unfavorable hemodynamics, with a high fixed pulmonary vascular resistance, and who do not respond to acute vasodilator testing, chronic vasodilator treatment can have adverse effects and precipitate or worsen right-sided heart failure. Acute responsiveness is usually assessed by giving incremental doses of prostacyclin, from 2 to 12 ng/kg/min, but a response is sometimes achieved only at a dose of 20 ng/kg/min or higher.[69] Children tolerate higher doses of prostacyclin than do adults. Alternative drugs used for testing include acetylcholine, NO, and sometimes adenosine. A positive response is taken as a decrease in mean pulmonary arterial pressure of 20% or more with no fall in cardiac index. Children show a positive response to acute vasodilator testing more frequently than do adults, 41% as compared with 12%.[90] Positive responders are treated long term with calcium channel blockers, and preferably with intravenous prostacyclin. Unfortunately, there is no evidence at present that prostacyclin can be given by inhalation as reliably and effectively as when given intravenously. Some patients who do not respond to acute vasodilator therapy can respond satisfactorily to chronic therapy but need close supervision. Also, some patients who do not respond to oral chronic vasodilator therapy can be treated with intravenous prostacyclin, with good clinical and hemodynamic effect and increased survival.[94]

Most patients treated with intravenous prostacyclin have been adults, but despite the obvious logistical problems, infants and young children can be managed satisfactorily. Problems include abrupt interruption of the infusion, which is usually noticed very rapidly, causing fatigue and occasionally syncope.[90,92] Rarely, death supervenes, presumably because of a pulmonary hypertensive crisis. Less dramatic complications include discomfort at the catheter site, bleeding, infection, and thrombotic episodes. Painful periostitis, particularly of the jaw, often occurs. Patients can become very tolerant of prostacyclin, requiring constant, aggressive, upward adjustment of their dosage. Clinical and hemodynamic improvement is generally sustained. Some patients treated as a bridge to transplantation have improved to such an extent that they are being treated with long-term intravenous prostacyclin rather than undergoing transplantation.[69] In these patients prostacyclin appears to be acting primarily by structurally remodeling the pulmonary vasculature rather than acting solely as a pulmonary vasodilator. The duration of treatment is not known but it should be continued for years. Additional conventional therapy includes diuretic drugs, but this can prejudice cardiac output by reducing the preload. Digoxin can sometimes help those in right-sided heart failure. Antiarrhythmic drugs are occasionally necessary. Other treatment strategies include supplemental domiciliary oxygen.[60]

Atrial septectomy can improve survival in those with recurrent syncope who have a bad prognosis.[66] In exercise-induced syncope, the systemic circulation dilates, and cardiac output cannot be sustained. But in the presence of a right-to-left shunt at atrial level, output is maintained, and the right-sided heart chambers are decompressed. After blade atrial septectomy, the 1- and 2-year survival rate in adult series improved from 54% and 42%, respectively, to 87% and 76%. Syncope was abolished. Atrial septectomy has also been carried out safely in children with primary pulmonary hypertension.

Save for those patients who can be satisfactorily managed on long-term intravenous prostacyclin, the only treatment that can be offered patients with primary pulmonary hypertension is transplantation. To date, transplantation has been performed predominantly in adolescents and adults. Primary pulmonary hypertension does not occur in the transplanted lung, suggesting that primary pulmonary hypertension is a disease intrinsic to the pulmonary circulation, not just a response to an abnormal and/or excessive circulating product.

PULMONARY HYPERTENSION IN THE NEWBORN

Failure of the pulmonary vascular resistance to fall normally after birth leads to persistent right-to-left shunting through fetal channels. Harvey first described the normal fetal circulation in 1628 and described persistence of the fetal circulation in the "unripe births of mankind."[95] Not until 1950 was this flow pattern associated with pulmonary hypertension.[96] In 1952, injection of contrast material into the umbilical vein showed that the foramen ovale had either failed to close or had reopened in asphyxiated infants, demonstrating the lability of the newborn pulmonary circulation.[97] Rowe described the association between right-to-left atrial or ductal shunting in congenital heart disease with pulmonary hypertension in 1959.[98] Regardless of etiology, PPHN is associated with failure of the pulmonary circulation to adapt normally to extrauterine life. Fewer than 20% of instances are idiopathic. PPHN is associated with many disorders including fetal, intrapartum, and postpartum asphyxia; parenchymal lung disease; and certain types of congenital heart disease, such as obstructed total anomalous pulmonary venous connection, left ventricular inflow or outflow tract obstruction, and obligatory left-to-right shunts. Despite this diversity, in all infants with PPHN, a persistently raised pulmonary vascular resistance causes right-to-left shunting through the foramen ovale, ductus arteriosus, or both to produce cyanosis. The pulmonary vasculature is excessively labile, and the structural features are those of an unadapted pulmonary vasculature. The pathogenesis is not understood, but it seems likely that similar defects in the cellular mechanisms determining the postnatal fall in pulmonary vascular resistance are present in idiopathic PPHN and in the diverse conditions with which the disorder can be associated. The severity of the illness and the likely outcome are related to the nature of the underlying disease or abnormality.

PPHN can be successfully modeled in several animal species, providing insight into many of the basic mechanisms involved in the pathogenesis of this condition and yielding information that can be applied more widely to other types of pulmonary hypertension. The following pages summarize current knowledge of the human disease and then describe the relevant experimental findings.

PATHOLOGIC AND HEMODYNAMIC FINDINGS

In neonates who die during the first days of life with PPHN, the intrapulmonary arterial wall structure is similar to that seen in fetal life—the pulmonary vasculature is unadapted. Characteristically, there are many clusters of undilated precapillary arteries. In those who survive for a few days, the medial smooth muscle cells differentiate into a more contractile phenotype than normal, and connective tissue deposition, predominantly elastin and collagen type I, is excessive. The vessels appear to have become fixed in an incompletely dilated state. These changes imply modulation of the cell phenotypes. The pulmonary arterial smooth muscle cell contractile cytoskeleton is excessively dense and composed of α- and γ-actin isoforms, the SM1 and SM2 myosin heavy chain isoforms and the actin-associated proteins caldesmon and calponin, which help regulate contraction. The pericytes and intermediate cells in the walls of arteries, which accompany respiratory bronchioli and alveolar ducts and lie within the alveolar walls, differentiate into smooth muscle cells, and muscle is then said to show abnormal extension along the arterial pathway. The vessel wall is innervated by sympathetic-like vasoconstrictor nerves.[99] Changes are present throughout the lung and are common to all forms of PPHN, idiopathic and secondary, regardless of etiology. In neonates with idiopathic PPHN, when the pulmonary circulation is itself at fault in failing to adapt, the presence of abnormally thick-walled vessels in those dying soon after birth prompted the suggestion that the intrapulmonary arteries may become excessively thick walled during fetal life.[100] When pulmonary hypertension results from lung disease, such as meconium aspiration, the vascular changes are most severe in the regions of lung showing the greatest parenchymal damage. The vascular changes in preterm infants are similar to those seen in term infants, and airway structure is commensurate with gestational age. In addition, many of these infants are mechanically ventilated. This process distorts the geometry of the peripheral airways, and the alveolar ducts may be dilated, and the alveoli flattened.

Neonates with PPHN are cyanotic and may have signs of respiratory distress. Cross-sectional echocardiography and Doppler interrogation rapidly determine the intracardiac anatomy, demonstrate the sites and the magnitude of the right-to-left shunt, and give an estimate of the pulmonary arterial pressure.

MANAGEMENT

The management of PPHN entails treating any underlying abnormality, optimizing ventilation, and dilating the pulmonary vasculature. Previously, tolazoline and prostacyclin were the most commonly used vasodilator drugs. Neither is selective for the pulmonary circulation, and therefore both systemic and pulmonary vascular resistance are decreased. By contrast, NO given by inhalation selectively dilates the pulmonary vasculature. Infants with parenchymal lung disease or developmental abnormalities of the lung may require high-frequency oscillatory or jet ventilation and exogenous surfactant to increase the uniform delivery of NO to atelectatic and underventilated peripheral airways. The dose of NO is titrated to the clinical response to achieve the lowest therapeutic dose possible. NO is immediately inactivated on entering the blood stream and binding to hemoglobin, so it cannot compromise the systemic circulation. It combines, however, with hemoglobin to produce methemoglobin, and in high concentration it injures the lung, oxidizes to the toxic gas nitrogen dioxide, and combines with superoxide to form the free radical peroxynitrate. It may prove possible to reduce the dose of NO by giving a phosphodiesterase inhibitor such as dipyridamole to block the breakdown of cGMP. Except for children with congenital heart disease who usually require surgery, NO is extremely effective. Failure to sustain an improvement can occur in those with pulmonary hypoplasia and dysplasia.[101]

PATHOGENESIS

The mechanisms responsible for achieving a normal fall in pulmonary vascular resistance at birth are poorly understood (see Chapter 7). They include ventilation, an increase in oxygen tension, the preterm reduction in vasoconstrictor leukotrienes, an increase in bradykinin, and the release of prostacyclin associated with the onset of breathing.[102–107] The NO pathway appears to play a crucial role in determining the vasoreactivity of the transitional circulation.[103] In the mature pulmonary circulation the interaction between healthy endothelial and smooth muscle cells produces a balance between relaxation and contraction, slightly in favor of relaxation because of the basal release of endothelium-derived NO (Fig. 46–9).[108] In theory, therefore, failure to achieve a satisfactory reduction in pulmonary arterial pressure at birth could involve a failure of endothelium-dependent or endothelium-independent relaxation, a primary structural abnormality in the target smooth muscle cell, or an excess of vasoconstrictor agonists such as endothelin and thromboxane. PPHN may represent a persistence of the fetal state because a normal vasoconstrictor mechanism inhibiting relaxation persists inappropriately after birth or because a vasodilator mechanism is inadequate or fails to appear at birth. The primary abnormality probably varies.

The rationale for giving NO to neonates with PPHN is that they have reduced endothelial release of NO and other relaxant factors, such as prostacyclin. The NO is also attempting to relax pulmonary arteries that fail to remodel normally after birth and become progressively more abnormal with time. The newborn pulmonary vasculature responds vigorously to an increase in pressure. The medial smooth muscle cells of pulmonary hypertensive newborn calves and rats show an increase in cell proliferation and DNA synthesis.[109, 110] The vessel wall normally contains a multiplicity of smooth muscle cell phenotypes expressing different contractile and cytoskeletal proteins and receptors. Most of these cells, however, normally have a predominantly synthetic phenotype at birth, and in PPHN, connective tissue deposition is rapid and excessive. The gene expression for tropoelastin and type I procollagen remains abnormally high after birth, and elastin and collagen synthesis and content and steady-state tropoelastin collagen I, III, and IV levels are increased.[111–113] In the adventitia, fibroproliferative changes are marked and precede those in the media. Experimental neonatal hypoxia causes a six-fold increase in ^{3}H-thymidine labeling within 24 hours and labeling increased 60-fold in response to hyperoxia,[114–116] a finding that has worrying implications for the treatment of sick infants. Remodeling of a vessel wall implies connective tissue degradation as well as synthesis. Neonatal pulmonary hypertension is associated with increased activation of the proteolytic enzyme endogenous vascular elastase.[117–119] This elastase is thought to enhance smooth muscle cell proliferation and migration and increase matrix production, changes that lead to vessel wall thickening.[120]

Pulmonary hypertension alters the expression and release of several growth factors, promotors, and inhibitors. Expression of insulin-like growth factor-1 (IGF-1) and IGF-2 increases and expression of TGFβ1 decreases.[121, 122] Circulating levels of endothelin are elevated in human and experimental PPHN,[123, 124] and the transcriptional rate of the preproendothelin gene is increased in hypoxic cultured endothelial cells, thus raising the steady-state level of messenger RNA expression.[125] Eicosanoid production, prostacyclin (PGI$_2$), and prostaglandin E$_2$ are diminished.[126]

Receptors link vascular structure and function, and PPHN alters the density and distribution of many vasoactive receptors and changes their signal transduction pathways, modifying the changes that normally take place after birth. For example, the density of vasoconstrictor endothelin type A (ET$_A$) receptors on the pulmonary arterial smooth muscle cells of chronically hypoxic newborn pigs increases.[124] The vasodilator endothelial endothelin type B (ET$_B$) receptors, which normally appear transiently at 3 days, fail to appear. Activation of these endothelial receptors causes relaxation.[127]

Experimental fetal intervention, either chronic fetal hypoxemia or ductus constriction or ligation, can lead to PPHN[128, 129] and is associated with impaired NO-dependent vasodilatation and a decrease in NO synthase activity and protein and gene expression.[130] Ductus constriction increases plasma endothelin-1 (ET-1) concentration, and produces ET$_A$ receptor–mediated vasoconstriction and decreased ET$_B$ receptor–mediated vasodilatation.[131] PPHN caused by chronic hypoxia from birth impairs endothelium-dependent and endothelium-independent relaxation mediated via the NO pathway (Fig. 46–11). It prevents the normal postnatal establishment of both the receptor-mediated relaxant response to acetylcholine and bradykinin and the non–receptor-dependent response to the calcium ionophore A23187 in isolated pulmonary arteries from newborn piglets.[132] It inhibits the established response in animals first allowed to adapt normally to extrauterine life before being exposed to hypoxia. These and other studies on fetal and newborn animals document a reduction in the gene and protein expression of NO synthesis.[130, 133] NO release continues but at a lower level than normal,[132] and an excess of reactive oxygen species might be responsible for inactivating much of the NO produced. NO synthase activates soluble guanylate cyclase. When endothelium-independent relaxation was studied, the basal generation of cGMP was sustained in animals kept in an hypoxic environment, and cGMP generation increased appropriately on stimulation with exogenous NO and zaprinast, a phosphodiesterase inhibitor. Nevertheless, relaxation was impaired.[132] This suggests a block in the relaxation pathway distal to the generation of cGMP. The pulmonary arterial smooth muscle cells of chronically hypoxic newborn piglets are excessively depolarized, a feature that can make cells insensitive to the relaxing effect of cGMP.[134] These experimental studies suggest that the NO pathway is usually less effective in the normal fetal and newborn lung and that PPHN disturbs signal transduction pathways, which have less reserve and are more precarious than those of the mature pulmonary circulation. Fortunately, other relaxant pathways appear to function well during the first days of life and to be more resistant to chronic hypoxia. Atrial natriuretic peptide activates particularly guanylate cyclase, NO activates soluble guanylate cyclase, and newborn vessels, normal and hypoxic, relax well to atrial natriuretic peptide. Also, the relaxant response to the adenosine triphosphate (ATP)–sensitive potassium channel agonist levcromakalim is not impaired. Thus, chronic hypoxia selectively impairs certain relaxation pathways while sparing others. In the adult rat lung, smooth muscle cells of different phenotypes show a predominance of different potassium channels.[135] Within the vessel wall, radioligand binding studies show that not all smooth muscle cells have the same receptors. The relation between the effect of chronic hypoxia on the different pulmonary arterial smooth muscle cell phenotypes of the newborn lung and the reactivity of each of these phenotypes is yet to be established.

As noted earlier in this chapter, the regulation of pulmonary vascular tone is disturbed in young infants with pulmonary hypertensive congenital heart disease. Experimental studies in which an aortopulmonary shunt was inserted in utero caused impaired endothelium-dependent vasodilatation at 4 weeks of age, increased basal NO activity, increased plasma ET-1 concentration, ET$_A$ receptor gene expression and vasoconstriction, and reduced ET$_B$ receptor gene expression and vasodilatation.[136–138]

Failure of the pulmonary circulation to adapt normally to extrauterine life probably involves potassium channel regulation of the smooth muscle membrane. In the adult lung, hypoxia causes vasoconstriction by inhibition of the outward potassium current, which causes membrane depolarization leading to calcium influx through voltage-gated calcium channels.[139] In the fetus, hypoxic vasoconstriction results from inhibition of a calcium-sensitive potassium channel, although some smooth muscle cells carry the delayed rectifier channels more commonly seen in resistance than conduit arteries.[135] Were we to understand the circumstances under which one type of channel was inactivated, we might exploit the use of an alternative channel.

Many of the agonists that influence relaxation and contraction also influence smooth muscle cell proliferation

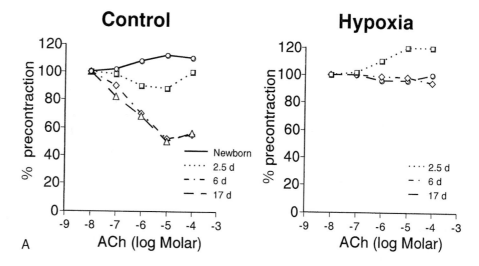

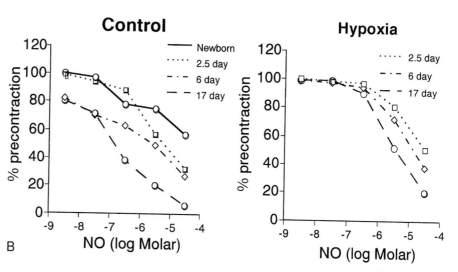

FIGURE 46–11

A, Response to acetylcholine (ACh) of normal newborn isolated porcine intrapulmonary arteries: cumulative concentration dose-response curves after $PGF_{2\alpha}$-induced contraction in arterial rings with endothelium at birth, 2.5 days, 6 days, and 17 days of age. The right-hand panel shows the response to ACh in pulmonary hypertensive vessels, after exposure to chronic hypobaric hypoxia (50.8 kPa), either from birth to 2.5 days, 3 to 6 days, or 14 to 17 days of age. B, Response to exogenous nitric oxide (NO) in normal isolated porcine intrapulmonary arteries at the ages given in A, from normal and hypertensive animals.

(see Fig. 46–10). Conversely, certain growth factors can act as contractile agonists. The smooth muscle cell is both the origin and target of many of these activities, and the characteristics of this cell (e.g., its phenotype) determine its response. As noted previously, not all the cells are alike. There is a gradient of differentiation from the subendothelium to the adventitia, such that the concentration of contractile myofilaments is always greater in the outermost cell layers. In addition, the media contains nests of cells that have quite a different phenotype. Hypertensive newborn pulmonary arteries have a high replication rate, a persistently high level of extracellular matrix gene expression, and impaired relaxant properties. Whether these problems reflect the activities of one or of several smooth muscle cell phenotypes is not yet established, but the cumulative response determines structural remodeling and reactivity. In theory, therapeutic regimens aimed at maximizing relaxation using long-term NO, NO donors, or supplementation with L-arginine might also modify structural remodeling, as prostacyclin treatment is thought to do in primary pulmonary hypertension. We focus clinically on maximizing endothelium-dependent relaxation rather than contemplating the necessity of reducing contraction, because we have the means at our disposal to replace or supplement endogenous NO with the exogenous substance. However,

endothelin receptor antagonists attenuate the pulmonary hypertensive response to experimental hypoxia,[140] and endothelin has both a vasoconstrictor and a mitogenic effect. Ultimately, our aim must be to control excessive reactivity and structural remodeling using therapeutic agents that exploit the interactions between the signaling pathways controlling these events.

THE FUTURE: WHERE DO WE GO FROM HERE?

Our understanding of normal adaptation to extrauterine life and early postnatal development is so deficient that it is difficult to identify the early crucial factors that are altered by persistent pulmonary hypertension and that instigate the cascade of abnormal structural and functional changes, which become increasingly difficult to reverse with the passage of time. Also, the direct effects of pulmonary hypertension must be distinguished from the effects of treatment. We need to understand (1) how pulmonary hypertension alters the endothelial sensing of oxygen tension, stress, and strain; (2) how it alters the contractile and cytoskeletal apparatus of pulmonary vascular smooth muscle cells; and (3) how these and other abnormalities of structural remodeling integrate and translate into functional disturbances. Future early therapy may be directed toward angiogenesis, possibly using VEGF. Understanding the potential for structural and functional recovery will determine what we can hope to achieve in practice. Clinical and experimental studies indicate that abnormal pulmonary vascular remodeling fails to resolve as completely in newborns as it does in adults and that the response to a subsequent hypertensive insult results in a disproportionately aggressive response. These observations suggest persistent abnormalities in gene expression and signal transduction, which we must understand if we are to modulate them therapeutically to reverse abnormal remodeling and ensure the resumption and continuation of normal development.

PULMONARY HYPERTENSION IN RHEUMATIC HEART DISEASE

In developing countries, rheumatic heart disease is a common cause of pulmonary hypertension. In a study of 100 Indian patients with mitral stenosis, 42 were younger than 20 years of age.[141] In a 1991 study of 125 children up to 12 years of age, 75% had moderate to severe pulmonary venous and arterial hypertension, and critical mitral stenosis was present in 69% at operation.[142] In India, some children develop mitral stenosis very rapidly after having rheumatic fever and require a valvotomy by 6 years of age or younger. The pulmonary vascular abnormalities in children with rheumatic mitral stenosis are generally more severe than those in adults.[143] Regardless of age or onset of symptoms (5 years of age or younger), the capillaries and the small vessels proximal and distal to them are more severely diseased than are the larger vessels. The capillary endothelial basement membranes are thickened at the blood-gas barrier, a finding compatible with the well-documented reduction in diffusing capacity in adult patients. Intra-acinar and, to a lesser extent, preacinar and postacinar vessels have increased muscularity, severe circumferential intimal fibrosis, and abnormally thick and dense connective tissue. In a minority of patients, the lesions resemble those seen in pulmonary vascular obstructive disease associated with congenital heart disease. Pulmonary arterial pressure nonetheless falls after valvotomy, indicating the need for early relief of mitral valve obstruction. Persistent abnormalities of respiratory function in adults after a mitral valvotomy have frequently been attributed to chronic obstructive airway disease. However, children who contract rheumatic fever in early childhood and suffer multiple episodes of active carditis can develop pulmonary hypertension while the airways are still growing, and deposition of excessive connective tissue may impair airway growth.

REFERENCES

1. Wood P: The Eisenmenger syndrome or pulmonary hypertension with reversed central shunt. Br Med J 2:701, 755, 1958.
2. Wood P: Diseases of the Heart and Circulation, 3rd ed. London, Eyre & Spottiswoode, 1968, pp 976–977.
3. Rabinovitch M, Keane JF, Fellows KE, et al: Quantitative analysis of the pulmonary wedge angiogram in congenital heart defects. Correlation with hemodynamic data and morphometric findings in lung biopsy tissue. Circulation 63:152, 1981.
4. Bush A, Busst C, Booth K, et al: Does prostacyclin enhance the selective pulmonary vasodilator effect of oxygen in children with congenital heart disease? Circulation 74:135, 1986.
5. Winberg P, Lundell BP, Gustafsson LE: Effect of inhaled nitric oxide on raised pulmonary vascular resistance in children with congenital heart disease. Br Heart J 73:282, 1994.
6. Roberts JDJ, Lang P, Bigatello LM, et al: Inhaled nitric oxide in congenital heart disease. Circulation 87:447, 1993.
7. Celermajer DS, Cullen S, Deanfield JE: Impairment of endothelium-dependent pulmonary artery relaxation in children with congenital heart disease and abnormal pulmonary hemodynamics. Circulation 87:440, 1993.
8. Clabby ML, Canter CE, Moller JH, et al: Hemodynamic data and survival in children with pulmonary hypertension. J Am Coll Cardiol 30:554, 1997.
9. Hall SM, Haworth SG: Onset and evolution of pulmonary vascular disease in young children: Abnormal postnatal remodelling studied in lung biopsies. J Pathol 166:183, 1992.
10. Allen K, Haworth SG: Cytoskeletal features of immature pulmonary vascular smooth muscle cells and the influence of pulmonary hypertension on normal human development. J Pathol 158:311, 1989.
11. Rabinovitch M, Mecham B, Davidson J, et al: Elastase activity and the pathophysiology of pulmonary hypertension. Eur Respir Rev 3:591, 1993.
12. Haworth SG: Pulmonary vascular disease in different types of congenital heart disease. Implications for interpretation of lung biopsy findings in early childhood. Br Heart J 52:557, 1984.
13. Haworth SG, Radley-Smith R, Yacoub M: Lung biopsy findings in transposition of the great arteries with ventricular septal defect: Potentially reversible pulmonary vascular disease is not always synonymous with operability. J Am Coll Cardiol 9:327, 1987.
14. Haworth SG: Pulmonary vascular disease in ventricular septal defect: Structural and functional correlations in lung biopsies from 85 patients, with outcome of intra-cardiac repair. J Pathol 152:157, 1987.
15. Haworth SG, Hall SM: Occlusion of intra-acinar pulmonary arteries in pulmonary hypertensive congenital heart disease. Int J Cardiol 13:207, 1986.
16. Ku DD, Zaleski JK, Liu S, et al: Vascular endothelial growth factor induces EDRF-dependent relaxation in coronary arteries. Am J Physiol 265:H586, 1993.
17. Leung DW, Cachianes G, Kuang WJ, et al: Vascular endothelial growth factor stimulates collateral formation by inducing arterial cell proliferation in a rabbit ischemic hindlimb. Science 246:1306, 1989.
18. Jones PL, Cowan KN, Rabinovitch M: Tenascin-C, proliferation and subendothelial fibronectin in progressive pulmonary vascular disease. Am J Pathol 150:1349, 1997.
19. Heath D, Du Shane JW, Wood EH, et al: The structure of the pulmonary trunk at different ages and in cases of pulmonary hypertension and pulmonary stenosis. J Pathol Bacteriol 77:443, 1959.
20. Heath D, Edwards JE: The pathology of hypertensive pulmonary vascular disease. A description of six grades of structural changes in the pulmonary artery with special reference to congenital cardiac septal defect. Circulation 18:533, 1958.
21. Heath D, Helmholz F, Burchell HB, et al: Graded pulmonary vascular changes in cases of atrial and ventricular septal defect and patent ductus arteriosus. Circulation 18:1155, 1958.
22. Heath D, Helmholz HF, Burchell HB, et al: Relationship between structural changes in the small pulmonary arteries and the immediate reversibility of pulmonary hypertension following closure of ventricular and atrial septal defects. Circulation 18:1167, 1958.
23. Wagenvoort CA, Wagenvoort N: Pathology of Pulmonary Hypertension. New York, John Wiley & Sons, 1977, pp 121–125.
24. Rabinovitch M, Haworth SG, Castaneda AR, et al: Lung biopsy in congenital heart disease: A morphometric approach to pulmonary vascular disease. Circulation 58:1107, 1978.
25. Haworth SG, Sauer U, Buhlmeyer K, et al: Development of the pulmonary circulation in ventricular septal defect: A quantitative structural study. Am J Cardiol 40:781, 1977.
26. Leanage R, Agnetti A, Graham G, et al: Factors influencing survival after balloon atrial septostomy for complete transposition of the great arteries. Br Heart J 45:559, 1981.

27. Ferencz C: Transposition of the great vessels. Pathophysiologic considerations based upon a study of the lungs. Circulation 33:232, 1966.

28. Newfeld EA, Paul MH, Muster AJ, et al: Pulmonary vascular disease in complete transposition of the great arteries. A study of 200 patients. Am J Cardiol 34:75, 1974.

29. Haworth S: Pulmonary vascular bed in children with complete atrioventricular septal defect: Relation between structural and haemodynamic abnormalities. Am J Cardiol 57:833, 1986.

30. Newfeld EA, Sher M, Paul MH, et al: Pulmonary vascular disease in complete atrioventricular canal defect. Am J Cardiol 39:721, 1977.

31. Haworth SG: Pulmonary vascular disease in secundum atrial septal defect in childhood. Am J Cardiol 51:265, 1983.

32. Haworth SG: Total anomalous pulmonary venous return. Prenatal damage to pulmonary vascular bed and extrapulmonary veins. Br Heart J 48:513, 1982.

33. Neill CA, Ferencz C, Sabiston DC, et al: The familial occurrence of hypoplastic right lung with systemic arterial supply and venous drainage "scimitar syndrome." Johns Hopkins Med J 107:1, 1960.

34. Haworth SG, Sauer U, Buhlmeyer K: Pulmonary hypertension in scimitar syndrome in infancy. Br Heart J 50:182, 1983.

35. Najm HK, Williams WG, Coles JG, et al: Scimitar syndrome: Twenty years' experience and results of repair. J Thorac Cardiovasc Surg 112:1168, 1996.

36. Fontan F, Baudet E: Surgical repair of tricuspid atresia. Thorax 26:240, 1971.

37. Gale AW, Danielson GK, McGoon DC, et al: Modified Fontan operation for univentricular heart and complicated congenital lesions. J Thorac Cardiovasc Surg 78:831, 1979.

38. Seghaye MC, Serraf A, Planche C: Endogenous nitric oxide production and atrial natriuretic peptide biological activity in infants undergoing cardiac operations. Crit Care Med 25:1063, 1997.

39. Adatia I, Barrow SE, Stratton PD, et al: Thromboxane A2 and prostacyclin biosynthesis in children and adolescents with pulmonary vascular disease. Circulation 88:2117, 1993.

40. Komai H, Adatia IT, Elliott MJ, et al: Increased plasma levels of endothelin-1 after cardiopulmonary bypass in patients with pulmonary hypertension and congenital heart disease. J Thorac Cardiovasc Surg 106:473, 1993.

41. Adatia I, Haworth SG: Circulating endothelin in children with congenital heart disease. Br Heart J 69:233, 1993.

42. Reves JG, Karp RB, Buttner EE, et al: Neuronal and adrenomedullary catecholamine release in response to cardiopulmonary bypass in man. Circulation 66:49, 1982.

43. Adatia I, Barrow SE, Stratton PD, et al: Effect of intracardiac repair on thromboxane A2 and prostacyclin biosynthesis in children with a left to right shunt. Br Heart J 72:452, 1994.

44. Angdin M, Settergren G: Acetylcholine reactivity in the pulmonary artery during cardiac surgery in patients with ischemic or valvular heart disease. J Cardiothorac Vasc Anesth 11:458, 1997.

45. Hiramatsu T, Imai Y, Takanashi Y, et al: Time course of endothelin-1 and nitrate anion levels after cardiopulmonary bypass in congenital heart defects. Ann Thorac Surg 63:648, 1997.

46. Kirshbom PM, Jacobs MT, Tsui SSL, et al: Effects of cardiopulmonary bypass and circulatory arrest on endothelium-dependent vasodilatation in the lung. J Thorac Cardiovasc Surg 111:1248, 1996.

47. Morita K, Ihnken K, Buckberg GD, et al: Pulmonary vasoconstriction due to impaired nitric oxide production after cardiopulmonary bypass. Ann Thorac Surg 61:1775, 1996.

48. Schreiber MD, Heymann MA, Soifer SJ: Increased arterial pH, not decreased PaCO2, attenuates hypoxia-induced pulmonary vasoconstriction in newborn lambs. Pediatr Res 20:113, 1986.

49. Dworetz AR, Moya FR, Sabo B, et al: Survival of infants with persistent pulmonary hypertension without extracorporeal membrane oxygenation. Pediatrics 84:1, 1989.

50. Beghetti M, Habre W, Friedli B, et al: Continuous low dose inhaled nitric oxide for treatment of severe pulmonary hypertension after cardiac surgery in paediatric patients. Br Heart J 73:65, 1995.

51. Betit P, Adatia I, Benjamin P, et al: Inhaled nitric oxide: Evaluation of a continuous titration delivery technique for infant mechanical and manual ventilation. Respir Care 40:706, 1995.

52. Goldman AP, Haworth SG, Macrae DJ: Does inhaled nitric oxide suppress endogenous nitric oxide production? Cardiovasc Thorac Surg 112:541, 1996.

53. Fullerton DA, Jaggers J, Piedalue F, et al: Effective control of refractory pulmonary hypertension after cardiac operations. J Thorac Cardiovasc Surg 113:368, 1997.

54. Atz AM, Adatia I, Wessel DL: Rebound pulmonary hypertension after inhalation of nitric oxide. Ann Thorac Surg 62:1759, 1996.

55. Dotsch J, Demirakca S, Hamm R, et al: Extracorporeal circulation increases nitric oxide–induced methemoglobinemia in vivo and in vitro. Crit Care Med 25:1153, 1997.

56. Haraldsson A, Kieler-Jensen N, Ricksten SE: Inhaled prostacyclin for treatment of pulmonary hypertension after cardiac surgery or heart transplantation: A pharmacodynamic study. J Cardiothorac Vasc Anesth 10:864, 1997.

57. Hislop A, Wigglesworth JS, Desai R: Alveolar development in the human fetus and infant. Early Hum Dev 13:1, 1986.

58. Rabinovitch M, Keane JF, Norwood WI, et al: Vascular structure in lung tissue obtained at biopsy correlated with pulmonary hemodynamic findings after repair of congenital heart defects. Circulation 69:655, 1984.

59. Friedli B, Kidd BSL, Mustard WT, et al: Ventricular septal defect with increased pulmonary vascular resistance. Late results of surgical closure. Am J Cardiol 33:403, 1974.

60. Bowyer JJ, Busst CM, Denison DM, et al: Effect of long term oxygen treatment at home in children with pulmonary vascular disease. Br Heart J 55:385, 1986.

61. Wessel DL, Adatia I, Thompson JE, et al: Delivery and monitoring of inhaled nitric oxide in patients with pulmonary hypertension. Crit Care Med 22:930, 1994.

62. Riley MS, Porszasz J, Miranda J, et al: Exhaled nitric oxide during exercise in primary pulmonary hypertension and pulmonary fibrosis. Chest 111:44, 1997.

63. Adatia I, Perry S, Landzberg M, et al: Inhaled nitric oxide and hemodynamic evaluation of patients with pulmonary hypertension before transplantation. J Am Coll Cardiol 25:1656, 1995.

64. Hayward CS, Rogers P, Keogh AM, et al: Inhaled nitric oxide in cardiac failure: Vascular versus ventricular effects. J Cardiovasc Pharmacol 27:80, 1996.

65. Hopkins WE, Ochoa LL, Richardson GW, et al: Comparison of the hemodynamics and survival of adults with severe primary pulmonary hypertension or Eisenmenger syndrome. J Heart Lung Transplant 15:100, 1996.

66. Kerstein D, Levy PS, Hsu DT, et al: Blade balloon atrial septostomy in patients with severe primary pulmonary hypertension. Circulation 91:2028, 1995.

67. Barst RJ, Long W, Gersony W: Long-term vasodilator treatment improves survival in children with primary pulmonary hypertension. Cardiol Young 3:89, 1993.

68. The International Primary Pulmonary Hypertension Study Group: The international primary pulmonary hypertension study (IPPHS). Chest 105:37S, 1994.

69. Barst RJ: Primary pulmonary hypertension in children. *In* Rubin LJ, Rich S (eds): Primary Pulmonary Hypertension. New York, Marcel Dekker, 1997, pp 179–225.

70. Rich S, Dantzker DR, Ayres SM: Primary pulmonary hypertension: A national prospective study. Ann Intern Med 107:216, 1987.

71. Langleben D: Familial primary pulmonary hypertension. Chest 105:13S, 1994.

72. Lloyd JE, Primm RK, Newman JH: Familial primary pulmonary hypertension: Clinical patterns. Am Rev Respir Dis 129:194, 1984.

73. Lloyd JE, Butler MG, Foroud TM, et al: Genetic anticipation and abnormal gender ratio at birth in familial primary pulmonary hypertension. Am J Respir Crit Care Med 152:93, 1995.

74. Nichols WC, Koller DL, Slovis B, et al: Localization of the gene for familial primary pulmonary hypertension to chromosome 2q31–32. Nat Genet 15:277, 1997.

75. Subramanian N, Bakthaviziam A, Sukamar IP, et al: Primary pulmonary hypertension. A clinicopathological study of 11 cases. Indian Heart J 26:171, 1974.

76. Gurtner HP: Aminorex and pulmonary hypertension. Cor Vasa 27:160, 1985.

77. Polos PG, Wolfe D, Harley RA: Pulmonary hypertension and human immuno-deficiency virus infection: Two reports and a review of the literature. Chest 101:474, 1992.

78. Asherson RA, Higenbottam TW, Dinh Xuan AT, et al: Pulmonary hypertension in a lupus clinic: Experience with twenty-four patients. J Rheumatol 17:1292, 1990.

79. Weir EK, Reeve HL, Huang JM, et al: Anorexic agents aminorex, fenfluramine, and dexfenfluramine inhibit potassium current in rat pulmonary vascular smooth muscle and cause pulmonary vasoconstriction. Circulation 94:2216, 1996.

80. Winters W, Joseph R, Learner N: Primary pulmonary hypertension and Raynaud's phenomenon. Arch Intern Med 114:821, 1964.

81. Morse JH, Barst RJ, Fotino M: Familial pulmonary hypertension: Immunogenetic findings in four Caucasian kindreds. Am Rev Resp Dis 145:787, 1992.

82. Barst RJ, Flaster ER, Menon A, et al: Evidence for the association of unexplained pulmonary hypertension in children with the major histocompatibility complex. Circulation 85:249, 1992.

83. Stewart DJ, Levy RD, Cernacek P, et al: Increased plasma endothelin-1 in pulmonary hypertension: Marker or mediator of disease? Ann Intern Med 114:464, 1991.

84. Christman BW, McPherson CD, Newman JH: Thromboxane receptor blockade prevents pulmonary hypertension induced by heparin-protamine reactions in awake sheep. N Engl J Med 327:70, 1991.

85. Eisenberg PR, Lucore C, Kaufmann E: Fibrinopeptide A levels indicative of pulmonary vascular thrombosis in patients with primary pulmonary hypertension. Circulation 82:841, 1990.

86. Fuster V, Steele PM, Edwards WD, et al: Primary pulmonary hypertension: Natural history and the importance of thrombosis. Circulation 70:580, 1984.

87. Mikkilineni S, Barst RJ, Cropp GJ: Pulmonary function in primary pulmonary hypertension. Pediatr Res 27:359A, 1990.

88. Rhodes J, Barst RJ, Garofano RP, et al: Hemodynamic correlates of exercise function in patients with primary pulmonary hypertension. J Am Coll Cardiol 18:1738, 1991.

89. D'Angelo A, Della Valle P, Crippa L, et al: Autoimmune protein S deficiency in a boy with severe thromboembolic disease. N Engl J Med 328:1753, 1993.

90. Barst RJ: Treatment of primary pulmonary hypertension with continuous intravenous prostacyclin. Heart 77:299, 1997.

91. McLaughlin VV, Genthner DE, Panella MM, et al: Reduction in pulmonary vascular resistance with long-term epoprostenol (prostacyclin) therapy in primary pulmonary hypertension. N Engl J Med 338:273, 1998.

92. Barst RJ, Rubin LJ, Long WA, et al: A comparison of continuous intravenous epoprostenol (prostacyclin) with conventional treatment for primary pulmonary hypertension. N Engl J Med 334:296, 1996.

93. Barst RJ: Pharmacologically induced pulmonary vasodilatation in children and young adults with primary pulmonary hypertension. Chest 98:497, 1986.

94. Barst RJ, Rubin LJ, McGoon MD, et al: Survival in primary pulmonary hypertension with long-term continuous intravenous prostacyclin. Ann Intern Med 121:409, 1994.

95. Harvey W: Exercitatio anatomica de motu cordis et sanguinis in animalibus. Francofurti: Fitzeri. 1628.

96. Novelo S, Limon-Lason R, Bouchard F: Un nouveau syndrome avec cyanose congenitale: La persistence du canal arterial avec hypertension pulmonaire. (Abstract) Paris Premier Congres Mondial de Cardiologie (1950), 1995.

97. Lind J, Wegelius E: Changes in the circulation at birth. Acta Pediatr 42:495, 1952.

98. Rowe RD: Clinical observation of transitional circulations. *In* Oliver TK (ed): Adaptation to Extrauterine Life. Report of Thirty-First Ross Conference on Paediatric Research. Columbus, OH, Ross Laboratories, 1959, p 339.

99. Allen KM, Wharton J, Polak JM, et al: A study of nerves containing peptides in the pulmonary vasculature of healthy infants and children and of those with pulmonary hypertension. Br Heart J 62:353, 1989.

100. Haworth SG, Reid L: Persistent fetal circulation: Newly recognised structural features. J Pediatr 88:614, 1976.

101. Goldman AP, Tasker RC, Haworth SG, et al: Four patterns of response to inhaled nitric oxide for primary pulmonary hypertension of the newborn. Pediatrics 98:706, 1996.

102. Liu SF, Hislop AA, Haworth SG, et al: Developmental changes in endothelium-dependent pulmonary vasodilatation in pigs. Br J Pharmacol 106:324, 1992.

103. Abman SH, Chatfield BA, Hall SL, et al: Role of endothelium-derived relaxing factor during transition of pulmonary circulation at birth. Am J Physiol 259:H1921, 1990.

104. Cassin S: Role of prostaglandins, thromboxanes and leukotrienes in the control of the pulmonary circulation in the fetus and newborn. Semin Perinatol 11:53, 1987.

105. Dawes GS: Fetal and Neonatal Physiology. St. Louis, Mosby–Year Book, 1968, p 167.

106. Kaapa P, Seppanen M, Kero P, et al: Pulmonary haemodynamics after synthetic surfactant replacement in neonatal RDS. J Pediatr 123:115, 1993.

107. Soifer SJ, Loitz RD, Roman C, et al: Leukotriene end organ antagonists increase pulmonary blood flow in fetal lambs. Am J Physiol 249:H570, 1985.

108. Cooper CJ, Landzberg MJ, Anderson TJ, et al: Role of nitric oxide in the local regulation of pulmonary vascular resistance in humans. Circulation 93:266, 1996.

109. Orton E, LaRue S, Ensley B, et al: Bromodeoxyuridine labelling and DNA content of pulmonary arterial medial cells from normal and hypoxia exposed calves. Am J Vet Res 53:1925, 1992.

110. Meyrick B, Reid L: Normal postnatal development of the media of the rat hilar pulmonary artery and its remodelling by chronic hypoxia. Lab Invest 46:505, 1982.

111. Mecham R, Stenmark K, Parks W: Role of the vascular smooth muscle in connective tissue production during development and disease. Chest 99:43S, 1991.

112. Mecham R, Whitehouse L, Wrenn D, et al: Smooth muscle mediated connective tissue remodeling in pulmonary hypertension. Science 237:423, 1987.

113. Crouch E, Parks W, Rosenbaum J, et al: Regulation of collagen production by medial smooth muscle cells in hypoxic pulmonary hypertension. Am Rev Respir Dis 140:1045, 1989.

114. Jones R, Adler C, Farber F: Lung vascular cell proliferation in hyperoxic pulmonary hypertension and on return to air: [³H]Thymidine pulse-labeling of intimal, medial, and adventitial cells in microvessels and at the hilum. Am Rev Respir Dis 140:1471, 1989.

115. Meyrick B, Reid L: Hypoxia and incorporation of [³H]-thymidine by cells of the rat pulmonary arteries and alveolar wall. Am J Pathol 96:51, 1979.

116. Coflesky J, Adler K, Woodcock-Mitchell J, et al: Proliferative changes in the pulmonary arterial wall during short-term hyperoxic injury to the lung. Am J Pathol 132:563, 1988.

117. Zhu L, Wigle D, Hinek A, et al: The endogenous vascular elastase that governs development and progression of monocrotaline-induced pulmonary hypertension in rats is a novel enzyme related to the serine proteinase adipsin. J Clin Invest 94:1163, 1994.

118. Todorovich-Hunter L, Dodo H, Ye C, et al: Increased pulmonary artery elastolytic activity in adult rats with monocrotaline-induced progressive hypertensive pulmonary vascular disease compared with infant rats with nonprogressive disease. Am Rev Respir Dis 146:213, 1992.

119. Maruyama K, Ye C, Woo M, et al: Chronic hypoxic pulmonary hypertension in rats and increased elastolytic activity. Am J Physiol 261:H1716, 1991.

120. Ikiw R, Todorovich-Hunter L, Maruyama K, et al: SC-39026, a serine elastase inhibitor, prevents muscularization of peripheral arteries, suggesting a mechanism of monocrotaline-induced pulmonary hypertension in rats. Circ Res 64:814, 1989.

121. Botney MD, Parks WC, Crouch EC, et al: Transforming growth factor-B1 is decreased in remodeling hypertensive bovine pulmonary arteries. J Clin Invest 89:1629, 1992.

122. Perkett E, Badesch D, Roessler M, et al: Insulinlike growth factor-1 and pulmonary hypertension induced by continuous air embolization in sheep. Am J Respir Cell Mol Biol 6:82, 1992.

123. Rosenberg AA, Kennaugh J, Koppenhafer SL, et al: Elevated immunoreactive endothelin-1 levels in newborn infants with persistent pulmonary hypertension. J Pediatr 123:109, 1993.

124. Noguchi Y, Hislop AA, Haworth SG: Influence of hypoxia on endothelin-1 binding sites in neonatal porcine pulmonary vasculature. Am J Physiol 272:H669, 1997.

125. Kourembanas S, Marsden P, McQuillan L, et al: Hypoxia induces endothelin gene expression and secretion in cultured human endothelium. J Clin Invest 88:1054, 1991.

126. Badesch D, Orton E, Zapp L, et al: Decreased arterial wall prostaglandin production in neonatal calves with severe chronic pulmonary hypertension. Am J Respir Cell Mol Biol 1:489, 1989.

127. Fukuroda T, Fujikawa T, Ozaki S, et al: Clearance of circulating endothelin-1 by ETB receptors in rats. Biochem Biophys Res Commun 199:1461, 1994.

128. Soifer SJ, Kaslow D, Roman C, et al: Umbilical cord compression produces pulmonary hypertension in newborn lambs: A model to study the pathophysiology of persistent pulmonary hypertension of the newborn. J Dev Physiol 9:239, 1997.

129. Morin FC: Ligating the ductus arteriosus before birth causes persistent pulmonary hypertension in the newborn lamb. Pediatr Res 25:245, 1989.

130. Shaul PW, Yuhanna IS, German Z: Pulmonary endothelial NO synthase gene expression is decreased in fetal lambs with pulmonary hypertension. Am J Physiol 272:L1005, 1997.

131. Ivy DD, Ziegler JW, Dubus MF: Chronic intrauterine pulmonary hypertension alters endothelin receptor activity in the ovine fetal lung. Pediatr Res 39:435, 1996.

132. Tulloh RMR, Hislop AA, Boels PJ, et al: Chronic hypoxia inhibits postnatal maturation of porcine intrapulmonary artery relaxation. Am J Physiol 272:H2436, 1997.

133. Hislop AA, Springall DR, Oliveira H, et al: Endothelial nitric oxide synthase in hypoxic newborn porcine pulmonary vessels. Arch Dis Child 76:F16, 1997.

134. Rapoport RM, Schwartz K, Murad F: Effects of Na+, K+-pump inhibitors and membrane depolarizing agents on acetylcholine-induced endothelium-dependent relaxation and cyclic GMP accumulation in rat aorta. Eur J Pharmacol 110:203, 1985.

135. Weir EK, Reeve HL, Cornfield DN, et al: Diversity of response in vascular smooth muscle cells to changes in oxygen tension. Kidney Int 51:462, 1997.

136. Reddy VM, Meyrick B, Wong J: In utero placement of aortopulmonary shunts: A model of postnatal pulmonary hypertension with increased pulmonary blood flow in lambs. Circulation 92:606, 1995.

137. Reddy VM, Wong J, Liddicoat JR: Altered endothelium-dependent vasoactive responses in lambs with pulmonary hypertension and increased pulmonary blood flow. Am J Physiol 271:H562, 1996.

138. Wong J, Reddy VM, Hendricks K: Altered endothelin-1 vasoactive responses in lambs with pulmonary hypertension and increased pulmonary blood flow. Am J Physiol 269:H1965, 1995.

139. Post JM, Hume JR, Archer SL, et al: Direct role for potassium channel inhibition in hypoxic pulmonary vasoconstriction. Am J Physiol 262:C882, 1992.

140. Oparil S, Chen SJ, Meng QC, et al: Endothelin-A receptor antagonist prevents acute hypoxia-induced pulmonary hypertension in the rat. Am J Physiol 268:L95, 1995.

141. Tandon HD, Kasturi J: Pulmonary vascular changes associated with isolated mitral stenosis in India. Br Heart J 37:26, 1975.

142. Shrivastava S, Tandon R: Severity of rheumatic mitral stenosis in children. Int J Cardiol 30:163, 1991.

143. Haworth SG, Hall SM, Patel M: Peripheral pulmonary vascular and airway abnormalities in adolescents with rheumatic mitral stenosis. Int J Cardiol 18:405, 1988.

CHAPTER 47
KAWASAKI DISEASE

HIROHISA KATO

Kawasaki disease (KD), or mucocutaneous lymph node syndrome, occurs in infants and children as an acute systemic vasculitis syndrome of unknown etiology; it mainly affects small and medium-sized arteries, particularly the coronary arteries.[1] The cardiovascular problems in KD are related to coronary arterial lesions: aneurysmal formation, thrombotic occlusion, progression to coronary artery disease, and premature atherosclerosis.[2] This disease was first described by Dr. Tomisaku Kawasaki in Japan.[3,4] Subsequently, it has been recognized not only in Japan but throughout the world, and it is now a leading cause of acquired heart disease in children in North America and Japan.

EPIDEMIOLOGY

The epidemiology in Japan, where KD is most prevalent, has been well documented[5] and may be summarized as follows. The incidence has increased since 1968, and the number of patients affected now totals more than 110,000. KD affects more than 5000 children each year in Japan, and the incidence is 70 to 90 per 100,000 children younger than 4 years. The age distribution is from 1 month with a peak at 1 year; 50% of patients are younger than 2 years, and occurrence after 10 years of age is rare. Boys are affected more often than are girls, with a ratio of 1.5.

KD is now widely prevalent in Asia, North America, South America, Europe, and Australia. Asians are more susceptible (5 to 10 times) than are whites.[6] There is a wide distribution with no geographic difference between urban and rural areas or south and north. Seasonal variation is not distinct, but there are small peaks in winter-spring. The recurrence rate is about 3.3%, and 1 to 2% of siblings are affected. Time-space clustering and outbreaks in a community are recognized, but there is no evidence of person-to-person transmission. In 1979, 1982, and 1986, there were large outbreaks in Japan, but there have been none since 1991.

ETIOLOGY AND PATHOGENESIS

The etiology of KD remains unknown despite extensive investigation. On the basis of clinical features and epidemiologic data, KD is now considered to be either of infectious origin with an unknown agent or an infection-triggered immune disorder. A variety of possible causative agents, such as bacteria, fungi, mycoplasma, rickettsiae, and viruses, have been proposed.

KD has clinical similarities to scarlet fever and toxic shock syndrome, both caused by toxin-producing bacteria. These toxins are superantigens capable of stimulating T cells carrying particular variable regions of the T cell receptor β chain. A study on peripheral blood T cells in KD has shown that T cells expressing T cell receptor variable regions Vβ2 and Vβ8 were selectively expanded.[7] These observations suggest that KD may be caused by a toxin (superantigen)-producing microorganism, including viruses. On the basis of these observations, Leung and coworkers[8] suggested that the expansion of Vβ2$^+$ T cells in most patients with KD may be caused by a new clone of toxic shock syndrome toxin–secreting *Staphylococcus aureus* found on bacterial cultures from patients with KD. Other studies do not support this theory.[9,10]

Yersinia pseudotuberculosis appears to be an etiologic agent of KD,[11] although only a small group of KD patients can be attributed to this organism. Interestingly, a product with superantigen properties has been identified from *Y. pseudotuberculosis.*[12] *Streptococcus sanguis* has been associated with KD. This bacterial strain produces glucan, a potent stimulator of the immune system, although only under specific conditions.[13] *Propionibacterium acnes* isolated from the cervical lymph node of KD patients has produced a cytotoxic protein like the bacterial exotoxin,[14,15] but its etiologic role remains to be determined.

Epstein-Barr virus (EBV) can rarely induce a clinical picture mimicking KD.[16] Three of 37 patients with chronic active EBV infection developed coronary lesions similar to those in KD. Epidemiologic, serologic, and virologic studies, however, do not support EBV as a causative agent of KD. Retroviruses received transient attention because of reverse transcriptase activity in cultured peripheral blood mononuclear cells from KD patients.[17] These findings have not been confirmed.

The acute phase of KD is associated with increased production of tumor necrosis factor α (TNFα), interleukin (IL)-1β, interferon α (IFN-α), and IL-6. TNFα, IL-1β, and IFN-α induce activation antigens and adhesion molecules, such as endothelial leukocyte adhesion molecule 1 and intercellular adhesion molecule 1, on endothelial cells, and TNFα and IFN-α cause endothelial injury in in vitro studies.[18] Leung and associates[19] have proposed a hypothesis that antiendothelial antibodies cause endothelial injury in KD, based on the findings that circulating autoantibodies in KD are cytotoxic against human umbilical vein endothelial cells treated with TNFα, IL-1β, or IFN-α. Coronary artery endothelial cells in KD actually expressed activation antigens in a necropsy study.[20]

Many hypotheses on the etiology and pathogenesis of KD have been proposed, but a host-microbial relationship specific to KD has not been identified. KD is widely scattered in the community, is self-limited, has multiorgan involvement, can recur, and has a tendency for epidemics every 3 to 4 years. These findings suggest that this disease may be caused in some susceptible children by a common infectious agent.

PATHOLOGY

On the basis of Hamashima's analyses of 37 KD autopsies, the Japanese Kawasaki Disease Research Committee reported the following pathomorphologic findings.[21, 22] KD is an acute inflammatory disease with systemic angiitis distinguishable from classic periarteritis nodosa of the Kussmaul-Maier type, a progressive and recurrent angiitis with marked fibrinoid necrosis but with rare pulmonary vasculitis. In contrast, KD is an acute inflammatory disease lasting about 7 weeks with rare and mild fibrinoid necrosis. Infantile polyarteritis nodosa resembles KD in many pathologic aspects,[23] but further studies are needed to identify the distinctive features. Coronary aneurysm is usually present at autopsy in infantile polyarteritis nodosa.

The course of angiitis can be classified into four stages according to the duration of illness:

- Stage 1 (1 to 2 weeks of illness): Perivasculitis and vasculitis of the microvessels (arterioles, capillaries, and venules), small arteries, and veins. Inflammation of intima, externa, and perivascular areas in the medium-sized and large arteries. Edema and inflammation with leukocytes and lymphocytes.
- Stage 2 (2 to 4 weeks of illness): Less inflammation in the microvessels, small arteries, and veins than in stage 1. Inflammatory changes of intima, media, externa, and perivascular areas in the medium-sized arteries with focal panvasculitis. Aneurysms with thrombi and stenosis in the medium-sized arteries, especially in the coronary arteries. Panvasculitis is rarely seen in the large arteries. Edema (exudative stage), infiltration with monocytes or necrosis (infiltrative stage), and cellular granulation with increase of capillaries.
- Stage 3 (4 to 7 weeks of illness): Subsidence of inflammation in the microvessels, small arteries, and veins. Granulation in the medium-sized arteries.
- Stage 4 (more than 7 weeks of illness): Scar formation and intimal thickening with aneurysm, thrombi, and stenosis in the medium-sized arteries (generally no acute inflammation in the vessels). These findings may persist until adult age and were observed in some autopsied patients who died more than 10 years after the illness.

Myocarditis (interstitial myocarditis with mild necrosis) involving the conduction system, pericarditis, endocarditis, cholecystitis, cholangitis, pancreatic ductitis, sialadenitis, meningitis, and lymphadenitis are frequently seen during the illness.

CLINICAL MANIFESTATIONS AND DIAGNOSIS OF KAWASAKI DISEASE

The diagnosis of KD is made according to the diagnostic guidelines prepared by the Research Committee (Table 47–1) because of the absence of a specific laboratory test.

The principal diagnostic criteria of KD are persistent fever, conjunctival injection, inflamed oropharyngeal mucosa, changes in the peripheral extremities, erythematous rash, and cervical lymphadenopathy. At least five items of six principal diagnostic criteria should be satisfied to establish a diagnosis of KD. Patients with four of the diagnostic criteria can be diagnosed with KD when coronary aneurysms are recognized by two-dimensional echocardiography or coronary angiography. Patients in early infancy

---

TABLE 47–1

DIAGNOSTIC GUIDELINES FOR KAWASAKI DISEASE

PRINCIPAL SYMPTOMS
1. Fever persisting for at least 5 days
2. Changes in peripheral extremities
   Initial stage: reddening of palms and soles, indurative edema
   Convalescent stage: membranous desquamation from fingertips
3. Polymorphous exanthema
4. Bilateral conjunctival congestion
5. Changes in lips and oral cavity: reddening of lips, strawberry tongue, diffuse injection of oral and pharyngeal mucosa
6. Acute nonpurulent cervical lymphadenopathy

At least five principal symptoms should be satisfied for the diagnosis of Kawasaki disease to be made. However, patients with four of the principal symptoms can be diagnosed as having Kawasaki disease when coronary aneurysm is recognized by two-dimensional echocardiography or coronary angiography.

OTHER SIGNIFICANT SYMPTOMS OR FINDINGS
The following symptoms and findings should be clinically considered:
1. Cardiovascular auscultation (heart murmur, gallop rhythm, distant heart sounds), electrocardiographic changes (prolonged PR-QT intervals, abnormal Q wave, low-voltage ST-T changes, arrhythmias), chest radiograph findings (cardiomegaly), two-dimensional echocardiographic findings (pericardial effusion, coronary aneurysms), aneurysm of peripheral arteries other than coronary (e.g., axillary), angina pectoris or myocardial infarction
2. Gastrointestinal tract: diarrhea, vomiting, abdominal pain, hydrops of gallbladder, paralytic ileus, mild jaundice, slight increase of serum transaminase
3. Blood: leukocytosis with shift to the left, thrombocytosis, increased erythrocyte sedimentation rates, positive C-reactive protein, hypoalbuminemia, increased α_2-globulin, slight decrease in erythrocyte and hemoglobin levels
4. Urine: proteinuria, increase of leukocytes in urine sediment
5. Skin: redness and crust at the site of bacille Calmette-Guérin inoculation, small pustules, transverse furrows of the fingernails
6. Respiratory: cough, rhinorrhea, abnormal shadow on chest radiograph
7. Joint: pain, swelling
8. Neurologic: pleocytosis of mononuclear cells in cerebrospinal fluid, convulsion, unconsciousness, facial palsy, paralysis of the extremities

REMARKS
1. For changes in peripheral extremities, the convalescent stage is considered important.
2. Male-to-female ratio: 1.3–1.5 : 1; patients younger than 5 years of age: 80–85%; fatality rate: 0.3–0.5%
3. Recurrence rate: 2–3%; proportion of siblings: 1–2%

Prepared by the Japan Kawasaki Disease Research Committee: Diagnostic Guidelines of Kawasaki Disease, 4th rev. ed. Tokyo, 1984.

DIAGNOSTIC CRITERIA

Fever lasting >5 days, >40°C, refractory to antipyretics

Within first 3 days:
Engorged bulbar conjunctival vessels
Acute, nonpurulent cervical adenopathy; one node >1.5 cm, painful
Oropharyngeal erythema, dry cracked lips, strawberry tongue

After 3 days:
Polymorphous erythematous maculopapular rash, starting with red palms and soles and moving to the trunk
Red, swollen, indurated hands and feet; after 2 to 3 weeks, desquamation of hands and feet

---

(younger than 6 months) or older children (older than 6 years) often demonstrate atypical symptoms.[24]

Every 2 years, national surveys of KD are conducted in Japan. Data are collected in (1) definite cases of KD, (2) atypical cases, and (3) probable cases. Definite KD, defined before, represents 85% of the total number. Atypical cases, defined as four of the six principal diagnostic criteria and coronary aneurysms on two-dimensional echocardiography, occur in 3.5%. Atypical cases occur more commonly at an age younger than 6 months or older than 5 years and may develop severe coronary artery lesions. Probable cases, defined as four principal diagnostic criteria, but diagnosed as KD after exclusion of other disease and coronary aneurysms, occur in 11.5%. Their prognosis is good.

The principal and initial symptom is high fever. This finding, which is key to the diagnosis, usually ranges from 38 to 41°C and lasts at least 5 days and as long as 3 to 4 weeks. The fever is usually remittent, with a pattern that is not spiking like that in juvenile rheumatoid arthritis. Antibiotics and antipyretics have little apparent effect in reducing the fever. A high dose of immune globulin, however, has an antipyretic effect.

Bilateral congestion of ocular conjunctivae appears within 2 to 3 days after the onset of fever and consists chiefly of discrete engorgement of the bulbar conjunctival vessels. There is neither conjunctival discharge nor corneal ulceration.

Oral changes consisting of dryness, redness, fissuring of lips, strawberry tongue, and diffuse redness of oral and pharyngeal mucosa appear within 2 or 3 days of illness. These findings usually disappear within a week, but redness of the lips sometimes lasts 3 or 4 weeks.

Lymphadenopathy is prominent at or just after the onset of fever, with nodes more than 1.5 cm in diameter and usually unilateral and single. The enlarged lymph nodes are usually nonerythematous and nonpurulent but painful. At the initial stage of the disease, some patients are misdiagnosed with mumps because of the pain. The axillary and inguinal lymph nodes are usually not enlarged.

An erythematous rash, seen in almost all patients, appears on the third to fifth day of illness. It usually starts on the extremities with pronounced reddening of the palms and soles and spreads over the trunk within a couple of days. Characteristically, the rash is a nonspecific, polymorphous maculopapular erythema in many patients; but in some, a diffuse scarlatiniform or erythema multiforme rash is evident. The rash usually has no vesicles or crusts. In a small number of patients, especially infants, the erythematous rash is associated with small vesicles that contain neutrophils and lymphocytes, but bacterial organisms have never been cultured. Intense erythema and desquamation of the skin of the scrotum and perineum are common.

Changes in the hands and feet are characteristic and appear in about 80% of the patients. Three or 4 days after the onset of fever, the hands and feet become diffusely indurative, swollen, and firm. At the same time, the palms and soles become diffusely erythematous or deep purplish red. In some patients, the erythematous changes appear without the indurative edema. Two or 3 weeks after the onset of the disease, when erythema and indurative edema have disappeared and the patient is no longer febrile, a characteristic skin desquamation appears; it begins at the junction of the tip of the nail and digit. This is one of the most important features of KD. Desquamation of the toes is usually delayed, compared with that of the fingers. Desquamation never appears on arms, legs, or trunk. Other significant symptoms and laboratory findings are indicated in Table 47–1.

DIFFERENTIAL DIAGNOSIS

- Infections due to streptococci (scarlet fever), staphylococci (toxic shock syndrome), *Haemophilus*, mononucleosis, enteroviruses, measles, arboviruses
- Drug allergies, hypersensitivity reactions (erythema multiforme, Stevens-Johnson syndrome)
- Acute flare-up of other forms of vasculitis (e.g., systemic lupus erythematosus, polyarteritis nodosa)

CARDIOVASCULAR SPECTRUM AND CARDIAC EVALUATION

The evaluation of the coronary arterial lesions in KD during the acute stage of illness is important. This is usually done by two-dimensional echocardiography and coronary angiography. Serial two-dimensional echocardiography is the most useful and essential method to evaluate coronary aneurysms.[25] If a patient reveals abnormal findings in the serial studies, coronary angiography is indicated.[26]

The evaluation of coronary arterial morphology is particularly important in KD. In our experience using two-dimensional echocardiography, it is possible to correctly diagnose left main coronary artery aneurysms with 98% sensitivity and 95% specificity compared with angiography. The echocardiographic evaluation for right coronary artery lesions is less sensitive. False-negative diagnoses were mainly due to isolated small peripheral coronary artery aneurysms, which occurred rarely. On two-dimensional echocardiography, coronary artery dilatation appears at approximately 10 days of illness, and about 40% of patients reveal coronary artery dilatation at this time (Fig. 47–1). Two thirds of these, however, demonstrate only a transient

2-D (two-dimensional)
echocardiography

Selective coronary
angiography (CAG)

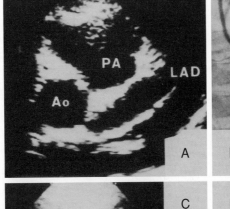

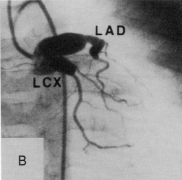

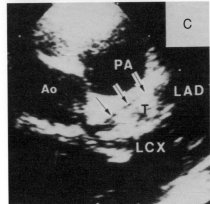

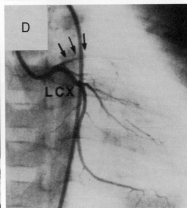

FIGURE 47–1

Serial echocardiography and coronary angiography of giant coronary aneurysm and thrombus formation. *A, B,* Two-dimensional echocardiography and coronary angiography at 1 month of illness demonstrated giant aneurysms in the left main trunk, the left anterior descending artery (LAD), and the circumflex artery (LCX). Ao = aorta; PA = pulmonary artery. *C, D,* Ten months later, two-dimensional echocardiography demonstrated massive, dense abnormal echo in the left main trunk (*arrows*), which suggested massive thrombotic formation (T) in the coronary aneurysm. At that time, coronary angiography showed the decreased size and a severe obstruction of the coronary aneurysm.

dilatation, and regression occurs within 3 to 5 weeks from the onset of illness. Acute massive thrombus formation can also be diagnosed by serial two-dimensional echocardiography, and then thrombolytic treatment with urokinase or tissue plasminogen activator (t-PA) is indicated. The evaluation of stenotic lesions of the coronary artery by two-dimensional echocardiography is more difficult but is possible with use of a high-frequency transducer and careful examination. The critical points in evaluation by two-dimensional echocardiography are the loss of the uniformity of the lumen of arteries, an irregular arterial wall, and a dense echo in the coronary arterial wall.

Selective coronary artery angiography is the most accurate method of defining the presence and severity of coronary arterial abnormalities in KD (see Fig. 47–1). The indications for coronary angiography include abnormal findings on two-dimensional echocardiography, symptoms or signs of ischemia, auscultatory evidence of valvar regurgitation, evidence of cardiac dysfunction, and the need for intracoronary thrombolytic treatment. If patients have a severe coronary lesion on coronary angiography, other systemic vascular involvement, such as in the axillary, iliac, renal, and intrathoracic arteries, should be evaluated. Because coronary artery aneurysms tend to regress and stenotic lesions progress usually within 2 years from the onset of illness, repeated coronary angiography is essential, especially in patients with a coronary aneurysm.[26] Regression of coronary aneurysms is diagnosed when follow-up coronary angiography demonstrates completely normal coronary arteries in a patient with previous coronary

aneurysms (Fig. 47–2). The aneurysms must have disappeared and the entire coronary arterial system have a smooth wall. This condition can be diagnosed by coronary angiography; however, two-dimensional echocardiography may miss mildly abnormal findings that subsequently progress to coronary artery disease. Coronary angiography is important and essential for evaluating stenotic obstructive lesions of the coronary arteries and assessing the collateral circulation.

The clinical feasibility of intravascular ultrasound imaging of coronary arteries in patients with KD to assess the long-term pathologic process in vivo has been described.[27] At the site of a regressed aneurysm, there is marked thickening of the intima. The portion of the coronary artery with a normal angiographic appearance showed normal findings except in the region near the regressed aneurysm, which showed mild intimal thickening. This technology can provide new information about the morphology, tissue characterization, and pathology of the coronary arteries late in the course of KD.

EVALUATING MYOCARDIAL ISCHEMIA

Because the morbidity and mortality of this disease mostly depend on the extent of associated coronary artery disease, myocardial ischemia must be assessed during the follow-up. Two-dimensional echocardiography can detect coronary aneurysms, but evaluating the significance of stenotic lesions by this method is unsatisfactory. Similarly, electrocardiographic sensitivity for detecting myocardial ischemia

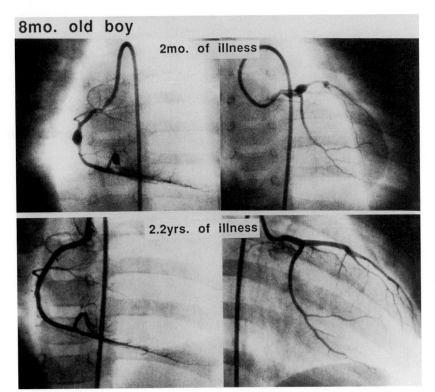

8mo. old boy

2mo. of illness

2.2yrs. of illness

FIGURE 47–2

Regression of coronary aneurysms. *Upper,* Eight-month-old boy with four coronary aneurysms in both right and left coronary arteries. *Lower,* Two years later. Follow-up coronary angiography demonstrated regression of aneurysms, which included the disappearance of aneurysms and no irregular arterial wall in the entire coronary artery system.

is inadequate. Coronary angiography is accurate for assessing coronary artery involvement, but repeated evaluation is often difficult because it is an invasive technique.

Although an exercise stress test can detect myocardial ischemia and this noninvasive technique is easy to repeat, the sensitivity of this technique is low, even in patients with significant coronary stenosis, and the test is difficult to perform in young children. Myocardial single-photon emission computed tomography (SPECT) using pharmacologic stress (i.e., dipyridamole infusion) is considered the most accurate diagnostic method for identifying myocardial ischemia, especially in children when an exercise test cannot be performed. Because pharmacologic stress SPECT study provides quantitative analysis, changes in the severity of myocardial ischemia can be assessed by serial studies. Kamiya[28] reported the sensitivity of detecting myocardial ischemia by various methods in KD patients having significant coronary stenosis (>75%). The most sensitive method was dipyridamole stress SPECT (85% sensitivity). In contrast, the sensitivity of treadmill exercise test remained less than 50%.[29]

MYOCARDIAL INFARCTION AND DEATH

The main cause of death in KD is acute myocardial infarction (MI). It occurred in 22 of our patients (1.3%), 9 of whom died (0.5%). A study of 104 fatal instances of KD in Japan suggests that 56.7% of the patients died of an acute MI, and 18% died of congestive cardiac failure caused by ischemia. Five patients died from rupture of a coronary aneurysm. In the 1970s, the fatality rate was about 2%, but it declined to 0.2% in Japan during the 1990s.[5] Late deaths several years after acute KD have increased recently; these deaths may occur at any time with obstructive lesions.

My colleagues and I analyzed 195 KD patients with MI from a nationwide survey in Japan.[30] MI mostly occurred within a year of illness. Attacks of MI are relatively more frequent at night when the patient is sleeping or resting; the primary manifestations are shock with pallor, restlessness, vomiting, and abdominal pain. Chest pain was more frequently recognized in the survivors and in children older than 4 years. An asymptomatic MI was seen in 37% of the 195 patients. Twenty-two percent died from the first attack; 16% of the survivors from the first attack had a second MI. Fatality was 63% in the second attack and 83% in the third attack. From the coronary angiographic studies in the patients with an MI, most of the patients who died had an obstruction in the left main coronary artery or in both the right main coronary artery and the anterior descending artery. In survivors, one-vessel obstruction, particularly in the right coronary artery, was frequently recognized.

The early recognition and treatment of acute MI are critical. Recurrence of MI is observed in about 20% of the patients who have had a previous MI. Because the mortality of recurrent MI is high, careful management is needed for such patients. Patients with complications after MI, such as ventricular aneurysm, papillary muscle dysfunction, heart failure, severe arrhythmias, and postinfarction angina, are managed by medical or operative approaches.

SYSTEMIC ARTERY INVOLVEMENT

Although the coronary arteries are the most important sites in KD, aneurysms in other arteries, such as the axillary, iliac, and renal arteries, were observed in 1.6% of the patients.[31] Prognosis of systemic artery aneurysms is generally favorable, but renovascular hypertension may develop in a patient with a renal artery lesion, and intrathoracic arterial lesions may cause difficulty during coronary bypass surgery. Digital gangrenous changes can occur.[32]

VALVAR HEART DISEASE, MYOCARDITIS, AND PERICARDITIS

Valvar heart disease appears in 1% of the patients and usually involves the mitral valve and rarely the aortic valve. My colleagues and I demonstrated acute mitral regurgitation in 15 of 1664 patients (0.9%); it eventually disappeared after a few months to several years in half of the patients. The regurgitation may be from either valvulitis or papillary muscle dysfunction caused by ischemia.[33] We had four patients with aortic regurgitation (0.24%), which appeared after the acute or subacute stage of illness and became severe several years later in some patients.[34] Pericarditis or pericardial effusion appeared in 15.7% of the patients during the acute phase; it was mostly subclinical and disappeared within 1 or 2 weeks. There have been no reports of its progression to chronic or constrictive pericarditis. Massive pericardial effusion and cardiac tamponade were rare. Relatively mild myocarditis was observed in 36% of patients during the acute phase, especially in the first and second weeks of illness, regardless of the presence of coronary aneurysms. A gallop rhythm, distant heart sounds, ST-T segment changes, or decreased voltage of R waves on electrocardiography may suggest myocarditis. In many instances, cardiac enzyme levels, such as creatine kinase, did not change significantly. Cardiomegaly or decreased ejection fraction of the left ventricle caused by myocarditis was noted in some patients. Myocarditis generally followed as the acute course resolved and seldom developed into a chronic cardiomyopathy. These incidences are summarized in Table 47–2.

LONG-TERM CARDIOVASCULAR SEQUELAE AND NATURAL HISTORY

FATE OF CORONARY ANEURYSMS

The dominant issue in KD is the clinical history and fate of coronary aneurysms.[35] My colleagues and I observed 594 consecutive patients with acute KD between 1973 and 1983, and this cohort has been followed up for 10 to 21 years.[31] In all patients, we evaluated the coronary lesions

TABLE 47–2		
CARDIOVASCULAR SPECTRUM IN KAWASAKI DISEASE		
Coronary artery		
Transient dilatation in acute stage	256/1042	(24.6%)
Coronary aneurysm	273/1664	(16.4)
Immune globulin treatment selected by Harada's score (1991–1995)	20/309	(6.5)
Systemic artery aneurysms (axillary, iliac, renal)	27/1664	(1.6)
Mitral regurgitation	15/1664	(0.9)
Aortic regurgitation	4/1664	(0.24)
Pericarditis or pericardial effusion	214/1355	(15.7)
Myocarditis	602/1664	(36.1)
Myocardial infarction	22/1664	(1.3)
Fatal cases	9/1664	(0.54)

Data from Kurume University, Kurume, Japan: 1973–1995.

by coronary angiography just after the acute stage. One hundred and forty-six patients (24.6%) were diagnosed as having coronary aneurysms. A second angiogram was performed 1 to 2 years later in all 146 patients with a coronary aneurysm, and 72 (49.3%) of the 146 showed regression of the aneurysm (Fig. 47–3). This suggests a strong tendency for coronary aneurysms in KD to regress. None of the patients with regression of coronary aneurysms had cardiac symptoms in the long-term follow-up. The results of their electrocardiography, exercise stress test, thallium myocardial scintigraphy, and left ventricular function studies were all within normal limits. In contrast, by 10 to 21 years after the onset of the illness, stenosis in the coronary aneurysms had developed in 28 patients. MI occurred in 11 patients, 5 of whom died. From this study, it is estimated that about 4% of patients with KD may develop ischemic heart disease.

My coworkers and I studied the time and the incidence of regression or progression to obstructive lesions from the onset of KD by use of the Kaplan-Meyer life table method. Regression of coronary aneurysms mostly occurred within 2 years of the onset of illness, whereas the obstructive lesions developed in 2 years and gradually increased subsequently.

We investigated factors that could affect the prognosis of coronary aneurysms.[36] The risk factors for development of coronary aneurysms into ischemic heart disease are aneurysms with a diameter more than 8 mm or a large diffuse or saccular shape, prolonged fever for more than 21 days, and age at onset older than 2 years. Takahashi and colleagues[37] reported that regression of coronary aneurysms was more likely to occur in patients younger than 1 year and in girls. In 26 of our patients with a giant coronary aneurysm, stenotic lesions developed in 12, and no regression occurred in our follow-up study. Thus, giant coronary aneurysms present a critical problem because they have a strong potential for progression to ischemic heart disease. The incidence of giant coronary aneurysms was 17.8% in the patients with a coronary aneurysm and 4.4% among all KD patients in the series.

The pathologic mechanism of regression of aneurysms is marked proliferation of intima without massive thrombus formation. The proliferation consists of rich, smooth muscle cells and well-regenerated endothelium covering a superficial thrombus.[38] Hemodynamic forces may regulate such arteries to maintain adequate lumina. It is uncertain whether intimal thickening eventually develops into an obstructive lesion, but it may be possible in the later stages of illness.[39] From our 10 to 21 years of follow-up study, none of the patients who had regressed aneurysms developed ischemic heart disease. Our experience may indicate that a stenotic lesion does not develop, at least within one or two decades, in patients with complete regression of coronary aneurysms.

LONG-TERM ISSUE OF KAWASAKI VASCULITIS

Pathology of the coronary arteries in KD several years after the acute episode demonstrates marked intimal proliferation and, in some patients, calcification and deposits of protein-like material and hyalinized degeneration in the thickened intima that resembles arteriosclerotic lesions.

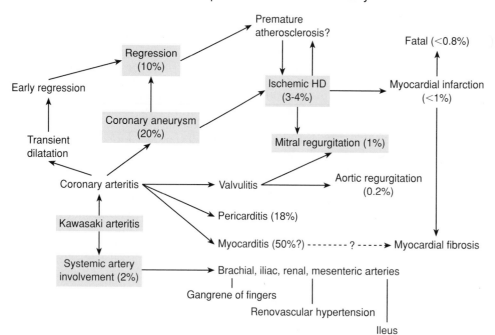

Cardiovascular Spectrum and Natural History

FIGURE 47–3

Natural history of cardiovascular lesions of Kawasaki disease. HD = heart disease.

An important issue is whether these coronary arterial lesions may develop into atherosclerotic coronary artery disease of adulthood.[35]

We studied the distensibility of the coronary arterial wall by intracoronary infusion of isosorbide dinitrate.[40] Persistent aneurysms or stenotic lesions demonstrated poor distensibility. By contrast, in patients with a regressed aneurysm at an early stage, such as 1 or 2 years from the onset, there were no significant differences from normal. Patients studied at a longer time after the acute episode, such as 8 years, showed lower distensibility. These results suggest that the coronary artery may become stiff even with a regressed aneurysm. Our intravascular ultrasound study of coronary arteries after KD demonstrated marked thickening of intima and calcification in the coronary aneurysms, similar to those of arteriosclerotic lesions.[27] Reduced reactivity to nitroglycerin has been demonstrated years later in coronary arteries that appeared to be normal by intravascular ultrasound study.[41] In fact, decreased endothelial function has been observed in the brachial arteries of subjects studied 5 to 17 years after the acute illness.[42]

It has now been more than 25 years since the first description of KD as a new clinical entity, and a number of the early KD children are now adults. My coworkers and I surveyed these adults to investigate coronary sequelae that may be due to the earlier KD and to determine their cardiac status.[43] Questionnaires were sent to adult cardiologists in all 354 major hospitals throughout Japan. Twenty-one adult patients with coronary lesions having a definite or suspected history of KD and 109 other patients with coronary aneurysms who had no documented history of KD were found. Of these 21, there were 17 men and 4 women whose ages ranged from 20 to 63 years (mean, 34 years). Nineteen of the patients who were diagnosed as having sepsis, pneumonia, viral syndrome, or fever of un-

known origin became ill before Dr. Kawasaki's first description. As adults, there was acute MI in five patients, old MI in six, angina pectoris in nine, and dilated cardiomyopathy in one. Burns and associates[44] also reported such adult patients from the literature.

Some patients with coronary artery sequelae of KD have already mixed into the group of young adults with ischemic heart disease. Abnormal Q waves or mitral regurgitation of unknown origin in the younger adults is important. Coronary angiographic findings are essential for recognition of preceding KD, and these include the presence of multiple aneurysms with stenoses frequently associated with calcification. Familial hypercholesterolemia or collagen vascular disease should be excluded. The coronary artery sequelae of KD may be an important cause of ischemic heart disease in young adults.

TREATMENT AND MANAGEMENT

TREATMENT IN THE ACUTE STAGE

The combination of aspirin and high-dose immune globulin is the major therapeutic strategy in acute KD.[45] In 1984, high-dose immune globulin treatment was found to be effective by Furusho and colleagues[46] in Japan. This was confirmed subsequently by a multicenter, randomized trial.[47] These two studies indicate that 400 mg/kg/day of immune globulin for 4 or 5 days is effective in preventing coronary aneurysms. Immune globulin treatment is now the most effective treatment; however, the optimal dose and indications for this treatment remain controversial. A single large dose of 2 g/kg has been reported to be much more effective.[48]

As mentioned before, coronary aneurysms develop in less than 20% of KD patients. If patients who develop

---

HARADA'S SCORING SYSTEM

White blood cell count above $12,000/mm^3$
Platelet count below $350,000/mm^3$
C-reactive protein level more than 3+
Hematocrit below 35%
Serum albumin concentration below 3.5 mg/dl
Age younger than 12 months
Sex: male

---

coronary aneurysms could be predicted and patients for immune globulin treatment selected, it would be more effective and reduce medical expenses. Harada's scoring system[49] may be useful for selecting the patients at high risk for development of coronary artery aneurysms and thus appropriate for treatment with immune globulin. Immune globulin treatment is indicated when more than four of the seven features are present.

Another problem is that coronary artery aneurysms may develop in a small number of patients with KD even with high-dose immune globulin treatment. Repeated immune globulin treatment of 1 g/kg may be indicated. Wright and coworkers[50] recommended pulsed high-dose corticosteroids for such globulin-resistant patients.

Aspirin is also an important and basic drug in KD for its antipyretic, anti-inflammatory, and antiplatelet effects. The optimal dose remains controversial.[45, 51] For the effects of aspirin on the platelet aggregation in KD, a low dose (30 mg/kg) can be used successfully to reduce the platelet aggregation that increases during the second and third weeks of the illness. A higher dose of aspirin (100 mg/kg), such as used in collagen vascular disease, did not have significant further effects on platelet aggregation. Biosynthesis of thromboxane B_2 was completely blocked in both groups. Plasma 6-keto prostaglandin $F_{1\alpha}$, a metabolite of prostacyclin that has potent antiaggregatory effect on platelets, was also blocked in a number of patients in the high-dose group. The finding suggests that high-dose aspirin may have a disadvantage for preventing thrombotic formation in some patients. Hepatic dysfunction occurred in much higher frequency in the high-dose group. In these patients, aspirin and substituted flurbiprofen were discontinued. The absorption of aspirin may decrease in the acute stage of KD. For these reasons, my colleagues and I recommend aspirin 30 mg/kg during the acute stage and 5 mg/kg in the convalescent stage.[52]

LONG-TERM MANAGEMENT

The long-term management of patients with KD depends on the degree of coronary arterial involvement. Low-dose aspirin (5 mg/kg/day in a single dose) is basic treatment in the convalescent phase, and it continues up to 6 to 8 weeks in patients without coronary abnormalities. If coronary arterial abnormalities are detected, low-dose aspirin should be continued until such coronary abnormalities resolve. Coronary angiography is recommended in children in whom cardiovascular abnormalities have been found by two-dimensional echocardiography. Because the risk of progression to ischemic heart disease is high, particularly in those with giant aneurysms, these patients should be managed by a pediatric cardiologist. My coworkers and I recommend the combination of aspirin and warfarin for patients with a giant coronary artery aneurysm. A β blocker may be indicated for patients with ischemic symptoms. Table 47–3 indicates recommendations for long-term management of this disease.

When symptoms of MI are noted, the patient should be hospitalized immediately, given oxygen, and prescribed bedrest. Vital signs, electrocardiograms, and central venous pressure should be monitored; mechanical ventilation should be given if necessary. Because the main cause of acute MI in KD is acute thrombotic occlusion in postaneurysmal stenosis, thrombolytic treatment and anticoagulation therapy are important during an acute MI. Intravenous administration of t-PA, intracoronary infusion of

---

TABLE 47–3

THERAPEUTIC RECOMMENDATIONS

ACUTE PHASE

Aspirin	30 mg/kg (divided in two) for 2 weeks and reduced to 5 mg/kg/day once a day for 2 months
IVIG	2 g/kg single dose for 12 hr or 400 mg/kg/day for 5 days
No response to IVIG	Add 1 g/kg single dose

CONVALESCENCE PHASE

Aspirin	5 mg/kg/day single dose for patient with coronary aneurysm
Warfarin or dipyridamole	In combination with aspirin for patient with giant aneurysm

CHRONIC TREATMENT

Aspirin	Continue 5 mg/kg single dose
β blocker	May be indicated for patient with ischemic symptoms
Thrombolytic therapy	Intravenous t-PA 0.5 mg/kg for 1 hr
	Intracoronary urokinase 10,000 IU/kg followed by IV heparin

PTCA, stent, atherectomy, or rotational ablation (Rotablator) may be effective in some patients.
Surgery is indicated for (1) patient with ischemic symptoms, (2) patient with severe multivessel obstruction, (3) severe obstruction in left main coronary artery, and (4) severe valvar disease.

IVIG = intravenous immune globulin; t-PA = tissue plasminogen activator; PTCA = percutaneous transluminal coronary angioplasty.

urokinase, and heparin should be given as indicated in Table 47–3. Intracoronary infusion of urokinase within 6 hours after the onset of MI is the most effective method of thrombolysis.[53] When an acute MI is recognized, pediatricians should use t-PA immediately intravenously and refer the patient to a cardiac center. Vasodilators, nitroglycerin, and diuretics are used in addition to catecholamines for cardiogenic shock and heart failure. Cardiac pacing, administration of lidocaine, and defibrillation are occasionally necessary for a severe arrhythmia.

Interventional catheterization of coronary arteries in KD has occasionally been performed. The long-term results are unknown. Balloon angioplasty is effective in some patients within 6 to 8 years of the acute episode but has not been as effective as in atherosclerotic coronary arteries because of elastic recoil and stiffness of the coronary arteries.[54] Recently, my colleagues and I have successfully performed coronary rotational ablation for long-term severe stenosis of a coronary artery in selected patients. Stent implantation may be useful in some patients.

Coronary bypass surgery may be indicated in patients with serious coronary artery lesions.[55] Bypass grafting with use of an intrathoracic artery is recommended for left coronary artery bypass, because the long-term patency is much more favorable (3 years, 77.1%) compared with saphenous vein grafts (3 years, 53.8%). The gastroepiploic artery is suitable for right coronary artery bypass grafting because it is usually large and has stable blood flow even in younger children. Current indications for operation are three-vessel obstruction, severe occlusion of the left main coronary arterial trunk, and severe occlusion in both left anterior descending artery and right coronary arteries.[56] If the patients are asymptomatic but demonstrate significant ischemic findings by exercise stress testing or thallium myocardial scintigraphy, operation may be indicated. A native, intrathoracic arterial graft is preferable because it can grow with age. Infants and children younger than 4 years present technical difficulties for a bypass operation. Viability of the myocardium should be evaluated by thallium myocardial scintigraphy. Cardiac transplantation has been performed in several patients in the United States and United Kingdom.[57] It may be indicated in rare patients who have severe diffuse myocardial fibrosis due to ischemia or previous multivessel bypass operation with difficult revascularization.

REFERENCES

1. Kato H, Koike S, Yamamoto M, et al: Coronary aneurysms in infants and young children with acute febrile mucocutaneous lymph node syndrome. J Pediatr 86:892, 1975.
2. Kato H, Akagi T, Sugimura T, et al: Kawasaki disease. Coron Artery Dis 6:194, 1995.
3. Kawasaki T: Acute febrile mucocutaneous syndrome with lymphoid involvement with specific desquamation of the fingers and toes in children. Arerugi Jpn J Allergol (Tokyo) 16:178, 1967.
4. Kawasaki T, Kosaki F, Okawa S, et al: A new infantile acute febrile mucocutaneous lymph node syndrome prevailing in Japan. Pediatrics 54:271, 1974.
5. Yanagawa H, Yashiro M, Nakamura T, et al: Results of twelve nationwide epidemiological incidence surveys of Kawasaki disease in Japan. Arch Pediatr Adolesc Med 149:779, 1995.
6. Yanagawa H, Nakamura T: Global epidemiology of Kawasaki disease. In Kato H (ed): Kawasaki Disease. Amsterdam, Elsevier, 1995, pp 90–100.
7. Abe J, Kotzin BL, Jujo K, et al: Selective expansion of T cells expressing T-cell receptor variable regions Vβ2 and Vβ8 in Kawasaki disease. Proc Natl Acad Sci U S A 89:4066, 1982.
8. Leung DYM, Meissner HC, Fulton DR, et al: Toxic shock syndrome toxin-secreting Staphylococcus aureus in Kawasaki syndrome. Lancet 342:1385, 1993.
9. Sakaguchi M, Kato H, Nishiyori A, et al: Characterization of CD4+ T helper cells in patients with Kawasaki disease: Preferential production of TNF-α by Vβ2 and Vβ8 CD4+ T helper cells. Clin Exp Immunol 99:276, 1995.
10. Pietra BA, De Inocencio J, Giannini EH, Hirsch R: TCR Vβ family repertoire and T cell activation markers in Kawasaki disease. J Immunol 153:1881, 1994.
11. Sato K, Ouichi K, Taki M: Yersinia pseudotuberculosis infection in children, resembling Izumi fever and Kawasaki syndrome. Pediatr Infect Dis J 2:123, 1983.
12. Uchiyama T, Miyoshi-Akiyama T, Kato H, et al: Superantigenic properties of a novel mitogenic substance produced by Yersinia pseudotuberculosis isolated from patients manifesting acute and systemic symptoms. J Immunol 151:4407, 1993.
13. Furusho K, Sato K, Kajino Y: A significance of glucan produced by Streptococcus sanguis. Prog Med 11:75, 1992.
14. Kato H, Fujimato T, Inoue O, et al: Variant strain of Propionibacterium acnes: A clue to the aetiology of Kawasaki disease. Lancet 2:1383, 1983.
15. Tomita S, Kato H, Fujimoto T, et al: Cytopathogenic protein in filtrates from cultures of Propionibacterium acnes isolated from patients with Kawasaki disease. Br Med J 295:1229, 1987.
16. Kikuta H, Mizuno F, Osato T: Kawasaki disease and an unusual primary infection with Epstein-Barr virus. Pediatrics 73:413, 1984.
17. Burns JC, Geha RS, Schneeberger EE, et al: Polymerase activity in lymphocyte culture supernatants from patients with Kawasaki disease. Nature 323:814, 1986.
18. Furukawa S, Matsubara T, Jutoh K, et al: Peripheral blood monocyte/macrophages and serum tumor necrosis factor in Kawasaki disease. Clin Immunol Immunopathol 48:247, 1988.
19. Leung DYM, Collins T, LaPierre LA, et al: Immunoglobulin M antibodies present in the acute phase of Kawasaki syndrome lyse cultured vascular endothelial cells stimulated by gamma interferon. J Clin Invest 77:1428, 1986.
20. Terai M, Kohno Y, Nanba M, et al: Class II antigen expression in the coronary artery endothelium in Kawasaki disease. Hum Pathol 21:231, 1990.
21. Fujiwara H, Hamashima Y: Pathology of the heart in Kawasaki disease. Pediatrics 61:100, 1978.
22. Naoe S, Shibuya K, Takahashi K, et al: Pathological observations concerning the cardiovascular lesions in Kawasaki disease. Cardiol Young 3:212, 1991.
23. Landing BH, Larson EJ: Are infantile periarteritis nodosa with coronary artery involvement and fetal mucocutaneous lymph node syndrome the same? Comparison of 20 patients from North America with patients from Hawaii and Japan. Pediatrics 59:651, 1977.
24. Burns JC, Wiggins JW Jr, Toews WH, et al: Clinical spectrum of Kawasaki disease in infants younger than 6 months of age. J Pediatr 109:759, 1986.
25. Dajani AS, Taubert KA, Takahashi M, et al: Guidelines for long-term management of patients with Kawasaki disease. Committee Report of Council on Cardiovascular Disease in the Young, American Heart Association. Circulation 89:916, 1994.
26. Kato H, Ichinose E, Yoshioka F, et al: Fate of coronary aneurysms in Kawasaki disease: Serial coronary angiography and long-term follow-up study. Am J Cardiol 49:1758, 1982.
27. Sugimura T, Kato H, Inoue O, et al: Intravascular ultrasound of coronary arteries in children: Assessment of the wall morphology and the lumen after Kawasaki disease. Circulation 89:258, 1994.
28. Kamiya T: How to evaluate the myocardial ischemia in Kawasaki disease. In Kato H (ed): Kawasaki Disease. Amsterdam, Elsevier, 1995, pp 447–450.
29. Fukuda T: Myocardial ischemia in Kawasaki disease: Evaluation by dipyridamole stress thallium-201 myocardial imaging and exercise test. Kurume Med J 39:245, 1992.
30. Kato H, Ichinose E, Kawasaki T: Myocardial infarction in Kawasaki disease: Clinical analyses in 195 cases. J Pediatr 108:923, 1986.

31. Kato H, Sugimura T, Akagi T, et al: Long-term consequences of Kawasaki disease: A 10- to 21-year follow-up study of 594 patients. Circulation 94:1379, 1996.
32. Tomita S, Chung K, Mas M, et al: Peripheral gangrene associated with Kawasaki disease. Clin Infect Dis 14:121, 1992.
33. Akagi T, Kato H, Inoue O, Sato N: Valvular heart disease in Kawasaki syndrome: Incidence and natural history. Am Heart J 120:366, 1990.
34. Gidding SS, Shulman ST, Ilbawi M, et al: Mucocutaneous lymph node syndrome (Kawasaki disease): Delayed aortic and mitral insufficiency secondary to valvulitis. J Am Coll Cardiol 7:894, 1986.
35. Kato H: Long-term consequences of Kawasaki disease: Pediatrics to adults. In Kato H (ed): Kawasaki Disease. Amsterdam, Elsevier, 1996, pp 557–566.
36. Ichinose E, Inoue O, Hiyoshi Y, Kato H: Fate of coronary aneurysms in Kawasaki disease: Analysis of prognostic factors. In Doyle EF, Engle MA, Gersony WM, et al (eds): Pediatric Cardiology. New York, Springer-Verlag, 1986, pp 1099–1101.
37. Takahashi M, Mason W, Lewis AB: Regression of coronary aneurysms in patients with Kawasaki syndrome. Circulation 75:387, 1987.
38. Sasaguri Y, Kato H: Regression of aneurysms in Kawasaki disease: A pathologic study. J Pediatr 100:225, 1982.
39. Suzuki A, Kamiya T, Arakaki Y, et al: Fate of coronary arterial aneurysms in Kawasaki disease. Am J Cardiol 74:822, 1994.
40. Sugimura T, Kato H, Inoue O, et al: Vasodilatory response of the coronary arteries after Kawasaki disease: Evaluation by intracoronary injection of isosorbide dinitrate. J Pediatr 121:684, 1992.
41. Suzuki A, Yamagishi M, Kimura K, et al: Functional behavior and morphology of the coronary wall in patients with Kawasaki disease assessed by intravascular ultrasound. J Am Coll Cardiol 27:291, 1996.
42. Dhillon R, Clarkson P, Donald AE, et al: Endothelial dysfunction later after Kawasaki disease. Circulation 94:2103, 1996.
43. Kato H, Inoue O, Kawasaki T, et al: Adult coronary artery disease probably due to childhood Kawasaki disease. Lancet 340:1127, 1992.
44. Burns JC, Shike H, Gordon JB, et al: Sequelae of Kawasaki disease in adolescents and young adults. J Am Coll Cardiol 28:253, 1996.
45. Dajani AS, Taubert KA, Takahashi M, et al: Diagnosis and therapy of Kawasaki disease in children. Committee Report of Council on Cardiovascular Disease in the Young, American Heart Association. Circulation 87:1776, 1993.
46. Furusho K, Kamiya T, Nakano H, et al: High-dose intravenous gammaglobulin for Kawasaki disease. Lancet 2:1055, 1984.
47. Newburger JW, Takahashi M, Burns JC, et al: The treatment of Kawasaki syndrome with intravenous gamma globulin. N Engl J Med 315:341, 1986.
48. Newburger JW, Takahashi M, Beiser AS, et al: A single intravenous infusion of gamma globulin as compared with four infusions in the treatment of acute Kawasaki syndrome. N Engl J Med 324:1633, 1991.
49. Harada K: Intravenous γ-globulin treatment in Kawasaki disease. Acta Paediatr Jpn 33:805, 1991.
50. Wright DA, Newburger JW, Baker A, Sundel RP: Treatment of immune globulin–resistant Kawasaki disease with pulsed doses of corticosteroids. J Pediatr 128:146, 1996.
51. Kato H, Koike S, Yokoyama T: Kawasaki disease: Effect of treatment on coronary artery involvement. Pediatrics 63:175, 1979.
52. Akagi T, Kato H, Inoue O, Sato N: Salicylate treatment in Kawasaki disease: High dose or low dose? Eur J Pediatr 150:642, 1991.
53. Kato H, Inoue O, Ichinose E, et al: Intracoronary urokinase in Kawasaki disease: Treatment and prevention of myocardial infarction. Acta Paediatr Jpn 33:27, 1991.
54. Ino T, Akimoto K, Ohkubo M, et al: Application of percutaneous transluminal coronary angioplasty to coronary arterial stenosis in Kawasaki disease. Circulation 93:1709, 1996.
55. Kitamura S, Kawachi K, Oyama C, et al: Severe Kawasaki heart disease treated with an internal mammary artery graft in pediatric patients. J Thorac Cardiovasc Surg 89:860, 1985.
56. Kato H, Inoue O, Akagi T: Kawasaki disease: Cardiac problems and management. Pediatr Rev 9:209, 1988.
57. Checchia P, Pahl E, Rosenfeld E, et al: The worldwide experience with cardiac transplantation for Kawasaki disease. In Kato H (ed): Kawasaki Disease. Amsterdam, Elsevier, 1996, pp 522–526.

CHAPTER 48

RHEUMATIC FEVER

ELIA M. AYOUB

Rheumatic fever is one of the nonpurulent complications of group A streptococcal pharyngitis. Its acute manifestations include inflammation of the joints, the heart, and, less commonly, the brain and the skin. Involvement of the heart is by far the most serious of these manifestations, and the morbidity of the disease is directly related to the occurrence of this complication. Rheumatic fever is classified as a connective tissue or collagen vascular disease. It is unique among collagen vascular diseases in that a well-defined infection, a group A streptococcal pharyngitis, acts as the precipitating event that leads to the clinical expression of the disease. Because of this established relationship, we are able to prevent rheumatic fever by treating the streptococcal pharyngitis. In addition, we can prevent recurrence of rheumatic fever in individuals who have acquired the disease previously by prescribing prophylactic antibiotics to these patients to prevent them from acquiring streptococcal pharyngitis.

Once common in the United States and western Europe, the incidence of rheumatic fever has declined steadily, starting in the middle part of the 20th century. The manifestations of the disease, particularly cardiac involvement, are less severe than those seen in an earlier period.[1] This is attributable in part to the institution of prophylactic measures that reduce recurrences of the disease and prevent cumulative cardiac damage. However, the disease is still highly prevalent in underdeveloped countries, where it remains the leading cause of acquired cardiac valvar disease in children and adolescents. The resurgence of rheumatic fever that was witnessed in the United States during the mid-1980s should prompt physicians to remain alert to the occurrence of this disease and be familiar with its manifestations, diagnosis, and treatment.[2]

EPIDEMIOLOGY

Group A streptococcal infection of the upper respiratory tract is a required antecedent to the occurrence of acute rheumatic fever. Rheumatic fever does not occur in all individuals after such an infection. Only 2 to 3% of previously healthy individuals with untreated streptococcal pharyngitis develop this complication. Although data are not available to determine whether systemic infection by group A streptococci at a site other than the respiratory tract leads to rheumatic fever in a susceptible individual, epidemiologic studies indicate that infection of the skin by group A streptococci, such as in impetigo, can lead to the occurrence of glomerulonephritis but not to rheu-

matic fever.[3] Rheumatic fever can be prevented in most individuals by appropriate treatment of streptococcal pharyngitis.

Acute rheumatic fever occurs most commonly in children between the ages of 5 and 15 years. This age incidence parallels that of streptococcal pharyngitis. In the United States, rheumatic fever is rarely encountered in children younger than 5 years. In developing countries, rheumatic fever with severe cardiac involvement occurs in children who are 3 to 5 years old. Earlier studies suggested that rheumatic fever was more common in girls, but our experience shows no difference in the incidence of the disease with gender.

Environmental factors influence the incidence of rheumatic fever in certain populations. Socioeconomic status, accessibility of health care, and crowding at home or site of work appear to play a role in determining the incidence of rheumatic fever by influencing the incidence of streptococcal infection within a population.[4,5] Crowding at site of work would explain the declining incidence of rheumatic fever after high school and the increased risk encountered in certain adult populations, such as military recruits, industrial workers in developing countries, and parents of school-aged children, particularly those living in crowded homes.

Ethnic and racial differences in the incidence and prevalence of rheumatic fever have been described. These differences were initially ascribed to socioeconomic factors, but additional information revealed differences unrelated to these factors. The incidence of rheumatic fever in the Maori population in New Zealand is 10-fold higher than that of the non-Maori population in that country,[6,7] independent of socioeconomic factors. Similarly, the incidence of rheumatic fever in the Samoan population in Hawaii is about 20 times higher than that of the Chinese population of these islands.[8] In the United States, rheumatic fever is more common in blacks, Hispanic Americans, and Native Americans than in whites. Cardiac involvement is more severe in blacks than in whites.[9] Socioeconomic factors may contribute to some of the differences between ethnic groups in the United States.

The steady decline in the incidence of rheumatic fever in the United States was interrupted in 1985 by a resurgence of the disease in certain areas.[2] The first report of this resurgence came in 1985 from Utah, where a substantial increase in the number of children with acute rheumatic fever occurred.[10] Similar reports from other areas of the country followed.[11–19] In two areas, Utah and Pennsylvania, the increased number of patients with rheumatic fever declined gradually during the subsequent years.[20–22] The resurgence of rheumatic fever in these areas, although unimpressive in absolute numbers, yielded important data regarding the epidemiology of the disease. In some areas, the children involved were from high- to middle-income families with ready access to medical care.[10] Most affected children did not have a history of a sore throat and did not seek attention for such an ailment before the onset of rheumatic fever.[2–10] Streptococcal isolates recovered from some of these patients and their siblings revealed predominance of certain M serotypes that produced highly mucoid colonies on culture with sheep blood agar. This phenotypic characteristic was reminiscent of isolates recovered during the high incidence of rheumatic fever in this country a half a century ago.

PATHOGENESIS

The pathogenesis of rheumatic fever involves an interaction between the group A streptococcus and the immune system of the host (Fig. 48–1). Each component possesses certain attributes that are necessary to allow this interaction. Current knowledge of the factors involved in the pathogenesis of rheumatic fever is detailed as follows.

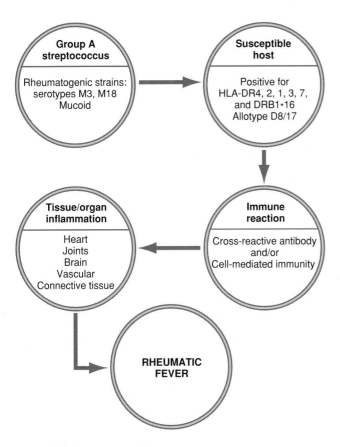

FIGURE 48–1

Outline of pathogenesis of rheumatic fever. (Adapted from Ayoub EM: Acute rheumatic fever. *In* Emmanouilides GC, Allen HD, Riemenschneider TA, Gutgesell HP [eds]: Heart Disease in Infants, Children and Adolescents: Including the Fetus and Young Adult, 5th ed. Baltimore, Williams & Wilkins, 1995, pp 1400–1416.)

MICROBIAL FACTORS

The Group A Streptococcus

The identification of streptococci as a cause of pharyngitis and scarlet fever around the turn of the 20th century stimulated further studies into the biology of this organism. Classification of streptococci based on the type of hemolysis as α-hemolytic, β-hemolytic, and γ streptococci was followed by the serologic identification of different groups among the β-hemolytic streptococci.

CELLULAR COMPONENTS

In her pioneering work, Lancefield classified β-hemolytic streptococci into 20 different groups (A to H, K to V) on the basis of differences in chemical composition and immunologic specificity of the cell-wall polysaccharide.[23]

Additional studies revealed that group A streptococci could be subdivided into serotypes on the basis of differences in the chemical composition of another cell-wall structure, the M protein. About 120 different serotypes exist among group A streptococci, of which only 80 types (M1 to M80) have been serologically identified. Despite differences in their M protein, all group A streptococci share in the identity of the cell-wall polysaccharide and some of the other cellular components and products.

The M protein is the primary component of the fimbriae that traverse the cell wall and extend beyond the surface of the cell. Its free distal terminal end consists of a hypervariable region that imparts antigenic type specificity to the M proteins of the various serotypes encountered among group A streptococci. M protein is considered a major virulence factor of group A streptococci because of its ability to retard and inhibit phagocytosis by host cells. Group A streptococci lacking the M protein are readily ingested and killed by host phagocytes. The antiphagocytic activity of the M protein is abrogated by antibody to the specific M protein, the type-specific antibody. Immunity to group A streptococcal infection is predicted on the presence of type-specific antibodies to the M protein of group A streptococci.

Particular interest in the M protein was aroused by its association with the nonpurulent complications of group A streptococcal infection. Early observations indicated that certain M protein serotypes (M1, M4, M12, M25, and M49) were associated with outbreaks of poststreptococcal glomerulonephritis. No such association was established with rheumatic fever until the resurgence of the disease in the 1980s. At that time, strains recovered from children with rheumatic fever or from their siblings were found to belong to serotypes M1, M3, M5, M6, M18, M19, and M24, particularly strains that produced mucoid colonies on culture with blood agar.[24] Subsequent studies indicated that the primary serotypes that were associated with rheumatic fever were limited to serotypes M3 and M18.[25] These two serotypes together with serotype M1 were associated with severe invasive group A streptococcal infections such as necrotizing fasciitis and streptococcal toxic shock syndrome.[25,26] Bessen and colleagues[27] described the association of rheumatic fever with serotypes that have conserved portions of the C-terminal portion of the M protein exposed on the cell surface (class I) and the absence of such an association with M protein serotypes that do not have these exposed portions (class II).

The importance of these observations is enhanced by prior studies indicating that the M protein plays a major role in the pathogenesis of rheumatic fever. Several epitopes within this molecule have been shown to cross-react antigenically with human myocardium, particularly myosin, and brain tissue.[28] In addition, studies suggest that the M protein may act as a "superantigen."[29] Thus, this streptococcal molecule has the capacity to elicit antibodies that could cross-react with the host tissue or stimulate cell-mediated immunity and lead to the inflammation observed in the organs affected during acute rheumatic fever.

EXTRACELLULAR PRODUCTS OF GROUP A STREPTOCOCCUS

A number of extracellular products are excreted by group A streptococci during growth in vitro and in vivo (Table 48–1). Most are proteins with defined enzymatic functions. The streptolysins are hemolysins responsible for the hydrolysis of the erythrocyte membranes; hemolysis can be either partial (α hemolysis) or complete (β hemolysis). Both of these products are cytotoxic to a variety of mammalian cells, including myocytes. In contrast to streptolysin S, which is nonimmunogenic in humans, streptolysin O and most of the other streptococcal products are immunogenic. The extracellular streptococcal products include four deoxyribonuclease (DNase) isozymes (A, B, C, D), of which DNase B is most commonly produced by group A streptococci. DNases are produced by other β-hemolytic streptococci, such as group C, which produces DNase C, commonly known as streptodornase.

The streptococcal pyrogenic exotoxins (SPEs) are extracellular products that have a potential role in invasive streptococcal infections. The SPEs include three previously described SPEs (A, B, and C) and two newly recognized ones, SPEF (mitogenic factor, MF) and the streptococcal superantigen SSA.[30–33] Although some investigators have suggested that SPEs play a role in the pathogenesis of invasive group A streptococcal diseases and toxic shock syndrome, the role of SPEs in the pathogenesis of rheumatic fever remains to be explored.

Streptococcal Antibody Tests

Most antibody tests for the streptococcal extracellular products (see Table 48–1) depend on the ability of the antibodies to neutralize the specific activity of these enzymatic products. The antibody titer is the reverse of the dilution required to neutralize a specific amount of the enzyme. The earliest of the tests for the extracellular products is the antistreptolysin O (ASO) test described by Todd.[34] This test, which has proved to be reproducible and reliable, has become the standard streptococcal antibody test used worldwide. Other tests included the antistreptokinase and antihyaluronidase tests, which have not proved to be as reproducible as the ASO test. The anti–DNase B test, which was established more recently, has proved equal in reliability to the ASO test and is currently used as an adjunct to it to provide evidence of group A streptococcal infection.[35, 36] The streptozyme antibody test is a slide agglutination test directed against a mixture of streptococcal antigens. Unlike the other tests, it is not a neutralizing antibody test. Although this test gained popularity because of its ease of performance, its lack of specificity and reproducibility makes it unreliable as a definitive test for the

TABLE 48–1

GROUP A STREPTOCOCCAL ANTIGENS AND CORRESPONDING ANTIBODY TESTS

Streptococcal Antigen	Antibody Test
EXTRACELLULAR PRODUCT	
Streptolysin O	ASO
Streptokinase	ASK
Hyaluronidase	ASH
Deoxyribonuclease B	Anti–DNase B
Nicotinamide adenine dinucleotidase	Anti–NADase
Multiple	Streptozyme
CELLULAR COMPONENT	
Type-specific M protein	Type-specific antibody
Group-specific polysaccharide	Anti–A-carbohydrate

ASO = antistreptolysin O; ASK = antistreptokinase; ASH = antistreptococcal hyaluronidase; DNase B = deoxyribonuclease B; NADase = nicotinamide adenine dinucleotidase.

From Ayoub EM: Streptococcal antibody tests in rheumatic fever. Clin Immunol Newsl 3:107, 1982.

confirmation of antecedent group A streptococcal infection.[37]

The antibody response to the streptococcal antigens is initiated after the acute infection and reaches its peak 3 to 4 weeks thereafter. The antibody level remains at this peak for 6 to 12 months, after which it declines to normal levels. Because of the ubiquity of group A streptococcal infections, normal individuals have low levels of antibody to many of the streptococcal antigens. The determination of whether an antibody titer is elevated depends on whether it exceeds the "upper limit of normal titer" that is established for a normal population of comparable age in the same geographic area. This titer is usually not exceeded by 15 to 20% of the normal population. Patients with acute streptococcal infection usually have normal antibody titers. However, evidence of such an infection can be established by obtaining titers on a serum sample procured during convalescence, that is, 3 to 4 weeks after the acute infection, which corresponds to the peak of the antibody response. A significant rise in antibody titer of two dilutions or more, or 0.2 log if the 0.1 log dilution system is used, is accepted as proof of a recent group A streptococcal infection. Streptococcal antibody tests are generally not used for the diagnosis of an acute infection, in which cultures are usually positive for the streptococcus. Their primary use is in the diagnosis of nonpurulent complications of group A streptococcal infections, such as poststreptococcal glomerulonephritis and acute rheumatic fever. Because these complications occur after a period of latency of 10 to 20 days from the inciting streptococcal infection, throat cultures are negative in most patients.[38] By then, the antibody response is near its peak level, and most patients with these nonpurulent complications should have an elevated antibody titer to one or more of the streptococcal antigens. Performance of antibody tests on a single serum sample obtained at the time of presentation is usually sufficient to document an antecedent streptococcal infection in most patients with acute rheumatic fever. Documentation of a rise in antibody titer on a serum sample obtained at a later interval may be needed in an occasional patient.

Not all group A streptococcal infections lead to an antibody response to all streptococcal antigens. Studies have shown that patients with postimpetigo nephritis have a feeble ASO but a good anti–DNase B response.[39] In contrast, most patients with streptococcal pharyngitis have equally good ASO and anti–DNase B responses. In addition, not all patients with the nonpurulent complications of streptococcal pharyngitis have an ASO or anti–DNase B response. As shown in Table 48–2, 83% of patients with acute rheumatic fever will have an elevated ASO titer during the course of their illness. A similar percentage will have an elevated anti–DNase B titer. A number of those with normal ASO titers, however, will have elevated anti–DNase B titers, so the frequency of an elevated titer to one of these tests rises to about 92%, if both tests are performed on the same serum sample.[36] That is why it is recommended that both tests be performed for a patient with suspected acute rheumatic fever if one of these test responses is normal.

Antibody tests to the cellular components include the type-specific antibody test, which is directed against the M protein, and the antibody to the group A streptococcal carbohydrate, anti–A-CHO. The anti–A-CHO antibody test is of interest because of the unique response of patients with rheumatic mitral insufficiency to this antigen.[36,40–42] Our studies indicate that these patients maintain a high level of this antibody for several years after their acute disease (Fig. 48–2). This contrasts with patients who have rheumatic fever without valvar disease, such as patients with arthritis or Sydenham chorea, or patients who have only transient carditis and valvulitis; these patients experience only a short-lasting rise in this antibody with return of titers to normal within 24 months after the acute illness. Patients with chronic rheumatic mitral insufficiency who have prolonged persistence of the anti–A-CHO do not manifest persistence of antibodies to other streptococcal antigens, such as the ASO or anti–DNase B. The persistence of the anti–A-CHO has been helpful in differentiating rheumatic from nonrheumatic mitral insufficiency in which a history of acute rheumatic fever cannot be documented.

HOST FACTORS

The importance of host factors in determining susceptibility to rheumatic fever was emphasized by the fact that only 2 to 3% of normal individuals acquire rheumatic fever after streptococcal pharyngitis, whereas as many as 75% of individuals who had a prior fever episode of rheumatic fever experience a recurrence of their disease after such an infection.[43] Studies documenting the familial occurrence

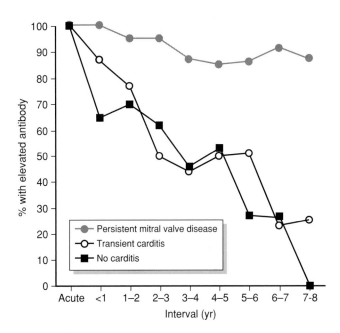

FIGURE 48–2

Persistent elevation of anti–A-CHO in patients with chronic rheumatic mitral insufficiency (persistent carditis). Note decline of this antibody in patients with transient carditis and those with no carditis. (Adapted from Ayoub EM, Shulman ST: Pattern of antibody response to the streptococcal group A carbohydrate in rheumatic patients with or without carditis. *In* Read SE, Zabriskie JB [eds]: Streptococcal Disease and the Immune Response. New York, Academic Press, 1980, pp 649–659.)

of the disease led some investigators to conclude that susceptibility to rheumatic fever was due to a single recessive gene.[44,45] Additional observations that support the role of host prevalence of this disease in certain populations and ethnic groups are discussed earlier.

Studies have provided more concrete evidence for host susceptibility to rheumatic fever. These include the presence of the 8/17 alloantigen on the B cells of more than 95% of patients with rheumatic fever[46] and the association of certain HLA-DR alleles with rheumatic fever (Table 48–3).[47–56] The latter finding is of particular interest in view of current knowledge on the role of HLA-DR antigens in modulating the immune response[57] and is particularly relevant to our observation of the peculiar immune response of patients with rheumatic mitral disease to the streptococcal group A carbohydrate and its association with inheritance of specific HLA-DR alleles, DR4, DR2,

TABLE 48–2

PERCENTAGE OF PATIENTS WITH ACUTE RHEUMATIC FEVER SHOWING AN ELEVATED ANTIBODY TITER*

Group	ASO (%)	Anti–DNase B (%)	ASO and Anti–DNase B (%)
Normal control subjects	19	19	30
Acute rheumatic fever	83	82	92
Sydenham chorea (isolated)	67	40	80

*Results with ASO, anti–DNase B, or both tests.
ASO = antistreptolysin O; DNase B = deoxyribonuclease B.
Adapted from Ayoub EM, Wannamaker LW: Evaluation of the streptococcal deoxyribonuclease B and diphosphopyridine nucleotidase antibody tests in acute rheumatic fever and acute glomerulonephritis. Reproduced with permission from Pediatrics, Vol 29, Page 527, 1962.

TABLE 48–3

SIGNIFICANT ASSOCIATIONS OF HLA-DR ANTIGENS WITH RHEUMATIC FEVER

Study	Location	No. of Patients	Ethnicity	HLA Class II Antigen Association	Percentage Positive	
					Controls	Patients
Ayoub et al[47]	Florida, USA	24	White	DR4	32	63
		48	Black	DR2	23	54
Anastasiou-Nana et al[48]	Utah, USA	33	White	DR4	32	52
Jhinghan et al[49]	New Delhi, India	134	Indian	DR3	26	50
Rajapakse et al[50]	Saudi Arabia	40	Arab	DR4	12	65
Maharaj et al[51]	Durbam, South Africa	120	Black	DR1	3	13
Taneja et al[52]	India	54	Indian	Dqw2	32	63
Guilherme et al[53]	São Paulo, Brazil	40	Brazilian	DR7	26	58
Ozkan et al[54]	Turkey	107	Turkish	DR3	23	49
				DR7	33	57
Weidebach et al[55]	São Paulo, Brazil	24	Brazilian	DR16	34	83
				Drw53		
Ahmed et al[56]	Florida, USA	33	White	DRB1°16	4	15

and DRB1.[47,56] The significance of this association is enhanced by studies in laboratory animals showing that the immune response to the streptococcal group A carbohydrate is genetically controlled.[58–62]

IMMUNOLOGIC MECHANISM OF TISSUE INJURY

Earlier theories regarding the mechanism of tissue injury in rheumatic fever suggested either invasion of tissue by the streptococcus or damage to tissue induced by streptococcal toxins. Attempts to confirm these theories have failed. The period of latency between the inciting infection and the onset of the clinical manifestations of tissue inflammation suggested that an immunologic mechanism may be responsible for the inflammatory reaction that leads to tissue injury. To link such a mechanism with the streptococcal infection, the possibility of antigenic mimicry between the group A streptococcus and host tissue has been investigated. Antigenic cross-reactivity has been found between the streptococcal M protein and cardiac sarcolemma.[61] Additional work confirmed the presence of circulating antibody that reacted with cardiac tissue and antibody deposits in cardiac tissue of patients with rheumatic heart disease.[62] Subsequent studies have reported shared epitopes between other streptococcal components and host tissue, including the streptococcal protoplasmic membrane and cardiac tissue, the group-specific polysaccharide and valvar glycoprotein, the hyaluronate capsule and articular cartilage, and the M protein and neuronal tissue of the caudate and subthalamic nuclei of human brain.[63–67]

On the basis of these findings, tissue injury in rheumatic fever may be due to the formation of reactive antibodies, induced by the streptococcal infection, that cross-react with host tissue. Although such a mechanism would provide a feasible explanation for the pathogenesis of tissue injury in this disease, a number of observations suggested that an alternative mechanism may be involved. If cross-reactive antibody is the mediator of tissue injury, why do patients with streptococcal pharyngitis or poststreptococcal glomerulonephritis who have high levels of these circulating cross-reactive antibodies escape injury to cardiac or neuronal tissue? Furthermore, studies in laboratory ani-

mals showed that antibodies to myosin failed to react with intact heart tissue and that passive transfer of these antibodies did not induce cardiac inflammation.[68] In experimental models of autoimmune myocarditis, adoptive transfer of the disease was accomplished with T cells and not with autoantibodies from affected animals.[69] Additional studies on the potential role of cell-mediated immunity in the pathogenesis of rheumatic fever revealed that peripheral blood mononuclear cells from patients with acute rheumatic carditis were cytotoxic to cultured myocardial cells.[70,71] These observations suggest that the immunologic mechanism involved in tissue damage in rheumatic fever may in fact be cell mediated rather than humoral.

PATHOLOGY

Rheumatic fever shares with other collagen vascular diseases the basic pathologic process of a diffuse vasculitis. Although cardiac involvement may be interpreted as a primary manifestation of this process, *erythema marginatum*, the rash that is characteristic of rheumatic fever, is more representative of the process. The vasculitis in the affected tissues is a proliferation of endothelial cells of small vessels.[72] The other primary organs involved include the joints and the brain. Cardiac inflammation, however, leads to the most characteristic and serious organ involvement in rheumatic fever. In the absence of carditis, rheumatic fever is a self-limited disease.

Cardiac inflammation may involve any of the tissues of the heart. During the acute disease, inflammation of the myocardium predominates. This is associated with inflammation of the endocardium, which may persist chronically, leading to the characteristic changes affecting valve tissue. Isolated pericarditis is rare in acute rheumatic fever, but pericarditis may occur in conjunction with severe myocarditis and often signals the presence of severe pancarditis. The histologic changes associated with cardiac inflammation are nonspecific and do not correlate with the severity of the clinical manifestations of carditis. Early stages of acute carditis are associated with minimal histologic changes. Cardiac dilatation and impairment of ventricular contraction may be most prominent, however, at this stage. Progression of the inflammation leads to more evident exudative and proliferative changes. Edema of the tissue occurs along with cellular infiltration. Lymphocytes and plasma cells predominate, with few granulocytes. The lymphocytes consist of activated CD4$^+$ cells.[73] Fibrin and globulin along with fibrinoid and eosinophilic granular substance that is derived from degenerating collagen are seen in the tissue. Aschoff's body formation, the pathognomonic lesion of rheumatic carditis, follows the acute inflammatory stage.[74] The Aschoff body consists of a perivascular infiltrate of large cells with basophilic cytoplasm and polymorphous nuclei that are arranged in a rosette around an avascular center of fibrinoid. Aschoff's body formation occurs in the subacute and chronic stage of carditis. It may be seen in any area of the myocardium but is most commonly found in the interventricular septum, the wall of the left ventricle, and the left atrial appendage.[72] The presence of Aschoff's bodies is limited to the heart; this lesion is not encountered in other organs.

Inflammation of valve tissue is the hallmark of rheumatic carditis. Rheumatic fever causes 76% of isolated mitral valve disease but only 13% of isolated aortic disease.[75] Multiple cardiac valve involvement represents a rheumatic etiology 97% of the time. Valve inflammation is associated with small, pink fleshy vegetations of platelet origin on the valve edges; they are on the atrial side of the mitral valve and the ventricular side of the aortic valve.

Arthritis and pericarditis are part of serositis in rheumatic fever. The inflammatory process consists of a fibrinous exudate and is associated with degeneration of the synovial lining of the joint. Pathologic changes associated with involvement of the neuronal tissue of the basal ganglia and caudate nuclei in Sydenham chorea consist of cellular degenerative changes and perivascular infiltration by mononuclear cells. Changes in the joints and brain are usually completely reversible.

CLINICAL MANIFESTATIONS

The manifestations of acute rheumatic fever are protean and overlap with a number of other collagen vascular diseases. Jones[76] originally divided the clinical manifestations of acute rheumatic fever into major and minor manifestations on the basis of their relative specificity for the disease. The major manifestations include arthritis, carditis, Sydenham chorea, erythema marginatum, and subcutaneous nodules. A patient with acute rheumatic fever may present with one or more of these manifestations. The minor manifestations, which have been modified repeatedly, are nonspecific. The major and minor manifestations form the basis of the Jones criteria for the diagnosis of an initial attack of acute rheumatic fever (Table 48–4).[77]

MAJOR MANIFESTATIONS

Arthritis

Arthritis is encountered in about 65% of patients with acute rheumatic fever. It is the most common but the least specific of the major manifestations of the disease. Arthritis usually affects the large joints—knees, ankles, wrists,

TABLE 48–4

GUIDELINES FOR THE DIAGNOSIS OF AN INITIAL ATTACK OF RHEUMATIC FEVER*

MAJOR MANIFESTATIONS
Carditis
Polyarthritis
Chorea
Erythema marginatum
Subcutaneous nodules

MINOR MANIFESTATIONS
Clinical
    Arthralgia
    Fever
Laboratory
    Elevated acute-phase reactants
        Elevated white blood cell count
        Erythrocyte sedimentation rate
        C-reactive protein
    Prolonged PR interval

SUPPORTING EVIDENCE OF ANTECEDENT GROUP A STREPTOCOCCAL INFECTION
Elevated or rising streptococcal antibody titer
Positive throat culture or rapid streptococcal antigen test result

*The presence of two major manifestations or of one major and two minor manifestations indicates a high probability of acute rheumatic fever, if supported by evidence of preceding group A streptococcal infection.
Adapted from Dajani AS, Ayoub EM, Bierman FZ, et al: Guidelines for the diagnosis of rheumatic fever: Jones criteria, updated 1992. JAMA 87:302, 1992.

and elbows. Small peripheral joints are rarely involved. The affected joint manifests the cardinal signs of inflammation with pain, swelling, heat, and redness. Pain is present at rest and is accentuated by motion of the joint. The severity of arthritis, however, is variable. Some patients with severe arthritis of the lower extremities may be unable to walk; this presentation has been called pseudoparalysis. Arthritis in acute rheumatic fever is asymmetric and migratory in nature; the migratory nature of arthritis in rheumatic fever is highly characteristic of this disease. A patient may have severe arthritis in a large joint for a few hours that resolves spontaneously and reappears shortly thereafter in another large joint. One characteristic of the arthritis in rheumatic fever is its prompt responsiveness to salicylates. A diagnosis of acute rheumatic fever should be questioned in patients without other major manifestations of the disease and whose arthritis persists for more than 2 to 3 days after initiation of salicylate therapy. Even without salicylate therapy, arthritis of acute rheumatic fever usually resolves after 2 to 3 weeks. If the patient has persistence of arthritis despite salicylate therapy and has evidence of antecedent group A streptococcal infection, the possibility of poststreptococcal reactive arthritis should be considered.[56]

Carditis

Cardiac involvement in acute rheumatic fever is the major cause of serious or prolonged morbidity and mortality due to this disease. Rheumatic heart disease remains the most common cause of acquired heart disease in children and young adults worldwide. About 50% of patients with acute rheumatic fever have cardiac involvement. A higher incidence of carditis was reported from different locations during the 1980s resurgence of rheumatic fever in this country.[10] The high incidence of cardiac involvement in rheumatic fever reported in young children from developing countries is related to the fact that patients with cardiac disease compose the bulk of patients who are brought to the attention of the physician or of children found to have cardiac murmurs during school surveys. Although rheumatic carditis is not uncommon in children younger than 5 years in developing countries, this presentation is rare in Western countries. An insidious form of carditis may be seen occasionally in the United States in children younger than 6 years.[78]

Some physicians regard cardiac involvement and mitral insufficiency as pathognomonic of rheumatic fever. Carditis with mitral valve involvement, however, has been reported in association with Kawasaki disease and after occurrence of rickettsial, viral, and mycoplasmal infections.

The severity of cardiac involvement is variable. Some patients have subtle clinical findings with a soft-grade murmur that could be missed on auscultation, as occurs in patients with Sydenham chorea. Careful examination along with echocardiography is needed to establish the presence of carditis in these patients. On occasion, carditis follows arthritis during the initial presentation of acute rheumatic fever. In such patients, the interval between the onset of arthritis and of carditis rarely exceeds 7 to 10 days. Late-onset carditis probably represents progression of mild carditis that was missed initially on auscultation.

Myocarditis can be clinically detected by tachycardia if the patient is afebrile and resting. Manifestations of myocarditis include an arrhythmia and varying degrees of heart block, which can be confirmed by performing an electrocardiogram. The latter abnormality is common in rheumatic myocarditis and is reflected by a prolonged PR interval. Other signs of rheumatic myocarditis include nonspecific pathologic murmur, particularly that of mitral insufficiency; progressive cardiac enlargement on radiologic examination; and evidence of congestive cardiac failure. The last finding reflects severe carditis, and its occurrence with pericarditis indicates life-threatening pancarditis.

Endocarditis is inflammation of the leaflets and chordae of the valves. Valvulitis is the most common lesion seen in rheumatic carditis, and mitral valve insufficiency is its most characteristic manifestation. Our experience indicates that isolated mitral valve disease occurs in 65% of patients with rheumatic carditis, isolated aortic valve disease occurs in only 6%, and simultaneous involvement of both valves occurs in 29%. Therefore, the mitral valve is affected either alone or in conjunction with other valves in 94% of patients. Involvement of the pulmonic or tricuspid valves is uncommon in rheumatic fever.

Acute valvar disease is associated with insufficiency. Auscultatory signs of mitral valve insufficiency include smooth, high-frequency apical holosystolic murmur, with radiation to the left axilla. More severe mitral insufficiency is associated with a low-frequency, mid-to-late diastolic murmur indicative of relative mitral stenosis. This murmur reflects the turbulence generated by the large volume of blood passing through the mitral valve into the left ventricle during its filling phase. This murmur sounds like the Carey Coombs murmur, which occurs in the absence of mitral incompetence, and is due to turbulence from thickening of the inflamed mitral valve as well as small vegetations on the valve margins. Auscultatory findings indicative of aortic insufficiency include a high-pitched early diastolic murmur that starts with the aortic component of the second heart sound and is loudest over the third intercostal space. It is best heard with the diaphragm of the stethoscope, with the patient in the upright position or leaning forward and holding the breath during expiration. The murmur may be faint or of such high frequency that it is missed. With severe insufficiency of the aortic valve, the murmur becomes louder and is associated with a diastolic thrill. This lesion may be associated with an increased pulse pressure due to the aortic runoff lesion as reflected by bounding peripheral pulses. Mitral or aortic stenosis, other than relative mitral valve stenosis, is uncommon during acute rheumatic fever and develops with chronic valvar disease. Its presence in a patient presenting with acute rheumatic fever should suggest a recurrence of the superimposed damage on a previously existing lesion.

Congestive cardiac failure may accompany severe valvar disease or myocarditis. This complication occurs in about 5% of patients with acute rheumatic heart disease, usually in younger children. Cardiac enlargement may be associated with dilatation of the ventricles from severe myocarditis or may be due to severe hemodynamic changes resulting from valvar disease. Enlargement of the cardiac silhouette can also indicate pericarditis and pericardial effusion. Pericarditis is often associated with a friction rub reflecting the rubbing of the inflamed visceral and parietal pericardial surfaces. The friction rub is a scratching sound, best heard over the midprecordium with the patient in the upright position, and it may disappear with excessive accumulation of pericardial fluid. Pericarditis in patients with acute rheumatic fever is an ominous sign indicative of pancarditis and its associated high mortality. Pericarditis in the absence of endocarditis is usually not due to rheumatic fever.

COURSE OF RHEUMATIC FEVER

The progression of acute carditis into chronic rheumatic heart disease is related to the severity of the carditis and subsequent recurrences of rheumatic fever. The latter factor has been influenced by the institution of antimicrobial prophylaxis to prevent recurrent attacks of rheumatic fever. In a study carried out before the era of prophylaxis, Bland and Jones[79] reported that one fourth of patients who initially had no clinical evidence of cardiac involvement developed rheumatic heart disease on follow-up by the end of 10 years, and 44% developed rheumatic heart disease insidiously at the end of 20 years of follow-up. The majority of the patients had mitral stenosis. Other studies[80–83] have shown that chronic rheumatic heart disease and mitral stenosis are directly related to the frequency of subsequent recurrences of rheumatic fever episodes.

With the advent of prophylaxis, the frequency of chronic rheumatic heart disease became related primarily to the severity of the initial carditis. In a major study[84] regarding the effect of antimicrobial prophylaxis on the evolution of cardiac disease, rheumatic heart disease developed at the end of 5 years in only 4% of the patients who had no carditis initially and in 18% of children with mild carditis initially, but it developed in 70% of patients with severe carditis initially. The influence of prophylaxis on the course of rheumatic heart disease is seen in a study by Tompkins and associates.[85] In this study, the resolution of clinical findings of rheumatic heart disease occurred in 50% of patients during the first 2 years of follow-up and in 70% of patients by the end of 8 to 9 years of follow-up in those patients who were compliant with antimicrobial prophylaxis.

Sydenham Chorea

Also known as St. Vitus' dance, Sydenham chorea represents involvement of the neuronal tissue of the basal ganglia and the caudate nucleus. Sydenham chorea is the third most common major manifestation of acute rheumatic fever. It occurs in about 15% of patients and in recent outbreaks was observed to occur in as many as 30%.[2] Sydenham chorea is unique among the manifestations of acute rheumatic fever in that the period of latency between the streptococcal infection and the onset of the clinical symptoms of chorea ranges between 3 and 6 months and sometimes up to 12 months.

The clinical findings include involuntary and purposeless movements, with muscle incoordination of the extremities. Signs that are characteristic of choreiform activity include hyperextension of the fingers, "spooning" when the arms are extended, pronation of the hands when the arms are raised vertically, irregular contractions of the muscles of the hands when the patient presses the hand of the examiner ("milkmaid's grip"), wavering of the upward stroke when drawing a vertical line, gross fasciculations of the tongue when it is extended ("wormian tongue"), and inability to sustain phonation. A patient will demonstrate clumsiness when asked to perform fine manual tasks, such as buttoning or unbuttoning a shirt. In addition, patients may demonstrate emotional lability, easy frustration, and crying when stressed. The symptoms are often detected first at school because of clumsiness, poor writing, and uncontrollable fidgeting. These manifestations are self-limited and may resolve spontaneously in 2 to 4 weeks but may persist for several months or recur during a few years, even with therapy. Studies suggest that many patients with Sydenham chorea may eventually have obsessive-compulsive behavior.[86]

Erythema Marginatum

This rash occurs in about 5% of patients and is rarely encountered in other illnesses besides acute rheumatic fever. The lesions are macular and consist of an irregular serpiginous erythematous circle surrounding normal skin. The rash changes in size and shape and is often evanescent. It is not pruritic. The rash is on the trunk and the proximal part of the extremities, and it is particularly prominent in those areas where the thighs are in contact. It is rarely, if ever, found on the face. A faint rash can be made more prominent if warmth or friction is applied to the area.

Subcutaneous Nodules

These nodules occur in 2 to 3% of patients but are rarely encountered now. They are seen mostly in patients with chronic rheumatic heart disease, such as patients with valvar stenosis. Subcutaneous nodules are located on the extensor tendons in the extremities and are sometimes seen along the spine. The nodules are freely moveable, are nontender, and have a diameter of about 1 cm.

MINOR MANIFESTATIONS

The minor manifestations are nonspecific clinical and laboratory criteria that are encountered in a variety of conditions and other rheumatologic diseases. The two clinical manifestations are fever and arthralgia. The laboratory findings are abnormal acute-phase reactants, such as an elevated white blood cell count, erythrocyte sedimentation rate, or C-reactive protein level, and a prolonged PR interval on electrocardiography.

DIAGNOSIS

No single laboratory test can establish the diagnosis of acute rheumatic fever. The diagnosis is confirmed by using the Jones criteria (see Table 48–4). Finding two of the major manifestations or one major and two minor manifestations listed in the guidelines provides preliminary confirmation of the diagnosis. The revised Jones criteria listed in Table 48–4 constitute guidelines for the diagnosis of an *initial* attack of acute rheumatic fever. These criteria are not used to confirm a rheumatic etiology in a patient with chronic valvar disease. Note that failure to meet the Jones criteria does not exclude rheumatic fever.

To establish the diagnosis, evidence for antecedent group A streptococcal infection should be provided. This requirement is a sine que non for confirmation of the diagnosis of acute rheumatic fever. Supporting evidence of antecedent group A streptococcal infection can be procured by finding the organism on a throat culture or a rapid streptococcal antigen test. Alternatively, the occurrence of such an infection can be confirmed through serologic tests. Because of the interposed period of latency, most patients with acute rheumatic fever have a negative throat culture because of the elimination of the organism by host defenses.[38] This occurs even when the patient is not treated with antibiotics. In addition, a positive culture or a positive rapid test result may indicate prolonged carriage of the organism and not reflect a recent infection. Because of these limitations, the use of streptococcal antibody tests to provide evidence for antecedent group A streptococcal infection is more reliable. As discussed previously, the streptococcal antibodies are usually at a peak when the patient presents with acute rheumatic fever. A significantly elevated streptococcal antibody titer found in a serum sample obtained at that time provides the necessary evidence for antecedent group A streptococcal infection. To achieve this, an ASO test can be performed on the serum. If the ASO titer is normal, an anti–DNase B or another of the ancillary tests should be performed. If results of both tests are normal, one may opt to obtain another serum sample 2 weeks after the initial one and repeat these tests. Any doubt about the reliability of the results should prompt the physician to solicit help from a reference laboratory for the performance of these and other antibody tests. If the antibody titers remain normal, the diagnosis of acute rheumatic fever should be questioned.

TREATMENT

Patients suspected of having acute rheumatic fever should be hospitalized for evaluation and confirmation of diagnosis, assessment of cardiac status, and appropriate treatment. Laboratory studies should include complete blood

TABLE 48–5

PRIMARY STREPTOCOCCAL ERADICATING AND SECONDARY PROPHYLACTIC ANTIBIOTIC REGIMENS IN RHEUMATIC FEVER

Agent	Dose	Route	Duration
PRIMARY PREVENTION OF RHEUMATIC FEVER			
Benzathine penicillin G	1,200,000 U	Intramuscular	Once every 4 wk
Penicillin V	250 mg tid	Oral	10 days
Erythromycin estolate or ethylsuccinate	40 mg/kg/day (maximum, 1 g/day) in 3 or 4 divided doses	Oral	10 days
SECONDARY PREVENTION OF RHEUMATIC FEVER			
Benzathine penicillin G	1,200,000 U	Intramuscular	Once every 4 wk
Penicillin V	250 mg bid	Oral	Daily
Sulfadiazine	1.0 g once	Oral	Daily
Erythromycin ethylsuccinate	250 mg bid	Oral	Daily

Adapted from Dajani A, Taubert K, Ferrieri P, et al: Committee on Rheumatic Fever, Endocarditis, and Kawasaki Disease of the Council on Cardiovascular Disease in the Young: Treatment of acute streptococcal pharyngitis and prevention of rheumatic fever: A statement for health professionals. Reproduced with permission from Pediatrics, Vol 96, Page 758, 1995.

cell count, erythrocyte sedimentation rate, C-reactive protein measurement, throat culture, and streptococcal antibody tests. If resting tachycardia and cardiac murmurs are present, a chest radiograph, an electrocardiogram, and an echocardiogram should be obtained to assess the degree and severity of myocarditis and valvar disease. Patients with acute arthritis and myocarditis should be placed at bedrest. Confinement to bedrest should be limited to the stage of active myocarditis, but prolonged confinement to bedrest of a patient who has stable rheumatic cardiac disease is unnecessary.

ANTIBIOTIC THERAPY

All patients with acute rheumatic fever should receive, at admission, a course of antibiotics to eradicate streptococci (Table 48–5), even though the throat culture or rapid streptococcal test result is negative. The antibiotic of choice is penicillin. Erythromycin is used in patients who are allergic to penicillin. Alternatively, clindamycin or a first-generation cephalosporin may be used in patients who do not tolerate erythromycin. Sulfa drugs, although effective as prophylactic agents, are ineffective in eradicating the infecting organism and should not be used in patients with acute streptococcal pharyngitis or initially in patients with acute rheumatic fever.

TREATMENT OF ARTHRITIS

The arthritis of acute rheumatic fever is exquisitely sensitive to salicylates. In the absence of carditis, aspirin is given in a dose of 75 mg/kg/day in four divided doses. The dose may be increased to a maximum of 100 mg/kg/day if the response is not satisfactory. This is rarely needed, and a lack of response to this dose should question the diagnosis of acute rheumatic fever. Aspirin therapy is continued for 2 weeks, then tapered and discontinued during the next 2 to 3 weeks.

TREATMENT OF CARDITIS

Mild to moderate carditis can be treated effectively with salicylates in a dose of 80 to 100 mg/kg/day in four divided doses. This treatment should be continued for 4 to 8 weeks, depending on the response of the patient. The dose is then gradually tapered and discontinued during the next 4 weeks. In this interval, it is advisable to determine the salicylate level in the blood once weekly; this level should be maintained between 20 and 30 mg/dl. Liver enzyme abnormalities (alanine transaminase), which would indicate salicylate hepatotoxicity, should be assessed simultaneously, and salicylates should be discontinued if such abnormalities occur. Prednisone is reserved for patients with severe carditis, patients in cardiac failure, and particularly patients with pancarditis; in the patient with pancarditis, prednisone may be lifesaving. In addition to producing a more rapid anti-inflammatory response, the use of prednisone obviates sodium overload associated with administration of salicylates. Prednisone is given in a dose of 2 mg/kg in a single daily morning dose. This dose should rarely be administered for longer than 2 weeks and then be tapered and discontinued during the next 2 to 3 weeks. Aspirin in a dose of 80 to 100 mg/kg/day should be started 1 week before termination of prednisone therapy and administered as outlined in the mentioned regimen to avoid clinical and laboratory rebound.

Therapy for cardiac failure includes digitalis, parenteral inotropic agents (dobutamine, dopamine, or amrinone) or peripheral vasodilators (captopril or enalapril), and diuretics.[87] Digitalis is used with care in patients with acute myocarditis. Digoxin, preferred for children, is given in a total digitalizing dose of 0.02 to 0.03 mg/kg, with a maximal dose of 1.5 mg, and a maintenance dose of one fourth the digitalizing dose. If severe congestive cardiac failure is associated with aortic or mitral valve regurgitation and does not respond to medication, an operation to replace or repair the valve may be lifesaving. This can be done even if the clinical and laboratory features indicate severe acute inflammatory activity.

Acute-phase reactants can be used to monitor the response to therapy. The erythrocyte sedimentation rate can be misleadingly normal in patients in severe congestive cardiac failure. It may rise to higher levels as the patient's congestive cardiac failure resolves. Care should be taken not to misinterpret this rise as an indication of deterioration of the patient's disease. On occasion, the erythrocyte sedimentation rate remains high until the patient ambulates, and then it may fall.

SYDENHAM CHOREA

The manifestations of chorea vary considerably. Mild choreiform activity is self-limited and may be treated with simple rest in a quiet environment and avoidance of stress. More severe chorea has been treated with phenobarbital, 15 to 30 mg every 5 hours, or haloperidol starting with a dose of 0.5 mg every 8 hours and increasing the dose to a maximum of 2.0 mg depending on the response. The effectiveness of these agents has been variable. Valproate, 15 to 20 mg/kg/day, has been reported to be effective in the treatment of Sydenham chorea.[88] Salicylates and steroids are not indicated in patients with isolated Sydenham chorea.

ANTIBIOTIC PROPHYLACTIC THERAPY

Secondary prophylaxis should be given to prevent recurrent streptococcal pharyngitis and recurrences of rheumatic fever.[89] The more recurrences, the greater the risk of chronic valve damage. Separate antibiotic prophylaxis should also be prescribed to prevent infective endocarditis in patients with residual valvar disease.[90] Secondary prophylaxis is administered in the regimens outlined in Table 48–5. The various regimens have been shown to be of varying efficacy in preventing recurrences of streptococcal pharyngitis and rheumatic fever (Fig. 48–3). Because of these differences, monthly injections of long-acting benzathine penicillin, 1.2 million units, are recommended during the first 5 years after the acute episode of rheumatic fever in patients with cardiac involvement. Patients may then be changed to oral prophylaxis. Sulfonamides, although ineffective in streptococcal eradication or primary prevention of rheumatic fever, are effective prophylaxis against recurrence of the disease. Other penicillins and cephalosporins, although effective in eradication of streptococci from the pharynx, have not been tested for efficacy as secondary prophylactic agents.

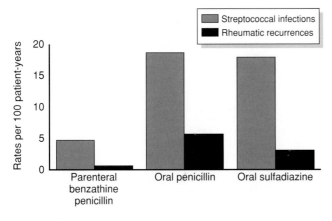

FIGURE 48–3

Rates of group A streptococcal pharyngitis and recurrences of rheumatic fever in patients receiving penicillin and sulfa prophylaxis. (Adapted from Taranta A, Gordis L: The prevention of rheumatic fever: Opportunities, frustrations and challenges. Cardiovasc Clin 4:1, 1972.)

The duration of prophylaxis has been addressed by an American Heart Association committee.[89] Prophylaxis should be continued until the age of 21 years or for a minimum of 5 years in patients who do not have cardiac involvement. Patients with residual rheumatic heart disease should receive prophylaxis for a minimum of 10 years or at least until the age of 40 years, depending on the duration of cardiac disease. Persistence of valvar abnormalities warrants lifelong prophylaxis. This should be continued even after operative repair. The importance of prophylaxis is illustrated in studies that have shown subsequent clinical resolution of cardiac disease in 70 to 80% of patients who were maintained with secondary prophylaxis after their initial episode of acute rheumatic fever.[84] Such information should be conveyed to patients to encourage compliance with prophylaxis.

REFERENCES

1. Stollerman GH: Rheumatogenic group A streptococci and the return of rheumatic fever. Adv Intern Med 35:1, 1990.
2. Ayoub EM: Resurgence of rheumatic fever in the United States. The changing picture of a preventable disease. Postgrad Med 92:133, 1992.
3. Wannamaker LW: Differences between streptococcal infections of the throat and of the skin. N Engl J Med 282:23, 1970.
4. Gordis L, Lilienfeld A, Rodriguez R: Studies in the epidemiology and preventability of rheumatic fever. I. Demographic factors and the incidence of acute attacks. J Chronic Dis 21:645, 1969.
5. Gordis L, Lilienfeld A, Rodriguez R: Studies in the epidemiology and preventability of rheumatic fever. II. Socio-economic factors and the incidence of acute attacks. J Chronic Dis 21:655, 1969.
6. Caughey DE, Douglas R, Wilson W, Hassall IB: HLA antigens in Europeans and Maoris with rheumatic fever and rheumatic heart disease. J Rheumatol 2:319, 1975.
7. Wannamaker LW: Changes and changing concepts in the biology of group A streptococci and in the epidemiology of streptococcal infections. Rev Infect Dis 1:967, 1979.
8. Chun LT, Reddy DV, Yamamoto LG: Rheumatic fever in children and adolescents in Hawaii. Pediatrics 79:549, 1987.
9. Markowitz M: The decline of rheumatic fever: Role of medical intervention. The Lewis W. Wannamaker Memorial Lecture. J Pediatr 106:545, 1985.
10. Veasy LG, Wiedmeier SE, Orsmond GS, et al: Resurgence of acute rheumatic fever in the intermountain area of the United States. N Engl J Med 316:421, 1987.
11. Wald ER, Dashefsky B, Feidt C, et al: Acute rheumatic fever in western Pennsylvania and the tristate area. Pediatrics 80:371, 1987.
12. Congeni B, Rizzo C, Congeni J: Outbreak of acute rheumatic fever in northeast Ohio. J Pediatr 111:176, 1987.
13. Hosier DM, Craenen JM, Teske DW: Resurgence of rheumatic fever. Am J Dis Child 141:730, 1987.
14. Griffiths SP, Gersony WM: Acute rheumatic fever in New York City (1969 to 1988): A comparative study of two decades. J Pediatr 116:882, 1990.
15. Westlake RM, Graham TP, Edwards KM: An outbreak of acute rheumatic fever in Tennessee. Pediatr Infect Dis J 9:97, 1990.
16. Eckerd JM, McJunkin JE: Recent increase in incidence of acute rheumatic fever in southern West Virginia. W V Med J 85:323, 1989.
17. Mason T, Fisher M, Kujala G: Acute rheumatic fever in West Virginia. Arch Intern Med 151:133, 1991.
18. Papadinos T, Escanmilla J, Garst P, et al: Acute rheumatic fever at a Navy training center San Diego, California. MMWR Morb Mortal Wkly Rep 37:101, 1988.
19. Sampson GL, Williams RG, House MD, et al: Acute rheumatic fever among Army trainees—Fort Leonard Wood, Missouri, 1987–1988. MMWR Morb Mortal Wkly Rep 37:519, 1988.
20. Veasy LG, Tani LY, Hill HR: Persistence of acute rheumatic fever in the intermountain area of the United States. J Pediatr 124:9, 1994.
21. Zangwill KM, Wald ER, Londino AV Jr: Acute rheumatic fever in western Pennsylvania: A persistent problem into the 1990s. J Pediatr 118:561, 1991.

22. Loeffler AM, Neches WH, Ortenzo M, et al: Identification of cases of acute rheumatic fever managed on an outpatient basis. Pediatr Infect Dis J 14:975, 1995.

23. Lancefield RC: A serological differentiation of human and other groups of hemolytic streptococci. J Exp Med 57:571, 1933.

24. Kaplan EL, Johnson DR, Cleary PP: Group A streptococcal serotypes isolated from patient and sibling contacts during the resurgence of rheumatic fever in the United States in the mid-1980's. J Infect Dis 159:101, 1989.

25. Johnson DR, Stevens DL, Kaplan EL: Epidemiologic analysis of group A streptococcal serotypes associated with severe systemic infections, rheumatic fever or uncomplicated pharyngitis. J Infect Dis 166:374, 1992.

26. Stevens DL, Tanner MH, Winship J, et al: Severe group A streptococcal infections associated with a toxic shock–like syndrome and scarlet fever toxin A. N Engl J Med 321:1, 1989.

27. Bessen D, Jones KF, Fischetti VA: Evidence for two distinct classes of streptococcal M protein and their relationship to rheumatic fever. J Exp Med 169:269, 1989.

28. Ayoub EM, Kaplan EL: Host-parasite interaction in the pathogenesis of rheumatic fever. J Rheumatol 18(suppl 30):6, 1991.

29. Tomai M, Kotb M, Majundar G, Beachey EH: Superantigenicity of streptococcal M protein. J Exp Med 172:359, 1990.

30. Hauser AR, Stevens DL, Kaplan EL, Schlievert PM: Molecular analysis of pyrogenic exotoxins from *Streptococcus pyogenes* isolates associated with toxic shock syndrome. J Clin Microbiol 29:1562, 1991.

31. Norrby-Teglund A, Newton D, Kotb M: Superantigenic properties of the group A streptococcal exotoxin SpeF (MF). Infect Immun 62:5227, 1994.

32. Mollick JA, Miller GG, Musser JM, et al: A novel superantigen isolated from pathogenic strains of *Streptococcus pyogenes* with aminoterminal homology to staphylococcal enterotoxins B and C. J Clin Invest 92:710, 1993.

33. Stevens DL: Streptococcal toxic-shock syndrome: Spectrum of disease, pathogenesis, and new concepts in treatment. Emerg Infect 1:69, 1995.

34. Todd EW: Antihaemolysin titers in haemolytic streptococcal infections and their significance in rheumatic fever. Br J Exp Pathol 13:248, 1932.

35. Ayoub EM, Wannamaker LW: Evaluation of the streptococcal deoxyribonuclease B and diphosphopyridine nucleotidase antibody tests in acute rheumatic fever and acute glomerulonephritis. Pediatrics 29:527, 1962.

36. Ayoub EM: Streptococcal antibody tests in rheumatic fever. Clin Immunol Newsl 3:107, 1982.

37. Gerber MA, Wright LL, Randolph MF: Streptozyme test for antibodies to group A streptococcal antigens. Pediatr Infect Dis J 6:36, 1987.

38. Ayoub EM: Immune response to group A streptococcal infections. Pediatr Infect Dis J 10(suppl):S15, 1991.

39. Kaplan EL, Anthony BF, Chapman SS, et al: The influence of the site of infection on the immune response to group A streptococci. J Clin Invest 49:1405, 1970.

40. Dudding BA, Ayoub EM: Persistence of streptococcal group A antibody in patients with rheumatic valvular disease. J Exp Med 128:1081, 1968.

41. Ayoub EM, Shulman ST: Pattern of antibody response to the streptococcal group A carbohydrate in rheumatic patients with or without carditis. *In* Read SE, Zabriskie JB (eds): Streptococcal Disease and the Immune Response. New York, Academic Press, 1980, pp 649–659.

42. Appleton RS, Victorica BE, Ayoub EM: Specificity of persistence of antibody to the streptococcal group A carbohydrate in rheumatic valvular heart disease. J Lab Clin Med 105:114, 1985.

43. Rammelkamp CH Jr: Epidemiology of streptococcal infections. Harvey Lect 51:113, 1956.

44. Read SE, Reid H, Poon-King T: HLAs and predisposition to the nonsuppurative sequelae of group A streptococcal infections. Transplant Proc 9:543, 1977.

45. Wilson MG, Schweitzer M: Pattern of hereditary susceptibility in rheumatic fever. Circulation 10:699, 1954.

46. Khanna AK, Buskirk DR, Williams RC, et al: Presence of non-HLA B cell antigen in rheumatic fever patients and their families as defined by a monoclonal antibody. J Clin Invest 83:1710, 1989.

47. Ayoub EM, Barrett DJ, Maclaren NK, Krischer JP: Association of class II human histocompatibility leukocyte antigens with rheumatic fever. J Clin Invest 77:2019, 1986.

48. Anastasiou-Nana MI, Anderson JL, Carlquist JF, Nanas JN: HLA-DR typing and lymphocyte subset evaluation in rheumatic heart disease: A search for immune response factors. Am Heart J 112:992, 1986.

49. Jhinghan B, Mehra NK, Reddy KS, et al: HLA, blood groups and secretor status in patients with established rheumatic fever and rheumatic heart disease. Tissue Antigens 27:172, 1986.

50. Rajapakse CNA, Halim K, Al-Orainey I, et al: A genetic marker for rheumatic heart disease. Br Heart J 58:659, 1987.

51. Maharaj B, Hammond MG, Bronsthapathy A, et al: HLA-A, B, DR, and DQ antigens in black patients with severe chronic rheumatic heart disease. Circulation 76:259, 1987.

52. Taneja V, Mehra NK, Reddy KS, et al: HLA-DR/DQ and reactivity to B cell alloantigen D8/17 in Indian patients with rheumatic heart disease. Circulation 80:335, 1989.

53. Guilherme L, Weidebach W, Kiss MH, et al: Association of human leukocyte class II antigens with rheumatic fever or rheumatic heart disease in a Brazilian population. Circulation 83:1995, 1991.

54. Ozkan M, Carin M, Sonmez G, et al: HLA antigens in Turkish race with rheumatic heart disease. Circulation 87:1974, 1993.

55. Weidebach W, Goldberg AC, Chiarella JM, et al: HLA class II antigens in rheumatic fever: Analysis of the DR locus by restriction fragment polymorphism and oligotyping. Hum Immunol 40:253, 1994.

56. Ahmed S, Ayoub EM, Scornik JC, et al: Poststreptococcal reactive arthritis: Clinical characteristics and association with HLA-DR alleles. Arthritis Rheum 41:1096, 1998.

57. Braciale TJ, Morrison LA, Sweetser MT, et al: Antigen presentation pathways to class I and class II MHC-restricted T lymphocytes. Immunol Rev 98:95, 1987.

58. Eichman K, Kindt TJ: The inheritance of individual antigenic specificity of rabbit antibodies to streptococcal carbohydrate. J Exp Med 134:532, 1971.

59. Klapper DG, Kindt TJ: Idiotypic cross-reactions among anti-streptococcal antibodies in an inbred rabbit population. Scand J Immunol 3:483, 1974.

60. Saszuki T, Kaneoka H, Nishimura Y, et al: An HLA-linked immune suppression gene in man. J Exp Med 152:297S, 1980.

61. Kaplan MH, Meyeserian M: An immunological cross reaction between group A streptococcal cells and human heart tissue. Lancet 1:706, 1962.

62. Kaplan MH, Suchy ML: Immunologic relation to streptococcal and tissue antigens II. Cross reactions of antisera to mammalian heart tissue and the cell wall constituent of certain strains of group A streptococci. J Exp Med 119:643, 1964.

63. Widdowson JP, Maxted WR, Pinney AM: An M-associated protein antigen (MAP) of group A streptococci. J Hyg (Lond) 69:553, 1971.

64. Zabriskie JB, Freimer EH: An immunological relationship between group A streptococci and mammalian muscle. J Exp Med 142:661, 1966.

65. Van de Rijn I, Zabriskie JB, McCarty M: Group A streptococcal antigens cross reactive with myocardium. Purification of heart reactive antibody and isolation and characterization of the streptococcal antigen. J Exp Med 146:579, 1977.

66. Dale JB, Beachey EH: Multiple heart–cross-reactive epitopes of streptococcal M proteins. J Exp Med 161:113, 1985.

67. Husby G, Van de Rijn I, Zabriskie JB, et al: Antibodies reacting with cytoplasm of the subthalamic and caudate nuclei neurons in chorea and acute rheumatic fever. J Exp Med 144:1094, 1976.

68. Neu N, Ploier B, Ofner C: Cardiac myosin–induced myocarditis. J Immunol 145:4094, 1990.

69. Smith SC, Allen PM: The role of T cells in myosin-induced autoimmune myocarditis. Clin Immunol Immunopathol 68:100, 1993.

70. Yang LC, Soprey PR, Wittner MK, et al: Streptococcal induced cell mediated immune destruction of cardiac myofibers in vitro. J Exp Med 146:344, 1977.

71. Hutto J, Ayoub EM: Cytotoxicity of lymphocytes from patients with rheumatic carditis to cardiac cells in vitro. *In* Read SE, Zabriskie JB (eds): Streptococcal Disease and the Immune Response. New York, Academic Press, 1980, pp 733–738.

72. Murphy GE: Nature of rheumatic heart disease. With special reference to myocardial disease and heart failure. Medicine (Baltimore) 39:289, 1960.

73. Raizada V, Williams RC, Chopra P, et al: Tissue distribution of lymphocytes in rheumatic heart valves as defined by monoclonal anti–T cell antibodies. Am J Med 74:90, 1983.
74. Aschoff L: Zur Myocardistisfrage. Dtsch Ges 8:46, 1904.
75. Roberts WC: Anatomically isolated aortic valvular disease; the case against it being of rheumatic etiology. Am J Med 49:151, 1970.
76. Jones TD: The diagnosis of rheumatic fever. JAMA 126:481, 1944.
77. Dajani AS, Ayoub EM, Bierman FZ, et al: Guidelines for the diagnosis of rheumatic fever: Jones criteria, updated 1992. JAMA 87:302, 1992.
78. Markovitz M, Gordis L: Rheumatic Fever. Philadelphia, WB Saunders, 1972, pp 51–60.
79. Bland EF, Jones TD: Rheumatic fever and rheumatic heart disease: A twenty-year report on 1000 patients followed since childhood. Circulation 4:836, 1951.
80. Ash R: The first 10 years of rheumatic infection in childhood. Am Heart J 36:89, 1948.
81. Wilson MG, Lubschez R: Longevity in rheumatic fever. Based on the experience of 1042 children observed over a period of 30 years. JAMA 238:794, 1948.
82. Walsh BJ, Bland EF, Jones TD: Pure mitral stenosis in young persons. Arch Intern Med 65:321, 1940.
83. Thomas GT: Five year follow-up on patients with rheumatic fever treated by bed rest, steroids or salicylate. Br Med J 1:1635, 1961.
84. United Kingdom and United States Joint Report: The evolution of rheumatic heart disease: Five year report of a cooperative clinical trial of ACTH, cortisone and aspirin. Circulation 22:503, 1960.
85. Tompkins DG, Boxerbaum B, Liebman J: Long-term prognosis of rheumatic fever patients receiving regular intramuscular benzathine penicillin. Circulation 45:543, 1972.
86. Swedo SE, Rapoport JL, Cheslow DL, et al: High prevalence of obsessive-compulsive symptoms in patients with Sydenham's chorea. Am J Psychiatry 145:246, 1989.
87. Ayoub EM: Rheumatic Fever. *In* Gessner IH, Victorica BE (eds): Pediatric Cardiology. A Problem Oriented Approach. Philadelphia, WB Saunders, 1993, pp 155–165.
88. Daoud AS, Zaki M, Shaki R, Al-Saleh Q: Effectiveness of sodium valproate in the treatment of Sydenham's chorea. Neurology 40:1140, 1990.
89. Dajani A, Taubert K, Ferrieri P, et al: Committee on Rheumatic Fever, Endocarditis, and Kawasaki Disease of the Council on Cardiovascular Disease in the Young: Treatment of acute streptococcal pharyngitis and prevention of rheumatic fever: A statement for health professionals. Pediatrics 96:758, 1995.
90. Dajani AS, Bisno AL, Chung KJ, et al: Prevention of bacterial endocarditis. Recommendations by the American Heart Association. Circulation 264:2929, 1990.

CHAPTER 49
CARDIOMYOPATHIES

JEFFREY A. TOWBIN

Cardiomyopathies are diseases of the heart muscle. When the term was introduced in 1957, it was used to identify a group of myocardial diseases not attributable to coronary artery disease.[1] The definition has been modified since then and now refers to structural or functional abnormalities of the myocardium that are not secondary to hypertension, valvar or congenital heart disease, or pulmonary vascular disease.

From a functional standpoint, cardiomyopathies are classified[2] into three categories:

1. Dilated cardiomyopathy (DCM), also called congestive cardiomyopathy, in which the left ventricle or both ventricles are enlarged and hypocontractile to variable degrees. Systolic dysfunction is a main clinical feature with resultant signs and symptoms of congestive heart failure.

2. Hypertrophic cardiomyopathies, formerly known as idiopathic hypertrophic subaortic stenosis, are characterized by left ventricular hypertrophy that may be asymmetric. Systolic function is usually preserved. Symptoms may result from left ventricular outflow tract obstruction, diastolic dysfunction, or arrhythmias resulting in sudden death.

3. Restrictive cardiomyopathies are recognized by markedly dilated atria, with generally normal ventricular dimensions and systolic function. Diastolic filling is impaired. Symptoms result from pulmonary and right-sided systemic venous congestion. Syncope may also be a presenting feature.

This chapter reviews the etiology, clinical presentation, diagnosis, management, and long-term outcomes of the three "functional" categories of cardiomyopathy as well as future directions of research and treatment in these disorders.

DILATED CARDIOMYOPATHY

ETIOLOGY

DCM is reported to be the most common form of cardiomyopathy, with an annual incidence of 2 to 8 affected individuals per 100,000 in the United States and Europe and an estimated prevalence of 36 per 100,000 population.[3] Reports of adult patients with DCM and congestive heart failure demonstrated the most common causes to be idiopathic (47%), myocarditis (12%), coronary artery disease (11%), and other identifiable causes in 30%.[3] In two studies of children of varying ages presenting with DCM, 2 to 15% had biopsy-proven myocarditis, whereas 85 to 90% had no cause identified.[4] In a group of 24 children who presented with DCM before the age of 2 years, 45% had myocarditis, 25% had endocardial fibroelastosis, and the remainder had no cause identified.[5] Familial forms of DCM have also been described in as many as 20 to 30% of patients having DCM.[6,7]

Autosomal dominant transmission is the most frequent inheritance pattern in familial DCM (FDCM).[6–9] Autosomal recessive, X-linked, and mitochondrial inheritance patterns have also been described.[8,9] Although no specific gene or gene product has been identified for autosomal dominant DCM, several studies suggest that HLA-DR4 and HLA-DQB1 loci on chromosome 6 may be genetic markers for susceptibility to DCM.[10,11] A possible correlation between autoimmunity and the development of cardiomyopathy exists because genetic control of portions of the immune system may be located in that region.[12,13] Several immune regulatory abnormalities have been identified in DCM, including humoral and cellular autoimmune reactivity against myocytes, decreased natural killer cell activity, and abnormal suppressor cell activity, thus suggesting that immune defects may be important etiologic factors in the development of DCM.[14] Despite the apparent association between HLA loci, the immune system, and DCM, further research is necessary to prove that these are involved in causing some forms of DCM.

To date, five genes have been mapped to chromosomal positions in families with autosomal dominant FDCM. In addition, two genes have been localized for X-linked DCM (XLCM). Towbin and colleagues[15] mapped the gene responsible for XLCM, a rapidly progressive disorder of teenage boys, to Xp21 within the dystrophin locus. Abnormalities of the dystrophin gene are known to cause Duchenne's and Becker's muscular dystrophies, both of which are skeletal muscle disorders with associated DCM. Multiple causative mutations in XLCM have been described.[16–18] Barth's syndrome (cardioskeletal myopathy), a second XLCM that presents in male infants, has been localized to Xq28.[19] Barth's syndrome is usually rapidly fatal and presents in early infancy with DCM, skeletal muscle disease, neutropenia, 3-methylglutaconic aciduria, and abnormal mitochondria.[20] The gene, G4.5, has been identified, and mutations have been described.[21] Other metabolic, toxic, and infectious causes of DCM are listed in Table 49–1.[9,10,22,23]

TABLE 49–1

CAUSES OF DILATED CARDIOMYOPATHY

FAMILIAL DILATED CARDIOMYOPATHY	**SENSITIVITY/TOXIC REACTIONS**
Cardioskeletal myopathy, X-linked (Barth's syndrome)	Sulfonamides
Familial idiopathic dilated cardiomyopathy	Penicillin
X-linked cardiomyopathy (XLCM)	Anthracyclines
Familial conduction defect with dilated cardiomyopathy	Chloramphenicol
Arrhythmogenic right ventricular dysplasia	Alcoholic cardiomyopathy
	Hemochromatosis
GENERAL SYSTEM DISEASES	
Systemic lupus erythematosus	**METABOLIC**
Juvenile rheumatoid arthritis	*Endocrine*
Polyarteritis nodosa	Thyrotoxicosis
Kawasaki disease	Hypothyroidism
	Diabetic cardiomyopathy
TACHYARRHYTHMIAS	Hypoglycemia
Supraventricular tachycardia	Pheochromocytoma
Atrial flutter	Neuroblastoma
Ventricular tachycardia	Catecholamine cardiomyopathy
	Hypocalcemia
INFECTIOUS MYOCARDITIS	Hypophosphatemia
Viral	*Familial Storage Disease*
Bacterial	Glycogen storage disease
Fungal	Type IV (Andersen's)
Protozoal	Type V (McArdle's)
Rickettsial	Type VI (Hers')
Spirochetal	Mucopolysaccharidoses
	Hurler's syndrome (type I)
HEREDOFAMILIAL DISORDERS	Sanfilippo's syndrome (type III)
Muscular dystrophies/myopathies	Morquio's syndrome (type IV)
Duchenne's and Becker's muscular dystrophies	Maroteaux-Lamy syndrome (type VI)
Emery-Dreifuss muscular dystrophy	Sphingolipidoses
Myotonic dystrophy (Steinert's)	Niemann-Pick disease
Limb-girdle muscular dystrophy (Erb's)	Farber's disease
Autosomal recessive muscular dystrophy	Gaucher's disease
Kugelberg-Welander spinal muscular atrophy	Tay-Sachs disease
Nemaline myopathy	G_{M1} gangliosidosis
Myotubular (centronuclear) myopathy	Sandhoff's disease (G_{M2})
Minicore-multicore myopathy	Refsum's disease
	Nutritional
MITOCHONDRIAL SYNDROMES	Kwashiorkor (protein deficiency)
Kearns-Sayre	Beriberi (thiamine deficiency)
MELAS	Selenium deficiency
NADH–coenzyme Q reductase deficiency	Carnitine deficiency
MERRF	β-Ketolase deficiency
Left ventricular noncompaction	Hypertaurinuria
	Acyl-CoA dehydrogenase deficiency
CONGENITAL CARDIOVASCULAR DISEASE	Propionicacidemia
Critical aortic stenosis of infancy	
Anomalous left coronary artery	**OTHER**
Ebstein anomaly	Hemolytic-uremic syndrome
Postoperative congenital heart disease	Reye's syndrome
Arteriovenous malformation	Peripartum cardiomyopathy
	Osteogenesis imperfecta

MELAS = mitochondrial encephalomyopathy, lactic acidosis, and stroke-like symptoms; MERRF = myoclonus epilepsy with ragged red fibers.

PATHOLOGY

On inspection of the heart, the chief morphologic feature is biventricular dilatation; the atria are generally enlarged as well.[23] Mural thrombi may be present in the cardiac chambers. The heart is globular; the myocardium is pale and sometimes mottled. The endocardium is usually thin and translucent[24]; however, focal sclerosis may be seen. The heart weight is increased, indicating hypertrophy, and the coronary arteries are normal.

Histologic features classically include myocyte hypertrophy and degeneration; varying degrees of interstitial fibrosis are seen.[23, 25] Occasional small clusters of lympho-

cytes may be present[26]; if so, it is necessary to differentiate this disorder from myocarditis, in which the lymphocytes are associated with areas of myocyte damage and necrosis.[27] Nonspecific ultrastructural changes in the mitochondria, T tubules, and Z bands have been described by electron microscopy.

PATHOPHYSIOLOGY

Abnormally depressed contractile function manifests as decreased shortening fraction, ejection fraction, and cardiac output. This decline in forward flow parameters results in pooling of intracavitary blood and a secondary increase in end-diastolic volume, end-diastolic pressure, and ventricular filling pressure.[23] To maintain an adequate cardiac output, the ventricles dilate and the myocardium hypertrophies to some degree. The dilatation results in increased wall tension, thereby increasing oxygen consumption and decreasing myocardial efficiency. As cardiac output diminishes, renal blood flow decreases. These features typically progress slowly, and therefore increases in atrial and venous compliance result in mild pulmonary edema and systemic venous congestion. In children with acute decompensation, significant pulmonary edema and systemic venous congestion occur.

In association with the limitation of ventricular pumping, neurohumoral mechanisms are increasingly activated, particularly the renin-angiotensin system and sympathetic nervous system. Activation of these systems contributes to peripheral vascular changes and the full-blown clinical picture of congestive heart failure.

Fibrosis of the ventricular myocardium may occur, resulting in an irritable focus that causes ventricular arrhythmias[28] as well as worsening of systolic function and diastolic dysfunction.

CLINICAL PRESENTATION

When an adequate cardiac output cannot be maintained, signs and symptoms of congestive heart failure develop.[28–30] Symptoms and signs may be subtle initially. Children or parents may notice decreasing exercise tolerance and dyspnea with exertion. In infants, this may be manifested as tachypnea that is more pronounced with feeding, resulting in decreased oral intake and failure to thrive. Palpitations and syncope or near-syncope may be reported in up to 13% of children.[28] Obtaining a thorough family history and echocardiograms from first-degree relatives is important to verify whether familial inheritance occurs. Signs and symptoms may be unmasked by a superimposed infectious illness that results in further cardiac decompensation.

PHYSICAL EXAMINATION

As with symptoms, there can be a wide spectrum of findings on physical examination.[28–30] Griffin and coworkers[31] reported that 70 to 80% of patients present with signs of congestive heart failure. Tachypnea and tachycardia are frequent. The skin may appear pale. Cyanosis is uncommon unless circulatory collapse is imminent. Peripheral pulses are often weak with normal to low blood pressure and a narrow pulse pressure. The extremities may be cool with decreased peripheral perfusion.

Auscultation of the lungs may reveal diminished breath sounds posteriorly on the left if there is compression atelectasis from the enlarged heart. Rales may occasionally be heard in this area in association with the atelectasis, but otherwise rales are rare in infants and small children even in the face of pulmonary edema on chest radiography. Mild to marked intercostal retractions may be present.

Evaluation of the heart usually reveals a displaced apical impulse. The heart sounds may be muffled, and a prominent diastolic filling sound that produces a gallop rhythm (S_3) may be heard. Murmurs may be absent, but

mitral regurgitation (due to a dilated mitral valve annulus or papillary muscle dysfunction) may be heard.

Examination of the abdomen commonly reveals hepatomegaly. Other signs of systemic venous congestion include neck vein distention and peripheral edema, which are more common in the older child or young adult than in infants.

DIAGNOSTIC STUDIES

Radiography

Chest films typically reveal cardiomegaly due to left atrial and left ventricular enlargement. Pulmonary venous congestion is often present and may progress to frank pulmonary edema (Fig. 49–1). Atelectasis of the lower lobe of the left lung may occur because of compression of the left main stem bronchus by the dilated left atrium. Pleural effusions may be present.

Electrocardiography and Holter Monitoring

The electrocardiogram in most patients shows sinus tachycardia. Nonspecific ST-T wave changes, left ventricular hypertrophy, right and left atrial enlargement, and right ventricular hypertrophy are common.[28–30] Friedman and associates[28] found arrhythmias in 46% of the children with DCM who underwent Holter monitoring, with atrial arrhythmias being more common than ventricular arrhythmias. Greenwood and colleagues,[30] however, reported ventricular arrhythmias to be more common than atrial arrhythmias.

Echocardiography

Echocardiographic features of DCM include dilatation of the left ventricle and left atrium with a decreased shortening fraction and ejection fraction,[23] decreased mean circumferential fiber shortening, and increased ratio of left ventricular pre-ejection period to ejection time (PEP/LVET).[32,33]

By two-dimensional echocardiography, global cardiac hypocontractility is usually seen; regional wall motion ab-

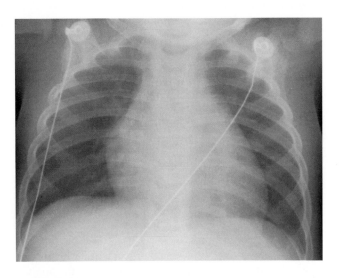

FIGURE 49–1

Chest film of a young child with dilated cardiomyopathy. The cardiac size is enlarged (cardiomegaly) with mildly congested lung markings.

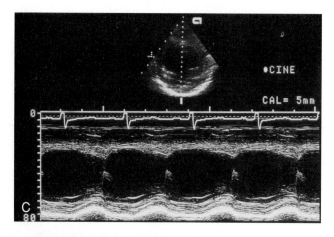

M-mode imaging shows the dilated left ventricle and poor fractional shortening. The parasternal short-axis two-dimensional echocardiographic frame being measured is seen above the M-mode image.

normalities are less common. The coronary artery origins should be identified to exclude anomalous left coronary artery arising from the pulmonary artery as the cause of cardiac dysfunction. Pericardial effusion may be present, and intracardiac thrombi have been reported in as many as 23% of children.[29] Color and pulse Doppler echocardiography frequently demonstrate mitral regurgitation (Fig. 49–2). Decreased aortic flow velocity from diminished cardiac output and abnormal mitral inflow patterns due to diastolic dysfunction may be seen.

Cardiac Catheterization and Biopsy

Because DCM can be diagnosed by echocardiography, cardiac catheterization, angiography, and biopsy are deferred in some centers until the patient has become stabilized. Catheterization can be useful (1) to exclude anomalous left coronary artery because this may be missed by echocardiography, (2) to predict etiology and prognosis if the biopsy shows myocarditis or metabolic abnormalities, or (3) to evaluate for cardiac transplantation.

Hemodynamic measurements generally reveal elevated left ventricular end-diastolic, left atrial, and pulmonary capillary wedge pressures; cardiac output is usually diminished. Angiography demonstrates left ventricular dilatation and reduced ejection fraction, normal coronary artery origins and course, and mitral regurgitation.

In DCM, endomyocardial biopsy typically shows variable degrees of myocyte hypertrophy and fibrosis, without significant lymphocytic infiltrate. Biopsies can be useful for detecting myocarditis as well as mitochondrial or infiltrative diseases,[9, 34–36] either by histologic examination[25–27] or polymerase chain reaction.[37, 38] This may have a significant impact on prognosis and treatment.[39]

Blood and Urine Studies

In infants and young children, other studies may be helpful to identify the etiology. Examination of urine for organic and amino acids[36, 40] may be useful, particularly if 3-methylglutaconic aciduria is found (i.e., Barth's syndrome).[20] Blood studies for lactate, calcium, magnesium,

carnitine/acylcarnitine, pyruvate, urea (blood urea nitrogen), creatinine, and electrolyte determinations are useful. Molecular analysis for dystrophin mutations and *G4.5* mutations may also be diagnostic.[8, 9]

MOLECULAR GENETICS

The only genes thus far identified in FDCM are those for two X-linked disorders, Barth's syndrome and XLCM. In Barth's syndrome, the gene *G4.5*, a novel gene located at Xq28, has been identified as the disease-causing gene.[21] This gene encodes a novel protein group known as tafazzins, named after a masochistic comic character from an Italian television sports show. These proteins appear to be important in myocyte membrane stabilization. Mutations resulting in truncated proteins have been found.

Towbin and coworkers[15] described the association of dystrophin abnormalities and XLCM. Dystrophin, the abnormal protein causing Duchenne's and Becker's muscular dystrophies, is a membrane-stabilizing protein that attaches an integral membrane glycoprotein complex; when mutated, this defective protein causes a wide spectrum of skeletal muscle and cardiac dysfunction.[8, 9] Multiple mutations in dystrophin have been identified in XLCM patients, particularly mutations in the 5' end of the gene.[16–18]

Genes for autosomal dominant FDCM have been localized. Four genes for a pure form of FDCM have been localized to chromosomes 9q13-q22,[41] 1q32,[42] 10q21-q23,[43] and 2q31.[43a] In the family mapped to 10q21-q23, mitral valve prolapse was associated with DCM. Two genes have also been localized for autosomal dominant DCM with conduction defects. Kass and associates[44] mapped a gene to 1p1-q1, and Olson and Keating[45] found linkage at 3p22-p25. These genes remain elusive. However, mutations in actin (chromosome 15q14)[45a] have been identified.

Other genetic forms of DCM have also been analyzed at the molecular level.[22, 36, 40] Deficiencies of enzymes required for efficient myocardial fatty acid β-oxidation have been described, including abnormalities in the plasma membrane carnitine transporter CPTII (carnitine palmitoyltransferase), carnitine/acylcarnitine translocase deficiency, long-chain 3-hydroxyacyl-CoA dehydrogenase deficiency, and very long chain acyl-CoA dehydrogenase deficiency.

DIFFERENTIAL DIAGNOSIS

The causes of DCM are varied (see Table 49–1), and the differential diagnosis is age dependent (Table 49–2). In infants and young children, the causes of DCM are typically more severe than in older children and adults and more frequently include other systemic abnormalities.

TREATMENT

Medical

If no identifiable and treatable cause of the DCM is found, therapy typically is supportive and consists of an anticongestive regimen, control of significant arrhythmias, and minimizing the risk of thromboembolic complications. Children who present critically ill frequently require intubation and mechanical ventilation.

TABLE 49–2

DILATED CARDIOMYOPATHY: DIFFERENTIAL DIAGNOSIS BASED ON AGE

<1 Year Old	>1 Year Old, <10 Years Old	>10 Years Old
Myocarditis	Familial dilated cardiomyopathy (autosomal dominant)	Familial dilated cardiomyopathy (autosomal dominant)
Endocardial fibroelastosis	Barth's syndrome	X-linked dilated cardiomyopathy
Barth's syndrome	Myocarditis	Myocarditis
Carnitine deficiency	Arrhythmogenic right ventricular dysplasia	Supraventricular tachycardia
Selenium deficiency	Endocardial fibroelastosis	Congenital heart disease (e.g., Ebstein's)
Anomalous left coronary artery from pulmonary artery	Carnitine deficiency	Postoperative congenital heart disease
Kawasaki disease	Selenium deficiency	Mitochondrial cardiomyopathy
Critical aortic stenosis	Anomalous left coronary artery from pulmonary artery	Chagas' disease
Supraventricular tachycardia	Kawasaki disease	Arrhythmogenic right ventricular dysplasia
Arteriovenous malformation (especially vein of Galen)	Supraventricular tachycardia	Eosinophilic cardiomyopathy
Calcium deficiency	Toxicity (doxorubicin)	Toxicity (doxorubicin)
Hypoglycemia	β-Ketothiolase deficiency	Pheochromocytoma
Left ventricular noncompaction	Ipecac toxicity	Duchenne's and Becker's muscular dystrophies
Mitochondrial cardiomyopathy	Systemic lupus erythematosus	Emery-Dreifuss muscular dystrophy
Nemaline myopathy	Polyarteritis nodosa	Hemochromatosis
Minicore-multicore myopathy	Hemolytic-uremic syndrome	Limb-girdle muscular dystrophy
Myotubular myopathy	Mitochondrial cardiomyopathy	Myotonic dystrophy
	Nemaline myopathy	Peripartum cardiomyopathy
	Minicore-multicore myopathy	Alcoholic cardiomyopathy
	Myotubular myopathy	

Intravenous inotropic support is used to improve cardiac function and output during episodes of decompensation. The mainstays of therapy have been dobutamine and dopamine.[46] Dopamine is begun in renal doses to enhance renal perfusion and diuresis. Myocardial phosphodiesterase inhibitors, such as amrinone or milrinone,[47] possess positive inotropic effects, have afterload-reducing properties, and improve left ventricular relaxation. They are useful when a combination of these effects is desired. Nitroprusside can also be used for afterload reduction but may have a greater blood pressure effect.

When the patient is well enough to begin oral medications, digoxin is usually instituted as intravenous inotropic agents are weaned. Oral captopril or enalapril should also be started as intravenous afterload-reducing agents are being decreased. β-Adrenergic blocking agents have been used in adults[48] and may become useful in children.

Diuretic therapy is used to enhance diuresis and is given intravenously initially to patients requiring inpatient therapy. Electrolytes should be monitored closely, because the combination of multiple drugs, poor myocardial function, and electrolyte imbalances may produce significant arrhythmias. Diuretic therapy can be changed to the oral route when the signs of pulmonary and systemic venous congestion have decreased and the likelihood of good absorption from oral therapy has increased.

Arrhythmias are common in children with DCM.[28–30] Sometimes all the treatment that is required is medical management of congestive heart failure to improve cardiac function and normalization of electrolyte imbalances. If significant arrhythmias persist, antiarrhythmic therapy is warranted. Many antiarrhythmic drugs adversely affect ventricular function and may be proarrhythmic. These factors must be taken into account in choosing antiarrhythmic therapy. For maintenance therapy of significant arrhythmias, amiodarone is effective and relatively safe in children.[49] If symptomatic bradyarrhythmias occur, temporary pacing may be necessary during the acute phase of illness.

Permanent pacing occasionally may be necessary.[50] Elective pacing to optimize atrioventricular synchrony and ventricular filling is investigational.

The utility of immunosuppressive agents in DCM, including steroids, cyclosporine, and azathioprine, remains unproven.[51]

Intracavitary thrombus formation and systemic embolization have been reported in young patients with DCM, and anticoagulation should be considered. If a thrombus is identified, patients are usually anticoagulated with heparin and then switched to warfarin. If a thrombus is not seen, antiplatelet drugs (aspirin, dipyridamole) may be useful in preventing thrombus formation.

In children with a metabolic cause of DCM, careful attention to biochemical derangement is important.[36] Correction of metabolic acidosis and diagnosis of the underlying cause are paramount. Oral feeding should be discontinued until stabilization has occurred. Intravenous fluid and dextrose replacement should be considered to provide energy and reduce the ongoing catabolic process.

Surgical

Despite maximal medical therapy, some patients continue to deteriorate. Children with acute and severe decompensation may require therapy with a ventricular assist device, intra-aortic balloon counterpropulsion, or extracorporeal membrane oxygenation.

Because some patients are not suitable transplant candidates, additional operative options are being investigated to support the failing heart. Dynamic cardiomyoplasty, a procedure in which the latissimus dorsi muscle is wrapped around the heart and electrically stimulated to synchronize with cardiac contraction, was first used clinically in 1985.[52] The left ventricular remodeling procedure developed by Dr. Randas Batista in Brazil has recently been attempted in adult patients with some success. This procedure includes removing a wedge of left ventricular myocardium to decrease the left ventricular size to improve function.

What role these procedures will have in the management of end-stage DCM in children requires further studies.

PROGNOSIS

In infants and children presenting with DCM, there are four possible outcomes[4,5,28–31,53]: complete resolution, improvement, death, and requirement for cardiac transplantation or other surgical option. Review of the available studies in children suggests that approximately one third die, one third improve but have some residual cardiac dysfunction, and one third recover completely. In children, 1-year survival ranges from 63 to 70%, 5-year survival from 34 to 66%; 10- to 11-year survival is 50%. Mortality is highest during the first 1 to 2 years after presentation.

Congestive heart failure is the most common cause of death, although sudden death also occurs. The time from presentation to approximately 6 months after diagnosis appears most critical in terms of defining outcome. In those who are going to recover or improve, signs of improvement are generally seen during the initial 6 months, although continued improvement may be seen for as long as 2 years. The first 6 months is also the time frame in which most deaths occur, with survival declining gradually thereafter. Although isolated prognostic indicators are difficult to identify, the persistence of signs and symptoms of congestive heart failure despite maximal medical therapy, and persistently low functional parameters on echocardiography (including ejection fraction and fractional shortening), should prompt the consideration of cardiac transplantation sooner rather than later.[33]

FUTURE DIRECTIONS

Diagnosis

The future advances in the diagnosis of FDCM are likely to come as a result of the molecular genetic understanding of this disease. As the genes responsible for FDCM become known and mutations are identified, genetic testing could become available. Analysis of individuals with DCM by mutation screening and polymerase chain reaction for viruses should better enable etiologic diagnosis to be reached in a larger number of children. Furthermore, the development of the recently funded National Institutes of Health Pediatric Cardiomyopathy Registry should enable clinicians to interact to evaluate children in a standard way.

Therapy

The left ventricular remodeling operation could add another dimension to the operative treatment of children with DCM, thereby avoiding early transplantation. In addition, the development of small assist devices could become reality, allowing stabilization of critically ill children. Finally, the potential use of β-blockers as medical therapy for children with DCM is on the horizon and could add another therapeutic agent to the clinical armamentarium.

MYOCARDITIS

Myocarditis is characterized by inflammatory infiltration of the myocardium associated with necrosis or degeneration of adjacent myocytes not typical of the ischemic damage

TABLE 49–3

INFECTIOUS CAUSES OF MYOCARDITIS

VIRAL	BACTERIAL
Adenovirus	Diphtheria
Enterovirus	Meningococcal
Coxsackievirus A	Pneumococcal
Coxsackievirus B	Gonococcal
Echovirus	**FUNGAL**
Cytomegalovirus	Candidiasis
Herpes simplex virus	Aspergillosis
Epstein-Barr virus	**PROTOZOAL**
Mumps virus	American trypanosomiasis (Chagas' disease)
Rubella virus	
Rubeola virus	Toxoplasmosis
Parvovirus	**SPIROCHETAL**
Influenza virus	Lyme disease
Human immunodeficiency virus	**RICKETTSIAL**
Hepatitis C virus	Rocky Mountain spotted fever
MYCOPLASMA	
Mycoplasma pneumoniae	

associated with coronary artery disease.[27,39] The underlying cause of myocarditis may be infectious, toxic, associated with connective tissue disorders, or other processes (see Table 49–1). The most common infectious etiology is viral, and many different viruses have been associated with myocarditis (Table 49–3). It is believed that myocarditis is a significant cause of idiopathic DCM.[54]

EPIDEMIOLOGY

Although epidemics have been reported, the disease is usually sporadic.[55,56] Coxsackievirus B has been most commonly reported as the causal agent, although culturing virus from the heart has been achieved only rarely. The spread of coxsackievirus B is by the fecal-oral or airborne route and is most common in the spring and summer but may be seen year-round. Young children, particularly infants, are most commonly affected. More recently, adenovirus has been shown to be a common cause of myocarditis in children.[38] Adenovirus infections occur sporadically throughout the year as well as in epidemics during winter, spring, and early summer.[56]

CLINICAL PRESENTATION

Children most commonly present with acute myocarditis, a disorder heralded by signs and symptoms of congestive heart failure that may rapidly lead to cardiovascular collapse.[56] Infants usually are pale and clammy, are irritable or somnolent, and have increasingly uncomfortable respiratory effort. On examination, they are tachypneic and tachycardic at rest. The cardiac examination demonstrates a gallop rhythm, and a mitral regurgitant murmur may be heard at the apex. The pulses are typically thready, and perfusion appears to be poor. Commonly, there is a modest degree of hepatomegaly. Rales are usually absent in small children. Older children generally present with breathlessness and signs of heart failure. Syncope may occur.

Children may give a history of recent viral-type illness, although a significant number of patients have not been ill. Infectious contacts may or may not be known.

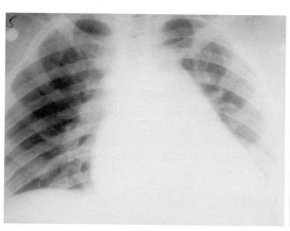
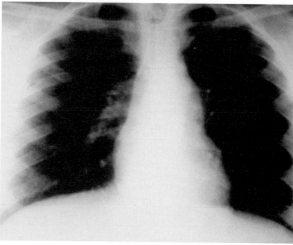

FIGURE 49–3

Chest radiographs obtained from a child with histopathologic evidence of myocarditis. The left panel demonstrates severe cardiomegaly and pulmonary vascular congestion. The right panel, which was obtained 3 months later, demonstrates normal cardiopericardial silhouette size and normal pulmonary vascular markings consistent with resolution of the child's cardiac dysfunction.

DIAGNOSTIC STUDIES

Chest Radiography

Cardiomegaly and pulmonary venous engorgement, with or without evidence of pneumonitis, are common. If the child improves with time and therapeutic intervention, the chest radiograph becomes normal (Fig. 49–3).

Electrocardiography

Classically, the surface electrocardiogram demonstrates low voltage of the QRS complexes in the limb leads (<5 mm total amplitude) with inverted T waves and absent or small Q waves in leads V_5 and V_6. Sinus tachycardia is the rule, although bradycardia may be evident. Premature ventricular complexes and supraventricular tachycardia have been reported to be the most common rhythm disturbances, although ventricular tachycardia[57,58] and complete atrioventricular block[56] also occur.

Echocardiography

The echocardiogram demonstrates left ventricular dilatation and depressed ventricular function. The atria (particularly the left atrium) may also appear mildly dilated. A pericardial effusion may be found. Doppler and color Doppler evaluation may demonstrate mitral regurgitation (Fig. 49–4).

Cardiac Catheterization and Endomyocardial Biopsy

Hemodynamic evaluation typically shows elevated ventricular end-diastolic pressures and reduced cardiac index.

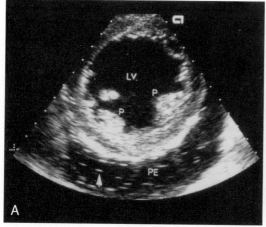
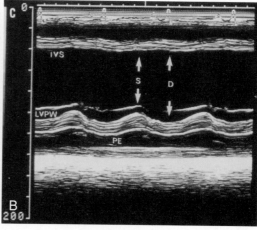

FIGURE 49–4

A, Parasternal short-axis view showing the dilated left ventricle (LV) cavity and pericardial effusion (PE). The two papillary muscles (P) are also shown. B, M-mode image obtained from the echocardiographic view shown in A. Note the interventricular septum (IVS), left ventricular posterior wall (LVPW), and pericardial effusion (PE). The left ventricular end-diastolic dimension (D) and end-systolic dimension (S) are measured to determine the shortening fraction, which is poor.

TABLE 49–4

DALLAS CRITERIA

General definition	Myocardial cell injury with degeneration or necrosis with inflammatory infiltrate not due to ischemia
Active myocarditis	Both myocyte degeneration or necrosis and definite cellular infiltrate with or without fibrosis
Borderline myocarditis	Definite cellular infiltrate without myocyte injury
Persistent myocarditis	Continued active myocarditis on repeated right ventricular endomyocardial biopsy
Resolving/resolved myocarditis	Diminished or absent infiltrate with evidence of connective tissue healing

Endomyocardial biopsy is used for histopathologic evaluation by light microscopy and electron microscopy, culture, and molecular analysis. Histopathologic analysis typically follows the Dallas criteria (Table 49–4), which rely on the amount of lymphocytic infiltrate, fibrosis, myocyte necrosis, and edema (Fig. 49–5).[27] Unfortunately, this approach yields a diagnosis in only 50% of patients.[59,60]

Viral Culture and Serology

Viral, bacterial, and fungal cultures are usually obtained from nasopharyngeal and stool specimens as well as from the myocardium. Blood cultures are generally useless for viral diagnosis because the virus is usually cleared before clinical presentation. If the culture is positive from peripheral sites, a presumptive etiologic diagnosis may be rendered. Serologic identification requires a four-fold increase in antibody titers on serial analysis.

Molecular Methods

In the 1980s, Bowles and colleagues[61] first described the use of in situ hybridization studies using probes designed to sequences of coxsackievirus to analyze myocardium.

They were able to show a high percentage of hybridization-positive samples (up to 50%) and suggested that coxsackievirus was indeed a common cause of myocarditis. In addition, they were able to show coxsackievirus probe hybridization in patients with idiopathic DCM and inferred that previous subclinical infection resulted in the cardiomyopathy.[61,62]

More recently, polymerase chain reaction has been used to analyze endomyocardial biopsy and autopsy specimens for viral sequences.[38,63,64] This rapid amplification process is highly sensitive and has been shown to identify coxsackieviral and adenoviral sequences in up to 30 to 50% of myocardial specimens studied (Fig. 49–6).

THERAPY

Patients with myocarditis and congestive heart failure require standard anticongestive therapy. If the patient is acutely ill, therapy should be given by the intravenous route and consists of dobutamine, low-dose dopamine to improve renal perfusion, afterload-reducing agents such as milrinone, and diuretics. Intubation and mechanical ventilation may be necessary as well. In rare instances, ventricular assist devices or intra-aortic balloon pump may be needed for circulatory support. In more stable patients, oral therapy with digoxin, afterload-reducing agents such as captopril or enalapril, and diuretics are used.

Therapy for treatment of the inflammatory response is controversial. Some centers advocate the use of steroids, whereas others use immunosuppressive agents such as cyclosporine or azathioprine.[65,66] More recently, intravenous immunoglobulin has been used.[67] Results have been mixed.

FUTURE DIRECTIONS

Diagnosis

Polymerase chain reaction is currently available in a small number of laboratories but will become available commercially, thereby enabling clinicians to evaluate children with

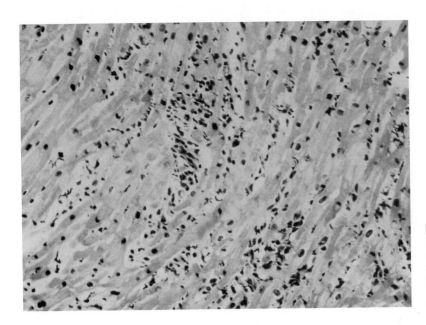

FIGURE 49–5

Histologic appearance of lymphocytic myocarditis in this right ventricular endomyocardial biopsy specimen obtained from the child with new-onset heart failure whose chest radiograph is seen in Figure 49–3. Note the lymphocytic inflammatory infiltrate and myocyte necrosis.

Paraffin-fixed Cardiac Tissue Adenovirus Myocarditis

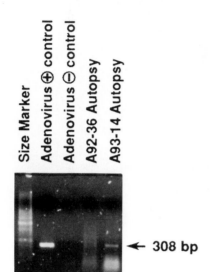

FIGURE 49–6

Polymerase chain reaction (PCR) identification of adenovirus in the myocardium of a child who died of myocarditis. This agarose gel of a PCR product obtained from the paraffin-fixed right ventricular autopsy specimen shows the 308–base pair sequence expected for adenoviral genome. Note the size marker in the first lane (left) and the adenovirus positive (+) control, which also has the 308–base pair product, in the second lane. The negative (−) control lane and another patient are devoid of a band.

myocarditis better. The expansion of the number of viruses able to be studied will further expand the etiologic diagnosis of myocarditis in children and lead to better understanding of the disease. Improvements in the understanding of the immune response in these patients are likely to follow.

Therapy

Intravenous γ-globulin is currently an experimental therapy being used by several institutions and appears to be promising. Another potential novel therapy to be investigated is mass vaccination for the more common viral agents.

HYPERTROPHIC CARDIOMYOPATHY

Hypertrophic cardiomyopathy (HCM) is a heterogeneous clinical disorder with myriad morphologic, clinical, and pathophysiologic features. Initially recognized in 1868, multiple descriptions of HCM were reported before the classic description of the pathology of HCM by Teare[68] appeared in 1958. The diagnosis of hypertrophic heart disease may be considered only after the exclusion of systemic hypertension, coronary artery disease, aortic valve disease, coarctation of the aorta, and congenital heart diseases predisposing to hypertrophy.[2,3] It is discussed fully in Chapter 35.

RESTRICTIVE CARDIOMYOPATHY

Restrictive cardiomyopathy (RCM) is uncommon, accounting for 5% of cardiomyopathies in children at two large pediatric institutions.[69–71] Restrictive cardiomyopathies are characterized by diastolic ventricular dysfunction with elevated left (and at times right) ventricular end-diastolic pressures, normal or nearly normal systolic function, and no significant ventricular dilatation.[72]

ETIOLOGY AND PATHOLOGY

Multiple causes of RCM have been described in adults and are listed in Table 49–5. The pathology and histology vary with the underlying disease process. In the idiopathic form of RCM, the ventricular cavity size is normal or nearly normal; the ventricular septal and free wall thicknesses are usually normal but may be mildly increased. Histochemical stains show variable degrees of myocyte hypertrophy, interstitial fibrosis, and myocytolysis.

CLINICAL PRESENTATION AND DIAGNOSTIC EVALUATION

The most common presenting signs and symptoms in children with RCM include dyspnea that is frequently exacerbated by an intercurrent respiratory illness, fatigue, syncope, and sudden death. Abnormal findings on physical examination include hepatomegaly, ascites, and an S_3 or S_4 gallop. In the three largest series in children, consisting of a combined total of 28 children, 4 of the 28 had a family history positive for cardiomyopathy, 2 of whom presented solely because of the family history.

Chest radiography usually reveals cardiomegaly. Pulmonary venous congestion is common and may be an indicator of poor prognosis. The most common abnormalities on electrocardiography are atrial enlargement and ST-T wave abnormalities. The most striking finding on echocardiography is massive atrial dilatation (Fig. 49–7). The ventricular cavity sizes are usually normal, although mild dilatation is occasionally seen. The ventricular wall thicknesses are usually normal, although mild left ventricular hypertrophy has been described as well as mild asymmetric septal hypertrophy.[73]

Doppler assessment may reveal short mitral deceleration time, consistently longer duration of pulmonary vein

TABLE 49–5

ETIOLOGY OF RESTRICTIVE CARDIOMYOPATHIES IN CHILDREN AND ADULTS

Myocardial	Endomyocardial
Idiopathic	Endomyocardial fibrosis
Scleroderma	Hypereosinophilic (Löffler's) syndrome
Amyloidosis	Carcinoid
Sarcoidosis	Metastatic malignant neoplasms
Gaucher's disease	Radiation
Hurler's disease	Anthracycline toxicity
Hemochromatosis	Pseudoxanthoma elasticum
Glycogen storage diseases	
Minicore-multicore myopathy	

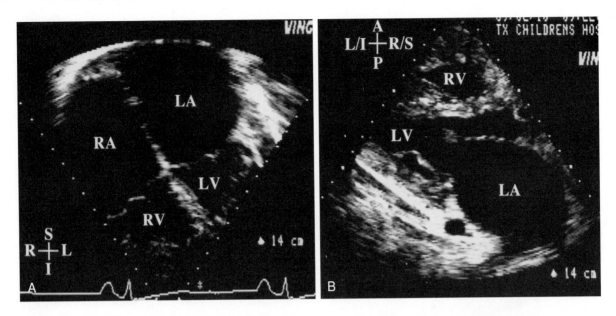

FIGURE 49–7

A, Apical four-chamber echocardiographic view of a child with restrictive cardiomyopathy. Note the extremely dilated atria and normal-sized ventricles (which appear to be small because of the large atrial dimensions). The electrocardiographic strip at the bottom demonstrates a giant P wave as well. *B,* Echocardiogram (parasternal long-axis view) in a child with restrictive cardiomyopathy. Note the giant left atrium and normal-sized left and right ventricles. LA = left atrium; LV = left ventricle; RA = right atrium; RV = right ventricle.

atrial reversal than of the mitral A wave, and increased velocity and duration of pulmonary vein atrial reversal.[71] The major hemodynamic problem in RCM is restriction to ventricular filling, and the diastolic pressure curve reflects this abnormality during cardiac catheterization. The diastolic pressure curve generally exhibits one of two patterns. In the first, the pressure is elevated at the onset of diastole and rises further with ventricular filling. The second shows a prominent *y* descent in early diastole, followed by an abrupt rise during the rapid filling phase, producing the "square root" or "dip and plateau" pattern. The first pattern can also be seen in cardiac tamponade, and the second may be seen in constrictive pericarditis (see also Chapter 51). Elevation in pulmonary artery pressure is common, and markedly elevated pulmonary vascular resistance can occur within 1 to 4 years of diagnosis. Endomyocardial biopsy reveals myofiber hypertrophy and mild to moderate interstitial fibrosis.

TREATMENT

Treatment of RCM is nonspecific and directed at alleviation of symptoms. In general, medical therapy does not improve survival. Diuretics are usually helpful in reducing pulmonary and systemic venous congestion. Because there is restriction to ventricular filling, care must be taken to avoid excessive reduction of preload. Afterload-reducing agents have not been useful, and in the limited available data, calcium channel blockers have not been beneficial. Some calcium channel blockers have substantial vasodilator properties as well, which could be deleterious in some circumstances. Inotropic agents have also not been beneficial. Adrenergic agonists and phosphodiesterase inhibitors have the ability to improve left ventricular relaxation. These agents are effective only in patients who have con-

current systolic dysfunction. Chatterjee[74] reported that in patients with RCM and overt and severe clinical heart failure, pharmacotherapy is uniformly ineffective, with cardiac transplantation being the most effective therapy. Atrial thrombi or embolic events were detected in 7 of the 28 children reported in the three series. Therefore, anticoagulation or antiplatelet therapy appears warranted. Pacing has been reported for symptomatic bradycardia or conduction disturbances. Elective pacing as a therapeutic intervention has not been reported in children. Transplantation remains the treatment of choice and should be considered at the time of diagnosis.

PROGNOSIS

The prognosis for children with RCM is poor.[69–71] The actuarial survival rate 2 years from the time of diagnosis is 44 to 50%. A markedly elevated pulmonary vascular resistance can develop within 1 to 4 years of presentation, precluding heart transplantation and necessitating heart-lung transplantation. Cetta and colleagues[71] suggested that those who present with dyspnea and radiographic evidence of pulmonary venous congestion have a particularly poor prognosis.

ARRHYTHMOGENIC CARDIOMYOPATHY/ARRHYTHMOGENIC RIGHT VENTRICULAR DYSPLASIA

The pathologic condition known as arrhythmogenic right ventricular dysplasia (ARVD) was first reported in 1978 by Frank and coworkers,[75] who described areas of dysplasia, predominantly in the right ventricular free wall in patients with this condition. A spectrum of right ventricular involvement occurs, from no functional impairment in some

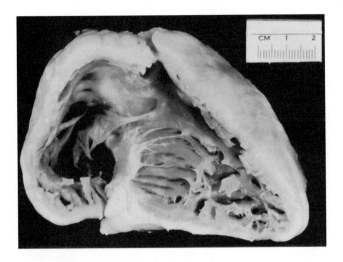

FIGURE 49–8

Gross anatomy of arrhythmogenic right ventricular dysplasia. There is thinning of the right ventricular free wall in the infundibulum and apex as well as dysplastic areas of endocardium.

patients to severe impairment in others. Classically, the patients present with syncope or palpitations secondary to ventricular tachycardia of the left bundle branch block morphology, originating from the dysplastic areas.[76]

PATHOLOGY

Pathologic specimens show an element of right ventricular enlargement, frequently with visible aneurysms and thinning of the right ventricular free wall in the region of the infundibulum, apex, or inferior wall (Fig. 49–8).[77] These areas of dysplasia are white, thickened, and sclerotic on the endocardial surface. Histologic sections show a variable reduction in myofibril numbers and interstitial infiltration by lipoid cells, histiocytes, and lymphocytes (Fig. 49–9). The few remaining myofibrils in the dysplastic region are hypertrophied or show signs of degeneration. The histologic appearance depends on the extent of secondary changes.[78] It is the fibrosis and fatty infiltration that are pathogno-

monic of ARVD; all layers of the free wall are affected. The degree of wall thinning cannot be used as a diagnostic criterion because the amount of adipose infiltration determines the thickness of the free wall.

Originally, the left ventricle was not thought to be involved pathologically. In some ways, this continues to be true, in that the right ventricle not only is the site of the primary tachycardia initiation but also shows the most functional and pathologic change. Now, however, left ventricular involvement is also recognized.

PREVALENCE

At present, it is difficult to assess the prevalence of ARVD. Because clinically evident right ventricular dysfunction is seen uncommonly, reporting is based primarily on the presentation of the arrhythmia and not the right-sided failure. Patients therefore will be missed if the arrhythmia precedes demonstrable right ventricular dysplasia.

Among patients with "idiopathic" right ventricular tachycardia, 24 to 30% may have ARVD on presentation. In one Italian study, ARVD accounted for 20% of sudden deaths in young people.[79] There are insufficient data to state conclusively that the prevalence is similar in adults and children. More males than females have been reported with the disease.

ETIOLOGY

No cohesive theory concerning the etiology of ARVD has been developed.[80] Several studies have reported an association with an infectious illness. No infectious agent has consistently been identified. Infection with coxsackievirus B3 and other viruses has been reported. One could speculate that in susceptible individuals, a preceding viral infection could lead to a gradual destruction of myocytes and fatty infiltration of the remaining stroma.

Familial occurrence is now widely recognized. Family members of suspected patients should be screened. Recently, genes for ARVD have been mapped to chromosome 14 (14q23 and 14q12-q22)[81,82] and chromosome 1 (1q42-q43)[83]; none of these genes has been elucidated.

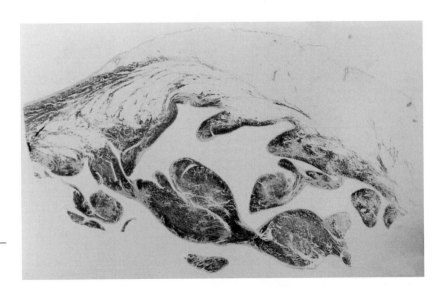

FIGURE 49–9

Histologic examination in arrhythmogenic right ventricular dysplasia shows fatty infiltration within the right ventricular tissue.

Certain features of ARVD are similar to Uhl's anomaly.[84] Although investigators have, in fact, speculated that Uhl's anomaly may be a severe form of ARVD, the clinical presentations of the two are different, and Uhl's anomaly has no adipose infiltration.

CLINICAL FINDINGS

The clinical picture seems to be independent of age. Whereas the typical patient is male and in the third decade of life, the age spectrum ranges from the first year of life to the ninth decade. The presentation is one of abrupt onset of syncopal episodes, palpitations, or ventricular tachycardia, often associated with exercise. The mean time from onset of symptoms to diagnosis can be as long as 7 years. Sudden death may be the initial (and final) presentation. The physical examination is usually normal. When findings are abnormal, diastolic filling sounds are most frequent (20%), whereas prominence of the left anterior thorax is seen in less than 10% of patients. An irregular rhythm is usually reported on physical examination. Presentation with right ventricular failure has been reported in less than 2% of patients.

DIAGNOSTIC STUDIES

Chest Radiography
The chest radiograph is normal in the absence of right ventricular failure. Although a cardiothoracic ratio of greater than 50% occurs in more than half of the older patients, this is not so in children. Pulmonary vascular markings are usually normal.

Electrocardiography
The electrocardiogram is often helpful in the diagnosis (Fig. 49–10).[77] It usually shows sinus rhythm, with frequent ventricular premature depolarizations of left bundle branch block morphology. The QRS, P wave, and T wave frontal plane axes are normal. Although precordial QRS morphology is normal, a pattern of incomplete right bundle branch block is seen in up to 30% of patients. The most striking and constant feature is the inversion of T waves in leads V_1 through V_4. Whereas this sign is highly suggestive of ARVD in the adult, it may be normal in children younger than 12 years.

Ventricular post-excitation waves, so-called epsilon waves, are found in the ST segments of the right precordial leads in 30% of adult patients. By increasing the gain or by using signal-averaging techniques, these potentials—which arise from areas with markedly delayed depolarization—can be made visible in nearly all patients. Epsilon waves are thought to be a marker for a myocardium that is at risk for re-entry tachycardia. The farther from the QRS these potentials are found, the more specific they may be for ARVD. When present, ventricular tachycardia is characterized by a left bundle branch block morphology (see Fig. 49–10), a rate in the range of 170 to 300 beats per minute (average 250), and a QRS axis that is normal to rightward.

Noninvasive Imaging
As for the identification of ARVD, the noninvasive evaluation of ventricular morphology and function is now helpful[85] but may not detect all patients in childhood. Echocardiographic imaging of right ventricular outpouching,

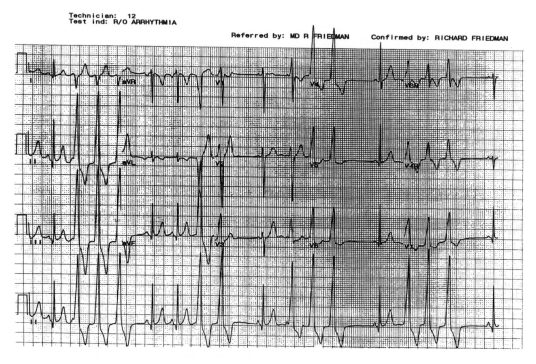

FIGURE 49–10

Electrocardiogram in arrhythmogenic right ventricular dysplasia. Note the sinus tachycardia in this 16-year-old as well as the frequent premature ventricular beats and brief run of ventricular tachycardia with a left bundle branch pattern.

diffuse dysfunction, or dilatation may be a sensitive approach. Global dysfunction and regional wall motion abnormalities may also be identified by radionuclide angiography.[86]

Cardiac Catheterization

If ARVD is suspected (e.g., ventricular tachycardia in a "normal heart") and not found on echocardiography, cardiac catheterization (especially with angiography) should be considered. At catheterization, the pressure may be normal in all four cardiac chambers. If abnormal, the most common finding is an elevation of the right atrial *a* wave; in patients with severe right ventricular dysfunction, it can exceed the pulmonary artery diastolic pressure. The major role of catheterization is to show right ventricular dyskinesis on ventriculography. Right ventricular dilatation is the rule in adults although it is less common in children, in whom segmental dilatation with paradoxical motion of the outflow tract is more common. The hallmark of the disease is the systolic bulging of the right ventricular free wall. The "triangle of dysplasia," as described by Marcus and coworkers,[77] includes the anterior infundibulum, the right ventricular apex, and the diaphragmatic free wall. Hemodynamic and angiographic assessment of left ventricular function should be carried out at catheterization. Endomyocardial biopsy of the right ventricular septum should be performed during catheterization as well,[78] because classic pathologic changes are seen in as many as 90% of patients who have right ventricular dyskinesis. In patients with ventricular tachycardia of right ventricular origin, the endomyocardial biopsy can be used to diagnose ARVD even in the absence of right ventricular dyskinesis.

Electrophysiology Study

Invasive electrophysiologic investigation is usually not essential for diagnosis. Atrial and atrioventricular node conduction times are often prolonged minimally. Although epsilon waves can be recorded in half the patients, it is usually necessary to place the catheter at the site of the dysplasia to be successful. The major roles of electrophysiologic testing, then, are to confirm that the tachycardia has its origin in the right ventricle, to map the location of initiation, and to evaluate the efficacy of various antiarrhythmic agents.

TREATMENT

Treatment focuses on control of the arrhythmia. Propranolol, sotalol, procainamide, disopyramide, and amiodarone have been efficacious in some patients, although a combination of these drugs is frequently required. In one series, 12 of 24 patients required operative intervention to stop frequent episodes of ventricular tachycardia. Although previous treatment with single and double antiarrhythmic medications had been successful in relieving symptoms, breakthrough tachycardia was the rule in these patients. The operation generally consists of an initial mapping of the epicardial surface for the area of initiation and then the performance of a simple ventriculotomy and cryoablation with or without local excision. Right ventricular disconnection has been performed,[87] but poor results have occurred in children.

NATURAL HISTORY

The natural history of ARVD requires further elucidation. Although sudden death has occurred in about 5% of the reported patients, most of these patients were either untreated or previously undiagnosed. Sudden death in childhood occurs, as does death from congestive failure, but it is uncommon. In an autopsy series from Italy, a large percentage of young adults who died suddenly had ARVD at autopsy.[79] There is some debate, as well, as to whether antiarrhythmic treatment will reduce the incidence of sudden death. The usual course appears to be one of slow deterioration in right ventricular function and a reduction in the efficacy of antiarrhythmic treatment.

REFERENCES

1. Brigden W: Uncommon myocardial diseases. The noncoronary cardiomyopathies. Lancet 2:1179, 1957.
2. Report of the 1995 World Health Organization/International Society and Federation of Cardiology: Task force on the definition and classification of cardiomyopathy. Circulation 93:841, 1988.
3. Manolio TA, Baughman KL, Rodenheffer R, et al: Prevalence and etiology of idiopathic dilated cardiomyopathy (summary of a National Heart, Lung, and Blood Institute workshop). Am J Cardiol 69:1458, 1992.
4. Wiles HB, McArthur PD, Taylor AB, et al: Prognostic features of children with idiopathic dilated cardiomyopathy. Am J Cardiol 68:1372, 1991.
5. Matitiau A, Perez-Atayde A, Sanders SP, et al: Infantile dilated cardiomyopathy. Relation of outcome to left ventricular mechanics, hemodynamics, and histology at the time of presentation. Circulation 90:1310, 1994.
6. Michels VV, Moll PP, Miller FA, et al: The frequency of familial dilated cardiomyopathy in a series of patients with idiopathic dilated cardiomyopathy. N Engl J Med 326:77, 1992.
7. Keeling PJ, McKenna WJ: Clinical genetics of dilated cardiomyopathy. Herz 19:91, 1994.
8. Towbin JA: Molecular genetic aspects of cardiomyopathy. Biochem Med Metab Biol 49:285, 1993.
9. Towbin JA, Roberts R: Cardiovascular diseases due to genetic abnormalities. *In* Schlant RC, Alexander RW (eds): Hurst's The Heart, 8th ed. New York, McGraw-Hill, 1994, p 1725.
10. Carlquist JF, Menlove RL, Murray MB, et al: HLA class II (DR and DQ) antigen associations in idiopathic dilated cardiomyopathy. Validation study and meta-analysis of published HLA association studies. Circulation 83:515, 1991.
11. Limas CJ, Limas C: HLA-DR antigen linkage of anti-beta receptor antibodies in idiopathic dilated and ischemic cardiomyopathy. Br Heart J 67:402, 1992.
12. Limas CJ, Limas C, Boudoulas H: *HLA-DQA1* and *-DQB1* gene haplotypes in familial cardiomyopathy. Am J Cardiol 74:510, 1994.
13. Caforio AL, Keeling PJ, Zachara E, et al: Evidence from family studies for autoimmunity in dilated cardiomyopathy. Lancet 334:773, 1994.
14. Kühl U, Noutsias M, Seeberg B, Schultheiss HP: Immunological analysis for a chronic intramyocardial inflammatory process in dilated cardiomyopathy. Heart 75:295, 1996.
15. Towbin JA, Hejtmancik JF, Brink P, et al: X-linked dilated cardiomyopathy: Molecular genetic evidence of linkage to the Duchenne muscular dystrophy (dystrophin) gene at the Xp21 locus. Circulation 87:1854, 1993.
16. Muntoni F, Cau M, Ganau A, et al: Brief report: Deletion of the dystrophin muscle-promoter region associated with X-linked dilated cardiomyopathy. N Engl J Med 329:921, 1993.
17. Milasin J, Muntoni F, Severini GM, et al: A point mutation in the 5′ splice site of the dystrophin gene first intron responsible for X-linked dilated cardiomyopathy. Hum Mol Genet 5:73, 1996.
18. Ortiz-Lopez R, Su J, Goytia V, Towbin JA: Evidence for a dystrophin missense mutation as a cause of X-linked dilated cardiomyopathy (XLCM). Circulation 95:2434, 1997.

19. Bolhuis PA, Hensels GW, Hulsebos TJ, et al: Mapping of the locus for X-linked cardioskeletal myopathy with neutropenia and abnormal mitochondria (Barth syndrome) to Xq28. Am J Hum Genet 48:481, 1991.

20. Kelley RI, Cheatham JP, Clark BJ, et al: X-linked dilated cardiomyopathy with neutropenia, growth retardation, and 3-methylglutaconic aciduria. J Pediatr 119:738, 1991.

21. Bione S, D'Adamo P, Maestrini E, et al: A novel X-linked gene, G4.5 is responsible for Barth syndrome. Nat Genet 12:385, 1996.

22. Kelly DP, Strauss AW: Inherited cardiomyopathies. N Engl J Med 330:913, 1994.

23. Gilbert EM, Bristow MR: Idiopathic dilated cardiomyopathy. *In* Schlant RC, Alexander RW (eds): Hurst's The Heart, 8th ed. New York, McGraw-Hill, 1994, p 1609.

24. Doshi R, Lodge KV: Idiopathic cardiomyopathy in infants. Arch Dis Child 48:431, 1973.

25. Lewis AB, Neustein HB, Takahashi M, Lurie PR: Findings on endomyocardial biopsy in infants and children with dilated cardiomyopathy. Am J Cardiol 55:143, 1985.

26. Tazelaar HD, Billingham ME: Leukocytic infiltrates in idiopathic dilated cardiomyopathy: A source of confusion with active myocarditis. Am J Surg Pathol 10:405, 1986.

27. Aretz HT, Billingham ME, Edwards WD, et al: Myocarditis: A histopathologic definition and classification. Am J Cardiovasc Pathol 1:3, 1987.

28. Friedman RA, Moak JP, Garson A Jr: Clinical course of idiopathic dilated cardiomyopathy in children. J Am Coll Cardiol 18:152, 1991.

29. Taliercio CP, Seward JB, Driscoll DJ, et al: Idiopathic dilated cardiomyopathy in the young: Clinical profile and natural history. J Am Coll Cardiol 6:1126, 1985.

30. Greenwood RD, Nadas AS, Fyler DC: The clinical course of primary myocardial disease in infants and children. Am Heart J 92:549, 1976.

31. Griffin ML, Hernandez A, Martin TC, et al: Dilated cardiomyopathy in infants and children. J Am Coll Cardiol 11:139, 1988.

32. Ghafour AD, Gutgesell HP: Echocardiographic evaluation of left ventricular function in children with congestive cardiomyopathy. Am J Cardiol 44:1332, 1979.

33. Lewis AB: Prognostic value of echocardiography in children with idiopathic dilated cardiomyopathy. Am Heart J 128:133, 1994.

34. Roberts WC, Ferrans VJ: Pathologic anatomy of the cardiomyopathies. Idiopathic dilated and hypertrophic types, infiltrative types, and endomyocardial disease with and without eosinophilia. Hum Pathol 6:287, 1975.

35. Kohlschuitter A, Hausdorf G: Primary (genetic) cardiomyopathies in infancy: A survey of possible disorders and guidelines for diagnosis. Eur J Pediatr 145:454, 1986.

36. Schwartz ML, Cox GF, Lin AE, et al: Clinical approach to genetic cardiomyopathy in children. Circulation 94:2021, 1996.

37. Towbin JA: Polymerase chain reaction and its uses as a diagnostic tool for cardiovascular disease. Trends Cardiovasc Med 5:175, 1995.

38. Martin AB, Webber S, Fricker FJ, et al: Acute myocarditis. Rapid diagnosis by PCR in children. Circulation 90:330, 1994.

39. Fenoglio JJ, Ursell PC, Kellogg CF, et al: Diagnosis and classification of myocarditis by endomyocardial biopsy. N Engl J Med 308:12, 1983.

40. Strauss AW: Defects of mitochondrial proteins and pediatric heart disease. Prog Pediatr Cardiol 6:83, 1996.

41. Krajinovic M, Pinamonti B, Sinagra G, et al: Linkage of familial dilated cardiomyopathy to chromosome 9. Am J Hum Genet 57:846, 1995.

42. Durand J-B, Bachinski LL, Bieling L, et al: Localization of a gene responsible for familial dilated cardiomyopathy to chromosome 1q32. Circulation 92:3387, 1995.

43. Bowles KR, Gajarski R, Porter P, et al: Gene mapping of familial autosomal dominant dilated cardiomyopathy to chromosome 10q21-23. J Clin Invest 98:1355, 1996.

43a. Sin BL, Nimura H, Osborne JA, et al: Familial dilated cardiomyopathy locus maps to chromosome 2q31. Circulation 99:1022, 1999.

44. Kass S, MacRae C, Graber HL, et al: A gene defect that causes conduction system disease and dilated cardiomyopathy maps to chromosome 1p1-1q1. Nat Genet 7:546, 1994.

45. Olson TM, Keating MT: Mapping a cardiomyopathy locus to chromosome 3p22-p25. J Clin Invest 97:528, 1996.

45a. Olson TM, Michels VV, Thibodeau SN, et al: Actin mutations in dilated cardiomyopathy, a heritable form of heart failure. Science 280:751, 1998.

46. Om A, Hess ML: Inotrophic therapy of the failing myocardium. Clin Cardiol 16:5, 1992.

47. Konstam MA, Cody RJ: Short-term use of intravenous milrinone for heart failure. Am J Cardiol 75:822, 1995.

48. Bristow MR: Pathophysiologic and pharmacologic rationales for clinical management of chronic heart failure with beta-blocking agents. Am J Cardiol 71:12C, 1993.

49. Guccione P, Paul T, Garson A Jr: Long-term follow-up of amiodarone therapy in the young: Continued efficacy, unimpaired growth, moderate side effects. J Am Coll Cardiol 15:1118, 1990.

50. Nishimura RA, Hayes DL, Holmes DR, Tajik AJ: Mechanism of hemodynamic improvement by dual-chamber pacing for severe left ventricular dysfunction: An acute Doppler and catheterization hemodynamic study. J Am Coll Cardiol 25:281, 1995.

51. Parrillo JE, Cunnion RE, Epstein SE, et al: A prospective, randomized controlled trial of prednisone for dilated cardiomyopathy. N Engl J Med 321:1061, 1989.

52. Carpenter A, Chachques JC: Myocardial substitution with a stimulated skeletal muscle: First successful clinical case. Lancet 1:1267, 1985.

53. Lewis AB, Chabot M: Outcome of infants and children with dilated cardiomyopathy. Am J Cardiol 68:365, 1991.

54. Billingham ME, Tazelaar HD: The morphological progression of viral myocarditis. Postgrad Med J 62:581, 1986.

55. Herskowitz A, Campbell S, Decker J, et al: Demographic features and prevalence of idiopathic myocarditis in patients undergoing endomyocardial biopsy. Am J Cardiol 71:982, 1993.

56. Friedman RA: Viral myocarditis in children. Current diagnosis and treatment. Cardiol Rev 3:164, 1995.

57. Wiles HB, Gillette PC, Harley RA: Cardiomyopathy and myocarditis in children with ventricular ectopic rhythm. J Am Coll Cardiol 20:359, 1992.

58. Friedman RA, Kearney DL, Moak JP: Persistence of ventricular arrhythmia after resolution of occult myocarditis in children and young adults. J Am Coll Cardiol 24:780, 1994.

59. Hauck AJ, Kearney DL, Edwards WD: Evaluation of postmortem endomyocardial biopsy specimens from 38 patients with lymphocytic myocarditis: Implications for the role of sampling error. Mayo Clin Proc 64:1235, 1988.

60. Chow LH, Radio SJ, Sears TD, McManus BM: Insensitivity of right ventricular endomyocardial biopsy in the diagnosis of myocarditis. J Am Coll Cardiol 14:915, 1989.

61. Bowles NE, Richardson PJ, Olsen EGJ, Archard LC: Detection of Coxsackie-B-virus specific RNA sequences in myocardial biopsy samples from patients with myocarditis and dilated cardiomyopathy. Lancet 1:1120, 1986.

62. Bowles NE, Rose ML, Taylor P, et al: End-stage dilated cardiomyopathy: Persistence of enterovirus DNA in myocardium at cardiac transplantation and lack of immune response. Circulation 80:1128, 1989.

63. Jin O, Sole MJ, Butany JW, et al: Detection of enterovirus RNA in myocardial biopsies from patients with myocarditis and cardiomyopathy using gene amplification by polymerase chain reaction. Circulation 82:8, 1990.

64. Griffin L, Kearney D, Ni J, et al: Analysis of formalin-fixed and frozen myocardial autopsy samples for viral genome in childhood myocarditis and dilated cardiomyopathy with endocardial fibroelastosis using polymerase chain reaction (PCR). Cardiovasc Pathol 4:3, 1995.

65. Jones SR, Herskowitz A, Hutchins GM, Baughman KL: Effects of immunosuppressive therapy in biopsy-proved myocarditis and borderline myocarditis on left ventricular function. Am J Cardiol 68:370, 1991.

66. Mason JW, O'Connell JB, Herskowitz A, et al: A clinical trial of immunosuppressive therapy for myocarditis. N Engl J Med 333:269, 1995.

67. Drucker NA, Colan SD, Lewis AB, et al: Gamma-globulin treatment of acute myocarditis in the pediatric population. Circulation 89:252, 1994.

68. Teare D: Asymmetrical hypertrophy of the heart in young adults. Br Heart J 20:1, 1958.

69. Lewis AB: Clinical profile and outcome of restrictive cardiomyopathy in children. Am Heart J 123:1589, 1992.

70. Denfield SW, Bricker JT, Gajarski R, et al: Restrictive cardiomyopathies in childhood: Etiologies and natural history. Tex Heart Inst J 24:38, 1997.

71. Cetta F, O'Leary PW, Seward JB, Driscoll DJ: Idiopathic restrictive cardiomyopathy in childhood: Diagnostic features and clinical course. Mayo Clin Proc 70:634, 1995.

72. Shabetai R: Restrictive cardiomyopathy. *In* Schlant RC, Alexander RW (eds): Hurst's The Heart, 8th ed. New York, McGraw-Hill, 1994, p 1637.

73. Sutton JM, Sayan CD, Reitz BA, Baughman KL: Hypertrophic restrictive cardiomyopathy. Heart Failure 4:55, 1988.

74. Chatterjee K: Diastolic ventricular failure: A clinician's approach. ACC Curr J Rev, March/April:50, 1995.

75. Frank R, Fontaine G, Vedee J, et al: Electrocardiologie de quatre cas de dysplasie ventriculaire droite arythmogenique. Arch Mal Coeur 71:963, 1978.

76. McKenna WJ, Thiene G, Nava A, et al: Diagnosis of arrhythmogenic right ventricular dysplasia/cardiomyopathy. Task Force of the Working Group Myocardial and Pericardial Disease of the European Society of Cardiology and of the Scientific Council on Cardiomyopathies of the International Society and Federation of Cardiology. Br Heart J 71:215, 1994.

77. Marcus FI, Fontaine G, Guiraudon G, et al: Right ventricular dysplasia: A report of 24 adult cases. Circulation 65:384, 1982.

78. Hasumi M, Sekiguchi M, Hiroe M, et al: Endomyocardial biopsy approach to patients with ventricular tachycardia with special reference to arrhythmogenic right ventricular dysplasia. Jpn Circ J 51:242, 1987.

79. Thiene G, Nava A, Corrado D, et al: Right ventricular cardiomyopathy and sudden death in young people. N Engl J Med 318:129, 1988.

80. Basso C, Thiene G, Corrado D, et al: Arrhythmogenic right ventricular cardiomyopathy. Dysplasia, dystrophy, or myocarditis. Circulation 94:983, 1996.

81. Rampazzo A, Nava A, Danieli GA, et al: The gene for arrhythmogenic right ventricular cardiomyopathy maps to chromosome 14q23-q24. Hum Mol Genet 3:959, 1994.

82. Severini GM, Krajinovic M, Pinamonti B, et al: A new locus for arrhythmogenic right ventricular dysplasia on the long arm of chromosome 14. Genomics 31:193, 1996.

83. Rampazzo A, Nava A, Erne P, et al: A new locus for arrhythmogenic right ventricular cardiomyopathy (*ARVD2*) maps to chromosome 1q42-q43. Hum Mol Genet 4:2151, 1995.

84. Uhl HSM: Previously undescribed congenital malformation of the heart: Almost total absence of the myocardium of the right ventricle. Bull Johns Hopkins Hosp 91:197, 1952.

85. Robertson JH, Bardy GH, German LD, et al: Comparison of two-dimensional echocardiographic and angiographic findings in arrhythmogenic right ventricular dysplasia. Am J Cardiol 55:1506, 1985.

86. LeGuludec D, Slama MS, Frank R, et al: Evaluation of radionuclide angiography in diagnosis of arrhythmogenic right ventricular cardiomyopathy. J Am Coll Cardiol 26:1476, 1995.

87. Guiraudon GM, Klein GJ, Gulamhusein SS, et al: Total disconnection of the right ventricular free wall: Surgical treatment of right ventricular tachycardia associated with right ventricular dysplasia. Circulation 67:463, 1983.

CHAPTER 50

INFECTIVE ENDOCARDITIS

KATHRYN A. TAUBERT   ADNAN S. DAJANI

Infective endocarditis (IE) is an infection of the endothelial (endocardial) surface of the heart valves (native or prosthetic), mural endocardium, or great vessels. Infection can also occur on intracardiac patches, indwelling catheters, and surgically constructed shunts. IE can be caused by bacteria, fungi, rickettsiae, or viruses, although most instances are due to bacterial infection.

Endocarditis is relatively rare in children. It is a serious and sometimes fatal complication of structural heart disease and can also occur in a normal heart. In the preantibiotic era, mortality was virtually 100%. Advances in antimicrobial prophylaxis and treatment of the disease and the development of better diagnostic and operative techniques have reduced the morbidity and mortality substantially, although even today mortality rates are 15 to 25%.

EPIDEMIOLOGY

Various groups since the 1930s have reported an incidence of IE in hospitalized children of between 1 in 4500 and 1 in 1280, with the incidence apparently increasing between the 1950s and the 1980s.[1-3] This increase in the incidence is due to several factors,[4] including

- greater number of patients undergoing operation;
- advances in the treatment of complex congenital cardiac anomalies;
- increased use of prosthetic material;
- aggressive management in neonatal and pediatric intensive care units;
- use of immunosuppressive agents; and
- intravenous drug abuse in older age groups.

In the United States, IE in children most often occurs in an individual with an underlying structural cardiac abnormality.[5,6] Children with structural cardiac abnormalities can develop endocarditis at any age. Several reviews indicate that about half of reported instances of endocarditis are in children 10 years of age or older.[7-9] Approximately 32,000 children are born in the United States each year with a cardiac malformation.[10] Improvement in the treatment of complex anomalies has increased the life expectancy of many of these individuals. Indeed, endocarditis is an important problem for adults with congenital heart disease.[11] A pooled analysis of data from 20 published studies regarding the underlying cardiac abnormality in 884 children with IE is shown in Table 50–1.[12]

Although rheumatic heart disease was an important risk factor for the development of endocarditis in earlier decades of this century, the incidence of rheumatic fever and rheumatic heart disease in the United States has declined in the past few decades. In the preantibiotic era, one third to one half of instances of IE were in children with rheumatic heart disease.[2,13] Today, however, in developed countries, rheumatic heart disease is the underlying cardiac abnormality in less than 10% of instances of IE.[9,12,14,15] In developing countries, however, rheumatic heart disease remains an important underlying cardiac lesion for the development of endocarditis.[16-20]

IE has been reported in neonates, especially premature neonates, with increasing frequency, and it is usually associated with indwelling arterial and central venous catheters.[14,21-23] Most of these instances of endocarditis are right-sided.

PATHOGENESIS

For IE to develop, two independent events are normally required: a damaged area of endothelium, and bacteremia caused by adherent organisms. Normal undamaged endothelium is not conducive to bacterial colonization. Endothelium can be damaged by an abnormally high velocity jet stream that results in turbulent blood flow. A model developed by Rodbard[24] to delineate the hemodynamic mechanisms responsible for the development of endocarditis showed that endothelial damage and bacterial deposition can occur in a low-pressure area immediately distal to an obstruction, such as coarctation of the aorta, regurgitant mitral or aortic valve, or ventricular septal defect. Thus, endothelium on the ventricular side of a regurgitant aortic valve would be damaged, and the right ventricular wall (or right-sided heart valves) would be damaged from the jet created by a ventricular septal defect. Endothelium can also be damaged by direct trauma from intracardiac devices, such as an indwelling catheter, or from an intracardiac operation.

Trauma to the endothelium can induce thrombogenesis (deposition of fibrin and platelets), which leads to a sterile lesion known as nonbacterial thrombotic endocarditis (NBTE). This lesion is more receptive to colonization by bacteria than is normal undamaged endothelium and serves as a nidus for subsequent infection. After bacteremia with an organism that can adhere to the NTBE, a vegetation can ensue. Certain bacteria are more likely than others to adhere and are also more able to avoid eradication by the host's defenses.[25] The adherence of streptococci may be related in part to the extracellular pro-

TABLE 50–1

UNDERLYING HEART DISEASE IN CHILDREN WITH INFECTIVE ENDOCARDITIS

Disease	No.	Percentage of Total
Congenital heart disease		
Acyanotic heart lesions		
Ventricular septal defect	194	21.8
Ventricular septal defect and other	18	2.0
Patent ductus arteriosus	25	2.8
Aortic stenosis	89	10.0
Subvalvar aortic stenosis	9	1.0
Coarctation of aorta	25	2.8
Pulmonary stenosis	21	2.4
Atrioventricular defect	16	1.8
Atrial septal defect	11	1.2
Mitral valve abnormality	16	1.8
Mitral valve prolapse	8	0.9
Cyanotic heart lesions		
Tetralogy of Fallot	143	16.0
Transposition of great vessels	35	3.9
Truncus arteriosus	8	0.9
Tricuspid atresia	9	1.0
Pulmonary atresia	8	0.9
Single ventricle	9	1.0
Other	79	8.9
Rheumatic heart disease	86	9.7
No heart disease	75	8.4
Total	884	

From Berkowitz FE: Infective endocarditis. *In* Nichols DG, Cameron DE, Greeley WJ, et al (eds): Critical Heart Disease in Infants and Children. St. Louis, Mosby–Year Book, 1995, p 961.

duction of the polysaccharide dextran, which facilitates adherence.[26] The vegetation itself is composed of fibrin, platelets, red blood cells, a few white blood cells, and the microorganisms, which can grow to a concentration that is achievable in pure culture in a Petri dish.

MICROBIOLOGY

Most instances of endocarditis are caused by a limited number of microorganisms. The most logical explanation relates to bacterial adherence. An in vitro study demonstrated that bacteria frequently responsible for endocarditis, such as viridans streptococci, readily adhered to canine or human cardiac valves, whereas gram-negative organisms, which infrequently cause endocarditis, adhered poorly to valves.[25]

In most series of endocarditis in children, gram-positive cocci account for at least two thirds of recoverable bacteria. Table 50–2 summarizes endocarditis in children in 20 pediatric series.[12] Viridans streptococci were responsible for about one third of the instances of endocarditis in this series. Staphylococci (*Staphylococcus aureus* and coagulase-negative staphylococci) were the second largest group, accounting for 30%. Gram-negative organisms less frequently cause endocarditis in children. Neonates, immunocompromised patients, and intravenous drug abusers, however, are at an increased risk for gram-negative bacterial endocarditis. The slow-growing fastidious gram-negative bacilli in the HACEK group (*Haemophilus, Actinobacillus, Cardiobacterium, Eikenella, Kingella*) can also cause endocarditis in

TABLE 50–2

MICROORGANISMS CAUSING INFECTIVE ENDOCARDITIS IN CHILDREN

Microorganism	No.	Percentage
Viridans streptococci	289	31.3
Other streptococci and enterococci	55	5.9
Streptococcus pneumoniae	18	1.9
Staphylococcus aureus	225	24.4
Coagulase-negative staphylococcus	46	4.9
HACEK plus diphtheroids	50	5.4
Gram-negative bacilli	45	4.8
Fungi	14	1.5
Others	28	3.0
Negative cultures	152	16.4
Total	922	100

HACEK = *Haemophilus, Actinobacillus, Cardiobacterium, Eikenella,* and *Kingella.*

From Berkowitz FE: Infective endocarditis. *In* Nichols DG, Cameron DE, Greeley WJ, et al (eds): Critical Heart Disease in Infants and Children. St. Louis, Mosby–Year Book, 1995, p 964.

children. They frequently affect damaged cardiac valves and often cause emboli. Other gram-negative bacilli, such as *Neisseria gonorrhoeae,* can cause endocarditis presenting as an acute illness, affecting previously normal valves, and commonly resulting in valvar destruction. In intravenous drug abusers, the most commonly isolated organism is *S. aureus.* Other organisms include *Pseudomonas* and other gram-negative bacilli and fungi (predominantly *Candida* species).[27]

In prosthetic valve endocarditis (PVE), the organisms differ according to whether endocarditis occurs within the first year after operation or later. Infection during the first year is primarily due to coagulase-negative staphylococci related to contamination during the operative procedure or nosocomially acquired.[28] *S. aureus,* gram-negative bacilli, diphtheroids, and *Candida* species are also common causes of PVE during this period. The coagulase-negative staphylococci recovered within the first year of operation are frequently resistant to methicillin and all other β-lactams. In contrast, infection occurring more than 1 year after operation is caused by organisms similar to ones in native valve endocarditis.[28]

Fungal endocarditis is rare in children and has a high morbidity and mortality even with intensive treatment.[29–32] It was responsible for 1.5% of the endocarditis in Table 50–2. It is difficult to diagnose and treat, and complications, especially embolization, are frequent.[33] The most frequently recovered fungal organism is *Candida albicans;* other organisms include *Aspergillus* species, *Torulopsis glabrata,* other *Candida* species, and other fungi.[31,32] Fungal endocarditis usually occurs in intravenous drug abusers and patients undergoing cardiac valve replacement.[31] It also occurs in immunocompromised patients and in neonates. In neonates, fungal endocarditis may be a complication of prolonged use of indwelling venous catheters, prolonged hyperalimentation, and broad-spectrum antibiotic use.[34–36]

In the series in Table 50–2, about 16% of instances of endocarditis were culture-negative. There are many possible reasons, particularly previous treatment with antibiotics.[37] Physicians should carefully evaluate such patients

TABLE 50–3

DUKE CRITERIA FOR DIAGNOSIS OF INFECTIVE ENDOCARDITIS

DEFINITE INFECTIVE ENDOCARDITIS

Pathologic criteria
  Microorganisms: demonstrated by culture or histology in a vegetation,
    or in a vegetation that has embolized, or in an intracardiac abscess,
    or
  Pathologic lesions: vegetation or intracardiac abscess present,
    confirmed by histology showing active endocarditis

Clinical criteria, using specific definitions listed in Table 50–4
  2 major criteria, *or*
  1 major and 3 minor criteria, *or*
  5 minor criteria

POSSIBLE INFECTIVE ENDOCARDITIS

Findings consistent with infective endocarditis that fall short of
  "definite" but not "rejected"

REJECTED

Firm alternative diagnosis for manifestations of endocarditis, *or*
Resolution of manifestations of endocarditis, with antibiotic therapy for
  4 days or less, *or*
No pathologic evidence of infective endocarditis at surgery or autopsy,
  after antibiotic therapy for 4 days or less

Reprinted from American Journal of Medicine, Volume 96, Durack DT, Lukes AS, Bright DK: New criteria for diagnosis of infective endocarditis: Utilization of specific echocardiographic findings, Pages 200–209, Copyright 1994, with permission from Excerpta Medica Inc.

for the possibility of other diseases. (See the section on culture-negative endocarditis.)

DIAGNOSIS

Criteria for the clinical diagnosis of IE have been developed over the years. Since 1981, the von Reyn criteria (also referred to as the Beth Israel criteria) have been the most widely used.[38] More recently, new criteria were developed by Durack and associates[39] from Duke University. These so-called Duke criteria are listed in Table 50–3 and defined in Table 50–4. There are two major criteria and six minor criteria. There are three diagnostic categories—definite, possible, and rejected. The clinical criteria can be used to establish a definitive diagnosis of IE when two major criteria, one major plus three minor criteria, or five minor criteria are met. The Duke criteria are more effective than the von Reyn criteria in establishing a diagnosis of IE in both adults[40–42] and children.[43]

CLINICAL FEATURES

Symptoms of endocarditis usually arise within 2 weeks of the initiating bacteremia.[44] They are usually related to cardiac complications caused by the infection, persistent bacteremia, systemic embolization, or immunopathologic reactions by the patient. Endocarditis can mimic many disorders, including other infectious diseases, lymphoma, leukemia, and connective tissue diseases. Endocarditis should be part of the differential diagnosis in patients with an underlying cardiac abnormality who have unexplained fever or other unusual illness that could be related to endocarditis.

Fever is the most common finding in patients with endocarditis, with the exception of neonates. Fever is usually low grade, reaching a maximal temperature of 39°C. In endocarditis caused by virulent bacteria such as *S. aureus*, however, there is spiking fever. Other nonspecific symptoms include myalgia, arthralgia, anorexia, night sweats, headache, and malaise. Because symptoms are usually mild, the diagnosis of IE is often not made until 2 to 4 weeks after the infection starts. By this time, vegetations are well established and difficult to eradicate.

Splenomegaly occurs less commonly in recent reports than it did previously. Enlargement of the spleen is reported in 15 to 50% of patients and is more common in patients with endocarditis of longer duration.

New or changing cardiac murmurs are usually heard except in patients with tricuspid or mural endocarditis.[45, 46] Murmurs may not be heard at the initial examination. Frequent auscultation is essential because it may be difficult to recognize a new or changing murmur in a patient with a pre-existing murmur. Careful and frequent auscultation is necessary to assist not only with the diagnosis but also with the patient's medical or operative management. Congestive heart failure is a serious complication of endocarditis and is primarily the result of valvar destruction or rupture of the chordae tendineae. Surgery to correct valvar dysfunction is often necessary and results in marked reduction in morbidity and mortality.

The classic peripheral manifestations of endocarditis occur less frequently today than had been reported and are absent in endocarditis involving the tricuspid valve. Petechiae are the most common but least specific manifestations and are found on the palpebral conjunctiva, the buccal and palatal mucosa, and the extremities. Splinter hemorrhages, which resemble a splinter underneath the nail in the nail bed, are also a nonspecific finding in endocarditis. They are more helpful diagnostically if they are present in the proximal rather than the distal nail bed. Osler's nodes are small, tender, purple, subcutaneous nodules that develop in the digits and persist for hours or days. They are not pathognomonic and may be seen in other disorders, such as systemic lupus erythematosus and disseminated gonococcal infections, and distal to infected arterial catheters. Janeway's lesions are small, erythematous or hemorrhagic, macular lesions on the palms and soles; unlike Osler's nodes, they are nontender. Roth's spots (also known as Litten's sign) are oval retinal hemorrhages with pale centers and are relatively rare.

Neurologic manifestations are found in about 20% of children with endocarditis.[12] They are associated with increased mortality and are more frequent in patients with *S. aureus* endocarditis. Neurologic complications include cerebral emboli, mycotic aneurysms, cerebritis, brain abscess, cerebral hemorrhage, and, less commonly, meningitis.

Embolic manifestations occur in some children with endocarditis, usually in association with infections that produce large bulky vegetations. Clinically recognized emboli are found most commonly in the pulmonary or cerebral circulations. Endocarditis involving the left side of the heart commonly results in peripheral embolization, lead-

TABLE 50–4

DEFINITIONS OF TERMS USED IN THE DUKE CRITERIA FOR THE DIAGNOSIS
OF INFECTIVE ENDOCARDITIS

MAJOR CRITERIA

1. Positive blood culture for IE
   A. Typical microorganism consistent with IE from two separate blood cultures as noted below:
      i. viridans streptococci,° *Streptococcus bovis*, or HACEK group *or*
      ii. community-acquired *Staphylococcus aureus* or enterococci, in the absence of a primary focus
   B. Microorganisms consistent with IE from persistently positive blood cultures defined as
      i. at least two positive cultures of blood samples drawn >12 hours apart *or*
      ii. all of three or a majority of four or more separate cultures of blood (with first and last sample drawn at least 1 hour apart)
2. Evidence of endocardial involvement
   A. Positive echocardiogram for IE defined as
      i. oscillating intracardiac mass on valve or supporting structures, in the path of regurgitant jets, or on implanted material in the absence of an alternative anatomic explanation, *or*
      ii. myocardial abscess, *or*
      iii. new partial dehiscence of prosthetic valve
   B. New valvar regurgitation (worsening or changing of pre-existing murmur not sufficient)

MINOR CRITERIA

1. Predisposition: predisposing heart condition or intravenous drug use
2. Fever: temperature ≥38.0°C
3. Vascular phenomena: major arterial emboli, septic pulmonary infarcts, mycotic aneurysm, intracranial hemorrhage, conjunctival hemorrhages, and Janeway's lesions
4. Immunologic phenomena: glomerulonephritis, Osler's nodes, Roth's spots, and rheumatoid factor
5. Microbiologic evidence: positive blood culture but does not meet a major criterion as noted in Table 50–3† or serologic evidence of active infection with organism consistent with IE
6. Echocardiographic findings: consistent with IE but do not meet a major criterion above

---

HACEK = *Haemophilus* species, *Actinobacillus actinomycetemcomitans*, *Cardiobacterium hominis*, *Eikenella* species, and *Kingella kingae*; IE = infective endocarditis.
°Includes nutritional variant strains.
†Excludes single positive cultures for coagulase-negative staphylococci and organisms that do not cause endocarditis.
Reprinted from American Journal of Medicine, Volume 96, Durack DT, Lukes AS, Bright DK: New criteria for diagnosis of infective endocarditis: Utilization of specific echocardiographic findings, Pages 200–209, Copyright 1994, with permission from Excerpta Medica Inc.

---

ing to ischemia, infarction, or mycotic aneurysms (aneurysms caused by growth of the organism in the vessel wall). Specific clinical findings depend on the localization of the emboli. Mycotic aneurysms may be silent but can rupture or thrombose months after IE has been cured. Embolization from the right side may be no less frequent, but such emboli are not easily appreciated clinically because of filtration by the lungs. Sometimes they cause an erroneous diagnosis of pneumonitis. However, large infected emboli may complicate endocarditis of the tricuspid valve, primarily in infants with IE secondary to indwelling catheters and in intravenous drug users. Embolic events may be an indication for surgical intervention. In patients with suspected embolic events, serial echocardiography can localize vegetations and define the changes that occur with time.

Renal involvement occurs in some patients with endocarditis. Renal dysfunction is usually secondary to hemodynamic changes. Renal emboli may be asymptomatic or cause flank pain, may result in gross or microscopic hematuria, but rarely result in significant renal dysfunction. Renal insufficiency may also occur from immune complex glomerulonephritis, particularly in patients with endocarditis caused by less virulent bacteria, such as coagulase-negative staphylococci. Azotemia may result from immune complex nephritis, but it usually improves after appropriate antimicrobial therapy.

LABORATORY FEATURES

BLOOD CULTURES

A positive blood culture is a valuable aid in making the diagnosis of endocarditis. Although a positive blood culture in a child with underlying or predisposing cardiac lesions does not necessarily indicate endocarditis, one must consider such a diagnosis. Blood cultures should be obtained in a child with a predisposition for endocarditis and persistent unexplained fever.

It is impossible to specify the exact number of cultures that should be obtained in each situation. The collection of three sets of blood cultures during a 24-hour period detects more than 97% of instances of bacterial endocarditis.[47] Once the etiologic agent has been identified, appropriate antimicrobial therapy can be begun. In some situations, making careful observations and obtaining more blood cultures before initiating antibiotic therapy are appropriate. In severely ill patients, three blood cultures should be obtained during a 1- to 2-hour period and antibiotic therapy instituted.

The bacteremia of endocarditis is often low grade and continuous.[48] Therefore, it is of no advantage to obtain blood cultures at any particular body temperature. Furthermore, the more blood that is collected, the better the chance of growing the bacteria. At least 20 ml of blood is usually collected from an adult patient, but this is not possible in a small child. As large a volume as is reasonable (preferably 3 to 5 ml) should be obtained. Either arterial or venous blood can be used, and samples should be drawn through venipuncture, not through an indwelling catheter. These samples should be taken after carefully sterilizing the venipuncture sites, as if for minor surgery. It is important to take blood from more than one site to reduce the risk of confusion by a skin contaminant. The microbiology laboratory should be consulted about the optimal volumes of blood and culture medium.

CULTURE-NEGATIVE ENDOCARDITIS

Culture-negative endocarditis refers to the situation in which the individual has IE but blood cultures are persistently negative. Blood cultures can be negative for a variety of reasons.[48a] Previous antimicrobial therapy is a major cause of a negative blood culture.[49] Blood cultures should become positive after cessation of the antimicrobial therapy; they remain negative for a longer time after prolonged prior antibiotic treatment.[48] The antibiotic can be removed from the blood with use of a resin device.[47]

On occasion, a patient is clinically suspected of having endocarditis, has not received antibiotics, yet has a negative blood culture. True culture-negative endocarditis is uncommon. The data in Table 50–2 show that 16.4% in this series had negative cultures, although this number included children who had received antimicrobial therapy and data from reports of several decades ago when blood culture techniques were unsophisticated by today's standards. In the absence of prior antimicrobial therapy, the incidence of endocarditis with a negative blood culture is 5% or less.[50] Many of these individuals demonstrate subsequent proof of endocarditis, either from culture of an infected embolus or from vegetations removed in the operating room or at necropsy. Some microorganisms capable of causing endocarditis are difficult to grow in culture with use of standard laboratory techniques, and prolonged incubation, special media, or other special techniques are needed.[37,47,50] Consultation with a clinical microbiologist is invaluable in seeking unusual and fastidious organisms. Microorganisms reported to cause culture-negative endocarditis include fastidious bacteria such as the nutritionally deficient streptococcus, fungi, HACEK organisms, *Coxiella burnetii*, and *Chlamydia*.[37,50,51]

OTHER LABORATORY TESTS

A variety of other laboratory tests, although nonspecific, can help support the diagnosis of endocarditis. Acute-phase reactants and the erythrocyte sedimentation rate are commonly elevated. Anemia is also common but may be missed if there was preceding polycythemia. It may be absent acutely but usually appears or worsens in long-standing infection. Leukocytosis may be present, although it is not a prominent feature of fungal endocarditis. Rheumatoid factor is present in as many as half of individuals with endocarditis, especially if it is of long duration.[48,52] Circulating immune complexes (CICs), formed by an antibody-antigen interaction, are found in the sera of most patients with IE, especially in those whose illness is of longer duration.[3,48,53] CICs are associated with arthritis and acute or chronic glomerulonephritis.[53,54] Levels of CICs usually fall with successful antibiotic treatment of IE and thus may be used to monitor therapy. Urinalysis may show proteinuria and macroscopic or microscopic hematuria.

ECHOCARDIOGRAPHY

Studies have evaluated the role of echocardiography to establish the diagnosis of endocarditis in adults[55,56] and children[3,5,22,57–60] with suspected IE. Two-dimensional echocardiography has a sensitivity in children of up to 80%.[3,5,57–61] Neither sensitivity nor specificity of echocardiography is 100%, so that a normal echocardiogram does not exclude endocarditis. Echocardiography is more helpful in children with normal cardiac anatomy or with isolated valvar abnormalities than in children with more complex congenital anomalies.[22] The application of the Duke criteria[39] for the diagnosis of IE in children has demonstrated that in addition to a positive blood culture, echocardiography plays a major role in the diagnosis.[43]

Transesophageal echocardiography (TEE) has been increasingly used in diagnosing endocarditis in adults, showing superior sensitivity for detecting vegetations compared with transthoracic echocardiography (TTE).[55,56] In adults, TEE is able to detect smaller vegetations (1 to 1.5 mm) than is TTE (2 mm). Studies of the usefulness of TEE in children with endocarditis have not been published.

In addition to detecting vegetations, echocardiography is also useful for evaluating valvar and extravalvar complications of IE and aiding in decision-making concerning the necessity and timing of cardiac operation. For more complete guidelines on the use of echocardiography in the diagnosis of IE, the reader is referred to the 1997 American College of Cardiology/American Heart Association Guidelines for the clinical use of echocardiography.[62]

ANTIMICROBIAL TREATMENT

Eradication of infecting organisms in patients with endocarditis is the target of antibiotic therapy. A prolonged period of therapy (at least 2 weeks, and often 4 to 6 weeks) is necessary for several reasons. Organisms are imbedded within the fibrin-platelet matrix (which impedes the entry of host phagocytic cells into the vegetation); they exist in high concentrations with relatively low rates of bacterial metabolism and cell division,[63,64] which result in decreased susceptibility to antibiotics.[64]

It is important to establish the microbiologic diagnosis before therapy is begun. This allows susceptibility testing and determination of minimal inhibitory concentration (MIC) and minimal bactericidal concentration (MBC). The MIC is the minimal concentration of antibiotic that inhibits growth in vitro, whereas the MBC is the minimal concentration of antibiotic that achieves a 99.9% decrease in the number of bacteria at 24 hours. These data assist in choosing the most appropriate antibiotic regimen.[65] Peak and trough serum levels should be monitored when potentially toxic antibiotics, such as vancomycin and aminoglycoside, are used. This ensures that levels are adequate and below the toxic range.

Bactericidal, rather than bacteriostatic, antibiotics should be chosen whenever possible to lessen the possibility of treatment failures or relapses. When combinations of antibiotics are employed, they can be tested in the laboratory for synergistic bactericidal activity, for example, the combination of penicillin G with gentamicin against enterococci or α-hemolytic streptococci.[65–67] Parenteral administration is recommended because of the need to achieve high serum levels of the antibiotics. In infants and small children, intravenous antibiotics are preferred over intramuscular agents because of the small muscle mass. In addition, intramuscular injections can be painful. Use of heparin lock devices for intravenous therapy in older children allows them more mobility and activity. Outpatient treatment of endocarditis can be considered in selected patients after initial treatment in the hospital and after hemodynamic stability and the patient's (or parent's) compliance are confirmed. It is increasingly used in adults[68]; however, it has not been generally recommended in children.

Blood cultures should be repeated often to assess the adequacy of the antibiotic regimen and to document the cessation of bacteremia. Bacteremia generally resolves within several days of beginning appropriate therapy. Patients with endocarditis require close follow-up. Obtaining occasional blood cultures at 1 and 2 months after completion of treatment is important, because most relapses occur during this period.[69]

Cardiovascular surgery may be lifesaving in some patients with IE. Decisions for operative intervention must be individualized. Indications for operation include progressive cardiac failure, valvar obstruction, suppurative complications around or near an infected valve, fungal endocarditis, persistent bacteremia, and significant embolic events,[70–72] especially when the aortic or mitral valve is involved. Medical management of progressive valvar damage and resulting cardiac failure is dangerous. Operation should not be delayed solely because a full course of antibiotic therapy has not been completed.

A detailed set of recommendations for antibiotic treatment of gram-positive bacterial endocarditis in the adult population has been made by the American Heart Association.[73] Table 50–5 is modeled after these guidelines. Antimicrobial treatment of endocarditis caused by the various gram-positive organisms is detailed in the following.

STREPTOCOCCAL AND ENTEROCOCCAL ENDOCARDITIS ON NATIVE OR PROSTHETIC CARDIAC VALVES (Table 50–5)

Streptococci are the most common organisms causing IE in children (see Table 50–2). Most of these organisms are viridans streptococci; the rest are *Streptococcus bovis* (nonenterococcal group D streptococci) or *Streptococcus pyogenes* (group A streptococci). Penicillin-susceptible streptococci have MIC to penicillin of less than 0.1 μg/ml. For patients who are able to take penicillin, two therapeutic regimens are associated with high cure rates (see Table 50–5).

A 4-week regimen of intravenous aqueous crystalline penicillin G cures up to 98%.[74] This regimen is preferred for children with impairment of renal function or of the eighth nerve. In adults, 4 weeks of therapy with once-daily ceftriaxone is also recommended[73] with bacteriologic cure rate of 98%,[75] but there are no data on the use of ceftriaxone in the treatment of pediatric IE.

A 2-week combined penicillin and aminoglycoside regimen has become increasingly popular and results in bacteriologic cure rates as high as 98%.[76] Synergy between penicillin G and aminoglycosides has been demonstrated in vitro and in experimental endocarditis.[66,67,77] This 2-week regimen is appropriate for uncomplicated instances of native valve IE but is not recommended for patients who have had endocarditis for more than 3 months or for those

---

TABLE 50–5

TREATMENT REGIMENS FOR ENDOCARDITIS CAUSED BY STREPTOCOCCI AND ENTEROCOCCI

Organism	Antimicrobial Agent	Dosage (per kg/24 h)	Maximal Dose (per 24 h)	Frequency of Administration	Duration
For patients not penicillin allergic					
Penicillin susceptible (MIC < 0.1 μg/ml)	Penicillin G *or*	200,000 U IV	18 million U	Continuous or q 4–6 hr	4 wk
	Penicillin G	200,000 U IV	18 million U	q 4–6 hr	2 wk
	plus gentamicin°	6 mg IM or IV	80 mg	q 8 hr	2 wk
Relatively resistant to penicillin (MIC 0.1–0.5 μg/ml)	Penicillin G	300,000 U IV	18 million U	q 4–6 hr	4 wk
	plus gentamicin°	6 mg IM or IV	80 mg	q 8 hr	2 wk
Enterococci or other resistant streptococci (MIC > 0.5 μg/ml)	Ampicillin	300 mg IV	12 g	q 4–6 hr	4–6 wk†
	plus gentamicin°	6 mg IM or IV	80 mg	q 8 hr	4–6 wk†
For penicillin-allergic patients					
MIC < 0.5 μg/ml	Vancomycin°	40 mg IV	2 g	q 6–12 hr	4 wk
MIC > 0.5 μg/ml	Vancomycin°	40 mg IV	2 g	q 6–12 hr	4–6 wk†
	plus gentamicin°	6 mg IM or IV	80 mg	q 8 hr	4–6 wk†

MIC = minimal inhibitory concentration.
°Dosing of gentamicin or vancomycin on a milligram per kilogram basis will produce higher serum concentrations in obese patients than in lean patients.
†Four weeks of therapy is recommended for patients with symptoms less than 3 months in duration; 6 weeks of therapy is recommended for patients with symptoms longer than 3 months in duration.

who have extracardiac foci of infection, intracardiac abscesses, or mycotic aneurysm. It is also inappropriate for children at risk for adverse events caused by gentamicin therapy.

For patients who are allergic to β-lactam antibiotics, vancomycin therapy is recommended (see Table 50–5). Each dose of this antibiotic should be infused during 1 to 2 hours to reduce the risk of the histamine-release "red man" syndrome. Children "allergic" to penicillins, but without a clear-cut history of an anaphylactic reaction, may be candidates for penicillin desensitization.

On occasion, the infection may be due to streptococci that are relatively resistant to penicillin (MIC between 0.1 μg/ml and 0.5 μg/ml). For these, the recommended treatment regimen is 4 weeks of penicillin combined with gentamicin for the first 2 weeks. For children who are allergic to β-lactams, vancomycin should be used.

Enterococcal endocarditis is uncommon in children. Treatment is difficult because of the relative resistance of enterococci to penicillin, expanded-spectrum penicillins, and vancomycin and their variable resistance to aminoglycosides.[78,79] The treatment regimen requires combination therapy of penicillin G or ampicillin with gentamicin for at least 4 and preferably 6 weeks.[73,78] For patients allergic to penicillins (but without a history of anaphylactic-type reaction), penicillin desensitization can be considered. If desensitization is not considered feasible, vancomycin plus gentamicin for 4 to 6 weeks is recommended. Nutritionally variant streptococci or streptococci with MIC greater than 0.5 μg/ml should be treated with the regimens listed for enterococci.

These recommendations are for native valve endocarditis. If the infection involves a prosthetic cardiac valve, 6 weeks of penicillin combined with gentamicin for at least the first 2 weeks is recommended.[80] If the infection is caused by "relatively penicillin resistant" streptococci or enterococci, the penicillin treatment may last for 8 weeks. The vancomycin plus gentamicin regimen is recommended for penicillin-allergic individuals who are not desensitized to penicillins.

STAPHYLOCOCCAL ENDOCARDITIS ON NATIVE VALVES
(Table 50–6)

Staphylococci are coagulase-positive (*S. aureus*) or coagulase-negative (*S. epidermidis* and various other species). Most staphylococci are highly resistant to penicillin G and ampicillin because of production of β-lactamases,[81] one form of which is termed penicillinase. Staphylococci sensitive to penicillinase-resistant penicillins are termed methicillin susceptible. Antibiotic therapy for staphylococcal endocarditis involving a native valve (or other native cardiac tissue) must include a semisynthetic, penicillinase-resistant penicillin (nafcillin or oxacillin) administered intravenously for 4 to 6 weeks. The 6-week regimen is preferable and is more commonly used. Gentamicin may be added for the first 3 to 5 days, and this may accelerate the killing of the bacteria. For patients allergic to penicillins, vancomycin for 4 to 6 weeks is recommended. In adults, cephalosporins are also recommended as an alternative in β-lactam–allergic patients, with or without gentamicin for the first 3 to 5 days.[73] Cephalosporins should not be used in patients with a history of an anaphylactic-type reaction to penicillin.

Some coagulase-negative staphylococci and *S. aureus* strains are methicillin resistant. Therefore, patients with IE from these organisms cannot receive nafcillin, oxacillin, or a cephalosporin. In vitro tests of antimicrobial susceptibility may suggest that cephalosporins are effective, but these organisms are indeed resistant to cephalosporins, and they should not be used as therapeutic agents. Patients with methicillin-resistant staphylococcal endocarditis should be treated for 4 to 6 weeks with vancomycin.

STAPHYLOCOCCAL ENDOCARDITIS ON INTRACARDIAC PROSTHETIC MATERIAL (Table 50–6)

Staphylococcal endocarditis on a prosthetic cardiac valve or other cardiac prosthetic material is usually nosocomially acquired. Most infections are from methicillin-resistant organisms, especially if the endocarditis develops within 1 year of

TABLE 50–6
TREATMENT REGIMENS FOR ENDOCARDITIS CAUSED BY STAPHYLOCOCCI

Organism	Antimicrobial Agent	Dosage (per kg/24 h)	Maximal Dose (per 24 h)	Frequency of Administration	Duration
STAPHYLOCOCCAL NATIVE VALVE ENDOCARDITIS					
Methicillin susceptible	Nafcillin or oxacillin	200 mg IV	12 g	q 4–6 hr	4–6 wk
	± gentamicin°	6 mg IM or IV	80 mg	q 8 hr	3–5 days
Penicillin allergic or methicillin resistant (including coagulase-negative staphylococci)	Vancomycin°	40 mg IV	2 g	q 6–12 hr	4–6 wk
STAPHYLOCOCCAL PROSTHETIC VALVE ENDOCARDITIS					
Methicillin susceptible	Nafcillin or oxacillin	200 mg IV	12 g	q 4–6 hr	≥6 wk
	with rifampin	20 mg orally	600 mg	q 8 hr	≥6 wk
	and with gentamicin°	6 mg IM or IV	80 mg	q 8 hr	2 wk
Methicillin resistant	Vancomycin°	40 mg IV	2 g	q 6–12 hr	≥6 wk
	with rifampin	20 mg orally	600 mg	q 8 hr	≥6 wk
	and with gentamicin°	6 mg IM or IV	80 mg	q 8 hr	2 wk

°For specific dosing issues concerning gentamicin and vancomycin, see footnotes on Table 50–5.

a cardiac operation.[80] Treatment requires a minimum of 6 weeks of vancomycin plus rifampin, with gentamicin for the first 2 weeks. If the bacteria are methicillin susceptible, nafcillin or oxacillin can replace vancomycin. For further recommendations on the treatment of staphylococcal endocarditis on intracardiac prosthetic material, the reader is referred to the American Heart Association guidelines.[73]

Staphylococcal bacteremia in patients with indwelling venous catheters or lines may be treated for 10 to 14 days with appropriate antibiotics after removal of the catheter as long as the patient is not severely ill and has no signs of organ involvement.

GRAM-NEGATIVE BACTERIAL ENDOCARDITIS

Gram-negative bacteria are an infrequent cause of endocarditis in children (see Table 50–2). The gram-negative bacteria most commonly causing endocarditis in children are the HACEK group of fastidious coccobacilli (*Haemophilus parainfluenzae, Haemophilus aphrophilus, Actinobacillus actinomycetemcomitans, Cardiobacterium hominis, Eikenella corrodens,* and *Kingella kingae*). Recommended therapy for the HACEK group is a 4-week course of ampicillin plus gentamicin, or ceftriaxone or another third-generation cephalosporin.[73]

Other gram-negative organisms, such as *Escherichia coli, Pseudomonas aeruginosa,* or *Serratia marcescens,* are occasionally noted. Most patients with these organisms are intravenous drug abusers, although a postoperative cardiac patient, an immunocompromised individual, or a neonate may occasionally have endocarditis with one of these organisms. Therapy must be individualized, guided by identification of the organism and antimicrobial susceptibility testing. Most experience has been with a broad-spectrum penicillin, such as ticarcillin, or a cephalosporin, such as cefotaxime or ceftazidime, combined with an aminoglycoside, such as gentamicin or amikacin.[82] At least 6 weeks of therapy is recommended.

Gonococcal endocarditis can be treated successfully with high-dose penicillin, provided that the organism is penicillin susceptible. For penicillin-resistant organisms, an appropriate third-generation cephalosporin is recommended.

FUNGAL ENDOCARDITIS

The prognosis in fungal endocarditis is poor and associated with high mortality and morbidity. Few patients survived when the entire treatment was with antifungal agents. Valve replacement operation in conjunction with antifungal agents is usually required.[31] Operation is best performed after 10 days of medical therapy if the patient's hemodynamic status permits but earlier if there are embolic phenomena.

Amphotericin B remains the first-line antifungal agent for medical therapy. A "test" dose of 0.1 mg/kg of amphotericin B (maximum, 1 mg) is administered initially. If it is well tolerated, it is followed by a dose of 0.5 mg/kg for 1 day and then 1 mg/kg/day as the maintenance dose. The minimal duration of therapy should be 6 to 8 weeks. Renal function and serum potassium concentration should be carefully monitored.

PROSTHETIC VALVE ENDOCARDITIS

Infection of a prosthetic cardiac valve occurs in between 1% and 4% of all patients at some time during the life span of the prosthesis.[28] Antibiotic therapy for patients with an infected prosthetic cardiac valve or other prosthetic material must be appropriate for the specific infecting agent. Therapy is given for 6 weeks or longer. Treatment regimens for a prosthetic valve infected with streptococci, staphylococci, or enterococci are discussed in the preceding sections.

Prosthetic valve endocarditis caused by diphtheroids is best treated with penicillin and gentamicin, or with vancomycin for penicillin-allergic patients.[80] Duration of therapy should be 6 weeks.

Therapy for prosthetic valve endocarditis caused by gram-negative bacilli must be based on the results of in vitro MIC and MBC tests and in vitro evaluation of antimicrobial synergy. Common regimens include a third-generation cephalosporin or a broad-spectrum penicillin with gentamicin for at least 6 to 8 weeks.

Experience with prosthetic valve endocarditis, derived mainly in adults, has emphasized that early replacement of the infected valve may lower the high mortality rate associated with such infections.[28] The timing of replacement of an infected prosthesis must be individualized. Some recommend that most or all patients with staphylococcal or early-onset prosthetic valve endocarditis should undergo replacement of the infected prosthetic valve. Indications for cardiac operation during active infection of a prosthetic valve include moderate to severe heart failure, significant valvar obstruction, fungal endocarditis, persistent bacteremia despite appropriate antibiotics for 10 to 14 days, an unstable prosthesis, ruptured sinus of Valsalva or ventricular septum, and recurrent major emboli.[28] Less definite indications for surgery include a single major embolus, bacteriologic relapse after an appropriate course of therapy, echocardiographic demonstration of a large vegetation, and extension of infection to an annular abscess or myocardial abscess.[28]

CULTURE-NEGATIVE ENDOCARDITIS

Treatment of culture-negative endocarditis is difficult. If blood cultures remain negative after careful work-up and specialized laboratory techniques, patients with native valve endocarditis should be treated with a penicillinase-resistant penicillin (nafcillin or oxacillin) and gentamicin. Some experts recommend adding penicillin to this regimen.[12] If the infection involves a prosthetic cardiac valve, vancomycin should be added to the regimen.[80] For penicillin-allergic individuals, vancomycin and gentamicin should be used. Discontinuation of the aminoglycoside after 2 weeks may be considered if there has been a substantial response to therapy. Treatment should be continued for 6 full weeks.[83]

PREVENTION

Prevention of endocarditis is desirable whenever possible. However, there has been no prospective study in patients with underlying structural cardiac disease to determine definitively whether prophylactic antibiotics provide protection against development of endocarditis during bacteremia-inducing procedures. Further, only a minority of instances of endocarditis (20% or less) are attributable to an invasive procedure, and only about half of individuals who develop endocarditis have an underlying cardiac anomaly for which prophylaxis would have been given. Durack[84] estimated that less than 500 instances of endocarditis per year in the United States could be prevented by use of a fully effective prophylactic regimen, but he also pointed out that prevention of even this small number remains desirable because of the substantial morbidity and mortality of the disease. Antimicrobial prophylaxis represents the accepted standard of practice in most countries, and the most widely used guidelines in the United States are those issued by the American Heart Association.[85] Their recommendations are based on analyses of the literature regarding procedure-related endocarditis, including in vitro susceptibility data of pathogens causing endocarditis, data from prophylactic studies in animal models of endocarditis, and retrospective analyses of human endocarditis cases in terms of antibiotic prophylaxis usage patterns and apparent prophylaxis failures.[85] These recommendations should not be viewed as the standard of care in all situations or as a substitute for clinical judgment.

Not all situations in which a bacteremia may occur are readily identifiable. Also, some bacteremias occur spontaneously on a daily basis (chewing of food, teeth brushing) and cannot logically be prevented. Most native valve endocarditis is caused by organisms that originate from the oral cavity. Therefore, children at risk for endocarditis should establish and maintain the best possible oral health to reduce potential sources of bacteremia. Individuals with cyanosis often have spongy, friable gums.[11] Optimal tooth care is especially important in these patients.

Antibiotic prophylaxis is recommended for children at risk who are undergoing procedures likely to cause a bacteremia with organisms that cause endocarditis. Recommendations listed here are based on those issued by the American Heart Association.[85] Certain cardiac conditions are associated with endocarditis more often than others are. Endocarditis prophylaxis is recommended for individuals who have a higher risk for development of endocarditis than that of the general population. Prophylaxis is especially important for children, in whom endocarditis is associated with high morbidity and mortality. Table 50–7 stratifies cardiac conditions into high-, moderate-, and negligible-risk categories.

Individuals in the high-risk category are at a much higher risk than the general population for development of severe endocardial infection that is often associated with substantial morbidity and mortality. On the other hand, individuals in the negligible-risk category have no greater risk for development of endocarditis than does the general population. Most congenital and acquired cardiac malformations and valvar dysfunction, however, fall into the moderate-risk category. The risk for development of endocarditis is greater for some of these conditions than for others, but they are all associated with a risk greater than that of the general population.[86] Some conditions (such as atrial septal defect, ventricular septal defect, and patent ductus

TABLE 50–7

CARDIAC CONDITIONS

ENDOCARDITIS PROPHYLAXIS RECOMMENDED
High-Risk Category
Prosthetic cardiac valves, including bioprosthetic and homograft valves
Previous bacterial endocarditis
Complex cyanotic congenital heart disease (e.g., single ventricle states, transposition of the great arteries, tetralogy of Fallot)
Surgically constructed systemic-pulmonary shunts or conduits

Moderate-Risk Category
Most other congenital cardiac malformations (other than above and below)
Acquired valvar dysfunction (e.g., rheumatic heart disease)
Hypertrophic cardiomyopathy
Mitral valve prolapse with valvar regurgitation or thickened leaflets*

ENDOCARDITIS PROPHYLAXIS NOT RECOMMENDED
Negligible-Risk Category
Isolated secundum atrial septal defect
Surgical repair without residua beyond 6 months of atrial septal defect, ventricular septal defect, or patent ductus arteriosus
Previous coronary artery bypass graft surgery
Mitral valve prolapse without valvar regurgitation*
Physiologic, functional, or innocent heart murmurs
Previous Kawasaki disease without valvar dysfunction
Previous rheumatic fever without valvar dysfunction
Cardiac pacemakers and implanted defibrillators

*See text for further details.

arteriosus), once successfully corrected, no longer require prophylaxis after a 6-month healing period.

Mitral valve prolapse poses problems in terms of the need for endocarditis prophylaxis. Individuals with a prolapsed mitral valve and a murmur of valvar regurgitation are at increased risk for the development of endocarditis and are placed in the moderate-risk category[85–87] (see Chapter 44). Patients in whom regurgitation has not been demonstrated are not at higher risk than the general population and are in a negligible-risk category. Several pediatric cardiologists believe that a careful evaluation of valve morphology and function is needed in children who have isolated clinical findings (such as a midsystolic click), because this may be the only indication of an important abnormality requiring prophylaxis.[9]

TABLE 50–8

COMMON PROCEDURES FOR WHICH PROPHYLAXIS IS RECOMMENDED*

Dental extractions
Initial placement of orthodontic bands
Cleaning or scaling where bleeding is anticipated
Surgical operations involving respiratory mucosa
Bronchoscopy with a rigid bronchoscope
Sclerotherapy for esophageal varices
Esophageal stricture dilatation
Endoscopic retrograde cholangiography with biliary obstruction
Biliary tract surgery
Surgical operations that involve intestinal mucosa
Cystoscopy
Urethral dilatation

*This table is not meant to be all-inclusive. For a more complete list of procedures for which prophylaxis is or is not recommended, see the American Heart Association guidelines.[85]

TABLE 50–9		
PROPHYLACTIC REGIMENS FOR DENTAL, ORAL, RESPIRATORY TRACT, OR ESOPHAGEAL PROCEDURES		
Situation	Agent	Regimen
Standard general prophylaxis	Amoxicillin	50 mg/kg (not to exceed 2 g) PO 1 hr before procedure°
Unable to take oral medications	Ampicillin	50 mg/kg (not to exceed 2 g) IM or IV within 30 min before procedure°
Penicillin allergic	Clindamycin	20 mg/kg (not to exceed 600 mg) PO 1 hr before procedure°
	or	
	Cephalexin† or cefadroxil†	50 mg/kg (not to exceed 2 g) PO 1 hr before procedure°
	or	
	Azithromycin or clarithromycin	15 mg/kg (not to exceed 500 mg) PO 1 hr before procedure°
Penicillin allergic and unable to take oral medications	Clindamycin	20 mg/kg (not to exceed 600 mg) IV within 30 min before procedure°
	or	
	Cefazolin†	25 mg/kg (not to exceed 1 g) IM or IV within 30 min before procedure°

°For patients in the high-risk category for endocarditis, half the dose may be repeated 6 hours after the initial dose (except for azithromycin—a second dose is not necessary).

†Cephalosporins should not be used in individuals with immediate-type hypersensitivity reaction (urticaria, angioedema, or anaphylaxis) to penicillins.

TABLE 50–10		
PROPHYLACTIC REGIMENS FOR GENITOURINARY TRACT OR GASTROINTESTINAL (EXCLUDING ESOPHAGEAL) PROCEDURES		
Situation	Agents*	Regimen
High-risk patients	Ampicillin plus gentamicin	Ampicillin 50 mg/kg IM or IV (not to exceed 2 g) plus gentamicin 1.5 mg/kg (not to exceed 120 mg) within 30 min before starting the procedure Six hours later, ampicillin 25 mg/kg (not to exceed 1 g) IM or IV or amoxicillin 25 mg/kg (not to exceed 1 g) PO
High-risk patients allergic to ampicillin or amoxicillin	Vancomycin plus gentamicin	Vancomycin 20 mg/kg (not to exceed 1 g) IV during 1–2 hr plus gentamicin 1.5 mg/kg IV or IM (not to exceed 120 mg) Complete injection or infusion within 30 min before starting the procedure
Medium-risk patients	Amoxicillin *or* Ampicillin	Amoxicillin 50 mg/kg (not to exceed 2 g) PO 1 hr before procedure Ampicillin 50 mg/kg (not to exceed 2 g) IM or IV within 30 min before starting the procedure
Medium-risk patients allergic to ampicillin or amoxicillin	Vancomycin	Vancomycin 20 mg/kg (not to exceed 1 g) IV during 1–2 hr Complete infusion within 30 min before starting procedure

*No second dose of vancomycin or gentamicin is recommended.

Certain procedures cause bacteremias with organisms commonly associated with endocarditis. These are outlined in Table 50–8.

Antibiotic regimens for endocarditis prophylaxis are listed in Tables 50–9 and 50–10. If a patient is already taking an antibiotic when he or she has a procedure that requires endocarditis prophylaxis, an antibiotic from a different class should be chosen for prophylaxis rather than increasing the dose of the current antibiotic.

The need for prophylaxis may change after operative or other reparative procedures.[86,88,89] For example, successful closure of atrial septal defect, ventricular septal defect, or patent ductus arteriosus reduces the patient's long-term risk for development of endocarditis, and after a 6-month healing period, prophylaxis is no longer required. Other procedures, such as balloon dilatation or repair of complex cardiac malformation, do not alter the patient's long-term risk for endocarditis. Still other procedures, such as replacement of a native cardiac valve with a prosthetic valve or aortic valve surgery,[90] actually put the patient in a higher risk category.[86,88]

REFERENCES

1. Johnson DH, Rosenthal A, Nadas AS: Bacterial endocarditis in children under 2 years of age. Am J Dis Child 129:183, 1975.
2. Zakrewski T, Keith JD: Bacterial endocarditis in infants and children. J Pediatr 67:1179, 1965.
3. Van Hare GF, Ben-Shachar G, Liebman J, et al: Infective endocarditis in infants and children during the past 10 years: A decade of change. Am Heart J 107:1235, 1984.
4. Harris SL: Definitions and demographic characteristics. *In* Kaye D (ed): Infective Endocarditis, 2nd ed. New York, Raven Press, 1992, p 1.
5. Coutlee F, Carceller A, Deschamps L, et al: The evolving pattern of pediatric endocarditis from 1960 to 1985. Can J Cardiol 6:164, 1990.
6. Kramer HH, Bourgenis M, Liersch R, et al: Current clinical aspects of bacterial endocarditis in infancy, childhood, and adolescence. Eur J Pediatr 140:253, 1983.
7. Kaplan EL, Rich H, Gersony W, Manning J: A collaborative study of infective endocarditis in the pediatric age group: An overview. *In* Kaplan EL, Taranta AV (eds): Infective Endocarditis—An American Heart Association Symposium. Dallas, American Heart Association, 1977, p 51. Monograph No. 52.
8. Johnson CM, Rhodes KH: Pediatric endocarditis. Mayo Clin Proc 57:86, 1982.

9. Awadallah SM, Kavey R-EW, Byrum CJ, et al: The changing pattern of infective endocarditis in childhood. Am J Cardiol 68:90, 1991.

10. American Heart Association: 1997 Heart and Stroke Statistical Update. Dallas, American Heart Association, 1997, p 18.

11. Dodo H, Child JS: Infective endocarditis in congenital heart disease. Cardiol Clin 14:383, 1996.

12. Berkowitz FE: Infective endocarditis. In Nichols DG, Cameron DE, Greeley WJ, et al (eds): Critical Heart Disease in Infants and Children. St. Louis, Mosby–Year Book, 1995, p 961.

13. Blumenthal S, Griffiths SP, Morgan BC: Bacterial endocarditis in children with heart disease: A review based on the literature and experience with 58 cases. Pediatrics 26:993, 1960.

14. Baltimore RS: Infective endocarditis in children. Pediatr Infect Dis J 11:907, 1992.

15. Normand J, Bozio A, Etienne J, et al: Changing patterns and prognosis of infective endocarditis in childhood. Eur Heart J 16(suppl B):28, 1995.

16. Berkowitz FE, Dansky R: Infective endocarditis in black South African children: Report of 10 cases with some unusual features. Pediatr Infect Dis J 8:787, 1989.

17. Bhandara S, Kaul U, Shrivastava S, et al: Infective endocarditis in children. Indian J Pediatr 51:529, 1984.

18. Somers K, Patel AK, Steiner I, et al: Infective endocarditis: An African experience. Br Heart J 34:1107, 1972.

19. Hugo-Hamman CT, de Moor MM, Human DG: Infective endocarditis in South African children. J Trop Pediatr 35:154, 1989.

20. Moethilalh R, Coovadia HM: Infective endocarditis in thirteen children: A retrospective study (1974–1981). Ann Trop Paediatr 2:57, 1982.

21. Noel GJ, O'Loughlin JE, Edelson PJ: Neonatal Staphylococcus epidermidis right-sided endocarditis: Description of five catheterized infants. Pediatrics 82:234, 1988.

22. Saiman L, Prince A, Gersony WM: Pediatric infective endocarditis in the modern era. J Pediatr 122:847, 1993.

23. Millard DD, Shulman ST: The changing spectrum of neonatal endocarditis. Clin Perinatol 15:587, 1988.

24. Rodbard S: Blood velocity and endocarditis. Circulation 27:18, 1963.

25. Gould K, Ramirez-Ronda CH, Holmes RK, Sanford JP: Adherence of bacteria to heart valves in vitro. J Clin Invest 56:1364, 1975.

26. Scheld WM, Valone JA, Sande MA: Bacterial adherence in the pathogenesis of endocarditis: Interaction of bacterial dextran, platelets, and fibrin. J Clin Invest 61:1394, 1978.

27. Sande MA, Lee BL, Mills J, Chambers HF: Endocarditis in intravenous drug users. In Kaye D (ed): Infective Endocarditis, 2nd ed. New York, Raven Press, 1992, p 345.

28. Douglas JL, Cobbs CG: Prosthetic valve endocarditis. In Kaye D (ed): Infective Endocarditis, 2nd ed. New York, Raven Press, 1992, p 375.

29. Andriole VT, Kravetz HM, Roberts WC, Utz JP: Candida endocarditis. Am J Med 32:251, 1962.

30. Seelig MS, Goldberg P, Kozinn PJ, Berger AR: Fungal endocarditis: Patients at risk and their treatment. Postgrad Med J 55:632, 1979.

31. Moyer DV, Edwards JE: Fungal endocarditis. In Kaye D (ed): Infective Endocarditis, 2nd ed. New York, Raven Press, 1992, p 299.

32. Rubinstein E, Noreiga ER, Simberkoff MS, et al: Fungal endocarditis: Analysis of twenty-four cases and review of the literature. Medicine (Baltimore) 54:331, 1975.

33. Gulmen S, Anderson WR: Candida endocarditis with distal aortic embolization. Minn Med 60:469, 1977.

34. Johnson DE, Bass JL, Thompson TR, et al: Candida septicemia and a right atrial mass in infancy secondary to umbilical vein catheterization. Am J Dis Child 135:275, 1981.

35. Dato VM, Dajani AS: Candidemia in children with central venous catheters: Role of catheter removal and amphotericin B therapy. Pediatr Infect Dis J 9:309, 1990.

36. Mayayo E, Moralejo J, Camps J, Guarro J: Fungal endocarditis in premature infants: Case report and review. Clin Infect Dis 22:366, 1996.

37. Van Scoy RE: Culture-negative endocarditis. Mayo Clin Proc 57:149, 1982.

38. von Reyn CF, Levy BS, Arbeit RD, et al: Infective endocarditis: An analysis based on strict case definitions. Ann Intern Med 94:505, 1981.

39. Durack DT, Lukes AS, Bright DK: New criteria for diagnosis of infective endocarditis: Utilization of specific echocardiographic findings. Am J Med 96:200, 1994.

40. Bayer AS, Ward JL, Ginzton LE, Shapiro SM: Evaluation of new clinical criteria for the diagnosis of infective endocarditis. Am J Med 96:211, 1994.

41. Olaison L, Hogevik H: Comparison of the von Reyn and Duke criteria for the diagnosis of infective endocarditis: A critical analysis of 161 episodes. Scand J Infect Dis 28:399, 1996.

42. Hoen B, Selton-Suty C, Danchin N, et al: Evaluation of the Duke criteria versus the Beth Israel criteria for the diagnosis of infective endocarditis. Clin Infect Dis 21:905, 1995.

43. Stockheim JA, Chadwick EG, Kessler S, et al: Are the Duke criteria superior to the Beth Israelect criteria for the diagnosis of infective endocarditis in children? Clin Infect Dis 27:1451, 1998.

44. Starkebaum M, Durack D, Beeson P: The "incubation period" of bacterial endocarditis. Yale J Biol Med 50:49, 1977.

45. Weinstein L, Rubin RH: Infective endocarditis—1973. Prog Cardiovasc Dis 274:199, 1973.

46. Bain RC, Edwards JE, Scheiffen CH, et al: Right sided bacterial endocarditis and endarteritis: Clinical and pathologic studies. Am J Med 24:98, 1958.

47. Washington JA II: The role of microbiology laboratory in the diagnosis and antimicrobial treatment of infective endocarditis. Mayo Clin Proc 57:22, 1982.

48. Kaye KM, Kaye D: Laboratory findings including blood cultures. In Kaye D (ed): Infective Endocarditis, 2nd ed. New York, Raven Press, 1992, p 117.

48a. Bayer AS, Bolger AF, Taubert KA, et al: Diagnosis and management of infective endocarditis and its complications. Circulation 98:2936, 1998.

49. Hoen B, Selton-Suty C, Lacassin F, et al: Infective endocarditis in patients with negative blood cultures: Analysis of 88 cases from a one-year nationwide survey in France. Clin Infect Dis 20:501, 1995.

50. Tunkel AR, Kaye D: Endocarditis with negative blood cultures. N Engl J Med 326:1215, 1992.

51. Roberts KB, Sidlak MJ: Satellite streptococci: A major cause of negative blood cultures in bacterial endocarditis? JAMA 241:2293, 1979.

52. Messner RP, Laxdal T, Quie PG, Williams R: Rheumatoid factors in subacute bacterial endocarditis: Bacterium, duration of disease or genetic predisposition? Ann Intern Med 68:746, 1968.

53. Bayer AS, Theofilopoulos AN, Eisenberg R, et al: Circulating immune complexes in infective endocarditis. N Engl J Med 295:1500, 1976.

54. Kauffman RH, Thompson J, Valentijn RM, et al: The clinical implications and the pathogenetic significance of circulating immune complexes in infective endocarditis. Am J Med 71:17, 1981.

55. Sokil AB: Cardiac imaging in infective endocarditis. In Kaye D (ed): Infective Endocarditis, 2nd ed. New York, Raven Press, 1992, p 125.

56. Aragam JR, Weyman AE: Echocardiographic findings in infective endocarditis. In Weyman AE (ed): Principles and Practice of Echocardiography, 2nd ed. Philadelphia, Lea & Febiger, 1994, p 1178.

57. Dillon T, Meyer RA, Korfhagen JC, et al: Management of infective endocarditis using echocardiography. J Pediatr 96:552, 1980.

58. Kavey REW, Frank DM, Byrum CJ, et al: Two-dimensional echocardiographic assessment of infective endocarditis in children. Am J Dis Child 137:851, 1983.

59. Bricker JT, Latson LA, Huhta JC, Gutgesell HP: Echocardiographic evaluation of infective endocarditis in children. Clin Pediatr (Phila) 24:312, 1985.

60. Sable CA, Rome JJ, Martin GR, et al: Indications for echocardiography in the diagnosis of infective endocarditis in children. Am J Cardiol 75:801, 1995.

61. Berger M, Delfin LA, Jelveh M, et al: Two-dimensional echocardiographic findings in right-sided infective endocarditis. Circulation 61:855, 1980.

62. Cheitlin MD, Alpert JS, Armstrong WF, et al: ACC/AHA Guidelines for the clinical application of echocardiography: A report of the American College of Cardiology/American Heart Association Task Force on Practice Guidelines (Committee on Clinical Application of Echocardiography). Circulation 95:1686, 1997.

63. Durack DT, Beeson PB: Experimental bacterial endocarditis. I: Colonization of a sterile vegetation. Br J Exp Pathol 53:44, 1972.

64. Durack DT, Beeson PB: Experimental bacterial endocarditis. II: Survival of bacteria in endocardial vegetations. Br J Exp Pathol 53:50, 1972.

65. Baldassarre JS, Kaye D: Principles and overview of antibiotic therapy. In Kaye D (ed): Infective Endocarditis, 2nd ed. New York, Raven Press, 1992, p 169.

66. Sande MA, Irvin RG: Penicillin-aminoglycoside synergy in experimental *Streptococcus viridans* endocarditis. J Infect Dis 129:572, 1974.

67. Wolfe JC, Johnson WD Jr: Penicillin-sensitive streptococcal endocarditis: In vitro and clinical observations on penicillin-streptomycin therapy. Ann Intern Med 81:178, 1974.

68. Patton JP: Infective endocarditis: Economic considerations. *In* Kaye D (ed): Infective Endocarditis, 2nd ed. New York, Raven Press, 1992, p 413.

69. Santoro J, Ingerman M: Response to therapy: Relapses and reinfections. *In* Kaye D (ed): Infective Endocarditis, 2nd ed. New York, Raven Press, 1992, p 423.

70. Douglas JL, Dismukes WE: Surgical therapy of infective endocarditis on natural valves. *In* Kaye D (ed): Infective Endocarditis, 2nd ed. New York, Raven Press, 1992, p 397.

71. Citak M, Rees A, Mavroudis C: Surgical management of infective endocarditis in children. Ann Thorac Surg 54:755, 1992.

72. Tolan RW Jr, Kleiman MB, Frank M, et al: Operative intervention in active endocarditis in children: Report of a series of cases and review. Clin Infect Dis 14:852, 1992.

73. Wilson W, Karchmer AW, Dajani AS, et al: Antibiotic treatment of adults with infective endocarditis due to streptococci, enterococci, staphylococci, and HACEK microorganisms. JAMA 274:1706, 1995.

74. Karchmer AW, Moellering RC Jr, Maki DG, et al: Single-antibiotic therapy for streptococcal endocarditis. JAMA 241:1801, 1979.

75. Francioli P, Etienne J, Hoigne R, et al: Treatment of streptococcal endocarditis with a single daily dose of ceftriaxone sodium for 4 weeks: Efficacy and outpatient treatment feasibility. JAMA 267:264, 1992.

76. Wilson WR, Thompson RL, Wilkowske CJ, et al: Short-term therapy for streptococcal infective endocarditis: Combined intramuscular administration of penicillin and streptomycin. JAMA 245:360, 1981.

77. Sande MA, Scheld WM: Combination antibiotic therapy of bacterial endocarditis. Ann Intern Med 92:390, 1980.

78. Eliopoulos GM: Enterococcal endocarditis. *In* Kaye D (ed): Infective Endocarditis, 2nd ed. New York, Raven Press, 1992, p 209.

79. Eliopoulos GM: Aminoglycoside resistant enterococcal endocarditis. Med Clin North Am 17:117, 1993.

80. Karchmer AW, Gibbons GW: Infection of prosthetic heart valves and vascular grafts. *In* Bisno AL, Waldvogel FA (eds): Infections Associated With Indwelling Medical Devices, 2nd ed. Washington, DC, American Society for Microbiology, 1994, p 213.

81. Karchmer AW: Staphylococcal endocarditis. *In* Kaye D (ed): Infective Endocarditis, 2nd ed. New York, Raven Press, 1992, p 225.

82. Geraci JE, Wilson WR: Endocarditis due to gram-negative bacteria: Report of 56 cases. Mayo Clin Proc 57:145, 1982.

83. Pesanti EL, Smith IM: Infective endocarditis with negative blood cultures: An analysis of 52 cases. Am J Med 66:43, 1979.

84. Durack DT: Prevention of infective endocarditis. N Engl J Med 332:38, 1995.

85. Dajani AS, Taubert KA, Wilson W, et al: Prevention of bacterial endocarditis. Recommendations by the American Heart Association. JAMA 277:1974, 1997.

86. Steckelberg JM, Wilson WR: Risk factors for infective endocarditis. Infect Dis Clin North Am 7:9, 1993.

87. Child JS: Risks for and prevention of infective endocarditis. Cardiol Clin 14:327, 1996.

88. Gersony WM, Hayes CJ, Driscoll DJ: Bacterial endocarditis in patients with aortic stenosis, pulmonary stenosis, or ventricular septal defect. Circulation 87(suppl I):I-121, 1993.

89. Moller JH, Anderson RC: 1,000 consecutive children with a cardiac malformation with 26- to 37-year follow-up. Am J Cardiol 70:661, 1992.

90. Morris CD, Reller MD, Menashe VD: Thirty-year incidence of infective endocarditis after surgery for congenital heart defect. JAMA 279:599, 1998.

CHAPTER 51
PERICARDIAL DISEASE

TODD T. NOWLEN   J. TIMOTHY BRICKER

The pericardium is composed of two layers, visceral and parietal, that completely surround the heart and juxtacardiac vessels. The pericardium restricts diastolic volume and maintains the position of the heart; it also protects the heart from the spread of inflammation, adhesions, infection, and malignant neoplasms from contiguous structures.[1] The responses of the pericardium include dilatation in pericardial effusion with or without tamponade, acute and chronic inflammation, adhesion formation, and fibrosis with and without constriction. The visceral pericardium is a single serous layer covering the entire surface of the heart and extending a short distance onto the great vessels. It contains no fibrous component because it must be able to contract and distend easily. The parietal pericardium has three layers. The inner serous layer is continuous with the serous layer of the visceral pericardium and is separated from it by a potential space, the pericardial cavity. A small amount of serous fluid normally exists between the two layers and decreases friction, allowing free movement of the heart within the pericardial cavity. The middle layer of the parietal pericardium is fibrous tissue, and the outer layer is epicardial connective tissue.[2] The parietal pericardium is mostly collagenous with little elastic tissue and therefore limits the diastolic dimension of the heart. Slow accumulation of fluid is well tolerated by stretching and growth of the parietal pericardium, but rapid accumulation is poorly tolerated and may result in cardiac tamponade. The pericardium is firmly anchored within the thoracic cavity with attachments anteriorly to the sternum, inferiorly to the diaphragm, and posteriorly to the thoracic vertebrae, esophagus, and aorta. Innervation is by the phrenic and vagus nerves. Localized pain is referred to the trapezius ridge by the phrenic nerve and is pathognomonic; however, pain indicative of pericardial disease is often caused by irritation of contiguous structures and felt elsewhere.[3] Lymphatics drain to anterior and posterior lymph nodes. Pericardial fluid has fibrinolytic activity (produced by the serous lining), which may decrease intrapericardial clotting and adhesion formation.[1] In addition, complement and prostacyclin production may contribute to a defensive mechanism.[4,5]

In this chapter, acute pericarditis and its various causes, conditions causing pericardial effusion, postpericardiotomy syndrome, congenital pericardial anomalies, and constrictive pericarditis are discussed.

ACUTE PERICARDITIS

HISTORY

The classic presentation of acute pericarditis is precordial or substernal chest pain described as squeezing, sharp, or dull. The pain is worsened in the supine position. The child assumes the most comfortable position of sitting upright and leaning forward; often the patient refuses to lie down for examination. The pain is worsened with inspiration, coughing, and movement. Chest pain is not found in all patients, however, particularly in small children.[6–8] Respiratory distress is usually associated with a pulmonary condition or cardiac tamponade. If the effusion has collected quickly, the signs of tamponade may be seen (see later), and the patient may complain of abdominal pain from hepatic distention.

PHYSICAL EXAMINATION

A friction rub, pathognomonic of acute pericarditis, is believed to result from friction between the inflamed pericardial surfaces. The rub, a high-frequency sandpaper-like sound that may have several components, is often described as to-and-fro or triphasic. It may not correlate with the cardiac cycle and can be heard during both systole and diastole. It is usually heard between the left sternal border and the cardiac apex and is loudest with the patient leaning forward; it must be searched for with the patient in multiple positions. The rub may be intermittent, and its absence does not exclude pericarditis. Maneuvers that bring the heart closer to the chest wall, such as leaning forward, kneeling, and inspiration, should increase the loudness of the rub. Pressing with the bell of the stethoscope firmly against the chest wall more closely approximates the visceral and parietal pericardium, increases the pain, amplifies the rub, and decreases the risk of a rub's being confused with movement of the skin underneath the stethoscope. When an effusion is large, the rub may disappear, and the heart sounds become muffled. A rub can be present during tamponade, however, and may be caused by friction between the inflamed pericardium and the surrounding structures. Fever is a common presenting sign of pericarditis and suggests an infectious etiology.

Pulsus paradoxus is characteristic of pericardial effusion with tamponade and is defined as a decrease in blood pressure of more than 10 mm Hg during inspiration. During inspiration, there is normally a decrease in systolic blood pressure (4 to 6 mm Hg) secondary to increased pulmonary venous capacitance and the decreased intrathoracic pressure (Fig. 51–1). With a pericardial effusion, the left ventricular diastolic volume is restricted by the increased pericardial pressure, decreased pulmonary venous return, and shifting of the interventricular septum from right to left. Pulsus paradoxus should be measured with the patient supine. A blood pressure cuff is inflated until the radial pulse is no longer palpable. With slow release of pressure, listen for the initial Korotkoff sounds. With inspiration, the Korotkoff sounds disappear (particularly if pulsus paradoxus is present). Cuff pressure is slowly released until the Korotkoff sounds are heard throughout the respiratory cycle. In a normal patient, the systemic pressure falls 4 to 6 mm Hg with inspiration. If the pressure falls more than 10 mm Hg, pulsus paradoxus is present.

Tamponade, which is compression of the heart from the surrounding fluid-filled pericardium, restricts atrial and ventricular filling and results in decreased cardiac output. Acute accumulation of fluid within the pericardial cavity may result in tamponade. Gradual increases in pericardial volume due to pericardial effusions, chronic dilated cardiomyopathy, shunt lesions, or chronic valve insufficiency are accommodated by stretching and growth of the pericardium. Large pericardial effusions that accumulate slowly without an increase in pericardial pressure are tolerated well until they reach a critical point beyond which the pericardium no longer distends. Classically, tamponade is described by Beck's triad, which includes hypotension, distant heart sounds, and elevated central venous pressure with jugular venous distention.[9] There are also pulsus paradoxus, tachycardia, narrow pulse pressure, and dyspnea. Tachycardia out of proportion to the fever or clinical state may occur with pericarditis and myocarditis and precede tamponade. Initially, during tamponade, cardiac output is maintained by an increased ejection fraction and tachycardia. As these mechanisms can no longer sustain cardiac output, systemic vascular resistance rises to maintain blood pressure, and pulse pressure narrows. Decreased coronary perfusion eventually results in myocardial dysfunction and further decreases in cardiac output and hypotension. Patients may demonstrate Kussmaul's sign, a paradoxical rise in venous pressure with inspiration (see Fig. 51–1). During inspiration, intrathoracic pressure normally falls and increases venous return to the right side of the heart. With tamponade, tension within the pericardium limits expansion of the right atrium and results in a paradoxical rise in venous pressure during inspiration.

CHEST RADIOGRAPHY

The radiographic appearance of the heart and pulmonary vasculature in pericarditis depends on the etiology and duration of symptoms. The cardiac silhouette does not correlate with hemodynamic effects, and the absence of cardiomegaly does not exclude pericarditis or pericardial

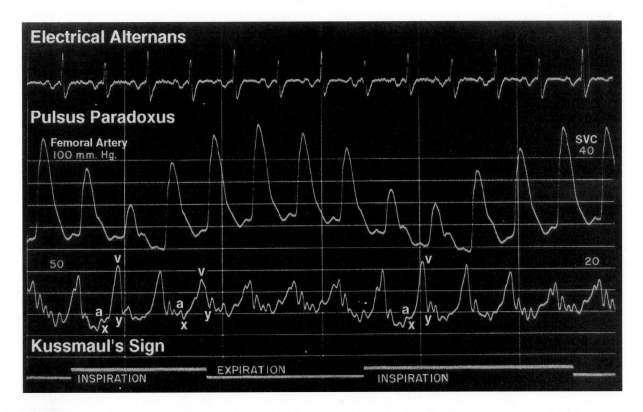

FIGURE 51–1

Electrical alternans, pulsus paradoxus, and Kussmaul's sign. Electrical alternans: alternating large and small QRS complexes. Pulsus paradoxus: exaggerated respiratory variation in femoral artery pressure (expiratory systolic pressure = 116 mm Hg, inspiratory systolic pressure = 80 mm Hg). Kussmaul's sign: paradoxical inspiratory rise in venous pressure (note large V wave). SVC = superior vena cava.

effusion. In acute pericarditis with a small effusion, the heart may not appear enlarged. Tamponade may occur without cardiac enlargement if the effusion has collected quickly without time for the pericardium to accommodate. With a large effusion, the cardiac silhouette may assume a triangular or "water bottle" shape, and pulmonary vascular markings are normal.

The chest film may suggest a cause of pericarditis, such as bacterial pneumonia, tuberculosis, or neoplastic disease. Pericardial effusion should always be considered in the differential diagnosis of an x-ray film that demonstrates an increased cardiac silhouette with normal pulmonary vascular markings. This same radiographic picture may help differentiate pericarditis from myocarditis with myocardial dysfunction in which there is pulmonary venous prominence and pulmonary edema.

ELECTROCARDIOGRAPHY

Several electrocardiographic findings occur in pericarditis. Pericarditis is the most frequent cause of ST elevation in children. Absence of electrocardiographic changes does not exclude pericarditis.[10] Changes in the electrocardiogram seen in pericarditis may be related to pressure exerted against the epicardium by pericardial fluid or by actual inflammatory changes in the epicardium. Low voltage in all leads can result from the insulating effect of the fluid-fibrin that surrounds the heart. This is typically seen with the chronic pericarditis of connective tissue disease. "Electrical alternans," a cyclical variation of the QRS amplitude, occurs in some patients and may be caused by the rotational or pendular motion of the heart within the fluid-filled pericardial space (see Fig. 51–1). Serial electrocardiograms may give an indication of myocardial involvement and alert the clinician to the rare patient with an arrhythmia.[11]

Spodick[12] described four changes in pericarditis. In stage 1, ST segment elevation, thought to be due to subepicardial myocarditis, occurs in the leads facing the epicardium (I, II, aVF, V_3 through V_6). Leads without epicardial representation (aVR and V_1) may show reciprocal ST depression and possible depression of the PR segment if atrial tissue is inflamed. ST changes in pericarditis can be differentiated from those seen in myocardial infarction. In myocardial infarction, only a few leads are affected, whereas in pericarditis, many leads are frequently affected; and there is frequently inversion of the T waves, whereas the T wave remains upright in the early stages of pericarditis. In stage 2, the ST segment begins to normalize, the amplitude of the T wave diminishes, and the PR segment becomes depressed. In stage 3, the ST segment is normal with symmetric T wave inversion in the leads that previously demonstrated ST elevation (may demonstrate a diphasic T wave). Stage 4 is characterized by normalization of the electrocardiogram. The T wave abnormalities may persist, however, and do not indicate active disease. A study of 19 patients performed by Ginzton and Lakes[13] suggests that a ratio of the amplitudes of the ST segment over the T wave in V_6 greater than 0.25 is predictive of pericarditis, although this has not been demonstrated in children.

ECHOCARDIOGRAPHY

The echocardiogram is now the primary tool used to assess possible myocardial, structural, and effusive causes of cardiomegaly. If the pericardial effusion is small, it is detected posteriorly between the epicardium and the parietal pericardium only during systole. As the volume of the effusion increases, fluid can be detected both posteriorly and anteriorly throughout the cardiac cycle. With a large effusion, the heart may swing within the fluid-filled cavity. Dilatation of the venae cavae and loss of respiratory variation may be noted. Abnormal septal motion is sometimes present.

A finding of concern is right atrial and right ventricular collapse, which suggests tamponade. Buckling of the right atrial wall into the right atrium starts abruptly in ventricular diastole and continues for a variable portion of systole. Right ventricular collapse is seen as abnormal posterior motion of the anterior free wall of the right ventricle during early to mid diastole.[14] No current echocardiographic criteria are specific for tamponade.[14] The echocardiogram may also show within the pericardial cavity echogenic matter that represents adhesions, clots, fibrinous material, metastases, or epicardial fat.

CARDIAC CATHETERIZATION

A pericardial effusion may be found during catheterization by noting a distance between the right cardiac border and the position of a catheter tip placed adjacent to the lateral wall of the right atrium. As pericardial fluid accumulates, diastolic pressures rise and equalize in the four chambers of the heart. Right ventricular and pulmonary artery pressures are also moderately elevated. Femoral artery and right atrial tracings will show pulsus paradoxus and Kussmaul's sign. In some patients, a square root sign is found in diastolic pressures of both ventricles.

OTHER DIAGNOSTIC MODALITIES

Other diagnostic modalities may be useful. Computed tomography and magnetic resonance imaging can detect pericardial thickening, calcification, and other pericardial masses.[15, 16] In constrictive disease, calcifications may be seen that are difficult to diagnose echocardiographically. In older children, computed tomography may be able to differentiate anterior and posterior adipose tissue from a pericardial effusion. Most children, however, have little epicardial adipose tissue, and the pericardium may be difficult to discern. Complete or partial absence of the pericardium may be detected by computed tomography.[17] Nuclear medicine techniques detecting leukocyte infiltration of the pericardium with gallium Ga 67 and indium In 111 scans have had some success.[18, 19]

DIFFERENTIAL DIAGNOSIS

Myocarditis and pericarditis often coexist and may be difficult to separate. In myocarditis, the degree of myocardial dysfunction is generally greater. If the chest radiograph shows an enlarged cardiac silhouette, the patient with myocarditis but not pericarditis may demonstrate significant pulmonary edema secondary to the myocardial dysfunction. An echocardiogram is necessary to evaluate an effusion and can accurately measure cardiac function.

MANAGEMENT

In a patient with tamponade, fluid administration increases diastolic filling pressure temporarily and provides emergency stabilization. Vasopressor therapy, vasodilators, digitalis, and diuretic therapy are each hazardous in a patient with cardiac tamponade. Pericardiocentesis should be performed. It may be diagnostic, therapeutic, and lifesaving. Pericardiocentesis is generally needed with suspected tamponade, with bacterial pericarditis, and in immunocompromised hosts or when the etiology of the effusion is unclear after less invasive testing. In some patients, pericardial biopsy may be necessary.

Emergency pericardiocentesis should be performed in symptomatic patients. Removal of a small amount of fluid may decrease pericardial pressure enough to alleviate symptoms temporarily. When possible, pericardiocentesis is best performed in an intensive care unit under echocardiographic guidance or in a cardiac catheterization laboratory under fluoroscopic guidance. The patient is placed in a 30-degree head-up position and is adequately sedated; recommended sedatives include benzodiazepines and ketamine. Anesthetics that decrease the heart rate or depress myocardial function (such as halothane) are contraindicated.[20] The electrocardiogram, blood pressure, and oximetry measurements are continuously monitored. Nearly complete drainage of the pericardial effusion can sometimes be achieved. A drainage catheter may be left in place with intermittent low-pressure drainage.[21] Complications include arrhythmias, myocardial puncture, coronary artery or vein laceration, hemopericardium-tamponade, pneumothorax, aortic injury, laceration of the internal mammary artery, hepatic laceration, and death.

Pericardial fluid studies can include cell count and differential; glucose and protein concentrations; histologic examination of cells with a cell block preparation; latex aggregation for bacterial antigens; Gram's stain and acid-fast bacilli stain; bacterial (aerobic, anaerobic, and tuberculosis), viral, and fungal cultures; and fluid for polymerase chain reaction analysis. If tuberculosis is considered, fluid may be sent for measurement of adenosine deaminase activity because of the long period for tuberculosis culture to grow.[22] Unstained slides are retained for possible later re-evaluation. Triglycerides can be measured in suspected chylopericardium. Purulent material may be too thick to drain or may be loculated. Multiple attempts at drainage are contraindicated, and operative drainage might be needed. Operation may need to be performed in patients with persistent or recurrent effusion. The approach (left anterolateral thoracotomy versus subxiphoid approach) and extent of pericardial removal (window versus pericardiectomy) are controversial. Care must be taken to avoid the phrenic nerves. There has been subxiphoid pericardial biopsy and drainage, but this approach has limited use in pediatrics.[23]

The erythrocyte sedimentation rate may be elevated as an indicator of inflammation. Cardiac enzyme activities may be mildly elevated in pericarditis associated with myocarditis.

ETIOLOGY

Acute pericarditis results from a number of infectious agents.

Viral Pericarditis

Many instances of pericarditis were historically labeled idiopathic but are now presumed to have a viral etiology. This represents the most common form of pericarditis in childhood. The presentation often follows by 10 days or 2 weeks an upper respiratory infection or gastrointestinal illness.[24] Patients present with classic precordial pain and rub and often complain of abdominal pain. Fever is usually present. The patient with viral pericarditis generally appears to be less toxic than the patient with bacterial pericarditis and has a lower body temperature.[24] Patients appear more toxic, however, if the pericarditis occurs in conjunction with myocarditis. Although tamponade is rare, patients must be observed closely in the initial period.

Diagnosis can be established with standard diagnostic techniques. Peripheral blood counts reveal a normal white blood cell count or a relative lymphocytosis. Pericardiocentesis should be performed if the cause is in question and for all symptomatic patients. Pericardial fluid is serous or serosanguineous and shows a predominance of lymphocytes, although polymorphonuclear cells may predominate early in the course of the illness.[24] Specific viral causes can be diagnosed by isolating the virus from the pericardial, nasopharyngeal, or stool culture or by a rise in viral titers. The polymerase chain reaction and in situ hybridization techniques have also allowed specific diagnosis.[25–27] Shimizu and colleagues[27] detected adenovirus and enterovirus by polymerase chain reaction analysis in the myocardium and liver, respectively, in two of eight infants with pericarditis who died suddenly and unexpectedly. Coxsackie B viruses have been demonstrated most frequently, although 14 different nonpoliovirus enteroviruses (coxsackieviruses A and B, echovirus) have been demonstrated (Table 51–1).[28] A pericardial effusion has been documented in 26 to 58% of patients with acquired immunodeficiency syndrome (AIDS)[29,30]; in fact, AIDS is the most common cause of pericardial effusion in some internal medicine services.

TABLE 51–1

VIRAL CAUSES OF PERICARDITIS

Enteroviruses (primarily coxsackievirus B)
Adenovirus
Influenza viruses A and B
Rubella virus
Mumps virus
Epstein-Barr virus (mononucleosis)
Measles virus
Cytomegalovirus
Respiratory syncytial virus
Herpesvirus
Hepatitis B virus
Human immunodeficiency virus

Treatment of most patients is symptomatic and includes bedrest and anti-inflammatory agents. Steroid therapy is indicated if nonsteroidal agents fail and if bacterial pericarditis has been excluded. There is no convincing evidence of reduced long-term sequelae with steroid use. Resolution usually occurs in days to weeks, with complete resolution in approximately 3 to 4 weeks. Patients may rarely become steroid dependent. Constrictive pericarditis is a rare late sequel of viral and idiopathic pericarditis.

Bacterial Pericarditis

Bacterial pericarditis is a rare, serious form of pericarditis. Patients generally appear more toxic than in other forms of pericarditis. Bacterial pericarditis occurs most frequently in the very young; nearly half of all purulent pericarditis occurs before the age of 18 to 24 months.[7,31,32] In one series, approximately two thirds of the patients presented in shock.[32] Patients present with the classic symptoms of precordial pain, rub, muffled heart sounds, and decreased cardiac output. High temperature is characteristic, along with dyspnea, tachypnea, and tachycardia out of proportion to the fever. Tamponade is more likely with bacterial than with viral pericarditis. Bacterial pericarditis is often secondary to dissemination from another site, by the hematogenous route but sometimes through contiguous structures. The most common associated site is the lung (*Staphylococcus aureus*, *Haemophilus influenzae*, and *Streptococcus pneumoniae*), although septic arthritis, osteomyelitis, meningitis, or soft tissue infection may be the primary site.[31] Bacterial pericarditis is usually culture-positive, although culture-negative pericarditis may be found in the patient who received antibiotics before pericardiocentesis. The pericardial fluid reveals a predominance of polymorphonuclear cells, although this is a nonspecific finding seen also with early viral pericarditis and tuberculous pericarditis. Latex agglutination of pericardial fluid, serum, or urine has been useful in the patient pretreated with antibiotics. If *S. aureus* is considered, appropriate studies might demonstrate teichoic acid antibodies.[33] The organism is also usually isolated from the blood.[34] Thoracentesis or lung aspiration may reveal the etiologic agent when it is associated with empyema or pneumonia.

Before the antibiotic era, the most common organisms were pneumococcus and streptococcus.[24] *S. aureus* is now the most common bacterial factor in the postantibiotic era and is associated with pneumonia, septic arthritis, osteomyelitis, and soft tissue infections.[6,31,32] It is the organism recovered most frequently when purulent pericarditis develops within 3 months of a cardiac operation.[24] *S. aureus* is a necrotizing infection, and patients appear toxic. In addition, *S. aureus* often releases an exotoxin that produces hemodynamic instability and increased risk of death. *S. aureus* pericarditis after varicella infection has been demonstrated.[34] *H. influenzae* type b has been the second most common cause of bacterial pericarditis (often associated with pneumonia and meningitis).[6,31,35] This may change now that *H. influenzae* b vaccine is being given. Other less common organisms are listed in Table 51–2. Anaerobic bacteria should be considered with an associated lung abscess, intra-abdominal infection, or penetrating or blunt chest trauma.[24,36–38]

TABLE 51–2
BACTERIAL CAUSES OF PERICARDITIS
Staphylococcus aureus
Haemophilus influenzae type b
Streptococcus pneumoniae
Streptococci
Neisseria meningitidis
Neisseria gonorrhoeae
Campylobacter fetus
Pseudomonas aeruginosa
Mycoplasma pneumoniae
Mycoplasma hominis
Legionella
Francisella tularensis
Chlamydia psittaci
Nocardia asteroides
Brucella
Yersinia
Salmonella
Actinomyces
Mycobacterium tuberculosis
Escherichia coli
Listeria monocytogenes
Pasteurella multocida
Anaerobes
Enteric bacilli
Klebsiella

Before culture results are obtained, initial treatment should consist of broad-spectrum antibiotic coverage against *S. aureus* and *H. influenzae*. An intravenous penicillinase-resistant penicillin (methicillin, nafcillin, or oxacillin) provides coverage for *S. aureus*. Vancomycin should be considered in areas with a high prevalence of methicillin-resistant *S. aureus*. Ampicillin (in geographic regions of low resistance) or a third-generation cephalosporin, such as cefotaxime or ceftriaxone, is effective against *H. influenzae*, pneumococci, streptococci, and meningococci.[24] An aminoglycoside should be added if pericarditis occurs after operation, is associated with a genitourinary tract infection, or is in an immunocompromised host. Specific therapy can be instituted once the organism is identified. Treatment duration varies according to the organism; *S. aureus* pericarditis is usually treated for 4 weeks, infection with other pathogens for 3 to 4 weeks. Antimicrobial therapy alone is insufficient and must be combined with surgical drainage. Mortality in the preantibiotic era approached 100%,[8] but studies demonstrate a 92 to 98% survival with medical and surgical therapy.[32,39] Factors affecting the outcome include delay in diagnosis, absence of early surgical drainage, inadequate drainage, degree of myocardial involvement, cardiac tamponade, septicemia, young age, and staphylococcal disease.[33] Constrictive pericarditis is a concern as a complication of pneumococcal, staphylococcal, and *H. influenzae* infections.

Tuberculous Pericarditis

Mycobacterium tuberculosis was once a common cause of acute pericarditis in children in the United States. Now it is associated more commonly with chronic pericarditis and pericarditis in developing countries. The presentation is of insidious onset with a long duration of symptoms of weight loss, malaise, low-grade fever, night sweats, and dyspnea in conjunction with chest pain. A subacute presentation may be associated with symptoms of pericardial tamponade.

Tuberculous pericarditis often results as a complication of miliary tuberculosis with direct invasion or by lymphatic spread from mediastinal lymph nodes. Hematogenous dissemination, however, may occur rarely in the absence of pulmonary infiltrates. Most patients have a positive Mantoux tuberculin skin test response. Pericardial fluid is serofibrinous or hemorrhagic with predominance of lymphocytes. Acid-fast bacilli are not reliably seen in the pericardial fluid, and fluorochrome staining may be more useful than traditional carbolfuchsin technique.[40] Pericardial biopsy helps confirm the diagnosis. Cultures often take 6 weeks to grow, and antituberculous therapy must be begun before definitive proof of etiology. Before the development of antituberculous drugs, *M. tuberculosis* pericarditis had a mortality of 80 to 90% acutely, with many of the survivors dying of constrictive pericarditis or miliary tuberculosis.[41]

Treatment is with multidrug therapy because of the high prevalence of multidrug-resistant tuberculosis. Therapy may include isoniazid, pyrazinamide, rifampin, and possibly streptomycin for 9 to 18 months.[24] Steroids are a useful adjunct to reduce pericarditis inflammation and increase fluid resorption.[42] The development of inflammatory and caseous material makes extensive pericardiectomy difficult and dangerous if it is performed early in the course of therapy. If possible, surgical removal of the pericardium should be deferred for 6 to 12 weeks to reduce inflammation and allow the formation of a pericardial peel to facilitate removal.[43] Constrictive pericarditis results from the inflammatory process of tuberculosis. Tuberculosis is a major cause of constrictive pericarditis worldwide.

Human Immunodeficiency Virus and Other Infections

In adults, human immunodeficiency virus (HIV) has been associated particularly with tuberculosis in Africa.[44] In retrospective reports of pericardial effusion or pericardiocentesis, it is the most frequent underlying disease in adults.[45] Other reported causes of pericardial effusion in adults with HIV infection are listed in Table 51–3. In adults, a markedly shortened survival occurs once a pericardial effusion is diagnosed.[46] In children, pericardial effusion without tamponade occurs in 26% of patients with HIV infection.[29] No pericardial fluid cultures yielded any infectious agents. Another study reported a pericardial effusion in 58% of children with HIV infection.[30] Half of the children with a pericardial effusion had a normal chest radiograph, two developed tamponade, and 69% had associated cardiac abnormalities including ventricular dilatation or hypertrophy, myocarditis, and pericarditis. A pericardial effusion was also highly correlated with pleural effusion

TABLE 51–3

CAUSES OF PERICARDIAL EFFUSION IN HUMAN IMMUNODEFICIENCY VIRUS INFECTION

Mycobacterium avium
Cytomegalovirus
Staphylococcus aureus
Streptococcus pneumoniae
Nocardia asteroides
Cryptococcus neoformans
Herpes simplex
Kaposi's sarcoma
B cell lymphoma

TABLE 51–4

OTHER INFECTIOUS CAUSES OF PERICARDITIS

Protozoal	*Toxoplasma gondii*
Parasitic	*Entamoeba histolytica, Echinococcus*
Spirochetal	Syphilis, leptospirosis
Rickettsial	Typhus, Q fever
Fungal	*Candida, Aspergillus, Blastomyces, Coccidioides, Histoplasma, Cryptococcus*

and ascites. Cultures of the pericardial fluid or pericardium either yielded no growth of any infectious agent (*S. aureus, Staphylococcus epidermidis, Pseudomonas aeruginosa*, enterococcus, *Mycobacterium avium*) or were contaminated. A patient with HIV-associated *P. aeruginosa* pericarditis with tamponade has been described.[47]

Numerous other infectious causes have been documented, with immunocompromised hosts at particular risk (Table 51–4).

OTHER CAUSES OF PERICARDIAL EFFUSION

Pericardial effusion occurs as a complication of other systemic conditions.[48]

RENAL FAILURE

Pericarditis is associated with end-stage renal disease (uremic pericarditis). It occurs before dialysis and even while the patient is receiving dialysis. It has been reported in 5 to 18% of patients stabilized by dialysis,[49] and a prevalence of 33% was found in adult autopsy examination.[50] Pericarditis is usually noted during the first 3 months of dialysis but may occur anytime[51] and may be large enough to cause tamponade. No significant biochemical finding has been demonstrated in uremic patients with pericarditis.[51] The pericardial fluid is usually serous, although it may become hemorrhagic because of abnormal hemostasis or repetitive heparin use. Full heparinization may precipitate pericardial hemorrhage and acute tamponade. Fibrinous pericardial fluid has been reported.[52] Pericardiocentesis should be performed in symptomatic patients or those with suspected infectious etiology.

Treatment includes increased frequency of dialysis and may be effective alone in 60% of patients.[51] In addition, nonsteroidal anti-inflammatory agents, systemic corticosteroids, and intrapericardial steroids have been effective in reducing the effusion. Aggressive dialysis, however, may exacerbate the cardiovascular effects of a pericardial effusion by causing acute hypovolemia. Peritoneal dialysis may be associated with a lower risk of tamponade.[53] Constrictive pericarditis occurs rarely, and pericardiectomy may be necessary.[51]

KAWASAKI DISEASE

In one third of patients with Kawasaki disease, a small asymptomatic pericardial effusion develops that usually resolves by the second week of illness.[54] Special treatment is usually not indicated. Acute pericardial tamponade may rarely occur from rupture of a coronary artery aneurysm.

DRUG-INDUCED PERICARDITIS

Several drugs cause pericarditis (Table 51–5). Antinuclear antibodies may develop, and the patient may progress to a lupus-like syndrome[55] including pericarditis that can be severe enough to cause tamponade. Cessation of the drug and therapy with anti-inflammatory agents are generally adequate to treat the pericarditis, although constrictive pericarditis has been described after procainamide, hydralazine, or methysergide administration. Anticoagulants and thrombolytics may cause pericardial bleeding in an inflamed pericardial sac and lead to adhesions and constriction.[55] Hypersensitivity reactions to penicillin and cromolyn sodium have also been associated with pericardial effusion.[55]

NEONATAL PERICARDIAL EFFUSION

Pericardial effusion in a fetus or neonate, often in association with pleural effusion and ascites, indicates nonimmune and immune hydrops fetalis. Cardiac factors include arrhythmias, structural heart disease, and myocardial dysfunction. Isolated pericardial effusion is rare and is usually caused by bacterial sepsis associated with a septic focus (usually pulmonary) (Table 51–6).[56] Treatment is aimed at the underlying cause, and pericardiocentesis and pericardiectomy should be performed as necessary.

HYPOTHYROIDISM

An asymptomatic pericardial effusion can occur in patients with hypothyroidism and is often present in patients with Down syndrome.[57] Asymptomatic pericardial effusions have been seen in up to 88% of adult patients, 72% of children, and 47% of infants with hypothyroidism.[57,58] The typical patient has bradycardia because of the hypothyroid state, unlike the tachycardia seen in patients with inflammatory pericarditis. The pericardial fluid is high in protein and mucopolysaccharides, and it is rarely large enough to cause tamponade because of the slow fluid accumulation.[57] The pericardial fluid usually resorbs and the cardiac silhouette returns to normal after thyroid hormone therapy.

CHYLOPERICARDIUM

Chylous pericardial effusion is associated with thoracic surgery, mediastinal masses, cystic hygromas, radiation therapy, and pancreatitis, or it may be idiopathic. Some authors suggest that idiopathic chylous pericardial effusion

---

TABLE 51–6

RARE CAUSES OF PERICARDIAL EFFUSION IN A NEONATE

Bacterial pericarditis
   Staphylococcus aureus
   Escherichia coli
   Haemophilus influenzae
   Salmonella wichita
   Klebsiella
   Pseudomonas aeruginosa
   Candida species
   Mycoplasma hominis
Intrapericardial teratoma
Maternal lupus
Congenital diaphragmatic defects
Chylopericardium
Central venous catheter perforation of the right atrium
Viral pericarditis
Chronic granulomatous disease

---

may be secondary to a direct communication of the pericardium and the thoracic duct.[59] There is often an associated pleural effusion. The effusion is milky in color with elevated triglyceride levels (often greater than 100 mg/dl) and protein concentration greater than 3 g/dl. Treatment includes a low-fat diet with emphasis on medium-chain triglycerides and eliminating the cause of the effusion by pericardiectomy and thoracic duct ligation.[60] Pleuroperitoneal shunts have been performed with some success.[60] Tamponade and constriction have also been reported.[60]

TRAUMA

Blunt and penetrating cardiac trauma can result in pericardial effusion even without initial cardiac injury. Asymptomatic effusions may be detected by echocardiography. Traumatic cardiac tamponade rarely presents with all the classic features of Beck's triad (see earlier). Treatment is based on symptoms, and symptomatic patients require emergency pericardiocentesis. A chronic pericarditis similar to postpericardiotomy syndrome may develop, with effusion lasting 1 to 4 weeks. Treatment with anti-inflammatory agents is usually effective. Myocardial rupture (atrial, ventricular, or great vessel) is associated with tamponade, although many of these patients will have associated pericardial lacerations resulting in exsanguinating hemorrhage. Penetrating cardiac injury due to stab and gunshot wounds can be rapidly fatal and can also be iatrogenic, occurring during procedures such as cardiac catheterization, central venous line placement, and pericardiocentesis. Infectious pericarditis can also occur; reported organisms include *Streptococcus sanguis, S. epidermidis, S. aureus, P. aeruginosa,* and enterococci.[36–38] Acute asymptomatic pericardial effusion responsive to anti-inflammatory agents and tamponade have also been reported in adults and children after endocardial and epicardial pacemaker lead placement[61,62] as well as after radiofrequency ablation.[63]

NEOPLASTIC DISEASE

Primary or secondary tumors in the pericardium are rare. The rare primary pericardial neoplasms include lymphoma, malignant teratoma, mesothelioma, and angiosarcomas.[64] Most pericardial neoplasms result from a metas-

---

TABLE 51–5

DRUGS THAT CAUSE PERICARDITIS

Chemotherapy
Procainamide
Hydralazine
Phenytoin
Cyclosporine
Methysergide
Isoniazid
Penicillin
Cromolyn sodium

tasis and include Hodgkin's disease, non-Hodgkin's lymphoma, leukemia, neuroblastoma, Wilms' tumor, soft tissue and bone sarcomas, Kaposi's sarcoma, and malignant melanoma.[64,65] In adults, cancer of the lung is the source in one third of patients with neoplastic pericardial disease; breast cancer is the second most common type.[64] Included in the differential diagnosis of pericardial neoplasms are congenital pericardial abnormalities (see later). Echocardiography may demonstrate masses within the pericardial space; however, computed tomography and magnetic resonance imaging are the most useful to delineate the masses completely.[15] Hydrops fetalis with tamponade secondary to an intrapericardial teratoma has been described.[66]

A pericardial effusion may be noted before or after treatment of childhood cancer. Pericarditis has been associated with doxorubicin, dactinomycin, and other chemotherapeutic agents that are often combined with radiation therapy. Anthracyclines enhance radiation damage, and the risk of pericardial involvement increases with the use of mediastinal irradiation. The irradiation effect is related to dose, volume, and fraction size. Postirradiation pericarditis has been demonstrated in 3 to 7% of patients after radiation therapy,[67,68] with the onset of symptoms between 2 months and 2.5 years after irradiation.[68,69] Pericarditis may range from asymptomatic and self-limited to chronic and constrictive.[70] Early treatment of Hodgkin's disease included high doses of radiation with an incidence of pericarditis as high as 29%.[69] With current techniques, changes are limited to late pericardial thickening.[70] Mild effusions can be treated symptomatically; corticosteroids are required in some patients. Symptomatic effusions require pericardiocentesis. Tetracycline and other sclerosing agents have been used with success.[71] Patients with chronic or constrictive pericarditis may require pericardiectomy.

POSTPERICARDIOTOMY SYNDROME

Postpericardiotomy syndrome is characterized by fever beyond the first few days after an operation involving the pericardium. There is pericardial and pleural inflammation (with associated pleural and pericardial effusions) resulting in chest pain that is often worsened by movement or inspiration. In children, the temperature is usually 38 to 39°C but occasionally reaches 40°C. In the small child, this condition may be manifest as irritability, malaise, decreased appetite, and occasionally arthralgias. Physical examination reveals a rub, relative tachycardia, and evidence of fluid retention (weight gain, hepatic congestion). Signs and symptoms of tamponade are rare but must be checked for. The etiology remains speculative, but the syndrome may be due to an autoimmune reaction to damaged myocardium, pericardium, or blood in the pericardial sac; it may share a common pathogenesis with pericardial effusions after cardiac trauma, pacemaker lead placement, and Dressler's syndrome (post–myocardial infarction syndrome).[72-74] Another theory suggests that it is secondary to a new or reactivated viral infection.[75] The incidence has been estimated at 27 to 45% and usually occurs as a single episode,[75,76] although it has been reported to recur weeks to years later. Children younger than 2 years seem to be less commonly affected.[75] Postpericardiotomy syndrome may occur after any cardiac surgery but may be more frequent after repair of tetralogy of Fallot, ventricular septal defects with pulmonary stenosis, and atrial septal defect.[75]

Laboratory evaluation reveals nonspecific indicators of inflammation with an elevated erythrocyte sedimentation rate and C-reactive protein. There is often an elevated white blood cell count with neutrophilia (10,000 to 30,000 white blood cells/mm³).[77] The chest radiograph is typical for a pericardial effusion. The electrocardiogram typically reveals nonspecific T wave abnormalities and may demonstrate T wave flattening or inversion.[77] An echocardiogram often reveals an effusion but is not diagnostic of postpericardiotomy syndrome. The effusion may be detected as early as postoperative day 2, is present in nearly all patients by postoperative day 5, and reaches maximal size by postoperative day 10.[76,78] Postpericardiotomy syndrome is typically a benign, self-limited illness. Treatment is usually limited to diuretics for fluid retention and anti-inflammatory agents. Historically, aspirin has been used (30 to 75 mg/kg/day in four divided doses for 1 month and then tapered). Indomethacin has been effective in adults. In severe disease, for patients with large effusions, or for patients refractory to nonsteroidal agents, prednisone (2 mg/kg/day with a maximum of 60 mg for the first week and then tapered) has been demonstrated to be effective.[79] Although tamponade is rare, patients may require pericardiocentesis, and pericardiectomy may be necessary in patients with recurrent effusions.

AUTOIMMUNE AND CONNECTIVE TISSUE DISEASES

Autoimmune and connective tissue diseases have been associated with pericardial inflammation and effusions (Table 51–7) (see also Chapter 60).

CONGENITAL ABNORMALITIES OF THE PERICARDIUM

ABSENCE OF THE PERICARDIUM

Partial or total absence of the pericardium is rare and is often detected incidentally at autopsy or thoracic surgery. Although typically asymptomatic, it may be associated with significant symptoms. An estimated 67% are left-sided defects and result from the premature atrophy of the left

TABLE 51–7
AUTOIMMUNE DISEASES ASSOCIATED WITH PERICARDIAL EFFUSION
Systemic lupus erythematosus
Juvenile rheumatoid arthritis
Dermatomyositis
Periarteritis nodosa
Mixed connective tissue diseases
Wegener's granulomatosis
Takayasu's arteritis
Inflammatory bowel disease
Spondyloarthropathies

duct of Cuvier during development.[80–82] Patients may complain of nonspecific chronic chest pain, lightheadedness, syncope, or dyspnea. The patient may experience symptoms of sudden death associated with herniation and entrapment of the left atrium, the left atrial appendage, the right atrium, or even the ventricles through the defect. Torsion of the great vessels, arrhythmias, or compression of a coronary artery, atrium, or ventricle along the edge of the defect may also occur. Thirty percent of patients have an associated cardiac malformation or other anomaly (Table 51–8).[80, 83, 84]

Physical examination generally is nonspecific but may reveal prominent precordial activity with a leftward shift of the apical impulse. There may also be a systolic ejection murmur along the left sternal border that is the result of distortion of the highly mobile heart. Chest radiography may reveal shifting of the heart toward the side of the defect; the trachea remains in the midline. There may be increased mobility in the lateral decubitus positions. Herniation of the left atrial appendage may be noted along the left cardiac border. The electrocardiogram may reveal right bundle branch block (complete or incomplete), right axis deviation, or sinus bradycardia.[80, 84] Echocardiography may demonstrate unusual echocardiographic windows, cardiac hypermobility, abnormal ventricular septal motion, and abnormal swinging of the heart,[81] but it may not be able to identify the defect. Magnetic resonance imaging or computed tomography is often able to delineate the defect.[15, 17, 82, 83]

Treatment depends on the size of the defect and the extent of symptoms. Patients with a history of herniation or with a small or moderate defect are at increased risk of herniation and strangulation and should undergo surgical repair. Operation may include pericardioplasty, patch closure, or extension of the defect with pericardiectomy. Complete absence of the pericardium rarely requires treatment.

PERICARDIAL CYSTS

Pericardial cysts are congenital anomalies that are thought to result from failure of fetal lacunae to coalesce into the pericardial coelom. They are typically discovered during routine chest radiography. Although they are usually asymptomatic, they may become secondarily infected or rarely cause bronchial compression. Two thirds appear as rounded densities near the right costophrenic angle, but they may occur anywhere on the pericardium.[85] Most cysts are asymptomatic, but they may be associated with chest pain, dyspnea, cough, and arrhythmias.

TABLE 51–8
ANOMALIES ASSOCIATED WITH PERICARDIAL DEFECTS
Atrial septal defect
Mitral stenosis
Patent ductus arteriosus
Tetralogy of Fallot
Pulmonary sequestration
Bronchogenic cyst
Tricuspid insufficiency
Pectus excavatum or diaphragmatic hernia

TABLE 51–9
DIFFERENTIAL DIAGNOSIS OF PERICARDIAL CYST
Teratoma
Hemangioma
Fibroma
Bronchogenic cyst
Extralobar sequestration
Lymphangioma
Lipoma
Neurogenic tumor
Sarcoma
Abscess

Treatment is usually unnecessary in an asymptomatic patient, and diagnosis can be confirmed by computed tomography or magnetic resonance imaging.[15] In a symptomatic patient or in a patient in whom the diagnosis is uncertain, aspiration may be performed, which reveals clear fluid.[86] The differential diagnosis includes a number of conditions (Table 51–9).[49, 85, 86]

CONSTRICTIVE PERICARDITIS AND RESTRICTIVE CARDIOMYOPATHY

Constrictive pericarditis is characterized by a thickened, fibrotic, and sometimes calcified pericardium that restricts ventricular filling. Constrictive pericarditis is described most frequently in adults and may be the endpoint after infectious pericarditis (bacterial or viral), connective tissue disorders, trauma (penetrating and nonpenetrating), neoplastic disease, radiation therapy, rare genetic and metabolic disorders (mulibrey nanism), surgery, pacemaker implantation, end-stage renal disease, and idiopathic pericarditis, or it may have no recognized antecedent.[61, 87–89] A relationship has been described between atrial septal defect and constrictive pericarditis, some in children; the reason for this is unknown.[90] Transient cardiac constriction has followed acute idiopathic and bacterial pericarditis.[8, 88, 89] Tuberculous pericarditis is the most frequent cause worldwide, but constriction may occur after any episode of pericarditis (frequently after pneumococcal, staphylococcal, or *H. influenzae* infection). Constrictive pericarditis has been reported to occur as early as the eighth day,[91] but acute constriction usually develops within weeks. With pericardial constriction, diastolic expansion of the ventricles is restricted, producing hemodynamic compromise. Early diastolic function is normal, but mid and late diastolic filling is decreased by the noncompliant pericardium; systolic function remains normal. Elevated central venous and pulmonary capillary wedge pressure results from the reduced compliance. Pathologic findings include a thickened pericardium with focal inflammation. The underlying myocardium may be atrophic secondary to the overlying thickened pericardium. Constriction is typically a diffuse process affecting all parts of the pericardium equally; however, there have been reports of localized constriction. This may result from inadequate pericardiectomy, and a calcified band may be seen on the chest radiograph. Regional constriction has been reported to affect the right ventricular outflow tract, the pulmonary artery, the aortic root, or the atrioventricular grooves, producing mitral or tricuspid stenosis.[87,88]

The patient may complain of exercise intolerance, dyspnea, chest pain, fatigue, weight gain, and syncope. Physical examination may reveal jugular and hepatic congestion, pedal edema, ascites, and signs of decreased cardiac output with severe constriction. Splenomegaly, mild prolongation of the prothrombin time, lymphopenia, and hypoproteinemia secondary to protein-losing enteropathy are rare complications of constrictive pericarditis.[92,93] Auscultation may reveal a precordial knock, an early diastolic sound that corresponds to the abrupt cessation of ventricular filling.[94] The chest radiograph may be normal. Fifty percent of patients demonstrate pericardial calcifications or pleural fluid.[87] A chest radiograph with persistent heart failure when the cardiac silhouette is decreasing suggests constrictive pericarditis. The electrocardiogram may demonstrate low-voltage QRS complexes and ST-T abnormalities.[87] The echocardiogram may reveal pericardial thickening, but there are currently no specific indicators of constrictive pericarditis. The pericardium is immobile with tethering to the myocardium. The superior and inferior venae cavae may be dilated, suggestive of elevated central venous pressures. Paradoxical septal motion or inspiratory bowing of the interventricular septa into the left-sided chambers may be present.[88] Doppler examination may reveal respiratory variation in right- and left-sided heart filling (Fig. 51–2). With inspiration, mitral valve peak E velocity decreases and tricuspid valve peak E velocity increases.[95,96] In constrictive pericarditis (as with tamponade), cardiac catheterization demonstrates that right and left atrial pressures, ventricular end-diastolic pressure, and pulmonary arterial wedge pressure are elevated and equal. Ventricular waveforms demonstrate the square root sign, an early diastolic drop in pressure followed by a plateau phase due to rapid early diastolic filling and subsequent restriction in filling. Magnetic resonance imaging and computed tomography are also sensitive tools for assessment of pericardial thickness and may be able to differentiate between pericardial thickening and the infiltrative process of restrictive cardiomyopathy.[16] The treatment of constrictive pericarditis is total pericardiectomy, although Allaria and colleagues[97] suggest that operation not be performed if the patient responds to medical management. Unfortunately, there are currently no data able to predict when constriction is irreversible or how long operation may be delayed. Dupuis and coworkers[32] found no constriction in children after combined medical and surgical therapy for bacterial pericarditis. The response to pericardiectomy may be imperfect because of underlying myocardial damage.

Restrictive cardiomyopathy is an infiltrative process (amyloidosis, hemochromatosis, endomyocardial fibrosis, eosinophilic cardiomyopathy, and idiopathic) characterized by abnormal diastolic function with preserved systolic function.[98] Although the clinical pictures of constrictive pericarditis and restrictive cardiomyopathy are similar, differentiation is necessary because of differences in management and prognosis. A history of previous pericarditis or disease with known pericardial association suggests constrictive pericarditis, whereas systemic disease suggests restrictive disease.

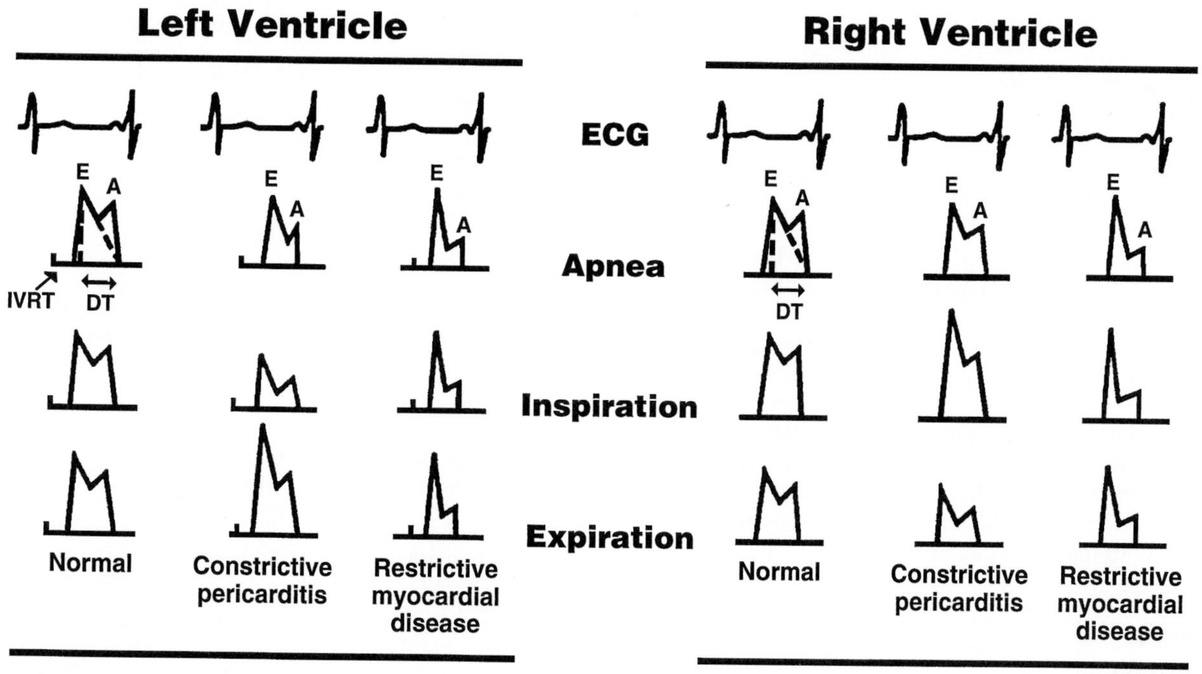

FIGURE 51–2

Diagram of inflow velocities into left ventricle (*left*) and right ventricle (*right*), comparing normal, constrictive pericarditis, and restrictive myocardial disease during various respiratory phases. Isovolumetric relaxation time (IVRT), deceleration time (DT), peak early (E), and peak late (A) velocities are shown. In constrictive pericarditis, there is marked respiratory variation. In restrictive myocardial disease, there is an increased E/A ratio, little respiratory variation, and shortened DT. (Modified from Klein AL, Cohen GI: Doppler echocardiographic assessment of constrictive pericarditis, cardiac amyloidosis, and cardiac tamponade. Cleve Clin J Med 59:278, 1992.)

The physical examination is usually noncontributory unless there is a residual rub or distinct precordial knock suggesting constrictive pericarditis. In constrictive pericarditis, Kussmaul's sign (rise in right atrial pressure with inspiration) and pulsus paradoxus (exaggerated decline in systolic blood pressure during inspiration) are found in 80% and 20% of patients, respectively, but they are generally absent in restrictive cardiomyopathy.[99] Cardiac catheterization has been used to help differentiate between constrictive and restrictive cardiac disease. Endomyocardial biopsy may demonstrate the infiltrative process of a restrictive cardiomyopathy, but a normal biopsy result does not exclude either diagnosis.

Three commonly used hemodynamic criteria are as follows[100]:

- Equalization of right and left ventricular end-diastolic pressures (e.g., a difference of under 5 mm Hg) suggests constrictive pericarditis.
- Right ventricular systolic pressure is elevated by 50 mm Hg or less in constrictive pericarditis, by more than 50 mm Hg in restrictive cardiomyopathy.
- Right ventricular end-diastolic pressure is greater than one third of systolic pressure in constrictive pericarditis but less than one third in restrictive cardiomyopathy.

Volume infusion during a cardiac catheterization has also been used to help distinguish the two causes. Right and left ventricular end-diastolic pressures increase to the same degree in constrictive pericarditis, but the left ventricular end-diastolic pressure rises more in restrictive cardiomyopathy. This method of differentiation has not been prospectively studied, however.[100]

Numerous echocardiographic studies have attempted to differentiate constrictive pericarditis from restrictive cardiomyopathy.[88,96,98] These studies suggest normal wall thickness in constrictive pericarditis and, conversely, increased wall thickness with restrictive cardiomyopathy (prominent thickening of the interatrial septum and cardiac valves in amyloidosis). In addition, pericardial thickening and calcification may be detected in constrictive pericarditis, and a "granular or sparkling" texture of the myocardium may be noted in amyloidosis. Doppler evaluation demonstrates in constrictive pericarditis an increased inspiratory right ventricular inflow velocity and decreased inspiratory left ventricular inflow velocity, whereas little inspiratory-expiratory change is noted with restrictive cardiomyopathy (Fig. 51–2).[96] Constrictive pericarditis additionally demonstrates expiratory augmentation of hepatic vein diastolic flow reversal, whereas augmentation is during inspiration in restrictive cardiomyopathy.[98] To date, no technique is totally reliable, and pericardiectomy may be necessary to make the diagnosis.

REFERENCES

1. Spodick DH: Macrophysiology, microphysiology, and anatomy of the pericardium: A synopsis (Review). Am Heart J 124:1046, 1992.
2. Ishihara T, Ferrans VJ, Jones M, et al: Histologic and ultrastructural features of normal human parietal pericardium. Am J Cardiol 46:744, 1980.
3. Spodick DH: Acute, clinically noneffusive ("dry") pericarditis. In Spodick DH (ed): The Pericardium: A Comprehensive Textbook, Vol 1. New York, Marcel Dekker, 1997, p 94.
4. Kinney E, Wynn J, Hinton DM, et al: Pericardial-fluid complement: Normal values. Am J Clin Pathol 72:972, 1979.
5. Herman AG, Claeys M, Moncada S, Vane JR: Prostacyclin production by rabbit aorta, pericardium, pleura, peritoneum and dura mater. Arch Int Pharmacodyn Ther 236:303, 1978.
6. Gersony WM, McCracken GH Jr: Purulent pericarditis in infancy (Review). Pediatrics 40:224, 1967.
7. Okoroma EO, Perry LW, Scott LP 3d: Acute bacterial pericarditis in children: Report of 25 cases. Am Heart J 90:709, 1975.
8. Benzing G III, Kaplan S: Purulent pericarditis. Am J Dis Child 106:289, 1963.
9. Beck CS: Two cardiac compression triads. JAMA 104:714, 1935.
10. Garson A Jr: The Electrocardiogram in Infants and Children: A Systematic Approach. Philadelphia, Lea & Febiger, 1983.
11. Spodick DH: Frequency of arrhythmias in acute pericarditis determined by Holter monitoring. Am J Cardiol 53:842, 1984.
12. Spodick DH: The electrocardiogram in acute pericarditis. In Spodick DH (ed): Acute Pericarditis. New York, Grune & Stratton, 1959, p 17.
13. Ginzton LE, Laks MM: The differential diagnosis of acute pericarditis from the normal variant: New electrocardiographic criteria. Circulation 65:1004, 1982.
14. Fowler NO: Cardiac tamponade. A clinical or an echocardiographic diagnosis? Circulation 87:1738, 1993.
15. Hoit BD: Imaging the pericardium. Cardiol Clin 8:587, 1990.
16. Soulen RL: Magnetic resonance imaging of great vessel, myocardial, and pericardial disease. Circulation 84 (suppl):I-311, 1991.
17. Baim RS, MacDonald IL, Wise DJ, Lenkei SC: Computed tomography of absent left pericardium. Radiology 135:127, 1980.
18. Bufalino VJ, Robinson JA, Henkin R, et al: Gallium-67 scanning: A new diagnostic approach to the post-pericardiotomy syndrome. Am Heart J 106:1138, 1983.
19. Greenberg ML, Niebulski HI, Uretsky BF, et al: Occult purulent pericarditis detected by indium-111 leukocyte imaging. Chest 85:701, 1984.
20. Wyler F, Knusli D, Rutishauser M, et al: Pericarditis purulenta in children. Helv Paediatr Acta 32:135, 1977.
21. Kopecky SL, Callahan JA, Tajik AJ, Seward JB: Percutaneous pericardial catheter drainage: Report of 42 consecutive cases. Am J Cardiol 58:633, 1986.
22. Komsuoglu B, Goldeli O, Kulan K, Komsuoglu SS: The diagnostic and prognostic value of adenosine deaminase in tuberculous pericarditis. Eur Heart J 16:1126, 1995.
23. Corey GR, Campbell PT, Van Trigt P, et al: Etiology of large pericardial effusions. Am J Med 95:209, 1993.
24. Pinsky WW, Friedman RA, Jubelirer DP, Nihill MR: Infectious pericarditis. In Feigin RD, Cherry JD (eds): Textbook of Pediatric Infectious Diseases, Vol 1, 3rd ed. Philadelphia, WB Saunders, 1992, p 377.
25. Satoh T, Kojima M, Ohshima K: Demonstration of the Epstein-Barr genome by the polymerase chain reaction and in situ hybridisation in a patient with viral pericarditis. Br Heart J 69:563, 1993.
26. Fujioka S, Koide H, Kitaura Y, et al: Molecular detection and differentiation of enteroviruses in endomyocardial biopsies and pericardial effusions from dilated cardiomyopathy and myocarditis. Am Heart J 131:760, 1996.
27. Shimizu C, Rambaud C, Cheron G, et al: Molecular identification of viruses in sudden infant death associated with myocarditis and pericarditis. Pediatr Infect Dis J 14:584, 1995.
28. Cherry JD: Enteroviruses: Polioviruses (poliomyelitis), coxsackieviruses, echoviruses, and enteroviruses. In Feigin RD, Cherry JD (eds): Textbook of Pediatric Infectious Diseases, Vol 2, 3rd ed. Philadelphia, WB Saunders, 1992, p 1705.
29. Lipshultz SE, Chanock S, Sanders SP, et al: Cardiovascular manifestations of human immunodeficiency virus infection in infants and children. Am J Cardiol 63:1489, 1989.
30. Mast HL, Haller JO, Schiller MS, Anderson VM: Pericardial effusion and its relationship to cardiac disease in children with acquired immunodeficiency syndrome. Pediatr Radiol 22:548, 1992.
31. Feldman WE: Bacterial etiology and mortality of purulent pericarditis in pediatric patients. Review of 162 cases. Am J Dis Child 133:641, 1979.

32. Dupuis C, Gronnier P, Kachaner J, et al: Bacterial pericarditis in infancy and childhood. Am J Cardiol 74:807, 1994.

33. Pinsky WW, Friedman RA: Pericarditis. *In* Garson A Jr, Bricker JT, McNamara DG (eds): The Science and Practice of Pediatric Cardiology, Vol 2. Philadelphia, Lea & Febiger, 1990, p 1590.

34. Kopec JS, Grifka RG, Karpawich PP: Isolated staphylococcal pericarditis following varicella in an adolescent: An unusual age-associated complication. Pediatr Emerg Care 6:38, 1990.

35. Echeverria P, Smith EW, Ingram D, et al: *Hemophilus influenzae* b pericarditis in children. Pediatrics 56:808, 1975.

36. Callanan DL, Morriss MJ, Kaplan SL, Park I: Constrictive pericarditis due to *Streptococcus sanguis*. South Med J 74:377, 1981.

37. Sato TT, Geary RL, Ashbaugh DG, Jurkovich GJ: Diagnosis and management of pericardial abscess in trauma patients. Am J Surg 165:637, 1993.

38. Van Vooren JP, Thys JP, Vanderhoeft P: Purulent pericarditis resulting from blunt chest trauma (Letter). J Thorac Cardiovasc Surg 100:932, 1990.

39. Majid AA, Omar A: Diagnosis and management of purulent pericarditis. Experience with pericardiectomy. J Thorac Cardiovasc Surg 102:413, 1991.

40. Nelson CT, Taber LH: Diagnosis of tuberculous pericarditis with a fluorochrome stain. Pediatr Infect Dis J 14:1004, 1995.

41. Schepers GW: Tuberculous pericarditis. Am J Cardiol 9:248, 1962.

42. Strang JI: Rapid resolution of tuberculous pericardial effusions with high dose prednisone and anti-tuberculous drugs. J Infect 28:251, 1994.

43. Hugo-Hamman CT, Scher H, De Moor MM: Tuberculous pericarditis in children: A review of 44 cases. Pediatr Infect Dis J 13:13, 1994.

44. Pozniak AL, Weinberg J, Mahari M, et al: Tuberculous pericardial effusion associated with HIV infection: A sign of disseminated disease. Tuber Lung Dis 75:297, 1994.

45. Hsia J, Ross AM: Pericardial effusion and pericardiocentesis in human immunodeficiency virus infection. Am J Cardiol 74:94, 1994.

46. Heidenreich PA, Eisenberg MJ, Kee LL, et al: Pericardial effusion in AIDS. Incidence and survival. Circulation 92:3229, 1995.

47. Tumaliuan JA, Stambouly JJ, Schiff RJ, et al: *Pseudomonas* pericarditis and tamponade in an infant with human immunodeficiency virus infection. Arch Pediatr Adolesc Med 151:207, 1997.

48. Rheuban KS: Diseases of the pericardium. *In* Emmanouilides GC, Riemenschneider TA, Allen HD, Gutgesell HP (eds): Moss and Adams Heart Disease in Infants, Children, and Adolescents: Including the Fetus and Young Adult, Vol 2, 5th ed. Baltimore, Williams & Wilkins, 1995, p 1531.

49. Gruskin AB, Baluarte HJ, Dabbagh S: Hemodialysis and peritoneal dialysis. *In* Edelmann CM Jr (ed): Pediatric Kidney Disease, Vol 1, 2nd ed. Boston, Little, Brown, 1992, p 827.

50. Ansari A, Kaupke CJ, Vaziri ND, et al: Cardiac pathology in patients with end-stage renal disease maintained on hemodialysis. Int J Artif Organs 16:31, 1993.

51. Marini PV, Hull AR: Uremic pericarditis: A review of incidence and management (Review). Kidney Int Suppl 163, 1975.

52. Baldwin JJ, Edwards JE: Uremic pericarditis as a cause of cardiac tamponade. Circulation 53:896, 1976.

53. Cohen GF, Burgess JH, Kaye M: Peritoneal dialysis for the treatment of pericarditis in patients on chronic hemodialysis. Can Med Assoc J 102:1365, 1970.

54. Cullen S, Duff DF, Denham B, Ward OC: Cardiovascular manifestations in Kawasaki disease. Ir J Med Sci 158:253, 1989.

55. Spodick DH: Drug- and toxin-related pericardial disease. *In* Spodick DH (ed): The Pericardium: A Comprehensive Textbook, Vol 1. New York, Marcel Dekker, 1997, p 411.

56. Marcy SM, Overturf GD: Focal bacterial infections. *In* Remington JS, Klein JO (eds): Infectious Diseases of the Fetus and Newborn Infant, Vol 1, 4th ed. Philadelphia, WB Saunders, 1995, p 935.

57. Bereket A, Yang TF, Dey S, et al: Cardiac decompensation due to massive pericardial effusion. A manifestation of hypothyroidism in children with Down's syndrome. Clin Pediatr (Phila) 33:749, 1994.

58. Kabadi UM, Kumar SP: Pericardial effusion in primary hypothyroidism. Am Heart J 120:1393, 1990.

59. Fruehwald C, Weber H, Mannheimer E, et al: Chylopericardium: A rare cause of pericardial effusion. Lymphology 17:89, 1984.

60. Chan BB, Murphy MC, Rodgers BM: Management of chylopericardium. J Pediatr Surg 25:1185, 1990.

61. Greene TO, Portnow AS, Huang SK: Acute pericarditis resulting from an endocardial active fixation screw-in atrial lead [see comments]. Pacing Clin Electrophysiol 17:21, 1994.

62. Peters RW, Scheinman MM, Raskin S, Thomas AN: Unusual complications of epicardial pacemakers. Recurrent pericarditis, cardiac tamponade and pericardial constriction. Am J Cardiol 45:1088, 1980.

63. Crozier I, Greenslade J, Haslett G, Ikram H: Radiofrequency ablation of anomalous cardiac pathways: Initial experience. N Z Med J 106:118, 1993.

64. Hancock EW: Neoplastic pericardial disease. Cardiol Clin 8:673, 1990.

65. Chan HS, Sonley MJ, Moes CA, et al: Primary and secondary tumors of childhood involving the heart, pericardium, and great vessels. A report of 75 cases and review of the literature. Cancer 56:825, 1985.

66. Rheuban KS, McDaniel NL, Feldman PS, et al: Intrapericardial teratoma causing nonimmune hydrops fetalis and pericardial tamponade: A case report. Pediatr Cardiol 12:54, 1991.

67. Stewart JR, Fajardo LF: Dose response in human and experimental radiation-induced heart disease. Application of the nominal standard dose (NSD) concept. Radiology 99:403, 1971.

68. Mill WB, Baglan RJ, Kurichety P, et al: Symptomatic radiation-induced pericarditis in Hodgkin's disease. Int J Radiat Oncol Biol Phys 10:2061, 1984.

69. Byhardt R, Brace K, Ruckdeschel J, et al: Dose and treatment factors in radiation-related pericardial effusion associated with the mantle technique for Hodgkin's disease. Cancer 35:795, 1975.

70. Green DM, Gingell RL, Pearce J, et al: The effect of mediastinal irradiation on cardiac function of patients treated during childhood and adolescence for Hodgkin's disease. J Clin Oncol 5:239, 1987.

71. Lange B, D'Angio G, Ross AJ III, et al: Oncologic emergencies. *In* Pizzo PA, Poplack DG (eds): Principles and Practice of Pediatric Oncology, vol 1, 2nd ed. Philadelphia, JB Lippincott, 1989, p 951.

72. Engle MA, McCabe JC, Ebert PA, Zabriskie J: The postpericardiotomy syndrome and antiheart antibodies. Circulation 49:401, 1974.

73. McCabe JC, Ebert PA, Engle MA, Zabriskie JB: Circulating heart-reactive antibodies in the postpericardiotomy syndrome. J Surg Res 14:158, 1973.

74. Dressler W: A post myocardial infarction syndrome: Preliminary report of complication resembling idiopathic, recurrent, benign pericarditis. JAMA 160:1379, 1956.

75. Engle MA, Zabriskie JB, Senterfit LB, et al: Viral illness and the postpericardiotomy syndrome. A prospective study in children. Circulation 62:1151, 1980.

76. Clapp SK, Garson A Jr, Gutgesell HP, et al: Postoperative pericardial effusion and its relation to postpericardiotomy syndrome. Pediatrics 66:585, 1980.

77. Kirsh MM, McIntosh K, Kahn DR, Sloan H: Postpericardiotomy syndromes. Ann Thorac Surg 9:158, 1970.

78. Weitzman LB, Tinker WP, Kronzon I, et al: The incidence and natural history of pericardial effusion after cardiac surgery—an echocardiographic study. Circulation 69:506, 1984.

79. Wilson NJ, Webber SA, Patterson MW, et al: Double-blind placebo-controlled trial of corticosteroids in children with postpericardiotomy syndrome. Pediatr Cardiol 15:62, 1994.

80. van Son JA, Danielson GK, Schaff HV, et al: Congenital partial and complete absence of the pericardium. Mayo Clin Proc 68:743, 1993.

81. Connolly HM, Click RL, Schattenberg TT, et al: Congenital absence of the pericardium: Echocardiography as a diagnostic tool. J Am Soc Echocardiogr 8:87, 1995.

82. Schiavone WA, O'Donnell JK: Congenital absence of the left portion of parietal pericardium demonstrated by nuclear magnetic resonance imaging. Am J Cardiol 55:1439, 1985.

83. Gehlmann HR, van Ingen GJ: Symptomatic congenital complete absence of the left pericardium. Case report and review of the literature. Eur Heart J 10:670, 1989.

84. Nasser WK, Helmen C, Tavel ME, et al: Congenital absence of the left pericardium. Clinical, electrocardiographic, radiographic, hemodynamic, and angiographic findings in six cases. Circulation 41:469, 1970.

85. Feigin DS, Fenoglio JJ, McAllister HA, Madewell JE: Pericardial cysts. A radiologic-pathologic correlation and review. Radiology 125:15, 1977.

86. Nath PH, Sanders C, Holley HC, McElvein RB: Percutaneous fine needle aspiration in the diagnosis and management of mediastinal cysts in adults. South Med J 81:1225, 1988.

87. Hirschmann JV: Pericardial constriction. Am Heart J 96:110, 1978.

88. Fowler NO: Constrictive pericarditis: Its history and current status. Clin Cardiol 18:341, 1995.

89. Sagrista-Sauleda J, Permanyer-Miralda G, Candell-Riera J, et al: Transient cardiac constriction: An unrecognized pattern of evolution in effusive acute idiopathic pericarditis. Am J Cardiol 59:961, 1987.

90. Harada K, Seki I, Okuni M: Constrictive pericarditis with atrial septal defect in children. Jpn Heart J 19:531, 1978.

91. Rubenstein JJ, Goldblatt A, Daggett WM: Acute constriction complicating purulent pericarditis in infancy. Am J Dis Child 124:591, 1972.

92. Simcha A, Taylor JF: Constrictive pericarditis in childhood. Arch Dis Child 46:515, 1971.

93. Nelson DL, Blaese RM, Strober W, et al: Constrictive pericarditis, intestinal lymphangiectasia, and reversible immunologic deficiency. J Pediatr 86:548, 1975.

94. Connolly DC, Mann RJ: Dominic J. Corrigan (1802–1880) and his description of the pericardial knock. Mayo Clinic Proc 55:771, 1980.

95. Hatle LK, Appleton CP, Popp RL: Differentiation of constrictive pericarditis and restrictive cardiomyopathy by Doppler echocardiography [see comments]. Circulation 79:357, 1989.

96. Klein AL, Cohen GI: Doppler echocardiographic assessment of constrictive pericarditis, cardiac amyloidosis, and cardiac tamponade. Cleve Clin J Med 59:278, 1992.

97. Allaria A, Michelli D, Capelli H, et al: Transient cardiac constriction following purulent pericarditis. Eur J Pediatr 151:250, 1992.

98. Kushwaha SS, Fallon JT, Fuster V: Restrictive cardiomyopathy. N Engl J Med 336:267, 1997.

99. Benotti JR, Grossman W: Restrictive cardiomyopathy. Annu Rev Med 35:113, 1984.

100. Vaitkus PT, Kussmaul WG: Constrictive pericarditis versus restrictive cardiomyopathy: A reappraisal and update of diagnostic criteria. Am Heart J 122:1431, 1991.

CHAPTER 52

HYPERLIPIDEMIA IN CHILDREN AND ADOLESCENTS

RONALD M. LAUER   LINDA SNETSELAAR   LINDA E. MUHONEN

There is now convincing evidence that the atherosclerotic process begins in children and adolescents.[1–4] Although lipid and lipoprotein levels in children and adolescents are related to the extent of the early atherosclerotic process, other risk factors in youth should be addressed with equal attention. Specifically, smoking should be discouraged, hypertension should be identified and treated, obesity should be avoided and reduced, exercise should be encouraged, and diabetes mellitus should be identified and treated.[5] This chapter discusses only lipids and lipoproteins, their relationship to the atherosclerotic process, and their medical management.

LIPIDS AND LIPOPROTEINS

Cholesterol and triglycerides are water-insoluble lipids that are transported in the blood by lipoproteins. Lipoproteins can be classified into four categories: low-density lipoproteins (LDL), very low density lipoproteins (VLDL), high-density lipoproteins (HDL), and chylomicrons. Apolipoproteins are made up of large lipid complexes and apoproteins, the ligands that react with receptor sites in cells. Apolipoproteins together with phospholipids serve to solubilize triglycerides and proteins in different lipoproteins. The principal lipoprotein associated with LDL is apolipoprotein (apo) B-100; apo A-I and apo A-II are associated with HDL. The complex of apo B-100 and LDL is the primary transporter of plasma cholesterol. High levels of LDL-cholesterol are associated with increased risk for cardiovascular disease. HDL-cholesterol acts through reverse transport to remove cholesterol from the cells and deliver it to the liver for catabolism; this lipoprotein has a protective effect against atherosclerotic cardiovascular disease. VLDL serves as the main carrier for triglycerides, which are the carrier or storage form of fatty acids in the tissues and plasma. Chylomicrons are the triglycerides of dietary origin. They are lipid complexes consisting of three fatty acids linked to a glycerol molecule by an ester bond.

In many large epidemiologic studies, elevated LDL-cholesterol levels and low HDL-cholesterol levels are associated with accelerated atherosclerosis in adult populations.[6] For a more complete description of lipoprotein abnormalities, the reader is referred to reference 7.

The link between lipid disorders and cardiovascular disease is the atherosclerotic plaque, a cap of intimal, lipid-containing cells (macrophages and modified smooth muscle cells) with some collagen covering a deeper deposit of extracellular lipid and cell debris. T lymphocytes are present. Subsequently, there may be calcification, cell necrosis, and rupture of or hemorrhage into the plaque; these changes result in overlying thrombosis. These lesions may narrow or occlude coronary, renal, or cerebral arteries and in the aorta lead to embolism of cholesterol crystals or thrombi.

OXIDIZED LDL-CHOLESTEROL

Oxidation mediates atherogenicity of LDL. Oxidized LDL-cholesterol (oxLDL) can affect many components of the atherogenic process, including vasomotor properties and thrombosis as well as lesion initiation and progression itself. OxLDL is immunogenic, and autoantibodies to epitopes of oxLDL, such as malondialdehyde (MDA)–lysine, are found in serum and recognize material in atheromatous tissue.[8, 9] Salonen and colleagues[10] compared antibodies to oxLDL and native LDL in serum samples of 30 Finnish men with accelerated progression of carotid atherosclerosis and 30 matched control subjects without progression. Neither group had antibody binding to native LDL. A titer was defined as the ratio of antibody binding to MDA-LDL/antibody binding to native LDL. Atherosclerotic patients had a significantly higher antibody titer to MDA-LDL (2.67 versus 2.06, $P = .003$). These differences remained significant after correction for smoking, LDL-cholesterol level, and serum copper concentrations. In addition, in vivo human resistance vessel endothelial function is inversely related to oxLDL antibodies; smoking potentiates this relationship in hypercholesterolemia.[11]

15-Lipoxygenase is one of the principal mammalian enzymes that can oxidize polyunsaturated fatty acids in intact lipoproteins and in membrane phospholipids in situ.[12] In animal studies, there is a massive induction of 15-lipoxygenase activity in vascular tissues by hypercholesterolemia.[12, 13] Epitopes of oxLDL are found in macrophage-rich areas of the human fatty streak as well as in more advanced human atherosclerotic lesions. Using in situ hybridization and immunostaining techniques, Yla-Herttuala and associates[13] have shown that 15-lipoxygenase messenger ribonucleic acid (mRNA) and protein colocalize to the same macrophage areas, and these same lesions express abundant mRNA for the acetyl LDL receptor but no detectable mRNA for the LDL receptor. This indicates that atherogenesis in human arteries may be linked to macrophage-induced oxidative modification of LDL, mediated by 15-lipoxygenase, leading to subsequent macrophage uptake, partly by way of the acetyl LDL receptor.

Paraoxonase is an enzyme exclusively bound to HDL in human serum.[14] Paraoxonase purified from human HDL prevents the accumulation of lipoperoxides in LDL.[15] Serum paraoxonase activity is significantly lower in individuals with familial hypercholesterolemia or insulin-dependent diabetes, in whom total cholesterol and apo B as well as triglyceride levels are increased.[16,17] Paraoxonase is an HDL-associated enzyme capable of hydrolyzing lipid peroxides. There are two isoforms (A and B), and the B allele is associated with excess coronary heart disease in non–insulin-dependent diabetics.[18,19] Chronic hyperglycemia and the production of advanced glycosylation end products predispose to lipid oxidation.[20]

SIGNIFICANCE OF LIPIDS AND LIPOPROTEINS IN CHILDREN AND ADOLESCENTS

In adult population studies, elevated cholesterol levels are important predictors of occlusive atherosclerotic vascular disease. Drug trials of cholesterol-lowering agents have shown major reduction in coronary heart disease rates. Because no long-term longitudinal studies of populations of children have been carried out to observe the predictive value of childhood blood cholesterol levels and because no long-term studies of drug therapy beginning in childhood have been performed, the significance of cholesterol levels in the general population of infants, children, and adolescents must be inferred from less direct evidence than in adults.

PATHOLOGIC STUDIES

Studies showing coronary atherosclerosis in U.S. soldiers killed at war have helped recognize the importance of the development of atherosclerosis in early adulthood.[21,22] The International Atherosclerosis Project (IAP) undertook an extensive study of atherosclerosis in 14 countries and found a wide range in the prevalence and mean extent of atherosclerotic lesions in different populations.[23] Strong and McGill[24] investigated coronary and aortic lesions in younger subjects included in the IAP and found that most aortas by 10 years of age had fatty streaks, and there were fewer coronary fatty streaks in this population of 10- to 14-year-olds. Although not all fatty streaks in children progress to more complex lesions, more advanced microscopic lesions that precede the fibrous plaque are seen in the coronary arteries of children at puberty and occur in 65% of children between 12 and 14 years of age.[25]

Research relating serum cholesterol levels to the extent of early arterial lesions of atherosclerosis in children has been reported in the Bogalusa Heart Study.[4,26] Aortic fatty streaks were related to antemortem levels of both total cholesterol and LDL-cholesterol independent of race, sex, and age and were negatively correlated with the ratio of HDL-cholesterol to LDL-cholesterol and VLDL-cholesterol. An extensive study involving 15- to 34-year-old traumatic death victims from across the United States found associations between serum LDL-cholesterol plus VLDL-cholesterol, HDL-cholesterol, and thiocyanate levels and the extent of the atherosclerotic process.[27] For additional descriptions of the pathologic evaluation of the atherosclerotic process, the reader is referred to other reviews.[28]

GENETIC DISORDERS

Several human genetic dyslipolipidemias have in common raised concentrations of cholesterol-rich lipoproteins, resulting from specific gene mutations. These disorders are characterized by severe atherosclerosis and often by the occurrence of coronary heart disease at a young age.

Familial Hypercholesterolemia

Familial hypercholesterolemia (FH) is a dominantly inherited defect in the LDL receptor that causes faulty LDL uptake and metabolism. The heterozygous form is the most commonly encountered dyslipoproteinemia in children and adolescents, affecting 1 in 500 persons. In some countries where the population has been maintained with little inbreeding, the rates of FH are higher; examples are the French-Canadians, Afrikaners, and Norwegians. More than 200 different mutations of the LDL receptor have been reported.[29,30]

A number of clinical findings determine whether a child or adolescent with primary elevation of LDL-cholesterol has FH. An evaluation of the family members is particularly helpful. For example, one of the parents and one of two siblings of an FH child will have elevated total cholesterol and LDL-cholesterol levels. The triglyceride levels are usually normal (below the 95th percentile). Children and adolescents with FH often have LDL-cholesterol levels above 160 mg/dl, with average levels about 240 mg/dl.[31,32] Parents with FH often have tendon xanthomas. Tendon xanthomas are rarely found before 10 years of age, however, and only 10 to 15% of these patients develop xanthomas in the second decade. When present, they are in the Achilles tendon and the extensor tendons of the hands. The clinical manifestations of occlusive vascular disease are extremely rare in FH heterozygous children and adolescents.[32] The development of coronary heart disease in approximately half of the fathers by age 50 years and in mothers by age 60 years, however, provides a strong rationale for the early detection and treatment of children and adolescents with FH.[29]

The homozygous form of FH is rare, affecting 1 in a million in the population. Affected children have cholesterol levels that average about 700 mg/dl, and many may be above 1000 mg/dl.[33] The profoundly elevated LDL-cholesterol levels in these children result in physical signs, such as planar xanthomas, that are present by age 5 years. These are in the webbing of the hands, over the elbows, and over the buttocks. Tendon xanthomas, corneal arcus, and clinically significant coronary heart disease are often present by 10 years of age, and aortic stenosis due to atherosclerosis in the valve is often present.[33]

Familial Combined Hyperlipidemia

Familial combined hyperlipidemia is a more frequent lipid disorder than FH among the adult population and is due to increased LDL production. The phenotypic expression of this dyslipoproteinemia is infrequent, however, and results in mild dyslipoproteinemia in children and adolescents. This disorder is thought to be transmitted as an autosomal dominant trait, but no specific genetic markers have been found.

Familial Hypertriglyceridemia

Familial hypertriglyceridemia with a normal LDL-cholesterol level is a disorder of triglyceride-rich lipoproteins that is a result of the abnormal production of VLDL-cholesterol. Familial hypertriglyceridemia does not predispose individuals to premature coronary heart disease. This disease is thought to be an autosomal dominant trait carried by approximately 10% of the population. Triglyceride levels generally run between 2.2 mmol/L (200 mg/dl) and 5.6 mmol/L (500 mg/dl), and a low HDL-cholesterol level is often seen.

Hypertriglyceridemia may be due to a deficiency in lipoprotein lipase[34] or apo C-II[35]; the decreased removal of VLDL particles results in the high triglyceride levels. Inherited deficiency of lipoprotein lipase, the enzyme responsible for catabolism of triglycerides in triglyceride-rich lipoproteins, results in a profound increase in chylomicrons. Deficiency of lipoprotein lipase or apo C-II manifests in the same manner clinically. A child or adolescent with this disorder may present with eruptive xanthomas over the mucous membranes or buttocks. Lipemia retinalis and hepatosplenomegaly may also be present. The lipid profile shows marked elevation in chylomicrons and triglycerides. Other disease processes include hypothyroidism, alcoholism, diabetic ketoacidosis, and pancreatitis.

A less common form of triglyceride-rich lipoprotein abnormality combines elevations of both chylomicrons and VLDL. This disease can cause pancreatitis, abdominal pain, glucose intolerance, and hyperuricemia.

Familial Dysbetalipoproteinemia

Familial dysbetalipoproteinemia is due to an underlying defect in apo E.[36] This disorder results in an accumulation of remnants of VLDL and chylomicrons. Clinical manifestations include palmar and tuberous xanthomas. More than 90% of individuals with this disease are homozygous for apo E-2. Both triglyceride and cholesterol levels are elevated; however, this disorder is not usually seen in childhood.

Familial Decreased HDL

Other primary disorders of lipid and lipoprotein metabolism have deficiencies of HDL-cholesterol. Hypoalphalipoproteinemia involves a low HDL-cholesterol level most often with normal triglyceride and LDL levels. In these families with low HDL-cholesterol levels, however, some affected members have elevated levels of triglycerides accompanying the low levels of HDL-cholesterol. With high triglyceride levels (>1.7 mmol/L; 150 mg/dl), the low HDL levels may not be a primary defect but rather a result of the hypertriglyceridemia.[37] Abnormalities in the genes for the major lipoprotein of HDL, apo A-I, have been detected in some families with hypoalphalipoproteinemia.[38–40]

EPIDEMIOLOGIC STUDIES

Many epidemiologic studies have established elevated blood cholesterol levels, specifically LDL-cholesterol levels, as one of several major risk factors for coronary heart disease in men and women, including the elderly. These investigations include case-control studies; comparisons of populations with low and high rates of coronary heart disease; migrant studies; and international studies of diet, atherosclerosis, cholesterol levels, and coronary heart disease.[41, 42]

Especially noteworthy are the findings of many prospective, observational studies within populations, such as the Framingham Heart Study,[43] the Honolulu Heart Program,[44] the British Regional Heart Study,[45] and studies of men screened for the Multiple Risk Factor Intervention Trial.[46–49] Such studies have consistently shown the blood cholesterol level to be a powerful and independent predictor of coronary heart disease. On the average, each 1% rise in cholesterol level is associated with an approximate 2% increase in risk of coronary heart disease. Davis and coworkers[50] suggested that this relationship has been underestimated because of failure to take into account intraindividual variations in cholesterol levels and that in fact each 1% rise in blood cholesterol level is associated with an approximate 3% increase in risk. The level of HDL-cholesterol, in contrast, is inversely and independently related to coronary heart disease in both sexes and at all ages.[51]

International Comparisons

In children, the major nutritional determinant of differences in serum total cholesterol levels between countries appears to be the proportion of saturated fat in the diet.[52–54] For example (Table 52–1), in countries such as the Philippines, Italy, and Ghana, saturated fat constitutes about 10% or less of the dietary energy intake, and the serum cholesterol level of boys aged 7 to 9 years is generally below 4.1 mmol/L (159 mg/dl).[52, 55, 56] These countries also often have lower dietary cholesterol intakes. From countries such as the United States, the Netherlands, and Finland, higher intakes are noted, the saturated fat intake varies between 13.5 and 17.7% of energy intake, and the average serum cholesterol levels are equal to or greater than 4.3 mmol/L (167 mg/dl).

Although blood cholesterol levels are lowest in countries in which nutrition is not optimal and growth is delayed, there are many industrialized countries (such as

TABLE 52–1

DIETARY SATURATED FAT AND CHOLESTEROL INTAKE AND SERUM TOTAL CHOLESTEROL IN BOYS AGED 7 TO 9 YEARS IN SIX COUNTRIES

| Country | Dietary Intake | | Serum Total Cholesterol (mmol/L [mg/dl]) |
	Saturated Fat (% of energy)	Cholesterol (mg/1000 calories)	
Philippines	9.3	97	3.8 (147)
Italy	10.4	159	4.1 (159)
Ghana	10.5	48	3.3 (128)
United States	13.5	151	4.3 (167)
Netherlands	15.1	142	4.5 (174)
Finland	17.7	157	4.9 (190)

United States data from National Health and Nutrition Examination Survey (NHANES): dietary intake data from NHANES-II,[56] serum cholesterol levels from NHANES-I.[55] Other data from Knuiman et al.[52]

Adapted from National Cholesterol Education Program: Report of the Expert Panel on Blood Cholesterol Levels in Children and Adolescents. Pediatrics 89:525, 1992. Used with permission of the American Academy of Pediatrics.

Portugal, Israel, and Italy) in which children have lower cholesterol levels and in which normal growth is maintained.[52,57,58] In general, higher serum cholesterol levels in children are associated with higher levels in middle-aged adults in the same country and with higher mortality rates of coronary heart disease in the adult population.

Animal Studies

Studies in laboratory animals have demonstrated that high blood cholesterol levels promote atherosclerosis.[41] Many species develop atherosclerosis when fed diets that raise their total cholesterol and LDL-cholesterol levels. Hypercholesterolemic animals develop intimal lesions that progress from fatty streaks to complicated ulcerated plaques resembling those of human atherosclerosis.[59,60] Studies in adolescent nonhuman primates show that they develop fatty streaks and fibrous plaques after a high-cholesterol, high–saturated fatty acid diet, but less extensive than in adult animals.[61,62] Severe atherosclerosis in monkeys regresses when blood cholesterol level is lowered for an extended period by diet or drugs.[41,63,64]

These studies support the view of a causal relationship between LDL-cholesterol and atherosclerosis. They also indicate that atherosclerosis may be reversible.

Familial Aggregation

Coronary heart disease occurs more frequently in adult members of families in which the children's levels of cholesterol, triglycerides, LDL-cholesterol, and apo B or combinations thereof are elevated. The cholesterol levels in the children and adolescents aggregate with their family members. The prevalence of coronary heart disease in adult relatives is significantly increased among children with high cholesterol levels compared with schoolchildren who have normal cholesterol levels.[65–68] In addition, when the progeny of young (<55 years of age) ischemic heart disease victims are examined, more than half have dyslipoproteinemia. Familial aggregation of blood lipid and lipoprotein levels is the result, in part, of a shared environment as well as genetic factors.

Tracking of Cholesterol Levels from Childhood to Adulthood

Children with high cholesterol levels have a greater risk of having elevated cholesterol levels as adults than does the general population. Rank order of cholesterol levels in childhood is maintained ("tracking"), but not as consistently as rank order of height and weight.[69–72] Lauer and Clarke[73] showed that of children aged 5 to 18 years who had cholesterol levels greater than the 90th percentile on two occasions, 75% had higher than desirable levels (≥5.2 mmol/L; 200 mg/dl), and 25% had desirable levels (<5.2 mmol/L; 200 mg/dl) at ages 20 to 25 years. Because 5.2 mmol/L (200 mg/dl) is approximately the 75th percentile for adults in their 20s, this percentage of individuals with levels at or greater than 5.2 mmol/L (200 mg/dl) is about three times the percentage expected for the general population. Quite a few children with cholesterol levels greater than the 90th percentile on two occasions did not qualify for individual medical care, as defined by the National Cholesterol Education Program, when they became adults.[6]

Adult Clinical Trials

Clinical trials in adult populations have provided convincing evidence that lowering cholesterol levels through the use of medication or diet reduces coronary risk.[74–78] Angiographic trials of cholesterol lowering have reported that progression of atherosclerotic lesions can definitely be slowed, and regression occurs in some patients after lipid lowering.[79–84] No studies provide direct evidence that lowering blood cholesterol levels in children and adolescents will reduce their risk of coronary heart disease in adulthood. Such studies may never be possible because they would involve large numbers of children for several decades. The available evidence, however, strongly suggests that the benefit of reducing cholesterol levels in childhood will be realized in adulthood.

STRATEGIES FOR LOWERING CHOLESTEROL IN CHILDREN AND ADOLESCENTS

Two strategies have been suggested for lowering cholesterol levels in children and adolescents to prevent or retard the atherosclerotic process: a population or public health approach and an individualized approach.

THE POPULATION APPROACH

The population approach aims to lower the average population levels of cholesterol in children and adolescents by encouraging the adoption of lower saturated fat, total fat, and cholesterol intake. Because infants need higher fat intake for adequate growth and development, reduction in dietary fat is not appropriate at this age. Children ages 2 to 5 years are selective in their food choices. Thus, it has been recommended that children older than 2 years gradually adopt a diet that by about 5 years of age contains no more than 30% of calories from fat. The following nutrient pattern is recommended: 10% of total calories from saturated fatty acid, no more than 30% percent of total calories as total fat, and dietary cholesterol intake of less than 300 mg/day. As children begin to consume fewer calories from fat, these calories should be replaced by more grain products, fruits, vegetables, low-fat milk products, beans, lean red meat, poultry, fish, and other protein-rich foods.

Changes in diet are designed as the principal means of preventing coronary heart disease. The aim is to lower the average level of blood cholesterol in all children and adolescents through population-wide changes in nutrient intake and eating patterns. These recommendations are directed to groups that influence the eating patterns of children and adolescents, including schools, health professionals, government agencies, the food industry, and the mass media. The advantage of this approach is that even a small reduction in mean total cholesterol and LDL-cholesterol levels in children and adolescents, if carried into adult life, could substantially decrease the incidence of coronary heart disease.[85] The United States Department of Agriculture 1985 Food Consumption Survey indicated that children and adolescents consume 35 to 36% of calories from total fat and 14% from saturated fat, with a cholesterol intake of 193 to 296 mg/day.[86,87] More recent U.S. population–based data from the third National

Health and Nutrition Examination Survey for persons 2 to 19 years of age indicate that mean intakes of total fat and saturated fat are 34% and 12%, respectively, with a mean cholesterol intake of approximately 270 mg/day.[88] Because concerns have been expressed that some parents and their children may overinterpret the need to restrict their fat intakes, a lower limit of 15% of total calories from fat has been suggested by the World Health Organization.[89]

THE INDIVIDUALIZED APPROACH

The individualized approach to cholesterol lowering calls on the cooperative effort of health care professionals to identify and treat children and adolescents at highest risk of having elevated blood cholesterol levels as adults and increased risk of coronary heart disease.

Selective Screening
Children and adolescents who have a family history of premature cardiovascular disease or have at least one parent with a high blood cholesterol level are those at increased risk of an elevated blood cholesterol level and an increased risk of coronary heart disease as adults. Selective screening is recommended for these children and adolescents in the context of their regular health care (Figs. 52–1 and 52–2). This focus is because of strong evidence of familial aggregation of coronary heart disease, high blood cholesterol level, and other risk factors. The lipid and lipoprotein levels described herein are based on high laboratory standards in established lipid laboratories maintaining quality control. Thus, measurements that are to be used to identify children at risk should be carried out in such laboratories.

The following specific recommendations are made for selective screening of children and adolescents in the context of their continuing health care:

- Screen children and adolescents whose parents or grandparents, at age 55 years or younger, underwent diagnostic coronary arteriography and were found to have coronary atherosclerosis. This includes those who have undergone balloon angioplasty or coronary artery bypass surgery.
- Screen the offspring of a parent who has been found to have a blood cholesterol level of 240 mg/dl or higher.
- For children and adolescents whose parental history is unobtainable, particularly for those with other risk factors, physicians may choose to measure cholesterol levels to identify those in need of individual nutritional and medical advice.

Optional cholesterol testing by practicing physicians may be appropriate in certain children who are judged to be at higher risk for coronary heart disease independent of family history. For example, adolescents who smoke, or consume excessive amounts of saturated fats and cholesterol, and who are overweight may also deserve testing at

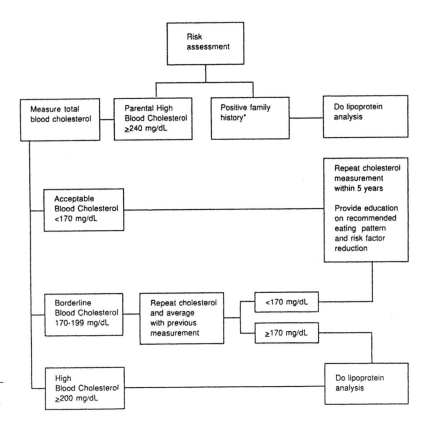

FIGURE 52–1

Selective screening of children and adolescents. Algorithm for risk assessment. (From the National Cholesterol Education Program: Report of the Expert Panel on Blood Cholesterol in Children and Adolescents. Bethesda, MD, US Department of Health and Human Services, Public Health Service, National Institutes of Health, National Heart, Lung, and Blood Institute, National Cholesterol Education Program, 1991. NIH publication 91-2732.)

* Defined as a history of premature (before age 55 years) cardiovascular disease in a parent or grandparent

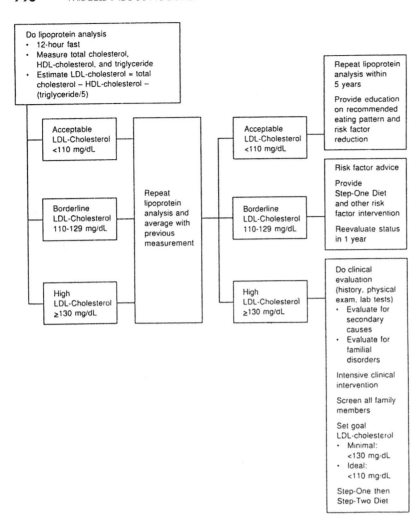

Selective screening of children and adolescents. Algorithm for classification, education, and follow-up on LDL-cholesterol determined in Figure 52–1. (From the National Cholesterol Education Program: Report of the Expert Panel on Blood Cholesterol in Children and Adolescents. Bethesda, MD, US Department of Health and Human Services, Public Health Service, National Institutes of Health, National Heart, Lung, and Blood Institute, National Cholesterol Education Program, 1991. NIH publication 91-2732.)

the discretion of their physician. For parents who do not know their cholesterol levels, pediatricians should arrange that their levels be measured.

What Should Be Measured

The focus of the individualized approach is to detect and treat the hypercholesterolemic child or adolescent whose elevated LDL-cholesterol level is likely to signify increased risk in adulthood. The screening protocol varies according to the reason for testing. This protocol is suggested to limit the greater expense of lipoprotein analyses.

If screening is being done because a parent has a cholesterol level in excess of 240 mg/dl, the initial test should be a measurement of total cholesterol (Table 52–2). If the child's level is above 200 mg/dl, a lipoprotein analysis should be carried out to measure HDL-cholesterol and LDL-cholesterol levels. If the total cholesterol level is borderline (170 to 199 mg/dl), a second measurement of total cholesterol should be taken and averaged with the first. If the average is borderline or high, a lipoprotein analysis should be carried out.

If the patient is being tested because of a documented family history of premature cardiovascular disease, the initial test should be a lipoprotein analysis, which requires a 12-hour fast.

Management

Once a lipoprotein analysis is obtained, it should be repeated to determine the average LDL-cholesterol level, which directs the steps for risk assessment and treatment. Follow-up of the LDL-cholesterol determinations is as follows:

- Acceptable LDL-cholesterol (<110 mg/dl): If the average LDL-cholesterol level is in the acceptable range, provide education on the eating pattern recommended for all children and adolescents and on other risk factors; repeat lipoprotein analysis in 5 years.

TABLE 52–2

CLASSIFICATION OF TOTAL AND LDL-CHOLESTEROL LEVELS IN CHILDREN AND ADOLESCENTS*

Category	Total Cholesterol (mg/dl)	LDL-Cholesterol (mg/dl)
Acceptable	<170	<110
Borderline	170–199	110–129
High	≥200	≥130

*From families with hypercholesterolemia or premature cardiovascular disease. Adapted from National Cholesterol Education Program: Report of the Expert Panel on Blood Cholesterol Levels in Children and Adolescents. Pediatrics 89:525, 1992. Used with permission of the American Academy of Pediatrics.

<table>
<tr><td colspan="2">TABLE 52–3</td></tr>
</table>

CAUSES OF SECONDARY HYPERCHOLESTEROLEMIA

EXOGENOUS

Drugs: corticosteroids, isotretinoin (Accutane), thiazides, anticonvulsants, β blockers, anabolic steroids, certain oral contraceptives
Alcohol
Obesity

ENDOCRINE AND METABOLIC

Hypothyroidism
Diabetes mellitus
Lipodystrophy
Pregnancy
Idiopathic hypercalcemia

STORAGE DISEASES

Glycogen storage disease
Sphingolipidoses

OBSTRUCTIVE LIVER DISEASE

Biliary atresia
Biliary cirrhosis

CHRONIC RENAL DISEASE

Nephrotic syndrome

OTHERS

Anorexia nervosa
Progeria
Collagen disease
Klinefelter's syndrome

Adapted from National Cholesterol Education Program: Report of the Expert Panel on Blood Cholesterol Levels in Children and Adolescents. Pediatrics 89:525, 1992. Used with permission of the American Academy of Pediatrics.

- Borderline LDL-cholesterol (110 to 129 mg/dl): If the average LDL-cholesterol level is borderline, provide risk factor advice; initiate the Step-One Diet (see later) and other risk factor intervention; re-evaluate in 1 year.
- High LDL-cholesterol (≥130 mg/dl): If the average LDL-cholesterol level is high, evaluate for secondary causes and familial disorders (Table 52–3); screen all family members; initiate the Step-One Diet, followed if necessary by the Step-Two Diet.

TREATMENT OF DYSLIPIDEMIA

DIET THERAPY

The general aim of diet therapy in children is to reduce elevated blood cholesterol levels while maintaining a nutritionally adequate eating pattern. The emphasis is on decreasing the level of saturated fat, total fat, and cholesterol and on consuming only enough calories to achieve or maintain desirable body weight. Diet therapy includes two steps (Table 52–4).

Methods of Diet Therapy

NUTRITIONAL HISTORY

It is important initially to identify current eating practices, including where meals and snacks are eaten (at home or away), how they are prepared, and when they are eaten. Family lifestyle provides clues to the frequency of meals away from home and use of commercially prepared foods. To analyze a child's eating habits fully, request that the child or parent and other care providers record the child's food intake for a week. This is best carried out by a professional who is trained in nutrient data collection.

Because children often cannot keep adequate dietary records, parents are useful sources of information but may be unaware of all the foods their child eats away from home. The Diet Intervention Study in Children (DISC) used three 24-hour recalls as one method of determining intake in children.[90] Eck and coworkers[91] conducted food recalls of children aged 4 to 9.5 years by interviewing the child and both parents together. This "consensus recall" provided more accurate information than interviewing individuals separately. Food records should be kept by parents or care providers (daycare workers, babysitters) who have been instructed in measuring and recording food eaten. Older children and adolescents can be instructed in keeping their own food records.

The interview focuses on helping the child and family determine how to achieve dietary change. A detailed description of the skills needed to use this type of counseling has been developed in DISC.[90]

Monitoring and follow-up are important components in implementation of the Step-One and Step-Two Diets. This is described in detail in the National Cholesterol Education Program's Report of the Expert Panel on Blood Cholesterol Levels in Children and Adolescents.[92]

Nutritionists who are involved in the care of children should use computerized nutrient programs with frequently updated fatty acid and dietary cholesterol values, which are helpful for dietary assessment. The foods recalled or written on a food record are entered, and the re-

<table>
<tr><td colspan="3">TABLE 52–4</td></tr>
</table>

CHARACTERISTICS OF STEP-ONE AND STEP-TWO DIETS FOR LOWERING BLOOD CHOLESTEROL

	Recommended Intake	
Nutrient	Step-One Diet	Step-Two Diet
Total fat	Average of no more than 30% of total calories	Same
Saturated fatty acids	Less than 10% of total calories	Less than 7% of total calories
Polyunsaturated fatty acids	Up to 10% of total calories	Same
Monounsaturated fatty acids	Remaining total fat calories	Same
Cholesterol	Less than 300 mg/day	Less than 200 mg/day
Carbohydrates	About 55% of total calories	Same
Protein	About 15–20% of total calories	Same
Calories	To promote normal growth and development and to reach or maintain desirable body weight	Same

Adapted from National Cholesterol Education Program: Report of the Expert Panel on Blood Cholesterol Levels in Children and Adolescents. Pediatrics 89:525, 1992. Used with permission of the American Academy of Pediatrics.

sulting analysis provides immediate detailed information about dietary intake.

ADHERENCE ISSUES FOR THE FAMILY AND CHILD

An elevated blood cholesterol level in a child or adolescent often points to established high-fat eating patterns. To reduce blood cholesterol levels, alternative food choices are necessary. The best support for the child with a high blood cholesterol level is a home environment in which everyone older than approximately 5 years follows the recommended population eating pattern. This includes reducing saturated fat, total fat, and dietary cholesterol and presenting foods in a positive, noncoercive manner.

DRUG THERAPY

Several algorithms for drug therapy in children have been recommended.[92, 93] We present herein the recommendations of the U.S. National Cholesterol Education Program's Expert Panel on Blood Cholesterol in Children and Adolescents.

There are few clinical trials involving the use of drug therapy in children or adolescents. Before initiating medication, the clinician must consider the potential adverse effects for childhood growth and development as well as the drug's known side effects. Because most drugs have not been thoroughly tested and thereby approved in pediatric populations, their use should be limited in this age group.

The National Cholesterol Education Program's guidelines restrict drug therapy to children older than 10 years who have had an insufficient response to an adequate trial of diet therapy for 6 to 12 months:

- LDL-cholesterol level remains at 190 mg/dl or higher There is a positive family history of premature cardiovascular disease (before 55 years of age).
- LDL-cholesterol level remains at 160 mg/dl or higher Two or more other risk factors (Table 52–5) are present in the child or adolescent after vigorous attempts have been made to control these risk factors.

The drugs that are currently recommended for the treatment of hypercholesterolemia and high LDL-cholesterol levels in children are the bile acid sequestrants in the intestinal lumen. They have proven efficacy, relative freedom from side effects, and apparent safety in children. The dose starts with 1 package (9 g) daily but may be increased to 4 packages per day for the most severely affected children (Table 52–6).

Many children and adolescents are unable to continue with daily doses of bile acid sequestrants because of their unwillingness to ingest the resin suspension. In these circumstances, some have recommended the use of hydroxymethylglutaryl–coenzyme A (HMG-CoA) reductase inhibitors. In large drug trials in adult populations, these drugs reduce LDL-cholesterol levels and result in a significant decrease not only in coronary heart disease mortality but also in all-cause mortality.[94–96] In the Canadian multicenter trial of lovastatin in boys older than 16 years at doses ranging from 10 to 40 mg/day, a reduction of 21 to 36% plasma LDL-cholesterol was observed.[94]

Because of their potential side effects, nicotinic acid, HMG-CoA reductase inhibitors, probucol, gemfibrozil, D-thyroxine, and p-aminosalicyclic acid are not recommended for routine use in younger children.

OTHER FORMS OF THERAPY

Both regular alcohol consumption[97] and exercise[98] have been shown to have a beneficial effect on HDL-cholesterol levels in adults. Because the regular consumption of alcohol in youth is associated with other deleterious outcomes, we do not recommend its use as a preventive agent. Antioxidants (e.g., vitamins E and C) are presently being examined for their preventive effects. At present, there is insufficient evidence to warrant their use as dietary supplements.

FUTURE PROSPECTS

The role of the endothelium and its interaction with coagulation factors and lipids in encouraging or retarding atheroma are being actively explored. Families with a high frequency of coronary atheroma may have hyperfibrinogenemia or mutations of coagulation factors V and VII or a platelet glycoprotein receptor. They may also have certain apolipoprotein polymorphisms. Many of the factors already mentioned as important in the etiology of atheroma (obesity, hypertension, diabetes) are familial, and they and factors like smoking or lack of exercise impair endothelial function. The role of estrogens in preventing coronary

---

TABLE 52–5

OTHER RISK FACTORS THAT CONTRIBUTE TO EARLIER ONSET OF CORONARY HEART DISEASE

Family history of premature coronary heart disease, cerebrovascular disease, or occlusive peripheral vascular disease (definite onset before the age of 55 years in siblings, parent, or sibling of parent)
Cigarette smoking
Elevated blood pressure
Low HDL-cholesterol concentration (<35 mg/dl)
Severe obesity (≥95th percentile for weight and height)

Adapted from National Cholesterol Education Program: Report of the Expert Panel on Blood Cholesterol Levels in Children and Adolescents. Pediatrics 89:525, 1992. Used with permission of the American Academy of Pediatrics.

TABLE 52–6

INITIAL DOSAGE SCHEDULE FOR TREATMENT OF FAMILIAL HYPERCHOLESTEROLEMIC CHILDREN AND ADOLESCENTS WITH A BILE ACID SEQUESTRANT*

Dose†	Total Cholesterol (TC) and LDL-Cholesterol (LDL-C) Levels After Diet (mg/dl)	
	TC	LDL-C
1	<245	<195
2	245–300	195–235
3	301–345	236–280
4	>345	

*These are generally recommended doses and may require adjustment based on the patient's response.
†One dose is the equivalent of a 9-g packet of cholestyramine (containing 4 g cholestyramine and 5 g filler), 1 bar of cholestyramine, or 5 g of colestipol.
Adapted from National Cholesterol Education Program: Report of the Expert Panel on Blood Cholesterol Levels in Children and Adolescents. Pediatrics 89:525, 1992. Used with permission of the American Academy of Pediatrics.

atheroma in premenopausal women is also under intense investigation, as much for its basic mechanisms as for its preventive use in older women.

The roles of antioxidants like α-tocopherol, certain flavonoids found in red wines, lycopene found in tomatoes and red grapefruit, and vitamin C are presently being examined for their preventive effects. At present, there is insufficient evidence to warrant their use as dietary supplements. Another factor that has been implicated strongly in the etiology of atheroma is hyperhomocystinemia. As yet, there is no evidence that lowering blood homocystine concentrations by supplementary vitamin B_6, vitamin B_{12}, and folic acid will decrease the incidence of atheroma. Nevertheless, in the future, it is likely that other types of treatments will be added to the primary ones of dietary restriction of fats and calories and drug therapy to lower blood lipid concentrations.

ACKNOWLEDGMENT

Material in this statement is adapted from the Report of the Expert Panel on Blood Cholesterol in Children and Adolescents of the National Cholesterol Education Program.[92]

REFERENCES

1. PDAY Research Group: Relationship of atherosclerosis in young men to serum lipoprotein cholesterol concentration and smoking: A preliminary report from the Pathological Determinants of Atherosclerosis in Youth (PDAY) Research Group. JAMA 264:3018, 1990.
2. Davies H: Atherogenesis and the coronary arteries in childhood. Int J Cardiol 28:283, 1990.
3. Haust MD: The genesis of atherosclerosis in the pediatric age-group. Pediatr Pathol 10:253, 1990.
4. Newman WPI, Freedman DS, Voors AW, et al: Relation of serum lipoprotein levels and systolic blood pressure to early atherosclerosis: The Bogalusa Heart Study. N Engl J Med 314:138, 1986.
5. Strong WB, Deckelbaum RJ, Gidding SS, et al: Integrated cardiovascular health promotion in childhood. A statement for health professionals from the Subcommittee on Atherosclerosis and Hypertension in Childhood of the Council on Cardiovascular Disease in the Young, American Heart Association. Circulation 85:1638, 1992.
6. National Cholesterol Education Program: Report of the Expert Panel on Detection, Evaluation, and Treatment of High Blood Cholesterol in Adults (Adult Treatment Panel II). Bethesda, MD, US Department of Health and Human Services, National Institutes of Health, National Heart, Lung and Blood Institute, 1993. NIH publication 9-3095.
7. Kwiterovich PO: Disorders of lipid and lipoprotein metabolism. In Rudolph AM, Hoffman JIE, Rudolph CD (eds): Pediatrics, 20th ed. Norwalk, CT, Appleton & Lange, 1996, p 343.
8. Steinberg D, Witztum JL: Lipoproteins and atherogenesis. JAMA 264:3047, 1990.
9. Sigal E, Laughton CW, Mulkins MA: Oxidation, lipoxygenase, and atherogenesis. Ann N Y Acad Sci 714:211, 1995.
10. Salonen JT, Yla-Herttuala S, Yamamoto R, et al: Autoantibody against oxidized LDL and progression of carotid atherosclerosis. Lancet 339:883, 1992.
11. Heitzer T, Yla-Herttuala S, Luoma J, et al: Cigarette smoking potentiates endothelial dysfunction of forearm resistance vessels in patients with hypercholesterolemia. Role of oxidized LDL. Circulation 93:1346, 1996.
12. Bailey JM, Makheja AN, Lee R, et al: Systemic activation of 15-lipoxygenase in heart, lung, and vascular tissues by hypercholesterolemia: Relationship to lipoprotein oxidation and atherogenesis. Atherosclerosis 113:247, 1995.
13. Yla-Herttuala S, Luoma J, Viita HV, et al: Transfer of 15-lipoxygenase gene into rabbit iliac arteries results in appearance of oxidation-specific lipid-protein adducts characteristic of oxidized low density lipoprotein. J Clin Invest 95:2692, 1995.
14. Blatter MC, James RWE, Messmer S, et al: Identification of distinct high-density lipoprotein subspecies defined by lipoprotein-associated protein K-45: Identity of K-45 with paraoxonase. Eur J Biochem 211:871, 1993.
15. Mackness MI, Arrol S, Durrington PN: Paraoxonase prevents accumulation of lipoperoxides in low-density lipoprotein. FEBS Lett 286:152, 1991.
16. Chisolm GM, Irwin KC, Penn MS: Lipoprotein oxidation and lipoprotein-induced cell injury in diabetes. Diabetes 39:1420, 1990.
17. Mackness MI, Harty D, Bhatnagar D, et al: Serum paraoxonase activity in familial hypercholesterolemia and insulin-dependent diabetes mellitus. Atherosclerosis 86:193, 1991.
18. Ruiz J, Blanche H, James RW, et al: Gin-Arg192 polymorphism of paraoxonase and coronary heart disease in type 2 diabetes. Lancet 346:869, 1995.
19. Adkins S, Gan KN, Mody M, et al: Molecular basis for polymorphic forms of human serum paraoxonase/arylesterase: Glutamine of arginine at position 191 for the respective allozymes. Am J Hum Genet 52:598, 1993.
20. Hunt JV, Smith CCT, Wolff SP: Auto-oxidative glycosylation and possible involvement of peroxides and free radicals in LDL modification by glucose. Diabetes 39:1420, 1990.
21. Enos WF Jr, Beyer JC, Holmes RH: Pathogenesis of coronary disease in American soldiers killed in Korea. JAMA 158:912, 1955.
22. McNamara JJ, Molot MA, Stremple JF, et al: Coronary artery disease in combat casualties in Vietnam. JAMA 216:1185, 1971.
23. Tejada C, Strong JP, Montenegro MR, et al: Distribution of coronary and aortic atherosclerosis by geographic location, race and sex. Lab Invest 18:509, 1968.
24. Strong JP, McGill HC Jr: The pediatric aspects of atherosclerosis. J Atherosclerosis Res 9:251, 1969.
25. Stary HC: Evolution and progression of atherosclerotic lesions in coronary arteries of children and young adults. Arteriosclerosis 9(suppl I):I–19, 1989.
26. Freedman DS, Newman WP III, Tracy RE, et al: Black-white differences in aortic fatty streaks in adolescence and early adulthood: The Bogalusa Study. Circulation 77:856, 1988.
27. Newman WP III, Wattigney W, Berenson GS: Autopsy studies in U.S. children and adolescents. Relationship of risk factors to atherosclerotic lesions. Ann N Y Acad Sci 623:16, 1991.
28. Ross R: The pathogenesis of atherosclerosis: A perspective for the 1990's. Nature 362:801, 1993.
29. Goldstein JL, Brown MS: Familial hypercholesterolemia. In Scriver CR, Beaudet AL, Sly WS, et al (eds): The Metabolic Basis of Inherited Disease, 6th ed. New York, McGraw-Hill, 1989, p 1215.
30. Leren TP, Solberg K, Rodningen OK, et al: Two founder mutations in the LDL receptor gene in Norwegian familial hypercholesterolemia subjects. Atherosclerosis 111:175, 1994.
31. Kwiterovich PO Jr: Pediatric implications of heterozygous familial hypercholesterolemia. Screening and dietary treatment. Arteriosclerosis 9(suppl I):I–111, 1989.
32. Kwiterovich PO Jr, Fredrickson DS, Levy RI: Familial hypercholesterolemia (one form of familial type II hyperlipoproteinemia). A study of its biochemical, genetic, and clinical presentation in childhood. J Clin Invest 53:1237, 1974.
33. Sprecher DL, Schaefer EJ, Kent KM, et al: Cardiovascular features of homozygous familial hypercholesterolemia: Analysis of 16 patients. Am J Cardiol 54:20, 1984.
34. Brunzell JD: Familial lipoprotein lipase deficiency and other causes of the chylomicronemia syndrome. In Scriver CR, Beaudet AL, Sly WS, et al (eds): The Metabolic Basis of Inherited Disease, 6th ed. New York, McGraw-Hill, 1989, p 1165.
35. Cox DW, Wills DE, Quan F, Ray PN: A deletion of one nucleotide results in functional deficiency of apolipoprotein CII (apo CII). J Med Genet 25:649, 1988.
36. Mahley RW, Rall SC Jr: Type III hyperlipoproteinemia (dysbeta-lipoproteinemia): Role of apolipoprotein E in normal and abnormal lipoprotein metabolism. In Scriver CR, Beaudet AL, Sly WE, et al (eds): The Metabolic Basis of Inherited Disease, 6th ed. New York, McGraw-Hill, 1989, p 1195.
37. Deckelbaum RJ, Granot E, Oschry Y, et al: Plasma triglyceride determines structure-composition in low and high density lipoproteins. Arteriosclerosis 4:225, 1984.

38. Schaefer EJ: Clinical, biochemical, and genetic features in familial disorders of high density lipoprotein deficiency. Arteriosclerosis 4:303, 1984.

39. Breslow JL: Genetic basis of lipoprotein disorders. J Clin Invest 84:373, 1989.

40. Assman G: Genes and dyslipoproteinaemias. Eur Heart J 11(suppl H):4, 1990.

41. LaRosa JC, Hunninghake D, Bush D, et al: The cholesterol facts. A summary of the evidence relating dietary fats, serum cholesterol, and coronary heart disease. A joint statement by the American Heart Association and the National Heart, Lung, and Blood Institute. Circulation 81:1721, 1990.

42. Stamler J: Lectures on Preventive Cardiology. New York, Grune & Stratton, 1967.

43. Castelli WP, Garrison RJ, Wilson PWF, et al: Incidence of coronary heart disease and lipoprotein cholesterol levels. The Framingham Study. JAMA 256:2835, 1986.

44. Kagan A, McGee DL, Yano K, et al: Serum cholesterol and mortality in a Japanese-American population: The Honolulu Heart Program. Am J Epidemiol 114:11, 1981.

45. Pocock SJ, Shaper AG, Phillips AN, et al: High density lipoprotein cholesterol is not a major risk factor for ischaemic heart disease in British men. Br Med J 292:515, 1986.

46. Kannel WB, Neaton JD, Wentworth D, et al: Overall and coronary heart disease mortality rates in relation to major risk factors in 325,348 men screened for the MRFIT. Am Heart J 112:825, 1986.

47. Stamler J, Wentworth D, Neaton JD: Is relationship between serum cholesterol and risk of premature death from coronary heart disease continuous and graded? Findings in 356,222 primary screens of the Multiple Risk Factor Intervention Trial (MRFIT). JAMA 256:2823, 1986.

48. Multiple Risk Factor Intervention Trial Research Group: Mortality rates after 10.5 years for participants in the Multiple Risk Factor Intervention Trial: Findings related to a priori hypotheses of the trial. JAMA 263:1795, 1990.

49. Martin MJ, Hulley SB, Browner WS, et al: Serum cholesterol, blood pressure, and mortality: Implications from a cohort of 361,662 men. Lancet 2:933, 1986.

50. Davis CE, Rifkind BM, Brenner H, et al: A single cholesterol measurement underestimates the risk for coronary heart disease. An empirical example from the Lipid Research Clinics Mortality Follow-up Study. JAMA 264:3044, 1990.

51. Gordon DJ, Rifkind BM: High-density lipoprotein: The clinical implications of recent studies. N Engl J Med 321:1311, 1989.

52. Knuiman JT, Westenbrink S, van der Heyden L, et al: Determinants of total and high density lipoprotein cholesterol in boys from Finland, the Netherlands, Italy, the Philippines and Ghana with special reference to diet. Hum Nutr Clin Nutr 37:237, 1983.

53. Blackburn H: Diet and atherosclerosis: Epidemiologic evidence and public health implications. Prev Med 12:2, 1983.

54. Knuiman JT, West CE, Katan MB, et al: Total cholesterol and high density lipoprotein cholesterol levels in populations differing in fat and carbohydrate intake. Arteriosclerosis 7:612, 1987.

55. National Health Survey: Total Serum Cholesterol Levels in Children 4–17 Years, United States, 1971–1974. Data from the National Health Survey. Hyattsville, MD, US Department of Health, Education, and Welfare, Public Health Service, National Center for Health Statistics, 1978. DHEW publication PHS 78-1655.

56. National Center for Health Statistics, Carroll MD, Abraham S, et al: Dietary Intake Source Data: United States 1976–80. Vital and Health Statistics. Hyattsville, MD, US Department of Health and Human Services, Public Health Service, National Center for Health Statistics, 1983. DHHS publication PHS 83-1681. Series 11, No. 231.

57. Knuiman JT, Hermus RJJ, Hautvast JGAJ: Serum total and high density lipoprotein (HDL) cholesterol concentrations in rural and urban boys from 16 countries. Atherosclerosis 36:529, 1980.

58. Halfon S-T, Rifkind BM, Harlap S, et al: Plasma lipids and lipoproteins in adult Jews of different origins: The Jerusalem Lipid Research Clinic Prevalence Study. Isr J Med Sci 18:1113, 1982.

59. Taylor CB, Patton DE, Cox GE: Atherosclerosis in rhesus monkeys. VI. Fatal myocardial infarction in a monkey fed fat and cholesterol. Arch Pathol 76:404, 1963.

60. Bullock BC, Lehner NDM, Clarkson TB, et al: Comparative primate atherosclerosis. I. Tissue cholesterol concentration and pathologic anatomy. Exp Mol Pathol 22:151, 1975.

61. Clarkson TB, Bond MG, Bullock BC, et al: A study of atherosclerosis regression in *Macaca mulatta*. IV. Changes in coronary arteries from animals with atherosclerosis induced for 19 months and then regressed for 24 or 48 months at plasma cholesterol concentrations of 300 or 200 mg/dL. Exp Mol Pathol 34:345, 1981.

62. Clarkson TB, Bond MG, Bullock BC, et al: A study of atherosclerosis regression in *Macaca mulatta*. V. Changes in abdominal aorta and carotid and coronary arteries from animals with atherosclerosis induced for 38 months and then regressed for 24 or 48 months at plasma cholesterol concentrations of 300 or 200 mg/dL. Exp Mol Pathol 41:96, 1984.

63. Armstrong ML: Regression of atherosclerosis. Atherosclerosis Rev 1:137, 1976.

64. Malinow MR: Experimental models of atherosclerosis regression. Atherosclerosis 48:105, 1983.

65. Hennekens CH, Jesse MJ, Klein BE, et al: Cholesterol among children of men with myocardial infarction. Pediatrics 58:211, 1976.

66. Schrott HG, Clarke WR, Abrahams P, et al: Coronary artery disease mortality in relatives of hypertriglyceridemic school children: The Muscatine Study. Circulation 65:300, 1982.

67. Moll PP, Sing CF, Weidman WH, et al: Total cholesterol and lipoproteins in school children: Prediction of coronary heart disease in adult relatives. Circulation 67:127, 1983.

68. Lee J, Lauer RM, Clarke WR: Lipoproteins in the progeny of young men with coronary artery disease: Children with increased risk. Pediatrics 78:330, 1986.

69. Clark DA, Allen MF, Wilson FH: Longitudinal study of serum lipids. 12-Year report. Am J Clin Nutr 20:743, 1967.

70. Clarke WR, Schrott HG, Leaverton PE, et al: Tracking of blood lipids and blood pressures in school age children: The Muscatine Study. Circulation 58:626, 1978.

71. Laskarzewski PM, Morrison JA, deGroot I, et al: Lipid and lipoprotein tracking in 108 children over a four-year period. Pediatrics 64:584, 1979.

72. Freedman DS, Shear CL, Srinivasan SR, et al: Tracking of serum lipids and lipoproteins in children over an 8-year period: The Bogalusa Heart Study. Prev Med 14:203, 1985.

73. Lauer RM, Clarke WR: Use of cholesterol measurements in childhood for the prediction of adult hypercholesterolemia: The Muscatine Study. JAMA 264:3034, 1990.

74. Lipid Research Clinics Program: The Lipid Research Clinics Coronary Primary Prevention Trial results. I. Reduction in incidence of coronary heart disease. JAMA 251:351, 1984.

75. Lipid Research Clinics Program: The Lipid Research Clinics Coronary Primary Prevention Trial results. II. The relationship of reduction in incidence of coronary heart disease to cholesterol lowering. JAMA 251:365, 1984.

76. Frick MH, Elo MO, Haapa K, et al: Helsinki Heart Study: Primary-prevention trial with gemfibrozil in middle-aged men with dyslipidemia. Safety of treatment, changes in risk factors, and incidence of coronary heart disease. N Engl J Med 317:1237, 1987.

77. Canner PL, Berge KG, Wenger NK, et al: Fifteen year mortality in Coronary Drug Project patients: Long-term benefit with niacin. J Am Coll Cardiol 8:1245, 1986.

78. Carlson LA, Rosenhamer G: Reduction of mortality in the Stockholm Ischaemic Heart Disease Secondary Prevention Study by combined treatment with clofibrate and nicotinic acid. Acta Med Scand 223:405, 1988.

79. Brensike JF, Levy RI, Kelsey SF, et al: Effects of therapy with cholestyramine on progression of coronary arteriosclerosis: Results of the NHLBI Type II Coronary Intervention Study. Circulation 69:313, 1984.

80. Blankenhorn DH, Nessim SA, Johnson RL, et al: Beneficial effects of combined colestipol-niacin therapy on coronary atherosclerosis and coronary venous bypass grafts. JAMA 257:3233, 1987.

81. Buchwald H, Varco RL, Matts JP, et al: Effect of partial ileal bypass surgery on mortality and morbidity from coronary heart disease in patients with hypercholesterolemia. Report of the Program on the Surgical Control of the Hyperlipidemias (POSCH). N Engl J Med 323:946, 1990.

82. Brown G, Albers JJ, Fisher LD, et al: Regression of coronary artery disease as a result of intensive lipid-lowering therapy in men with high levels of apolipoprotein B. N Engl J Med 323:1289, 1990.

83. Kane JP, Malloy MJ, Ports TA, et al: Regression of coronary atherosclerosis during treatment of familial hypercholesterolemia with combined drug regimens. JAMA 264:3007, 1990.

84. Ornish D, Brown SE, Scherwitz LW, et al: Can lifestyle changes reverse coronary heart disease? The Lifestyle Heart Trial. Lancet 336:129, 1990.

85. Rose G: Sick individuals and sick populations. Int J Epidemiol 14:32, 1985.

86. Nationwide Food Consumptive Survey. Continuing survey of food intakes by individuals: Women 19–50 years and their children 1–5 years. Hyattsville, MD, US Department of Agriculture, Human Nutrition Information Service, Nutrition Monitoring Division, 1985. NFCS, CSFII Report No. 85–1.

87. Nationwide Food Consumption Survey Continuing Survey of Food Intakes by Individuals: Men 19–50 Years. Hyattsville, MD, US Department of Agriculture, Human Nutrition Information Service, Nutrition Monitoring Division, 1985. NFCS, CSFII Report No. 85-3.

88. McDowell MA, Briefel RR, Alairno K, et al: Energy and Macronutrient Intakes of Persons Ages 2 months and Over in the United States: Third National Health and Nutrition Examination Survey, Phase 1, 1988–91. Washington, DC, US Department of Health and Human Services, Public Health Service, Centers for Disease Control and Prevention, National Center for Health Statistics, 1994. No. 255.

89. Fats and Oils in Human Nutrition: Report of a Joint Expert Consultation. Rome, World Health Organization/Food and Agriculture Organization of the United Nations, 1994. Paper 57.

90. DISC Collaborative Research Group (Lauer RM, chairman): The efficacy and safety of lowering dietary intake of total fat, saturated fat, and cholesterol in children with elevated LDL-cholesterol: The Dietary Intervention Study in Children (DISC). JAMA 273:1429, 1995.

91. Eck LH, Klesges RC, Hanson CL: Recall of a child's intake from meals: Are parents accurate? J Am Diet Assoc 89:784, 1989.

92. National Cholesterol Education Program: Report of the Expert Panel on Blood Cholesterol Levels in Children and Adolescents. Pediatrics 89:525, 1992.

93. Ose L, Tonstad S: The detection and management of dyslipidemia in children and adolescents. Acta Paediatr 84:1213, 1995.

94. Lambert M, Lupien PJ, Gagne C, et al: Treatment of familial hypercholesterolemia in children and adolescents: Effect of lovastatin. Canadian Lovastatin in Children Study Group. Pediatrics 97:619, 1996.

95. Ducobu J, Brasseur D, Chaudron JM, et al: Simvistatin use in children. Lancet 339:1488, 1992.

96. Sinzinger H, Schmid P, Pirich CH, et al: Treatment of hypercholesterolemia in children. Lancet 340:548, 1992.

97. Hanna EZ, Chow SP, Grant BF: The relationship between drinking and heart disease morbidity in the US: Results of the National Health Interview Survey. Alcohol Clin Exp Res 21:111, 1997.

98. Pate RR, Pratt M, Blair SN, et al: Physical activity and public health: A recommendation from the Centers for Disease Control and Prevention and the American College of Sports Medicine. JAMA 273:402, 1995.

CHAPTER 53

HYPERTENSION IN CHILDREN AND ADOLESCENTS

BONITA FALKNER   ROBERT H. SADOWSKI

Hypertension is an important clinical problem that can occur during childhood, from infancy through adolescence. Abnormal elevation of blood pressure during childhood is a clinical sign that may indicate an underlying cardiovascular, endocrine, or renal disorder. High blood pressure in these situations is considered secondary hypertension. Abnormal elevation of blood pressure may also be regarded as a disease, termed essential or primary hypertension. Essential hypertension had generally been considered to be a problem of adults. As more clinical and epidemiologic knowledge has developed, the perspective on the origin and expression of primary hypertension has shifted, with more attention directed toward the young. Whether hypertension is detected in childhood or later adulthood, the consequences of sustained blood pressure elevation render hypertension a significant health problem both for populations from a public health perspective and for an individual patient.

BACKGROUND AND DEFINITION OF HYPERTENSION IN THE YOUNG

Before 1977, hypertension was not considered a problem relevant to the pediatric population, except in rare patients with extreme elevations of blood pressure. Blood pressure measurement was not a part of the routine pediatric examination. In the absence of routine measurement of blood pressure in children, there was neither understanding of the normal range of blood pressure in the young nor standard measurement methodology. In lieu of definitive criteria, the adult standard of 140/90 mm Hg was also applied to children. Children who were detected with this degree of blood pressure elevation were usually symptomatic and had, by current standards, severe hypertension. A National Task Force was established by the National Heart, Lung, and Blood Institute and was charged with evaluating the available data on blood pressure in children. Their report,[1] based on an examination of data from about 5000 children, was published in 1977 and provided the first set of normative values for blood pressure in children aged 4 through 18 years. The blood pressure distribution curves in a population of healthy children demonstrated a progressive rise in the blood pressure level with increasing age throughout childhood. These data made it clear that the normal range of blood pressure in children was well below the standard adult level of 140/90 mm Hg. By use of the 95th percentile for age and sex as the level to define higher than normal blood pressure, a more appropriate definition of hypertension during childhood began to emerge. The Task Force report provided guidelines for methods to measure blood pressure in young children, with attention to cuff size. The report also provided recommendations for evaluating children detected with hypertension, defined as blood pressure consistently greater than the 95th percentile for age and sex.

During the following decade, several epidemiologic studies provided additional data with regard to childhood blood pressure. A Second Task Force examined data from a much larger population of more than 70,000 healthy children that included African Americans, Mexican Americans, and whites. The 1987 report[2] presented more refined blood pressure distribution curves from birth through 18 years of age. These curves gave a clear view of the normal range of blood pressure throughout childhood. The data verified the normal rise in blood pressure that accompanies growth. These data substantiated a definition of normal blood pressure as blood pressure level below the 90th percentile for age and sex, of high blood pressure as blood pressure level greater than the 95th percentile for age and sex. Blood pressure levels between the 90th and 95th percentiles were termed high-normal. Analysis of the larger data in the second report suggested that children having blood pressure consistently at the higher portion of the normal distribution may be at risk for hypertension.

This Second Task Force report also recommended that measurement of blood pressure be a routine part of well-child care. Beginning at the age of 3 years, all children should have blood pressure, as well as height and weight, measured during regular health assessments. Also, regardless of age, all sick children and adolescents should have their blood pressure measured. This practice has generally been adopted by health care providers. Regular blood pressure measurement in the young adds to our understanding that the risk for primary hypertension can be detected in the young.

The national blood pressure data in childhood were reexamined by a Third Task Force, and additional refinement of the blood pressure distribution curves was presented in a 1996 report.[3] With expansion of the available epidemiologic data and reanalysis of these data, it became apparent that the strongest correlate of blood pressure in children and adolescents is height. Children of a given age have a broad variation in height, so that accurate assessment of blood pressure in a child requires adjustment for height as well as for age and sex. Therefore, the current reference values for blood pressure level in childhood are provided for age, sex, and height. Figure 53–1 provides the

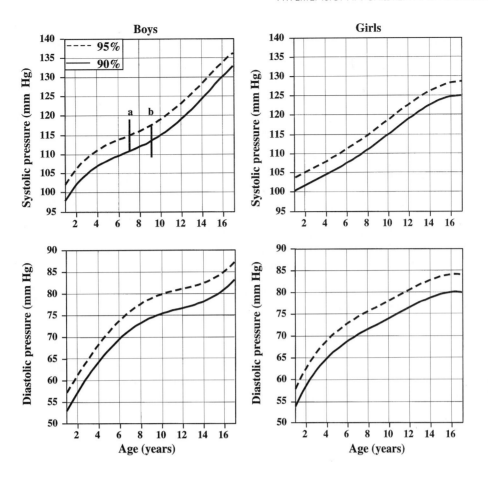

FIGURE 53–1

The 90th and 95th percentiles for systolic and diastolic blood pressure are shown for boys and girls aged 1 to 17 years who are at the 50th percentile for height.

For systolic pressures in boys, pressures for the 95th and 5th height percentiles are respectively 4 mm Hg above and below pressures for the 50th height percentile.

For diastolic pressures in boys, pressures for the 95th and 5th height percentiles are respectively 2 mm Hg above and below pressures for the 50th height percentile.

For systolic pressures in girls, pressures for the 95th and 5th heigth percentiles are respectively 3 mm Hg above and below pressures for the 50th height percentile.

For diastolic pressures in girls, pressures for the 95th and 5th height percentiles are respectively 2 to 3 mm Hg above and 1 to 2 mm Hg below pressures for the 50th height percentile.

If a 9-year-old boy has a systolic pressure of 113 mm Hg, that is the 90th pressure percentile if he is at the 50th percentile for height, but at the 95th pressure percentile if he is at the 5th percentile for height (upper end of line *b*) and below the 90th pressure percentile if he is at the 95th percentile for height (lower end of line *b*). A 7-year-old boy with a systolic pressure of 115 mm Hg is at the 95th pressure percentile if his height percentile is the 50th, but only at the 90th pressure percentile if he is at the 95th percentile for height (lower end of line *a*) and above the 95th pressure percentile if he is at the 5th percentile for height (upper end of line *a*).

For girls, systolic pressures can be interpreted in almost the same way. For diastolic pressures, the effects of height are not large enough to change pressures from the 90th to the 95th percentile or vice versa.

(From Zubrow AB, Hulman S, Kushner H, Falkner B: Determinants of blood pressure in infants admitted to neonatal intensive care units: A prospective multicenter study. J Perinatol 15:470, 1995.)

blood pressure levels at the 90th and 95th percentiles for boys and girls according to age and height percentile. These reference values for blood pressure in the young prevent misclassification of tall children as hypertensive and prevent missing detection of high blood pressure in short children.

The reference values are used in the following way. First, the child's height is measured and plotted on standard growth curves. The appropriate height percentile for age and sex is determined. The child's blood pressure is measured by methods appropriate for children (see later). The child's systolic blood pressure and diastolic blood pressure are compared with the reference blood pressure levels according to the child's sex, age, and height percentile. The child is normotensive if both systolic and diastolic blood pressures are less than the 90th percentile. If either systolic or diastolic blood pressure is above the 95th percentile, the child may be hypertensive. If either systolic or diastolic blood pressure is between the 90th and 95th percentiles, the child has high-normal blood pressure. For example, a 7-year-old girl whose height is 47.6 inches (121 cm) is at the 50th percentile for height on the standard pediatric growth chart. For her age and height, the 90th percentile for systolic blood pressure is 111 mm Hg, and the

95th percentile is 115 mm Hg (see Fig. 53–1); the 90th percentile for diastolic blood pressure is 71 mm Hg, and the 95th percentile is 75 mm Hg. If her measured blood pressure is 118/68 mm Hg, she could be hypertensive. However, a single measurement of blood pressure in the elevated range is not sufficient to diagnose hypertension in childhood. Unless the blood pressure is extremely elevated or the child is symptomatic, multiple measurements of blood pressure on several occasions are necessary to verify a diagnosis of hypertension.

Measurement of diastolic blood pressure in children is sometimes difficult. The determination of diastolic blood pressure depends on which Korotkoff sound is considered the most accurate estimate of diastolic blood pressure. The fourth Korotkoff sound (K4) is defined as the muffling of the auscultated pulsation; the fifth Korotkoff sound (K5) is defined as the disappearance of the auscultated pulsation. In adults, K5 is used to determine the diastolic blood pressure. However, in younger children, there may be a wide gap between K4, the muffling of the Korotkoff sounds, and K5, the disappearance of the Korotkoff sounds. In some children, K5 may be heard to nearly 0 mm Hg. Because of the large difference between K4 and K5 in some children, K4 had been the recommended measure of diastolic blood pressure in children younger than 13 years, and K5 had been the recommended measure of diastolic blood pressure in adolescents age 13 years and older. In the Task Force report, however, K5 was recommended as the measure of diastolic blood pressure. The available data were considered sufficient to derive accurate blood pressure distribution based on K5 for diastolic blood pressure. In measurement of blood pressure, K5 is more easily distinguishable than is K4. In children who do have a large difference between K4 and K5, elevated diastolic blood pressure is rarely an issue. Therefore, to detect elevated diastolic blood pressure, K5 is regarded as an accurate measure of diastolic blood pressure in children as well as in adolescents and adults. More clinical observation and prospective data are necessary to decide whether K4 or K5 is a more reliable predictor of risk for future hypertension.

NEWBORN BLOOD PRESSURE

There are limited data on blood pressure in neonates. Early reports that examined the level of blood pressure in neonates were based on single measurements of blood pressure.[4–6] A few reports that described the relationship of blood pressure with birth weight in large numbers of infants[7,8] indicated a direct relationship between blood pressure and birth weight. These reports, however, showed wide variability in the data. Hulman and colleagues[9] examined blood pressure in healthy neonates on the day of birth and repeatedly on consecutive days in the nursery. There was a rapid and consistent increase in blood pressure during the first 5 days of life, which reflects a hemodynamic transition from intrauterine to extrauterine life. These observations were replicated in a larger study of newborn infants including a broad range of birth weight and gestational age.[10]

There is a direct relationship of blood pressure with both birth weight and gestational age at birth. In all infants, regardless of birth weight or gestational age at birth,

there is a transition, reflected by an increase in blood pressure, lasting 5 days. Subsequently, there is a direct relationship of blood pressure with weight or gestational age. Figure 53–2 provides the mean systolic blood pressure level with the 95% confidence bands for infants in the neonatal period, according to their postconceptional age (gestational age plus chronologic age in weeks). This figure is a useful reference in evaluating blood pressure in the neonatal period.

MEASUREMENT TECHNIQUE

Figure 53–1 provides reference blood pressure levels on which determination is made of normotension, high-normal blood pressure, and hypertension in children and adolescents. Use of these reference values depends on measurement of blood pressure by a standardized method.

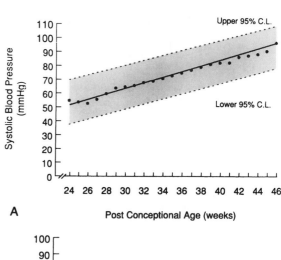

A

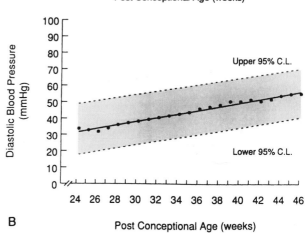

B

FIGURE 53–2

Postconceptional age (gestational age in weeks + weeks after delivery) is computed daily for each infant (8566 daily records) and regressed against mean systolic blood pressure (A) and diastolic blood pressure (B) for that day. Regression lines and equations are presented in terms of postconceptional weeks, which is more useful clinically. Regression equations are systolic blood pressure = (0.255 · postconceptional age in weeks · 7) + 6.34, r = 0.61, P < .0001, and diastolic blood pressure = (0.151 · postconceptional age in weeks · 7) + 3.32, r = 0.46, P < .0001. Observed means of systolic blood pressure and diastolic blood pressure for each postconceptional week are also plotted. C.L. = confidence limits. (A, B from Zubrow AB, Hulman S, Kushner H, Falkner B: Determinants of blood pressure in infants admitted to neonatal intensive care units: A prospective multicenter study. J Perinatol 15:470, 1995.)

The values are based on blood pressure measurements obtained by auscultation with an inflatable blood pressure cuff. This method is recommended for screening and standard office measurement of blood pressure. Similar tables based on oscillometric or other instrumentation for blood pressure measurement are unavailable because of insufficient data. The auscultatory method for measuring blood pressure is also recommended because the instruments for measurement are inexpensive and easily available. The automated instruments have appropriate clinical use in hospital settings, in critical care units, and for neonates, in whom the measurement of blood pressure by auscultation is particularly difficult.

Blood pressure should be measured in a calm and controlled environment after the patient has been seated for 3 to 5 minutes. Ideally, the blood pressure should be measured twice and the average of the values used to estimate the blood pressure level.[3] With the patient seated and the right arm at the level of the heart, the stethoscope is placed over the brachial artery, approximately 2 cm superior to the cubital fossa and just inferior to the cuff. The cuff used for a patient must be appropriately sized. In fact, most errors in measurement occur because the blood pressure cuff used is not appropriately sized for the individual patient. The cuff name (e.g., "infant," "child") may not correctly designate the appropriate cuff for a child of the designated age range. The bladder, not the cloth covering, is the key determinant of correct size. For each child, the bladder width of the cuff should be approximately 40% of the arm circumference midway between the olecranon and the acromion. This size of cuff bladder will cover 80 to 100% of the circumference of the arm. This ensures that the brachial artery is completely compressed during inflation, and it avoids premature blood flow through the artery during deflation of the bladder.[3] A cuff that is too small for a patient will result in falsely elevated readings; however, a cuff that appears somewhat large for a patient will not obscure elevated values.[2] Most errors in blood pressure measurement occur in obese patients or fully muscular adolescent boys when too small a cuff is used. Oversized adult cuffs may be necessary in obese or large muscular adolescents. Careful attention to correct cuff size is key to accurate assessment of blood pressure in children and adolescents.

SECONDARY HYPERTENSION IN CHILDHOOD

The prevalence of secondary forms of hypertension is greater during childhood than in any other period of life. In one report about hypertensive children younger than 10 years, 90% had identifiable or secondary causes, and only 10% were attributed to essential hypertension.[11] In contrast, in another series that included both children and adolescents, the prevalence of secondary hypertension in the adolescents was 65%, that of essential hypertension 35%.[12] Thus, secondary causes of hypertension predominate during childhood, and the expression of essential hypertension increases with age.

Although a younger age at the time of detection should raise the suspicion of a secondary cause of hypertension, the degree of elevation of the blood pressure is also important. Table 53–1 provides estimates of blood pressure lev-

TABLE 53–1

CLASSIFICATION OF HYPERTENSION BY AGE GROUP

Age Group	Significant Hypertension (mm Hg)	Severe Hypertension (mm Hg)
Newborn		
7 days	Systolic BP ≥96	Systolic BP ≥106
8–30 days	Systolic BP ≥104	Systolic BP ≥110
Infant	Systolic BP ≥112	Systolic BP ≥118
(<2 yr)	Diastolic BP ≥74	Diastolic BP ≥82
Children	Systolic BP ≥116	Systolic BP ≥124
(3–5 yr)	Diastolic BP ≥76	Diastolic BP ≥84
Children	Systolic BP ≥122	Systolic BP ≥130
(6–9 yr)	Diastolic BP ≥78	Diastolic BP ≥86
Children	Systolic BP ≥126	Systolic BP ≥134
(10–12 yr)	Diastolic BP ≥82	Diastolic BP ≥90
Adolescents	Systolic BP ≥136	Systolic BP ≥144
(13–15 yr)	Diastolic BP ≥86	Diastolic BP ≥92
Adolescents	Systolic BP ≥142	Systolic BP ≥150
(16–18 yr)	Diastolic BP ≥92	Diastolic BP ≥98

BP = blood pressure.
From Task Force on Blood Pressure Control in Children: Report of the Second Task Force on Blood Pressure Control in Children, 1987. Pediatrics 79:1, 1987. Used with permission of the American Academy of Pediatrics.

els considered to indicate significant and severe hypertension in children of different ages.[2] When significant or severe hypertension is documented in childhood, a secondary cause should be strongly considered. For example, a 4-year-old with a blood pressure of 126/84 has severe hypertension and requires a careful evaluation to uncover a probable secondary etiology. A general rule to guide the evaluation of high blood pressure in the pediatric population is that the higher the blood pressure and the younger the child, the more likely a secondary cause is responsible.[2]

Unlike in adults, for whom endocrine and renovascular disorders predominate as secondary causes, the dominant cause of secondary hypertension in children is renal disease. Although renovascular, cardiovascular, endocrine, neurogenic, and pharmacologic abnormalities do cause hypertension in children, these categories account for far fewer subjects. Some of the more common causes of secondary hypertension in the pediatric population are shown in Table 53–2. Although many pathologic states have been associated with hypertension in childhood, most can be attributed to renal disease.

Moreover, within the pediatric age range, certain causes of hypertension are typically seen at particular ages. Knowing which causes of hypertension predominate at various ages can therefore aid in constructing a differential diagnosis and focus an evaluation.

Infants

Although hypertension is uncommon in the neonatal period, certain infants are at increased risk for hypertension. For example, newborn infants with a history of umbilical artery catheterization are at risk for thromboembolic events, leading to abnormalities in renal blood flow, sometimes acute renal failure, and resultant hypertension.[13,14] Those who have developed bronchopulmonary dysplasia may also develop hypertension, sometimes related to steroid use and sodium retention.[15]

TABLE 53–2

ACUTE AND CHRONIC CAUSES OF HYPERTENSION

Cause	Acute Hypertension	Chronic Hypertension	
Renal	Postinfectious glomerulonephritis Schönlein-Henoch purpura Hemolytic-uremic syndrome Acute tubular necrosis	Focal segmental glomerulosclerosis Chronic glomerulonephritis Crescentic glomerulonephritis Collagen vascular diseases Alport's syndrome Reflux nephropathy	IgA nephropathy Interstitial nephritis Polycystic kidney disease Medullary cystic disease Hydronephrosis Hypoplastic kidney
Endocrine		Pheochromocytoma Primary aldosteronism	Hyperthyroidism (systolic)
Vascular	Renal or renovascular trauma	Coarctation of the aorta Renal artery stenosis Takayasu's arteritis	Arteriovenous fistula Tuberous sclerosis
Neurogenic	Increased intracranial pressure Guillain-Barré syndrome	Dysautonomia	
Drugs	Cocaine Phencyclidine amphetamines Jimsonweed	Nonsteroidal anti-inflammatory drugs Corticosteroids Alcohol Appetite suppressants	Anabolic steroids Oral contraceptives Nicotine
Miscellaneous	Burns Orthopedic surgery Urologic surgery	Heavy metal poisoning	
Syndromes		Williams' (renovascular lesions) Turner's (coarctation or renovascular) Tuberous sclerosis (cystic renal) Neurofibromatosis (renovascular) Adrenogenital	

In general, the most frequent detectable causes of neonatal hypertension include renal artery stenosis, renal artery thrombosis, congenital renal malformations, coarctation of the aorta, and bronchopulmonary dysplasia.[2] In some neonates with hypertension, however, the diagnostic evaluation fails to identify a cause. Nevertheless, these infants require blood pressure control and monitoring.

Children

From infancy to 6 years of age, renal parenchymal diseases, coarctation of the aorta, and renal artery stenosis are the most frequent diagnoses. From 6 to 10 years of age, renal artery stenosis and renal parenchymal diseases are the most common causes of elevated diastolic pressure. Essential hypertension, causing milder elevations in blood pressure, also begins to occur in this age range.

During childhood, an acute elevation in blood pressure can also be seen with renal diseases such as hemolytic-uremic syndrome and acute postinfectious glomerulonephritis. These acute elevations may require prompt intervention and in-hospital management. Some conditions can also cause permanent renal dysfunction, resulting in chronic hypertension.

Adolescents

In adolescents, renal parenchymal diseases are the leading cause of hypertension. The other major cause of hypertension during the teenage years is essential hypertension. The renal diseases during adolescence are varied. More chronic diseases, such as chronic pyelonephritis, reflux nephropathy, and focal segmental glomerulosclerosis, may manifest during adolescence. Renal disease associated with systemic illnesses, such as systemic lupus erythematosus, may also occur during these years.

There are other important aggravating, if not causative, factors related to hypertension in adolescents. Any form of nicotine, whether cigarette smoking or smokeless tobacco,[16,17] may contribute to elevated blood pressure. Illicit substance use, especially cocaine and amphetamine-related compounds, may also cause hypertension. To achieve rapid increases in muscle strength and bulk, some teenage athletes use anabolic steroids, which commonly result in blood pressure elevation.[18] Other substances associated with hypertension in adolescents include appetite suppressants (both over-the-counter and prescription), oral contraceptive pills, and ethanol when it is used excessively.

One often-missed diagnosis in children and adolescents is coarctation of the aorta. In a retrospective review of coarctation diagnosed in children older than 1 year,[19] specific diagnosis was made before referral to a pediatric cardiologist in only 2 of 50 patients (4%). In these patients, whose mean age at the time of diagnosis was 8.4 years, the most consistent physical examination findings were a murmur and a systolic blood pressure gradient of more than 10 mm Hg between the arms and legs. Ninety-four percent of the children had systolic blood pressure in an upper extremity that was greater than the 95th percentile. Lower extremity pulses were absent in only 9 of 50 (18%). Had the absence of lower extremity pulses been used as the sole criterion for diagnosis, 82% of the children would have been missed. Ing and associates[19] concluded that an arm-to-leg blood pressure differential is the most reliable and specific physical examination sign of coarctation of the aorta. The results of this review, as well as of previous ones,[20,21] indicate that child health providers may be missing coarctation during infancy and early childhood. This is especially of concern because early childhood repair of coarctation has been associated with an improved long-term outcome.

ESSENTIAL HYPERTENSION IN CHILDREN AND ADOLESCENTS

Essential hypertension of adulthood has its roots in childhood. This concept has been inferred from blood pressure tracking studies,[22–28] which suggest that children with elevated blood pressure will continue to have elevated blood pressure as adults. Therefore, an important aspect of blood pressure surveillance in the young is to distinguish whether elevated blood pressure signals an underlying disease, as a form of secondary hypertension, or is an early expression of primary or essential hypertension.

Children and adolescents with essential hypertension generally demonstrate several clinical characteristics or risk factors associated with the elevated blood pressure. The degree of blood pressure elevation is generally mild, approximating the 95th percentile. The blood pressure levels obtained on repeated measurements often exhibit considerable variability over time. Thus, on one occasion, the systolic or diastolic blood pressure may be at or above the 95th percentile. On a repeated measurement a few months later, the blood pressure may be at or just below the 90th percentile. Several laboratory and observational studies have also demonstrated marked cardiovascular responses to stress, including heightened heart rate and blood pressure responses to stimuli.[29–32] A consistent clinical observation in children exhibiting mild essential hypertension is a strong family history of hypertension. A history of hypertension in parents or grandparents is almost always detected in these children.[23,33,34]

In both children and adults, body weight and increases in body weight correlate with blood pressure.[35,36] Essential hypertension in children is frequently associated with obesity. The obesity appears to contribute to the elevation in blood pressure because even a modest reduction in excess adiposity in these children is accompanied by a reduction in blood pressure.[37,38] The cluster of mild blood pressure elevation, a family history of hypertension, and obesity is a typical pattern in children and adolescents having essential hypertension. Obesity is not always present, particularly in adolescent boys expressing mild blood pressure elevation and a family history of hypertension. These children and adolescents should be considered at risk for development of chronic hypertension and may benefit from lifestyle changes to reduce their cardiovascular risk.

During the past two decades, the literature on hypertension and cardiovascular disease in adults has focused on the overlap of hypertension, non–insulin-dependent diabetes mellitus, atherosclerosis, and obesity. This constellation within individuals and within populations has been described as the insulin resistance syndrome.[39–41] The metabolic aspect of the syndrome is a tissue resistance to the glucose-regulatory action of insulin. To achieve metabolic control of glucose, greater amounts of insulin are required, and relative hyperinsulinemia results. Theoretical explanations to link insulin resistance with high blood pres-

sure include the effect of insulin on sodium transport, on the sympathetic nervous system, and on vascular growth factors. Hyperinsulinemia may also have an effect on lipoprotein metabolism, resulting in elevations in low-density lipoproteins and reductions in high-density lipoproteins in the plasma. Children as well as adults may express characteristics of the insulin resistance syndrome.[38,42,43] Some investigators have detected the insulin resistance syndrome in nonobese offspring of hypertensive parents,[44,45] indicating a hereditary component to the syndrome. The characteristics of the insulin resistance syndrome are also congruent with the overweight child's having a strong family history of hypertension or early heart disease. These children often have higher than normal plasma lipid levels. Although these children are not at risk for immediate adverse effects of the higher than normal blood pressure, they should be considered at risk for future cardiovascular disease. Efforts to control excess adiposity, modify diet, and increase physical activity are likely to benefit these children. These health behaviors improve insulin action.

The cause of essential hypertension is believed to be multifactorial and the outcome of an interplay of genetic and environmental factors. In the past decade, a number of reports have proposed another possible contributing cause to later hypertension and cardiac disease in adulthood. This concept is based on an association of hypertension and ischemic heart disease in adults with a lower recorded birth weight. It has been proposed that lower birth weight, within the normal range of birth weights and gestational ages, reflects alteration in the intrauterine nutritional environment. The impairment in optimal fetal growth effects an alteration in organ structure and an impairment in organ function in later life.[46,47] Higher blood pressure is considered to be the link between compromised intrauterine growth and the long-term risk for cardiovascular disease.[46] Despite the reports, based on retrospective data, that support the low birth weight–high blood pressure hypothesis,[46–49] this concept is in conflict with the body of data in childhood as well as in adulthood that consistently demonstrates a direct relationship between body weight and blood pressure.[22,50,51] Furthermore, the observation of blood pressure tracking in childhood[22,24,27,28] is in conflict with the low birth weight–high blood pressure hypothesis. Despite the appeal of this novel concept, investigations are necessary to obtain prospective data and rigorously examine the relationship of intrauterine nutritional environment and fetal growth effect on blood pressure with the risk for cardiovascular disease in later life.

At present, the prevalence of childhood obesity is increasing.[52] Obesity does have an adverse effect on risk for cardiovascular disease and warrants attention for prevention and health promotion.

EVALUATION OF HYPERTENSION IN CHILDREN AND ADOLESCENTS

Once sustained hypertension in a child is established by several elevated blood pressure measurements, decisions must be made regarding the extent of further evaluation. The evaluation is usually dictated by the type of hypertension the patient is considered to have. In general, when a secondary cause is suspected, an extensive, comprehensive array of studies may be necessary. On the other hand, when the patient's elevated blood pressure is more likely to be an early expression of essential hypertension, a few screening studies may be sufficient. The key, then, is to determine whether the characteristics of a patient's presentation indicate essential hypertension or reflect a secondary, potentially correctable cause.

Children in whom a secondary cause of hypertension is possible often have certain characteristics. Specifically, children with significant or severe hypertension (see Table 53–1) generally have an identifiable underlying cause. As noted before, the higher the blood pressure and the younger the child, the more likely a secondary cause is present. A 2-month-old infant with a blood pressure of 120/82, for example, has severe hypertension, probably resulting from a secondary cause, and requires a thorough evaluation to identify the etiology of the hypertension. On the other hand, a 12-year-old with the same blood pressure of 120/82 has, depending on his or her height percentile, mild elevation in blood pressure and is less likely to have a secondary cause.

In addition, a particular symptom complex revealed in the history should also prompt a thorough investigation for physical abnormalities. In these patients, the nature and direction of the evaluation are dictated by the particular symptom complex or physical examination findings. For instance, a 16-year-old girl with declining school performance, weight loss, tachycardia, emotional lability, and a "fullness" of her thyroid requires a focused evaluation for hyperthyroidism. Any pediatric patient who is hypertensive and is not growing normally should also undergo an evaluation for secondary causes. Although it is often difficult to determine the precise onset of hypertension from the history, the sudden onset of elevated blood pressure in a previously normotensive child should always prompt a search for secondary causes. Further, evidence of target organ injury implies a level of severity or chronicity of hypertension that mandates a survey for secondary causes. When no family history of hypertension exists, the likelihood of the child's having essential hypertension decreases. Absence of a family history of hypertension should increase the level of suspicion for an underlying disorder and widen the extent of the evaluation.

In contrast, another set of findings tends to characterize children and adolescents with essential hypertension. These characteristics include slight to mild elevations in blood pressure, a strong family history of essential hypertension, elevated resting heart rate, variable blood pressure readings on repeated measurement, and obesity. Clusters of these characteristics often help to identify children with essential hypertension. If no other abnormalities are found on history or physical examination, these children and adolescents require less extensive evaluations than do those in whom secondary causes are suspected. For example, an obese 15-year-old girl with a blood pressure of 148/96 mm Hg, two parents with primary hypertension, and no additional findings on history or physical examination usually will not require invasive studies or an extensive evaluation. However, a slender 8-year-old girl with a blood pressure of 148/96 mm Hg (see Table 53–1) and no family history of hypertension requires a thorough evaluation for secondary causes. Although the focus of follow-up is different, both children require monitoring and management to control blood pressure. The 15-year-old requires few diagnostic studies. On the other hand, the 8-year-old requires careful examination and diagnostic studies to determine an etiology.

MEDICAL HISTORY

The major thrust of the history and physical examination is detection of clues that suggest that the elevated blood pressure may be secondary or essential. Because certain diseases present more acutely and others are chronic in onset, it is also helpful to determine whether the hypertension is long-standing or of acute onset. The information obtained from the medical history and physical examination assists in determining the extent and direction of the evaluation.

The family history is particularly important. In both first- and second-degree relatives, a history of essential hypertension, myocardial infarction, stroke, renal disease, diabetes, and obesity should be obtained. It is particularly relevant for a hypertensive child of relatives who had an onset at an early age of any of these conditions. For instance, if parents had early-onset coronary artery disease, their children may be at high risk for lipid abnormalities. Parents should also be asked about conditions in family members that are inheritable and have hypertension as a component (e.g., polycystic kidney disease, neurofibromatosis, pheochromocytoma). Another recently recognized familial type of hypertension is glucocorticoid-remediable aldosteronism, an autosomal dominant condition, which should be considered when multiple family members have early-onset hypertension associated with hypokalemia or stroke.[53,54]

Details regarding the child's hospitalizations and operations should be obtained. In younger children with hypertension, the neonatal history is especially important. A history of prolonged mechanical ventilation or umbilical artery catheterization may suggest bronchopulmonary dysplasia or a thromboembolic complication, respectively. A history of urinary tract infections is important because there may be associated reflux nephropathy, renal scarring, and resultant hypertension.

A history of medication use can be helpful. Patients may not consider over-the-counter preparations as medications and therefore need to be specifically asked. The most commonly misused products are cold preparations containing pseudoephedrine or phenylpropanolamine.[55,56] Adolescents need to be discreetly questioned about the use of "street" drugs, smokeless tobacco, oral contraceptive pills, cigarette smoking, diet aids, ethanol, and anabolic steroids. It may also be helpful to gather information about the patient's usual diet, level of activity, and lifestyle.

The review of systems should be directed at uncovering chronic symptoms and establishing whether any symptoms associated with hypertension-causing diseases are present. For example, the complex of headaches, palpitations, weight loss, and excessive sweating suggests pheochromocytoma.

PHYSICAL EXAMINATION

The physical examination for a hypertensive child should be comprehensive. Special mention is made of several key points.

The correct technique in taking the blood pressure is essential. Particular attention should be paid to using the correct cuff size. On the basis of the height percentile, the systolic and diastolic blood pressure percentiles are determined from Figure 53–1. To determine whether a child is underweight or overweight, the child's weight and accompanying percentile ranking for age are compared with his or her height percentile.

To rule out coarctation of the aorta, evaluation of every child for hypertension should include upper and lower extremity blood pressure measurements taken with appropriately sized cuffs. For example, the cuffs appropriate for thigh measurements in adolescents or overweight children often need to be large and oversized. The leg blood pressure levels are normally slightly higher than the arm blood pressure levels. A child with coarctation will have systolic hypertension in an upper extremity, sometimes absent or decreased femoral or other lower extremity pulses, and, more reliably, a blood pressure differential greater than 10 mm Hg between the upper and lower extremities.[19] In older infants and children, extensive collateral circulation may have developed so that femoral pulses are still easily palpated. During simultaneous palpation of the radial and femoral pulses, however, a delay in the femoral pulse timing can sometimes be detected.[21]

An assessment of the child's general growth rate and pattern should be made. A decrease in the weight or height percentile may indicate a more chronic or insidious disease process associated with hypertension. Abnormalities in growth that are associated with hypertension can be seen with chronic renal disease, hyperthyroidism (causing primarily systolic hypertension), pheochromocytoma, adrenal disorders, and certain genetic abnormalities such as Turner's syndrome.

Finally, clues on physical examination that might suggest a particular secondary etiology should be sought. On physical examination, the cause of the hypertension should be looked for by body region.[57] For instance, abnormal facies or dysmorphic features may suggest a syndrome. Some syndromes are linked with specific lesions causing hypertension; for example, both Turner's and Williams' syndromes are associated with renovascular or cardiac lesions that cause hypertension. A retinal examination should be performed to determine the presence of hypertensive vessel injury. Auscultation of the abdomen should also be performed because renal vascular lesions may sometimes have an audible abdominal bruit. Skin lesions are sometimes the first manifestations of disorders such as tuberous sclerosis and systemic lupus erythematosus.

DIAGNOSTIC TESTING

If the history and physical examination provide clues for a specific underlying cause of the hypertension, such as an endocrine or cardiac disorder, the testing should be directed to the area of clinical suspicion. Other important historical information, such as a history of urinary tract infections, might dictate studies to evaluate vesicoureteral reflux and renal scarring.

In the absence of clues, renal parenchymal disease should be considered a likely etiology because this is the most frequent cause of secondary hypertension in the pediatric population. The initial evaluation of children with possible secondary hypertension should therefore include a screen for renal abnormalities. This screen should include a full urinalysis, electrolyte determinations, creatinine concentration, complete blood count, urine culture, and renal ultrasound examination.

In addition, the other important component of the initial evaluation is an assessment of target organ injury. The presence of target organ injury provides a measure of chronicity and severity (characteristics sometimes difficult to ascertain from the history) and will later aid in deciding whether pharmacologic therapy should be instituted. This is best accomplished with echocardiography or an ophthalmologic evaluation. Echocardiography is a sensitive means to detect interventricular septal and posterior ventricular wall thickening.[58–61] Chest radiography and electrocardiography are much less sensitive measures of left ventricular hypertrophy. Not as well appreciated is the usefulness of a thorough ophthalmologic examination. In a study of 97 children and adolescents with essential hypertension, Daniels and associates[62] found that 51% displayed retinal abnormalities. The usefulness of microalbuminuria, sometimes used as a marker for renal injury in adults,[63] has not been determined for children.

The remainder of the evaluation is directed by specific findings on history and physical examination as well as by results of initial screening studies. The 24-hour ambulatory blood pressure monitoring has become increasingly used in the evaluation of adults with hypertension.[64] Standards for ambulatory blood pressure values in children and adolescents, however, have not been firmly established. Therefore, the 1996 Working Group did not recommend its routine use in children. Some data are available,[65] though, and may be helpful in providing comparison values for particular patients. For example, in children or adolescents with intermittent significant elevations in blood pressure, ambulatory blood pressure monitoring may prove useful in determining how consistently blood pressure readings are elevated during a 24-hour period and aid in assessing the urgency for implementing pharmacologic therapy.

MANAGEMENT OF HYPERTENSION IN CHILDREN AND ADOLESCENTS

In adults, control of hypertension reduces morbidity and mortality.[66, 67] The same long-term data are unavailable for the pediatric population. On the basis of inferences from blood pressure tracking studies, which suggest that a child with elevated blood pressure will continue to display elevated blood pressure as an adult,[22–28] intervention is indicated in hypertensive children and adolescents.[3]

NONPHARMACOLOGIC APPROACHES

Children and adolescents with a mild elevation of blood pressure (blood pressure values in the high-normal category) and without end-organ damage, or with probable early essential hypertension, should begin treatment with nonpharmacologic interventions. Nonpharmacologic approaches include weight reduction, exercise, and diet modification.

Obesity is often associated with mild hypertension in childhood and adolescence, and weight reduction has been shown to benefit this population. With a program of both behavior modification and parental involvement, Brownell and coworkers[68] showed that weight loss in obese adolescents was associated with a significant decrease in blood pressure. Exercise training alone both in school-aged children and in adolescents also lowers both systolic and diastolic blood pressures.[69, 70] Compared with a regimen of caloric restriction alone, Rocchini and colleagues[37] showed that a program integrating both caloric restriction and exercise produced the greatest decrease in blood pressure as well as a reversal of structural changes in forearm resistance vessels. In fact, the rate of age-related increase in blood pressure can be decreased by an increase in aerobic fitness or a decrease in body mass index.[71]

Weight reduction can be extraordinarily frustrating and is usually best accomplished in conjunction with comprehensive programs that combine the input of a nutritionist with dietary education, emotional support, information about exercise, and family involvement. Power weightlifting, an understudied area of exercise training, should probably be discouraged in hypertensive adolescents because of its potential, with Valsalva maneuvers and improper breathing techniques, to markedly elevate blood pressure.

Participation in other sports should, in most subjects, be encouraged, though, as long as blood pressure is under reasonable control, regular monitoring of blood pressure occurs, and a thorough examination has been conducted to exclude cardiac conditions.[18]

The guidelines for dietary modifications in the pediatric population are less clear than in adults. There may be, as in adults, a subset of hypertensive children who are "salt sensitive."[38] Yet the data with regard to children and the effects of salt on blood pressure are not as definitive as in adults. In general, significant correlations have not been demonstrated between sodium intake and blood pressure in children and adolescents. There does seem to be, however, a subset of adolescents who demonstrate blood pressure sensitivity to salt as well as other risk factors for hypertension. Sodium most likely acts not as an isolated factor but rather in conjunction with other factors to influence blood pressure. Because the usual dietary intake of sodium for most children and adolescents in the United States far exceeds nutrient requirements, it may be reasonable to restrict sodium intake to less than 4 g per day by decreasing fast food consumption and refraining from adding salt to cooked foods.[72]

TABLE 53–3

ANTIHYPERTENSIVE DRUG THERAPY FOR CHRONIC HYPERTENSION IN CHILDREN

Drug*	Dose (mg/kg/day)		Dosing Interval
	Initial	Maximum	
ADRENERGIC BLOCKING AGENTS			
α/β Blocker			
Labetalol	1	3	q 6–12 hr
α Blocker			
Prazosin	0.05–0.1	0.5	q 6–8 hr
β-Adrenergic blockers			
Atenolol	1	8	q 12–24 hr
Propranolol	1	8	q 6–12 hr
α AGONIST			
Clonidine	0.05–0.1†	0.5–0.6‡	q 6 hr
CALCIUM ANTAGONISTS			
Nifedipine	0.25	3	q 4–6 hr
Nifedipine XL	0.25	3	q 12–24 hr
CONVERTING ENZYME INHIBITORS			
Captopril			
Children	1.5	6	q 8 hr
Neonates	0.03–0.15	2	q 8–24 hr
Enalapril	0.15	Not established	q 12–24 hr
DIURETICS			
Bumetanide	0.02–0.05	0.3	q 4–12 hr
Furosemide	1	12	q 4–12 hr
Hydrochlorothiazide	1	2–3	q 12 hr
Metolazone	0.1	3	q 12–24 hr
Spironolactone	1	3	q 6–12 hr
Triamterene	2	3	q 6–12 hr
VASODILATORS			
Hydralazine	0.75	7.5	q 6 hr
Minoxidil	0.1–0.2	1	q 12 hr

*Listed in alphabetical order by drug class. Other drugs are available in some classes, but data on dosage in children have not been published.

†Total initial dose in milligrams.

‡Total daily dose in milligrams.

Adapted from National High Blood Pressure Education Program Working Group Report on Hypertension Control in Children and Adolescents: The Update on the 1987 Task Force Report on High Blood Pressure in Children and Adolescents: A Working Group Report from the National High Blood Pressure Education Program. Pediatrics 98:649, 1996. Used with permission of the American Academy of Pediatrics.

Our current understanding with regard to potassium and calcium intake and their effects on blood pressure is even less definitive. Some evidence exists to suggest that a diet high in potassium and calcium may help to lower blood pressure,[73] yet no study has definitively shown this effect in children or adolescents.

PHARMACOLOGIC THERAPY

If nonpharmacologic approaches have been unsuccessful or a child is symptomatic, has severe hypertension, or has end-organ damage, pharmacologic therapy is indicated. In addition, there is suggestive evidence that a child with diabetes mellitus or slowly progressive renal disease may benefit from the "renal protective" effects of low doses of certain antihypertensive medications.

Most of the medications used for adults are also used for children. However, efficacy data, as well as long-term safety data, are limited for the pediatric population. Consequently, few of the medications currently used in practice have ever been approved by the Food and Drug Administration for use in children. As a result, a few selected medications from each class of antihypertensives have been used, with each practitioner's experience serving as the guide. The choice of antihypertensive medication must be individualized and depends on the child's age and lifestyle, the etiology of the hypertension, the degree of blood pressure elevation, adverse effects, and concomitant medical conditions. In most patients, therapy is begun with a single agent. The dose is titrated upward until control of the blood pressure is attained. Blood pressure control, in most instances, is defined as maintenance of diastolic pressure below the 90th percentile. If control cannot be achieved by use of the maximal dose of a single agent, a second medication can be added or, alternatively, another agent from a different class selected. The more commonly used medications for antihypertensive therapy in children are listed in Table 53–3 for chronic hypertension and in Table 53–4 for acute, hypertensive emergencies. The dosing recommendations for children have been largely based on experience of practitioners, not on large, multicenter trials.

The stepped care approach, once the guideline for antihypertensive therapy in adults, is no longer recommended for all patients, adults or children. For example, diuretics are rarely chosen as first-line agents, except occasionally in the salt-sensitive, obese patient. The benefits of thiazide diuretics may be offset by their effects on lipids. β-Adrenergic blockers, such as propranolol and atenolol, are good choices in some nonasthmatic children yet are not well tolerated by athletes, in whom exercise tolerance may be decreased, or in adolescent boys, who may experience sexual difficulties. More frequently, first-line medications are either angiotensin-converting enzyme (ACE) inhibitors or calcium channel blockers. ACE inhibitors rarely cause side effects (e.g., cough, rash, neutropenia) in children and are usually well tolerated; some formulations have the advantage of once-a-day dosing. Not only are they effective at controlling blood pressure, but they may have beneficial effects on renal function, peripheral vasculature, and cardiac function.[74] Importantly, children with diabetes and those with chronic renal disease may be at special risk for progressive renal deterioration and may benefit from the

TABLE 53–4

ANTIHYPERTENSIVE DRUG THERAPY FOR HYPERTENSIVE EMERGENCIES IN CHILDREN

Drug	Dose
Nifedipine	0.25–0.5 mg/kg orally prn May be repeated 2 times, if no response
Sodium nitroprusside	0.5–1 µg/kg/min IV initially May be increased stepwise to 8 µg/kg/min maximum
Labetalol	0.2–1 mg/kg/dose IV; may be increased incrementally to 1 mg/kg/dose until response achieved 0.25–2 mg/kg/hr maintenance, either bolus or IV infusion
Esmolol	500–600 µg/kg IV loading dose in 1–2 min, then 200 µg/kg/min May be increased by 50–100 µg/kg q 5–10 min to maximum of 1000 µg/kg
Diazoxide	1–5 mg/kg/dose IV bolus up to maximum of 150 mg/dose
Hydralazine	0.2–0.4 mg/kg IV prn May be repeated 2 times if no response
Minoxidil	0.1–0.2 mg/kg orally

Adapted from National High Blood Pressure Education Program Working Group Report on Hypertension Control in Children and Adolescents: The Update on the 1987 Task Force Report on High Blood Pressure in Children and Adolescents: A Working Group Report from the National High Blood Pressure Education Program. Pediatrics 98:649, 1996. Used with permission of the American Academy of Pediatrics.

renal protective effects of low doses of ACE inhibitors.[75, 76] Because of their vasodilator effects on the efferent arteriole, ACE inhibitors can severely reduce glomerular filtration and should therefore be used with caution in patients with renal artery stenosis, a solitary kidney, or a transplanted kidney.[77] ACE inhibitors are also contraindicated during pregnancy because of teratogenic effects on the lungs, kidneys, and brain of the fetus.[78] Therefore, these agents should be used with special caution in adolescent girls.

Of the calcium channel blockers, nifedipine is most commonly used in pediatrics. The appropriate dose prescribed for small children is often lower than the strength of available capsules, so that nifedipine is more practical to dose in older children and adolescents. Both short-acting and longer-acting forms are available. Although the short-acting forms have adverse effects in some adults,[79, 80] the same data are unavailable in children. Until more information becomes available, short-acting calcium channel blockers should be used on a limited basis for children with acute hypertension. When calcium channel blockers are needed for blood pressure control in chronic hypertension, long-acting preparations are preferred, provided that the correct dosage preparation can be used.

FUTURE DIRECTIONS

Although secondary hypertension may involve a more elaborate and extensive work-up than does essential hypertension, the child with essential hypertension also requires close and prolonged follow-up. Indeed, considering the long-term morbidity and mortality associated with essential hypertension, major efforts of all health care providers for children and adolescents are needed to focus on blood pressure control. Essential hypertension, no doubt, will be found to encompass several distinct pathophysiologic entities, each with its own genetic basis and management approach. With continuing research, the knowledge on hypertension in the young as well as in adults will continue to expand.

REFERENCES

1. National Heart, Lung, and Blood Institute: Report of the Task Force on Blood Pressure Control in Children. Pediatrics 59:797, 1977.
2. Task Force on Blood Pressure Control in Children: Report of the Second Task Force on Blood Pressure Control in Children, 1988. Pediatrics 79:1, 1987.
3. National High Blood Pressure Education Program Working Group Report on Hypertension Control in Children and Adolescents: The Update on the 1987 Task Force Report on High Blood Pressure in Children and Adolescents: A Working Group Report from the National High Blood Pressure Education Program. Pediatrics 98:649, 1996.
4. deSwiet M, Fayers P, Shinebourne EA: Blood pressure survey in a population of newborn infants. Br Med J 2:9, 1976.
5. Schachter J, Kuller LH, Perfetti C: Blood pressure during the first five years of life: Relation to ethnic group (black or white) and to parental hypertension. Am J Epidemiol 119:541, 1984.
6. Zinner SH, Rosner B, Oh WO: Significance of blood pressure in infancy. Hypertension 7:411, 1985.
7. Versmold HT, Kitterman JA, Phibbs RH, et al: Aortic blood pressure during the first 12 hours of life in infants with birth weight 610 to 4220 grams. Pediatrics 67:607, 1981.
8. Tan KL: Blood pressure in full-term healthy neonates. Clin Pediatr 26:21, 1987.
9. Hulman S, Edwards R, Chen Y, et al: Blood pressure patterns in the first three days of life. J Perinatol 11:231, 1991.
10. Zubrow AB, Hulman S, Kushner H, Falkner B: Determinants of blood pressure in infants admitted to neonatal intensive care units: A prospective multicenter study. J Perinatol 15:470, 1995.
11. Hanna JD, Chan JCM, Gill JR Jr: Hypertension and the kidney. J Pediatr 118:327, 1991.
12. Arar MY, Hogg RJ, Arant BS Jr, Seikaly MG: Etiology of sustained hypertension in children in the southwestern United States. Pediatr Nephrol 8:186, 1994.
13. Plumer LB, Kaplan GW, Mendoza SA: Hypertension in infants—a complication of umbilical arterial catheterization. J Pediatr 89:802, 1976.
14. Vailas GN, Brouillette RT, Scott JP, et al: Neonatal aortic thrombosis. Recent experience. J Pediatr 109:101, 1986.
15. Abman SH, Warady BA, Lum GM, Koops BL: Systemic hypertension in infants with bronchopulmonary dysplasia. J Pediatr 104:928, 1984.
16. Adelman RD: Smokeless tobacco and hypertension in an adolescent. Pediatrics 79:837, 1987.
17. Blachley JD, Knochel JP: Tobacco chewer's hypokalemia: Licorice revisited. N Engl J Med 302:784, 1980.
18. Committee on Sports Medicine and Fitness: Athletic participation by children and adolescents who have systemic hypertension. Pediatrics 99:637, 1997.
19. Ing FF, Starc TJ, Griffiths SP, Gersony WM: Early diagnosis of coarctation of the aorta in children: A continuing dilemma. Pediatrics 99:904, 1996.
20. Strafford MA, Griffiths SP, Gersony WM: Coarctation of the aorta: A study in delayed detection. Pediatrics 69:159, 1982.
21. Thoele DG, Muster AJ, Paul MH: Recognition of coarctation of the aorta. Am J Dis Child 141:1201, 1987.
22. Lauer RM, Clarke WR, Beaglehole R: Level, trend, and variability of blood pressure during childhood. The Muscatine Study. Circulation 69:242, 1984.
23. Shear CL, Burke GL, Freedman DS, Berenson GS: Value of childhood blood pressure measurements and family history in predicting future blood pressure status: Results from 8 years of follow-up in the Bogalusa Heart Study. Pediatrics 77:862, 1986.
24. Michels V, Bergstralh E, Hoverman V, et al: Tracking and prediction of blood pressure in children. Mayo Clin Proc 62:875, 1987.
25. Julius S, Jamerson K, Mejia A, et al: The association of borderline hypertension with target organ changes and higher coronary risk. Tecumseh Blood Pressure Study. JAMA 264:354, 1990.
26. Mahoney LT, Clarke WR, Burns TL, Lauer RM: Childhood predictors of high blood pressure. Am J Hypertens 4:6085, 1991.
27. Nelson M, Ragland D, Syme S: Longitudinal prediction of adult blood pressure from juvenile blood pressure levels. Am J Epidemiol 136:633, 1992.
28. Lauer RM, Clarke WR, Maloney LT, Witt J: Childhood predictors for high adult blood pressure: The Muscatine Study. Pediatr Clin North Am 40:23, 1993.
29. Falkner B, Onesti G, Angelakos ET, et al: Cardiovascular response to mental stress in normal adolescents with hypertensive parents. Hypertension 1:23, 1979.
30. Warren P, Fischbein C: Identification of labile hypertension in children and hypertensive parents. Conn Med 44:77, 1980.
31. Matthews KA, Manuck SB, Saab PG: Cardiovascular responses of adolescents during a naturally occurring stressor and their behavioral and psychophysiological predictors. Psychophysiology 23:198, 1984.
32. Falkner B, Kushner H: Racial differences in stress induced reactivity in young adults. Health Psychol 8:613, 1989.
33. Falkner B, Lowenthal DT: Dynamic exercise response in hypertensive adolescents. Int J Pediatr Nephrol 1:161, 1980.
34. Munger R, Prineas R, Gomez-Marin O: Persistent elevation of blood pressure among children with a family history of hypertension: The Minneapolis Children's Blood Pressure Study. J Hypertens 6:647, 1988.
35. Report of the Hypertension Task Force: Current Research and Recommendations from the Task Force Reports on Therapy, Pregnancy, Obesity, Vol 9. Washington, DC, US Department of Health, Education and Welfare, 1979. Publication (NIH) 79-1631.
36. Havlik R, Hubert H, Fabsity R, Feinleib M: Weight and hypertension. Ann Intern Med 98:855, 1983.
37. Rocchini AP, Katch V, Anderson J, et al: Blood pressure in obese adolescents: Effect of weight loss. Pediatrics 82:16, 1988.
38. Rocchini AP, Key J, Bondie D, et al: The effect of weight loss on the sensitivity of blood pressure to sodium in obese adolescents. N Engl J Med 321:580, 1989.
39. DeFronzo R, Tobin J, Andres R: Glucose clamp technique: A method for quantifying insulin secretion and resistance. Am J Physiol 237:E214, 1979.
40. Ferrannini E, Buzzigoli G, Bonadonna R, et al: Insulin resistance in essential hypertension. N Engl J Med 317:350, 1987.
41. Reaven GM: Role of insulin resistance in human disease. Diabetes 37:1595, 1988.
42. Berenson GS, Wattigney WA, Bao W, et al: Epidemiology of early primary hypertension and implications for prevention: The Bogalusa Heart Study. J Hum Hypertens 8:303, 1994.
43. Falkner B, Hulman S, Tannenbaum J, Kushner H: Insulin resistance and blood pressure in young black men. Hypertension 16:36, 1990.
44. Ferrari P, Weidmann P, Shaw S, et al: Altered insulin sensitivity, hyperinsulinemia, and dyslipidemia in individuals with a hypertensive parent. Am J Med 91:589, 1991.
45. Grunfeld B, Balzareti M, Romo M, et al: Hyperinsulinemia in normotensive offspring of hypertensive parents. Hypertension 23(suppl I):12, 1994.
46. Barker DJP, Osmond C, Golding J, et al: Growth in utero, blood pressure in childhood and adult life, and mortality from cardiovascular disease. Br Med J 298:564, 1989.
47. Law CM, Shiell AW: Is blood pressure inversely related to birth weight? The strength of evidence from a systematic review of the literature. J Hypertens 14:935, 1996.
48. Barker DJP, Gluckman PD, Godfrey KM, et al: Fetal nutrition and cardiovascular disease in adult life. Lancet 341:938, 1993.
49. Osmond C, Barker DJP, Winter PD, et al: Early growth and death from cardiovascular disease in women. Br Med J 307:1519, 1993.
50. Harlan WR, Cornoni Huntley J, Leaverton PE: Blood pressure in childhood. National Health Examination Survey. Hypertension 1:566, 1979.

51. Katz SH, Hediger MC, Schall HI, et al: Blood pressure, growth and maturation from childhood to adolescence. Hypertension 2(suppl): I-55, 1980.
52. Troiano RP, Flegal KM, Kuczmarski RJ, et al: Overweight prevalence and trends for children and adolescents. Arch Pediatr Adolesc Med 149:1085, 1995.
53. Rich GM, Ulick S, Cook S, et al: Glucocorticoid-remediable aldosteronism in a large kindred: Clinical spectrum and diagnosis using a characteristic biochemical phenotype. Ann Intern Med 116:813, 1992.
54. Lifton RP, Dluhy RG, Powers M, et al: Hereditary hypertension caused by chimeric gene duplications and ectopic expression of aldosterone synthase. Nat Genet 2:66, 1992.
55. Kroenke K, Omori DM, Simmons JO, et al: The safety of phenylpropanolamine in patients with stable hypertension. Ann Intern Med 111:1043, 1989.
56. Lake CR, Gallant S, Masson E, Miller P: Adverse drug effects attributed to phenylpropanolamine: A review of 142 case reports. Am J Med 89:195, 1990.
57. Hurley JK: A pediatrician's approach to the evaluation of hypertension. Pediatr Ann 18:542, 1989.
58. Laird WP, Fixler DE: Left ventricular hypertrophy in adolescents with elevated blood pressure: Assessment by chest roentgenography, electrocardiography and echocardiography. Pediatrics 67:255, 1981.
59. Shieken RM, Clark WR, Lauer RM: Left ventricular hypertrophy in children with blood pressures in the upper quintile of the distribution: The Muscatine Study. Hypertension 3:669, 1981.
60. Zahka KG, Neill CA, Kidd L, et al: Cardiac involvement in adolescent hypertension. Hypertension 3:664, 1981.
61. Culpepper WS, Sodt PC, Messerli FH, et al: Cardiac status in juvenile borderline hypertension. Ann Intern Med 98:1, 1983.
62. Daniels SR, Lipman MJ, Burke MJ, Loggie JM: The prevalence of retinal vascular abnormalities in children and adolescents with essential hypertension. Am J Ophthalmol 111:205, 1991.
63. Yudkin JS, Forrest RD, Jackson CA: Microalbuminuria as predictor of vascular disease in non-diabetic subjects. Lancet 2:530, 1988.
64. Townsend RR, Ford V: Ambulatory blood pressure monitoring: Coming of age in nephrology. J Am Soc Nephrol 7:2279, 1996.
65. Harshfield GA, Alpert BS, Pulliam DA, et al: Ambulatory blood pressure recordings in children and adolescents. Pediatrics 94:180, 1994.
66. Kannel WB, Doyle JT, Ostfeld AM, et al: Optimal resources for primary prevention of atherosclerotic diseases. Circulation 70:155A, 1984.
67. Dannenberg AL, Drizd T, Horan MJ: Progress in the battle against hypertension. Hypertension 10:226, 1987.
68. Brownell KD, Kelman JH, Stunkard AJ: Treatment of obese children with and without their mothers: Changes in weight and blood pressure. Pediatrics 71:515, 1983.
69. Hagberg JM, Goldring D, Ehsani AA, et al: Effect of exercise training on the blood pressure and hemodynamic features of hypertensive adolescents. Am J Cardiol 52:763, 1983.
70. Hansen HS, Froberg K, Hyldebrandt N, Nielson JR: A controlled study of eight months of physical training and reduction of blood pressure in children: The Odense School-Child Study. Br Med J 303:682, 1991.
71. Shea S, Basch CE, Gutin B, et al: The rate of increase in blood pressure in children 5 years of age is related to changes in aerobic fitness and body mass index. Pediatrics 94:465, 1994.
72. Falkner B, Michel S: Blood pressure response to sodium in children and adolescents. Am J Clin Nutr 65(suppl):618S, 1997.
73. Sinaiko AR, Gomez-Marin O, Prineas RJ: Effect of low sodium diet or potassium supplementation on adolescent blood pressure. Hypertension 21:989, 1993.
74. Doyle AE: Angiotensin-converting enzyme (ACE) inhibition: Benefits beyond blood pressure control. Am J Med 92:1S, 1992.
75. Krolewski AS, Canessa M, Warram JH, et al: Predisposition to hypertension and susceptibility to renal disease in insulin-dependent diabetes mellitus. N Engl J Med 318:140, 1988.
76. National High Blood Pressure Education Program: Working Group report on hypertension and diabetes. Hypertension 23:145, 1994.
77. Hricik DE, Dunn MJ: Angiotensin-converting enzyme inhibitor–induced renal failure: Causes, consequences, and diagnostic uses. J Am Soc Nephrol 1:845, 1990.
78. Pryde PG, Sedman AB, Nugent CE, Barr M: Angiotensin-converting enzyme inhibitor fetopathy. J Am Soc Nephrol 3:1575, 1993.
79. Furberg CD, Psaty BM, Meyer JV: Nifedipine: dose-related increase in mortality in patients with coronary heart disease. Circulation 92:1326, 1995.
80. National Heart, Lung, and Blood Institute: New Analyses Regarding the Safety of Calcium-Channel Blockers: A Statement for Health Professionals from the National Heart, Lung, and Blood Institute. Bethesda, MD, National Institutes of Health, 1995.

NORMAN S. TALNER   JAMES J. MCGOVERN   MICHAEL P. CARBONI

The clinical syndrome of congestive heart failure as encountered in pediatric age groups, including the fetus, represents the inability of the heart and circulation to meet the metabolic demands of the growing organism. This can occur from excessive loading conditions (pressure or volume) imposed on the myocardium, alterations in the contractile process itself (depressed inotropic or lusitropic state), or a combination of mechanical and contractile element factors. The clinical picture that emerges may consist of signs of pulmonary venous congestion (pulmonary edema) and systemic venous congestion (primarily hepatic); evidence of the operation of various adaptive mechanisms is found in heart rate changes, vasoconstrictor tone, and the development of myocardial hypertrophy. The clinical syndrome has variable expressions in the fetus, infant, older child, and adolescent; when encountered, it represents a high-risk situation that demands prompt recognition, accurate diagnosis, and appropriate management strategies.

The major components of this review are the causative factors based on the altered physiologic state, the hemodynamic basis for the clinical expression, and the adaptive and maladaptive responses that can take place. This is followed by a presentation of clinical-physiologic correlations, which then sets the stage for a consideration of current diagnosis and management approaches, at first in general terms that relate to pharmacologic interventions and key supportive measures, and finally in specific therapeutic schema for the more common clinical encounters in which congestive heart failure represents the major therapeutic challenge.

CAUSES OF HEART FAILURE

The heart failure syndrome may arise from diverse causes. Cardiac malformations account for most congestive heart failure in infancy.[1-3] In a fetus, nonimmune hydrops fetalis, the clinical expression of heart failure in utero, is usually associated with tachyarrhythmias and inflammatory diseases (parvovirus) and only rarely with cardiac malformations. In the older child and adolescent, although relatively rare, cardiac failure may arise as a long-term sequel of heart operations performed earlier; in the natural history of certain valve malformations; and with inflammatory disease, endocrine disorders, familial cardiomyopathies, chronic diseases of the large and small airways, hematologic problems, drugs, and tachyarrhythmias or bradyarrhythmias. Table 54–1 lists the common and rare causes of heart failure in the various age groups.

From the physiologic standpoint, all of these causes of heart failure may be classified on the basis of the fundamental alterations in loading conditions imposed on the developing myocardium or alterations in the basic function of the contractile element that may impair systolic and diastolic function. This can be appreciated most readily by considering the pressure-volume relations of the myocardium under various loading conditions as well as when the contractile element function is impaired or the diastolic function is compromised, keeping in mind the maturational aspects of cardiovascular function that may be taking place simultaneously.

FUNDAMENTAL HEMODYNAMIC MECHANISMS

DEVELOPMENTAL ASPECTS

The normal maturing cardiovascular system operates at a high diastolic volume, and thus diastolic reserve in the infant may be less than in the adult.[4] The myocardial response to an acute increase in afterload in the neonate appears impaired—a factor that relates to a diminished ability to increase tension as afterload is raised.[5,6] Although the developing myocardium may respond appropriately to sympathetic stimulation, contractile reserve is limited.[7,8] An increase in heart rate through the sympathetic nervous system, however, is the dominant mechanism to augment or maintain cardiac output at all ages.

The mechanical properties of the developing myocardium also differ from those of an adult.[9] Ventricular compliance is decreased, exhibiting a greater resting tension for any increment in stretch. Excitation-contraction coupling studies in the developing mammal also indicate that calcium ion movement from extracellular sites to the contractile elements plays a greater role in the excitatory process than does release of calcium from the sarcoplasmic reticulum (see Chapter 3).[10]

THE VENTRICULAR PRESSURE-VOLUME DIAGRAM

Within the framework of the developing cardiovascular system, the various conditions that may lead to the clinical expression of congestive heart failure can be analyzed by the ventricular pressure-volume diagram.[11,12] In this approach, four types of cardiac failure have been recognized. The first two types are expressed when an increased workload, either pressure or volume, is presented to a normal

TABLE 54–1

ETIOLOGY OF HEART FAILURE: COMMON AND RARE CAUSES AT VARIOUS AGES

Common	Rare
FETUS Tachyarrhythmias Anemia—parvovirus	Atrioventricular valve regurgitation Arteriovenous malformation Hemolytic disease Heart block Premature closure of foramen ovale Endomyocardial disease Cardiac tumors Pulmonary lymphangiectasia Fetal-maternal transfusion
AT BIRTH Birth asphyxia Tricuspid regurgitation Tachyarrhythmia	Arteriovenous malformation Myocarditis Pulmonary regurgitation Hyperviscosity Premature closure of foramen ovale Premature closure of ductus arteriosus
FIRST WEEK OF LIFE Patent ductus arteriosus (preterm) Hypoplastic left heart Obstructed pulmonary venous return Tachyarrhythmias Tricuspid regurgitation Critical aortic stenosis Critical pulmonic stenosis	Common mixing lesions (truncus, single ventricle) Persistent pulmonary hypertension Myocarditis Myocardial and pericardial tumor Systemic hypertension (renal) Thyroid disease—hyperthyroidism, hypothyroidism Parathyroid disease Infant of diabetic mother Adrenal insufficiency Sepsis Postoperative Norwood procedure Obstructive airway disease Cardiomyopathy Heart block
1 WEEK TO 3 MONTHS Coarctation L→R shunt (ventricular septal defect, patent ductus arteriosus, atrioventricular septal defect) Common mixing lesion Tachyarrhythmias Postoperative cardiopulmonary bypass	Anomalous left coronary artery from pulmonary artery Anomalous pulmonary venous return (nonobstructive) Myocarditis Systemic hypertension Adrenal insufficiency Familial cardiomyopathy Pompe's disease Mitochondrial cardiomyopathy Atrial septal defect Carnitine deficiency

LATE-ONSET HEART FAILURE (ALL RELATIVELY RARE)
Preoperative—congenital
  Tricuspid regurgitation
  Mitral regurgitation
  Aortic regurgitation
  Heart block
  Subaortic obstruction
  Pulmonary atresia and ventricular septal defect with large collaterals
Postoperative—congenital
  Obstructed right ventricle–pulmonary artery conduit
  Fontan's procedure
  Mustard-Senning operation
  Pulmonary regurgitation
  Large aortic-pulmonary shunt
Acquired
  Primary pulmonary hypertension
  Myopericarditis
  Rheumatic heart disease
  Collagen vascular diseases
  Kawasaki disease
  Airway obstructive disease
  Cystic fibrosis
  Systemic hypertension
  Sepsis
  Cardiomyopathies (hypertrophic, dilated, restrictive)
  Neuromuscular diseases
  Tachyarrhythmias
  Drugs—anthracyclines, ipecac
  Anemias—sickle, thalassemia	

myocardium. This results in elevated filling pressures and, as a consequence, clinical signs of pulmonary venous congestion (interstitial or alveolar edema) or systemic venous congestion (notably hepatomegaly). Figure 54–1A (type I, volume overload) depicts the pressure-volume relations with pure augmentation of volume as might take place with a large-volume left-to-right shunt, valvar regurgitation, anemia, or a systemic arteriovenous fistula.

The pressure-volume relationship in pure pressure overload is shown in Figure 54–1B (type I, pressure overload). Pressure overload heart failure in pediatric patients may arise from semilunar valve stenosis, coarctation of the aorta, and pathologic elevations of pulmonary or systemic vascular resistance. The increase in afterload diminishes stroke volume. To restore stroke volume, diastolic filling increases along the same end-diastolic pressure-volume relation, which results in an increase in diastolic pressure. This elevation in diastolic pressure is transmitted to the pulmonary or systemic venous system with the development of congestive symptoms. If the source of the pressure overload is at the level of left ventricular outflow or the proximal arterial system, clinical signs of forward heart failure develop. Ventricular stroke work is increased as shown by a larger area included in the pressure-volume diagram. Wall stress and myocardial oxygen consumption are increased until compensatory ventricular hypertrophy develops. The hypertrophic response tends to minimize these changes; wall stress and myocardial oxygen consumption per 100 g of muscle tend to normalize, although total oxygen consumption remains elevated owing to the increase in muscle mass.

The third pathophysiologic mechanism causing heart failure is systolic dysfunction as depicted in Figure 54–1D (type II, loss of contractility). Myocarditis, global myocar-

dial ischemia from disorders of the coronary circulation, inborn errors of metabolism such as storage disorders or defects in the oxidation of fatty acids, and tachyarrhythmia-induced cardiomyopathies are only a few examples of processes that lead to impaired systolic function and the development of congestive heart failure. Decreased contractility leads to a decrease in the slope of the end-systolic pressure-volume relationship. The ventricle is unable to generate an appropriate amount of force at a given end-diastolic volume and pressure to maintain an adequate stroke volume. In an attempt to normalize stroke volume, the ventricle dilates to increase end-diastolic pressure and volume by the Frank-Starling mechanism. The decrease in size of the pressure-volume loop reflects a lower amount of stroke work. In pure systolic failure, the end-diastolic pressure-volume relationship is unchanged. The ventricle dilates to the point of creating clinical signs of venous congestion, and this is accompanied by an inability to augment cardiac output. This leads to poor tissue perfusion, particularly with stress (exercise).

Diastolic dysfunction represents the fourth pathophysiologic mechanism that may be associated with the development of signs of congestive heart failure. Hypertrophic, restrictive, and infiltrative processes as well as constrictive pericarditis can lead to abnormalities in diastolic function (decreased compliance). Figure 54–1C (type III, restriction to filling) shows the pressure-volume diagram with pure diastolic dysfunction. The end-diastolic pressure-volume loop is shifted to the left. This leads to a higher end-diastolic pressure for a given volume with a subsequent decrease in stroke volume. With use of the Frank-Starling mechanism, end-diastolic volumes and pressures are increased and lead to venous congestion.

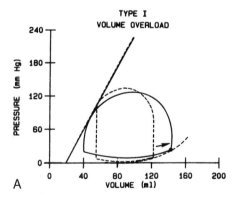

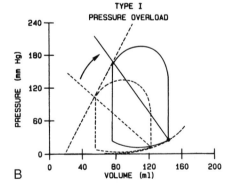

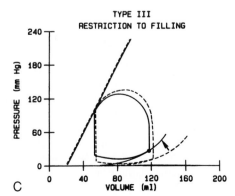

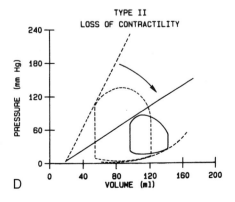

FIGURE 54–1

Pressure-volume diagrams. *A,* Volume overload (type I). *B,* Pressure overload (type I). *C,* Restriction to ventricular filling (type III). *D,* Loss of contractility (type II). Each panel compares a normal pressure-volume loop (*dashed lines*) with a loop from a patient in heart failure (*solid lines*). (Adapted from Cardiac Contraction and the Pressure-Volume Relationship by Kiichi Sagawa and Lowell Maughan, et al. Copyright © 1988 by Oxford University Press, Inc. Used by permission of Oxford University Press, Inc.)

ADAPTIVE MECHANISMS

A cardiologist must understand the important contribution of the major neurohormonal mechanisms that play a key role in the pathophysiologic process of congestive heart failure, particularly in its later stages. Although these neurohormonal responses represent an attempt to preserve cardiovascular homeostasis, activation of the adrenergic and renin-angiotensin-aldosterone systems may also play a role in the progressive deterioration of cardiac function.[13, 14] This can best be illustrated in the dilated cardiomyopathies but may also influence the natural history of certain volume- and pressure-loading situations as well.

ADRENERGIC SYSTEMS

Chronic stimulation of the sympathetic nervous system due to stretching of atrial and ventricular mechanoreceptors accompanies the clinical syndrome of congestive heart failure. Infants and children who are in cardiac failure have increased plasma levels of circulating catecholamines and increased catecholamine metabolites in their urine.[15, 16] The major hemodynamic consequences of chronic adrenergic stimulation include sinus tachycardia, an increase in vasomotor tone, and an initial positive inotropic effect. In addition, sympathetic cholinergic nerve endings that innervate sweat glands are affected.

In heart failure, the compensatory adrenergic stimulation of heart rate and myocardial contractility, although initially favorable, eventually lead to adverse myocardial effects. Catecholamines are toxic to cardiac muscle, perhaps by producing calcium overload or by inhibiting the synthesis of contractile proteins.[17] An additional adverse effect of chronic sympathetic stimulation is the desensitization of the myocardial adrenergic pathway.[18, 19] This has been associated with a decrease in the density of β-adrenergic receptors on the surfaces of the myocardial cell,[20] a finding shown in the myocardial cells of pediatric patients who were in cardiac failure.[21] The decline in β_1-adrenergic receptors is a major contributor to the functional loss of the catecholamine-mediated positive inotropic response. Another desensitization effect is the uncoupling of β_2 receptors from the receptor–G protein–adenylate cyclase complex, with resulting diminished activation of adenylate cyclase and a decline in muscle contraction on exposure to β-agonists.[22] Therefore, chronic activation of adrenergic systems, initially adaptive, may harm myocardial performance.

On the basis of these observations, β-receptor blockade now provides a new avenue of approach to the management of congestive heart failure in a patient with a dilated cardiomyopathy. Therapy is aimed at modulating these adverse effects (see later).

ANGIOTENSIN II

Angiotensin II also participates in hemodynamic responses that are initially adaptive but become maladaptive during time.[23] Angiotensin II, acting as an extracellular messenger, binds to specific receptors on the surface of the plasma cell membrane. A complex signaling cascade ensues, which causes a trophic response in blood vessels that results only in contraction of vascular smooth muscle and a trophic response, both in blood vessels and in the myocardium, that is independent of its hemodynamic effects. Mechanical stretch of cardiac myocytes, as might be induced by cardiac dilatation, causes release of angiotensin II secretory granules in the myocyte that act to initiate the hypertrophic response.[24] Of interest is the finding that angiotensin II can act directly on myocardial fibroblasts to promote fibrosis.[25] Thus, although the hypertrophic response is adaptive by attempting to restore wall stress to normal, by initiating fibrosis and altering ventricular compliance, angiotensin II occupies a maladaptive role as well. In addition, angiotensin is involved in the production of aldosterone, a key factor in salt and water retention.[26–28]

These observations are key to the importance of angiotensin-converting enzyme (ACE) inhibitors in a therapeutic attempt to vasodilate and modulate the ventricular remodeling process and thereby forestall the development of maladaptive hypertrophy and myocardial fibrosis (see later).

OTHER POTENTIAL ADAPTIVE OR MALADAPTIVE NEUROHORMONAL MECHANISMS

Although the adrenergic systems and angiotensin II appear to be the principal neurohormonal mechanisms that operate in the clinical milieu of congestive heart failure, other mechanisms have been implicated, although their precise role remains to be defined.

ARGININE VASOPRESSIN

The plasma levels of arginine vasopressin (AVP), a potent vasoconstrictor, are increased in patients in cardiac failure.[29] This finding suggests that AVP may occupy a role in the development of increased vascular resistance. Vasopressin is a nonapeptide synthesized in the hypothalamus and released from axonal terminals in the posterior pituitary gland. The primary stimuli for AVP release in heart failure are mono-osmotic, with afferent signals to the central nervous system arising from alterations in volume and pressure status.[30] Baroreceptor abnormalities appear to be the major contributors to the elevated plasma AVP levels in heart failure.[31] Studies in infants with cardiac failure and left ventricular outflow tract obstruction imply that impaired flow to sinoaortic and ventricular baroreceptors contributes to the release of AVP.[32]

NEUROPEPTIDE Y

This neuropeptide is present in abundance in sympathetic perivascular nerves throughout the circulation and central nervous system. Neuropeptide Y (NPY) is released during periods of intense sympathetic stimulation and results in vasoconstriction and myocardial depression.[33] Studies in patients with heart failure revealed increased resting levels of NPY that failed to increase further with exercise.[34] The neuropeptide is modulated by G_i guanosine triphosphate–binding protein, a factor that is known to be enhanced in myocardial failure.[35] Thus, the increased plasma levels of NPY could contribute to a negative inotropic state that would be facilitated by increased G_i activity.

ENDOTHELIN

The local vasoconstrictor hormone endothelin may also occupy a role in the pathophysiologic process of congestive heart failure. Because the endothelium has both a vasodilator and a vasoconstrictor function, either increased production of endothelin or inhibition of nitric oxide, the vasodilator factor, would potentiate the maladaptive vasoconstrictor response as has been observed in experimental heart failure.[36]

ATRIAL NATRIURETIC FACTOR

The peptide hormone atrial natriuretic factor (ANF) has assumed major importance in volume and blood pressure regulation. An increase in atrial stretch by volume appears to be the signal that stimulates its release.[37] The major responses to its release are natriuresis, diuresis, and vasodilatation. ANF also appears to interact with other modulators of volume control, including the renin-angiotensin-aldosterone axis, sympathetic nervous system, and AVP.[38] Children with heart failure accompanied by increased pulmonary blood flow, elevated left atrial pressure, and pulmonary arterial hypertension have been found to have elevated levels of ANF.[39]

ENDOTHELIUM-DERIVED RELAXING FACTORS

The actual vasodilating substance derived from the endothelium is most likely nitric oxide, although other factors may be involved. This vasodilator response is impaired in experimental congestive heart failure and therefore may contribute to the elevation in systemic vascular resistance observed in heart failure.[40]

VASOACTIVE INTESTINAL PEPTIDE

Vasoactive intestinal peptide (VIP) is structurally related to secretin and glucagon. It is a vasodilator with positive inotropic properties. Of interest, the myocardial concentration of VIP is reduced in patients with heart failure and rises when patients are prescribed ACE inhibitors.[41]

TUMOR NECROSIS FACTOR

The tumor necrosis factor (cachectin) is a cytokine produced by myocytes. This factor is increased in chronic cardiac failure associated with cachexia, and levels correlate with marked activation of the renin-angiotensin system.[42]

RED BLOOD CELL ADAPTION

A compensatory mechanism that permits improved oxygen delivery to the tissues by an increase in oxygen unloading resides in the red blood cell. A rightward shift in the oxyhemoglobin dissociation curve by the 2,3-diphosphoglycerate (2,3-DPG) mechanism results in an increase in P_{50} (oxygen tension at 50% oxygen saturation), which favors the pressure head for oxygen delivery. Increased levels of 2,3-DPG have been found in infants in cardiac failure. After repair of the cardiac anomaly, these values return to normal as oxygen delivery to the tissues improves.[43] This compensatory mechanism is absent in preterm infants and neonates who have a high proportion of fetal hemoglobin.

CLINICAL-PHYSIOLOGIC CORRELATES

The net effect of the impaired myocardial performance described in the preceding section is the appearance of the classical clinical signs and symptoms of congestive heart failure, despite the operation of various adaptive mechanisms.

The clinical expression of congestive heart failure represents an admixture of components that may reflect pulmonary and systemic congestion, the contractile status of the myocardium, loading conditions, perfusion status, and the operation of the various adaptive mechanisms. These components and the fundamental mechanisms involved are shown in Table 54–2.

The clinical picture of heart failure as exhibited by a fetus warrants special attention. In contrast to the rare occurrence of peripheral edema and ascites postnatally, congestive heart failure in a fetus is dominated by excessive fluid accumulation. Hydrops fetalis can be defined as the accumulation of fluid in pericardial, pleural, and peritoneal spaces as well as generalized edema that results from an imbalance in fetal fluid homeostasis.[44] This imbalance may be a manifestation of fetal congestive heart failure and can arise from tachyarrhythmias or bradyarrhythmias and certain cardiac malformations, notably those with marked atrioventricular valve regurgitation. During an episode of supraventricular tachycardia, ventricular filling is compromised, resulting in increased atrial volumes and pressures that elevate systemic venous pressures and produce hepatic congestion and dysfunction.[45] Hepatic dysfunction may cause hypoalbuminemia and a decrease in oncotic pressure, further favoring fluid transudation. Significant atrioventricular valve regurgitation increases atrial volumes and pressures with a concomitant increase in diastolic filling volumes that are presented to the fetal ventricles.[46]

DIAGNOSTIC AIDS

The diagnosis of congestive heart failure rests primarily on clinical grounds and is supported by various laboratory tests aimed at defining the nature of the specific disease process, functional status of the myocardium, accompanying blood gas and electrolyte abnormalities, and any contributing conditions (inflammatory, metabolic, or toxic).

RADIOGRAPHIC FINDINGS

The chest film is important in assessing cardiac size because enlargement provides direct evidence of cardiac involvement. In addition to cardiac size, the pulmonary vascular markings confirm the pulmonary venous congestion and the status of pulmonary blood flow and lung parenchyma, as discussed in Chapter 10. A normal cardiac size may be seen in a patient with prominent venous mark-

TABLE 54-2

THE CARDINAL SIGNS AND SYMPTOMS OF CONGESTIVE HEART FAILURE AND THEIR MECHANISMS OF PRODUCTION

Signs and Symptoms	Mechanisms
Pulmonary venous congestion	↑ Left-sided filling pressure
Tachypnea	Interstitial pulmonary edema
Wheezing	Bronchiolar edema
Crepitant rales	Alveolar edema
Feeding difficulties	↑ Work of breathing
Irritability	↓ Oxygen transport
Systemic venous congestion	↑ Right-sided filling pressure
Hepatomegaly	Hepatic venous congestion
Peripheral edema—may be only facial	↑ Fluid transudation, ↑ aldosterone
Impaired cardiac output	Decreased inotropic state
↓ Precordial activity	↓ Inotropic function
↓ Arterial pulsations	↓ Systemic perfusion
↓ Capillary refill	↓ Systemic perfusion
Volume loading	Chamber dilatation
↑ Precordial activity	Preserved inotropic state
Gallop sounds	↑ Ventricular filling
Pressure loading	↑ Afterload
Gallop sounds	↓ Compliance
Murmurs	Poststenotic turbulence
Adaptive changes	↑ Neurohormonal responses
Tachycardia	↑ β_1-Adrenergic activity
Pallor	↑ α_1 and angiotensin response (vasoconstriction)
Low urine output	↓ Renal perfusion
Growth failure	↑ Metabolic demands
Sweating	↑ Sympathetic and cholinergic stimulation

ings when there is obstruction to pulmonary venous return and anomalous pulmonary venous connections.

ELECTROCARDIOGRAPHIC FINDINGS

Although the electrocardiogram is of little aid in diagnosing congestive heart failure, it may provide supportive data as to etiology. For example, low QRS voltages and ST-T wave changes suggest myocardial-pericardial disease, and an infarct pattern may be observed with coronary artery abnormalities. The major contribution of the electrocardiogram is to define a specific tachyarrhythmia (supraventricular tachycardia, ventricular tachycardia, atrial fibrillation) or heart block producing or exacerbating clinical signs of congestive heart failure.

ECHOCARDIOGRAPHY AND DOPPLER INTERROGATION

Cardiac ultrasound techniques with Doppler analysis now offer a noninvasive means to establish not only the correct anatomic diagnosis but also the functional status of the myocardium. The echocardiogram also occupies a prominent role in differentiating cardiac from pulmonary conditions. In addition, these studies permit follow-up assessment of the response to various therapeutic interventions.

The assessment of systolic and diastolic ventricular function consists of a number of valuable determinations by use of ultrasound and Doppler techniques.[47,48] With the echo Doppler approach, ejection-phase indices including ejection fraction and shortening fraction can be deter-

mined. These parameters are load dependent and thus vary with volume of ventricular filling and changes in afterload. Consequently, the cardiologist should use load-independent indices of ventricular function, specifically the end-systolic wall stress determination.[49] This approach offers a clinician the possibility of separating the effects of abnormal loading conditions from alterations in ventricular contractility.

Ultrasound evaluation has also been helpful in assessing diastolic function. Diastolic filling is evaluated by the mitral valve inflow patterns.[50,51]

The diagnosis of fetal hydrops is established by ultrasonic demonstration of generalized skin thickening and fluid accumulation in pericardial, pleural, or peritoneal spaces. By definition, fetal hydrops is fluid in two of these spaces or in one space plus skin thickening (edema).[52] Pericardial effusion predominates when hydrops results from a cardiac anomaly. Fetal cardiomegaly may also be determined during ultrasound examination by measuring the cardiothoracic ratio.[53] Dilatation of the atria or ventricles may be reflected in an increase in this ratio.

Pulsed Doppler flow analysis has demonstrated the frequent association of atrioventricular valve regurgitation with a cardiac malformation and nonimmune hydrops.[54] Ventricular filling pressures are markedly increased because the fetal ventricular myocardium is relatively restrictive. Similar flow studies in the human fetus have suggested that the fetal ventricle primarily fills during atrial contraction.[55] These observations imply that a fetal ventricle depends more on active, rather than passive, diastolic filling.

BLOOD GAS VALUES AND pH

Certain patterns of blood gas alterations and pH have been observed in infants with clinical signs of acute or chronic congestive heart failure.[56,57] For example, an infant with an acutely developing low cardiac output syndrome usually shows a metabolic acidosis with a lactic acidemia. The PaO_2 in these infants may not be markedly diminished. Of interest is the response of pH and $PaCO_2$ in infants with hypoplastic left heart syndrome to the hyperoxia test. As the ductus arteriosus constricts in response to the increase in arterial oxygen tension, there is a further compromise in systemic blood flow, and pH falls. $PaCO_2$ decreases as the respiratory rate increases. Arterial oxygen tension rises consequent to increased pulmonary blood flow and the decrease in systemic venous return.

In contrast, infants and children who develop signs of congestive heart failure during a longer time tend to have a lowered $PaCO_2$ and nearly normal pH; PaO_2, although not normal, may be only slightly decreased. If there is a complicating infection or lobar emphysema or atelectasis, there may be a more pronounced fall in PaO_2, and $PaCO_2$ may become elevated, so that respiratory failure then complicates the picture of congestive heart failure.

SERUM ELECTROLYTE CONCENTRATIONS

Pediatric patients in cardiac failure who are receiving therapy[57] may develop hyponatremia (less than 125 mEq/L), associated with an increase in water retention relative to sodium and the limited ability of the patient to handle a water load, and hypochloremia (see later).

When perfusion is impaired, potassium levels become elevated as this ion is released from intracellular sites. Similarly, lactic acid concentration rises with tissue hypoxia.

RED BLOOD CELL COUNTS

A decrease in red blood cell count may accentuate the left-to-right shunt in patients with a ventricular or great artery communication on the basis of decreasing blood viscosity, which lowers pulmonary vascular resistance. Anemia by itself (less than 8.0 g/dl) stimulates a high cardiac output state and lowered systemic vascular resistance. An elevated hemoglobin level and hematocrit, on the other hand, increase pulmonary vascular resistance and decrease the left-to-right shunt.

GLUCOSE AND CALCIUM DETERMINATIONS

Hypoglycemia has been noted in infants in cardiac failure[58] from depletion of hepatic glycogen stores. Hypocalcemia has been reported as a cause of left ventricular dysfunction in neonates and is reversible with calcium therapy.[59]

CREATINE KINASE MB FRACTION AND TROPONIN T

These determinations now provide biochemical evidence for myocardial ischemic changes, particularly as they relate to birth asphyxia or coronary artery malformations.[60,61]

CARDIAC CATHETERIZATION

Although not used as frequently as in the past, cardiac catheterization offers important functional data and can demonstrate intracardiac or extracardiac malformations that may complicate the clinical expression of congestive failure. Myocardial biopsy offers a new approach to specific diagnosis, such as inflammatory disease or metabolic disorders.[62] When myocarditis is suspected on clinical grounds, the diagnosis may be confirmed by myocardial biopsy. The polymerase chain reaction provides a means for isolating the offending viral agent.[63] In a patient with dilated cardiomyopathy, evaluation of biopsy specimens, including genetic analysis, may provide data permitting the diagnosis of specific metabolic causes, such as carnitine deficiency.

In most instances, the clinical evaluation supported by certain laboratory aids, particularly chest radiography and cardiac ultrasonography, permits a definitive diagnosis. Difficulties occasionally arise in infants with signs of respiratory distress, when a cardiac anomaly has to be distinguished from pulmonary disease or disorders of the pulmonary vascular bed (see Chapter 17). Here again, ultrasound examination provides key data. Other measures, such as the hyperoxia test, although helpful, do not clearly distinguish a cardiac problem from a disorder involving the lung or pulmonary circulation. Furthermore, infants with congestive heart failure may have complicating pulmonary problems. For example, in a patient with a large-volume left-to-right shunt, the dilated pulmonary artery under high pressure and an enlarged, distended left atrium and left ventricle may compress the major bronchi and produce atelectasis or obstructive emphysema.[64] On the other hand, chronic obstructive disease of the airways may be associated with the development of pulmonary edema.

In summary, clinical appraisal aided by radiographic evidence of cardiac enlargement and pulmonary or systemic venous congestion should permit the diagnosis of congestive heart failure. Echo Doppler studies are able to define the specific disorder or malformation present as well as the functional status of the myopericardium, particularly the nature of the loading condition.

MANAGEMENT STRATEGIES

The management of a pediatric patient in congestive heart failure rests on a solid foundation of precise anatomic and functional diagnosis with appropriate attention to complicating factors such as infection, anemia, rhythm disturbances, and malnutrition. The clinician must recognize the available therapeutic options, including surgical repair and transplantation. In this section, we present the pharmacologic approaches that improve the contractility of the myocardium, lessen or decrease loading conditions, and diminish pulmonary venous and systemic venous congestion. In addition, we introduce some general and specific supportive measures, including methods to improve nutrition, pulmonary toilet, positioning, oxygen administration, and ventilation, as well as the potential use of mechanical-assist devices as in the postoperative state or as a bridge to cardiac transplantation.

PHARMACOLOGIC TREATMENT

Inotropic Agents for Use on a Chronic Basis

DIGITALIS GLYCOSIDES. The digitalis glycosides continue to be the most widely used inotropic agents to treat congestive heart failure on a chronic basis, although their use in an acute situation and in specific lesions has been questioned. Attention has recently been directed to some therapeutic benefits resulting from their ability to inhibit sympathetic nerve traffic and thus decrease metabolic demands.[65]

Mode of Action. The increase in contractility occurs when digitalis glycosides bind to their receptor site, the sodium pump (Na+,K+-ATPase), and inhibit pump action.[66] As a result, intracellular sodium increases, stimulating calcium entry into the cell by the sodium-calcium exchange mechanism. Myocardial contractility is enhanced thereby. The net positive result in a patient with congestive heart failure is increased cardiac output. The other effects of digitalis glycosides include parasympathetic activation, which produces cardiac slowing and inhibition of atrioventricular nodal conduction. Digitalis is also a primary diuretic agent.

Administration. The cardiac glycoside digoxin can be given parenterally or orally, depending on the severity of the heart failure. Dosage depends on age (Appendix 1). Although loading doses have been advocated, many patients are started on maintenance doses to achieve digitalization, thereby greatly simplifying management. Parents must be instructed carefully in how to measure the medications, timing of administration, and potential side effects. The medication must be stored out of reach of siblings. All calculated doses should be checked carefully to avoid a potentially lethal dosage.

Serum Digoxin Levels. There has been little use of digoxin blood level measurement by cardiologists, and more attention has been focused on clinical response and the monitored electrocardiogram. When, however, there may be potential drug interactions, hepatic or renal complications, or electrolyte disorders, determining serum digoxin levels may be helpful.[67] Drug interactions elevating serum digoxin levels result from quinidine, verapamil, amiodarone, β blockers, tetracycline, and erythromycin. Low serum digoxin levels have been noted with rifampin, kaolin-pectin, neomycin, and cholestyramine.

MILRINONE. Milrinone resembles amrinone in site of action (phosphodiesterase inhibition) and has an advantage because it can be administered orally.[68] Regardless of route of administration, positive inotropic and vasodilatory effects occur with minimal effects on blood pressure and heart rate.

Inotropic Agents for Acute Low-Output Cardiac Failure

DOPAMINE. Dopamine is a catecholamine-like inotropic agent that has been widely used to manage severe acute congestive heart failure and cardiogenic shock. This agent occupies a key role in the management of pediatric patients with low cardiac output after open heart surgery.[69]

Mode of Action. Dopamine is a precursor of norepinephrine and releases the catecholamine from cardiac adrenergic receptor sites (β_1, β_2 effects). In the peripheral vasculature, however, the principal activity is on dopaminergic receptors, which inhibit norepinephrine release and thereby produce vasodilatation. This effect appears at low doses and is associated with augmentation of renal and coronary perfusion. At high doses, dopamine causes α-receptor stimulation with vasoconstriction and limitation of renal blood flow.

Administration. Dopamine must be given intravenously with the patient carefully monitored for blood pressure, heart rate, urine output, and electrocardiographic changes. Weaning should be gradual with echocardiographic assessment to ensure that the improved contractile state is maintained.

DOBUTAMINE. Dobutamine is a synthetic analogue of dopamine and produces β_1 stimulating effects of contractility rather than heart rate. In contrast to dopamine, this drug does not produce direct release of norepinephrine or affect dopamine receptors.[70] In addition to its effect on myocardial contractility, dobutamine is a mild vasodilator. Because dobutamine directly stimulates the β_1 receptor, available norepinephrine stores are unnecessary to produce the desired positive inotropic effect. Dobutamine must be used with caution in conjunction with dopamine in managing severe acute low cardiac output states associated with decreased myocardial contractile state. In children, dobutamine consistently increases cardiac output, decreases systemic vascular resistance, and minimally alters blood pressure and heart rate.[71] Like dopamine, it must be given by an infusion pump with appropriate monitoring of the patient.

EPINEPHRINE. Epinephrine produces mixed β-receptor stimulation and α-mediated effects as well. In postoperative states in which intense vasoconstriction occurs, epinephrine may dilate vascular beds and thus, coupled with its potent inotropic effects, be suitable for the management of an acute low cardiac output state.

AMRINONE. Amrinone belongs to the class of nonglycosidal, noncatecholamine agents that exert their inotropic and vasodilator effect by inhibiting phosphodiesterase.[72] In patients with congestive heart failure, vasodilatation may dominate the pharmacologic response with variable effects on contractility. This drug must be administered by infusion pump with appropriate monitoring of the patient. Blood platelets should be checked and the drug discontinued if the platelet count falls below 150,000/mm^3. This inotrope may be particularly useful in patients with severe congestive heart failure (dilated cardiomyopathy) who have received prolonged treatment with β_1 stimulants, such as dopamine, that has desensitized the β_1 receptor.

Diuretics

Diuretics remain the principal therapeutic agents to control pulmonary and systemic venous congestion. The kidneys respond to the apparent volume deficit of cardiac failure by increasing sodium reabsorption, which then leads to volume expansion and the potential for congestion of the pulmonary and systemic circulations. The fundamental aim of therapy is to increase renal perfusion with use of the agents described in the previous section and to increase sodium transport in the kidney to distal diluting sites. Diuretic agents are designed to maximize sodium loss by increasing renal excretion of sodium and other ions. This is achieved by inhibiting the tubular reabsorption of sodium at various sites along the nephron.[73,74] In the ensuing discussion, the various types of diuretics are considered in reference to their primary site of action in the renal tubular transport processes.

LOOP DIURETICS. The loop diuretics include furosemide, bumetanide, and ethacrynic acid, which act on the medullary and cortical segments of the ascending limbs of the loop of Henle to block sodium and chloride reabsorption.[75] Loop diuretics inhibit the sodium-potassium-chloride cotransporter that is concerned with the transport of chloride ion across the lining cells of the ascending loop of Henle. This results in maintenance in the tubular lumen of sodium, potassium, chloride, and hydrogen ions, which are then lost in the urine. As such, there is the potential for hyponatremia, hypokalemia, hypochloremia, and metabolic alkalosis. There is also hypercalciuria.

DIURETIC AGENTS AFFECTING THE CORTICAL DILUTING SEGMENT. Included in this grouping are the thiazides and metolazone. These agents block sodium and chloride reabsorption in the area of renal tubule concerned with the generation of free water: the cortical diluting segment of the ascending limb and the proximal portion of the distal convoluted tubule. As a result of this action, more sodium reaches the distal tubules, where it can be exchanged with potassium. In addition, thiazides increase the active excretion of potassium ion. By acting at different sites than the loop diuretics, these drugs may produce additive effects on electrolyte losses. In contrast to loop diuretics, thiazides decrease renal calcium excretion.

Although metolazone is categorized with thiazide diuretics, it may produce a profound diuresis when administered as a single daily dose. Because of the risk of excessive volume depletion,[76] this medication should be given in the hospital under close medical observation.

POTASSIUM-SPARING DIURETIC AGENTS. Spironolactone is the principal potassium-sparing agent that has been used in infants and children with congestive heart failure. This drug acts on the distal tubule to inhibit sodium-potassium exchange at the site of aldosterone activity. This impairs the reabsorption of sodium and the excretion of potassium hydrogen ions, thus sparing potassium loss. The principal use of spironolactone is in conjunction with a loop diuretic to minimize potassium losses. On the other hand, when ACE inhibitors are being used, spironolactone should be discontinued to avoid hyperkalemia.

COMPLICATIONS OF PROLONGED DIURETIC TREATMENT
HYPONATREMIA. The development of hyponatremia reflects increased renal sodium losses in the face of an inability to excrete free water.[77] There may also be an increase in AVP antidiuretic hormone activity and increased activity of angiotensin II. Management of this complication includes restriction of water intake in combination with furosemide and an ACE inhibitor.

METABOLIC ALKALOSIS. This abnormality is observed frequently when loop diuretics are administered for a prolonged time and results from excessive loss of potassium.

HYPOKALEMIA. The risk of hypokalemia is present when loop diuretics are given intravenously in high doses, and the low blood potassium level may precipitate cardiac arrhythmias and digitalis intoxication. This complication can usually be avoided by providing potassium supplements or using potassium-sparing diuretics or ACE inhibitors.

VOLUME CONTRACTION. Significant depletion of intravascular volume may occur, particularly when the more potent diuretics, such as furosemide or metolazone, are administered. When these agents are used, frequent checks of perfusion status and serum electrolyte, creatinine, and urea nitrogen concentrations are required if this serious complication is to be avoided. Furosemide used for long periods carries the risk of renal stones as a consequence of chronic hypercalciuria.

Vasodilators

Pharmacologic interventions to manipulate ventricular loading conditions represent major advances in the treatment of congestive heart failure. Vasodilator drugs now occupy a prominent role in the treatment of infants with cardiac failure secondary to a large left-to-right shunt, postoperative low-output states, severe atrioventricular valve and semilunar valve regurgitation, and dilated cardiomyopathy.[78,79] These medications are used in conjunction with inotropic agents (improve pump function) and diuretics (decrease pulmonary and systemic congestion), with the focus being to augment function by altering resistances in the precapillary and postcapillary vascular beds and to change afterload and preload conditions, thereby improving cardiovascular performance.

ACE INHIBITORS. In the treatment of chronic severe congestive heart failure, such as with a dilated cardiomyopathy, the ACE inhibitors are now favored; their principal role is to inhibit the maladaptive neurohormonal responses initiated by the renin-angiotensin-aldosterone axis. A number of well-controlled studies have documented that the outcome in dilated cardiomyopathy has been improved markedly with the addition of ACE inhibition in conjunction with cardiac glycosides and diuretics.[80–82] In addition to their vasodilating effect, inhibiting angiotensin alters ventricular remodeling, as previously noted. Increased production of bradykinin may also occupy an important role in the decrease in afterload. When ACE inhibitors are given, blood pressure must be carefully monitored, particularly during the initial phases of therapy. Neutropenia may occur, so blood counts should be obtained as part of the monitoring process. As mentioned previously, potassium supplements and potassium-sparing diuretics should not be used with ACE inhibition. Those agents occasionally cause blood urea to rise by virtue of having more effect on post-glomerular rather than preglomerular arterioles.

Captopril and enalapril decrease the left-to-right shunt in infants with a large communication at the ventricular level and improve the hemodynamic status of patients with severe congestive but not restrictive cardiomyopathy.[83–87]

SODIUM NITROPRUSSIDE. Sodium nitroprusside is the most frequently used vasodilator in acute situations, such as after cardiopulmonary bypass when manipulation of afterload is required.[88] Nitroprusside dilates smooth muscle of both arterioles and venules, and it acts to decrease filling pressures and systemic and pulmonary vascular resistances. The mode of action is probably by releasing nitric oxide. Attention must be directed to intravascular volume and to the possibility of the development of cyanide toxicity if it is given for more than 48 hours.

Other vasodilators have been used previously in the management of cardiac failure but have largely been replaced by the ACE inhibitors for chronic use and nitroprusside for acute use. These agents include hydralazine, a directly acting dilator; prazosin, an adrenergic blocking agent; and nifedipine, a calcium channel blocker.[89] The last may have a therapeutic role in the management of pulmonary hypertensive crises, but not when inotropic support is required.

β-Receptor Blockage

Low-dose β-receptor blockade has been added to the treatment of dilated cardiomyopathy with encouraging results on the basis of a number of well-controlled studies in adults.[90, 91] This therapeutic approach is based on the potential of these agents to interfere with the deleterious effects of increased sympathoadrenal activity. Workload improves without an increase in myocardial oxygen consumption; in addition, ventricular relaxation is enhanced. Exercise capacity has also been enhanced. Obviously, these drugs must be used with caution because myocardial performance may deteriorate initially, before improvement is noted. Some newer selective β_1-blockers, such as bucindolol and metoprolol, appear to produce the most encouraging therapeutic effects.[92, 93] Up-regulation of β-receptors has been described in patients with dilated cardiomyopathy undergoing treatment with these agents, thereby restoring responsiveness to inotropic interventions.

SUPPORTIVE MEASURES

Nutrition

In managing an infant or child with congestive failure, adequate calories and fluid must be provided to permit weight stabilization or, ideally, to allow weight gain. An important criterion for successful treatment of an infant, in particular, is the ability to resume nearly normal growth. As previously cited, growth limitation represents an adaptive mechanism to limit metabolic demands and preserve vital organ function. Frequent small feedings are tolerated reasonably well in infants. If not, intermittent or continuous gavage feedings are recommended. The increased metabolic rate of infants in congestive heart failure requires a higher than normal intake if growth is to occur.[94] The required calorie intake may be as high as 150 kcal/kg/day for infants. Lower calorie requirements are necessary for those older than 1 year. Measurement of oxygen consumption offers a way of calculating calorie requirements.

Infant formulas should be concentrated to 26 to 30 kcal per ounce of body weight to provide adequate calorie intake while limiting, to some extent, fluid intake. Severe fluid restriction is not indicated, nor should diets low in sodium be instituted. The instruction of parents in proper feeding techniques requires a supportive nursing staff, because feeding of the infant or child in cardiac failure can be frustrating. Before discharge from hospital care, feeding by the parents should be instituted to build their confidence when management takes place at home.

Positioning

Positioning the infant or child in a semiupright position may lessen pulmonary congestion and decrease the work of breathing. Attention should be directed to pulmonary toilet with measures such as suctioning, chest physiotherapy, and postural drainage.

Supplemental Oxygen

Oxygen is required for certain patients if pulse oximetry indicates compromise of blood oxygenation. A few words of caution, however, are indicated. In a large-volume left-to-right shunt, oxygen decreases pulmonary vascular resistance and raises systemic vascular resistance. These changes increase left-to-right shunting. In an infant with a lesion that has ductus-dependent systemic blood flow, oxygen may close the ductus. This further compromises systemic perfusion.

Ventilation

On occasion, respiratory failure accompanies cardiac failure, particularly in an infant with pulmonary overcirculation. A superimposed pulmonary infection, such as from respiratory syncytial virus, may precipitate this complication. Intubation and positive-pressure ventilation usually normalize the blood gas tensions and pH and lessen metabolic demands. Respiratory failure usually signifies that surgical intervention will be needed once stabilization is attained.

Bed Rest

In an older patient with congestive heart failure, bed rest remains an important component of management, particularly during the acute phase or when an exacerbation occurs. This is of special importance in a patient with myocarditis. There must be adequate time for sleep, some limitation of disturbing interventions, and the availability of a television screen and computer games for entertainment. Parental support is needed, and arrangements for home schooling should be made for an older child and adolescent. Resumption of activity should be carefully monitored.

MECHANICAL SUPPORT DEVICES

Mechanical circulatory support takes a number of forms, including intra-aortic balloon pump counterpulsation, extracorporeal membrane oxygenation, ventricular-assist devices, and abdominal compression devices. This subject has been reviewed as it applies to the pediatric patient and is briefly summarized here.[95–97]

Intra-aortic Balloon Counterpulsation

Intra-aortic balloon counterpulsation has been widely used in adults refractory to management of acute low-output cardiac failure. This modality has also been introduced after cardiopulmonary bypass procedures for pediatric patients who cannot be weaned from support.[98,99] The balloon pump functions by decreasing the workload on the left ventricle by forward displacement of blood volume and increasing blood pressure during diastole, thus improving systemic and coronary blood flow. Patients in end-stage heart failure awaiting transplantation have also received balloon counterpulsation.

There are technical problems related to catheter size and insertion in small patients. Heart rate tracking presents some difficulties, especially if an arrhythmia is present. Another major drawback for infants, in particular, is the greater arterial compliance that can result in decreased effectiveness. Nevertheless, intra-aortic balloon counterpulsation remains a viable option for patients with end-stage cardiomyopathy and for patients who, despite inotropic agents and vasodilators, cannot maintain a satisfactory cardiac output.

Extracorporeal Membrane Oxygenation

This approach has been used for a number of years in children with pulmonary disorders and ventilatory failure.[100,101] As a form of partial cardiopulmonary bypass, it can provide some ventricular support, although concern has been raised that extracorporeal membrane oxygenation may not decompress the left side of the heart. This results in an increase in wall stress and a greater ventricular workload.

The pediatric experience has been in the stabilization of infants with cardiac malformations before surgery or in the postoperative state as a bridge to cardiac transplantation.

Ventricular-Assist Devices

These devices are in their developmental stages for infants and children.[102] In adults, the principal use has been in patients who cannot be weaned from cardiopulmonary bypass and as a bridge to cardiac transplantation.

Abdominal Compression Devices

Methods of abdominal compression have been used to treat right-sided heart failure in children.[103] Antishock air trousers connected to a pneumatic pump that delivers phasic compression to the lower body at 1-minute cycles is one such approach. Another method uses a ventilator reservoir bag connected to a volume respirator and placed under a cloth wrapped tightly around the child's abdomen. A similar method involves a large blood pressure cuff wrapped around the patient's waist. The cuff is then attached to a ventilator, and the cycled inflation of the cuff causes an increase in systemic venous return. These devices decrease right-sided volume overload and augment forward blood flow through the pulmonary circulation. These abdominal compression devices appear useful in right-sided congestive failure as might follow a Fontan operation.

PARENT-STAFF CONFERENCES

Medical and nursing staff must discuss with the parents the nature of the underlying condition and what the term *heart failure* means for the particular child. We tend to avoid the use of this term, if possible, and use other terms, such as lung congestion, liver congestion, and impaired pumping ability, because the connotation of "failure" is distressing to a concerned parent. The staff should stress that the heart may be functioning well but because of the underlying abnormality, there may be overcirculation to the lungs with lung congestion and liver congestion as well. A definitive plan of action should be elaborated with alternatives offered, depending on the clinical response of the patient.

SPECIFIC MANAGEMENT SCHEMA

In this section, four typical clinical problems associated with heart failure are discussed, and the method of appropriate management is presented.

ACUTE LOW CARDIAC OUTPUT DEVELOPING WITH COARCTATION OF THE AORTA

The clinical picture in a neonate younger than 2 weeks with critical coarctation of the aorta represents a situation demanding prompt recognition and stabilization before surgical repair or balloon dilatation. The sudden development of tachypnea and pallor with diminished pulses in this age group should immediately raise the suspicion of a lesion such as coarctation with ductus-dependent systemic blood flow.[104,105] These neonates require a venous access route so that prostaglandin E_1 can be given to dilate the ductus arteriosus and volume support provided. Because prostaglandin E_1 may produce apnea, the infant should be intubated and ventilated.

The symptoms of coarctation develop when the ductus constricts and the left ventricle is then subjected to an acute increase in afterload. The left ventricle can only dilate, and impaired contractility quickly ensues. These neonates require prompt inotropic support with a titratable agent such as dopamine. The clinical picture may be complicated by metabolic acidosis, as a reflection of the limited systemic perfusion. This is all reversible if prostaglandin E_1 can dilate the ductus arteriosus, minimizing the left ventricular obstruction by placing the infant in its fetal circulatory state (minus the placenta). Perfusion improves, the pH returns to normal, and ventricular systolic function is enhanced. When the neonate stabilizes, surgical repair of the coarctation or balloon dilatation of the obstructive area can take place. This approach has markedly improved the morbidity and mortality of coarctation in neonates. The pertinent management strategies in this type of presentation are summarized in Table 54–3.

TABLE 54–3
LOW PERFUSION STATE: COARCTATION OF THE AORTA
Venous access: ensure adequate vascular volume
Improve contractility and cardiac output: dopamine
Attempt to open ductus: prostaglandin E_1
Positive-pressure ventilation
Correct pH: sodium bicarbonate
When stable: surgical repair or possibly balloon dilatation

A LARGE-VOLUME LEFT-TO-RIGHT SHUNT (VENTRICULAR SEPTAL DEFECT, ATRIOVENTRICULAR SEPTAL DEFECT)

In this clinical situation, a 3-week-old to 2-month-old irritable tachypneic infant has poor feeding, a rapid heart rate, and a hyperdynamic precordium. A chest radiograph reveals an enlarged heart with prominent pulmonary vascular markings. Echocardiographic assessment reveals a large communication at the ventricular level with dilated cardiac chambers and normal ventricular contractility. The therapeutic challenge is to manage the pulmonary edema, limit the left-to-right shunt, provide nutrition, and allow the infant to grow in the hope that the defect may become smaller in time. To accomplish this, diuretic therapy with furosemide is initiated, and attempts are made to provide adequate calorie intake by concentrating the formula and offering frequent small-volume feedings, possibly by the nasogastric route. The use of digoxin in this situation is controversial because ventricular contractility is normal.[106, 107] We believe, however, that digoxin is indicated not primarily for its inotropic effect but for its ability to produce sympathoadrenal withdrawal and thereby lessen metabolic demands while preserving myocardial pumping function.

Two additional approaches can decrease the left-to-right shunt. The first uses a vasodilator; ACE inhibitors are now most common, although hydralazine has been used in the past. By decreasing the left-to-right shunt and favoring systemic blood flow, a dramatic clinical improvement may occur. A second approach is to transfuse red blood cells to raise the hemoglobin level to 12 to 14 g/dl, which also decreases pulmonary blood flow while preserving oxygen transport to the tissues.[108]

If there is evidence of respiratory failure ($PaCO_2 > 50$ mm Hg), mechanical ventilation with positive end-expiratory pressure may be required. This decreases metabolic requirements, lessens pulmonary edema, and aids in stabilizing the infant before operation.

In the management of this clinical problem, interventions may only make the patient a better candidate for surgical repair. If control of heart failure with resumption of growth cannot be achieved, operation is certainly indicated, sooner rather than later.

Table 54–4 summarizes our current management approach to the infant in congestive heart failure from a large-volume left-to-right shunt.

ACUTE LOW CARDIAC OUTPUT STATE AFTER A CARDIOPULMONARY BYPASS PROCEDURE

Another acute low cardiac output state may occur after cardiopulmonary bypass, even when repair has been excellent. Myocardial and circulatory support measures are required to ensure survival of the patient. This state has been labeled "stunned" myocardium and is associated with periods of myocardial ischemia that occur during the operation.[109] Echocardiographic studies of these patients provide evidence of decreased ventricular shortening and impaired diastolic function. Filling pressures tend to be elevated; oxygen extraction from the poorly perfused tissue is increased. Metabolic acidosis, with increased lactic acid concentration, may also develop.

Management of this situation requires prompt recognition and institution of inotropic support with titratable agents such as dopamine, dobutamine, or epinephrine after ensuring that there is adequate filling volume. Vasodilatation with sodium nitroprusside is valuable to decrease afterload and lessen the workload of the compromised ventricle. Ventilation must be continued to lessen pulmonary venous congestion and decrease metabolic demands. Careful attention must be paid when the patient is weaned from inotropes to ensure that improved contractility is maintained. Close monitoring is also required as the infant or child is weaned from ventilatory support, because signs of congestive heart failure may reappear when negative-pressure breathing takes place. In patients who cannot be weaned from bypass, various mechanical support devices (as cited before) have been used to maintain a satisfactory cardiac output until ventricular contractility improves. A management schema for the low-perfusion state that accompanies a cardiopulmonary bypass procedure is shown in Table 54–5.

DILATED CARDIOMYOPATHY

Congestive heart failure resulting from a dilated cardiomyopathy presents the pediatric cardiologist with a challenge. This patient may be any age with a myopathy arising from any one of a number of causes. Management is aimed at improving ventricular contractility, decreasing filling pressures and volumes, lessening pulmonary and systemic venous congestion, and preventing thromboembolic and arrhythmia complications. The endpoint may be a

---

TABLE 54–4

LARGE-VOLUME LEFT-TO-RIGHT SHUNT: VENTRICULAR SEPTAL DEFECT, ATRIOVENTRICULAR SEPTAL DEFECT

↓ Pulmonary and systemic venous congestion: furosemide
Pulmonary toilet: positioning, suction, chest percussion
Treat secondary infection: antibiotics
↓ Adrenergic background and maintain contractility: digoxin
↓ Left-to-right shunt: angiotensin-converting enzyme inhibitor, raise hemoglobin level
Attention to nutrition: concentrate formula, gavage feedings
Ventilation: if $PaCO_2 > 50$ mm Hg
Surgical repair: failure to improve clinically and resume growth

---

TABLE 54–5

LOW CARDIAC OUTPUT STATE AFTER CARDIOPULMONARY BYPASS PROCEDURE

Ensure adequate intravascular volume
Rule out cardiac tamponade: ultrasound evaluation and Doppler interrogation
Check for adequacy of repair: echo Doppler study
Improve myocardial contractility: dopamine, dobutamine, or epinephrine
Vasodilatation: sodium nitroprusside
Continue ventilation
Wean slowly: monitor perfusion when patient goes to unassisted ventilation and inotropes are discontinued
Poor response to above: mechanical-assist devices

TABLE 54–6

CHRONIC CONGESTIVE HEART FAILURE: DILATED
CARDIOMYOPATHY

Improve myocardial contractility: digoxin
Decrease venous congestion: furosemide
Vasodilatation: angiotensin-converting enzyme inhibition
Modify ventricular remodeling: angiotensin-converting enzyme
    inhibition
Decrease adrenergic drive: β_1 blockade, metoprolol
Anticoagulation: warfarin (Coumadin)
Antiarrhythmics: as indicated
Consider mechanical-assist devices as bridge to transplantation

---

mechanical-assist device as a bridge to transplantation unless cardiovascular performance improves. The current
therapeutic approach to a patient with a dilated cardiomyopathy is based on large controlled studies in primarily
adult populations.[80–82] The approach includes digoxin for
inotropic support, furosemide to provide control of pulmonary edema and systemic venous congestion, and ACE
inhibition to induce vasodilatation and modulation of the
ventricular remodeling process. Patients treated in this
fashion have improved exercise performance and lessened
morbidity and mortality. Nevertheless, return of normal
function is an exception.

β-Receptor blockade has been introduced into the drug
regimens. Relatively large controlled studies in adults appear to indicate substantial benefits from this approach
(see earlier).[91] The pediatric experience is limited, however. On the basis of adult experience and anecdotal pediatric reports, β-receptor blockade warrants cautious introduction into a pediatric cardiologist's armamentarium for a
patient with a dilated cardiomyopathy who is refractory to
the standard drug regimens. Informed consent is necessary. Table 54–6 summarizes the management schema for
chronic dilated cardiomyopathy.

OTHER SPECIFIC INTERVENTIONS

A few special therapeutic interventions aimed at specific
disease processes warrant citation. These include giving
digoxin or other antiarrhythmics to the mother to control a
supraventricular tachyarrhythmia in the fetus,[110] pacing
for heart block associated with compromised cardiac output, immune globulin for acute myocarditis,[111] transfusions for heart failure associated with anemia, and carnitine replacement for documented disorders of fatty acid
metabolism.[112] There is now experimental evidence that
probucol, a lipid-lowering drug with strong antioxidant
properties, may protect against doxorubicin-induced cardiomyopathy without interfering with the antitumor actions of the drug.[113]

MANAGEMENT OF DIASTOLIC HEART FAILURE

Diastolic heart failure rarely occurs in an isolated form but
may certainly accompany systolic failure. Pure diastolic
heart failure is defined hemodynamically as an elevated
end-diastolic pressure in the presence of a normal ventricular volume.[114] The ejection fraction is also normal. Unfortunately, therapy for this functional impairment is rarely
successful. β-Receptor and calcium channel blocking
agents have been tried with limited success. ACE inhibitors have also been used with the aim being to minimize myocardial fibrosis.[112] All of these agents have been
most effective in the treatment of systemic hypertension,
in which they appear to inhibit the maladaptive components of the ventricular hypertrophic response. Paramount
in any consideration of pure impairment of lusitropic function, however, is the importance of ruling out constrictive
pericarditis as the causative factor producing clinical signs
of systemic venous congestion.

FUTURE DIRECTIONS

As outlined by Katz,[115] heart failure was traditionally
viewed in terms of disturbed organ physiology. Later, focus
was placed on cellular biochemistry, which enhanced our
understanding of calcium cycling that is responsible for excitation-contraction coupling and how this process becomes impaired when the myocardium fails. Recently, the
focus has again shifted, this time to the growth processes
that accompany hypertrophy in the hemodynamically
overloaded myocardium, with special emphasis on altered
gene expression.

This new area that looks at disordered cell growth and
proliferation will be expanded with the potential development of new therapeutic agents targeted against maladaptive processes, thus prolonging survival and perhaps avoiding transplantation. In addition, we can expect further
elucidation of the role of intracellular Ca^{2+} handling in
cardiac failure, with studies of the recovery kinetics of
Ca^{2+} release mechanisms and the sequestration capacity
of the sarcoplasmic reticulum. These investigations also offer the potential for new pharmacologic interventions that
may modify systolic and diastolic performance. At the
same time, we should see improvement in cardiovascular
repair procedures, with operations being performed at a
younger age or possibly in the fetus. Myocardial preservation techniques will undoubtedly be improved and should
diminish the problems associated with myocardial stunning. Finally, innovative methods will be forthcoming that
will prevent transplant rejection and allow more transplants to be undertaken.

ACKNOWLEDGMENT

The authors wish to thank Ms. Barbara Shaw for her secretarial assistance in the preparation of this manuscript.

REFERENCES

1. Moller JH, Moodie DS, Blees M, et al: Symptomatic heart disease
   in infants. Comparison of three studies performed during
   1969–1987. Pediatr Cardiol 16:216, 1995.
2. Fyler DC, Buckley LP, Hellenbrand WE, et al: Report of the New
   England Regional Infant Cardiac Program. Pediatrics 65:375, 1980.

3. Scott DJ, Rigby ML, Miller GAH, et al: The presentation of symptomatic heart disease in infancy based on 10 years experience (1973–1982): Implications for the provision of services. Br Heart J 52:248, 1984.

4. Teitel D, Sidi D, Chin T, et al: Developmental changes in myocardial contractile reserve in the lamb. Pediatr Res 19:948, 1985.

5. Downing SE, Talner NS, Gardner TH: Ventricular function in the newborn lamb. Am J Physiol 208:931, 1965.

6. Nassar R, Reedy MC, Anderson PAW: Developmental changes in the ultrastructure and sarcomere shortening of the isolated cardiac myocyte. Circ Res 61:465, 1987.

7. Downing SE, Talner NS, Campbell AGM, et al: Influence of cardiac sympathetic nerve stimulation on ventricular function in the newborn lamb. Circ Res 25:417, 1969.

8. Lebowitz EA, Novick JS, Rudolph AM: Development of myocardial sympathetic innervation in the fetal lamb. Pediatr Res 6:887, 1972.

9. Friedman WF: The intrinsic properties of the developing heart. In Sonnenblick E, Lesch M, Friedman WF (eds): Neonatal Heart Disease. New York, Grune & Stratton, 1973, p 21.

10. Klitzner TS, Friedman WF: A diminished role for the sarcoplasmic reticulum in newborn myocardial contraction. Pediatr Res 26:98, 1989.

11. Sagawa K, Maughan L, Suga H, Sunagawa K: Clinical use and limitation of end-systolic pressure-volume relationship. In Sagawa K, Maughan L, Suga H, Sunagawa K (eds): Cardiac Contraction and the Pressure-Volume Relationship. New York, Oxford University Press, 1988, p 314.

12. Sagawa K: The ventricular pressure-volume diagram revisited. Circ Res 43:677, 1978.

13. Francis GS, Goldsmith SR, Levine TB, et al: The neurohumoral axis in congestive heart failure. Ann Intern Med 101:370, 1984.

14. Bristow MR, Kantrowitz NE, Ginsburg R, Fowler MB: β-Adrenergic function in heart muscle disease and heart failure. J Mol Cell Cardiol 17:41, 1985.

15. Ross RD, Daniels SR, Schwartz DC, et al: Plasma norepinephrine levels in infants and children in congestive heart failure. Am J Cardiol 39:911, 1987.

16. Lees MH: Catecholamine metabolite excretion of infants with heart failure. J Pediatr 69:259, 1966.

17. Rona G: Catecholamine cardiotoxicity. J Mol Cell Cardiol 17:291, 1985.

18. Ungerer M, Bohn M, Elce JS, et al: Altered expression of β-adrenergic receptor kinase and β$_1$-adrenergic receptors in the failing human heart. Circulation 87:454, 1993.

19. Bristow MR, Ginsburg R, Minohe W, et al: Decreased catecholamine sensitivity and β-adrenergic receptor density in failing human hearts. N Engl J Med 307:205, 1982.

20. Wu JR, Chang HR, Huang TY, et al: Reduction in lymphocyte beta-adrenergic receptor density in infants and children with heart failure secondary to congenital heart disease. Am J Cardiol 77:170, 1996.

21. Kozlik R, Kramer HH, Wicht H, et al: Beta-adrenoreceptor density on mononuclear leukocytes and right atrial myocardium in infants and children with congenital heart disease. Klin Wochenschr 69:910, 1991.

22. Benovic JL, Bouvier M, Caron MG, Lefkowitz RJ: Regulation of adenylyl cyclase–coupled β-adrenergic receptors. Annu Rev Cell Biol 4:405, 1988.

23. Katz AM: Angiotensin-II: Hemodynamic regulator or growth factor? J Mol Cell Cardiol 22:739, 1990.

24. Everett AD, Tufro-McReddie A, Fisher A, Gomez RA: Angiotensin receptor regulates hypertrophy and transforming growth factor-β1 expression. Hypertension 23:587, 1994.

25. Brecher P: Angiotensin-II and cardiac fibrosis. Trends Cardiovasc Med 6:193, 1996.

26. Brown JJ, Davies DL, Johnson VW, et al: Renin relationships in congestive heart failure, treated and untreated. Am Heart J 80:329, 1970.

27. Dzau VJ, Colucci WS, Hollenberg NK, Williams GH: Relation of renin-angiotensin-aldosterone system to clinical state in congestive heart failure. Circulation 63:645, 1981.

28. Baylen BG, Johnson G, Tsang R, et al: The occurrence of hyperaldosteronism in infants with congestive heart failure. Am J Cardiol 45:305, 1980.

29. Goldsmith SR, Francis GS, Cowley AW, et al: Increased plasma arginine vasopressin levels in patients with congestive heart failure. J Am Coll Cardiol 1:1385, 1983.

30. Schrier RW, Berl T, Anderson RJ: Osmotic and nonosmotic control of vasopressin release. Am J Physiol 236:F321, 1979.

31. Share L: Role of vasopressin in cardiovascular regulation. Physiol Rev 68:1248, 1988.

32. Stewart JM, Zeballos GA, Wool PK, et al: Variable arginine vasopressin levels in neonatal congestive heart failure. J Am Coll Cardiol 11:645, 1988.

33. Lehmann J: Neuropeptide Y: An overview. Drug Dev Res 19:329, 1990.

34. Maisel AS, Scottna, Motulsky HJ, et al: Elevation of plasma neuropeptide Y levels in congestive heart failure. Am J Med 86:43, 1989.

35. Hermann J, Scholz H, Doring V, et al: Increase in myocardial Gi-proteins in heart failure. Lancet 2:936, 1988.

36. Margulies KB, Hildebrad FL, Lerman A, et al: Increased endothelin in experimental heart failure. Circulation 82:2226, 1990.

37. Edwards BS, Zimmerman RS, Schwab TR, et al: Atrial stretch, not pressure is the principal determinant controlling the acute release of atrial natriuretic factor. Circ Res 62:191, 1988.

38. Scriven TA, Burnett JC: Effects of synthetic atrial natriuretic peptide on renal function and renin release in acute experimental heart failure. Circulation 72:892, 1985.

39. Kikuchi K, Nishioka K, Ueda J, et al: Relationship between atrial natriuretic polypeptide concentration and hemodynamic measurements in children with congenital heart diseases. J Pediatr 111:335, 1987.

40. Kubo SH, Rector TS, Bank AJ, et al: Endothelium dependent vasodilation is attenuated in patients with heart failure. Circulation 84:1589, 1991.

41. Woie L, Dickstein K, Kaada B: Increase in vasoactive intestinal polypeptides (VIP) by the angiotensin converting enzyme (ACE) inhibitor lisinopril in congestive heart failure. Relation to haemodynamic and hormonal changes. Gen Pharmacol 18:577, 1987.

42. Levine B, Kalman J, Mayer L, et al: Elevated circulating levels of tumor necrosis factor in severe chronic heart failure. N Engl J Med 323:236, 1990.

43. Versmold HT, Linderkamp O, Dohlemann C, et al: Oxygen transport in congenital heart disease: Influence of fetal hemoglobin, red cell pH, and 2,3-diphosphoglycerate. Pediatr Res 10:566, 1976.

44. Hutchison AA: Pathophysiology of hydrops fetalis. In Long WA (ed): Fetal and Neonatal Cardiology. Philadelphia, WB Saunders, 1990, p 197.

45. Stevens DC, Hilliard JK, Schreiner RL, et al: Supraventricular tachycardia with edema, ascites and hydrops in fetal sheep. Am J Obstet Gynecol 142:316, 1982.

46. Silverman NS, Kleinman CS, Rudolph AM, et al: Fetal atrioventricular valve insufficiency associated with nonimmune hydrops. A two-dimensional echocardiographic and pulsed Doppler ultrasound study. Circulation 72:825, 1985.

47. Borow KM, Green LH, Grossman W, et al: Left ventricular end-systolic stress-shortening and stress-length relations in humans: Normal values and sensitivity in inotropic state. Am J Cardiol 50:1301, 1982.

48. Marshall SA, Levine RA, Weyman AE: Echocardiography in cardiac research. In Fozzard HH, Jennings RB, Haber E, Katz AM: The Heart and Cardiovascular System, Scientific Foundations. New York, Raven Press, 1991, p 745.

49. Borow KM, Propper R, Bierman FZ, et al: The left ventricular end-systolic pressure dimension relation in patients with thalassemia major. Circulation 66:980, 1982.

50. Rokey R, Kuo LC, Zoghbi WH, et al: Determination of parameters of left ventricular diastolic filling with pulsed Doppler echocardiography: Comparison with cineangiography. Circulation 71:543, 1985.

51. Snider AR, Meliones JN, Minich L: Doppler echocardiographic evaluation of diastolic dysfunction in children. In Gaasch W, LeWinter MM: Left Ventricular Diastolic Dysfunction and Heart Failure. Philadelphia, Lea & Febiger, 1994, p 408.

52. Apkon M: Pathophysiology of hydrops fetalis. Semin Perinatol 19:437, 1995.

53. Kleinman CS, Donnerstein RL, De Vore GR, et al: Fetal echocardiography for evaluation of in utero congestive heart failure. N Engl J Med 306:568, 1982.

54. Hornberger LK, Sahn DJ, Leinman CS, et al: Tricuspid valve disease with significant tricuspid insufficiency in the fetus: Diagnosis and outcome. J Am Coll Cardiol 17:167, 1991.

55. Reed KL, Sahn DS, Scagnelli WS, et al: Doppler echocardiographic studies of diastolic function in the human fetal heart: Changes during gestation. J Am Coll Cardiol 8:391, 1986.

56. Talner NS, Sanyal SK, Halloran KW, et al: Congestive heart failure in infancy: Abnormalities in blood gases and acid-base equilibrium. Pediatrics 35:20, 1965.

57. Talner NS: Heart failure. In Emmanouilides GC, Riemenschneider TA, Allen HA, Gutgesell HP (eds): Moss & Adams Heart Disease in Infants, Children and Adolescents, 5th ed. Baltimore, Williams & Wilkins, 1995, p 1746.

58. Benzing G III, Schubert W, Hug G, et al: Simultaneous hypoglycemia and acute congestive heart failure. Circulation 40:209, 1969.

59. Burnard ED, James LS: Failure of the heart after cardiac asphyxia at birth. Pediatrics 28:545, 1961.

60. Bucciarelli R, Nelson RM, Egan EA III, et al: Transient tricuspid insufficiency of the newborn: A form of myocardial dysfunction in stressed newborns. Pediatrics 59:330, 1977.

61. Adams JE III, Bodor GS, Davila-Roman VG, et al: Cardiac troponin-I: A marker with high specificity for cardiac injury. Circulation 88:101, 1993.

62. Webber SA, Boyle GJ, Jaffe R, et al: Role of right ventricular endomyocardial biopsy in infants and children with suspected or possible myocarditis. Br Heart J 72:360, 1994.

63. Martin AB, Webber S, Fricker FJ: Acute myocarditis: Rapid diagnosis by polymerase chain reaction (PCR) in children. Circulation 90:330, 1994.

64. Stanger P, Lucas R, Edwards J: Anatomic factors causing respiratory distress in a cyanotic cardiac disease: Special reference to bronchial obstruction. Pediatrics 44:760, 1969.

65. Ferguson DW, Berg WJ, Sanders JS, et al: Sympathoinhibitory responses in digitalis glycosides in heart failure patients. Direct evidence from sympathetic neural recordings. Circulation 80:65, 1989.

66. Akera T, Brody TM: The role of Na^+,K^+-ATPase in the inotropic action of digitalis. Pharmacol Rev 29:110, 1978.

67. Hayes CJ, Butler VP Jr, Gersony WM: Serum digoxin studies in infants and children. Pediatrics 52:561, 1973.

68. Baim DS, McDowell AV, Cherniles J, et al: Evaluation of a new bipyridine inotropic agent—milrinone—in patients with severe congestive heart failure. N Engl J Med 309:748, 1983.

69. Bhatt-Mehta V, Nahata MC: Dopamine and dobutamine in pediatric therapy. Pharmacology 9:303, 1989.

70. Opie LH: Drugs for the Heart, 3rd ed. Philadelphia, WB Saunders, 1991, p 142.

71. Driscoll DJ, Gillette PC, Duff DF, et al: Hemodynamic effects of dobutamine in children. Am J Cardiol 43:581, 1979.

72. LeJemtel TH, Keung E, Sonnenblick EH, et al: Amrinone: A new non-glycosidic non-adrenergic cardiotonic agent effective in the treatment of intractable myocardial failure in man. Circulation 59:1098, 1979.

73. Thier SO: Diuretic mechanisms as a guide to therapy. Hosp Pract 22:61, 1987.

74. Breyer J, Jacobson HR: Molecular mechanisms of diuretic agents. Annu Rev Med 41:265, 1990.

75. Brater DC, Chennavasin P, Day B, et al: Bumetanide and furosemide. Clin Pharmacol Ther 34:207, 1983.

76. Kiyingi A, Field MJ, Pawsey CC, et al: Metolazone in treatment of severe refractory congestive cardiac failure. Lancet 335:29, 1990.

77. Defronzo RA, Thier SO: Pathophysiologic approach to hyponatremia. Arch Intern Med 140:897, 1980.

78. Friedman WF, George BL: Medical progress—treatment of congestive heart failure by altering loading conditions of the heart. J Pediatr 106:697, 1985.

79. Artman M, Graham TP: Guidelines for vasodilator therapy of congestive heart failure in infants and children. Am Heart J 113:994, 1987.

80. The Captopril Multicenter Research Group: A cooperative multicenter study of captopril in congestive heart failure: Hemodynamic effects and long-term response. Am Heart J 110:439, 1985.

81. The Consensus Trial Study Group: Effects of enalapril on mortality in severe congestive heart failure: Results of the cooperative North Scandinavia enalapril survival study (consensus). N Engl J Med 316:1429, 1987.

82. The SOLVD Investigators: Effect of enalapril on survival in patients with reduced ejection fractions and congestive heart failure. N Engl J Med 325:293, 1991.

83. Webster MW, Neutze JM, Calder AL: Acute hemodynamic effects of converting enzyme inhibition in children with intracardiac shunts. Pediatr Cardiol 13:129, 1992.

84. Montigny M, Davignon A, Fouron JC, et al: Captopril in infants in congestive heart failure secondary to a large ventricular left-to-right shunt. Am J Cardiol 63:631, 1989.

85. Lewis AB, Chabot M: The effect of treatment with angiotensin converting enzyme inhibitors on survival of pediatric patients with dilated cardiomyopathy. Pediatr Cardiol 14:9, 1993.

86. Stern H, Weil J, Genz T, et al: Captopril in children with dilated cardiomyopathy: Acute and long-term effects in a prospective study of hemodynamic and hormonal effects. Pediatr Cardiol 11:22, 1990.

87. Bengur AR, Beekman RH, Rocchini AP, et al: Acute hemodynamic effects of captopril in children with a congestive or restrictive cardiomyopathy. Circulation 83:523, 1991.

88. Benzing G III, Helmsworth JA, Schrieber JT, et al: Nitroprusside after open heart surgery. Circulation 54:467, 1976.

89. Beekman RH, Rocchini AP, Dick M II, et al: Vasodilator therapy in children: Acute and chronic effects in children with left ventricular dysfunction or mitral regurgitation. Pediatrics 73:43, 1984.

90. Anderson JL, Gilbert EM, O'Connell JB, et al: Long term (2 year) beneficial effects of beta receptor blockade with bucindolol in patients with dilated cardiomyopathy. J Am Coll Cardiol 17:1373, 1991.

91. Eichhorn EJ: Paradox of beta-adrenergic blockade for the management of congestive heart failure. Am J Med 92:527, 1992.

92. Bristow MR: Physiologic and pharmacologic rationales for clinical management of chronic heart failure with beta-blocking agents. Am J Cardiol 71:12C, 1993.

93. Shaddy RE, Olsen SL, Bristow MR, et al: Efficacy and safety of metopril in the treatment of doxorubicin-induced cardiomyopathy in pediatric patients. Am Heart J 129:197, 1995.

94. Lees MH, Bristow JD, Griswold HE, et al: Relative hypermetabolism in infants with congenital heart disease and undernutrition. Pediatrics 36:183, 1965.

95. Pennington DG, Swartz MT: Circulatory support in infants and children. Ann Thorac Surg 55:233, 1993.

96. Jensen C, Hill C: Mechanical support for congestive heart failure in infants and children. Crit Care Nurs Clin North Am 6:165, 1994.

97. Veasy LG, Blalock RC, Orth JL, et al: Intra-aortic balloon pumping in infants and children. Circulation 68:1095, 1983.

98. Dunn JM: The use of intra-aortic balloon pumping in pediatric patients. Cardiac Assists 5:2, 1989.

99. Park JK, Hsu DT, Gersony WM: Intra-aortic balloon pump management of refractory congestive heart failure in children. Pediatr Cardiol 14:19, 1993.

100. Raithel SC, Pennington DG, Boegner E, et al: Extracorporeal membrane oxygenation in children after heart surgery. Circulation 86:305, 1992.

101. delNido PJ, Armitage JM, Fricker FJ, et al: Extracorporeal membrane oxygenation support as a bridge to pediatric heart transplantation. Circulation 90:66, 1994.

102. Takano H, Nakatani T, Tanaka Y: Clinical experience with ventricular assist systems in Japan. Ann Thorac Surg 55:250, 1993.

103. Heckjr HA, Doty DB: Assisted circulation by phasic external lower body compression. Circulation 64:118, 1981.

104. Rudolph AM, Heymann MA, Spitznas U: Hemodynamic considerations in the development of narrowing of the aorta. Am J Cardiol 30:514, 1972.

105. Talner NS, Berman MA: Postnatal development of coarctation of the aorta. The role of the ductus arteriosus. Pediatrics 56:559, 1975.

106. Alpert BS, Barfield JA, Taylor WJ: Reappraisal of digitalis in infants with left-to-right shunts and heart failure. J Pediatr 106:66, 1985.

107. Kimball TR, Daniels SR, Meyer RD, et al: Effect of digoxin on contractility and symptoms in infants with a large ventricular septal defect. N Engl J Med 208:363, 1983.

108. Lister G, Hellenbrand WE, Kleinman CS, et al: Physiologic effects of increasing hemoglobin concentration in left-to-right shunting in infants with ventricular septal defects. N Engl J Med 306:502, 1982.

109. Braunwald E, Kloner I: The stunned myocardium: Prolonged ischemic ventricular dysfunction. Circulation 66:1146, 1982.

110. Kleinman CS, Copel JA, Weinstein EM, et al: In utero diagnosis and treatment of fetal supraventricular tachycardia. Semin Perinatol 9:113, 1985.

111. Drucker NA, Colan SD, Lewis AB, et al: Gammaglobulin treatment of acute myocarditis in the pediatric population. Circulation 89:252, 1994.

112. Waber LJ, Valle D, Neill D, et al: Carnitine deficiency presenting as familial cardiomyopathy: A treatable defect in carnitine transport. J Pediatr 101:700, 1982.

113. Siveski-Iliskovic N, Hill M, Chow DA, Singal PK: Probucol protects against Adriamycin cardiomyopathy without interfering with its antitumor effect. Circulation 91:10, 1997.

114. Levine HJ, Gaasch W: Clinical recognition and treatment of diastolic dysfunction and heart failure. *In* Gaasch W, LeWinter MM: Left Ventricular Diastolic Dysfunction and Heart Failure. Philadelphia, Lea & Febiger, 1991, p 439.

115. Katz AM: The cardiomyopathy of overload: An unnatural growth response in the hypertrophied heart. Ann Intern Med 121:363, 1994.

CHAPTER 55
ARRHYTHMIAS

VICTORIA VETTER

ELECTROPHYSIOLOGIC MECHANISMS OF PEDIATRIC ARRHYTHMIAS

Cardiac arrhythmias result from abnormal impulse formation, abnormal impulse conduction, or a combination of both[1-3] (Table 55–1).

All cardiac fibers are excitable. Certain cells in the specialized conducting system in the sinus and atrioventricular (AV) nodes depolarize spontaneously until threshold potential is attained and an action potential is initiated. This ability to depolarize spontaneously is called automaticity. In automatic fibers, the outward potassium current decreases or an inward sodium current increases with time, resulting in gradual depolarization. The rate at which normally automatic cells fire is controlled primarily by the activity of the autonomic nervous system and secondarily by changes in the local environment, including potassium concentration, pH, PO_2, and extracellular calcium concentration. The action potentials of both the sinus and the AV nodes are secondary to slow inward calcium channel–dependent currents.

Abnormal automaticity occurs when the normal sinus pacemaker is depressed or ectopic pacemakers compete with the sinus node. Depression of sinus node automaticity by an increase in vagal activity may shift the site of origin of the cardiac impulse to other automatic cells proximal to the AV node or to cells in the His-Purkinje system that are not strongly influenced by vagal activity. Similarly, there may be an increase in automaticity at an ectopic site as a result of a local increase in sympathetic efferent activity or a local change in the cells that decreases membrane potential as from ischemia or stretch. Ectopic atrial tachycardia and automatic ventricular tachycardia (VT) are manifestations of abnormal automaticity. Sympathetic stimulation or catecholamine excess may result in ectopic impulse initiation that competes with a normal sinus node. Triggered activity results from a second depolarization that either occurs during repolarization (early afterdepolarization) or occurs after repolarization (delayed afterdepolarization). With delayed afterdepolarization, the slope of phase 4 is increased as the rate of stimulus is increased. This mechanism may be responsible for digoxin toxic rhythms[4] and some VTs. Early afterdepolarizations can be associated with hypoxia, ischemia, hypokalemia, cesium, catecholamines, and some antiarrhythmic drugs with proarrhythmic effects, such as the class I agents. Early afterdepolarizations may be responsible for the torsades de pointes type of ventricular arrhythmia, especially that associated with antiarrhythmic agents.

Abnormal impulse conduction is another mechanism that is responsible for arrhythmias. Conduction velocity of the cardiac impulse is determined by the level of resting membrane potential, the amplitude and upstroke velocity of the action potential, and the passive or cable properties of the fibers themselves.[5] Abnormal conduction occurs when conduction proceeds along abnormal pathways, as in preexcitation, such as in Wolff-Parkinson-White (WPW) syndrome and other reentrant pathways, or when normal conduction is blocked as in sinoatrial block or AV conduction block.

Reentry is a form of abnormal impulse conduction. Three conditions are required for reentry to occur: (1) closed circuit of conduction, (2) unidirectional block in the circuit, and (3) slow conduction. A closed circuit and reentry may exist in the sinus node, atrium, AV node, accessory pathways, or Purkinje fibers of the ventricle. Reentry within the AV node illustrates this concept. Mines first described AV nodal reentry in 1913,[6] and Moe and colleagues[7] described dual AV nodal pathways in 1956. By convention, dual pathways have been labeled alpha and beta. The alpha pathway is slower conducting but has a shorter refractory period than the faster-conducting beta pathway. The application of this concept to human supraventricular tachycardia (SVT) is shown in Figure 55–1.[8] During sinus rhythm (*panel A*), the atrial impulse traverses the faster-conducting beta pathway to produce a single QRS complex. The impulse simultaneously travels down the alpha (slow) pathway, reaching the His bundle shortly after it has been depolarized and rendered refractory by the impulse that was conducted down the beta pathway. In response to an atrial premature depolarization (*panel B*), the impulse is blocked in the beta pathway as a result of its longer refractory period and proceeds slowly down the alpha pathway. If conduction down the alpha pathway is slow enough to allow the previously refractory beta pathway time to recover, an atrial echo results. If the alpha pathway has sufficient time to recover, sustained AV nodal reentrant tachycardia (AVNRT) results. If conduction delay and refractoriness in both pathways are appropriate, a continuously circulating wave front of electrical activity ensues, resulting in a reentrant tachycardia. AV nodal reentry probably involves the approaches to the AV node rather than only the AV node. Simultaneous abnormalities of impulse generation and conduction result in abnormal rhythms, such as parasystole.[9]

TABLE 55-1

MECHANISMS OF ARRHYTHMIAS

Disorders of Impulse Formation

Enhanced automaticity
  Sinus tachycardia
Abnormal automaticity
  Automatic or ectopic atrial tachycardia
  Automatic ventricular tachycardia
Triggered activity
  Early afterdepolarizations: pause-dependent torsades de pointes
  Delayed afterdepolarizations: digoxin toxicity, ventricular tachycardia

Disorders of Impulse Conduction

Reentry
  Sinus node reentry
  Intra-atrial reentry, atrial flutter, atrial fibrillation
  WPW syndrome with AV reentry, atriofascicular, nodofascicular, nodoventricular
  AV reentry with concealed accessory pathways
  AV nodal reentry
  Bundle branch reentrant VT
  Reentrant VT

VT = ventricular tachycardia; AV = atrioventricular; WPW = Wolff-Parkinson-White syndrome.

ELECTROPHYSIOLOGY

CARDIAC ACTION POTENTIAL

The cardiac action potential (Fig. 55-2)[8] has five phases: phase 0—upstroke or rapid depolarization; phase 1—early rapid repolarization; phase 2—plateau; phase 3—final rapid repolarization; and phase 4—resting membrane potential and diastolic depolarization. The phases result from passive fluxes of ions through specific channels and are regulated by their individual electrochemical gradients resulting from active ion pumps and exchange mechanisms. Each ion has its own specific channel. Sodium and calcium channels provide the depolarizing currents, and potassium channels, the repolarizing currents. Sodium channels are referred to as fast channels, and calcium channels are referred to as slow channels, although the rapidity relates to the increased numbers of sodium channels.[3, 10]

A typical atrial or ventricular cardiac myocardial cell has a resting membrane potential of -90 mV with respect to the outside of the cell as a result of the high permeability of K^+, which is the major ion that determines the resting potential. Sodium is pumped out of the cell, and K^+ is pumped into the cell by the Na^+/K^+ pump against their electrochemical gradients, allowing intracellular K^+ to remain high and intracellular Na^+ low. In diastole, the cell membrane is permeable to K^+ and is relatively impermeable to Na^+, Cl^-, and Ca^{2+}. The rapid Na^+ current is responsible for activation of the atrial and ventricular myocardial cells. The slow Ca^{2+} current is responsible for activation in depolarized cells exhibiting the slow response and for activation in sinus and AV nodal cells.[11, 12]

PHASE 0—UPSTROKE OR RAPID DEPOLARIZATION. The rapid upstroke in atrial and ventricular muscle and His-Purkinje fibers of the action potential is caused by a sudden increase in the membrane conductance to Na^+, generating a fast sodium current. The increase in Na^+ con-

Atrium

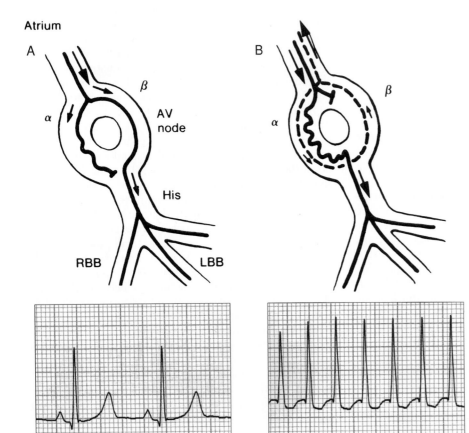

FIGURE 55-1

Schematic of dual pathways of atrioventricular (AV) node. *A,* Normal conduction, resulting in normal sinus rhythm. *B,* Reentrant circuit, resulting in AV nodal reentrant SVT. RBB = right bundle branch; LBB = left bundle branch. (Adapted from Vetter VL: Arrhythmias. *In* Holbrook PR [ed]: Textbook of Pediatric Critical Care. Philadelphia, WB Saunders, 1993, p 384.)

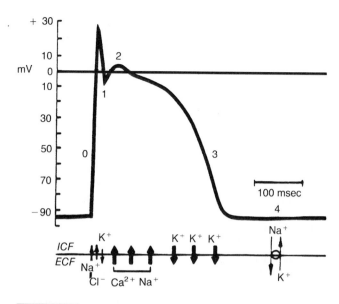

FIGURE 55–2

Schematic of action potential of ventricular myocardium showing ionic fluxes and phases of depolarization and repolarization. ICF = intracellular fluid; ECF = extracellular fluid. (From Vetter VL: Arrhythmias. *In* Holbrook PR [ed]: Textbook of Pediatric Critical Care. Philadelphia, WB Saunders, 1993, p 384.)

ductance results from the opening of voltage-gated Na^+ channels with rapid depolarization opening the channels, whereas maintained depolarization inactivates them. The steady-state availability of Na^+ channels is regulated by resting potential such that at -90 mV, more than 80% of Na^+ channels are available for activation, whereas at -60 mV (a level present in ischemic myocardium), only 10 to 20% of Na^+ channels are available for activation. Larger Na^+ currents producing rapid upstroke velocity and resulting in more rapidly propagating waveforms are seen in myocardium with high (-90 mV) resting potential. Tissues with lower resting potential, such as the sinus and AV nodes and ischemic tissue, have slower velocity and propagating waveforms. During phase 0, when the membrane is depolarized to potentials positive to -40 mV, a slower inward current is activated that is carried by the opening of Ca^{2+} channels.

PHASE 1—EARLY RAPID REPOLARIZATION. Rapid repolarization of the membrane to zero millivolts occurs with partial inactivation of the rapid inward Na^+ current and activation of a transient outward K^+ current and possibly a Cl^- current at potentials positive to zero millivolts. A slow inward Ca^{2+} current is activated at membrane potentials positive to -40 mV mediated by highly selective Ca^{2+} channels, which inactivate slowly, maintaining the plateau. Phases 0 and 1 occur during inscription of the QRS complex of the electrocardiogram (ECG).

PHASE 2—PLATEAU. The plateau phase lasts several hundred milliseconds, during which time conductance of the membrane to all ions is low. The primary inward current supporting the plateau is the Ca^{2+} current. Compared with the resting state, Na^+ and Ca^{2+} conductance are significantly enhanced and K^+ permeability is markedly di-

minished during the plateau phase. The Ca^{2+} current provides the trigger for the release of Ca^{2+} from the sarcoplasmic reticulum, resulting in activation of myofilaments providing the link between excitation and contraction. At the end of phase 2, when a sufficient number of Na^+ and Ca^{2+} channels are inactivated, the cell becomes inexcitable, and the absolute or effective refractory period occurs. As the membrane becomes partially repolarized and more Na^+ channels become available, a phase known as the relative refractory period occurs. Although an action potential may be initiated during this interval, its rate of rise and velocity of propagation are slow, and the action potential duration is shorter. This results in slow aberrant conduction or block. Phase 2 occurs during the ST segment of the ECG.

PHASE 3—FINAL RAPID REPOLARIZATION. Repolarization occurs with inactivation of the inward Ca^{2+} current and activation of an outward K^+ current (delayed rectifier), resulting in a net efflux of positive charges shifting the membrane toward a more negative potential. This results in the activation of inwardly rectifying K^+ current, which is the dominant current of the resting membrane.

PHASE 4—RESTING MEMBRANE POTENTIAL AND DIASTOLIC DEPOLARIZATION. In atrial and ventricular muscle cells, the resting membrane potential remains stable throughout diastole, controlled by the inwardly rectifying K^+ channel. In pacemaker cells, the membrane potential gradually depolarizes, resulting in a spontaneous action potential when the threshold level is reached. The slow diastolic, or phase 4, depolarization is affected by numerous factors. The slope of diastolic depolarization determines the rate of pacemaker firing. For example, sympathetic stimulation (catecholamines) increases the slope of phase 4, or diastolic depolarization, whereas parasympathetic stimulation (acetylcholine) decreases the slope. Many ionic currents control the pacemaker potential.

Antiarrhythmic agents affect resting membrane potential, threshold potential, and phase 4 depolarization.[13]

SPECIFIC ARRHYTHMIAS

GENERAL PRINCIPLES

Appropriate management of arrhythmia disturbance in an infant or child requires correct and rapid diagnosis of the specific type of arrhythmia.

When an abnormal rhythm is suspected, a 12-lead ECG should be obtained. The ECG should be examined to determine whether the heart rate is abnormally high or low and whether the mechanism is of sinus or abnormal origin. The relationship of the P wave to the QRS, the P wave axis, the PR interval, and the QRS duration and axis should be considered in differentiating between sinus and abnormal rhythm.

A rapid or slow rhythm with a normal P wave axis and PR interval is most likely of sinus origin. The normal heart rate ranges for age are given in Table 55–2.[14]

If the rhythm is not of sinus origin, the physician must determine its origin. Is it supraventricular or ventricular?

TABLE 55–2

NORMAL HEART RATES

Age	Resting Heart Rate (bpm)
<1 day	94–155
1–7 days	90–165
8–30 days	105–185
1–3 months	115–180
3–6 months	105–185
6–12 months	105–175
1–3 years	90–160
3–5 years	65–145
5–8 years	65–135
8–12 years	55–125
12–16 years	55–120

Data from Davignon A, Rautaharju P, Boisselle E, et al: ECG standards for children. Pediatr Cardiol 1:133, 1979.

TABLE 55–3

WIDE QRS–COMPLEX TACHYCARDIA

Supraventricular Origin

Antidromic supraventricular tachycardia
Atrial flutter or fibrillation with aberrancy
Nodofascicular or nodoventricular accessory pathways with reciprocating tachycardia
Orthodromic reciprocating tachycardia with aberrancy
Supraventricular tachycardia with pre-existing bundle branch block

Ventricular Origin

Ventricular tachycardia

Although most narrow-complex tachycardias are of supraventricular origin and most wide-complex tachycardias are of ventricular origin, wide-complex tachycardias do include a number of conditions (Table 55–3).[15] The other confounding issue is that many ventricular rhythms in infants have a QRS complex that is only 80 or 90 milliseconds in duration, making the distinction between wide and narrow complex difficult until sinus rhythm is present for comparison. Many patients who have had a cardiac operation have right bundle branch block (RBBB) or left bundle branch block (LBBB). Sinus tachycardia in these patients, especially if associated with first-degree AV block, appears as a wide QRS tachycardia with a P wave that is difficult or impossible to visualize and is often on top of the T wave.

NONCRITICAL ARRHYTHMIAS

Certain arrhythmias are critical because they produce hemodynamic instability, and others, because of their potential to do so. Before instituting a therapy that may complicate or worsen the patient's condition, the physician must be certain that the clinical problem warrants intervention.

Premature ventricular contractions do not need intervention unless they are frequent enough to interfere with the cardiac output, are closely coupled, frequently fall on the T wave in a patient judged to be vulnerable to such occurrences (long QT syndrome [LQTS]), or occur in runs that result in hemodynamic instability.

Premature atrial contractions or premature junctional contractions rarely require intervention unless they are

blocked and cause bradycardia in an infant or induce frequent episodes of SVT.

First- and second-degree AV block can usually be observed without necessitating intervention unless symptoms or long pauses occur, a medication is found to be responsible, or progression to high-grade second-degree block or third-degree block is noted.

CHRONIC OR CRITICAL ARRHYTHMIAS

Arrhythmias become critical because of their hemodynamic effects. Certain arrhythmias are likely to produce instability and are discussed in the following sections. Others require attention because of their recurrence, frequency, or interference with daily activities.

Supraventricular Tachycardia
ELECTROCARDIOGRAPHIC MANIFESTATIONS
Paroxysmal SVT, previously known as paroxysmal atrial tachycardia, is the most common significant arrhythmia in children. Supraventricular tachycardia describes a group of arrhythmias with similar electrocardiographic manifestations but different mechanisms and includes AV reentry secondary to an accessory pathway (AVRT), atrioventricular nodal reentrant tachycardia (AVNRT), primary atrial tachycardia, and junctional ectopic tachycardia (JET). A typical example of SVT is shown in Figure 55–3. The rate of the tachycardia in infants ranges from 220 to 320 bpm and in older children ranges from 150 to 250 bpm. In most instances, SVT presents as a narrow-complex tachycardia. Sometimes, a wide QRS from aberrancy may occur during the first few complexes of the tachycardia, with a narrow-complex SVT subsequently occurring at a similar or slightly faster rate. With a wide QRS tachycardia, change in rate may help identify the site of an accessory pathway, if that is the mechanism of the tachycardia (Fig. 55–4). A bundle branch block on the same side as the reentrant accessory pathway prolongs the cycle length of the tachycardia. Other causes of wide-QRS SVT are listed in Table 55–3.

Atrioventricular block may occur during atrial tachycardia or AVNRT. Atrioventricular reentrant tachycardia requires 1:1 AV conduction, which usually occurs in AVNRT as well. In many instances, this characteristic distinguishes these forms of SVT from automatic or primary atrial tachycardia, JET, and VT. Supraventricular tachycardia terminates suddenly, either in the anterograde limb (after a P wave) or in the retrograde limb (after the QRS with no P wave) of the circuit. When adenosine or verapamil is used to cause block in the AV node, the tachycardia blocks in the AV node after the P wave is inscribed. Rarely, 2:1 AV conduction occurs in AVNRT. The reentrant circuit in AVNRT is confined to the AV node and contiguous atrium such that the ventricle and most of the atrium are not necessary for the continuation of the tachycardia. In AVRT, the ventricle and His-Purkinje system are integral parts of the circuit. Atrioventricular reentrant tachycardia and AVNRT may have electrocardiographic manifestations of rapid ventriculoatrial (VA) conduction, resulting in a short VA interval with a short RP interval and sometimes an obscured P wave, or a long RP interval (slow VA conduction) and a P wave that is visible but with a vector that indicates it is not

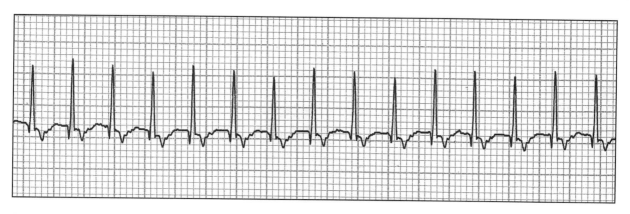

FIGURE 55–3

Lead II electrocardiographic rhythm strip showing supraventricular tachycardia at a rate of 225 beats. Narrow QRS complexes and retrograde inverted P wave.

from the sinoatrial node. With AVNRT, the RP is short in the typical form, and the P wave may not be visible or may be seen in the terminal portion of the QRS complex or early ST segment, particularly in lead V_1 (Fig. 55–5). The atypical form of AVNRT with slow retrograde conduction has a longer RP interval. In most instances, AVRT has a visible P wave in the ST segment of the T wave from the retrograde VA conduction.

Children with a form of SVT known as permanent junctional reciprocating tachycardia (PJRT) have a normal PR interval and a long RP interval. The P wave axis is inverted in leads II, III, and aVF (Fig. 55–6). A negative P wave in lead I suggests a left atrial insertion site of the accessory pathway but does not rule out a primary left atrial tachycardia. Most SVTs are paroxysmal, starting and stopping suddenly, often preceded by a premature atrial or ventricular contraction or less frequently by sinus acceleration.[16]

Atrioventricular reentrant tachycardia is more likely than AVNRT to be started by premature ventricular contractions.

In SVT secondary to AVNRT or AVRT with a concealed accessory pathway, the ECG shows a normal PR interval and P wave axis and a normal QRS duration and axis when the patient is in sinus rhythm. If the PR interval is short with a narrow QRS duration, an atriofascicular pathway should be suspected. A short PR interval with a slurred upstroke or downstroke to the QRS (delta wave) and a wide QRS signifies the WPW anomaly.

CLINICAL CORRELATIONS

The incidence of SVT is estimated to be one in 250 to 1000 children.[17] It occurs most commonly in males younger than 4 months of age. Predisposing factors or associations are present in more than half of the patients and include

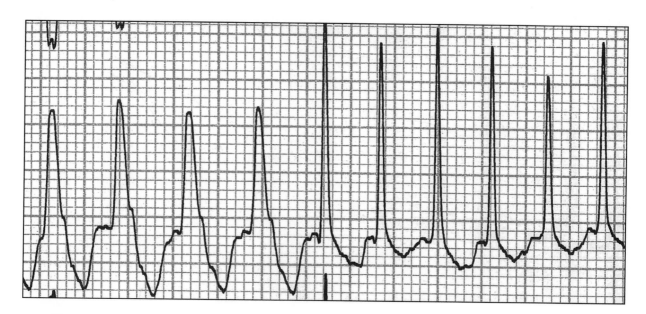

FIGURE 55–4

Example of bundle branch aberrancy occurring at initiation of supraventricular tachycardia. Narrow QRS tachycardia is faster, indicating location of accessory pathway in same ventricle as bundle branch block.

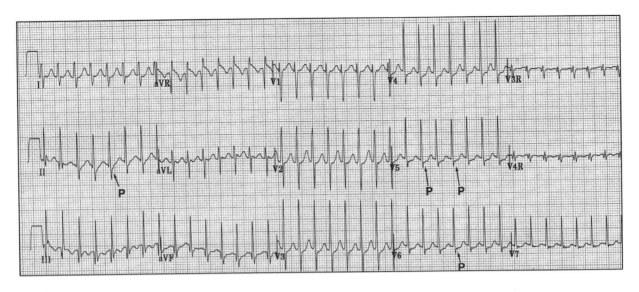

FIGURE 55–5

Electrocardiographic example of atrioventricular nodal reentrant supraventricular tachycardia at a rate of 214 beats per minute. P wave in ST segment immediately after QRS complex.

infection, fever, and drug exposure (20 to 24%); WPW syndrome (10 to 22%); and congenital heart disease (20 to 23%). Ventricular septal defect, Ebstein anomaly of the tricuspid valve, corrected transposition of the great arteries, and cardiomyopathies are the most common unoperated lesions associated with SVT. The most common postoperative congenital heart lesions are complete transposition of the great arteries, atrial septal defect, and AV septal defect. Supraventricular tachycardia is also common in those with a Fontan repair. The 40 to 50% of patients without an asso-

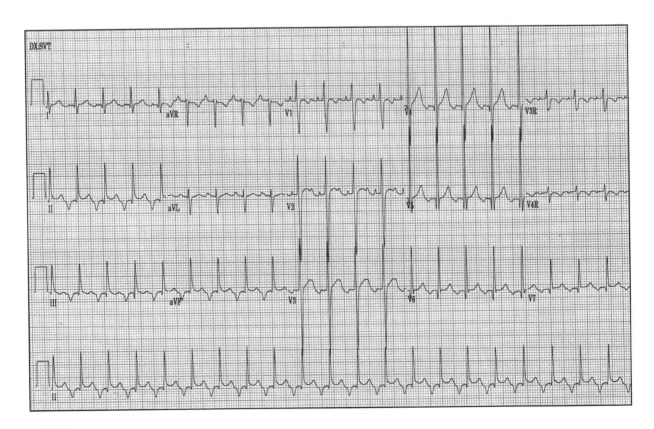

FIGURE 55–6

Example of the permanent junctional reciprocating tachycardia form of supraventricular tachycardia. Negative retrograde P waves in leads II, III, aVF and V_5, V_6, V_7, as well as long RP interval.

ciated condition are considered to have idiopathic SVT, but most have a concealed accessory pathway or AV nodal reentry.

In SVT, congestive heart failure occurs most commonly in infants younger than 4 months of age and is unlikely to occur in children with a normal heart during the first 24 hours of the tachycardia. Children with an extremely fast rate or underlying abnormalities of the heart or other systems are less tolerant of the arrhythmia and may present with congestive heart failure sooner after the onset of SVT.

SIGNS AND SYMPTOMS

Children with SVT experience palpitations, generally described as a rapid heart rate with sudden onset and either sudden or gradual cessation. Although the SVT stops suddenly, the catecholamine elevation that often accompanies SVT may increase the underlying sinus rate sufficiently that the sinus rate remains elevated to 130 to 160 beats per minute (bpm) after the SVT stops. The perceived tachycardia subsides gradually as the sinus tachycardia slows. Children with SVT have throbbing or pain in their neck and a sensation of fluttering or pain in their chest. They may have abdominal pain, which may be associated with nausea or vomiting. These patients may feel dizzy or lightheaded or may lose consciousness (syncope) as a result of the hypotension that accompanies the SVT.

The signs of SVT include tachycardia of 200 to 320 bpm in the infant and 150 to 300 bpm in the child or adolescent. Tachypnea, dyspnea, pallor and diaphoresis, poor feeding, irritability, and lethargy may occur in an infant in congestive heart failure resulting from SVT. In addition, older children may develop exercise intolerance and easy fatigability.

SPECIFIC MECHANISMS OF SUPRAVENTRICULAR TACHYCARDIA

Electrophysiologic mechanisms of SVT include reentry, as discussed earlier, or enhanced automaticity of the atrial or AV junctional tissues. The most common mechanisms of

supraventricular arrhythmias in children include concealed bypass tracts with SVT,[18] WPW syndrome with SVT,[19] AVNRT, atrial ectopic tachycardia, and JET. Atrial flutter or fibrillation, not uncommon in children, is discussed separately.

The mechanism of SVT is somewhat age dependent. Gillette[20] reported that more than 90% of infants had AV reentrant SVT secondary to an accessory pathway. In adolescents, he found that one third had AVNRT, and most of the remainder had AVRT.[20] In another study of 137 patients, the mechanism of SVT was an accessory connection in 73% (48% of these had preexcitation), primary atrial tachycardia in 14%, and AV nodal reentry in 13%. SVT utilizing an accessory pathway or atrial tachycardia was found in all age groups. AV nodal reentry was rare before 2 years of age.[21] Using esophageal electrophysiologic studies (EPSs), Crosson and associates[22] reported that only 6 of 52 infants (mean age, 2 months) met the criteria for AVNRT.

ACCESSORY PATHWAYS

With regard to accessory pathways, those that conduct anterograde with a short PR interval and a delta wave are said to have the WPW syndrome or a manifest accessory pathway (Fig. 55–7). Early activation of the ventricle, referred to as preexcitation, occurs with WPW. Pathways associated with WPW generally conduct in both anterograde and retrograde directions. When the conduction is only in the retrograde (VA) direction, the pathway is termed *concealed*. Occasionally, preexcitation may be intermittently visible anterograde, and these pathways are labeled *latent*. These pathways are frequently slow but in the face of autonomic stimulation may accelerate and become manifest.

Accessory connections are thought to be atrial tissue that crosses the AV groove along the tricuspid or mitral annulus, except in the region of mitral-aortic fibrous continuity. These pathways provide abnormal continuity between the atrium and the ventricle and are believed to develop from AV ring tissue during early cardiac development. Accessory pathways are classified according to anatomic loca-

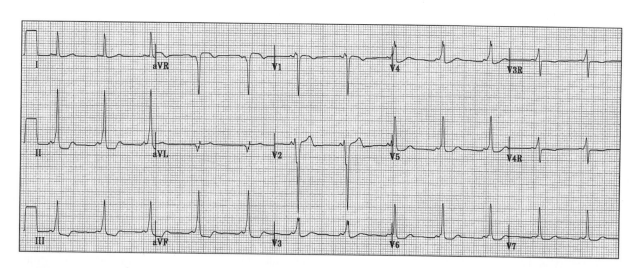

FIGURE 55–7

Electrocardiogram of Wolff-Parkinson-White syndrome secondary to right anterior accessory pathway. Short PR interval, delta waves, and wide QRS morphology.

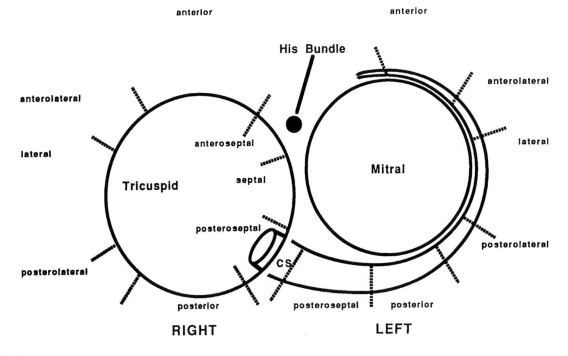

FIGURE 55–8

Schematic of location of accessory atrioventricular pathways in the left anterior oblique view. (From Naccarelli GV: Catheterablation for the treatment of tachyarrhythmias. *In* Willerson JT, Cohn JN [eds]: Cardiovascular Medicine. New York, Churchill Livingstone, 1995, p 1453.)

tion along the AV ring (Fig. 55–8).[23] The most common locations in children are left lateral and posterior septal. Anterior septal is the least common location.

WOLFF-PARKINSON-WHITE SYNDROME

Wolff-Parkinson-White syndrome occurs in about 0.1% of children. Supraventricular tachycardia associated with the WPW syndrome occurs most commonly at younger than 1 month of age. A cardiac anomaly occurs in approximately one fifth to one third of these patients.[24] A positive family history has been reported.[25] Of children who have SVT after infancy, preexcitation has been noted in sinus rhythm in 22 to 50% of patients.[26, 27]

A number of algorithms have been developed to predict the location of the accessory pathway from the surface ECG.[28–32] This is most effective when the patient's rhythm is completely preexcited. The method that we have found most accurate in children is that described by Chiang and coworkers,[32] which uses the vector of the delta wave at 40 milliseconds in a stepwise fashion in leads V_2, III, V_1, and aVF.

The typical WPW complex is not seen in most episodes of SVT associated with these pathways because the tachycardia is initiated by a premature complex that blocks in the accessory pathway and is conducted anterograde through the AV node and retrograde through the accessory pathway. A continuation of this circuit results in an orthodromic AV reciprocating SVT with a narrow QRS–complex tachycardia. Thus, reentrant SVT in the WPW syndrome is analogous to AV nodal reentrant SVT, with the bypass tract functioning like a beta pathway (fast conduction, long refractory period) and the AV node functioning like an alpha pathway (slow conduction, short refractory period). In ap-

proximately 10% of these children, the route of reentry is reversed, and the bypass tract forms the anterograde limb, with the AV node forming the retrograde limb of the reentrant circuit. These tachycardias are referred to as *antidromic* and present as a wide-QRS tachycardia that may be difficult to distinguish from VT (Fig. 55–9). More than half of children with antidromic SVT have more than one accessory pathway.[15] When more than one pathway is present, both can participate in the circuit without the use of the AV node. Patients with orthodromic SVT, especially in the initial complexes of the tachycardia, commonly have bundle branch aberrancy morphology.

Multiple pathways are more likely to occur on the right side. The most common combination has right free wall and posteroseptal locations. Right-sided pathways tend to be subendocardial, whereas left-sided pathways are more likely to be subepicardial. Pathways may cross the annulus in an oblique or serpentine fashion, the latter possibly being responsible for the occasional accessory pathway that has decremental conduction. Most accessory pathways have set conduction and refractory characteristics that do not depend on the patient's heart rate.

Electrophysiologic studies of children with WPW syndrome illustrate some interesting differences between children and adults with WPW.[33] The anterograde bypass tract refractory periods are the same as or longer than those of adults. Short refractory periods of less than 200 milliseconds are unusual in children. Retrograde bypass tract refractory periods are similar to or longer than those of adults. The tachycardia rates are faster in children than in adults because their AV nodal refractory periods are shorter and most SVTs associated with WPW syndrome use the AV node for the anterograde pathway. Although

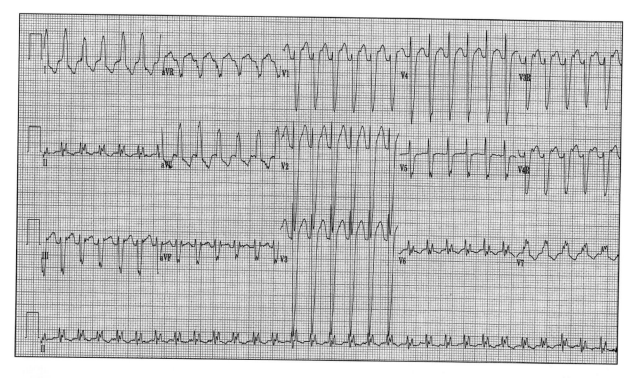

FIGURE 55–9

Electrocardiogram of antidromic supraventricular tachycardia at 190 beats per minute in a patient with Wolff-Parkinson-White syndrome. Wide QRS complexes and retrograde P wave (lead II). The accessory pathway was in the right midseptal position.

atrial fibrillation occurs commonly in adults with WPW, it is less common in children, and when it occurs, it is often after 10 years of age. Atrial fibrillation is dangerous because a pathway with a short refractory period and rapid conduction allows rapid conduction of the impulse to the ventricle, with resultant hemodynamic deterioration or ventricular fibrillation[34–36] (Fig. 55–10).

Asymptomatic Wolff-Parkinson-White Syndrome

Adults with asymptomatic WPW appear to be at low risk for serious problems, but this may not be so in children.[37] In Klein's study, three previously asymptomatic pediatric patients had ventricular fibrillation as the initial presentation at 8, 9, and 16 years of age. In a study of 42 children with WPW who had a cardiac arrest, the cardiac arrest was

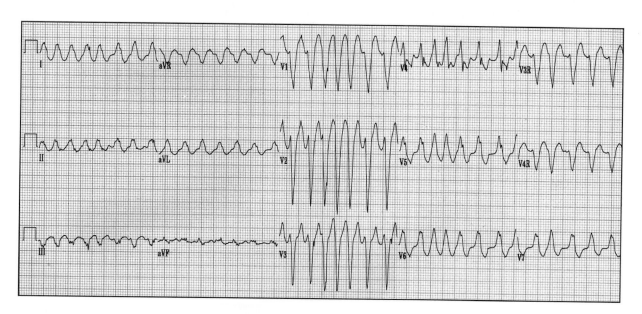

FIGURE 55–10

Example of atrial fibrillation in patient with Wolff-Parkinson-White syndrome. Irregular rhythm and wide QRS complexes with rapid ventricular response.

the presenting symptom in 20 (48%).[38] The incidence of cardiac arrest (3 to 4%) among children with asymptomatic or symptomatic WPW syndrome is higher than the incidence of sudden death (1 to 2%) in adults and may be as high as 12% in those with short R-R intervals during atrial fibrillation.

Among 60 children referred for surgical treatment of WPW syndrome, 10 had experienced a cardiac arrest, which was the initial manifestation in 8 of these.[39] Only 2 of the 10 had prior syncope. From other studies, a short R-R interval (<220 milliseconds) during atrial fibrillation was sensitive, but not predictive, and was more sensitive than a prior clinical history. The risk of sudden death did not correlate with the presence or absence of symptoms such as syncope. Another study found that a R-R interval during atrial fibrillation of 220 milliseconds or less was associated with syncope.[40] Thus, the conduction characteristics of the accessory pathway may be the best method of identifying high-risk patients.

OTHER FORMS OF PREEXCITATION

Other types of pathways may result in early activation or preexcitation of the ventricle (Fig. 55–11). Preexcitation may occur from pathways at sites such as nodoventricular and nodofascicular pathways that provide direct continuity between the AV node and the distal bundle branch or ventricular myocardium.[41] These patients have normal ECGs at rest that preexcite at faster rates or during SVT, resulting in an LBBB pattern.[42] Earliest ventricular activation in these patients is observed at the right ventricular apex. A nodoventricular connection may be a bystander during AVNRT but a wide QRS is inscribed. Fasciculoventricular connections arising from the His bundle or bundle branches are less common. The degree of preexcitation remains relatively fixed whether in sinus rhythm or tachycardia.

The most common variant of preexcitation is by an atriofascicular pathway, which is the anterograde limb, and the normal His-Purkinje AV nodal system is the retrograde limb. These pathways cross the tricuspid annulus in the right anterior region and conduct only anterograde in a decremental fashion. The ventricular insertion is in the region of right bundle branch. These pathways show right ventricular preexcitation with anterograde decremental conduction, but with no retrograde conduction over the accessory connection.[43]

These fibers have been labeled Mahaim fibers, with the original belief being that they exited from the AV node and inserted into the ventricle or fascicle.[41] With information gained from radiofrequency ablation (RFA), it is now believed that Mahaim fibers should be used to describe atriofascicular fibers and not nodoventricular and nodofascicular connections. In sinus rhythm, the QRS complex associated with atriofascicular pathways appears normal, with a widening of the QRS or evidence of preexcitation only with premature atrial stimulation or during SVT, when an LBBB morphology and left axis deviation are evident.[42] As with all AVRT, a 1:1 AV relationship must be present. These pathways have a significant association with Ebstein anomaly.[43–45]

LOWN-GANONG-LEVINE SYNDROME

The electrocardiographic pattern of short PR interval and normal QRS duration has been known as Lown-Ganong-Levine syndrome. This condition is believed to be secondary to a nondecremental bypass tract, which inserts into the AV node. A variety of pathways resulting in this ECG pattern have been described.[46,47] Many no longer use the term Lown-Ganong-Levin syndrome.

CONCEALED ACCESSORY PATHWAYS

A concealed bypass tract, sometimes referred to as concealed WPW syndrome, indicates that the bypass tract is utilized only as the retrograde limb of the reentrant circuit during SVT and not during normal sinus rhythm.[48] The resting ECG shows no delta wave because anterograde conduction does not occur over this tract. When accessory pathways form part of the reentrant circuit, the atrium is always depolarized after the ventricle, and the ECG during SVT reveals a retrograde P wave in SVT, associated with a concealed accessory pathway. The P wave may be difficult to identify because it occurs during the T wave. The RP interval is usually less than the PR interval. The locations of concealed accessory pathways are similar to those associ-

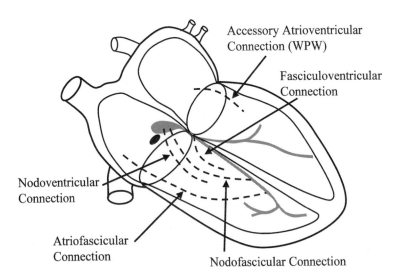

FIGURE 55–11

Schematic of atrioventricular (AV) conduction system with potential accessory AV connections bypassing that system.

ated with manifest accessory pathways or WPW syndrome. In 1977, a study by Gillette[18] describing the location of concealed bypass tracts found 60% in the left atrium, 30% in the right atrium, and 10% in the septum.

An unusual form of SVT known as PJRT has a slow retrograde pathway and therefore a long RP interval compared with the faster anterograde pathway, as evidenced by a shorter PR interval (see Fig. 55–6).[49] Premature beats may be unnecessary to initiate this tachycardia, which may occur after sinus tachycardia or simply during sinus rhythm.

It is not unusual for infants or young children to have delayed appearance of delta waves on the surface ECG. Pathways initially thought to be concealed may later present as manifest WPW syndrome.[50]

ATRIOVENTRICULAR NODAL REENTRY
Information gleaned from surgical ablation or RFA suggests that the reentry circuit in AV nodal reentry involves the approaches to the AV node, most likely atrial muscle several millimeters from the compact AV node.[51,52] The fast pathway is thought to be in the anteroseptal right AV ring close to the AV node. The slow pathway seems to be posterior to the AV node in the posteroseptal-to-midseptal region of the AV ring. Rarely, the fast pathway can be in this region. Before ablation is performed, the physician must take care to differentiate and locate these pathways precisely.[53]

Typical AVNRT utilizes the slow pathway as the anterograde limb and utilizes the fast pathway as the retrograde limb, resulting in a relatively obscure retrograde P wave. Retrograde P waves may not be seen in this type of SVT because atrial and ventricular activation occur almost simultaneously. If the P wave is visible, it is closely related to the preceding QRS complex. A VA interval in these types of tachycardia is less than 60 milliseconds.[54] Atypical AVNRT, which is much less common, reverses the typical circuit, using the fast pathway anterograde and the slow pathway retrograde with a retrograde P wave that is apparent on the ECG. Electrocardiographic characteristics are similar to those in PJRT. In one study, AV nodal reentry was the second most common type of SVT in children, occurring in 24%, and was the most common type in children older than 5 years.[55] Ablation studies have allowed increased understanding of differences between AV nodal physiology in children and adults. Silka and colleagues[56] found that almost one third of children with AVNRT did not have evidence of dual AV nodal pathways. Atypical fast-slow form of AVNRT was more common in the group of patients without dual AV nodal physiology. A study of the electrophysiology of the AV node suggested that maturational changes occur with age.[57] Dual AV nodal pathways were present in 15% of patients younger than 13 years and in 44% of patients older than 13 years.[57] These differences may be responsible for the increased incidence of AVNRT in older children and adults.

Young people with AVNRT typically have faster heart rates than their adult counterparts, often greater than 250 bpm. Although occasionally associated with syncope or presyncope, these episodes are rarely life-threatening, but they may disrupt daily activities.

SINUS NODE REENTRY
Sinus node reentry is uncommon in children but may mimic sinus tachycardia. The ECG presentation is that of a sinus tachycardia, but onset and offset may be sudden. It has been reported after an operation for a cardiac malformation. β-Blockers are the most effective treatment for this arrhythmia. If sinus node automaticity is abnormal, a pacemaker may be needed to provide an adequate heart rate.

PROGNOSIS OF SUPRAVENTRICULAR TACHYCARDIA
For infants, recurrences occurred in about 20 to 30%, but if SVT presentated after 5 years of age, 78% had recurrences. In addition, up to a third of infants with WPW syndrome lose the accessory connection with age.

ELECTROPHYSIOLOGIC STUDY OF SUPRAVENTRICULAR TACHYCARDIA
Although the ECG during SVT may suggest the mechanism, an electrophysiologic study (EPS) may be needed to determine the precise mechanism of the tachycardia, if it is determined that this information is necessary. The EPS may be utilized to locate the site of the accessory pathway in both WPW syndrome and concealed accessory pathway SVT. It is also utilized to determine the refractory period of the accessory pathway, to induce the SVT, and to determine the ventricular response to atrial fibrillation when it can be induced in patients with WPW syndrome.[58]

The indications to study SVT are shown in Box 55–1.

BOX 55–1. INDICATIONS FOR ELECTROPHYSIOLOGIC STUDY IN SUPRAVENTRICULAR TACHYCARDIA (SVT)

1. Syncope or cardiac arrest associated with SVT
2. WPW syndrome
   Atrial fibrillation, usually with rapid ventricular response
   New presentation in patients over 6–8 years
   Refractory SVT
   Unacceptable side effects of medicine
   Determination of risk: refractory period of accessory pathway, inducibility of atrial fibrillation
   For radiofrequency ablation
3. AVRT, concealed accessory pathway, or AVNRT
   Refractory SVT
   Unacceptable side effects of medicine
   Syncope, presyncope, other symptoms
   For radiofrequency ablation
4. To test medication efficacy or guide medical therapy in refractory SVT
5. To document SVT in patients with known SVT before or after medication withdrawal

WPW = Wolff-Parkinson-White; AVRT = atrioventricular reentrant tachycardia; AVNRT = atrioventricular nodal reentrant tachycardia.

TREATMENT OF SUPRAVENTRICULAR TACHYCARDIA

Emergency Treatment

Because the mechanism of SVT can usually be identified, treatment can be chosen for the specific form of SVT.[59] The treatment of any cardiac arrhythmia is determined by the clinical status of the patient. Thus, the type of treatment chosen for the patient in shock is different from that given to the patient who is asymptomatic and has only a fast heart rate (Box 55–2). When the SVT is due to AV reentry, any intervention that interrupts the critical relationship of conduction and refractoriness between the two limbs of the reentrant circuit can interrupt the tachycardia. Carotid sinus pressure or the Valsalva maneuver is infrequently successful in children, but should be attempted. In children, a headstand often successfully interrupts the tachycardia. More commonly, especially in infants, application of ice or ice-water bag directly to the center of the infant's face recruits the diving reflex and stops the SVT.[60]

A rapid pharmacologic treatment that is now available is adenosine. Its effect usually occurs within 10 seconds, and it has a short half-life, with side effects lasting less than a minute and rarely being serious.[61] It is effective in 80 to 100% of patients, but success rates are lower in neonates.[62] The mean reported effective doses have been 132 to 173 µg/kg as an intravenous bolus.[63] Our starting dose is 100 µg/kg, increasing by 50- to 100-µg increments up to 400 µg/kg. The maximum dose is 12 mg. Higher doses may be necessary in the presence of caffeine or theophylline. Dipyridamole potentiates adenosine.

The rapidity of delivering the bolus is the most important factor in administering this drug. Effective results have been reported with interosseous administration,[64] but the intravenous route is preferred. The few serious reported adverse side effects include atrial fibrillation, high-grade AV block, VT or other complex ventricular arrhythmias, asystole, apnea, or bronchospasm. There appears to be a proadrenergic effect, which may result in postinfusion acceleration of arrhythmias, such as atrial flutter, that do not convert. For these reasons, use adenosine in children in a setting where emergency care, including cardioversion and cardiopulmonary resuscitation, can be accomplished. Adenosine may be used in acutely ill patients, but its use should not delay immediate cardioversion in severely compromised patients.

For those patients who become acidotic or hypotensive, immediate synchronized direct-current cardioversion is advised with a dosage of 1 to 2 watt-sec/kg. The dosage may be repeatedly doubled until the treatment is effective or a level of 10 watt-sec/kg is reached. The patient should be given a sedative or a short-acting anesthetic, and preparation should be made for airway support and ventilation should these be needed. The underlying acidosis should be treated and adequate ventilation and oxygenation of the patient provided because cardioversion may be unsuccessful with hypoxia and acid-base imbalance. Cardioversion should not be delayed to make these corrections but should be performed immediately in emergency situations. It is best to utilize adult paddles when possible in children weighing more than 10 kg to optimize current flow.[65] Digoxin administration should not prevent the use of cardioversion when needed. Evidence of digoxin toxicity, such as ventricular arrhythmias, may be treated with intravenous lidocaine (1 mg/kg). Once the patient's rhythm has converted and an ECG in sinus rhythm has been obtained, long-term treatment should be initiated immediately.

Children with mild-to-moderate congestive heart failure may be treated initially with adenosine if vagal maneuvers are unsuccessful. Pharmacologic agents, such as digoxin, amiodarone, and procainamide, may be used (Table 55–4). The intravenous route is preferred for digoxin in the critically ill patient or in any infant. The digitalizing dose intervals may be given as frequently as 2- to 4-hour intervals, depending on the patient's status. Although digoxin toxic rhythms may not be noted as easily by this type of rapid digitalization, the need to convert the tachycardia takes precedence. If the tachycardia persists after three doses, one to two additional doses equivalent to one fourth of the total digitalizing dose may be given. Vagal stimulation or adenosine may be effective after digitalization if such treatment was ineffective before. The maintenance dose of digoxin should be determined according to the total digitalizing dose required and is one eighth of the total digitalizing dose twice daily.

BOX 55–2. EMERGENCY TREATMENT OF SUPRAVENTRICULAR TACHYCARDIA

A. Asymptomatic
1. Ice, vagal maneuvers
2. IV adenosine
3. Pharmacologic agents
    a. IV digoxin
    b. Oral β-blocking agents
    c. Oral class I agents
B. Mild congestive heart failure
1. Ice, vagal maneuvers
2. IV adenosine
3. Pharmacologic agents
    a. IV digoxin
    b. Oral β-blocking agents
    c. Oral class I agents
    d. Oral amiodarone or sotalol
C. Moderate congestive heart failure
1. Ice, vagal maneuvers
2. IV adenosine
3. Pharmacologic agents—if IV access
    a. IV digoxin
    b. IV amiodarone
4. Pacing (esophageal or intracardiac)—if no IV access or for infants
5. Cardioversion, synchronized
D. Severe congestive heart failure
1. IV adenosine if IV access
2. Cardioversion, synchronized
3. Pacing, esophageal or intracardiac
4. Pharmacologic agents
    a. IV digoxin
    b. IV amiodarone

IV = intravenous.

TABLE 55–4

PHARMACOLOGIC AGENTS FOR EMERGENCY TREATMENT OF SUPRAVENTRICULAR TACHYCARDIA

Agent	Initial Intravenous Treatment
Adenosine	50–100 µg/kg, increase by 50-µg/kg increments q 2 min to 400 µg/kg or 12 mg maximal dose
Amiodarone	5 mg/kg over 1 hour, followed by 5- to 10-µg/kg/min infusion
Digoxin	Dose is age dependent.
	Give in 3 doses (½ TDD, ¼ TDD, ¼ TDD)
	Preterm infant: 10–15 µg/kg TDD
	Term newborn-adolescent:
	22–30 µg/kg TDD to maximal TDD of 1–1.5 mg
	Oral maintenance: 10 µg/kg/day q 12 h
Esmolol	IV load: 200–500 µg/kg/min over 2–4 min. May increase in 50- to 100-µg/kg/min increments (maximum dose: 1000 µg/kg/min)
	Maintenance infusion: 50–200 µg/kg/min
Procainamide	5 mg/kg over 5–10 min or 10–15 mg/kg over 30–45 min
	Infusion: 20–100 µg/kg/min
Propranolol	0.05–0.1 mg/kg over 5 min q 6 h
Phenylephrine	100-µg/kg bolus
	Infusion: 10 µg/kg/min
Verapamil	0.05–0.30 mg/kg over 3–5 min
	Maximal dose: 10 mg

TDD = total digitalizing dose; IV = intravenous.

Esmolol or propranolol, which may further depress cardiac function, should be used with caution in the critically ill child and should be avoided in the patient with pronounced congestive heart failure. When cardiac function is not compromised, a slow intravenous dose may be given. A shorter-acting β-blocker, such as esmolol, is preferable in this setting, although few data are available in children. The advantage of this β-blocker is its very short distribution half-life of 2 minutes and its elimination half-life of 9 minutes. Steady state is reached in 5 minutes. Propranolol or esmolol may be effective in treating SVT associated with accessory pathways by slowing the AV nodal limb of the circuit without affecting the accessory pathway.[66] In the absence of congestive heart failure, WPW syndrome is preferably treated with β-blockers, and digoxin should be avoided. However, with moderate-to-severe congestive heart failure, digoxin can be used initially (unless atrial flutter or fibrillation is present in association with WPW/SVT), with a switch to a β-blocker once the heart failure has resolved.

Amiodarone is now available for intravenous use and is being used increasingly for the emergency treatment of SVT. In studies of intravenous amiodarone, 60 to 71% of patients had elimination of their SVT, and 80 to 94% had improvement.[67,68] The median therapeutic effect occurred in 1 day (range, 1 hour to 5 days). Thirty-four percent responded within 2 hours of the initial bolus. The predominant adverse effects include hypotension, bradycardia, and decreased left ventricular function. In spite of these potential problems, patients who have undergone surgery or those with congestive heart failure from their SVT tolerate intravenous amiodarone well. The hypotension generally responds to stopping or slowing the infusion for a short period of time and giving a fluid bolus.

The class I agent procainamide may be given intravenously and terminates the SVT by blocking retrograde conduction in the fast pathway of the AV node or in the accessory pathway when it is a part of the circuit. Procainamide can result in second-degree or complete heart block or in a proarrhythmic state, incessant SVT, or a new arrhythmia. QT prolongation can occur and has been associated with a torsades de pointes type of ventricular tachycardia. Procainamide is a myocardial depressant and can cause hypotension and bradycardia. When an atrial arrhythmia is being treated, procainamide should be used in combination with an agent that blocks the AV node, such as digoxin or a β-blocker, to prevent an increased ventricular response and a higher ventricular rate as the atrial rate slows. Procainamide is particularly effective with SVT of the PJRT variety.

Phenylephrine is infrequently used but may be effective by raising the blood pressure and thus recruiting the baroreceptor-vagal reflexes. Termination usually occurs in the anterograde slow pathway.[69]

In any form of wide QRS-tachycardia, both digoxin and verapamil should be avoided because of the association of WPW syndrome with antidromic SVT and the possibility of accelerating the tachycardia with life-threatening results.

Although verapamil is an effective treatment of SVT in adults, serious problems have occurred with its use in children, particularly in patients younger than 1 year and in those with severe congestive heart failure. Use of verapamil in infants has resulted in cardiovascular collapse and death.[70,71] Pretreatment with calcium does not prevent this complication in all patients. For these reasons, we generally avoid using verapamil in patients younger than 3 years.

Even in older patients, we would use other regimens before giving verapamil. Adenosine is more rapid in its action, has much lower risk, and is preferred. The dose of verapamil for older patients is 0.1 to 0.3 mg/kg, given slowly intravenously. The maximum dose is 10 mg.

Both digoxin and verapamil should be avoided in patients with a wide-QRS tachycardia and when WPW syndrome with atrial fibrillation is considered as a possible cause, to avoid acceleration of the ventricular response and resultant ventricular fibrillation, unless one knows that the accessory pathway refractory period is relatively long and is unaffected by these drugs. Digoxin and verapamil have been shown to shorten the refractory period of an accessory pathway, facilitating the conduction of electrical impulses to the ventricle, especially in atrial fibrillation.[34–36] In patients with WPW syndrome and congestive heart failure secondary to the arrhythmias, digoxin may be used under careful ECG monitoring. If the congestive heart failure resolves after conversion to sinus rhythm, the therapy may be changed to another antiarrhythmic agent. If digoxin is continued, its effect on the accessory pathway characteristics should be assessed.

Esophageal, transthoracic, or intracardiac overdrive pacing may be used to convert SVT to sinus rhythm.[72] Use of the transvenous method involves placing an intracardiac catheter with pacing of the atrium at a rate slightly higher than the rate of the tachycardia. Cessation of pacing often results in resumption of sinus rhythm. A less invasive

TABLE 55-5

LONG-TERM ANTIARRHYTHMIC AGENTS FOR SUPRAVENTRICULAR AND VENTRICULAR TACHYCARDIA

Arrhythmia	Agent	Dose (Oral)	Level
SVT	Digoxin	Dose is age dependent Give in 3 doses (½ TDD, ¼ TDD, ¼ TDD) Preterm infant: 10–20 μg/kg TDD Term newborn-adolescent: 30–40 μg/kg TDD oral to maximal TDD of 1–1.5 mg oral (IV ¾ of PO dose) Oral maintenance: 10 μg/kg/day q 12 h	1–2.5 ng/ml
	Verapamil	2–8 mg/kg tid	100–300 ng/ml
SVT or VT	Propranolol	0.5–2 mg/kg/day q 6 h	50–100 μg/L
	Nadolol	0.25–1 mg/kg/day q 12 h	0.03–0.13 μg/ml
	Atenolol	0.5–1 mg/kg q d	
	Procainamide	20–100 mg/kg/day q 4–6 h	PA: 4–10 mg/L; NAPA = 4–8 mg/L
	Quinidine	20–60 mg/kg/day q 6–8 h	2–5 mg/L
	Disopyramide	5–15 mg/kg/day q 6 h	2–4 μg/ml
	Flecainide	50–200 mg/m^2/day or 3–6 mg/kg/day q 12 h	0.2–1.0 mg/L
	Amiodarone	Loading dose: 10–20 mg/kg/day q 12 h × 7 days Maintenance: 5–10 mg/kg q d	RT$_3$ < 90 ng/dl
	Sotalol	2–8 mg/kg/day q 12 h	
VT	Phenytoin	Loading dose: 10–20 mg/kg/day q 12 h × 2 d Maintenance: 5–10 mg/kg/day q 12 h	10–20 μg/ml
	Mexiletine	5–15 mg/kg/day q 8 h	0.5–2.0 μg/ml

SVT = supraventricular tachycardia; VT = ventricular tachycardia; IV = intravenous; TDD = total digitalizing dose; PA = procainamide; NAPA = N-acetylprocainamide; RT$_3$ = reverse triiodothyronine; PO = oral.

method of overdrive pacing involves an esophageal pacing catheter used in the same manner to capture the atrial rhythm and to interrupt the reentrant circuit.[73] It is effective in most instances of AV reciprocating tachycardia and in more than half of the instances of atrial flutter. After postoperative cardiac surgery, epicardial transthoracic wires may be used for pacing to terminate the tachycardia. Some patients may have a pacemaker, which is triggered to overdrive pace tachycardias, and others may have a pacemaker that can be activated by the patient or physician to overdrive pace the tachycardia.

As soon as the patient converts from the SVT, an ECG in sinus rhythm should be obtained. This allows determination of the presence of the WPW pattern or other abnormalities that affect the choice of long-term therapy. After conversion, one of the long-term treatment regimens shown in Table 55–5 should be instituted to prevent recurrence of the arrhythmia. The doses and levels of the various drugs used in the long-term treatment of SVT are shown.

Long-Term Treatment

The aim of long-term treatment is to prevent recurrence of the tachycardia. With AVRT and AVNRT, interruption of the AV nodal portion of the circuit terminates or prevents the recurrence of the tachycardia. Treatment of AV nodal reentrant SVT consists of drugs that primarily affect the AV node, such as digoxin, propranolol, and verapamil. Alternatively, one could perform slow-pathway modification of the AV node or the approaches to the AV node by use of radiofrequency energy. AV reentrant tachycardia may be treated with drugs that affect either the AV node or the ac-

cessory pathway or with RFA. Medical therapy for AV nodal reentrant SVT has usually included digoxin, β-blockers, and verapamil. Class I agents and amiodarone, as well as newer agents, such as sotalol and propafenone, have been used. The preferred medical treatment of AV nodal SVT or SVT utilizing a concealed bypass tract is digoxin.[74] It is effective by prolonging AV nodal conduction and refractoriness in both the fast (beta) and slow (alpha) pathways. When refractoriness of the fast pathway is prolonged more than conduction down the slow pathway, SVT cannot be initiated. Class I or class III antiarrhythmic agents may be more effective in some patients with WPW syndrome because these agents affect the accessory pathway and the AV node.[75] A combination of accessory pathway and AV nodal effects may be necessary in some refractory tachycardias. β-Blockers (class II agents) are the preferred treatment for AV reentrant tachycardia associated with the WPW syndrome. Other effective agents include class IA (procainamide), IC (flecainide or propafenone), and III (amiodarone or sotalol). As previously discussed, digoxin is avoided long term if possible: short-term treatment is appropriate in the infant with WPW syndrome with congestive heart failure until a switch to a β-blocker can be made after cardiac function has improved.

The development of the technique of RFA has revolutionized the long-term treatment of SVT and is discussed subsequently.

Long-term management decisions regarding SVT depend on many factors, including age; symptoms at presentation; potential of threatening symptoms; effect of the tachycardia on the patient's lifestyle; other associated cardiac diseases; other medical conditions or diseases; results of previous treatment, including control of the tachycardia; side effects of the medication; tolerance of the patient and family to either the tachycardia or medications; and preferences of the patient, family, and physician. The natural history of the arrhythmia and the potential for significant life-threatening events should be considered. Older patients with infrequent recurrences and short episodes that can be self-terminated may not require long-term treatment.

We recommend treatment of SVT in infants for the first year of life, regardless of the mechanism. If there is no evidence of WPW syndrome at the end of the first year and no recurrences of the tachycardia within the previous 3 to 6 months, digoxin is discontinued at that time or over the next 6 months. In the presence of the WPW pattern antiarrhythmic medication is continued because of the likelihood of recurrence of tachycardia in WPW syndrome. If these patients with WPW syndrome have no recurrences over the subsequent 12 months, the medication is stopped or weaned.

Controversy remains as to whether treatment is effective in preventing recurrences, especially in infants,[76, 77] because 40 to 80% have recurrences during drug therapy.[78] For older children and adolescents, many treatment options are available for the various types of SVT. First, the physician must decide whether or not to treat the condition. The decision to treat is clear in patients with life-threatening events or serious symptoms, such as syncope and presyncope. With life-threatening symptoms, we recommend the use of RFA, or surgery, if RFA cannot be successfully performed. If this mode of treatment is not chosen, the pharmacologic treatment should be tested in the electrophysiologic laboratory. In patients with a life-threatening event, the medication should effectively suppress the SVT. Medications only suppress the tachycardia and do not obliterate it. Asymptomatic children who have rapid, potentially threatening tachycardias should be treated identically to the patients described earlier with significant symptoms.

When there are moderate symptoms, frequent recurrences, and either physiologic or psychological impairment caused by the SVT, we recommend either long-term pharmacologic treatment or RFA. Radiofrequency ablation is usually the primary option in children older than 8 to 9 years, but medication is indicated in younger children unless there are extenuating circumstances. Currently, the risk of RFA is slightly increased in children younger than 4 years, but as more experience is gained, RFA may be recommended routinely at an earlier age. Each treatment decision should be individualized, using general guidelines, by specialists familiar with the treatment of these arrhythmias and the side effects of the medications or risks of the RFA procedure.

When the first episode in children is either self-limited and non–life-threatening or attributable to an external cause, such as a decongestant or anesthetic agent, it is reasonable to wait for a subsequent episode before initiating long-term treatment. In these patients, one must consider the ability of the patient to report or recognize another episode, the ability of the family to recognize the episode and respond appropriately, the proximity of appropriate care, and the potential risks of the tachycardia. We are more likely to treat a tachycardia of greater than 250 bpm

in a young child than a tachycardia of 160 bpm in a school-aged child.

Generally, long-term treatment is given in order to achieve therapeutic blood levels. In asymptomatic SVT in older children or adolescents, a rapidly acting antiarrhythmic agent, such as procainamide, can be given at the onset of the tachycardia to interrupt the SVT. This is effective only in a small group of patients sensitive to that medication who can tolerate the SVT until the therapeutic level is achieved and who do not immediately revert back to their tachycardia.

SPECIFIC DRUGS FOR CHRONIC SUPRAVENTRICULAR TACHYCARDIA

Digoxin. The method of digitalization has been previously described. Once the child's condition has improved, the tachycardia controlled, and the digitalizing doses given, we often change to oral medications for maintenance. We never digitalize by simply starting the maintenance dose, because side effects still occur, but often at a later time, when the infant is out of the hospital and is not being observed. To achieve a slower digitalization, one may separate the digitalization doses into four quarter doses or use longer dosing intervals.

β-Blockers. β-Blockers are the second most commonly used drugs to treat SVT in infants and are used primarily in the presence of WPW syndrome. In young children, hypoglycemia may occur, especially when normal alimentation is not occurring, as with an intercurrent illness. A child or infant should be given some nutrition before receiving this medication. Likewise, adolescents and older children should be advised not to skip meals, although their increased glycogen stores provide protection from the more severe symptoms. Nadolol or atenolol may be used effectively for SVT in children.

Amiodarone. Amiodarone is an effective long-term treatment in children with SVT and in infants with refractory SVT.[79] Generally, we have been able to wean amiodarone after 1 year with no more likelihood of recurrences than in children who were treated with less potent medications, such as digoxin or a β-blocker. Amiodarone may be used as a bridge to control refractory SVT until the child is of an acceptable age for RFA. The most serious side effects, such as pulmonary toxicity, tend to occur in older adults, so short-term therapy with amiodarone should not be avoided on this basis. Careful surveillance for hepatic, ocular, and thyroid toxicity should be practiced. Avoidance of sun exposure and use of sunscreens are necessary.

Most antiarrhythmics can be used in children with SVT (see Table 55–5). Reports of efficacy with drug combinations have been reported.[80–82]

Newer Medications. Flecainide, propafenone, and sotalol have been used effectively for AVNRT and AVRT, but all have proarrhythmic effects. Flecainide appears to be most effective in treating AVRT (73%), PJRT (100%), and the automatic tachycardias (automatic atrial tachycardia [81%] and JET [83%]). Concerns have been raised about the use of flecainide in light of the Cardiac Arrhythmia Suppression Trial in adults.[83] The proarrhythmic potential of this drug has been seen in children but appears to be quite low in children with SVT and a normal heart.[84] Propafenone is most effective with AVRT (70%) and JET

(100%).[85,86] Sotalol is effective for SVT (89%) and automatic atrial tachycardia (86%).[87,88]

Surgical Treatment

Since its first report,[89] surgical ablation has been very successful in eliminating the accessory pathway in 80 to 100% of patients. Today, surgical ablation is reserved primarily for patients in whom RFA has failed or is not possible because of structural cardiovascular abnormalities.

Radiofrequency Ablation

GENERAL PRINCIPLES. Transvenous RFA has been used to treat children and adults with a cardiac arrhythmia.[90–93] Radiofrequency energy is a low-voltage, high-frequency (radiofrequency) alternating current at a frequency of 30 kHz to 300 MHz. Most contemporary radiofrequency generators used for cardiac ablation deliver 300 to 1000 kHz of alternating current to produce thermal injury. The current is delivered to the cardiac tissue through a steerable electrode catheter and a unipolar delivery system. Through an active 2- to 4-mm tip, a high current density is directed at the cardiac tissue interface. The other pole is a passive dispersive or ground electrode on the skin under the patient's left scapula. The electrical field coming from the catheter tip results in resistive heating of the local tissue in the area of the catheter tip and tissue desiccation and necrosis. The greatest heat occurs at the point of greatest current density at the catheter tip–tissue interface. Living tissue is permanently destroyed at 45 to 50°C. Biologic effects of RFA include thermal effects on the plasma membrane, the cytoskeleton of the cell, and the nucleus. Additional effects are noted on cellular metabolism and on the microvasculature and include inflammatory responses. Electrical effects cause transient changes in membrane ion permeability.

Catheters allow measurement of the temperature at the tip of the catheter. The extent of the induced lesion depends on current density at the catheter tip, size of the electrode, tissue contact, impedance of the tissue, and degree of tissue heating. Temperatures in the 50 to 65°C range generally have been successful in our pediatric patients. The maximal lesion size is achieved within 30 to 60 seconds; extending the duration beyond 60 to 90 seconds does not increase success or lesion growth. The maximal width of the lesion is achieved before the maximal depth. The time to induce 50% of lesion width is 5 to 10 seconds for lesion diameter but 30 seconds for lesion depth.[94] Ninety percent of tissue injury is achieved within 30 seconds. Likewise, steady-state temperature for tissue death can generally be achieved within 10 to 15 seconds at the contact point and 40 to 50 seconds at the borders of the lesion.[95] Lesion size averages 3 to 5 mm wide and 1 to 3 mm deep.[96,97] At the border zone of the lesion, either extension of damage or reversibility may occur, resulting either in recurrence of an arrhythmia that appeared to be successfully ablated or disappearance of an arrhythmia that was not thought to be successfully ablated after the ablation. Temperatures greater than 100°C result in boiling and coagulum formation at the tip of the catheter. Vaporization may occur, and cardiac perforation is possible. Rapid increases in impedance also occur. In these instances, radiofrequency energy should be stopped immediately. The power required to achieve a successful lesion is generally between 10 to 50 W.

Radiofrequency catheter ablation has been used successfully in children for various arrhythmias, but most commonly for WPW syndrome, concealed accessory pathways, and AV nodal reentry.[98–100] It is also used for atrial arrhythmias, including atrial ectopic tachycardias, atrial flutter, and ventricular arrhythmias.

Before RFA is performed, patients should not receive antiarrhythmic drugs for an adequate period of time to allow elimination of the drug so that the patient's electrophysiologic status can be thoroughly evaluated. A complete EPS is performed, with a special emphasis on the mechanism of the tachycardia and the location of the accessory pathway.

In children, prolonged exposure to radiation is a concern because of the increased sensitivity to radiation of younger cells and the potential for later growth of the lesion, particularly when RFA is performed in infants or small children.[101]

HISTORY AND CLINICAL REPORTS OF RADIOFREQUENCY ABLATION IN CHILDREN. Radiofrequency ablation was first described in children in 1991.[92,93] Subsequently, more than 5000 procedures have been entered in the Pediatric Radiofrequency Ablation Registry, and results of RFA have been described in numerous studies[98–100,102–108] and in the Pediatric Radiofrequency Ablation Registry.[106] The success rate is now 90% for accessory pathways, 96% for AVNRT, 64% for VT, 76% for atrial flutter, and 88% for ectopic atrial tachycardia. Higher success is associated with left accessory pathways, AVNRT, and greater operator experience, and lower success, with right-sided pathways, VT, higher body weight, associated heart disease, and age of 4 years or younger.[109] Major complications occur in 3.2% and include death (0.11%),[110] AV block,[111] emboli, deep vein thrombosis, brachial plexus injury, perforation, pericardial effusion, tamponade, pulmonary embolism, and hemothorax. Minor complications include hematoma and chest pain. Late recurrences have been reported in 5 to 20% of patients.

The most common indications for RFA include life-threatening symptoms: syncope or near-syncope associated with arrhythmias, seizures with tachyarrhythmias, or resuscitation from cardiac arrest; medically refractory tachycardia; adverse drug effects; tachycardia-induced ventricular dysfunction; impending congenital heart surgery; and patient choice.

In contrast to antiarrhythmic therapy, which suppresses but does not cure the tachycardia, RFA provides a method for cure. It improves quality of life in patients in whom a successful ablation is achieved, alleviating symptoms both from the arrhythmia and from medication side effects. It is also cost effective.[112,113]

RADIOFREQUENCY ABLATION OF SPECIFIC CONDITIONS

Wolff-Parkinson-White/Manifest Accessory Pathway. In most instances, preexcitation is identified before the EPS. Once AV reentrant SVT has been documented as the mechanism of the tachycardia, the characteristics of the pathway assessed, and the general location determined, the pathway location should be precisely mapped.[103, 114–119] When the suspected successful location is identified, the radiofrequency generator is turned on and the desired power and/or temperature achieved. After an apparently successful lesion is produced, a repeat EPS is performed both with and without isoproterenol to look for evidence of the pathway as well as initiation of SVT. This EPS should be performed immediately after the RFA as well as on two to three occasions up to 1 hour after the successful treatment. As long as the catheters are in the heart, especially on the left side, we maintain the activated clotting time at greater than 250 seconds.

Loss of the delta wave is insufficient evidence to declare ablation successful because retrograde conduction may still be present and may result in SVT. Adenosine infusion may be used to evaluate the success of accessory pathway ablation by demonstrating latent anterograde pathway conduction once AV nodal conduction is blocked. High-grade AV block after adenosine indicates absence of accessory pathway conduction.[120]

In children, septal and right free wall pathway ablation has been more difficult to achieve and perform than ablation of left free wall pathways or AV nodal modifications. Right free wall pathways require more fluoroscopy time and more applications of energy.[106, 121]

Concealed Accessory Pathways. A concealed accessory pathway is an AV connection that is not seen on the surface ECG. It is utilized as the retrograde limb of the SVT circuit, and the AV node is used as the anterograde limb. No delta wave is present in sinus rhythm. During EPS, one needs to initiate SVT or find eccentric retrograde conduction with ventricular pacing to identify an accessory pathway. The earliest retrograde sites in SVT or ventricular pacing can be used to identify a potentially successful site, with the physician looking for the closest VA interval and the earliest retrograde atrial activation.[114, 122, 123] Ablation should be performed during SVT or with ventricular pacing. The postablation testing should be similar to that used with WPW syndrome, but adenosine is unnecessary.

A special type of concealed accessory pathway is that responsible for PJRT. This pathway has been found in the right or left posterior septal space, has decremental properties, and has been successfully treated with RFA.[124–128] Other sites include right anterior, right anteroseptal, and left posterior locations.[129] Patients with PJRT may have multiple pathways.[130]

Atrioventricular Nodal Reentrant Supraventricular Tachycardia. Atrioventricular nodal reentrant tachycardia accounts for 10% of SVT in infants and young children[22] and 20% of SVT in adolescents.[21] Given a success rate of 95% and a low incidence of complete AV block with a low slow pathway modification, strong consideration to RFA should be given for the adolescent. The risk is no higher in a child than in an adult.[121]

This form of SVT utilizes differential conduction in the approaches to or in the perinodal atrial tissue near the AV node to allow the formation of a reentrant circuit in the area of the AV node, resulting in SVT.[131–133] Surgical experience suggested that fast-conducting fibers are located superiorly in the anterior septum, extending from the AV node toward the tendon of Todaro and the foramen ovale. The slowly conducting fibers are located inferiorly in the

posterior septum, extending along the tricuspid annulus toward the coronary sinus ostium.[134] Experience with RFA in these area has confirmed the location of the "fast" and "slow" pathways.[52, 135–139]

Atrioventricular nodal reentrant tachycardia can be diagnosed by EPS. Although dual AV nodal pathways, as evidenced by discontinuous AV nodal curves or a jump in the AH interval with decremental atrial premature beats, is a hallmark of AV nodal reentry, Silka and colleagues[56] reported that children with AVNRT may not always have evidence of dual AV nodal pathways. With AVNRT, anterograde conduction is through the slow pathway and retrograde conduction through the fast pathway in 90% of patients (slow-fast).[52] In the remaining 10%, conduction may be either fast-slow or slow-slow.[56, 139, 140]

The standard technique used for AVNRT is slow pathway modification, which is generally located along the inferoposterior septal region of the tricuspid valve annulus just anterior to the coronary sinus ostium.

Success is associated with periods of accelerated junctional rhythm.[141, 142] In children, Rhodes and associates[143] described successful AV nodal slow pathway modifications at lower temperatures (mean, 54°C) than have generally been recommended. Successful ablation should eliminate inducible SVT. Although elimination of dual AV nodal pathway physiology is preferable, it is not required for a successful ablation. Conversely, in children, Silka and coworkers[140] showed that atypical AVNRT was still inducible after elimination of dual pathways.

In a small number of patients, the fast pathway may be in the posterior septum.[53] In these patients, unexpected AV block may occur with application of the usual slow-pathway modification techniques. Care must be taken to map the characteristics and the location of the slow and fast pathways carefully before applying radiofrequency energy.

In the Pediatric Radiofrequency Ablation Registry, there has been a 96% success rate. The freedom from recurrence at 3 years was 77%, and the incidence of AV block was 1.6%.[106, 111]

Supraventricular Arrhythmias in Patients With Congenital Heart Disease. Patients with a cardiac anomaly may have an accessory pathway—either manifest (WPW) or concealed, or a postoperative atrial arrhythmia. Because of the increased time required to ablate the arrhythmia surgically in combination with congenital heart surgery and a resultant increase in morbidity and mortality, RFA has been recommended before surgical repair, when possible, to prevent postoperative arrhythmias.[144] In patients with a cardiac anomaly, multiple pathways were common and were frequently associated with the tricuspid valve.[145] Success was achieved in 60%, but the recurrence rate was higher than in those with a normal heart.[146] The approach to the accessory pathway may be made more difficult by the cardiac anomaly. In some lesions, such as those requiring the Fontan repair, the operation may prevent future access to the pathway.

Atrial Flutter

ELECTROCARDIOGRAPHIC MANIFESTATIONS

Atrial flutter is defined by its characteristic ECG manifestations of negative saw-toothed flutter waves best seen in

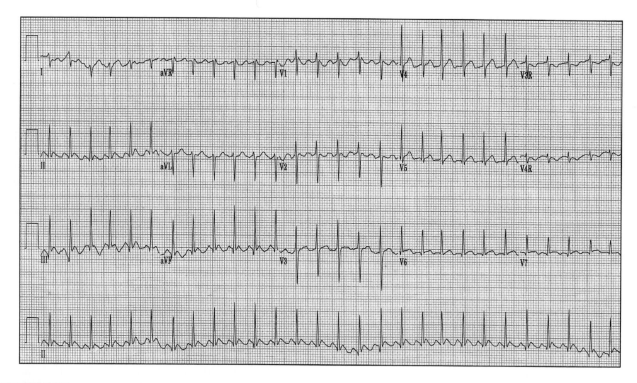

FIGURE 55–12

Electrocardiographic example of atrial flutter with 2 : 1 atrioventricular conduction. Flutter waves are best seen in the lead II.

leads II, III, and aVF; biphasic flutter waves in leads I and V6; and upright waves in lead V1 (Fig. 55–12). At times, the flutter waves are less distinct. Atrial flutter consists of rapid, regular atrial excitation at rates of 280 to 480 bpm, but rates as high as 500 bpm may be seen in infants. The ventricular response is related to AV nodal conduction, which may allow 1 : 1, 2 : 1, or greater than 3 to 4:1 AV conduction. The term *atrial flutter* may be used to refer to reentrant atrial arrhythmias that do not have the distinct saw-toothed appearance or an atrial rate of 300 bpm. These atrial arrhythmias may be faster or slower and may result from "atypical" reentrant circuits often created by atrial surgery. These tachycardias are often referred to as intra-atrial reentry, primary atrial tachycardia, or atypical atrial flutter.

CLINICAL CORRELATIONS

In children, atrial flutter occurs in three distinct groups: (1) the fetal or neonatal patient,[147, 148] (2) the patient with acquired heart disease or unoperated congenital heart disease, and (3) the patient with postoperative congenital heart disease.[149, 150] When noted in utero, hydrops fetalis may develop in 11 to 40%.[151]

Atrial flutter represents 15 to 55% of all fetal tachyarrhythmias with associated structural heart disease in 21%. The atrial rate is often as high as 300 to 500 bpm. The rhythm is often irregular because of variable AV block with 2 to 4:1 AV conduction. Fetal flutter can be recognized on fetal echocardiography by the rapid atrial wall contraction associated with a slower but rapid ventricular contraction. The initial medical treatment should be digitalization of the infant or of the mother and the fetus.[152, 153] Digitalis increases AV block, which slows the ventricular rate and

improves cardiac function. Conversion to sinus rhythm may occur. Other agents, including procainamide, quinidine, flecainide, propranolol, and amiodarone, also have been used to treat the fetus in atrial flutter, most commonly by giving medication to the mother.[154] In the presence of hydrops, direct infusion of antiarrhythmic medication into the fetal umbilical vessels has been successful. In a viable fetus, early delivery may be necessary if medication is unsuccessful.

Most infants with atrial flutter have a normal heart. Those who respond initially to medical management usually have a good prognosis, but those requiring multiple drugs and emergency delivery may do poorly even after birth, especially if an associated cardiac malformation is present.

Postoperative atrial flutter is most commonly seen after intra-atrial repair of complete transposition, repair of an atrial septal defect, or Fontan repair.[149, 155–157] In this group of patients, the P wave may be difficult to distinguish. It is also common in lesions with associated AV valve regurgitation.

TREATMENT

Pharmacologic Treatment

Adenosine may be helpful in confirming the diagnosis of atrial flutter by increasing the degree of AV block and uncovering the flutter waves; conversion to sinus rhythm is not expected. Immediately after adenosine, the degree of AV conduction may be increased, speeding up the ventricular response secondary to increased circulating catecholamines.

As with other arrhythmias, the mode of therapy is determined by the patient's status. Immediate synchronous cardioversion should be performed if the infant or child is in severe congestive heart failure. Digoxin should be used to maintain sinus rhythm. If adequate digoxin has been given and is ineffective in maintaining sinus rhythm, a second drug should be added and cardioversion performed if atrial flutter persists. In children, especially in acute situations, intravenous procainamide or intravenous amiodarone is recommended. Infants frequently require higher than expected doses of procainamide to obtain therapeutic levels; plasma concentrations are helpful in determining the appropriate dose. Once the rhythm is converted, the patient may be changed to the oral formulation. If the child is too young to take the capsule or sustained-release tablet, the intravenous form of procainamide may be used orally. A suspension made from the powder in the capsule often results in erratic absorption and failure to maintain adequate levels. Other class I agents have been successful in treating atrial flutter but should not be given unless an AV nodal blocking agent is used concomitantly. Propafenone has shown a 20 to 50% success rate in treating atrial flutter.[85, 158] Sotalol has been reported to be successful in 60% of patients.[87] Chronic intractable atrial flutter may require amiodarone, which has been successful in 80 to 97% of patients. If amiodarone is used in a patient with sinus node dysfunction or marked AV nodal dysfunction, a pacemaker should be in place to provide an adequate escape rhythm.[159]

Atrial pacing techniques, either esophageal or intracardiac, may be used to convert the rhythm. Esophageal pacing is effective in only 50% of patients. Intracardiac pacing is usually effective but may result in conversion from atrial flutter to atrial fibrillation, which may require cardioversion.[160] New antitachycardia pacemakers are a helpful adjunct in selected patients with refractory atrial flutter.[161] Patients must be carefully selected and tested because atrial pacing may cause deterioration to more life-threatening rhythms.[160]

Radiofrequency Ablation

In patients without congenital heart disease, atrial flutter usually results from a counterclockwise reentry circuit in the right atrium. The circuit includes the atrial septum and the right atrial free wall, originating just inferior or posterior to the coronary sinus ostium, proceeding superiorly in the atrial septum to the right atrial free wall, then inferiorly toward the tricuspid annulus and medially between the inferior vena cava and the tricuspid annulus, where low-amplitude fragmented electrical activity is noted, along with an area of slow conduction.[162–165] In patients with typical atrial flutter, a zone of slow conduction is present in the isthmus of atrial tissue between the inferior vena cava and the tricuspid valve or between the tricuspid valve and the coronary sinus. A number of electrophysiologic techniques have been described to target an appropriate area for catheter ablation.[162–166] Successful sites are usually inferior or posterior to the coronary sinus ostium and anterior to the isthmus between the inferior vena cava and the tricuspid annulus.

In children who have undergone surgery, atrial flutter appears to be secondary to a reentry mechanism within the atrial muscle. This type of tachycardia is more appropriately termed *intra-atrial reentrant tachycardia*. The atrial

rates are commonly 250 bpm or slower. This type of atypical atrial flutter occurs primarily in patients who have had cardiac surgery involving atrial tissue, often with multiple suture lines. Reentry may be due to critical slowing in areas of slow conduction or to reentry around fixed anatomic obstacles or postsurgical suture lines.[167, 168] Successful ablation depends on identification of areas of early activation relative to the surface ECG flutter waves, critical zones of slow conduction, and areas of exit from the circuit. Attempts at ablation of atrial flutter have been reported,[99, 169] with early success but late recurrences. Multiple circuits were present in these.[167] Techniques similar to those used in typical atrial flutter are used for successful ablation of intra-atrial reentrant tachycardia.[168, 170]

Atrial Fibrillation

Atrial fibrillation is less common than atrial flutter in children.[171] The atrial rate is rapid and irregular from 400 to 700 bpm. The ventricular rhythm is irregular secondary to variable AV block. Although apparent flutter waves may be seen intermittently, the atrial rate is irregular, and the atrial morphology is variable. Atrial fibrillation occurs in association with many conditions (Table 55–6).[172]

TREATMENT

Digoxin is the initial treatment to slow the AV conduction and to increase the degree of AV block. Atrial fibrillation may be converted to sinus rhythm. Intravenous procainamide may be used for conversion to normal sinus rhythm in an acute situation when the patient is hemodynamically stable and cardioversion is not required. Normally, digoxin should be given before class I agents to prevent a paradoxical increase in ventricular rate as the atrial rate is slowed and more atrial impulses are conducted through the AV node.

Atrial fibrillation is associated with the WPW syndrome and may be life-threatening because of rapid conduction to the ventricle, resulting in a rapid ventricular response and possible ventricular fibrillation.[173] Digoxin should be avoided in these patients with atrial fibrillation and WPW syndrome because of its potential to shorten the refractory period of the accessory pathway.[35, 36] β-Blockers may be used in combination with class I agents, such as procainamide and quinidine. Amiodarone or sotalol may be effective in some instances. Esophageal or intracardiac pacing is ineffective, and electrical cardioversion may be required. Although positive results have been obtained

TABLE 55–6
CONDITIONS ASSOCIATED WITH ATRIAL FIBRILLATION
Rheumatic heart disease
Cardiac malformations
Ebstein anomaly
Tricuspid atresia
Atrial septal defects
AV valve regurgitation
Acquired heart disease
Cardiomyopathies
Idiopathic
Adolescents

AV = atrioventricular.

with RFA of atrial fibrillation in a very select group of adults, no published data are available in children.

Patients with atrial fibrillation and atrial flutter have a significant incidence of thromboembolism, although the specific risk in children is unknown. In patients with a cardiac malformation and possible right-to-left shunting, the risks may be considerable. These patients should have an echocardiogram to rule out intracardiac thrombi and should undergo anticoagulation with heparin if the onset is very recent (within hours). Transesophageal echocardiography may define atrial thrombi better than transthoracic echocardiography. Patients with chronic atrial fibrillation should receive anticoagulation with either aspirin or warfarin derivatives.

Automatic Atrial Tachycardia or Ectopic Atrial Tachycardia

Automatic atrial tachycardia or ectopic atrial tachycardia arises from a site in the atrium other than the sinus node[174,175] and represented 18% of SVT in a study on the electrophysiologic mechanisms of SVT.[17,176] The P wave axis and morphology and PR interval are different from that present during sinus rhythm, but for sites located close to the sinus node, they may appear similar to sinus rhythm (Fig. 55–13). First- or second-degree AV block may occur without interruption of the tachycardia. Characteristic acceleration (warm-up) is seen, and the rate of the tachycardia responds to autonomic influences or exercise. Cool-down or slowing may occur before termination. Ectopic foci may occur anywhere but are most commonly seen in the atrial appendages and around the orifices of the pulmonary veins. Right atrial sites are slightly more common than left atrial sites. Tachycardias from the automatic ectopic focus tend to be chronic and incessant and may result in a cardiomyopathy. Congestive heart failure is common and may be the presenting feature.[177] Presentation is more common in children younger than 6 years, although it is not uncommon in adolescents or preadolescents with a

TABLE 55–7
CONDITIONS OR EVENTS ASSOCIATED WITH ECTOPIC ATRIAL TACHYCARDIA

Myocarditis
Chronic cardiomyopathy
AV valve regurgitation
Atrial dilatation
Postoperative atrial surgery
   Intra-atrial repair of complete transposition
   Fontan repair

AV = atrioventricular.

structurally normal heart.[176] Although the cause is rarely identifiable and is attributed to abnormal automaticity, this arrhythmia may be associated with various conditions (Table 55–7).

Usual heart rates in older children range from 110 to 160 bpm. The tachycardia rate varies during the day, accelerating with sympathetic stimuli to rates as high as 300 bpm. Patients may be unaware of the tachycardia, presumably because of its incessant nature.

Electrophysiologic criteria for the diagnosis of atrial tachycardia help to differentiate this arrhythmia from the reentrant SVTs. Ectopic atrial tachycardia is not induced or terminated by programmed electrical stimulation. In most instances, adenosine results in AV block with continuation of atrial tachycardia.

TREATMENT

Pharmacologic Treatment

Treatment of ectopic or automatic atrial tachycardia is difficult. The response from the usual first-line drugs that are effective in other forms of SVT is suboptimal.[178] Digoxin and propranolol may slow the rate but rarely convert the rhythm to a sinus mechanism. Because of the association of congestive heart failure, digoxin is the first drug given. Digoxin improves symptoms and slows the tachycardia

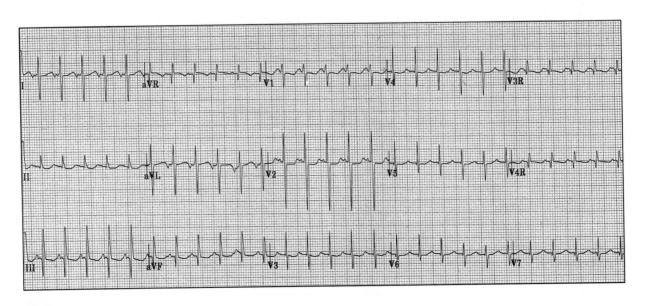

FIGURE 55–13

Electrocardiogram from a patient with ectopic atrial tachycardia. P wave axis is 119 degrees. Ectopic site was around the left upper pulmonary vein.

slightly but is rarely effective alone. β-Blockers and other medications may be effective but must be used with caution in patients with depressed ventricular function. Class IA agents have been effective in slowing the tachycardia to rates that allow cardiac function to improve markedly. Procainamide may be given intravenously initially and changed to the oral form if effective. Class IC agents, such as flecainide and propafenone, may be effective.[179, 180] Class III agents, particularly amiodarone and sotalol, have been effective in some patients.[174, 181, 182] Because some of these drugs depress cardiac function, they may not be indicated in patients with congestive heart failure. In patients refractory to other forms of treatment, amiodarone has been effective in suppressing the ectopic focus and allowing return of normal sinus rhythm. Cardioversion or atrial pacing is ineffective because the ectopic rhythm resumes immediately. Surgical or catheter ablation may be necessary in patients who are refractory to medical management.[183, 184] Because of the difficulty of controlling this arrhythmia and its tendency to result in a cardiomyopathy, surgical ablation has been attempted with 83% success but with some degree of recurrence, especially for right atrial sites.[185] Radiofrequency ablation has been used to treat atrial ectopic tachycardia. Spontaneous resolution does occur in some patients.

Radiofrequency Ablation

Because of the difficulty of controlling ectopic atrial tachycardia, the need for long-term medical therapy, and the success of surgical ablation, RFA techniques have been applied to this arrhythmia.[170, 186, 187]

In the latest tabulation of the Pediatric Radiofrequency Ablation Registry, 98 left atrial sites had been ablated with a 93% success rate, and 145 right atrial sites had been ablated with an 88% success rate. Although freedom from recurrence was 84% at the end of the first year, by the third year, freedom from recurrence was 64%, and by the fifth year, it was 58%. (Kugler JD/Pediatric Radiofrequency Ablation Registry: Personal communication, 1998).

Multifocal Atrial Tachycardia

Multifocal atrial tachycardia, also known as chaotic atrial tachycardia, is an uncommon form of atrial tachycardia whose precise mechanism has been poorly defined, although multiple reentrant circuits and triggered automaticity have been suggested. The ECG is characterized by three or more distinct P wave morphologies. The P-P and R-R intervals are irregular, with variable PR intervals, and the arrhythmia may be misdiagnosed as atrial fibrillation (Fig. 55–14). This tachycardia has been reported in young infants with and without structural heart disease; one third to one half have various types of cardiac anomalies or other medical conditions. Spontaneous resolution frequently occurs.[188] Multifocal atrial tachycardia may be associated with junctional or sinus bradycardia, making therapy more difficult. Premature atrial contractions are common.

Many of these patients have sustained atrial tachycardia. Such patients or those with symptoms of cardiac dysfunction may be the only ones to require long-term treatment.[189] Generally, digoxin has been ineffective in controlling the arrhythmia, but it may be helpful in instances of decreased cardiac function. Sudden death occurred with a 17% incidence in series of Yeager and colleagues[190]; two of the deaths were secondary to bradycardia.

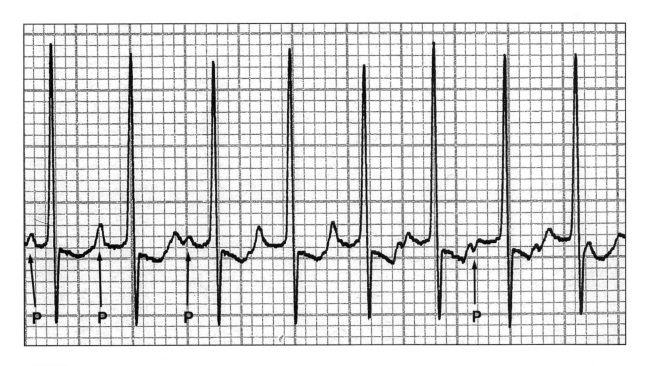

FIGURE 55–14

Lead II electrocardiographic rhythm strip illustrating chaotic atrial tachycardia at a rate of 205 beats per minute. Four different P wave morphologies are noted.

Because this tachycardia tends to resolve over months, care must be taken in the choice of antiarrhythmics so as not to enhance the tendency toward bradycardia. Drugs that slow the ventricular response, such as digoxin and propranolol, or those that decrease automaticity, such as the class IA or IC and class III agents, may be useful. Attempts to use adenosine, overdrive pacing, or direct-current cardioversion are unsuccessful because the arrhythmia does not convert or immediately recurs.

Junctional Ectopic Tachycardia

The ECG in junctional ectopic tachycardia (JET) (Fig. 55–15) shows a narrow QRS with a slower atrial rate than ventricular rate and AV dissociation. As with automatic atrial tachycardia, pacing or cardioversion is ineffective in treating the tachycardia.

JET occurs in two distinctly separate settings.[191] The first type occurs in infants in a familial form and may be associated with a cardiac malformation in as many as 50% of patients.[191] The second type occurs in the immediate postoperative period after a cardiac operation.[192] Both forms may occur at heart rates exceeding 200 bpm. The mechanism is suspected to be enhanced automaticity, but little specific information is available. In the congenital form of JET, digoxin should be used initially. If the rate does not slow sufficiently, the addition of a class IA agent may be effective. Amiodarone has been the most successful drug in treating this group of patients, controlling the tachycardia in up to 80% of patients. Sudden death has been reported in this group of patients.[193] Because the sinus node is suppressed by these drugs and sudden death associated with asystole has occurred, a pacemaker may be needed if amiodarone is used. Radiofrequency energy has been used in this group of patients.[194, 195] We reserve RFA for persistent or medically refractory JET. After several years, some of our patients with JET have been weaned from medications with no residual arrhythmias or only slow junctional ectopic rhythms.

The postoperative occurrence of JET or accelerated junctional rhythm may be fatal but generally is transient or self-limited within 24 to 72 hours.[192, 196, 197] Junctional ectopic tachycardia, often at rates greater than 250 bpm, is seen most commonly after repair of tetralogy of Fallot or Fontan repair. In the acute postoperative setting, numerous modalities have been used, including digoxin, intravenous amiodarone, class IA agents, surface cooling, and paired pacing. Waldo and coworkers[198] described a technique of paired ventricular pacing to decrease the effective ventricular rate and increase the cardiac output. Propafenone has had limited success. We have found intravenous amiodarone to be most effective in this setting. If the rate can be slowed and the patient supported for 24 to 72 hours, the JET resolves and normal sinus rhythm resumes. No long-term sequelae of this arrhythmia have been identified, but systematic studies have not been reported.

Ventricular Tachycardia

In children, ventricular arrhythmias are less common than supraventricular arrhythmias but are occurring more frequently after operations for cardiac anomalies, particularly as survival after complex operations increases.[199] Improved methods of surveillance and diagnosis of arrhythmias have allowed recognition of other causes of ventricular tachycardia (VT) in children, with the most common being the LQTS, cardiomyopathy, myocarditis, and VT in patients with a structurally normal heart.

ELECTROCARDIOGRAPHIC MANIFESTATIONS

The electrocardiographic diagnosis of VT is recognized by a wide QRS tachycardia and AV dissociation (Fig. 55–16). Ventricular tachycardia is defined as three or more consecutive wide premature QRS complexes. Other mechanisms of wide-QRS tachycardia have been described, but until proved otherwise, a wide-QRS tachycardia must be considered to be a VT. Ventricular tachycardia must be differentiated from other forms of wide-QRS tachycardias (Fig. 55–17; see Table 55–3). The rates of VT in children vary from 120 to 300 bpm. The T wave vector diverges from the QRS vector, but opposite polarity does not occur in every lead. Left bundle branch block is the most common QRS morphology, but RBBB or alternating right and LBBB may occur. Atrioventricular dissociation suggests VT, but 1:1 VA conduction is common, especially in young children. Fusion beats are noted frequently at the onset or termination of the VT. Tachycardia morphology similar to that

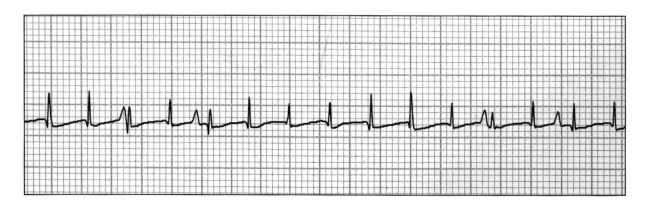

FIGURE 55-15

Lead II electrocardiographic rhythm strip illustrating junctional ectopic tachycardia. The ventricular (junctional) rate is 220 beats per minute (bpm). The atrial rate is 125 bpm.

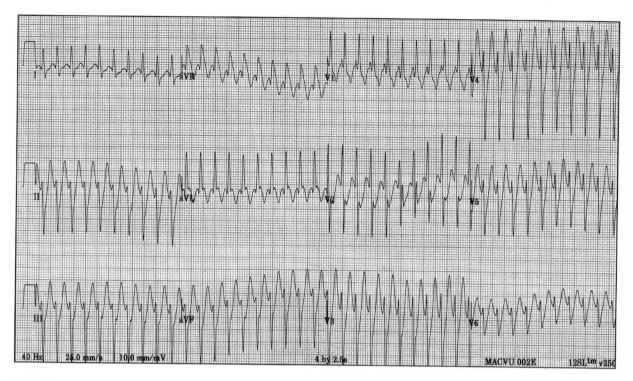

Example of ventricular tachycardia in a 2-year-old patient. Ventricular rate is 240 beats per minute. Wide QRS and inferior frontal axis.

of isolated premature ventricular contractions suggests VT. Ventricular tachycardia may be sustained (>30 consecutive complexes) or nonsustained (3 to 30 consecutive complexes). Further differentiation is made according to the morphology, with VT being described as monomorphic or polymorphic. Two types of polymorphic VT have been described: torsades de pointes and bidirectional VT (Fig. 55–18). Bidirectional VT has been associated with digoxin toxicity, familial hyperkalemic paralysis, or catecholamine sensitivity. The ECG shows beat-to-beat variation in the QRS axis.[200] Torsades de pointes is associated with the LQTS and receives its name from its twisting, undulating nature.

CLINICAL CORRELATIONS

Presentation of patients with VT varies and depends largely on the underlying cause, myocardial function, and cardiac structure. In one study of patients with VT and a structurally normal heart, 48% presented in infancy, and 58% of these were younger than 6 months. Associated findings were heart failure in 30%, hemodynamic compromise or collapse in 23%, and in utero diagnosis in 18%. In 30%, VT was an incidental diagnosis. No specific cause was found in 50%, and cardiomyopathy or myocarditis (20%) was the most common cause identified.[201]

CLINICAL SIGNS AND SYMPTOMS

The symptoms appear to be rate related, with symptoms being most common in patients with rates of greater than 150 bpm. Except for those patients with underlying cardiac disease, patients with VT have symptoms similar to those with SVT, with the degree of symptoms relating more to the rate than to the mechanism of tachycardia. Symptoms include dyspnea, shortness of breath, chest or abdominal pain, palpitations, dizziness, syncope, and cardiac arrest or sudden death. Older children may exhibit exercise intolerance or easy fatigability. Infants may feed poorly and be irritable or lethargic. Patients with VT and heart disease usually have symptoms, but only one third with a normal heart and VT have symptoms. Sudden death occurs most commonly with an abnormal heart[202] but has been reported in patients with a normal heart.[203,204] Signs include tachypnea, hypotension with accompanying pallor and diaphoresis, and signs of congestive heart failure. Although VT usually has a sudden onset, it may occur during exercise and be difficult to perceive. It may gradually warm up or increase in rate.

ETIOLOGY

Causes of acute VT, unassociated with cardiac malformations, are listed in Table 55–8, and the causes of chronic or recurrent VT are listed in Table 55–9. Commonly, a specific cause cannot be identified in children.[201,203,205,206]

MECHANISMS OF VENTRICULAR TACHYCARDIA

Ventricular tachycardia results from reentry, triggered automaticity, or abnormal automaticity. The mechanisms of VT in children include reentry in 60% and abnormal automaticity in 40%.[207] Digoxin toxicity and torsades de pointes result from triggered automaticity. Reentry is most often the mechanism in cardiac patients who have undergone surgery and is related to reentry circuits that develop around suture lines or scars, including ventriculotomies.

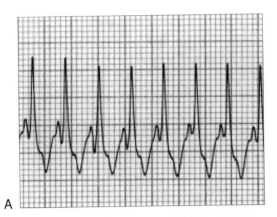

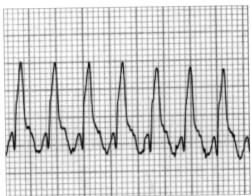

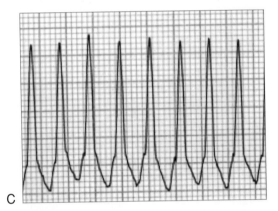

FIGURE 55–17

Electrocardiographic lead V$_1$ during wide-QRS tachycardia in three patients. *A* is from a 2-year-old patient with ventricular tachycardia. *B* is from a 13-year-old patient with supraventricular tachycardia with aberrancy. *C* is from a 10-year-old patient with atrial flutter.

TABLE 55–8

CAUSES OF ACUTE VENTRICULAR TACHYCARDIA

Metabolic

Hypoxia
Acidosis
Hypoglycemia
Hypocalcemia
Hypokalemia
Hyperkalemia

Trauma

Blunt: cardiac contusion
Thoracic surgery
Cardiac catheters

Myocardial Ischemia

Abnormal coronaries/infarction
Kawasaki disease

Hyperlipidemia

Infectious

Myocarditis
Pericarditis
Rheumatic fever

Drugs/Toxins

General anesthetics
Antiarrhythmics
Caffeine
Nicotine
Sympathomimetics/catecholamine infusions
Psychotropic agents: tricyclic antidepressants/phenothiazines
Cocaine
Digoxin toxicity

Idiopathic

SPECIFIC ASSOCIATED CONDITIONS

Accelerated Ventricular Rhythm

An accelerated ventricular rhythm originates from the ventricle and has the characteristics of VT, but the cardiac rate is only slightly higher than the underlying sinus rhythm, usually being less than 120 bpm except in neonates. It occurs most commonly in neonates and in patients with a normal heart. This arrhythmia is self-limited, resolving from 2 weeks to 3 months after birth. These early ventricular arrhythmias probably relate to developmental factors associated with the autonomic nervous system. In children, this arrhythmia is generally considered benign, even in the patient who has a cardiac anomaly.[208, 209] In older children, this arrhythmia may relate to unidentified viral infections resulting in myocarditis that affects only the conduction system. Such patients generally require no therapy but

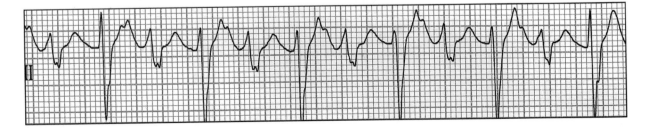

FIGURE 55–18

Electrocardiographic example of bidirectional ventricular tachycardia. Two distinctly different wide QRS morphologies.

TABLE 55–9
ETIOLOGY OF CHRONIC VENTRICULAR TACHYCARDIA

Congenital heart disease	Ebstein anomaly
	Tetralogy of Fallot, absent PV leaflets
	Aortic valve disease, AI/AS
	Mitral valve prolapse
	Hypertrophic cardiomyopathy/IHSS
	Coronary artery anomalies
	Eisenmenger's syndrome, pulmonary hypertension
Postoperative CHD	Tetralogy of Fallot, DORV
	Ventricular septal defects
	AV septal defects
	Aortic stenosis or insufficiency
	Single ventricle complexes after Fontan repair
	D-TGA after intraatrial repair
Cardiomyopathies	Hypertrophic
	RV dysplasia
	Postviral
	Connective tissue disease: SLE
	Marfan's syndrome
	Muscular dystrophy, Friedreich's ataxia
Acquired heart disease	Rheumatic heart disease
	Lyme disease
	Myocarditis
	Kawasaki disease
Tumors and infiltrates	Rhabdomyoma
	Hemosiderosis: thalassemia, sickle cell disease
	Oncocytic cardiomyopathy
	Leukemia
Idiopathic/structurally normal heart	RV outflow tract VT
	LV septal VT/fascicular tachycardia
Primary arrhythmias	LQTS
	Congenital complete heart block
	Familial VT
Other	Myocardial ischemia/infarction

PV = pulmonary valve; AI = aortic insufficiency; AS = aortic stenosis; DORV = double-outlet left ventricle; AV = atrioventricular; D-TGA = D-transposition of the great arteries; SLE = systemic lupus erythematosus; RV = right ventricular; VT = ventricular tachycardia; LV = left ventricular; LQTS = long QT syndrome; CHD = coronary heart disease; IHSS = idiopathic hypertrophic subaortic stenosis.

should be monitored because, occasionally, patients have acceleration of the ventricular rhythm to a much higher rate and experience symptoms. This arrhythmia is also seen around puberty and again probably relates to autonomic and hormonally mediated factors. In addition, accelerated ventricular rhythms have been associated with metabolic abnormalities, medication, right ventricular dysplasia, and myocardial infarction.[209] Treatment of this arrhythmia and restriction of activity are not required in most patients, especially those with a normal heart.

Long QT Syndrome

The LQTS is an inherited condition characterized by syncope, seizures, and sudden death, associated in most individuals with a prolongation of the QT interval on the ECG (Fig. 55–19).[210] These patients often also have bizarre or notched T waves and prominent U waves or T wave alternans. They experience life-threatening VT, known as torsades de pointes, or ventricular fibrillation. This syndrome includes the Jervell and Lange-Nielsen syndrome, described in 1957, associated with congenital deafness and believed to demonstrate an autosomal recessive inheritance,[211] and the Romano-Ward syndrome, described in 1963 and 1964, demonstrating autosomal dominant inheritance without a hearing deficit.[212, 213]

In 1993, a group of 287 children with LQTS were reviewed from numerous medical centers.[214] The presentation was cardiac arrest (9%), syncope (26%), seizures (10%), and presyncope or palpitations (6%). Eighty-eight percent had exercise-related symptoms. Thirty-nine percent were identified because of family history or identification of other family members with the syndrome. Thirty-nine percent of the patients were asymptomatic at presentation. Of these asymptomatic patients, 4% experienced sudden death, compared with 9% of the overall group. The strongest predictors of sudden death were QTc

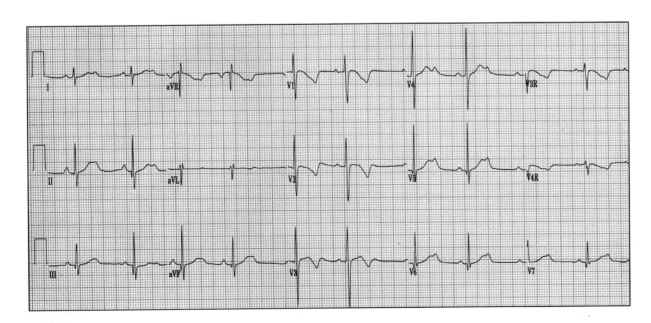

FIGURE 55–19

Fifteen-lead electrocardiogram of 12-year-old patient with long QT syndrome. The QT interval measures 500 milliseconds. Broad, notched T waves.

greater than 0.60 second and noncompliance with recommended medical therapy.

Schwartz and associates[215] provided diagnostic criteria and suggested a scale for identifying these patients. These criteria involve measurement of the QT interval and a careful history for syncope, seizures, and arrhythmias in the patients and their families. A family history of early or sudden death is extremely important in making the diagnosis. Additional studies, such as 24-hour monitoring and exercise stress testing, may provide helpful information in the form of significantly prolonged QT intervals, especially during recovery from exercise, or with the development of polymorphic ventricular arrhythmias during or after exercise. Bradycardia is common, and some patients experience or present with second-degree AV block. The latter is more common in neonates who may have second- or third-degree AV block[216] but may occur in older children, especially with exercise. The use of provocative testing, such as isoproterenol and epinephrine infusions, remains controversial.[217,218]

One series reported sudden death occurring in 73% of patients without treatment.[219] Others have reported sudden death in 21% of symptomatic patients in the first year after presenting with syncope. Treatment with β-blockers can lower the mortality to 6%.[210] The sudden death is secondary to ventricular arrhythmias (torsades de pointes) (Fig. 55–20), which frequently degenerates to ventricular fibrillation.[220]

A high level of suspicion is needed to diagnose these patients. Any patient who presents with VT, especially of the polymorphic or torsades de pointes type or in association with physical or emotional stress, should have corrected QT intervals determined. A complete history may reveal a family history of sudden death in young relatives or a history of syncope or seizures associated with exercise or emotional stress.

Some studies have identified genetic abnormalities that encode for proteins modulating potassium and sodium ion channels and have suggested that these abnormalities are the cause of this syndrome.[221–224] These abnormalities in channel function alter cardiac repolarization and increase the risk for ventricular arrhythmias (see Chapter 2).

Not all families with known LQTS have shown linkage to the identified loci, suggesting additional genes yet to be discovered. In addition to these genes that affect ionic channels, which alter the repolarization phase of the cardiac action potential and result in the development of ventricular arrhythmias, an imbalance or an oversensitivity of the myocardium to sympathetic stimulation appears to play a role in the development of ventricular arrhythmias.

CLINICAL ASSOCIATIONS OF GENETIC FINDINGS. Typical T wave changes have been associated with specific genetic mutations,[225] as shown in Figure 55–21. Overlap exists with all T wave patterns seen with each genetic abnormality, limiting the specificity of this finding. Patients with LQTS linked to chromosome 3 have more cardiac events at rest or during sleep, and patients with LQTS linked to chromosome 7 experience more events during exercise or stress.

The study by Vincent and associates[226] indicated that some patients may be genetic carriers for this syndrome without manifesting significant prolongation of the QT interval. Some noncarriers (15%) have abnormal prolongation of the QTc interval above 0.44 second. A QTc of greater than 0.47 second had a 100% positive predictive value in gene carriers. At QTc intervals of greater than 0.47 second, there were no false positive results in this study. Only 6% of gene carriers had QTc intervals of less than 0.44 second.[226] These genetic tests may make it possible to identify more specifically many patients with the LQTS.

Diagnosis

Diagnosis is made by a careful history of the individual's episodes and a complete family history, with the physician looking for sudden unexplained death, syncopal episodes, unusual seizure disorders, or hearing deficits. Careful evaluation of the ECG and 24-hour ambulatory monitoring are essential. The QTc interval is measured by use of Bazett's formula[227]: the longest QT interval in any lead is divided by the square root of the preceding R-R interval. The measurement should be manually made and calculated because the computerized values are frequently incorrect. We use a value of greater than 0.45 second in any lead as abnormal on the resting or exercise ECG. On the Holter monitor, because different filters are used, a value of greater than 0.50 second is considered abnormal. Although

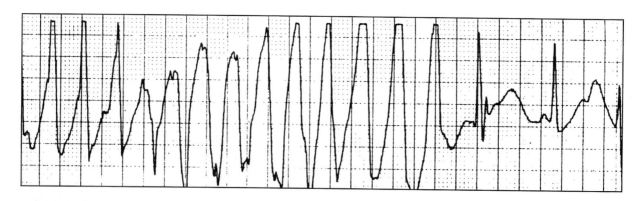

FIGURE 55–20
Electrocardiographic rhythm strip from a patient with long QT syndrome illustrating torsades de pointes. This ventricular tachycardia is rapid, irregular and polymorphic, changing axis around the more narrow fourth complex.

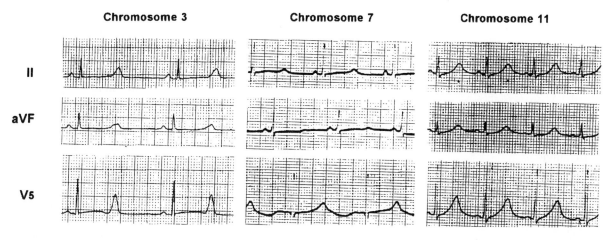

Chromosome 3   **Chromosome 7**   **Chromosome 11**

II

aVF

V5

FIGURE 55–21

Electrocardiographic recordings from leads II, aVF and V5 in three patients with long QT syndrome, linked to chromosomes 3, 7, and 11. The patient with chromosome 3 linkage has late-onset T waves with a QTc of 570 milliseconds. The patient with chromosome 7 linkage has low-amplitude T waves and a QTc of 583 milliseconds. The patients with chromosome 11 linkage has early-onset broad T waves and a QTc of 573 milliseconds. (From Moss AJ, Zareba W, Benhorin J, et al: ECG T-wave patterns in genetically distinct forms of the hereditary long QT syndrome. Circulation 92:2929–2934, 1995.)

numerous methods have been proposed for calculating the QTc in the presence of sinus arrhythmia,[228] we make every attempt to record an ECG not in sinus arrhythmia. Provocative testing, including exercise stress testing and isoproterenol or epinephrine infusion, may help to identify these patients. We use a value of greater than 0.50 second as abnormal on isoproterenol testing. T wave abnormalities,[229] in addition to QTc prolongation or the development of ventricular arrhythmias during these provocative tests, may be seen in these patients. Exercise generally obliterates sinus arrhythmia, and an electrocardiographic recording can be obtained in which a reasonable QTc calculation can be made. The recovery period with heart rates around 120 to 130 bpm seems to demonstrate the greatest degree of QTc prolongation in many patients.

Clinical research efforts continue to identify risk predictors for syncope and sudden death. High-risk electrocardiographic markers have included QTc greater than 0.60 second, T wave alternans, and QTc dispersion.[230, 231] Dispersion of the QT interval has been correlated with high risk in LQTS patients.[214, 229, 230, 232] QT dispersion, which indicates heterogeneity of repolarization, could predispose to the development of torsades de pointes. In Priori and colleagues' study,[230] patients not responding to a β-blocker had a significantly higher dispersion of repolarization than did responders. In Shah and associates study,[232] patients with long QT who are at high risk for developing critical ventricular arrhythmias had a QT or JT dispersion of at least 55 milliseconds.[232]

EARLY AFTERDEPOLARIZATIONS. Early afterdepolarizations have been recorded with the use of monophasic action potentials in congenital and acquired LQTS.[233–235] Excessive prolongation of the action potential duration could result in reactivation of l-type calcium channels, leading to afterdepolarizations. Catecholamines also enhance the development of early afterdepolarizations.[233, 236–238] These early afterdepolarizations are likely to play a role in the development of torsades de pointes or VT.

TREATMENT. Emergency treatment of these patients includes lidocaine and cardioversion. In addition, temporary atrial or ventricular pacing at a rate 10 to 20% faster than the underlying sinus rate may be needed to control the arrhythmia, especially in patients with underlying bradycardia, a common association.[239] Intravenous propranolol and phenytoin have also been used successfully. The class I agents, which are known to prolong the QT interval in normal patients, should be avoided in long QT patients. In fact, a number of drugs may produce this form of VT (Box 55–3). This phenomenon is thought to be related to QTc prolongation with associated bradycardia and/or ventricular arrhythmias. Temporary pacing and removal of the offending agent are effective therapies.

The standard treatment in this condition is a β-blocker, usually either propranolol or nadolol. Although the use of long-acting propranolol or atenolol has been suggested, once-daily dosing leads to the lowest levels being present in early morning hours, a high-risk time for some patients. Therefore, we suggest twice-daily dosing, at least, in this group of patients. One study suggested an unfavorable result with atenolol.[240] The dose of β-blocker varies and is usually greater per kilogram in younger patients. Most teenagers require 10 to 20 mg of nadolol twice daily. We titrate the appropriate dose according to the heart rate response to maximal exercise testing, aiming for a blunted maximal heart rate response on therapy consisting of 150 to 160 bpm. Our patients are followed-up yearly or twice yearly with exercise stress tests and Holter monitoring to look for adequacy of treatment and/or development of significant ventricular arrhythmias.

Patients who do not respond to β-blockers may be treated with mexiletine, pacing, or phenytoin. Rarely, other antiarrhythmics may be helpful, but those known to prolong the QT interval should be avoided.

Left stellate ganglionectomy has been used but has variable success and is controversial.[241–244]

Permanent pacing has been an effective adjunctive treatment, especially in those with severe bradycardia ei-

BOX 55–3. PHARMACOLOGIC AGENTS THAT PROLONG QT INTERVALS AND DRUGS TO AVOID IN LONG QT SYNDROME PATIENTS*

ANTIARRHYTHMIC AGENTS
Quinidine
Procainamide
Flecainide
Disopyramide
Amiodarone
Sotalol
Ibutilide
Dofetilide
Moricizine
Tocainide

ANTIHISTAMINES
Terfenadine
Astemizole
Diphenhydramine
Fexofenadine
Clemastine

ANTIBIOTICS/ANTIFUNGAL AGENTS
Erythromycin
Azithromycin (Zithromax)
Clarithromycin (Biaxin)
Trimethoprim
Sulfamethoxazole
Pentamidine
Amantadine
Chloroquine
Halofantrine
Clindamycin
Ketoconazole
Fluconazole
Itraconazole

PSYCHOTROPIC DRUGS
Tricyclic antidepressants
  Amitriptyline (Elavil), clomipramine (Anafranil), doxepin (Sinequan), desipramine (Norpramin), imipramine (Tofranil), and others
Phenothiazines
  Chlorpromazine (Thorazine), prochlorperazine (Compazine), thioridazine (Mellaril), and others
Haloperidol
Risperidone
Pimozide
Fluroxamine (Luvox)
Carbamazepine (Tegretol)

OTHER
Cisapride
Ketanserin
Bepridil
Probucol
Tamoxifen
Fludrocortisone
Diuretics
Epinephrine
Caffeine

*Partial list.

ther from the syndrome itself or from the β-blocker therapy.[245,246] The rate of the pacing should be at least 10 to 20% higher than the sinus rate and in severe disease should control the patient's rhythm as much of the time as possible. In these instances, episodes of torsades de pointes may be reduced or eliminated.

In patients who have had cardiac arrest or frequent or significant syncope associated with ventricular arrhythmias, we recommend the implantation of an automatic implantable cardioverter-defibrillator. These devices recognize VT or fibrillation according to programmed criteria and provide a series of shocks to convert the patient to sinus rhythm. Because of the size of the device, it has limited use in smaller children, but improved technology will eventually allow even the smallest child to receive this treatment. This therapy must be considered seriously because follow-up and possible false discharges can significantly affect a child's life and lifestyle. Groh and colleagues[247] reported on 35 patients with LQTS who had implanted cardioverter-defibrillators and were followed up for a mean of 31 months. The major indication for implantation was aborted sudden death. Sixty percent of patients had at least one appropriate discharge in the follow-up period. Two patients had multiple discharges and required additional therapy. No patients died. These results were similar to those reported earlier by Silka and associates.[248]

A greater understanding of the molecular mechanisms of LQTS has prompted studies to identify more specific or gene-directed therapies.[249] The sodium channel blocker mexiletine has been used[250] and the QT interval has been decreased in patients with LQTS linked to chromosome 3. Sato and associates[251] used a potassium channel opener, nicorandil, in a patient with LQTS. Trials are underway with potassium supplementation and spironolactone.

Competitive athletics should be avoided in many patients with LQTS, particularly those with symptoms or arrhythmias. As more "carriers," or asymptomatic patients, are discovered, who have only a prolonged QT interval and no family history of sudden death or ventricular arrhythmias, individual exercise and sports participation recommendations may be made. The most important aspect of the care is continued surveillance. Young family members may have normal QT intervals on initial evaluation, but these intervals may change with age. Thus, we recommend periodic ECGs and appropriate 24-hour and exercise electrocardiography.

Myocarditis
Patients with myocarditis present another special problem; 14 to 50% of these patients have ventricular ectopy.[252,253] Steroid therapy has helped some patients.[254] The most common causes of viral myocarditis are coxsackievirus A and B and adenovirus. Often, these patients have diminished myocardial function and require inotropic support to maintain cardiac output. An agent with the least arrhythmogenic characteristics, such as dobutamine, should be chosen. Ventricular arrhythmias may occur in patients with myocarditis and associated complete heart block with slow escape rhythms. In these instances, increasing the heart rate with a temporary transvenous pacemaker may be all that is needed to control the ventricular arrhythmia. Pressor agents should not be used merely to increase the heart

rate in the absence of hemodynamic impairment, because of the arrhythmogenic potential in this subset of patients.

Many patients with myocarditis present with a ventricular arrhythmia, usually single premature ventricular contractions or nonsustained VT and only mild or no impairment of ventricular function. In these instances, the ventricular arrhythmia may require no treatment or may need suppression if it is potentially threatening or impairing ventricular function. We have used β-blockade or mexiletine successfully in these patients.

Postoperative Ventricular Tachycardia

With few exceptions, patients who undergo intracardiac surgery risk the development of postoperative arrhythmias and conduction defects.[255] Postoperative VT is more likely to occur with long-standing right ventricular hypertension, healing of a ventriculotomy scar under pressure, postoperative volume overload of the right ventricle, residual left ventricular pressure overload, or a previous ventriculotomy. The most common lesion associated with VT is tetralogy of Fallot,[256, 257] but VT follows a number of types of repairs.[258] In addition, 10 to 15% of patients after intra-atrial repair of complete transposition or Fontan repair present with ventricular arrhythmias. Sudden death occurs in 5 to 10%.[259, 260]

In tetralogy of Fallot, risk factors associated with the development of VT and sudden death include older age at repair, longer postoperative period, right ventricular systolic pressure of greater than 60 mm Hg at rest, right ventricular end-diastolic pressure of greater than 10 mm Hg at rest, depressed right ventricular systolic function, moderate-to-severe pulmonary or tricuspid regurgitation, and QRS duration of greater than 0.18 second.[256, 261–263]

Abnormal results on signal-averaged electrograms with late potentials are associated with the development of VT.[264] Ventriculotomy, myocardial resection, and subsequent scarring may provide the electrophysiologic substrate of slow conduction and block that predisposes the patient to develop reentrant arrhythmias. Pathologic studies in patients with tetralogy of Fallot who have died suddenly have revealed extensive fibrosis of the right ventricular myocardium at the ventriculotomy site, right ventricular outflow tract, and septum.[265] Serious ventricular arrhythmias occasionally occur despite good hemodynamic results, although sudden death occurs most commonly in patients with VT associated with poor hemodynamics.

ELECTROPHYSIOLOGIC STUDIES IN POSTOPERATIVE PATIENTS. Electrophysiologic studies have been used to evaluate the propensity of postoperative patients to develop VT, to evaluate specific pharmacologic therapies, to locate the site of origin of the arrhythmia in patients who are candidates for ablative therapy,[266–268] and to help determine the need for implantation of an automatic cardioverter-defibrillator.[269] Fifteen percent of patients have inducible VT after repair of tetralogy of Fallot.

The site of origin of the VT has been localized to the right ventricular outflow tract in most instances and to the ventricular septum in others.[267, 270] The VT in these patients can be reproducibly initiated and terminated at EPS and has been presumed to be reentrant.[271] Factors associated with inducibility include right ventricular systolic or volume overload and a longer period from the time of op-

eration.[272] Continuous electrical activity has been noted in these patients in the right ventricular outflow tract.[267] Fragmented, prolonged, low-amplitude electrographic findings from the right ventricle have been reported and occur more commonly in patients with VT.[255]

Early repair has been reported to decrease the incidence of VT.[271, 273, 274]

MANAGEMENT AND PROGNOSIS OF PATIENTS WITH POSTOPERATIVE VENTRICULAR TACHYCARDIA. Because of the high incidence of ventricular arrhythmias in patients who have undergone surgery, their precise role in the occurrence of sudden death is unclear. After tetralogy repair, exercise stress testing or ambulatory monitoring uncovers a 25 to 70% incidence of ventricular arrhythmias. In 1985, Garson and coworkers[275] suggested that treatment of greater than 10 premature ventricular contractions per hour on ambulatory monitoring had decreased the incidence of sudden death in their population. Conversely, Sullivan and colleagues[276] have reported no increase in the incidence of sudden death by not treating similar patients. The presence of frequent or complex ventricular ectopy probably identifies a high-risk group, but at present, our ability to identify further those patients at highest risk is limited.

Although there is no agreement about the indications for treatment, we treat patients with clinical episodes of VT, with symptoms and inducible VT, with complex ventricular arrhythmias and abnormal hemodynamics, and/or with significant symptoms and abnormal hemodynamics. We use the EPS to determine the efficacy of specific drug regimens or the need for an implantable cardioverter-defibrillator in patients in whom drug therapy is ineffective or in those with hemodynamic deterioration.

The most commonly used drug regimens include β-blockers, mexiletine, and class IA or IC agents. In the 1970s, phenytoin was found to be an effective drug in this population, but mexiletine is now more commonly used. Amiodarone is an effective drug in some refractory patients. Surgical or catheter ablation has also been used effectively.

Ventricular Tachycardia and Tumors

Ventricular tachycardia is associated with cardiac rhabdomyomas. An incessant form of VT has been reported in infants and young children secondary to myocardial hamartomas that have been treated successfully with surgical ablation.[277] Aggressive medical management, including combination drug therapy, may be used to control this type of VT. Rhabdomyomas may regress. A more diffuse infiltrative type of disease known as *histiocytoid* or *oncocytic cardiomyopathy of infancy* manifests as incessant VT in infancy and is usually fatal.[278]

Ventricular Tachycardia and Mitral Valve Prolapse

In adults, the incidence of sudden death associated with mitral valve prolapse is 1.4%.[279] There are also reports of sudden death in children and adolescents with mitral valve prolapse, especially in athletes.[280] Sudden death is proposed to be secondary to ventricular arrhythmias.[281] Twenty-four-hour monitoring has revealed premature ventricular contractions or more complex ventricular arrhythmias in as many as 46% of children with mitral valve prolapse.[282] Twenty-three percent of these arrhythmias were considered life-threatening. Exercise stress testing revealed serious ventricular arrhythmias in 20% of patients. When indicated, β-blockers have been the drugs of choice for control of these arrhythmias, although we have found few of these arrhythmias to be clinically significant or life-threatening in our patients.

Ventricular Tachycardia and Cardiomyopathies

There is a high incidence of sudden death, presumably from ventricular arrhythmias, in children with hypertophic obstructive cardiomyopathy.[283-286] Hypertrophic cardiomyopathy is the most common cause of sudden death in young competitive athletes.[283,287] A family history of sudden death, ventricular arrhythmias on 24-hour ambulatory monitoring, previous syncope, extensive generalized hypertrophy, or ventricular systolic or diastolic dysfunction may identify a high-risk population.[286] Two events that predict subsequent sudden death include a combination of inducible sustained VT at EPS and a history of cardiac arrest or syncope.[288] Unfortunately, many high-risk patients do not have inducible VT. Fractionation of electrograms with programmed stimulation may be a marker for high-risk patients.[289] Asymptomatic VT on a Holter recording may be predictive.[290] Treatment includes antiarrhythmic therapy,[291-293] pacemakers,[294,295] myotomy/myectomy,[296] and implantable defibrillators.[248,297] Genetic identification of hypertrophic cardiomyopathy may increase understanding and identify high-risk patients (see Chapters 35 and 49).[298] Specific genetic mutations are associated with a higher incidence of sudden death.[299,300]

Ventricular Tachycardia and Structurally Normal Heart

In structurally normal hearts, two sites have been associated with VT. The first is in the right ventricular outflow tract, most commonly in the anteroseptal region, but also in the anterolateral and anterior regions.[301,302] The morphology of the VT on ECG is LBBB pattern, most commonly with an inferior axis but also with a superior or rightward axis. Right bundle branch block pattern with superior or rightward axis is also seen. Both sustained and nonsustained VTs occur. In 40 to 80% of selected patients, the tachycardia may be induced as nonsustained or sustained VT by programmed electrical stimulation with or without isoproterenol. The second site is in the mid-to-inferior portion of the left ventricular septum. The morphology of the VT is generally RBBB with left axis deviation. It can also be induced. Ventricular tachycardia from the basal aspect of the superior left ventricular septum can present as repetitive monomorphic VT, revealing a dominant R wave pattern in V_1, an inferior axis, and a precordial R wave transition at or before lead V_2.[303] These VTs may respond to verapamil or adenosine, suggesting a triggered mechanism.[304] Both forms of VT are amenable to RFA,[302,303,305,306] with a higher success rate in the right ventricular tachycardias.

TREATMENT AND EVALUATION OF VENTRICULAR TACHYCARDIA

Emergency Treatment

Ventricular tachycardia should be treated as an emergency unless the rate is slow and the patient is stable. If an extracardiac cause, such as an electrolyte abnormality or acidosis, has been identified, the underlying abnormality should be corrected. This usually converts the ventricular arrhythmia to sinus rhythm. In patients with cardiac compromise, intravenous lidocaine at 1 mg/kg should be given immediately. If the lidocaine is effective, a continuous infusion of lidocaine at 10 to 50 μg/kg/min should be started to maintain an adequate level of lidocaine. Lidocaine levels should be carefully monitored to prevent toxicity.

Synchronized cardioversion at 2 to 5 watt-sec/kg should be performed if the lidocaine does not result in immediate conversion or if an intravenous site is unavailable.

Procainamide has been used to treat acute episodes of VT. Because of its negative inotropic effects, the patients must be monitored carefully during the infusion. Amiodarone is also effective when given intravenously for VT. Drugs used in emergent therapy are shown in Table 55–10.

TABLE 55–10

EMERGENCY TREATMENT OF VENTRICULAR TACHYCARDIA

Initial Treatment	Dosage	Level
Lidocaine	1–2 mg/kg IV bolus every 5–15 min IV infusion: 20–50 μg/kg/min	1.5–5.0 mg/L
Cardioversion	1–5 watt-sec/kg Double if ineffective	

Secondary Treatment	IV Dosage	Level
Procainamide	5 mg/kg over 5–10 min or 15 mg/kg over 30–45 min Infusion: 20–100 μg/kg/min	NAPA: 4–10 mg/L PA: 4–8 mg/L
Propranolol	0.05–0.1 mg/kg over 5 min q 6 h	
Phenytoin	3–5 mg/kg over 5 min, not to exceed 1 mg/kg/min	10–20 μg/ml
Bretylium	5-mg/kg bolus every 15 min Infusion: 5–10 mg/kg over 10 min every 6 h	
Amiodarone	5 mg/kg over 1 h, followed by 5- to 10-μg/kg/min infusion	
Magnesium	0.25 mEq/kg over 1 min, followed by 1 mEq/kg over 5 h to achieve Mg^{2+} level of 3–4 mg/dl	

NAPA = N-acetylprocainamide; PA = procainamide; IV = intravenous.

Rapid ventricular pacing may convert the rhythm to sinus if pharmacologic therapy fails or is contraindicated.

Long-Term Treatment

Once the VT has been converted, choice of an appropriate long-term regimen is essential to maintain stability of the patient. The drugs most commonly used are shown in Table 55–5. If lidocaine has been successful, it may be given until adequate levels of a long-term drug have been reached or the acute causative agent is no longer present. When changing to mexiletine, the lidocaine should be gradually weaned as the mexiletine is loaded in order to prevent combined toxicity of these two drugs because their side effects are similar. Propranolol or other β-blockers are especially effective in patients whose arrhythmia is sensitive to sympathetic or adrenergic stimuli.[307] The class I agents and amiodarone are effective in more refractory arrhythmias.[79,308]

Because sudden death occurs in up to 30% of patients with VT and a cardiac anomaly, such patients should be placed on a long-term regimen. These life-threatening arrhythmias are most commonly seen in association with tetralogy of Fallot; anomalies with long-standing ventricular pressure overload, such as single ventricle or complete transposition after intra-atrial repair; and conditions with abnormal myocardium, such as Ebstein or hypertrophic subaortic stenosis. In patients who have just undergone surgery, this arrhythmia is poorly tolerated but generally responds to lidocaine and correction of other underlying hemodynamic and metabolic abnormalities. Patients with early postoperative VT are likely to develop this arrhythmia in the late postoperative period, so long-term therapy is recommended. A thorough investigation is needed to exclude underlying hemodynamic abnormalities because VT is tolerated less well in this group of patients. Mexiletine and β-blockers provide effective long-term therapy in patients after tetralogy of Fallot repair.[309] Class I agents and amiodarone may be effective in refractory patients. Electrophysiologic study may help guide medical therapy[266,267] or, in patients refractory to drug therapy, may determine the site of origin of the tachycardia and direct treatment by surgical ablation or RFA. Patients with life-threatening episodes or those refractory to medical or ablative therapy may require implantation of a cardioverter-defibrillator.

Electrophysiologic Study

The specific indications used for performance of EPSs in children with VT are shown in Box 55–4. Intracardiac recordings during VT show the absence of His bundle deflections consistently preceding ventricular depolarizations, with atrial capture at more rapid rates than the tachycardia normalizing the QRS complex. One of the most significant differences between adults and children is in the different mechanisms responsible for VT.[207] In adults, more than 90% have inducible VT. In children, only 30 to 50% have inducible or reentrant VT, and the rest have triggered or automatic VT. Most inducible VT in children is associated with cardiac anomalies.

Radiofrequency Ablation

In children, the categories of VT that are amenable to RFA include those in a structurally normal heart that originate

---

> ### BOX 55–4. INDICATIONS FOR ELECTROPHYSIOLOGIC STUDY IN VENTRICULAR TACHYCARDIA (VT)
>
> 1. Documented VT > 150 bpm or wide-QRS tachycardia, except in association with acute metabolic or electrolyte abnormalities, myocarditis, or LQTS. Value of EPS in cardiomyopathies has not been determined but may be helpful in selected patients.
> 2. Nonsustained VT or complex premature ventricular arrhythmias in a patient with an abnormal heart.
> 3. Suspected VT in the presence of syncope or cardiac arrest of unknown etiology.
> 4. Symptoms suggestive of VT in vulnerable patient with an abnormal heart, e.g., postoperative tetralogy of Fallot, hypertrophic cardiomyopathy.
> 5. Follow-up of patient with inducible, documented VT to test efficacy of chronic medication.
> 6. For radiofrequency ablation in selected patients.

LQTS = long QT syndrome; EPS = electrophysiologic study.

---

primarily in the right ventricular outflow tract or in the left ventricular septum. The technique of ablation involves identifying an intracardiac electrogram from an activation site during VT that is earlier than on any surface ventricular electrogram. At this site, pace mapping is performed to identify an ECG result that has the same morphology with pacing as the clinical VT.[302,310,311]

The other category of patients with VT that is amenable to RFA are those who have postoperative VT, particularly in the right ventricular outflow tract.[267] Scarring from the right ventriculotomy or infundibular resection allows a zone of slow conduction that produces the substrate for reentry.[265] Successful ablation sites in these patients include those with earliest activation during VT, areas of slow conduction with low amplitude, fractionated electrograms, and sites that produce a pace map identical to that of the clinical or inducible VT.[312–314] One report has noted success in 15 of 16 patients with postoperative tetralogy of Fallot.[315] In the Pediatric Radiofrequency Ablation Registry, 134 patients with VT had an ablation with 64% success.[106]

PROGNOSIS OF VENTRICULAR TACHYCARDIA

The prognosis of VT depends on the underlying condition. Reviews of VT in children have reported an incidence of death of 10 to 47%.[199] A higher incidence occurs in those with an underlying structural or postoperative cardiac anomaly and poor hemodynamic results. Sudden death has been reported in patients with VT and a normal heart. Sudden death occurs in 6 to 8% of patients. With a normal heart spontaneous resolution of VT may occur, especially in the neonate or young child. The outlook for infants and children with VT is excellent if the VT can be controlled with treatment.[201]

Bradycardia

Patients present with a slow ventricular rate because of abnormalities of impulse formation in the sinus node or block of conduction through the atrium or AV node. This may result from a primary abnormality or autonomic nervous system influences. Bradycardia occurs when subsidiary pacemakers fail to take over when the sinus node fails. A relatively common cause of bradycardia in the neonate is blocked premature atrial contractions. With blocked premature atrial contractions, the medical treatment of choice is digoxin, which suppresses the premature atrial contractions and increases the ventricular rate; treatment is needed only if the rate is low enough to produce symptoms or signs of low cardiac output or decreased cardiac function.

If the patient with bradycardia is symptomatic, temporary pacing or pharmacologic agents may be used to increase the rate (Table 55–11).

SINUS BRADYCARDIA

Symptomatic sinus bradycardia may occur in a wide range of clinical settings and systemic diseases (Table 55–12). Therapy for the underlying disorder is indicated. The QTc interval should be determined in all infants with marked sinus bradycardia because sinus slowing often accompanies the congenital LQTS. Cardiac surgical procedures may damage the sinus node, as in intra-atrial repair for complete transposition or Fontan repair, and result in sinus node dysfunction and marked sinus bradycardia.[155,316]

Support of the heart rate and blood pressure with pharmacologic or inotropic agents or temporary pacing may be

TABLE 55–12
ETIOLOGY OF SINUS BRADYCARDIA AND SINUS TACHYCARDIA

Sinus Tachycardia	Sinus Bradycardia
Fever, infection	Hypothermia
Anemia	Increased intracranial pressure
Hypoxia	Meningitis
Hypotension	Q fever, Chagas' disease
Dehydration, hypovolemia	Hypothyroidism
Fear, anxiety	Drugs: digoxin, β-blockers, morphine
Myocarditis	Anorexia
Hyperthyroidism	Obstructive jaundice
Drugs: sympathomimetic, other	
Pheochromocytoma	

necessary with extreme slowing. In patients with sinus bradycardia, temporary pacing can generally be achieved by the transesophageal route because of the proximity of the esophagus to the atrium.

SINUS NODE DYSFUNCTION

Sinus node dysfunction may be manifested by either bradycardia or alternating bradycardia and tachycardia. The most common arrhythmias include sinus bradycardia, sinus arrest, and pause with junctional escape rhythms (Fig. 55–22), wandering atrial pacemakers, severe sinus arrhythmia, sinoatrial block, SVT, and atrial flutter or fibrillation. Syncopal episodes may occur. Although sinus node dysfunction occurs in children without associated illness, it commonly occurs in inflammatory illnesses, such as a viral myocarditis, or after atrial surgery.[317,318] Congenital causes include LQTS, asplenia syndrome, and rare familial instances.

TREATMENT OF BRADYCARDIA
General Principles

Acute medical therapy consists of atropine (0.02 to 0.04 mg/kg given intravenously) or isoproterenol (0.01 to 2.0 μg/kg/min). Temporary atrial pacing may be performed by the transcutaneous, esophageal, or intracardiac routes. Long-term medical therapy is rarely indicated, and persis-

TABLE 55–11
PHARMACOLOGIC TREATMENT OF BRADYCARDIA AND ATRIOVENTRICULAR BLOCK

Drug	Dosage
Atropine	0.02–0.04 mg/kg IV (maximum: 1–2 mg)
Epinephrine	0.01–0.5 mg/kg (0.1 ml/kg of 1:10,000 dilution) (0.01 ml/kg of 1:1000 dilution) IV bolus Infusion: 0.1–2.0 μg/kg/min
Isoproterenol	Infusion: 0.01–2.0 μg/kg/min

IV = intravenously.

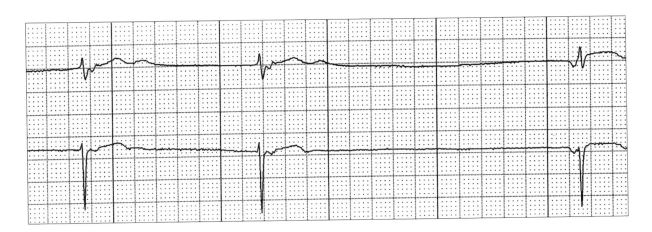

FIGURE 55–22
Electrocardiographic tracing from a 24-hour ambulatory monitor in a patient with intra-atrial repair of complete transposition revealing prolonged pause of 2.92 seconds. Intrinsic rhythm is junctional at 36 beats per minute.

tent symptomatic bradycardia should be treated by permanent pacing.

IMPLANTABLE PACEMAKERS

Use of permanent pacemakers was first reported in children in the early 1960s.[319–322] Subsequently, there have been steady advances in lead and generator technology. The programmability and miniaturization of the generators have significantly increased their use in children.[323–326]

Children in whom pacemakers are implanted generally fall into three categories: (1) those with congenital complete heart block,[327] (2) those with postoperative or acquired heart block,[328–331] and (3) those with postoperative or acquired sinus node dysfunction.[332,333] Indications for pacemaker implantation are shown in Table 55–13.[159,334] The classification system is separated into three classes: (1) those for whom there is general agreement that a pacemaker is needed, (2) those with possible indications but for whom some controversy exists, and (3) those in whom there is general agreement that a pacemaker is not necessary. New data may lead to periodic revisions of these recommendations. For example, asymptomatic patients with congenital complete heart block and awake rates of less than 50 bpm and evidence of escape pacemaker instability have a high incidence of sudden death and possibly should be a class 1 indication.[319,335] Other new indications should include LQTS with bradycardia or uncontrolled arrhythmias, and congenital AV block with prolonged QT intervals.

Once the decision has been made to implant the pacemaker, the lead route and the type of pacing system should be selected. Initial lead systems were epicardial, but high thresholds resulted in pacemaker failure or early generator battery depletion, especially in children who required higher cardiac rates than adults.[336] Once transvenous lead systems were developed, it became possible to place pacemakers without a thoracotomy.[337,338] Intracardiac thresholds were much lower, improving the longevity of the pacemaker. Esperer and coworkers[339] reported that the rate of lead-related complications was 35% and did not differ significantly between the epicardially and endocardially paced group. Epicardially paced children have a higher rate of exit block. Endocardial leads are more likely to dislocate.[339] The newer steroid eluting leads available in both endocardial and epicardial systems have markedly decreased thresholds and should significantly decrease problems with exit block. They can be implanted through a minimally invasive subxiphoid or small left thoracotomy for placement of both atrial and ventricular leads.

We do not advise intracardiac leads in very small children, although it is technically possible to use them. Thrombosis or narrowing of the venous system occurs in many of these patients.[340–342] Because most require a pacemaker for 60 or more years, obstruction of the venous system at an early age is undesirable and complicates later pacing. Transvenous leads are a potential source for emboli in patients with a right-to-left shunt or sluggish circulation as after a Fontan repair. We do not use them in such patients.

Pacemakers are available in both single- and dual-chamber systems. Dual-chamber pacemakers provide AV synchrony and may improve cardiac output.[343] Various programmable functions are used. The classification system used to describe these functions is shown in Table 55–14.[344] The first letter in the code identifies the chamber paced; the second, the chamber sensed; the third, the pacemaker's response to the sensed event, which is either inhibition or triggering; and the fourth and fifth relate to different types of programmability functions. The most common modes used in children are the single-chamber VVI or VVIR or AAI or AAIR, and the dual-chamber, the DDD or DDDR modes. Rate-responsive pacemakers allow the patient to benefit from an increased heart rate in the presence of sinus node dysfunction. Many newer pacemakers provide the

---

TABLE 55–13

INDICATIONS FOR PERMANENT PACING IN CHILDREN AND ADOLESCENTS

CLASS I

1. Advanced second- or third-degree AV [atrioventricular] block associated with symptomatic bradycardia, congestive heart failure, or low cardiac output. *(Level of evidence: C)*
2. Sinus node dysfunction with correlation of symptoms during age-inappropriate bradycardia. The definition of bradycardia varies with the patient's age and expected heart rate. *(Level of evidence: B)*
3. Postoperative advanced second- or third-degree AV block that is not expected to resolve or persists at least 7 days after cardiac surgery. *(Level of evidence: B, C)*
4. Congenital third-degree AV block with a wide QRS escape rhythm or ventricular dysfunction. *(Level of evidence: B)*
5. Congenital third-degree AV block in the infant with a ventricular rate <50 to 55 bpm or with congenital heart disease and a ventricular rate <70 bpm, *(Level of evidence: B, C)*
6. Sustained pause-dependent ventricular tachycardia, with or without prolonged QT, in which the efficacy of pacing is thoroughly documented. *(Level of evidence: B)*

CLASS IIa

1. Bradycardia-tachycardia syndrome with need for long-term antiarrhythmic treatment other than digitalis. *(Level of evidence: C)*
2. Congenital third-degree AV block beyond the first year of life with an average heart rate <50 bpm or abrupt pauses in ventricular rate that are two or three times the basic cycle length. *(Level of evidence: B)*
3. Long QT syndrome with 2:1 AV or third-degree AV block *(Level of evidence: B)*
4. Asymptomatic sinus bradycardia in the child with complex congenital heart disease with resting heart rate <35 bpm or pauses in ventricular rate >3 seconds. (Level of evidence: C)

CLASS IIb

1. Transient postoperative third-degree AV block that reverts to sinus rhythm with residual bifascicular block. *(Level of evidence: C)*
2. Congenital third-degree AV block in the asymptomatic neonate, child, or adolescent with an acceptable rate, narrow QRS complex, and normal ventricular function. *(Level of evidence: B)*
3. Asymptomatic sinus bradycardia in the adolescent with congenital heart disease with resting heart rate <35 bpm or pauses in ventricular rate >3 seconds. *(Level of evidence: C)*

CLASS III

1. Transient postoperative AV block with return of normal AV conduction within 7 days. *(Level of evidence: B)*
2. Asymptomatic postoperative bifascicular block with or without first-degree AV block. *(Level of evidence: C)*
3. Asymptomatic type I second-degree AV block. *(Level of evidence: C)*
4. Asymptomatic sinus bradycardia in the adolescent with longest RR interval <3 seconds and minimum heart rate >40 bpm. *(Level of evidence: C)*

TABLE 55–14

PACEMAKER CLASSIFICATION SYSTEM

NASPE/BPEG Generic Pacemaker Code

Letter Position Category	I	II	III	IV	V
	Chamber paced	Chamber sensed	Response to sensing	Programmability, rate modulation	Antitachyarrhythmic functions
	O, none	O, none	O, none	O, none	O, none
	A, atrium	A, atrium	I, inhibited	R°, sensor triggered	P, pacing
	V, ventricle	V, ventricle	T, triggered	M, multiprogrammable	D, both O + P
	D, dual (A + V)	D, dual (A + V)	D, dual (I + T)	C, communicating	S, shock
				P, simple programmable	

°R, only designation of fourth and fifth letters commonly used.

NASPE, North American Society of Pacing and Electrophysiology; BPEG, British Pacing and Electrophysiology Group.

From Bernstein AD, Camm AJ, Fletcher R, et al: The NASPE/BPEG generic pacemaker code for antibradyarrhythmia and adaptive-rate pacing and antitachyarrhythmia devices. PACE 10:794, 1987.

ability to perform temporary rapid pacing and/or noninvasive programmed electrophysiologic testing.

Other special pacemakers include the atrial antitachycardia pacemaker. This pacemaker is effective in patients with bradycardia-tachycardia syndrome. It has been used in children with sick sinus syndrome and atrial flutter that is unresponsive to medication.[345] The risk of acceleration of the atrial tachycardia or degeneration to a more serious rhythm is present and should lead to caution in the use of this pacemaker.[160]

The implantable cardioverter-defibrillator has been used in children. Silka and coworkers identified 177 patients younger than 20 years of age who had an implantable cardioverter-defibrillator.[248] Follow-up was obtained on 125 of these patients. The most common indications for placement included survival of sudden cardiac death (76%), drug-refractory VT (10%), and syncope with inducible VT (10%). The associated cardiovascular conditions were hypertrophic or dilated cardiomyopathy (54%), LQTS (26%),[247] and cardiac malformation (18%). Sixty-eight percent of patients experienced an appropriate discharge during follow-up. Nine deaths occurred during the period of follow-up. The use of transvenous nonthoracotomy leads has made implantation less invasive, but epicardial patches are still necessary in smaller children as a result of the size of the transvenous lead system.[346]

Pacemaker Follow-Up. Pacemakers should be monitored in a systematic and organized fashion. These follow-up visits aid in the detection of pacemaker malfunction or battery depletion and determine the settings to provide optimal pacemaker benefit and longevity. Most pacemaker companies recommend schedules for pacemaker transtelephonic checks after implantation. These schedules may need to be altered for children, depending on their particular condition and the degree of pacemaker dependency. These transtelephonic checks are insufficient for follow-up of pacemakers in children. Careful surveillance for wire fracture, impedance changes, and threshold changes require on-site visits with the pediatric cardiology pacemaker specialist. At these visits, pacemaker thresholds, sensitivity, graphic analysis of rate ranges over time, and other information can be assessed to determine the best settings for the optimal func-

tion of the pacemaker. In addition, Holter monitoring and exercise stress tests can be used to assess proper function and to determine the most appropriate settings.

Atrioventricular Block

FIRST-DEGREE ATRIOVENTRICULAR BLOCK

First-degree heart block reflects slowed conduction from the sinus node to the ventricle and is manifested by a prolonged PR interval. It is encountered with digitalis intoxication; inflammatory cardiac diseases, such as viral myocarditis, rheumatic fever, and Kawasaki disease; and certain cardiac malformations. It also occurs after cardiac operation (Table 55–15).

Electrophysiologic studies in children have generally localized the delay to the AV node.[347] Delay in the His-Purkinje system with prolongation of the HV interval may be more significant, indicating a predisposition to the development of complete heart block.

SECOND-DEGREE ATRIOVENTRICULAR BLOCK

Second-degree AV block is the failure of some atrial impulses to traverse the AV node. Two forms are identified. In one, a progressive increase in the PR interval occurs with an eventual dropped QRS complex, as in Wenckebach's AV block (Mobitz I). In the other, a sudden failure of AV conduction occurs without preceding slowing of AV conduction (Mobitz II) (Fig. 55–23). Atrioventricular block may develop with digitalis intoxication; inflammatory cardiac diseases, such as viral myocarditis, rheumatic fever, and collagen vascular diseases; Kawasaki disease; neuromuscular,

TABLE 55–15

CONGENITAL HEART DEFECTS ASSOCIATED WITH ATRIOVENTRICULAR BLOCK

Ebstein anomaly of the tricuspid valve
L-transposition of the great arteries
Primum/secundum atrial septal defect
Postoperative cardiac anomalies
  VSD, AV septal defect, tetralogy of Fallot
  Aortic valve replacement/valvotomy
  Mitral valve replacement/valvotomy
  IHSS resection

VSD = ventricular septal defect; AV = atrioventricular; IHSS = idiopathic hypertrophic subaortic stenosis.

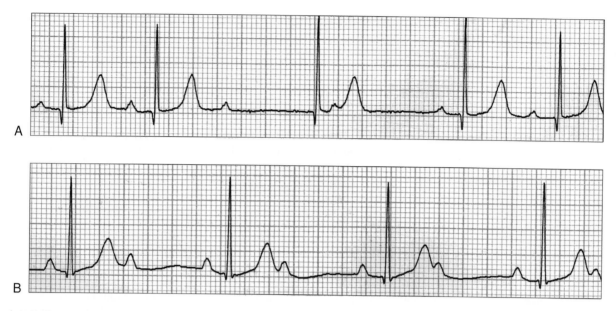

FIGURE 55–23

Electrocardiographic example of second-degree atrioventricular (AV) block. *A,* Mobitz type I (Wenkebach's) second-degree AV block. *B,* Mobitz type II AV block with 2:1 AV conduction.

metabolic or hematologic disorders; cardiac tumors; cardiac sclerosis; or certain cardiac malformations.[348,349]

The delay may be in either the AV node or the His-Purkinje system, the latter being more significant and likely to progress to complete heart block. Second-degree AV block is generally asymptomatic, but if the ventricular rate is low, especially in a patient with compromised myocardial function, the cardiac output may be insufficient. If a higher rate is needed, pharmacologic agents, such as atropine, may be helpful, especially if the block is in the AV node and is partially mediated by vagal influences. Isoproterenol may increase the heart rate by increasing the rate of the escape pacemaker. Acutely, temporary transcutaneous or transvenous pacing may be necessary. For persistent symptomatic or high-grade AV block, permanent pacing may be needed. Second-degree AV block may progress to complete AV block.[348,349]

COMPLETE HEART BLOCK

Complete heart block is total failure of the AV junctional area to conduct the electrical impulse from the atria to the ventricles (Fig. 55–24). This is the most common cause of significant bradycardia in children. The atrial rate is faster than the ventricular rate, which is usually 40 to 80 bpm. The QRS morphology and the heart rate vary according to the location of the escape pacemaker. The higher the origin of the pacemaker, the faster the ventricular rate and the narrower the QRS complex. Wider QRS escape complexes usually originate from the His bundle or below. The usual ventricular rate in the neonate is 60 to 80 bpm.

Complete heart block may be either congenital or acquired and occurs in 1 per 20,000 live births. Acquired heart block results from the same cause as second-degree AV block. In a series of 599 patients with congenital complete heart block followed up for more than 10 years, two thirds had a normal heart, and 92% were alive.[350] The greatest risk of death was during the first weeks of life, with half of the deaths occurring during the first year. Highest risk was associated with cardiac anomalies, cardiomegaly, ventricular bradycardia of less than 55 bpm, and atrial tachycardia of greater than 140 bpm in infants.

A strong association has been noted with maternal connective tissue disease, with an 85% prevalence in the mothers of affected infants.[351–353] Only half of these af-

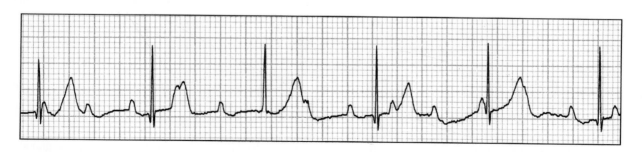

FIGURE 55–24

Electrocardiographic example of complete or third-degree atrioventricular block in a 5-month-old patient. Complete AV dissociation is present. The atrial rate is 136 beats per minute (bpm), and the ventricular rate is 68 bpm.

fected mothers are symptomatic from their underlying condition, whereas the other half are asymptomatic but serologically positive. A mother with systemic lupus erythematosus has a 1 in 20 risk of having a child with complete heart block if she is anti-Ro positive.[354] Maternal immunoglobulin G antibodies to soluble tissue ribonucleoprotein antigens, found in the cytoplasm or nucleus of human cells (anti-Ro:SS-A and anti-La:SS-B), cross the placenta after the 12th to 16th week of gestation. This transfer of antibodies results in an inflammatory response in the fetal heart, particularly the conduction system, which destroys the AV node.[352,354-359] Buyon and colleagues[360] demonstrated increased risk when the maternal antibodies target specific portions of the ribonuclear complex, particularly the 48-kDa La (SS-B), the 52-kDa Ro (SS-A), and the 60-kDa Ro (SS-A). The highest risk was reactivity to both the 48-kDa La (SS-B) and the 52-kDa Ro (SS-A) components. Because of this immunologic factor, dexamethasone and plasmapheresis have been recommended as effective treatments in the mother with an affected fetus.[361,362] Although the heart block has not resolved with this treatment, the clinical course of the fetus is improved.

Cardiac abnormalities are present in one third of infants with congenital complete heart block. With associated cardiac malformations, often corrected transposition or heterotaxy, mortality during the first year was 29%.[350]

Some infants are diagnosed in utero because of low fetal heart rates, which usually develop after the 17th week of gestation. Fetal echocardiography may show fetal hydrops in 15 to 61% anomalies, the higher incidence being associated with structural cardiac anomalies, especially AV valve regurgitation. The survival with hydrops is less than 10% unless the fetus can be delivered immediately. The outlook is relatively good if the fetal heart rate is greater than 55 bpm and the heart is normal.

Some infants with congenital complete heart block show findings of congestive heart failure. A subset develop severe congestive heart failure and cardiovascular collapse. These distressed infants require intubation and ventilation, treatment of acidosis, and catecholamine support of heart rate and blood pressure. In emergencies, immediate transthoracic pacing should be performed. The transcutaneous pacemaker may be effective for short-term emergency situations but should be replaced with another pacing method as soon as possible. Placement of a temporary transvenous pacemaker, through either the umbilical vein or the femoral vein, is preferred. Although infants with a ventricular rate lower than 50 bpm or with higher rates with an associated cardiac malformation or cardiomyopathy may require pacing, this decision should not be made on the basis of rate alone.

Older children with complete heart block may develop exercise intolerance, easy fatigability, or syncope. Some patients with congenital complete heart block need a pacemaker, but many do not require this until an older age.[335] Pacemakers may be placed because of associated ventricular arrhythmias, during either sleep or exercise, easy fatigability, exercise intolerance, syncope, or presyncope.[327,363,364] Sudden death has been associated with severe bradycardia; ventricular ectopy, especially with exercise; prolonged pauses; increased QRS width; prolongation of the QTc interval[365]; and junctional recovery time of

greater than 3 seconds.[366] In a study of patients with congenital heart block followed up for more than 30 years, only 10% did not require a pacemaker. The incidence of sudden death was 20%. Mitral regurgitation and prolonged QTc interval were poor prognostic findings. Pacemakers were recommended, even in asymptomatic adults.[335]

In one study, the site of block was located above the His bundle in 61%, below the His bundle in 11%, and within the His bundle in 17%.[367] In this study, 26% received permanent pacemakers, and mortality was 15%.

Acquired heart block associated with other inflammatory disease, such as viral myocarditis, Lyme disease, and rheumatic fever, may be transient and may require only temporary pacing.

Cardiac lesions that are complex or have an unusual course of the AV conduction system[368] may have postoperative block. Temporary pacing is often performed for 7 to 10 days. Permanent pacing is indicated if sinus rhythm does not return, because of the high incidence of sudden death if such patients are not paced.[369] Even the return of sinus rhythm does not ensure that heart block will not return subsequently, and thus close follow-up is indicated.

After ventricular septal defect repair, the presence of RBBB and left anterior hemiblock is 7 to 17%, with a 1% incidence of complete heart block.[370] Complete heart block has developed as late as 14 years after repair.[371] Complete heart block occurs more commonly after repair of an AV septal defect,[372] probably because of the unusual course of the conduction system, and may occur in up to 7%.

Corrected transposition of the great arteries is associated with AV conduction disturbances ranging from first-degree to complete heart block in 30 to 60% of patients. These conduction disturbances may be present at birth, develop insidiously, or may occur during or after the correction of associated malformation. The AV bundle and conduction system cross the pulmonary outflow tract and descend along the anterior rim of the ventricular septal defect or along the right margin of the foramen between the main and outflow chambers in patients with a single ventricle with an outflow chamber. Careful attention and intraoperative mapping have decreased the incidence of this form of postoperative block.

TREATMENT OF ATRIOVENTRICULAR BLOCK

Treatment of AV block is similar to that for bradycardia except that atrial pacing will not increase the heart rate in the presence of second- and third-degree AV block, and dual-chamber or ventricular pacing is required.

Other Conduction Disturbances: Bundle Branch Block

When activation in the conduction system is delayed in the His-Purkinje system, the QRS duration is prolonged. Common patterns include the RBBB pattern: wide QRS with slurred S in leads I and V_6 and a slurred R' in leads III, aVR, and V_1 with a large terminal deflection in lead V_1, or LBBB: wide QRS, bizarre QRS morphology in leads V_5 and V_6 with a large terminal deflection in lead V_6, and a QS or rS complex in leads V_1 and V_2 (Fig. 55–25). Incomplete RBBB is a term to describe an rSR' pattern in lead V_1 without QRS prolongation sufficient to qualify for RBBB. Abnormalities in intraventricular conduction may be con-

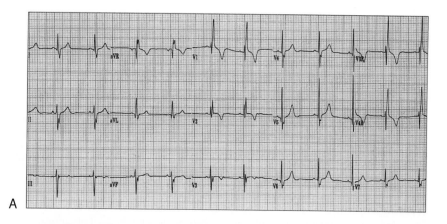

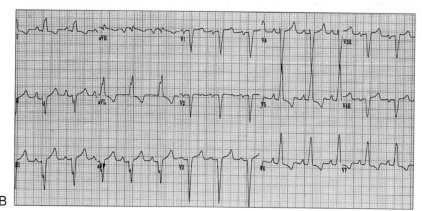

FIGURE 55–25

Fifteen-lead electrocardiograms. *A,* right bundle branch block morphology. *B,* left bundle branch block morphology.

genital or acquired. Congenital RBBB may be inherited[373] or associated with Ebstein's anomaly of the tricuspid valve.[374] Children with Kearns-Sayre syndrome[375] have RBBB that progresses to complete heart block; prophylactic placement of a pacemaker is recommended in such patients to prevent sudden death. Postoperative RBBB is common after repair of many cardiac anomalies[328] and is either central or peripheral in location.[376] Some patients with coexistent left anterior hemiblock and RBBB in postoperative patients, especially after repair of tetralogy of Fallot,[377,378] are susceptible to the development of complete heart block. At the present time, close follow-up is recommended.

CONGENITAL HEART DISEASE

A variety of cardiac malformations are associated with a cardiac arrhythmia. These are discussed in chapters dealing with the individual lesions.

POSTOPERATIVE ARRHYTHMIAS

The correction of specific cardiac anomalies predisposes to the development of specific arrhythmias.[379] The significant postoperative arrhythmias include SVT, atrial flutter, accelerated junctional rhythm, VT, sick sinus syndrome, and complete heart block.[380]

Supraventricular arrhythmias are more common in lesions requiring extensive atrial surgery or after repair with elevated preoperative or postoperative atrial pressure.

Intra-atrial repairs are associated with sick sinus syndrome and SVT, especially atrial flutter.[155,316] Supraventricular arrhythmias are associated with sudden death in 2 to 8% of these patients.[381–384] As these patients age, ventricular arrhythmias are being reported more frequently.[385]

Early operative repair may prevent problems such as fibrosis, subendocardial ischemia, and ventricular hypertrophy that are associated with long-standing ventricular hypertension and chronic hypoxemia. Likewise, systematic follow-up with early repair of residual defects should diminish the abnormal hemodynamics associated arrhythmogenic sequelae.

Improvements in surgical techniques and myocardial protection may prevent late sequelae resulting in ventricular dysfunction and arrhythmias. Modifications or alternative procedures, such as the arterial switch repair for complete transposition, may dramatically change the arrhythmias associated with specific congenital heart lesions.

Systematic follow-up with aggressive identification and appropriate treatment should minimize the serious and life-threatening nature of many of these arrhythmias.

ACQUIRED HEART DISEASE AND CONDITIONS ASSOCIATED WITH ARRHYTHMIAS

INFLAMMATORY AND INFECTIOUS DISORDERS

A variety of acquired infections and inflammatory disorders are associated with arrhythmias. These include viral myocarditis,[386,387] rheumatic fever,[388] Lyme disease,[389] and Kawasaki disease.[390]

ELECTROLYTE IMBALANCES

Abnormalities in electrolyte concentrations may affect cardiac rate, rhythm, and automaticity and may lead to arrhythmias. Potassium and calcium abnormalities are the most common electrolyte abnormalities resulting in abnormal rhythms, although alterations in magnesium and acid-base balance also may produce arrhythmias.[391,392] Any patient with significant unexplained arrhythmia should have serum electrolyte levels determined. Electrocardiographic changes may be characteristic and lead to suspicion of a specific electrolyte abnormality.

HYPERKALEMIA. Electrocardiographic abnormalities of hyperkalemia correlate roughly with serum levels.[393] Peaked T waves are seen at a serum concentration of 5 to 6 mEq/L, and the QRS widens when the concentration exceeds 6 mEq/L. At concentrations greater than 7 mEq/L, the QT interval increases, the QRS widens, P wave amplitude decreases, P wave duration increases, and the PR interval increases. At concentrations greater than 8 to 9 mEq/L, P waves disappear, the ventricular rate becomes irregular, and severe bradycardia with sinus arrest, block, or idioventricular rhythms occur, often with a sinusoidal wave pattern. Ventricular fibrillation or asystole occurs at serum concentrations greater than 12 to 14 mEq/L. The myocardial toxicity of hyperkalemia is enhanced by low serum calcium levels.

HYPOKALEMIA. Potassium concentrations of less than 2.7 mEq/L produce a U wave with an amplitude of more than 1 mm, as well as ST segment depression greater than 0.5 mm. The QT interval prolongs and the T wave flattens with progressive hypokalemia. The PR interval prolongs and intraventricular conduction delays with a widened QRS complex. P wave and QRS amplitude may increase with marked hypokalemia. Arrhythmias associated with low serum potassium levels include ectopic atrial and ventricular complexes, ectopic or automatic atrial tachycardia with block, AV dissociation, second-degree AV block, VT, and ventricular fibrillation. Hypokalemic patients receiving digoxin are particularly susceptible to digoxin toxic arrhythmias related to the combined effects on automaticity and conduction.[394]

HYPOCALCEMIA. The ECG changes correlate with ionized calcium levels, the degree of QT prolongation (ST segment prolongation) being proportional to the degree of hypocalcemia. Associated arrhythmias include SVT and second-degree or complete heart block. The effects of potassium and calcium on myocardial cells are antagonistic. Calcium should be administered cautiously to patients taking digoxin, with continuous cardiac monitoring because of the possibility of precipitating digoxin toxic rhythms.

HYPERCALCEMIA. Calcium levels greater than 12 mg/dl result in a shortened QT interval, a shortened ST segment, and normal or prominent U waves. More marked hypercalcemia may produce PR and QRS prolongation and second-degree or complete heart block. Elevated levels of serum calcium decrease the effect of hyperkalemia and potentiate digoxin toxicity.

HYPOMAGNESEMIA. Low magnesium levels are frequently associated with hypokalemia or hypocalcemia, with the ECG abnormalities reflecting the combined effects of these aberrations. Arrhythmias have included ectopic complexes and ventricular fibrillation.[395]

HYPERMAGNESEMIA. Magnesium levels of 3 to 5 mEq/L are associated with delays in AV and intraventricular conduction.

DRUGS, TOXINS, AND ANESTHETIC AGENTS

Accidental ingestions are common in young children. Many ingested agents result in arrhythmias (Table 55–16). The general procedures for acute poisoning should be followed, but specific arrhythmias must be recognized and treated appropriately. With tricyclic antidepressant toxicity, in addition to the usual antiarrhythmics, the anticholinesterase physostigmine is indicated to treat life-threatening arrhythmias, which are usually VT, atrial flutter, or fibrillation.[396] Intravenous lidocaine and β-blockers may also be indicated.

A number of factors related to general anesthesia and surgery may result in cardiac arrhythmias.[397] These factors include abnormal blood gas levels, electrolyte imbalances, endotracheal intubation with exaggeration of vagal reflexes, central nervous system or sympathetic nervous system involvement or stimulation, dental surgery with autonomic nervous system stimulation, pre-existing cardiac disease, and placement of wires or catheters in the heart.

TRAUMA

Blunt Trauma

Cardiac contusion from blunt trauma is unusual in children but may occur without obvious chest wall injury. Precordial chest pain is the most common symptom. Evidence of myocardial injury may be evident on the ECG as ST-T wave changes and abnormal Q waves. Premature ventricular contractions are the most common arrhythmia.[398]

TABLE 55–16

DRUGS, TOXINS, AND ANESTHETIC AGENTS THAT CONTRIBUTE TO THE DEVELOPMENT OF ARRHYTHMIAS

Agent	Common Arrhythmias
Tricyclic antidepressants	Atrial flutter or fibrillation
	Ventricular tachycardia or fibrillation
	Atrioventricular block
	Asystole
Phenylephrine	Ventricular arrhythmia
	Bradycardia
	Supraventricular tachycardia
Sympathomimetic amines	Supraventricular tachycardia
Antihistamine-decongestant preparations	
Volatile hydrocarbons	Ventricular fibrillation
Benzene	
Cocaine/crack	Ventricular tachycardia
	Ventricular fibrillation
Anesthetic agents	Ventricular arrhythmia
Halothane	
Enflurane	
Ketamine	

Other reported arrhythmias include SVT, VT, AV block, or bundle branch block, and ventricular fibrillation.[399]

Electrical Trauma

Accidental electrocution in children may result in ventricular fibrillation.[400] Low levels of electrical shock that may not produce ventricular fibrillation may result in frequent ventricular premature complexes, VT, and evidence of myocardial damage on an ECG.

ELECTROPHARMACOLOGY OF ANTIARRHYTHMIC AGENTS

GENERAL PRINCIPLES

Determination of the site of origin and the electrophysiologic mechanism of an arrhythmia guides selection of pharmacologic therapy, based on the types of tissue affected by the agent and its ability to interfere with the specific underlying mechanism of the arrhythmia. Antiarrhythmic agents may be grouped according to their mechanisms of action and electrophysiologic properties or by the types of arrhythmias they are used to treat. In the 1960s, Vaughan-Williams[401, 402] developed a classification of antiarrhythmic drugs based on their electrophysiologic properties (Box 55–5). Although many drugs have multiple actions, this scheme is helpful for the understanding of drug actions and selection of drugs that may be effective in the treatment of specific arrhythmias. Antiarrhythmic agents are grouped by their blocking actions on sodium, potassium, or calcium channels or by their ability to block adrenoreceptors. The action of these drugs on a normal fiber differs from their actions on a damaged fiber or a fiber exposed to external factors, such as hypoxia, acid-base or electrolyte imbalance, or variable heart rates.[13] It is important to keep in mind the effects of the various agents on cardiovascular function, and on interactions with the autonomic nervous system and other major organ systems. Many drugs have metabolites that may behave differently from the parent compound.

Antiarrhythmic drugs are believed to interact with receptors in the membrane channels when these channels are in the rested, activated, or inactivated states.[403] When the drug is bound to the receptor, the channel cannot conduct. These interactions vary with the rate of association and dissociation of the drug and may be voltage or time dependent.

In general, most cited drug levels are trough levels and should be obtained just before the next dose. Digoxin levels are steady state and should be obtained 6 to 12 hours after a dose. Levels should not absolutely direct therapy but in some instances may be an adjunct to help guide therapy and evaluate possible toxicities.

A few of the more commonly used antiarrhythmics are discussed later as representative examples.

CLASS I ANTIARRHYTHMIC AGENTS

Class IA agents act on the Na^+ channel and interfere with reactivation of these channels, prolonging the action potential duration and effective refractory periods in atrial, ventricular, and Purkinje cells.[404] They also decrease

---

BOX 55–5. CLASSIFICATION OF ANTIARRHYTHMIC AGENTS

Class	Drug	Action
IA	Procainamide Quinidine Disopyramide	Block fast Na^+ channel[404] Decrease maximum rate of rise of phase 0 (Vmax) and prolong refractoriness and slow conduction
B	Lidocaine Phenytoin Mexiletine	No change in Vmax Shorten action potential duration Shorten effective refractory period
C	Flecainide Propafenone	Reduce Vmax; slow conduction more than prolongation of refractoriness
II	β-Adrenergic blockers Propranolol Nadolol Atenolol Acebutolol Esmolol	Block adrenoreceptors[435]
III	Amiodarone Bretylium Sotalol	Block K^+ channels[436] Prolong repolarization
IV	Calcium channel blockers Verapamil	Block slow calcium channel
Other	Digoxin Adenosine	

Adapted from Vaughan-Williams EM: A classification of antiarrhythmic actions reassessed after a decade of new drugs. J Clin Pharmacol 24:129, 1984; and Vaughan-Williams EM: Classification of antiarrhythmic drugs. J Pharmacol Ther 1:115, 1975.

---

membrane responsiveness and conduction velocity without changing resting membrane potential. These drugs decrease automaticity by decreasing the slope of phase 4 depolarization, except at high concentrations, when phase 4 depolarization is increased and automaticity enhanced.[405] These drugs also have a vagolytic action, with a resultant increase in sinus rate and AV conduction. In patients with sinus node dysfunction, sinus node automaticity may be depressed. Atrioventricular nodal and His-Purkinje conduction times may be prolonged. Because of a property referred to as use dependence, more channels are blocked at faster rates. These drugs are effective in treating AVRTs related to accessory pathways because they prolong refractoriness and slow conduction in the accessory pathway. When class IA agents are used to treat atrial tachycardias, such as atrial flutter and fibrillation, digoxin or propranolol should be used first to block AV nodal conduction. Slowing of the atrial flutter rate in combination with improved AV nodal conduction (secondary to vagolytic effects of class IA agents) may increase the ventricular response and result in hemodynamic deterioration if AV nodal blockade is not present. Class IA agents affect the ECG by prolonging the PR interval, the QRS duration, and the QTc interval. Because of their ability to suppress abnormal automaticity, they may be effective in treating automatic atrial tachycardias, JET, and VT.

The major metabolite of procainamide, N-acetylprocainamide, is an active antiarrhythmic agent but differs from procainamide in that it does not suppress the rate of phase 4 depolarization and does not alter resting membrane potential, action potential, or rate of rise of phase 0.[406] It does prolong action potential duration. Compared with quinidine and disopyramide, procainamide has less vagolytic effect but greater local anesthetic effect.

Side effects of procainamide include a lupus-like syndrome that is generally reversible; gastrointestinal symptoms, especially diarrhea; confusion, disorientation, and depression; blood dyscrasias; decreased myocardial function; and hypotension.

Cardiac side effects include significant QTc prolongation, which is associated with proarrhythmic events (occurrence of new arrhythmia or production of an incessant existing arrhythmia), especially a torsades de pointes type of polymorphic VT.[407] This type of proarrhythmia occurs less frequently in children than in adults and less commonly with procainamide than with quinidine. An increase in the QTc of greater than 30% or more than 0.5 seconds should be considered a harbinger of possible proarrhythmia, and the class IA agent should be stopped or the dosage reduced appropriately. In addition to ventricular arrhythmias, AV block may occur.

Young children may require high doses of procainamide to maintain adequate blood levels. Dosages of up to 150 mg/kg/day may be given to infants under careful monitoring of blood levels and side effects. Consistent levels are obtained by the intravenous route, but the infusion must be continuous because the intravenous half-life is short. The best oral absorption in children too young to take the capsule or tablet is from oral administration of the intravenous form. In our experience, absorption from a suspension of the oral powder (from the capsule) has been erratic and levels difficult to maintain. Levels should be obtained after five doses (half-lives) and the dosage adjusted appropriately to obtain a therapeutic response with as little toxicity as possible.

Quinidine

Quinidine exerts α-adrenoreceptor blocking effects that decrease peripheral vascular resistance and cause hypotension. Because these effects are pronounced when the drug is given intravenously, the parenteral route is generally not used. Therefore, quinidine is rarely used in children in emergencies. Its oral dosage formulation also limits its use in smaller children.

The most common side effects are gastrointestinal, consisting of abdominal pain, diarrhea, and anorexia. Central nervous system toxicity includes visual disturbances, hearing loss, confusion, and delirium referred to as *cinchonism*.

ECG effects are similar to those of procainamide, although quinidine seems to have a higher incidence of proarrhythmia and QTc prolongation in children than does procainamide, especially in children who have undergone a cardiac operation.[150]

Quinidine-induced syncope is associated with the development of polymorphic VT or torsades de pointes.[408] Quinidine- or procainamide-induced torsades de pointes is treated by increasing the heart rate by pacing, usually atrial.[245] If pacing cannot be achieved, isoproterenol may be used cautiously.[409] Intravenous magnesium has also been used.[395]

Disopyramide

Disopyramide is a class I agent that decreases phase 4 diastolic depolarization, decreases the upstroke of phase 0, and increases the action potential duration of normal cardiac cells. The effective refractory period of the atrium is prolonged, as is conduction in accessory pathways. Disopyramide exhibits anticholinergic activity. The primary indication has been for the treatment of ventricular arrhythmias.

Side effects include significant negative inotropic activity such that this drug should generally not be used in patients with decreased ventricular function. Atrioventricular block may occur, limiting use in patients with second- or third-degree AV block. Prolongation of the QT interval occurs. Other side effects include hypoglycemia, dry mouth, urinary hesitancy, constipation, dizziness, headache, blurred vision, and malaise. Gastrointestinal side effects of anorexia, nausea, diarrhea, and vomiting may occur.

CLASS IB ANTIARRHYTHMIC AGENTS

Lidocaine

Lidocaine is the most commonly used class IB agent in the acute setting and is the most effective agent for the treatment of ventricular arrhythmias. Lidocaine suppresses normal and abnormal automaticity in Purkinje fibers, including early and late afterdepolarizations.[410] It shortens the action potential duration to a greater extent than it shortens the effective refractory period. Its effect is greater in association with acidosis, high potassium level, and decreased membrane potential, as in ischemic states.

Major side effects involve the gastrointestinal and central nervous systems. When used as a constant infusion, levels should be monitored because they correlate with side effects. With high levels, drowsiness, agitation, slurred speech, tinnitus, disorientation, seizures, coma, and paresthesias may occur.

Mexiletine

Mexiletine's action is similar to that of lidocaine, but it may be given orally. Therefore, it is used as maintenance therapy in patients in whom lidocaine has been effective emergently but who need a long-term oral therapy. Mexiletine depresses the rate of rise of phase 0 of the action potential and depresses Purkinje fiber automaticity.[411] Mexiletine has been effective in treating ventricular arrhythmias after tetralogy of Fallot repair and in association with β-blockers in the congenital LQTS.[412]

The major side effects are gastrointestinal and consist of nausea and abdominal pain. Many of these may be avoided by giving the drug after a meal. Central nervous system effects are primarily dizziness, headache, visual disturbance, tremor, and convulsions. Blood dyscrasias and hepatic toxicity may occur. Cardiac effects are infrequent but may be manifested as bradycardia.

Phenytoin

Phenytoin has electrophysiologic actions similar to those of lidocaine and mexiletine. It may increase phase 0 upstroke velocity and may be effective in digoxin toxicity by suppressing afterdepolarizations and treating digoxin-related ventricular arrhythmias.[413] It is effective in the congenital LQTS and after repair of tetralogy of Fallot.[414]

Side effects include myocardial depression after rapid intravenous infusion. Allergic reactions manifested by a rash are relatively common. Central nervous system effects include ataxia, nystagmus, drowsiness, and coma.

CLASS IC ANTIARRHYTHMIC AGENTS

Flecainide

Flecainide is the most commonly used class IC agent. Its role is that of maintenance therapy after short-term treatment of SVT or VT. In children, it has been used with greatest efficacy in the treatment of SVT associated with accessory pathways, especially PJRT.[179,415] In this setting, it appears to be relatively safe in the treatment of reentrant SVT.[416] Nevertheless, its use must be carefully monitored because of its potential to cause proarrhythmia, torsades de pointes types of polymorphic VT, and sudden death, as noted in adults treated for ventricular arrhythmias after myocardial infarction. Concerns have been raised about its use in children with a cardiac malformation and atrial flutter.

Flecainide blocks the rapid sodium channel, decreasing Vmax. Purkinje fiber action potential durations are decreased, whereas those of ventricular myocardium are increased. Conduction is reduced in all tissues.

The proarrhythmic actions are the most serious side effects. Careful ECG monitoring must be employed for several days in the hospital when this drug is initiated. Flecainide is a negative inotrope and should be used cautiously and only after careful consideration in patients with depressed ventricular function. Because of its effect on conduction, patients with AV conduction system delays or damage may experience heart block while using this drug. Central nervous system effects include blurred vision, dizziness, and headache.

Propafenone

Propafenone is a sodium channel blocking agent, slowing conduction by decreasing Vmax of the action potential. It has mild β-adrenergic and calcium channel blocking activity. The β-blocking activity is one fortieth of the activity of propranolol.[417] This β-blocking activity may counter the proarrhythmic potential of the class IC activity.[418] Propafenone may be more proarrhythmic in the presence of structural heart disease. Overall, a 2% proarrhythmic effect has been reported. Its metabolites are potent sodium channel blockers. Metabolism is genetically determined,

and 10% of the population are poor metabolizers with slow clearance.[419] Propafenone has been most effective in automatic junctional or atrial tachycardia or in SVT secondary to accessory AV pathways.[85,86,420,421] It is less effective in patients with atrial flutter or structural heart disease.

Propafenone may increase digoxin levels. Side effects are neurologic (dizziness, headaches, tremor, and taste disturbances), gastrointestinal (anorexia, nausea and vomiting, constipation, transient hepatic enzyme elevation), and cardiac (bradycardia, heart failure, and proarrhythmia). Prolongation of the PR interval and QRS are common.[420] Caution should be used in patients with congestive heart failure because of the negative inotropic effects. The incidence of proarrhythmia is lower with propafenone than with other class IC agents.[85]

CLASS II ANTIARRHYTHMIC AGENTS

β-Blocking Agents

The β-adrenoreceptor blocking agents most commonly used to treat arrhythmias in children are propranolol, nadolol, and atenolol.[422] β-Blockers act by competitive inhibition of catecholamine binding at β-receptor sites. Higher concentrations exert a local anesthetic effect that depresses the inward sodium current and membrane responsiveness in Purkinje fibers. Propranolol slows automaticity in fibers, especially automaticity that occurs in response to adrenergic stimulation. β-Blockers slow sinus rate and prolong the PR interval by slowing AV nodal conduction.

β-Blockers are negative inotropes and may decrease ventricular function and worsen congestive heart failure in some patients. This effect may occur particularly if propranolol is given intravenously. The intravenous dose is one tenth of the oral dose.

Other side effects include hypoglycemia; gastrointestinal symptoms of abdominal pain, diarrhea, and anorexia; and bronchospasm. Atrioventricular block and sinus bradycardia may occur.

CLASS III ANTIARRHYTHMIC AGENTS

Amiodarone

Amiodarone prolongs action potential duration by blocking potassium channels and prolonging repolarization.[423,424] At faster rates, Vmax is reduced. These effects result in prolonged refractoriness and slowed conduction. Amiodarone blocks inactivated sodium channels, decreases automaticity, and blocks α- and β-receptors. Amiodarone is generally given orally because its effects on conduction and refractoriness are less when the intravenous route is utilized. This may be related to the fact that the concentration of amiodarone in the myocardium is 15 to 50 times that in the plasma after long-term use. Thus, the onset of its effect after oral administration is 2 to 3 days at the earliest and may be 1 to 3 weeks. Elimination is extremely slow after therapy is stopped (mean, 53 days).

In children, amiodarone is effective in suppressing refractory arrhythmias, especially VT (79%), atrial flutter (80 to 97%), and JET (68%), and has an overall effectiveness of 60 to 80%.[79]

Although side effects are less likely to occur in children than in adults, significant side effects exist, and this drug should be used cautiously. The most significant side effect in adults of pulmonary fibrosis has rarely been reported in children. Liver function abnormalities, photosensitivity, bluish-gray skin discoloration, corneal deposits, and thyroid dysfunction (both hypothyroidism and hyperthyroidism) are among the more commonly noted effects. Because amiodarone inhibits the conversion of thyroxine to triiodothyroxine, reverse triiodothyroxine level is elevated. Levels of reverse triiodothyroxine of greater than 90 ng/dl have correlated with a greater likelihood of toxicities.

Cardiac side effects include marked sinus bradycardia, AV block, and polymorphic VT. Patients with sinus node dysfunction or AV nodal disease may need a pacemaker when amiodarone is introduced because of its profound effects on all areas of the conduction system. Electrocardiographic effects include PR, QRS, and QTc prolongation.

Bretylium

Bretylium is concentrated in sympathetic ganglia and postganglionic adrenergic nerve terminals. Initially, it causes norepinephrine release but subsequently prevents this release.[425,426] Initial norepinephrine release may aggravate some arrhythmias. Prolonged administration prolongs action potential duration and refractoriness. Bretylium increases ventricular fibrillation thresholds, thus exerting an antifibrillatory effect. Bretylium is used in recurrent ventricular fibrillation or VT after lidocaine, procainamide, and β-blockers have failed.

Hypotension may occur because the efferent limb of the baroreceptor reflex is blocked. Gastrointestinal side effects include nausea and vomiting.

Sotalol

Sotalol hydrochloride is a noncardioselective β-blocking agent with additional class III antiarrhythmic properties, prolonging the action potential duration by inhibiting the rapid component of the outward delayed rectifying (I_{Kr}) potassium current and increasing the refractory period in all cardiac tissues. It lacks intrinsic sympathomimetic and membrane stabilizing activity.[427] The QTc interval is increased.

Sotalol may be effective in patients who have not responded to conventional therapy with class II agents. Sotalol is less successful in treating VT in children than in adults.[87] The incidence of proarrhythmia is 3 to 5% in adults and up to 10% in children.[88,428] Sotalol is most effective in treating AV reentrant SVT and atrial ectopic tachycardia in children. Patients with bradycardia from sinus node dysfunction may require pacing if sotalol is required, especially after a cardiac operation.

The side effects include bradycardia, hypotension, worsening congestive heart failure, fatigue, bronchospasm, and proarrhythmic effects.

CLASS IV ANTIARRHYTHMIC AGENTS

Verapamil

The calcium channel blocker most commonly used to treat arrhythmias is verapamil. Its electrophysiologic effect is to block the slow inward calcium current. It is most effective in decreasing the slope of diastolic depolarization in sinus node cells and reducing the rate of rise of phase 0, maximum diastolic potential, and action potential amplitude in sinus and AV nodal cells.[429] Therefore, it slows AV nodal conduction and prolongs AV nodal refractoriness.

Verapamil suppresses early and late afterdepolarizations. Verapamil is most effective in treating AV nodal SVT or AV reentrant SVT in older children and adolescents. One form of exercise-related VT is responsive to verapamil.[430]

Verapamil, by virtue of its calcium channel blockade, interferes with excitation-contraction coupling and depresses myocardial function. This effect is especially pronounced in infants and young children, in whom cardiovascular collapse and death have been reported.[70] Intravenous verapamil is not recommended for use in children younger than 1 year or in those with impaired ventricular function. Pretreatment with calcium does not prevent this occurrence. In patients with atrial flutter or fibrillation and WPW syndrome, verapamil may result in an increased ventricular response over the accessory pathway and should be avoided in this setting.[34] Bradycardia and AV block may occur.

ADDITIONAL AGENTS FOR TREATMENT OF SUPRAVENTRICULAR TACHYCARDIA

Adenosine

Adenosine decreases automaticity and slows conduction in the sinus and AV nodes.[431] It terminates AVRT by blocking the impulse in the AV node.[432] Its extremely short half-life (<10 seconds) makes it a very attractive drug for use in children because its side effects are short-lived and repetitive doses may be given, starting at 50 to 100 µg/kg and increasing by 50 µg/kg at 2-minute intervals to a maximum dose of 400 µg/kg or 12 mg until an effect has occurred. The dose is given by rapid intravenous bolus and flushed with saline.

Side effects include transient shortness of breath, bronchospasm, hypotension, flushing, and irritability. Atrioventricular block, marked sinus bradycardia, and atrial or ventricular arrhythmias may occur. Although these effects are generally transient, support of the patient's circulation and ventilation may be necessary until a normal rhythm resumes.

Digitalis

Digitalis is a cardiac glycoside, and digoxin is the most commonly used form in children. Digoxin has a direct effect on myocardial cells and indirect effects mediated by the parasympathetic nervous system.[433,434] Digoxin slows the sinus rate by both a direct and an indirect effect. The AV nodal effects result in slowing of conduction and prolongation of the effective refractory period. The direct effects on the AV node are to decrease maximum diastolic potential, action potential amplitude, and rate of rise of phase 0. The slope of phase 4 depolarization is increased, resulting in ectopic rhythms in toxic states.

Digoxin is most effective in the treatment of AV nodal reentrant SVT or AV reentrant SVT utilizing a concealed accessory pathway. It should be avoided in patients with manifest accessory pathways (WPW) because it may decrease the refractory period of the accessory pathway, increasing the ventricular response to atrial fibrillation.[35, 36] In patients with WPW syndrome in whom digoxin is used long term, usually for the treatment of congestive heart failure associated with acquired or congenital cardiac abnormalities, the effect of digoxin on the refractory period of the accessory pathway should be evaluated by EPS.

Amiodarone, quinidine, and flecainide increase digoxin levels. Digoxin doses must be decreased and levels monitored during concomitant use of these drugs.

Cardiac side effects include sinus bradycardia or sinus arrest, junctional rhythm, AV block, and ventricular arrhythmias. Gastrointestinal side effects include anorexia, nausea, vomiting, diarrhea, and abdominal pain. Central nervous system side effects include headaches, confusion, visual changes, lethargy, and irritability.

FUTURE DIRECTIONS IN THE TREATMENT OF CARDIAC ARRHYTHMIAS IN PEDIATRICS

Over the past five decades, much has been learned about arrhythmias in infants and children. Pharmacologic advances have improved the control of tachyarrhythmias. Radiofrequency ablation has revolutionized the treatment of SVT and other arrhythmias. Newer surgical approaches and techniques have lessened the incidence of postoperative arrhythmias. We are at the early understanding of the molecular genetic causes and the molecular mechanisms of many arrhythmias. Advances in these areas will provide new directions for the treatment and cure of many difficult arrhythmias.

REFERENCES

1. Zipes DP, Jolife J: Cardiac Electrophysiology and Arrhythmias. New York, Grune & Stratton, 1985.
2. Wit AL: Cellular electrophysiologic mechanisms of cardiac arrhythmias. Ann N Y Acad Sci 432:1, 1984.
3. Hoffman BF, Cranefield PF: Electrophysiology of the Heart. New York, McGraw-Hill, 1960.
4. Ferrier GR: Digitalis arrhythmias: Role of oscillatory afterpotentials. Prog Cardiovasc Dis 19:459, 1977.
5. Weidmann S: Passive properties of cardiac fibers. In Rosen MR, Janse MJ, Wit AL (eds): Cardiac Electrophysiology: A Textbook: In Honor of Brian S. Hoffman, M.D. Mt. Kisco, NY, Futura, 1990, p 29.
6. Mines GR: On dynamic equilibrium in the heart. J Physiol 46:349, 1913.
7. Moe GK, Preston JB, Burlington H: Physiologic evidence for a dual AV transmission system. Circulation 4:357, 1956.
8. Vetter VL: Arrhythmias. In Holbrook PR (ed): Textbook of Pediatric Critical Care. Philadelphia, WB Saunders, 1993, p 384.
9. Singer DH, Lazzara R, Hoffman BF: Interrelationships between automaticity and conduction in Purkinje fibers. Circulation 21:537, 1967.
10. Zipes DP: Genesis of cardiac arrhythmias: Electrophysiologic considerations. In Braunwald E (ed): Heart Disease, A Textbook of Cardiovascular Medicine. Philadelphia, WB Saunders, 1988, p 581.
11. Reuter H: The dependence of slow inward current in Purkinje fibers on the extracellular calcium concentration. J Physiol (Lond) 192:479, 1967.
12. Cranefield PF: The Conduction of the Cardiac Impulse. New York, Futura, 1975.
13. Zipes DP: Management of cardiac arrhythmias: Pharmacological, electrical, and surgical techniques. In Braunwald E (ed): Heart Disease, A Textbook of Cardiovascular Medicine. Philadelphia, WB Saunders, 1988, p 621.
14. Davignon A, Rautaharju P, Boisselle E, et al: ECG standards for children. Pediatr Cardiol 1:133, 1979.
15. Benson DW Jr, Smith WM, Dunnigan A, et al: Mechanisms of regular, wide QRS tachycardia in infants and children. Am J Cardiol 49:1778, 1982.
16. Dunnigan A, Benditt DG, Benson DW Jr: Modes of onset ("initiating events") for paroxysmal atrial tachycardia in infants. Am J Cardiol 57:1280, 1986.
17. Ludomirsky A, Garson A Jr: Supraventricular tachycardia. In Garson A Jr, Gillette PC (eds): Pediatric Arrhythmias: Electrophysiology and Pacing. Philadelphia, WB Saunders, 1990, p 380.
18. Gillette PC: Concealed anomalous cardiac conduction pathways: A frequent cause of supraventricular tachycardia. Am J Cardiol 40:848, 1977.
19. Deal BJ, Keane JF, Gillette PC, et al: WPW syndrome with supraventricular tachycardia during infancy: Management and follow-up. J Am Coll Cardiol 5:130, 1985.
20. Gillette PC: The mechanisms of supraventricular tachycardia in children. Circulation 54:133, 1976.
21. Ko JK, Deal BJ, Strasburger JF, et al: Supraventricular tachycardia mechanisms and their age distribution in pediatric patients. Am J Cardiol 69:1028, 1992.
22. Crosson JE, Hesslein PS, Thilenius OG, et al: AV node reentry tachycardia in infants. PACE 18:2144, 1995.
23. Naccarelli GV: Catheter ablation for the treatment of tachyarrhythmias. In Willerson JT, Cohn JN (eds): Cardiovascular Medicine. New York, Churchill Livingstone, 1995, p 1453.
24. Mantakas ME, McCue CM, Miller WW: Natural history of Wolff-Parkinson-White syndrome discovered in infancy. Am J Cardiol 41:1097, 1978.
25. McIntire MS, Freed AE: Wolff-Parkinson-White syndrome: Report of a case in a mother and infant. Am J Dis Child 89:743, 1955.
26. Garson A Jr, Gillette PC, McNamara DG: Supraventricular tachycardia in children: Clinical features, response to treatment and long-term follow-up in 217 patients. J Pediatr 98:875, 1981.
27. Lundberg A: Paroxysmal atrial tachycardia in infancy: Long-term follow-up study of 49 subjects. Pediatrics 70:638, 1982.
28. Gallagher JJ, Pritchett EC, Sealy WC, et al: The preexcitation syndrome. Prog Cardiovasc Dis 20:285, 1978.
29. Arruda M, Wang X, McClelland J, et al: ECG algorithm for predicting sites of successful radiofrequency ablation of accessory pathways. PACE 16(suppl):865, 1993.
30. Fitzpatrick AP, Gonzales RP, Lesh MD, et al: New algorithm for the localization of accessory atrioventricular connections using a baseline electrocardiogram. J Am Coll Cardiol 23:107, 1994.
31. Xie B, Heald SC, Bashir Y, et al: Localization of accessory pathways from the 12-lead electrocardiogram using a new algorithm. Am J Cardiol 74:161, 1994.
32. Chiang CE, Chen SA, Teo WS, et al: An accurate stepwise electrocardiographic algorithm for localization of accessory pathways in patients with Wolff-Parkinson-White syndrome from a comprehensive analysis of delta waves and R/S ratio during sinus rhythm. Am J Cardiol 76:40, 1995.
33. Gillette PC, Garson AJ, Kugler JD: Wolff-Parkinson-White syndrome in children: Electrophysiologic and pharmacologic characteristics. Circulation 60:1487, 1979.
34. Gulamhusein S, Ko P, Klein GJ: Ventricular fibrillation following verapamil in the Wolff-Parkinson-White syndrome. Am Heart J 106:145, 1983.
35. Byrym C, Wahl RA, Behrendt DM, et al: Ventricular fibrillation associated with the use of digitalis in a newborn infant with Wolff-Parkinson-White syndrome. J Pediatr 101:400, 1982.
36. Sellers TD, Bashore TM, Gallagher JJ: Digitalis in the pre-excitation syndrome: Analysis during atrial fibrillation. Circulation 56:260, 1977.
37. Klein GJ, Bashore TM, Sellers TD, et al: Ventricular fibrillation in the Wolff-Parkinson-White syndrome. N Engl J Med 301:1080, 1979.
38. Deal BJ, Dick M, Beerman L, et al: Cardiac arrest in young patients with Wolff-Parkinson-White syndrome. PACE 18:815, 1995.
39. Bromberg BI, Lindsay BD, Cain ME, et al: Impact of clinical history and electrophysiologic characterization of accessory pathways on management strategies to reduce sudden death among children

with Wolff-Parkinson-White syndrome. J Am Coll Cardiol 27:690, 1996.

40. Paul T, Guccione P, Garson A Jr: Relation of syncope in young patients with Wolff-Parkinson-White syndrome to rapid ventricular response during atrial fibrillation. Am J Cardiol 65:318, 1990.

41. Mahaim I, Winston MR: Recherches d'anatomie comparée et de pathologie experimentale sur les connexions hautes du faisceau de His-Tawara. Cardiologia 5:189, 1941.

42. Bardy GH, German LD, Packer DL, et al: Mechanisms of tachycardia using a nodofascicular Mahaim fiber. Am J Cardiol 54:1140, 1984.

43. Klein GJ, Guiradon GM, Kerr CR, et al: "Nodoventricular" accessory pathway: Evidence for a distinct accessory atrioventricular pathway with atrioventricular node-like properties. J Am Coll Cardiol 11:1035, 1988.

44. Smith WM, Gallagher JJ, Kerr CR, et al: The electrophysiologic basis and management of symptomatic recurrent tachycardia in patients with Ebstein's anomaly of the tricuspid valve. Am J Cardiol 49:1223, 1982.

45. Benditt DG, Milstein S: Nodoventricular accessory connections: A misnomer or a structural functional spectrum. J Cardiovasc Electrophysiol 1:321, 1990.

46. Lown B, Ganong WF, Levine SA: The syndrome of short P-R interval, normal QRS complex and paroxysmal rapid heart action. Circulation 5:693, 1952.

47. Benditt DG, Pritchet ELC, Smith WM, et al: Characteristics of atrioventricular conduction and the spectrum of arrhythmias in Lown-Ganong-Levine syndrome. Circulation 57:454, 1978.

48. Spurell RAJ, Krikler DM, Sowton E: Concealed bypasses of the atrioventricular mode in patients with paroxysmal supraventricular tachycardia revealed by intracardiac electrical stimulation and verapamil. Am J Cardiol 33:590, 1974.

49. Critelli G, Gallagher JJ, Monda V, et al: Anatomic and electrophysiologic substrate of the permanent form of junctional reciprocating tachycardia. J Am Coll Cardiol 4:601, 1984.

50. Wolff GS, Han J, Gurran J: Wolff-Parkinson-White syndrome in the neonate. Am J Cardiol 41:559, 1978.

51. McGuire MA, Janse MJ, Ross DL: "AV nodal" reentry: AV nodal, AV junctional or atrionodal reentry? J Cardiovasc Electrophysiol 4:573, 1993.

52. Jackman WM, Beckman KJ, McClelland JH, et al: Treatment of supraventricular tachycardia due to atrioventricular nodal reentry by radiofrequency catheter ablation of slow pathway conduction. N Engl J Med 327:313, 1992.

53. Engelstein ED, Stein KM, Markowitz SM, et al: Posterior fast atrioventricular node pathways: Implications for radiofrequency catheter ablation of atrioventricular node reentrant tachycardia. J Am Coll Cardiol 27:1098, 1996.

54. Benditt DG, Pritchett ELC, Smith WM, et al: Ventriculoatrial intervals: Diagnostic use in paroxysmal supraventricular tachycardia. Ann Intern Med 91:161, 1979.

55. Garson A Jr, Gillette PC: Electrophysiologic studies of supraventricular tachycardia in children: I. Clinical electrophysiologic correlations. Am Heart J 102:383, 1981.

56. Silka MJ, Kron J, Halperin BD, et al: Mechanisms of AV node reentrant tachycardia in young patients with and without dual AV node physiology. PACE 17:2129, 1994.

57. Cohen MI, Wieand TS, Rhodes LA, et al: Electrophysiologic properties of the AV node in pediatric patients. J Am Coll Cardiol 29:403, 1997.

58. Vetter VL: The pediatric electrophysiologic study. In Liebman J, Plonsey R, Rudy Y (eds): Pediatric and Fundamental Electrocardiography. Philadelphia, Martinus Nijhoff Publishing, 1987, pp 161–184.

59. Vetter VL: Management of arrhythmias in children: Unusual features. In Dreifus LS (ed): Cardiac Arrhythmias. Philadelphia, FA Davis, 1985, p 329.

60. Bisset GSI, Gaum W, Kaplan S: The ice bag: A new technique for interruption of supraventricular tachycardia. J Pediatr 97:593, 1980.

61. Overholt ED, Rheuban KS, Gutgesell HP, et al: Usefulness of adenosine for arrhythmias in infants and children. Am J Cardiol 61:925, 1988.

62. Dorostkar PC, Dick M II, Serwer GQ: Failure of adenosine to terminate supraventricular tachycardia in neonates. Am J Cardiol 72:501, 1993.

63. Crosson JE, Etheridge SP, Milstein S, et al: Therapeutic and diagnostic utility of adenosine during tachycardia evaluation in children. Am J Cardiol 74:155, 1994.

64. Friedman FD: Intraosseous adenosine for the termination of supraventricular tachycardia in an infant. Ann Emerg Med 28:356, 1996.

65. Adkins DL, Kerber RE: Pediatric defibrillation: Current flow is improved by using "adult" electrode paddles. Pediatrics 94:90, 1994.

66. Rosen KM, Barwolf C, Ehsani A, et al: Effects of lidocaine and propranolol on the normal and anomalous pathways in patients with pre-excitation. Am J Cardiol 30:801, 1972.

67. Perry JC, Fenrich AL, Hulse JE, et al: Pediatric use of intravenous amiodarone: Efficacy and safety in critically ill patients from a multicenter protocol. J Am Coll Cardiol 27:1246, 1996.

68. Figa FH, Gow RM, Hamilton RM, et al: Clinical efficacy and safety of intravenous amiodarone in infants and children. Am J Cardiol 74:573, 1994.

69. Klein HO, Hoffman BF: Cessation of paroxysmal supraventricular tachycardia by parasympathomimetic interventions. Ann Intern Med 81:48, 1974.

70. Epstein MC, Kiel EA, Victorica BE: Cardiac decompensation following verapamil therapy in infants with supraventricular tachycardia. Pediatrics 75:737, 1985.

71. Abinader E, Borochowitz Z, Berger A: A hemodynamic complication of verapamil therapy in a neonate. Hebw Paediatr Acta 36:451, 1981.

72. Lister JW, Cohen LS, Bernstein WH, et al: Treatment of supraventricular tachycardia by rapid atrial stimulation. Circulation 38:1044, 1968.

73. Benson DW Jr, Dunnigan A, Sterba A, et al: Atrial pacing from the esophagus in the diagnosis and management of tachycardia and palpitations. J Pediatr 102:40, 1983.

74. Wellens HJJ, Durer DR, Liem KL, et al: Effects of digitalis in patients with paroxysmal atrioventricular nodal tachycardia. Circulation 52:779, 1975.

75. Wellens HJJ, Durer DR: Effect of procainamide, quinidine and ajmaline in the Wolff-Parkinson-White syndrome. Circulation 30:114, 1974.

76. Benson DW, Jr., Deal BJ: Primary treatment of supraventricular tachycardia in infants and children. Progr Pediatr Cardiol 4:209, 1995.

77. Ludomirsky A, Garson A Jr: Supraventricular tachycardia. In Garson A Jr, Bricker JT, McNamara DG (eds): The Science and Practice of Pediatric Cardiology. Malvern, PA, Lea & Febiger, 1990, p 1809.

78. Franklin WH, Deal BJ, Strasburger JF, et al: Do infants have medically refractory supraventricular tachycardia (Abstract)? J Am Coll Cardiol 23:250A, 1994.

79. Garson A Jr, Gillette PC, McVoy P: Amiodarone treatment of critical arrhythmias in children and young adults. J Am Coll Cardiol 4:749, 1984.

80. Yee R, Gulamhusein SS, Klein GJ: Combined verapamil and propranolol for supraventricular tachycardia. Am J Cardiol 53:757, 1984.

81. Pongiglione G, Strasburger JF, Deal BJ, et al: Use of amiodarone for short-term and adjuvant therapy in young patients. Am J Cardiol 68:603, 1991.

82. Perry JC, McQuinn RL, Smith RT, et al: Flecainide for resistant arrhythmias in the young: efficacy and pharmacokinetics. J Am Coll Cardiol 14:185, 1989.

83. Cardiac Arrhythmia Suppression Trial (CAST) Investigators: Preliminary report: Effect of encainide and flecainide on mortality in a randomized trial of arrhythmia suppression after myocardial infarction. N Engl J Med 321:406, 1989.

84. Fish FA, Gillette PC, Benson DW Jr: Proarrhythmia, cardiac arrest and death in young patients receiving encainide and flecainide. J Am Coll Cardiol 18:356, 1991.

85. Guccione P, Drago F, DiDonato RM, et al: Oral propafenone therapy for children with arrhythmias: Efficacy and adverse effects in midterm follow-up. Am Heart J 122:1022, 1991.

86. Janousek J, Paul T, Reimer A, et al: Usefulness of propafenone for supraventricular arrhythmias in infants and children. Am J Cardiol 72:294, 1993.

87. Maragnès P, Tipple M, Fournier A: Effectiveness of oral sotalol for treatment of pediatric arrhythmias. Am J Cardiol 69:751, 1992.

88. Pfammatter JP, Paul T, Lehmann C, et al: Efficacy and proarrhythmia of oral sotalol in pediatric patients. J Am Coll Cardiol 26:1002, 1995.

89. Cobb FR, Blumenschein SD, Sealy WC, et al: Successful surgical interruption of the bundle of Kent in a patient with Wolff-Parkinson-White syndrome. Circulation 38:1018, 1968.

90. Lavergne T, Guize LJ, Le Heuzey JY, et al: Transvenous ablation of the atrio-ventricular junction in human with high-frequency energy. J Am Coll Cardiol 9:99A, 1987.

91. Sebag CI, Guize LJ, Le Heuzey JY, et al: Transcatheter radiofrequency modification of atrioventricular conduction for refractory supraventricular tachycardia. Circulation 78:305, 1988.

92. Van Hare GF, Lesh MD, Scheinman M, et al: Percutaneous radiofrequency catheter ablation for supraventricular arrhythmias in children. J Am Coll Cardiol 17:1474, 1991.

93. Dick M II, O'Connor BK, Serwer GA, et al: Use of radiofrequency current to ablate accessory connections in children. Circulation 84:2318, 1991.

94. Haines DE: Determinants of lesion size during radiofrequency catheter ablation: The role of electrode-tissue contact pressure and duration of energy delivery. J Cardiovasc Electrophysiol 2:509, 1991.

95. Hindricks G, Haverkamp W, Gulker H, et al: Improved prediction of lesion size by monitoring catheter tip temperature. Eur Heart J 10:972, 1989.

96. Hindricks G, Haverkamp W, Gulker H, et al: Radiofrequency coagulation of ventricular myocardium: Improved prediction of lesion size by monitoring catheter tip temperature. Eur Heart J 10:972, 1989.

97. Hindricks G, Haverkamp W: Determinants of radiofrequency induced lesion size. In Huang SKS (ed): Radiofrequency Catheter Ablation of Cardiac Arrhythmias: Basic Concepts and Clinical Applications. Armonk, NY, Futura, 1994, p 97.

98. Van Hare GF: Radiofrequency catheter ablation of cardiac arrhythmias in pediatric patients. Adv Pediatr 41:83, 1994.

99. Case CL, Gillette PC, Oslizlok PC, et al: Radiofrequency catheter ablation of incessant, medically resistant supraventricular tachycardia in infants and small children. J Am Coll Cardiol 20:1405, 1992.

100. Saul JP, Hulse JE, De W, et al: Catheter ablation of accessory atrioventricular pathways in young patients: Use of long vascular sheaths, the transseptal approach and a retrograde left posterior parallel approach. J Am Coll Cardiol 21:571, 1993.

101. Saul JP, Hulse JE, Papagiannis J, et al: Late enlargement of radiofrequency lesions in infant lambs. Circulation 90:492, 1994.

102. Bromberg BI, Dick M II, Scott WA, et al: Transcatheter electrical ablation of accessory pathways in children. PACE 12:1787, 1989.

103. Van Hare GF, Witherell CL, Lesh MD: Follow-up of radiofrequency catheter ablation in children: Results in 100 consecutive patients. J Am Coll Cardiol 23:1651, 1994.

104. Schlüter M, Kuck KH: Radiofrequency current for catheter ablation of accessory atrioventricular connections in children and adolescents: Emphasis on the single-catheter technique. Pediatrics 89:930, 1992.

105. Walsh EP, Saul JP: Transcatheter ablation for pediatric tachyarrhythmias using radiofrequency electrical energy. Pediatr Ann 20:386, 1991.

106. Kugler JD, Danford DA, Houston K, Felix G: Radiofrequency catheter ablation for paroxysmal supraventricular tachycardia in children without structural heart disease. Pediatric EP Society, Radiofrequency Catheter Ablation Registry. Am J Cardiol 80:1438, 1977.

107. Kugler JD: Radiofrequency catheter ablation in children and adolescents: Early results in 189 patients from 13 centers. PACE 15:589, 1992.

108. Kugler JD, Danford DA, Deal BJ, et al: Radiofrequency catheter ablation for tachyarrhythmias in children and adolescents. N Engl J Med 330:1481, 1994.

109. Kugler JD, Danford DA, Felix G, et al: Follow-up of pediatric radiofrequency catheter ablation registry patients. Circulation 92(suppl I):765, 1995.

110. Scheinman MM: NASPE survey on catheter ablation. PACE 18:1474, 1995.

111. Schaffer MS, Silka MJ, Ross BA, et al: Inadvertent atrioventricular block during radiofrequency catheter ablation. Circulation 94:3214, 1996.

112. Case CL, Gillette PC, Crawford FA, et al: Comparison of medical care costs between successful radiofrequency catheter ablation and surgical ablation of accessory pathways in the pediatric age group. Am J Cardiol 73:600, 1994.

113. Hogenhuis W, Stevens SK, Wang P, et al: Cost-effectiveness of radiofrequency ablation compared with other strategies in Wolff-Parkinson-White syndrome. Circulation 88:437, 1993.

114. Calkins H, Sousa J, El-Atassi R, et al: Diagnosis and cure of the Wolff-Parkinson-White syndrome or paroxysmal supraventricular tachycardia during a single electrophysiologic test. N Engl J Med 324:1612, 1991.

115. Jackman WM, Wang X, Friday KJ, et al: Catheter ablation of accessory atrioventricular pathways (Wolff-Parkinson-White syndrome) by radiofrequency current. N Engl J Med 324:1605, 1991.

116. Huang SK: Advances in applications of radiofrequency current to catheter ablation therapy. PACE 14:28, 1991.

117. Lesh MD, Van Hare GF, Schamp DJ, et al: Curative percutaneous catheter ablation using radiofrequency energy for accessory pathways in all locations: Results in 100 consecutive patients. J Am Coll Cardiol 19:1303, 1992.

118. Lesh MD, Van Hare GF, Scheinman MM, et al: A comparison of the retrograde and transseptal methods for ablation of left free-wall accessory pathways. J Am Coll Cardiol 22:542, 1993.

119. Grimm W, Miller J, Josephson ME: Successful and unsuccessful sites of radiofrequency catheter ablation of accessory atrioventricular connections. Am Heart J 128:77, 1994.

120. Keim S, Curtis AB, Belardinelli L, et al: Adenosine-induced atrioventricular block: A rapid and reliable method to assess surgical and radiofrequency catheter ablation of accessory atrioventricular pathways. J Am Coll Cardiol 19:1005, 1992.

121. Park JK, Halperin BD, McAnulty JH, et al: Comparison of radiofrequency catheter ablation procedures in children, adolescents, and adults and the impact of accessory pathway location. Am J Cardiol 74:786, 1994.

122. Warin J, Haissaguerre M, Lemetayer P, et al: Catheter ablation of accessory pathways with a direct approach: Results in 35 patients. Circulation 78:800, 1988.

123. Miller JM, Rosenthal ME, Gottlieb CD, et al: Usefulness of the delta HA interval to accurately distinguish atrioventricular nodal reentry from orthodromic septal bypass tract tachycardias. Am J Cardiol 68:1037, 1991.

124. Morady F, Scheinman MM, Kou WH, et al: Long-term results of catheter ablation of a posteroseptal accessory atrioventricular connection in 48 patients. Circulation 79:1160, 1989.

125. Gang ES, Oseran D, Rosenthal M, et al: Closed chest catheter ablation of an accessory pathway in a patient with permanent junctional reciprocating tachycardia. J Am Coll Cardiol 6:1167, 1985.

126. Haissaguerre M, Montserrat P, Warin JF, et al: Catheter ablation of left posteroseptal accessory pathways and of long RP tachycardias with a right endocardial approach. Eur Heart J 12:845, 1991.

127. Smith RT, Gillette PC, Massumi A, et al: Transcatheter ablative techniques for treatment of the permanent form of junctional reciprocating tachycardia in young patients. J Am Coll Cardiol 8:385, 1986.

128. Chien WW, Cohen TJ, Lee MA, et al: Electrophysiological findings and long-term follow-up of patients with the permanent form of junctional reciprocating tachycardia treated by catheter ablation. Circulation 85:1329, 1992.

129. Ticho BS, Saul P, Hulse JE, et al: Variable location of accessory pathways associated with the permanent form of junctional reciprocating tachycardia and confirmation with radiofrequency ablation. Am J Cardiol 70:1559, 1992.

130. Shih HT, Miles WM, Klein LS, et al: Multiple accessory pathways in the permanent form of junctional reciprocating tachycardia. Am J Cardiol 73:361, 1994.

131. Holman WL, Ikeshita M, Lease JG, et al: Alteration of antegrade atrioventricular conduction by cryoablation of periatrioventricular nodal tissue. J Thorac Cardiovasc Surg 88:67, 1984.

132. Cox JL, Holman WL, Cain ME: Cyrosurgical treatment of atrioventricular node reentrant tachycardia. Circulation 76:1329, 1987.

133. Ross DL, Johnson DC, Deniss R, et al: Curative surgery for atrioventricular junctional ("AV nodal") reentrant tachycardia. J Am Coll Cardiol 6:1383, 1985.

134. Kay GN, Plumb VJ: Selective slow pathway ablation (posterior approach) for treatment of atrioventricular nodal reentrant tachycar-

dia. *In* Huang SKS (ed): Radiofrequency Catheter Ablation of Cardiac Arrhythmias. Armonk, NY, Futura, 1994, p 171.

135. Jazayeri MR, Hempe SL, Sra JS, et al: Selective transcatheter ablation of the fast and slow pathways using radiofrequency energy in patients with atrioventricular nodal reentrant tachycardia. Circulation 85:1318, 1992.

136. Kay GN, Epstein AE, Dailey SM, et al: Selective radiofrequency ablation of the slow pathway for the treatment of atrioventricular nodal reentrant tachycardia: Evidence for involvement of perinodal myocardium within the reentrant circuit. Circulation 85:1675, 1992.

137. Haissaguerre M, Warin J, Le Metayer P, et al: Closed-chest ablation of retrograde conduction in patients with atrioventricular nodal reentrant tachycardia. N Engl J Med 320:426, 1989.

138. Epstein LM, Scheinman MM, Langberg JJ, et al: Percutaneous catheter modification of the atrioventricular node: A potential cure for atrioventricular nodal reentrant tachycardia. Circulation 80:757, 1989.

139. Jackman WM, Nakagawa H, Heidbüchel H, et al: Three forms of atrioventricular nodal (junctional) reentrant tachycardia: Differential diagnosis, electrophysiological characteristics, and implications for anatomy of the reentrant circuit. *In* Zipes DP, Jalife J (eds): Cardiac Electrophysiology: From Cell to Bedside. Philadelphia, WB Saunders, 1995, p 620.

140. Silka MJ, Kron J, Park JK, et al: Atypical forms of supraventricular tachycardia due to atrioventricular node reentry in children after radiofrequency modification of slow pathway conduction. J Am Coll Cardiol 23:1363, 1994.

141. Wang X, McClelland JH, Beckman KJ, et al: Accelerated junctional rhythm during slow pathway ablation. Circulation 84(suppl 2):II–582, 1991.

142. Baker JH, Plumb VJ, Epstein AE, et al: Selective ablation of the slow AV nodal pathway: Predictors of recurrent AV nodal reentrant tachycardia. Circulation 86:I–521, 1992.

143. Rhodes LA, Wieand TS, Vetter VL: Low temperature and low energy radiofrequency modification of atrioventricular node slow pathway in pediatric patients. J Am Coll Cardiol 29(suppl A):357A, 1997.

144. Van Hare GF, Lesh MD: Catheter ablation of accessory pathways as preparation for congenital heart disease surgery. Circulation 84:II–223, 1991.

145. Van Hare GF, Lesh MD, Stanger P: Radiofrequency catheter ablation of supraventricular arrhythmias in patients with congenital heart disease: Results and technical considerations. J Am Coll Cardiol 22:883, 1993.

146. Levine JC, Walsh EP, Saul JP: Radiofrequency ablation of accessory pathways associated with congenital heart disease including heterotaxy syndrome. Am J Cardiol 72:689, 1993.

147. Dunnigan A, Benson DW Jr, Benditt DG: Atrial flutter in infancy: Diagnosis, clinical features, and treatment. Pediatrics 75:725, 1985.

148. Mendelsohn A, Dick M II, Serwer GA: Natural history of isolated atrial flutter in infancy. J Pediatr 119:386, 1991.

149. Vetter VL, Tanner CS, Horowitz LN: Inducible atrial flutter after the Mustard repair of complete transposition of the great arteries. Am J Cardiol 61:428, 1988.

150. Garson A Jr, Bink-Boelkens M, Hesslein PS: Atrial flutter in the young: A collaborative study of 380 cases. J Am Coll Cardiol 6:871, 1985.

151. Soyeur DJ: Atrial flutter in the human fetus: Diagnosis, hemodynamic consequences, and therapy. J Cardiovasc Electrophysiol 7:989, 1996.

152. Kleinman CS, Copel JA, Weinstein EM, et al: In utero diagnosis and treatment of fetal supraventricular tachycardia. Semin Perinatol 9:113, 1985.

153. Ito S, Magee L, Smallhorn J: Drug therapy for fetal arrhythmias. Clin Perinatol 21:543, 1994.

154. Ward RM: Drug therapy of the fetus. J Clin Pharmacol 33:780, 1993.

155. Kürer CC, Tanner CS, Vetter VL: Electrophysiologic findings after Fontan repair of functional single ventricle. J Am Coll Cardiol 17:174, 1991.

156. Gewillig M, Wyse RK, de Leval MR, et al: Early and late arrhythmias after the Fontan operation: Predisposing factors and clinical consequences. Br Heart J 67:72, 1992.

157. Balaji S, Gewillig M, Bull C, et al: Arrhythmias after the Fontan procedure: Comparison of total cavopulmonary connection and atriopulmonary connection. Circulation 84:III–162, 1991.

158. Reimer A, Paul T, Kallfelz H: Efficacy and safety of intravenous and oral propafenone in pediatric cardiac dysrhythmias. Am J Cardiol 68:741, 1991.

159. Dreifus LS, Fisch C, Griffin JC, et al: Guidelines for implantation of cardiac pacemakers and antiarrhythmic devices: A report of the American College of Cardiology/American Heart Association Task Force on Assessment of Diagnostic and Therapeutic Cardiovascular Procedures (Committee on Pacemaker Implantation). J Am Coll Cardiol 18:1, 1991.

160. Rhodes LA, Walsh EP, Gamble WJ, et al: Benefits and potential risks of atrial antitachycardia pacing after repair of congenital heart disease. PACE 18:1005, 1995.

161. Fisher JD, Johnston DR, Kim SG, et al: Implantable pacers for tachycardia termination: Stimulation techniques and long-term efficacy. PACE 9:1325, 1986.

162. Feld GK: Catheter ablation for the treatment of atrial tachycardia. Prog Cardiovasc Dis 37:205, 1995.

163. Feld GK, Fleck RP, Chen P, et al: Radiofrequency catheter ablation for the treatment of human type 1 atrial flutter: Identification of a critical zone in the reentrant circuit by endocardial mapping techniques. Circulation 86:1233, 1992.

164. Disertori M, Inama G, Vergara G, et al: Evidence of a reentry circuit in the common type of atrial flutter in man. Circulation 67:434, 1983.

165. Klein GJ, Guiradon GM, Sharma AD, et al: Demonstration of macroreentry and feasibility of operative therapy in the common type of atrial flutter. Am J Cardiol 57:587, 1986.

166. Feld GK: Ablation of human type 1 atrial flutter. *In* Huang SKS (ed): Radiofrequency Catheter Ablation of Cardiac Arrhythmias: Basic Concepts and Clinical Applications. Armonk, NY, Futura, 1994, p 459.

167. Triedman JK, Saul JP, Weindling SN, et al: Radiofrequency ablation of intra-atrial reentrant tachycardia after surgical palliation of congenital heart disease. Circulation 91:707, 1995.

168. Kalman JM, Van Hare GF, Olgin JE, et al: Ablation of "incisional" reentrant atrial tachycardia complicating surgery for congenital heart disease: Use of entrainment to define a critical isthmus of conduction. Circulation 93:502, 1996.

169. Case CL, Gillette PC, Douglas DE, et al: Radiofrequency catheter ablation of atrial flutter in a patient with postoperative congenital heart disease. Am Heart J 126:715, 1993.

170. Lesh MD, Van Hare GF, Epstein LM, et al: Radiofrequency catheter ablation of atrial arrhythmias: Results and mechanisms. Circulation 89:1074, 1994.

171. Radford DJ, Izukawa T: Atrial fibrillation in children. Pediatrics 59:250, 1977.

172. Stafford WJ, Trohman RG, Bilsker M, et al: Cardiac arrest in an adolescent with atrial fibrillation and hypertrophic cardiomyopathy. J Am Coll Cardiol 7:701, 1986.

173. Dreifus LS, Wellens HJJ, Watanabe Y, et al: Sinus bradycardia and atrial fibrillation associated with the Wolff-Parkinson-White syndrome. Am J Cardiol 38:149, 1976.

174. Bernuth GV, Engelhardt W, Kramer HH, et al: Atrial automatic tachycardia in infancy and childhood. Eur Heart J 13:1410, 1992.

175. Keane JF, Plauth WH, Nadas AS: Chronic ectopic tachycardia of infancy and childhood. Am Heart J 84:748, 1972.

176. Gillette PC, Garson A Jr: Electrophysiologic and pharmacologic characteristics of automatic ectopic atrial tachycardia. Circulation 56:571, 1977.

177. Gillette PC, Smith RT, Garson A Jr, et al: Chronic supraventricular tachycardia: A curable cause of congestive cardiomyopathy. JAMA 253:391, 1985.

178. Mehta AV, Sanchez GR, Sacks EJ, et al: Ectopic automatic atrial tachycardia in children: Clinical characteristics, management and follow-up. J Am Coll Cardiol 11:379, 1988.

179. Perry JC, McQuinn R, Smith RT: Flecainide acetate for resistant arrhythmias in the young: Efficacy and pharmacokinetics. J Am Coll Cardiol 14:185, 1989.

180. Zeigler VL, Gillette PC, Ross B, et al: Flecainide for supraventricular and ventricular arrhythmias in children and young adults. Clin Prog Electrophysiol Pacing 4:328, 1986.

181. Coumel P, Fidelle J: Amiodarone in the treatment of cardiac arrhythmias in children: One hundred thirty-five cases. Am Heart J 100:1063, 1992.

182. Colloridi V, Perri C, Ventriglia F, et al: Oral sotalol in pediatric atrial ectopic tachycardia. Am Heart J 123:254, 1992.

183. Gillette PC, Garson AJ, Hesslein PS, et al: Successful surgical treatment of atrial, junctional and ventricular tachycardia unassociated with accessory connections in infants and children. Am Heart J 102:984, 1981.

184. Margolis PO, Roman CA, Moulton KP, et al: Radiofrequency catheter ablation of left and right ectopic atrial tachycardia (Abstract). Circulation 82:718, 1991.

185. Ott DA, Gillette PC, Garson A Jr, et al: Surgical management of refractory supraventricular tachycardia in infants and children. J Am Coll Cardiol 5:124, 1985.

186. Silka MJ, Gillette PC, Garson A Jr, et al: Transvenous catheter ablation of a right atrial automatic ectopic tachycardia. J Am Coll Cardiol 5:999, 1997.

187. Walsh EP, Saul JP, Hulse JE, et al: Transcatheter ablation of ectopic atrial tachycardia in young patients using radiofrequency current. Circulation 86:1138, 1992.

188. Liberthson RR, Colan SD: Multifocal or chaotic atrial rhythm. Pediatr Cardiol 2:179, 1982.

189. Bissett GSI, Seigel SF, Gaum WE, et al: Chaotic atrial tachycardia in childhood. Am Heart J 101:268, 1981.

190. Yeager SB, Hougen TJ, Levy AM: Sudden death in infants with chaotic atrial rhythm. Am J Dis Child 138:689, 1984.

191. Garson A Jr, Gillette PC: Junctional ectopic tachycardia in children: Electrocardiography, electrophysiology and pharmacologic response. Am J Cardiol 44:298, 1979.

192. Case CL, Gillette PC: Automatic atrial and junctional tachycardias in the pediatric patient: Strategies for diagnosis and management. PACE 16:1323, 1993.

193. Villain E, Vetter VL, Garcia JM, et al: Evolving concepts in the management of junctional ectopic tachycardia: A multicenter study. Circulation 81:1544, 1990.

194. Van Hare GF, Velvis H, Langberg JJ: Successful transcatheter ablation of congenital junctional ectopic tachycardia in a ten-month-old infant using radiofrequency energy. PACE 13:730, 1990.

195. Rychik J, Marchlinski F, Sweeten TL, et al: Transcatheter radiofrequency ablation of congenital junctional ectopic tachycardia in a neonate. Pediatr Cardiol 17:220, 1996.

196. Balaji S, Sullivan I, Deanfield JE, et al: Moderate hypothermia in the management of resistant automatic tachycardias in children. Br Heart J 66:221, 1991.

197. Till JA, Rowland E: Atrial pacing as an adjunct to the management of post-surgical His bundle tachycardia. Br Heart J 66:225, 1991.

198. Waldo AL, Krongrad E, Kupersmith J, et al: Ventricular paired pacing to control rapid ventricular heart rate following open heart surgery: Observations on ectopic automaticity. Report of a case in a four-month-old patient. Circulation 53:176, 1976.

199. Vetter VL: Ventricular arrhythmias in pediatric patients with and without congenital heart disease. In Horowitz LN (ed): Current Management of Arrhythmias. Philadelphia, BC Decker, 1990, p 208.

200. Benson DW Jr, Gallagher JJ, Sterba R, et al: Catecholamine induced double tachycardia: Case report in a child. PACE 3:96, 1980.

201. Davis AM, Gow RM, McCrindle BW, et al: Clinical spectrum, therapeutic management, and follow-up of ventricular tachycardia in infants and young children. Am Heart J 131:186, 1996.

202. Garson A Jr, Smith RT, Moak JP, et al: Ventricular arrhythmias and sudden death in children. J Am Coll Cardiol 5:130B, 1985.

203. Fulton DR, Kyung JC, Burton ST: Ventricular tachycardia in children without heart disease. Am J Cardiol 55:1328, 1985.

204. Deal BJ, Scott MM, Scagliotti D, et al: Ventricular tachycardia in a young population without overt heart disease. Circulation 73:1111, 1986.

205. Rocchini AP, Chun PO, Dick M: Ventricular tachycardia in children. Am J Cardiol 47:1091, 1981.

206. Noh CI, Gillette PC, Case CL, et al: Clinical and electrophysiological characteristics of ventricular tachycardia in children with normal hearts. Am Heart J 120:1326, 1990.

207. Vetter VL, Josephson ME, Horowitz LN: Idiopathic recurrent sustained ventricular tachycardia in children and adolescents. Am J Cardiol 47:315, 1981.

208. Nakagawa M, Yoshihara T, Matsumura A, et al: Accelerated idioventricular rhythm in three newborn infants with congenital heart disease. Chest 104:322, 1993.

209. MacLellan-Tolbert SG, Porter CJ: Accelerated idioventricular rhythm: A benign arrhythmia in childhood. Pediatrics 96:122, 1995.

210. Schwartz PJ: Idiopathic long QT syndrome: Progress and questions. Am Heart J 109:399, 1985.

211. Jervell A, Lange-Nielsen F: Congenital deaf-mutism, functional heart diseases, with prolongation of the QT interval and sudden death. Am Heart J 54:59, 1957.

212. Romano C, Gemme G, Pongiglione R: Aritmie cardiache rare dell'età pediatrica. II. Accessi sincopali della fibrillazione ventricolare parossista. Clin Pediatr (Bologna) 45:565, 1963.

213. Ward O: A new familial cardiac syndrome in children. J Irish Med Assoc 54:103, 1964.

214. Garson A Jr, Dick M II, Fournier A, et al: The long QT syndrome in children: An international study of 287 patients. Circulation 87:1866, 1993.

215. Schwartz PJ, Moss AJ, Vincent GM, et al: Diagnostic criteria for the long QT syndrome: An update. Circulation 88:782, 1993.

216. Scott WA, Dick M II: Two:one atrioventricular block in infants with congenital long Q-T syndrome. Am J Cardiol 60:1409, 1987.

217. Vetter VL, Berul CI, Sweeten TL: Response of corrected QT intervals to exercise, pacing and isoproterenol. Cardiol Young 3(suppl 1):63, 1993.

218. Callans DJ, Schwartzman D, Marchlinski FE: Is an isoproternol induced QT abnormality specific to patients with the long QT syndrome? Circulation 94:I–432, 1996.

219. Moss AJ, Schwartz PJ, Crompton RS, et al: The long QT syndrome: A prospective international study. Circulation 71:17, 1985.

220. Kay GN, Plumb VJ, Araiegas JG, et al: Torsades de pointes: The long-short initiating sequence and other clinical features: Observations in 32 patients. J Am Coll Cardiol 2:806, 1983.

221. Keating M, Atkinson D, Dunn C, et al: Linkage of a cardiac arrhythmia, the long QT syndrome, and the Harvey ras-1 gene. Science 252:704, 1991.

222. Jiang C, Atkinson D, Towbin JA, et al: Two long QT syndrome loci map to chromosomes 3 and 7 with evidence for further heterogeneity. Nat Genet 8:141, 1994.

223. Curran ME, Splawski I, Timothy KW, et al: A molecular basis for cardiac arrhythmia: HERG mutations cause long QT syndrome. Cell 80:795, 1995.

224. Schott J, Charpentier F, Peltier S, et al: Mapping of a gene for long QT syndrome to chromosome 4q25-27. Am J Hum Genet 57:1114, 1995.

225. Moss AJ, Zareba W, Benhorin J, et al: ECG-T wave patterns in genetically distinct forms of the hereditary long QT syndrome. Circulation 92:2929, 1995.

226. Vincent GM, Timothy KW, Leppert M, et al: The spectrum of symptoms and QT intervals in carriers of the gene for the long QT syndrome. N Engl J Med 327:846, 1992.

227. Bazett HC: An analysis of the time-relations of electrocardiograms. Heart 7:353, 1920.

228. Garson A Jr: How to measure the QT interval: What is normal? Am J Cardiol 72:14B, 1993.

229. Malfatto G, Beria G, Sala S, et al: Quantitative analysis of T wave abnormalities and their prognostic implications in the idiopathic long QT syndrome. J Am Coll Cardiol 23:296, 1994.

230. Priori SG, Napolitano C, Diehl L, et al: Dispersion of QT interval: A marker of therapeutic efficacy in the idiopathic long QT syndrome. Circulation 89:1681, 1994.

231. Moss AJ: Measurement of the QT interval and the risk associated with QT$_c$ interval prolongation: A review. Am J Cardiol 72:23B, 1993.

232. Shah MJ, Wieand TS, Rhodes LA, et al: QT and JT dispersion in children with long QT syndrome. J Cardiovasc Electrophysiol 8:642, 1997.

233. Shimizu W, Ohe T, Kurita T, et al: Early afterdepolarizations induced by isoproterenol in patients with congenital long QT syndrome. Circulation 84:1915, 1991.

234. Zhou JT, Zheng LR, Liu WY, et al: Early afterdepolarizations in the familial long QTU syndrome. J Cardiovasc Electrophysiol 3:431, 1992.

235. Bonatti V, Rolli A, Botti G: Recording of monophasic action potentials of the right ventricle in long QT syndrome complicated by severe ventricular arrhythmias. Eur Heart J 4:168, 1983.

236. Shimizu W, Ohe T, Kurita T, et al: Epinephrine-induced ventricular premature complexes due to early afterdepolarizations and effects of verapamil and propranolol in a patient with congenital long QT syndrome. J Cardiovasc Electrophysiol 5:438, 1994.

237. Shimizu W, Ohe T, Kurita T, et al: Effects of verapamil and propranolol on early afterdepolarizations and ventricular arrhythmias induced by epinephrine in congenital long QT syndrome. J Am Coll Cardiol 26:1299, 1995.

238. Schechter E, Anderson J, Prabhu S, et al: Epinephrine infusion in the congenital long-QT syndrome. J Am Coll Cardiol 7:155A, 1986.

239. Crawford MH, Karliner JS, O'Rouke RA, et al: Prolonged QT interval syndrome: Successful treatment with combined ventricular pacing and propranolol. Chest 68:369, 1975.

240. Trippel DL, Gillette PC: Atenolol in children with ventricular arrhythmias. Am Heart J 119:1312, 1990.

241. Locati EH, Schwartz PJ, Moss AJ, et al: Long-term survival after left cervico-thoracic sympathectomy in high risk long Q-T syndrome patients with refractory ventricular arrhythmias. J Am Coll Cardiol 7:235A, 1986.

242. Packer DL, Coltori F, Smith MS, et al: Sudden death after left stellectomy in the long Q-T syndrome. Am J Cardiol 54:1365, 1984.

243. Ouriel K, Moss AJ: Long QT syndrome: An indication for cervicothoracic sympathectomy. Cardiovasc Surg 3:475, 1995.

244. Schwartz PJ, Locati EH, Moss AJ, et al: Left cardiac sympathetic denervation in the therapy of congenital long QT syndrome: A worldwide report. Circulation 84:503, 1991.

245. Eldar M, Griffin JC, Abbott JA: Permanent cardiac pacing in patients with the long QT syndrome. J Am Coll Cardiol 10:600, 1987.

246. Moss AJ, Liu JE, Gottlieb S, et al: Efficacy of permanent pacing in the management of high-risk patients with long QT syndrome. Circulation 84:1524, 1991.

247. Groh WJ, Silka MJ, Oliver RP, et al: Use of implantable cardioverter-defibrillators in the congenital long QT syndrome. Am J Cardiol 78:703, 1996.

248. Silka MJ, Kron J, Dunnigan A, et al: Sudden cardiac death and the use of implantable cardioverter-defibrillators in pediatric patients. Circulation 87:800, 1993.

249. Roden DM, Lazzara R, Rosen M, et al: Multiple mechanisms in the long-QT syndrome: Current knowledge, gaps, and future directions. Circulation 94:1996, 1996.

250. Schwartz PJ, Priori SG, Locati EH, et al: Long QT syndrome patients with mutations of the SCN5A and HERG genes have differential responses to Na$^+$ channel blockade and to increases in heart rate. Circulation 92:3381, 1995.

251. Sato T, Hata Y, Yamamoto M, et al: Early afterdepolarizations abolished by potassium channel opener in a patient with idiopathic long QT syndrome. J Cardiovasc Electrophysiol 6:279, 1995.

252. Balaji S, Wiles HB, Sens MA, et al: Immunosuppressive treatment for myocarditis and borderline myocarditis in children with ventricular ectopic rhythm. Br Heart J 72:354, 1994.

253. Wiles HB, Gillette PC, Harley RA, et al: Cardiomyopathy and myocarditis in children with ventricular ectopic rhythm. J Am Coll Cardiol 20:359, 1992.

254. Ino T, Okubo M, Akimoto K, et al: Corticosteroid therapy for ventricular tachycardia in children with silent lymphocytic myocarditis. J Pediatr 126:304, 1995.

255. Vetter VL, Horowitz LN: Electrophysiologic residua and sequelae of surgery for congenital heart defects. Am J Cardiol 50:588, 1982.

256. Garson A Jr, Nihill MR, McNamara DG, et al: Status of the adult and adolescent after repair of tetralogy of Fallot. Circulation 59:1232, 1979.

257. Gillette PC, Yeoman MA, Mullins CE, et al: Sudden death after repair of tetralogy of Fallot. Circulation 56:566, 1977.

258. Vetter VL: Ventricular arrhythmias in patients with congenital heart disease. In Greenspon AJ, Waxman HL (eds): Contemporary Management of Ventricular Arrhythmias. Philadelphia, FA Davis, 1991, pp 255–273.

259. Girod DA, Fontan F, Deville C, et al: Long-term results after the Fontan operation for tricuspid atresia. Circulation 75:605, 1987.

260. Fontan F, Deville C, Quaegebeur J, et al: Repair of tricuspid atresia in 100 patients. J Thorac Cardiovasc Surg 85:647, 1983.

261. Deanfield JE, McKenna WJ, Presbitero P, et al: Ventricular arrhythmia in unrepaired tetralogy of Fallot: Relation to age, timing of repair and hemodynamic status. Br Heart J 52:77, 1984.

262. Vaksmann G, Fournier A, Davignon A, et al: Frequency and prognosis of arrhythmias after operative "correction" of tetralogy of Fallot. Am J Cardiol 66:346, 1990.

263. Gatzoulis MA, Till JA, Somerville J, et al: Congenital heart disease: Mechanoelectrical interaction in tetralogy of Fallot: QRS prolongation relates to right ventricular size and predicts malignant ventricular arrhythmias and sudden death. Circulation 92:231, 1995.

264. Zimmermann M, Friedli B, Adamec R, et al: Ventricular late potentials and induced ventricular arrhythmias after surgical repair of tetralogy of Fallot. Am J Cardiol 67:873, 1991.

265. Deanfield JE, Ho S, Anderson RH, et al: Late sudden death after repair of tetralogy of Fallot: A clinicopathologic study. Circulation 67:626, 1983.

266. Garson A Jr, Porter CJ, Gillette PC, et al: Induction of ventricular tachycardia during electrophysiologic study after repair of tetralogy of Fallot. J Am Coll Cardiol 1:1493, 1983.

267. Horowitz LN, Vetter VL, Harken AH, et al: Electrophysiologic characteristics of sustained ventricular tachycardia occurring after repair of tetralogy of Fallot. Am J Cardiol 46:446, 1980.

268. Deal BJ, Scagliotti D, Miller SM, et al: Electrophysiologic drug testing in symptomatic ventricular arrhythmias after repair of tetralogy of Fallot. Am J Cardiol 59:1380, 1987.

269. Chandar JS, Wolff GS, Garson A Jr, et al: Ventricular arrhythmias in postoperative tetralogy of Fallot. Am J Cardiol 65:655, 1990.

270. Kugler JD, Pinsky WW, Cheatham JP, et al: Sustained ventricular tachycardia after repair of tetralogy of Fallot: New electrophysiologic findings. Am J Cardiol 51:1137, 1983.

271. Vetter VL: Postoperative arrhythmias after surgery for congenital heart defects. In Zipes DP (ed): Cardiology in Review. Baltimore, Williams & Wilkins, 1994, p 83.

272. Marie PY, Marçon F, Brunotte F, et al: Right ventricular overload and induced sustained ventricular tachycardia in operatively "repaired" tetralogy of Fallot. Am J Cardiol 69:785, 1992.

273. Walsh EP, Rockenmacher S, Keane JF, et al: Late results in patients with tetralogy of Fallot repaired during infancy. Circulation 77:1062, 1988.

274. Joffe H, Georgakopoulos D, Celermajer DS, et al: Late ventricular arrhythmia is rare after early repair of tetralogy of Fallot. J Am Coll Cardiol 23:1146, 1994.

275. Garson A Jr, Randall DC, Gillette PC, et al: Prevention of sudden death after repair of tetralogy of Fallot: Treatment of ventricular arrhythmias. J Am Coll Cardiol 6:221, 1985.

276. Sullivan I, Presbitero P, Gooch VM, et al: Is ventricular arrhythmias in repaired tetralogy of Fallot an effect of operation or a consequence of the course of the disease? Br Heart J 58:40, 1987.

277. Garson A Jr, Gillette PC, Titus JL, et al: Surgical treatment of ventricular tachycardia in infants. N Engl J Med 310:1443, 1984.

278. Malhotra V, Ferrans VJ, Virmani R: Infantile histiocytoid cardiomyopathy: Three cases and literature review. Am Heart J 128:1009, 1994.

279. Jeresaty RM: Sudden death in the mitral valve prolapse click syndrome. Am J Cardiol 37:317, 1976.

280. Maron BJ, Roberts WC, McAllister HA, et al: Sudden death in young athletes. Circulation 62:218, 1980.

281. Swartz MH, Teichholz LE, Donoso E: Mitral valve prolapse: A review of associated arrhythmias. Am J Med 62:377, 1977.

282. Kavey RW, Sondheimer HM, Blackman MS: Detection of dysrhythmia in pediatric patients with mitral valve prolapse. Circulation 62:582, 1980.

283. Maron BJ, Roberts WC, Epstein SE: Sudden death in hypertrophic cardiomyopathy: A profile of 78 patients. Circulation 65:1388, 1982.

284. McKenna WJ, Deanfield JE, Faruqui A, et al: Prognosis in hypertrophic cardiomyopathy: Role of age and clinical, electrocardiographic and hemodynamic features. Am J Cardiol 47:532, 1981.

285. Maron BJ, Savage DD, Wolfson JK, et al: Prognostic significance of 24 hour ambulatory electrocardiographic monitoring in patients with hypertrophic cardiomyopathy: A prospective study. Am J Cardiol 48:252, 1981.

286. McKenna WJ, England D, Doi YL, et al: Arrhythmias in hypertrophic cardiomyopathy: I. Influence on prognosis. Br Heart J 46:168, 1981.

287. Maron BJ, Fananapazir L: Sudden cardiac death in hypertrophic cardiomyopathy. Circulation 85:I–57, 1992.

288. Fananapazir L, Chang AC, Epstein SE, et al: Prognostic determinants in hypertrophic cardiomyopathy: Prospective evaluation of a therapeutic strategy based on clinical, Holter, hemodynamic, and electrophysiological findings. Circulation 86:730, 1992.

289. Saumarez RC: Electrophysiological investigation of patients with hypertrophic cardiomyopathy: Evidence that slowed intraventricular conduction is associated with an increased risk of sudden death. Br Heart J 72(suppl):S19, 1994.

290. McKenna WJ, Franklin RCG, Nihoyannopoulos P, et al: Arrhythmia and prognosis in infants, children and adolescents with hypertrophic cardiomyopathy. J Am Coll Cardiol 11:147, 1988.

291. Pelliccia F, Cianfrocca C, Romeo F, et al: Hypertrophic cardiomyopathy: Long-term effects of propranolol versus verapamil in pre-

venting sudden death in "low-risk" patients. Cardiovasc Drugs Ther 4:1515, 1990.

292. Rosing DR, Condit JR, Maron BJ, et al: Verapamil therapy: A new approach to the pharmacologic treatment of hypertrophic cardiomyopathy: III. Effects of long-term administration. Am J Cardiol 48:545, 1981.

293. McKenna WJ, Oakley CM, Krikler DM, et al: Improved survival with amiodarone in patients with hypertrophic cardiomyopathy and ventricular tachycardia. Br Heart J 53:412, 1985.

294. Fananapazir L, Cannon ROI, Tripodi D, et al: Impact of dual-chamber permanent pacing in patients with obstructive hypertrophic cardiomyopathy with symptoms refractory to verapamil and beta-adrenergic blocker therapy. Circulation 85:2148, 1992.

295. Jeanrenaud X, Goy JJ, Kappenberger L: Effects of dual-chamber pacing in hypertrophic obstructive cardiomyopathy. Lancet 339:1318, 1992.

296. Cohn LH, Trehan H, Collins JJ Jr: Long-term follow-up of patients undergoing myotomy/myectomy for obstructive hypertrophic cardiomyopathy. Am J Cardiol 70:657, 1992.

297. Morrow AG, Koch JP, Maron BJ, et al: Left ventricular myotomy and myectomy in patients with obstructive hypertrophic cardiomyopathy and previous cardiac arrest. Am J Cardiol 46:313, 1980.

298. Marian AJ: Sudden cardiac death in patients with hypertrophic cardiomyopathy: From bench to bedside with an emphasis on genetic markers. Clin Cardiol 18:189, 1995.

299. Epstein ND, Cohn GM, Cyran F, et al: Differences in clinical expression of hypertrophic cardiomyopathy associated with two distinct mutations in the β-myosin heavy chain gene: A 908 Leu-Val mutation and a 403 Arg-Gln mutation. Circulation 86:345, 1992.

300. Watkins H, Rosenzweig A, Hwang D, et al: Characteristics and prognostic implications of myosin missense mutations in familial hypertrophic cardiomyopathy. N Engl J Med 326:1108, 1992.

301. Klein LS, Zipes DP, Miles WM: Ablation of ventricular tachycardia in patients without coronary artery disease and ventricular tachycardia due to bundle branch reentry. In Huang SKS (ed): Radiofrequency Catheter Ablation of Cardiac Arrhythmias: Basic Concepts and Clinical Applications. Armonk, NY, Futura, 1994, p 479.

302. Klein LS, Shih H, Hackett FK, et al: Radiofrequency catheter ablation of ventricular tachycardia in patients without structural heart disease. Circulation 85:1666, 1992.

303. Callans DJ, Menz V, Schwartzman D, et al: Repetitive monomorphic tachycardia from the left ventricular outflow tract: Electrocardiographic patterns consistent with a left ventricular site of origin. J Am Coll Cardiol 29:1023, 1997.

304. Lauer MR, Liem LB, Young C, et al: Cellular and clinical electrophysiology of verapamil-sensitive ventricular tachycardias. J Cardiovasc Electrophysiol 3:500, 1992.

305. Wen M, Yeh S, Wang C, et al: Radiofrequency ablation therapy in idiopathic left ventricular tachycardia with no obvious structural heart disease. Circulation 89:1690, 1994.

306. Coggins DL, Lee RJ, Sweeney J, et al: Radiofrequency catheter ablation as a cure for idiopathic tachycardia of both left and right ventricular origin. J Am Coll Cardiol 23:1333, 1994.

307. Kornbluth A, Frishman WH, Ackerman M: β-Adrenergic blockade in children. Cardiol Clin 5:629, 1987.

308. Moak JR, Smith RT, Garson AJ: Newer antiarrhythmic drugs in children. Am Heart J 113:179, 1986.

309. Malcolm ID, Stubington D, Gibbons JE: Mexiletine for ventricular arrhythmia after repair of tetralogy of Fallot. Can Med Assoc J 123:530, 1980.

310. Morady F, Kadish AH, DiCarlo L, et al: Long-term results of catheter ablation of idiopathic right ventricular tachycardia. Circulation 82:2093, 1990.

311. Gursoy S, Brugada J, Souza O, et al: Radiofrequency ablation of symptomatic benign ventricular arrhythmias. PACE 15:738, 1992.

312. Burton ME, Leon AR: Radiofrequency catheter ablation of right ventricular outflow tract tachycardia late after complete repair of tetralogy of Fallot using the pace mapping technique. PACE 16:2319, 1993.

313. Goldner BG, Cooper R, Blau W, et al: Radiofrequency catheter ablation as a primary therapy for treatment of ventricular tachycardia in a patient after repair of tetralogy of Fallot. PACE 17:1441, 1994.

314. Biblo LA, Carlson MD: Transcatheter radiofrequency ablation of ventricular tachycardia following surgical correction of tetralogy of Fallot. PACE 17:1556, 1994.

315. Gonska B, Cao K, Raab J, et al: Radiofrequency catheter ablation of right ventricular tachycardia late after repair of congenital heart defects. Circulation 94:1902, 1996.

316. Vetter VL, Tanner CS, Horowitz LN: Electrophysiologic consequences of the Mustard repair of d-transposition of the great arteries. J Am Coll Cardiol 10:265, 1987.

317. Yabek SM, Jamakani JM: Sinus node dysfunction in children, adolescents and young adults. Pediatrics 61:593, 1978.

318. Greenwood RD, Rosenthal A, Sloss LJ, et al: Sick sinus syndrome after surgery for congenital heart disease. Circulation 52:208, 1975.

319. Kugler JD, Danford DA: Pacemakers in children: An update. Am Heart J 17:665, 1989.

320. Taber RE, Estoye LR, Green ER, et al: Treatment of congenital and acquired heart block with an implantable pacemaker. Circulation 29:182, 1964.

321. Kangos JJ, Griffiths SP, Blumenthal S: Congenital complete heart block: A classification and experience with 18 patients. Am J Cardiol 20:632, 1967.

322. Glenn WW, De Leuchtenberg N, Van Heeckeren DW, et al: Heart block in children: Treatment with a radiofrequency pacemaker. J Thorac Cardiovasc Surg 58:361, 1969.

323. Furman S, Young D: Cardiac pacing in children and adolescents. Am J Cardiol 39:550, 1977.

324. Young D: Permanent pacemaker implantation in children: Current status and future considerations. PACE 4:61, 1981.

325. Beder SD, Hanisch DG, Cohen MH, et al: Cardiac pacing in children: A 15-year experience. Am Heart J 109:152, 1985.

326. Goldman BS, Williams WG, Hill T, et al: Permanent cardiac pacing after open heart surgery: Congenital heart disease. PACE 8:732, 1985.

327. Karpawich PP, Gillette PC, Garson A Jr, et al: Congenital complete atrioventricular block: Clinical and electrophysiologic predictors of need for pacemaker insertion. Am J Cardiol 48:1098, 1981.

328. Krongrad E: Prognosis for patients with congenital heart disease and postoperative intraventricular conduction defects. Circulation 57:867, 1978.

329. Daicoff GR, Aslami A, Tobias JA, et al: Management of postoperative complete heart block in infants and children. Chest 66:639, 1974.

330. Driscoll DJ, Gillette PC, Hallman GL, et al: Management of surgical complete AV block in children. Am J Cardiol 43:1175, 1979.

331. Hofschire PJ, Nicoloff DM, Moller JH: Postoperative complete heart block in 64 children treated with and without cardiac pacing. Am J Cardiol 39:559, 1977.

332. Flinn CJ, Wolff GS, Dick M II, et al: Cardiac rhythm after the Mustard operation for complete transposition of the great arteries. Circulation 310:1635, 1984.

333. Smith RT Jr: Pacemakers for children. In Gillette PC, Garson A, Jr (eds): Pediatric Arrhythmias: Electrophysiology and Pacing. Philadelphia, WB Saunders, 1990, p 532.

334. Frye RL, Collins JJ Jr, DeSanctis RW, et al: Guidelines for permanent cardiac pacemaker implantation: A report of the joint American College of Cardiology/American Heart Association Task Force on Assessment of Cardiovascular Procedures (Subcommittee on Pacemaker Implantation). Circulation 70:331A, 1984.

335. Michaëlsson M, Jonzon A, Riesenfeld T: Isolated congenital complete atrioventricular block in adult life. Circulation 92:442, 1995.

336. Williams WG, Hesslein PS, Kormos R: Exit block in children with pacemakers. Clin Prog Electrophysiol Pacing 4:478, 1986.

337. Gillette PC, Shannon C, Blair H, et al: Transvenous pacing in pediatric patients. Am Heart J 105:843, 1983.

338. Epstein ML, Knauf DG, Alexander JA: Long-term follow-up of transvenous cardiac pacing in children. Am J Cardiol 57:889, 1986.

339. Esperer HD, Singer H, Riede FT, et al: Permanent epicardial and transvenous single- and dual-chamber cardiac pacing in children. Thorac Cardiovasc Surg 41:21, 1993.

340. Molina JE, Dunnigan AC, Crosson JE: Implantation of transvenous pacemakers in infants and small children. Ann Thorac Surg 59:689, 1995.

341. Ward DE, Jones S, Shinebourne EA: Long-term transvenous pacing in children weighing less than 10 kg. Circulation 72(suppl 3):340, 1985.

342. Walsh C, McAlister H, Andrews C, et al: Pacemaker implantation in children: A 21-year experience. PACE 11(suppl 2):1940, 1988.

343. Karpawich PP, Perry BL, Farooki ZQ, et al: Pacing in children and young adults with nonsurgical atrioventricular block: Comparison of

single-rate ventricular and dual-chamber modes. Am Heart J 113:316, 1987.

344. Bernstein AD, Camm AJ, Fletcher R, et al: The NASPE/BPEG generic pacemaker code for antibradyarrhythmia and adaptive-rate pacing and antitachyarrhythmia devices. PACE 10:794, 1987.

345. Gillette PC, Ziegler VL, Case CL, et al: Atrial antitachycardia pacing in children and young adults. Am Heart J 122:844, 1997.

346. Kron J, Silka MJ, Ohm OJ, et al: Preliminary experience with nonthoracotomy implantable cardioverter defibrillators in young patients. PACE 17:26, 1994.

347. Gillette PC, Reitman MJ, Gutgesell HP, et al: Intracardiac electrocardiography in children and young adults. Am Heart J 89:36, 1975.

348. Young D, Eisenberg R, Fish B, et al: Wenckebach atrioventricular block (Mobitz type 1) in children and adolescents. Am J Cardiol 40:393, 1977.

349. Kelly DT, Brodsky SJ, Krovetz LJ: Mobitz type II atrioventricular block in children. Pediatrics 79:972, 1971.

350. Michaëlsson M, Engle MA: Congenital complete heart block: An international study of the natural history. In Engle MA (ed): Pediatric Cardiology. Philadelphia, FA Davis, 1972, p 85.

351. Chameides L, Truex RC, Vetter VL, et al: Association of maternal systemic lupus erythematosus with congenital complete heart block. N Engl J Med 297:1204, 1977.

352. Scott JS, Maddison PJ, Taylor PV, et al: Connective-tissue disease, antibodies to ribonucleoprotein, and congenital heart block. N Engl J Med 309:209, 1983.

353. McCue CM, Mantakas ME, Tingelstad JB, et al: Congenital heart block in newborns of mothers with connective tissue disease. Circulation 56:82, 1977.

354. Ramsey-Goldman R, Hom D, Deng J, et al: Anti-SS-A antibodies and fetal outcome in maternal systemic lupus erythematosus. Arthritis Rheum 29:1269, 1986.

355. Harley JB, Kaine JL, Fox OF, et al: Ro(SS-A) antibody antigen in a patient with congenital complete heart block. Arthritis Rheum 28:1321, 1985.

356. Taylor PV, Scott JS, Gerlis LM, et al: Maternal antibodies against fetal cardiac antigens in congenital complete heart block. N Engl J Med 315:667, 1986.

357. Lee LA, Coulter S, Erner S, et al: Cardiac immunoglobulin deposition and congenital heart block associated with maternal anti-Ro autoantibodies. Am J Med 83:793, 1987.

358. Litsey SE, Noonan JA, O'Connor WN, et al: Maternal connective tissue disease and congenital heart block: Demonstration of immunoglobulin in cardiac tissue. N Engl J Med 312:98, 1985.

359. Reed BR, Lee LA, Harmon C, et al: Autoantibodies to SS-A/Ro in infants with congenital heart block. J Pediatr 6:889, 1983.

360. Buyon JP, Winchester RJ, Slade SG, et al: Identification of mothers at risk for congenital heart block and other neonatal lupus syndromes in their children: Comparison of enzyme-linked immunosorbent assay and immunoblot for measurement of anti-SS-A/Ro and anti-SS-B/La antibodies. Arthritis Rheum 36:1263, 1993.

361. Buyon JP, Swersky SH, Fox HE, et al: Intrauterine therapy for presumptive fetal myocarditis with acquired heart block due to system lupus erythematosus. Arthritis Rheum 30:44, 1987.

362. Buyon JP, Winchester R: Congenital complete heart block: A human model of passively acquired autoimmune injury. Arthritis Rheum 33:609, 1990.

363. Levy AM, Camon AJ, Keane JF: Multiple arrhythmias detected during nocturnal monitoring in patients with congenital complete heart block. Circulation 55:247, 1977.

364. Dewey RC, Capeles MA, Levy AM: Use of ambulatory electrocardiographic monitoring to identify high-risk patients with congenital complete heart block. N Engl J Med 316:835, 1987.

365. Sholler GF, Walsh EP: Congenital complete heart block in patients without anatomic cardiac defects. Am Heart J 118:1193, 1989.

366. Benson DW Jr, Spach MS, Edwards SB, et al: Heart block in children: Evaluation of subsidiary ventricular pacemaker recovery times and ECG tape recordings. Pediatr Cardiol 2:39, 1982.

367. Pinsky WW, Gillette PC, Garson A Jr, et al: Diagnosis, management, and long-term results of patients with congenital complete atrioventricular block. Pediatrics 69:728, 1982.

368. Fryda RJ, Kaplan S, Helmsworth JA: Postoperative complete heart block in children. Br Heart J 22:456, 1971.

369. Lillehei CW, Sellers RD, Bonabeau R, et al: Chronic postsurgical complete heart block. J Thorac Cardiovasc Surg 46:436, 1963.

370. Kulbertus HE, Coyne JJ, Hallidie-Smith KA: Conduction disturbances before and after surgical closure of ventricular septal defect. Am Heart J 77:123, 1969.

371. Moss AJ, Klyman G, Emmanouilides GC: Late onset of complete heart block. Am J Cardiol 30:884, 1972.

372. Levy MJ, Cuello L, Tuna N, et al: Atrioventricularis communis. Am J Cardiol 14:587, 1964.

373. Esscher E, Hardell L, Michaëlsson M: Familial, isolated, complete right bundle branch block. Br Heart J 37:745, 1976.

374. Giuliani ER, Fuster V, Brandenburg RO, et al: Ebstein's anomaly: The clinical features and natural history of Ebstein's anomaly of the tricuspid valve. Mayo Clin Proc 54:163, 1979.

375. Gallastegui J, Hariman RF, Handler B, et al: Cardiac involvement in the Kearns-Sayre syndrome. Am J Cardiol 60:385, 1987.

376. Horowitz LN, Alexander JA, Edmonds LH: Postoperative right bundle branch block: Identification of three levels of block. Circulation 60:319, 1980.

377. Quattlebaum TG, Varghese PJ, Neill CA, et al: Sudden death among postoperative patients with tetralogy of Fallot. Circulation 54:289, 1976.

378. Friedli B, Bolens M, Taktak M: Conduction disturbances after correction of tetralogy of Fallot: Are electrophysiologic studies of prognostic value? J Am Coll Cardiol 11:162, 1988.

379. Vetter VL: What every pediatrician needs to know about arrhythmias in children who have had cardiac surgery. Pediatr Ann 20:378, 1991.

380. Vetter VL: Postoperative pediatric electrocardiographic and electrophysiologic sequelae. In Liebman J, Plonsey R, Rudy Y (eds): Pediatric and Fundamental Electrocardiography. Boston, Martinus Nijhoff Publishing, 1987, p 187.

381. Champsaur GL, Sokol DM, Trusler GA, et al: Repair of transposition of the great arteries in 123 pediatric patients. Circulation 47:1032, 1973.

382. Saalouke MG, Rios J, Perry LW, et al: Electrophysiologic studies after Mustard's operation for d-transposition of the great vessels. Am J Cardiol 41:1104, 1978.

383. Vetter VL: Sudden death in infants, children and adolescents. In Josephson ME (ed): Sudden Cardiac Death. Philadelphia, FA Davis, 1985, p 301.

384. Garson A Jr, McNamara DG: Sudden death in a pediatric cardiology population 1958 to 1983: Relation to prior arrhythmias. J Am Coll Cardiol 5:134B, 1985.

385. Scagliotti D, Strasberg N, Duffy CE, et al: Inducible polymorphous ventricular tachycardia following Mustard operation for transposition of the great arteries. Pediatr Cardiol 5:39, 1984.

386. Karjalainen J, Viitasals M, Kala R, et al: 24 hour electrocardiogram recordings in mild acute infectious myocarditis. Ann Clin Res 16:34, 1984.

387. Vikerfors T, Stjerna A, Icen P, et al: Acute myocarditis: Serologic diagnosis, clinical findings and follow-up. Acta Med Scand 223:45, 1988.

388. Clarke M, Keith JD: Atrioventricular conduction in acute rheumatic fever. Br Heart J 34:472, 1972.

389. Belani K, Regelmann WE: Lyme disease in children. Rheum Dis Clin North Am 15:679, 1989.

390. Kegel SM, Dorsey TJ, Rowen M, et al: Cardiac death in mucocutaneous lymph node syndrome. Am J Cardiol 40:282, 1977.

391. Surawicz B: Role of electrolytes in the etiology and management of cardiac arrhythmias. Prog Cardiovasc Dis 8:364, 1966.

392. Surawicz B: Electrolyte solutions. In Horowitz LN (ed): Current Management of Arrhythmias. Philadelphia, BC Decker, 1991, p 322.

393. Ettinger PO, Regan TJ, Oldewurtel H: Hyperkalemia, cardiac conduction and the electrocardiogram: A review. Am Heart J 88:360, 1974.

394. Williams JF, Klocke FJ, Braunwald E: Studies on digitalis XIII: A comparison of the effects of potassium on the inotropic and arrhythmia producing actions of ouabain. J Clin Invest 45:346, 1966.

395. Tzivoni D, Keren A, Cohen AM: Magnesium therapy for torsades de pointes. Am J Cardiol 53:528, 1984.

396. Slovis TL, Oh JE, Teitelbaum DT: Physostigmine therapy in acute tricyclic antidepressant poisoning. Clin Toxicol 4:451, 1971.

397. Scheffer GJ, Jonges R, Holley HS, et al: Effects of halothane on the conduction system of the heart in humans. Anesth Analg 69:721, 1989.

398. Dowd DM, Krug S: Pediatric blunt cardiac injury: Epidemiology, clinical features, and diagnosis. J Trauma 40:61, 1996.

399. Tellez DW, Hardin WDJ, Takahashi M, et al: Blunt cardiac injury in children. J Pediatr Surg 22:1123, 1987.

400. Langan MNS, Horowitz LN: Cardiac surgery and cardiac trauma. In Horowitz LN (ed): Current Management of Arrhythmias. Philadelphia, BC Decker, 1991, p 272.

401. Vaughan-Williams EM: Classification of antiarrhythmic drugs. J Pharmacol Ther 1:115, 1975.

402. Vaughan-Williams EM: A classification of antiarrhythmic actions reassessed after a decade of new drugs. J Clin Pharmacol 24:129, 1984.

403. Bean BP, Cohen CJ, Tsien RW: Lidocaine block of cardiac channels. J Gen Physiol 81:613, 1983.

404. Grant AO, Starmer CF, Strauss HC: Antiarrhythmic drug action: Blockade of the inward sodium current. Circulation 55:427, 1984.

405. Hoffman BF, Rosen MR, Wit AL: Electrophysiology and pharmacology of cardiac arrhythmias: VII. Cardiac effects of quinidine and procainamide. Am Heart J 90:117, 1975.

406. Giardina EG: Procainamide: Clinical pharmacology and efficacy against ventricular arrhythmias. Ann N Y Acad Sci 432:117, 1984.

407. Strasberg B, Schlarovsky S, Erdberg A: Procainamide-induced polymorphous ventricular tachycardia. Am J Cardiol 47:1309, 1981.

408. Smith WM, Gallagher JJ: "Les torsades de pointes": An unusual ventricular arrhythmia. Ann Intern Med 93:578, 1980.

409. Sclarovsky S, Strasberg BL, Lewin RF: Polymorphous ventricular tachycardia: Clinical features and treatment. Am J Cardiol 44:339, 1979.

410. Binah O, Rosen MR: The cellular mechanisms of cardiac antiarrhythmic drug action. Ann N Y Acad Sci 432:31, 1984.

411. Singh B, Vaughan-Williams EM: Investigations of the mode of action of a new antidysrhythmic drug, KO 1173. Br J Pharmacol 44:1, 1972.

412. Monk JP, Brogden RN: Mexiletine: A review of its pharmacodynamic and pharmacokinetic properties, and therapeutic use in the treatment of arrhythmias. Drugs 40:374, 1990. [Published erratum in Drugs 41:377, 1991.]

413. Bigger JT, Strauss HC: Digitalis toxicity: Drug interactions promoting toxicity and the management of toxicity. Semin Drug Treat 2:147, 1972.

414. Garson A Jr, Kugler JD, Gillette PC: Control of late postoperative arrhythmias with phenytoin in young patients. Am J Cardiol 46:290, 1980.

415. Chang AC, Zappalla FR, Kurer CC: Clinical outcome in children with the permanent form of junctional reciprocating tachycardia. J Am Coll Cardiol 15:176A, 1990.

416. Fish FA, Gillette PC, Benson DW: Proarrhythmia, cardiac arrest and death in young patients receiving encainide or flecainide. The Pediatric Electrophysiology Group. J Am Coll Cardiol 18:356, 1991.

417. McLeod AA, Stiles GL, Shand DG: Demonstration of beta adrenoceptor blockade by propafenone hydrochloride: Clinical pharmacologic, radioligand binding and adenylate cyclase activation studies. J Pharmacol Exp Ther 228:461, 1984.

418. Kishore AGR, Camm AJ: Guidelines for the use of propafenone in treating supraventricular arrhythmias. Drugs 50:250, 1995.

419. Siddoway LA, Thompson KA, McAllister CB, et al: Polymorphism of propafenone metabolism and disposition in man: Clinical and pharmacokinetic consequences. Circulation 75:785, 1987.

420. Paul T, Reimer A, Janousek J, et al: Efficacy and safety of propafenone in congenital junctional ectopic tachycardia. J Am Coll Cardiol 20:911, 1992.

421. Paul T, Janousek J: New antiarrhythmic drugs in pediatric use: Propafenone. Pediatr Cardiol 15:190, 1994.

422. Gillette PC, Garson AJ, Eterovic E: Oral propranolol treatment in infants and children. J Pediatr 92:141, 1978.

423. Naccarelli GV, Rinkenberger RL, Dougherty AH, Giebel RA: Amiodarone: Pharmacology and antiarrhythmic and adverse effects. Pharmacotherapy 5:298, 1985.

424. Yabek SM, Kato R, Singh BN: Acute effects of amiodarone on the electrophysiologic properties of isolated neonatal and adult cardiac fibers. J Am Coll Cardiol 5:1109, 1985.

425. Leveque PE: Antiarrhythmic action of bretylium. Nature 207:203, 1965.

426. Heissenbuttel RH, Bigger JT: Bretylium tosylate: a newly available antiarrhythmic drug for ventricular arrhythmias. Ann Intern Med 91:229, 1979.

427. Sanguinetti MC, Jurkiewicz NK: Two components of cardiac delayed rectifier K+ current. J Gen Physiol 96:195, 1990.

428. Hohnloser SH, Woosley RL: Sotalol. N Engl J Med 331:31, 1994.

429. Rosen MR, Wit AL, Hoffman BF: Electrophysiology and pharmacology of cardiac arrhythmias: VI. Cardiac effects of verapamil. Am Heart J 89:665, 1975.

430. Woelfel A, Foster JR, McAllister RG, et al: Efficacy of verapamil in exercise-induced ventricular tachycardia. Am J Cardiol 56:292, 1985.

431. Pelleg A: Cardiac cellular electrophysiologic actions of adenosine and adenosine triphosphate. Am Heart J 110:688, 1985.

432. DiMarco JP, Sellers TD, Berne RM, et al: Adenosine: Electrophysiologic effects and therapeutic use for terminating paroxysmal supraventricular tachycardia. Circulation 68:1254, 1983.

433. Fozzard HA, Sheets MF: Cellular mechanisms of action of cardiac glycosides. J Am Coll Cardiol 5:10A, 1985.

434. Watanabe AM: Digitalis and autonomic nervous system. J Am Coll Cardiol 5:35A, 1985.

435. Koch-Weser J, Frishman WH: Beta-adrenoreceptor antagonist: New drugs and new indications. N Engl J Med 305:500, 1981.

436. Singh BN, Vaughan-Williams EM: The effect of amiodarone, a new antianginal drug on cardiac muscle. Br J Pharmacol 39:657, 1970.

CHAPTER 56
SYNCOPE

LARRY A. RHODES

Syncope, a sudden transient loss of consciousness and postural control, is the chief complaint in 1% of all pediatric emergency department admissions.[1] The basic mechanism is transient cerebral ischemia. Although the syndrome is often benign, the patient may sustain injury. Syncope often recurs unpredictably and leads to tremendous anxiety in patients and their parents. Although syncope may be the presenting symptom of a more complex medical problem, such as a cardiac arrhythmia, structural cardiac anomaly, or neurologic disorder, most adolescents who present with syncope have no overt causes. Physicians evaluating patients with syncope must determine whether it is benign or a marker of a more life-threatening condition. This section offers a brief review of the differential diagnosis of syncope in this age group and then concentrates on evaluating and treating neurocardiogenic syncope.

INCIDENCE

Up to 15% of children experience syncope.[2–4] Driscoll and colleagues[5] reported the incidence of syncope in patients seeking medical attention in the Rochester, Minnesota, area between 1987 and 1991 as 125.8 per 100,000. The incidence was higher in girls (166.3) than in boys (92.9), and the peak age range for syncope was 15 to 19 years.

CAUSES OF SYNCOPE

These are listed in Table 56–1. All the causes except noncardiovascular and three of the four vascular causes (cerebrovascular diseases, subclavian steal, and basilar artery migraine) produce varying degrees of bradycardia and hypotension, so that cerebral blood flow is reduced as part of a general decrease in cardiac output. Most of the noncardiovascular and cerebrovascular causes, except for hysteria, produce a local decrease in cerebral blood flow.

NEUROCARDIOGENIC SYNCOPE

Various cardiac conditions that obstruct blood flow through the heart can cause syncope (see Table 56–1). Most pediatric patients with syncope have a form of neurocardiogenic syncope.

Neurocardiogenic syncope results from inappropriate output from the autonomic nervous system leading to symptomatic changes in blood pressure and heart rate. This typically occurs while the patient is standing. It also develops during emotional stress, such as during speaking performances, or after noxious stimuli, such as phlebotomy. Many patients have a prodrome of dizziness before the syncopal event. Others complain of an aura, such as flashing lights, changes in hearing, tunnel vision, or nausea. The blood pressure falls, the heart rate slows, and the subject becomes pale and loses consciousness. Myoclonic jerks are common, but true tonic-clonic seizures are rare.

PATHOPHYSIOLOGY

A possible trigger for syncope in patients with neurocardiogenic syncope is venous pooling in the lower extremities while standing. In an adult, approximately 500 ml of intravenous volume is displaced into the lower extremities during standing.[6] This translates to approximately 10 ml per kilogram in the child.[7] With venous pooling, there is a decrease in the central venous volume and a corresponding decrease in left ventricular preload. The normal response to decreased ventricular filling is reduced stretching of left ventricular mechanoreceptors, commonly referred to as C fibers.[8] The resultant decreased output from the C fibers leads to a reflex elevation in sympathetic tone and an increase in heart rate and peripheral vascular resistance.[8–10] These mechanoreceptors originate in both atrial and ventricular tissues.[5,6] The atrial afferents are myelinated and arise from the junction of the vena cava and pulmonary veins with the atrium,[9] and they appear to be sensitive to central volume changes and insensitive to myocardial contractility.[8,10] The ventricular afferents are unmyelinated C fibers sensitive to contractility and end-diastolic pressure.[9] When there is decreased stretching, there is less output from these fibers back to the brain stem, leading to a reflex increase in sympathetic output.[8–10]

The heart rate and blood pressure responses that accompany standing have been evaluated in children by Dambrink and coworkers.[11] In normal children, standing leads to an initial decrease in systolic and diastolic blood pressures followed by an increase in both pressures and an increase in heart rate. As the child continues to stand, the systolic blood pressure returns to baseline with the diastolic blood pressure and heart rate remaining elevated as long as 2 minutes. In individuals prone to syncope, the act of standing produces a more exaggerated decrease in systolic and diastolic blood pressure and, in some, a paradoxical decrease in heart rate.

In patients with neurocardiogenic syncope, this reflex is abnormal. These patients experience a decrease in sympathetic tone and an increase in parasympathetic tone lead-

TABLE 56–1

CAUSES OF SYNCOPE

Vasodepressor (neurocardiogenic) syncope: most common cause
Orthostatic hypotension: failure of normal postural reflexes
    Decreased central blood volume
        Prolonged standing
        Poor muscle tone (e.g., after prolonged recumbency)
        Severe fluid or blood loss without replacement
    Autonomic insufficiency
        Peripheral neuritis
        Central autonomic failure: Shy-Drager syndrome
        Idiopathic: Bradbury-Eggleston syndrome
        Spinal cord lesions
    Drugs
        Vasodilators
        Sympatholytic drugs (e.g., antihypertensives)
        Nitrates
        Antidepressants (e.g., tricyclic antidepressants)
        Sedatives and narcotics
Other vascular causes
    Cerebrovascular diseases
    Subclavian steal
    Carotid sinus hypersensitivity
    Basilar artery migraine
Cardiac causes
    Obstruction
        Aortic stenosis
        Hypertrophic cardiomyopathy
        Left atrial myxoma
        Tetralogy of Fallot
        Severe pulmonary hypertension without shunts
        Acute pulmonary embolism
    Arrhythmia
        Tachycardia
        Supraventricular
        Ventricular
    Bradycardia
        Sinus node dysfunction
        Atrioventricular block
    Pacemaker malfunction
    Long QT syndrome
Other cardiac causes
    Abnormal origin or course of coronary arteries
    Cardiac tamponade
Vagal syncope
    Micturition
    Deglutition
    Glossopharyngeal neuralgia
    Postgastrectomy (dumping) syndrome
Noncardiovascular
    Hyperventilation
    Hysteria
    Atypical seizures
    Cough syncope

ing to hypotension and bradycardia.[8] The exact abnormality in the reflex is not fully understood. One proposed mechanism is that a decrease in left ventricular preload leads to an increase in contractility, which then raises the intracavitary pressure. This pressure increase stimulates the left ventricular mechanoreceptors and in turn elevates parasympathetic tone.[8] The role of left ventricular mechanoreceptors in this reflex has been demonstrated in work by Oberg and Thoren,[12] in which they documented an initial decline followed by a marked increase in ventricular mechanoreceptor activity in cats subjected to experimental hemorrhage or occlusion of inferior vena cava blood flow leading to decreased ventricular filling. They proposed that the underfilled left ventricle becam. distorted, activating

the mechanoreceptors, which in turn fed back to the brain stem, causing a reflex withdrawal of sympathetic outflow and an increase in parasympathetic output.[12] Similar mechanisms may operate in the syncope that occurs in some patients with left or right ventricular outflow obstruction. A variation of this hypothesis suggests that there may be an initial increase in sympathetic tone contributing to this reflex. This is supported by the finding that patients with neurocardiogenic syncope often have an increase in heart rate and arterial blood pressure immediately before the syncopal episode[13–15] and increased levels of urinary catecholamines before the event.[16]

A second possible mechanism for syncope may be central triggers that lead to bradycardia and hypotension. Neurohormonal agents other than catecholamines may play an important role in leading to the depressor response in neurally mediated syncope. Perna and associates[17] have demonstrated increased levels of β-endorphin in patients with vasodepressor syncope. These increased levels were also seen in hemorrhagic shock.[18,19] Evans and colleagues[18] found that hypotension could be prevented in hemorrhagic shock by giving naloxone intracisternally. Serotonin, a central mediator, may also play a role in neurocardiogenic syncope. Animal studies have suggested that serotonin may lead to the depressor response seen in hemorrhage.[20] In a study by Abboud and Thames,[9] it was shown that intracerebrovascular serotonin induces hypotension and changes in renal sympathetic nerve activity and may also be acting centrally to inhibit sympathetic activity, thereby contributing to syncope.

EVALUATION OF THE PATIENT WITH SYNCOPE
(Fig. 56–1)

HISTORY

The evaluation of a child or adolescent with syncope begins with a thorough medical history. The history should include a precise, detailed account of events around the episode. Important points include any prodrome such as nausea, vomiting, palpitations, visual aura, decreased hearing, or dizziness. A complete history may be difficult to obtain from a patient because of amnesia around the event. If so, try to obtain witness accounts. Helpful information includes an assessment of the patient's appearance, such as pallor or cyanosis before and during the event. An estimation of the duration of the syncopal episode is also important. In general, neurocardiogenic syncope is brief in contrast to syncope from arrhythmias. Document abnormal movements such as seizure activity or abnormal posturing during the period of unconsciousness. The patient's mental status after the episode may be helpful in developing a differential diagnosis. Other important historical data are illness around the time of the event, oral intake in the preceding 24 hours, medications, and previous similar events.

A key element of the past medical history is a careful account of medications the patient may be using, including over-the-counter drugs, recreational drugs, and prescription medications. History of prior medical problems, including psychological illness, is obtained. A complete review of systems with special concentration on the cardio-

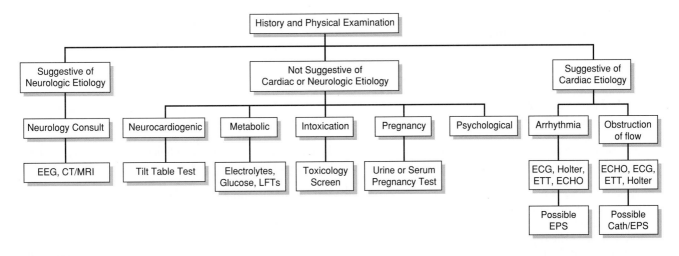

FIGURE 56-1

Scheme for evaluation of the patient with syncope. CT/MRI = computed tomography/magnetic resonance imaging; ECG = electrocardiography; ECHO = echocardiography; EEG = electroencephalography; EPS = electrophysiologic study; ETT = exercise tolerance testing; LFTs = liver function tests.

vascular and neurologic systems is made. A detailed family history should also be obtained, particularly history of neurologic disorders, hypertrophic cardiomyopathy, cardiac malformations, long QT syndrome, arrhythmias, and psychological disorders. The social history is important in assessing whether there is a possibility for substance abuse, pregnancy, or factors leading to a conversion reaction.

PHYSICAL EXAMINATION

A complete physical examination is performed on a patient with syncope. On the examination during and immediately after syncope, document the patient's heart rate, blood pressure, and respiratory effort and evaluate motor movements consistent with a seizure disorder. The physical examination after the event includes a complete evaluation of vital signs with measurement of blood pressure and heart rate while the patient is supine and standing to exclude orthostatic hypotension or tachycardia. Signs of trauma or drug abuse are sought. Neurologic examination should be complete, with particular attention to the fundus, looking for papilledema or other signs of increased intracranial pressure. Cardiovascular examination includes palpation of the patient's pulses for rhythm and quality. A complete auscultatory examination evaluates rhythm, quality of the first and second heart sounds, and presence of cardiac murmurs. This examination should be performed in both a sitting and a supine position, with use of standing, squatting, and the Valsalva maneuver to enhance findings consistent with mitral valve prolapse or hypertrophic cardiomyopathy. Particular attention is given to the second heart sound as a screen for pulmonary hypertension.

LABORATORY TESTS

Further testing is directed toward the patient's specific symptoms and physical examination findings. If a neurologic cause is being considered, a complete evaluation by a pediatric neurologist is indicated. If substance abuse or intoxication is suspected, a toxicology screen is performed. Other possible laboratory evaluations include serum electrolyte, blood urea nitrogen, creatinine, and glucose determinations as a screen for metabolic abnormalities as well as serum or urine concentration of human chorionic gonadotropin β subunit to exclude pregnancy.

A 12-lead electrocardiogram is reviewed for bradycardia, tachycardia, and conduction abnormalities such as heart block. PR, QRS, and QT, with the QT interval corrected for heart rate, should be measured. If syncope is associated with activity, an exercise stress test should be performed. If there is a question of an arrhythmia, a 24-hour ambulatory monitoring (Holter) should be performed. A complete electrophysiologic study is considered if the Holter monitoring suggests an arrhythmia. In patients in whom the history suggests neurocardiogenic syncope, a tilt table evaluation should be performed.

The remainder of this section deals with the evaluation and treatment of patients with neurocardiogenic syncope.

TILT TABLE TESTING

Even though the exact mechanism of neurocardiogenic syncope is incompletely defined, venous pooling related to assuming an upright posture may be a common trigger. For that reason, tilt table testing is used to evaluate patients with possible neurocardiogenic syncope. There have been numerous reports on the use of upright tilting in the evaluation of syncope in children and adolescents.[21-26] Although there is marked institutional variation in the specific protocols, all include upright posture to obtain necessary pooling of blood in the lower extremities.

Procedure

Tilt table evaluations are usually outpatient procedures performed with the patient in a fasting state. The patient is brought into a quiet room, and heart rate and blood pressure are monitored. Intravenous access is obtained for administration of medications such as isoproterenol or for volume resuscitation. Some institutions use an arterial line to monitor the blood pressure,[27–29] but a sphygmomanometer or automatic blood pressure monitoring equipment is usually used. The patient lies flat for 10 to 30 minutes to reach a steady state and is then placed in an upright tilt; the heart rate and blood pressure are continuously monitored. If symptoms occur during the upright tilt, the patient is returned to a supine position and allowed to recover. Some centers measure serum catecholamine levels immediately before and after syncope.[27,28] If the patient is asymptomatic during the initial tilt, the procedure may be repeated with an infusion of isoproterenol ranging from 0.02 to 2.0 μg/kg/min. Other autonomic testing, such as carotid or ocular massage, the Valsalva maneuver, and the diving reflex, is occasionally performed during the tilt table procedure. At the completion of the test, the patient is placed in a supine position and allowed to recover. The patient is usually discharged on the day of the test without hospitalization.

The use of isoproterenol in the evaluation of patients with neurocardiogenic syncope remains somewhat controversial. It may increase the sensitivity of the test. The proposed mechanism of action of isoproterenol is its positive inotropic property leading to increased contractility and subsequent stimulation of the left ventricular mechanoreceptors triggering the aforementioned abnormal autonomic reflex. The high yield of positive results in tilt table evaluations performed with isoproterenol infusion has led to concerns about its specificity. Kapoor and Brant[30] studied a group of patients with syncope of unknown etiology and two separate control groups of normal individuals. A similar tilt table test protocol was used for symptomatic individuals and one control group. The protocol included an upright tilt at 80 degrees for 15 minutes and the addition of an isoproterenol infusion (1 to 5 μg/min) if patients remained asymptomatic during initial tilt. The second control group was tested with a modified protocol in which patients who were asymptomatic during the initial tilt received isoproterenol but were rested in the supine position before each incremental increase in the isoproterenol infusion. The study showed that regardless of the isoproterenol infusion protocol used, positive test results were produced in all three groups (75% in the symptomatic group, 65% in the first control group, and 45% in the second control group). The findings of this study suggest that isoproterenol may increase the sensitivity of upright tilt testing in symptomatic patients but definitely hinders the specificity.

Response Patterns to Tilt Table Testing

The possible abnormal responses leading to symptoms during tilt table testing in patients being evaluated for recurrent syncope have been divided into cardioinhibitory, vasodepressor, and mixed. The cardioinhibitory response has been defined as an abrupt decrease in heart rate of at least 50% from baseline. The vasodepressor response is defined as a 50% or greater decrease in systolic or mean blood pressure from baseline. Mixed response is a combination of cardioinhibitory and vasodepressor responses.

Grubb and colleagues[31] established five subgroups of responses to tilt table testing:

1. neurocardiogenic: an abrupt decrease in blood pressure with or without bradycardia

2. dysautonomic: a gradual decrease in blood pressure leading to syncope

3. postural orthostatic tachycardia syndrome: an excessive heart rate increase to maintain an adequate blood pressure to prevent syncope (a response that may be related to chronic fatigue syndrome[32])

4. cerebral: syncope secondary to vasoconstriction without systemic hypotension[33]

5. psychogenic: syncope without a change in heart rate, blood pressure, electroencephalographic activity, or cranial blood flow[34]

Validity of Tilt Table Testing Results

A variety of protocols are used in tilt table testing. These variations have led to speculation about the sensitivity and specificity of the test. Specificity has ranged from 40 to 92%,[22,35,36] which may reflect the various protocols. Specificity varies according to the angle of inclination.[35] Tilt table tests performed at 80 degrees had a specificity of only 40%. This increased to 71% when testing was done at 70 degrees and 65% at 60 degrees. Specificity could be increased to more than 85% if the test was performed for only 10 minutes at 60 degrees or 70 degrees.[35]

TREATMENT

This section discusses the treatment of children and adolescents with neurocardiogenic syncope.

The primary method of treatment has been volume expansion; some patients respond to increasing their fluid intake, and no other medical intervention is needed. This often requires an intake of 3 to 4 L/day in an adolescent. Most patients in this age group do not have a thirst drive that prompts them to ingest this amount of fluid. The physician, parents, and patient must be creative to find ways to increase fluid intake. Controversy exists about the most appropriate fluid. There are proponents of the use of electrolyte-rich fluids, such as sport drinks. Caffeine-containing drinks should be avoided because of their effects analogous to those of isoproterenol, which may exaggerate the abnormal autonomic reflex. Patients should also avoid drinking fluids that are high in calories and fat, such as whole milk.

If increasing fluids alone does not work, salt or fludrocortisone may be added. Fludrocortisone (Florinef) is a mineralocorticoid steroid that stimulates the retention of sodium chloride and intravascular volume. Fludrocortisone prevented syncope in 90% of children and adolescents in one study.[22] With the use of salt, fludrocortisone, and increased fluid intake, significant changes in serum electrolyte concentrations may require monitoring and possible intervention. Serum sodium and potassium concentrations are generally well maintained, but serum bicarbonate levels are often elevated.[37] A decrease in proximal tubular sodium reabsorption resulting from the expansion in extracellular volume may increase sodium reabsorption in the distal nephron in exchange for potassium and hydrogen ions and cause metabolic alkalosis.[38] The mild abnormality is not thought to be important enough to modify treatment.[37] Hypertension and weight gain associated with the additional salt and fluid retention may result. Hypertension has not been found, but weight gain has been demonstrated.[33] This change in body weight may be secondary to normal growth of adolescence or related to increased fluid intake as well as fluid retention. Weight increase may hinder successful treatment because patients in this age group are often sensitive to even minor increases in their weight.

A second treatment approach is β-adrenergic blockers. Theoretically, β blockers, being negative inotropic agents, may offset the increased ventricular contractility seen as part of the abnormal reflex in neurocardiogenic syncope. They may also block the effect of circulating epinephrine, which may act as a central trigger for the abnormal reflex. The efficacy of β blockers in preventing recurrent syncope in adults has varied from 71 to 100%.[22, 24, 39–46] β Blockers are generally well tolerated in children. They must be used with caution in patients with reactive airway disease. Side effects include depression, decrease in school performance, and fatigue.

Disopyramide (Norpace), a type IA antiarrhythmic medication, has also been used in patients with neurocardiogenic syncope.[47] Because it is a potent negative inotrope, it may work like β blockers in decreasing contractility by hindering the initiation of the reflex. Disopyramide also has anticholinergic properties, which could, hypothetically, prevent the bradycardia associated with a cardioinhibitory episode. Disopyramide may also increase peripheral vascular resistance.[47–49] The efficacy of disopyramide ranges from 73 to 90% in mostly adult series.[44, 45, 50, 51] A disadvantage of disopyramide is that it may be proarrhythmic. Type I antiarrhythmics (sodium channel blockers) prolong the QT interval, increasing the risk for development of torsades de pointes.

α-Adrenergic agonists, such as phenylephrine and pseudoephedrine, are another class of medications used to treat neurocardiogenic syncope in young people. Decreased venous return to the heart while standing may be related to venodilatation and venous pooling. These agents increase venous tone by direct sympathetic stimulation. Systemic hypotension may also be blocked by arterial vasoconstriction, leading to an increase in systemic vascular resistance.[25] These potential advantages have been verified in a study performed in a group of children with neurocardiogenic syncope documented by tilt table testing whose responses were subsequently negative when they were tested after an infusion of phenylephrine. These patients were subsequently treated with pseudoephedrine with no recurrence of symptoms during follow-up.[51] Headaches, palpitations, tremors, insomnia, restlessness, and hypertension were not reported with the use of pseudoephedrine.[51] The efficacy ranged from 94 to 100%.[25, 52, 53]

The final class of medications used in the treatment of neurocardiogenic syncope is the serotonin uptake inhibitors, including fluoxetine hydrochloride (Prozac) and sertraline hydrochloride (Zoloft). These agents have antidepressant properties and have been used in patients with neurocardiogenic syncope refractory to conventional medications.[54] The elimination of the vasodepressor response by depletion or receptor blockade of serotonin has been well described in animal models of acute hemorrhage.[19, 55] Although the exact mechanism of action of serotonin uptake inhibition in the treatment of neurocardiogenic syncope is not fully understood, it is probably related to a similar abolition of the serotonin-mediated vasodepressor response. On the basis of findings in patients with clinical depression treated with fluoxetine hydrochloride[56] in which the symptoms of neurocardiogenic syncope were alleviated, Grubb and coworkers[54] studied the effects of sertraline hydrochloride therapy in pediatric patients with neurocardiogenic syncope whose conventional therapy had failed. A beneficial response to treatment with sertraline hydrochloride was found in 53% of the patients. Side effects reported included nausea, diarrhea, headache, and mild insomnia.[54]

The final therapeutic option is the use of pacing in patients with recurrent syncope. Pacing in patients with neurocardiogenic syncope is a class II indication as described by the American College of Cardiology/American Heart Association 1991 guidelines.[57] The use of pacemakers in patients with neurocardiogenic syncope remains controversial. In pediatric patients, neurocardiogenic syncope is not generally life-threatening and often responds to medical intervention. Most young people who have symptoms of neurocardiogenic syncope outgrow their propensity to this abnormal reflex. Although bradycardia is often present, the more dominant abnormality is the vasodepressor response leading to significant hypotension.

REFERENCES

1. Pratt JL, Fleisher GR: Syncope in children and adolescents. Pediatr Emerg Care 5:80, 1989.
2. Scott WA: Evaluating the child with syncope. Pediatr Ann 20:350, 1991.
3. Ruckman RN: Cardiac causes of syncope. Pediatr Rev 9:101, 1987.
4. Strasberg B, Sagie A, Rechavia E, et al: The noninvasive evaluation of syncope of suspected cardiovascular origin. Am Heart J 117:160, 1989.
5. Driscoll DJ, Jacobsen SJ, Porter CJ, Wollan PC: Syncope in children and adolescents. J Am Coll Cardiol 29:1039, 1997.
6. Ibrahim MM, Tarazi RC, Dustan HG: Orthostatic hypotension: Mechanisms and management. Am Heart J 90:513, 1975.
7. Freed MD: Advances in the diagnosis and therapy of syncope and palpitations in children. Curr Opin Pediatr 6:368, 1994.
8. Thoren P: Role of cardiac vagal C-fibers in cardiovascular control. Rev Physiol Biochem Pharmacol 86:1, 1979.
9. Abboud FM, Thames MD: Interaction of cardiovascular reflexes in circulatory control. In Shepherd JT, Abboud FM (eds): Handbook of Physiology. Bethesda, MD, American Physiological Society, 1983, p 675.
10. Donald ED, Shepherd JT: Reflexes from the heart and lungs. Physiological curiosities or important regulatory mechanisms. Cardiovasc Res 12:449, 1978.
11. Dambrink JHA, Imholz BPM, Karemaker JM, Wieling W: Circulatory adaptation to orthostatic stress in healthy 10–14-year-old children investigated in a general practice. Clin Sci 81:51, 1991.
12. Oberg B, Thoren P: Increased activity in left ventricular receptors during hemorrhage or occlusion of caval veins in the cat. A possible cause of the vasovagal reaction. Acta Physiol Scand 85:164, 1972.
13. Sra JS, Murthy V, Natale A, et al: Circulatory and catecholamine changes during head-up tilt in neurocardiogenic (vasovagal) syncope. Am J Cardiol 73:33, 1994.
14. Graham DT, Kabler JD, Lunsford L Jr: Vasovagal fainting: A diphasic response. Psychosom Med 23:493, 1961.
15. Glick G, Yu PN: Hemodynamic changes during spontaneous vasovagal reactions. Am J Med 34:43, 1963.
16. Chosey JJ, Graham DT: Catecholamines in vasovagal fainting. J Psychosom Res 9:189, 1965.
17. Perna GP, Ficola V, Salvatori MP, et al: Increase of plasma beta endorphins in vasodepressor syncope. Am J Cardiol 65:929, 1990.
18. Evans RG, Ludbrook J, Potocnik SJ: Intracisternal naloxone and cardiac nerve blockade prevent vasodilatation during simulated haemorrhage in awake rabbits. J Physiol (Lond) 409:1, 1989.
19. Rutter PC, Potocnik SJ, Ludbrook J: Sympathoadrenal mechanisms in cardiovascular responses to naloxone after hemorrhage in conscious rabbits. Circ Res 63:165, 1988.

20. Morgan DA, Thoren P, Wilczynski EA, et al: Serotonergic mechanisms mediate renal sympathoinhibition during severe hemorrhage in rats. Am J Physiol 255:H496, 1988.

21. Kenny RA, Ingram A, Bayliss J, Sutton R: Head up tilt: A useful tool for investigating unexplained syncope. Lancet 2:1352, 1986.

22. Grubb BP, Temesy-Armos P, Moore J, et al: The use of head upright tilt table testing in the evaluation and management of syncope in children and adolescents. Pacing Clin Electrophysiol 15:742, 1992.

23. Fish FA, Strasburger JF, Benson DW Jr: Reproducibility of a symptomatic response to upright tilt in young patients with unexplained syncope. Am J Cardiol 70:605, 1992.

24. Blanc JJ, Corbel C, Mansourati J, Genet L: Evaluation of beta-adrenergic blockade therapy in vasovagal syncope reproduced by head-up tilt test. Arch Mal Coeur Vaiss 84:1453, 1991.

25. Strieper MJ, Campbell RM: Efficacy of alpha-adrenergic agonist therapy for prevention of pediatric neurocardiogenic syncope. J Am Coll Cardiol 22:594, 1993.

26. Thilenius OG, Quinones JA, Husayni TS, Novak J: Tilt test for diagnosis of unexplained syncope in pediatric patients. Pediatrics 87:334, 1991.

27. Perry JC, Garson A Jr: The child with recurrent syncope: Autonomic function testing and beta-adrenergic hyposensitivity. J Am Coll Cardiol 17:1168, 1991.

28. Balaji S, Oslizlok PC, Allen MC, et al: Neurocardiogenic syncope in children with a normal heart. J Am Coll Cardiol 23:779, 1994.

29. Pongiglione G, Fish FA, Strasburger JF, Benson DW Jr: Heart rate and blood pressure response to upright tilt in young patients with unexplained syncope. J Am Coll Cardiol 16:165, 1990.

30. Kapoor WN, Brant N: Evaluation of syncope by upright tilt testing with isoproterenol. Ann Intern Med 116:358, 1992.

31. Grubb BP, Kosinski D: Tilt table testing: Concepts and limitations. Pacing Clin Electrophysiol 20(pt II):781, 1997.

32. Bou-Holaigh I, Rowe P, Kan T, Calkins H: The relationship between neurally mediated hypotension and chronic fatigue syndrome. JAMA 274:961, 1995.

33. Fredman CS, Bierman KM, Patel V, et al: Transcranial Doppler ultrasonography during head upright tilt table testing. Ann Intern Med 123:848, 1995.

34. Grubb BP, Wolfe D, Gerard G: Syncope and seizures of psychogenic origin: Identification with head upright tilt table testing. Clin Cardiol 15:834, 1992.

35. Lewis DA, Zlotocha J, Henke L, Dhala A: Specificity of head-up tilt testing in adolescents: Effects of various degrees of tilt challenge in normal control subjects. J Am Coll Cardiol 30:1057, 1997.

36. Natale A, Akhtar M, Jazayeri M, et al: Provocation of hypotension during head-up tilt testing in subjects with no history of syncope or presyncope. Circulation 92:54, 1995.

37. Salim MA, DiSessa TG: Serum electrolytes in children with neurocardiogenic syncope treated with fludrocortisone and salt. Am J Cardiol 78:228, 1996.

38. Shapiro JI, Kaehny WD: Pathogenesis and management of metabolic acidosis and alkalosis. In Schrier RW (ed): Renal and Electrolyte Disorders, 4th ed. Boston, Little, Brown, 1992, p 161.

39. Grubb BP, Temesy-Armos P, Hahn H, Elliot L: Utility of upright tilt table–testing in the evaluation and management of syncope of unknown origin. Am J Med 90:8, 1991.

40. Muller G, Deal BJ, Strasburger JF, Benson DW Jr: Usefulness of metoprolol for unexplained syncope and positive response to tilt testing in young persons. Am J Cardiol 71:592, 1993.

41. Brignole M, Menozzi C, Gianfranchi L, et al: A controlled trial of acute and long-term medical therapy in tilt induced neurally mediated syncope. Am J Cardiol 70:399, 1992.

42. Leor J, Rotstein Z, Vered Z, et al: Absence of tachycardia during tilt test predicts failure of beta-blocker therapy in patients with neurocardiogenic syncope. Am Heart J 127:1539, 1994.

43. Natale A, Sra J, Dhala A, et al: Efficacy of different treatment strategies for neurocardiogenic syncope. Pacing Clin Electrophysiol 18:655, 1995.

44. Sra JS, Anderson AJ, Sheikh SH, et al: Unexplained syncope evaluated by electrophysiologic studies and head-up tilt testing. Ann Intern Med 114:1013, 1991.

45. Scott WA, Pongiglione G, Bromberg BJ, et al: Randomized comparison of atenolol and fludrocortisone acetate in the treatment of pediatric neurally mediated syncope. Am J Cardiol 76:400, 1995.

46. Cox MM, Perlman BA, Mayor MR, et al: Acute and long-term beta-adrenergic blockade for patients with neurocardiogenic syncope. J Am Coll Cardiol 26:1293, 1995.

47. Morady F, Scheinman MM, Desei J: Disopyramide. Ann Intern Med 96:337, 1982.

48. Befeler B: The hemodynamic effects of Norpace (Part I). Angiology 26(pt 2):99, 1975.

49. Willis PW III: The hemodynamic effects of Norpace (Part II). Angiology 26(pt 2):102, 1975.

50. Morillo CA, Leitch JW, Yee R, Klein GJ: A placebo-controlled trial of intravenous and oral disopyramide for prevention of neurally mediated syncope induced by head-up tilt. J Am Coll Cardiol 22:1843, 1993.

51. Milstein S, Buetikofer J, Dunnigan A, et al: Usefulness of disopyramide for prevention of upright tilt-induced hypotension-bradycardia. Am J Cardiol 65:1339, 1990.

52. Raviele A, Gasparini G, DiPede F, et al: Usefulness of head-up tilt test in evaluating patients with syncope of unknown origin and negative electrophysiologic study. Am J Cardiol 65:1322, 1990.

53. Moya A, Permanyer-Miralda G, Sagrista-Sauleda J, et al: Limitations of head-up tilt test for evaluating the efficacy of therapeutic interventions in patients with vasovagal syncope. Results of a controlled study of etilefrine versus placebo. J Am Coll Cardiol 25:65, 1995.

54. Grubb BP, Samoil D, Kosinski D, et al: Use of sertraline hydrochloride in the treatment of refractory neurocardiogenic syncope in children and adolescents. J Am Coll Cardiol 24:490, 1994.

55. Elam RF, Bergman F, Feverstein G: The use on anti-serotonergic agents for the treatment of acute hypovolemia in conscious mammals. Am J Physiol 260:H305, 1991.

56. Grubb BP, Wolfe DA, Samoil D, et al: Usefulness of fluoxetine hydrochloride for prevention of resistant upright tilt induced syncope. Pacing Clin Electrophysiol 16(pt 1):458, 1993.

57. Dreifus LS, Fisch C, Griffin JC, et al: Guidelines for implantation of cardiac pacemakers and antiarrhythmia devices. A report of the American College of Cardiology/American Heart Association Task Force on Assessment of Diagnostic and Therapeutic Cardiovascular Procedures. J Am Coll Cardiol 18:1, 1991.

CHAPTER 57.

SUDDEN CARDIAC DEATH IN THE YOUNG ATHLETE AND THE PREPARTICIPATION CARDIOVASCULAR EVALUATION

BARRY J. MARON

During the past few years, interest and concern have heightened considerably in the medical community and the lay public regarding causes of sudden and unexpected death in young trained athletes.[1] The underlying cardiovascular diseases responsible for sudden death in athletes and others participating in sporting activities have been studied and clarified considerably.[1–13] The risks associated with participation in organized competitive sports are diverse and range from sudden collapse due to underlying (and usually unsuspected) cardiovascular disease[2–13] to nonpenetrating chest blows.[14,15] Recognition that athletic field deaths may be due to a variety of detectable cardiovascular lesions has also stimulated intense interest in preparticipation screening in high-school and college-aged athletes[16] and in criteria for eligibility and disqualification from competitive sports.[17]

DEFINITIONS

A competitive athlete has been defined as one who participates in an organized team or individual sport that requires regular competition against others as a central component, places a high premium on excellence and achievement, and requires vigorous and intense training in a systematic fashion.[18] This definition is somewhat arbitrary because many individuals participate in "recreational" sports in a truly competitive fashion.

CAUSES OF SUDDEN DEATH IN YOUNG ATHLETES

Autopsy-based studies have documented the cardiovascular diseases responsible for sudden death in young competitive athletes or youthful asymptomatic individuals with active lifestyles.[2–13] These structural abnormalities are in-

Portions of this text have been adapted from Maron BJ, Thompson PD, Puffer JC, et al: Cardiovascular preparticipation screening of competitive athletes. A statement for health professionals from the Sudden Death Committee (clinical cardiology) and Congenital Cardiac Defects Committee (cardiovascular disease in the young), American Heart Association. Circulation 94(4):850–856, 1996.

dependent of the normal physiologic adaptations in cardiac dimension evident in many trained athletes, usually consisting of increased left ventricular end-diastolic cavity dimension or occasionally wall thickness.[19–22]

It is also important to be cautious in assigning strict prevalence figures for the relative occurrence of various cardiovascular diseases in studies of sudden death in athletes; biases in the selection of patients and other limitations unavoidably influence the acquisition of such data in the absence of a systematic national registry. Indeed, the available published studies differ with regard to the methods used to document cardiovascular diagnosis and are derived from a variety of databases.

Even with these considerations in mind, most sudden deaths in young athletes (<35 years) are due to a variety of primarily congenital cardiovascular diseases (more than 20 in number) (Table 57–1).[2] Indeed, virtually any disease capable of causing sudden death in young people may potentially do so in young competitive athletes. Although these conditions may be relatively common among young athletes dying suddenly, each is uncommon within the general population.

The single most common cardiovascular abnormality among the causes of sudden death in young athletes is hypertrophic cardiomyopathy (HCM), usually in the nonobstructive form[23–27] and accounting for about 35% of such catastrophes (see Table 57–1). HCM is a primary and familial cardiac malformation with heterogeneous clinical and morphologic expression, complex pathophysiologic mechanisms, and diverse clinical course for which five disease-causing mutations in genes encoding proteins of the cardiac sarcomere have been reported (see Chapters 35 and 49). Within the general population, HCM is a relatively common genetically transmitted cardiovascular malformation occurring in about 0.2%.[28]

On the basis of referral center data,[26,27,29] sudden death in HCM is most common in children and young adults, usually in individuals who have previously been asymptomatic (or only mildly symptomatic); therefore, such catastrophes are often the first clinical manifestations of disease.[30] Although most patients die while they are sedentary or during mild exertion,[29] many collapse during or just after vigorous physical activity.[2,29] This observation as well as the evidence that HCM is the most common cause of sudden death in young competitive athletes[2,3,5–7,10,11] (and that athletes

TABLE 57–1

CARDIOVASCULAR ABNORMALITIES IN 134 YOUNG COMPETITIVE ATHLETES WITH SUDDEN DEATH

Primary Cardiovascular Lesions	No. (%) of Athletes	Median Age (Range) (Years)
Hypertrophic cardiomyopathy	48 (36.0)	17.0 (13–28)
Unexplained increase in cardiac mass ("possible hypertrophic cardiomyopathy")	14 (10.0)	17.0 (14–24)
Aberrant coronary arteries	17° (13.0)	15.0 (12–23)
Other coronary anomalies	8 (6.0)	17.5 (14–40)
Ruptured aortic aneurysm	6 (5.0)	17.0 (16–31)
Tunneled LAD coronary artery	6 (5.0)	17.5 (14–20)
Aortic valve stenosis	5 (4.0)	14.0 (14–17)
Consistent with myocarditis	4 (3.0)	15.5 (13–16)
Idiopathic myocardial scarring	4 (3.0)	20.0 (14–27)
Idiopathic dilated cardiomyopathy	4 (3.0)	18.0 (18–21)
ARVD	4 (3.0)	16.0 (15–17)
Mitral valve prolapse	3 (2.0)	16.0 (15–23)
Atherosclerotic coronary artery disease	3 (2.0)	19.0 (14–28)
Other congenital heart diseases	2 (1.5)	13.5 (12–15)
Long QT syndrome	1 (0.5)	—
Sarcoidosis	1 (0.5)	—
Sickle cell trait	1† (0.5)	—
"Normal" heart	3‡ (2.0)	18.0 (16–21)

LAD = left anterior descending; ARVD = arrhythmogenic right ventricular dysplasia.

°Anomalous origin of the left main coronary artery from the right sinus of Valsalva in 13, anomalous origin of right coronary artery from left sinus of Valsalva in 2, anomalous origin of the left main coronary artery (from between the left and posterior cusps) with acute-angled take-off in one, and origin of left anterior descending coronary from pulmonary trunk in one.

†Judged to be the probable cause of death in the absence of any identifiable structural cardiovascular abnormality.[83]

‡Absence of structural heart disease on standard autopsy examination.

From Maron BJ, Shirani J, Poline LC, et al: Sudden death in young competitive athletes: Clinical, demographic and pathological profiles. JAMA 276:199–208, 1996. Copyright 1996 American Medical Association.

with HCM who collapse usually do so during training or competition[2]) supports the view that intense physical activity represents a trigger for sudden death and that it is prudent to recommend the disqualification of athletes with HCM from intense competitive sports.[17]

The clinical diagnosis of HCM has been based on the definition (by two-dimensional echocardiography) of the most characteristic morphologic feature of the disease, that is, asymmetric thickening of the left ventricular wall associated with a nondilated cavity in the absence of another cardiac or systemic disease capable of producing the magnitude of hypertrophy present (e.g., systemic hypertension or aortic stenosis)[31–33] (see Chapter 35). Because the nonobstructive form of HCM is predominant,[23, 31] the well-described features of dynamic obstruction to left ventricular outflow are not required for diagnosis.[23]

On the basis of both echocardiographic and necropsy analyses in large numbers of patients, the HCM disease spectrum is characterized by vast structural diversity with regard to the patterns and extent of left ventricular hypertrophy[31, 34, 35] (see Chapter 35). Indeed, virtually all possible patterns of left ventricular hypertrophy occur in HCM, and no single phenotypic expression can be considered classic or typical of this disease. However, the HCM phenotype is not invariably expressed as a greatly thickened left ventricle, and some patients show only a mild increase of 15 mm or less, including a few genetically affected adults with normal thicknesses (≤ 12 mm).[36, 37]

Some young athletes with segmental hypertrophy of the anterior ventricular septum (wall thicknesses, 13 to 15 mm), consistent with a relatively mild morphologic expression of HCM, may be difficult to distinguish from extreme expressions of physiologic left ventricular hypertrophy that represent an adaptation to athletic training (i.e., athlete's heart).[38] In asymptomatic, trained athletes within this mor-

phologic *gray zone*, the differential diagnosis between physiologic athlete's heart and HCM can often be resolved by clinical assessment and noninvasive testing (Fig. 57–1).[38]

Second in importance and frequency to HCM as a cause of sudden death is a spectrum of congenital vascular malformations of the coronary arterial tree (occurring in about 20% of young athletic field deaths), the most common of which appears to be anomalous origin of the left main coronary artery from the right (anterior) sinus of Valsalva[39–42] (see Chapter 39). Such coronary artery anomalies are difficult to detect because they may not be readily identifiable by conventional noninvasive imaging technology or simply because the clinical index of suspicion is not sufficiently high.

Patients with anomalous left main coronary from the right sinus of Valsalva may die suddenly as the first manifestation of their disease (usually before 35 years of age), although one third experience angina or syncope or even acute myocardial infarction. Most of these events are related to exertion. Indeed, occurrence of one or more episodes of exertional syncope in a young athlete should necessitate the exclusion of this coronary anomaly. Also, in youthful athletes, it is possible to identify or raise a strong suspicion of anomalous left main coronary artery by use of conventional cross-sectional two-dimensional or transesophageal echocardiography (see Chapter 39), which can subsequently lead to definitive confirmation with coronary arteriography. These considerations are particularly important because this malformation is rarely identified during life but nevertheless is amenable to corrective surgery.

Other unusual variants of coronary arterial anatomy may be rare causes of exercise-related sudden deaths in young athletic individuals.[39–42] These include hypoplasia of the right coronary and left circumflex arteries, the left anterior descending or right coronary artery emanating from the pulmonary trunk, virtual absence of the left coronary artery,

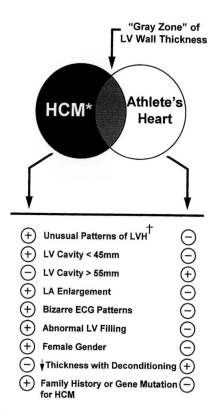

"Gray Zone" of LV Wall Thickness

HCM*   Athlete's Heart

(+) Unusual Patterns of LVH†   (−)
(+) LV Cavity < 45mm   (−)
(−) LV Cavity > 55mm   (+)
(+) LA Enlargement   (−)
(+) Bizarre ECG Patterns   (−)
(+) Abnormal LV Filling   (−)
(+) Female Gender   (−)
(−) ↓Thickness with Deconditioning   (+)
(+) Family History or Gene Mutation for HCM   (−)

FIGURE 57–1

Chart showing criteria used to distinguish hypertrophic cardiomyopathy (HCM) from athlete's heart when the left ventricular (LV) wall thickness is within the shaded gray zone of overlap (13 to 15 mm), consistent with both diagnoses. °Assumed to be the nonobstructive form of HCM in this discussion, because substantial mitral valve systolic anterior motion would confirm the diagnosis of HCM in an athlete. †May involve a variety of abnormalities, including heterogeneous distribution of left ventricular hypertrophy (LVH) in which asymmetry is prominent, and adjacent regions may be of greatly different thicknesses, with sharp transitions evident between segments; also, patterns in which the anterior ventricular septum is spared from the hypertrophic process and the region of predominant thickening may be in the posterior portion of the septum or the anterolateral or posterior free wall or even the left ventricular apex. ↓ = decreased; LA = left atrial. (From Maron BJ, Pelliccia A, Spirito P: Cardiac disease in young trained athletes. Insights into methods for distinguishing athlete's heart from structural heart disease, with particular emphasis on hypertrophic cardiomyopathy. Circulation 91:1596–1601, 1995. Copyright American Medical Association.)

and coronary arterial intussusception producing occlusion of the coronary lumen.

Less common causes of sudden death in young athletes are myocarditis, dilated cardiomyopathy, aortic dissection and rupture due to Marfan's syndrome, sarcoidosis, mitral valve prolapse, aortic valve stenosis, atherosclerotic coronary artery disease, long QT syndrome, and arrhythmogenic right ventricular dysplasia (ARVD) (see Table 57–1). ARVD, an unusual, often familial condition that may be associated with important ventricular or supraventricular arrhythmias, has been cited as a cause of sudden death in the young[4,43,44] (see Chapters 2 and 49). Corrado and associates[4] reported ARVD to be the most common cause of sudden death in athletes in the Veneto region in northeastern Italy. Although this disease is also a component of our experience with athletic field deaths, its frequency is clearly in the range of less than 5% in reports from North America.[2,3,5] The explanation for such discrepancies is un-

certain, although it is possible that the difference reflects a unique genetic substrate in that particular region of Italy. Furthermore, the relatively low frequency with which HCM is apparently responsible for sudden death in Italian athletes is probably due to the long-standing and systematic Italian national program for the cardiovascular assessment of competitive athletes,[45] which appears to identify and disqualify disproportionate numbers of trained athletes with HCM (compared with ARVD, which is much more difficult to identify clinically).[46]

A spectrum of occult abnormalities in the cardiac conduction system (in the absence of other structural cardiac abnormalities) may be responsible for sudden death in competitive athletes and other young people with otherwise structurally normal hearts.[6,8–10,12,13,47] Thiene and colleagues[8] described three young athletes with a variety of atrioventricular conduction system abnormalities that the authors suggested were responsible for lethal arrhythmias, including one with accessory atrioventricular pathways. James and associates[9] and Burke and coworkers[47] described morphologic abnormalities of the small intramural artery to the sinoatrial node, consisting of thickened vessel wall and narrowed lumen, which they incriminated as the determinant of sudden death and probably the cause of degeneration, scarring, and hemorrhage present in the surrounding conducting tissue. We have also identified similar morphologic alterations of intramural arteries (to either the sinoatrial or atrioventricular nodes) in a small number of the young athletes dying with HCM or left ventricular hypertrophy apparently not part of the HCM disease spectrum.[6,10]

On occasion, athletes may die suddenly without evidence of structural cardiovascular disease, even after careful gross and microscopic examination of the heart. In such instances (about 2% of our series) (see Table 57–1),[2] it may not be possible to exclude noncardiac factors (like drug abuse) as responsible for the catastrophe or to know whether careful inspection of the specialized conducting system and associated vasculature with serial sectioning (which is not part of the standard medical examiner's protocol) would have revealed occult but clinically relevant abnormalities.[12] Some of these deaths may be due to primary ventricular arrhythmia in the absence of cardiac morphologic abnormalities,[48,49] previously unidentified Wolff-Parkinson-White syndrome, rare diseases in which structural abnormalities of the heart are characteristically lacking at necropsy such as long QT syndrome,[50,51] or possibly exercise-induced coronary spasm or undetected segmental forms of right ventricular dysplasia.

Major coronary arteries "tunneled" within left ventricular myocardium (i.e., myocardial "bridges") may constitute a potentially lethal anatomic variant that may cause sudden unexpected death in otherwise healthy young individuals during exertion or stress[2,52,53] (see Chapter 39). Such tunneled coronary arteries (usually the left anterior descending) are completely surrounded by myocardium for at least a portion of their course (about 1 to 3 cm); in certain susceptible individuals, such an artery may be subjected to a critical degree of compression, resulting in myocardial ischemia (even in the absence of hemodynamically significant atherosclerotic narrowing). Indeed, in about 5% of our athletic field deaths, a tunneled left anterior descending coronary artery was present in the absence of any other structural anomaly.[2] Also, the chronic ingestion of agents

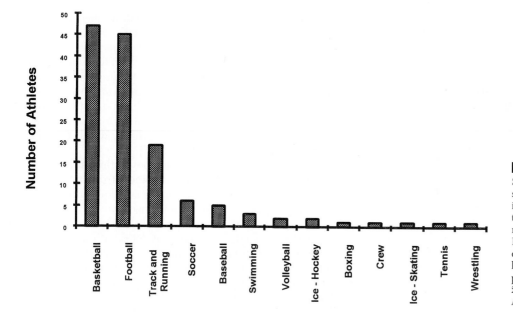

FIGURE 57–2

Sports engaged in at the time of sudden death in 134 young competitive athletes. Those competing in track events were either distance runners or sprinters. (From Maron BJ, Shirani J, Poliac LC, et al: Sudden death in young competitive athletes: Clinical, demographic and pathological profiles. JAMA 276:199–208, 1996. Copyright 1996 American Medical Association.)

such as cocaine may have important adverse cardiovascular consequences that can produce clinicopathologic profiles of acute myocardial infarction and myocarditis.[54–56]

PREVALENCE AND SIGNIFICANCE OF THE PROBLEM

Sudden unexpected death due to cardiovascular disease during competitive sports is rare in high-school students participating in organized interscholastic sports (i.e., about 1 per 200,000 participants per academic year or 1 per 70,000 participants during a 3-year high-school period[57]; somewhat higher estimates of the risk for sudden death have been reported for apparently healthy males, joggers, and marathon racers, usually due to atherosclerotic coronary artery disease.[58–60] Such estimates suggest that the intense and persistent public interest in these tragic events is perhaps disproportionate to their significance in the population. However, the emotional and social impact of athletic field catastrophes remains high.

Despite its low event rate, sudden death in young athletes continues to represent an important medical issue. Indeed, it is an important responsibility of the medical community to create a fully informed public and also, when it is prudent and practical, to pursue early detection of the causes of catastrophic events in young athletes as well as initiate preventive measures. Because such events are uncommon relative to the vast numbers of athletes participating safely in sports, information about athletic field deaths should not raise undue anxiety among youthful athletes and their families and thereby inhibit participation in sports.

DEMOGRAPHICS

On the basis of data assembled primarily from broad-based U.S. populations,[2,3,5–7,10] a profile of young competitive athletes who die suddenly has emerged. Such athletes par-ticipated in a large number and variety of sports, with the most frequent being basketball and football (about 70%), not only reflecting the high participation level in these popular team sports but also their intensity (Fig. 57–2). Most athletic field deaths occur in men (about 90%); relative infrequency in women probably reflects a lower participation level, sometimes less intense levels of training, and the fact that some diseases most commonly accounting for sudden death in athletes are recognized less frequently in women (e.g., HCM). Most athletes are of high-school age at the time of death (about 60%); however, other sudden deaths occur in young athletes who have achieved collegiate or even professional levels of competition.

Most athletes who die suddenly, regardless of their particular underlying disease, have been free of cardiovascular symptoms and are usually not suspected of harboring a cardiovascular abnormality. Sudden collapse usually occurs with exercise, predominantly in the late afternoon and early evening hours corresponding to peak periods of competition and training, particularly in organized team sports such as football and basketball (Fig. 57–3).[2] The predilection for sudden death late in the day is similar in athletes with HCM and in those athletes with other lesions. This observation for athletes with HCM contrasts strikingly with prior reports in patients with HCM (who were not competitive athletes) for whom a bimodal pattern of circadian variability during the 24-hour day was evident, including a prominent early to midmorning peak, similar to that described in patients with coronary artery disease (i.e., with sudden death, acute myocardial infarction, or angina) (see Fig. 57–3).[61]

Although most sudden deaths reported in competitive athletes have been in white men, a substantial proportion (>40%) are black athletes.[2,62] Indeed, HCM represents a common cause of sudden death in young black men (see Fig. 57–4).[2] This substantial occurrence of HCM-related sudden death in young black male athletes contrasts sharply with the infrequent identification of black patients with HCM in hospital-based populations. These data emphasize that it is less likely for young black men to receive a relatively sophisticated cardiovascular diagnosis such as HCM, compared with their white counterparts. Consequently, black athletes with HCM are also less likely to be disqualified from competition in accordance with the recommendations of the 26th Bethesda Conference[17] to reduce their risk for sudden death.

MECHANISMS AND RESUSCITATION

Although the precise mechanism ultimately responsible for sudden death in young athletes depends on the particular disease state involved, in most victims (including athletes with HCM), cardiac arrest results from electrical instability due to ventricular tachyarrhythmias. There are a number of unusual exceptions,[40,63] the most common being Marfan's syndrome, in which death is due to a ruptured aorta.[2,6,7,10]

Regardless of mechanism, few athletes with cardiovascular disease who collapse on an athletic field are successfully resuscitated. Routine access to automatic external defibrillators at athletic events may result in the survival of greater numbers of such athletes. However, the rarity of these events also represents an obstacle to efficient resuscitation practice.

SCREENING AND PREPARTICIPATION DETECTION OF CARDIOVASCULAR ABNORMALITIES

PERSPECTIVES

The detection of a pre-existing cardiovascular abnormality with the potential for significant morbidity or sudden death is an important objective of the widespread practice of preparticipation screening of high-school and college-aged

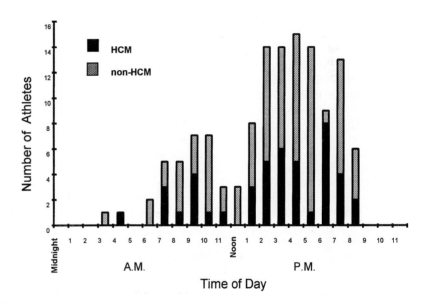

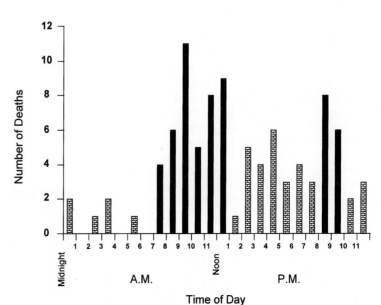

FIGURE 57–3

Hourly distribution of sudden cardiac deaths. *Top,* Histogram showing time of death for 127 competitive athletes with either HCM (bold portion of bars) or a variety of other predominantly congenital cardiovascular malformations (lighter portions of bars). Time of death was predominantly in the late afternoon and early evening, corresponding largely to the time of training and competition. (From Maron BJ, Shirani J, Poliac LC, et al: Sudden death in young competitive athletes: Clinical, demographic and pathological profiles. JAMA 276:199–208, 1996. Copyright 1996 American Medical Association.) *Bottom,* In contrast, histogram shown for 94 nonathlete patients with HCM demonstrating a prominent early morning peak between 7 AM and 1 PM and a secondary peak in the early evening (most evident between 8 PM and 10 PM). (From Maron BJ, Kogan J, Proschan MA, et al: Circadian variability in the occurrence of sudden cardiac death in patients with hypertrophic cardiomyopathy. J Am Coll Cardiol 23:1405, 1994.)

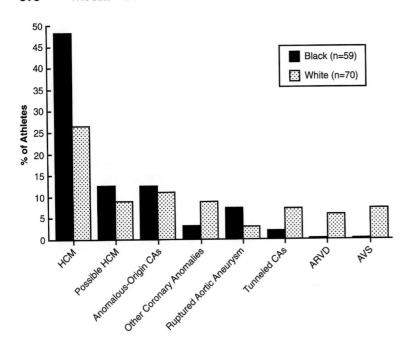

FIGURE 57–4

Effect of race on cardiovascular causes of sudden death in competitive athletes. ARVD = arrhythmogenic right ventricular dysplasia; AVS = aortic valve stenosis; CAs = coronary anomalies; HCM = hypertrophic cardiomyopathy. (From Maron BJ, Shirani J, Poliac LC, et al: Sudden death in young competitive athletes: Clinical, demographic and pathological profiles. JAMA 276:199–208, 1996. Copyright 1996 American Medical Association.)

athletes. There seems to be a general consensus that within a benevolent society, a responsibility exists on the part of physicians to initiate prudent efforts for the identification of life-threatening diseases in athletes to minimize the cardiovascular risks associated with sport and to protect the health of such individuals.[1, 16, 17]

Athletic screening has traditionally been performed in the context of a personal and family history and physical examination. Screening recommendations are predicated on the probability that intense athletic training is likely to increase the risk for sudden cardiac death (or disease progression) in trained athletes with clinically important underlying structural heart disease, although it is presently not possible to quantify that risk with precision, nor to know definitively to which individual athletes these considerations apply.

PRIOR SCREENING EFFORTS

To date, there have been relatively few reports of prospective cardiovascular screening efforts in large athletic populations.[64–69] Most of these studies have implemented noninvasive testing (i.e., conventional or limited echocardiography, 12-lead electrocardiography [ECG]) in high-school or collegiate athletes. The populations screened (usually during a 1-year period) have ranged in size from 250 to 2000 athletes. Few definitive examples of potentially lethal cardiovascular abnormalities have been detected. One retrospective analysis[2] showed that cardiovascular disease was suspected by preparticipation history and physical screening in only 3% of 115 high-school and collegiate athletes who ultimately died suddenly of these abnormalities (Fig. 57–5).

LIMITATIONS

One obstacle to large population screening strategies for competitive athletes is the rarity of the lesions responsible for sudden cardiac death. The several congenital malformations relevant to athletic screening (including HCM) may account for a combined prevalence of only 0.3% or less within the general athletic population. The large reservoir of competitive athletes constitutes a second major obstacle[5, 16, 57]; the total number of trained and truly competitive athletes in the United States every year is probably in the range of 8 to 10 million.

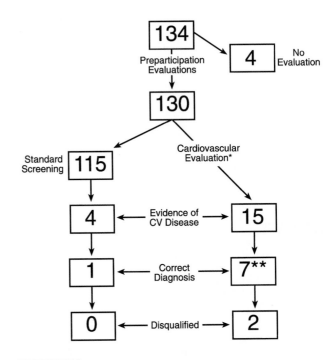

FIGURE 57–5

Flow diagram showing impact of preparticipation history and physical examination on the detection of structural cardiovascular (CV) disease (which caused sudden death) as well as subsequent disqualification from competitive athletics. *Cardiovascular evaluation with testing (independent of standard school or institutional preparticipation screening) was performed in 15 athletes because of symptoms, family history, heart murmur, or physical findings suggestive of heart disease, of whom 7 had heart disease (**). (From Maron BJ, Shirani J, Poliac LC, et al: Sudden death in young competitive athletes: Clinical, demographic and pathological profiles. JAMA 276:199–208, 1996. Copyright 1996 American Medical Association.)

CUSTOMARY PRACTICE AND LEGAL CONSIDERATIONS

The law enables the medical profession to establish the bounds of appropriate management of athletes by the physician; indeed, it is the medical standard that is ultimately translated into the legal standard for malpractice purposes. Although educational institutions and professional teams are required to use reasonable care in conducting their athletic programs, there is currently no clear legal precedent regarding their duty to conduct preparticipation screening of athletes for the purpose of detecting medically significant abnormalities.[16] Indeed, at present, no lawsuits have been brought forward alleging negligence in the failure either to perform cardiovascular screening or to diagnose cardiac disease in young competitive athletes. In the absence of binding requirements established by state law or athletic governing bodies, most institutions and teams presently rely on the team physician (or other medical personnel) to determine the appropriate medical screening procedures.[16, 70, 71]

A physician who has medically cleared an athlete to participate in competitive sports is not necessarily legally liable for an injury or death caused by an undetected cardiovascular condition.[16] Malpractice liability for failure to discover a latent, asymptomatic cardiovascular condition requires proof that a physician deviated from customary or accepted medical practice in his or her specialty in performing the preparticipation screening of athletes and that use of established diagnostic criteria and techniques would have disclosed the medical condition.

Currently, there are no universally accepted standards for the screening of high-school and college athletes in the United States, nor are there approved certification procedures for the health care professionals who perform such screening examinations.[16] Some form of medical clearance by a physician or other trained health care worker, usually consisting of a history and physical examination, presently appears customary for most high-school athletes. Standards may be mandated by state legislative action or be the responsibility of individual state high-school athletic associations or school districts. There is no agreement among the states, however, as to the precise format of preparticipation medical evaluations. Indeed, almost 40% of the states either do not require this process or have no recommended standard history and physical forms to serve as a guide to examiners, or the medical clearance forms are judged to be generally inadequate when they are evaluated against the specific screening recommendations proposed by the 1996 American Heart Association consensus panel.[16] Some states require only a signature to provide clearance for an athlete to compete in organized sports. In a number of states, nonphysician health care workers are sanctioned to perform athletic screening examinations, including chiropractors (in 10 states) and advanced nurse practitioners or physician assistants (in 16 states).

EXPECTATIONS

Preparticipation screening by history and physical examination alone does not have sufficient power to guarantee detection of many critical cardiovascular abnormalities in large populations of young trained athletes. Indeed, significant aortic valvar stenosis is probably the lesion most likely to be detected during routine screening because of its characteristically loud heart murmur. Identification of HCM by the standard screening history or physical examination is unreliable because most patients have the nonobstructive form of this disease, characteristically expressed by no or only a soft heart murmur.[23–27] Furthermore, most athletes (or patients) with HCM do not experience exertional syncope or have a family history of the disease or premature sudden death, and therefore this disease is not easily detected by the preparticipation history.[23–27] Most of the lesions considered here as potentially responsible for sudden death in young athletes are challenging to detect, even with echocardiography, ECG, or other noninvasive tests incorporated into the screening process (e.g., a variety of congenital coronary anomalies, particularly anomalous origin of left main coronary artery from the right sinus of Valsalva).

Despite these major limitations, simple history and physical examination screening is theoretically of value by virtue of its capability for raising the suspicion of cardiovascular disease in some at-risk athletes. For example, genetic diseases such as HCM, Marfan's syndrome, and some instances of ARVD and premature atherosclerotic coronary artery disease can be suggested by the family history alone or by virtue of transient symptoms from the personal history. Physical examination may identify the stigmata of Marfan's syndrome, lesions associated with left ventricular outflow obstruction by a loud heart murmur (aortic valvar stenosis and some patients with HCM), systemic hypertension, as well as often raise suspicion of diseases such as dilated cardiomyopathy and myocarditis. Although data are lacking with regard to the efficacy of large-scale screening trials in the United States,[16] the potential for detecting cardiovascular disease has not been fully achieved because of the imperfections in the current screening methods.

NONINVASIVE SCREENING TESTS

Echocardiography

The addition of noninvasive diagnostic tests to the screening process has the potential to enhance the detection of certain cardiovascular defects in young athletes. For example, the two-dimensional echocardiogram is the principal diagnostic tool for clinical recognition of HCM by demonstrating otherwise unexplained asymmetric left ventricular wall thickening.[31–35] Comprehensive and routine screening for HCM by laboratory genetic testing for a variety of known disease-causing mutations is not yet practical or feasible for large populations.

Echocardiography could also be expected to detect other relevant abnormalities associated with sudden death in young athletes, such as valvar heart disease (e.g., mitral valve prolapse and aortic stenosis), aortic root dilatation, and left ventricular dysfunction (e.g., due to myocarditis or dilated cardiomyopathy). Echocardiography will not identify all important lesions, however, and some relevant cardiovascular diseases may be beyond detection with any screening method. For example, identification of many congenital coronary artery anomalies usually requires sophisticated laboratory examination including coronary arteriography, although it is possible in selected young athletes for important anomalies (i.e., left main coronary artery from the right sinus of Valsalva) to be strongly suggested or even identified by transthoracic or transesophageal two-dimensional echocardiography.[72–76] ARVD usually cannot be reliably diagnosed solely with echocardiography and ECG; the best available noninvasive test for this disease is probably magnetic resonance imaging, which is both expensive and not universally available.[77]

Cost-efficiency issues are important in assessing the feasibility of applying expensive noninvasive testing to the screening of large athletic populations.[16,77–79] The costs are probably prohibitive, usually ranging from about $400 to $1000 per echocardiographic study (average, about $600). If the occurrence of HCM in a young athletic population is assumed to be 1 per 500, even at $500 per study it would theoretically cost $250,000 to detect even one previously undiagnosed patient.

Screening protocols that incorporate noninvasive testing at greatly reduced cost have been described.[64–66,68,78,79] However, these efforts have been in unique circumstances in which equipment was donated and professional expenses were waived for all but technician-related costs. Some investigators have also suggested an inexpensive shortened-format echocardiogram for population screening (limited to parasternal views; about 2 minutes in duration).[64,69] Although such individual initiatives are laudable, public service projects based largely on volunteerism usually cannot be sustained on a consistent basis because priorities for the use of available resources often change; therefore, such efforts are unlikely to be implemented on a scale necessary to consistently provide effective screening to 5,000,000 high-school and 500,000 collegiate athletes every year.[16]

Another important limitation is the potential for false-positive or false-negative test results with echocardiography. False-positive results arise from the assignment of borderline left ventricular wall thicknesses (or particularly enlarged cavity size) and ultimately require formulation of a differential diagnosis between normal but extreme physiologic adaptations of athlete's heart and pathologic conditions such as HCM or other cardiomyopathies.[38] Indeed, such clinical dilemmas (which cannot always be resolved definitively in individual athletes) generate substantial emotional, financial, and medical burdens for the athlete, family, team, and institution by virtue of the uncertainty created and also the requirement for further testing. False-negative screening results may also occur when athletes with HCM are encountered at a point of incomplete phenotypic expression during adolescence[80]; in individuals with HCM younger than 15 years, left ventricular hypertrophy is often absent or mild. Therefore, the echocardiographic findings (and phenotypic expression) may not yet be diagnostic at the time of preparticipation screening.

Electrocardiography

The 12-lead ECG has been proposed as a more practical and cost-efficient alternative to echocardiography for population-based screening.[46,66,67] Indeed, the ECG is abnormal in about 90 to 95% of patients with HCM[81] and has been shown to be a powerful tool for detection in an Italian population.[46] It may be abnormal in other potentially lethal structural lesions, such as the coronary artery anomalies, and will usually identify the important (but uncommon) long QT syndrome.[50,51] A certain proportion of genetically affected relatives in families with long QT syndrome, however, may have little or no phenotypic expression on the ECG.[50]

As a primary screening test, the ECG lacks the imaging capability of the echocardiogram for recognition of structural cardiovascular malformations. The ECG also has low specificity as a screening test in athletic populations because of the high frequency of ECG alterations associated with the normal physiologic adaptations to training of the athlete's heart.[82] In preparticipation screening, about 20 to 25% of athletes examined will have an ECG pattern that ultimately stimulates echocardiographic study.[66] Finally, elite athletes not infrequently demonstrate distinctly abnormal ECG patterns indistinguishable from pathologic conditions, even in the absence of structural heart disease and without evidence of a morphologic adaptation to training.[83] These false-positive test results complicate efforts to use the 12-lead ECG as a primary screening tool in athletic populations.

CONSENSUS GUIDELINES

An American Heart Association expert consensus panel[16] has recommended a standard preparticipation screening approach to detect relevant cardiovascular lesions and a more systematic approach to enhance the likelihood that such potentially lethal abnormalities will be identified (see Appendix). However, no available screening design can detect all important lesions or affected athletes. Consequently, medical clearance for sports does not necessarily connote the absence of cardiovascular disease.

ELIGIBILITY CONSIDERATIONS FOR ATHLETES WITH KNOWN CARDIOVASCULAR DISEASE

When a cardiovascular abnormality is identified in a competitive athlete, the following considerations arise: (1) the magnitude of risk for sudden cardiac death associated with continued participation in competitive sports and (2) the criteria to be implemented for determining whether individual athletes should be withdrawn from sports competition. Recommendations for athletic eligibility or disqualification, taking into account the severity of the cardiovascular abnormality and the nature of the sports training and competition, are available.[17] These recommendations are predicated on the likelihood that intense athletic training and competition will increase the risk for sudden cardiac death (or disease progression) in trained athletes with clinically important underlying structural heart disease, although it is not possible at present to quantify that risk in precise terms. Consequently, temporary or permanent withdrawal of selected athletes from participation in certain intense competitive sports is probably both prudent and beneficial.

REFERENCES

1. Maron BJ: Sudden death in young athletes: Lessons from the Hank Gathers affair. N Engl J Med 329:55, 1993.

2. Maron BJ, Shirani J, Poliac LC, et al: Sudden death in young competitive athletes: Clinical, demographic and pathological profiles. JAMA 276:199, 1996.
3. Burke AP, Farb A, Virmani R, et al: Sports-related and non–sports-related sudden cardiac death in young athletes. Am Heart J 121:568, 1991.
4. Corrado D, Thiene G, Nava A, et al: Sudden death in young competitive athletes. Clinicopathologic correlates in 22 cases. Am J Med 39:588, 1990.
5. Van Camp SP, Bloor CM, Mueller FO, et al: Nontraumatic sports death in high school and college athletes. Med Sci Sports Exerc 27:641, 1995.
6. Maron BJ, Roberts WC, McAllister HA, et al: Sudden death in young athletes. Circulation 62:218, 1980.
7. Liberthson RR: Sudden death from cardiac causes in children and young adults. N Engl J Med 334:1039, 1996.
8. Thiene G, Pennelli N, Rossi L: Cardiac conduction system abnormalities as a possible cause of sudden death in young athletes. Hum Pathol 14:706, 1983.
9. James TN, Froggatt P, Marshall TK: Sudden death in young athletes. Ann Intern Med 67:1013, 1967.
10. Maron BJ, Epstein SE, Roberts WC: Causes of sudden death in the competitive athlete. J Am Coll Cardiol 7:204, 1986.
11. Topaz O, Edwards JE: Pathologic features of sudden death in children, adolescents, and young adults. Chest 87:476, 1985.
12. Bharati S, Lev M: Congenital abnormalities of the conduction system in sudden death in young adults. J Am Coll Cardiol 8:1096, 1986.
13. Corrado D, Thiene G, Cocco P, Frescura C: Non-atherosclerotic coronary artery disease and sudden death in the young. Br Heart J 68:601, 1992.
14. Maron BJ, Poliac LV, Kaplan JA, Mueller FO: Blunt impact to the chest leading to sudden death from cardiac arrest during sports activities. N Engl J Med 33:337, 1995.
15. Link MS, Wang PJ, Pandian NG, et al: An experimental model of sudden death due to low-energy chest wall impact (commotio cordis). N Engl J Med 338:1805, 1998.
16. Maron BJ, Thompson PD, Puffer JC, et al: Cardiovascular preparticipation screening of competitive athletes. Circulation 94:850, 1996.
17. Maron BJ, Mitchell JH: 26th Bethesda Conference. Recommendations for determining eligibilty for competition in athletes with cardiovascular abnormalities. J Am Coll Cardiol 24:845, 1994.
18. Maron BJ, Mitchell JH: Revised eligibility recommendations for competitive athletes with cardiovascular abnormalities. (Introduction to 26th Bethesda Conference.) J Am Coll Cardiol 24:848, 1994.
19. Huston TP, Puffer JC, Rodney WM: The athletic heart syndrome. N Engl J Med 313:24, 1985.
20. Maron BJ: Structural features of the athlete heart as defined by echocardiography. J Am Coll Cardiol 7:190, 1986.
21. Pelliccia A, Maron BJ, Spataro A, et al: The upper limit of physiologic cardiac hypertrophy in highly trained elite athletes. N Engl J Med 324:295, 1991.
22. Pelliccia A, Maron BJ, Culasso F, et al: Athlete's heart in women: Echocardiographic characterization of highly trained elite female athletes. JAMA 276:211, 1996.
23. Maron BJ, Bonow RO, Cannon RO, et al: Hypertrophic cardiomyopathy: Interrelation of clinical manifestations, pathophysiology, and therapy. N Engl J Med 316:780, 884, 1987.
24. Wigle ED, Sasson Z, Henderson MA, et al: Hypertrophic cardiomyopathy: The importance of the site and extent of hypertrophy—a review. Prog Cardiovasc Dis 28:1, 1985.
25. Louie EK, Edwards LC: Hypertrophic cardiomyopathy. Prog Cardiovasc Dis 36:275, 1994.
26. Spirito P, Seidman CE, McKenna WJ, Maron BJ: The management of hypertrophic cardiomyopathy. N Engl J Med 336:775, 1997.
27. Maron BJ: Hypertrophic cardiomyopathy. Lancet 350:127, 1997.
28. Maron BJ, Gardin JM, Flack JM, et al: Assessment of the prevalence of hypertrophic cardiomyopathy in a general population of young adults: Echocardiographic analysis of 4111 subjects in the CARDIA study. Circulation 92:785, 1995.
29. Maron BJ, Roberts WC, Epstein SE: Sudden death in hypertrophic cardiomyopathy: Profile of 78 patients. Circulation 65:1388, 1982.
30. Maron BJ, Roberts WC, Edwards JE, et al: Sudden death in patients with hypertrophic cardiomyopathy: Characterization of 26 patients without functional limitation. Am J Cardiol 41:803, 1978.
31. Klues HG, Schiffers A, Maron BJ: Phenotypic spectrum and patterns of left ventricular hypertrophy in hypertrophic cardiomyopathy: Morphologic observations and significance as assessed by two-dimensional echocardiography in 600 patients. J Am Coll Cardiol 26:1699, 1995.
32. Maron BJ, Epstein SE: Hypertrophic cardiomyopathy: A discussion of nomenclature. Am J Cardiol 43:1242, 1979.
33. Maron BJ, Gottdiener JS, Epstein SE: Patterns and significance of the distribution of left ventricular hypertrophy in hypertrophic cardiomyopathy: A wide-angle, two-dimensional echocardiographic study of 125 patients. Am J Cardiol 48:418, 1981.
34. Shapiro LM, McKenna WJ: Distribution of left ventricular hypertrophy in hypertrophic cardiomyopathy: A two-dimensional echocardiographic study. J Am Coll Cardiol 2:437, 1983.
35. Maron BJ, Gross BW, Stark SI: Extreme left ventricular hypertrophy. Circulation 92:3748, 1995.
36. Solomon SD, Wolff S, Watkins H, et al: Left ventricular hypertrophy and morphology in familial hypertrophic cardiomyopathy associated with mutations of the beta-myosin heavy chain gene. J Am Coll Cardiol 22:498, 1993.
37. Charron P, Dubourg O, Desnos M, et al: Diagnostic value of electrocardiography and echocardiography for familial hypertrophic cardiomyopathy in a genotyped adult population. Circulation 96:214, 1997.
38. Maron BJ, Pelliccia A, Spirito P: Cardiac disease in young trained athletes: Insights into methods for distinguishing athlete's heart from structural heart disease with particular emphasis on hypertrophic cardiomyopathy. Circulation 91:1596, 1995.
39. Menke DM, Waller BF, Pless JE: Hypoplastic coronary arteries and high take-off position of the right coronary ostium. A fatal combination of congenital coronary artery anomalies in an amateur athlete. Chest 88:299, 1985.
40. Roberts WC, Silver MA, Sapala JC: Intussusception of a coronary artery associated with sudden death in a college football player. Am J Cardiol 57:179, 1986.
41. Choi JH, Kornblum RN: Pete Maravich's incredible heart. J Forensic Sci 41:981, 1990.
42. Roberts WC, Glick BN: Congenital hypoplasia of both right and left circumflex coronary arteries. Am J Cardiol 70:121, 1992.
43. McKenna WJ, Thiene G, Nava A, et al: Diagnosis of arrhythmogenic right ventricular dysplasia/cardiomyopathy. Br Heart J 71:215, 1994.
44. Basso C, Thiene G, Corrado D, et al: Arrhythmogenic right ventricular cardiomyopathy: Dysplasia, dystrophy or myocarditis? Circulation 94:983, 1996.
45. Pelliccia A, Maron BJ: Preparticipation cardiovascular evaluation of the competitive athlete: Perspectives from the 30 year Italian experience. Am J Cardiol 75:827, 1995.
46. Corrado D, Basso C, Schiaron M, Thiene G: Screening for hypertrophic cardiomyopathy in young athletes. N Engl J Med 339:364, 1998.
47. Burke AP, Subramanian R, Smialek J, Virmani R: Nonatherosclerotic narrowing of the atrioventricular node artery and sudden death. J Am Coll Cardiol 21:117, 1993.
48. Benson DW, Benditt DG, Anderson RW, et al: Cardiac arrest in young, ostensibly healthy patients: Clinical, hemodynamic and electrophysiologic findings. Am J Cardiol 52:65, 1983.
49. Fan W, Peter CT: Survival and incidence of appropriate shocks in implantable cardioverter defibrillator recipients who have no detectable structural heart disease. Am J Cardiol 74:687, 1994.
50. Vincent GM, Timothy KW, Leppert M, Keating M: The spectrum of symptoms and QT intervals in carriers of the gene for the long-QT syndrome. N Engl J Med 327:846, 1992.
51. Moss AJ, Schwartz PJ, Crampton RS, et al: The long QT syndrome: Prospective longitudinal study of 328 families. Circulation 84:1136, 1991.
52. Morales AR, Romanelli R, Boucek RJ: The mural left anterior descending coronary artery, strenuous exercise and sudden death. Circulation 62:230, 1980.
53. Schwarz ER, Lues HG, vom Dahl J, et al: Functional angiographic and intracoronary Doppler flow characteristics in symptomatic patients with myocardial bridging: Effect of short-term intravenous beta-blocker medication. J Am Coll Cardiol 27:1637, 1996.
54. Virmani R, Robinowitz M, Smialek JE, Smyth DF: Cardiovascular effects of cocaine: An autopsy study of 40 patients. Am Heart J 115:1068, 1988.
55. Isner JM, Estes NAM III, Thompson PD, et al: Acute cardiac events temporarily related to cocaine abuse. N Engl J Med 315:1438, 1986.
56. Kloner RA, Hale S, Alkekr K, Rezkalla S: The effects of acute and chronic cocaine use on the heart. Circulation 85:407, 1992.

57. Maron BJ, Gohman TE, Aeppli D: Prevalence of sudden cardiac death during competitive sports activities in Minnesota high school athletes. J Am Coll Cardiol 32:1881, 1998.

58. Maron BJ, Poliac LC, Roberts WC: Risk for sudden cardiac death associated with marathon running. J Am Coll Cardiol 28:428, 1996.

59. Siscovick DS, Weiss NS, Fletcher RH, Lasky T: The incidence of primary cardiac arrest during vigorous exercise. N Engl J Med 311:874, 1984.

60. Thompson PD, Funk EJ, Carleton RA, Sturner WQ: Incidence of death during jogging in Rhode Island from 1975 through 1980. JAMA 247:2535, 1982.

61. Maron BJ, Kogan J, Proschan MA, et al: Circadian variability in the occurrence of sudden cardiac death in patients with hypertrophic cardiomyopathy. J Am Coll Cardiol 23:1405, 1994.

62. Maron BJ, Poliac LC, Mathenge R: Hypertrophic cardiomyopathy as an important cause of sudden cardiac death on the athletic field in African-American athletes (Abstract). J Am Coll Cardiol 29(suppl A):462A, 1997.

63. Sherrid MV, Mieres J, Mogtader A, et al: Onset during exercise of spontaneous coronary artery dissection and sudden death. Occurrence in a trained athlete: Case report and review of prior cases. Chest 108:284, 1995.

64. Weidenbener EJ, Krauss MD, Waller BF, Taliercio CP: Incorporation of screening echocardiography in the preparticipation exam. Clin J Sport Med 5:86, 1995.

65. Lewis JF, Maron BJ, Diggs JA, et al: Preparticipation echocardiographic screening for cardiovascular disease in a large, predominantly Black population of collegiate athletes. Am J Cardiol 64:1029, 1989.

66. Maron BJ, Bodison SA, Wesley YE, et al: Results of screening a large group of intercollegiate competitive athletes for cardiovascular disease. J Am Coll Cardiol 10:1214, 1987.

67. LaCorte MA, Boxer RA, Gottesfeld IB, et al: EKG screening program for school athletes. Clin Cardiol 12:41, 1989.

68. Murray PM, Cantwell JD, Heith DL, Shoop J: The role of limited echocardiography in screening athletes. Am J Cardiol 76:849, 1995.

69. Feinstein RA, Colvin E, Oh MK: Echocardiographic screening as part of a preparticipation examination. Clin J Sport Med 3:149, 1993.

70. Mitten MJ: Team physicians and competitive athletes: Allocating legal responsibility for athletic injuries. U Pitt L Rev 55:129, 1993.

71. Knapp v Northwestern University; 101 F3d 473 (7th Cir. November 22, 1996) United States Court of Appeals; No. 96–3450.

72. Maron BJ, Leon MB, Swain JA, et al: Prospective identification by two-dimensional echocardiography of anomalous origin of the left main coronary artery from the right sinus of Valsalva. Am J Cardiol 68:140, 1991.

73. Jureidini SB, Eaton C, Williams J, et al: Transthoracic two-dimensional and color flow echocardiographic diagnosis of aberrant left coronary artery. Am Heart J 127:438, 1994.

74. Salloum JA, Thomas D, Evans J: Transesophageal echocardiography in diagnosis of aberrant coronary artery. Int J Cardiol 32:106, 1991.

75. Alam M, Brymer J, Smith S: Transesophageal echocardiographic diagnosis of anomalous left coronary artery from the right aortic sinus. Chest 103:1617, 1993.

76. Gaither NS, Rogan KM, Stajduhr K, et al: Anomalous origin and course of coronary arteries in adults: Identification and improved imaging utilizing transesophageal echocardiography. Am Heart J 122:69, 1991.

77. Ricci C, Longo R, Pagnan L, et al: Magnetic resonance imaging in right ventricular dysplasia. Am J Cardiol 70:1589, 1992.

78. Risser WL, Hoffman HM, Gordon BG Jr, Green LW: A cost-benefit analysis of preparticipation sports examination of adolescent athletes. J Sch Health 55:270, 1985.

79. Epstein SE, Maron BJ: Sudden death and the competitive athlete: Perspectives on preparticipation screening studies. J Am Coll Cardiol 7:220, 1986.

80. Maron BJ, Spirito P, Wesley YE, Arce J: Development and progression of left ventricular hypertrophy in children with hypertrophic cardiomyopathy. N Engl J Med 315:610, 1986.

81. Maron BJ, Wolfson JK, Ciró E, Spirito P: Relation of electrocardiographic abnormalities and patterns of left ventricular hypertrophy identified by two-dimensional echocardiography in patients with hypertrophic cardiomyopathy. Am J Cardiol 51:189, 1980.

82. Zehender M, Meinertz T, Keul J, Just H: ECG variants and cardiac arrhythmias in athletes: Clinical relevance and prognostic importance. Am Heart J 119:1378, 1990.

83. Pelliccia A, Cullasso F, Di Paolo FM, et al: Clinical significance of abnormal electrocardiographic patterns in elite athletes: The impact of gender and cardiac morphologic adaptations to training (Abstract). Circulation 94:I-326, 1996.

CHAPTER 58

CONNECTIVE TISSUE DISEASES

MARY ELLA M. PIERPONT   AMY S. HENTGES

Connective tissue consists of collagen and elastic fibers and the ground substance in which they are embedded—glycosoaminoglycans and small amounts of proteins such as fibronectin. Disorders of formation or degradation of any of these components can produce cardiovascular disease. Their effects on the cardiovascular system are mainly on the cardiac valves and the arteries, both large and small, but sometimes primary myocardial dysfunction occurs. Two important connective tissue disorders, Marfan syndrome and Ehlers-Danlos syndrome (EDS), are described in detail, and osteogenesis imperfecta, pseudoxanthoma elasticum, and the mucopolysaccharides are described in brief.

MARFAN SYNDROME

Marfan syndrome, a common connective tissue disorder, is an autosomal dominant disease caused by mutations in the fibrillin gene (FBN1) on chromosome 15. Fibrillin is an important constituent of the extracellular microfibrils that serve as support for the formation of elastin networks in connective tissue. Mutations in FBN1 are associated with the variable cardiovascular, ocular, and skeletal features of Marfan syndrome.[1]

PATHOLOGY

Fibrillin is a large glycoprotein secreted from connective tissue cells, is extracellularly processed, and forms aggregates.[2] It is a key component of the microfibril, which is organized into fiber bundles in tissues. Microfibrils interact with elastin in elastic tissues, such as the aorta and ligaments. They also serve as an anchor in nonelastic tissues, such as ciliary zonules and tendons.[3] Individuals with Marfan syndrome often have mutations in FBN1 that cause abnormalities of secretion, decreased synthesis, or decreased deposition of fibrillin into the microfibril matrix, thus adversely affecting the function of tissues containing fibrillin.[4] Studies have shown that individuals whose fibroblasts have reduced fibrillin deposition have more severe cardiac complications at earlier ages.[5]

Although many organs contain elastic tissues, the most severe pathology in Marfan syndrome is in the cardiovascular system. Blood vessels, cardiac valves, and myocardium all contain substantial elastic fibers. The most common pathologic finding is dilatation or aneurysm of arterial vessels, including the ascending aorta, main pulmonary artery, distal pulmonary arteries, and coronary arteries.

Ascending aortic dilatation begins within the sinuses of Valsalva in infancy or childhood and is usually progressive. Microscopic examination of the ascending aorta typically reveals aortic elastic media disruption caused by separation of muscle fibers by abnormal fibrous elements.[6] These changes, termed cystic medial necrosis, are not specific to Marfan syndrome. The aortic media disruption leads to aneurysmal dilatation of the sinuses of Valsalva and the aortic arch. Increasing aortic root dilatation may result in aortic insufficiency due to separation of the aortic valve commissures and valve failure.[6] When the ascending aorta is dilated, risk of aortic rupture and dissecting aneurysm increases. Dissecting aneurysms usually start immediately above the aortic valve and extend through the aortic arch into the descending aorta. In 10 to 20% of patients, the coronary arteries develop aneurysms that may rupture into the pericardial sac or mediastinum and be fatal.[7]

Mitral valve prolapse (ballooning) and dysplasia with or without regurgitation commonly occur in patients with Marfan syndrome.[8] The mitral leaflets undergo a fibromyxoid thickening, and the chordae tendineae may be abnormally elongated or fused, producing prolapse and mitral insufficiency.[9–11] The leaflets are frequently redundant (Fig. 58–1),[12] and calcification of the mitral annulus can occur before the age of 40 years. Another valvar abnormality in patients with Marfan syndrome is bicuspid aortic valve, which had an incidence of 9.7% in one study compared with that of 2% in the normal population.[13] Other less common cardiac manifestations include tricuspid valve prolapse with or without regurgitation, ventricular hypertrophy with areas of fibrosis and necrosis, atrial dilatation, and conduction abnormalities.[6] Degenerative changes in arteries that supply the sinoauricular node or atrioventricular node are thought to lead to conduction disturbances.[14]

HEMODYNAMICS

Cardiovascular complications of Marfan syndrome manifest over time as the weakened aorta is stressed. The aorta of adults with Marfan syndrome has decreased distensibility, increased stiffness, and a faster pulse-wave velocity.[15] These changes indicate loss of the normal elastic properties of the aorta. Children with Marfan syndrome have aortic distensibility and aortic stiffness values similar to the normal adult population, indicating that these changes occur with long-term stress on the aorta.[16]

With continued stress, the aorta gradually dilates, resulting in failure of the aortic leaflets to close completely,

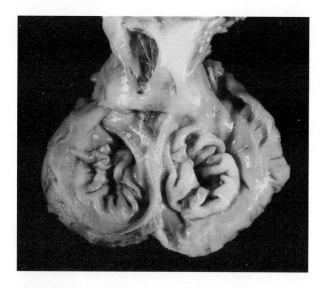

FIGURE 58–1

Gross specimen of the heart of a 10-day-old premature infant with Marfan syndrome. Redundant prolapsed atrioventricular valves. Tricuspid valve on the left and mitral valve on the right. (From Day DL, Burke BA: Pulmonary emphysema in a neonate with Marfan syndrome. Pediatr Radiol 16:518–521, 1986.)

valvar regurgitation, increased left ventricular end-diastolic volume, and reflex increase in contractility because of the Frank-Starling mechanism. These hemodynamic changes cause even more stress on the aorta and an increased risk of tears and dissection of the aortic wall.[8] Mitral valve insufficiency, common in children with Marfan syndrome, can lead to left ventricular enlargement, left atrial enlargement, and eventually myocardial dysfunction due to volume overload.[17]

CLINICAL MANIFESTATIONS

Clinical features of Marfan syndrome are evident in the tissues containing microfibrils, including the skeletal, ocular, pulmonary, skin, and cardiac systems. Current criteria for the clinical diagnosis of Marfan syndrome are described in Table 58–1.[18] The most frequent skeletal features include scoliosis; tall, thin habitus; pectus deformities (including excavatum or carinatum); flat feet; arachnodactyly; and joint hypermobility. Lens dislocation (upward) and myopia are common ocular findings. Pulmonary features include spontaneous pneumothorax and emphysema. Marfan syndrome has also been associated with an increased prevalence of obstructive sleep apnea[19] and bronchial hyper-reactivity.[20] Cutaneous features include striae and inguinal hernias. Dural ectasias are occasionally seen.

Cardiac manifestations of Marfan syndrome in children and young adults include mitral and aortic valve abnormalities, aortic dilatation, and aortic dissection. Murmurs of mitral valve prolapse and insufficiency are more common than aortic lesions in children.[21] The late-systolic murmur of mitral valve prolapse is heard at the cardiac apex, usually associated with a midsystolic to late-systolic click. There is often a musical quality to the murmur. If mitral insufficiency has become more significant, an apical pansystolic murmur is present. Symptoms associated with mitral valve prolapse include dyspnea, chest pain, palpitations, and lightheadedness. More than 50% of patients with mitral valve prolapse have various cardiac arrhythmias including supraventricular and ventricular tachyarrhythmias and abnormal atrioventricular conduction, but these arrhythmias rarely result in sustained ventricular tachycardia or sudden death.[22–24]

Aortic dilatation is present in approximately 50% of children and 70 to 80% of adults with Marfan syndrome.[3, 25] Early aortic root dilatation is frequently clinically silent.[17] More generalized aortic dilatation, extending from the aortic annulus into the supra-aortic ridge and proximal ascending aorta, is associated with a more serious outcome.[26] Progressive aortic root enlargement during the second decade of life may lead to aortic regurgitation. Dissection of the aorta occurs much more frequently in a dilated aortic root but can occur in a nondilated aortic root.[27] Aortic dissection occurs suddenly, usually progresses distally, and is accompanied by severe anterior or posterior chest pain.[3] The pain may radiate to the jaw, or occasionally, the dissection may be painless.[28] Aortic dissection has been described in a child as young as 5 years of age.[29]

Marfan syndrome is usually identified in late childhood or adolescence. In the last 10 years, however, more individuals with infantile Marfan syndrome have been described. These infants have a more pronounced facial phenotypic appearance, have more severe cardiac involvement, and are more likely to have de novo sporadic mutations of *FBN1* rather than familial mutations. These children often have serious cardiac pathology at birth, congenital contractures, arachnodactyly, hyperextensible joints, anterior chest deformity, and ocular anomalies. A characteristic facies with high-arched palate, micrognathia, malar hypoplasia, large deep-set eyes, frontal bossing, and dolichocephaly is present.[30] Severe neonatal pulmonary emphysema in the absence of thoracic cage deformity has been described in infants with severe Marfan syndrome.[12, 31] Cardiac findings may include mitral valve prolapse, pulmonary artery dilatation, hemorrhoidal appearance of the mitral and tricuspid valves (see Fig. 58–1), severe valvar regurgitation, and aortic root dilatation, which is progressive early in childhood. In severely affected infants, mitral valve prolapse and regurgitation are usually the most common cause of morbidity and mortality.[32] In adolescents and adults, the most common cause of morbidity and mortality is dissection or rupture of the aorta.[33, 34]

ELECTROCARDIOGRAPHIC FEATURES

Children and adolescents with Marfan syndrome frequently have a normal electrocardiogram (ECG). The QRS axis is normal in most patients but can be deviated to the right, indeterminate, or superiorly oriented in the presence of significant scoliosis or pectus deformities.[21] The most frequent ECG abnormalities include left ventricular hypertrophy or dilatation due to valvar abnormalities. First-degree atrioventricular block and inverted T waves associated with ST depression in leads II, III, and aVF are also common. T wave inversion may occur transiently and may indicate papillary muscle dysfunction in patients with

TABLE 58–1

MARFAN SYNDROME DIAGNOSTIC CRITERIA*

Organ System	Major Criteria	Minor Criteria	Criteria for System Involvement
Skeletal†	Pectus carinatum Pectus excavatum requiring surgery Reduced upper to lower segment ratio or arm span to height ratio greater than 1.05 Wrist thumb signs Scoliosis of >20 degrees or spondylolisthesis Reduced extension at elbows (<170 degrees) Medial displacement of the medial malleolus causing pes planus Protrusio acetabulae of any degree	Pectus excavatum of moderate severity Joint hypermobility Highly arched palate with crowding of teeth Facial appearance (dolichocephaly, malar hypoplasia, enophthalmos, retrognathia, downslanting palpebral fissures)	2 major criteria, or 1 major plus 2 minor
Ocular	Ectopia lentis	Abnormally flat cornea Increased axial length of globe Hypoplastic iris or hypoplastic ciliary muscle causing decreased miosis	2 minor
Cardiovascular	Dilatation of ascending aorta with or without aortic regurgitation and involving at least the sinuses of Valsalva Dissection of ascending aorta	Mitral valve prolapse ± regurgitation Dilatation of the main pulmonary artery, in the absence of valvar or peripheral pulmonic stenosis or other obvious cause, <age 40 yr Calcification of mitral annulus, <age 40 yr Dilatation or dissection of descending thoracic or abdominal aorta, <age 50 yr	1 major or 1 minor
Pulmonary	None	Spontaneous pneumothorax Apical blebs	1 minor
Skin and integument	None	Striae atrophicae not associated with marked weight changes, pregnancy, or repetitive stress Recurrent or incisional hernia	1 minor
Dura	Lumbosacral dural ectasia by computed tomography or magnetic resonance imaging	None	1 major
Family and genetic history	Having a parent, child, or sibling who meets these diagnostic criteria independently Presence of a mutation in *FBN1* Presence of a linkage haplotype around *FBN1* associated with Marfan syndrome in the family	None	1 major

*For the index case:
If the family and genetic history is not contributory, one major criterion in at least two different organ systems and involvement of a third organ system.
If a mutation known to cause Marfan syndrome in others is detected, one major criterion in an organ system and involvement of a second organ system.
For a relative of an index case:
Presence of a major criterion in the family history and one major criterion in an organ system and involvement of a second organ system.
†Presence of at least four major criteria is necessary to count as presence of "one major criterion" in the skeletal system.
Data from De Paepe A, Devereux RB, Dietz HC, et al: Revised diagnostic criteria for the Marfan syndrome. Am J Med Genet 62:417, 1996.

systolic click-murmur.[21] Twenty-four-hour ambulatory ECG monitoring in adults with Marfan syndrome has demonstrated a higher than normal prevalence of atrial or ventricular premature beats, prolonged atrioventricular conduction time, longer QT intervals, and ST segment depression.[35] The major dysrhythmias reported in Marfan syndrome are short runs of paroxysmal supraventricular tachycardia, atrial flutter, atrial fibrillation, complete or incomplete atrioventricular block, and Wolff-Parkinson-White syndrome.[36]

RADIOLOGIC FEATURES

Chest radiography may be normal in children with Marfan syndrome, even in those with cardiac disease. The usefulness of chest radiographs resides in identifying the severity of skeletal abnormalities such as kyphoscoliosis and pectus deformities.[21] A chest radiograph may provide suspicion of aortic dissection with an abnormal ascending aortic silhou-ette but is often not diagnostic.[37] Mild degrees of aortic root enlargement are usually not evident on a routine chest radiograph. Magnetic resonance imaging (Fig. 58–2) is useful for more extensive visualization of the aorta and can show advanced aortic root enlargement, aortic dissection, or aortic aneurysms in atypical locations.[38] Echocardiography, however, is the most efficient and best means of serial aortic root evaluation.

CARDIAC CATHETERIZATION

Cardiac catheterization and selective angiography are useful in assessing cardiac function and characterizing cardiac pathology. Aortography (Fig. 58–3) can give information about aortic dilatation and can diagnose aortic dissection with visualization of a double lumen or an intimal flap.[39] Advantages include the ability to detect complications of aortic dissection, such as aortic insufficiency, thrombus in the false lumen, and involvement of branch vessels.[39] Aortography

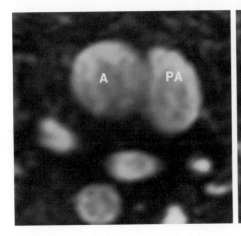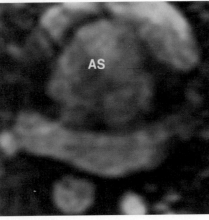

FIGURE 58–2

Magnetic resonance imaging of the thoracic aorta in a 17-year-old boy with Marfan syndrome. *Left,* Cross-section view at the level of the sinotubular ridge showing an aorta of the upper limits of normal size. *Right,* Cross-section of the aorta at the level of the sinuses of Valsalva showing aortic root dilatation measuring 46 mm. A = aorta; PA = pulmonary artery; AS = sinuses of Valsalva.

can also quantitate the severity of regurgitant lesions, outline the anatomy of the great arteries, and detect coexisting congenital cardiovascular malformations.[21] Left ventriculography typically shows mitral valve prolapse that may appear scalloped and may be associated with mitral insufficiency. Cardiac catheterization has limited sensitivity, and risks are involved in using contrast agents, although complications are rare.

ECHOCARDIOGRAPHIC FEATURES

Echocardiography is the most rapid and sensitive diagnostic tool for the assessment of cardiovascular lesions associated with Marfan syndrome. It provides serial measurements of the aortic root dimension, which can direct the management of cardiovascular disease in these patients (Fig. 58–4). One of the earliest changes in Marfan syndrome is the bulging of the sinuses of Valsalva, which in the short-axis view resembles a cloverleaf. Transthoracic echocardiography can identify aortic dilatation, aortic dissection, valvar prolapse and regurgitation, and other cardiac anomalies. The image quality may be compromised by obesity, chest wall deformities, or emphysema.[39] The aortic arch and descending aorta are difficult to image with this method. Transesophageal echocardiography allows visualization of the entire thoracic aorta,[40] definition of aortic dissection, better visualization of cardiac structures and abnormalities, and visualization of the proximal coronary arteries.[41] Color Doppler flow mapping allows identification of the true and false lumina in aortic dissection.[40]

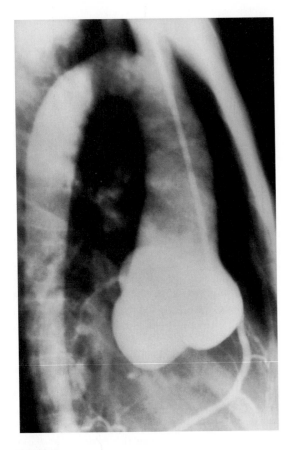

FIGURE 58–3

Lateral projection of an aortogram showing the enlarged ascending aorta and the prominent sinuses of Valsalva.

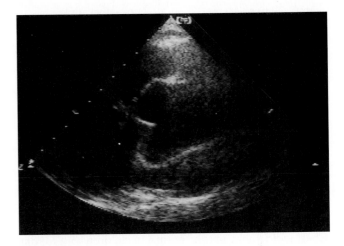

FIGURE 58–4

Two-dimensional echocardiogram, long-axis view, showing an enlarged aortic root with sinuses of Valsalva measuring 50 mm in a 17-year-old boy with Marfan syndrome.

This technique can be used to evaluate the aorta in individuals who are difficult to image by the transthoracic mode.

CLINICAL MANAGEMENT AND PROGNOSIS

Since 1972, long-term survival of individuals with Marfan syndrome has improved because of early detection and treatment of cardiovascular manifestations. Life expectancy has increased 25%, from 32 ± 10.4 years in 1972[34] to 41 ± 18 years in 1995.[42] This increase is likely due to early and improved cardiovascular surgery, β-blocker therapy, increased diagnosis of mild disease, and a general increase in population life expectancy.[42] Early death in Marfan syndrome is most commonly precipitated by aortic dissection, chronic aortic regurgitation, or severe mitral regurgitation.[34] Progression of these cardiac lesions may be either rapid or slow. Sudden death may occur in patients without known cardiac disease.[43]

Effective management of the cardiovascular manifestations include prophylactic surgical replacement of the aortic root, use of negative inotropic drugs, and symptomatic treatment. β-Blockers reduce the inotropic force of the heart and decrease the impact of ejected blood on the aortic wall, thereby slowing aortic root dilatation.[44] β-Adrenergic blockade with propranolol slows the rate of aortic dilatation and reduces the development of aortic complications in adults and adolescents with mild to moderate aortic dilatation.[45] Atenolol, the drug of choice for this condition, has greater cardiac selectivity, a long half-life, and minimal adverse side effects. Atenolol therapy is associated with a reduced rate of aortic dilatation in children.[16,46,47] It has been recommended that β-blockers be administered to children when the aortic root size exceeds the upper range of normal (95th percentile).[44]

Echocardiographic aortic root measurements should be obtained at least annually. If the aortic root is 5.0 cm wide or more, the frequency of echocardiography should increase to every 3 to 4 months.[48] If the aortic root reaches a diameter of 5.5 cm or more, elective aortic replacement with a composite graft is recommended because of the increased risk of aortic dissection. Factors influencing a decision for surgical repair include increasing left ventricular end-diastolic dimension, aortic regurgitation of more than moderate severity, severe mitral regurgitation, a family history of dissection, and a future need to undergo major operative procedures, as for treatment of scoliosis.[49]

In children, aortic root replacement should be considered when its diameter equals approximately twice the average measurement for that age group and is actively dilating.[50] The procedure of choice is composite graft repair with a prosthesis containing an aortic valve.[51] Children younger than 8 years could be considered for replacement of their aortic root with an aortic homograft because of technical or anticoagulant concerns.[49]

Increased survival of surgical patients since 1979 is associated with composite graft repair of the aorta with reimplantation of the coronary arteries.[33] The "button" technique or the Bentall procedure is associated with the best long-term results.[51] Patients with aortic dissection at the time of surgery are more likely to require a subsequent aortic operation than are patients who undergo elective composite graft repair of an aortic aneurysm.[52] Follow-up of the thoracic and abdominal aorta for late dilatation and dissection is essential after aortic root repair.[53]

In children younger than 18 years, the most common surgical indication is aortic root dilatation (81%).[54] Cardiac failure due to severe mitral valve regurgitation is the most common indication for surgery in the preadolescent years.[8] Mitral valve repair, or valve replacement when necessary, is the optimal surgical approach to mitral regurgitation, and early follow-up results are satisfactory.[32]

Children and young adults with Marfan syndrome should be evaluated for noncardiac manifestations of this condition. Regular assessment for lens dislocation and myopia is important. Myopia may be progressive and severe.[3] Prophylaxis for infective endocarditis is indicated in patients with cardiac involvement including aortic root dilatation and valvar abnormalities. Joint laxity and scoliosis can be treated with bracing or surgical stabilization. Significant pectus deformities should be repaired late in adolescence if possible when skeletal maturity is nearly complete.[49]

Patients and their families should be counseled about the prognosis, lifestyle changes, and hereditary nature of Marfan syndrome. Participation in contact sports and hard labor should be avoided to reduce the risk of cardiac, skeletal, and ophthalmic problems.[3] Avoidance of contact sports is necessary because of heightened susceptibility to transverse tears in the weakened aorta.[49] Activities that increase systolic blood pressure such as weightlifting and isometric exercises or those that increase pressure and volume loads in the heart such as endurance exercises should not be undertaken.[55]

Young women with Marfan syndrome should be counseled on the possible complications of pregnancy with this syndrome and the 50% risk of transmission of the disease. The hemodynamic stresses of pregnancy can damage an already weakened or dilated aorta. In one study, 6 of 36 women with a normal aortic root size had an aortic dissection or increased aortic dilatation related to their pregnancy.[56] The risk is substantially increased for women with aortic root measurements larger than 4 cm or if the aortic root has been steadily dilating.[57] Aortic events can occur throughout the pregnancy or after delivery, so frequent monitoring of aortic root size is advised.[56] For patients with aortic dissection, rapid dilatation, or other cardiac abnormalities, cesarean section is the preferred method of delivery.[58] β-Blocker therapy may be started or continued throughout pregnancy to prevent aortic root dilatation.[59]

GENETICS AND DIFFERENTIAL DIAGNOSIS

Marfan syndrome is caused by mutations in *FBN1* on chromosome 15q21 and has autosomal dominant transmission in families.[60] Twenty-five percent of all patients with Marfan syndrome have a new mutation with no known family history.[61] Allelic heterogeneity or different mutations in *FBN1* may play a role in the vast range of clinical severity seen among individuals and families affected with Marfan syndrome. Additionally, relatives who share the same mutation can show marked phenotypic variability, suggesting the importance of genetic and environmental modifiers.[62] The severely affected infantile patients are usually the result of spontaneous mutations of *FBN1*.[6] Genetic analysis has shown clustering of mutations involved in infantile Marfan syndrome in exons 24 to 26 and exon 32.[63]

The pathogenic mechanism and etiology of Marfan syndrome are not fully understood. Evidence suggests that Marfan syndrome may be due to a dominant negative effect. Mutant fibrillin proteins can interfere with the formation of stable microfibrils and impair microfibril integrity, thus producing manifestations in the various body systems containing microfibrils. A second genetic locus for Marfan syndrome has been proposed on chromosome 3p24,[64] but some questions remain concerning the correct diagnosis of this family.[3] One large family with cardiovascular and skeletal manifestations of Marfan syndrome has been described without linkage to either *FBN1* or a second fibrillin gene, *FBN2*.[65] This suggests that more than one gene can produce phenotypes similar to Marfan syndrome. Syndromes with overlapping phenotypes may be due to mutations relating to microfibril formation and function. Mutations in *FBN1* have also been associated with familial ascending aortic aneurysms,[66] dominant ectopia lentis,[67] isolated skeletal features of Marfan syndrome,[4] and Shprintzen-Goldberg syndrome.[68]

The differential diagnosis of Marfan syndrome includes congenital contractural arachnodactyly, homocystinuria, Shprintzen-Goldberg syndrome, and familial aortic aneurysms or dissections. Children with congenital contractural arachnodactyly (Beals' syndrome) have dolichostenomelia with arachnodactyly, camptodactyly, joint contractures, and "crumpled" ears. Other findings include myopia, ulnar deviation of the fingers, and progressive scoliosis. Cardiac manifestations include mitral valve prolapse with regurgitation, atrial septal defect, ventricular septal defect, and hypoplasia of the aorta.[69] This syndrome is characterized by autosomal dominant inheritance of mutations in *FBN2* located on 5q23.[70]

Homocystinuria is an autosomal recessive disorder due to cystathionine β-synthase deficiency or defects of folate and cobalamin metabolism. Individuals have dislocated lenses (downward), myopia, tall stature, arachnodactyly, sternal deformities, scoliosis, and learning disability. Cardiovascular features include thromboembolic events such as strokes, acute myocardial infarctions, and pulmonary emboli occurring in childhood or as an adult.[71] These patients are usually fair-haired and blue-eyed, and their joints often have limited mobility.

Findings in Shprintzen-Goldberg syndrome include craniosynostosis, ocular proptosis, micrognathia, high-arched palate, pectus deformities, arachnodactyly, camptodactyly, and mental deficiencies. Less common features are mitral valve prolapse, aortic dilatation, scoliosis, hypermobile joints, and myopia.[72] The etiology of this syndrome is unknown, although individuals with Shprintzen-Goldberg syndrome and *FBN1* mutations have been described, suggesting a role for fibrillin-1 in early craniofacial and central nervous system development.[68]

Familial thoracic aortic aneurysms and dissections have been previously described.[73–75] Aortic pathology looks histologically similar to that in Marfan syndrome, but individuals lack the skeletal and ocular changes of Marfan syndrome. Patients often present with aortic disease (either dilatation or dissection), multiple affected family members, and marked variability in the age at onset. The transmission is autosomal dominant with decreased penetrance. In some families, mutations in the type III procollagen gene (*COL3A1*) have been found,[75] whereas other families have no mutations detected in *COL3A1*, *FBN1*, or a second Marfan-like syndrome locus at 3p24.[73] Some individuals with aortic root dilatation, but without arachnodactyly or ocular features of Marfan syndrome, have *FBN1* mutations, emphasizing that marked variation in expression may occur in Marfan syndrome.[76]

Most patients with familial thoracic aortic aneurysms and dissections have aortic dilatation before dissection. Histologic examination of aortic tissue of affected individuals reveals cystic medial necrosis, loss and fragmentation of elastic fibers, increased deposits of mucopolysaccharide-like material, and normal microfibrillar fiber arrays. Echocardiographic follow-up and surgical recommendations are similar to those for patients with Marfan syndrome. Although most of the dissections have occurred beyond middle age, deaths have occurred in children aged 10 to 15 years.[74]

EHLERS-DANLOS SYNDROME

EDS encompasses a wide range of phenotypic expressions, and, in the past, 10 or more types were described based on clinical presentation, inheritance patterns, and biochemical abnormalities.[77] Reclassification has yielded seven major types: classical, hypermobility, vascular, kyphoscoliosis, arthrochalasia, dermatosparaxis, and other.[78]

EDS is one of the most frequently inherited connective tissue disorders.[79] Patients may have fragility of the skin and blood vessels, skin hyperelasticity, hypermobile joints, and subcutaneous nodules. Bruising occurs easily, and atrophic scarring occurs over bony prominences. The internal organs may be fragile as well. No one feature is common to all types of EDS, and patients with some of the mentioned characteristics may not meet the criteria for any one type.[80] Inheritance may be autosomal dominant, autosomal recessive, or X-linked recessive depending on the type. Cardiac anomalies have been described in several types, and these types of EDS are the focus of this section.

EHLERS-DANLOS SYNDROME TYPES I, II, AND III

EDS types I and II (classical) and III (hypermobility) are the most common forms of this disease, and each has autosomal dominant transmission. These types differ in their severity and degree of involvement of different systems.

Pathology

EDS types I, II, and III show similar dermal pathology including large, irregular-shaped collagen fibrils and smaller than normal collagen bundles.[81–83] The skin is thin with decreased collagen content and increased elastin.[84] It is believed that skin hyperextensibility is due to a defective "wickerwork" of structurally normal collagen fiber bundles. The connective tissue in muscles is quite sparse, barely holding the muscle bundles together.[85]

Clinical Manifestations

Patients with the classical EDS types I and II show skin hyperextensibility, generalized joint hypermobility, bruisability, flat feet, wide atrophic scarring, and tissue fragility. Facial features may include a narrow maxilla, wide nasal bridge, and epicanthal folds. EDS type II exhibits these traits in a much milder form. EDS type I is usually more severe in its clinical manifestations and shows an increased tendency for hemorrhage but can vary in its expression. EDS type I may show connective tissue pseudotumors or calcified spheroids under the skin, varicose veins, hernias, and rupture of the arteries, colon, or uterus, although this is rare. Premature birth due to early rupture of fetal membranes has been seen in EDS type I.[85]

EDS type III has less apparent skin manifestations but severe generalized joint hypermobility with dislocation, hemarthroses, and precocious arthritis as sequelae.[79] Infantile muscular hypotonia, delayed walking, chronic pain, and joint dislocations have been seen in all three types.[86] Infants with suspected EDS are difficult to assess because skin hyperextensibility, bruising, and skin scarring tendencies do not usually become apparent until the child is 1 year of age.[85]

Cardiac manifestations in EDS types I to III have not been well defined. Congenital cardiac lesions have been associated with these types of EDS,[87] but an increased risk has not been established. Mitral valve prolapse and enlarged sinuses of Valsalva are more common in hospitalized patients with EDS types I to III, but the risk of these abnormalities does not seem to be increased in healthy patients with these types.[88] Aortic arch dilatation has also been described in EDS.[89] Aneurysms, dissecting aneurysms, and rupture of blood vessels have been noted in EDS type I, but they are rare.[85]

Diagnostic Testing

Chest radiograph and ECG are usually normal, but conduction abnormalities have been reported. Echocardiography may show mitral valve prolapse, tricuspid valve prolapse, mitral regurgitation, tricuspid regurgitation, or congenital cardiac abnormality. Cardiac catheterization and angiography can usually be performed without vascular complications as in EDS type IV (discussed later). Enlarged sinuses of Valsalva and right ventricular outflow abnormalities have occurred in a few selected patients.[87]

Management and Prognosis

Life expectancy is normal for EDS types I to III.[79] Children with marked skin fragility should wear protective gear to avoid excessive scarring. Children may experience more falls due to joint laxity, and increased bruising and scarring may lead to suspicion of child abuse.[90] Surgery may be more difficult due to tissue fragility, and the surgical problem can often recur.[85] Surgery should be performed only when necessary because of tissue fragility and problems with wound healing. Stitches should be left in place twice as long as usual.

Counseling regarding avoidance of trauma in EDS types I and II because of the risk of hemorrhage should be undertaken. Sports with heavy joint strain should be discouraged in children with joint laxity. Increased risk of major pregnancy complications is not usually present with these types of EDS, although postpartum hemorrhage, uterine or bladder prolapse, cervical incompetence, and premature delivery have been reported.[91, 92] Affected parents have a 50% risk of transmitting the disorder. If aortic root dilatation is found, periodic evaluation by echocardiography is recommended. If the aortic root becomes excessively large, surgical replacement with a composite graft may be indicated to prevent rupture or dissection.

Genetics

EDS types I, II, and III are dominantly inherited, but the exact biochemical etiologies are unknown. Mutations in *COL5A1* and *COL5A2* have been found in some patients with EDS types I and II, suggesting a causal role of collagen type V.[93, 94] Collagen type V mutations have not been found in all individuals or families with EDS types I and II. Mutations in collagen types I, II, and III are not involved in EDS types I, II, and III.[95–97]

EHLERS-DANLOS SYNDROME TYPE IV

EDS type IV, the vascular type, is a potentially life-threatening disease associated with an abnormality of type III collagen.[78] The affected organs have tissues that contain type III collagen, including large and medium-sized blood vessel walls, the dermis, the gastrointestinal tract, and the uterus.[98] The pattern of inheritance is autosomal dominant.

Pathology

Because large and medium-sized arterial vessels contain 40% type III collagen, a deficiency in type III collagen formation leads to fragile arterial walls. Abnormal structure, synthesis, or secretion accounts for the reduced amounts or absence of type III collagen in tissues and leads to their fragility.[99] Any major artery can be affected, and multiple vessel involvement is common.[100] Microangiopathy with bleeding, aneurysm, and increased transcapillary diffusion has been demonstrated in two patients.[101] Rupture of major arteries can occur spontaneously or after minor trauma in the cranium, abdomen, or extremities.[102] Other vascular complications include aneurysmal dilatation (Fig. 58–5) with degeneration and rupture or dissection, arteriovenous fistulae, and myocardial infarction.[103–105] Arterial vessel walls in patients with EDS type IV have reduced total collagen content and thin walls with fragmented elastic fibers.[106] The heart itself has little type III collagen and is not directly involved in this syndrome.[98] However, the coronary arteries can show aneurysms, dissection, or rupture, thus adversely affecting the heart.[107–109]

Clinical Manifestations

Clinical presentation of patients with EDS type IV is not uniform, and often manifestations become more frequent with increasing age. Complications can occur at any age, including the neonatal period.[110] Patients usually have severe skin fragility and bruisability, but skin hyperextensibility is minimal. The skin is translucent with prominent venous patterning and shows premature aging changes over the hands and feet. The skin may have poor wound-healing ability and show abnormal scarring.[111] Coagulation studies

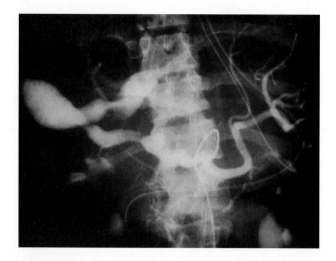

FIGURE 58–5

Celiac artery injection of contrast material in a patient with Ehlers-Danlos type IV. (Courtesy of JH Moller, MD.)

are usually normal in EDS type IV,[85,107] although early reports documented a coagulation factor or platelet abnormality in selected patients.[112,113] Joint hypermobility is often present in the small joints of the hands and feet. A typical facial appearance has been described including prominent eyes, pinched nose, hollow cheeks, thin lips, and firm ear pinnae with minimal lobes. Other clinical findings include inguinal hernias, congenital club foot, chronic pain, and periodontal disease.[86,114] Infants with EDS type IV can present with premature birth, low birth weight, failure to thrive, and congenital dislocation of the hips.[111] Life-threatening events usually occur after puberty and include rupture of arteries, hollow viscus organs, or a gravid uterus.[85]

Diagnostic Testing

Chest radiographs may show a very large aneurysm of major blood vessels. ECGs are usually normal but may show evidence of a myocardial infarction, although this is rare.[105,109] Echocardiograms usually do not show an increased occurrence of mitral valve prolapse or dilatation of the aortic root, although some reports have found mitral valve prolapse in selected patients with EDS type IV.[88,115] Invasive vascular imaging may be hazardous. For example, angiography is associated with a 67% complication rate and a 17% death rate.[107] A more recent report cited a 16.7% morbidity and 5.6% mortality rate associated with angiography.[116] If angiography must be performed, the smallest possible catheter with a soft tip should be used.[117] Less invasive techniques should be attempted first to diagnose vascular complications. These include computed tomography, magnetic resonance angiography, and digital subtraction angiography using intravenous infusion.[116]

Management and Prognosis

The natural history of this disease may follow a stormy course. Patients may or may not show clinical features as mentioned earlier, although easy bruisability is common. Most deaths are caused by spontaneous rupture of arterial vessels.[85] Other vascular complications, such as carotid-

cavernous sinus fistulae, aneurysms, hematomas, intracranial aneurysms with secondary hemorrhage, or extensive bleeding after a simple operative procedure, may occur.[102,117] Serious nonvascular complications include spontaneous rupture of the colon, pneumothorax, and complications during pregnancy.[111,118] Bowel rupture usually occurs in the distal colon, and repair can be difficult, with many patients experiencing recurrent colonic perforations or anastomotic leaks. The recommended treatment of colon perforation is total abdominal colectomy and end ileostomy to prevent such complications.[116] Pregnancy carries a 25% risk of death with such complications as rupture of the uterus, bowel, aorta, and vena cava; vaginal lacerations; and postpartum uterine hemorrhage.[119] Various catastrophic events can occur in different individuals within a family or sequentially in one person.[120]

Effective treatment for this disease is minimal, and a conservative approach is stressed. Surgical procedures on patients with EDS type IV have a high potential for complications or death due to increased vascular fragility.[121] Repair of the vascular structures after rupture or diagnostic puncture is difficult, with ligation often being necessary. Bypass grafting should be considered when ligation is impossible.[103,107] Nonoperative management of these patients should be attempted when possible because operative mortality has been reported at 19%.[107] External compression with bedrest and careful monitoring may be used in patients with peripheral vascular hemorrhage if they are stable.[116] Noninvasive investigative techniques such as Doppler, computed tomography, or magnetic resonance imaging should be used for diagnostic purposes when possible. Anticoagulant therapy is not recommended because the risk of bruising and bleeding is increased.[102] Aspirin and nonsteroidal anti-inflammatory drugs could possibly promote hemorrhage due to leaky vessels and should be avoided.[85]

The prognosis of EDS type IV is poor with or without surgery. Most patients die of arterial complications in the third through the fifth decades of life.[122] Complications can occur in childhood, and sudden infant death in association with EDS type IV has been reported.[110] Unfortunately, many patients remain undiagnosed until a catastrophic, spontaneous rupture of an artery or the bowel occurs. In one study, only 5 of 31 patients had signs or symptoms suggesting EDS.[107] Patients known to have EDS type IV who develop acute abdominal or chest pain should be suspected of having bowel rupture or a vascular catastrophe and treated accordingly.[117]

Patients with EDS type IV should be informed of the possible complications of their disease and encouraged to tell physicians caring for them about their condition so that appropriate precautions can be taken. Counseling regarding autosomal dominant transmission of the disease and avoidance of potentially harmful situations, especially in regard to employment and recreation, should be undertaken. In children, care must be taken to avoid minor trauma as arterial vessels may be easily ruptured.

Genetics

EDS type IV is caused by mutations in the *COL3A1* gene on chromosome 2q31–q32.3, resulting in abnormal type III collagen.[123] Half of these mutations are spontaneous with no family history of the disease.[124] EDS type IV shows autosomal dominant transmission. The clinical diagnosis of EDS type IV is confirmed by demonstration of defects in type III collagen metabolism in cultured skin fibroblasts.[125]

OTHER TYPES OF EHLERS-DANLOS SYNDROME

There are few reports of the other EDS types. Cardiovascular manifestations have been reported in EDS type VI, type X, and unspecified types.[126] EDS type VI (kyphoscoliosis type) is an autosomal recessive condition due to a deficiency of lysyl hydroxylase, a collagen-modifying enzyme.[127] Its major features include retinal detachment, rupture of the ocular globe, muscular hypotonia, generalized joint laxity, and progressive kyphoscoliosis.[78] Rupture of cerebral arteries and a dissecting aortic aneurysm have been reported with this type.[128,129]

EDS type X (classified now in the other types of EDS) is due to an abnormality of fibronectin, and its pattern of inheritance is uncertain because only one kindred has been described.[130] Clinical manifestations of the proposita include joint hyperextensibility, thin hyperextensible skin, easy bruisability, petechiae, mitral valve prolapse, and an enlarged aortic root diameter.[131] Beighton[126] described a variety of cardiac abnormalities in EDS (types not specified) including mitral regurgitation, aortic stenosis and regurgitation, right-sided aortic arch, widening of the ascending aorta, and numerous apical systolic murmurs. Because cardiac manifestations are unpredictable and the incidence is unknown, echocardiographic study of patients with EDS is suggested.

OTHER CONNECTIVE TISSUE DISEASES AFFECTING THE HEART (Editor's Addendum)

OSTEOGENESIS IMPERFECTA

This group of diseases is due to abnormal formation of type I collagen because of a mutation in chromosome 17 or occasionally in chromosome 7. Type I collagen is the major collagen in bone, which bears the brunt of the disease, but it also occurs in arterial walls and cardiac valves.[132,133] Patients with this disorder may therefore have aortic root dilatation or dysfunction of mitral or aortic valves.[134,135] Mitral valve prolapse occurs, but probably not more frequently than in the normal population. Premature coronary artery disease occurs rarely.

PSEUDOXANTHOMA ELASTICUM

This rare disorder of elastic tissue has both autosomal dominant and recessive forms and is associated with mutations on chromosome 16p3.1.[136] Fragmentation and calcification of elastic fibers are present. The disease affects the skin, which shows yellow papules and a crinkled appearance ("plucked chicken skin"). Retinal angiomatoid streaks develop and may interfere with vision. Arterial involvement is widespread and may result in gastrointestinal or other bleeding, renal vascular hypertension, intermittent claudication, or angina pectoris. Mitral valve prolapse is common.[137,138] Severe coronary arterial disease has been recorded in children as young as 8 years of age.[139,140] Restrictive cardiomyopathy has been described.[141] A few patients may have left ventricular hypertrophy, even in the absence of skin changes.

MUCOPOLYSACCHARIDOSES

Sulfated mucopolysaccharides (glycosoaminoglycans) are long polymers present in most cells and intercellular ground substance. Failure to hydrolyze the terminal galactosamine (in dermatan sulfate) or glucosamine (in heparan and keratin sulfate) results in excessive accumulation of mucopolysaccharide chains. This accumulation is often prominent in cardiac valves, leading to aortic or mitral incompetence.[142-145] The lumina of coronary or pulmonary arteries may be severely narrowed.[143,144,146] Occasionally, primary myocardial dysfunction occurs.[147,148] These changes are most marked in Hurler's syndrome (α-L-iduronidase deficiency, due to mutation at chromosome 4p16.3) and the Maroteaux-Lamy syndrome (galactosamine-4-sulfate deficiency, due to mutation at chromosome 5q11–q13), and less severe in the Scheie syndrome (α-L-iduronidase deficiency, also due to mutation at chromosome 4p16.3), all of which are autosomal recessive disorders. The Hunter syndrome is X-linked (iduronate 2-sulfatase deficiency, due to mutation at chromosome Xq27.3), and valve infiltration and dysfunction are prominent and indeed the main causes of death. There are both severe and less severe forms of this syndrome, with the average age at death being 12 and 22 years, respectively. Diagnosis of the different mucopolysaccharidoses is made by identification of a combination of typical physical features, assaying cells or tissues for the specific enzyme, or by polymerase chain reaction techniques to determine the mutation.

REFERENCES

1. Dietz HC, Cutting GR, Maslen CL, et al: Marfan syndrome caused by a recurrent de novo missense mutation in the fibrillin gene. Nature 352:337, 1991.
2. Sakai LY, Keene DR, Glanville RW, et al: Purification and partial characterization of fibrillin, a cysteine-rich structural component of connective tissue microfibrils. J Biol Chem 266:14763, 1991.
3. Gray JR, Davies SJ: Marfan syndrome. J Med Genet 33:403, 1996.
4. Milewicz DM, Grossfield J, Cao SN, et al: A mutation in *FBN1* disrupts profibrillin processing and results in isolated skeletal features of the Marfan syndrome. J Clin Invest 95:2373, 1995.
5. Aoyama T, Francke U, Gasner C, Furthmayr H: Fibrillin abnormalities and prognosis in Marfan syndrome and related disorders. Am J Med Genet 58:169, 1995.
6. Geva T, Sanders SP, Diogenes MS, et al: Two-dimensional and Doppler echocardiographic and pathologic characteristics of the infantile Marfan syndrome. Am J Cardiol 65:1230, 1990.
7. Hirst AE Jr, Johns VJ Jr, Kime SW Jr: Dissecting aneurysms of the aorta: A review of 505 cases. Medicine 37:217, 1958.
8. Dietz HC, Ramirez F, Sakai LY: Marfan's syndrome and other microfibrillar diseases. *In* Harris H, Hirschhorn K (eds): Advances in Human Genetics. New York, Plenum Press, 1994, p 153–186.
9. Raghib G, Jue KL, Anderson RC, Edwards JE: Marfan's syndrome with mitral insufficiency. Am J Cardiol 16:127, 1965.
10. Grondin CM, Steinberg CL, Edwards JE: Dissecting aneurysm complicating Marfan's syndrome (arachnodactyly) in a mother and son. Am Heart J 77:301, 1969.

11. Bowden DH, Favara BE, Donahoe JL: Marfan's syndrome: Accelerated course in childhood associated with lesions of mitral valve and pulmonary artery. Am Heart J 69:96, 1965.

12. Day DL, Burke BA: Pulmonary emphysema in a neonate with Marfan syndrome. Pediatr Radiol 16:518, 1986.

13. El Habbel MH: Cardiovascular manifestations of Marfan's syndrome in the young. Am Heart J 123:752, 1992.

14. James TN, Frame B, Schatz IJ: Pathology of cardiac conduction system in Marfan's syndrome. Arch Intern Med 114:339, 1964.

15. Hirata K, Triposkiadis F, Sparks E: The Marfan syndrome: Abnormal aortic elastic properties. J Am Coll Cardiol 18:57, 1991.

16. Reed CM, Fox ME, Alpert BS: Aortic biomechanical properties in pediatric patients with the Marfan syndrome, and the effects of atenolol. Am J Cardiol 71:606, 1993.

17. Hirata K, Triposkiadis F, Sparks E, et al: The Marfan syndrome: Cardiovascular physical findings and diagnostic correlates. Am Heart J 123:743, 1992.

18. De Paepe A, Devereux RB, Dietz HC, et al: Revised diagnostic criteria for the Marfan syndrome. Am J Med Genet 62:417, 1996.

19. Cistulli PA, Sullivan CE: Sleep apnea in Marfan's syndrome, increased upper airway collapsibility during sleep. Chest 108:631, 1995.

20. König P, Boxer R, Morrison J, Pletcher B: Bronchial hyperreactivity in children with Marfan syndrome. Pediatr Pulmonol 11:29, 1991.

21. Phornphutkul C, Rosenthal A, Nadas AS: Cardiac manifestations of Marfan syndrome in infancy and childhood. Circulation 47:587, 1973.

22. Pratt CM, Young JB, Wierman AM, et al: Complex ventricular arrhythmias associated with mitral valve prolapse syndrome. Am J Med 80:626, 1986.

23. Josephson ME, Horwitz LN, Kastor J: Paroxysmal supraventricular tachycardia in patients with mitral valve prolapse. Circulation 57:111, 1978.

24. Ware JA, Margo SA, Luck JC, et al: Conduction system abnormalities in symptomatic mitral valve prolapse: An electrophysiologic analysis of 60 patients. Am J Cardiol 53:1075, 1984.

25. Hwa J, Richards JG, Huang H, et al: The natural history of aortic dilation in the Marfan syndrome. Med J Aust 158:558, 1993.

26. Roman MJ, Rosen SE, Kramer-Fox R, Devereux RB: Prognostic significance of the pattern of aortic root dilation in the Marfan syndrome. J Am Coll Cardiol 22:1470, 1993.

27. Roberts WC, Honig HS: The spectrum of cardiovascular disease in the Marfan syndrome. A clinico-morphologic study of 18 necropsy patients and comparison to 151 previously reported necropsy patients. Am Heart J 104:115, 1982.

28. Gott VL, Pyeritz RE, Magovern GJ, et al: Surgical treatment of aneurysms of the ascending aorta in the Marfan syndrome. Results of composite-graft repair in 50 patients. N Engl J Med 314:1070, 1986.

29. Ruiz ME, Sty JR, Wells RG: Aortic dissection in a 5-year-old girl with Marfan's syndrome. Arch Pediatr Adolesc Med 150:440, 1996.

30. Morse RP, Rockenmacher S, Pyeritz RE, et al: Diagnosis and management of infantile Marfan syndrome. Pediatrics 86:888, 1990.

31. Dominguez R, Weisgrau RA, Santamaria M: Pulmonary hyperinflation and emphysema in infants with the Marfan syndrome. Pediatr Radiol 17:365, 1987.

32. Gillinov AM, Hulyalkar A, Cameron DE, et al: Mitral valve operation in patients with the Marfan syndrome. J Thorac Cardiovasc Surg 107:724, 1994.

33. Marsalese DL, Moodie DA, Vacante M, et al: Marfan's syndrome: Natural history and long-term follow-up of cardiovascular involvement. J Am Coll Cardiol 14:422, 1989.

34. Murdoch JL, Walker BA, Halpern BL, et al: Life expectancy and causes of death in the Marfan syndrome. N Engl J Med 286:804, 1972.

35. Savolainen A, Kupari M, Toivonen L, et al: Abnormal ambulatory electrocardiographic findings in patients with the Marfan syndrome. J Intern Med 241:221, 1997.

36. Cipolloni PB, Shane SR, Marshall RJ: Chronic atrial flutter in brothers with the Marfan syndrome. Circulation 31:572, 1965.

37. Patton DJ, Galliani CA, Johnson WH Jr, Hedlund GL: Sudden death in Marfan syndrome. AJR Am J Roentgenol 165:160, 1995.

38. Boxer RA, LaCorte MA, Singh S, et al: Evaluation of the aorta in the Marfan syndrome by magnetic resonance imaging. Am Heart J 111:1001, 1985.

39. Cigarroa JE, Isselbacher EM, DeSanctis RW, Eagle KA: Diagnostic imaging in the evaluation of suspected aortic dissection. N Engl J Med 328:35, 1993.

40. Simpson IA, de Belder MA, Treasure T, et al: Cardiovascular manifestations of Marfan's syndrome: Improved evaluation by transoesophageal echocardiography. Br Heart J 69:104, 1993.

41. Ballal RS, Nanda NC, Gatewood R, et al: Usefulness of transesophageal echocardiography in assessment of aortic dissection. Circulation 84:1903, 1991.

42. Silverman DI, Burton KJ, Gray J, et al: Life expectancy in the Marfan syndrome. Am J Cardiol 75:157, 1995.

43. Bain MA, Zumwalt RE, van der Bel-Khan J: Marfan syndrome presenting as aortic rupture in a young athlete: Sudden unexpected death? Am J Forensic Med Pathol 8:334, 1987.

44. Reed CM, Alpert BS: Assessment of ventricular performance after chronic beta-adrenergic blockade in the Marfan syndrome. Am J Cardiol 70:541, 1992.

45. Shores J, Berger KR, Murphy EA, Pyeritz RE: Progression of aortic dilation and the benefit of long-term beta-adrenergic blocade in Marfan's syndrome. N Engl J Med 330:1335, 1994.

46. Salim MA, Alpert BS, Ward JC, Pyertiz RE: Effect of beta-adrenergic blockade on aortic root rate of dilation in the Marfan syndrome. Am J Cardiol 74:629, 1994.

47. Alpert BS, Reed CM, Ward JC, et al: Atenolol reduces aortic growth in the Marfan syndrome (Abstract). Pediatr Res 29:14A, 1991.

48. Antman EM: Current diagnosis and prescription for Marfan syndrome: When to operate. J Card Surg 9(suppl):174, 1994.

49. Pyeritz RE: Marfan syndrome: Current and future clinical and genetic management of cardiovascular manifestations. Semin Thorac Cardiovasc Surg 5:11, 1993.

50. Child AH: Marfan syndrome-current medical and genetic knowledge: How to treat and when. J Card Surg 12:131, 1997.

51. Bachet J, Termingon JL, Goudot B, et al: Aortic root replacement with a composite graft. Eur J Cardiothorac Surg 10:207, 1996.

52. Finkbohner R, Johnston D, Crawford S, et al: Marfan syndrome: Long-term survival and complications after aortic aneurysm repair. Circulation 91:728, 1995.

53. Gott VL, Cameron DE, Reitz BA, Pyeritz RE: Current diagnosis and prescription for the Marfan syndrome: Aortic root and valve replacement. J Card Surg 9(suppl):177, 1994.

54. Gillinov AM, Zehr KJ, Redmond JM, et al: Cardiac operations in children with Marfan's syndrome: Indications and results. Ann Thorac Surg 64:1140, 1997.

55. Kronisch RL, Flowers FM, Ball RT: Medicolegal challenges of advising at-risk patients. The example of Marfan's syndrome. Physician Sports Med 22:37, 1994.

56. Lipscomb KJ, Smith JC, Clarke B, et al: Outcome of pregnancy in women with Marfan's syndrome. Br J Obstet Gynaecol 104:201, 1997.

57. Pyeritz RE: Maternal and fetal complications of pregnancy in the Marfan syndrome. Am J Med 71:784, 1981.

58. Elkayam U, Ostrzega E, Shotan A, Mehra A: Cardiovascular problems in pregnant women with the Marfan syndrome. Ann Intern Med 123:117, 1995.

59. Child AH: Management of pregnancy in Marfan syndrome, Ehlers-Danlos syndrome, and other heritable connective tissue disorders. *In* Oakley C (ed): Heart Disease in Pregnancy. London, Br Med J Pub Group, 1997, p 153–179.

60. Kainulainen K, Steinmann B, Collins F, et al: Marfan syndrome: No evidence for heterogeneity in different populations, and more precise mapping of the gene. Am J Hum Genet 49:662, 1991.

61. Dietz HC, Pyeritz RE: Mutations in human gene for fibrillin-1 (*FBN1*) in the Marfan syndrome and related disorders. Hum Mol Genet 4:1799, 1995.

62. Dietz HC, Pyeritz RE, Francomano CA, et al: Marfan phenotype variability in a family segregating a missense mutation in the EGF-like motif of the fibrillin gene. J Clin Invest 89:1674, 1992.

63. Hayward C, Brock DJH: Fibrillin-1 mutations in Marfan syndrome and other type-1 fibrillinopathies. Hum Mutat 10:415, 1997.

64. Collod G, Babron MC, Jondau G, et al: A second locus for Marfan syndrome maps to chromosome 3p24.2–p25. Nat Genet 8:264, 1994.

65. Boileau C, Jondeau G, Babron MC, et al: Autosomal dominant Marfan-like connective-tissue disorder with aortic dilation and skeletal anomalies not linked to the fibrillin genes. Am J Hum Genet 53:46, 1993.

66. Francke U, Berg MA, Tynan MA, et al: A gly1127ser mutation in an EGF-like domain of the fibrillin-1 gene is a risk factor for ascending aortic aneurysm and dissection. Am J Hum Genet 56:1287, 1995.

67. Booms P, Vetter U, Robinson PN: A novel FBN1 gene mutation in an EGF-like motif in a patient with ectopia lentis. Eur J Pediatr 155:739, 1996.

68. Sood S, Eldadah ZA, Krause WL, et al: Mutation in fibrillin-1 and the Marfanoid-craniosynostosis (Shprintzen-Goldberg) syndrome. Nat Genet 12:209, 1996.

69. Anderson RA, Koch S, Camerini-Otero D: Cardiovascular findings in congenital contractural arachnodactyly: Report of an affected kindred. Am J Med Genet 18:265, 1984.

70. Putnam EA, Zhang H, Ramirez F, Milewicz DM: Fibrillin-2 (FBN2) mutations result in the Marfan-like disorder, congenital contractural arachnodactyly. Nat Genet 11:456, 1995.

71. Skovby F: The homocystinurias. In Royce P, Steinmann B (eds): Connective Tissue and Its Heritable Disorders. New York, Wiley-Liss, 1993, p 469–486.

72. Gorlin RJ, Cohen MM Jr, Lewin LS: Syndromes with craniosynostosis: Miscellaneous syndromes. In Gorlin RJ, Cohen MM Jr, Lewin LS (eds): Syndromes of the Head and Neck, 3rd ed. New York, Oxford University Press, 1990, p 541–564.

73. Milewicz DM, Chen H, Park ES, et al: Reduced penetrance and variable expressivity of familial thoracic aortic aneurysms/dissections. Am J Cardiol 82:474, 1998.

74. Nicod P, Bloor C, Godfrey M, et al: Familial aortic dissecting aneurysm. J Am Coll Cardiol 13:811, 1989.

75. Kontusaari S, Tromp G, Kuivaniemi H, et al: A mutation in the gene for type III procollagen (COL3A1) in a family with aortic aneurysms. J Clin Invest 86:1465, 1990.

76. Milewicz DM, Michael K, Fisher N, et al: Fibrillin-1 (FBN1) mutations in patients with thoracic aortic aneurysms. Circulation 94:2708, 1996.

77. Beighton P, de Paepe A, Danks D, et al: International nosology of heritable disorders of connective tissue, Berlin, 1986. Am J Med Genet 29:581, 1988.

78. Beighton P, De Paepe A, Steinmann B, et al: Ehlers-Danlos syndromes: Revised nosology, Villefranche, 1997. Am J Med Genet 77:31, 1998.

79. Hollister DW: Heritable disorders of connective tissue: Ehlers-Danlos syndrome. Pediatr Clin North Am 25:575, 1978.

80. Beighton P: The Ehlers-Danlos Syndrome. London, William Heinemann, 1970.

81. Sevenich M, Schultz-Ehrenburg U, Orfanos CE: Ehlers-Danlos syndrome: A disease of fibroblasts and collagen fibrils. Arch Dermatol Res 267:237, 1980.

82. Vogel A, Holbrook KA, Steinmann B, et al: Abnormal collagen fibril structure in the gravis form (type I) of the Ehlers-Danlos syndrome. Lab Invest 40:201, 1979.

83. Byers PH, Holbrook KA: Molecular basis of clinical heterogeneity in the Ehlers-Danlos syndrome. Ann N Y Acad Sci 460:298, 1985.

84. Wechsler HL, Fisher ER: Ehlers-Danlos syndrome. Pathologic, histochemical and electron microscopic observations. Arch Pathol 77:613, 1964.

85. Steinmann B, Royce PM, Superti-Furga A: The Ehlers-Danlos syndrome. In Royce P, Steinmann B (eds): Connective Tissue and Its Heritable Disorders. New York, Wiley-Liss, 1993, p 351–407.

86. Sacheti A, Szemere J, Bernstein B, et al: Chronic pain is a manifestation of the Ehlers-Danlos syndrome. J Pain Symptom Manage 14:88, 1997.

87. Leier CV, Call TD, Fulkerson PK, Wooley CF: The spectrum of cardiac defects in the Ehlers-Danlos syndrome, types I and III. Ann Intern Med 92(pt 1):171, 1980.

88. Dolan AL, Mishra MB, Chambers JB, Grahame R: Clinical and echocardiographic survey of the Ehlers-Danlos syndrome. Br J Rheumatol 36:459, 1997.

89. Shohet I, Rosenbaum I, Frand M, et al: Cardiovascular complications in the Ehlers-Danlos syndrome with minimal external findings. Clin Genet 31:148, 1987.

90. Owen SM, Durst RD: Ehlers-Danlos syndrome simulating child abuse. Arch Dermatol 120:97, 1984.

91. Snyder RR, Gilstrap LC, Hauth JC: Ehlers-Danlos syndrome and pregnancy. Obstet Gynecol 61:649, 1983.

92. Hordnes K: Ehlers-Danlos syndrome and delivery. Acta Obstet Gynecol Scand 73:671, 1994.

93. Michalickova K, Susic M, Willing MC, et al: Mutations of the alpha2(V) chain of type V collagen impair matrix assembly and produce Ehlers-Danlos syndrome type I. Hum Mol Genet 7:249, 1998.

94. De Paepe A, Nuytinck L, Hausser I, et al: Mutations in the COL5A1 gene are causal in the Ehlers-Danlos syndromes I and II. Am J Hum Genet 60:547, 1997.

95. Sokolov BP, Prytkov AN, Tromp G, et al: Exclusion of COL1A1, COL1A2, and COL3A1 genes as candidate genes for Ehlers-Danlos syndrome type I in one large family. Hum Genet 88:125, 1991.

96. Wordsworth BP, Ogilvie DJ, Sykes BC: Segregation analysis of the structural genes of the major fibrillar collagens provides further evidence of molecular heterogeneity in type II Ehlers-Danlos syndrome. Br J Rheumatol 30:173, 1991.

97. Wordsworth P, Ogilvie D, Smith R, Sykes B: Exclusion of the alpha1(II) collagen structural gene as the mutant locus in type II Ehlers-Danlos syndrome. Ann Rheum Dis 44:431, 1985.

98. Kivirikko KI: Collagens and their abnormalities in a wide spectrum of diseases. Ann Med 25:113, 1993.

99. Byers PH: Ehlers-Danlos syndrome: Recent advances and current understanding of the clinical and genetic heterogeneity. J Invest Dermatol 103:47S, 1994.

100. Lauwers G, Nevelsteen A, Daenen G, et al: Ehlers-Danlos syndrome type IV: A heterogenous disease. Ann Vasc Surg 11:178, 1997.

101. Superti-Furga A, Saesseli B, Steinmann B, Bollinger A: Microangiopathy in Ehlers-Danlos syndrome type IV. Int J Microcirc Clin Exp 11:241, 1992.

102. North KN, Whiteman DAH, Pepin MG, Byers PH: Cerebrovascular complications in Ehlers-Danlos syndrome type IV. Ann Neurol 38:960, 1995.

103. Hunter GC, Malone JM, Moore WS, et al: Vascular manifestations in patients with Ehlers-Danlos syndrome. Arch Surg 117:495, 1982.

104. Lach B, Nair SG: Spontaneous carotid cavernous fistula and multiple arterial dissections in type IV Ehlers-Danlos syndrome. J Neurosurg 66:462, 1987.

105. Kitazono T, Imaizumi T, Imayama S, et al: Two cases of myocardial infarction in type 4 Ehlers-Danlos syndrome. Chest 95:1274, 1989.

106. Crowther MA, Lach B, Dunmore PJ, Roach MR: Vascular collagen fibril morphology in type IV Ehlers-Danlos syndrome. Connect Tissue Res 25:209, 1991.

107. Cikrit DF, Miles JH, Silver D: Spontaneous arterial perforation: The Ehlers-Danlos specter. J Vasc Surg 5:248, 1987.

108. Eriksen UH, Aunsholt NA, Nielsen TT: Enormous right coronary arterial aneurysm in a patient with type IV Ehlers-Danlos syndrome. Int J Cardiol 35:259, 1992.

109. Ades LC, Waltham RD, Chiodo AA, Bateman JF: Myocardial infarction resulting from coronary artery dissection in an adolescent with Ehlers-Danlos syndrome type IV due to a type III collagen mutation. Br Heart J 74:112, 1995.

110. Byard RW, Keeley FW, Smith CR: Type IV Ehlers-Danlos syndrome presenting as sudden infant death. Am J Clin Pathol 93:579, 1990.

111. Pope FM, Narcisi P, Nicholls AC, et al: Clinical presentations of Ehlers Danlos syndrome type IV. Arch Dis Child 63:1016, 1988.

112. Kashiwagi H, Riddle JM, Abraham JP: Functional and ultrastructural abnormalities of platelets in Ehlers-Danlos syndrome. Ann Intern Med 63:249, 1965.

113. Day HJ, Xarafonetis CJD: Coagulation studies in four patients with Ehlers-Danlos syndrome. Am J Med Sci 242:565, 1961.

114. Hartsfield JK Jr, Kousseff BG: Phenotypic overlap of Ehlers-Danlos syndrome types IV and VIII. Am J Med Genet 37:465, 1990.

115. Jaffe AS, Geltman EM, Rodey GE, Uitto J: Mitral valve prolapse: A consistent manifestation of type IV Ehlers-Danlos syndrome. Circulation 64:121, 1981.

116. Freeman RK, Swegle J, Sise MJ: The surgical complications of Ehlers-Danlos syndrome. Am Surg 62:869, 1994.

117. Bergqvist D: Ehlers-Danlos type IV syndrome. A review from a vascular surgical point of view. Eur J Surg 162:163, 1996.

118. Ayres JG, Pope FM, Reidy JF, Clark TFH: Abnormalities of the lungs and thoracic cage in the Ehlers-Danlos syndrome. Thorax 40:300, 1985.

119. Rudd NL, Holbrook KA, Nimrod C, et al: Pregnancy complications in type IV of Ehlers-Danlos syndrome. Lancet 1:50, 1983.

120. Sparkman RS: Ehlers-Danlos syndrome type IV: Dramatic, deceptive, and deadly. Am J Surg 147:703, 1984.

121. Mattar SG, Kumar AG, Lumsden AB: Vascular complications in Ehlers-Danlos syndrome. Am Surg 60:827, 1994.

122. Pepin MG, Superti-Furga A, Beyers PH: Natural history of Ehlers-Danlos syndrome type IV (EDS type IV): Review of 137 cases (Abstract). Am J Hum Genet 51:A44, 1992.

123. Porey S, Falk CT: Report of the committee on the genetic constitution of chromosome 2. Cytogenet Cell Genet 51:91, 1989.

124. Superti-Furga A, Steinmann B, Ramirez F, Byers PH: Molecular defects of type III procollagen in Ehlers-Danlos syndrome type IV. Hum Genet 82:104, 1989.

125. Tsipouras P, Ramirex F: Genetic disorders of collagen. J Med Genet 24:2, 1987.

126. Beighton P: Cardiac abnormalities in the Ehlers-Danlos syndrome. Br Heart J 31:227, 1969.

127. Pinnell SR, Krane SM, Zenzora JE, Glimcher MJ: A heritable disorder of connective tissue: Hydroxylysine-deficient collagen disease. N Engl J Med 286:1013, 1972.

128. Sussman M, Lichtenstein JR, Nigra TP, et al: Hydroxylysine-deficient collagen in a patient with a form of Ehlers-Danlos syndrome. J Bone Joint Surg Am 56:1228, 1974.

129. Pemberton JW, Freeman HM, Schepens CL: Familial retinal detachment and the Ehlers-Danlos syndrome. Arch Opthalmol 76:817, 1966.

130. Arneson MA, Hammerschmidt DE, Furcht LT, King RA: A new form of Ehlers-Danlos syndrome: Fibronectin corrects defective platelet function. JAMA 244:144, 1980.

131. Hammerschmidt DE, Arneson MA, Larson SL, et al: Maternal Ehlers-Danlos syndrome type X. JAMA 248:2487, 1982.

132. Cole WG: The molecular pathology of osteogenesis imperfecta. Clin Orthop 343:235, 1997.

133. Kocher MS, Shapiro F: Osteogenesis imperfecta. J Am Acad Orthop Surg 6:225, 1998.

134. Pyeritz RE, Levin LS: Aortic root dilatation and valvular dysfunction in osteogenesis imperfecta. Circulation 69:311, 1981.

135. Stein D, Kloster FE: Valvular heart disease in osteogenesis imperfecta. Am Heart J 94:637, 1977.

136. Struk B, Neldne KH, Rao VS, et al: Mapping of both autosomal recessive and dominant variants of pseudoxanthoma elasticum to chromosome 16p13.1. Hum Mol Genet 6:1823, 1997.

137. Lebwohl MG, Distefano D, Prioleau PG, et al: Pseudoxanthoma elasticum and mitral-valve prolapse. N Engl J Med 307:228, 1982.

138. Liberfarb R, Goldblatt A: Prevalence of mitral-valve prolapse in the Stickler syndrome. Am J Med Genet 24:387, 1986.

139. Kevorkian JP, Masquet C, Kural-Menasche S, et al: New report of severe coronary artery disease in an eighteen-year-old girl with pseudoxanthoma elasticum. Case report and review of the literature. Angiology 48:735, 1997.

140. Lebwohl M, Halperin J, Phelps RG: Brief report: Occult pseudoxanthoma elasticum in patients with premature cardiovascular disease. N Engl J Med 329:1237, 1993.

141. Challenor VF, Conway N, Monro JL: The surgical treatment of restrictive cardiomyopathy in pseudoxanthoma elasticum. Br Heart J 59:266, 1988.

142. Gross DM, Williams JC, Caprioli C, et al: Echocardiographic abnormalities in the mucopolysaccharide storage diseases. Am J Cardiol 61:170, 1988.

143. Krovetz LJ, Lorincz AE, Schiebler GL: Cardiovascular manifestations of the Hurler syndrome: Hemodynamic and angiocardiographic observations in 15 patients. Circulation 31:132, 1965.

144. Wraith JE, Rogers JG, Danks DM: The mucopolysaccharidoses. Aust Paediatr 23:239, 1987.

145. Young D, Harper PS: The natural history of the severe form of Hunter's syndrome: A study based on 52 cases. Dev Med Child Neurol 25:481, 1983.

146. Brosius FC, Roberts WC: Coronary artery disease in the Hurler syndrome: Qualitative and quantitative analysis of the extent of coronary narrowing at necropsy in six children. Am J Cardiol 47:649, 1981.

147. Donaldson MD, Pennock CA, Berry PJ, et al: Hurler syndrome with cardiomyopathy in infancy. J Pediatr 114:430, 1989.

148. Whitley CB: The mucopolysaccharidoses. *In* Beighton P (ed): McKusick's Heritable Disorders of Connective Tissue, New York, Mosby–Year Book, 1993, p 367–499.

CHAPTER 59
CARDIAC TUMORS

JACK L. TITUS   JESSE E. EDWARDS

Tumors and tumor-like conditions of the heart and pericardium are rare. Some cardiac tumors are hamartomas, and others are heterotopias (choristomas) related to abnormality in development of the heart.

CLASSIFICATION AND FREQUENCIES

Reported frequencies of primary cardiac tumors in general autopsy series range from 0.001% (1 per 100,000) to 0.03% (1 per 30,000).[1,2] In general, secondary (metastatic) tumors of the heart and pericardium are significantly more frequent than primary tumors by a ratio between 100:1 and 1000:1.

The primary cardiac tumors that occur most often in children are (in order of frequency) the benign tumors rhabdomyoma, fibroma, myxoma, teratoma (mainly pericardial), hemangioma, atrioventricular (AV) nodal tumor (AV nodal cystic tumor, "mesothelioma"), and arrhythmogenic hamartoma (histiocytoid cardiomyopathy, Purkinje cell tumor). In infants and children, other benign tumors or tumor-like conditions such as lipoma, fibrolipoma, bronchogenic cyst (not teratoma), hemangioma, and lymphangioma are even more rare. Malignant primary cardiac tumors in the young occur with one-fourth the frequency of benign tumors. They are usually sarcomas, most often rhabdomyosarcoma,[1,2] but fibrosarcoma, angiosarcoma, leiomyosarcoma, and malignant teratoma also occur, as do unclassified lesions.

CLINICAL FEATURES

Clinical features of cardiac tumors in infants and children vary from clinically silent lesions without signs or symptoms to those mimicking congenital malformations of the cardiovascular system, collagen vascular disease, infective endocarditis, or viral pericarditis. Rarely, sudden unexpected death may be the first symptom. Cardiovascular tumors may be identified in utero for various reasons, including incidental to a fetal ultrasound examination, a fetal cardiac arrhythmia, nonimmune hydrops fetalis, or a family history of conditions such as tuberous sclerosis in which a cardiac tumor or tumor-like conditions involving the heart may occur.

Cardiac tumors may cause congestive heart failure by different mechanisms. Among these are compression of the great veins by large pericardial masses or effusions, a large volume of cardiac muscle replaced by tumor, and obstruction of inflow or outflow of cardiac chambers by a tumor that may distort or almost occlude a valve or an inflow or outflow tract. In addition to the usual signs and symptoms of heart failure, afflicted patients may have syncope, anginal chest pain, and a variety of heart murmurs.

When pulmonary venous return to the left atrium is obstructed or embolization of tumor or thrombus from right-sided tumors is present in the pulmonary arterial bed, pulmonary hypertension may develop. Glomerulomegaly, juxtaglomerular hyperplasia with excessive erythropoietin production, and polycythemia may result. Polycythemia may also result from chronic hypoxemia or from right-to-left shunting. Turbulence may cause destruction of formed blood elements, leading to thrombocytopenia and hemolytic anemia in some patients with "mobile" intracardiac tumors.

Embolization of tumor, mostly from left atrial myxomas, may occur to the brain, kidneys, spleen, extremities, and coronary arteries. Aneurysm or infarct may result from tumor emboli and may be fatal. Pulmonary embolism from right-sided tumors may lead to pulmonary hypertension.

Fever, malaise, weight loss, polymyositis, Raynaud's phenomenon, hepatic dysfunction, hyperglobulinemia, and elevated sedimentation rate may be manifestations of cardiac myxoma. These manifestations, often associated with peripheral embolism, suggest collagen vascular disease or infective endocarditis. Systemic symptoms have been related to autoimmune reactions and an altered response to tumor breakdown products, tissue necrosis, or hemorrhage. Cytokines, such as interleukin-6, may play a role in the genesis of some of these constitutional manifestations.

Tachyarrhythmias are relatively common with cardiac tumors. They may be supraventricular or ventricular in origin. The myocardial tumor itself may be the source of an arrhythmia. Involvement of the cardiac conduction system, as with the AV nodal hamartomatous tumor (mesothelioma of the AV node), may cause heart block, Stokes-Adams syncope, or sudden unexpected death. Sudden death may also result from arrhythmia, rupture of an aneurysm secondary to tumor embolization, embolic occlusion of a coronary artery or a valve, or tumor emboli of sufficient number or size to a critical organ.

PRIMARY BENIGN CARDIAC TUMORS

Important familial, syndromic, and genetic features relate to some cardiovascular tumors, specifically cardiac rhabdomyoma, lipoma, fibroma, and myxoma.[2]

RHABDOMYOMA

Rhabdomyoma (Fig. 59–1A) is a cardiac myocytic hamartoma (thus, a congenital tumor) composed of large, vacuolated, glycogen-rich cardiac muscle cells that form a well-circumscribed but not truly encapsulated nodule in the myocardium. It is the most common cardiac tumor in infants and children. The tumor cells are abnormal myocytes but are not Purkinje cell derivatives. Although the cells contain large amounts of glycogen, the tumor is not a form of glycogen storage disease.

Typically, the tumor cells are larger than adjacent myocytes. Sparse cytoplasm of cardiac muscle type is often concentrated about the large bland nucleus. Cytoplasmic extensions from the central perinuclear cytoplasm toward the periphery of the cell cross the glycogen-rich vacuolated cytoplasm, creating the appearance termed spider cell (Fig. 59–1B).

These congenital tumors may be small (<1 mm) or large (3 to 8 cm), and they may be single or multiple in the heart. Although they may be in any chamber, they are most common in the left ventricle and ventricular septum. The tumors may be entirely intramural or may project into a chamber as a large mass that may obstruct inflow or outflow tracts.

Cardiac rhabdomyomas are common in patients with tuberous sclerosis, the hamartomatous-neoplastic condition with the classic triad of seizures, mental retardation, and angiofibromas. At least 50% (and probably a higher number) of patients with rhabdomyoma have tuberous sclerosis. Apparent decrease of the frequency of cardiac rhabdomyoma in older patients with tuberous sclerosis is probably related to the known spontaneous regression of rhabdomyoma.

Many cardiac rhabdomyomas are isolated. A smaller number are associated with structural congenital cardiac anomalies. In the sporadic disease (i.e., no major associated developmental abnormality), the clinical presentation includes significant obstructions to blood flow that simulate tricuspid, pulmonic, mitral, or aortic atresia or severe stenosis. Arrhythmias may result from the rhabdomyoma. The sporadic tumors are single in about half of patients so that surgical excision for cure may be feasible. Surgically excised tumors do not regrow. Even without total excision, resection of the intracavitary obstructing part of the tumor may be beneficial.

The prognosis for untreated cardiac rhabdomyoma is poor. More than half die in the first month of life, and about three fourths or more of untreated patients die in the first year of life.

FIBROMA

Fibroma is the second most common cardiac tumor in children. It is a benign, usually discrete tumor mass composed of mature fibroblasts and collagen. Usually, fibroma is solitary; rarely, two tumors may be present. Both genders and all ages are affected, but 80% are in children. It has been reported in neonates in association with other abnormalities.[2] Signs and symptoms relate to size and location of the tumor. Arrhythmias and sudden death have been related to involvement of the cardiac conduction system. Heart failure may result from replacement of myocardium by tumor, obstruction of inflow or outflow of the ventricle, or compromise of the ventricular cavity. Locations in decreasing order of frequency are ventricular septum, anterior and lateral wall of left ventricle, posterior wall of left ventricle, and right ventricle.[2] The atria are rarely involved.

Partial excision of tumors obstructing inflow or outflow of a ventricular chamber may result in long-term survival. Spontaneous regression has been described. Large intramural tumors of the left ventricle have been successfully resected, and ablation of re-entrant ventricular tachycardia due to a left ventricular fibroma has been reported. Once resected, the lesions usually do not recur. Fibromas rarely

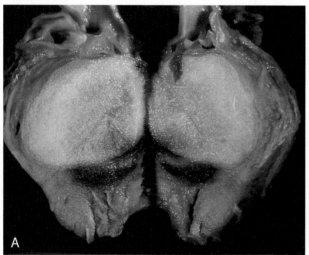
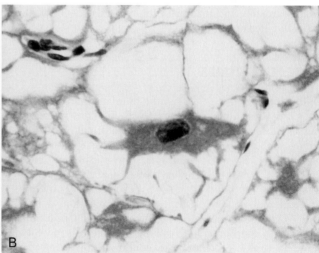

FIGURE 59–1

A, Cut surface of the ventricular septum demonstrates a large rhabdomyoma of the ventricular system. *B*, Photomicrograph of this tumor demonstrates typical "spider cell" (*center*) (hematoxylin-eosin stain).

occur in association with congenital cardiovascular malformations, and when they do, the association appears to be coincidental. A 14% frequency of cardiac fibroma is found in the Gorlin syndrome of nevoid basal cell carcinoma.[2]

The tumors are more or less round, fibrous, yellow to white masses that may be focally calcified. On the cut surface, a whorled appearance is often seen (Fig. 59–2). The lesions are usually well demarcated from adjacent myocardium and easily shelled out, but many have margins "pushing" into the myocardium in an infiltrating fashion.

In infants and children, plump fibroblasts are present on histologic examination in a slightly myxoid stroma with mature collagen. With age, tumor cellularity decreases and mature collagen, often with a whorled appearance, increases. Blood vessels in the tumor are usually small and few. Myocardial cells surrounding the lesion have hypertrophy.

Most authors regard the cardiac fibroma as a hamartoma, not a true neoplasm, because partial resection may not be followed by recurrence. Patients with typical cardiac fibromas do not have generalized fibromatosis, but this tumor might be a form of isolated fibromatosis.[2]

MYXOMA

Myxoma ranks third in frequency of benign primary cardiac tumors in children, although it is the most common cardiac tumor in adults, in whom it accounts for about half of all primary cardiac tumors and 75 to 80% in operative series.[1] The histogenesis of this tumor is uncertain; it is not derived from organization of a thrombus, and it is histologically distinct from the usual soft tissue myxoma.[1,2]

Cardiac myxomas occur on endocardial surfaces. They vary in shape, size, basilar attachments, and color, depending on the prominence of different tissues in the matrix. Myxomas are usually pedunculated (Fig. 59–3), often arising from a relatively narrow stalk, and commonly form a polypoid, friable mass in the cardiac chamber. Some have

smooth surfaces and a broad base. Most myxomas are soft, gelatinous, and gray-white or red-purple. Large foci of hemorrhage or apparent infarction with fibrosis are often present (Fig. 59–3). Focal calcifications are common (Fig. 59–3). Fibrin thrombi may be present focally on the surface of some tumors. The average size of myxomas varies from 1 cm to approximately 6 cm, although larger tumors with a maximum dimension of 15 cm have been observed in adults.

The histologic hallmark is the cardiac myxoma cell (so-called lepidic cell) in the myxomatous matrix of the tumor. The cells are polygonal (polyhedral) or stellate, with a small amount of eosinophilic or amphophilic cytoplasm and bland nuclei without mitoses. Cellularity of myxomas varies greatly, both among tumors and within the same tumor.

The myxoid stroma usually has some collagen and reticular or elastic fibers. Extramedullary hematopoiesis may be found. The myxoid stroma is composed of chondroitin sulfate A and C, with lesser amounts of hyaluronic acid.

Electron microscopic studies show that the cardiac myxoma cell resembles a multipotential mesenchymal cell, with a well-developed Golgi apparatus and prominent rough endoplasmic reticulum. Immunohistochemical staining of the gland-like structures demonstrates cytokeratin, epithelial membrane antigen, and carcinoembryonic antigen. The glands in some myxomas may represent entrapped endodermal (foregut) rests. These and other immunohistochemical findings have been interpreted to confirm the neoplastic nature of myxomas originating from multipotential cells that have differentiated along different mesenchymal lines.

More than 90% of myxomas are in the atria, with most (70 to 75%) in the left atrium. The infrequent ventricular tumors are divided equally between right and left ventricles. In the atria, 90% of myxomas originate from the atrial

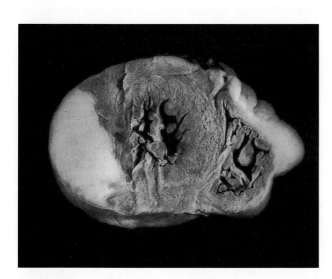

FIGURE 59–2

A large left ventricular fibroma (white area) occupies the left ventricular lateral wall.

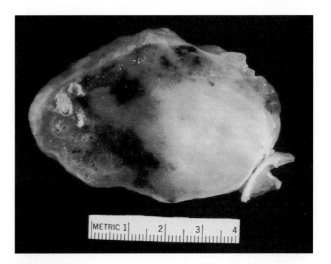

FIGURE 59–3

Cut surface of a large left atrial myxoma has foci of calcium (white material near surface toward 9 o'clock), foci of hemorrhage (dark material), cysts, and a large area of nearly acellular matrix (white area of right half of tumor). A cuff of atrial septum on the right of the tumor at 4 o'clock shows attachment of the tumor to the septum.

septum in the region opposite the fossa ovalis, whereas only 10% of ventricular tumors are on the ventricular septum. Cardiac myxomas originating from cardiac valves have been reported in small numbers, but the existence of true myxomas of valves has been disputed, although a few appear to be convincing examples.

Clinical presentation is usually one of three types: obstructive (usually mitral valvar); embolic; and constitutional, often resembling a collagen vascular disease.[2] Calcified and petrified tumors may be found incidental to routine cardiac radiography in adults. In children, the symptoms and signs may mimic congenital cardiac malformations.

In children, the gender distribution of cardiac myxomas is about equal. The tumors have been found at any age, including the newborn period. A left atrial myxoma may cause injury of the mitral valve, leading to fibrotic repair and deformity of the valve as a result of a "wrecker-ball" phenomenon of the mobile, pedunculated tumor.

Among cardiac tumors, the myxoma is associated with several specific syndromes. These include a familial form (the Carney complex), the LAMB (lentigenes of face and vulva, atrial myxoma, mucocutaneous myxoma, blue nevi) syndrome, and the NAME (nevi, atrial myxoma, ephelis) syndrome. The syndromic myxomas occur at younger ages than do the apparently sporadic tumors.

TERATOMA

Teratomas of the heart are rare, and most are intrapericardial rather than myocardial. By definition, they contain endodermal, mesodermal, and ectodermal elements. If only one or two germ cell layers are represented, the tumor may be a bronchogenic cyst rather than a teratoma.

In infants and children, two thirds of patients with intrapericardial teratoma are female. In contrast to adults, pediatric patients usually have respiratory distress, pericardial tamponade, and often cyanosis.

A few cardiac teratomas are entirely intramyocardial. All or nearly all reported teratomas occur in neonates or young children, most of whom die of the effects of the tumor. Sudden death may occur when the tumor is in the ventricular septum, as it usually is. The ventricular septal tumor may bulge into the right or less often the left ventricle. Different tissue cells line the cysts present in teratomas; the intervening solid areas have a myxoid stroma with multiple different tissues in both intramyocardial and intrapericardial teratomas.

Intrapericardial teratomas are huge, multicystic tumors that displace the heart. They are usually on the right side of the heart, displacing the heart leftward. An arterial blood supply comes from the aorta.

In both locations, cardiac teratomas are most often histologically benign lesions. With teratomas in either site, however, malignant foci are germ cell derivatives, such as embryonal carcinoma, choriocarcinoma, squamous carcinoma arising in the teratoma, and endodermal sinus tumor.

Surgical excision has been successful for pericardial teratomas. Partial resection has been beneficial for intramyocardial tumors even if complete removal could not be accomplished.

HEMANGIOMA

Hemangiomas are benign tumors of blood vessels that are classified histologically as cavernous (composed of dilated thin-walled vessels), capillary, and arteriovenous (composed of dysplastic arteries and veins) types. Cardiac hemangiomas often have features of all three types. They are rare cardiac tumors constituting 5 to 10% of benign cardiac tumors.[1] About 15% involve the epicardium or pericardium.

In the heart, these tumors occur at all ages and appear to be more frequent in males. Most often, they are asymptomatic and found incidentally at surgery or autopsy. They have been reported to cause, or to be associated with, arrhythmias, heart failure, outflow obstruction, and coronary arterial insufficiency. Cardiac hemangiomas may be found in any cardiac chamber. Surgical resection has been reported in several patients.[1]

ATRIOVENTRICULAR NODAL TUMOR

AV nodal tumor and cystic tumor of the AV node are the preferred terms for this tumor. The historical term mesothelioma is considered to be inaccurate. Most evidence today suggests that these tumors are of endodermal origin.[1,2] It is the only known tumor of the cardiac conduction system. AV nodal tumors have been reported at all ages, including the neonatal period. It has been reported more frequently in females by a ratio of 3:1. Clinical manifestations include heart block, Stokes-Adams syndrome, ventricular fibrillation (palpitations), angina, congestive heart failure, and sudden unexpected death. Reported associated congenital anomalies in children include hydrocephalus, ventricular septal defect, and multicystic ovaries.

The tumors often are not suspected at gross morphologic examination of the heart and are found only by specific study of the cardiac conduction system. Sometimes an area of thickening or a small nodule may be noted in the floor of the right atrium near the expected site of the AV node. Histologic sections through this area demonstrate the cystic tumor (Fig. 59–4).

On histologic examination, nests of cells form small cysts that contain seromucoid fluid. The lining cells are cuboidal, squamous, or transitional and sometimes layered. The irregularly shaped nests and cysts may "invade" or displace or replace contiguous myocardium. Both the AV node and the junctional zone of node–His bundle are often replaced in whole or in part by the tumor. Although most are diagnosed at autopsy in patients who had known heart block or suffered sudden unexpected death, there is one report of apparently successful surgical excision.[1]

ARRHYTHMOGENIC HAMARTOMA

Arrhythmogenic hamartomas (histiocytoid cardiomyopathy) are generally multiple, small, tumor-like lesions associated with recurrent episodes of life-threatening tachyarrhythmias.[3] The lesions are usually found in neonates or infants from birth to about 4 years of age, as a result of electrophysiologic study (with surgical removal or electrical ablation) or in infants who suffered sudden death.

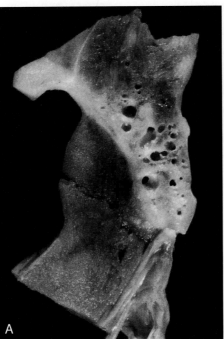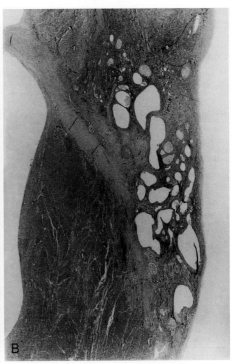

A, Block of tissue from the atrioventricular (AV) septum viewed from posterior (inferior) side of block with AV nodal tumor. Atrial septum is upper, and ventricular septum is lower, with a small amount of tricuspid valve and chordae tendineae. The cystic tissue (tumor) replaces the AV node. *B*, Histologic section from the tissue block shows cystic tumor on the right side of the AV septum *(right)* occupying region of AV node. Ventricular septal myocardium is below the fibrous (gray) tissue of the AV ring on the left and midportion of the photograph (hematoxylin-eosin stain).

The tumor nodules are small, usually less than 2 to 3 mm in size, yellow-white, soft lesions scattered in the myocardium, endocardium, and epicardium in different patients. The left ventricle is nearly always involved. The nodules are usually well circumscribed, but sometimes the tumor cells are scattered among adjacent normal myocytes. The cells are not rhabdomyoma cells, nor are they derived from histiocytes. At this time, the majority view is that the cells are derived from embryonic cardiac myocytes or Purkinje cells,[1–3] thus being a type of hamartoma.

OTHER BENIGN TUMORS

Other benign tumors or tumor-like conditions of the heart occur rarely in children.[2] They are often found incidental to some study and may or may not be the cause of dysfunction. Those that have caused intracardiac obstruction are lipoma (not lipomatous hypertrophy of the atrial septum), fibrolipoma, bronchogenic cyst (not a teratoma), pericardial hemangioma, and inflammatory pseudotumor. Papillary fibroelastoma and paraganglioma are rarely if ever found in children. Pericardial cysts (diverticula) that occur especially at the right costophrenic angle are usually asymptomatic.

PRIMARY MALIGNANT CARDIAC TUMORS

Primary malignant tumors of the heart occur in children less frequently than benign tumors by a ratio of about 1:4. Virtually all are sarcomatous tumors; of those that can be classified as to cell type, rhabdomyosarcoma is most frequent. Angiosarcoma, malignant fibrous histiocytoma, fibrosarcoma, leiomyosarcoma, and myxosarcoma have been recognized. Cardiac myxosarcoma is not considered to be a malignant form of the common cardiac myxoma. Surgical excision of cardiac sarcomas is rarely curative, but short-term palliation is possible.[1] At this time, chemotherapy and radiation treatments do not appear to have long-term benefit. Heart-lung transplantation has been done in a few patients.

Malignant tumors of the pericardium reported in infants and children include fibrosarcoma and malignant mesothelioma. Both of these tumors are bulky and widespread in the pericardium. These tumors are fatal.

METASTATIC (SECONDARY) CARDIAC TUMORS

Metastatic (secondary) tumors of the heart and pericardium are found in about 15% of autopsies of pediatric patients with disseminated malignant neoplasms.[1] In adults, the frequency of types of cardiac metastatic tumors nearly parallels that of the specific tumor in the general population with the exception that three relatively uncommon tumors have a disproportionate frequency of cardiac (heart and pericardium) metastatic deposits; these are malignant melanoma, malignant germ cell tumor, and malignant thymoma.

At one center, the most frequent types of tumors in children with metastatic (secondary) spread to the heart and pericardium were reported to be Wilms' tumor, non-Hodgkin's lymphoma, and neuroblastoma, and, at another center, leukemia-lymphoma, osteosarcoma, and Wilms' tumor.[2] Differences probably relate to different populations of patients. The wide variety of cardiac and pericardial functional abnormalities that may result from cardiac metastatic tumor are beyond the scope of this chapter.

PRIMARY TUMORS OF THE GREAT VESSELS

Primary tumors of the great vessels (aorta, pulmonary artery, venae cavae) are derived from vascular smooth muscles in 70% of patients, whether benign or malignant. These are rare in children.[2] Two thirds of primary tumors of the great vessels arise in great veins. Primary tumors of the great arteries are usually malignant (sarcoma), and the pulmonary artery is more often the site than is the aorta; apparent successful surgical treatment of pulmonary arterial sarcomas has been reported in at least two patients.[2]

REFERENCES

1. Burke A, Virmani R: Tumors of the Heart and Great Vessels. Atlas of Tumor Pathology, Series 3, Fascicle 16. Washington, DC, Armed Forces Institute of Pathology, 1996.
2. Burke B, Edwards JE, Titus JL: Tumors and tumor-like lesions of the heart and great vessels in the young. *In* Advances in Pathology and Laboratory Medicine, Vol 5. St. Louis, Mosby–Year Book, 1993, p 357.
3. Kearney DL, Titus JL, Hawkins EP, et al: Pathologic features of myocardial hamartomas causing childhood tachyarrhythmias. Circulation 75:705, 1987.

CHAPTER 60
CARDIAC INVOLVEMENT IN VASCULITIS AND OTHER RHEUMATIC DISEASES

HELEN M. EMERY   JULIEN I. E. HOFFMAN

Childhood rheumatic diseases are a miscellaneous group of diseases that have in common noninfectious inflammatory processes causing damage to soft tissues and blood vessels. Most are uncommon in childhood and are infrequently the cause of cardiac problems; nevertheless, any of these diseases can affect the pericardial, myocardial, and endocardial layers of the heart as well as extramyocardial and intramyocardial blood vessels. Therefore, these conditions should be considered in unexplained myocardial ischemia or cardiac dysfunction at any age. This discussion includes the cardiovascular findings in juvenile rheumatoid arthritis (JRA), the spondyloarthopathies, systemic lupus erythematosus (SLE) and antiphospholipid antibody syndrome, dermatomyositis, scleroderma, mixed connective tissue disease, and the vasculitic syndromes.

JUVENILE RHEUMATOID ARTHRITIS

This is the most common childhood rheumatic disease, affecting 1 in 1000 children at some time before the 17th birthday. The synovium is the main target for immune attack, but other organ systems can be affected. The disease has been classified into several patterns, each of which has different risks for cardiovascular complications.

Systemic-onset JRA is characterized by high spiking fevers (generally above 103°F with return to baseline between fever spikes), an evanescent rash most prominent during the fevers, and multiple-joint arthritis. This pattern accounts for approximately 10% of patients with JRA, may begin from infancy to young adulthood, and affects boys slightly more frequently than girls. Laboratory studies usually show anemia, elevated white blood cell and platelet counts, and increased erythrocyte sedimentation rate, but test results for rheumatoid factors and antinuclear antibodies are usually negative. Fatigue, weight loss, lymphadenopathy, and hepatosplenomegaly are common accompanying signs and symptoms.

Pericarditis and pleuritis are found in more than one third of children with active systemic-onset JRA,[1,2] although symptoms and signs may be subtle; for example, a child may complain of shoulder or back pain, may avoid lying down, may take shallow breaths to avoid pleuritic pain, or may have tachycardia out of proportion to fever and anemia. Rubs may be absent if fluid separates the serous layers, and distant heart sounds may reflect the size of the effusion. Fortunately, tamponade or constrictive changes are rare.

Whereas electrocardiographic changes may be present, the optimal diagnostic study is the echocardiogram.

Myocarditis is rare in systemic-onset JRA (<1%) and may cause cardiac failure. Arrhythmias and even complete heart block have been reported.[3] Valvar involvement is extremely rare, although aortic and mitral insufficiency have been described.[4–6]

The cardiac features of systemic JRA usually do not respond to nonsteroidal anti-inflammatory agents, but management with steroids, either orally or as an intravenous pulse of 20 mg/kg (maximum, 1 g), is usually effective, especially acutely. Other agents, such as immunosuppressive agents or intravenous immune globulin, may be needed for control of ongoing active disease to reduce long-term steroid side effects. Cardiac failure, if detected, should be managed with steroids and diuretics if possible, because the inflamed myocardium may be sensitive to the effects of digoxin.

Pauciarticular JRA (fewer than five affected joints and absence of classic systemic pattern) accounts for about half of children with this disease and may be divided into two groups:

1. Younger age at onset (generally younger than 5 years), female predominant category. These children are not at risk for cardiovascular complications.
2. Older age at onset (usually older than 7 years), male predominant category. These children have peripheral arthritis and enthesitis (inflammation of sites of tendon attachment to bones, e.g., Achilles tendinitis). They are frequently HLA-B27 positive and often have a family history of HLA-B27–associated diseases. Over time, some patients develop sacroiliitis and other classic findings of ankylosing spondylitis. Although aortic root inflammation and aortic valve insufficiency are usually identified only in older patients with long-standing disease, this complication has been reported in adolescents.[7]

Polyarticular JRA (five or more affected joints and absence of classic systemic findings) accounts for about 40% of JRA and can also be divided into two groups on the basis of presence or absence of rheumatoid factor:

1. Those who are seropositive for rheumatoid factor (about 10% of all children with JRA) are generally older at onset, and their disease can be considered typical of adult-type disease that happens to begin during childhood years. Its course tends to be aggressive and is often accompanied

by rheumatoid nodules; although rare, cardiac findings have included myocarditis and valvulitis.[6,8,9] Small-vessel necrotizing vasculitis has also been reported in this group.[4]

2. Children who have multiple-joint disease but do not have rheumatoid factor are generally younger, have a more benign course, and are unlikely to have cardiac involvement.

SYSTEMIC LUPUS ERYTHEMATOSUS

SLE is a disease predominantly of young preteen and teenage girls and is characterized by the formation of autoantibodies. Most childhood-onset SLE is not drug induced, although anticonvulsants and some cardiac medications (e.g., procainamide) can result in a transient lupus picture that, in contrast to the spontaneous form, usually spares the kidneys but often causes pericarditis and hemolytic anemia without lowering complement levels or raising antibodies to double-stranded DNA. The presence of antihistone antibodies may be helpful in differentiating drug-induced from spontaneous SLE.

SLE is diagnosed by meeting 4 of the 11 clinical criteria: malar rash; discoid rash; mucous membrane ulceration; photosensitivity; arthritis; nephritis (casts or proteinuria); hematologic abnormalities (including leukopenia, hemolytic anemia, thrombocytopenia); central nervous system involvement (seizures or psychosis); serositis (pleuritis or pericarditis); presence of antinuclear antibodies; other serologic abnormalities (Smith antibodies, double-stranded DNA antibodies, or false-positive VDRL test result). SLE can, however, cause many other problems not specific enough to be listed as criteria.

Cardiovascular complications include Raynaud's phenomenon in about 25% of childhood patients (sometimes resulting in digital necrosis) and a less common immune complex–mediated vasculitis that affects medium and small arteries throughout the body with occasional serious consequences, such as pulmonary hemorrhage, mesenteric arteritis, pancreatitis, transverse myelitis, and stroke.

Pericarditis is common, occurring in about 30% of patients, but may be asymptomatic. It seldom produces tamponade or constriction, although creation of a pericardial window is occasionally required for chronic or resistant effusion.

Myocardial involvement from myocarditis or small arterial disease occurs in about 25% of patients, resulting in cardiomegaly, cardiac failure, or arrhythmias. Coronary flow reserve may be markedly reduced.[10] On occasion, the extramural coronary arteries are affected.

Valve lesions are prominent in SLE.[11–13] Classic Libman-Sacks lesions, nonbacterial vegetations 2 to 4 mm in diameter on the mitral or less often other valves, can sometimes be detected echocardiographically. They may result in regurgitant or stenotic murmurs but seldom cause severe valve dysfunction. These lesions are susceptible to infective endocarditis, and antibiotic prophylaxis should be recommended as for valves damaged by rheumatic fever. Libman-Sacks lesions have also been associated with the risk of microthrombi and cerebral ischemic events. In rare patients, the valves are thickened, and incompetence may be severe.[14]

Pulmonary hypertension can occur.[15,16] Although usually mild, it can progress and cause death. Contributing factors include recurrent pulmonary embolism, in situ thrombosis, vasculitis, and vasoconstriction associated with a Raynaud-like syndrome.

Conduction defects including partial or complete heart block may occur beyond the neonatal period but are rare.

Premature atherosclerosis has been observed,[17] resulting in cardiac ischemia and sometimes overt myocardial infarction and death. In fact, coronary artery occlusion has become one of the leading causes of death in patients with SLE now that other aspects of lupus, such as renal disease, can be controlled more effectively. Many risk factors contribute to the increased incidence, for example, dyslipoproteinemia associated with SLE and with steroid use, hypertension and hypercholesterolemia that result from nephritis and nephrotic syndrome, vasculitis associated with endothelial damage and premature plaque formation, diabetes from either steroid use or antibodies to insulin or insulin receptors, and antiphospholipid antibodies and their associated thrombotic tendencies.

Optimal interventions to prevent and manage this atherosclerotic complication have not been defined. Some studies support the role of hydroxychloroquine in controlling vasculitis and dyslipoproteinemia, and low-dose aspirin is usually recommended for patients with known antiphospholipid antibodies.

Antiphospholipid antibodies are found in a high percentage of patients with SLE. They have been implicated in several disease manifestations, including thrombocytopenia; thrombotic events, such as deep vein thrombosis and pulmonary emboli; pulmonary hypertension; strokes; hepatic and renal vein thromboses; fetal loss; cutaneous findings of livedo reticularis; and abnormal laboratory findings including false-positive VDRL test results and prolonged coagulation studies, such as partial thromboplastin time (PTT) and Russell viper venom time (RVVT), all tests that use a phospholipid-rich substrate.

Primary antiphospholipid syndrome may occur independently of SLE. Laboratory studies detect the antibody (prolonged PTT or RVVT uncorrected by mixing with normal serum, or positive anticardiolipin antibodies) accompanied by clinical events consistent with this antibody (thrombotic events, recurrent fetal loss, thrombocytopenia, or livedo reticularis) in patients with insufficient other criteria to fulfill the diagnosis of SLE.[18,19]

Treatment of antiphospholipid antibody syndrome is not well defined. In general, for patients in whom antibodies are detected but not causing complications, low-dose aspirin is recommended unless it is contraindicated by conditions such as thrombocytopenia. For patients who have a thrombotic event, immediate heparinization is recommended, although the PTT is an unreliable marker for assessing anticoagulation because of antibody interference. Warfarin (Coumadin) should be used for long-term anticoagulation with the goal of achieving an international normalized ratio of approximately 3.[20] The role of immunosuppression with either steroids or other agents has not been clarified, although in pregnancy, low-dose aspirin appears to be as effective as and safer than steroids in preventing fetal loss.[21]

NEONATAL SYSTEMIC LUPUS ERYTHEMATOSUS AND COMPLETE CONGENITAL HEART BLOCK

Antibodies are transferred to the fetus from the maternal circulation primarily in the latter half of the pregnancy. If a mother with SLE has autoantibodies, these cross the placenta and may damage the fetus, whether or not the mother has problems caused by these antibodies. One common neonatal lupus syndrome is caused by anti-Ro antibodies (also known as SS-A antibodies), which appear to bind to the atrioventricular node, stimulating an inflammatory response leading to fibrous destruction and congenital heart block (see Chapter 55). The immature conduction system seems to be at particular risk from the 18th to the 22nd week of gestation. In more than one third of all patients with congenital heart block, these maternal antibodies can be found, although the mother is frequently asymptomatic and unaware that she has autoantibodies or SLE. Having one affected child does not mean that subsequent children will be affected.

Clinically, these fetuses may develop cardiac failure and nonimmune hydrops, and they are likely to need permanent pacemakers. Endocardial fibroelastosis and rarely other cardiac defects have been reported in infants of mothers with SLE.

Management of women who have had a previously affected child, or a fetus who appears to be affected, is not established. Trials of betamethasone or intravenous immune globulin have been initiated in an effort to block antibody transfer or reduce the inflammatory response following individual reports of successful interventions.[22, 23]

JUVENILE DERMATOMYOSITIS

Childhood dermatomyositis differs in many aspects from its adult-onset counterpart, particularly in the frequent vascular involvement, the lack of association with malignant disease, and the good prognosis if it is identified early and treated aggressively.

Clinical criteria include muscle weakness affecting striated muscle (proximal more than distal) and a purple (lilac, heliotrope) rash over the eyelids, sometimes over the face and "shawl" area of the neck and back, and over the extensor surfaces of the extremities and knuckles. Evidence of muscle inflammation is shown by elevated muscle enzymes, abnormal electromyographic findings, or muscle biopsy. Arthralgias, arthritis, dysphagia and aspiration episodes, and rarely respiratory failure may also occur. The associated vasculitis primarily targets the intestinal tract with significant risk of abdominal pain, hemorrhage, and perforation, although vessels in the lungs (pulmonary hemorrhage), skin, and central nervous system (retinal vasculitis) may also be affected. Renal involvement almost never occurs, unlike in other vasculitic syndromes. This vasculitis appears to be immune complex mediated.

Because heart muscle is striated, cardiac involvement occurs rarely. The resultant myocarditis may be severe enough to cause arrhythmias or death; occasionally, pericarditis has been reported.[24, 25] Caution must be used in interpreting fractionated creatinine kinase (CK) levels in this disease, because the MB fraction is elevated by regen-

erating skeletal as well as cardiac muscle and does not necessarily reflect myocardial damage.[26, 27]

Treatment is steroids and if necessary immunosuppressive agents, such as methotrexate or cyclosporine, as well as intensive supportive measures to control airway and gastrointestinal complications if required.

PROGRESSIVE SYSTEMIC SCLEROSIS (SCLERODERMA) AND CREST SYNDROME

This disease is uncommon in children.[28] Characteristically, there is thickening of the skin with joint stiffness, Raynaud's syndrome, and lower esophageal dysmotility. Pulmonary fibrosis and renal involvement with hypertension are frequent.[29–32] Fibrosis in skin and other organs results from increased collagen deposition, possibly mediated by factors released by endothelial cells and in the extracellular matrix. Although childhood series are small, cardiac involvement seems to be more frequent than in adults. When present, it is due to small-vessel vasculitis, fibrosis, or pulmonary hypertension, resulting in ventricular hypertrophy and dysfunction.[33, 34] On 24-hour continuous monitoring, arrhythmias secondary to conduction system scarring are reported in one third of patients. Decreases in myocardial perfusion can be documented on thallium scans. Cardiopulmonary involvement is the main cause of death in childhood progressive systemic sclerosis.

CREST syndrome (calcinosis, Raynaud's syndrome, esophageal dysfunction, sclerodactyly, and telangiectasia) is regarded as a more benign variant of scleroderma and may be distinguished by the presence of anticentromere antibodies. Late pulmonary hypertension is the major cause of death.

Management of scleroderma has been unsatisfying. Numerous agents designed for either inhibition of collagen cross-linkage (D-penicillamine) or immunosuppression (steroids, cyclophosphamide, azathioprine, cyclosporine) do not seem to prevent the progression of the disease with any consistency. Preventing Raynaud's phenomenon with calcium channel blockers seems to improve coronary and pulmonary blood flow. Supportive measures including preventing esophageal reflux and the use of H_2 blockers appear to decrease pulmonary complications. Careful control of renal complications by using angiotensin-converting enzyme inhibitors has significantly improved the outcome of patients with scleroderma. If pulmonary hypertension is suspected, attempts at afterload reduction may reduce the risk of right ventricular failure.

WEGENER'S GRANULOMATOSIS

This is a necrotizing granulomatous vasculitis affecting the upper airways, lungs, and kidneys. Although uncommon in children,[35] the diagnosis should be suspected in children with sinusitis, airway or lung disease (often cavitating lung lesions or pulmonary hemorrhage), and renal disease. Cardiac complications are unusual but include pericarditis, myocardial dysfunction from the vasculitis, and aortic incompetence.[36–39]

CHURG-STRAUSS SYNDROME

This is a syndrome of an eosinophilic necrotizing vasculitis occurring in allergic subjects. The patients usually have asthma and increased blood eosinophils. The vasculitis affects mainly the lung, gastrointestinal tract, kidneys, and heart. Heart failure or myocardial infarction due to coronary vasculitis has been reported in young adults.[40, 41]

PRIMARY VASCULITIDES IN CHILDREN

The classification of vasculitis is the source of much confusion and discussion, and it will continue to be so until there is a better biologic understanding of the disease processes. Currently, vasculitides may be classified into primary (those thought not to be secondary to another disease process) and secondary (to conditions such as SLE and dermatomyositis). Primary vasculitis is usually classified according to the size of the vessels that are mainly affected: large, medium, and small vessels. Most of them can, however, affect more than one size of vessel, although one size usually predominates. A classification of the vasculitides appears in Table 60–1.[42]

The two most common forms of vasculitis in children are Henoch-Schönlein purpura, an immunoglobulin A–mediated small-vessel vasculitis that targets primarily skin, kidneys, and the gastrointestinal tract and seldom causes cardiac problems; and Kawasaki disease, a vasculitis of medium-sized vessels with significant risk of both short- and long-term cardiac effects (discussed in Chapter 47).

GENERAL ASPECTS

Almost all primary vasculitides begin acutely with an inflammatory infiltrate. In some, this follows deposition in the vessel wall of immune complexes. These complexes attract polymorphonuclear leukocytes through complement-activated chemotactic factors, and the white blood cells in turn release lysosomal enzymes that damage the vessel wall. Subsequently, the acute inflammatory cells are replaced by proliferating fibroblasts and endothelial cells. The result is the chronic disease phase, characterized by fibrosis and narrowing or even occlusion of the arteries, sometimes thrombosis, and formation of macroaneurysms or microaneurysms.

In the acute phase, these diseases present with many features in common and may be difficult to diagnose until specific features develop or a biopsy is done. Nonspecific features are fatigue, malaise, weight loss, fever, night sweats, myalgia, arthralgia, arthritis, chest pain from pleurisy or pericarditis, neurologic symptoms like seizures and paresthesias or pareses, abdominal pain, and headaches from local vascular changes or hypertension. There are also nonspecific laboratory findings: anemia, leukocytosis, and a raised erythrocyte sedimentation rate. In addition, there may be findings that indicate involvement of an organ but not the cause of the disease. Examples are hematuria and proteinuria with renal involvement, elevated transaminases with liver involvement, and hemoptysis with pulmonary involvement.

TABLE 60–1

CAUSES OF SYSTEMIC VASCULITIS

DIRECT INFECTIOUS (e.g., Rocky Mountain spotted fever)

NONINFECTIOUS

Large vessels
  Giant cell (temporal) arteritis
  Takayasu's arteritis° †
Medium-sized vessels
  Polyarteritis nodosa‡
  Kawasaki syndrome° ‡
Small vessels
  ANCA associated
    Microscopic polyangiitis (p-ANCA)
    Wegener's granulomatosis (c-ANCA)†
    Churg-Strauss syndrome‡
    Drug induced
  Immune complex associated
    Henoch-Schönlein purpura°
    Cryoglobulinemic vasculitis
    Systemic lupus erythematosus° ‡
    Rheumatoid vasculitis° ‡
    Sjögren's syndrome
    Hypocomplementemic urticarial vasculitis
    Behçet's disease
    Goodpasture's syndrome
    Serum sickness
    Drug induced
    Infection induced
  Paraneoplastic
    Lymphoproliferative
    Myeloproliferative
    Carcinoma induced
  Inflammatory bowel disease
  Miscellaneous
    Progressive systemic sclerosis (scleroderma)†
    Dermatomyositis†

ANCA = antineutrophil cytoplasmic antibodies: p-, perinuclear; c-, cytoplasmic.
°Relatively common in childhood.
†Coronary artery involvement occasional.
‡Coronary artery involvement common.
Adapted with permission from Jennette JC, Falk RJ: Small-vessel vasculitis. N Engl J Med 337:1512–1523, 1997. Copyright © 1997 Massachusetts Medical Society. All rights reserved.

Cardiac involvement occurs in several ways. Vasculitides affecting large or medium-sized arteries may narrow or thrombose extramural coronary arteries and produce angina or myocardial infarction. Vasculitides affecting small intramyocardial arteries impair local blood flow and cause patchy myocardial necrosis and fibrosis. These changes, if extensive, produce nonspecific electrocardiographic changes, some arrhythmias, occasional conduction defects (including complete heart block), and varying degrees of ventricular hypertrophy and myocardial dysfunction that can end in congestive heart failure. Some of these diseases cause pericarditis or myocarditis, possibly by direct tissue damage rather than indirectly through vasculitis. A few of these diseases, notably Takayasu's syndrome, SLE, and rheumatoid arthritis, produce lesions of the valves, mainly the aortic valve. Finally, many of these diseases affect pulmonary arteries and cause pulmonary hypertension.

TREATMENT

In the absence of known causes or the inability to remove them, treatment is empirical. Corticosteroids have been valuable, but the known complications of their prolonged administration in high doses have led to the search for alternative therapies. Antimitotic agents like cyclophosphamide and methotrexate have been of great value, either alone or in allowing reduction of the steroid dose. In a few vasculitides that are associated with viruses (e.g., polyarteritis nodosa), antiviral therapy has been helpful. Trials of plasmapheresis show limited success.

Prognosis for children with vasculitis appears significantly better than that in adults. Some children can be withdrawn completely from medication after a couple of years of treatment.[43,44]

Diseases of Large Arteries

TAKAYASU'S SYNDROME

This syndrome was first described in 1946 when Takayasu, a Japanese ophthalmologist, described an unusual vascular pattern in the retina; this pattern was confirmed by another ophthalmologist who also noted that his patients had absent pulses in the arms. Absence of pulses is a common finding that has led to the alternative name of pulseless disease. The syndrome is due to a giant cell arteritis that is confined to larger arteries ranging in size from coronary arteries to the aorta. It affects predominantly young teenage girls but can begin in young children or as late as 66 years of age. The syndrome appears to be particularly frequent in Japan, India, and Mexico but occurs worldwide.[45-51] In the United States, the incidence has been estimated at about 2.6 per million per year,[52] and the prevalence is about 1 per 1000.[53]

Pathology

Acutely, there are granulomatous changes in the intima, media, and adventitia of the large arteries, with many giant cells present.[52,54,55] The media may degenerate. Later, there is fibrosis of the intima and adventitia, and stenosis or aneurysms occur. The histopathologic process may be indistinguishable from that found in Horton's disease (temporal arteritis), a disease that occurs almost exclusively after the age of 60 years, usually affects the temporal arteries and occasionally the arteries of the upper body, and may be associated with polymyalgia rheumatica.

Arterial stenoses develop and are frequently localized to the origins of the arteries from the aorta and less often distally, although narrowing of the midportions of the subclavian arteries is almost pathognomonic. Coronary arteries are stenosed in about 15% of patients.[53] Aneurysms of major arteries occur in 10 to 30% of patients.[53,56] The aorta has a thickened wall and is diffusely narrowed. Sometimes the aortic valve is involved in the pathologic change, and severe aortic incompetence ensues.[57,58] Distal pulmonary artery branches are affected,[59] usually in the chronic phase of the disease, but initial pulmonary artery involvement has been reported.[60] Thrombosis is not prominent, although occasional association with the antiphospholipid syndrome has been reported. The disease is currently classified as type I, aortic arch and its branches affected; type II, like type I but including descending thoracic aorta; type III, descending thoracic aorta and abdominal aorta; type IV, abdominal aorta only; and type V, aortic arch, descending thoracic aorta, and abdominal aorta. There are some differences in the arteries affected in different countries. Types I and II predominate in Japan, and types IV and V

predominate in India[47,61]; in South Africa, types II and IV predominate.[46] In all countries, the renal arteries are commonly involved.

Etiology and Pathogenesis

No definite cause has been found for Takayasu's syndrome. The syndrome is most common in countries where tuberculosis is frequent, but whether this is a causal relationship has not been defined. Certain HLA-1 types seem to occur more frequently in patients with the syndrome, but because the predominant HLA types in Takayasu's syndrome seem to vary in different parts of the world, it is difficult to show a direct causal relationship. Efforts to find specific antigens or antibodies have been unsuccessful.

The syndrome has an acute onset and a more prolonged chronic phase. Acute changes are nonspecific as described earlier. Then, as the vascular damage becomes chronic, the acute inflammatory change is followed by fibrosis and constriction of the arteries or aneurysm formation. The acute and chronic phases may overlap, but sometimes no acute phase is apparent.

Clinical Presentation

It is difficult to diagnose the disease in its acute, nonspecific phase until overt signs of vascular occlusion occur. In the chronic phase, there may be symptoms of cerebrovascular insufficiency, such as syncope or dizziness, sometimes associated with a subclavian steal; amaurosis fugax; intermittent claudication of the arms or legs; myocardial ischemia due to coronary artery narrowing; abdominal symptoms due to mesenteric artery narrowing; or headache due to renal hypertension. On examination, there may be absence of pulses in the neck, arms, or legs; hypertension; bruits over the narrowed arteries; aortic incompetence; and a diagnostic circular anastomosis around the optic disk.

Diagnosis

In the acute phase, there are no specific laboratory tests, but the aortic wall may be found to be thickened by magnetic resonance imaging or computed tomography,[62-64] and some patients may have weakly positive test responses for antinuclear antibody and rheumatoid factor. Angiography with or without digital subtraction is not useful until stenoses or aneurysms occur.[65] In the chronic phase, echocardiography is useful in evaluating the heart and valves, and it may detect stenoses or aneurysms, although not with 100% sensitivity. Magnetic resonance angiography and conventional angiography are the major diagnostic tools.[66]

Treatment

Both local and general treatments have been used. In the acute phase, prednisone, 1 to 2 mg/kg/day for at least 1 month, may help to abolish systemic signs and symptoms. It should probably be given in young patients even in the absence of acute features because of the likelihood of subclinical inflammation. Prednisone should be tapered after 3 months. If it cannot be tapered or if it fails to suppress the acute phase, then cyclophosphamide, 2 mg/kg/day, can be added.[67] Low-dose methotrexate (10 to 30 mg/m²/wk) has been used successfully.[68] If the arterial narrowing is critical, as in some carotid, coronary, or renal arterial disease, blood flow to the territory of the affected artery needs to be increased. In some patients, it has been possible to dilate the narrowed segment with a balloon.[69] If this is not possible, bypass surgery may be required.[56,70–73] Should there be hypertension, it must be controlled until the renal artery stenosis has been relieved.

Diseases of Medium-Sized Arteries

KAWASAKI SYNDROME

Kawasaki syndrome is described in detail in Chapter 47.

POLYARTERITIS NODOSA

This is a focal, segmental necrotizing vasculitis that affects medium-sized and small arteries, mainly in the kidneys, muscle, and nervous system. It is rare in children.[74–76] The acute phase shows necrosis of the arterial wall with fibrinoid necrosis and an inflammatory infiltrate.[55] Tissue damage is associated with thrombosis and aneurysm formation. In the chronic phase, there is proliferation of fibrous tissue and endothelial cells, and vessels are narrowed or occluded. Coronary arteritis, myocardial infarction, and pericarditis may occur. It occasionally affects the lung, mainly by thromboembolism.[31]

Classic polyarteritis nodosa has been distinguished from microscopic polyangiitis, which shows similar pathologic changes confined to small vessels.[77,78] This type is more likely to cause vasculitis of small pulmonary and coronary arteries and to be positive for perinuclear antineutrophil cytoplasmic antibodies.

The cause is unknown. In adults, there is a striking association with hepatitis B surface antigen.

Children of any age may get the disease, but the mean age at onset is 10 to 11 years.[75,76] The presentation of the acute illness is protean, as described before, but hypertension and a specific rash are prominent. Hematuria and albuminuria may occur, and there may be renal insufficiency. Liver transaminases may be elevated. Acute-phase reactants are increased. Cardiac findings range from electrocardiographic abnormalities, to mild ventricular dysfunction with mild or moderate mitral or tricuspid incompetence, to frank myocardial infarction. Pulmonary hypertension or hemorrhage may occur.

Diagnosis is made by biopsy of the skin, kidney, sural nerve, or muscle or by characteristic angiographic changes of microaneurysms and stenoses of small and medium-sized arteries.

Treatment is with prednisone, 1 to 2 mg/kg/day for 1 month, with tapering of the dose thereafter. Cyclophosphamide and other immunosuppressive agents have been used in an effort to control steroid side effects, although efficacy has not been proved in controlled studies. With hepatitis B or C antigens, therapy with antiviral agents has been tried.

REFERENCES

1. Leitman PS, Bywaters EGL: Pericarditis in juvenile rheumatoid arthritis. Pediatrics 32:855, 1963.
2. Bernstein B, Takahashi M, Hanson V: Cardiac involvement in juvenile rheumatoid arthritis. J Pediatr 85:313, 1974.
3. Goldenberg J, Ferraz MB, Pessoa AP, et al: Symptomatic cardiac involvement in juvenile rheumatoid arthritis. Int J Cardiol 34:57, 1992.
4. Lebowitz WB: The heart in rheumatoid arthritis (rheumatoid disease). A clinical and pathological study of sixty-two cases. Ann Intern Med 58:102, 1963.
5. Roberts WC, Kehoe JA, Carpenter DF, Golden A: Cardiac valvular lesions in rheumatoid arthritis. Arch Intern Med 122:141, 1968.
6. Kramer PH, Imboden JB Jr, Waldman FM, et al: Severe aortic insufficiency in juvenile chronic arthritis. Am J Med 74:1088, 1983.
7. Cosh JA, Lever JV: The aortic valve. In Ansell BM, Simkin PA (eds): The Heart and Rheumatic Disease. London, Butterworth, 1984, pp 83–119.
8. Delgado EA, Petty RE, Malleson PN, et al: Aortic valve insufficiency and coronary artery narrowing in a child with polyarticular juvenile rheumatoid arthritis. J Rheumatol 15:144, 1988.
9. Leak AM, Millar-Craig MW, Ansell BM: Aortic regurgitation in seropositive juvenile arthritis. Ann Rheum Dis 40:229, 1981.
10. Strauer BE, Brune I, Schenk H, et al: Lupus cardiomyopathy: Cardiac mechanics, hemodynamics, and coronary blood flow in uncomplicated systemic lupus erythematosus. Am Heart J 92:715, 1976.
11. Leung WH, Wong KL, Lau CP, et al: Cardiac abnormalities in systemic lupus erythematosus: A prospective M-mode, cross-sectional and Doppler echocardiographic study. Int J Cardiol 27:367, 1990.
12. Roldan CA, Shively BK, Lau CC, et al: Systemic lupus erythematosus valve disease by transesophageal echocardiography and the role of antiphospholipid antibodies [see comments]. J Am Coll Cardiol 20:1127, 1992.
13. Straaton KV, Chatham WW, Reveille JD, et al: Clinically significant valvular heart disease in systemic lupus erythematosus. Am J Med 85:645, 1988.
14. Galve E, Candell-Riera J, Pigrau C, et al: Prevalence, morphologic types, and evolution of cardiac valvular disease in systemic lupus erythematosus. N Engl J Med 319:817, 1988.
15. Clausen KP, Geer JC: Hypertensive pulmonary arteritis. Am J Dis Child 118:718, 1969.
16. Fuster V, Steele PM, Edwards WD, et al: Primary pulmonary hypertension: Natural history and the importance of thrombosis. Circulation 70:580, 1984.
17. Bulkley BH, Roberts WC: The heart in systemic lupus erythematosus and the changes induced in it by corticosteroid therapy. A study of 36 necropsy patients. Am J Med 58:243, 1975.
18. Hojnik M, George J, Ziporen L, Shoenfeld Y: Heart valve involvement (Libman-Sacks endocarditis) in the antiphospholipid syndrome. Circulation 93:1579, 1996.
19. Ravelli A, Martini A: Antiphospholipid antibody syndrome in pediatric patients. Rheum Dis Clin North Am 23:657, 1997.
20. Khamashta MA, Cuadrado MJ, Mujic F, et al: The management of thrombosis in the antiphospholipid-antibody syndrome [see comments]. N Engl J Med 332:993, 1995.
21. Cowchock S: Treatment of antiphospholipid syndrome in pregnancy. Lupus 7(suppl 2):S95, 1998.
22. Copel JA, Buyon JP, Kleinman CS: Successful in utero therapy of fetal heart block [see comments]. Am J Obstet Gynecol 173:1384, 1995.
23. Buyon JP: Neonatal lupus. Curr Opin Rheumatol 8:485, 1996.
24. Pereira RM, Lerner S, Maeda WT, et al: Pericardial tamponade in juvenile dermatomyositis. Clin Cardiol 15:301, 1992.
25. Yale SH, Adlakha A, Stanton MS: Dermatomyositis with pericardial tamponade and polymyositis with pericardial effusion. Am Heart J 126:997, 1993.
26. Michels H: Course of mixed connective tissue disease in children. Ann Med 29:359, 1997.
27. Shehata R, al-Mayouf S, al-Dalaan A, et al: Juvenile dermatomyositis: Clinical profile and disease course in 25 patients. Clin Exp Rheumatol 17:115, 1999.
28. Goldenberg J, Pinto-Pessoa A, Odete-Hilario M, et al: Infantile scleroderma. Apropos of 11 cases [in French]. Rev Rhum Ed Fr 60:131, 1993.
29. White B: Clinical approach to scleroderma. Semin Cutan Med Surg 17:213, 1998.
30. Steen VD: Clinical manifestations of systemic sclerosis. Semin Cutan Med Surg 17:48, 1998.
31. Feigin DS: Vasculitis in the lung. J Thorac Imaging 3:33, 1988.
32. Koh ET, Lee P, Gladman DD, Abu-Shakra M: Pulmonary hypertension in systemic sclerosis: An analysis of 17 patients. Br J Rheumatol 35:989, 1996.

33. Kahan A, Devaux JY, Amor B, et al: Nifedipine and thallium-201 myocardial perfusion in progressive systemic sclerosis. N Engl J Med 314:1397, 1986.

34. Murata I, Takenaka K, Shinohara S, et al: Diversity of myocardial involvement in systemic sclerosis: An 8-year study of 95 Japanese patients. Am Heart J 135:960, 1998.

35. Rottem M, Fauci AS, Hallahan CW, et al: Wegener granulomatosis in children and adolescents: Clinical presentation and outcome. J Pediatr 122:26, 1993.

36. Hoffman GS, Kerr GS, Leavitt RY, et al: Wegener granulomatosis: An analysis of 158 patients [see comments]. Ann Intern Med 116:488, 1992.

37. Grant SC, Levy RD, Venning MC, et al: Wegener's granulomatosis and the heart. Br Heart J 71:82, 1994.

38. Delevaux I, Hoen B, Selton-Suty C, Canton P: Relapsing congestive cardiomyopathy in Wegener's granulomatosis. Mayo Clin Proc 72:848, 1997.

39. Fox AD, Robbins SE: Aortic valvulitis complicating Wegener's granulomatosis. Thorax 49:1176, 1994.

40. Kozak M, Gill EA, Green LS: The Churg-Strauss syndrome. A case report with angiographically documented coronary involvement and a review of the literature. Chest 107:578, 1995.

41. Hellemans S, Dens J, Knockaert D: Coronary involvement in the Churg-Strauss syndrome. Heart 77:576, 1997.

42. Jennette JC, Falk RJ: Small-vessel vasculitis. N Engl J Med 337:1512, 1997.

43. Blanco R, Martínez-Taboada VM, Rodríguez-Valverde V, García-Fuentes M: Cutaneous vasculitis in children and adults. Associated diseases and etiologic factors in 303 patients. Medicine (Baltimore) 77:403, 1998.

44. Dillon MJ: Childhood vasculitis. Lupus 7:259, 1998.

45. Dabague J, Reyes PA: Takayasu arteritis in Mexico: A 38-year clinical perspective through literature review. Int J Cardiol 54(suppl):S103, 1996.

46. Hahn D, Thomson PD, Kala U, et al: A review of Takayasu's arteritis in children in Gauteng, South Africa. Pediatr Nephrol 12:668, 1998.

47. Jain S, Kumari S, Ganguly NK, Sharma BK: Current status of Takayasu arteritis in India. Int J Cardiol 54(suppl):S111, 1996.

48. Lupi-Herrera E, Sánchez-Torres G, Marcushamer J, et al: Takayasu's arteritis. Clinical study of 107 cases. Am Heart J 93:94, 1977.

49. Moriwaki R, Noda M, Yajima M, et al: Clinical manifestations of Takayasu arteritis in India and Japan—new classification of angiographic findings. Angiology 48:369, 1997.

50. Rosenthal T, Morag B, Rubinstein Z, Itzchak Y: Takayasu arteritis in Israel—update. Int J Cardiol 54(suppl):S137, 1996.

51. Sharma BK, Jain S, Radotra BD: An autopsy study of Takayasu arteritis in India. Int J Cardiol 66(suppl 1):S85, 1998.

52. Hall S, Barr W, Lie JT, et al: Takayasu arteritis. A study of 32 North American patients. Medicine (Baltimore) 64:89, 1985.

53. Brantley BD, Forman MB, Virmani R: Diagnosis and treatment of Takayasu's arteritis. Prim Cardiol 16:47, 1990.

54. Arend WP, Michel BA, Bloch DA, et al: The American College of Rheumatology 1990 criteria for the classification of Takayasu arteritis. Arthritis Rheum 33:1129, 1990.

55. Lie JT: Illustrated histopathologic classification criteria for selected vasculitis syndromes. American College of Rheumatology Subcommittee on Classification of Vasculitis. Arthritis Rheum 33:1074, 1990.

56. Regina G, Fullone M, Testini M, et al: Aneurysms of the supra-aortic trunks in Takayasu's disease. Report of two cases. J Cardiovasc Surg (Torino) 39:757, 1998.

57. Ohteki H, Itoh T, Natsuaki M, et al: Aortic valve replacement for Takayasu's arteritis. J Thorac Cardiovasc Surg 104:482, 1992.

58. Ravelli A, Pedroni E, Perrone S, et al: Aortic valve regurgitation as the presenting sign of Takayasu arteritis. Eur J Pediatr 158:281, 1999.

59. Ogawa Y, Hayashi K, Sakamoto I, Matsunaga N: Pulmonary arterial lesions in Takayasu arteritis: Relationship of inflammatory activity to scintigraphic findings and sequential changes. Ann Nucl Med 10:219, 1996.

60. Nakabayashi K, Kurata N, Nangi N, et al: Pulmonary artery involvement as first manifestation in three cases of Takayasu arteritis. Int J Cardiol 54(suppl):S177, 1996.

61. Sharma BK, Jain S, Suri S, Numano F: Diagnostic criteria for Takayasu arteritis. Int J Cardiol 54(suppl):S141, 1996.

62. Hayashi K, Fukushima T, Matsunaga N, Hombo Z: Takayasu's arteritis: Decrease in aortic wall thickening following steroid therapy, documented by CT. Br J Radiol 59:281, 1986.

63. Tanigawa K, Eguchi K, Kitamura Y, et al: Magnetic resonance imaging detection of aortic and pulmonary artery wall thickening in the acute stage of Takayasu arteritis. Improvement of clinical and radiologic findings after steroid therapy. Arthritis Rheum 35:476, 1992.

64. Choe YH, Lee WR: Magnetic resonance imaging diagnosis of Takayasu arteritis. Int J Cardiol 66(suppl 1):S175, 1998.

65. Matsunaga N, Hayashi K, Aikawa H, et al: Digital subtraction angiography in Takayasu arteritis. Acta Radiol 28:247, 1987.

66. Oneson SR, Lewin JS, Smith AS: MR angiography of Takayasu arteritis. J Comput Assist Tomogr 16:478, 1992.

67. Shelhamer JH, Volkman DJ, Parrillo JE, et al: Takayasu's arteritis and its therapy. Ann Intern Med 103:121, 1985.

68. Shetty AK, Stopa AR, Gedalia A: Low-dose methotrexate as a steroid-sparing agent in a child with Takayasu's arteritis. Clin Exp Rheumatol 16:335, 1998.

69. Tyagi S, Singh B, Kaul UA, et al: Balloon angioplasty for renovascular hypertension in Takayasu's arteritis. Am Heart J 125:1386, 1993.

70. Abad C: Coronary artery bypass surgery for patients with left main coronary lesions due to Takayasu's arteritis. Eur J Cardiothorac Surg 9:661, 1995.

71. Amano J, Suzuki A: Coronary artery involvement in Takayasu's arteritis. Collective review and guideline for surgical treatment. J Thorac Cardiovasc Surg 102:554, 1991.

72. Amano J, Suzuki A: Surgical treatment of cardiac involvement in Takayasu arteritis. Heart Vessels Suppl 7:168, 1992.

73. Duncan JM, Cooley DA: Surgical considerations in aortitis with special emphasis on Takayasu's arteritis. Tex Heart Inst J 10:233, 1983.

74. Ozen S, Besbas N, Saatci U, Bakkaloglu A: Diagnostic criteria for polyarteritis nodosa in childhood. J Pediatr 120:206, 1992.

75. Günal N, Kara N, Cakar N, et al: Cardiac involvement in childhood polyarteritis nodosa. Int J Cardiol 60:257, 1997.

76. Maeda M, Kobayashi M, Okamoto S, et al: Clinical observation of 14 cases of childhood polyarteritis nodosa in Japan. Acta Paediatr Jpn 39:277, 1997.

77. Lhote F, Cohen P, Guillevin L: Polyarteritis nodosa, microscopic polyangiitis and Churg-Strauss syndrome. Lupus 7:238, 1998.

78. Guillevin L, Durand-Gasselin B, Cevallos R, et al: Microscopic polyangiitis: Clinical and laboratory findings in eighty-five patients. Arthritis Rheum 42:421, 1999.

CHAPTER 61
POSTOPERATIVE PROBLEMS

RALPH S. MOSCA   THOMAS J. KULIK

In infants and children after a cardiac operation, a number of issues may arise that require attention. Two of these problems, cardiac failure and low output (Chapter 54) and arrhythmias (Chapter 55) are discussed separately. In this chapter, more general postoperative problems are considered.

CARE OF WOUNDS

Postoperative wound healing represents the normal response to injury. Wound healing consists of three sequential yet overlapping events: an inflammatory phase, a proliferative phase, and a remodeling phase. The inflammatory phase begins immediately after injury and persists for 8 to 10 days; it consists of vasoconstriction, clot formation, and the initiation of the inflammatory response that will result in wound healing. Epithelialization, accomplished by the migration of epithelial cells from the basal layer across the wound, occurs within 24 to 48 hours in a surgically coapted wound. The proliferative phase (day 4 to 3 weeks) involves fibroblast proliferation and angiogenesis, replacing the fibrin-fibronectin matrix with collagen and ground substance. Collagen accumulation reaches a maximum at 2 to 3 weeks after injury. After a state of collagen content equilibrium has been reached, the remodeling phase (3 weeks to 12 months) begins. As the collagen is remodeled and reorganized, the tensile strength increases.

We recommend that thoracotomy and chest tube wounds be kept clean and dry, but no other special care is generally provided. Because epithelialization is complete by 48 hours, there is no need to protect the wound from water beyond this time, but prolonged immersion in water is avoided for 7 days postoperatively (or 1 day after stitch removal, whichever is longer). Gentle washing of the wound helps to remove any blood and protein (which provide an excellent culture medium for skin bacteria). Excess water must be removed to prevent maceration of wound edges. Families should be instructed to report promptly signs of wound infection (erythema, purulent drainage, dehiscence).

The strength of the wound varies with time, the type of suture material used, and the degree of mobility and stress on the area involved. At 1 to 2 weeks after operation, when skin sutures are removed, the wound has only regained a portion of its eventual strength and will disrupt with a minor stress. A wound regains 50% of its eventual strength by 6 weeks, and thus heavy lifting and other similar activities should be avoided for 6 to 8 weeks after operation. The thoracotomy scar is sensitive to sunburn for about 6 to 8 months and needs protection when it is exposed to sunlight, as in sunbathing or swimming.

POSTOPERATIVE FEVER

Fever, the elevation of the core body temperature above normal daily fluctuations, has many potential causes after a cardiac operation. Two of particular concern are low cardiac output and infection, although postoperative fever can also be caused by noninfectious inflammation, such as postpericardiotomy syndrome. Low cardiac output as a cause of postoperative fever is an issue in an intensive care unit, because it is predominantly limited to the early postoperative period. Postoperative fever secondary to infection in pediatric cardiac patients can be localized in most patients to the lungs, to the surgical wound, to the presence of an intravascular device, to a urinary catheter, or to cardiac structures.

LUNG

The lungs can be a source of fever from atelectasis or infection. Pulmonary atelectasis represents the most common cause of fever during the initial 24 hours after operation. In infants and children, therapy consists of chest physiotherapy, nasotracheal suctioning as needed, coughing, deep breathing, and early postoperative ambulation when appropriate. A pulmonary infection may be caused by a preexisting subclinical infection, the introduction of nosocomial organisms through an endotracheal tube, or aspiration. The treatment of pneumonia is enhanced when the causative bacteria can be identified in the tracheal aspirate, although this is not always possible. A third-generation cephalosporin, such as ceftriaxone, is an appropriate antibiotic when the identity of the organism is unknown.

WOUND INFECTIONS

Wound infections are another common cause of postoperative fever. Major and minor sternal wound complications occur in 7% of adult patients who undergo a cardiac operation; however, serious deep mediastinal infections occur less frequently (0.5%).[1,2] Most sternal wound infections are caused by staphylococci, strongly suggesting operating room contamination. Gram-negative infection suggests seeding in the intensive care unit. Infections caused by unusual organisms such as *Serratia, Pseudomonas,* or methicillin-resistant *Staphylococcus aureus,* especially when they occur in clusters, imply a common contaminating source. Polymicrobial infections or fungal infections are often associated with a systemic disease producing immunosuppression, low cardiac output syndrome, or multiorgan failure.

Early diagnosis is important, but this can be difficult especially in infants and children. Early signs of infection may include a low-grade fever and irritability as well as wound erythema, tenderness, and seropurulent drainage. Sternal instability with purulent drainage definitively establishes the diagnosis of a deep sternal infection. Often these findings are only evident by the 10th to 14th postoperative day and may occur after several weeks. In some patients, blood cultures are positive before local signs are present. Computed tomography and radioisotope studies are expensive, nonspecific, and nondiagnostic methods to evaluate this problem.

INFECTIONS FROM AN INTRAVASCULAR CATHETER

Bacteremia from an intravascular catheter is a major consideration in the evaluation of a postoperative fever. Typically, fever secondary to a catheter-related infection has an abrupt onset and often exceeds 39°C. A positive blood culture establishes the diagnosis, although, especially in patients already receiving antibiotics, blood cultures may fail to reveal a bona fide infection. Therapy consists of removal of the catheter, although sterilization of the catheter by use of intravenous antibiotics and low-dose thrombolytic agents through the catheter is sometimes possible. (With gram-negative or fungal infections, the likelihood of sterilization is remote.) Antibiotic therapy for 24 to 48 hours after catheter removal is usually adequate. If defervescence does not occur after catheter removal and antibiotics, other possibilities should be considered: incorrect diagnosis (the catheter was not the cause of the fever); the infection has spread to additional sites (i.e., endocarditis); septic thrombophlebitis at the site of the catheter placement has occurred.

ENDOCARDITIS

Infective endocarditis refers to the invasion of the endocardial surface of the heart by microorganisms, most often affecting the native cardiac structures or intravascular prosthetic material (such as prosthetic valves) (see Chapter 50). The most common structural abnormalities that predispose to infective endocarditis include ventricular septal defect, tetralogy of Fallot, and aortic stenosis. Endocarditis involving native cardiac tissue is most often due to streptococci (50 to 75%) or staphylococci (25%). In adults, endocarditis involving *prosthetic material* (e.g., a mechanical heart valve) accounts for 5 to 15% of infective endocarditis, and it is further subdefined as early (less than 60 days) or late (more than 60 days) after insertion of the prosthesis. The risk of endocarditis involving prosthetic material shows an early peak at 6 weeks after operation and then declines during the next 12 to 14 months. *Staphylococcus epidermidis* and *S. aureus* infections usually occur early and are more virulent and more often lethal. Late endocarditis related to prosthetic material occurs in an inci-

dence of approximately 0.2 to 0.5% per patient per year and is most often caused by *Streptococcus viridans* or *S. epidermidis.* Homograft valves are unique in that they do not have this risk of early infection, although they have approximately the same risk of late infection as that of a prosthetic valve.

The clinical manifestations of infective endocarditis vary. Most patients present with a febrile illness associated with nonspecific symptoms, such as shaking chills, night sweats, fatigue, diffuse arthralgia, myalgias, and anorexia. A new cardiac murmur or change in an old murmur may be found. Clinically apparent emboli appear in 15 to 30% of patients. Leukocytosis may occur, although anemia and a normal white blood cell count are frequent. To establish a definitive diagnosis, the involved microorganism must be demonstrated by blood cultures. Blood cultures are positive in 95% of patients not already receiving antibiotics. Echocardiography can be helpful in delineating vegetations as small as 5 mm in diameter, evaluating the degree of valve dysfunction, and identifying valve ring abscesses.

The treatment of infective endocarditis requires the sterilization of the vegetation, mandating appropriate antibiotics to achieve bactericidal levels, usually for 6 weeks (see Chapter 50). Late endocarditis associated with prosthetic material is usually caused by *S. epidermidis* or streptococci and can be cured with antibiotics alone approximately 75% of the time. In general, infections involving left-sided cardiac structures tend not to respond as well, regardless of the organism.

Operative intervention is necessary for infective endocarditis when it is complicated by congestive heart failure due to valve dysfunction, myocardial abscess, uncontrolled infection despite proper antimicrobial therapy, dehiscence of prosthetic valve or material, and infections caused by fungal or gram-negative organisms. Relative indications for operations include the presence of intracardiac prosthetic material, recurrent emboli, large vegetations, and infections caused by *S. aureus.*

The morbidity and mortality of operative intervention for infective endocarditis are multifactorial and dependent on the patient's condition, the virulence of the involved microorganisms, the extent of the infection, and its proximity to vital cardiac structures. Current reviews of the surgical treatment of infective endocarditis in children report approximately a 7% hospital mortality.[3] Significant postoperative complications include residual or recurrent infection, semilunar or atrioventricular valve insufficiency, and heart block.

An aggressive combined medical and surgical approach improves survival of the patient. The optimal timing of surgery in the pediatric patient with infective endocarditis must consider the patient's clinical condition, weight, available surgical options, and durability of the proposed therapy.

URINARY CATHETERS

Accurate, hour by hour quantification of urine output is important in estimating adequacy of systemic perfusion, and hence urinary catheters are routinely placed in essentially all patients undergoing cardiac operations. Antibiotic prophylaxis is generally not provided for placement of the catheter. Because urinary catheters are associated with urinary tract infections, it is important that they be removed as soon as is feasible after surgery. In addition, patients who have or had a urinary catheter with fever or symptoms suggestive of a urinary tract infection should have prompt evaluation with a urinalysis and urine culture.

TREATMENT OF WOUND INFECTIONS

The treatment of sternal wound infections depends on the depth of penetration. Antibiotics are a critical adjunct but when used alone to treat deep infections are associated with a mortality of 40 to 75% in adults.[2] Once a wound infection is suspected, multiple blood cultures should be obtained and the patient prescribed broad-spectrum intravenous antibiotics until identification of the causative organism makes more focused antibiotic therapy possible. Superficial wound infections are treated by opening the wound to achieve adequate drainage and a short course of antibiotic therapy.

The treatment of a deep sternal infection, characterized by instability of the sternum, is urgent operative drainage, removal of necrotic tissue and foreign bodies, and obliteration of any dead space. The duration of antibiotic therapy is controversial and ranges from 1 to 6 weeks. Unlike infection in most adult patients, which requires either a period of open wound treatment or sternal débridement and flap reconstruction as a one-stage procedure, post-sternotomy wound infections in infants and children can be treated by opening the wound, minimal débridement of necrotic tissue, and adequate drainage of the pericardial space followed by primary sternal closure and loose approximation of the skin and subcutaneous tissue. Myocutaneous flap closure of the wound is reserved for those in whom this initial therapy fails or those who require additional maneuvers to obliterate the dead space.

POSTPERICARDIOTOMY SYNDROME

Postpericardiotomy syndrome is a febrile illness presenting beyond the first postoperative week and characterized by malaise, irritability, pleuropericardial pain, and decreased appetite. It is the most common inflammatory syndrome after a cardiac operation, affecting 10 to 30% of adult patients and 3 to 5% of children younger than 2 years.[4] Although self-limited and rarely fatal, it can prolong recovery and must be differentiated from other postoperative complications.

DIAGNOSIS

Young children generally present 1 to 3 weeks after a cardiac operation in which the pericardium is opened. The fever usually ranges from 38 to 40°C, and there are accompanying vague symptoms of fatigue, malaise, irritability, nonspecific chest pain, and anorexia. Common physical findings include a pericardial friction rub, tachycardia, and evidence of hepatic congestion. On occasion, a pleural effusion, most commonly on the left side, may be present. Those uncommon patients who progress to pericardial

tamponade display the signs and symptoms of hepatic congestion, abdominal pain, nausea, and vomiting typical of this condition.

Laboratory findings include a chest radiograph demonstrating an enlarged cardiac silhouette and widening of the mediastinum as well as pleural effusion. The electrocardiogram may be helpful and display changes consistent with pericardial irritation, that is, ST segment elevation and flattening or inversion of the T waves in the limb and lateral precordial leads. Evidence of an inflammatory process may be reflected by a neutrophilic leukocytosis and elevation of acute-phase reactants (sedimentation rate and C-reactive protein). Echocardiography demonstrates a pericardial effusion. Although sensitive, this test is not specific because 50% of children after pericardiotomy and a cardiac operation have a small pericardial effusion at the time of discharge from the hospital. If present, the effusion persists throughout the course of the illness and resolves with the symptoms. Postpericardiotomy syndrome is usually a single illness; however, recurrences have been reported months later.

TREATMENT

Postpericardiotomy syndrome is usually self-limited and generally requires only supportive therapy. Diuretics are often used in patients with signs of fluid retention and for pleural as well as pericardial effusions that are not causing hemodynamic compromise. Aspirin (30 to 75 mg/kg/day) may be employed for a 4- to 6-week course. *Most severe cases may be treated with steroids.* A 2- to 3-week course of prednisone (beginning at 2 mg/kg/day and tapering to zero) hastens the recovery of children with postpericardiotomy syndrome. Intercurrent infection should be excluded before the initiation of steroid therapy.

The rare patient with hemodynamic compromise from a large pericardial effusion may require pericardiocentesis. It may be difficult to remove sufficient fluid to relieve symptoms; some of the fluid is often loculated. Recurrent pericardial effusions may be treated more definitively with a pericardial window or partial pericardiectomy.

EXERCISE ADVICE AND RETURN TO WORK OR SCHOOL

There are two issues regarding recommendations for permissible exercise after a cardiac operation: the exercise restrictions required because of the operation itself, and the exercise restrictions indicated on account of a residual cardiac lesion. In regard to the first issue, practices vary widely, as does the response of the individual to an operation. We restrict children from activities that might injure the chest (e.g., bicycle riding, skiing) for 4 to 6 weeks after sternotomy or thoracotomy. Activity is otherwise permitted as tolerated. We generally allow 2 weeks of recovery before return to school, although some children—especially those who had repair of a simple lesion—may be ready for school sooner. For adults, we recommend avoiding heavy lifting (>10 lb), and activity with significant potential for chest trauma, for 6 to 8 weeks. Adults can return to driving an automobile in 2 weeks, if this is comfortable for them. Adult patients often take longer to return to work than do children to school and may require 6 weeks of recuperation.

The extent of exercise limitation on account of a residual cardiac condition is the more important issue because these recommendations may apply for the patient's entire lifetime. Unfortunately, the information necessary for a rational approach to this issue is limited. Because young children tend to limit their activities to an intensity they tolerate (and because it would be a nightmare to try to limit them anyway), exercise limitations are rarely advised. For older children and adolescents, the issue of exercise restrictions related to the presence of cardiac lesions was addressed in a policy statement.[5] These guidelines serve as a reasonable guide for recommendations regarding appropriate exercise. One increasingly large group of patients not specifically covered in these recommendations is that of patients who have had a Fontan procedure. Considerable hemodynamic variation exists among these patients, although in general they have low maximal cardiac output with exercise.[6] It is reasonable not to impose a fixed restriction on such patients but to recognize that strenuous activities are not possible for many of these patients.

MEDICATIONS

With the possible exception of oral analgesics, there are no medications routinely prescribed in postoperative patients. Certain medications, such as digoxin and diuretics, are commonly used in these patients, but there should be specific indication for their use. Many patients do not require them. It is unclear whether to prescribe digoxin for pediatric cardiac patients who were in congestive heart failure before repair of the responsible lesion (e.g., ventricular septal defect). Similarly, whether digoxin is indicated in patients after tetralogy of Fallot repair (to ameliorate the right ventricular dysfunction) is a matter of controversy.

Because of the risk of intracardiac thrombus formation, many centers prescribe anticoagulation for patients after Fontan palliation. Whether all such patients require anticoagulation is unclear; some centers reserve anticoagulation for those at highest risk of thrombus formation (e.g., patients with low cardiac output or high venous pressure).[7] Patients with a modified Blalock-Taussig shunt (using a Gore-Tex tube graft) are often treated with low-dose aspirin in hopes of decreasing the chance of shunt thrombosis.

The recommendations about prophylaxis of subacute bacterial endocarditis (SBE), discussed in Chapter 50, apply to most postoperative patients. Whether SBE prophylaxis is perpetually required for patients with complete closure of ventricular septal defect is unclear: some practitioners discontinue such prophylaxis after 6 months (after which time the patch has presumably endothelialized), whereas others prescribe prophylaxis indefinitely. Our practice has been to recommend SBE prophylaxis for intravascular devices (e.g., atrial septal defect closure devices or coils for closure of patent ductus arteriosus) for 6 months after placement of the device (presuming complete closure of any lesion associated with a jet lesion). Most agree that SBE prophylaxis is no longer required 6 months after atrial septal defect or ductal ligation.

FOLLOW-UP

A postoperative patient requires outpatient follow-up. The timing of the first postoperative visit depends on the type of operation, age and physical condition of the patient, duration of postoperative stay, presence of postoperative complications (e.g., pleural or pericardial effusions), and availability of pediatric and cardiologic care in the patient's community. Because patients are often discharged soon after operation, earlier follow-up is often necessary to be certain that the patient is making a satisfactory recovery. We routinely see (or recommend follow-up with the referring physician) postoperative patients 2 weeks after operation to check on general well-being and to inspect incisions. The frequency of follow-up after the initial visit will be determined by the factors noted before. The "unnatural" history of repaired congenital cardiac lesions is still being learned, and late sequelae may occur with even the most straightforward defects (e.g., atrial arrhythmias after atrial septal defect repair, or recanalization of a ligated patent ductus arteriosus). Virtually all patients with a congenital cardiac anomaly should be seen periodically throughout their life by a cardiologist with knowledge of congenital heart disease.

OTHER ISSUES

DISCHARGE STUDIES

A chest radiograph is often obtained to identify pleural effusion or evidence of a large pericardial effusion. These findings do not necessarily mandate therapy if they are unassociated with physical signs or symptoms but might influence the follow-up. Most patients should have a chest radiograph within 48 hours of discharge. Echocardiography should be performed in most postoperative patients, especially those with a complex malformation. Unappreciated residual lesions can be detected, systolic ventricular function may be estimated, and the presence of pericardial fluid is ascertained. Oxygen saturation should be obtained and recorded in a patient with a systemic–pulmonary artery anastomosis. Blood sodium and potassium concentrations should be measured in patients receiving a significant amount of diuretics.

FEEDING

Many infants may be hemodynamically stable and doing well after operation but taking insufficient calories for adequate growth. Nasogastric feeding at home can be an important adjunct to other medical therapy in these infants. Extensive education of the patient's parents, while in the hospital, as well as follow-up by a home care nurse is necessary in these instances.

AIR TRANSPORTATION

Flight in commercial airlines may entail exposure to ambient pressure equivalent to approximately 8000 feet in altitude.[8] This results in pulmonary venous desaturation and the potential for hypoxia-related pulmonary vasoconstriction. As a result, it has been recommended that patients with cyanotic congenital heart disease be provided supplemental oxygen during the flight.[9] This seems a reasonable rule for patients with significant cyanosis, although it is difficult to see how patients adapted to altitudes equivalent to those experienced in an airplane would suffer from the absence of supplemental oxygen. One study found relatively little effect of airline travel on oxygen saturation in adults with a cyanotic cardiac malformation.[10]

REFERENCES

1. The Parisian Mediastinitis Study Group: Risk factors for deep sternal wound infection after sternotomy; a prospective multicenter study. J Thorac Cardiovasc Surg 111:1200, 1996.
2. Rutledge R, Applebaum RE, Kim BJ: Mediastinal infection after open heart surgery. Surgery 97:88, 1985.
3. Nomura F, Penny DJ, Menahem S, et al: Surgical treatment for infective endocarditis in infancy and childhood. Ann Thorac Surg 60:90, 1995.
4. Engle MA, Zabriskie JB, Senterfit LB, et al: Viral illness and the post pericardiotomy syndrome. A prospective study in children. Circulation 62:1151, 1980.
5. Gutgesell HP, Gessner IH, Vetter VL, et al: Recreational and occupational recommendations for young patients with heart disease. A statement for physicians by the committee on congenital cardiac defects of the Council on Cardiovascular Disease in the Young, American Heart Association. Circulation 74:1195A, 1986.
6. Gewillig MH, Lundstrom UR, Bull C, et al: Exercise responses in patients with congenital heart disease after Fontan repair: Patterns and determinants of performance. J Am Coll Cardiol 15:1425, 1990.
7. Jonas RA: Intracardiac thrombus after the Fontan procedure (Editorial). J Thorac Cardiovasc Surg 110:1502, 1995.
8. Liebman J, Lucas R, Moss A, et al: Airline travel for children with chronic pulmonary disease. Pediatrics 57:408, 1976.
9. AMA Commission on Emergency Medical Services: Medical aspects of transportation aboard commercial aircraft. JAMA 253:1007, 1982.
10. Harinck E, Hutter PA, Hoorntije TM, et al: Air travel and adults with cyanotic congenital heart disease. Circulation 93:272, 1996.

CHAPTER 62
NEUROLOGIC PROBLEMS IN CHILDHOOD HEART DISEASE

ADRÉ J. du PLESSIS   JANE W. NEWBURGER

Dramatic improvements in the survival of patients with congenital heart disease have been accompanied by the recognition that this population manifests a high prevalence of neurologic and developmental abnormalities, including mental retardation and lifelong language and learning problems.[1] The factors underlying this morbidity are complex, multifactorial, and probably cumulative. Neurologic abnormalities among children with cardiac disease are sometimes mediated by known chromosome abnormalities (e.g., trisomy 21, chromosome 22q11 microdeletion) or by inherited disorders of metabolism or neuromuscular degeneration. Other neurologic abnormalities are acquired, either from sequelae of congenital heart disease itself or from its therapies.

Although neurologic complications of open heart surgery have been the focus of most recent clinical investigations, brain injury among patients with congenital heart disease may be caused by severe chronic hypoxemia or congestive heart failure, episodes of arrhythmia or cardiac arrest, thromboembolic events unrelated to operation, poor nutritional status, and central nervous system infection. Both the mechanisms and the clinical profile of acquired neurologic injury in patients with a cardiac malformation have changed in recent years, largely owing to the advent of prostaglandin therapy for ductus-dependent lesions and dramatic advances in infant cardiac surgery.

CEREBRAL DYSGENESIS

The prevalence of cerebral dysgenesis in children with congenital heart disease ranges from 10 to 29% in autopsy studies and varies with the underlying cardiac lesion.[2–4] Infants with hypoplastic left heart syndrome appear to be at particular risk for associated developmental cerebral abnormalities, which range in severity from microdysgenesis to gross malformations like holoprosencephaly.[2] With increasing availability and use of neuroimaging, the association between cardiac anomalies and brain dysgenesis will become more clearly defined.

These dysgenetic lesions may present in the neonatal period with seizures, alterations in level of consciousness, and abnormalities in motor tone. Conversely, brain abnormalities may remain clinically occult until later infancy and childhood, when they present with developmental delay, epilepsy, and cerebral palsy. Thus, cerebral dysgenesis

should be considered in any child with congenital heart disease and neurologic manifestations.

NEONATAL INTRACRANIAL HEMORRHAGE

Many of the previously lethal congenital cardiac conditions that presented with shock and acidosis in the neonatal period are now amenable to early correction or palliation; survivors may manifest the long-term neurologic consequences of neonatal hemodynamic compromise. Perhaps as a consequence of hemodynamic instability, the risk period for intraventricular-periventricular hemorrhage[5] characteristic of premature infants appears to extend further into maturity in infants with a cardiac anomaly. Cranial ultrasonography has demonstrated such hemorrhage in 24% of term infants with congenital heart disease.[6]

The diagnosis of intraventricular-periventricular hemorrhage in a neonate with congenital heart disease complicates operative planning. In these infants, the use of anticoagulation, the increase in fibrinolytic activity,[7] and the variation in cerebral perfusion pressure during cardiopulmonary bypass each may predispose to extension of intraventricular-periventricular hemorrhage or hemorrhagic transformation of ischemic lesions. The timing and management of cardiac surgery in infants with intraventricular-periventricular hemorrhage attempt to balance the risks of extension of hemorrhage during a cardiac operation against those of ischemia-reperfusion injury and further hemorrhagic extension during the persistent cardiorespiratory instability associated with an uncorrected cardiac malformation. Factors that must be considered include the severity of the cardiac illness, the expected complexity of the operation, and the severity of the intracranial hemorrhage. Hemorrhage confined to the subependymal region should not delay operation. It is probably advisable to delay cardiopulmonary bypass for at least 1 week in infants with intraventricular hemorrhage, preferably longer in those with intraparenchymal hemorrhage.

THE PERIOPERATIVE PERIOD

CARDIOPULMONARY BYPASS TECHNIQUES

An important portion of acquired brain injury among patients with congenital cardiac anomalies is attributable to perioperative events, particularly the support techniques used to protect vital organs during cardiac repair.[8] Sources of brain injury from cardiopulmonary bypass itself include hypoperfusion, macroemboli, and microemboli, both particulate and gaseous. The incidence of focal neurologic abnormalities after cardiopulmonary bypass in adults is 5%, with approximately 1% having persistent functional disability; retinal abnormalities detected by retinal fluorescein angiography and reflective of microembolic events appear to be nearly universal.[9] One pediatric study found that 14% of patients with complete transposition had evidence of cerebral infarction, usually small, after the arterial switch operation.[10]

Neurocognitive morbidity can be documented in most adults undergoing a cardiac operation, although long-term sequelae are usually mild.[11] In children with a cardiac anomaly who have undergone open heart surgery, cognitive deficits are also common, but maturational changes together with multiple preoperative and postoperative risk factors make it difficult to ascertain the extent to which these are strictly attributable to intraoperative events.[10, 12, 13] The risk of brain injury related to cardiopulmonary bypass in infants and children may be influenced by many variables, including the duration of total support, the depth of hypothermia, the rate and duration of core cooling,[14] the type of pH management chosen during core cooling (alpha-stat versus pH-stat),[15] the degree of hemodilution,[16] the duration of total circulatory arrest,[10, 12, 17] the type of oxygenator (bubble versus membrane), the use of arterial filtration, and other aspects of the biochemical milieu.[18, 19]

POSTOPERATIVE DELAYED RECOVERY OF CONSCIOUSNESS

In most instances of inappropriately delayed recovery of mental status after operation, no clear cause is established. Although hypoxic-ischemic reperfusion injury is often suspected, it is important to exclude postoperative hepatic or renal impairment resulting in accumulation of toxic metabolites or impaired metabolism or excretion of sedating drugs. Prolonged use of neuromuscular blocking agents may be associated with delayed recovery of motor function,[20–22] which if severe may mimic a state of impaired consciousness. As discussed later, a significant minority of infants develop postoperative seizures, which may recur serially and are often clinically silent.[17] A persistent depression of consciousness warrants consideration of occult seizures or a prolonged postictal state.

POSTOPERATIVE SEIZURES

Seizures are probably the most common neurologic complication of infant open heart surgery and are clinically manifest in up to 15% of patients in the early postoperative period.[17,23,24] Prospective long-term video electroencephalographic monitoring has demonstrated a significantly higher incidence of electrographic seizure activity in this early postoperative period, frequently without typical behavioral seizure manifestations.[17] Postoperative seizures may have a number of possible etiologic factors; of greatest concern to long-term outcome are those resulting from

hypoxic-ischemic reperfusion injury due to either generalized cerebral hypoperfusion or focal vasocclusive disease. More commonly, however, these early postoperative seizures remain cryptogenic and are often referred to as post-pump seizures. Although these post-pump seizures are often assumed to be related to hypoxic-ischemic reperfusion injury, they differ in several respects from other forms of such seizures. First, post-pump seizures typically occur later after injury than, for instance, those occurring after birth asphyxia. Whereas most asphyxial seizures have their onset within the first 12 hours after birth, post-pump seizures are first seen most commonly during the second postoperative 24 hours. Second, although post-pump seizures are associated with later neurologic and developmental dysfunction,[10] they nonetheless carry a less devastating prognosis than do asphyxial seizures, in which as many as 50% of infants are left with neurologic disability.[25–27] The delayed onset of these post-pump seizures and their more favorable outcome may reflect the neuroprotective effective of hypothermia during cardiopulmonary bypass.[28]

Post-pump seizures, as monitored by continuous electroencephalography, follow a fairly typical clinical course and appear confined to a relatively narrow time window. After their onset, usually between 24 and 48 hours postoperatively, these seizures tend to occur serially and often evolve to status epilepticus. The tendency toward further seizures persists for several days and then appears to decrease rapidly. The clinical manifestations of these electroencephalographic seizures depend, in part, on the presence of sedating and paralyzing drugs. Even in the absence of such medications, clinical manifestations may be minimal, confined to paroxysmal changes in autonomic function and pupillary size. Convulsive activity, when it is evident, is often focal or multifocal. Highly focal electroencephalographic abnormalities may reflect an underlying stroke, and hence indicate the need for neuroimaging.

Therapy for postoperative seizures includes intravenous anticonvulsant drugs in addition to identifying and correcting reversible causes, such as hypoglycemia, hypomagnesemia, and hypocalcemia.[29, 30] The potential for some anticonvulsants to cause myocardial or rhythm disturbances necessitates careful cardiorespiratory monitoring, particularly during the induction phase of anticonvulsant drug therapy.[31] Because post-pump seizures are usually self-limited, anticonvulsant therapy can often be successfully withdrawn before hospital discharge.

The prognosis of postoperative seizures varies with the underlying cause. In the majority, the cause is unclear and is often assumed to reflect intraoperative cerebral hypoxia-ischemia. These so-called post-pump seizures were previously regarded as benign, transient events. A prospective study using continuous video electroencephalography demonstrated a significant association between post-pump seizures and worse neurologic and developmental outcome at ages 1 year[10] and 4 years.[12] None of these patients had developed epilepsy by age 4 years, however. Among those infants for whom seizures have a specific cause, long-term outcome is related to etiology. For instance, in patients for whom seizures are a presenting symptom of cerebral dysgenesis, poor long-term outcome is nearly universal and epilepsy is a common sequel. In patients in whom seizures result from stroke, the risk of subsequent epilepsy ranges from 19 to 28%.[32,33] In this group, the epilepsy risk relates to age at the time of stroke and the latency to first seizure after the stroke; in a neonate, the risk for subsequent epilepsy is low,[34] whereas longer latency to first seizure is associated with greater incidence of epilepsy.[33] These features may guide decisions regarding duration of anticonvulsant therapy.

MOVEMENT DISORDERS

Soon after the advent of deep hypothermic cardiac surgery, striking movement disorders were reported[35,36]; approximately 100 patients have been described during the last three decades.[35,37–47] Although the incidence in different series has ranged from 0.5%[48] to 19%,[38] underdiagnosis and underreporting of these dyskinesias are such that the true incidence is unknown. Despite their relative rarity, these movement disorders are often dramatic, frequently intractable, and, particularly if severe, associated with a substantial mortality. Although choreoathetosis is the most frequent form of dyskinesia complicating a cardiac operation, other movement disorders have been described, including oculogyric crises[48] and parkinsonism.[49]

The appearance of postoperative movement disorders is typically preceded by a latency period of 2 to 7 days, during which neurologic recovery from operation appears uncomplicated. The dyskinesia is usually heralded by the subacute onset of delirium, with marked irritability, insomnia, confusion, and disorientation, followed shortly by abnormal involuntary movements. These movements begin in the distal extremities and orofacial muscles, progressing proximally to involve the girdle muscles and trunk; in severe instances, violent ballismic thrashing may develop. The abnormal movements are present during wakefulness, peak with distress, and resolve during periods of sleep. In addition, an apraxia of oculomotor and oromotor function develops, with a loss of feeding and expressive language skills. A supranuclear ophthalmoplegia often becomes apparent, with a loss of voluntary gaze but sparing of reflex extraocular movements; these patients do not appear to look at parents or caretakers and show minimal facial signs of recognition, thereby arousing concerns about blindness. The onset of involuntary movements is usually followed by a period of deterioration lasting about 1 week, a plateau period of 1 to 2 weeks during which the movements remain relatively constant, and finally a recovery phase of more variable duration.

Diagnosis of postoperative hyperkinetic syndromes is clinical; to date, adjunctive neurodiagnostic tests have been useful only to exclude other disorders. Neuroimaging studies, including computed tomography (CT) and magnetic resonance imaging (MRI), have shown nonspecific changes, most commonly diffuse cerebral atrophy. Focal abnormalities are rare.[43–45,47] Single-photon emission computed tomography (SPECT) functional brain imaging studies have shown a high incidence of both cortical and subcortical perfusion defects even in the absence of structural defects on CT and MRI.[50] Electroencephalographic studies are commonly normal or show diffuse slowing; ictal activity is not seen during these movements. Autopsy studies are limited and the neuropathologic findings are inconsistent,[39,51] ranging from normal to extensive degrees of neuronal loss and gliosis, particularly focused in the external globus pallidus.[51] Typical features of infarction are characteristically absent.

The prognosis of these conditions depends largely on their initial severity. Mild ones tend to resolve within weeks to months, but more severe instances have an associated mortality approaching 40% and a high incidence of persistent neurodevelopmental deficits in survivors.[47] Only approximately 10% of survivors in the severe group demonstrate normal neurologic outcome.[47] Common residual deficits include generalized hypotonia, developmental delay, and expressive language impairment. However, these reports are anecdotal, and detailed long-term follow-up is lacking.

The mechanisms underlying these movement disorders after a cardiac operation have remained elusive.[52–54] Despite the absence of a unifying mechanism, a number of risk factors have been identified. Children at particular risk include those with a cyanotic cardiac malformation, especially with systemic-to-pulmonary collaterals from the head and neck; age at operation older than 9 months; and excessively short cooling periods before attenuation of intraoperative blood flow. Some authors have suggested deep hypothermia itself as a cause.[41] Several reports have cited prolonged use of fentanyl and midazolam as a cause of postoperative dyskinesias. These drug-related dyskinesias tend to be relatively mild and to resolve during a period of weeks.[55–57]

CEREBROVASCULAR ACCIDENT (STROKE)

Congenital heart disease is the most common condition associated with stroke in childhood, being present in 25 to 30% of cases.[32,58,59] Stroke of cardiac origin, that is, cardiogenic stroke, has three broad mechanisms. First, arterial emboli may be generated from an intracardiac embolic source (cardioembolic stroke). Second, emboli may arise from a systemic venous or right-sided heart source and bypass the pulmonary circulation through a right-to-left shunt (paradoxical embolic stroke). Finally, cerebral venous thrombosis may result from a combination of central venous hypertension, venous stasis, and polycythemia. Risk factors for cardiogenic stroke include altered vascular surface, stasis, and hypercoagulability and paradoxical vascular pathways.

Open heart surgery presents multiple risk factors for stroke. During cardiopulmonary bypass, particulate and gaseous emboli originating from the cardiopulmonary bypass apparatus or operative field enter the systemic circulation directly.[60–63] Improvements in bypass circuits, particularly the switch from bubble to membrane oxygenators, have decreased the incidence of macroembolization; reduction in microembolic load is suggested by a smaller total ischemic area assessed with retinal fluorescein angiography after use of membrane oxygenators compared with bubble oxygenators.[9] Although bypass-related cerebral injury in adults is related primarily to atheromatous emboli or fixed cerebrovascular stenoses, such injury in infants results most commonly from global hypoperfusion during periods of decreased or arrested systemic blood flow. A further potential mechanism of intraoperative vascular injury may relate to the often marked inflammatory response triggered by the extensive and prolonged exposure between bypass blood and artificial surfaces.[64–66] These factors are known to trigger complex cascades, including endothelium-leukocyte interactions.[67–70] Stroke in the early postoperative period may present with focal motor weakness and speech and visual dysfunction. Seizures are a particularly common presentation of stroke in young infants.[32, 71]

Patients with congenital heart disease are also at risk for stroke from factors outside the operating room. Cardiac catheterization poses a risk of both particulate and gaseous emboli, particularly in cyanotic patients who are at risk for paradoxical embolization. In patients with cardiomyopathy, cerebral emboli can derive from intracardiac thrombus. Similarly, embolic stroke may occur in patients with a left atrial clot who convert to normal sinus rhythm from atrial fibrillation, prompting the recommendation for either transesophageal echocardiography or anticoagulation before planned cardioversions. Vascular surfaces may promote thrombosis secondary to endothelial injury or to the presence of prosthetic tissue, especially in an area of vascular stasis.[72–74] Patients with a left-sided prosthetic valve are at risk for thromboembolic complications. Those with left-sided infective endocarditis may have septic cerebral emboli and occasional intracranial mycotic aneurysms (see later).

A number of risk factors for stroke converge in patients undergoing the Fontan procedure, a common palliative operation for patients with single-ventricle physiology. In a retrospective review of 645 patients after the Fontan operation, the incidence of stroke was reported to be 2.6%.[72] The risk of stroke extends for 3[72] to 15 years[74] and may be higher among patients in whom a baffle leak or fenestration permits right-to-left shunting.

Stroke prevention may be regarded as primary (i.e., treatment of high-risk patients to prevent a first stroke) or secondary (i.e., aimed at preventing stroke recurrence).[75] Because there have been no prospective trials related to childhood stroke, preventive stroke management in children with a cardiac anomaly is based almost entirely on studies in adults. Most pediatric cardiologists use prophylactic anticoagulant therapy in children with a prosthetic heart valve, dilated cardiomyopathy, and intracardiac thrombus on echocardiography. The need for stroke prophylaxis in individual patients should consider risk factors such as elevated right atrial pressure, intracardiac prosthetic material, and a right-to-left shunt in children requiring prolonged bedrest. Because of the relatively high risk of stroke after the Fontan operation, many cardiologists administer antithrombotic therapy for at least several months in these patients, particularly those with a "fenestrated" baffle. Secondary stroke prophylaxis aims to balance the risk of recurrent embolism and that of hemorrhagic transformation of a bland infarction.

HEADACHES

Headaches in patients with a cardiac malformation commonly require evaluation. Acute severe headache should always raise the question of subarachnoid hemorrhage, particularly in patients with a history of coarctation of the aorta. In addition, patients with severe polycythemia tend to experience more frequent headaches. Raised central venous pressure, as may be seen after the Fontan procedure or the bidirectional Glenn procedure, may result in increased cerebral venous pressure, which by itself may be associated with headaches. However, such raised central venous pressure may also impair absorption of cerebrospinal fluid, resulting in communicating hydrocephalus[76] with elevated intracranial pressure and headache.

Headache is the most common presenting feature[77] in the otherwise often subtle clinical presentation of brain abscess (see later). Papilledema is a common clinical finding in brain abscess and may also be seen with communicating hydrocephalus. Before the direct measurement of cerebrospinal fluid pressure by lumbar puncture, a brain abscess should be excluded by neuroimaging (MRI or CT scan with contrast enhancement) to exclude a mass effect before a lumbar puncture is performed.

INFECTIOUS ENDOCARDITIS

Children with a cardiac anomaly are at increased risk for infectious endocarditis with its protean neurologic manifestations. These include meningitis, brain abscess, seizures, and, most commonly, cerebrovascular injury. Despite modern antibiotic advances, approximately one third of the children with infectious endocarditis have neurologic complications, approximately half of which are embolic in origin.[78] Not only are cerebrovascular complications the most common form of neurologic injury in endocarditis, but they also carry the highest mortality, reaching 80 to 90% with hemorrhage of mycotic aneurysms.[79] The high risk of hemorrhagic transformation of septic infarction or the direct subarachnoid hemorrhage through mycotic aneurysms contraindicates the use of anticoagulation in children with infectious endocarditis and cerebrovascular disease.[80]

BRAIN ABSCESS

Cyanotic cardiac malformation constitutes a major predisposing factor for brain abscess,[81] with an incidence ranging from 2 to 6%.[82] Conversely, congenital heart disease is present in almost half of childhood brain abscess,[83] with tetralogy of Fallot being the most common underlying cardiac lesion. Arterial oxygenation is inversely correlated with the incidence, morbidity, and mortality of brain abscess in congenital heart disease.[82] The incidence of brain abscess among patients with a cardiac anomaly has recently decreased markedly, primarily because of earlier corrective operation.

In cyanotic patients with polycythemia, periods of systemic illness and dehydration may critically disturb cerebral microvascular perfusion with subsequent localized areas of ischemia. Organisms bypassing the pulmonary filtration system may gain direct access to the brain, where they breach the disrupted blood-brain barrier, passing into necrotic areas to form focal septic cerebritis and, subsequently, frank cerebral abscess. Seventy-five percent of brain abscesses are supratentorial, predominantly occurring in the distribution of the middle cerebral artery. Posterior fossa abscesses, less common, are more dangerous; cerebellar abscesses may remain clinically silent until the onset of a rapid deterioration from tonsillar herniation and brain stem compression. Cerebral abscesses are multifocal in about 20% of patients.

In children with a cardiac anomaly, brain abscess is rare before the age of 2 years.[84] The clinical manifestations of brain abscess result from a combination of intracranial hypertension, focal neurologic injury, and sepsis. Headache is the predominant and usual presenting symptom. The initial presentation is often subtle, the course slowly progressive. On occasion, the presentation may be abrupt, for example, when the presenting symptom is a seizure. The common early symptoms are headache and vomiting, present in 50% and 72% of patients, respectively.[77] Personality changes and irritability occur early. Fever is relatively infrequent, being absent in up to 75% of patients at presentation, and peripheral leukocytosis may be minimal. The cerebrospinal fluid, which should be obtained only after exclusion of a significant mass effect by brain imaging, may have elevated protein but often only mild leukocytosis. The diagnosis of brain abscess is best confirmed by contrast-enhanced CT or MRI scan. By CT scan, brain abscess presents as an area of hypodensity with contrast ring enhancement; marked cerebral edema often surrounds the abscess. Although diagnostic and therapeutic advances have reduced the mortality of brain abscess from 40%[84] to 10%,[85] the 35 to 45% prevalence of neurologic sequelae in survivors has remained largely unchanged.[83,85] Epilepsy develops in up to 30% of survivors, often after many years.[83]

The optimal management of brain abscess remains controversial.[85] Operation is still widely considered the definitive first-line treatment. Whether direct resection or aspiration of the abscess under CT guidance is the preferable approach is uncertain. Advances in both antibiotic therapy and neuroimaging have allowed more conservative antibiotic management to be monitored closely by brain scans[86,87]; this approach may be particularly effective early in patients with focal cerebritis without rapid progression. With or without surgery, high-dose antibiotic therapy should be administered for at least 6 weeks. Mixed aerobic and anaerobic streptococci and staphylococci are the most common causative organisms.[88] Although earlier initial antibiotic regimens have now been largely superseded by third-generation cephalosporins together with antistaphylococcal and anaerobic agents, subsequent therapy should be guided by culture results, when they are available. In immunosuppressed patients (e.g., after cardiac transplantation), other lower virulence organisms as well as fungi (e.g., *Aspergillus*) and parasites (e.g., *Toxoplasma*) should be considered.

Because the clinical presentation of brain abscess may closely resemble that of aseptic stroke in up to 30% of patients,[89] it has been suggested that children with a cyanotic cardiac malformation and a stroke-like presentation be managed with antibiotics until a brain abscess is excluded.[89]

SYDENHAM CHOREA

Sydenham chorea is the major neurologic complication of acute rheumatic fever and in earlier years was the most common form of acquired chorea in childhood. For details, see Chapter 48.

FUTURE DIRECTIONS

Reparative infant cardiac surgery, with its necessity for use of cardiopulmonary bypass techniques and "planned" ischemia-reperfusion injury, provides an unparalleled opportunity for prospective clinical trials of neuroprotective agents. Techniques targeting the inhibition of cellular injury mediated by excitotoxicity and free radical damage have exciting potential applications in cardiac surgery. In addition, new neurodiagnostic techniques are likely to facilitate the early identification of infants at risk for brain injury, the timely institution of neuroprotective agents, and the evaluation of such agents in clinical trials.

REFERENCES

1. Ferry PC: Neurologic sequelae of open-heart surgery in children. An "irritating question." Am J Dis Child 144:369, 1990.
2. Glauser T, Rorke L, Weinberg P, et al: Congenital brain anomalies associated with hypoplastic left heart syndrome. Pediatrics 85:984, 1990.
3. Jones M: Anomalies of the brain and congenital heart disease. A study of 52 necropsy cases. Pediatr Pathol 11:721, 1991.
4. Terplan K: Brain changes in newborns, infants and children with congenital heart disease in association with cardiac surgery. Additional observations. J Neurosurg 212:225, 1976.
5. Volpe JJ: Intracranial hemorrhage. In Neurology of the Newborn. Philadelphia, WB Saunders, 1994, p 373.
6. van Houten J, Rothman A, Bejar R: Echoencephalographic (ECHO) findings in infants with congenital heart disease (CHD). Pediatr Res 33:376A, 1993.
7. Giuliani R, Szwarcer E, Aquino E, et al: Fibrin-dependent fibrinolytic activity during extracorporeal circulation. Thromb Res 61:369, 1991.
8. Ferry PC: Neurologic sequelae of cardiac surgery in children. Am J Dis Child 141:309, 1987.
9. Blauth C: Retinal fluorescein angiography in the assessment of microembolism during cardiopulmonary bypass. In Smith P, Taylor K (eds): Cardiac Surgery and the Brain. London, Edward Arnold, 1993, p 165.
10. Bellinger DC, Jonas RA, Rappaport LA, et al: Developmental and neurologic status of children after heart surgery with hypothermic circulatory arrest or low-flow cardiopulmonary bypass. N Engl J Med 332:549, 1995.
11. Shaw PJ: The neurologic sequelae of cardiopulmonary bypass: The Newcastle experience. In Smith P, Taylor K (eds): Cardiac Surgery and the Brain. London, Edward Arnold, 1993, p 24.
12. Newburger JW, Wypij D, Kuban KCK, et al: Four year neurodevelopmental status: The Boston Circulatory Arrest Study. Circulation 94(suppl):I-173, 1996.
13. Wernovsky G, Stiles KM, Gauvreau K, et al: Cognitive development following the Fontan operation. Circulation 92(suppl):I-121, 1995.
14. Bellinger DC, Wernovsky G, Rappaport LA, et al: Cognitive development of children following early repair of transposition of the great arteries using deep hypothermic circulatory arrest. Pediatrics 87:701, 1991.
15. du Plessis AJ, Jonas RA, Wypij D, et al: Perioperative effects of alpha-stat versus pH-stat strategies for deep hypothermic cardiopulmonary bypass in infants. J Thorac Cardiovasc Surg 114:991, 1997.

16. Shin-oka T, Shuma-Tim D, Jonas RA, et al: Higher hematocrit improves cerebral outcome after deep hypothermic circulatory arrest. J Thorac Cardiovasc Surg 112:1610, 1996.

17. Newburger JW, Jonas RA, Wernovsky G, et al: A comparison of the perioperative neurologic effects of hypothermic circulatory arrest versus low-flow cardiopulmonary bypass in infant heart surgery. N Engl J Med 329:1057, 1993.

18. Kirklin JW: Hypothermia, circulatory arrest, and cardiopulmonary bypass. In Kirklin JW, Barratt-Boyes BG (eds): Cardiac Surgery. New York, Churchill Livingstone, 1993, p 61.

19. Jonas RA: Problems of deep hypothermic circulatory arrest and low-flow perfusion. With particular reference to the paediatric population. In Smith P, Taylor K (eds): Cardiac Surgery and the Brain. London, Edward Arnold, 1993, p 95.

20. Gooch J, Suchyta M, Balbierz J, et al: Prolonged paralysis after treatment with neuromuscular junction blocking agents. Crit Care Med 19:1125, 1991.

21. Partridge B, Abrams J, Bazemore C, et al: Prolonged neuromuscular blockade after long-term infusion of vecuronium bromide in the intensive care unit. Crit Care Med 18:1577, 1990.

22. Waitling S, Dasta J: Prolonged paralysis in intensive care unit patients after use of neuromuscular blocking agents: A review of the literature. Crit Care Med 22:884, 1994.

23. Ehyai A, Fenichel G, Bender H: Incidence and prognosis of seizures in infants after cardiac surgery with profound hypothermia and circulatory arrest. JAMA 252:3165, 1984.

24. Miller G, Eggli K, Contant C, et al: Postoperative neurologic complications after open heart surgery on young infants. Arch Pediatr Adolesc Med 149:764, 1995.

25. Andre M, Matisse N, Vert P: Prognosis of neonatal seizures. In Waterlain C, Vert P (eds): Neonatal Seizures. New York, Raven Press, 1990, p 61.

26. Bergman I, Painter M, Hirsch R, et al: Outcome in neonates with convulsions treated in an intensive care unit. Ann Neurol 14:642, 1983.

27. Volpe J: Neonatal seizures. In Neurology of the Newborn. Philadelphia, WB Saunders, 1994, p 172.

28. Dietrich W, Busto R, Alonso O, et al: Intraischemic but not postischemic brain hypothermia protects chronically following global forebrain ischemia in rats. J Cereb Blood Flow Metab 13:541, 1993.

29. Lynch N, Rust R: Natural history and outcome of neonatal hypocalcemic and hypomagnesemic seizures. Pediatr Neurol 11:23, 1994.

30. Satur C, Jennings A, Walker D: Hypomagnesemia and fits complicating pediatric cardiac surgery. Ann Clin Biochem 30:315, 1993.

31. Cranford R, Leppik I, Patrick B, et al: Intravenous phenytoin: Clinical and pharmacological aspects. Neurology 28:874, 1978.

32. Lanska M, Lanska D, Horwitz S, et al: Presentation, clinical course and outcome of childhood stroke. Pediatr Neurol 7:333, 1991.

33. Yang J, Park Y, Hartlage P: Seizures associated with stroke in childhood. Pediatr Neurol 12:136, 1995.

34. Levy S, Abroms I, Marshall P, et al: Seizures and cerebral infarction in the full-term newborn. Ann Neurol 17:366, 1985.

35. Bergouignan M, Fontan F, Trarieux M: Syndromes choreiformes de l'enfant au cours d'interventions cardio-chirurgicales sous hypothermie profonde. Rev Neurol 105:48, 1961.

36. Bjork V, Hultquist G: Contraindications to profound hypothermia in open-heart surgery. J Thorac Cardiovasc Surg 44:1, 1962.

37. Barratt-Boyes BG: Choreoathetosis as a complication of cardiopulmonary bypass. Ann Thorac Surg 50:693, 1990.

38. Brunberg JA, Doty DB, Reilly EL: Choreoathetosis in infants following cardiac surgery with deep hypothermic and circulatory arrest. J Pediatr 84:232, 1974.

39. Chaves E, Scaltsas-Persson I: Severe choreoathetosis (CA) following congenital heart disease (CHD) surgery (Abstract). Neurology 38:284, 1988.

40. Curless R, Katz D, Perryman R, et al: Choreoathetosis after surgery for congenital heart disease. J Pediatr 124:737, 1994.

41. DeLeon S, Ilbawa M, Arcilla R, et al: Choreoathetosis after deep hypothermia without circulatory arrest. Ann Thorac Surg 50:714, 1990.

42. Donaldson D, Fullerton D, Gollub R, et al: Choreoathetosis in children after cardiac surgery. Neurology 40:337, 1990.

43. Huntley D, Al-Mateen M, Menkes J: Unusual dyskinesia complicating cardiopulmonary bypass surgery. Dev Med Child Neurol 35:631, 1993.

44. Medlock M, Cruse R, Winek S, et al: A 10-year experience with postpump chorea. Ann Neurol 34:820, 1993.

45. Robinson RO, Samuels M, Pohl KRE: Choreic syndrome after cardiac surgery. Arch Dis Child 63:1466, 1988.

46. Wical B, Tomasi L: A distinctive neurologic syndrome after profound hypothermia. Pediatr Neurol 6:202, 1990.

47. Wong PC, Barlow CF, Hickey PR, et al: Factors associated with choreoathetosis after cardiopulmonary bypass in children with congenital heart disease. Circulation 86(suppl):II-118, 1992.

48. Wessel D, du Plessis AJ: Choreoathetosis. In Volpe J (ed): Brain Injury and Pediatric Cardiac Surgery. Boston, Butterworth-Heinemann, 1995, p 353.

49. Straussberg R, Shahar E, Gat R, et al: Delayed parkinsonism associated with hypotension in a child undergoing open-heart surgery. Dev Med Child Neurol 35:1007, 1993.

50. du Plessis AJ, Treves S, Hickey P, et al: Regional cerebral perfusion abnormalities after cardiac operations. Thorac Cardiovasc Surg 107:1036, 1994.

51. Kupsky W, Drozd M, Barlow C: Selective injury of the globus pallidus in children with post-cardiac surgery choreic syndrome. Dev Med Child Neurol 37:135, 1995.

52. Greenmyre T, Penney J, Young A, et al: Evidence for transient perinatal glutamatergic innervation of globus pallidus. J Neurosci 7:1022, 1987.

53. Johnston M, Redmond J, Gillinov A, et al: Neuroprotective strategies in a model of selective neuronal necrosis from hypothermic circulatory arrest. In Moskowitz M, Caplan L (eds): Cerebrovascular Diseases. Boston, Butterworth-Heinemann, 1995, p 165.

54. Redmond J, Gillinov A, Zehr K, et al: Glutamate excitotoxicity: A mechanism of neurologic injury associated with hypothermic circulatory arrest. J Thorac Cardiovasc Surg 107:776, 1994.

55. Bergman I, Steeves M, Burckart G, et al: Reversible neurologic abnormalities associated with prolonged intravenous midazolam and fentanyl administration. J Pediatr 119:644, 1991.

56. Lane J, Tennison M, Lawless S, et al: Movement disorder after withdrawal of fentanyl infusion. J Pediatr 119:649, 1991.

57. Petzinger G, Mayer SA, Przedborski S: Fentanyl-induced dyskinesias. Mov Disord 10:679, 1995.

58. Riela A, Roach E: Etiology of stroke in children. J Child Neurol 8:201, 1993.

59. Schoenberg B, Mellinger J, Schoenberg D: Cardiovascular disease in infants and children: A study of incidence, clinical features, and survival. Neurology 28:763, 1978.

60. Boyajian R, Sobel D, DeLaria G, et al: Embolic stroke as a sequelae of cardiopulmonary bypass. J Neuroimaging 3:1, 1993.

61. Moody D, Bell M, Challa V, et al: Brain microemboli during cardiac surgery or aortography. Ann Neurol 28:477, 1990.

62. Padayachee T, Parsons S, Theobold R, et al: The detection of microemboli in the middle cerebral artery during cardiopulmonary bypass: A transcranial Doppler ultrasound investigation using membrane and bubble oxygenators. Ann Thorac Surg 44:298, 1987.

63. Solis R, Kennedy P, Beall A, et al: Cardiopulmonary bypass: Microembolization and platelet aggregation. Circulation 52:103, 1975.

64. Kirklin JK, Westaby S, Blackstone EH, et al: Complement and the damaging effects of cardiopulmonary bypass. J Thorac Cardiovasc Surg 86:845, 1983.

65. Millar A, Armstrong L, van der Linden J, et al: Cytokine production and hemofiltration in children undergoing cardiopulmonary bypass. Ann Thorac Surg 56(suppl):1499, 1993.

66. Steinberg J, Kapelanski D, Olson J, et al: Cytokine and complement levels in patients undergoing cardiopulmonary bypass. J Thorac Cardiovasc Surg 106:1008, 1993.

67. del Zoppo G: Microvascular changes during cerebral ischemia and reperfusion. Cerebrovasc Brain Metab Rev 6:47, 1994.

68. Elliott M, Finn A: Interaction between neutrophils and endothelium. Ann Thorac Surg 56:1503, 1993.

69. Feuerstein G, Liu T, Barone F: Cytokines, inflammation, and brain injury. Role of tumor necrosis factor-α. Cerebrovasc Brain Metab Rev 6:341, 1994.

70. Lucchesi B: Complement activation, neutrophils, and oxygen radicals in reperfusion injury. Stroke 24(suppl):I41, 1993.

71. Clancy R, Malin S, Laraque D, et al: Focal motor seizures heralding stroke in full-term infants. Am J Dis Child 139:601, 1985.

72. du Plessis A, Chang A, Wessel D, et al: Cerebrovascular accidents following the Fontan procedure. Pediatr Neurol 12:230, 1995.

73. Rosenthal D, Bulbul Z, Friedman A, et al: Thrombosis of the pulmonary artery stump after distal ligation. J Thorac Cardiovasc Surg 110:1563, 1995.

74. Rosenthal D, Friedman A, Kleinman C, et al: Thromboembolic complications after Fontan operations. Circulation 92:287, 1995.

75. Anderson D: Cardioembolic stroke: Primary and secondary prevention. Postgrad Med 90:67, 1991.

76. Rosman P, Shands K: Hydrocephalus caused by increased intracranial venous pressure: A clinicopathological study. Ann Neurol 3:445, 1978.

77. Aicardi J: Disease of the Nervous System in Childhood. London, MacKeith Press, 1992, p 590.

78. Saiman L, Prince A, Gersony W: Pediatric infective endocarditis in the modern era. J Pediatr 122:847, 1993.

79. Jones H, Sieker R: Neurologic manifestations of infective endocarditis. Brain 122:1295, 1989.

80. Pruitt A, Rubin R, Karchmer A, et al: Neurologic complications of bacterial endocarditis. Medicine (Baltimore) 57:329, 1978.

81. Tyler R, Clark D: Cerebrovascular accidents in patients with congenital heart disease. Arch Neurol Psychiatry 77:483, 1957.

82. Shu-yuan Y: Brain abscess associated with congenital heart disease. Surg Neurol 31:129, 1989.

83. Aebi C, Kaufmann F, Schaad U: Brain abscess in childhood: Long-term experiences. Eur J Pediatr 150:282, 1991.

84. Kagawa M, Takeshita M, Yato S, et al: Brain abscess in congenital heart disease. J Neurosurg 58:913, 1983.

85. Dodge P, Pomeroy S: Parameningeal infections (including brain abscess, epidural abscess, subdural empyema). *In* Feigin R, Cherry J (eds): Textbook of Pediatric Infectious Diseases. Philadelphia, WB Saunders, 1992, p 455.

86. Berg B, Franklin G, Cuneo R, et al: Nonsurgical cure of brain abscess: Early diagnosis and follow-up with computerized tomography. Ann Neurol 3:474, 1978.

87. Rosenblum M, Hoff J, Norman D, et al: Nonoperative treatment of brain abscess in selected high-risk patients. J Neurosurg 52:217, 1980.

88. Ghosh S, Chandy M, Abraham J: Brain abscess and congenital heart disease. J Indian Med Assoc 88:312, 1988.

89. Kurlan R, Griggs R: Cyanotic congenital heart disease with suspected stroke. Should all patients receive antibiotics? Arch Neurol 40:209, 1983.

CHAPTER 63
COMPLICATIONS IN CHRONIC CYANOTIC HEART DISEASE

ELIZABETH A. BRAUNLIN

Current knowledge and techniques in pediatric cardiology and cardiovascular surgery permit repair of most cyanotic congenital cardiac anomalies in infancy and childhood with permanent relief of cyanosis. There are, however, at least two groups of patients with cardiac malformations who have permanent cyanosis: those with irreparable cyanotic cardiac anomalies (e.g., tetralogy of Fallot with pulmonary atresia and multiple small bronchial arteries) and those adults with cyanotic cardiac anomalies for whom the advances in knowledge came too late. Complications of chronic hypoxemia affect all organ systems.

NEUROPSYCHOLOGIC EFFECTS

Brain abscess and cerebral embolism are well-described sequelae of cyanotic congenital cardiac disease and are discussed in Chapter 62. Cyanotic children have significantly lower intelligence quotients than have children with acyanotic cardiac anomalies. The difference is small, and both fall within the normal range.[1] This difference persists regardless of sex, race, social class, or severity of the malformation and occurs before operative intervention. Cognitive function also appears inversely related to age at surgical repair.[2] The mechanism responsible for these findings is unknown but may be related to the development of white matter gliosis because of cyanosis, to recurrent unrecognized small cerebrovascular events, or to other reasons not presently understood.

HEMATOLOGIC EFFECTS

Chronic cyanosis causes tissue hypoxia that activates specialized renal sensor cells to produce erythropoietin. This chemical messenger induces the bone marrow to increase red cell mass and is thus responsible for the erythrocytosis of cyanotic cardiac malformations.

Erythrocytosis in the iron-replete individual is seldom associated with symptoms (i.e., stroke) if the hematocrit is less than 65%.[3] If the hematocrit rises above 70%, symptoms of hyperviscosity may occur. These include headache, dizziness, fatigue, myalgias, visual disturbances, altered mentation, paresthesia of fingers and toes or lips, and tinnitus. Phlebotomy is recommended for symptomatic individuals only, even if the hematocrit is in excess of 70%.[3] In clinical practice, evidence-based policies regarding this issue are often absent.[4] Repeated phlebotomies may be associated with the development of iron deficiency anemia. Replacement of red cell volume taken during phlebotomy, optimally by colloid, is recommended[3,4] to prevent hemodynamic instability. Care must be taken with phlebotomy in cyanotic patients with decreased pulmonary blood flow because their blood volume is already reduced.

Iron deficiency is particularly hazardous in individuals with a cyanotic cardiac condition because of its effect on red cell shape and rigidity. Iron deficiency causes the erythrocyte to change from a flexible biconcave disk to a spherical microcyte that is rigid and larger than capillary diameters. This change in shape alone increases the viscosity of blood regardless of hematocrit. Iatrogenic iron deficiency from repeated phlebotomies in asymptomatic cyanotic patients can increase the risk of stroke or thrombosis by this mechanism.

Abnormal bleeding in cyanotic individuals can be modest (easy bruising, gingival bleeding) or life-threatening (hemoptysis, trauma). Abnormalities in coagulation remain poorly defined but appear to be more common with increasing hematocrit.[5] Thrombocytopenia is the most commonly identified abnormality; excessive concentrations of factors V and VIII and occasionally low levels of factors II, VII, IX, and X occur in individuals whose hematocrits are 70% or greater.[5] Deficiency of large von Willebrand's factor multimeric forms has been identified. Thrombocytopenia occurs because of right-to-left intracardiac shunting. Megakaryocytes escape the normal fragmentation that occurs in the lung. Abnormalities in factor levels may be due to decreased production from hepatic dysfunction as a result of hypoxia and polycythemia rather than increased consumption from an active intravascular coagulopathy.

Regardless of etiology, treatment of patients with aspirin or nonsteroidal anti-inflammatory agents should be avoided because both inhibit platelet function and increase the risk of significant bleeding. Conversely, drugs such as desmopressin that increase levels of circulating factor VIII have proved useful perioperatively or with significant hemoptysis or epistaxis.

RENAL EFFECTS

Long-standing cyanosis induces morphologic changes in the kidney including enlarged hypercellular glomeruli with thickened basement membranes, focal interstitial fibrosis, tubular atrophy, and hyalinization of afferent and efferent arterioles.[6] As a result, patients with cyanotic congenital heart disease may develop a glomerulopathy associated with significant proteinuria and impaired renal function.[7] The development of pathologic proteinuria is directly related to higher erythrocyte count and to the age of the patient. Patients older than 20 years are most often affected, and those younger than 10 years are uncommonly affected. At higher levels of proteinuria, creatinine clearance is likely to be decreased, especially with cardiac failure. Electrophoresis of urinary proteins reveals an unselective glomerular proteinuria with a molecular mass range of 41 to 400 kDa consistent with a glomerular abnormality in most patients.[7]

Hyperuricemia occurs frequently in adolescents and adults with cyanotic forms of congenital heart disease in a manner similar to that for proteinuria.[8] Serum uric acid level correlates directly and significantly with both age and severity of erythrocytosis. Serum uric acid level is significantly higher for individuals taking furosemide than for those not receiving this medication. In those older than 15 years with hyperuricemia (serum uric acid levels above 8 mg/dl), 24-hour urinary uric acid excretion, uric acid clearance, and fractional excretion of uric acid values are notably lower than normal. A decrease in creatinine clearance and proteinuria has been noted in these patients by age 13 years before development of hyperuricemia.[8]

Hyperuricemia in cyanotic patients reflects increased purine catabolism.[8] The accumulation of adenosine monophosphate (a purine-based compound) in organs during hypoxia due to suppression of aerobic metabolic pathways represents a likely source of increased purine load.[8]

Symptoms such as uric acid kidney stones, soft tissue urate deposits, and acute gouty arthritis have been reported but are uncommon in individuals with cyanotic cardiac anomalies.[3] Treatment with colchicine is effective in reducing symptoms but may lead to nausea, vomiting, and dehydration. Nonsteroidal anti-inflammatory drugs are less effective and will affect underlying hemostatic abnormalities.[3] In recurrent symptomatic hyperuricemia, treatment with probenecid or sulfinpyrazone (uricosuric agents) or allopurinol is recommended.[3]

CARDIOPULMONARY EFFECTS

Cardiac contractility is highly dependent on aerobic metabolic pathways. Experimentally, profound hypoxemia produces a rapid decline in high-energy phosphates within the heart, disappearance of myocardial glycogen, and production of lactic acid.[9] Myocardial dysfunction is frequently found in individuals with long-standing cyanotic cardiac disease, although the mechanisms responsible are incompletely understood. Contractile dysfunction has been linked to impaired free fatty acid metabolism of the ventricle in cyanotic individuals[10] and to lower activity levels of aerobic enzymes within both the atrium and ventricle of cyanotic hearts compared with normal control hearts.[11] Infarction or fibrosis of the subendocardium and papillary muscles can occur in individuals with chronic hypoxemia.[12]

Vulnerability of the human myocardium to injury by free radicals is postulated to be responsible for the decreased ventricular function often present after cardiopulmonary bypass in patients with tetralogy of Fallot[13] and may be another cause of ventricular dysfunction in cyanotic individuals. Under normal conditions, free radicals are generated in small quantities by all cells. Antioxidant enzymes—superoxide dismutase, catalase, glutathione peroxidase—are present in myocardial tissue to scavenge these highly reactive compounds and prevent tissue damage. In patients with tetralogy of Fallot, these enzyme levels are directly related to the level of preoperative arterial oxygen tension, with the lowest protective levels occurring in most hypoxemic patients. Data suggest that the sudden increase in arterial oxygen tension occurring with cardiopulmonary bypass provides an increased load of free radicals that the free radical–scavenging mechanism of the cyanotic myocardium is unable to neutralize. The release of these free radicals produces myocardial injury that is more severe than that seen in the noncyanotic myocardium.[13] These data imply that the cyanotic myocardium may be more vulnerable to oxidative stress regardless of origin.

The control of ventilation in humans is through automatic and voluntary mechanisms. The carotid and aortic bodies are chemoreceptor cells that regulate the automatic responses to respiration. The most important physiologic stimulus to these receptors is arterial oxygen tension.[14] Both ventilation (primarily respiratory rate) and heart rate increase significantly in response to hypoxemia.[14] This response is attenuated by age in normal individuals. There may be loss of peripheral chemoreceptor sensitivity with central depression of ventilation in individuals with cyanotic cardiac disease as a result of lifelong hypoxemia.[15] If long-standing, the insensitivity to hypoxemia may be irreversible and exist even after relief of cyanosis.[15] Alteration of this protective mechanism by hypoxia is important when medications that have respiratory depression as one of their side effects are given.

Individuals with chronic cyanosis because of right-to-left intracardiac shunting have an abnormal response to exercise.[16] There is a significant inability to increase oxygen uptake above baseline values, and the time required to attain steady state is prolonged compared with that in acyanotic control subjects. The limited ability to increase oxygen consumption correlates well with reported physical activity tolerance of these individuals.[16]

MUSCULOSKELETAL EFFECTS

Individuals with a cardiac malformation have an increased incidence (4%) of scoliosis compared with that of the general population (1.1%) although the reason is unknown.[17] The incidence of scoliosis in individuals with cyanotic forms has been reported to be higher than in those with acyanotic malformations.[18]

Individuals with cyanotic cardiac anomalies have clubbing of the digits on both hands and feet, although the precise mechanism of these changes is unproven. It has been suggested that clubbing is due to the peripheral impaction in the fingers and toes of megakaryocytes and platelet clumps that have bypassed the pulmonary circulation because of the right-to-left intracardiac shunt. These platelets may release platelet-derived growth factor (PDGF), which is a general growth promoter and mitogen for mesenchymal cells.[18] The release of PDGF could account for findings of increased thickness of nail bed and pulp, increased vascular connective tissue, and cellular infiltration of pulp tissues.[18]

Abnormalities in skeletal muscle metabolism have also been found in individuals with a cyanotic cardiac anomaly. By use of ^{31}P nuclear magnetic resonance imaging during exercise, phosphocreatine depletion and cytosolic acidification were found to be increased in muscles of cyanotic individuals compared with those of acyanotic healthy control subjects. Recovery times of phosphocreatine, adenosine diphosphate, and phosphate were prolonged in cyanotic individuals when exercise ceased. This finding is consistent with a reduction in the effective maximal rate of oxidative adenosine triphosphate synthesis in these individuals compared with acyanotic control subjects.[19]

REFERENCES

1. Aram DM, Ekelman BL, Ben-Shachar G, Levinsohn MW: Intelligence and hypoxemia in children with congenital heart disease: Fact or artifact? J Am Coll Cardiol 6:889, 1985.
2. Newburger JW, Silbert AR, Buckley LP, Fyler DC: Cognitive function and age at repair of transposition of the great arteries in children. N Engl J Med 310:1495, 1984.
3. Perloff JK: Systemic complications of cyanosis in adults with congenital heart disease. Cardiol Clin 11:689, 1993.
4. Swan L, Birnie DH, Hillis WS: The haematological management of patients with cyanotic congenital heart disease. A time for consensus? Eur Heart J 18:1973, 1997.
5. Wedemeyer AL, Edson JR, Krivit W: Coagulation in cyanotic congenital heart disease. Am J Dis Child 124:656, 1972.
6. Spear GS: The glomerulus in cyanotic congenital heart disease and primary pulmonary hypertension. Nephron 1:238, 1964.
7. Krull F, Ehrich JHH, Wurster U, et al: Renal involvement in patients with congenital cyanotic heart disease. Acta Paediatr Scand 80:1214, 1991.
8. Hayabuchi Y, Matsuoka S, Akita H, Kuroda Y: Hyperuricaemia in cyanotic congenital heart disease. Eur J Pediatr 152:873, 1993.
9. Bing RJ: Cardiac metabolism. Physiol Rev 45:171, 1965.
10. Kondo C, Nakazawa M, Kusakabe K, Momma K: Myocardial dysfunction and depressed fatty acid metabolism in patients with cyanotic congenital heart disease. J Nucl Cardiol 3:30, 1996.
11. Samanek M, Bass A, Ostadal B, Hucin B: Energieliefernder Stoffwechsel des volumen- und hypoxiebelasteten Herzens bei Kindern. Wien Klin Wochenschr 101:21, 1989.
12. Franciosi RA, Blanc WA: Myocardial infarcts in infants and children. I. A necropsy study in congenital heart disease. J Pediatr 73:309, 1968.
13. Del Nido PJ, Mickle DA, Wilson GJ, et al: Evidence of myocardial free radical injury during elective repair of tetralogy of Fallot. Circulation 76 (suppl):V-174, 1987.
14. Kafer ER, Sugioka K: Respiratory and cardiovascular responses to hypoxemia and the effects of anesthesia. Int Anesthesiol Clin 19:85, 1981.
15. Sorensen SC, Severinghaus JW: Respiratory insensitivity to acute hypoxia persisting after correction of tetralogy of Fallot. J Appl Physiol 25:221, 1968.
16. Sietsema KE, Cooper DM, Perloff JK, et al: Dynamics of oxygen uptake during exercise in adults with cyanotic congenital heart disease. Circulation 73:1137, 1986.
17. Roth A, Rosenthal A, Hall JE, Mizel M: Scoliosis and congenital heart disease. Clin Orthop 93:95, 1973.
18. Dickinson CJ: The aetiology of clubbing and hypertrophic osteoarthropathy. Eur J Clin Invest 23:330, 1993.
19. Adatia I, Kemp GJ, Taylor DJ, et al: Abnormalities in skeletal muscle metabolism in cyanotic patients with congenital heart disease: A ^{31}P nuclear magnetic resonance spectroscopy study. Clin Sci 85:105, 1993.

CHAPTER 64
PEDIATRIC CARDIAC TRANSPLANTATION

CHARLES E. CANTER

In 1968 the first recorded pediatric cardiac transplantation was performed in a 3-week-old infant with tricuspid atresia.[1] For the next 20 years, cardiac transplantation remained a heroic therapy for children. The development of effective maintenance immunosuppression protocols based on cyclosporine increased the success rate of adult cardiac transplantation and led to the application of transplantation to all forms of end-stage pediatric cardiac disease. Pediatric cardiac transplantation has since evolved from a medical curiosity to an accepted therapy for terminal cardiac disease in infants, children, and adolescents. Data from the International Society for Heart and Lung Transplantation Registry[2] indicate that approximately 200 pediatric transplantations are performed every year worldwide. Congenital heart disease has been the most common indication for cardiac transplantation in infants and children, followed by cardiomyopathy (Fig. 64–1). Congenital heart disease accounts for more than 75% of the transplantations in patients younger than 1 year of age but for only 30% of the transplantations in children older than 12 months of age. One-year survival rates for older children are approximately 80%,[2,3] similar to adult survival rates (Fig. 64–2).[2,4] One-year survival rates for infants are lower (approximately 70%),[2,5] although individual institutions[6,7] have reported survival rates for infants similar to those for adults. As with any new therapy, ultimate long-term survival is unknown. However, a 1997 multicenter study demonstrated that pediatric cardiac transplant recipients surviving 5 years had approximately an 80% actuarial 10-year survival rate and a 67% 15-year survival rate.[8]

Mortality with pediatric cardiac transplantation should be considered to begin after the patient is listed for cardiac transplantation. Although the number of pediatric cardiac transplants has plateaued in the past few years, the number of infants and children *listed* for cardiac transplantation in the United States has increased from 205 in 1988 to 497 in 1995 and, depending on age, the median waiting time for a donor increased from 40 to 200%.[9] The cardiac transplantation list in the United States is managed by the United Network for Organ Sharing and is stratified into status 1 (patients receiving intravenous inotropes in an intensive care unit or younger than 6 months of age) and status 2 (all others). In the period from 1993 to 1995, approximately 80% of status 1 infants and children underwent transplantation within 2 months of attaining this status level. Regardless of age, the 2-month mortality rate for children listed as status 1 was between 40 and 50% while awaiting cardiac transplantation versus 5% for children listed as status 2.[10]

Donor hearts are matched to recipients based on ABO compatibility, size, and distance as well as severity of illness. Studies of large populations of cardiac transplant recipients indicate a correlation between the survival of the patient and the number of HLA matches between the donor and recipient.[11] The increased risk of graft failure and death with long (greater than 4 to 5 hours) donor ischemic times[2] makes attempts at HLA matching of donors and recipients impractical. Donor hearts are routinely accepted with a small ventricular or atrial septal defect. Because brain death frequently leads to hypotension due to hypovolemia and loss of vasomotor tone, mild to moderate inotropic support in a potential donor does not make that heart unsuitable for transplantation.

PATIENT SELECTION

Cardiac transplantation is indicated in any child with cardiac abnormality who is refractory to maximal medical therapy and for whom there is no other surgical alternative that could restore a reasonable quality of life. The initial poor results with palliative procedures for hypoplastic left heart syndrome led to transplantation being used as a primary treatment[7,12–15] for that lesion. It has been used for complex cardiac malformations associated with heterotaxia, which have also been associated with poor survival after palliative operation.[16]

End-stage cardiac failure that can be treated only with inotropic support is a clear indication for evaluation for cardiac transplantation. The progression of cardiac failure in children who are not hospital bound is unpredictable. Natural history studies of pediatric cardiomyopathy[17–19] have not defined consistent predictors of mortality. Criteria for pediatric cardiac transplantation have been published (Table 64–1)[20–21] but are less well defined than those for adults. The use of maximum oxygen consumption has been a useful tool in adult transplant candidates; a maximum oxygen consumption of less than 10 ml/kg/min or less than 14 ml/kg/min with a major limitation in lifestyle is the generally accepted indication for transplantation. Maximum oxygen consumption is age dependent; a maximum oxygen consumption of 14 ml/kg/min is approximately 60% of oxygen consumption predicted for an active 60-year-old patient but only 30% of that predicted for a 20-year-old patient. For children as in young adults,[22] the use of percent predicted maximal oxygen consumption may be more significant in the assessment of cardiac status.

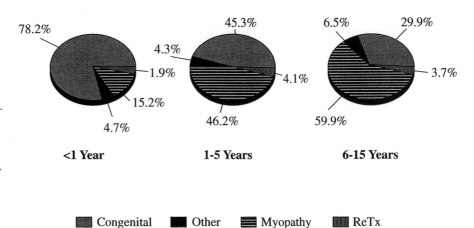

78.2%
4.3%
1.9%
15.2%
4.7%
<1 Year

45.3%
4.1%
46.2%
1-5 Years

6.5%   29.9%
3.7%
59.9%
6-15 Years

▨ Congenital   ■ Other   ▤ Myopathy   ▨ ReTx

FIGURE 64-1

Indications for pediatric cardiac transplantation by age and diagnosis from the registry of the International Society of Heart and Lung Transplantation (1982–1995). ReTx = retransplant. (From Hosenpud JD, Novick RJ, Bennett LE, et al: The Registry of the International Society for Heart and Lung Transplantation: Thirteenth official report—1996. J Heart Lung Transplant 15:655–674, 1996.)

Very few children with end-stage cardiac failure are not acceptable candidates for cardiac transplantation. The technical challenges of cardiac replacement in the face of congenital or acquired abnormalities of body situs, pulmonary arteries, atria, and systemic and pulmonary venous return have been overcome.[23–26] Transplant evaluations (Table 64–2) are designed to identify potential exclusion criteria such as irreversible disease in the lungs, liver, kidney, or central nervous system; active infection; severe psychological illness; or high titers of HLA antibodies that would attack and damage the graft (hyperacute rejection) within hours after transplantation. Because the genetic etiology of many pediatric cardiomyopathies is being identified,[27] a genetic or metabolic evaluation is an important part of transplant evaluation in children. A 1996 report[28] demonstrated that operations that use homograft material (e.g., valves, aorta, pulmonary artery) are associated with the development of high titers of HLA antibodies in the survivors. For patients with high antibody titers, transplantation has been performed successfully by using prospective cross-matching with the donor before transplantation or plasmapheresis[29] to lower the antibody titer in the perioperative period.

End-stage cardiac disease is frequently associated with elevated pulmonary artery pressure and resistance. As most donor hearts have been exposed only to normal pulmonary pressures, pulmonary hypertension may be associated with acute right ventricular failure and death in the immediate postoperative period. For this reason, a pulmonary vascular resistance of more than 6 Wood units or above 3 Wood units after treatment with vasodilators[20–21] or a transpulmonary gradient of more than 15 mm Hg[30] have been used as exclusion criteria in adults for cardiac transplantation and an indication for heart-lung transplantation. Experience with pediatric cardiac transplant recipients[31–32] suggests that pulmonary vascular resistance should be indexed to body surface area in infants and children and that the reactivity of the pulmonary vascular bed is a more important indicator of suitability for transplantation than the resting pulmonary vascular resistance. Furthermore, intensive treatment of cardiac failure over a period of weeks in a patient with an unacceptable pulmonary

Jan 1993 - Dec 1995
Death After Transplant

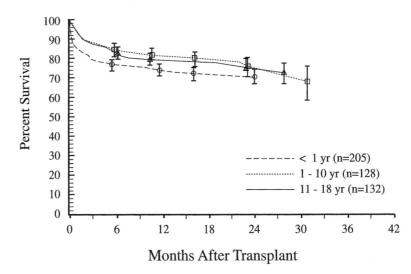

FIGURE 64-2

Actuarial survival curves for deaths of infants, children, and adolescents from the Pediatric Heart Transplant Study (PHTS). (Adapted from Shaddy RE, Naftel DC, Kirklin JK, et al: Outcome of cardiac transplantation in children. Survival in a contemporary multi-institutional experience. Pediatric Heart Transplant Study. Circulation 94[suppl II]:II69–II73, 1996; and Canter CE, Naftel D, Caldwell R, et al: Survival and risk factors for death after cardiac transplantation in infants. A multi-institutional study. The Pediatric Heart Transplant Study. Circulation 96:227–231, 1997.)

TABLE 64-1

TABLE 64-1

INDICATIONS FOR PEDIATRIC CARDIAC TRANSPLANTATION

1. Progressive deterioration of ventricular function or functional status, despite optimal medical care including treatment with digitalis, diuretics, and angiotensin-converting enzyme inhibitors
2. Complex cardiac malformations unamenable to conventional operative repair or palliation or a situation in which the surgical procedure carries a higher risk of mortality than that of transplantation
3. Growth failure secondary to cardiac disease
4. Malignant arrhythmias unresponsive to medical treatment, catheter ablation, or an automatic implantable defibrillator
5. Need for ongoing intravenous inotropic support
6. Unacceptably poor quality of life
7. Progressive pulmonary hypertension that would preclude cardiac transplantation at a later date

Adapted from O'Connell JB, Bourge RC, Costanzo-Nordin MR, et al: Cardiac transplantation: Recipient selection, donor procurement, and medical follow-up. Circulation 86:1061–1079, 1992.

vascular resistance on initial study can lower the pulmonary resistance to an acceptable level.[33] Pulmonary vascular resistance is usually not calculated in infant transplant candidates with lesions, such as hypoplastic left heart syndrome, that are associated with severe pulmonary hypertension before transplantation. Although irreversible pulmonary vascular disease has been reported in infant cardiac transplant recipients,[34] virtually all these recipients, including those who wait for many months, exhibit normal cardiac hemodynamics with long-term follow-up.[12]

MANAGEMENT AFTER TRANSPLANTATION

Cardiac transplantation is not a cure or a repair; it is a therapy that exchanges a fatal cardiac disease for a chronic disease. Lifelong immunosuppressant medications are required to prevent acute rejection of the heart. Multiple chronic immunosuppression protocols have been developed to prevent immunologic destruction of the transplanted organ.[35–38] These protocols share similar characteristics. The degree of immunosuppression is greatest in the first weeks and months after transplantation, and a calcineurin inhibitor (cyclosporine, tacrolimus [FK-506]) to block interleukin-2 secretion and subsequent T lymphocyte activation and proliferation is the cornerstone of chronic immunosuppressive therapy. Some protocols use powerful polyclonal (antilymphocyte globulin)[35] or monoclonal (OKT3)[14,36] antilymphocyte antibodies immediately after transplantation to induce immunotolerance in the recipient. Most protocols use multiple immunosuppressants to minimize toxic side effects of the medications, although some rely on monotherapy.[35,37] A common protocol is the combination of prednisone, azathioprine, and cyclosporine—so-called triple immunosuppression.[39] Table 64–3 demonstrates a typical triple immunosuppression protocol in which blood levels of cyclosporine and dosages of prednisone are gradually decreased. Prednisone can often be discontinued.[40] Mycophenolate mofetil[41] may replace azathioprine in immunosuppression protocols.

ACUTE REJECTION

Despite these combinations of immunosuppressant medications, episodes of acute rejection are common. Pediatric cardiac transplant recipients on the average experience one episode of rejection in the first 12 months after transplantation (Fig. 64–3),[12,42–45] although many will never have such an episode. Although neonatal recipients may be more immunotolerant of heart grafts,[46] clinical experience has provided conflicting results[42,44] of a decreased prevalence of rejection among neonates, infants, and children.

Acute rejection is generally characterized by myocardial infiltration, destruction, and ultimately dysfunction by both cellular and humoral immunologic mechanisms.[47] Although acute rejection is commonly not associated with symptoms, it is a primary cause of death during the first year after transplantation.[2–4] Thus, surveillance protocols have been developed to detect rejection and prevent graft

TABLE 64-2

PEDIATRIC CARDIAC TRANSPLANTATION EVALUATION PROTOCOL

Cardiology

Chest radiograph
Electrocardiogram
Echocardiogram
Exercise stress test including maximal oxygen consumption
Cardiac catheterization and angiography
    May include endomyocardial biopsy
    May include drug studies to manipulate cardiac index and pulmonary vascular resistance

Hematology

Complete blood cell count and differential count
Prothrombin and partial thromboplastin time

Blood Chemistry

Serum electrolytes, magnesium, calcium, phosphorus
Serum transaminases, bilirubin, albumin, total protein, alkaline phosphatase, cholesterol, triglycerides, uric acid, lactate dehydrogenase, creatine kinase

Renal

Urinalysis
Serum blood urea nitrogen and creatinine
24-hour urine collection for creatinine clearance

Pulmonary

Pulmonary function tests

Serology

CMV, EBV, varicella, herpes, hepatitis, HIV titers

Cultures

Bacterial + viral blood, throat, urine, stool,° sputum,° parasites,° fungus°

Immunology

HLA typing
Panel reactive antibody (titer + type of anti-HLA antibodies)

Neurology

Computed tomographic or magnetic resonance imaging scans°
Electroencephalogram°

Consultations

Neurology (also to exclude associated skeletal muscle disease)
Genetics
Psychology
Physical/occupational therapy
Dietetics
Social work
Financing/health insurance

CMV = cytomegalovirus; EBV = Epstein-Barr virus; HIV = human immunodeficiency virus; HLA = human leukocyte antigen.
°In selected patients.

TABLE 64–3

TABLE 64–3

TRIPLE THERAPY IMMUNOSUPPRESSION PROTOCOL

Presurgery

Methylprednisolone 10 mg/kg IV
Cyclosporine 10 mg/kg PO

Immediate Postoperative Period

Methylprednisolone 2 mg/kg IV q 8 hr × 3 doses, then prednisone 1
  mg/kg/day PO in divided doses
Cyclosporine infusion 0.5–1.5 mg/kg/day, target level 300 ng/ml whole
  blood
Azathioprine 1–2 mg/kg PO or IV

Maintenance

Prednisone 1 mg/kg/day, decrease to 0.2 mg/kg/day by 3 mo, stop by 6
  mo after transplantation
Azathioprine 1–2 mg/kg/day, adjust according to white blood cell count
Cyclosporine (PO) bid dosing, q 8 hr for infants <6 mo of age

Postoperative Month	Target Trough Level (ng/ml)
0–3	300
3–12	200–250
>12	150–200

IV = intravenous; PO = by mouth.

TABLE 64–4

STANDARDIZED NOMENCLATURE FOR DIAGNOSING ACUTE
REJECTION BY ENDOMYOCARDIAL BIOPSY*

Grade	Criteria
0	No rejection
1A	Mild rejection: focal perivascular or interstitial lymphocytic infiltrate without myocyte necrosis
1B	Mild rejection: diffuse but sparse lymphocytic infiltrate without myocyte necrosis
2	Focal moderate rejection: one focus only with aggressive lymphocytic infiltration and/or focal myocyte necrosis
3A	Moderate rejection: multifocal aggressive lymphocytic infiltrates and/or myocyte necrosis
3B	Borderline severe rejection: diffuse inflammatory process with necrosis
4	Severe rejection: diffuse aggressive polymorphous infiltrate consisting of edema, hemorrhage, and/or vasculitis, with myocyte necrosis

*As determined by the International Society for Heart and Lung Transplantation.

Adapted from Billingham ME, Cary NR, Hammond ME, et al: A working formulation for the standardization of nomenclature in the diagnosis of heart and lung rejection: Heart Rejection Study Group. The International Society for Heart and Lung Transplantation. J Heart Lung Transplant 9:587–593, 1990.

failure and patient death. The risk for rejection is greatest in the first 3 months after transplantation yet is uncommon 6 months after transplantation, assuming patient compliance with the immunosuppression regimen.[12, 42–44] Thus, surveillance for rejection is most intense during the first 3 months after transplantation and gradually decreases to an every-6-month schedule 18 months after transplantation. Endomyocardial biopsy has improved detection and treatment of acute rejection and is considered the "gold standard" for diagnosing rejection. Standardized grading systems (Table 64–4) have been formulated.[48] Biopsies demonstrating multifocal myocardial lymphocytic infiltration *and* myocardial necrosis are accepted as diagnostic of rejection requiring treatment. Immunofluorescence techniques[49] have been used to diagnose humorally related rejection, although some studies question their sensitivity and specificity.[50]

Endomyocardial biopsy techniques for rejection surveillance in infants and children have been developed; the complication rates are similar to those in adults.[51–53] Noninvasive pediatric rejection surveillance, however, has been successfully demonstrated, especially in infant recipients. Decreased appetite, irritability, gallop rhythm, enlarged cardiac silhouette on a chest radiograph, and decreased QRS voltages on an electrocardiogram have been used as signs of rejection.[54, 55] Serial echocardiography is an important tool in the noninvasive assessment of rejection.

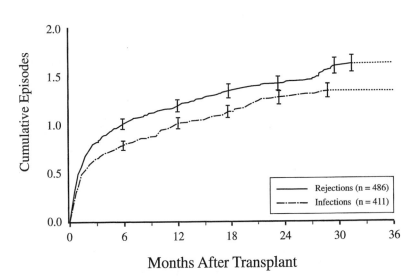

Jan 1993 - Dec 1995
All Institutions (n = 465)

FIGURE 64–3

Cumulative episodes of acute rejection and infection requiring hospitalization, intravenous medication, or both within the first 3 years after transplantation, from the Pediatric Heart Transplant Study database. (From Canter CE: Current outcomes in pediatric thoracic transplantation. ACC Cur J Rev 5:65, 1997.)

TABLE 64–5

SCORING SYSTEM FOR THE NONINVASIVE DIAGNOSIS OF REJECTION BY DIGITIZED M-MODE ECHOCARDIOGRAPHY

Parameter	Threshold	Weighted Score
Left ventricular volume (LVV)*	<65%	2
Left ventricular mass (LVM)*	>130%	1
LVV/LVM ratio	<45%	1
Left ventricular posterior wall thickening fraction	<70%	2
Interventricular septal thickening fraction	<25%	1
Maximum velocity of posterior wall† (diastole)	<11 (−1/sec)	1
Average velocity of left ventricular wall thinning	<25 mm/sec	1
Average velocity of left ventricular enlargement	<60 mm/sec	1
Mitral insufficiency	>1+	1

Rejection Grade

GRADE		CUMULATIVE SCORE
1	Normal	0
2	Probably normal	1–3
3	Probable rejection	4–6
	or new pericardial effusion	
	or new mitral regurgitation >2+	
4	Rejection	7–11
	or left ventricular shortening fraction <28% with normal septal thickening	

*Percentage of predicted normal for body surface area.
†Corrected for dimension at maximum velocity potential number.
Adapted from Boucek MM, Mathis CM, Boucek RJ, et al: Prospective evaluation of echocardiography for primary rejection surveillance after infant heart transplantation: Comparison with endomyocardial biopsy. J Heart Lung Transplant 13:66–73, 1994.

Acute rejection in children and adults is generally associated with increases in left ventricular mass and signs of diastolic dysfunction.[56–60] Decreased systolic function is a late finding in severe rejection episodes. In adults, Doppler evaluation of diastolic function is useful in the noninvasive diagnosis of rejection.[61, 62] Experience in children[63, 64] indicates that Doppler techniques may be less reliable. Protocols using digitized M-mode echocardiograms have been successfully employed in infants and children as a rejection surveillance technique.[65–68] Rejection is diagnosed via a scoring system of left ventricular structural and functional parameters (Table 64–5). Echocardiography has not been universally successful[58, 69] in the diagnosis of rejection. Hypoxic and ischemic myocardial injury early after transplantation[62] and steroid administration[70] may alter the echocardiographic characteristics of the allograft in a manner similar to acute rejection.

Acute rejection is treated by increasing immunosuppression. The intensity of immunosuppression depends on the degree of symptoms and patient's response to previous treatment. Pulses of high-dose steroids, polyclonal or monoclonal antilymphocytic antibody preparations, or both control most episodes of acute rejection. For patients who experience recurrent rejection, the addition of low-dose methotrexate is effective,[71, 72] as is total lymphocytic radiation[73, 74] for severely resistant patients. Antibody-related (humoral) rejection can be treated with plasmapheresis.[75, 76]

INFECTION

Infection is the other primary cause of death early after pediatric cardiac transplantation.[3, 4] Similar to rejection, serious infections most likely occur in the first 3 months after transplantation when immunosuppression is greatest.[76, 77] The intensity of immunosuppression and the degree of illness in a patient before transplantation increase the risk of serious infection after transplantation.[78]

Pediatric cardiac transplant recipients average one infection requiring hospitalization or treatment with intravenous medications in the first year after transplantation (see Fig. 64–3).[76] The same bacterial and viral pathogens accountable for infections after surgery for congenital cardiac anomalies are responsible for most of the infections after cardiac transplantation. Immunosuppression, however, increases the likelihood that infections may be due to fungi (*Candida, Aspergillus, Cryptococcus*), protozoa (*Pneumocystis*), or bacteria that are not generally considered pathogens. Typical signs and symptoms associated with infections (e.g., nuchal rigidity with meningitis) may not be present with infections in the immunocompromised patient. Prophylactic nystatin and trimethoprim-sulfamethoxazole are routinely given to prevent fungal or protozoal infections. Cytomegalovirus infection commonly occurs in cardiac transplant recipients as a result of primary exogenous infection, donor-recipient transfer of the virus, or reactivation of infection in the recipient during this time period. Infection may be asymptomatic but can be associated with pneumonitis or gastrointestinal disease.[79] Ganciclovir can be used as both prophylaxis and treatment of an established cytomegalovirus infection.[80, 81] Immunosuppressed patients should avoid live virus vaccines (e.g., oral polio, measles-mumps-rubella) and killed virus or protein vaccines such as diphtheria, pertussis, and tetanus. Salk polio, hepatitis B, *Haemophilus influenzae* type b, and influenza vaccines should be given. Varicella as a primary or reactivated infection (zoster) can be treated with oral or intravenous acyclovir. Because of potentially fatal varicella in immunocompromised children, varicella exposures should be treated with varicella-zoster immune globulin within 48 hours of the exposure.

LONG-TERM COMPLICATIONS

Transplanted hearts in infants and children increase in chamber size, wall thickness, and mass/volume ratios proportional to the increase in size of the recipient; thus, they appear to have the capacity to grow as the child ages.[82–84] Transplanted hearts are obviously denervated at the time of implantation. Partial reinnervation may occur with time,[85, 86] but the heart rate response to exercise is usually blunted. As in adult recipients, most pediatric cardiac transplant recipients have a lower than normal exercise capacity with exercise testing.[87] Sequential cardiac catheterization studies have also demonstrated hemodynamics consistent with a restrictive cardiomyopathy in long-term survivors of pediatric cardiac transplantation.[8, 88] Moderate to severe tricuspid regurgitation is also common in long-term cardiac transplant recipients, usually the result of trauma to the valve apparatus from repetitive endomyocardial biopsies.[89, 90]

Arrhythmias are common in a transplanted heart. Significant bradycardia may occur in the immediate postoperative period; it usually improves but may require permanent pacing.[91, 92] Right bundle branch block is typically present on a resting electrocardiogram, and isolated atrial or ventricular premature contractions at a greater frequency than that observed in normal hearts may be noted with a Holter monitor.[93, 94] Supraventricular and ventricular tachycardias may be a sign of rejection in pediatric recipients. However, supraventricular tachycardias that occur late after transplantation are usually not associated with rejection. Late ventricular tachyarrhythmias may be a sign of transplant coronary arteriopathy.[95, 96]

Many of the medical problems in cardiac transplant recipients can be attributed to side effects of immunosuppressive medications (Table 64–6). Hypertension is commonly associated with cyclosporine therapy. Cyclosporine is a potent renal vasoconstrictor, but chronic hypertension correlates poorly with changes in renal function.[39] Renal vasoconstriction with cyclosporine therapy does not appear to be attributable to sympathetic stimulation.[97] Hypertensive patients taking cyclosporine have low plasma renin levels, and blood pressure reduction is greater with calcium channel blockers compared with angiotensin-converting enzyme inhibitors, suggesting a renin-independent form of hypertension.[98] Calcium channel blockers are used most frequently as antihypertensive agents in cardiac transplant recipients, but diuretics, angiotensin-converting enzyme inhibitors, β-blockers, and α-blockers have been used alone or in combination therapy. The alternative calcineurin-inhibitor immunosuppressant tacrolimus (FK-506) may be less likely to be associated with hypertension compared with cyclosporine.[41]

Nephrotoxicity is also frequently observed with cyclosporine and tacrolimus therapy. Patients taking cyclosporine typically demonstrate a prerenal pattern to their azotemia, with a blood urea nitrogen level disproportionately elevated when compared with the level of serum creatinine. Renal tubular acidosis, hyperuricemia, and hyperkalemia can also be observed with cyclosporine therapy.[98] Cyclosporine overdose can be associated with acute renal failure that is reversible. Knowledge of the drugs that interact with cyclosporine (Table 64–7) is important to avoid acute toxicity or underimmunosuppression. Long-term administration of cyclosporine in pediatric heart transplant recipients has generally resulted in steady, gradual increases in serum blood urea nitrogen and creatinine levels.[8, 36, 99]

A year after transplantation, transplant coronary artery disease (allograft vasculopathy, accelerated atherosclerosis) becomes a leading cause of cardiac mortality and morbidity. In adults, angiographic evidence of transplant coronary artery disease is present in 50% of recipients 5 years after transplantation.[100, 101] Usually this lesion is a progressive, concentric myointimal proliferation that initially appears as intimal thickening and may lead to luminal occlusion. Transplant coronary artery disease involves the entire length of the vessel. In contrast, traditional atherosclerosis is usually characterized by focal lesions with asymmetric intimal proliferation in the proximal vessels. Unlike atherosclerosis, transplant coronary artery disease lesions rarely calcify and are unassociated with disruption of the internal elastic lamina. Transplant coronary artery disease may result from an immunologic injury to the coronary endothelial cells, leading to the stimulation of growth factors and cytokines resulting in intimal proliferation. Direct confirmation of immunologic endothelial injury is lacking. Circumstantial evidence supports this hypothesis, however. Endothelial cells express class I and II major histocompatibility complex antigens. The lesions are confined to the transplanted organ, and similar lesions have been observed in the vessels of transplanted kidneys.[102, 103]

Despite a reduction in the frequency of acute rejection with current immunosuppression protocols, the prevalence of transplant coronary disease has remained constant.[104] In

TABLE 64–6					
COMPLICATIONS OF IMMUNOSUPPRESSIVE AGENTS					
Complication	Cyclosporine	Steroids	Tacrolimus	Azathioprine	Mycophenolate Mofetil
Hypertension	+	+	+		
Nephrotoxicity	+		+		
Glucose intolerance		+	+		
Neurotoxicity	+		+		
Gingival hyperplasia	+				
Hirsutism	+				
Hyperlipidemia	+	+			
Coarse facies	+				
Hepatotoxicity	+			+	
Cholelithiasis	+				
Diarrhea, nausea					+

TABLE 64–7

CYCLOSPORINE DRUG INTERACTIONS

Drugs Increasing Cyclosporine Levels

Ketoconazole
Fluconazole
Erythromycin
Metoclopramide
Diltiazem
Verapamil

Drugs Decreasing Cyclosporine Levels

Phenobarbital
Phenytoin
Carbamazepine
Rifampin
Trimethoprim-sulfamethoxazole

adults, cytomegalovirus infections have been associated with development of coronary artery disease.[105, 106] Some studies have demonstrated a correlation with the degree of donor-recipient HLA antigen mismatch. Factors associated with the development of traditional atherosclerosis, such as hyperlipidemia, hypertension, and smoking, also affect the development of transplant coronary artery disease.[102, 103]

The manifestations of transplant coronary artery disease range from myocardial infarction and left ventricular dysfunction to sudden death. Because of variability in the reinnervation of the transplanted heart, myocardial infarction with transplant coronary artery disease is usually silent and not associated with angina. For these reasons, cardiac transplantation protocols routinely include coronary angiography performed on a yearly or biannual basis. The most frequent angiographic lesion is diffuse, rapid pruning of the vessel with distal obliteration of small vessels, although focal stenoses are occasionally observed.[107] Intravascular ultrasound techniques have demonstrated that angiography underestimates the presence and severity of transplant coronary artery disease.[108] Intravascular ultrasonography frequently demonstrates disease in angiographically normal vessels.

Transplant coronary artery disease has been documented in infant and childhood recipients. It may occur within the first year after transplantation, is demonstrable in recipients undergoing transplantation from infancy through adolescence, and is frequently associated with sudden death.[109–112] Unlike results with adults, recurrent rejection has been associated with transplant coronary artery disease in studies with children. Increasing the maintenance level of immunosuppression decreased the prevalence of coronary disease in pediatric recipients at one center.[113] Some angiographic studies[112] have observed less coronary disease in pediatric recipients than that observed in adults. Preliminary evidence regarding intravascular ultrasonography in pediatric-aged recipients revealed coronary disease to be a frequent finding in angiographically normal coronary arteries (Fig. 64–4), as well as some correlation of the degree of intimal thickening with time after transplantation.[114]

Once present, transplant coronary artery disease in adults progresses and is irreversible. Coronary angioplasty and bypass surgery can be employed for focal lesions. Prophylactic use of the calcium channel blocker diltiazem has been demonstrated in one controlled study to decrease pro-

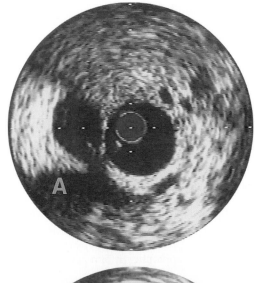

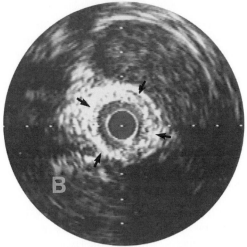

FIGURE 64–4

Two cross-sectional intravascular ultrasound sections of the left main coronary artery in two pediatric heart transplant recipients with normal coronary angiograms. *A*, No significant intimal proliferation in a 5-year-old transplant recipient who had undergone transplantation in the first month of life for hypoplastic left heart syndrome. *B*, Typical concentric moderately severe intimal proliferation *(arrows)* demonstrated in a 15-year-old patient who underwent transplantation at age 5. The *hashmarks* represent a distance of 1 mm. The dark circle surrounded by the white ring is the guidewire within the artery.

gressive reduction in luminal size after transplantation.[115] Pravastatin, a cholesterol-lowering agent, decreased the incidence of coronary disease 1 year after transplantation.[116] Retransplantation is probably the only definitive treatment for transplant coronary artery disease. Although survival with cardiac retransplantation is lower than that with primary transplantation, the survival rate for retransplantation performed for transplant coronary disease is similar to that for primary transplantation.[117]

Chronic immunosuppression is associated with an increased risk for development of neoplasms. The prevalence of neoplasms in various series of pediatric cardiac transplant patients has varied from 0.7 to 10%.[12, 43, 118, 119] The most common neoplasm observed after pediatric cardiac transplantation is lymphoproliferative disease. It most commonly occurs during the first months after transplantation and is usually associated with either a primary or a re-activated Ebstein-Barr virus infection. Lymphoproliferative disease is a heterogeneous disorder ranging from a plasmacytic hyperplasia lacking oncogene and tumor suppressor gene alterations to an aggressive metastatic immunoblastic lymphoma or multiple myeloma.[120] It may present as an isolated disease process in the oropharyngeal nodes, lungs, or gastrointestinal tract or as a disseminated multisystem disease that can involve the central nervous system. The more benign forms of lymphoproliferative disease respond to reduction of immunosuppression; however, chemotherapy, radiation therapy, or both have been used to treat more malignant variants. With long-term follow-up, neoplasm remains a major complication of cardiac transplantation. Non–Ebstein-Barr virus–related lymphomas, basal cell carcinomas, cervical carcinomas, and Kaposi's sarcoma have also been observed at higher frequency in transplant recipients than in the general population.[121]

HEART-LUNG AND LUNG TRANSPLANTATION

Pulmonary vascular disease associated with primary pulmonary hypertension, cardiac malformations, and cystic fibrosis is the primary condition leading to heart-lung and lung transplantation in children. The indications for pulmonary transplantation for pulmonary vascular disease are not clearly defined. The National Institutes of Health registry for primary pulmonary hypertension demonstrated an inverse correlation with duration of survival and magnitude of central venous pressure, pulmonary artery pressure, and pulmonary vascular resistance.[122] A smaller retrospective study demonstrated a similar relationship in pediatric patients with primary pulmonary hypertension or pulmonary vascular disease associated with cardiac malformations.[123] Waiting times for cadaveric lung donors can exceed 1 year, which has led some centers to use living-related donation of isolated lobes of the lung.[124]

Pediatric lung transplantation has a higher mortality rate than cardiac transplantation, with a 12-month survival rate of 60 to 70% (Fig. 64–5).[2, 125] Survival has improved,[2] with one center reporting a 1995 12-month survival rate approaching 80%.[126] Risk factors for mortality after lung transplantation in children have included the need for ventilator support before transplantation and multiple aortopulmonary artery collaterals.[2, 126] A history of multiple thoracotomies is probably a risk factor for intractable bleeding after pulmonary transplantation. Cardiac malformation and primary pulmonary hypertension are risk factors for poor survival rates in adult recipients but not in children.[2, 126]

The patterns of rejection and infection after lung transplantation resemble those observed after cardiac transplantation.[126] The transplanted lung, however, is more susceptible to infection because of its greater exposure to environmental pathogens. Bronchiolitis obliterans in pulmonary allografts is the counterpart to transplant coronary artery disease in cardiac allografts. Bronchiolitis obliterans can be a rapidly progressive disease leading to respiratory failure or may stabilize after an acute decrease in lung function. In pediatric-aged recipients, it has a prevalence of 25 to 30% and increases in prevalence with longer duration of follow-up.[125, 126] The prevalence of bronchiolitis obliterans in heart-lung recipients equals or is greater than its prevalence in isolated lung transplant recipients.[127, 128] Studies, however, have demonstrated that the prevalence of transplant coronary artery disease is less in heart-lung as opposed to heart transplant recipients.[129]

REFERENCES

1. Kantrowitz A, Haller JD, Joos H, et al: Transplantation of the heart in an infant and an adult. Am J Cardiol 22:782, 1968.
2. Hosenpud JD, Novick RJ, Bennett LE, et al: The Registry of the International Society for Heart and Lung Transplantation: Thirteenth official report—1996. J Heart Lung Transplant 15:655, 1996.
3. Shaddy RE, Naftel DC, Kirklin JK, et al: Outcome of cardiac transplantation in children. Survival in a contemporary multi-institutional experience. Pediatric Heart Transplant Study. Circulation 94(suppl II):II69, 1996.
4. Bourge RC, Naftel DC, Costanzo-Nordin MR, et al: Pretransplantation risk factors for death after heart transplantation: A multi-

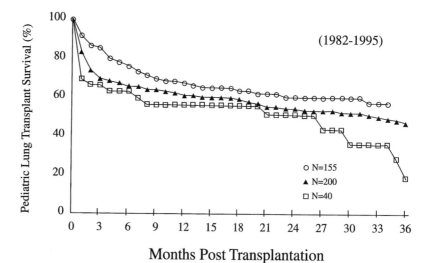

FIGURE 64–5

Actuarial survival of pediatric heart-lung and lung transplantation from the registry of the International Society for Heart and Lung Transplantation. (From Hosenpud JD, Novick RJ, Bennett LE, et al: The Registry of the International Society for Heart and Lung Transplantation: Thirteenth official report—1996. J Heart Lung Transplant 15:655–674, 1996.)

institutional study. The Transplant Cardiologists Research Database Group. J Heart Lung Transplant 12:549, 1993.

5. Canter C, Naftel D, Caldwell R, et al: Survival and risk factors for death after cardiac transplantation in infants. Circulation 96:227, 1997.

6. Bailey LL, Gundry SR, Razzouk AJ, et al: Bless the babies: One hundred fifteen late survivors of heart transplantation during the first year of life. J Thorac Cardiovasc Surg 105:805, 1993.

7. Canter CE, Moorhead S, Huddleston CB, Spray TL: Restrictive atrial communication as a determinant of outcome of cardiac transplantation for hypoplastic left heart syndrome. Circulation 88(part 2):456, 1993.

8. Sigfusson F, Fricker FJ, Bernstein D, et al: Long-term survivors of pediatric heart transplantation: A multicenter report of sixty-eight children who have survived longer than five years. J Pediatr 130:862, 1997.

9. 1996 Annual Report of the U.S. Scientific Registry for Transplant Recipients and the Organ Procurement and Transplant Network: Transplant data 1988–1995. UNOS, Richmond, VA and the Division of Transplantation, Bureau of Health Resources Development, Health Resources and Services Administration, U.S. Department of Health and Human Services, Rockville, MD.

10. Addonizio L, Naftel D, Fricker J, et al: Risk factors for pretransplant outcome in children listed for cardiac transplantation: A multi-institutional study (Abstract). J Heart Lung Transplant 14:S48, 1995.

11. Opelz G, Wujaciak T: The influence of HLA compatibility on graft survival after heart transplantation. N Engl J Med 330:816, 1994.

12. Razzouk AJ, Chinnock RE, Gundry SR, et al: Transplantation as a primary treatment for hypoplastic left heart syndrome: Intermediate-term results. Ann Thorac Surg 62:1, 1996.

13. Backer CL, Zales VR, Harrison HL, et al: Intermediate term results of infant orthotopic cardiac transplantation from two centers. J Thorac Cardiovasc Surg 101:826, 1991.

14. Turrentine MW, Kesler KA, Caldwell R, et al: Cardiac transplantation in infants and children. Ann Thorac Surg 57:546, 1994.

15. Starnes VA, Griffin ML, Pitlick PT, et al: Current approach to hypoplastic left heart syndrome. J Thorac Cardiovasc Surg 104:189, 1992.

16. Bailey LL: Heart transplantation techniques in complex congenital heart disease. J Heart Lung Transplant 12:S168, 1993.

17. Akagi T, Benson LT, Lightfoot NE, et al: Natural history of dilated cardiomyopathy in children. Am Heart J 121:1502, 1991.

18. Lewis AB, Chabot M: Outcome of infants and children with dilated cardiomyopathy. Am J Cardiol 68:365, 1991.

19. Friedman RA, Moak JP, Garson A Jr: Clinical course of idiopathic dilated cardiomyopathy in children. J Am Coll Cardiol 68:152, 1991.

20. O'Connell JB, Bourge RC, Costanzo-Nordin MR, et al: Cardiac transplantation: Recipient selection, donor procurement, and medical follow-up. Circulation 86:1061, 1992.

21. Mudge GH, Goldstein S, Addonizio LJ, et al: Task Force 3: Recipient guidelines/prioritization. 24th Bethesda conference: Cardiac transplantation. J Am Coll Cardiol 22:21, 1993.

22. Stelken AM, Younis LT, Jennison SH, et al: Prognostic value of cardiopulmonary exercise testing using percent achieved of predicted peak oxygen uptake for patients with ischemic and dilated cardiomyopathy. J Am Coll Cardiol 27:345, 1996.

23. Mayer JE, Perry S, O'Brien P, et al: Orthotopic heart transplantation for complex congenital heart disease. J Thorac Cardiovasc Surg 99:484, 1990.

24. Doty DB, Renlund DG, Caputo GR, et al: Cardiac transplantation in situs inversus. J Thorac Cardiovasc Surg 99:493, 1990.

25. Webber SA, Ficker FJ, Michaels M, et al: Orthotopic heart transplantation in children with congenital heart disease. Ann Thorac Surg 58:1664, 1994.

26. Cooper MM, Fuzesi L, Addonizio LJ, et al: Pediatric heart transplantation after operations involving the pulmonary arteries. J Thorac Cardiovasc Surg 102:386, 1991.

27. Schwartz ML, Cox GF, Lin AE, et al: Clinical approach to genetic cardiomyopathy in children. Circulation 94:2021, 1996.

28. Shaddy RE, Hunter DD, Osborn KA, et al: Prospective analysis of HLA immunogenicity of cryopreserved valved allografts used in pediatric heart surgery. Circulation 94:1063, 1996.

29. Ratkovec RM, Hammond EH, O'Connell JB, et al: Outcome of cardiac transplant recipients with a positive donor-specific crossmatch—preliminary results with plasmapheresis. Transplantation 54:651, 1992.

30. Bando K, Konishi H, Komatsu K, et al: Improved survival following pediatric cardiac transplantation in high-risk patients. Circulation 88:218, 1993.

31. Addonizio LJ, Gersony WM, Robbins RC, et al: Elevated pulmonary vascular resistance and cardiac transplantation. Circulation 76(suppl V):V52, 1987.

32. Gajarski RJ, Towbin JA, Bricker JT, et al: Intermediate follow-up of pediatric heart transplant recipients with elevated pulmonary vascular resistance index. J Am Coll Cardiol 23:1682, 1994.

33. Zales VR, Pahl E, Backer CL, et al: Pharmacologic reduction of pretransplantation pulmonary vascular resistance predicts outcome after pediatric heart transplantation. J Heart Lung Transplant 12:965, 1993.

34. Collins MH, Darragh RK, Caldwell RL, et al: Short-term survivors of pediatric heart transplantation: An autopsy study of their pulmonary vascular disease. J Heart Lung Transplant 14:1116, 1995.

35. Chiavarelli M, DeBegona JA, Vigesaa RE, et al: Heart transplantation in children. Adv Cardiac Surg 3:155, 1992.

36. Baum D, Bernstein D, Starnes VA, et al: Pediatric heart transplantation at Stanford: Results of a 15-year experience. Pediatrics 88:203, 1991.

37. Pham SM, Kormos RL, Hattler BG, et al: A prospective trial of tacrolimus (FK 506) in clinical heart transplantation: Intermediate term results. J Thorac Cardiovasc Surg 111:764, 1996.

38. Canter CE, Saffitz JE, Moorhead S, et al: Early results after pediatric cardiac transplantation with triple drug immunosuppression therapy. Am J Cardiol 71:971, 1993.

39. Olivari MT, Kubo SH, Braunlin EA, et al: Five-year experience with triple drug immunosuppressive therapy in cardiac transplantation. Circulation 82(suppl IV):IV276, 1990.

40. Canter CE, Moorhead S, Saffitz JE, et al: Steroid withdrawal in the pediatric heart transplant recipient initially treated with triple immunosuppression. J Heart Lung Transplant 13:74, 1994.

41. Renlund DG, Gopinatter SK, Kfoury AG, Taylor DO: Mycophenolate mofetil (MMF) in heart transplantation: Rejection prevention and treatment. Clin Transplant 10:136, 1996.

42. Rotondo K, Naftel D, Boucek R, et al: Allograft rejection following cardiac transplantation (C Tx) in infants and children: A multi-institutional study (Abstract). J Heart Lung Transplant 15:S80, 1996.

43. Armitage JM, Fricker FJ, del Nido P, et al: A decade (1982–1992) of pediatric cardiac transplantation and the impact of FK 506 immunosuppression. J Thorac Cardiovasc Surg 105:464, 1993.

44. Balzer DT, Moorhead S, Saffitz JE, et al: Utility of surveillance biopsies in infant heart transplant recipients. J Heart Lung Transplant 14:1095, 1995.

45. Canter CE: Current outcomes in pediatric thoracic transplantation. ACC Cur J Rev 5:65, 1997.

46. Nelson-Cannarella S: The unique newborn immune response. J Heart Lung Transplant 11:751, 1992.

47. Halloran PF, Miller LW: In vivo immunosuppressive mechanisms. J Heart Lung Transplant 15:959, 1996.

48. Billingham ME, Cary NR, Hammond ME, et al: A working formulation for the standardization of nomenclature in the diagnosis of heart and lung rejection: Heart Rejection Study Group. The International Study for Heart and Lung Transplantation. J Heart Lung Transplant 9:587, 1990.

49. Hammond EH, Hansen JK, Spencer LS, et al: Immunofluorescence of endomyocardial biopsy specimens: Methods and interpretation. J Heart Lung Transplant 12:S113, 1993.

50. Bonnaud DN, Lewis NP, Masek MA, Billingham ME: Reliability and usefulness of immunofluorescence in heart transplantation. J Heart Lung Transplant 14:163, 1995.

51. Zales VR, Crawford S, Backer CL, et al: Role of endomyocardial biopsy in rejection surveillance after heart transplantation in neonates and children. J Am Coll Cardiol 23:766, 1994.

52. Balzer D, Moorhead S, Saffitz JE, et al: Pediatric endomyocardial biopsy performed solely with echocardiographic guidance. J Am Soc Echocardiogr 6:510, 1993.

53. Yoshizato T, Edwards WD, Alboliras ET, et al: Safety and utility of endomyocardial biopsy in infants, children and adolescents: A review of 66 procedures in 53 patients. J Am Coll Cardiol 15:436, 1990.

54. Johnston J, Mathis C: Determination of rejection using noninvasive parameters after cardiac transplantation in very early infancy. Prog Cardiovasc Nursing 3:13, 1988.

55. Chinnock RE, Baum MF, Larsen R, Bailey L: Rejection management and long-term surveillance of the pediatric heart transplant recipient: The Loma Linda experience. J Heart Lung Transplant 12:S255, 1993.

56. Kawauchi M, Boucek MM, Gundry SR, et al: Changes in left ventricular mass with rejection after heart transplantation in infants. J Heart Lung Transplant 11:99, 1992.

57. Tantengco MV, Dodd D, Frist WH, et al: Echocardiographic abnormalities with acute cardiac allograft rejection in children: Correlation with endomyocardial biopsy. J Heart Lung Transplant 12:S203, 1993.

58. Santos-Ocampo SD, Sekarski TJ, Saffitz JE, et al: Echocardiographic characteristics of biopsy-proven cellular rejection in infant heart transplant recipients. J Heart Lung Transplant 15:25, 1996.

59. Hosenpud J: Noninvasive diagnosis of cardiac rejection. Circulation 85:370, 1992.

60. Valentine HA, Fowler MB, Hunt SA, et al: Changes in Doppler echocardiographic indexes of left ventricular function as potential markers of acute cardiac rejection. Circulation 76(suppl V):V86, 1987.

61. Valentine HA, Yeoh TK, Gibbons R, et al: Sensitivity and specificity of diastolic indexes for rejection surveillance: Temporal correlation with endomyocardial biopsy. J Heart Lung Transplant 10:757, 1991.

62. Valentine HA: Rejection surveillance by Doppler echocardiography. J Heart Lung Transplant 12:422, 1993.

63. Frommelt MA, Snider AR, Crowley DC, et al: Echocardiographic indexes of allograft rejection in pediatric cardiac transplant recipients. J Am Soc Echocardiogr 5:41, 1992.

64. Holzmann G, Gidding SS, Crawford SE, Zales VR: Usefulness of left ventricular inflow Doppler in predicting rejection in pediatric cardiac transplant recipients. Am J Cardiol 73:205, 1994.

65. Dodd DA, Brady LD, Carden KA, et al: Pattern of echocardiographic abnormalities with acute cardiac allograft rejection in adults: Correlation with endomyocardial biopsy. J Heart Lung Transplant 12:1009, 1993.

66. Boucek MM, Mathis CM, Boucek RJ, et al: Prospective evaluation of echocardiography for primary rejection surveillance after infant heart transplantation: Comparison with endomyocardial biopsy. J Heart Lung Transplant 13:66, 1994.

67. Boucek MM, Mathis CM, Kanakriyeh MS, et al: Serial echocardiographic evaluation of cardiac graft rejection after infant heart transplantation. J Heart Lung Transplant 12:824, 1993.

68. Loker J, Darragh R, Ensing G, Caldwell R: Echocardiographic analysis of rejection in the infant heart transplant recipient. J Heart Lung Transplant 13:1014, 1994.

69. Mannaerts HFJ, Balk AHMM, Simoons ML, et al: Changes in left ventricular function and wall thickness in heart transplant recipients and their relation to acute rejection: An assessment by digitised M mode echocardiography. Br Heart J 68:356, 1992.

70. Kimball TR, Witt SA, Daniels SR, et al: Frequency and significance of left ventricular thickening in transplanted hearts in children. Am J Cardiol 77:77, 1996.

71. Bouchart F, Gundry SR, Van Schaack-Gonzales J, et al: Methotrexate as rescue/adjunctive immunotherapy in infant and adult heart transplantation. J Heart Lung Transplant 12:427, 1993.

72. Shaddy RE, Bullock EA, Tani LY, et al: Methotrexate therapy in pediatric heart transplantation as treatment of recurrent mild to moderate acute cellular rejection. J Heart Lung Transplant 13:1009, 1994.

73. Hunt SA, Strober S, Hoppe RT, Stinson EB: Total lymphoid irradiation for treatment of intractable cardiac allograft rejection. J Heart Lung Transplant 10:211, 1991.

74. Kirklin JK, George JF, McGiffin DC, et al: Total lymphoid irradiation: Is there a role in pediatric heart transplantation? J Heart Lung Transplant 12:S293, 1993.

75. Olsen SL, Wagoner LE, Hammond EH, et al: Vascular rejection in heart transplantation: Clinical correlation, treatment options, and future considerations. J Heart Lung Transplant 12:S135, 1993.

76. Schowengardt K, Naftel D, Seib P, et al: Infection after pediatric heart transplantation: Results of a multiinstitutional study. The Pediatric Heart Transplant Group. J Heart Lung Transplant 16:1207, 1997.

77. Miller LW, Naftel DC, Bourge RC, et al: Infection after heart transplantation: A multi-institutional study. J Heart Lung Transplant 13:381, 1994.

78. Smart FW, Naftel DC, Costanzo MR, et al: Risk factors for early, cumulative, and fatal infections after heart transplantation: A multi-institutional study. J Heart Lung Transplant 15:329, 1996.

79. Kirklin JK, Naftel DC, Levine TB, et al: Cytomegalovirus after heart transplantation. Risk factors for infection and death: A multi-institutional study. J Heart Lung Transplant 13:394, 1994.

80. Keay S, Petersen E, Icenogle G, et al: Ganciclovir treatment of serious cytomegalovirus infection in heart and heart-lung recipients. J Infect Dis 10(suppl 3):S563, 1988.

81. Merigan TC, Renlund DG, Keay S, et al: A controlled trial of ganciclovir to prevent cytomegalovirus disease after heart transplantation. N Engl J Med 326:1182, 1992.

82. Bernstein D, Kolla S, Miner M, et al: Cardiac growth after pediatric heart transplantation. Circulation 85:1433, 1992.

83. Hirsch R, Huddleston CB, Mendeloff EN, et al: Infant and donor organ growth after heart transplantation in neonates with hypoplastic left heart syndrome. J Heart Lung Transplant 15:1093, 1996.

84. Zales VR, Wright KL, Pahl E, et al: Normal left ventricular muscle mass and mass/volume ratio after pediatric cardiac transplantation. Circulation 90(5 pt 2):II61, 1994.

85. Wilson RF, Laxson DD, Christensen BV, et al: Regional differences in sympathetic reinnervation after human orthotopic cardiac transplantation. Circulation 88:165, 1993.

86. Kaye DM, Esler M, Kingwell B, et al: Functional and neurochemical evidence for partial sympathetic reinnervation after cardiac transplantation in humans. Circulation 88:1110, 1993.

87. Hsu DT, Garofano RP, Douglas JM, et al: Exercise performance after pediatric heart transplantation. Circulation 88(5 pt 2):II238, 1993.

88. Pahl E, Miller SA, Griffith BP, Fricker FJ: Occult restrictive hemodynamics after pediatric heart transplantation. J Heart Lung Transplant 14:1109, 1995.

89. Hausen B, Albes JM, Rohde R, et al: Tricuspid valve regurgitation attributable to endomyocardial biopsies and rejection in heart transplantation. Ann Thorac Surg 59:1134, 1995.

90. Williams MJA, Lee M, DiSalvo TG, et al: Biopsy-induced flail tricuspid leaflet and tricuspid regurgitation following orthotopic cardiac transplantation. Am J Cardiol 77:1339, 1996.

91. Miyamoto Y, Curtiss EI, Kormos RL, et al: Bradyarrhythmia after heart transplantation. Incidence, time course and outcome. Circulation 82(suppl 5):IV313, 1992.

92. Raghavan C, Maloney JD, Nitta J, et al: Long-term follow-up of heart transplant recipients requiring permanent pacemakers. J Heart Lung Transplant 14:1081, 1995.

93. Sandhu JS, Curtiss EI, Follansbee WP, et al: The scalar electrocardiogram of the orthotopic heart transplant recipient. Am Heart J 119:917, 1990.

94. Alexopoulos D, Yusuf S, Bostock J, et al: Ventricular arrhythmias in long term survivors of orthotopic and heterotopic cardiac transplantation. Br Heart J 59:48, 1988.

95. Park JK, Hsu DT, Hordof AJ, Addonizio LJ: Arrhythmias in pediatric heart transplant recipients: Prevalence and association with death, coronary artery disease, and rejection. J Heart Lung Transplant 12:956, 1993.

96. Pavri BB, O'Nunain SS, Newell JB, et al: Prevalence and prognostic significance of atrial arrhythmias after orthotopic cardiac transplantation. J Am Coll Cardiol 25:1673, 1995.

97. Kaye D, Thompson J, Jennings G, Esler M: Cyclosporine therapy after cardiac transplantation causes hypertension and renal vasoconstriction without sympathetic activation. Circulation 88:1101, 1993.

98. Mason J: The pathophysiology of Sandimmune (cyclosporine) in man and animals. Pediatr Nephrol 4:554, 1990.

99. Greenberg A, Thompson ME, Griffith BJ, et al: Cyclosporine nephrotoxicity in cardiac allograft patients—a seven-year follow-up. Transplantation 50:589, 1990.

100. McGiffin DC, Savunen T, Kirklin JK, et al: Cardiac transplant coronary artery disease. J Thorac Cardiovasc Surg 109:1081, 1995.

101. Mullins PA, Cary NR, Sharples L, et al: Coronary occlusive disease and late graft failure after cardiac transplantation. Br Heart J 68:260, 1992.

102. Hosenpud JD, Shipley GD, Wagner CR: Cardiac allograft vasculopathy: Current concepts, recent developments, and future directions. J Heart Lung Transplant 11:9, 1992.

103. Ventura HO, Mehra MR, Smart FW, Stapleton DD: Cardiac allograft vasculopathy: Current concepts. Am Heart J 129:791, 1995.

104. Olivari MT, Homans DC, Wilson RF, et al: Coronary artery disease in cardiac transplant patients receiving triple-drug immunosuppressive therapy. Circulation 80(5 pt 2):III111, 1989.

105. Grattan MT, Moreno-Cabral CE, Starnes VA, et al: Cytomegalovirus infection is associated with cardiac allograft rejection and atherosclerosis. JAMA 261:3561, 1989.

106. McDonald K, Rector TS, Braunlin EA, et al: Association of coronary artery disease in transplant recipients with cytomegalovirus infection. Am J Cardiol 64:359, 1989.

107. Gao SZ, Alderman EL, Schroeder JS, et al: Accelerated coronary vascular disease in the heart transplant patient: Coronary arteriographic findings. J Am Coll Cardiol 17:449, 1991.

108. Rickenbacher PR, Pinto FJ, Chenzbraun A, et al: Incidence and severity of transplant coronary artery disease early and up to 15 years after transplantation as detected by intravascular ultrasound. J Am Coll Cardiol 25:171, 1995.

109. Braunlin EA, Hunter DW, Canter CE, et al: Coronary artery disease in pediatric cardiac transplant recipients receiving triple-drug immunosuppression. Circulation 84(suppl 5):III303, 1991.

110. Pahl E, Fricker FJ, Armitage J, et al: Coronary arteriosclerosis in pediatric heart transplant survivors: Limitation of long-term survival. J Pediatr 116:177, 1990.

111. Pahl E, Zales VR, Fricker FJ, Addonizio LJ: Posttransplant coronary artery disease in children. Circulation 90(suppl II):II56, 1994.

112. Bailey LL, Zuppan CW, Chinnock RE, et al: Graft vasculopathy among recipients of heart transplantation during the first 12 years of life. Transplant Proc 27:1921, 1995.

113. Addonizio LJ, Hsu DT, Douglas JF, et al: Decreasing incidence of coronary disease in pediatric cardiac transplant recipients using increased immunosuppression. Circulation 88(suppl 2):II224, 1993.

114. Balzer DT, Canter CE: Evaluation of graft vasculopathy with intravascular ultrasound in pediatric heart transplant recipients (Abstract). Circulation 94(suppl I):I65, 1996.

115. Schroeder JS, Gao SZ, Alderman EL, et al: A preliminary study of diltiazem in the prevention of coronary artery disease in heart-transplant recipients. N Engl J Med 328:164, 1993.

116. Kobashigawa JA, Katznelson S, Laks H, et al: Effect of pravastatin on outcomes after cardiac transplantation. N Engl J Med 333:621, 1995.

117. Karwande SV, Ensley RD, Renlund DG, et al: Cardiac retransplantation: A viable option? Ann Thorac Surg 54:840, 1992.

118. Addonizio LJ, Hsu DT, Smith CR, et al: Late complications in pediatric cardiac transplant recipients. Circulation 82(suppl IV):IV-295, 1990.

119. Bernstein D, Baum D, Berry G, et al: Neoplastic disorders after pediatric heart transplantation. Circulation 88(5 Pt 2):II230, 1993.

120. Knowles DM, Cesarman E, Chadburn A, et al: Correlative morphologic and molecular genetic analysis demonstrates three distinct categories of posttransplantation lymphoproliferative disorders. Blood 85:552, 1995.

121. Penn I: Incidence and treatment of neoplasia after transplantation. J Heart Lung Transplant 12:S328, 1993.

122. D'Alonzo GE, Barst RJ, Ayres SM, et al: Survival in patients with primary pulmonary hypertension. Ann Intern Med 115:343, 1991.

123. Clabby ML, Canter CE, Moller JH, Bridges ND: Hemodynamics and survival in children with pulmonary hypertension. J Am Coll Cardiol 30:354, 1997.

124. Starnes VA, Barr ML, Cohen RG, et al: Living-donor lobar lung transplantation experience: Intermediate results. J Thorac Cardiovasc Surg 112:1284, 1996.

125. Armitage JM, Kurland G, Michaels M, et al: Critical issues in pediatric lung transplantation. J Thorac Cardiovasc Surg 109:60, 1995.

126. Sweet SC, Spray TL, Huddleston CB, et al: Pediatric lung transplantation at St. Louis Children's Hospital 1990–1995. Am J Resp Crit Care Med 155:1027, 1997.

127. Conte JV, Robbins RC, Reichenspurner H, et al: Pediatric heart-lung transplantation: Intermediate-term results. J Heart Lung Transplant 15:692, 1996.

128. Whitehead B, Rees P, Sorenson K, et al: Incidence of obliterative bronchiolitis after heart-lung transplantation in children. J Heart Lung Transplant 13:903, 1994.

129. Lim TT, Botas J, Ross H, et al: Are heart-lung transplant recipients protected from developing transplant coronary artery disease? Circulation 94:1573, 1996.

MARCELO AUSLENDER   MICHAEL ARTMAN

LIST OF ABBREVIATIONS

AC	Adenylate cyclase
ACE	Angiotensin-converting enzyme
AET	Atrial ectopic tachycardia
AT-III	Antithrombin III
AV	Atrioventricular
BP	Blood pressure
cAMP	Cyclic adenosine monophosphate
cGMP	Cyclic guanosine monophosphate
CHF	Congestive heart failure
CNS	Central nervous system
CPR	Cardiopulmonary resuscitation
DA	Dopamine receptor
DIC	Disseminated intravascular coagulation
ECG	Electrocardiogram
EEG	Electroencephalogram
ERP	Effective refractory period
G_s	Stimulatory G protein
GABA	γ-Aminobutyric acid
GC	Guanylate cyclase
HMG-CoA	Hydroxymethylglutaryl–coenzyme A reductase
HR	Heart rate
ICU	Intensive care unit
INR	International normalized ratio
JET	Junctional ectopic tachycardia
NAPA	N-Acetylprocainamide
NO	Nitric oxide
PDE	Phosphodiesterase
PGE_1	Prostaglandin E_1
PICU	Pediatric intensive care unit
PJRT	Persistent junctional reciprocating tachycardia
PR	Per rectum
PTT	Partial thromboplastin time
SL	Sublingual
SND	Sinus node dysfunction
SR	Sarcoplasmic reticulum
SVT	Supraventricular tachycardia
TDD	Total digitalizing dose
TEE	Transesophageal echocardiogram
TnC	Troponin C
VF	Ventricular fibrillation
VT	Ventricular tachycardia

CALCULATION OF CONTINUOUS INFUSIONS (GENERAL FORMULA)

$$\text{Infusion rate (ml/hr)} = \frac{60 \text{ (min/hr)} \cdot \text{body weight (kg)} \cdot \text{dose (µg/kg/min)}}{\text{drug concentration (µg/ml)}}$$

$$\text{µg/kg/min} = (\text{µg of drug/ml of fluid}) \cdot (\text{ml/hr}) \div (60 \text{ min/hr}) \div \text{weight (kg)}$$

CALCULATION OF CONTINUOUS INFUSIONS*

Drug	Dose	Calculation	Infusion Rate
Dobutamine	2–20 µg/kg/min	6 × body wt (kg) = mg added to make 100 ml	1 ml/hr = 1 µg/kg/min
Dopamine	2–20 µg/kg/min	6 × body wt (kg) = mg added to make 100 ml	1 ml/hr = 1 µg/kg/min
Epinephrine	0.05–2 µg/kg/min	0.6 × body wt (kg) = mg added to make 100 ml	1 ml/hr = 0.1 µg/kg/min
Isoproterenol	0.05–2 µg/kg/min	0.6 × body wt (kg) = mg added to make 100 ml	1 ml/hr = 0.1 µg/kg/min
Lidocaine	20–50 µg/kg/min	60 × body wt (kg) = mg added to make 100 ml	1 ml/hr = 10 µg/kg/min
Nitroprusside	0.5–5 µg/kg/min	6 × body wt (kg) = mg added to make 100 ml	1 ml/hr = 1 µg/kg/min
Prostaglandin E_1	0.01–0.1 µg/kg/min	0.6 × body wt (kg) = mg added to make 100 ml	1 ml/hr = 0.1 µg/kg/min

*Patients weighing 30 kg or more or those requiring fluid restriction may need more concentrated solutions to deliver less fluid per hour.

PEDIATRIC EMERGENCY DRUG DOSAGES

Drug	Dose	Comments
Adenosine	50–400 μg/kg rapid IV bolus (maximal adult dose = 12 mg)	May repeat every 2–4 min with increasing dosage in increments of 50 μg/kg up to maximum of 300 μg/kg/dose (or to the adult maximal dose).
Albumin 5%	5–10 ml/kg, IV	May repeat as clinically indicated.
Atropine	0.02 mg/kg every 5 min (minimal dose = 0.1 mg) IV Maximal total dose: child = 1 mg; adolescent and adult = 2 mg	May be given by endotracheal tube after dilution to 1–2 ml with normal saline.
Bretylium	1st dose = 5 mg/kg; repeat dose = 10 mg/kg, IV	May produce hypotension. May repeat dose every 15–30 min during CPR. Maximal total dose: 30 mg/kg.
Calcium chloride Calcium gluconate	10–20 mg/kg/dose, IV 100 mg/kg/dose, IV	Role in resuscitation questionable. Should be used only when hyperkalemia, hypermagnesemia, hypocalcemia, or calcium channel blocker toxicity is present.
Dextrose 50%	0.5 g/kg (2 ml/kg of dextrose 25%), IV	Dilute to a 25% solution before giving.
Epinephrine	Neonate: 0.01–0.03 mg/kg every 5 min, IV Pediatric: 0.01 mg/kg every 5 min, IV Maximal dose: 0.5–1 mg, IV IV infusion: 0.05–1.5 μg/kg/min	May be given by endotracheal tube after dilution to 1–2 ml with normal saline. Do not mix with bicarbonate.
Etomidate	0.3–0.4 mg/kg	
Hetastarch	5–10 ml/kg, IV	Maximal dose = 1 g/kg/day (concentration = 60 g/L).
Lidocaine	0.5–1 mg/kg loading dose; may repeat to a total dose not greater than 3 mg/kg Infusion: 20–50 μg/kg/min	May be administered by endotracheal tube. Dilute to 1–2 ml with normal saline before endotracheal administration.
Morphine sulfate	0.1 mg/kg IV	
Mannitol	0.5–1 g/kg IV	
Midazolam	0.1 mg/kg IV	Short-acting benzodiazepine. Onset of action after IV dose 1–5 min. Can cause significant myocardial and respiratory depression.
Naloxone	Birth to 5 years or 20 kg: 0.01–0.1 mg/kg/dose >5 years or >20 kg: 0.4–2 mg/dose May repeat IV doses every 2–3 min	May be given by endotracheal tube after dilution to 1–2 ml with normal saline.
Nifedipine	0.25–0.5 mg/kg SL Maximal dose: 10 mg	
Nitroprusside	IV infusion: 0.5–5 μg/kg/min	Maximum 10 μg/kg/min.
Pancuronium	0.05–0.1 mg/kg IV	May repeat every 30–60 min as needed.
Prostaglandin E$_1$	IV infusion: 0.01–0.1 μg/kg/min	After ductus patency is established, infusion rate may be reduced. Side effects include apnea, hypotension, and fever.
Sodium bicarbonate	1 mEq/kg IV × 1 May repeat with 0.5 mEq/kg IV	Use only the 0.5 mEq/ml solution for neonates. NaHCO$_3$ should be used on the basis of documented metabolic acidosis. Routine use in cardiac arrest is not recommended.
Succinylcholine	1–2 mg/kg IV	In susceptible patients, may cause masseter muscle spasm and malignant hyperthermia.

PEDIATRIC EMERGENCY CARDIOVERSION/DEFIBRILLATION

Method	Treatment	Comments
DC shock	1–2 joules/kg	Use 0.5–1 joule/kg for cardioversion. For defibrillation, may require 2–4 joules/kg.

ACUTE NONCOMPENSATED HEART FAILURE

POOR DIASTOLIC FUNCTION

- Positive-pressure ventilation (in case of hemodynamic compromise) — ↓ Preload to RV →↓ RV wall tension →↓ afterload; ↓ LV afterload; ↓ Work of breathing and VO_2
- Low-dose sympathomimetic — Lusitropic effect of β-receptor stimulation; ↑ Contractility, inotropic effect
- Heart rate modulation — β-Blockers; Calcium channel blockers
- Inodilators — PDE III inhibitors — ↓ Afterload; ↑ cAMP → mild positive inotropy; ↑ cAMP → lusitropic effect
- Load modification
  - Preload and afterload — Nitroprusside, nitroglycerin, amrinone, milrinone
  - Preload — Diuretics { Loop diuretics; Thiazides; Osmotic agents }; Low-dose nitroglycerin

POOR SYSTOLIC FUNCTION

- Positive-pressure ventilation — Equivalent to vasodilator therapy, decreases afterload and improves cardiac output in preload-independent patients; Decreases work of breathing and VO_2, important in the pediatric patient unable to gain weight because of decompensated CHF
- Digoxin; Low-dose dobutamine — Improve cardiac output leading to decrease in sympathetic nervous system tone and upregulation of cardiac β receptors
- Inodilators — PDE III inhibitors — ↓ Afterload; ↑ Contractility; Less proarrhythmic than β-agonists
- Diuretics — Loop diuretics; Thiazides — ↓ Pulmonary and hepatic congestion; Mild vasodilatation; Improve symptoms
- Steroid pulse — Upregulation of β receptors
- β-Agonists
  - Positive effect — ↑ Contractility
  - Negative effect — ↑ Afterload (epinephrine, norepinephrine, high-dose dopamine); Proarrhythmic; ↑ Preload; ↑ VO_2

SUMMARY OF GENERAL CARDIOVASCULAR PHARMACOLOGY

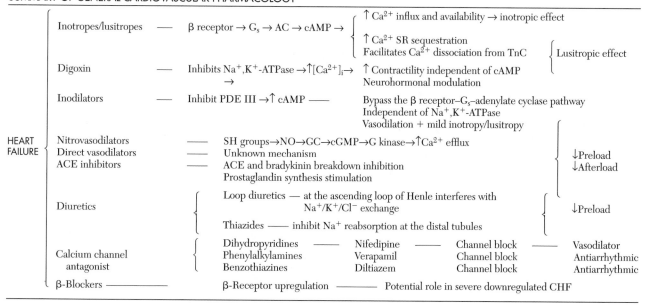

HEART FAILURE

- Inotropes/lusitropes — β receptor → G_s → AC → cAMP →
  - ↑ Ca^{2+} influx and availability → inotropic effect
  - ↑ Ca^{2+} SR sequestration; Facilitates Ca^{2+} dissociation from TnC } Lusitropic effect
- Digoxin — Inhibits Na^+,K^+-ATPase →↑$[Ca^{2+}]_i$→ → ↑ Contractility independent of cAMP; Neurohormonal modulation
- Inodilators — Inhibit PDE III →↑ cAMP — Bypass the β receptor–G_s–adenylate cyclase pathway; Independent of Na^+,K^+-ATPase; Vasodilation + mild inotropy/lusitropy
- Nitrovasodilators — SH groups→NO→GC→cGMP→G kinase→↑Ca^{2+} efflux
- Direct vasodilators — Unknown mechanism
- ACE inhibitors — ACE and bradykinin breakdown inhibition; Prostaglandin synthesis stimulation } ↓Preload; ↓Afterload
- Diuretics
  - Loop diuretics — at the ascending loop of Henle interferes with $Na^+/K^+/Cl^-$ exchange
  - Thiazides — inhibit Na^+ reabsorption at the distal tubules } ↓Preload
- Calcium channel antagonist
  - Dihydropyridines — Nifedipine — Channel block — Vasodilator
  - Phenylalkylamines — Verapamil — Channel block — Antiarrhythmic
  - Benzothiazines — Diltiazem — Channel block — Antiarrhythmic
- β-Blockers — β-Receptor upregulation — Potential role in severe downregulated CHF

GUIDELINES FOR DRUG DOSAGE

Diuretics

Drug	Receptor	Dose	Comments
LOOP DIURETICS			
Bumetanide	Inhibits the $Na^+/K^+/2Cl^-$ cotransport mechanism Weak inhibitor of carbonic anhydrase	Adults: 0.5–2.0 mg/dose PO (1–2 times/day) 0.5–1.0 mg/dose IV (maximum, 10 mg/day) Pediatrics: 0.01 mg/kg/dose IV (or PO) (maximum, 0.1 mg/kg/day) Neonates: 0.01–0.05 mg/kg/dose (IV or PO) qd or qd Infants and children: 0.015–0.1 mg/kg/dose (IV or PO) q 6 hr–qd (maximal dose = 10 mg/day) May be used as a continuous infusion	Hyperuricemia. Hypokalemia. Hypomagnesemia. Hyponatremia. Potential ototoxicity. Hypochloremic metabolic alkalosis. Hypercalciuria. Nephrocalcinosis.
Ethacrynic acid	Inhibits the $Na^+/K^+/2Cl^-$ cotransport mechanism	0.5–1.0 mg/kg IV (maximal dose = 50 mg) May repeat in 12–24 hr	
Furosemide	Inhibits the $Na^+/K^+/2Cl^-$ cotransport mechanism Weak inhibitor of carbonic anhydrase	Pediatrics: 1–2 mg/kg IV or 1–6 mg/kg PO q 6–12 hr (maximum, 12 mg/kg/day) Continuous infusion: 0.05 mg/kg/hr, titrate up to desired effect Adult: 20–80 mg/day q 6–12 hr, PO, IM, IV	
BENZOTHIAZIDES			
Chlorothiazide	Blockade of electroneutral Na^+/Cl^- cotransport	20–40 mg/kg/day PO bid 1–4 mg/dose IV q 6–12 hr	Synergistic effect when given before a loop diuretic; may aggravate existing diabetes mellitus. Intrahepatic cholestasis. Hyperlipidemia. Hypokalemia. Hypochloremic-metabolic alkalosis. Hyperuricemia.
Hydrochlorothiazide	Blockade of electroneutral Na^+/Cl^- cotransport	2–3 mg/kg/day PO in 2 divided doses Maximal adult dose = 200 mg/day	
Metolazone		Adults: 2.5–10 mg PO qd Pediatrics: 0.2–0.4 mg/kg PO qd	
OSMOTIC AGENT			
Mannitol		0.5–1 g/kg IV After urine flow is established, lower doses (0.25–0.5 g/kg) are recommended. Repeat every 6 hours as clinically indicated.	Can cause an acute expansion in the extracellular space, which can be hazardous in the patient with decompensated CHF.
ALDOSTERONE ANTAGONIST			
Spironolactone	Competitive antagonist of the actions of aldosterone	Adults: 25–200 mg/day PO Pediatrics: 1–3.5 mg/kg/day PO Administer in 1 or 2 daily doses	Potassium-sparing diuretic. Caution with ACE inhibitors (may cause hyperkalemia).
POTASSIUM-SPARING AGENTS			
Triamterene	Inhibit electrogenic entry of Na^+ → electrical potential across the tubules falls →↓ secretion of K^+	0.7–4 mg/kg/day PO Maximal dose = 300 mg/day	Can cause megaloblastic anemia.
Amiloride		0.07–0.4 mg/kg/day PO	Can cause megaloblastic anemia.

Vasodilators and Antihypertensives

Drug	Receptor	Dose	Comments
α- AND β-RECEPTOR BLOCKER			
Labetalol	α and β	0.25–1.0 mg/kg IV	May administer by continuous infusion (0.4–3.0 mg/kg/hr).
α-RECEPTOR BLOCKERS/ANTAGONISTS			
Phentolamine	α_1 and α_2	0.05–0.1 mg/kg/dose IV, IM; maximal single dose = 5 mg 2.5–15 µg/kg/min continuous infusion IV Most impressive effect in patients with pheochromocytoma	Treatment of extravasation (due to dopamine, dobutamine, norepinephrine, epinephrine, or phenylephrine). Dilute 5–10 mg in 10 ml normal saline and infiltrate area subcutaneously. Do not exceed 0.1–0.2 mg/kg or 5 mg total. Rapid development of tachyphylaxis.
Prazosin	α_1	Initial dose: 5 µg/kg PO May increase to 25 µg/kg/dose PO q 6–8 hr (maximal total daily dose = 20 mg)	Rapid development of tachyphylaxis. May develop orthostatic hypotension after first dose.
Tolazoline	α_1 and α_2	1 mg/kg/hr continuous infusion IV Maximum = 6 mg/kg/hr	Rapid development of tachyphylaxis. Monitor for gastrointestinal bleeding.
β-RECEPTOR BLOCKERS			
Atenolol	β_1-selective	1–2 mg/kg/day PO (single daily dose)	
Carvedilol	β_1 and β_2; α	Initial dose = 0.05 mg/kg/dose given bid (maximal initial dose = 3.125 mg PO bid) May titrate upward weekly to 0.4–0.5 mg/kg/dose given bid Do not exceed adult dose (3.125 mg PO bid initially; target dose, 25 to 50 mg PO bid)	Recently approved for use in adult patients with CHF; similar studies in children have not been completed. May cause decompensation during drug initiation or up-titration.
Esmolol	β_1-selective	75–300 µg/kg/min continuous infusion after 200–500 µg/kg loading dose during 2–4 min	Titrate dose up by 25–50 µg/kg/min increments. Given the short half-life (2.88 ± 2.67 min), load may be avoided altogether because steady state is reached in ±15 min.
Propranolol	β_1 and β_2	Initial oral dose: 0.5–1 mg/kg/day q 6–12 hr; increase slowly to a maximal dose of 8–10 mg/kg/day 0.01–0.05 mg/kg IV over 10 min; maximal dose: infants = 1 mg, children = 3 mg	Avoid in status asthmaticus or conduction defects. Use cautiously in CHF or diabetes.
Metoprolol	β_1-selective	1–2 mg/kg q 12 hr Maximal daily adult dose = 450 mg	
Acebutolol	β_1-selective Intrinsic sympathomimetic activity	200–400 mg/day (4–8 mg/kg) q 12 hr Maximal daily dose = 1200–2400 mg	
Nadolol	β_1 and β_2	40 mg/day (1–5 mg/kg) q 24 hr Maximal daily dose = 640 mg	As for propranolol.
Pindolol	β_1 and β_2 Intrinsic sympathomimetic activity	10 mg/day (0.3 mg/kg), q 12 hr Maximal daily dose = 30 mg	As for propranolol.
Timolol	β_1 and β_2	5–10 mg q 12 hr Maximal daily dose = 30 mg	As for propranolol.

Table continued on following page

GUIDELINES FOR DRUG DOSAGE (Continued)

Vasodilators and Antihypertensives (Continued)

Drug	Receptor	Dose	Comments
ACE INHIBITORS			
Captopril	ACE inhibition Bradykinin breakdown inhibition Increase prostaglandin production	Adults: 6.25–25 mg/dose PO q 8–12 hr Pediatrics: 0.1–0.5 mg/kg/dose PO q 8 hr Maximal pediatric dose = 4–6 mg/kg/24 hr (divided tid)	It appears that low doses are sufficient to inhibit ACE and that higher doses increase the duration but not the intensity of the inhibition. Permanent inhibition of ACE is not a prerequisite to adequate blood pressure control around-the-clock. Because ACE inhibitors are used at concentrations many times greater than the EC_{50}, even one with short half-life may remain effective during a long dosage interval.
Enalapril	Modulation of sympathetic activity Improved suppressed vagal activity	Adults: 2.5–5 mg/day PO; may increase to 10–40 mg/day Pediatrics: 0.1–0.4 mg/kg/day PO Administer qd or divide bid	ACE inhibitors must be introduced at low doses in patients with CHF owing to the potential development of symptomatic hypotension. In addition, patients with heart failure have a higher incidence of acute renal failure when prolonged and persistent inhibition of ACE is induced with high doses of long-acting ACE inhibitors. In these patients, a short-acting (captopril) or a low-dose long-acting ACE inhibitor is recommended.
Enalaprilat	Reduced incidence and severity of malignant arrhythmias, perhaps by preventing hypokalemia and reducing ventricular wall stress	Adults: 0.625–1.25 mg/dose IV q 6–8 hr Pediatrics: 0.005–0.01 mg/kg/dose IV q 8–24 hr	The conversion of prodrugs into their active forms is delayed in patients with liver disease or severe congestion due to heart failure (except for captopril and enalaprilat).
Lisinopril		0.08 mg/kg/day Maximal dose = 40 mg once daily 5 mg once daily	Hypotension, hypokalemia, and acute renal failure are complications related to ACE inhibition. The severity of renal failure and hypokalemia may be aggravated when ACE inhibitors are used in combination with nonsteroidal anti-inflammatory drugs (NSAID). The anti-hypertensive effects of ACE inhibition are blunted by concurrent treatment with NSAID.
Ramipril	Regression of ventricular hypertrophy	Maximal dose = 10 mg once daily	Captopril increases serum digoxin levels by 30%. Sulfhydryl (SH)–containing ACE inhibitors can restore the efficacy of nitrates by providing a source of SH (captopril)
Alacepril Benazepril Cilazapril Quinapril Fosinopril	Limited to no experience in pediatrics		
CENTRAL α_2-AGONISTS			
Clonidine		5–10 μg/kg/day PO divided tid or bid May increase gradually to maximum of 25 μg/kg/day Do not exceed adult maximum of 2.4 mg/day	Available as a transdermal patch (0.1, 0.2, or 0.3 mg/day for 7 days). Danger of severe rebound hypertension if chronic therapy is abruptly discontinued.
Methyldopa		Adults: 250–500 mg PO q 4–12 hr Pediatrics: 10 mg/kg/24 hr PO (divide bid or tid)	Pediatric dose may be increased to 60 mg/kg/24 hr.
DIRECT VASODILATOR			
Hydralazine		Adults: 5–20 mg IV or IM q 4–6 hr 10–25 mg PO q 6 hr Pediatrics: 0.1–0.5 mg/kg/dose IV (maximal IV dose = 20 mg) 0.25–0.75 mg/kg/dose PO	High doses give lupus-like syndrome. For chronic therapy, administer q 6–8 hr PO or q 4–6 hr IV. Maximal total daily dose = 200 mg.

Drug	Mechanism	Dose	Comments
K⁺ CHANNEL OPENERS			
Minoxidil		Initial dose: 0.1–0.2 mg/kg PO once/day (maximum, 5 mg) If necessary, increase to 0.25–1.0 mg/kg/day (maximal daily maintenance dose = 50 mg)	Monitor BP continuously and stop infusion when BP reaches target level.
Diazoxide		1–5 mg/kg slow IV during 30 min (does not require rapid bolus infusion) (maximal dose: 150 mg in a single injection)	May repeat 1–5 mg/kg slow IV × 2.
NITROVASODILATORS			
Nitroglycerin	SH groups → NO → GC → cGMP → protein kinase → ↑Ca²⁺ efflux	0.5–3.0 μg/kg/min IV	Maximum = 10 μg/kg/min.
Nitroprusside		0.5–3.0 μg/kg/min IV	Maximum = 10 μg/kg/min. Cyanide liberation and production of thiocyanate occur with the use of nitroprusside. Toxicity is rare when it is used in low dose (<2 μg/kg/min) or given for less than 3 days. Cyanide toxicity may be prevented by infusion of sodium thiosulfate.
CALCIUM CHANNEL BLOCKERS			
Nifedipine	L-type Ca²⁺ channel α₁ subunit	0.1–0.5 mg/kg PO q 8 hr	Maximum = 20 mg/dose.
Nicardipine		0.1 μg/kg/min	May cause flushing, tachycardia, and headache.
INODILATORS			
Amrinone	PDE III inhibition → ↑cAMP	Loading dose: 1–3 mg/kg IV during 30 min Continuous infusion: 5–10 μg/kg/min	Cannot be mixed with dextrose solutions. May cause thrombocytopenia.
Milrinone		Loading dose: 0.05–0.1 mg/kg IV during 15–30 min Continuous infusion: 0.5–0.75 μg/kg/min	Second generation, more potent than Amrinone with possibly fewer side effects.
PROSTAGLANDINS			
Prostaglandin E₁		Initial dose: 0.05 μg/kg/min May increase to 0.1–0.15 μg/kg/min	Lower doses (as low as 0.01 μg/kg/min) may be effective. Tapering to lowest effective dose is recommended. May cause apnea, hypotension, and fever.
Prostacyclin			Pulmonary vasodilator, not yet approved in the United States.
NO		Effective dose not well established Range 1–40 ppm, given by inhalation	Pulmonary vasodilator.

Table continued on following page

Inotropic Agents

Drug	Receptor	Dose	Comments
INODILATORS			
Amrinone	PDE III inhibition	Loading dose: 1–3 mg/kg IV during 30 min Continuous infusion: 5–10 µg/kg/min Cannot be mixed with dextrose solutions	The inotropic/lusitropic effect is less pronounced when the cAMP levels are depressed, as in chronic systolic heart failure. Thrombocytopenia is rare (2.4% incidence) or mild if it is given for short-term periods and the dose is kept ≤10 µg/kg/min (develops in 54 ± 15 hr).
Milrinone		Loading dose: 0.05–0.1 mg/kg IV during 15–30 min Continuous infusion: 0.5–0.75 µg/kg/min	The drug is metabolized by hepatic N-acetylation; half-life is 1.5 hr in fast acetylators, and 4.4 hr in slow acetylators; half-life increases to 6–8 hr in severe CHF In infants and children (1–15 yr), the half-life quoted to be 2.2–10.5 hr Second generation, more potent than Amrinone with possibly fewer side effects (i.e., thrombocytopenia).
DIGOXIN	Sarcolemmal Na$^+$, K$^+$-ATPase	Total digitalizing dose: Preterm infant: 6–10 µg/kg PO Term infant: 20–30 µg/kg PO 1–5 yr: 30–40 µg/kg PO 5–10 yr: 20–30 µg/kg PO Adults: 10–15 µg/kg PO Maintenance dose: 5–10 µg/kg/day PO	IV dose is approximately 80% of PO dose. Reduce dose in renal dysfunction. Narrow toxic/therapeutic ratio.
INOTROPES/LUSITROPES			
Dobutamine	β$_1$ and β$_2$	2–20 µg/kg/min continuous infusion IV	Can cause severe tachycardia, particularly in neonates. Good inotrope/lusitrope for CHF with poor systolic function and dilated ventricles.
Dopamine	DA$_1$, DA$_2$, β, and α ↑ Circulating norepinephrine	2–20 µg/kg/min continuous infusion IV	2–3 µg/kg/min, DA$_1$-DA$_2$ receptor actions predominate. ↑ Renal blood flow and sodium excretion. 4–8 µg/kg/min, β$_1$ > β$_2$ predominate, inotropic/lusitropic effect. >8 µg/kg/min, α$_1$ predominate and so afterload increases.
Epinephrine	β$_1$, β$_2$, α$_1$, and α$_2$	Acute: 0.1 ml/kg of 1 : 10,000 (0.01 mg/kg) Continuous IV infusion: 0.05–2 µg/kg/min At low doses <0.02 µg/kg/min, β effects predominate	Mostly used in patients with severe systolic failure, particularly after circulatory arrest. In severe shock at high doses, has less negative chronotropic effect than norepinephrine.
Isoproterenol	β$_1$ and β$_2$	0.05–1 µg/kg/min continuous infusion Rarely require >0.5 µg/kg/min	Rarely used for inotropic support. In the ICU, it is used mainly to accelerate the sinus node or the AV node conduction, as well as ventricular rate in AV block until a pacemaker is in place. In addition, it is an effective bronchodilator and pulmonary/systemic vasodilator.
Norepinephrine	α$_1$, α$_2$, and β$_1$	0.05–1 µg/kg/min continuous infusion IV Rarely require >0.5 µg/kg/min	Mostly used in severe shock.

Antiarrhythmic Agents

Drug	Receptor, Mechanism of Action	Dose	Comments
CLASS I: FAST NA⁺ CHANNEL BLOCKADE			
Class Ia Quinidine	Class Ia drugs: Moderate phase 0 depression Depress conduction Prolong repolarization ↑PR, QRS If QTc increases >30%, may produce toxicity	15–60 mg/kg/day PO; divide q 4–6 hr for sulfate and q 6–8 hr for gluconate Test dose: 2 mg/kg (for idiosyncratic reaction)	May produce torsades de pointes (due to acquired prolonged QT syndrome), AV block, SND, or increased ventricular ectopy. Potentiates nondepolarizing and depolarizing muscle relaxants. Verapamil, amiodarone, cimetidine increase quinidine levels. Phenytoin, phenobarbital decrease quinidine levels.
Procainamide		5–15 mg/kg slow IV (during 30 min) loading dose; then 20–100 μg/kg/min continuous IV; do not exceed 100 mg/dose during load; do not exceed 500 mg in 30 min PO: 20–40 mg/kg/24 hr in 6 divided doses (maximum = 60 mg/kg/24 hr or 4 g/24 hr)	During IV infusion, carefully monitor ECG (QT interval) and BP (may cause hypotension, do not administer faster than 20–30 mg/min; hypotension responds to fluid replacement). In patients with first-degree AV block, IV infusion must be closely monitored because of potential worsening of the degree of block. The elimination kinetics are age dependent, with longer half-life at younger age. Most arrhythmias respond to therapeutic levels between 4 and 8 μg/ml. NAPA, the active metabolite of procainamide, is a K⁺ channel blocker that displays class III activity. Therapeutic NAPA levels are 12–16 μg/ml.
Disopyramide		Adults: 100–150 mg PO q 6 hr or 200–300 mg PO q 12 hr (sustained-release form) Children: 5–15 mg/kg/day PO (4 divided doses); do not exceed adult dose	May produce syncope (due to acquired prolonged QT syndrome), AV block, SND, or increased ventricular ectopy. Negative inotropic effect.
Class Ib Lidocaine	Class Ib drugs: Minimal phase 0 depression Shorten repolarization No significant effect on ERP Moderate phase 0 depression	1–2 mg/kg IV loading dose; then 20–50 μg/kg/min continuous infusion IV Therapeutic range = 1.5–5 μg/ml Toxic >5 μg/ml	Reduce dose in severe CHF/low output (potent negative inotropic agent). May cause seizures, anxiety, euphoria, hallucinations.
Phenytoin		10–20 mg/kg slow IV loading dose; then 5–10 mg/kg/day PO or IV (divided bid)	
Mexiletine		1.4–5 mg/kg/day PO (divided tid)	

Table continued on following page

GUIDELINES FOR DRUG DOSAGE (Continued)

Antiarrhythmic Agents (Continued)

Drug	Receptor, Mechanism of Action	Dose	Comments
Class Ic			
Flecainide	Class Ic drugs: Marked phase 0 depression Prolong conduction Little effect on repolarization	Adults: 100–400 mg/day Pediatrics: 3–6 mg/kg/day PO (divided tid or bid) Half-life differs by patient's age: $t_{1/2}$ < 1 yr and >12 yr = 11–12 hr → dose bid $t_{1/2}$ 1–12 yr = 8–9 hr → dose tid Average effective dose: 50–200 mg/m²/day	Reserved for PJRT, SVT, VT (with normal hemodynamics); effective therapy for bypass tract–mediated tachycardia and abnormal enhanced automaticity (AET, JET). It is also effective in fetal tachycardia. Therapeutic range: 200–800 ng/ml. Levels should be obtained at steady state (at least 3 days) and when the patient is taking a regular diet. Absorption increases with decreased milk intake. Increases pacing thresholds; avoid if myocardial damage.
Propafenone		10 mg/kg/day PO (divided tid) 300–500 mg/m²/day PO, divided bid Therapeutic levels = 500–2000 ng/ml	May be useful in managing postoperative junctional ectopic tachycardia. Treatment of PJRT, SVT. Negative inotrope (mild β and Ca²⁺ blockade).
CLASS II: β-BLOCKERS			
Atenolol	β_1-selective ↓ HR, ↓ QT	0.5–1 mg/kg/day PO (single daily dose)	If therapy is discontinued, gradually taper over a 2-wk period. May produce fatigue, headache, nightmares.
Propranolol	Nonselective β-blockade Membrane-stabilizing activity ↓ HR	Initial oral dose: 0.5–1 mg/kg/day q 6–12 hr; increase slowly to a maximal dose of 8–10 mg/kg/day 0.01–0.05 mg/kg IV during 1 hr; maximum, 10 mg	May produce asthma exacerbation, fatigue, insomnia, depression. Negative inotrope.
Esmolol	Nonselective β-blockade	Pediatrics: loading dose of 200–500 µg/kg IV during 2–4 min; initial maintenance: 50–200 µg/kg/min Mean effective dose = 500–600 µg/kg/min	May increase in increments of 50–100 µg/kg/min up to maximum of 1 mg/kg/min. Given the short half-life (2.88 ± 2.67 min), load may be avoided altogether because steady state is reached in ±15 min.
Nadolol	Nonselective β-blockade	0.5–1 mg/kg/dose bid	
CLASS III: PROLONG REPOLARIZATION			
Amiodarone	α- and β-antagonist Ca²⁺ channel blockade K⁺ channel blockade	Loading dose: 10–20 mg/kg/day PO for 1–2 wk Maintenance: 5–10 mg/kg/day PO qd or 5 of 7 days/wk IV: Initial bolus of 5–10 mg/kg during 1 hr; if inadequate response, 5 mg/kg during 30–60 min, which can be repeated ×1; maximal total initial bolus = 20 mg/kg; infusion: 5–10 µg/kg/min Treat for at least 24 hr after resolution of arrhythmia	IV form reserved for resistant, life-threatening arrhythmias; high incidence of toxicity; may exacerbate SND. Amiodarone IV has been used successfully in the treatment of postoperative JET, life-threatening ventricular arrhythmias, and automatic atrial arrhythmias. IV infusion is associated with hypotension responsive to calcium and fluid replacement.
Bretylium		5 mg/kg IV, during 1 min; may repeat every 15–20 min for a maximal dose of 30 mg/kg Maintenance dose: 5 mg/kg q 6–8 hr	Treatment of arrhythmias associated with digoxin toxicity. Treatment of VF: 5 mg/kg, followed by DC cardioversion; if no response, repeat with 10 mg/kg followed by DC cardioversion (maximal total dose = 30 mg/kg). Causes postural hypotension.

Drug	Mechanism	Dose	Comments
Sotalol	Nonselective β-blockade, K⁺ channel blockade, ↓ HR, ↑ QTc	2–8 mg/kg/day PO (divided bid); maximum, 30–180 mg/m²/day	May cause prolongation of QTc (which can be aggravated by hypokalemia or hypomagnesemia) and risk of torsades de pointes. Avoid in asthma or conduction defects.
Magnesium		Adults: Magnesium sulfate 1–2 g IV followed by 0.5–1 g/hr. Children: 0.2–0.4 mEq/kg/ dose q 4–6 hr	Not adequate for prolonged therapy.
CLASS IV: CA²⁺ CHANNEL BLOCKERS Verapamil	L-type Ca²⁺ channel α₁ subunit	Adults: 2.5–10 mg IV during 2 min; may repeat in 15–30 min; 80–120 mg PO q 8 hr. Pediatrics: 0.05–0.2 mg/kg IV during 3–5 min; may repeat in 30 min (total dose not to exceed 0.3 mg/kg or 10 mg total); 2–8 mg/kg/day PO (divided tid or qid)	Contraindicated in infants (<12 mo). Myocardial depressant.
Diltiazem		Initial dose: 0.25 mg/kg during 2 min IV. If inappropriate response, administer a second dose of 0.35 mg/kg during 2 min IV, then begin IV continuous, infusion 5–15 mg/hr	After 24 hr, DC cardioversion if no resolution of atrial flutter. IV boluses should be repeated 15 min apart. Limited experience in infants and children.
CLASS V: CARDIAC GLYCOSIDES Digoxin	Sarcolemmal Na⁺,K⁺-ATPase	Digitalizing dose is age dependent. Give in 3 divided doses (½, ¼, ¼), spaced 8–12 hr. Preterm infant: 6–10 µg/kg PO. Term infant: 20–30 µg/kg PO. 1–5 yr: 30–40 µg/kg PO. 5–10 yr: 20–30 µg/kg PO. Adults: 10–15 µg/kg PO. Maximal TDD: 1–1.5 mg. IV dose: ¾ oral dose. Oral maintenance: 10 µg/kg/day q 12 hr	IV dose is approximately 75% of PO dose. Reduce dose in renal dysfunction. Narrow toxic/therapeutic ratio. If loading is omitted, steady state is reached in approximately 5–7 days (5 half-life times).
Antidigoxin Fab		Fab dose (mg) = (serum digoxin concentration in ng/ ml × 5.6 × body weight in kg/1000) × 64. If the steady-state serum digoxin concentration is unknown but reliable information is available on the amount ingested, the dose of Fab can be based on the fact that 40 mg (1 vial) of Fab bind approximately 0.66 mg of digoxin	Infuse IV during 15–30 min. Monitor serum potassium levels. Consider intradermal skin testing before infusion, especially in individuals at increased risk for hypersensitivity reaction.
CLASS VI: PURINERGIC AGONIST Adenosine	A₁ and A₂ adenosine receptor, ↑ AV refractoriness, ↓ AV conduction	Adults: 6 mg rapid IV bolus; may repeat using 12 mg rapid IV bolus. Pediatrics: 50–100 µg/kg rapid IV bolus; may repeat q 2–4 min in increments of 50 µg/kg; maximal single dose = 400 µg/kg or 12 mg total	Median effective pediatric dose = 150 µg/kg. Side effects are frequent but transient (hypotension, dyspnea). Reduce dose in patient with right-to-left shunt (↓first-pass) and in patients receiving dipyridamole.
DC SYNCHRONIZED CARDIOVERSION		SVT: 0.25–1.0 joule/kg synchronized. VT: 1.0–2.0 joule/kg synchronized. VF: 1.0–2.0 joule/kg nonsynchronized	

Table continued on following page

GUIDELINES FOR DRUG DOSAGE (Continued)

Drug	Receptor and Effects	Sedatives, Analgesics, and Paralytic Agents	
		Dose	Comments
BENZODIAZEPINES			
Midazolam	Benzodiazepine receptor (R) Benzodiazepines facilitate GABA binding to its R → opening of Cl^- channel → cell hyperpolarization → makes the cell more difficult to depolarize	0.05–0.2 mg/kg IM or IV; after loading dose, may administer by continuous infusion IV (0.1 mg/kg/hr) if prolonged conscious sedation is required 5–15 min 0.2–0.3 mg/kg intranasal; may repeat in 5–15 min	CNS effects peak at 5 min after infusion. Two metabolites, one of them active. Myocardial depressant; must be used with caution in patients with poor systolic function.
Diazepam		Adults: 0.5–10 mg PO or IV (tid) Pediatrics: 0.1 mg/kg IV q 4 hr Seizures: 0.05–0.3 mg/kg IV 0.5 mg/kg PR	Maximal effect immediately after injection. Permits close titration of effect, making it a good drug for endoscopic procedures. Long half-life; two active metabolites. Myocardial depressant.
Lorazepam		Status epilepticus: 0.1 mg/kg slow IV, PR (maximum, 4 mg); may repeat after 10 min with 0.05 mg/kg IV Sedation: 0.05–0.1 mg/kg q 4–6 hr	CNS effects even after IV infusion may take up to 30 min; no active metabolite. Myocardial depressant.
BENZODIAZEPINE ANTAGONIST			
Flumazenil	Benzodiazepine/GABA receptor antagonist	Children: initial dose of 0.01 mg/kg (maximal dose = 0.2 mg); then 5–10 µg/kg/hr to a maximal cumulative dose of 1 mg Adults: 0.2–0.3 mg IV; may be repeated at 1-min intervals up to a cumulative dose of 1–3 mg	Benzodiazepine receptor antagonist. Has a high clearance and short half-life, so the effects are short-lived and CNS depression may recur after initial response.
OPIATES Fentanyl	Receptor subtype μ receptor: Analgesia Miosis Respiratory depression ↓Response to CO_2 ↓Tidal volume	IV or IM single dose: 2–10 µg/kg 1–3 µg/kg/hr continuous infusion IV Dosage range based on desired degree of analgesia/ anesthesia May cause narcotic withdrawal when given for >5 days as continuous infusion	Short-acting potent sedative and analgesic. Little or no histamine release. May produce muscle rigidity and so impair ventilation (rarely seen with doses <5 µg/kg). May cause tics as withdrawal reaction.
Sufentanil Alfentanil	κ receptor: Spinal analgesia Miosis Sedation Hypotension		
Morphine	δ receptor: Hallucinations Respiratory depression ↑Vasomotor activity	0.05–0.2 mg/kg IV, IM, or SC 5–20 µg/kg/hr IV continuous infusion May cause narcotic withdrawal when given for >5 days as continuous infusion	μ > κ agonist activity; may cause hypotension by histamine release. Neonates need close monitoring after sedation with morphine because they can experience delayed respiratory depression.
Meperidine		1–2 mg/kg PO, IM, IV, or SC q 3–4 hr prn (maximal dose = 100–150 mg)	Produces histamine release. Has anticholinergic effects that may cause seizures. Less potent and shorter acting than morphine.
Codeine		0.5–1 mg/kg/dose q 4–6 hr prn; may be administered PO, IM, or SC (maximal single dose = 60 mg)	

Drug	Mechanism	Dose	Comments
OPIATE ANTAGONIST			
Naloxone	μ and κ competitive antagonist	0.01–0.1 mg/kg/dose IV Administer slowly by increments of 10 μg/kg to prevent sudden irritability	Because the duration of action is shorter than that of the opiate, opiate rebound may occur.
BARBITURATES			
Thiopental	Barbiturates potentiate GABA-induced increase in Cl− conductance; can produce mild sedation to general anesthesia Barbiturates with 5-phenyl substituent like phenobarbital have selective anticonvulsant activity	3–5 mg/kg IV slow infusion; onset of action in 30 sec; duration of sedation: <30 min	Not recommended for procedures lasting more than 15 min owing to high lipid solubility responsible for prolonged recovery. Avoid fast infusion; it causes hypotension and low cardiac output.
Pentobarbital		2–6 mg/kg IV slow infusion; rapid onset; duration of sedation: 2–4 hr Pentobarbital coma: Loading dose: 10–15 mg/kg during 1–2 hr Maintenance dose: start at 1 mg/kg/hr; may increase to 2–3 mg/kg/hr; maintain burst suppression in EEG Therapeutic range for coma: 20–40 μg/ml	Can cause dependency with chronic use. May cause arrhythmias, bradycardia, and hypotension.
Phenobarbital		Sedation: Children: 2 mg/kg tid PO, IM Adult: 30–120 mg/day in 2–3 divided doses, PO, IM Anticonvulsant: Loading dose: 15–20 mg/kg IV in single or divided doses Maintenance: neonates, 3–4 mg/kg/day qd PO IV; children <12 yr, 5 mg/kg/day bid or qd PO, IV; children >12 yr, 1–3 mg/kg/day bid or qd PO, IV	
OTHERS			
Acetaminophen		Adults: 325–650 mg q 4–6 hr prm Pediatrics: 1–3 yr, 60 mg/yr of age q 4–6 hr prm; 4–6 yr, 240–300 mg q 4–6 hr prm; 6–12 yr, 325 mg q 4–6 hr prm	May be administered orally or rectally.
Chloral hydrate	CNS unknown mechanism	25–75 mg/kg PO or PR; may repeat 30 min after initial dose (maximum, 100 mg/kg or 1 g)	Rapid onset due to chloral hydrate, and delayed action due to trichloroethanol (active metabolite). Contraindicated in patients with renal or hepatic failure. Can produce adverse reactions in patients receiving furosemide.
Chlorpromazine	DA and α CNS receptors	0.5–1 mg/kg/dose q 6 hr prm; may be administered PO, IV, IM, or PR	It is often used in combination with meperidine and promethazine ("lytic cocktail"); however, this combination can be substituted for more specific sedative/analgesic agents with fewer side effects.
Ibuprofen	↓Cyclooxygenase activity→↓synthesis of prostaglandins	4–10 mg/kg/dose PO q 6–8 hr Maximal dose = 30 mg/kg/day Adults: 400–800 mg/dose q 8 hr	
Ketamine	Dissociative anesthetic	0.5–2 mg/kg IV initially, supplement q 30–60 min prm with 0.25–2 mg/kg IV; 3–7 mg/kg IM	Effective drug for PICU or catheterization laboratory procedures, such as line placement. Although it provides centrally mediated cardiovascular stability, it is a direct myocardial depressant and can produce hypotension in critically ill patients. Not recommended for infants younger than 3 months.

Table continued on following page

GUIDELINES FOR DRUG DOSAGE (Continued)

Sedatives, Analgesics, and Paralytic Agents (Continued)

Drug	Receptor	Dose	Comments
Ketorolac	↓Cyclooxygenase activity→↓synthesis of prostaglandins	Pediatric dosing guidelines not well established	
Propofol	General anesthetic	Administer IV continuous infusion 1–2 mg/kg/hr can be used for short invasive procedures; initial dose of 1 mg/kg during 2 min may be necessary Doses as high as 8–12 mg/kg/hr may be necessary for the assisted ventilated patient (Pediatric dosing guidelines are not well established.); not recommended for children < 3 yr of age	Short-acting, rapidly metabolized drug that provides sedation for short invasive procedures (TEE) as well as during the management of the postoperative patient. On discontinuation of the drug, extubation is possible in approximately 20–40 min. It usually produces a transient drop in blood pressure during the loading phase that responds to fluid replacement. At low infusion rates, respiratory depression is rare (except in neonates and infants).
Promethazine		0.5–1 mg/kg/dose PO, IM, IV, PR; may repeat q 6 hr prn	
NEUROMUSCULAR BLOCKING AGENTS			
Succinylcholine	Depolarizing agent	1–2 mg/kg IV; onset: 30–60 sec; duration of action: 4–6 min 2.5–4 mg/kg IM; onset: 2–3 min; duration of action: 10–30 min	It is contraindicated in patients with signs of increased intracranial pressure, stroke, paraplegia, muscular dystrophies, myotonia, burns, and family history of malignant hyperthermia. In patients with Duchenne-type muscular dystrophy, it may cause rhabdomyolysis, hyperkalemia, and cardiac arrest. The most common use is for rapid-sequence endotracheal intubation in patients at increased risk of hypoxia or aspiration of stomach contents.
Vecuronium	Nondepolarizing agents	0.05–0.1 mg/kg/dose IV; may repeat q 1 hr prn	In children <1 yr, the recommended dose maintains neuromuscular blockade for an average of 60 min. In infants and adolescents, the effect lasts for an average of 18–37 min. Persistent paralysis after prolonged continuous infusion can be seen particularly in patients with renal or hepatic compromise. Vecuronium does not cause tachycardia.
Pancuronium		Pediatrics: 0.05–0.1 mg/kg IV	May repeat as often as every 30–60 min as needed. It may cause tachycardia and increase in blood pressure.
Atracurium		0.5 mg/kg IV Neuromuscular blockade can be maintained with a continuous infusion rate of 2–15 μg/kg/min	It undergoes spontaneous hydrolysis at the pH of the body fluids (the Hoffman elimination); therefore, there is no cumulative effect with multiple doses, and it can be used in patients with renal or hepatic failure.

Anticoagulants

Drug	Receptor	Dose	Comments
Heparin	Acts in conjunction with AT-III as an inhibitor of activated coagulation factors (XIIa, XIa, IXa, Xa, IIa). Inhibits the activation of prothrombin by Xa	IV infusion: loading dose of 50 U/kg, and then continuous infusion of 15–25 U/kg/hr. Mean infusion rate for children 1–16 yr: 20 U/kg/hr. IV intermittent: 50–100 U/kg q 4 hr	Monitoring test, PTT; half-life, 90 min. Heparin-induced bleeding can be reversed by protamine. To reverse recent heparin administration, an IV dose of 1 mg of protamine for every 100 U of heparin can be given. The dose of protamine may need to be repeated because heparin may dissociate from the salt complex. In addition, considering a heparin half-life of 60–90 min, the dose of protamine can be adjusted accordingly. Thrombocytopenia is an unwanted side effect that is seen in <6% of the patients 6–12 days after starting heparin therapy. It improves with discontinuation of therapy or changing the source of heparin. It is less frequent with low-molecular-weight heparin.
Warfarin sodium	Vitamin K antagonist → inhibits the synthesis of factors II, VII, IX, and X, protein C and protein S	Infants and children: Loading dose: 0.2 mg/kg PO, qd for 2 days (maximal dose = 10 mg). Maintenance: 0.1 mg/kg/day; range, 0.05–0.34 mg/kg/day. Adults: 5–15 mg/day for 2–5 days. Usual maintenance dose: 2–10 mg/day	Monitoring parameter, INR; target INR depends on the clinical condition (in general, 2–3); peak effect, 5–7 days; half-life, 42 hr. After warfarin therapy has been initiated, the PTT begins to prolong at 24 hours owing to loss of factor VII activity. This has clinical importance in patients with underlying protein C deficiency. In these patients, an acute reduction in protein C may have an actual thrombogenic effect. In these patients, warfarin therapy should be started with a 4- to 5-day overlap with heparin therapy.
ANTIPLATELETS			
Aspirin (acetylsalicylic acid)	Acetylation of cyclooxygenase → inhibition of thromboxane A_2	Antiplatelet dose: dosing range from 3–5 mg/kg/day to 5–10 mg/kg/day (maximal dose = 80 mg/day), given as single daily dose. Anti-inflammatory dose: Kawasaki: 80–100 mg/kg/day q 6 hr (must monitor levels); once fever resolves, 3–5 mg/kg/day qd (maximal dose = 80 mg/day)	Synergistic effect with dipyridamole.
Dipyridamole	Inhibits adenosine deaminase and phosphodiesterase → increases adenosine, cAMP → inhibit platelet aggregation	Children: 3–6 mg/kg/day tid. Adults: 75–400 mg/day tid-qid	Coronary vasodilator.
THROMBOLYTIC THERAPY			
Urokinase	Activates plasminogen to plasmin	For arterial and venous thrombosis or pulmonary embolism: Loading dose of 4400 U/kg during 10 min, and then 4400 U/kg/hr continuous infusion for 12–72 hr. Occluded catheter: 5000–10,000 U/ml, instill in catheter a volume equal to the internal volume of the catheter. Leave in the catheter for 1–4 hr, and then *aspirate out of the catheter*	Monitor fibrin degradation products and fibrinogen levels; half-life, 10–20 min. In neonates, higher doses may be needed because of lower levels of plasminogen.
Streptokinase	Activates plasminogen to plasmin	Loading dose of 3500–4000 U/kg, and then continuous infusion of 1000–1500 U/kg/hr	Safety and efficacy in children are not well established. Fever occurs in 20% of the patients.

Table continued on following page

GUIDELINES FOR DRUG DOSAGE (Continued)

Anticoagulants (Continued)

Drug	Receptor	Dose	Comments
AGENT THAT ENHANCES HEMOSTASIS			
ε-Aminocaproic acid	Inhibits conversion of plasminogen to plasmin	Loading dose: 100–200 mg/kg PO, IV Maintenance: 100 mg/kg/dose q 6 hr Maximal daily dose = 30 g	Contraindicated in DIC.

Drugs for Hyperlipidemias

Drug	Receptor	Dose	Comments
Cholestyramine	Forms nonabsorbable complex with bile acids in the intestine Inhibits enterohepatic reuptake of intestinal bile salts	Begin with 250–300 mg/kg/day PO divided tid May increase as tolerated up to 1–1.5 g/kg/day Do not exceed adult maximum of 32 g/day	Give mixed with water or juice.
Clofibrate		Adults: 2 g/day PO in 2–4 divided doses	Dosage, safety, and efficacy in children are not established.
Colestipol	Forms nonabsorbable complex with bile acids in the intestine Inhibits enterohepatic reuptake of intestinal bile salts	Begin with 250–500 mg/kg/day PO divided bid-qid May increase as tolerated, but do not exceed adult dose (15–30 g/day) Adults: 1.2 g/day PO divided bid	Give mixed with water, juice, soup, or cereal.
Gemfibrozil		Adults: 1.2 g/day PO divided bid	Dosage, safety, and efficacy in children are not established.
Lovastatin	HMG-CoA reductase inhibitor	Adults: 20–80 mg/day PO (qd or divided bid)	Not recommended in prepubertal children.
Nicotinic acid (niacin)	Inhibits synthesis of very low density lipoprotein	Adults: 2–7 g/day PO divided tid Pediatrics: 25–75 mg/kg/day PO divided tid	Pretreatment with aspirin may diminish cutaneous flushing.
Pravastatin	HMG-CoA reductase inhibitor	Adults: 20–40 mg PO (single daily dose)	Not recommended in prepubertal children.
Probucol		Adults: 500 mg PO bid	Dosage, safety, and efficacy in children are not established.
Simvastatin	HMG-CoA reductase inhibitor	Adults: 10–40 mg PO (single daily dose)	Not recommended in prepubertal children.

REFERENCES

Burnier M, Biollaz J: Pharmacokinetic optimisation of angiotensin converting enzyme inhibitor therapy. Clin Pharmacokinet 22:375, 1992.

Chernow B (ed): The Pharmacologic Approach to the Critically Ill Patient, 3rd ed. Baltimore, Williams & Wilkins, 1994.

Gillette PC, Garson A (eds): Pediatric Arrhythmias: Electrophysiology and Pacing. Philadelphia, WB Saunders, 1990.

Gronert BJ, Brandom BW: Neuromuscular blocking drugs in infants and children. Pediatr Clin North Am 41:73, 1994.

Hardman JG, Limbird LL, Molinoff PB, et al (eds): Goodman and Gilman's The Pharmacological Basis of Therapeutics, 9th ed [CD-ROM]. New York, McGraw-Hill, 1996.

Marx CM: Sedation and analgesia. *In* Blumer JL (ed): A Practical Guide to Pediatric Intensive Care. St. Louis, Mosby–Year Book, 1990, p 292.

Miller K: Pharmacological management of hypertension in pediatric patients. Drugs 48:868, 1994.

Taketomo CK, Hodding JH, Kraus DM: Pediatric Dosage Handbook, 3rd ed. Hudson, OH, Lexi-Comp, 1996.

Yaffe SJ, Aranda JV (eds): Pediatric Pharmacology: Therapeutic Principles in Practice, 2nd ed. Philadelphia, WB Saunders, 1992.

Note: Page numbers in *italics* indicate illustrations; page numbers followed by t refer to tables.